Drug Information Handbook

3rd Edition ❚❚ 1995-96

APhA

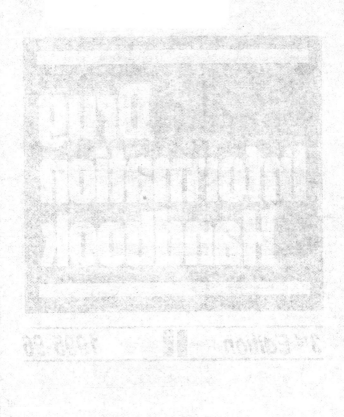

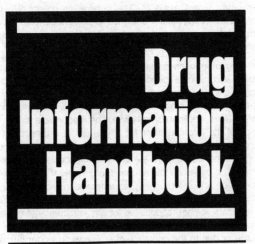

Drug Information Handbook

3rd Edition ‖ **1995-96**

Charles F. Lacy, RPh, PharmD
Drug Information Pharmacist
Cedars-Sinai Medical Center
Los Angeles, California

Lora L. Armstrong, RPh, BSPharm, BCPS
Director of Drug Information Services
The University of Chicago Hospitals
Chicago, Illinois

Naomi Ingrim, PharmD
Specialist in Poison Information
Central Texas Poison Center
Temple, TX

Leonard L. Lance, RPh, BSPharm
Pharmacist
Lexi-Comp, Inc
Hudson, Ohio

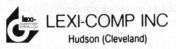 LEXI-COMP INC
Hudson (Cleveland)

AMERICAN PHARMACEUTICAL ASSOCIATION APhA

NOTICE

This handbook is intended to serve the user as a handy reference and not as a complete drug information resource. It does not include information on every therapeutic agent available. The publication covers 975 commonly used drugs and is specifically designed to present certain important aspects of drug data in a more concise format than is typically found in medical literature or product material supplied by manufacturers.

The nature of drug information is that it is constantly evolving because of ongoing research and clinical experience and is often subject to interpretation. While great care has been taken to ensure the accuracy of the information presented, the reader is advised that the authors, editors, reviewers, contributors, and publishers cannot be responsible for the continued currency of the information or for any errors or omissions in this book or for any consequences arising therefrom. Because of the dynamic nature of drug information, readers are advised that decisions regarding drug therapy must be based on the independent judgment of the clinician, changing information about a drug (eg, as reflected in the literature and manufacturer's most current product information), and changing medical practices. The editors are not responsible for any inaccuracy of quotation or for any false or misleading implication that may arise due to the text or formulas as used or due to the quotation of revisions no longer official.

The editors, authors, and contributors have written this book in their private capacities. No official support or endorsement by any federal or state agency or pharmaceutical company is intended or inferred.

The publishers have made every effort to trace the copyright holders for borrowed material. If they have inadvertently overlooked any, they will be pleased to make the necessary arrangements at the first opportunity.

If you have any suggestions or questions
regarding any information presented in this handbook,
please contact our drug information pharmacist at

1-800-837-LEXI

This manual was produced using the FormuLex™ Program —
A complete publishing service of Lexi-Comp Inc.

Lexi-Comp Inc.
1100 Terex Road
Hudson, Ohio 44236-3771
(216) 650-6506

ISBN 0-916589-31-5

TABLE OF CONTENTS

ABOUT THE AUTHORS

Charles F. Lacy, RPh, PharmD

Dr Lacy received his doctorate from the University of Southern California School of Pharmacy. With over 10 years of clinical experience at one of the nation's largest teaching hospitals, he has developed a reputation as an acknowledged expert in drug information and critical care drug therapy.

In his current capacity as Drug Information specialist at Cedar-Sinai Medical Center in Los Angeles, Dr Lacy plays an active role in the education and training of the medical, pharmacy, and nursing staff. He coordinates the Drug Information Center, the Medical Center's Intern Pharmacist Clinical Training Program, the Department's Continuing Education Program for pharmacists; maintains the Medical Center formulary program; and is editor of the Medical Center's *Drug Formulary Handbook* and the drug information newsletter — *Prescription*.

Presently, Dr Lacy holds teaching affiliations with the University of Southern California School of Pharmacy, the University of California at San Francisco School of Pharmacy, the University of the Pacific School of Pharmacy and the University of Alberta at Edmonton, School of Pharmacy and Health Sciences.

Dr Lacy is an active member of numerous professional associations including the American Society of Hospital Pharmacists (ASHP), the California Society of Hospital Pharmacists (CSHP), and the American College of Clinical Pharmacy (ACCP).

Lora L. Armstrong, RPh, BSPharm, BCPS

Lora L. Armstrong received her bachelor's degree in pharmacy from Ferris State University in 1982. With over 13 years of clinical experience at one of the nation's most prominent teaching institutions, she has developed a reputation as an acknowledged expert in drug information. Her interests involve the areas of critical care, hematology, oncology, infectious disease, and pharmacokinetics. Ms. Armstrong is a Board Certified Pharmacotherapy Specialist (BCPS).

In her current capacity as Director of Drug Information at the University of Chicago Hospitals (UCH), Ms Armstrong plays an active role in the education and training of the medical, pharmacy, and nursing staff. She coordinates the Drug Information Center, the medical center's Adverse Drug Reaction Monitoring Program, and the department's Continuing Education Program for pharmacists. She also maintains the hospital's strict formulary program and is editor of the *UCH Formulary of Accepted Drugs* and the drug information newsletter "Topics in Drug Therapy."

Ms Armstrong is an active member of the American Society of Hospital Pharmacists (ASHP), the American Pharmaceutical Association (APhA), and the American College of Clinical Pharmacy (ACCP). She is the APhA designated author for this handbook.

Naomi B. Ingrim, PharmD

Dr Ingrim received her PharmD degree from the University of Nebraska Medical Center - Omaha in 1980 and completed two residencies in Hospital Pharmacy Practice and in Drug Information, respectively in 1982 and 1983. Since that time she has held a variety of clinical, teaching, and management positions, broadening her expertise and further strengthening her drug information skills.

From 1984-89, she held positions at Scott and White Hospital in Temple, Texas as clinical pharmacist in drug information and pediatrics and as assistant professor in pediatrics with Texas A & M Medical School. During the following four years, she served as clinical pharmacy coordinator at

Egleston Children's Hospital at Emory University in Atlanta, Georgia and was cross-appointed with the Emory University Medical School Department of Pediatrics and Mercer University Southern School of Pharmacy. From 1991-93, she additionally served as the acting director of Egleston Hospital pharmacy department. In this capacity, Dr Ingrim directed the development of an active clinical program and staff, including a supportive drug information service/center. She has had much experience designing ADR, CQI, and DUE programs, teaching and public speaking, serving on hospital/national pharmacy organization committees, writing technical documents, and performing drug-related research.

Dr Ingrim is active in state pharmacy organizations, the American Society of Health-System Pharmacists (ASHP), and the American College of Clinical Pharmacists (ACCP).

Currently, Dr Ingrim enjoys increased time with her family, serving as a specialist in poison information at the Central Texas Poison Center and as a freelance consultant in drug information, clinical pharmacy practice, and expert system development.

Leonard L. Lance, RPh, BSPharm

Leonard L. (Bud) Lance has been directly involved in the pharmaceutical industry since receiving his bachelor's degree in pharmacy from Ohio Northern University 23 years ago. Upon graduation from ONU, Mr Lance spent four years as a navy pharmacist in various military assignments and was instrumental in the development and operation of the first whole hospital I.V. admixture program in a military (Portsmouth Naval Hospital) facility.

After completing his military service, he entered the retail pharmacy field and has managed both an independent and a home I.V. franchise pharmacy operation. Since the late 1970s Mr Lance has focused much of his interest on using computers to improve pharmacy service and to advance the dissemination of drug information to practitioners and other health care professionals.

As a result of his strong publishing interest, he serves in the capacity of pharmacy editor and technical advisor as well as pharmacy (information) database coordinator for Lexi-Comp. Along with the *Drug Information Handbook for the Allied Health Professional* edition, he provides technical support to Lexi-Comp's *Pediatric Dosage Handbook*, *Laboratory Test Handbook*, *Diagnostic Procedure Handbook*, and *Geriatric Dosage Handbook* publications. Mr Lance has also assisted approximately 100 major hospitals in producing their own formulary (pharmacy) publications through Lexi-Comp's custom publishing service.

Mr Lance is a member and past president (1984) of the Summit County Pharmaceutical Association (SCPA). He is also a member of the Ohio Pharmacists Association (OPA), the American Pharmaceutical Association (APhA), and the American Society of Hospital Pharmacists (ASHP).

PREFACE

Drug therapy literature is vast and rapidly changing. The format of this book responds to the tremendous challenge to develop a logical guide that can best direct therapy for the multitudes of disease states while remaining current, timely, and concise. The authors have extensively researched the literature and have arranged the information into this one-of-a-kind compendium. The ongoing editorial process continues to review and update the information. The material is presented concisely and consistently in a format which allows for rapid retrieval to facilitate decisions regarding drug therapy. This unique editorial process integrates hard-to-find clinical information like laboratory test interactions, reference range values for therapeutic drug monitoring, nursing implications, monitoring parameters, pediatric dosing, and recommendations for renal and/or hepatic impairment dosing. The format and content was developed to lend itself for use by all practitioners and students involved in drug therapy decisions. We have tried to emphasize fundamental clinical principles of drug therapy, while paying particular attention to providing timely, pertinent, and practical information.

ACKNOWLEDGMENTS

This handbook exists in its present form as a result of the concerted efforts of many individuals. The publisher and president of Lexi-Comp Inc, Robert D. Kerscher and the senior director of Programming and Publications, James P. Caro, American Pharmaceutical Association (APhA) deserve much of the credit for bringing the concept of such a book to fruition.

Other members of the Lexi-Comp staff whose contributions were invaluable and whose patience with the editors' enumerable drafts, revisions, deletions, additions, and enhancements was inexhaustible include: Lynn Coppinger, managing editor; John E. Janosik, PharmD; Diane Harbart, MT (ASCP), medical editor; Barbara F. Kerscher, production manager; Alexandra Hart, composition specialist; Jeanne Eads, Beth Daulbaugh, Julie Weekes, and Lisa Leukart, project managers; Jil R. Neuman, Jacqueline L. Mizer, and Tracey J. Reinecke, production assistants; Jeff J. Zaccagnini, Brian B. Vossler, and Jerry Reeves, sales managers; Edmund A. Harbart, vice-president, custom publishing division; and Jack L. Stones, vice-president, reference publishing division. The complex computer programming required for the typesetting of the book was provided by Dennis P. Smithers, Jay L. Katzen, David C. Marcus, Dale E. Jablonski, and Kenneth J. Hughes, system analysts, under the direction of Thury L. O'Connor, vice-president, and Alan R. Frasz, vice-president, information technologies.

Other APhA staff members whose contributions were important are Julian I. Graubart, director special projects, and James V. McGinnis, manager of art and production. A special thanks goes to Chris Lomax, PharmD, director of pharmacy, Children's Hospital, Los Angeles, who played a significant role in bringing APhA and Lexi-Comp together.

Much of the material contained in the book was a result of pharmacy contributors throughout the United States and Canada. Lexi-Comp has assisted many medical institutions to develop hospital-specific formulary manuals that contains clinical drug information as well as dosing. Working with these clinical pharmacists, hospital pharmacy and therapeutics committees, and hospital drug information centers, Lexi-Comp has developed an evolutionary drug database that reflects the practice of pharmacy in these major institutions.

In addition, the authors wish to thank their families, friends, and colleagues who supported them in their efforts to complete this handbook.

USE OF THE DRUG INFORMATION HANDBOOK

The *Drug Information Handbook, 3rd Edition* is divided into four sections.

The first section is a compilation of introductory text relating to the use of this book.

The drug information section of the handbook, in which all drugs are listed alphabetically, details information pertinent to each drug. Extensive cross-referencing is provided by brand names and synonyms.

The third section is an invaluable appendix section with charts, tables, nomograms, algorithms, and therapy guidelines.

The last section of this handbook is an index listing drugs in their unique therapeutic category.

Alphabetical Listing of Drugs

Drug information is presented in a consistent format and provides the following:

Generic Name	U.S. adopted name
Pronunciation Guide	
Related Information	Cross-reference to other relevant drug information found in the Appendix
Brand Names	Common trade names
Synonyms	Other names or accepted abbreviations for the generic drug
Use	Information pertaining to appropriate indications of the drug
Restrictions	DEA classification for federally scheduled controlled substances
Pregnancy Risk Factor	Five categories established by the FDA to indicate the potential of a systemically absorbed drug for causing birth defects
Pregnancy/Breast Feeding Implications	Related comments, warnings, or precautions are indicated
Contraindications	Information pertaining to inappropriate use of the drug
Warnings/Precautions	Hazardous conditions related to use of the drug and disease states or patient populations in which the drug should be cautiously used
Adverse Reactions	Side effects are grouped by percentage of incidence
Overdosage/Toxicology Drug Interactions Stability	Comments and/or considerations are offered when appropriate
Mechanism of Action	How the drug works in the body to elicit a response
Pharmacodynamics/ Kinetics	The magnitude of a drug's effect depends on the drug concentration at the site of action. The pharmacodynamics are expressed in terms of onset of action and duration of action. Pharmacokinetics are expressed in terms of absorption, distribution (including appearance in breast milk and crossing of the placenta), protein binding, metabolism, bioavailability, half-life, time to peak serum concentration, and elimination.
Usual Dosage	The amount of the drug to be typically given or taken during therapy

Administration	Information regarding the recommended final concentrations, rates for administration, and other guidelines relating to the administration of the drug
Monitoring Parameters	Laboratory tests and patient physical parameters that should be monitored for safety and efficacy of drug therapy are listed when appropriate
Reference Range	Therapeutic and toxic serum concentrations listed when appropriate
Test Interactions	Listing of assay interferences when relevant; (B) = Blood; (S) = Serum; (U) = Urine
Patient Information Nursing Implications	Comments and/or considerations are offered when appropriate
Additional Information	Information about sodium content and/or pertinent information about specific brands
Dosage Forms	Information with regard to form, strength, and availability of the drug
Extemporaneous Preparations	Directions for preparing liquid formulations from solid drug products. May include stability information and references when appropriate.

Appendix

The appendix offers a compilation of tables, guidelines, nomograms, algorithms, and conversion information which can often be helpful when considering patient care.

Therapeutic Category & Key Word Index

This index provides a useful listing of drugs by their therapeutic classification, as well as controlled substance information.

FDA PREGNANCY CATEGORIES

Throughout this book there is a field labeled Pregnancy Risk Factor (PRF) and the letter A, B, C, D or X immediately following which signifies a category. The FDA has established these five categories to indicate the potential of a systemically absorbed drug for causing birth defects. The key differentiation among the categories rests upon the reliability of documentation and the risk:benefit ratio. Pregnancy Category X is particularly notable in that if any data exists that may implicate a drug as a teratogen and the risk:benefit ratio is clearly negative, the drug is contraindicated during pregnancy.

These categories are summarized as follows:

A   Controlled studies in pregnant women fail to demonstrate a risk to the fetus in the first trimester with no evidence of risk in later trimesters. The possibility of fetal harm appears remote.

B   Either animal-reproduction studies have not demonstrated a fetal risk but there are no controlled studies in pregnant women, or animal-reproduction studies have shown an adverse effect (other than a decrease in fertility) that was not confirmed in controlled studies in women in the first trimester and there is no evidence of a risk in later trimesters.

C   Either studies in animals have revealed adverse effects on the fetus (teratogenic or embryocidal effects or other) and there are no controlled studies in women, or studies in women and animals are not available. Drugs should be given only if the potential benefits justify the potential risk to the fetus.

D   There is positive evidence of human fetal risk, but the benefits from use in pregnant women may be acceptable despite the risk (eg, if the drug is needed in a life-threatening situation or for a serious disease for which safer drugs cannot be used or are ineffective).

X   Studies in animals or human beings have demonstrated fetal abnormalities or there is evidence of fetal risk based on human experience, or both, and the risk of the use of the drug in pregnant women clearly outweighs any possible benefit. The drug is contraindicated in women who are or may become pregnant.

DRUGS IN PREGNANCY

Analgesics
Acceptable: Acetaminophen, meperidine, methadone
Controversial: Codeine, propoxyphene
Unacceptable: Nonsteroidal anti-inflammatory agents, salicylates, phenazopyridine

Antimicrobials
Acceptable: Penicillins, 1st and 2nd generation cephalosporins, erythromycin (base and EES), clotrimazole, miconazole, nystatin, isoniazid*, lindane
Controversial: 3rd generation cephalosporins, aminoglycosides, nitrofurantoin†
Unacceptable: Erythromycin estolate, chloramphenicol, sulfa, metronidazole, tetracyclines, acyclovir

ENT
Acceptable: Diphenhydramine*, dextromethorphan
Controversial: Pseudoephedrine
Unacceptable: Brompheniramine, cyproheptadine, dimenhydrinate

GI
Acceptable: Trimethobenzamide, antacids*, simethicone, other H$_2$ blockers, psyllium, bisacodyl, docusate
Controversial: Metoclopramide, prochlorperazine

---

*Do not use in first trimester
†Do not use in third trimester

Neurologic
  Controversial: Phenytoin, phenobarbital
  Unacceptable: Carbamazepine, valproic acid, ergotamine

Pulmonary
  Acceptable: Theophylline, metaproterenol, terbutaline, inhaled steroids
  Unacceptable: Epinephrine, oral steroids

Psych
  Acceptable: Hydroxyzine*, lithium*, haloperidol
  Controversial: Benzodiazepines, tricyclics, phenothiazines

Other
  Acceptable: Heparin, insulin
  Unacceptable: Warfarin, sulfonylureas

SAFE WRITING

Health professionals and their support personnel frequently produce hand-written copies of information they see in print; therefore, such information is subjected to even greater possibilities for error or misinterpretation on the part of others. Thus, particular care must be given to how drug names and strengths are expressed when creating written health care documents.

The following are a few examples of safe writing rules suggested by the Institute for Safe Medication Practices, Inc.*

1. There should be a space between a number and its units as it is easier to read. There should be no periods after the abbreviations mg or mL.

Correct	Incorrect
10 mg	10mg
100 mg	100mg

2. Never place a decimal and a zero after a whole number (2 mg is correct and 2.0 mg is incorrect). If the decimal point is not seen because it falls on a line or because individuals are working from copies where the decimal point is not seen, this causes a ten-fold overdose.

3. Just the opposite is true for numbers less than one. Always place a zero before a naked decimal (0.5 mL is correct, .5 mL is incorrect).

4. Never abbreviate the word unit. The handwritten U or u, looks like a 0 (zero), and may cause a tenfold overdose error to be made.

5. Q.D. is not a safe abbreviation for once daily, as when the Q is followed by a sloppy dot, it looks like QID which means four times daily.

6. O.D. is not a safe abbreviation for once daily, as it is properly interpreted as meaning "right eye" and has caused liquid medications such as saturated solution of potassium iodide and lugol's solution to be administered incorrectly. There is no safe abbreviation for once daily. It must be written out in full.

7. Do not use chemical names such as 6-mercaptopurine or 6-thioguanine, as 6 fold overdoses have been given when these were not recognized as chemical names. The proper names of these drugs are mercaptopurine or thioguanine.

8. Do not abbreviate drug names (5FC, 6MP, 5-ASA, MTX, HCTZ CPZ, PBZ, etc) as they are misinterpreted and cause error.

9. Do not use the apothecary system or symbols.

10. Do not abbreviate microgram as μg; instead use mcg as there is less likelihood of misinterpretation.

11. When writing an outpatient prescription, write a complete prescription. A complete prescription can prevent the prescriber, the pharmacist, and/or the patient from making a mistake and can eliminate the need for further clarification.

*From "Safe Writing" by Davis NM, PharmD and Cohen MR, MS, Lecturers and Consultants for Safe Medication Practices, 1143 Wright Drive, Huntingdon Valley, PA 19006. Phone: (215) 947-7566.

The legible prescriptions should contain:

    a.   patient's full name

    b.   for pediatric or geriatric patients: their age (or weight where applicable)

    c.   drug name, dosage form and strength; if a drug is new or rarely prescribed, print this information

    d.   number or amount to be dispensed

    e.   complete instructions for the patient, including the purpose of the medication

    f.   when there are recognized contraindications for a prescribed drug, indicate to the pharmacist that you are aware of this fact (ie, when prescribing a potassium salt for a patient receiving an ACE inhibitor, write "K serum leveling being monitored")

ALPHABETICAL
LISTING OF
DRUGS

A-200™ Pyrinate [OTC] *see* Pyrethrins *on page 959*

Abbokinase® *see* Urokinase *on page 1141*

Accupril® *see* Quinapril Hydrochloride *on page 965*

Accutane® *see* Isotretinoin *on page 602*

ACE *see* Captopril *on page 174*

Acebutolol Hydrochloride (a se byoo' toe lole)

Related Information
Beta-Blockers Comparison *on page 1257-1259*

Brand Names Sectral®

Use Treatment of hypertension, ventricular arrhythmias, angina

Pregnancy Risk Factor B

Contraindications Hypersensitivity to beta-blocking agents, avoid use in uncompensated congestive heart failure; cardiogenic shock; bradycardia or heart block; sinus node dysfunction; A-V conduction abnormalities. Although acebutolol primarily blocks $beta_1$-receptors, high doses can result in $beta_2$-receptor blockage. Use with caution in bronchospastic lung disease and renal dysfunction (especially the elderly).

Warnings/Precautions Abrupt withdrawal of beta-blockers may result in an exaggerated cardiac beta-adrenergic responsiveness. Symptomatology has included reports of tachycardia, hypertension, ischemia, angina, myocardial infarction, and sudden death. It is recommended that patients be tapered gradually off of beta-blockers over a 2-week period rather than via abrupt discontinuation.

Adverse Reactions
>10%: Fatigue

1% to 10%:
Cardiovascular: Chest pain, edema, bradycardia, hypotension
Central nervous system: Headache, dizziness, insomnia, depression, abnormal dreams
Dermatologic: Rash
Gastrointestinal: Constipation, diarrhea, dyspepsia, nausea, flatulence
Genitourinary: Micturition (frequency)
Neuromuscular & skeletal: Arthralgia, myalgia
Ocular: Abnormal vision
Respiratory: Dyspnea, rhinitis, cough

<1%:
Cardiovascular: Ventricular arrhythmias, heart block, heart failure
Central nervous system: Cold extremities
Gastrointestinal: Dry mouth, anorexia
Genitourinary: Impotence, urinary retention
Miscellaneous: Facial swelling

Overdosage/Toxicology
Symptoms of intoxication include cardiac disturbances, CNS toxicity, bronchospasm, hypoglycemia, and hyperkalemia. The most common cardiac symptoms include hypotension and bradycardia; atrioventricular block, intraventricular conduction disturbances, cardiogenic shock, and systole may occur with severe overdose, especially with membrane-depressant drugs (eg, propranolol); CNS effects include convulsions, coma, and respiratory arrest is commonly seen with propranolol and other membrane-depressant and lipid-soluble drugs

Treatment includes symptomatic treatment of seizures, hypotension, hyperkalemia and hypoglycemia; bradycardia and hypotension resistant to atropine, isoproterenol or pacing may respond to glucagon; wide QRS defects caused by the membrane-depressant poisoning may respond to hypertonic sodium bicarbonate; repeat-dose charcoal, hemoperfusion, or hemodialysis may be helpful in removal of only those beta-blockers with a small V_d, long half-life or low intrinsic clearance (acebutolol, atenolol, nadolol, sotalol)

Drug Interactions
Decreased effect of beta-blockers with aluminum salts, barbiturates, calcium salts, cholestyramine, colestipol, NSAIDs, penicillins (ampicillin), rifampin, salicylates and sulfinpyrazone due to decreased bioavailability and plasma levels

Beta-blockers may decrease the effect of sulfonylureas

Increased effect/toxicity of beta-blockers with calcium blockers (diltiazem, felodipine, nicardipine), contraceptives, flecainide, haloperidol (propranolol, hypotensive effects), H_2 antagonists (metoprolol, propranolol only by cimetidine, possibly ranitidine), hydralazine (metoprolol, propranolol), loop diuretics (propranolol, not atenolol), MAO inhibitors (metoprolol, nadolol, bradycardia), phenothiazines (propranolol), propafenone (metoprolol, propranolol), quinidine (in extensive metabolizers), ciprofloxacin, thyroid hormones (metoprolol, propranolol, when hypothyroid patient is converted to euthyroid state)

Beta-blockers may increase the effect/toxicity of flecainide, haloperidol (hypotensive effects), hydralazine, phenothiazines, acetaminophen, anticoagulants (propranolol, warfarin), benzodiazepines (not atenolol), clonidine (hypertensive crisis after or during withdrawal of either agent), epinephrine (initial hypertensive episode followed by bradycardia), nifedipine and verapamil lidocaine, ergots (peripheral ischemia), prazosin (postural hypotension)

Beta-blockers may affect the action or levels of ethanol, disopyramide, nondepolarizing muscle relaxants and theophylline although the effects are difficult to predict

Mechanism of Action Competitively blocks beta$_1$-adrenergic receptors with little or no effect on beta$_2$-receptors except at high doses; exhibits membrane stabilizing and intrinsic sympathomimetic activity

Pharmacodynamics/Kinetics
Absorption: Oral: Well absorbed (40%)
Protein binding: 5% to 15%
Metabolism: Extensive first-pass
Half-life: 6-7 hours average
Time to peak: 2-4 hours
Elimination: ~55% of dose excreted via bile into feces and 35% excreted into urine

Usual Dosage Oral:
Adults: 400-800 mg/day in 2 divided doses; maximum: 1200 mg/day
Elderly: Initial: 200-400 mg/day; dose reduction due to age related decrease in Cl$_{cr}$ will be necessary; do not exceed 800 mg/day

Dosing adjustment in renal impairment:
Cl$_{cr}$ 25-49 mL/minute/1.73 m^2: Reduce dose by 50%
Cl$_{cr}$ <25 mL/minute/1.73 m^2: Reduce dose by 75%
Dosing adjustment in hepatic impairment: Use with caution
Monitoring Parameters Blood pressure, orthostatic hypotension, heart rate, CNS effects, EKG
Test Interactions ↑ triglycerides, potassium, uric acid, cholesterol (S), glucose; ↓ HDL, ↑ thyroxine (S)
Patient Information Do not discontinue abruptly; consult pharmacist or physician before taking with other adrenergic drugs (eg, cold medications); notify physician if CHF symptoms become worse or if other side effects occur; take at the same time each day; use with caution while driving or performing tasks requiring alertness; may mask signs of hypoglycemia in diabetics; may be taken without regard to meals
Dosage Forms Capsule: 200 mg, 400 mg

**Acel-Imune® ** *see* Diphtheria and Tetanus Toxoids and Acellular Pertussis Vaccine *on page 354*

Acephen® [OTC] *see* Acetaminophen *on this page*

Acetaminophen (a seet a min' oh fen)
Related Information
Acetaminophen Toxicity Nomogram *on page 1384*
Brand Names Acephen® [OTC]; Aceta® [OTC]; Anacin-3® [OTC]; Apacet® [OTC]; Banesin® [OTC]; Dapa® [OTC]; Datril® [OTC]; Dorcol® [OTC]; Feverall™ [OTC]; Genapap® [OTC]; Halenol® [OTC]; Neopap® [OTC]; Panadol® [OTC]; Tempra® [OTC]; Tylenol® [OTC]; Valadol® [OTC]
Synonyms APAP; N-Acetyl-P-Aminophenol; Paracetamol
Use Treatment of mild to moderate pain and fever; does not have antirheumatic effects (analgesic)
Pregnancy Risk Factor B
Contraindications Patients with known G-6-PD deficiency; hypersensitivity to acetaminophen
Warnings/Precautions May cause severe hepatic toxicity on overdose; use with caution in patients with alcoholic liver disease; chronic daily dosing in adults of 5-8 g of acetaminophen over several weeks or 3-4 g/day of acetaminophen for 1 year have resulted in liver damage
Adverse Reactions
<1%:
Dermatologic: Rash and hypersensitivity reactions (rare)
Gastrointestinal: Nausea, vomiting
Hematologic: Blood dyscrasias (neutropenia, pancytopenia, leukopenia), anemia
Renal: Analgesic nephropathy, nephrotoxicity with chronic overdose
(Continued)

Acetaminophen *(Continued)*

Overdosage/Toxicology Symptoms of overdose include hepatic necrosis, transient azotemia, renal tubular necrosis with acute toxicity, anemia, and GI disturbances with chronic toxicity. Acetylcysteine 140 mg/kg orally (loading) followed by 70 mg/kg every 4 hours for 17 doses. Therapy should be initiated based upon laboratory analysis suggesting high probability of hepatotoxic potential. Activated charcoal is very effective at binding acetaminophen. Intravenous acetylcysteine should be reserved for patients unable to take oral forms.

Drug Interactions

Decreased effect: Rifampin can interact to reduce the analgesic effectiveness of acetaminophen

Increased toxicity: Barbiturates, carbamazepine, hydantoins, sulfinpyrazone can increase the hepatotoxic potential of acetaminophen; chronic ethanol abuse increases risk for acetaminophen toxicity

Mechanism of Action Inhibits the synthesis of prostaglandins in the central nervous system and peripherally blocks pain impulse generation; produces antipyresis from inhibition of hypothalamic heat-regulating center

Pharmacodynamics/Kinetics

Protein binding: 20% to 50%

Metabolism: At normal therapeutic dosages, the parent compound is metabolized in the liver to sulfate and glucuronide metabolites, while a small amount is metabolized by microsomal mixed function oxidases to a highly reactive intermediate (acetylimidoquinone) which is conjugated with glutathione and inactivated; at toxic doses (as little as 4 g in a single day) glutathione conjugation becomes insufficient to meet the metabolic demand causing an increase in acetylimidoquinone concentration, which is thought to cause hepatic cell necrosis

Half-life:

Neonates: 2-5 hours

Adults:

Normal renal function: 1-3 hours

End stage renal disease: 1-3 hours

Time to peak serum concentration: Oral: 10-60 minutes after normal doses, may be delayed in acute overdoses

Usual Dosage Oral, rectal (if fever not controlled with acetaminophen alone, give with full doses of aspirin on an every 4- to 6-hour schedule, if aspirin is not otherwise contraindicated):

Children <12 years: 10-15 mg/kg/dose every 4-6 hours as needed; do **not** exceed 5 doses (2.6 g) in 24 hours; alternatively, the following doses may be used. See table.

Acetaminophen Dosing

Age	Dosage (mg)	Age	Dosage (mg)
0-3 mo	40	4-5y	240
4-11 mo	80	6-8y	320
1-2 y	120	9-10y	400
2-3 y	160	11y	480

Adults: 325-650 mg every 4-6 hours or 1000 mg 3-4 times/day; do **not** exceed 4 g/day

Dosing interval in renal impairment:

Cl_{cr} 10-50 mL/minute: Administer every 6 hours

Cl_{cr} <10 mL/minute: Administer every 8 hours (metabolites accumulate)

Moderately dialyzable (20% to 50%)

Dosing adjustment/comments in hepatic impairment: Appears to be well tolerated in cirrhosis; serum levels may need monitoring with long-term use

Monitoring Parameters Relief of pain or fever

Reference Range

Therapeutic concentration: 10-30 µg/mL

Toxic concentration: >200 µg/mL

Toxic concentration with probable hepatotoxicity: >200 µg/mL at 4 hours or 50 µg/mL at 12 hours

Test Interactions ↑ chloride, bilirubin, uric acid, glucose, ammonia (B), chloride (S), uric acid (S), alkaline phosphatase (S), chloride (S); ↓ sodium, bicarbonate, calcium (S)

Nursing Implications Give with food

Suppositories: Do not freeze

Suspension, oral: Shake well before pouring a dose

Dosage Forms
Caplet: 160 mg, 325 mg, 500 mg
Drops: 48 mg/mL (15 mL); 60 mg/0.6 mL (15 mL)
Elixir: 120 mg/5 mL, 160 mg/5 mL, 167 mg/5 mL, 325 mg/5 mL
Liquid, oral: 160 mg/5 mL, 500 mg/15 mL
Solution: 100 mg/mL (15 mL); 120 mg/2.5 mL
Suppository, rectal: 120 mg, 125 mg, 300 mg, 325 mg, 650 mg
Tablet: 325 mg, 500 mg, 650 mg
Tablet, chewable: 80 mg, 160 mg

Acetaminophen and Codeine (a seet a min' oh fen)
Related Information
Acetaminophen Toxicity Nomogram *on page 1384*
Brand Names Capital® and Codeine; Phenaphen® With Codeine; Tylenol® With Codeine
Synonyms Codeine and Acetaminophen
Use Relief of mild to moderate pain
Restrictions C-III; C-V
Pregnancy Risk Factor C
Contraindications Hypersensitivity to acetaminophen, codeine phosphate, or similar compounds
Warnings/Precautions Use with caution in patients with hypersensitivity reactions to other phenanthrene derivative opioid agonists (morphine, hydrocodone, hydromorphone, levorphanol, oxycodone, oxymorphone); tablets contain metabisulfite which may cause allergic reactions
Adverse Reactions
>10%:
Central nervous system: Lightheadedness, dizziness, sedation
Gastrointestinal: Nausea, vomiting
Respiratory: Shortness of breath
1% to 10%:
Central nervous system: Euphoria, dysphoria
Dermatologic: Pruritus
Gastrointestinal: Constipation, abdominal pain
Miscellaneous: Histamine release
<1%:
Cardiovascular: Palpitations, hypotension, bradycardia, peripheral vasodilation
Central nervous system: Increased intracranial pressure
Endocrine & metabolic: Antidiuretic hormone release
Gastrointestinal: Biliary tract spasm
Genitourinary: Urinary retention
Ocular: Miosis
Respiratory: Respiratory depression
Miscellaneous: Physical and psychological dependence
Overdosage/Toxicology Symptoms of overdose include hepatic necrosis, blood dyscrasias, respiratory depression
Acetylcysteine 140 mg/kg orally (loading) followed by 70 mg/kg every 4 hours for 17 doses; therapy should be initiated based upon laboratory analysis suggesting high probability of hepatotoxic potential
Naloxone 2 mg I.V. (0.01 mg/kg for children) with repeat administration as necessary up to a total of 10 mg; can also be used to reverse the toxic effects of the opiate. Activated charcoal is effective at binding certain chemicals, and this is especially true for acetaminophen.
Drug Interactions Increased toxicity: CNS depressants, phenothiazines, tricyclic antidepressants, guanabenz, MAO inhibitors (may also → ↓ blood pressure)
Mechanism of Action Inhibits the synthesis of prostaglandins in the central nervous system and peripherally blocks pain impulse generation; produces antipyresis from inhibition of hypothalamic heat-regulating center; binds to opiate receptors in the CNS, causing inhibition of ascending pain pathways, altering the perception of and response to pain; causes cough supression by direct central action in the medulla; produces generalized CNS depression
Usual Dosage Doses should be adjusted according to severity of pain and response of the patient. Adult doses ≥60 mg codeine fail to give commensurate relief of pain but merely prolong analgesia and are associated with an appreciably increased incidence of side effects. Oral:

Children:
Analgesic: 0.5-1 mg codeine/kg/dose every 4-6 hours
Acetaminophen: 10-15 mg/kg/dose every 4 hours up to a maximum of 2.6 g/24 hours for children <12 years
3-6 years: 5 mL 3-4 times/day as needed of elixir
7-12 years: 10 mL 3-4 times/day as needed of elixir
(Continued)

Acetaminophen and Codeine *(Continued)*

>12 years: 15 mL every 4 hours as needed of elixir

Adults:
Antitussive: Based on codeine (15-30 mg/dose) every 4-6 hours
Analgesic: Based on codeine (30-60 mg/dose) every 4-6 hours
1-2 tablets every 4 hours to a maximum of 12 tablets/24 hours

Dosing adjustment in renal impairment: Refer to individual monographs for Acetaminophen and Codeine

Monitoring Parameters Relief of pain, respiratory and mental status, blood pressure, bowel function

Patient Information May cause drowsiness; do not exceed recommended dose; do not take for more than 10 days without physician's advice

Nursing Implications Observe patient for excessive sedation, respiratory depression, constipation

Dosage Forms
Capsule:
#2: Acetaminophen 325 mg and codeine phosphate 15 mg (C-III)
#3: Acetaminophen 325 mg and codeine phosphate 30 mg (C-III)
#4: Acetaminophen 325 mg and codeine phosphate 60 mg (C-III)
Elixir: Acetaminophen 120 mg and codeine phosphate 12 mg per 5 mL with alcohol 7% (C-V)
Suspension, oral, alcohol free: Acetaminophen 120 mg and codeine phosphate 12 mg per 5 mL (C-V)
Tablet: Acetaminophen 500 mg and codeine phosphate 30 mg (C-III); acetaminophen 650 mg and codeine phosphate 30 mg (C-III)
Tablet:
#1: Acetaminophen 300 mg and codeine phosphate 7.5 mg (C-III)
#2: Acetaminophen 300 mg and codeine phosphate 15 mg (C-III)
#3: Acetaminophen 300 mg and codeine phosphate 30 mg (C-III)
#4: Acetaminophen 300 mg and codeine phosphate 60 mg (C-III)

Acetaminophen and Hydrocodone *see* Hydrocodone and Acetaminophen *on page 543*

Acetaminophen and Oxycodone *see* Oxycodone and Acetaminophen *on page 826*

Acetaminophen Toxicity Nomogram *see page 1384*

Aceta® [OTC] *see* Acetaminophen *on page 17*

Acetazolamide *(a set a zole' a mide)*
Related Information
Glaucoma Drug Therapy Comparison *on page 1270*
Brand Names AK-Zol®; Diamox®; Diamox Sequels®
Use Lowers intraocular pressure to treat glaucoma, also as a diuretic, adjunct treatment of refractory seizures and acute altitude sickness; centrencephalic epilepsies (sustained release not recommended for anticonvulsant)
Pregnancy Risk Factor C
Pregnancy/Breast Feeding Implications
Despite widespread usage, no reports linking the use of acetazolamide with congenital defects have been located
The American Academy of Pediatrics considers acetazolamide to be compatible with breast feeding
Contraindications Hypersensitivity to sulfonamides or acetazolamide; patients with hepatic disease or insufficiency; patients with decreased sodium and/or potassium levels; patients with adrenocortical insufficiency, hyperchloremic acidosis, severe renal disease or dysfunction, or severe pulmonary obstruction; long-term use in noncongestive angle-closure glaucoma
Warnings/Precautions
Use in impaired hepatic function may result in coma; use with caution in patients with respiratory acidosis and diabetes mellitus; impairment of mental alertness and/or physical coordination may occur
I.M. administration is painful because of the alkaline pH of the drug
Drug may cause substantial increase in blood glucose in some diabetic patients; malaise and complaints of tiredness and myalgia are signs of excessive dosing and acidosis in the elderly
Adverse Reactions
>10%:
Gastrointestinal: Anorexia, diarrhea, malaise, metallic taste
Genitourinary: Increased urination
Neuromuscular & skeletal: Muscular weakness

<1%:
Central nervous system: Fever, fatigue, mental depression, drowsiness
Dermatologic: Rash
Endocrine & metabolic: Hyperchloremic metabolic acidosis, hypokalemia
Gastrointestinal: GI irritation, dryness of mouth
Genitourinary: Dysuria, renal calculi
Hematologic: Bone marrow suppression, blood dyscrasias, elevation of blood glucose
Neuromuscular & skeletal: Paresthesia
Ocular: Myopia
Miscellaneous: Black stools

Overdosage/Toxicology Symptoms of overdose include low blood sugar, tingling of lips and tongue, nausea, yawning, confusion, agitation, tachycardia, sweating, convulsions, stupor, and coma.

Hypoglycemia should be managed with 50 mL I.V. dextrose 50% followed immediately with a continuous infusion of 10% dextrose in water (administer at a rate sufficient enough to approach a serum glucose level of 100 mg/dL). The use of corticosteroids to treat the hypoglycemia is controversial, however, the addition of 100 mg of hydrocortisone to the dextrose infusion may prove helpful.

Drug Interactions
Decreased effect: Increased lithium excretion and altered excretion of other drugs by alkalinization of urine (such as amphetamines, quinidine, procainamide, methenamine, phenobarbital, salicylates); primidone serum concentrations may be decreased
Increased toxicity: Cyclosporine trough concentrations may be increased resulting in possible nephrotoxicity and neurotoxicity; salicylates use may result in carbonic anhydrase inhibitor accumulation and toxicity including CNS depression and metabolic acidosis; digitalis toxicity may occur if hypokalemia is untreated

Stability
Reconstitute with at least 5 mL sterile water to provide a solution containing not more than 100 mg/mL; further dilution in 50 mL of either D_5W or NS for I.V. infusion administration
Reconstituted solution may be stored under refrigeration (2°C to 8°C) for 1 week
Stability of IVPB solution: 5 days at room temperature (25°C) and 44 days at refrigeration (5°C)

Mechanism of Action Reversible inhibition of the enzyme carbonic anhydrase resulting in reduction of hydrogen ion secretion at renal tubule and an increased renal excretion of sodium, potassium, bicarbonate, and water to decrease production of aqueous humor; also inhibits carbonic anhydrase in central nervous system to retard abnormal and excessive discharge from CNS neurons

Pharmacodynamics/Kinetics
Onset of action:
Extended release capsule: 2 hours
I.V.: 2 minutes
Peak effect:
Extended release capsule: 3-6 hours
Tablet: 1-4 hours
I.V.: 15 minutes
Duration:
Extended release capsule: 18-24 hours
Tablet: 8-12 hours
I.V.: 4-5 hours
Distribution: Distributes into erythrocytes, kidneys; crosses blood-brain barrier; crosses placenta and distributes into milk to ~30% of plasma concentrations
Protein binding: 95%
Half-life: 2.4-5.8 hours
Elimination: 70% to 100% of I.V. or tablet dose is excreted unchanged in the urine within 24 hours

Usual Dosage Note: I.M. administration is not recommended because of pain secondary to the alkaline pH

Children:
Glaucoma:
Oral: 8-30 mg/kg/day or 300-900 mg/m²/day divided every 8 hours
I.M., I.V.: 20-40 mg/24 hours divided every 6 hours, not to exceed 1 g/day
Edema: Oral, I.M., I.V.: 5 mg/kg or 150 mg/m² once every day
Epilepsy: Oral: 8-30 mg/kg/day in 1-4 divided doses, not to exceed 1 g/day; sustained release capsule is not recommended for treatment of epilepsy
(Continued)

Acetazolamide *(Continued)*

Adults:

Glaucoma: Chronic simple (open-angle): Oral: 250 mg 1-4 times/day or 500 mg sustained release capsule twice daily

Elderly: Oral: Initial: 250 mg once or twice daily; use lowest effective dose possible

Secondary, acute (closed-angle): I.M., I.V.: 250-500 mg, may repeat in 2-4 hours to a maximum of 1 g/day

Edema: Oral, I.M., I.V.: 250-375 mg once daily

Epilepsy: Oral: 8-30 mg/kg/day in 1-4 divided doses, not to exceed 1 g/day; **sustained release capsule is not recommended for treatment of epilepsy**

Altitude sickness: Oral: 250 mg every 8-12 hours (or 500 mg extended release capsules every 12-24 hours)

Therapy should begin 24-48 hours before and continue during ascent and for at least 48 hours after arrival at the high altitude

Urine alkalinization: Oral: 5 mg/kg/dose repeated 2-3 times over 24 hours

Dosing adjustment in renal impairment:

Cl_{cr} 10-50 mL/minute: Administer every 12 hours

Cl_{cr} <10 mL/minute: Avoid use → ineffective

Moderately dialyzable (20% to 50%)

Administration Recommended rate of administration: 100-500 mg/minute for I.V. push and 4-8 hours for I.V. infusions

Monitoring Parameters Intraocular pressure, serum electrolytes, periodic CBC with differential

Test Interactions May cause false-positive results for urinary protein with Albustix®, Labstix®, Albutest®, Bumintest®

Patient Information Report numbness or tingling of extremities to physician; do not crush, chew, or swallow contents of long-acting capsule, but may be opened and sprinkled on soft food; ability to perform tasks requiring mental alertness and/or physical coordination may be impaired; take with food; drug may cause substantial increase in blood glucose in some diabetic patients

Additional Information Sodium content of 500 mg injection: 47.2 mg (2.05 mEq)

Dosage Forms

Capsule, sustained release: 500 mg

Injection: 500 mg

Tablet: 125 mg, 250 mg

Extemporaneous Preparations Tablets may be crushed and suspended in cherry, chocolate, raspberry, or other highly flavored carbohydrate syrup to a maximum concentration of 100 mg/mL; suspensions are stable for 7 days; stability data for compounding a 25 mg/mL oral suspension from crushed tablets is available in the following reference

Alexander KS, Haribhakti RP, and Parker GA, "Stability of Acetazolamide in Suspension Compound From Tablets," *Am J Hosp Pharm,* 1991, 48(6):1241-4.

Acetic Acid *(a see' tik)*

Brand Names VōSol®

Synonyms Ethanoic Acid

Use Irrigation of the bladder; treatment of superficial bacterial infections of the external auditory canal and vagina

Pregnancy Risk Factor C

Contraindications During transurethral procedures; hypersensitivity to drug or components

Warnings/Precautions Not for internal intake or I.V. infusion; topical use or irrigation use only; use of irrigation in patients with mucosal lesions of urinary bladder may cause irritation; systemic acidosis may result from absorption

Adverse Reactions

<1%:

Endocrine & metabolic: Systemic acidosis

Genitourinary: Urologic pain

Renal: Hematuria

Usual Dosage

Irrigation (note dosage of an irrigating solution depends on the capacity or surface area of the structure being irrigated):

For continuous irrigation of the urinary bladder with 0.25% acetic acid irrigation, the rate of administration will approximate the rate of urine flow; usually 500-1500 mL/24 hours

For periodic irrigation of an indwelling urinary catheter to maintain patency, about 50 mL of 0.25% acetic acid irrigation is required

Otic: Insert saturated wick; keep moist 24 hours; remove wick and instill 5 drops 3-4 times/day

Nursing Implications For continuous or intermittent irrigation of the urinary bladder, urine pH should be checked at least 4 times/day and the irrigation rate adjusted to maintain a pH of 4.5-5

Dosage Forms Solution:

Irrigation: 0.25% (1000 mL)

Otic: Acetic acid 2% in propylene glycol (15 mL, 30 mL, 60 mL)

Acetohexamide (a set oh hex' a mide)

Related Information

Hypoglycemic Agents Comparison *on page 1271*

Brand Names Dymelor®

Use Adjunct to diet for the management of mild to moderately severe, stable, noninsulin-dependent (type II) diabetes mellitus

Pregnancy Risk Factor D

Pregnancy/Breast Feeding Implications When administered near term, acetohexamide crosses the placenta and may persist in the neonatal serum for several days; despite lack of evidence of teratogenicity, acetohexamide should not be used in pregnancy

Contraindications Diabetes complicated by ketoacidosis, therapy of type I diabetes, hypersensitivity to sulfonylureas

Warnings/Precautions Advise patient to avoid alcohol or products containing alcohol; monitor for signs and symptoms of hypoglycemia (fatigue, excessive hunger, profuse sweating, or numbness of extremities)

Adverse Reactions

>10%:

Central nervous system: Headache, dizziness

Gastrointestinal: Constipation, diarrhea, heartburn, anorexia, epigastric fullness

1% to 10%: Dermatologic: Rash, hives, photosensitivity

<1%:

Endocrine & metabolic: Hypoglycemia

Hematologic: Aplastic anemia, hemolytic anemia, bone marrow depression, thrombocytopenia, agranulocytosis

Overdosage/Toxicology

Symptoms of overdose include low blood sugar, tingling of lips and tongue, nausea, yawning, confusion, agitation, tachycardia, sweating, convulsions, stupor, and coma

Hypoglycemia should be managed with 50 mL I.V. dextrose 50% followed immediately with a continuous infusion of 10% dextrose in water (administer at a rate sufficient enough to approach a serum glucose level of 100 mg/dL). The use of corticosteroids to treat the hypoglycemia is controversial, however, the addition of 100 mg of hydrocortisone to the dextrose infusion may prove helpful.

Drug Interactions

Monitor patient closely; large number of drugs interact with sulfonylureas

Decreased effect: Decreases hypoglycemic effect when coadministered with cholestyramine, diazoxide, hydantoins, rifampin, thiazides, loop or thiazide diuretics, and phenylbutazone

Increased effect: Increases hypoglycemia when coadministered with salicylates or beta-adrenergic blockers; MAO inhibitors; oral anticoagulants, NSAIDs, sulfonamides, phenylbutazone, insulin, clofibrate, fenfluramine, fluconazole, gemfibrozil, H_2 antagonists, methyldopa, tricyclic antidepressants

Mechanism of Action Believed to cause hypoglycemia by stimulating insulin release from the pancreatic beta cells; reduces glucose output from the liver (decreases gluconeogenesis); insulin sensitivity is increased at peripheral target sites (alters receptor sensitivity/receptor density); potentiates effects of ADH; may produce mild diuresis and significant uricosuric activity

Pharmacodynamics/Kinetics

Onset of effect: 1 hour

Peak hypoglycemic effects: 8-10 hours

Duration: 12-24 hours, prolonged with renal impairment

Distribution: Into breast milk

Protein binding: ~90% (ionic/nonionic)

Metabolism: In the liver to potent active metabolite

Half-life:

Parent compound: 0.8-2.4 hours

Metabolite: 5-6 hours

Elimination: Urinary excretion <40% as unchanged drug; metabolite, hydroxyhexamide is more potent and is excreted less rapidly; ~80% to 95% of dose excreted in urine within 24 hours; ~15% is excreted in bile

(Continued)

23

Acetohexamide *(Continued)*

Usual Dosage Adults: Oral (elderly patients may be more sensitive and should be started at a lower dosage initially): 250 mg to 1.5 g/day in 1-2 divided doses; doses >1.5 g/day are not recommended; if dose is ≤1 g, administer as a single daily dose

Dosing adjustment in renal impairment: Cl_{cr} <50 mL/minute: Avoid use; prolonged hypoglycemia occurs in azotemic patients

Dosing adjustment in hepatic impairment: Initiate therapy at lower than recommended doses

Monitoring Parameters Fasting blood glucose, urine glucose, hemoglobin A_{1c} or fructosamine

Reference Range Glucose fasting: Adults: 80-140 mg/dL; elderly: 100-180 mg/dL

Patient Information If nausea or stomach upset occurs, may be taken with food; take at the same time each day; avoid alcohol; avoid hypoglycemia, eat regularly, do not skip meals; keep sugar source with you

Nursing Implications Blood (preferred) and urine glucose concentrations should be monitored when therapy is started; normally takes 7 days to determine therapeutic response; patients who are anorexic or NPO may need to have their dose held to avoid hypoglycemia

Dosage Forms Tablet: 250 mg, 500 mg

Acetophenazine Maleate *(a set oh fen' a zeen)*

Brand Names Tindal®

Use Management of manifestations of psychotic disorders

Pregnancy Risk Factor C

Contraindications Blood dyscrasias and bone marrow depression, patients in coma or brain damage, known hypersensitivity to acetophenazine

Adverse Reactions

>10%:
  Cardiovascular: Hypotension, orthostatic hypotension
  Central nervous system: Pseudoparkinsonism, akathisia, dystonias, tardive dyskinesia (persistent), dizziness
  Gastrointestinal: Constipation
  Ocular: Pigmentary retinopathy
  Respiratory: Nasal congestion
  Miscellaneous: Decreased sweating

1% to 10%:
  Dermatologic: Increased sensitivity to sun, skin rash
  Endocrine & metabolic: Changes in menstrual cycle, ejaculatory disturbances, changes in libido, pain in breasts
  Gastrointestinal: Weight gain, nausea, vomiting, stomach pain
  Genitourinary: Difficulty in urination
  Neuromuscular & skeletal: Trembling of fingers

<1%:
  Central nervous system: Neuroleptic malignant syndrome (NMS)
  Dermatologic: Discoloration of skin (blue-gray)
  Endocrine & metabolic: Galactorrhea
  Genitourinary: Priapism
  Hematologic: Agranulocytosis, leukopenia
  Hepatic: Cholestatic jaundice, hepatotoxicity
  Ocular: Cornea and lens changes, pigmentary retinopathy
  Miscellaneous: Impairment of temperature regulation, lowering of seizures threshold

Overdosage/Toxicology

Seizures: I.V.: Diazepam 5-10 mg (adults), 0.25-0.4 mg/kg (children up to 5 years)
  Recurrence: Consider phenytoin or phenobarbital
Hypotension: I.V. fluids (10-20 mL/kg); place in Trendelenburg position; dopamine or levarterenol may be infused if no response
Arrhythmias: Lidocaine drip or phenytoin are considered drugs of choice
Documented torsade de pointes: Isoproterenol 2-10 mcg/minute (0.1-1 mcg/minute in children) magnesium sulfate

Mechanism of Action Antagonizes the effects of dopamine in the basal ganglia and limbic areas of the forebrain; this activity appears responsible for the antipsychotic efficacy, as well as the production of extrapyramidal symptoms; increases the secretion of prolactin and has a marked suppressive effect on the chemoreceptor trigger zone; also produces peripheral blockade of cholinergic neurons

Pharmacodynamics/Kinetics

Duration of effect: ~24 hours, permitting daily dosing

Absorption: Tissue saturation, particularly in high lipid tissues such as the central nervous system

Metabolism: Phenothiazines are extensively hepatically metabolized with major routes of metabolism including oxidative processes and glucuronidation

Half-life, elimination: Range: 20-40 hours

Elimination: From the plasma is not significant for the phenothiazines; elimination from tissue saturated sites such as the central nervous system is slow, with metabolites of some phenothiazines detected in urine for several months after discontinuation of the drug

Usual Dosage Adults: Oral: 20 mg 3 times/day up to 60-120 mg/day

Hospitalized schizophrenic patients may require doses as high as 400-600 mg/day

Not dialyzable (0% to 5%)

Reference Range Therapeutic plasma levels have not yet been established

Test Interactions ↑ cholesterol (S), glucose; ↓ uric acid (S)

Dosage Forms Tablet: 20 mg

Acetoxymethylprogesterone see Medroxyprogesterone Acetate on page 677

Acetylcholine Chloride (a se teel koe' leen)

Related Information

Glaucoma Drug Therapy Comparison on page 1270

Brand Names Miochol®

Use Produces complete miosis in cataract surgery, keratoplasty, iridectomy and other anterior segment surgery where rapid miosis is required

Pregnancy Risk Factor C

Pregnancy/Breast Feeding Implications Acetylcholine is used primarily in the eye and there are no reports of its use in pregnancy; because it is ionized at physiologic pH, transplacental passage would not be expected

Contraindications Hypersensitivity to acetylcholine chloride and any components; acute iritis and acute inflammatory disease of the anterior chamber

Warnings/Precautions Systemic effects rarely occur but can cause problems for patients with acute cardiac failure, bronchial asthma, peptic ulcer, hyperthyroidism, GI spasm, urinary tract obstruction, and Parkinson's disease; open under aseptic conditions only

Adverse Reactions

<1%:

Cardiovascular: Bradycardia, hypotension, flushing

Central nervous system: Headache

Ocular: Altered distance vision, decreased night vision, transient lenticular opacities

Respiratory: Breathing difficulty

Miscellaneous: Sweating

Overdosage/Toxicology Treatment includes flushing eyes with water or normal saline and supportive measures; if accidentally ingested, induce emesis or perform gastric lavage

Drug Interactions

Decreased effect possible with flurbiprofen and suprofen, ophthalmic

Increased effect may be prolonged or enhanced in patients receiving tacrine

Stability Prepare solution immediately before use and discard unused portion; acetylcholine solutions are unstable

Mechanism of Action Causes contraction of the sphincter muscles of the iris, resulting in miosis and contraction of the ciliary muscle, leading to accommodation spasm

Pharmacodynamics/Kinetics

Onset of miosis: Occurs promptly

Duration: ~10 minutes

Usual Dosage Adults: Intraocular: 0.5-2 mL of 1% injection (5-20 mg) instilled into anterior chamber before or after securing one or more sutures

Patient Information May sting on instillation; use caution while driving at night or performing hazardous tasks; do not touch dropper to eye

Nursing Implications Discard any solution that is not used; open under aseptic conditions only

Dosage Forms Powder, intraocular: 1:100 [10 mg/mL] (2 mL, 15 mL)

Acetylcysteine (a se teel sis' tay een)

Brand Names Mucomyst®; Mucosil™

Synonyms Mercapturic Acid; NAC; N-Acetylcysteine; N-Acetyl-L-cysteine

(Continued)

Acetylcysteine (Continued)

Use Adjunctive mucolytic therapy in patients with abnormal or viscid mucous secretions in acute and chronic bronchopulmonary diseases; pulmonary complications of surgery and cystic fibrosis; diagnostic bronchial studies; antidote for acute acetaminophen toxicity

Pregnancy Risk Factor B

Pregnancy/Breast Feeding Implications There are no adequate and well controlled studies in pregnant women; use if only clearly needed

Contraindications Known hypersensitivity to acetylcysteine

Warnings/Precautions If bronchospasm occurs, administer a bronchodilator; discontinue acetylcysteine if bronchospasm progresses; since increased bronchial secretions may develop after inhalation, percussion, postural drainage and suctioning should follow

Adverse Reactions
>10%:
Gastrointestinal: Vomiting
Miscellaneous: Unpleasant odor during administration
1% to 10%:
Central nervous system: Drowsiness, clamminess, chills
Gastrointestinal: Stomatitis, nausea
Hematologic: Hemoptysis
Local: Irritation
Respiratory: Bronchospasm, rhinorrhea
<1%: Dermatologic: Skin rash

Overdosage/Toxicology The treatment of acetylcysteine toxicity is usually aimed at reversing anaphylactoid symptoms or controlling nausea and vomiting. The use of epinephrine, antihistamines, and steroids may be beneficial.

Stability Store opened vials in the refrigerator, use within 96 hours; dilutions should be freshly prepared and used within 1 hour; light purple color of solution does **not** affect its mucolytic activity

Mechanism of Action Exerts mucolytic action through its free sulfhydryl group which opens up the disulfide bonds in the mucoproteins thus lowering mucous viscosity. The exact mechanism of action in acetaminophen toxicity is unknown; thought to act by providing substrate for conjugation with the toxic metabolite.

Pharmacodynamics/Kinetics
Oral:
Peak plasma levels: 1-2 hours
Distribution: 0.33-0.47 L/kg
Plasma protein binding: 50%
Onset of action: Inhalation: Mucus liquefaction occurs maximally within 5-10 minutes
Duration: Can persist for >1 hour
Half-life:
Reduced acetylcysteine: 2 hours
Total acetylcysteine: 5.5 hours

Usual Dosage
Acetaminophen poisoning (initiate treatment within 24 hours):
Children and Adults: Oral: 140 mg/kg; followed by 17 doses of 70 mg/kg every 4 hours or until acetaminophen assay reveals nontoxic levels; repeat dose if emesis occurs within 1 hour of administration
Inhalation: Acetylcysteine 10% and 20% solution (Mucomyst®) (dilute 20% solution with sodium chloride or sterile water for inhalation); 10% solution may be used undiluted
Infants: 1-2 mL of 20% solution or 2-4 mL 10% solution until nebulized given 3-4 times/day
Children: 3-5 mL of 5% to 10% solution nebulized given 3-4 times/day
Adolescents: 5-10 mL of 5% to 10% solution nebulized given 3-4 times/day
Note: Patients should receive an aerosolized bronchodilator 10-15 minutes prior to acetylcysteine

Meconium ileus equivalent: Children and Adults:
100-300 mL of 4% to 10% solution by irrigation or orally
or
5-30 mL of 10% solution 3-6 times/24 hours orally or rectally

Administration For treatment of acetaminophen overdosage, administer orally as a 5% solution
Dilute the 20% solution 1:3 with a cola, orange juice, or other soft drink
Use within 1 hour of preparation; unpleasant odor becomes less noticeable as treatment progresses

Reference Range Determine acetaminophen level as soon as possible, but no sooner than 4 hours after ingestion (to ensure peak levels have been obtained); administer for acetaminophen level >150 μg/mL; toxic concentration with probable hepatotoxicity: >200 μg/mL at 4 hours or 50 μg at 12 hours

Patient Information Clear airway by coughing deeply before aerosol treatment

Nursing Implications Assess patient for nausea, vomiting, and skin rash following oral administration for treatment of acetaminophen poisoning; intermittent aerosol treatments are commonly given when patient arises, before meals, and just before retiring at bedtime

Dosage Forms Solution, as sodium: 10% [100 mg/mL] (4 mL, 10 mL, 30 mL); 20% [200 mg/mL] (4 mL, 10 mL, 30 mL, 100 mL)

Acetylsalicylic Acid *see* Aspirin *on page 92*

Aches-N-Pain® [OTC] *see* Ibuprofen *on page 561*

Achromycin® *see* Tetracycline *on page 1069*

Achromycin® V *see* Tetracycline *on page 1069*

Aciclovir *see* Acyclovir *on next page*

Acidulated Phosphate Fluoride *see* Fluoride *on page 471*

A-Cillin® *see* Amoxicillin Trihydrate *on page 68*

Aclovate® *see* Alclometasone Dipropionate *on page 35*

Acrivastine and Pseudoephedrine (ak′ ri vas teen & soo doe e fed′ rin)

Related Information
Pseudoephedrine *on page 955*

Brand Names Semprex-D®

Synonyms Pseudoephedrine and Acrivastine

Use Temporary relief of nasal congestion, decongest sinus openings, running nose, itching of nose or throat, and itchy, watery eyes due to hay fever or other upper respiratory allergies

Pregnancy Risk Factor B

Contraindications MAO inhibitor therapy within 14 days of initiating therapy, severe hypertension, severe coronary artery disease, hypersensitivity to pseudoephedrine, acrivastine (or other alkylamine antihistamines), or any component, renal impairment (Cl_{cr} <48 mL/minute)

Warnings/Precautions Use with caution in patients >60 years of age; use with caution in patients with high blood pressure, ischemic heart disease, diabetes, increased intraocular pressure, GI or GU obstruction, asthma, thyroid disease, or prostatic hypertrophy; not recommended for use in children

Adverse Reactions
>10%: Central nervous system: Drowsiness, headache
1% to 10%:
  Cardiovascular: Tachycardia, palpitations
  Central nervous system: Nervousness, dizziness, insomnia, vertigo, lightheadedness, fatigue, weakness
  Gastrointestinal: Nausea, vomiting, dry mouth, diarrhea
  Genitourinary: Difficult urination
  Respiratory: Pharyngitis, cough increase
  Miscellaneous: Diaphoresis
<1%:
  Endocrine & metabolic: Dysmenorrhea
  Gastrointestinal: Dyspepsia

Overdosage/Toxicology Symptoms of overdose include trembling, tachycardia, stridor, loss of consciousness, and possible convulsions; there is no specific antidote for pseudoephedrine intoxication, and the bulk of the treatment is supportive. Hyperactivity and agitation usually respond to reduced sensory input, however, with extreme agitation haloperidol (2-5 mg I.M. for adults) may be required.

Hyperthermia is best treated with external cooling measures, or when severe or unresponsive, muscle paralysis with pancuronium may be needed. Hypertension is usually transient and generally does not require treatment unless severe. For diastolic blood pressure >110 mm Hg, a nitroprusside infusion should be initiated. Seizures usually respond to diazepam I.V. and/or phenytoin maintenance regimens.

Drug Interactions
Decreased effect of guanethidine, reserpine, methyldopa, and beta-blockers
Increased toxicity with MAO inhibitors (hypertensive crisis), sympathomimetics, CNS depressants, alcohol (sedation)

Mechanism of Action Refer to Pseudoephedrine monograph; acrivastine is an analogue of triprolidine and it is considered to be relatively less sedating than traditional antihistamines; believed to involve competitive blockade of H_1-receptor sites resulting in the inability of histamine to combine with its receptor sites and exert its usual effects on target cells
(Continued)

Acrivastine and Pseudoephedrine *(Continued)*

Usual Dosage Adults: 1 capsule 3-4 times/day
  Dosing comments in renal impairment: Do not use
Dosage Forms Capsule: Acrivastine 8 mg and pseudoephedrine hydrochloride 60 mg

ACT *see* Dactinomycin *on page 298*

Actagen® [OTC] *see* Triprolidine and Pseudoephedrine *on page 1131*

ACTH® *see* Corticotropin *on page 274*

Acthar® *see* Corticotropin *on page 274*

Acticort™ *see* Hydrocortisone *on page 546*

Actidose-Aqua® [OTC] *see* Charcoal *on page 214*

Actidose® With Sorbitol [OTC] *see* Charcoal *on page 214*

Actifed® [OTC] *see* Triprolidine and Pseudoephedrine *on page 1131*

Actigall™ *see* Ursodiol *on page 1143*

Actinex® *see* Masoprocol *on page 666*

Actinomycin D *see* Dactinomycin *on page 298*

Activase® *see* Alteplase *on page 46*

Activated Carbon *see* Charcoal *on page 214*

Activated Charcoal *see* Charcoal *on page 214*

Activated Dimethicone *see* Simethicone *on page 1006*

Activated Ergosterol *see* Ergocalciferol *on page 396*

Activated Methylpolysiloxane *see* Simethicone *on page 1006*

ACT® [OTC] *see* Fluoride *on page 471*

Acular® *see* Ketorolac Tromethamine *on page 612*

Acutrim® Precision Release® [OTC] *see* Phenylpropanolamine Hydrochloride *on page 876*

ACV *see* Acyclovir *on this page*

Acycloguanosine *see* Acyclovir *on this page*

Acyclovir *(ay sye′ kloe ver)*
  Related Information
    Antimicrobial Drugs of Choice *on page 1298-1302*
  Brand Names Zovirax®
  Synonyms Aciclovir; ACV; Acycloguanosine
  Use Treatment of initial and prophylaxis of recurrent mucosal and cutaneous herpes simplex (HSV-1 and HSV-2) infections; herpes simplex encephalitis; herpes zoster; genital herpes infection; varicella-zoster infections in healthy, nonpregnant persons >13 years of age, children <12 months of age who have a chronic skin or lung disorder or are receiving long-term aspirin therapy, and immunocompromised patients; for herpes zoster, acyclovir should be started within 72 hours of the appearance of the rash to be effective; acyclovir will not prevent postherpetic neuralgias
  Pregnancy Risk Factor C
  Contraindications Hypersensitivity to acyclovir
  Warnings/Precautions Use with caution in patients with pre-existing renal disease or in those receiving other nephrotoxic drugs concurrently; maintain adequate urine output during the first 2 hours after I.V. infusion; use with caution in patients with underlying neurologic abnormalities, serious hepatic or electrolyte abnormalities, or substantial hypoxia
  Adverse Reactions
    >10%:
      Central nervous system: Headache
      Local: Inflammation at injection site
    1% to 10%:
      Central nervous system: Lethargy, dizziness, seizures, confusion, agitation, coma
      Dermatologic: Rash
      Gastrointestinal: Nausea, vomiting
      Neuromuscular & skeletal: Tremor
      Renal: Impaired renal function
    <1%:
      Central nervous system: Mental depression, insomnia
      Gastrointestinal: Anorexia

Hepatic: LFT elevation
Miscellaneous: Sore throat

Overdosage/Toxicology Symptoms of overdose include elevated serum creatinine, renal failure. In the event of an overdose, sufficient urine flow must be maintained to avoid drug precipitation within the renal tubules. Hemodialysis has resulted in up to 60% reductions in serum acyclovir levels.

Drug Interactions Increased CNS side effects with zidovudine and probenecid

Stability Incompatible with blood products and protein-containing solutions; reconstituted solutions remain stable for 24 hours at room temperature; do not refrigerate reconstituted solutions as they may precipitate; in patients who require fluid restriction, a concentration of up to 10 mg/mL has been infused, however, concentrations >10 mg/mL (usual recommended concentration: <7 mg/mL in D_5W) increase the risk of phlebitis

Mechanism of Action Inhibits DNA synthesis and viral replication by competing with deoxyguanosine triphosphate for viral DNA polymerase and being incorporated into viral DNA

Pharmacodynamics/Kinetics

Absorption: Oral: 15% to 30%; food does not appear to affect absorption
Distribution: Widely distributed throughout the body including brain, kidney, lungs, liver, spleen, muscle, uterus, vagina, and CSF
Protein binding: <30%
Metabolism: Small amount of hepatic metabolism
Half-life, terminal phase:
 Neonates: 4 hours
 Children 1-12 years: 2-3 hours
 Adults: 3 hours
Time to peak serum concentration:
 Oral: Within 1.5-2 hours
 I.V.: Within 1 hour
Elimination: Primary route is the kidney (30% to 90% of a dose excreted unchanged); hemodialysis removes ~60% of the dose while removal by peritoneal dialysis is to a much lesser extent (supplemental dose recommended)

Usual Dosage

Dosing weight should be based on the smaller of lean body weight or total body weight
 Adult determination of lean body weight (LBW) in kg:
  LBW males: 50 kg + (2.3 kg x inches >5 feet)
  LBW females: 45 kg + (2.3 kg x inches >5 feet)

Treatment of herpes simplex virus infections: I.V.
 Neonates: 1500 mg/m²/day divided every 8 hours or 30 mg/kg/day divided every 8 hours for 10-14 days
 Children and Adults:
  Mucocutaneous HSV infection 750 mg/m²/day divided every 8 hours or 5 mg/kg/dose every 8 hours for 5-10 days
  HSV encephalitis: 1500 mg/m²/day divided every 8 hours for 5-10 days
  I.V.: 5 mg/kg/dose every 8 hours for 5-10 days
Treatment of herpes simplex virus infections: Adults:
 Oral: Treatment: 200 mg every 4 hours while awake (5 times/day)
 Topical: ½" ribbon of ointment for a 4" square surface area every 3 hours (6 times/day)
Treatment of varicella-zoster virus (chickenpox) infections:
 Oral:
  Children: 10-20 mg/kg/dose (up to 800 mg) 4 times/day for 5 days; begin treatment within the first 24 hours of rash onset
  Adults: 600-800 mg/dose every 4 hours while awake (5 times/day) for 7-10 days or 1000 mg every 6 hours for 5 days
 I.V.: Children and Adults: 1500 mg/m²/day divided every 8 hours or 10 mg/kg/dose every 8 hours for 7 days
Treatment of herpes zoster infections:
 Oral:
  Children (immunocompromised): 250-600 mg/m²/dose 4-5 times/day for 7-10 days
  Adults (immunocompromised): 800 mg every 4 hours (5 times/day) for 7-10 days
 I.V.: Children and Adults (immunocompromised): 7.5 mg/kg/dose every 8 hours
Prophylaxis in immunocompromised patients:
 Varicella zoster or herpes zoster in HIV-positive patients: Adults: Oral: 400 mg every 4 hours (5 times/day) for 7-10 days
 Bone marrow transplant recipients: Children and Adults: I.V.:
  Autologous patients who are HSV seropositive: 150 mg/m²/dose (5 mg/kg) every 12 hours; with clinical symptoms of herpes simplex: 150 mg/m²/dose every 8 hours

(Continued)

Acyclovir *(Continued)*

Autologous patients who are CMV seropositive: 500 mg/m²/dose (10 mg/kg) every 8 hours; for clinically symptomatic CMV infection, consider replacing acyclovir with ganciclovir

Prophylaxis of herpes simplex virus infections: Adults: 200 mg 3-4 times/day or 400 mg twice daily

Dosing adjustment in renal impairment:
Oral: HSV/varicella-zoster:
Cl_{cr} 10-25 mL/minute: Administer dose every 8 hours
Cl_{cr} <10 mL/minute: Administer dose every 12 hours
I.V.:
Cl_{cr} 25-50 mL/minute: 5-10 mg/kg/dose: Administer every 12 hours
Cl_{cr} 10-25 mL/minute: 5-10 mg/kg/dose: Administer every 24 hours
Cl_{cr} <10 mL/minute: 2.5-5 mg/kg/dose: Administer every 24 hours
Dialyzable (50% to 100%); administer dose postdialysis
Peritoneal dialysis effects: Dose as for Cl_{cr} <10 mL/minute
Continuous arterio-venous or venous-venous hemofiltration (CAVH/CAVHD) effects: Dose as for Cl_{cr} <10 mL/minute

Administration Infuse over 1 hour; maintain adequate hydration of patient; check and rotate infusion sites for phlebitis

Monitoring Parameters Urinalysis, BUN, serum creatinine, liver enzymes, CBC

Patient Information Patients are contagious only when viral shedding is occurring; recurrences tend to appear within 3 months of original infection; acyclovir is **not** a cure; avoid sexual intercourse when lesions are present; may take with food

Nursing Implications Wear gloves when applying ointment for self-protection

Additional Information Sodium content of 1 g: 4.2 mEq

Dosage Forms
Capsule: 200 mg
Injection: 500 mg (10 mL); 1000 mg (20 mL)
Ointment, topical: 5% [50 mg/g] (3 g, 15 g)
Suspension, oral (banana flavor): 40 mg/mL
Tablet: 800 mg

Adagen™ *see* Pegademase Bovine *on page 843*

Adalat® *see* Nifedipine *on page 794*

Adalat® CC *see* Nifedipine *on page 794*

Adamantanamine Hydrochloride *see* Amantadine Hydrochloride *on page 49*

Adapin® *see* Doxepin Hydrochloride *on page 369*

Adeflor® *see* Vitamin, Multiple *on page 1166*

Adenine Arabinoside *see* Vidarabine *on page 1156*

Adenocard® *see* Adenosine *on this page*

Adenosine *(a den' oh seen)*

Related Information
Antiarrhythmic Drugs *on page 1246-1248*

Brand Names Adenocard®

Synonyms 9-Beta-D-ribofuranosyladenine

Use Treatment of paroxysmal supraventricular tachycardia (PSVT) including that associated with accessory bypass tracts (Wolff-Parkinson-White syndrome); when clinically advisable, appropriate vagal maneuvers should be attempted prior to adenosine administration; not effective in atrial flutter, atrial fibrillation, or ventricular tachycardia

Pregnancy Risk Factor C

Pregnancy/Breast Feeding Implications Case reports (4) on administration during pregnancy have indicated no adverse effects on fetus or newborn attributable to adenosine

Contraindications Known hypersensitivity to adenosine; second or third degree A-V block or sick-sinus syndrome (except in patients with a functioning artificial pacemaker); atrial flutter, atrial fibrillation, and ventricular tachycardia (the drug is not effective in converting these arrhythmias to sinus rhythm)

Warnings/Precautions Patients with pre-existing S-A nodal dysfunction may experience prolonged sinus pauses after adenosine; there have been reports of atrial fibrillation/flutter in patients with PSVT associated with accessory conduction pathways after adenosine; adenosine decreases conduction through the A-V node and may produce a short lasting first, second, or third degree heart block. Because of the very short half-life, the effects are generally self limiting. At the time of conversion to normal sinus rhythm, a variety of new rhythms may appear on the EKG.

A limited number of patients with asthma have received adenosine and have not experienced exacerbation of their asthma. Be alert to the possibility that adenosine could produce bronchoconstriction in patients with asthma.

Adverse Reactions

>10%:
Cardiovascular: Facial flushing (18%), palpitations, chest pain, hypotension
Central nervous system: Headache
Respiratory: Shortness of breath/dyspnea (12%)
Miscellaneous: Sweating

1% to 10%:
Central nervous system: Dizziness, tingling in arms, numbness
Gastrointestinal: Nausea (3%)
Respiratory: Chest pressure (7%)

<1%:
Cardiovascular: Hypotension
Central nervous system: Lightheadedness, dizziness, apprehension, head pressure
Gastrointestinal: Metallic taste, tightness in throat, pressure in groin
Neuromuscular & skeletal: Heaviness in arms, neck and back pain
Ocular: Blurred vision
Respiratory: Hypoventilation
Miscellaneous: Sweating, burning sensation

Overdosage/Toxicology Since half-life of adenosine is <10 seconds, any adverse effects are rapidly self-limiting; intoxication is usually short-lived, since the half-life of the drug is very short. Treatment of prolonged effects requires individualization. Theophylline and other methylxanthines are competitive inhibitors of adenosine and may have a role in reversing its toxic effects.

Drug Interactions
Decreased effect: Methylxanthines antagonize effects
Increased effect: Dipyridamole potentiates effects of adenosine
Increased toxicity: Carbamazepine may increase heart block

Stability Do not refrigerate, precipitation may occur (may dissolve by warming to room temperature)

Mechanism of Action Slows conduction time through the A-V node, interrupting the re-entry pathways through the A-V node, restoring normal sinus rhythm

Pharmacodynamics/Kinetics
Onset: Clinical effects occur rapidly
Duration: Very brief
Metabolism: In the blood and tissue to inosine then to adenosine monophosphate (AMP) and hypoxanthine
Half-life: <10 seconds, thus adverse effects are usually rapidly self-limiting

Usual Dosage Rapid I.V. push (over 1-2 seconds):
Children: Pediatric advanced life support: Treatment of SVT: 0.1 mg/kg; if not effective, give 0.2 mg/kg; maximum single dose: 12 mg
Adults: 6 mg; if not effective within 1-2 minutes, 12 mg may be given; may repeat 12 mg bolus if needed; maximum single dose: 12 mg

Note: Patients who are receiving concomitant theophylline therapy may be less likely to respond to adenosine therapy
Note: Higher doses may be needed for administration via peripheral versus central vein

Administration Give rapid I.V. push (administered over a 1- to 2-second period), follow with flush; requires a cardiac monitor for administration

Monitoring Parameters EKG monitoring, heart rate, blood pressure, respirations

Nursing Implications Be alert for possible exacerbation of asthma in asthmatic patients

Dosage Forms Injection, preservative free: 3 mg/mL (2 mL)

ADH *see* Vasopressin *on page 1149*

Adipex-P® *see* Phentermine Hydrochloride *on page 872*

Adlone® *see* Methylprednisolone *on page 724*

ADR *see* Doxorubicin Hydrochloride *on page 370*

Adrenalin® *see* Epinephrine *on page 389*

Adrenaline *see* Epinephrine *on page 389*

Adrenergic Agonists, Cardiovascular Comparison *see page 1242*

Adrenocorticotropic Hormone *see* Corticotropin *on page 274*

Adriamycin PFS™ *see* Doxorubicin Hydrochloride *on page 370*

Adriamycin RDF™ *see* Doxorubicin Hydrochloride *on page 370*

Adrucil® *see* Fluorouracil *on page 473*

Adsorbent Charcoal *see* Charcoal *on page 214*

Adsorbocarpine® *see* Pilocarpine *on page 883*

Adsorbonac® [OTC] Ophthalmic *see* Sodium Chloride *on page 1012*

Advil® [OTC] *see* Ibuprofen *on page 561*

AeroBid® *see* Flunisolide *on page 468*

AeroBid-M® *see* Flunisolide *on page 468*

Aerolate® *see* Theophylline/Aminophylline *on page 1072*

Aerolate III® *see* Theophylline/Aminophylline *on page 1072*

Aerolate JR® *see* Theophylline/Aminophylline *on page 1072*

Aerolate SR® *see* Theophylline/Aminophylline *on page 1072*

Aeroseb-Dex® *see* Dexamethasone *on page 314*

Aeroseb-HC® *see* Hydrocortisone *on page 546*

Aerosporin® *see* Polymyxin B Sulfate *on page 901*

Afrinol® [OTC] *see* Pseudoephedrine *on page 955*

Afrin® Nasal Solution [OTC] *see* Oxymetazoline Hydrochloride *on page 829*

Aftate® [OTC] *see* Tolnaftate *on page 1106*

AgNO₃ *see* Silver Nitrate *on page 1004*

Agoral® Plain [OTC] *see* Mineral Oil *on page 743*

AHF *see* Antihemophilic Factor (Human) *on page 80*

A-HydroCort® *see* Hydrocortisone *on page 546*

Akarpine® *see* Pilocarpine *on page 883*

AKBeta® *see* Levobunolol Hydrochloride *on page 623*

AK-Chlor® *see* Chloramphenicol *on page 219*

AK-Con® *see* Naphazoline Hydrochloride *on page 775*

AK-Dex® *see* Dexamethasone *on page 314*

AK-Dilate® Ophthalmic Solution *see* Phenylephrine Hydrochloride *on page 874*

AK-Fluor *see* Fluorescein Sodium *on page 470*

AK-Homatropine® *see* Homatropine Hydrobromide *on page 537*

AK-Nefrin® Ophthalmic Solution *see* Phenylephrine Hydrochloride *on page 874*

AK-Pentolate® *see* Cyclopentolate Hydrochloride *on page 286*

AK-Poly-Bac® *see* Bacitracin and Polymyxin B *on page 112*

AK-Pred® *see* Prednisolone *on page 919*

AK-Spore H.C.® *see* Neomycin, Polymyxin B, and Hydrocortisone *on page 781*

AK-Spore® Ophthalmic Solution *see* Neomycin, Polymyxin B, and Gramicidin *on page 781*

AK-Sulf® *see* Sodium Sulfacetamide *on page 1018*

AK-Taine® *see* Proparacaine Hydrochloride *on page 943*

AK-Tracin® *see* Bacitracin *on page 111*

AK-Trol® *see* Neomycin, Polymyxin B, and Dexamethasone *on page 780*

AK-Zol® *see* Acetazolamide *on page 20*

Ala-Cort® *see* Hydrocortisone *on page 546*

Ala-Scalp™ *see* Hydrocortisone *on page 546*

Ala-Tet® *see* Tetracycline *on page 1069*

Alba-Dex® *see* Dexamethasone *on page 314*

Albalon® Liquifilm® *see* Naphazoline Hydrochloride *on page 775*

Albuminar® *see* Albumin, Human *on this page*

Albumin, Human (al byoo' min)
Brand Names Albuminar®; Albumisol®; Albutein®; Buminate®; Plasbumin®

Synonyms Normal Human Serum Albumin; Normal Serum Albumin (Human); Salt Poor Albumin; SPA

Use Plasma volume expansion and maintenance of cardiac output in the treatment of certain types of shock or impending shock; may be useful for burn patients, ARDS, and cardiopulmonary bypass; other uses considered by some investigators (but not proven) are retroperitoneal surgery, peritonitis, and ascites; unless the condition responsible for hypoproteinemia can be corrected, albumin can provide only symptomatic relief or supportive treatment; nutritional supplementation is not an appropriate indication for albumin

Pregnancy Risk Factor C

Contraindications Patients with severe anemia or cardiac failure, known hypersensitivity to albumin; avoid 25% concentration in preterm infants due to risk of idiopathic ventricular hypertrophy

Warnings/Precautions Use with caution in patients with hepatic or renal failure because of added protein load; rapid infusion of albumin solutions may cause vascular overload. All patients should be observed for signs of hypervolemia such as pulmonary edema. Use with caution in those patients for whom sodium restriction is necessary. Rapid infusion may cause hypotension.

Adverse Reactions
1% to 10%:
Cardiovascular: Precipitation of congestive heart failure or pulmonary edema, hypotension, tachycardia, hypervolemia
Central nervous system: Fever, chills
Dermatologic: Rash
Gastrointestinal: Nausea, vomiting

Overdosage/Toxicology Hypervolemia, congestive heart failure, pulmonary edema

Stability Do not use solution if it is turbid or contains a deposit; use within 4 hours after opening vial

Usual Dosage I.V.:
5% should be used in hypovolemic patients or intravascularly-depleted patients
25% should be used in patients in whom fluid and sodium intake must be minimized

Dose depends on condition of patient:
Children:
Emergency initial dose: 25 g
Nonemergencies: 25% to 50% of the adult dose
Adults: Usual dose: 25 g; no more than 250 g should be administered within 48 hours
Hypoproteinemia: 0.5-1 g/kg/dose; repeat every 1-2 days as calculated to replace ongoing losses
Hypovolemia: 0.5-1 g/kg/dose; repeat as needed; maximum dose: 6 g/kg/day

Administration Albumin administration must be completed within 6 hours after entering the 5% container, provided that administration is begun within 4 hours of entering the container; rapid infusion may cause vascular overload; albumin is best administered at a rate of 2-4 mL/minute; 25% albumin may be given at a rate of 1 mL/minute

Test Interactions ↑ alkaline phosphatase (S)

Additional Information Sodium content of 1 L: Both 5% and 25% albumin contain 130-160 mEq

Dosage Forms Injection: 5% [50 mg/mL] (50 mL, 250 mL, 500 mL, 1000 mL); 25% [250 mg/mL] (10 mL, 20 mL, 50 mL, 100 mL)

Albumisol® see Albumin, Human on previous page

Albutein® see Albumin, Human on previous page

Albuterol (al byoo' ter ole)
Brand Names Proventil®; Ventolin®; Volmax®

Synonyms Salbutamol

Use Bronchodilator in reversible airway obstruction due to asthma or COPD

Pregnancy Risk Factor C

Contraindications Hypersensitivity to albuterol, adrenergic amines or any ingredients

Warnings/Precautions Use with caution in patients with hyperthyroidism, diabetes mellitus, or sensitivity to sympathomimetic amines; cardiovascular disorders including coronary insufficiency or hypertension; excessive use may result in tolerance
(Continued)

Albuterol *(Continued)*

Some adverse reactions may occur more frequently in children 2-5 years of age than in adults and older children

Because of its minimal effect on beta$_1$-receptors and its relatively long duration of action, albuterol is a rational choice in the elderly when a beta agonist is indicated. All patients should utilize a spacer device when using a metered dose inhaler. Oral use should be avoided in the elderly due to adverse effects.

Adverse Reactions
>10%:
Cardiovascular: Tachycardia, palpitations, pounding heartbeat
Gastrointestinal: GI upset, nausea
1% to 10%:
Cardiovascular: Flushing of face, hypertension or hypotension
Central nervous system: Nervousness, CNS stimulation, hyperactivity, insomnia, dizziness, lightheadedness, drowsiness, headache, weakness
Gastrointestinal: Dry mouth, heartburn, vomiting, unusual taste
Genitourinary: Difficult urination
Neuromuscular & skeletal: Muscle cramping, tremor
Respiratory: Coughing
Miscellaneous: Increased sweating
<1%:
Neuromuscular & skeletal: Chest pain
Respiratory: Paradoxical bronchospasm
Miscellaneous: Loss of appetite, unusual paleness

Overdosage/Toxicology Symptoms of overdose include hypertension, tachycardia, angina, hypokalemia; hypokalemia and tachyarrhythmias: Prudent use of a cardioselective beta-adrenergic blocker (eg, atenolol or metoprolol); keep in mind the potential for induction of bronchoconstriction in an asthmatic. Dialysis has not been shown to be of value in the treatment of an overdose with this agent.

Drug Interactions
Decreased effect: Beta-adrenergic blockers (eg, propranolol)
Increased therapeutic effect: Inhaled ipratropium → ↑ duration of bronchodilation, nifedipine → ↑ FEV-1
Increased toxicity: Cardiovascular effects are potentiated in patients also receiving MAO inhibitors, tricyclic antidepressants, sympathomimetic agents (eg, amphetamine, dopamine, dobutamine), inhaled anesthetics (eg, enflurane)

Mechanism of Action Relaxes bronchial smooth muscle by action on beta$_2$-receptors with little effect on heart rate

Pharmacodynamics/Kinetics
Peak effect:
Oral: 2-3 hours
Nebulization/oral inhalation: Within 0.5-2 hours
Duration of action:
Oral: 4-6 hours
Nebulization/oral inhalation: 3-4 hours
Metabolism: By the liver to an inactive sulfate, with 28% appearing in the urine as unchanged drug
Half-life:
Inhalation: 3.8 hours
Oral: 2.7-5 hours
Elimination: 30% appears in urine as unchanged drug

Usual Dosage
Oral:
Children:
2-6 years: 0.1-0.2 mg/kg/dose 3 times/day; maximum dose not to exceed 12 mg/day (divided doses)
6-12 years: 2 mg/dose 3-4 times/day; maximum dose not to exceed 24 mg/day (divided doses)
Children >12 years and Adults: 2-4 mg/dose 3-4 times/day; maximum dose not to exceed 32 mg/day (divided doses)
Elderly: 2 mg 3-4 times/day; maximum: 8 mg 4 times/day

Inhalation MDI: 90 mcg/spray:
Children <12 years: 1-2 inhalations 4 times/day using a tube spacer
Children ≥12 years and Adults: 1-2 inhalations every 4-6 hours; maximum: 12 inhalations/day
Exercise-induced bronchospasm: 2 inhalations 15 minutes before exercising

Inhalation: Nebulization: 2.5 mg = 0.5 mL of the 0.5% inhalation solution to be diluted in 1-2.5 mL of NS **or** 0.01-0.05 mL/kg of 0.5% solution every 4-6 hours;

intensive care patients may require more frequent administration; minimum
dose: 0.1 mL; maximum dose: 1 mL diluted in 1-2 mL normal saline
<5 years: 1.25-2.5 mg every 4-6 hours as needed
>5 years: 2.5-5 mg every 4-6 hours as needed

Not removed by hemodialysis

Monitoring Parameters Heart rate, CNS stimulation, asthma symptoms, arterial
or capillary blood gases (if patients condition warrants)

Test Interactions ↑ renin (S), ↑ aldosterone (S)

Patient Information Do not exceed recommended dosage; rinse mouth with
water following each inhalation to help with dry throat and mouth; follow specific
instructions accompanying inhaler; if more than one inhalation is necessary, wait
at least 1 full minute between inhalations. May cause nervousness, restlessness,
insomnia - if these effects continue after dosage reduction, notify physician; also
notify physician if palpitations, tachycardia, chest pain, muscle tremors, dizziness, headache, flushing or if breathing difficulty persists.

Nursing Implications Before using, the inhaler must be shaken well; assess
lung sounds, pulse, and blood pressure before administration and during peak of
medication; observe patient for wheezing after administration, if this occurs, call
physician

Dosage Forms
Aerosol: 90 mcg/dose (17 g)
Capsule, oral inhalation: 0.5% (20 mL)
Solution:
  Inhalation: 0.5% (20 mL)
  Concentrate for nebulization: 0.5%
  Nebulization: 0.083% (3 mL)
Syrup, as sulfate (alcohol and sugar free): 2 mg/5 mL (480 mL)
Tablet, as sulfate: 2 mg, 4 mg
Tablet, extended release (Volmax®): 4 mg, 8 mg

Alcaine® see Proparacaine Hydrochloride on page 943

Alclometasone Dipropionate (al kloe met' a sone)
Brand Names Aclovate®
Use Treats inflammation of corticosteroid-responsive dermatosis (low potency
topical corticosteroid)
Pregnancy Risk Factor C
Contraindications Viral, fungal, or tubercular skin lesions, known hypersensitivity to alclometasone or any component
Warnings/Precautions Adverse systemic effects may occur when used on large
areas of the body, denuded areas, for prolonged periods of time, with an occlusive dressing, and/or in infants or small children
Adverse Reactions
1% to 10%: Topical: Itching, burning, erythema, dryness, irritation, papular
rashes
<1%: Topical: Hypertrichosis, acneiform eruptions, hypopigmentation, perioral
dermatitis, maceration of skin, skin atrophy, striae, miliaria
Overdosage/Toxicology Symptoms of overdose include cushingoid appearance (systemic), muscle weakness (systemic), osteoporosis (systemic) all with
long-term use only. When consumed in excessive quantities for prolonged
periods, systemic hypercorticism and adrenal suppression may occur; in those
cases, discontinuation and withdrawal of the corticosteroid should be done judiciously.
Stability Store between 2°C and 30°C (36°F and 86°F)
Mechanism of Action Stimulates the synthesis of enzymes needed to decrease
inflammation, suppress mitotic activity, and cause vasoconstriction
Usual Dosage Topical: Apply a thin film to the affected area 2-3 times/day
Patient Information Before applying, gently wash area to reduce risk of infection;
apply a thin film to cleansed area and rub in gently and thoroughly until medica-
tion vanishes; avoid exposure to sunlight, severe sunburn may occur
Nursing Implications For external use only; do not use on open wounds; apply
sparingly to occlusive dressings; should not be used in the presence of open or
weeping lesions
Dosage Forms
Cream: 0.05% (15 g, 45 g, 60 g)
Ointment, topical: 0.05% (15 g, 45 g, 60 g)

Alconefrin® Nasal Solution [OTC] see Phenylephrine Hydrochloride on
page 874

Aldactone® see Spironolactone on page 1025

Aldesleukin (al des loo' kin)

Related Information
Cancer Chemotherapy Regimens *on page 1218-1241*

Brand Names Proleukin®

Synonyms IL-2; Interleukin-2

Use Primarily investigated in tumors known to have a response to immunotherapy, such as melanoma and renal cell carcinoma; has been used in conjunction with LAK cells, TIL cells, IL-1, and interferon

Pregnancy Risk Factor C

Contraindications Known history of hypersensitivity to interleukin-2 or any component; patients with an abnormal thallium stress test or pulmonary function test; patients who have had an organ allograft; retreatment in patients who have experienced sustained ventricular tachycardia (≥5 beats), cardiac rhythm disturbances not controlled or unresponsive to management, recurrent chest pain with EKG changes (consistent with angina or myocardial infarction), intubation required >72 hours, pericardial tamponade; renal dysfunction requiring dialysis >72 hours, coma or toxic psychosis lasting >48 hours, repetitive or difficult to control seizures, bowel ischemia/perforation, GI bleeding requiring surgery

Warnings/Precautions Has been associated with capillary leak syndrome (CLS); CLS results in hypotension and reduced organ perfusion which may be severe and can result in death; therapy should be restricted to patients with normal cardiac and pulmonary functions as defined by thallium stress and formal pulmonary function testing; extreme caution should be used in patients with normal thallium stress tests and pulmonary functions tests who have a history of prior cardiac or pulmonary disease.

Intensive aldesleukin treatment is associated with impaired neutrophil function (reduced chemotaxis) and with an increased risk of disseminated infection, including sepsis and bacterial endocarditis, in treated patients. Consequently, pre-existing bacterial infections should be adequately treated prior to initiation of therapy. Additionally, all patients with indwelling central lines should receive antibiotic prophylaxis effective against *S. aureus*. Antibiotic prophylaxis which has been associated with a reduced incidence of staphylococcal infections in aldesleukin studies includes the use of oxacillin, nafcillin, ciprofloxacin, or vancomycin. Disseminated infections acquired in the course of treatment are a major contributor to treatment morbidity and use of antibiotic prophylaxis, and aggressive treatment of suspected and documented infections may reduce the morbidity of aldesleukin treatment.

Adverse Reactions
>10%:
  Cardiovascular: Sinus tachycardia, edema, arrhythmias, pulmonary congestion; hypotension (dose-limiting toxicity) which may require vasopressor support and hemodynamic changes resembling those seen in septic shock can be seen within 2 hours of administration; angina, acute myocardial infarction, SVT with hypotension has been reported
  Central nervous system: Dizziness, sensory dysfunction, fever, chills, fatigue, weakness, malaise; rigors which can be decreased or ameliorated with acetaminophen or a nonsteroidal agent and meperidine
  Dermatologic: Pruritus, erythema, rash, dry skin, exfoliative dermatitis
  Endocrine & metabolic: Hypomagnesemia, acidosis, hypocalcemia, hypophosphatemia
  Gastrointestinal: Nausea, vomiting, pain, weight gain, diarrhea, stomatitis, anorexia, GI bleeding
  Hematologic: Anemia, thrombocytopenia, leukopenia, coagulation disorders, elevated bilirubin, BUN, serum creatinine, transaminase, and alkaline phosphatase
  Hepatic: Jaundice
  Neuropsychiatric: Cognitive changes, disorientation, somnolence, paranoid delusion, and other behavioral changes; reversible and dose related
  Renal: Oliguria, anuria, proteinuria; renal failure (dose-limiting toxicity) manifested as oliguria noted within 24-48 hours of initiation of therapy; marked fluid retention, azotemia, and increased serum creatinine seen, which may return to baseline within 7 days of discontinuation of therapy
  Respiratory: Dyspnea, pulmonary edema
1% to 10%: Increase in vascular permeability: Capillary-leak syndrome manifested by severe peripheral edema, ascites, pulmonary infiltration, and pleural effusion; occurs in 2% to 4% of patients and is resolved after therapy ends
<1%:
  Cardiovascular: Congestive heart failure
  Central nervous system: Coma, seizures
  Dermatologic: Pruritus, macular erythema, alopecia

Endocrine & metabolic: Hypothyroidism, hypercalcemia, hypophosphatemia, hypocalcemia, hypomagnesemia, increased plasma levels of stress-related hormones

Gastrointestinal: Pancreatitis

Genitourinary: Urinary frequency

Hematologic: Anemia, thrombocytopenia, eosinophilia

Neuromuscular & skeletal: Arthritis, muscle spasm

Miscellaneous: Allergic reactions

Overdosage/Toxicology Side effects following the use of aldesleukin are dose related. Administration of more than the recommended dose has been associated with a more rapid onset of expected dose-limiting toxicities. Adverse reactions generally will reverse when the drug is stopped particularly because of its short serum half-life. Continuing symptoms should be treated supportively.

Drug Interactions

Decreased toxicity: Corticosteroids have been shown to decrease toxicity of IL-2, but have not been used since there is concern that they may reduce the efficacy of the lymphokine

Increased toxicity:

Aldesleukin may affect central nervous function; therefore, interactions could occur following concomitant administration of psychotropic drugs (eg, narcotics, analgesics, antiemetics, sedatives, tranquilizers)

Concomitant administration of drugs possessing nephrotoxic (eg, aminoglycosides, indomethacin), myelotoxic (eg, cytotoxic chemotherapy), cardiotoxic (eg, doxorubicin), or hepatotoxic (eg, methotrexate, asparaginase) effects with aldesleukin may increase toxicity in these organ systems. The safety and efficacy of aldesleukin in combination with chemotherapies has not been established.

Beta-blockers and other antihypertensives may potentiate the hypotension seen with Proleukin®

Stability

Store vials of lyophilized injection in a refrigerator at 2°C to 8°C (36°F to 46°F)

Reconstituted or diluted solution is stable for up to 48 hours at refrigerated and room temperatures 2°C to 25°C (36°F to 77°F); however, since this product contains no preservatives, the reconstituted and diluted solutions should be stored in the refrigerator

Compatible only with D_5W

Gently swirl, do not shake

Note: As with most biological proteins, solutions containing IL-2 should not be filtered. Filtration will result in significant loss of bioactivity; see table.

Recommendations for IL-2 (Aldesleukin - Proleukin™) Dilutions in D_5W*

Concentration (mcg/mL)	Concentration (million units/mL)	Stability Recommendation
<60	<1	Human serum albumin must be added to bag prior to addition of IL-2; these solutions are stable for 6 days at room temperature†
60-100	1-1.7	**These concentrations should not be utilized as they are unstable**
100-500	1.7-8.4	These solutions are stable for 6 days at room temperature†

*1.3 mg of IL-2 (aldesleukin - Proleukin™) is equivalent to 22 million units.

†Although stability is 6 days, IL-2 does not contain a preservative and 24-hour expiration dating should be used.

Volume of Human Serum Albumin to Be Added to IL-2 (Aldesleukin - Proleukin™) Infusions in D_5W

Volume of I.V. Diluent (mL)	Volume of 5% Human Serum Albumin to Be Added Prior to IL-2 Addition (mL)	Volume of 25% Human Serum Albumin to Be Added Prior to IL-2 Addition (mL)
50	1	0.2
100	2	0.4
150	3	0.6
200	4	0.8
250	5	1
500	10	2

(Continued)

Aldesleukin *(Continued)*

Concentrations of IL-2 which fall into the unstable (60-100 mcg/mL **or** 1-1.7 microunits/mL) range require addition of human serum albumin (final human serum albumin concentration of 0.1%) as shown in the table.

Mechanism of Action IL-2 promotes proliferation, differentiation, and recruitment of T and B cells, natural killer (NK) cells, and thymocytes; IL-2 also causes cytolytic activity in a subset of lymphocytes and subsequent interactions between the immune system and malignant cells; IL-2 can stimulate lymphokine-activated killer (LAK) cells and tumor-infiltrating lymphocytes (TIL) cells. LAK cells (which are derived from lymphocytes from a patient and incubated in IL-2) have the ability to lyse cells which are resistant to NK cells; TIL cells (which are derived from cancerous tissue from a patient and incubated in IL-2) have been shown to be 50% more effective than LAK cells.

Pharmacodynamics/Kinetics

Absorption: Oral: Not absorbed

Distribution: V_d: Has been noted to be 4-7 L; primarily into the plasma and then into a second compartment, the lymphocytes themselves

Bioavailability: I.M.: 37%

Half-life:

Initial: 6-13 minutes

Terminal: 20-120 minutes

Usual Dosage All orders should be written in million International units (million IU) (refer to individual protocols)

Adults: Metastatic renal cell carcinoma:

Treatment consists of two 5-day treatment cycles separated by a rest period. 600,000 units/kg (0.037 mg/kg)/dose administered every 8 hours by a 15-minute I.V. infusion for a total of 14 doses; following 9 days of rest, the schedule is repeated for another 14 doses, for a maximum of 28 doses per course.

Investigational regimen: I.V. continuous infusion: 4.5 million units/m²/day in 250-1000 mL of D_5W for 5 days

Dose modification: Hold or interrupt a dose rather than reducing dose; refer to protocol

Retreatment: Patients should be evaluated for response ~4 weeks after completion of a course of therapy and again immediately prior to the scheduled start of the next treatment course. Additional courses of treatment may be given to patients only if there is some tumor shrinkage following the last course and retreatment is not contraindicated. Each treatment course should be separated by a rest period of at least 7 weeks from the date of hospital discharge. Tumors have continued to regress up to 12 months following the initiation of therapy.

Administration Administer in D_5W **only; incompatible** with sodium chloride solutions

Management of symptoms related to vascular leak syndrome:

Actual body weight increases >10% above baseline, or rales or rhonchi are audible:

(1) Administer furosemide at dosage determined by patient response

(2) Administer dopamine hydrochloride 2-4 mcg/kg/minute to maintain renal blood flow and urine output

Patient has dyspnea at rest: Give supplemental oxygen by face mask

Patient has severe respiratory distress: Intubate patient and provide mechanical ventilation; administer ranitidine (as the hydrochloride salt), 50 mg I.V. every 8-12 hours as prophylaxis against stress ulcers

Monitoring Parameters

The following clinical evaluations are recommended for all patients prior to beginning treatment and then daily during drug administration:

Standard hematologic tests including CBC, differential, and platelet counts

Blood chemistries including electrolytes, renal and hepatic function tests

Chest x-rays

Daily monitoring during therapy should include vital signs (temperature, pulse, blood pressure, and respiration rate) and weight; in a patient with a decreased blood pressure, especially <90 mm Hg, constant cardiac monitoring for rhythm should be conducted. If an abnormal complex or rhythm is seen, an EKG should be performed; vital signs in these hypotension patients should be taken hourly and central venous pressure (CVP) checked.

During treatment, pulmonary function should be monitored on a regular basis by clinical examination, assessment of vital signs and pulse oximetry. Patients with dyspnea or clinical signs of respiratory impairment (tachypnea or rales) should be further assessed with arterial blood gas determination. These tests are to be repeated as often as clinically indicated.

Cardiac function is assessed daily by clinical examination and assessment of vital signs. Patients with signs or symptoms of chest pain, murmurs, gallops, irregular rhythm or palpitations should be further assessed with an EKG examination and CPK evaluation. If there is evidence of cardiac ischemia or congestive heart failure, a repeat thallium study should be done.

Additional Information
1 Cetus Unit = 6 International Units
1.1 mg = 18 x 10^6 International Units (or 3 x 10^6 Cetus Units)
1 Roche Unit (Teceleukin) = 3 International Units
Reimbursement Hot Line: 1-800-775-7533
Professional services [CETUS ONCOLOGY]: 1-800-238-8779

Dosage Forms Powder for injection, lyophilized: 22 x 10^6 IU [18 million IU/mL = 1.1 mg/mL when reconstituted]

Aldomet® see Methyldopa on page 719

Aleve® (OTC) see Naproxen on page 776

Alfenta® see Alfentanil Hydrochloride on this page

Alfentanil Hydrochloride (al fen' ta nill)
Related Information
Narcotic Agonist Comparison Charts on page 1274-1275
Brand Names Alfenta®
Use Analgesic adjunct given by continuous infusion or in incremental doses in maintenance of anesthesia with barbiturate or NO_2 or a primary anesthetic agent for the induction of anesthesia in patients undergoing general surgery in which endotracheal intubation and mechanical ventilation are required
Restrictions C-II
Pregnancy Risk Factor C
Contraindications Hypersensitivity to alfentanil hydrochloride or narcotics; increased intracranial pressure, severe respiratory depression
Warnings/Precautions Drug dependence, head injury, acute asthma and respiratory conditions; hypotension has occurred in neonates with respiratory distress syndrome; use caution when administering to patients with bradyarrhythmias; rapid I.V. infusion may result in skeletal muscle and chest wall rigidity → impaired ventilation → respiratory distress/arrest; inject slowly over 3-5 minutes; nondepolarizing skeletal muscle relaxant may be required. Alfentanil may produce more hypotension compared to fentanyl, therefore, be sure to administer slowly and ensure patient has adequate hydration.
Adverse Reactions
Hematologic: Antidiuretic hormone release
Ocular: Miosis

>10%:
Cardiovascular: Bradycardia, peripheral vasodilation
Central nervous system: Drowsiness, sedation, increased intracranial pressure
Gastrointestinal: Nausea, vomiting, constipation
1% to 10%:
Cardiovascular: Cardiac arrhythmias, orthostatic hypotension
Central nervous system: Confusion, CNS depression
Ocular: Blurred vision
<1%:
Central nervous system: Convulsions, mental depression, paradoxical CNS excitation or delirium, dizziness, dysesthesia
Dermatologic: Skin rash, hives, itching
Respiratory: Respiratory depression, bronchospasm, laryngospasm
Miscellaneous: Physical and psychological dependence with prolonged use, cold, clammy skin, biliary or urinary tract spasm
Overdosage/Toxicology Symptoms of overdose include miosis, respiratory depression, seizures, CNS depression; naloxone 2 mg I.V. (0.01 mg/kg for children) with repeat administration as necessary up to a total of 10 mg; may precipitate withdrawal
Drug Interactions
Decreased effect: Phenothiazines may antagonize the analgesic effect of opiate agonists
Increased effect: Dextroamphetamine may enhance the analgesic effect of morphine and other opiate agonists
Increased toxicity: CNS depressants (eg, benzodiazepines, barbiturates, phenothiazines, tricyclic antidepressants), erythromycin, reserpine, beta-blockers
Stability Dilute in D_5W, NS, or LR
(Continued)

39

Alfentanil Hydrochloride *(Continued)*

Mechanism of Action Binds with stereospecific receptors at many sites within the CNS, increases pain threshold, alters pain perception, inhibits ascending pain pathways; is an ultra short-acting narcotic

Pharmacodynamics/Kinetics

Distribution: V_d:
  Newborns, premature: 1 L/kg
  Children: 0.163-0.48 L/kg
  Adults: 0.46 L/kg
Half-life, elimination:
  Newborns, premature: 5.33-8.75 hours
  Children: 40-60 minutes
  Adults: 83-97 minutes

Usual Dosage Doses should be titrated to appropriate effects; wide range of doses is dependent upon desired degree of analgesia/anesthesia

Children <12 years: Dose not established
Adults: Dose should be based on ideal body weight. See table.

Alfentanil

Indication	Approximate Duration of Anesthesia (min)	Induction Period (Initial Dose) (mcg/kg)	Maintenance Period (Increments/ Infusion)	Total Dose (mcg/kg)	Effects
Incremental injection	≤30	8-20	3-5 mcg/kg or 0.5-1 mcg/kg/min	8-40	Spontaneously breathing or assisted ventilation when required.
	30-60	20-50	5-15 mcg/kg	Up to 75	Assisted or controlled ventilation required. Attenuation of response to laryngoscopy and intubation.
Continuous infusion	>45	50-75	0.5-3.0 mcg/kg/min average infusion rate 1-1.5 mcg/kg/min	Dependent on duration of procedure	Assisted or controlled ventilation required. Some attenuation of response to intubation and incision, with intraoperative stability.
Anesthetic induction	>45	130-245	0.5-1.5 mcg/kg/min or general anesthetic	Dependent on duration of procedure	Assisted or controlled ventilation required. Administer slowly (over three minutes). Concentration of inhalation agents reduced by 30%-50% for initial hour.

Monitoring Parameters Respiratory rate, blood pressure, heart rate
Reference Range 100-340 ng/mL (depending upon procedure)
Nursing Implications Monitor patient for CNS, respiratory depression, and urticaria
Dosage Forms Injection, preservative free: 500 mcg/mL (2 mL, 5 mL, 10 mL, 20 mL)

Alferon® N *see* Interferon Alfa-N3 *on page 585*

Alglucerase *(al glue′ cir race)*

Brand Names Ceredase®; Cerezyme®
Synonyms Glucocerebrosidase
Use Orphan drug for treatment of Gaucher's disease
Pregnancy Risk Factor C
Contraindications Hypersensitivity to any component
Warnings/Precautions Prepared from pooled human placental tissue that may contain the causative agents of some viral diseases
Adverse Reactions
  >10%: Local: Discomfort, burning, and swelling at the site of injection
  <1%:
    Central nervous system: Fever, chills
    Gastrointestinal: Abdominal discomfort, nausea, vomiting
Overdosage/Toxicology No obvious toxicity was detected after single doses of up to 234 units/kg
Stability Refrigerate (4°C), do not shake
Mechanism of Action Glucocerebrosidase is an enzyme prepared from human placental tissue. Gaucher's disease is an inherited metabolic disorder caused by

the defective activity of beta-glucosidase and the resultant accumulation of glucosyl ceramide laden macrophages in the liver, bone, and spleen; acts by replacing the missing enzyme associated with Gaucher's disease.

Usual Dosage Usually administered as a 20-60 units/kg I.V. infusion given with a frequency ranging from 3 times/week to once every 2 weeks

Administration Filter during administration

Patient Information Alglucerase should be stored under refrigeration (4°C), solutions should not be shaken

Dosage Forms Injection: 10 units/mL (5 mL); 80 units/mL (5 mL)

Alimenazine Tartrate *see* Trimeprazine Tartrate *on page 1124*

Alkaban-AQ® *see* Vinblastine Sulfate *on page 1157*

Alka-Mints® [OTC] *see* Calcium Carbonate *on page 161*

Alkeran® *see* Melphalan *on page 681*

Allbee® With C *see* Vitamin, Multiple *on page 1166*

Aller-Chlor® [OTC] *see* Chlorpheniramine Maleate *on page 229*

Allerest® 12 Hours Nasal Solution [OTC] *see* Oxymetazoline Hydrochloride *on page 829*

Allerest® Eye Drops [OTC] *see* Naphazoline Hydrochloride *on page 775*

Allerfrin® [OTC] *see* Triprolidine and Pseudoephedrine *on page 1131*

AllerMax® [OTC] *see* Diphenhydramine Hydrochloride *on page 351*

Allerphed® [OTC] *see* Triprolidine and Pseudoephedrine *on page 1131*

Allopurinol (al oh pure' i nole)
Brand Names Zyloprim®
Use Prevention of attacks of gouty arthritis and nephropathy; also used to treat secondary hyperuricemia which may occur during treatment of tumors or leukemia; prevent recurrent calcium oxalate calculi

Pregnancy Risk Factor C

Pregnancy/Breast Feeding Implications There are few reports describing the use of allopurinol during pregnancy; no adverse fetal outcomes attributable to allopurinol have been reported in humans

Contraindications Not to be used in pregnancy or lactation, or in patients with a previous severe allergy reaction to allopurinol or any component

Warnings/Precautions Do not use to treat asymptomatic hyperuricemia. Discontinue at first signs of rash; reduce dosage in renal insufficiency, reinstate with caution in patients who have had a previous mild allergic reaction, use with caution in children; monitor liver function and complete blood counts before initiating therapy and periodically during therapy, use with caution in patients taking diuretics concurrently.

Adverse Reactions
>10%: Dermatologic: Skin rash (usually maculopapular), exfoliative, urticarial or purpuric lesions
1% to 10%:
Central nervous system: Drowsiness, chills, fever
Dermatologic: Alopecia
Gastrointestinal: Nausea, vomiting, diarrhea, abdominal pain, gastritis, dyspepsia
Hepatic: Increased alkaline phosphatase, AST, and ALT, hepatomegaly, hyperbilirubinemia, and jaundice; hepatic necrosis has been reported
<1%:
Cardiovascular: Vasculitis
Central nervous system: Headache, somnolence, neuritis
Dermatologic: Toxic epidermal necrolysis and Stevens-Johnson syndrome have been reported
Hematologic: Bone marrow depression has been reported in patients receiving allopurinol with other myelosuppressive agents
Idiosyncratic: Reaction characterized by fever, chills, eosinophilia, arthralgia, nausea, and vomiting, leukopenia, leukocytosis
Local: Thrombophlebitis
Neuromuscular & skeletal: Peripheral neuropathy, paresthesia
Ocular: Cataracts
Renal: Renal impairment
Miscellaneous: Epistaxis

Overdosage/Toxicology If significant amounts of allopurinol are thought to have been absorbed, it is a theoretical possibility that oxypurinol stones could be
(Continued)

Allopurinol *(Continued)*

formed, but no record of such occurrence in overdose exists. Alkalinization of urine and forced diuresis can help prevent potential xanthine stone formation.

Drug Interactions
Decreased effect with alcohol
Increased toxicity:
    Allopurinol prolongs half-life of oral anticoagulants
    Allopurinol increases serum half-life of theophylline
    Allopurinol may compete for excretion in renal tubule with chlorpropamide and increase chlorpropamide's serum half-life
    Inhibits metabolism of azathioprine and mercaptopurine
    Thiazide diuretics enhance toxicity, monitor renal function
    Use with ampicillin or amoxicillin may increase the incidence of skin rash
    Urinary acidification with large amounts of vitamin C may increase kidney stone formation

Mechanism of Action Allopurinol inhibits xanthine oxidase, the enzyme responsible for the conversion of hypoxanthine to xanthine to uric acid. Allopurinol is metabolized to oxypurinol which is also an inhibitor of xanthine oxidase; allopurinol acts on purine catabolism, reducing the production of uric acid without disrupting the biosynthesis of vital purines.

Pharmacodynamics/Kinetics
Decreases in serum uric acid occur in 1-2 days with nadir achieved in 1-2 weeks
Absorption:
    Oral: ~80% of dose absorbed from GI tract; peak plasma concentrations are seen 30-120 minutes after administration
    Rectal: Poor and erratic
Distribution: V_d ~1.6 L/kg; distributes into breast milk
Protein binding: <1%
Metabolism: ~75% metabolized to active metabolites, chiefly oxypurinol
Half-life:
    Normal renal function:
    Parent drug: 1-3 hours
    Oxypurinol: 18-30 hours
    End stage renal disease: Half-life is prolonged
Elimination: Both allopurinol and oxypurinol are dialyzable; 10% may be eliminated by enterohepatic excretion; <10% excreted in urine unchanged; 45% to 65% excreted as oxypurinol

Usual Dosage Oral:
Children: 10 mg/kg/day in 2-3 divided doses or 200-300 mg/m^2/day in 2-4 divided doses, maximum: 600 mg/24 hours
    Alternative dosing:
        <6 years: 150 mg/day in 3 divided doses
        6-10 years: 300 mg/day in 2-3 divided doses
Children >10 years and Adults: Daily doses >300 mg should be administered in divided doses
Myeloproliferative neoplastic disorders: 200-800 mg/day in 2-3 divided doses for prevention of acute uric acid nephropathy for 2-3 days starting 1-2 days before chemotherapy
Gout: 200-300 mg/day (mild); 400-600 mg/day (severe); maximum dose: 800 mg/day

Dosing interval in renal impairment: Must be adjusted due to accumulation of allopurinol and metabolites; see table.

Adult Maintenance Doses of Allopurinol*

Creatinine Clearance (mL/min)	Maintenance Dose of Allopurinol (mg)
140	400 qd
120	350 qd
100	300 qd
80	250 qd
60	200 qd
40	150 qd
20	100 qd
10	100 q2d
0	100 q3d

*This table is based on a standard maintenance dose of 300 mg of allopurinol per day for a patient with a creatinine clearance of 100 mL/min.

Administer dose posthemodialysis or administer 50% supplemental dose

Monitoring Parameters CBC, serum uric acid levels, I & O, hepatic and renal function, especially at start of therapy

Reference Range Uric acid, serum: An increase occurs during childhood
Adults:
Male: 3.4-7 mg/dL or slightly more
Female: 2.4-6 mg/dL or slightly more
Values >7 mg/dL are sometimes arbitrarily regarded as hyperuricemia, but there is no sharp line between normals on the one hand, and the serum uric acid of those with clinical gout. Normal ranges cannot be adjusted for purine ingestion, but high purine diet increases uric acid. Uric acid may be increased with body size, exercise, and stress.

Patient Information Take after meals with plenty of fluid (at least 10-12 glasses of fluids per day); discontinue the drug and contact physician at first sign of rash, painful urination, blood in urine, irritation of the eyes, or swelling of the lips or mouth; may cause drowsiness; alcohol decreases effectiveness

Dosage Forms Tablet: 100 mg, 300 mg

Extemporaneous Preparations Crush tablets to make a 5 mg/mL suspension in simple syrup; stable 14 days under refrigeration.
Nahata MC and Hipple TF, *Pediatric Drug Formulations*, 1st ed, Harvey Whitney Books Co, 1990.

Alomide® *see* Lodoxamide Tromethamine *on page 644*

Alpha$_1$-PI *see* Alpha$_1$-Proteinase Inhibitor (Human) *on this page*

Alpha$_1$-Proteinase Inhibitor (Human) (alfa one pro' tee in ase in hi' bi tor)

Brand Names Prolastin®

Synonyms Alpha$_1$-PI

Use Congenital alpha$_1$-antitrypsin deficiency

Pregnancy Risk Factor C

Contraindications Selective IgA deficiencies with known antibody against IgA

Warnings/Precautions Plasma volume will increase after administration. Immunize against hepatitis B prior to administration. Do not mix solution with other drugs. Unused reconstituted product should be appropriately discarded; as a heat treated, pooled human plasma product, risk of hepatitis B or other virus transmission cannot be completely eliminated.

Adverse Reactions
<1%:
Central nervous system: Dizziness, lightheadedness, delayed fever <102°F
Hematologic: Leukocytosis

Stability
Alpha$_1$-proteinase inhibitor should be stored under refrigeration (2°C to 8°C;35°F to 46°F); freezing should be avoided as breakage of the diluent bottle might occur
Each bottle has the functional activity, as determined by inhibition of porcine pancreatic elastase, stated on the label of the bottle

Reconstitution directions:
Warm the unopened diluent and concentrate to room temperature
After removing the plastic flip-top caps, aseptically cleanse rubber stoppers of both bottles
Remove the protective cover from the plastic transfer needle cartridge with tamper-proof seal and penetrate the stopper of the diluent bottle
Remove the remaining portion of the plastic cartridge; invert the diluent bottle and penetrate the rubber seal on the concentrate bottle with the needle at an angle
The vacuum will draw the diluent into the concentrate bottle; for best results, and to avoid foaming, hold the diluent bottle at an angle to the concentrate bottle until the powder is completed dissolved
After removing the diluent bottle and transfer needle, gently swirl the concentrate bottle until the powder is completely dissolved
Swab top of reconstituted bottle of alpha$_1$-proteinase inhibitor again
Attach the sterile filter needle provided to syringe; with filter needle in place, insert syringe into reconstituted bottle and withdraw solution into syringe
To administer, replace filter needle with appropriate injection needle and follow procedure for I.V. administration
The contents of more than one bottle of alpha$_1$-proteinase inhibitor may be drawn into the same syringe before administration

Mechanism of Action Human alpha$_1$-proteinase inhibitor is prepared from the pooled human plasma of normal donors and is intended for use in the therapy of congenital alpha$_1$-antitrypsin deficiency. Alpha$_1$-antitrypsin (AAT) is the principal
(Continued)

Alpha$_1$-Proteinase Inhibitor (Human) *(Continued)*

protease inhibitor in the serum and exists as a single polypeptide glycoprotein. Production of AAT occurs in the liver hepatocyte and secretion occurs at a rate to maintain serum concentrations of 150-200 mg/dL. The major physiologic role of the antiprotease is that of combining with proteolytic enzymes to render them inactive. Several proteases can be inactivated by AAT including trypsin, chymotrypsin, coagulation factor XI, plasmin, thrombin, and neutrophil elastase.

Pharmacodynamics/Kinetics Half-life, elimination (parent compound): 4.5-5.2 days

Usual Dosage Adults: I.V.: 60 mg/kg once weekly (at a rate ≥0.08 mL/kg/minute)

Administration

Administer at a rate of 0.08 mL/kg/minute or greater intravenously; the recommended dosage of 80 mg/kg takes approximately 30 minutes to infuse

Administer within 3 hours after reconstitution

Additional Information Sodium content of 1 L after reconstitution: 100-210 mEq

Dosage Forms Injection: 500 mg alpha$_1$-PI (20 mL diluent); 1000 mg alpha $_1$-PI (40 mL diluent)

Alpha Chymotrypsin *see* Chymotrypsin, Alpha *on page 243*

Alphamin® *see* Hydroxocobalamin *on page 552*

Alphamul® [OTC] *see* Castor Oil *on page 190*

AlphaNine® *see* Factor IX Complex (Human) *on page 438*

Alphatrex® *see* Betamethasone *on page 129*

Alprazolam *(al pray' zoe lam)*

Related Information

Benzodiazepines Comparison *on page 1256*

Brand Names Xanax®

Use Treatment of anxiety; adjunct in the treatment of depression; management of panic attacks

Restrictions C-IV

Pregnancy Risk Factor D

Contraindications Hypersensitivity to alprazolam or any component; there may be a cross-sensitivity with other benzodiazepines; severe uncontrolled pain, narrow-angle glaucoma, severe respiratory depression, pre-existing CNS depression; not to be used in pregnancy or lactation

Warnings/Precautions Withdrawal symptoms including seizures have occurred 18 hours to 3 days after abrupt discontinuation; when discontinuing therapy, decrease daily dose by no more than 0.5 mg every 3 days; reduce dose in patients with significant hepatic disease. Not intended for management of anxieties and minor distresses associated with everyday life.

Adverse Reactions

>10%:

Cardiovascular: Tachycardia, chest pain

Central nervous system: Drowsiness, fatigue, impaired coordination, lightheadedness, memory impairment, insomnia, anxiety, depression, headache

Dermatologic: Rash

Endocrine & metabolic: Decreased libido

Gastrointestinal: Dry mouth, constipation, decreased salivation, constipation, nausea, vomiting, diarrhea, increased or decreased appetite

Neuromuscular & skeletal: Dysarthria

Ocular: Blurred vision

Miscellaneous: Sweating

1% to 10%:

Cardiovascular: Syncope, hypotension

Central nervous system: Confusion, nervousness, dizziness, akathisia

Dermatologic: Dermatitis

Gastrointestinal: Weight gain or loss

Neuromuscular & skeletal: Rigidity, tremor, muscle cramps

Otic: Tinnitus

Respiratory: Nasal congestion, hyperventilation

Miscellaneous: Increased salivation

Overdosage/Toxicology Symptoms of overdose include somnolence, confusion, coma, and diminished reflexes; treatment for benzodiazepine overdose is supportive. Rarely is mechanical ventilation required; flumazenil has been shown to selectively block the binding of benzodiazepines to CNS receptors, resulting in a reversal of benzodiazepine-induced sedation; however, its use may not alter the course of overdose.

Drug Interactions

Decreased therapeutic effect: Carbamazepine, disulfiram

Increased toxicity: Oral contraceptives, CNS depressants, cimetidine, lithium

Mechanism of Action Binds at stereospecific receptors at several sites within the central nervous system, including the limbic system, reticular formation; effects may be mediated through GABA

Pharmacodynamics/Kinetics
Distribution: V_d: 0.9-1.2 L/kg; distributes into breast milk
Protein binding: 80%
Metabolism: Extensive in the liver; major metabolite is inactive
Half-life: 12-15 hours
Time to peak serum concentration: Within 1-2 hours
Elimination: Excretion of metabolites and parent compound in urine

Usual Dosage Oral:
Children <18 years: Safety and dose have not been established
Adults: 0.25-0.5 mg 2-3 times/day, titrate dose upward; maximum: 4 mg/day

Dosing adjustment in hepatic impairment: Reduce dose by 50% to 60% or avoid in cirrhosis

Note: Treatment >4 months should be re-evaluated to determine the patient's need for the drug

Monitoring Parameters Respiratory and cardiovascular status

Test Interactions ↑ alkaline phosphatase

Patient Information Avoid alcohol and other CNS depressants; avoid activities needing good psychomotor coordination until CNS effects are known; drug may cause physical or psychological dependence; avoid abrupt discontinuation after prolonged use

Nursing Implications Assist with ambulation during beginning therapy, raise bed rails and keep room partially illuminated at night; monitor for CNS respiratory depression

Dosage Forms Tablet: 0.25 mg, 0.5 mg, 1 mg, 2 mg

Alprostadil (al pross' ta dil)

Brand Names Prostin VR Pediatric®

Synonyms PGE_1; Prostaglandin E_1

Use Temporary maintenance of patency of ductus arteriosus in neonates with ductal-dependent congenital heart disease until surgery can be performed. These defects include cyanotic (eg, pulmonary atresia, pulmonary stenosis, tricuspid atresia, Fallot's tetralogy, transposition of the great vessels) and acyanotic (eg, interruption of aortic arch, coarctation of aorta, hypoplastic left ventricle) heart disease

Investigational use: Treatment of pulmonary hypertension in infants and children with congenital heart defects with left-to-right shunts

Pregnancy Risk Factor X

Contraindications Hyaline membrane disease or persistent fetal circulation and when a dominant left-to-right shunt is present, respiratory distress syndrome

Warnings/Precautions Use cautiously in neonates with bleeding tendencies; apnea may occur in 10% to 12% of neonates with congenital heart defects, especially in those weighing <2 kg at birth; apnea usually appears during the first hour of drug infusion

Adverse Reactions
>10%:
  Cardiovascular: Flushing
  Central nervous system: Fever
  Respiratory: Apnea
1% to 10%:
  Cardiovascular: Bradycardia, hypotension, tachycardia, cardiac arrest, edema
  Central nervous system: Seizures
  Endocrine & metabolic: Hypokalemia
  Gastrointestinal: Diarrhea
  Hematologic: Disseminated intravascular coagulation
  Miscellaneous: Sepsis
<1%:
  Cardiovascular: Cerebral bleeding, congestive heart failure, second degree heart block, shock, supraventricular tachycardia, ventricular fibrillation
  Central nervous system: Hyperirritability, hypothermia, jitteriness, lethargy
  Endocrine & metabolic: Hypoglycemia, hyperkalemia
  Gastrointestinal: Gastric regurgitation
  Hematologic: Hyperemia, anemia, bleeding, thrombocytopenia
  Hepatic: Hyperbilirubinemia
  Neuromuscular & skeletal: Hyperextension of neck, stiffness
  Renal: Anuria, hematuria
  Respiratory: Bradypnea, bronchial wheezing
(Continued)

45

Alprostadil *(Continued)*

Miscellaneous: Peritonitis

Overdosage/Toxicology Symptoms of overdose include apnea, bradycardia, hypotension, and flushing; if hypotension or pyrexia occurs, the infusion rate should be reduced until the symptoms subside, while apnea or bradycardia requires drug discontinuation.

Stability Refrigerate ampuls; protect from freezing; prepare fresh solutions every 24 hours; **compatible** in D_5W, $D_{10}W$, and NS solutions

Mechanism of Action Causes vasodilation by means of direct effect on vascular and ductus arteriosus smooth muscle

Pharmacodynamics/Kinetics

Metabolism: ~75% metabolized by oxidation during single pass through the lungs

Half-life: 5-10 minutes

Elimination: Metabolites excreted in urine

Usual Dosage I.V. continuous infusion into a large vein, or alternatively through an umbilical artery catheter placed at the ductal opening: 0.05-0.1 mcg/kg/minute with therapeutic response, rate is reduced to lowest effective dosage; with unsatisfactory response, rate is increased gradually; maintenance: 0.01-0.4 mcg/kg/minute

PGE_1 is usually given at an infusion rate of 0.1 mcg/kg/minute, but it is often possible to reduce the dosage to $1/2$ or even $1/10$ without losing the therapeutic effect. The mixing schedule is shown in the table.

Add 1 Ampul (500 mcg) to:	Concentration (mcg/mL)	Infusion Rate	
		mL/min/kg Needed to Infuse 0.1 mcg/kg/min	mL/kg/24 h
250 mL	2	0.05	72
100 mL	5	0.02	28.8
50 mL	10	0.01	14.4
25 mL	20	0.005	7.2

Therapeutic response is indicated by increased pH in those with acidosis or by an increase in oxygenation (pO_2) usually evident within 30 minutes

Monitoring Parameters Arterial pressure, respiratory rate, heart rate, temperature

Patient Information Refrigerate

Nursing Implications Monitor arterial pressure; assess all vital functions; apnea and bradycardia may indicate overdose, stop infusion if occurring; infuse for the shortest time and at the lowest dose that will produce the desired effects. Flushing is usually a result of catheter malposition; central line preferred for I.V. administration.

Dosage Forms Injection: 500 mcg/mL (1 mL)

AL-R® [OTC] *see* Chlorpheniramine Maleate *on page 229*

Altace™ *see* Ramipril *on page 973*

Alteplase *(al' te place)*

Brand Names Activase®

Synonyms Tissue Plasminogen Activator, Recombinant; t-PA

Use Management of acute myocardial infarction for the lysis of thrombi in coronary arteries; management of acute massive pulmonary embolism (PE) in adults

Pregnancy Risk Factor C

Contraindications Active internal bleeding, history of cerebrovascular accident, intracranial neoplasm, aneurysm, or recent (within 2 months) intracranial or intraspinal surgery or trauma; patients with known bleeding diathesis, arteriovenous malformation, or severe uncontrolled hypertension

Warnings/Precautions Doses >150 mg have been associated with an increase of intracranial hemorrhage

Adverse Reactions

1% to 10%:

Cardiovascular: Hypotension

Central nervous system: Fever

Dermatologic: Ecchymosis

Gastrointestinal: GI hemorrhage, nausea, vomiting

Genitourinary: GU hemorrhage

<1%:

Hematologic: Retroperitoneal hemorrhage, gingival hemorrhage, intracranial hemorrhage rapid lysis of coronary artery thrombi by thrombolytic agents may be associated with reperfusion-related atrial and/or ventricular arrhythmias

Miscellaneous: Epistaxis

Overdosage/Toxicology Increased incidence of intracranial bleeding

Drug Interactions Increased effect: Anticoagulants, aspirin, ticlopidine, dipyridamole, and heparin are at least additive

Stability Refrigerate; must be used within 8 hours of reconstitution; alteplase is **incompatible** with dobutamine, dopamine, heparin, and nitroglycerin infusions; physically **compatible** with lidocaine, metoprolol, propranolol when administered via Y site; compatible with either D_5W or NS

Standard dose: 100 mg/100 mL 0.9% NaCl [total volume: 200 mL]

Mechanism of Action Initiates local fibrinolysis by binding to fibrin in a thrombus (clot) and converts entrapped plasminogen to plasmin

Pharmacodynamics/Kinetics Elimination: Cleared rapidly from circulating plasma at a rate of 550-650 mL/minute, primarily by the liver; >50% present in plasma is cleared within 5 minutes after the infusion has been terminated, and ~80% is cleared within 10 minutes

Usual Dosage

Coronary artery thrombi: I.V.: Front loading dose: Total dose is 100 mg over 1.5 hours (for patients who weigh <65 kg, use 1.25 mg/kg/total dose). Add this dose to a 100 mL bag of 0.9% sodium chloride for a total volume of 200 mL. Infuse 15 mg (30 mL) over 1-2 minutes; infuse 50 mg (100 mL) over 30 minutes. Begin heparin 5000-10,000 unit bolus followed by continuous infusion of 1000 units/hour. Infuse 35 mg/hour (70 mL) for next 2 hours.

Acute pulmonary embolism: 100 mg over 2 hours

Administration Do not use bacteriostatic water for reconstitution

Reference Range Not routinely measured; literature supports therapeutic levels of 0.52-1.8 mcg/mL

Nursing Implications Assess for hemorrhage during first hour of treatment

Dosage Forms Powder for injection, lyophilized: 20 mg [11.6 million units] (20 mL); 50 mg [29 million units] (50 mL)

ALternaGEL® [OTC] *see* Aluminum Hydroxide *on next page*

Altretamine (al tret' a meen)

Brand Names Hexalen®

Synonyms Hexamethylmelamine

Use Palliative treatment of persistent or recurrent ovarian cancer following first-line therapy with a cisplatin- or alkylating agent-based combination

Pregnancy Risk Factor D

Contraindications Hypersensitivity to altretamine, pre-existing severe bone marrow depression or severe neurologic toxicity

Warnings/Precautions The U.S. Food and Drug Administration (FDA) currently recommends that procedures for proper handling and disposal of antineoplastic agents be considered. Peripheral blood counts and neurologic examinations should be done routinely before and after drug therapy. Use with caution in patients previously treated with other myelosuppressive drugs or with pre-existing neurotoxicity; use with caution in patients with renal or hepatic dysfunction; altretamine may be slightly mutagenic.

Adverse Reactions

>10%:

Central nervous system: Peripheral sensory neuropathy, neurotoxicity

Gastrointestinal: Nausea, vomiting

Hematologic: Anemia, thrombocytopenia, leukopenia

1% to 10%:

Central nervous system: Seizures

Gastrointestinal: Anorexia, diarrhea, stomach cramps

Hepatic: Increased alkaline phosphatase

<1%:

Central nervous system: Dizziness, depression

Dermatologic: Rash, alopecia

Hematologic: Myelosuppression

Hepatic: Hepatotoxicity

Neuromuscular & skeletal: Tremor

Overdosage/Toxicology Symptoms of overdose include nausea, vomiting, peripheral neuropathy, severe bone marrow depression; after decontamination, treatment is supportive

(Continued)

Altretamine (Continued)

Drug Interactions

Decreased effect: Phenobarbital may increase metabolism of altretamine

Increased toxicity: May cause severe orthostatic hypotension when administered with MAO inhibitors; cimetidine may decrease metabolism of altretamine

Mechanism of Action Although altretamine clinical antitumor spectrum resembles that of alkylating agents, the drug has demonstrated activity in alkylator-resistant patients; probably requires hepatic microsomal mixed-function oxidase enzyme activation to become cytotoxic. The drug selectively inhibits the incorporation of radioactive thymidine and uridine into DNA and RNA, inhibiting DNA and RNA synthesis; metabolized to reactive intermediates which covalently bind to microsomal proteins and DNA. These reactive intermediates can spontaneously degrade to demethylated melamines and formaldehyde which are also cytotoxic.

Pharmacodynamics/Kinetics

Absorption: Oral: Well absorbed (75% to 89%)

Metabolism: Rapid and extensive demethylation in liver; high concentrations in liver and kidney, but low concentrations in other organs

Half-life: 13 hours

Peak plasma levels: 0.5-3 hours after dose

Elimination: In urine (<1% unchanged)

Usual Dosage Oral (refer to protocol):

Adults: 4-12 mg/kg/day in 3-4 divided doses for 21-90 days

Alternatively: 240-320 mg/m^2/day in 3-4 divided doses for 21 days, repeated every 6 weeks

Alternatively: 260 mg/m^2/day for 14-21 days of a 28-day cycle in 4 divided doses

Temporarily discontinue (for ≥14 days) & subsequently restart at 200 mg/m^2/day if any of the following occurs:

if GI intolerance unresponsive to symptom measures

WBC <2000/mm^3

granulocyte count <1000/mm^3

platelet count <75,000/mm^3

progressive neurotoxicity

Administration Administer orally; administer total daily dose as 4 divided oral doses after meals and at bedtime

Patient Information Report any numbness or tingling in extremities to physician; nausea and vomiting may occur and even begin up to weeks after therapy is stopped

Dosage Forms Capsule: 50 mg

Alu-Cap® [OTC] see Aluminum Hydroxide on this page

Aluminum Hydroxide (a loo' mi num hi drok' side)

Brand Names ALternaGEL® [OTC]; Alu-Cap® [OTC]; Alu-Tab® [OTC]; Amphojel® [OTC]; Dialume® [OTC]; Nephrox Suspension [OTC]

Use Treatment of hyperacidity; hyperphosphatemia

Pregnancy Risk Factor C

Contraindications Hypersensitivity to aluminum salts or drug dry components

Warnings/Precautions Hypophosphatemia may occur with prolonged administration or large doses; aluminum intoxication and osteomalacia may occur in patients with uremia. Use with caution in patients with congestive heart failure, renal failure, edema, cirrhosis, and low sodium diets, and patients who have recently suffered gastrointestinal hemorrhage; uremic patients not receiving dialysis may develop osteomalacia and osteoporosis due to phosphate depletion.

Elderly, due to disease and/or drug therapy, may be predisposed to constipation and fecal impaction. Careful evaluation of possible drug interactions must be done. When used as an antacid in ulcer treatment, consider buffer capacity (mEq/mL) to calculate dose; consider renal insufficiency as predisposition to aluminum toxicity.

Adverse Reactions

>10%: Gastrointestinal: Constipation, chalky taste, stomach cramps, fecal impaction

1% to 10%: Gastrointestinal: Nausea, vomiting, discoloration of feces (white speckles)

<1%: Endocrine & metabolic: Hypophosphatemia, hypomagnesemia

Overdosage/Toxicology Aluminum antacids may cause constipation, phosphate depletion, and bezoar or fecalith formation; in patients with renal failure, aluminum may accumulate to toxic levels.

Deferoxamine, traditionally used as an iron chelator, has been shown to increase urinary aluminum output

Deferoxamine chelation of aluminum has resulted in improvements of clinical symptoms and bone histology; however, remains an experimental treatment for aluminum poisoning and has a significant potential for adverse effects.

Drug Interactions Decreased effect: Tetracyclines, digoxin, indomethacin, or iron salts, isoniazid, allopurinol, benzodiazepines, corticosteroids, penicillamine, phenothiazines, ranitidine, ketoconazole, itraconazole

Usual Dosage Oral:

Peptic ulcer disease:
    Children: 5-15 mL/dose every 3-6 hours or 1 and 3 hours after meals and at bedtime
    Adults: 15-45 mL every 3-6 hours or 1 and 3 hours after meals and at bedtime

Prophylaxis against gastrointestinal bleeding:
    Infants: 2-5 mL/dose every 1-2 hours
    Children: 5-15 mL/dose every 1-2 hours
    Adults: 30-60 mL/dose every hour
    Titrate to maintain the gastric pH >5

Hyperphosphatemia:
    Children: 50-150 mg/kg/24 hours in divided doses every 4-6 hours, titrate dosage to maintain serum phosphorus within normal range
    Adults: 500-1800 mg, 3-6 times/day, between meals and at bedtime

Antacid: Adults: 30 mL 1 and 3 hours postprandial and at bedtime

Monitoring Parameters Monitor phosphorous levels periodically when patient is on chronic therapy

Test Interactions Decreases phosphorus, inorganic (S)

Patient Information Dilute dose in water or juice, shake well; chew tablets thoroughly before swallowing with water; do not take oral drugs within 1-2 hours of administration; notify physician if relief is not obtained or if there are any signs to suggest bleeding from the GI tract

Nursing Implications Used primarily as a phosphate binder; dose should be followed with water

Dosage Forms
    Capsule: 475 mg, 500 mg
    Gel: 600 mg/5 mL (360 mL)
    Suspension, oral: 320 mg/5 mL (500 mL)
    Tablet: 300 mg, 500 mg, 600 mg

Aluminum Sucrose Sulfate, Basic *see* Sucralfate *on page 1036*

Alupent® *see* Metaproterenol Sulfate *on page 697*

Alu-Tab® [OTC] *see* Aluminum Hydroxide *on previous page*

Amantadine Hydrochloride (a man' ta deen)

Related Information
    Antimicrobial Drugs of Choice *on page 1298-1302*

Brand Names Symadine®; Symmetrel®

Synonyms Adamantanamine Hydrochloride

Use Symptomatic and adjunct treatment of parkinsonism; prophylaxis and treatment of influenza A viral infection; treatment of drug-induced extrapyramidal symptoms

Pregnancy Risk Factor C

Contraindications Hypersensitivity to amantadine hydrochloride or any component

Warnings/Precautions Use with caution in patients with liver disease, a history of recurrent and eczematoid dermatitis, uncontrolled psychosis or severe psychoneurosis, seizures and in those receiving CNS stimulant drugs; when treating Parkinson's disease, do not discontinue abruptly. In many patients, the therapeutic benefits of amantadine are limited to a few months. Elderly patients may be more susceptible to the CNS effects (using 2 divided daily doses may minimize this effect).

Adverse Reactions
1% to 10%:
    Cardiovascular: Orthostatic hypotension, peripheral edema
    Central nervous system: Insomnia, depression, anxiety, irritability, dizziness, hallucinations, ataxia, headache, somnolence, nervousness, dream abnormality, agitation, fatigue
    Dermatologic: Livedo reticularis
    Gastrointestinal: Nausea, anorexia, constipation, diarrhea
    Miscellaneous: Dry mouth/nose
<1%:
    Cardiovascular: Congestive heart failure, hypertension
(Continued)

Amantadine Hydrochloride *(Continued)*

Central nervous system: Psychosis, weakness, slurred speech, euphoria, confusion, amnesia, instances of convulsions

Dermatologic: Skin rash, eczematoid dermatitis

Endocrine & metabolic: Decreased libido

Genitourinary: Urinary retention

Gastrointestinal: Vomiting

Hematologic: Leukopenia, neutropenia

Neuromuscular & skeletal: Hyperkinesis

Ocular: Visual disturbances, oculogyric episodes

Respiratory: Dyspnea

Overdosage/Toxicology Symptoms of overdose include nausea, vomiting, slurred speech, blurred vision, lethargy, hallucinations, seizures, myoclonic jerking; treatment should be directed at reducing the CNS stimulation and at maintaining cardiovascular function. Seizures can be treated with diazepam while a lidocaine infusion may be required for the cardiac dysrhythmias.

Drug Interactions

Increased effect: Drugs with anticholinergic or CNS stimulant activity

Increased toxicity/levels: Hydrochlorothiazide plus triamterene, amiloride

Stability Protect from freezing

Mechanism of Action As an antiviral, blocks the uncoating of influenza A virus preventing penetration of virus into host; antiparkinsonian activity may be due to its blocking the reuptake of dopamine into presynaptic neurons and causing direct stimulation of postsynaptic receptors

Pharmacodynamics/Kinetics

Onset of antidyskinetic action: Within 48 hours

Absorption: Well absorbed from GI tract

Distribution: To saliva, tear film, and nasal secretions; in animals, tissue (especially lung) concentrations higher than serum concentrations, crosses blood-brain barrier

V_d:

Normal: 4.4±0.2 L/kg

Renal failure: 5.1±0.2 L/kg

Protein binding:

Normal renal function: ~67%

Hemodialysis patients: ~59%

Metabolism: Not appreciable, small amounts of an acetyl metabolite identified

Half-life:

Normal renal function: 2-7 hours

End stage renal disease: 7-10 days

Time to peak: 1-4 hours

Elimination: 80% to 90% excreted unchanged in urine by glomerular filtration and tubular secretion

Usual Dosage

Children:

1-9 years: (<45 kg): 5-9 mg/kg/day in 1-2 divided doses to a maximum of 150 mg/day

10-12 years: 100-200 mg/day in 1-2 divided doses

Prophylaxis: Administer for 10-21 days following exposure if the vaccine is concurrently given or for 90 days following exposure if the vaccine is unavailable or contraindicated and re-exposure is possible

Adults:

Parkinson's disease: 100 mg twice daily

Influenza A viral infection: 200 mg/day in 1-2 divided doses

Prophylaxis: Minimum 10-day course of therapy following exposure if the vaccine is concurrently give or for 90 following exposure if the vaccine is unavailable or contraindicated and re-exposure is possible

Elderly patients should take the drug in 2 daily doses rather than a single dose to avoid adverse neurologic reactions

Dosing interval in renal impairment:

Cl_{cr} 50-60 mL/minute: Administer 200 mg alternating with 100 mg/day

Cl_{cr} 30-50 mL/minute: Administer 100 mg/day

Cl_{cr} 20-30 mL/minute: Administer 200 mg twice weekly

Cl_{cr} 10-20 mL/minute: Administer 100 mg 3 times/week

Cl_{cr} <10 mL/minute: Administer 200 mg alternating with 100 mg every 7 days

Slightly hemodialyzable (5% to 20%); no supplemental dose is needed in hemo- or peritoneal dialysis nor with continuous arterio-venous or venous-venous hemofiltration (CAVH/CAVHD) procedures

Monitoring Parameters Renal function, mental status, blood pressure

Patient Information Do not abruptly discontinue therapy, it may precipitate a parkinsonian crisis; may impair ability to perform activities requiring mental alertness or coordination; must take throughout flu season or for at least 10 days following vaccination for effective prophylaxis; take second dose of the day in early afternoon to decrease incidence of insomnia

Nursing Implications If insomnia occurs, the last daily dose should be given several hours before retiring; assess parkinsonian symptoms prior to and throughout course of therapy

Dosage Forms
Capsule: 100 mg
Solution, oral: 50 mg/5 mL

Amaphen® *see* Butalbital Compound *on page 153*

Ambien™ *see* Zolpidem Tartrate *on page 1177*

Amcill® *see* Ampicillin *on page 73*

Amcinonide (am sin' oh nide)

Related Information
Corticosteroids Comparisons *on page 1266-1268*

Brand Names Cyclocort®

Use Relief of the inflammatory and pruritic manifestations of corticosteroid-responsive dermatoses (high potency corticosteroid)

Pregnancy Risk Factor C

Contraindications Hypersensitivity to amcinonide or any component; use on the face, groin, or axilla

Warnings/Precautions Adverse systemic effects may occur when used on large areas of the body, denuded areas, for prolonged periods of time, with an occlusive dressing, and/or in infants or small children; occlusive dressings should not be used in presence of infection or weeping lesions

Adverse Reactions
1% to 10%: Topical: Itching, maceration of skin, skin atrophy, burning, erythema, dryness, irritation, papular rashes
<1%: Topical: Hypertrichosis, acneiform eruptions, hypopigmentation, perioral dermatitis, striae, miliaria

Overdosage/Toxicology Symptoms of overdose include cushingoid appearance (systemic), muscle weakness (systemic), osteoporosis (systemic) all with long-term use only. When consumed in excessive quantities for prolonged periods, systemic hypercorticism and adrenal suppression may occur; in those cases, discontinuation and withdrawal of the corticosteroid should be done judiciously.

Mechanism of Action Stimulates the synthesis of enzymes needed to decrease inflammation, suppress mitotic activity, and cause vasoconstriction

Pharmacodynamics/Kinetics
Absorption: Adequate through intact skin; increases with skin inflammation or occlusion
Metabolism: In the liver
Elimination: By the kidney and in bile

Usual Dosage Adults: Topical: Apply in a thin film 2-3 times/day

Patient Information Before applying, gently wash area to reduce risk of infection; apply a thin film to cleansed area and rub in gently and thoroughly until medication vanishes; avoid exposure to sunlight, severe sunburn may occur

Nursing Implications Assess for worsening of rash or fever

Dosage Forms
Cream: 0.1% (15 g, 30 g, 60 g)
Lotion: 0.1% (20 mL, 60 mL)
Ointment, topical: 0.1% (15 g, 30 g, 60 g)

Amcort® *see* Triamcinolone *on page 1112*

Amen® *see* Medroxyprogesterone Acetate *on page 677*

Americaine® [OTC] *see* Benzocaine *on page 121*

A-Methapred® *see* Methylprednisolone *on page 724*

Amethocaine Hydrochloride *see* Tetracaine Hydrochloride *on page 1068*

Amethopterin *see* Methotrexate *on page 711*

Amfepramone *see* Diethylpropion Hydrochloride *on page 333*

Amicar® *see* Aminocaproic Acid *on page 55*

Amidate® *see* Etomidate *on page 434*

Amikacin Sulfate (am i kay' sin)

Related Information
Antimicrobial Drugs of Choice *on page 1298-1302*

Brand Names Amikin®

Use Treatment of documented gram-negative enteric infection resistant to genta-micin and tobramycin (bone infections, respiratory tract infections, endocarditis, and septicemia); documented infection of mycobacterial organisms susceptible to amikacin including *Pseudomonas*, *Proteus*, *Serratia*, and gram-positive *Staph-ylococcus*

Pregnancy Risk Factor C

Contraindications Hypersensitivity to amikacin sulfate or any component; cross-sensitivity may exist with other aminoglycosides

Warnings/Precautions Dose and/or frequency of administration must be moni-tored and modified in patients with renal impairment; drug should be discontinued if signs of ototoxicity, nephrotoxicity, or hypersensitivity occur; ototoxicity is proportional to the amount of drug given and the duration of treatment; tinnitus or vertigo may be indications of vestibular injury and impending bilateral irreversible damage; renal damage is usually reversible

Adverse Reactions
1% to 10%:
  Central nervous system: Neurotoxicity
  Otic: Ototoxicity (auditory), ototoxicity (vestibular)
  Renal: Nephrotoxicity
<1%:
  Cardiovascular: Hypotension
  Central nervous system: Headache, drowsiness, weakness
  Dermatologic: Rash
  Gastrointestinal: Nausea, vomiting
  Hematologic: Eosinophilia
  Neuromuscular & skeletal: Paresthesia, tremor, arthralgia
  Respiratory: Difficulty in breathing
  Miscellaneous: Drug fever

Overdosage/Toxicology Symptoms of overdose include ototoxicity, nephrotox-icity, and neuromuscular toxicity; treatment of choice following a single acute overdose appears to be the maintenance of good urine output of at least 3 mL/kg/hour. Dialysis is of questionable value in the enhancement of aminoglyco-side elimination. If required, hemodialysis is preferred over peritoneal dialysis in patients with normal renal function.

Drug Interactions
Decreased effect of aminoglycoside: High concentrations of penicillins and/or cephalosporins (*in vitro* data)

Increased toxicity of aminoglycoside: Indomethacin I.V., amphotericin, loop diuretics, vancomycin, enflurane, methoxyflurane; increased toxicity of depolar-izing and nondepolarizing neuromuscular blocking agents and polypeptide antibiotics with administration of aminoglycosides

Stability Stable for 24 hours at room temperature and 2 days at refrigeration when mixed in D_5W, $D_51/4NS$, $D_51/2NS$, NS, LR

Mechanism of Action Inhibits protein synthesis in susceptible bacteria by binding to ribosomal subunits

Pharmacodynamics/Kinetics
Absorption: I.M.: May be delayed in the bedridden patient
Distribution: Crosses the placenta; primarily distributes into extracellular fluid (highly hydrophilic); penetrates the blood-brain barrier when meninges are inflamed
  Relative diffusion of antimicrobial agents from blood into cerebrospinal fluid (CSF): Good only with inflammation (exceeds usual MICs); ratio of CSF to blood level (%):
    Normal meninges: 10-20
    Inflamed meninges: 15-24
Half-life (dependent on renal function):
  Infants:
    Low birthweight (1-3 days): 7-9 hours
    Full term >7 days: 4-5 hours
  Children: 1.6-2.5 hours
  Adults:
    Normal renal function: 1.4-2.3 hours
    Anuria: End stage renal disease: 28-86 hours
Time to peak serum concentration:
  I.M.: Within 45-120 minutes
  I.V.: Within 30 minutes following 30-minute infusion
Elimination: 94% to 98% excreted unchanged in urine via glomerular filtration within 24 hours; clearance dependent on renal function and patient age

Usual Dosage Individualization is critical because of the low therapeutic index

Use of ideal body weight (IBW) for determining the mg/kg/dose appears to be more accurate than dosing on the basis of total body weight (TBW)
In morbid obesity, dosage requirement may best be estimated using a dosing weight of IBW + 0.4 (TBW - IBW)

Initial and periodic peak and trough plasma drug levels should be determined, particularly in critically ill patients with serious infections or in disease states known to significantly alter aminoglycoside pharmacokinetics (eg, cystic fibrosis, burns, or major surgery)

Once daily dosing: Higher peak serum drug concentration to MIC ratios, demonstrated aminoglycoside postantibiotic effect, decreased renal cortex drug uptake, and improved cost-time efficiency are supportive reasons for the use of once daily dosing regimens for aminoglycosides. Current research indicates these regimens to be as effective for nonlife-threatening infections, with no higher incidence of nephrotoxicity, than those requiring multiple daily doses. Doses are determined by calculating the entire day's dose via usual multiple dose calculation techniques and administering this quantity as a single dose. Doses are then adjusted to maintain mean serum concentrations above the MIC(s) of the causative organism(s). (Example: 4.5-6 mg/kg as a single dose, adjusted to achieve an average serum level of 3-4 mcg/mL). Further research is needed for universal recommendation in all patient populations and gram-negative disease.

Neonates: I.M., I.V.:
  <1200 g, 0-4 weeks: 7.5 mg/kg/dose every 12 hours
  Postnatal age ≤7 days:
    1200-2000 g: 7.5 mg/kg/dose every 12 hours
    >2000 g: 10 mg/kg/dose every 12 hours
  Postnatal age >7 days:
    1200-2000 g: 7.5 mg/kg/dose every 8-12 hours
    >2000 g: 10 mg/kg/dose every 8 hours
Infants, Children, and Adults: I.M., I.V.: 5-7.5 mg/kg/dose every 8 hours

Dosing interval in renal impairment: Some patients may require larger or more frequent doses if serum levels document the need (ie, cystic fibrosis or febrile granulocytopenic patients)
  Cl_{cr} ≥60 mL/minute: Administer every 8 hours
  Cl_{cr} 40-60 mL/minute: Administer every 12 hours
  Cl_{cr} 20-40 mL/minute: Administer every 24 hours
  Cl_{cr} 10-20 mL/minute: Administer every 48 hours
  Cl_{cr} <10 mL/minute: Administer every 72 hours
Dialyzable (50% to 100%)
Administer dose postdialysis or administer $2/3$ normal dose as a supplemental dose postdialysis and follow levels
Peritoneal dialysis effects: Dose as Cl_{cr} <10 mL/minute: Follow levels
Continuous arterio-venous or veno-venous hemodiafiltration (CAVH) effects: Dose as Cl_{cr} <10 mL/minute: Follow levels
Administration Administer I.M. injection in large muscle mass. Administer around-the-clock rather than 3 times/day, to promote less variation in peak and trough serum levels.
Monitoring Parameters Urinalysis, BUN, serum creatinine, appropriately timed peak and trough concentrations, vital signs, temperature, weight, I & O, hearing parameters (audiology testing warranted in extended treatment courses (>10 days))
Reference Range
  Sample size: 0.5-2 mL blood (red top tube) or 0.1-1 mL serum (separated)
  Therapeutic levels:
    Peak:
      Life-threatening infections: 25-30 µg/mL
      Serious infections: 20-25 µg/mL
      Urinary tract infections: 15-20 µg/mL
      Synergy against gram-positive organisms: 15-20 µg/mL
    Trough:
      Serious infections: 1-4 µg/mL
      Life-threatening infections: 4-8 µg/mL
  Toxic concentration: Peak: >35 µg/mL; Trough: >10 µg/mL
  Timing of serum samples: Draw peak 30 minutes after completion of 30-minute infusion or at 1 hour following initiation of infusion or I.M. injection; draw trough immediately before next dose
  The presence of fever may decrease peak levels; in vitro data indicate the presence of high concentrations of penicillins concurrent with sampling of aminoglycoside levels may result in inactivation (decreased values)
(Continued)

Amikacin Sulfate *(Continued)*

Patient Information Report loss of hearing, ringing or roaring in the ears, or feeling of fullness in head

Nursing Implications Aminoglycoside levels measured from blood taken from Silastic® central catheters can sometimes give falsely high readings (draw levels from alternate lumen or peripheral stick, if possible)

Additional Information Sodium content of 1 g: 29.9 mg (1.3 mEq)

Dosage Forms Injection: 50 mg/mL (2 mL); 250 mg/mL (2 mL, 4 mL)

Amikin® *see* Amikacin Sulfate *on page 51*

Amiloride Hydrochloride (a mill' oh ride)

Brand Names Midamor®

Use Counteracts potassium loss induced by other diuretics in the treatment of hypertension or edematous conditions including CHF, hepatic cirrhosis, and hypoaldosteronism; usually used in conjunction with more potent diuretics such as thiazides or loop diuretics

Investigational use: Cystic fibrosis

Pregnancy Risk Factor B

Contraindications Hyperkalemia, potassium supplementation and impaired renal function, hypersensitivity to amiloride or any component

Warnings/Precautions Use cautiously in patients with severe hepatic insufficiency; may cause hyperkalemia (serum levels >5.5 mEq/L) which, if uncorrected, is potentially fatal; medication should be discontinued if potassium level are >6.5 mEq/L

Adverse Reactions

1% to 10%:

Central nervous system: Headache, weakness, fatigability, dizziness

Endocrine & metabolic: Hyperkalemia, hyperchloremic metabolic acidosis, dehydration, hyponatremia, gynecomastia

Gastrointestinal: Nausea, diarrhea, vomiting, abdominal pain, gas pain, appetite changes, constipation

Genitourinary: Impotence

Neuromuscular & skeletal: Muscle cramps

Respiratory: Cough, dyspnea

<1%:

Cardiovascular: Angina pectoris, orthostatic hypotension, arrhythmias, palpitations, chest pain

Central nervous system: Vertigo, nervousness, insomnia, depression

Dermatologic: Skin rash or dryness, pruritus, alopecia

Endocrine & metabolic: Decreased libido

Gastrointestinal: GI bleeding, thirst, heartburn, flatulence, dyspepsia

Genitourinary: Urinary frequency, bladder spasms

Hepatic: Jaundice

Neuromuscular & skeletal: Joint pain, tremor, neck/shoulder pain, back pain

Ocular: Increased intraocular pressure

Renal: Polyuria, dysuria

Respiratory: Shortness of breath

Overdosage/Toxicology Clinical signs are consistent with dehydration and electrolyte disturbance; large amounts may result in life-threatening hyperkalemia (>6.5 mEq/L). This can be treated with I.V. glucose (dextrose 25% in water), with rapid-acting insulin, with concurrent I.V. sodium bicarbonate and, if needed, Kayexalate® oral or rectal solutions in sorbitol; persistent hyperkalemia may require dialysis.

Drug Interactions

Decreased effect of amiloride: Nonsteroidal anti-inflammatory agents

Increased risk of amiloride-associated hyperkalemia: Triamterene, spironolactone, angiotensin-converting enzyme (ACE) inhibitors, potassium preparations, indomethacin

Increased toxicity of amantadine and lithium by reduction of renal excretion

Mechanism of Action Interferes with potassium/sodium exchange (active transport) in the distal tubule, cortical collecting tubule and collecting duct by inhibiting sodium, potassium-ATPase; decreases calcium excretion; increases magnesium loss

Pharmacodynamics/Kinetics

Absorption: Oral: ~15% to 25%

Onset: 2 hours

Duration: 24 hours

Distribution: V_d: 350-380 L

Protein binding: 23%

Metabolism: No active metabolites

Half-life:
  Normal renal function: 6-9 hours
  End stage renal disease: 8-144 hours
Peak serum concentration: 6-10 hours
Elimination: Unchanged equally in the urine and the feces

Usual Dosage Oral:
  Children: Although safety and efficacy have not been established by the FDA in children, a dosage of 0.625 mg/kg/day has been used in children weighing 6-20 kg
  Adults: 5-10 mg/day (up to 20 mg)
  Elderly: Initial: 5 mg once daily or every other day

  Dosing adjustment in renal impairment:
    Cl_{cr} 10-50 mL/minute: Administer at 50% of normal dose
    Cl_{cr} <10 mL/minute: Avoid use
Monitoring Parameters I & O, daily weights, blood pressure, serum electrolytes, renal function
Test Interactions ↑ potassium (S)
Patient Information Take with food or milk; avoid salt substitutes; because of high potassium content, avoid bananas and oranges; report any muscle cramps, weakness, nausea, or dizziness; use caution operating machinery or performing other tasks requiring alertness
Nursing Implications Assess fluid status via daily weights, I & O ratios, standing and supine blood pressures; observe for hyperkalemia; if ordered once daily, dose should be given in the morning
Dosage Forms Tablet: 5 mg

2-Amino-6-Mercaptopurine *see* Thioguanine *on page 1081*

Aminobenzylpenicillin *see* Ampicillin *on page 73*

Aminocaproic Acid (a mee noe ka proe′ ik)
Brand Names Amicar®
Use Treatment of excessive bleeding from fibrinolysis
Pregnancy Risk Factor C
Contraindications Disseminated intravascular coagulation, hematuria of upper urinary tract
Warnings/Precautions Rapid I.V. administration of the undiluted drug is not recommended; aminocaproic acid may accumulate in patients with decreased renal function; do not use in hematuria of upper urinary tract origin unless possible benefits outweigh risks; use with caution in patients with cardiac, renal or hepatic disease; do not administer without a definite diagnosis of laboratory findings indicative of hyperfibrinolysis; should not be used in nursing women
Adverse Reactions
  1% to 10%:
    Cardiovascular: Hypotension, bradycardia, arrhythmia
    Central nervous system: Dizziness, headache, tinnitus, malaise, weakness, fatigue
    Dermatologic: Rash
    Gastrointestinal: GI irritation, nausea, cramps, diarrhea
    Hematologic: Decreased platelet function, elevated serum enzymes
    Neuromuscular & skeletal: Myopathy
    Respiratory: Nasal congestion
  <1%:
    Central nervous system: Convulsions
    Genitourinary: Ejaculation problems
    Neuromuscular & skeletal: Rhabdomyolysis
    Renal: Renal failure
Overdosage/Toxicology Nausea, diarrhea, delirium, hepatic necrosis, thrombo-embolism
Drug Interactions Increased toxic effect with oral contraceptives, estrogens
Mechanism of Action Competitively inhibits activation of plasminogen to plasmin, also, a lesser antiplasmin effect
Pharmacodynamics/Kinetics
  Oral:
    Peak effect: Within 2 hours
    Therapeutic effect: Within 1-72 hours after dose
  Distribution: Widely distributes through intravascular and extravascular compartments
  Metabolism: Minimal hepatic
  Half-life: 1-2 hours
  Elimination: 68% to 86% excreted as unchanged drug in urine within 12 hours
(Continued)

Aminocaproic Acid *(Continued)*

Usual Dosage In the management of acute bleeding syndromes, oral dosage regimens are the same as the I.V. dosage regimens in adults and children

Chronic bleeding: Oral, I.V.: 5-30 g/day in divided doses at 3- to 6-hour intervals

Acute bleeding syndrome:
Children: Oral, I.V.: 100 mg/kg or 3 g/m^2 during the first hour, followed by continuous infusion at the rate of 33.3 mg/kg/hour or 1 g/m^2/hour; total dosage should not exceed 18 g/m^2/24 hours
Traumatic hyphema: Oral: 100 mg/kg/dose every 6-8 hours
Adults:
Oral: For elevated fibrinolytic activity, give 5 g during first hour, followed by 1-1.25 g/hour for approximately 8 hours or until bleeding stops
I.V.: Give 4-5 g in 250 mL of diluent during first hour followed by continuous infusion at the rate of 1-1.25 g/hour in 50 mL of diluent, continue for 8 hours or until bleeding stops
Maximum daily dose: Oral, I.V.: 30 g

Dosing adjustment in renal impairment: Oliguria or ESRD: Reduce dose by 15% to 25%

Administration Administration by infusion using appropriate I.V. solution (dextrose 5% or 0.9% sodium chloride); rapid I.V. injection (IVP) should be avoided since hypotension, bradycardia, and arrhythmia may result. Aminocaproic acid may accumulate in patients with decreased renal function.

Monitoring Parameters Fibrinogen, fibrin split products, creatine phosphokinase (with long-term therapy)

Reference Range Therapeutic concentration: >130 µg/mL (concentration necessary for inhibition of fibrinolysis)

Test Interactions ↑ potassium, creatine phosphokinase [CPK] (S)

Patient Information Report any signs of bleeding; change positions slowly to minimize dizziness

Dosage Forms
Injection: 250 mg/mL (20 mL, 96 mL, 100 mL)
Syrup: 1.25 g/5 mL (480 mL)
Tablet: 500 mg

Amino-Cerv™ Vaginal Cream *see Urea on page 1139*

Aminoglutethimide *(a mee noe gloo teth′ i mide)*

Brand Names Cytadren®

Use Suppression of adrenal function in selected patients with Cushing's syndrome; also used successfully in postmenopausal patients with advanced breast carcinoma and in patients with metastatic prostate carcinoma as salvage (third-line hormonal agent)

Pregnancy Risk Factor D

Pregnancy/Breast Feeding Implications Suspected of causing virilization when given throughout pregnancy

Contraindications Hypersensitivity to aminoglutethimide or any component and glutethimide

Warnings/Precautions Monitor blood pressure in all patients at appropriate intervals; hypothyroidism may occur; **mineralocorticoid replacement therapy may be necessary in up to 50% of patients** (ie, fludrocortisone); if glucocorticoid replacement therapy is necessary, 20-30 mg of hydrocortisone daily in the morning will replace endogenous secretion (steroid replacement regimen is controversial - high-dose versus low-dose)

Adverse Reactions Most adverse effects will diminish in incidence and severity after the first 2-6 weeks

>10%:
Central nervous system: Headache, dizziness, drowsiness, and lethargy are frequent at the start of therapy, clumsiness
Dermatologic: Systemic lupus erythematosus, skin rash
Gastrointestinal: Nausea, vomiting, anorexia
Hepatic: Cholestatic jaundice
Neuromuscular & skeletal: Myalgia
Renal: Nephrotoxicity
Respiratory: Pulmonary alveolar damage
1% to 10%:
Cardiovascular: Hypotension and tachycardia, orthostatic hypotension
Central nervous system: Headache
Endocrine & metabolic: Hirsutism in females, adrenocortical insufficiency

Hematologic: Rare cases of neutropenia, leukopenia, thrombocytopenia, pancytopenia, and agranulocytosis have been reported

Neuromuscular & skeletal: Muscle pain

<1%: Endocrine & metabolic: Adrenal suppression, lipid abnormalities (hypercholesterolemia), hyperkalemia, hypothyroidism, goiter

Overdosage/Toxicology Symptoms of overdose include ataxia, somnolence, lethargy, dizziness, distress, fatigue, coma, hyperventilation, respiratory depression, hypovolemic shock; supportive treatment

Drug Interactions
Decreased effect:
Dexamethasone: Reported to increase metabolism
Digitoxin: Increased clearance of digitoxin after 3-8 weeks of aminoglutethimide therapy
Theophylline: Aminoglutethimide increases the metabolism of theophylline
Warfarin: Decrease in anticoagulant response to warfarin
Increased toxicity: Propranolol: Case report of enhanced aminoglutethimide toxicity (rash and lethargy)

Mechanism of Action Blocks the enzymatic conversion of cholesterol to delta-5-pregnenolone, thereby reducing the synthesis of adrenal glucocorticoids, mineralocorticoids, estrogens, aldosterone, and androgens

Pharmacodynamics/Kinetics
Onset of action (adrenal suppression): 3-5 days
Absorption: Oral: Well absorbed (90%)
Distribution: Crosses the placenta
Protein binding: Minimally bound to plasma proteins (20% to 25%)
Metabolism: Major metabolite is N-acetylaminoglutethimide
Half-life: 7-15 hours; shorter following multiple administrations than following single doses (induces hepatic enzymes increasing its own metabolism)
Elimination: 50% excreted unchanged in urine

Usual Dosage Adults: Oral: 250 mg every 6 hours may be increased at 1- to 2-week intervals to a total of 2 g/day; give in divided doses, 2-3 times/day to reduce incidence of nausea and vomiting

Dosing adjustment in renal impairment: Dose reduction may be necessary
Patient Information Masculinization can occur and is reversible after discontinuing treatment; may cause drowsiness or dizziness
Dosage Forms Tablet, scored: 250 mg

Amino-Opti-E® [OTC] see Vitamin E on page 1164

Aminophyllin™ see Theophylline/Aminophylline on page 1072

Aminophylline see Theophylline/Aminophylline on page 1072

Aminosalicylate Sodium (a mee noe sal i sill' ik)
Brand Names Sodium P.A.S.
Synonyms PAS
Use Treatment of tuberculosis with combination drugs
Pregnancy Risk Factor C
Contraindications Hypersensitivity to aminosalicylate sodium
Warnings/Precautions Use with caution in patients with hepatic or renal dysfunction, patients with gastric ulcer, patients with CHF, and patients who are sodium restricted
Adverse Reactions
1% to 10%: Gastrointestinal: Nausea, vomiting, diarrhea, abdominal pain
<1%:
Cardiovascular: Vasculitis
Central nervous system: Fever
Dermatologic: Skin eruptions
Endocrine & metabolic: Goiter with or without myxedema
Hematologic: Leukopenia, agranulocytosis, thrombocytopenia, hemolytic anemia
Hepatic: Jaundice, hepatitis

Overdosage/Toxicology Acute overdose results in crystalluria and renal failure, nausea, and vomiting; alkalinization of the urine with sodium bicarbonate and forced diuresis can prevent crystalluria and nephrotoxicity

Drug Interactions Decreased levels of digoxin and vitamin B_{12}

Mechanism of Action Aminosalicylic acid (PAS) is a highly specific bacteriostatic agent active against M. tuberculosis. Most strains of M. tuberculosis are sensitive to a concentration of 1 mcg/mL; structurally related to para-aminobenzoic acid (PABA) and its mechanism of action is thought to be similar to the sulfonamides, a competitive antagonism with PABA; disrupts plate biosynthesis in sensitive organisms.

(Continued)

Aminosalicylate Sodium (Continued)

Pharmacodynamics/Kinetics
Absorption: Readily absorbed >90%
Metabolism: >50% acetylated in liver
Elimination: >80% excreted through kidneys as parent drug and metabolites; elimination is reduced with renal dysfunction

Usual Dosage Oral:
Children: 150-300 mg/kg/day in 3-4 equally divided doses
Adults: 150 mg/kg/day in 2-3 equally divided doses (usually 12-14 g/day)

Dosing adjustment in renal impairment:
Cl_{cr} 10-50 mL/minute: Administer 50% to 75% of dose
Cl_{cr} <10 mL/minute: Administer 50% of dose

Administer after hemodialysis CAPD/CAVHD: Dose for Cl_{cr} <10 mL/minute

Patient Information Notify physician if persistent sore throat, fever, unusual bleeding or bruising, persistent nausea, vomiting, or abdominal pain occurs; do not stop taking before consulting your physician; take with food or meals; do not use products that are brown or purple; store in a cool, dry place away from sunlight

Nursing Implications Do not give if discolored; give with food or meals

Dosage Forms Tablet: 500 mg

5-Aminosalicylic Acid see Mesalamine on page 691

Amiodarone Hydrochloride (a mee' oh da rone)

Related Information
Antiarrhythmic Drugs on page 1246-1248

Brand Names Cordarone®

Use Management of resistant, life-threatening ventricular arrhythmias or supraventricular arrhythmias unresponsive to conventional therapy with less toxic agents

Pregnancy Risk Factor C

Contraindications Hypersensitivity to amiodarone; severe sinus node dysfunction, second and third degree A-V block, marked sinus bradycardia except if pacemaker is placed, thyroid disease, pregnancy and lactation

Warnings/Precautions Not considered first-line antiarrhythmic due to high incidence of significant and potentially fatal toxicity, especially with large doses; reserve for use in arrhythmias refractory to other therapy; hospitalize patients while loading dose is administered; use cautiously in elderly due to predisposition to toxicity

Adverse Reactions With large dosages (≥400 mg/day), adverse reactions occur in ~75% patients and require discontinuance in 5% to 20%

>10%:
Central nervous system: Ataxia, fatigue, malaise, dizziness, headache, insomnia, nightmares
Dermatologic: Photosensitivity
Gastrointestinal: Nausea, vomiting
Neuromuscular & skeletal: Tremor, paresthesias, muscle weakness
Respiratory: Pulmonary fibrosis (cough, fever, dyspnea, malaise), interstitial pneumonitis
Miscellaneous: Alveolitis
1% to 10%:
Cardiovascular: Congestive heart failure, cardiac arrhythmias (atropine-resistant bradycardia, heart block, sinus arrest, paroxysmal ventricular tachycardia), myocardial depression, flushing, edema
Endocrine & metabolic: Hypothyroidism or hyperthyroidism (less common), decreased libido
Gastrointestinal: Constipation, anorexia, abdominal pain
Hematologic: Coagulation abnormalities
Hepatic: Abnormal liver function tests
Ocular: Visual disturbances
Miscellaneous: Abnormal taste and smell, abnormal salivation
<1%:
Cardiovascular: Hypotension, vasculitis
Central nervous system: Pseudotumor cerebri
Dermatologic: Skin rash, alopecia, slate blue discoloration of skin, photosensitivity
Endocrine & metabolic: Hyperglycemia, hypertriglyceridemia
Genitourinary: Epididymitis
Hematologic: Thrombocytopenia
Hepatic: Cirrhosis, severe hepatic toxicity (potentially fatal hepatitis)

Ocular: Optic neuritis, corneal microdeposits, photophobia

Overdosage/Toxicology Symptoms include extensions of pharmacologic effect, sinus bradycardia and/or heart block, hypotension and Q-T prolongation; patients should be monitored for several days following ingestion. Intoxication with amiodarone necessitates EKG monitoring; bradycardia may be atropine resistant; injectable isoproterenol or a temporary pacemaker may be required.

Drug Interactions Cytochrome P-450 3A enzyme inhibitor

Amiodarone appears to interfere with the hepatic metabolism of several drugs resulting in significantly increased plasma concentrations; see table.

Amiodarone Common Drug Interactions

Drug	Interaction
Anticoagulants, oral	The effects of the anticoagulant is increased due to inhibition of its metabolism
β-adrenergic receptor antagonists	β -blocker effects are enhanced by amiodarone's inhibition of the β -blocker's hepatic metabolism
Calcium channel antagonists	Additive effects of both drugs resulting in a reduction in cardiac sinus conduction, atrioventricular nodal conduction and myocardial contractility
Digoxin	Digoxin concentrations may be increased with resultant increases in activity and potential for toxicity
Flecainide	Flecainide plasma concentrations are increased
Phenytoin	Phenytoin serum concentrations are increased due to reduction in phenytoin metabolism, with possible symptoms of phenytoin toxicity
Procainamide	Procainamide serum concentrations may be increased
Quinidine	Quinidine serum concentrations may be increased and can potentially cause fatal cardiac dysrhythmias

Mechanism of Action Class III antiarrhythmic agent which inhibits adrenergic stimulation, prolongs the action potential and refractory period in myocardial tissue; decreases A-V conduction and sinus node function

Pharmacodynamics/Kinetics

Onset of effect: 3 days to 3 weeks after starting therapy

Peak effect: 1 week to 5 months

Duration of effect after discontinuation of therapy: 7-50 days

Note: Mean onset of effect and duration after discontinuation may be shorter in children versus adults

Distribution: V_d: 66 L/kg (range: 18-148 L/kg); crosses placenta; distributes into breast milk in concentrations higher than maternal plasma concentrations

Protein binding: 96%

Metabolism: In liver, major metabolite active

Bioavailability: ~50%

Half-life: Oral chronic therapy: 40-55 days (range: 26-107 days); shortened in children versus adults

Elimination: Via biliary excretion; possible enterohepatic recirculation; <1% excreted unchanged in urine

Usual Dosage Oral:

Children (calculate doses for children <1 year on body surface area):

Loading dose: 10-15 mg/kg/day or 600-800 mg/1.73 m^2/day for 4-14 days or until adequate control of arrhythmia or prominent adverse effects occur (this loading dose may be given in 1-2 divided doses/day); dosage should then be reduced to 5 mg/kg/day or 200-400 mg/1.73 m^2/day given once daily for several weeks; if arrhythmia does not recur, reduce to lowest effective dosage possible; usual daily minimal dose: 2.5 mg/kg/day; maintenance doses may be given for 5 of 7 days/week

Adults: Ventricular arrhythmias: 800-1600 mg/day in 1-2 doses for 1-3 weeks, then 600-800 mg/day in 1-2 doses for 1 month; maintenance: 400 mg/day; lower doses are recommended for supraventricular arrhythmias

Dosing adjustment in hepatic impairment: Probably necessary in substantial hepatic impairment

(Continued)

Amiodarone Hydrochloride *(Continued)*

Not removed by hemodialysis or peritoneal dialysis (0% to 5%); no supplemental doses required

Monitoring Parameters Monitor heart rate (EKG) and rhythm throughout therapy; assess patient for signs of thyroid dysfunction (thyroid function tests and liver enzymes), lethargy, edema of the hands, feet, weight loss, and pulmonary toxicity (baseline pulmonary function tests)

Reference Range Therapeutic: 0.5-2.5 mg/L (SI: 1-4 µmol/L) (parent); desethyl metabolite is active and is present in equal concentration to parent drug

Test Interactions Thyroid function tests: Amiodarone partially inhibits the peripheral conversion of thyroxine (T_4) to tri-iodothyronine (T_3); serum T_4 and reverse tri-iodothyronine (RT_3) concentrations may be increased and serum T_3 may be decreased; most patients remain clinically euthyroid, however, clinical hypothyroidism or hyperthyroidism may occur

Patient Information Take with food; use sunscreen or stay out of sun to prevent burns; skin discoloration is reversible; photophobia may make sunglasses necessary; do not discontinue abruptly; regular blood work for thyroid functions tests and ophthalmologic exams are necessary; notify physician if persistent dry cough or shortness of breath occurs

Nursing Implications Muscle weakness may present a great hazard for ambulation; give with food

Dosage Forms Tablet: 200 mg (scored)

Amitone® [OTC] *see* Calcium Carbonate *on page 161*

Amitriptyline Hydrochloride *(a mee trip' ti leen)*

Related Information

Antidepressant Agents Comparison *on page 1250-1252*

Brand Names Elavil®; Endep®; Enovil®

Use Treatment of various forms of depression, often in conjunction with psychotherapy; analgesic for certain chronic and neuropathic pain, prophylaxis against migraine headaches

Pregnancy Risk Factor D

Contraindications Hypersensitivity to amitriptyline (cross-sensitivity with other tricyclics may occur); patients receiving MAO inhibitors within past 14 days; narrow-angle glaucoma; avoid use during pregnancy and lactation

Warnings/Precautions

Amitriptyline should not be abruptly discontinued in patients receiving high doses for prolonged periods

Use with caution in patients with cardiac conduction disturbances; an EKG prior to initiation of therapy is advised; use with caution in patients with a history of hyperthyroidism, renal or hepatic impairment

The most anticholinergic and sedating of the antidepressants; pronounced effects on the cardiovascular system (hypotension), hence, many psychiatrists agree it is best to avoid in the elderly

Adverse Reactions Anticholinergic effects may be pronounced; moderate to marked sedation can occur (tolerance to these effects usually occurs)

>10%:

Central nervous system: Dizziness, drowsiness, headache

Gastrointestinal: Dry mouth, constipation, increased appetite, nausea, weakness, unpleasant taste, weight gain

1% to 10%:

Cardiovascular: Hypotension, postural hypotension, arrhythmias, tachycardia, sudden death

Central nervous system: Nervousness, restlessness, parkinsonian syndrome, insomnia, sedation, weakness, fatigue, anxiety, impaired cognitive function, seizures have occurred occasionally, extrapyramidal symptoms are possible

Gastrointestinal: Diarrhea, heartburn, constipation

Genitourinary: Sexual function impairment, urinary retention

Neuromuscular & skeletal: Tremor

Ocular: Eye pain, blurred vision

Miscellaneous: Excessive sweating

<1%:

Central nervous system: Anxiety, seizures

Dermatologic: Alopecia, photosensitivity

Endocrine & metabolic: Breast enlargement, galactorrhea, rarely SIADH

Genitourinary: Testicular swelling

Hematologic: Leukopenia, eosinophilia, rarely agranulocytosis

Hepatic: Cholestatic jaundice, increased liver enzymes

Ocular: Increased intraocular pressure

Otic: Tinnitus

Miscellaneous: Trouble with gums, decreased lower esophageal sphincter tone may cause GE reflux; allergic reactions

Overdosage/Toxicology Symptoms of overdose include agitation, confusion, hallucinations, urinary retention, hypothermia, hypotension, ventricular seizures, tachycardia

Following initiation of essential overdose management, toxic symptoms should be treated. Ventricular arrhythmias often respond to phenytoin 15-20 mg/kg (adults) with concurrent systemic alkalinization (sodium bicarbonate 0.5-2 mEq/kg I.V.). Arrhythmias unresponsive to this therapy may respond to lidocaine 1 mg/kg I.V. followed by a titrated infusion. Physostigmine (1-2 mg I.V. slowly for adults or 0.5 mg I.V. slowly for children) may be indicated in reversing cardiac arrhythmias that are due to vagal blockade or for anticholinergic effects, but should only be used as a last measure in life-threatening situations. Seizures usually respond to diazepam I.V. boluses (5-10 mg for adults up to 30 mg or 0.25-0.4 mg/kg/dose for children up to 10 mg/dose). If seizures are unresponsive or recur, phenytoin or phenobarbital may be required.

Drug Interactions

Decreased effect: Phenobarbital may increase the metabolism of amitriptyline; amitriptyline blocks the uptake of guanethidine and thus prevents the hypotensive effect of guanethidine

Increased toxicity: Clonidine → hypertensive crisis; amitriptyline may be additive with or may potentiate the action of other CNS depressants such as sedatives or hypnotics; with MAO inhibitors, hyperpyrexia, hypertension, tachycardia, confusion, seizures, and **deaths have been reported**; amitriptyline may increase the prothrombin time in patients stabilized on warfarin; amitriptyline potentiates the pressor and cardiac effects of sympathomimetic agents such as isoproterenol, epinephrine, etc; cimetidine and methylphenidate may decrease the metabolism of amitriptyline; additive anticholinergic effects seen with other anticholinergic agents

Stability Protect injection and Elavil® 10 mg tablets from light

Mechanism of Action Increases the synaptic concentration of serotonin and/or norepinephrine in the central nervous system by inhibition of their reuptake by the presynaptic neuronal membrane

Pharmacodynamics/Kinetics

Onset of therapeutic effect: 7-21 days

Desired therapeutic effect (for depression) may take as long as 3-4 weeks, at that point dosage should be reduced to lowest effective level

When used for migraine headache prophylaxis, therapeutic effect may take as long as 6 weeks; a higher dosage may be required in a heavy smoker, because of increased metabolism

Distribution: Crosses placenta; enters breast milk

Metabolism: In the liver to nortriptyline (active), hydroxy derivatives, and conjugated derivatives; metabolism may be impaired in the elderly

Half-life: Adults: 9-25 hours (15-hour average)

Time to peak serum concentration: Within 4 hours

Elimination: Renal excretion of 18% as unchanged drug; small amounts eliminated in feces by bile

Usual Dosage

Children: Pain management: Oral: Initial: 0.1 mg/kg at bedtime, may advance as tolerated over 2-3 weeks to 0.5-2 mg/day at bedtime

Adolescents: Oral: Initial: 25-50 mg/day; may give in divided doses; increase gradually to 100 mg/day in divided doses

Adults:

Oral: 30-100 mg/day single dose at bedtime or in divided doses; dose may be gradually increased up to 300 mg/day; once symptoms are controlled, decrease gradually to lowest effective dose

I.M.: 20-30 mg 4 times/day

Dosing interval in hepatic impairment: Use with caution and monitor plasma levels and patient response

Nondialyzable

Monitoring Parameters Monitor blood pressure and pulse rate prior to and during initial therapy; evaluate mental status; monitor weight

Reference Range Therapeutic: Amitriptyline and nortriptyline 100-250 ng/mL (SI: 360-900 nmol/L); nortriptyline 50-150 ng/mL (SI: 190-570 nmol/L); Toxic: >0.5 µg/mL; plasma levels do not always correlate with clinical effectiveness

Test Interactions ↑ glucose

Patient Information Avoid alcohol ingestion; do not discontinue medication abruptly; may cause urine to turn blue-green; may cause drowsiness; full effect

(Continued)

Amitriptyline Hydrochloride *(Continued)*

may not occur for 3-6 weeks; dry mouth may be helped by sips of water, sugarless gum, or hard candy

Nursing Implications May increase appetite and possibly a craving for sweets

Dosage Forms
Injection: 10 mg/mL (10 mL)
Tablet: 10 mg, 25 mg, 50 mg, 75 mg, 100 mg, 150 mg

Amlodipine *(am loe' di peen)*

Related Information
Calcium Channel Blockers Cardiovascular Adverse Reactions *on page 1262*
Calcium Channel Blockers Central Nervous System Adverse Reactions *on page 1264*
Calcium Channel Blockers Comparative Actions *on page 1260*
Calcium Channel Blockers Comparative Pharmacokinetics *on page 1261*
Calcium Channel Blockers FDA-Approved Indications *on page 1263*
Calcium Channel Blockers Gastrointestinal and Miscellaneous Adverse Reactions *on page 1265*

Brand Names Norvasc®

Use Treatment of hypertension and angina

Pregnancy Risk Factor C

Pregnancy/Breast Feeding Implications Teratogenic and embryotoxic effects have been demonstrated in small animals. No well controlled studies have been conducted in pregnant women. Use in pregnancy only when clearly needed and when the benefits outweigh the potential hazard to the fetus.

Contraindications Hypersensitivity

Warnings/Precautions Use with caution and titrate dosages for patients with impaired renal or hepatic function; use caution when treating patients with congestive heart failure, sick-sinus syndrome, severe left ventricular dysfunction, hypertrophic cardiomyopathy (especially obstructive), concomitant therapy with beta-blockers or digoxin, edema, or increased intracranial pressure with cranial tumors; do not abruptly withdraw (may cause chest pain); elderly may experience hypotension and constipation more readily.

Adverse Reactions
>10%: Cardiovascular: Peripheral edema
1% to 10%:
Cardiovascular: Edema, flushing, palpitations
Central nervous system: Headache, fatigue, dizziness, somnolence
Dermatologic: Dermatitis, rash
Endocrine & metabolic: Sexual difficulties
Gastrointestinal: Nausea, abdominal pain
Respiratory: Shortness of breath
Neuromuscular & skeletal: Muscle cramps
<1%:
Cardiovascular: Hypotension, bradycardia, arrhythmias, abnormal EKG, ventricular extrasystoles
Dermatologic: Alopecia, petechiae
Gastrointestinal: Weight gain, anorexia
Neuromuscular & skeletal: Joint stiffness
Respiratory: Nasal congestion, cough
Miscellaneous: Sweating, epistaxis

Overdosage/Toxicology The primary cardiac symptoms of calcium blocker overdose includes hypotension and bradycardia. The hypotension is caused by peripheral vasodilation, myocardial depression, and bradycardia. Bradycardia results from sinus bradycardia, second- or third-degree atrioventricular block, or sinus arrest with junctional rhythm. Intraventricular conduction is usually not affected so QRS duration is normal (verapamil does prolong the P-R interval and bepridil prolongs the Q-T and may cause ventricular arrhythmias, including torsade de pointes).

The noncardiac symptoms include confusion, stupor, nausea, vomiting, metabolic acidosis, and hyperglycemia. Following initial gastric decontamination, if possible, repeated calcium administration may promptly reverse the depressed cardiac contractility (but not sinus node depression or peripheral vasodilation); glucagon, epinephrine, and amrinone may treat refractory hypotension; glucagon and epinephrine also increase the heart rate (outside the U.S., 4-aminopyridine may be available as an antidote); dialysis and hemoperfusion are not effective in enhancing elimination although repeat-dose activated charcoal may serve as an adjunct with sustained-release preparations.

Mechanism of Action Inhibits calcium ion from entering the "slow channels" or select voltage-sensitive areas of vascular smooth muscle and myocardium during depolarization, producing a relaxation of coronary vascular smooth muscle and coronary vasodilation; increases myocardial oxygen delivery in patients with vasospastic angina

Pharmacodynamics/Kinetics
Onset of action: 30-50 minutes
Peak effect: 6-12 hours
Duration: 24 hours
Absorption: Oral: Well absorbed
Protein binding: 93%
Metabolism: Hepatic, >90% to inactive compound
Bioavailability: 64% to 90%
Half-life: 30-50 hours
Elimination: Metabolite and parent drug excreted renally

Usual Dosage Adults: Oral: Initial dose: 2.5-5 mg once daily; usual dose: 5-10 mg once daily; maximum dose: 10 mg once daily

Hemodialysis and peritoneal dialysis does not enhance elimination; supplemental dose is not necessary.
Dosage adjustment in hepatic impairment: 2.5 mg once daily

Patient Information Do not discontinue abruptly; report any dizziness, shortness of breath, palpitations, or edema

Dosage Forms Tablet: 2.5 mg, 5 mg, 10 mg

Ammonium Chloride (a moe' nee um klor' ide)

Use Diuretic or systemic and urinary acidifying agent; treatment of hypochloremic states

Pregnancy Risk Factor C

Contraindications Severe hepatic and renal dysfunction; patients with primary respiratory acidosis

Warnings/Precautions Safety and efficacy not established in children, use with caution in infants

Adverse Reactions
1% to 10%:
Cardiovascular: Bradycardia
Central nervous system: Mental confusion, coma, headache
Dermatologic: Rash
Endocrine & metabolic: Metabolic acidosis secondary to hyperchloremia
Gastrointestinal: Gastric irritation, nausea, vomiting
Local: Pain at site of injection
Respiratory: Hyperventilation

Overdosage/Toxicology Symptoms of overdose include acidosis, headache, drowsiness, confusion, hyperventilation, hypokalemia; administer sodium bicarbonate or lactate to treat acidosis; supplemental potassium for hypokalemia

Mechanism of Action Increases acidity by increasing free hydrogen ion concentration

Pharmacodynamics/Kinetics
Absorption: Rapid from GI tract, complete within 3-6 hours
Metabolism: In the liver
Elimination: In urine

Usual Dosage Metabolic alkalosis: The following equations represent different methods of correction utilizing either the serum HCO_3^-, the serum chloride, or the base excess

Dosing of mEq NH_4Cl via the chloride-deficit method (hypochloremia):
Dose of mEq NH_4Cl = [0.2 L/kg x body weight (kg)] x [103 - observed serum chloride]; give 100% of dose over 12 hours, then re-evaluate
Note: 0.2 L/kg is the estimated chloride space and 103 is the average normal serum chloride concentration

Dosing of mEq NH_4Cl via the bicarbonate-excess method (refractory hypochloremic metabolic alkalosis):
Dose of NH_4Cl = [0.5 L/kg x body weight (kg) x (observed serum HCO_3^- - 24)]; give 50% of dose over 12 hours, then re-evaluate
Note: 0.5 L/kg is the estimated bicarbonate space and 24 is the average normal serum bicarbonate concentration

Dosing of mEq NH_4Cl via the base-excess method:
Dose of NH_4Cl = [0.3 L/kg x body weight (kg) x measured base excess (mEq/L)]; give 50% of dose over 12 hours, then re-evaluate
Note: 0.3 L/kg is the estimated extracellular bicarbonate and base excess is measured by the chemistry lab and reported with arterial blood gases

These equations will yield different requirements of ammonium chloride
(Continued)

Ammonium Chloride *(Continued)*

Equation #1 is inappropriate to use if the patient has severe metabolic alkalosis without hypochloremia or if the patient has uremia

Equation #3 is the most useful for the first estimation of ammonium chloride dosage

Children: Urinary acidifying agents: Oral, I.V.: 75 mg/kg/day in 4 divided doses; maximum daily dose: 6 g

Adults: Urinary acidifying agent/diuretic:

Oral: 2-3 g every 6 hours

I.V.: 1.5 g/dose every 6 hours

Administration Rapid I.V. injection may increase the likelihood of ammonia toxicity; rate should not exceed 1 mEq/kg/hour; 26.75% solution must be diluted prior to administration

Test Interactions ↑ ammonia (B); ↓ potassium (S), sodium (S)

Patient Information Take oral dose after meals

Dosage Forms

Injection: 26.75% [5 mEq/mL] (20 mL)

Tablet: 500 mg

Tablet, enteric coated: 500 mg

Amobarbital *(am oh bar' bi tal)*

Brand Names Amytal®

Synonyms Amylobarbitone

Use

Oral: Hypnotic in short-term treatment of insomnia, to reduce anxiety and provide sedation preoperatively

I.M., I.V.: Control status epilepticus or acute seizure episodes. Also used in catatonic, negativistic, or manic reactions and in "Amytal® Interviewing" for narcoanalysis.

Restrictions C-II

Pregnancy Risk Factor D

Contraindications Marked liver function impairment or latent porphyria; hypersensitivity to barbiturates; do not administer in presence of chronic or acute pain

Warnings/Precautions Safety has not been established in children <6 years of age; potential for drug dependency exists; avoid alcoholic beverages; use with caution in patients with CHF, hepatic or renal impairment, hypovolemic shock; when administered I.V., respiratory depression and hypotension are possible, have equipment and personnel available; this I.V. medication should be given only to hospitalized patients

Adverse Reactions

>10%:

Central nervous system: Dizziness, lightheadedness, "hangover" effect, drowsiness, CNS depression, fever

Local: Pain at injection site

1% to 10%:

Central nervous system: Confusion, mental depression, unusual excitement, nervousness, faint feeling, headache, insomnia, nightmares

Gastrointestinal: Nausea, vomiting, constipation

<1%:

Cardiovascular: Hypotension

Central nervous system: Hallucinations

Dermatologic: Skin rash, exfoliative dermatitis urticaria, Stevens-Johnson syndrome

Hematologic: Agranulocytosis, megaloblastic anemia, thrombocytopenia

Local: Thrombophlebitis

Respiratory: Respiratory depression, apnea, laryngospasm

Overdosage/Toxicology Symptoms of overdose include unsteady gait, slurred speech, confusion, jaundice, hypothermia, fever, hypotension; if hypotension occurs, administer I.V. fluids and place the patient in the Trendelenburg position. If unresponsive, an I.V. vasopressor (eg, dopamine, epinephrine) may be required. Forced alkaline diuresis is of no value in the treatment of intoxications with short-acting barbiturates. Charcoal hemoperfusion or hemodialysis may be useful in the harder to treat intoxications, especially in the presence of very high serum barbiturate levels.

Drug Interactions

Decreased effect: Cimetidine's tricyclic antidepressants and doxycycline's efficacy may be reduced with amobarbital

Increased toxicity when combined with other CNS depressants or antidepressants, respiratory and CNS depression may be additive

Stability Hydrolyzes when exposed to air; use contents of vial within 30 minutes after constitution; use only clear solution

Mechanism of Action Interferes with transmission of impulses from the thalamus to the cortex of the brain resulting in an imbalance in central inhibitory and facilitatory mechanisms

Pharmacodynamics/Kinetics

Onset of action:
  Oral: Within 1 hour
  I.V.: Within 5 minutes
Distribution: Readily crosses the placenta; small amounts appear in breast milk
Metabolism: Chiefly in the liver by microsomal enzymes
Half-life, biphasic:
  Initial: 40 minutes
  Terminal: 20 hours

Usual Dosage

Children: Oral:
  Sedation: 6 mg/kg/day divided every 6-8 hours
  Insomnia: 2 mg/kg or 70 mg/m^2/day in 4 equally divided doses
  Hypnotic: 2-3 mg/kg

Adults:
  Insomnia: Oral: 65-200 mg at bedtime
  Sedation: Oral: 30-50 mg 2-3 times/day
  Preanesthetic: Oral: 200 mg 1-2 hours before surgery
  Hypnotic:
    Oral: 65-200 mg at bedtime
    I.M., I.V.: 65-500 mg, should not exceed 500 mg I.M. or 1000 mg I.V.

Administration I.M. injection should be deep to prevent against pain, sterile abscess, and sloughing

Monitoring Parameters Vital signs should be monitored during injection and for several hours after administration

Reference Range
Therapeutic: 1-5 µg/mL (SI: 4-22 µmol/L)
Toxic: >10 µg/mL (SI: >44 µmol/L)
Lethal: >50 µg/mL

Test Interactions ↑ ammonia (B); ↓ bilirubin (S)

Patient Information Avoid alcohol ingestion; physical dependency may result when used for an extended period of time (1-3 months); do not try to get out of bed without assistance, will cause drowsiness

Nursing Implications Raise bed rails at night

Dosage Forms
Capsule, as sodium: 65 mg, 200 mg
Injection, as sodium: 250 mg, 500 mg
Tablet: 30 mg, 50 mg, 100 mg

Amonidrin® [OTC] *see* Guaifenesin *on page 515*

Amoxapine (a mox′ a peen)

Related Information
  Antidepressant Agents Comparison *on page 1250-1252*

Brand Names Asendin®

Use Treatment of neurotic and endogenous depression and mixed symptoms of anxiety and depression

Pregnancy Risk Factor C

Contraindications Hypersensitivity to amoxapine; cross-sensitivity with other tricyclics may occur; narrow-angle glaucoma; patients receiving MAO inhibitors within past 14 days

Warnings/Precautions Use with caution in patients with seizures, cardiac conduction disturbances, cardiovascular diseases, urinary retention, hyperthyroidism, or those receiving thyroid replacement; do not discontinue abruptly in patients receiving high doses chronically; tolerance develops in 1-3 months in some patients, close medical follow-up is essential

Adverse Reactions
>10%:
  Central nervous system: Dizziness, drowsiness, headache, weakness
  Gastrointestinal: Dry mouth, constipation, increased appetite, nausea, unpleasant taste, weight gain
1% to 10%:
  Cardiovascular: Arrhythmias, hypotension
  Central nervous system: Confusion, delirium, hallucinations, nervousness, restlessness, parkinsonian syndrome, insomnia, tardive dyskinesia
  Gastrointestinal: Diarrhea, heartburn
(Continued)

65

Amoxapine *(Continued)*

    Genitourinary: Difficult urination, sexual function impairment
    Neuromuscular & skeletal: Fine muscle tremors
    Ocular: Blurred vision, eye pain
    Miscellaneous: Excessive sweating
  <1%:
    Central nervous system: Anxiety, seizures, neuroleptic malignant syndrome
    Dermatologic: Photosensitivity, alopecia
    Endocrine & metabolic: Breast enlargement, galactorrhea, SIADH
    Genitourinary: Testicular swelling
    Hematologic: Agranulocytosis, leukopenia, eosinophilia
    Hepatic: Cholestatic jaundice, increased liver enzymes
    Ocular: Increased intraocular pressure
    Otic: Tinnitus
    Miscellaneous: Trouble with gums, decreased lower esophageal sphincter tone may cause GE reflux, allergic reactions

Overdosage/Toxicology Symptoms of overdose include grand mal convulsions, acidosis, coma, renal failure

Following initiation of essential overdose management, toxic symptoms should be treated. Ventricular arrhythmias often respond to phenytoin 15-20 mg/kg (adults) with concurrent systemic alkalinization (sodium bicarbonate 0.5-2 mEq/kg I.V.). Arrhythmias unresponsive to this therapy may respond to lidocaine 1 mg/kg I.V. followed by a titrated infusion. Physostigmine (1-2 mg I.V. slowly for adults or 0.5 mg I.V. slowly for children) may be indicated in reversing cardiac arrhythmias that are due to vagal blockade or for anticholinergic effects, but should only be used as a last measure in life-threatening situations. Seizures usually respond to diazepam I.V. boluses (5-10 mg for adults up to 30 mg or 0.25-0.4 mg/kg/dose for children up to 10 mg/dose). If seizures are unresponsive or recur, phenytoin or phenobarbital may be required.

Drug Interactions
Decreased effect of clonidine, guanethidine
Increased effect of CNS depressants, adrenergic agents, anticholinergic agents
Increased toxicity of MAO inhibitors (hyperpyrexia, tachycardia, hypertension, seizures and death may occur); similar interactions as with other tricyclics may occur

Mechanism of Action Reduces the reuptake of serotonin and norepinephrine and blocks the response of dopamine receptors to dopamine

Pharmacodynamics/Kinetics
Onset of antidepressant effect: Usually occurs after 1-2 weeks
Absorption: Oral: Rapidly and well absorbed
Distribution: V_d: 0.9-1.2 L/kg; distributes into breast milk
Protein binding: 80%
Metabolism: Extensive in the liver
Half-life:
  Parent drug: 11-16 hours
  Active metabolite (8-hydroxy): Adults: 30 hours
Time to peak serum concentration: Within 1-2 hours
Elimination: Excretion of metabolites and parent compound in urine

Usual Dosage Once symptoms are controlled, decrease gradually to lowest effective dose. Maintenance dose is usually given at bedtime to reduce daytime sedation. Oral:

Children: Not established in children <16 years of age
Adolescents: Initial: 25-50 mg/day; increase gradually to 100 mg/day; may give as divided doses or as a single dose at bedtime
Adults: Initial: 25 mg 2-3 times/day, if tolerated, dosage may be increased to 100 mg 2-3 times/day; may be given in a single bedtime dose when dosage <300 mg/day
Elderly: Initial: 25 mg at bedtime increased by 25 mg weekly for outpatients and every 3 days for inpatients if tolerated; usual dose: 50-150 mg/day, but doses up to 300 mg may be necessary

Maximum daily dose:
  Inpatient: 600 mg
  Outpatient: 400 mg

Monitoring Parameters Monitor blood pressure and pulse rate prior to and during initial therapy evaluate mental status; monitor weight

Reference Range Therapeutic: Amoxapine: 20-100 ng/mL (SI: 64-319 nmol/L); 8-OH amoxapine: 150-400 ng/mL (SI: 478-1275 nmol/L); both: 200-500 ng/mL (SI: 637-1594 nmol/L)

Test Interactions ↑ glucose

Patient Information Dry mouth may be helped by sips of water, sugarless gum, or hard candy; avoid alcohol; very important to maintain established dosage regimen; photosensitivity to sunlight can occur, do not discontinue abruptly; full effect may not occur for 3-4 weeks; full dosage may be taken at bedtime to avoid daytime sedation

Nursing Implications May increase appetite and possibly a craving for sweets; recognize signs of neuroleptic malignant syndrome and tardive dyskinesia

Dosage Forms Tablet: 25 mg, 50 mg, 100 mg, 150 mg

Amoxicillin and Clavulanate Potassium *see* Amoxicillin and Clavulanic Acid *on this page*

Amoxicillin and Clavulanic Acid (a mox i sill' in & klav yoo lan' ick)

Related Information
Antimicrobial Drugs of Choice *on page 1298-1302*

Brand Names Augmentin®

Synonyms Amoxicillin and Clavulanate Potassium

Use Treatment of otitis media, sinusitis, and infections caused by susceptible organisms involving the lower respiratory tract, skin and skin structure, and urinary tract; spectrum same as amoxicillin with additional coverage of beta-lactamase producing *B. catarrhalis*, *H. influenzae*, *N. gonorrhoeae*, and *S. aureus* (not MRSA). The expanded coverage of this combination makes it a useful alternative when amoxicillin resistance is present and patients cannot tolerate alternative treatments.

Pregnancy Risk Factor B

Contraindications Known hypersensitivity to amoxicillin, clavulanic acid, or penicillin; concomitant use of disulfiram

Warnings/Precautions In patients with renal impairment, doses and/or frequency of administration should be modified in response to the degree of renal impairment; high percentage of patients with infectious mononucleosis have developed rash during therapy; a low incidence of cross-allergy with cephalosporins exists; incidence of diarrhea is higher than with amoxicillin alone

Adverse Reactions
<1%:
Dermatologic: Rash, urticaria
Gastrointestinal: Nausea, vomiting, diarrhea
Genitourinary: Vaginitis

Overdosage/Toxicology Symptoms of penicillin overdose include neuromuscular hypersensitivity (agitation, hallucinations, asterixis, encephalopathy, confusion, and seizures) and electrolyte imbalance with potassium or sodium salts, especially in renal failure; hemodialysis may be helpful to aid in the removal of the drug from the blood, otherwise most treatment is supportive or symptom directed

Drug Interactions
Decreased effect: Efficacy of oral contraceptives may be reduced
Increased effect: Disulfiram, probenecid → ↑ amoxicillin levels, increased effect of anticoagulants
Increased toxicity: Allopurinol theoretically has an additive potential for amoxicillin rash

Stability Discard unused suspension after 10 days; reconstituted oral suspension should be kept in refrigerator; unit dose antibiotic oral syringes are stable for 48 hours

Mechanism of Action Interferes with bacterial cell wall synthesis during active multiplication, causing cell wall death and resultant bactericidal activity against susceptible bacteria. Clavulanic acid binds and inhibits beta-lactamases that inactivate amoxicillin resulting in amoxicillin having an expanded spectrum of activity.

Pharmacodynamics/Kinetics Amoxicillin pharmacokinetics are not affected by clavulanic acid
Absorption: Oral: Rapid and nearly complete; food does not interfere
Protein binding: 17% to 20%
Metabolism: Partial (Clavulanic acid is hepatically metabolized)
Half-life:
Neonates, full-term: 3.7 hours
Infants and Children: 1-2 hours
Adults with normal renal function: ~1 hour for both agents
Patients with Cl_{cr} <10 mL/minute: 7-21 hours
Time to peak: 2 hours (capsule) and 1 hour (suspension)
Elimination: Amoxicillin excreted primarily (80%) unchanged and clavulanic acid is excreted 30% to 40% unchanged in the urine (lower in neonates)

Usual Dosage Oral:
(Continued)

Amoxicillin and Clavulanic Acid *(Continued)*

Children ≤40 kg: 20-40 mg (amoxicillin)/kg/day in divided doses every 8 hours
Children >40 kg and Adults: 250-500 mg every 8 hours; maximum dose: 2 g/day

Dosing interval in renal impairment:
Cl$_{cr}$ 10-30 mL/minute: Administer every 12 hours
Cl$_{cr}$ <10 mL/minute: Administer every 24 hours
Hemodialysis effects: Moderately dialyzable (20% to 50%)
Amoxicillin/clavulanic acid: Administer dose after dialysis
Peritoneal dialysis effects: Moderately dialyzable (20% to 50%)
Amoxicillin: Administer 250 mg every 12 hours
Clavulanic acid: Dose for Cl$_{cr}$ <10 mL/minute

Continuous arterio-venous or veno-venous hemofiltration (CAVH) effects:
Amoxicillin: ~50 mg of amoxicillin/L of filtrate is removed
Clavulanic acid: Dose for Cl$_{cr}$ <10 mL/minute
Administration Administer around-the-clock rather than 3 times/day to promote less variation in peak and trough serum levels
Monitoring Parameters Assess patient at beginning and throughout therapy for infection; with prolonged therapy, monitor renal, hepatic, and hematologic function periodically
Test Interactions Urinary glucose (Benedict's solution, Clinitest®)
Patient Information Report diarrhea promptly; entire course of medication (10-14 days) should be taken to ensure eradication of organism; should be taken in equal intervals around-the-clock to maintain adequate blood levels; females should report onset of symptoms of candidal vaginitis; may interfere with the effects of oral contraceptives
Nursing Implications Two 250 mg tablets are not equivalent to a 500 mg tablet (both tablet sizes contain equivalent clavulanate); potassium content: 0.16 mEq of potassium per 31.25 mg of clavulanic acid
Dosage Forms
Suspension, oral:
125: Amoxicillin trihydrate 125 mg and clavulanic acid 31.25 mg per 5 mL (75 mL, 150 mL)
250: Amoxicillin trihydrate 250 mg and clavulanic acid 62.5 mg per 5 mL (75 mL, 150 mL)
Tablet:
Film coated:
250: Amoxicillin trihydrate 250 mg and clavulanic acid 125 mg
500: Amoxicillin trihydrate 500 mg and clavulanic acid 125 mg
Chewable:
125: Amoxicillin trihydrate 125 mg and clavulanic acid 31.25 mg
250: Amoxicillin trihydrate 250 mg and clavulanic acid 62.5 mg

Amoxicillin Trihydrate (a mox i sill' in)
Related Information
Antimicrobial Drugs of Choice *on page 1298-1302*
Prevention of Bacterial Endocarditis *on page 1285-1288*
Brand Names A-Cillin®; Amoxil®; Larotid®; Polymox®; Trimox®; Utimox®; Wymox®
Synonyms Amoxycillin; *p*-Hydroxyampicillin
Use Treatment of otitis media, sinusitis, and infections caused by susceptible organisms involving the respiratory tract, skin, and urinary tract; prophylaxis of bacterial endocarditis
Pregnancy Risk Factor B
Contraindications Hypersensitivity to amoxicillin, penicillin, or any component
Warnings/Precautions In patients with renal impairment, doses and/or frequency of administration should be modified in response to the degree of renal impairment; a high percentage of patients with infectious mononucleosis have developed rash during therapy with amoxicillin; a low incidence of cross-allergy with other beta-lactams and cephalosporins exists
Adverse Reactions
1% to 10%:
Central nervous system: Seizures, fever
Dermatologic: Rash (especially patients with mononucleosis)
Gastrointestinal: Diarrhea
Miscellaneous: Superinfection
Overdosage/Toxicology Symptoms of penicillin overdose include neuromuscular hypersensitivity (agitation, hallucinations, asterixis, encephalopathy, confusion, and seizures) and electrolyte imbalance with potassium or sodium salts, especially in renal failure; hemodialysis may be helpful to aid in the removal of

the drug from the blood, otherwise most treatment is supportive or symptom directed

Drug Interactions
Decreased effect: Efficacy of oral contraceptives may be reduced
Increased effect: Disulfiram, probenecid → ↑ amoxicillin levels
Increased toxicity: Allopurinol theoretically has an additive potential for amoxicillin rash

Stability Oral suspension remains stable for 7 days at room temperature or 14 days if refrigerated; unit dose antibiotic oral syringes are stable for 48 hours

Mechanism of Action Interferes with bacterial cell wall synthesis during active multiplication, causing cell wall death and resultant bactericidal activity against susceptible bacteria

Pharmacodynamics/Kinetics
Absorption: Oral: Rapid and nearly complete; food does not interfere
Protein binding: 17% to 20%
Ratio of CSF to blood:
Normal meninges: <1%
Inflamed meninges: 8% to 90%
Metabolism: Partial; renal excretion (80% as unchanged drug); lower in neonates
Half-life:
Neonates, full-term: 3.7 hours
Infants and Children: 1-2 hours
Adults with normal renal function: 0.7-1.4 hours
Patients with Cl_{cr} <10 mL/minute: 7-21 hours
Time to peak: 2 hours (capsule) and 1 hour (suspension)
Elimination: Renal excretion (80% as unchanged drug); lower in neonates

Usual Dosage Oral:
Children: 20-50 mg/kg/day in divided doses every 8 hours
Uncomplicated gonorrhea: ≥2 years: 50 mg/kg plus probenecid 25 mg/kg in a single dose; do not use this regimen in children <2 years of age, probenecid is contraindicated in this age group
Subacute bacterial endocarditis prophylaxis: 50 mg/kg 1 hour before procedure and 25 mg/kg 6 hours later
Adults: 250-500 mg every 8 hours; maximum dose: 2-3 g/day
Uncomplicated gonorrhea: 3 g plus probenecid 1 g in a single dose
Endocarditis prophylaxis: 3 g 1 hour before procedure and 1.5 g 6 hours later
Helicobacter pylori: Clinically effective treatment regimens include triple therapy with amoxicillin or tetracycline, metronidazole, and bismuth subsalicylate; amoxicillin, metronidazole, and an H_2-receptor antagonist. Adult dose: Oral: 250-500 mg 3 times/day

Dosing interval in renal impairment:
Cl_{cr} 10-50 mL/minute: Administer every 12 hours
Cl_{cr} <10 mL/minute: Administer every 24 hours
Moderately dialyzable (20% to 50%) by hemo- or peritoneal dialysis; approximately 50 mg of amoxicillin per liter of filtrate is removed by continuous arteriovenous or veno-venous hemofiltration (CAVH); dose as per Cl_{cr} <10 mL/minute guidelines

Administration Administer around-the-clock rather than 3 times/day to promote less variation in peak and trough serum levels

Monitoring Parameters With prolonged therapy, monitor renal, hepatic, and hematologic function periodically; assess patient at beginning and throughout therapy for infection

Test Interactions ↑ AST, ALT, protein

Patient Information Report diarrhea promptly; entire course of medication (10-14 days) should be taken to ensure eradication of organism; should be taken in equal intervals around-the-clock to maintain adequate blood levels; may interfere with oral contraceptives; females should report symptoms of vaginitis; pediatric drops may be placed on child's tongue or added to formula, milk, etc

Nursing Implications Obtain specimens for culture and sensitivity before the first dose

Dosage Forms
Capsule: 250 mg, 500 mg
Drops, pediatric: 50 mg/mL (15 mL, 30 mL)
Suspension, oral: 125 mg/5 mL (5 mL unit dose, 80 mL, 100 mL, 150 mL, 200 mL); 250 mg/5 mL (5 mL unit dose, 80 mL, 100 mL, 150 mL, 200 mL)
Tablet, chewable: 125 mg, 250 mg

Amoxil® *see* Amoxicillin Trihydrate *on previous page*

Amoxycillin *see* Amoxicillin Trihydrate *on previous page*

Amphetamine Sulfate (am fet' a meen)

Synonyms Racemic Amphetamine Sulfate

Use Treatment of narcolepsy; exogenous obesity; abnormal behavioral syndrome in children (minimal brain dysfunction); attention deficit hyperactive disorder (ADHD)

Restrictions C-II

Pregnancy Risk Factor C

Contraindications Patients with advanced arteriosclerosis, symptomatic cardiovascular disease, moderate to severe hypertension, hyperthyroidism, glaucoma, hypersensitivity, diabetes mellitus, agitated states, patients with a history of drug abuse, and during or within 14 days following MAO inhibitor therapy. Stimulant medications are contraindicated for use in children with attention deficit disorders and concomitant Tourette's syndrome or tics.

Warnings/Precautions Cardiovascular disease, nephritis, angina pectoris, hypertension, glaucoma, patients with a history of drug abuse, known hypersensitivity to amphetamine

Adverse Reactions

>10%:
Cardiovascular: Irregular heartbeat
Central nervous system: False feeling of well being, nervousness, restlessness, insomnia

1% to 10%:
Cardiovascular: Hypertension
Central nervous system: Mood or mental changes, dizziness, lightheadedness, headache
Endocrine & metabolic: Changes in libido
Gastrointestinal: Diarrhea, nausea, vomiting, stomach cramps, constipation, anorexia, weight loss dry mouth
Ocular: Blurred vision
Miscellaneous: Increased sweating

<1%:
Cardiovascular: Chest pain
Central nervous system: CNS stimulation (severe), Tourette's syndrome, hyperthermia, seizures, paranoia
Dermatologic: Skin rash, hives
Miscellaneous: Tolerance and withdrawal with prolonged use

Overdosage/Toxicology There is no specific antidote for amphetamine intoxication and the bulk of the treatment is supportive. Hyperactivity and agitation usually respond to reduced sensory input; however, with extreme agitation, haloperidol (2-5 mg I.M. for adults) may be required. Hyperthermia is best treated with external cooling measures, or when severe or unresponsive, muscle paralysis with pancuronium may be needed. Hypertension is usually transient and generally does not require treatment unless severe. For diastolic blood pressures >110 mm Hg, a nitroprusside infusion should be initiated. Seizures usually respond to diazepam IVP and/or phenytoin maintenance regimens.

Drug Interactions Increased toxicity of MAO inhibitors (hyperpyrexia, hypertension, arrhythmias, seizures, cerebral hemorrhage, and death has occurred)

Mechanism of Action The amphetamines are noncatechol sympathomimetic amines with pharmacologic actions similar to ephedrine. They require breakdown by monoamine oxidase for inactivation; produce central nervous system and respiratory stimulation, a pressor response, mydriasis, bronchodilation, and contraction of the urinary sphincter; thought to have a direct effect on both alpha- and beta-receptor sites in the peripheral system, as well as release stores of norepinephrine in adrenergic nerve terminals. The central nervous system action is thought to occur in the cerebral cortex and reticular-activating system. The anorexigenic effect is probably secondary to the CNS-stimulating effect; the site of action is probably the hypothalamic feeding center.

Usual Dosage Oral:

Narcolepsy:
Children:
6-12 years: 5 mg/day, increase by 5 mg at weekly intervals
>12 years: 10 mg/day, increase by 10 mg at weekly intervals
Adults: 5-60 mg/day in 2-3 divided doses

Attention deficit disorder: Children:
3-5 years: 2.5 mg/day, increase by 2.5 mg at weekly intervals
>6 years: 5 mg/day, increase by 5 mg at weekly intervals not to exceed 40 mg/day

Short-term adjunct to exogenous obesity: Children >12 years and Adults: 10 mg or 15 mg long-acting capsule daily, up to 30 mg/day; or 5-30 mg/day in divided doses (immediate release tablets only)

Reference Range Therapeutic: 20-30 ng/mL; Toxic: >200 ng/mL

Patient Information Take during day to avoid insomnia; do not discontinue abruptly, may cause physical and psychological dependence with prolonged use

Nursing Implications Monitor CNS, dose should not be given in evening or at bedtime

Dosage Forms Tablet: 5 mg, 10 mg

Amphojel® [OTC] *see* Aluminum Hydroxide *on page 48*

Amphotericin B (am foe ter′ i sin)

Related Information
Antifungal Agents *on page 1253-1254*

Brand Names Fungizone®

Use Treatment of severe systemic infections and meningitis caused by susceptible fungi such as *Candida* species, *Histoplasma capsulatum*, *Cryptococcus neoformans*, *Aspergillus* species, *Blastomyces dermatitidis*, *Torulopsis glabrata*, and *Coccidioides immitis*; fungal peritonitis; irrigant for bladder fungal infections; and topically for cutaneous and mucocutaneous candidal infections

Pregnancy Risk Factor B

Contraindications Hypersensitivity to amphotericin or any component

Warnings/Precautions Avoid additive toxicity with other nephrotoxic drugs; monitor BUN and serum creatinine levels frequently while therapy is increased and at least weekly thereafter. I.V. amphotericin is used primarily for the treatment of patients with progressive and potentially fatal fungal infections; topical preparations may stain clothing.

Adverse Reactions
>10%:
  Central nervous system: Fever, chills, headache, malaise, generalized pain
  Endocrine & metabolic: Hypokalemia, hypomagnesemia
  Gastrointestinal: Anorexia
  Hematologic: Anemia
  Renal: Nephrotoxicity
1% to 10%:
  Cardiovascular: Hypotension, hypertension, flushing
  Central nervous system: Delirium, arachnoiditis, pain along lumbar nerves
  Gastrointestinal: Nausea, vomiting
  Genitourinary: Urinary retention
  Hematologic: Leukocytosis, bone marrow depression
  Local: Thrombophlebitis
  Neuromuscular & skeletal: Paresthesia (especially with I.T. therapy)
  Renal: Renal tubular acidosis, renal failure
<1%:
  Cardiovascular: Cardiac arrest
  Central nervous system: Convulsions
  Dermatologic: Maculopapular rash
  Genitourinary: Anuria
  Hematologic: Coagulation defects, thrombocytopenia, agranulocytosis, leukopenia
  Hepatic: Acute liver failure
  Ocular: Vision changes
  Otic: Hearing loss
  Respiratory: Dyspnea

Overdosage/Toxicology Symptoms of overdose include renal dysfunction, anemia, thrombocytopenia, granulocytopenia, fever, nausea, and vomiting; treatment is supportive

Drug Interactions Increased toxicity: Cyclosporine and aminoglycosides (nephrotoxicity), corticosteroids (hypokalemia)

Stability
Reconstitute only with sterile water without preservatives, not bacteriostatic water. **Benzyl alcohol, sodium chloride, or other electrolyte solutions may cause precipitation.**
For I.V. infusion, an in-line filter (>1 micron mean pore diameter) may be used
Short-term exposure (<24 hours) to light during I.V. infusion does **not** appreciably affect potency
Reconstituted solutions with sterile water for injection and kept in the dark remain stable for 24 hours at room temperature and 1 week when refrigerated
Stability of parenteral admixture at room temperature (25°C): 24 hours; at refrigeration (4°C): 2 days
Standard diluent: Dose/500 mL D_5W
Minimum volume: 250 mL D_5W (concentrations should not exceed 0.1 mg/mL for peripheral administration or 1 mg/mL for central administration)
(Continued)

Amphotericin B *(Continued)*

Mechanism of Action Binds to ergosterol altering cell membrane permeability in susceptible fungi and causing leakage of cell components with subsequent cell death

Pharmacodynamics/Kinetics

Distribution: Minimal amounts enter the aqueous humor, bile, CSF (inflamed or noninflamed meninges), amniotic fluid, pericardial fluid, pleural fluid, and synovial fluid

Protein binding, plasma: 90% infusion

Half-life, biphasic:

Initial: 15-48 hours

Terminal: 15 days

Time to peak: Within 1 hour following a 4- to 6-hour dose

Usual Dosage

I.V.:

Infants and Children:

Test dose (not required): I.V.: 0.1 mg/kg/dose to a maximum of 1 mg; infuse over 30-60 minutes

Initial therapeutic dose: 0.25 mg/kg gradually increased, usually in 0.25 mg/kg increments on each subsequent day, until the desired daily dose is reached

Maintenance dose: 0.25-1 mg/kg/day given once daily; infuse over 2-6 hours. Once therapy has been established, amphotericin B can be administered on an every other day basis at 1-1.5 mg/kg/dose; cumulative dose: 1.5-2 g over 6-10 week

Adults:

Test dose (not required).: 1 mg infused over 20-30 minutes

Initial dose: 0.25 mg/kg administered over 2-6 hours, gradually increased on subsequent days to the desired level by 0.25 mg/kg increments per day; in critically ill patients, may initiate with 1-1.5 mg/kg/day with close observation

Maintenance dose: 0.25-1 mg/kg/day or 1.5 mg/kg over 4-6 hours every other day; do not exceed 1.5 mg/kg/day; cumulative dose: 1-4 g over 4-10 weeks

Duration of therapy varies with nature of infection: Histoplasmosis, *Cryptococcus*, or blastomycosis may be treated with total dose of 2-4 g

I.T.:

Children.: 25-100 mcg every 48-72 hours; increase to 500 mcg as tolerated

Adults: 25-300 mcg every 48-72 hours; increase to 500 mcg to 1 mg as tolerated

Topical: Apply to affected areas 2-4 times/day for 1-4 weeks of therapy depending on nature and severity of infection

Dosing adjustment in renal impairment: If renal dysfunction is due to the drug, the daily total can be decreased by 50% or the dose can be given every other day; I.V. therapy may take several months

Poorly dialyzed; no supplemental dosage necessary when using hemo- or peritoneal dialysis or CAVH/CAVHD

Administration in dialysate: Children and Adults: 1-2 mg/L of peritoneal dialysis fluid either with or without low-dose I.V. amphotericin B (a total dose of 2-10 mg/kg given over 7-14 days)

Administration via bladder Irrigation: Children and Adults:50 mg/day in 1 L of sterile water irrigation solution instilled over 24 hours for 2-7 days or until cultures are clear

Monitoring Parameters Electrolytes (especially potassium and magnesium), BUN, serum creatinine, liver function tests, temperature, CBC; monitor input and output; monitor for signs of hypokalemia (muscle weakness, cramping, drowsiness, EKG changes, etc)

Reference Range Therapeutic: 1-2 µg/mL (SI: 1-2.2 µmol/L)

Test Interactions ↑ BUN (S); ↓ magnesium, potassium (S)

Patient Information Amphotericin cream may slightly discolor skin and stain clothing; good personal hygiene may reduce the spread and recurrence of lesions; avoid covering topical applications with occlusive bandages; most skin lesions require 1-3 weeks of therapy; report any cramping, muscle weakness, or pain at or near injection site

Nursing Implications May premedicate patients with acetaminophen and diphenhydramine 30 minutes prior to the amphotericin infusion; meperidine (Demerol®) may help to reduce rigors; avoid rapid injection (usually 4- to 6-hour infusion required)

Dosage Forms

Cream: 3% (20 g)

Lotion: 3% (30 mL)
Ointment, topical: 3% (20 g)
Powder for injection, lyophilized: 50 mg

Ampicillin (am pi sill' in)

Related Information

Antimicrobial Drugs of Choice *on page 1298-1302*
Prevention of Bacterial Endocarditis *on page 1285-1288*

Brand Names Amcill®; Amplin®; Omnipen®; Penamp®; Polycillin®; Principen®; Totacillin®

Synonyms Aminobenzylpenicillin

Use Treatment of susceptible bacterial infections (nonbeta-lactamase-producing organisms); susceptible bacterial infections caused by streptococci, pneumococci, nonpenicillinase-producing staphylococci, *Listeria*, meningococci; some strains of *H. influenzae*, *Salmonella*, *Shigella*, *E. coli*, *Enterobacter*, and *Klebsiella*

Pregnancy Risk Factor B

Contraindications Known hypersensitivity to ampicillin or other penicillins

Warnings/Precautions Dosage adjustment may be necessary in patients with renal impairment; a low incidence of cross-allergy with other beta-lactams exists; high percentage of patients with infectious mononucleosis have developed rash during therapy with ampicillin. Appearance of a rash should be carefully evaluated to differentiate a nonallergic ampicillin rash from a hypersensitivity reaction. Ampicillin rash occurs in 5% to 10% of children receiving ampicillin and is a generalized dull red, maculopapular rash, generally appearing 3-14 days after the start of therapy. It normally begins on the trunk and spreads over most of the body. It may be most intense at pressure areas, elbows, and knees.

Adverse Reactions

>10%:
　Dermatologic: Rash (appearance of a rash should be carefully evaluated to differentiate a nonallergic ampicillin rash from a hypersensitivity reaction; incidence is higher in patients with viral infections, *Salmonella* infections, lymphocytic leukemia, or patients that have hyperuricemia)
　Gastrointestinal: Diarrhea, vomiting
　Miscellaneous: Oral candidiasis
1% to 10%: Gastrointestinal: Severe abdominal or stomach cramps and pain
<1%:
　Central nervous system: Penicillin encephalopathy, seizures
　Hematologic: Lymphocytic leukemia

Overdosage/Toxicology Symptoms of penicillin overdose include neuromuscular hypersensitivity (agitation, hallucinations, asterixis, encephalopathy, confusion, and seizures) and electrolyte imbalance with potassium or sodium salts, especially in renal failure; hemodialysis may be helpful to aid in the removal of the drug from the blood, otherwise most treatment is supportive or symptom directed

Drug Interactions

Decreased effect: Efficacy of oral contraceptives may be reduced
Increased effect: Disulfiram, probenecid → ↑ penicillin levels, increased effect of anticoagulants
Increased toxicity: Allopurinol theoretically has an additive potential for amoxicillin (ampicillin) rash

Stability Oral suspension is stable for 7 days at room temperature or for 14 days under refrigeration; solutions for I.M. or direct I.V. should be used within 1 hour; solutions for I.V. infusion will be inactivated by dextrose at room temperature; if dextrose-containing solutions are to be used, the resultant solution will only be stable for 2 hours versus 8 hours in the 0.9% sodium chloride injection. D_5W has limited stability.

Minimum volume: Concentration should not exceed 30 mg/mL due to concentration-dependent stability restrictions. Manufacturer may supply as either the anhydrous or the trihydrate form.
Stability of parenteral admixture in NS at room temperature (25°C): 8 hours
Stability of parenteral admixture in NS at refrigeration temperature (4°C): 2 days
Standard diluent: 500 mg/50 mL NS; 1 g/50 mL NS; 2 g/100 mL NS

Mechanism of Action Interferes with bacterial cell wall synthesis during active multiplication, causing cell wall death and resultant bactericidal activity against susceptible bacteria

Pharmacodynamics/Kinetics

Absorption: Oral: 50%
Distribution: Distributes into bile; penetration into CSF occurs with inflamed meninges only, good only with inflammation (exceeds usual MICs)
　Normal meninges: Nil
(Continued)

Ampicillin *(Continued)*

Inflamed meninges: 5-10
Protein binding: 15% to 25%
Half-life:
Neonates:
2-7 days: 4 hours
8-14 days: 2.8 hours
15-30 days: 1.7 hours
Children and Adults: 1-1.8 hours
Anuria/end stage renal disease: 7-20 hours
Time to peak: Oral: Within 1-2 hours
Elimination: ~90% of the drug excreted unchanged in the urine within 24 hours

Usual Dosage I.M., I.V.:
Neonates:
Postnatal age ≤7 days:
≤2000 g: Meningitis: 50 mg/kg/dose every 12 hours; other infections: 25 mg/kg/dose every 12 hours
>2000 g: Meningitis: 50 mg/kg/dose every 8 hours; other infections: 25 mg/kg/dose every 8 hours
Postnatal age >7 days:
<1200 g: Meningitis: 50 mg/kg/dose every 12 hours; other infections: 25 mg/kg/dose every 12 hours
1200-2000 g: Meningitis: 50 mg/kg/dose every 8 hours; other infections: 25 mg/kg/dose every 8 hours
>2000 g: Meningitis: 50 mg/kg/dose every 6 hours; other infections: 25 mg/kg/dose every 6 hours
Infants and Children: I.M., I.V.: 100-400 mg/kg/day in doses divided every 4-6 hours
Meningitis: 200 mg/kg/day in doses divided every 4-6 hours; maximum dose: 12 g/day
Children: Oral: 50-100 mg/kg/day in doses divided every 6 hours; maximum dose: 2-3 g/day
Adults:
Oral: 250-500 mg every 6 hours
I.M.: 500 mg to 1.5 g every 4-6 hours
I.V.: 500 mg to 3 g every 4-6 hours; maximum dose: 12 g/day
Sepsis/meningitis: 150-250 mg/kg/24 hours divided every 3-4 hours

Dosing interval in renal impairment:
Cl_{cr} 30-50 mL/minute: Administer every 6-8 hours
Cl_{cr} 10-30 mL/minute: Administer every 8-12 hours
Cl_{cr} <10 mL/minutes: Administer every 12 hours
Moderately dialyzable (20% to 50%)
Administer dose after dialysis
Peritoneal dialysis effects: Moderately dialyzable (20% to 50%)
Administer 250 mg every 12 hours
Continuous arterio-venous or veno-venous hemofiltration (CAVH) effects: ~50 mg of ampicillin/L of filtrate is removed

Administration Administer around-the-clock rather than 4 times/day to promote less variation in peak and trough serum levels

Test Interactions ↑ protein; urinary glucose (Benedict's solution, Clinitest®); ↑ positive Coombs' [direct]

Patient Information Refrigerate at 2°C to 8°C (36°F to 46°F); do not freeze

Nursing Implications Ampicillin and gentamicin should not be mixed in the same I.V. tubing or administered concurrently; give orally on an empty stomach (ie, 1 hour prior to, or 2 hours after meals) to increase total absorption.

Additional Information
Sodium content of 5 mL suspension (250 mg/5 mL): 10 mg (0.4 mEq)
Sodium content of 1 g: 66.7 mg (3 mEq)

Dosage Forms
Capsule, as anhydrous: 250 mg, 500 mg
Capsule, as trihydrate: 250 mg, 500 mg
Drops, pediatric, as trihydrate: 100 mg/mL (20 mL)
Injection, as sodium: 125 mg, 250 mg, 500 mg, 1 g, 2 g, 10 g
Suspension, oral, as trihydrate: 100 mg/mL (20 mL); 125 mg/5 mL (5 mL unit dose, 100 mL, 150 mL, 200 mL); 250 mg/5 mL (5 mL unit dose, 80 mL, 100 mL, 150 mL, 200 mL); 500 mg/5 mL (5 mL unit dose, 100 mL)

Ampicillin Sodium and Sulbactam Sodium (am pi sil' in so' dee um & sul' bak tam so' dee um)

Related Information
Antimicrobial Drugs of Choice *on page 1298-1302*

Brand Names Unasyn®

Synonyms Sulbactam and Ampicillin

Use Treatment of susceptible bacterial infections involved with skin and skin structure, intra-abdominal infections, gynecological infections; spectrum is that of ampicillin plus organisms producing beta-lactamases such as *S. aureus, H. influenzae, E. coli, Klebsiella, Acinetobacter, Enterobacter,* and anaerobes

Pregnancy Risk Factor B

Contraindications Hypersensitivity to ampicillin, sulbactam or any component, or penicillins

Warnings/Precautions Dosage adjustment may be necessary in patients with renal impairment; a low incidence of cross-allergy with other beta-lactams exists; high percentage of patients with infectious mononucleosis have developed rash during therapy with ampicillin. Appearance of a rash should be carefully evaluated to differentiate a nonallergic ampicillin rash from a hypersensitivity reaction. Ampicillin rash occurs in 5% to 10% of children receiving ampicillin and is a generalized dull red, maculopapular rash, generally appearing 3-14 days after the start of therapy. It normally begins on the trunk and spreads over most of the body. It may be most intense at pressure areas, elbows, and knees.

Adverse Reactions

>10%: Local: Pain at injection site (I.M.)

1% to 10%:

Dermatologic: Rash

Gastrointestinal: Diarrhea

Local: Pain at injection site (I.V.)

<1%:

Cardiovascular: Chest pain

Central nervous system: Fatigue, malaise, headache, chills

Dermatologic: Itching

Gastrointestinal: Nausea, vomiting, enterocolitis, pseudomembranous colitis

Hematologic: Decreased WBC, neutrophils, platelets, hemoglobin, and hematocrit

Hepatic: Increased liver enzymes

Local: Thrombophlebitis

Renal: Increased BUN and creatinine, dysuria

Miscellaneous: Hypersensitivity reactions, candidiasis, hairy tongue

Overdosage/Toxicology Symptoms of penicillin overdose include neuromuscular hypersensitivity (agitation, hallucinations, asterixis, encephalopathy, confusion, and seizures) and electrolyte imbalance with potassium or sodium salts, especially in renal failure; hemodialysis may be helpful to aid in the removal of the drug from the blood, otherwise most treatment is supportive or symptom directed

Drug Interactions

Decreased effect: Efficacy of oral contraceptives may be reduced

Increased effect: Disulfiram, probenecid results in increased amoxicillin levels

Increased toxicity: Allopurinol theoretically has had an additive potential for amoxicillin/ampicillin rash

Stability I.M. and direct I.V. administration: Use within 1 hour after preparation; reconstitute with sterile water for injection or 0.5% or 2% lidocaine hydrochloride injection (I.M.); sodium chloride 0.9% (NS) is the diluent of choice for I.V. piggyback use, solutions made in NS are stable up to 72 hours when refrigerated whereas dextrose solutions (same concentration) are stable for only 4 hours

Mechanism of Action Interferes with bacterial cell wall synthesis during active multiplication, causing cell wall death and resultant bactericidal activity against susceptible bacteria; addition of sulbactam, a beta-lactamase inhibitor, to ampicillin extends the spectrum of ampicillin to include beta-lactamase producing organisms

Pharmacodynamics/Kinetics

Distribution: Into bile, blister and tissue fluids; poor penetration into CSF with uninflamed meninges; higher concentrations attained with inflamed meninges

Protein binding:

Ampicillin: 28%

Sulbactam: 38%

Half-life: Ampicillin and sulbactam are similar: 1-1.8 hours and 1-1.3 hours, respectively in patients with normal renal function

Elimination: ~75% to 85% of both drugs are excreted unchanged in the urine within 8 hours following administration

Usual Dosage Unasyn® (ampicillin/sulbactam) is a combination product. Each 3 g vial contains 2 g of ampicillin and 1 g of sulbactam. Sulbactam has very little antibacterial activity by itself, but effectively extends the spectrum of ampicillin to include beta-lactamase producing strains that are resistant to ampicillin alone. Therefore, dosage recommendations for Unasyn® are based on the ampicillin component.

(Continued)

75

Ampicillin Sodium and Sulbactam Sodium *(Continued)*

I.M., I.V.:
Children: 100-200 mg ampicillin/kg/day divided every 6 hours; maximum dose: 8 g ampicillin/day
Adults: 1-2 g ampicillin every 6-8 hours; maximum dose: 8 g ampicillin/day

Dosing interval in renal impairment:
Cl_{cr} 15-29 mL/minute: Administer every 12 hours
Cl_{cr} 5-14 mL/minute: Administer every 24 hours

Administration Administer around-the-clock rather than 4 times/day to promote less variation in peak and trough serum levels

Monitoring Parameters With prolonged therapy, monitor hematologic, renal, and hepatic function

Test Interactions False-positive urinary glucose levels (Benedict's solution, Clinitest®)

Nursing Implications Ampicillin and gentamicin should not be mixed in the same I.V. tubing or administered concurrently

Dosage Forms Powder for injection: 1.5 g [ampicillin sodium 1 g and sulbactam sodium 0.5 g]; 3 g [ampicillin sodium 2 g and sulbactam sodium 1 g]

Amplin® *see* Ampicillin *on page 73*

AMPT *see* Metyrosine *on page 735*

Amrinone Lactate *(am' ri none)*

Related Information
Adrenergic Agonists, Cardiovascular Comparison *on page 1242*

Brand Names Inocor®

Use Treatment of low cardiac output states (sepsis, congestive heart failure); adjunctive therapy of pulmonary hypertension; normally prescribed for patients who have not responded well to therapy with digitalis, diuretics, and vasodilators

Pregnancy Risk Factor C

Contraindications Hypersensitivity to amrinone lactate or sulfites (contains sodium metabisulfite)

Warnings/Precautions Diuresis may result from improvement in cardiac output and may require dosage reduction of diuretics

Adverse Reactions
1% to 10%:
Gastrointestinal: Nausea
Cardiovascular: Arrhythmias, hypotension (may be infusion rate-related), ventricular and supraventricular arrhythmias
Hematologic: Thrombocytopenia (may be dose-related)
<1%:
Cardiovascular: Chest pain
Central nervous system: Fever
Gastrointestinal: Vomiting, abdominal pain, anorexia
Hepatic: Hepatotoxicity
Local: Pain or burning at injection site

Overdosage/Toxicology Symptoms of overdose includes hypotension (sometimes severe); there is no specific antidote for amrinone intoxication; treatment is supportive

Drug Interactions When furosemide is admixed with amrinone, a precipitate immediately forms; diuretics may cause significant hypovolemia and decrease filling pressure

Stability May be administered undiluted for I.V. bolus doses. For continuous infusion: Dilute with 0.45% or 0.9% sodium chloride to final concentration of 1-3 mg/mL; use within 24 hours; do not directly dilute with dextrose-containing solutions, chemical interaction occurs; may be administered I.V. into running dextrose infusions. Furosemide forms a precipitate when injected in I.V. lines containing amrinone.

Mechanism of Action Inhibits myocardial cyclic adenosine monophosphate (cAMP) phosphodiesterase activity and increases cellular levels of cAMP resulting in a positive inotropic effect and increased cardiac output; also possesses systemic and pulmonary vasodilator effects resulting in pre- and afterload reduction; slightly increases atrioventricular conduction

Pharmacodynamics/Kinetics
Onset of action: I.V.: Within 2-5 minutes
Peak effect: Within 10 minutes
Duration: Dose dependent (~30 minutes low dose, ~2 hours higher doses)
Distribution: V_d: 1.2 L/kg
Protein binding: 10% to 49%
Metabolism: Hepatic

Half-life:
Neonates 1-2 weeks: 22.2 hours
Infants 6-38 weeks: 6.8 hours; negative correlation of age with half-life in infants 4-38 weeks of age
Adults, normal volunteers: 3.6 hours
Adults with CHF: 5.8 hours
Elimination: 60% to 90% excreted as metabolites in urine within 24 hours

Usual Dosage Dosage is based on clinical response
Note: Dose should not exceed 10 mg/kg/24 hours

Neonates: 0.75 mg/kg I.V. bolus over 2-3 minutes followed by maintenance infusion 3-5 mcg/kg/minute; I.V. bolus may need to be repeated in 30 minutes

Children and Adults: 0.75 mg/kg I.V. bolus over 2-3 minutes followed by maintenance infusion 5-10 mcg/kg/minute; I.V. bolus may need to be repeated in 30 minutes

Dosing adjustment in renal failure: Cl_{cr} <10 mL/minute: Administer 50% to 75% of dose
Administration Should be administered solely via an I.V. pump
Monitoring Parameters Patients should be carefully monitored for hemodynamic response (hypotension) and potential adverse effects (ie, thrombocytopenia, hepatotoxicity, and GI effects); monitor cardiac index, stroke volume, systemic vascular resistance, and pulmonary vascular resistance (if Swan-Ganz catheter available); CVP, blood pressure and heart rate (every 5 minutes during infusion), fluids and electrolytes (especially potassium), fluid status, platelet count, CBC, liver function and renal function tests
Patient Information Make position changes slowly because of postural hypotension
Dosage Forms Injection: 5 mg/mL (20 mL)

Amvisc® *see* Sodium Hyaluronate *on page 1014*

Amyl Nitrite (am' il)

Synonyms Isoamyl Nitrite
Use Coronary vasodilator in angina pectoris; adjunct in treatment of cyanide poisoning; used to produce changes in the intensity of heart murmurs
Pregnancy Risk Factor C
Contraindications Severe anemia; hypersensitivity to nitrates
Warnings/Precautions Use with caution in patients with increased intracranial pressure, low systolic blood pressure, and coronary artery disease
Adverse Reactions
1% to 10%:
Cardiovascular: Postural hypotension, cutaneous flushing of head, neck, and clavicular area
Central nervous system: Headache
<1%:
Dermatologic: Skin rash
Hematologic: Hemolytic anemia
Overdosage/Toxicology Symptoms of overdose include hypotension; treatment includes general supportive measures for transient hypotension; I.V. fluids; Trendelenburg position, vasopressors
Drug Interactions Increased toxicity: Alcohol
Stability Store in cool place; protect from light
Pharmacodynamics/Kinetics
Onset of action: Angina relieved within 30 seconds
Duration: 3-15 minutes
Usual Dosage Adults: 1-6 inhalations from one capsule are usually sufficient to produce the desired effect
Administration Administer nasally; patient should not be sitting; crush ampul in woven covering between fingers and then hold under patients nostrils
Monitoring Parameters Monitor blood pressure during therapy
Patient Information Lie down during administration, crush ampul between fingers and then inhale through nostrils; may cause dizziness; call paramedics or have someone take you to the hospital immediately if pain is not relieved after 3 doses
Dosage Forms Inhalant, crushable glass perles: 0.3 mL

Amylobarbitone *see* Amobarbital *on page 64*
Amytal® *see* Amobarbital *on page 64*
Anacin-3® [OTC] *see* Acetaminophen *on page 17*

Anacin® [OTC] *see* Aspirin *on page 92*

Anadrol® *see* Oxymetholone *on page 830*

Anafranil® *see* Clomipramine Hydrochloride *on page 260*

Anaprox® *see* Naproxen *on page 776*

Anaspaz® *see* Hyoscyamine Sulfate *on page 559*

Anbesol® [OTC] *see* Benzocaine *on page 121*

Anbesol® Maximum Strength [OTC] *see* Benzocaine *on page 121*

Ancef® *see* Cefazolin Sodium *on page 194*

Ancobon® *see* Flucytosine *on page 462*

Andro® *see* Testosterone *on page 1063*

Andro-Cyp® *see* Testosterone *on page 1063*

Android® *see* Methyltestosterone *on page 726*

Andro-L.A.® *see* Testosterone *on page 1063*

Androlone® *see* Nandrolone *on page 774*

Androlone®-D *see* Nandrolone *on page 774*

Andronate® *see* Testosterone *on page 1063*

Andropository® *see* Testosterone *on page 1063*

Andryl® *see* Testosterone *on page 1063*

Anectine® Chloride *see* Succinylcholine Chloride *on page 1035*

Anectine® Flo-Pack® *see* Succinylcholine Chloride *on page 1035*

Anergan® *see* Promethazine Hydrochloride *on page 939*

Anestacon® *see* Lidocaine Hydrochloride *on page 633*

Aneurine Hydrochloride *see* Thiamine Hydrochloride *on page 1079*

Anexsia® *see* Hydrocodone and Acetaminophen *on page 543*

Angiotensin-Converting Enzyme Inhibitors, Comparative Pharmacokinetics *see page 1244*

Angiotensin-Converting Enzyme Inhibitors, Comparisons of Indications and Adult Dosages *see page 1243*

Anisotropine Methylbromide (an iss oh troe' peen)

Brand Names Valpin® 50

Use Adjunctive treatment of peptic ulcer

Pregnancy Risk Factor C

Contraindications Narrow-angle glaucoma, obstructive GI tract or uropathy, severe ulcerative colitis, myasthenia gravis, intestinal atony, hepatic disease, hypersensitivity

Warnings/Precautions Drug-induced heatstroke can develop in hot or humid climates

Adverse Reactions

>10%:

Cardiovascular: Palpitations

Gastrointestinal: Constipation

Miscellaneous: Decreased sweating, dry mouth, nose, throat, or skin

1% to 10%: Decreased flow of breast milk, decreased salivary secretion

<1%:

Cardiovascular: Orthostatic hypotension,

Central nervous system: Confusion, drowsiness, headache, loss of memory, weakness, tiredness

Dermatologic: Skin rash

Gastrointestinal: Bloated feeling, nausea, vomiting

Genitourinary: Decreased urination

Ocular: Increased intraocular pain, blurred vision, increased sensitivity to light

Overdosage/Toxicology Symptoms of overdose include blurred vision, dysphagia, urinary retention, tachycardia, hypertension. Anisotropine toxicity is caused by strong binding of the drug to cholinergic receptors. Anticholinesterase inhibitors reduce acetylcholinesterase, the enzyme that breaks down acetylcholine and thereby allows acetylcholine to accumulate and compete for receptor binding with this offending anticholinergic. For an overdose with severe life-threatening symptoms, physostigmine 1-2 mg (0.5 or 0.02 mg/kg for children) S.C. or I.V., slowly may be given to reverse these effects.

Mechanism of Action Blocks the action of acetylcholine at parasympathetic sites in smooth muscle, secretory glands, and the CNS; increases cardiac output, dries secretions, antagonizes histamine and serotonin

Pharmacodynamics/Kinetics
Absorption: Poor (~10%) from GI tract
Elimination: Principally in urine as unchanged drug and metabolites

Usual Dosage Adults: Oral: 50 mg 3 times/day

Administration Administer 30-60 minutes before meals

Monitoring Parameters Monitor patient's vital signs and I & O

Patient Information Dry mouth can be relieved by sugarless gum or hard candy; drink plenty of fluids

Dosage Forms Tablet: 50 mg

Anisoylated Plasminogen Streptokinase Activator Complex *see* Anistreplase *on this page*

Anistreplase (a niss' tre place)

Brand Names Eminase®

Synonyms Anisoylated Plasminogen Streptokinase Activator Complex; APSAC

Use Management of acute myocardial infarction (AMI) in adults; lysis of thrombi obstructing coronary arteries, reduction of infarct size; and reduction of mortality associated with AMI

Pregnancy Risk Factor C

Contraindications Active internal bleeding, history of CVA, intracranial neoplasma, known hypersensitivity to anistreplase or other kinases (streptokinase); history of cerebrovascular accident; recent intracranial surgery or trauma; arteriovenous malformation or aneurysm; severe uncontrolled hypertension

Adverse Reactions
>10%:
Cardiovascular: Arrhythmias, hypotension, perfusion arrhythmias
Hematologic: Bleeding or oozing from cuts
1% to 10%: Anaphylactic reaction
<1%:
Central nervous system: Headache, chills
Dermatologic: Rash
Gastrointestinal: Nausea, vomiting
Hematologic: Anemia, eye hemorrhage
Respiratory: Bronchospasm
Miscellaneous: Epistaxis, sweating

Drug Interactions Increased efficacy and bleeding potential: Anticoagulants (heparin, warfarin), antiplatelet agents (aspirin)

Stability Discard solution 30 minutes after reconstitution if not administered; do not shake solution

Mechanism of Action Activates the conversion of plasminogen to plasmin by forming a complex exposing plasminogen-activating site and cleavage of a peptide bond that converts plasminogen to plasmin; plasmin being capable of thrombolysis, by degrading fibrin, fibrinogen and other procoagulant proteins into soluble fragments, effective both outside and within the formed thrombus/embolus

Pharmacodynamics/Kinetics
Duration of action: Fibrinolytic effect persists for 4-6 hours following administration
Metabolism: Anistreplase is an acylated complex of streptokinase with lys-plasminogen; one of the purposes of this acylation is to extend the serum circulating time of anistreplase; because deacylation of the complex occurs more rapidly than dissociation, fibrinolytic activity is controlled by the rate of deacylation rather than of dissociation
Half-life: 70-120 minutes

Usual Dosage Adults: I.V.: 30 units injected over 2-5 minutes as soon as possible after onset of symptoms

Administration Can be given as a bolus; avoid I.M. injections and nonessential handling of patient after administration of drug

Nursing Implications Drug should not be used for any condition in which bleeding constitutes a significant hazard or would be particularly difficult to manage

Dosage Forms Powder for injection, lyophilized: 30 units

Anodynos-DHC® *see* Hydrocodone and Acetaminophen *on page 543*

Anoquan® *see* Butalbital Compound *on page 153*

Ansaid® *see* Flurbiprofen Sodium *on page 482*

Ansamycin *see* Rifabutin *on page 981*

Antabuse® *see* Disulfiram *on page 360*

Anthra-Derm® *see* Anthralin *on this page*

Anthralin (an' thra lin)

Brand Names Anthra-Derm®; Drithocreme®; Drithocreme® HP 1%; Dritho-Scalp®; Lasan™; Lasan HP-1™

Use Treatment of psoriasis (quiescent or chronic psoriasis)

Pregnancy Risk Factor C

Contraindications Hypersensitivity to anthralin or any component, acute psoriasis (acutely or actively inflamed psoriatic eruptions); use on the face

Warnings/Precautions If redness is observed, reduce frequency of dosage or discontinue application; avoid eye contact; should generally not be applied to intertriginous skin areas and high strengths should not be used on these sites; do not apply to face or genitalia; use caution in patients with renal disease and in those having extensive and prolonged applications; perform periodic urine tests for albuminuria.

Adverse Reactions

1% to 10%: Topical: Transient primary irritation of uninvolved skin; temporary discoloration of hair and fingernails, may stain skin, hair, or fabrics

<1%: Topical: Skin rash, excessive irritation

Drug Interactions Increased toxicity: Long-term use of topical corticosteroids may destabilize psoriasis, and withdrawal may also give rise to a "rebound" phenomenon, allow an interval of at least 1 week between the discontinuance of topical corticosteroids and the commencement of therapy

Mechanism of Action Reduction of the mitotic rate and proliferation of epidermal cells in psoriasis by inhibiting synthesis of nucleic protein from inhibition of DNA synthesis to affected areas

Usual Dosage Adults: Topical: Generally, apply once a day or as directed. The irritant potential of anthralin is directly related to the strength being used and each patient's individual tolerance. Always commence treatment for at least one week using the lowest strength possible.

Skin application: Apply sparingly only to psoriatic lesions and rub gently and carefully into the skin until absorbed. Avoid applying an excessive quantity which may cause unnecessary soiling and staining of the clothing or bed linen.

Scalp application: Comb hair to remove scalar debris and, after suitably parting, rub cream well into the lesions, taking care to prevent the cream from spreading onto the forehead

Remove by washing or showering; optimal period of contact will vary according to the strength used and the patient's response to treatment. Continue treatment until the skin is entirely clear (ie, when there is nothing to feel with the fingers and the texture is normal)

Patient Information For external use only; may discolor skin, hair, or fabrics; avoid sunlight to treated areas

Nursing Implications Wear gloves; can discolor skin, hair, or clothes

Dosage Forms

Cream: 0.1% (50 g, 65 g); 0.2% (65 g); 0.25% (50 g); 0.4% (65 g); 0.5% (50 g); 1% (50 g, 65 g)

Ointment, topical: 0.1% (42.5 g); 0.25% (42.5 g); 0.4% (60 g); 0.5% (42.5 g); 1% (42.5 g)

Antiarrhythmic Drugs *see page 1246*

AntibiOtic® *see* Neomycin, Polymyxin B, and Hydrocortisone *on page 781*

Antidepressant Agents Comparison *see page 1250*

Antidigoxin Fab Fragments *see* Digoxin Immune Fab *on page 342*

Antidiuretic Hormone *see* Vasopressin *on page 1149*

Antiemetics for Chemotherapy Induced Nausea and Vomiting *see page 1202*

Antifungal Agents *see page 1253*

Antihemophilic Factor (Human) (an tee hee moe fill' ik)

Brand Names Hemofil® M; Humate-P®; Koāte®-HP; Koāte®-HS; Monoclate-P®; Profilate® OSD; Profilate® SD

Synonyms AHF; Factor VIII

Use

Management of hemophilia A in patients whom a deficiency in factor VIII has been demonstrated

Can be of significant therapeutic value in patients with acquired factor VII inhibitors not exceeding 10 Bethesda units/mL

Unlabeled use: Can be of value in von Willebrand's disease

Pregnancy Risk Factor C

Contraindications Hypersensitivity to mouse protein (Monoclate-P®; Hemofil® M, Method M, Monoclonal Purified) and Antihemophilic Factor (Human); Method M, Monoclonal Purified contain trace amounts of mouse protein

Warnings/Precautions Risk of viral transmission is not totally eradicated. Risk of hepatitis: Because antihemophilic factor is prepared for pooled plasma, it may contain the causative agent of viral hepatitis. Antihemophilic factor contains trace amounts of blood groups A and B isohemagglutinins; when large or frequently repeated doses are given to individuals with blood groups A, B, and AB, the patient should be monitored for signs of progressive anemia and the possibility of intravascular hemolysis should be considered.

Adverse Reactions

<1%:

Cardiovascular: Flushing, tachycardia

Central nervous system: Headache

Gastrointestinal: Nausea, vomiting

Neuromuscular & skeletal: Paresthesia

Sensitivity reactions: Allergic vasomotor reactions, tightness in neck or chest

Overdosage/Toxicology Intravascular hemolysis

Stability Dried concentrate should be refrigerated (2°C to 8°C/36°F to 46°F) but may be stored at room temperature for up to 6 months depending upon specific product; if refrigerated, the dried concentrate and diluent should be warmed to room temperature before reconstitution; gently agitate or rotate vial after adding diluent, do not shake vigorously; do **not** refrigerate after reconstitution, a precipitation may occur; Method M, monoclonal purified products should be administered within 1 hour after reconstitution

Stability of parenteral admixture at room temperature (25°C): 24 hours, but it is recommended to administer within 3 hours after reconstitution

Mechanism of Action Protein (factor VIII) in normal plasma which is necessary for clot formation and maintenance of hemostasis; activates factor X in conjunction with activated factor IX; activated factor X converts prothrombin to thrombin, which converts fibrinogen to fibrin and with factor XIII forms a stable clot

Pharmacodynamics/Kinetics

Distribution: Does not readily cross the placenta

Half-life, biphasic: 4-24 hours with a mean of 12 hours (biphasic: 12 hours is usually used for dosing interval estimates)

Usual Dosage I.V.: Individualize dosage based on coagulation studies performed prior to and during treatment at regular intervals. One AHF unit is the activity present in 1 mL of normal pooled human plasma; dosage should be adjusted to actual vial size currently stocked in the pharmacy.

Hospitalized patients: 20-50 units/kg/dose; may be higher for special circumstances. Dose can be given every 12-24 hours and more frequently in special circumstances.

Formula to approximate percentage increase in plasma antihemophilic factor:

Units required = desired level increase (desired level - actual level) x plasma volume (mL)

Total blood volume (mL blood/kg) = 70 mL/kg (adults); 80 mL/kg (children)

Plasma volume = total blood volume (mL) x [1 - Hct (in decimals)]

Example: For a 70 kg adult with a Hct = 40% : plasma volume = [70 kg x 70 mL/kg] x [1 - 0.4] = 2940 mL

To calculate number of units of factor VIII needed to increase level to desired range (highly individualized and dependent on patient's condition):

Number of units = desired level increase [desired level - actual level] x plasma volume (in mL)

Example: For a 100% level in the above patient who has an actual level of 20% the number of units needed = [1 (for a 100% level) - 0.2] x 2940 mL = 2352 units

Administration I.V. administration only; maximum rate of administration is product dependent: Monoclate-P® 2 mL/minute; Humate-P® 4 mL/minute; administration of other products should not exceed 10 mL/minute; use filter needle to draw product into syringe

(Continued)

Antihemophilic Factor (Human) *(Continued)*

Monitoring Parameters Heart rate (before and during I.V. administration); antihemophilic factor levels prior to and during treatment; in patients with circulating inhibitors, the inhibitor level should be monitored

Reference Range

Average normal antihemophilic factor plasma activity ranges 50% to 150%

Level to prevent spontaneous hemorrhage: 5%

Required peak postinfusion AHF activity in blood (as % of normal or IU/dL plasma):

Early hemarthrosis or muscle bleed or oral bleed: 20% to 40%

More extensive hemarthrosis, muscle bleed, or hematoma: 30% to 60%

Life-threatening bleeds, such as head injury, throat bleed, severe abdominal pain

Minor surgery, including tooth extraction: 60% to 80%

Major surgery: 80% to 100% (pre- and postoperative)

Nursing Implications Reduce rate of administration or temporarily discontinue if patient becomes tachycardiac

Dosage Forms Injection: 10 mL, 20 mL, 30 mL

Antihemophilic Factor (Porcine) (an tee hee moe fil' ik fak' ter)

Brand Names Hyate®:C

Use Treatment of congenital hemophiliacs with antibodies to human factor VIII:C and also for previously nonhemophiliac patients with spontaneously acquired inhibitors to human factor VIII:C; patients with inhibitors who are bleeding or who are to undergo surgery

Pregnancy Risk Factor C

Contraindications Should not be used to treat patients who have previously suffered acute allergic reaction to antihemophilic factor (porcine)

Warnings/Precautions Rarely administration has been associated with anaphylaxis; adrenaline, hydrocortisone, and facilities for cardiopulmonary resuscitation should be available in case such a reaction occurs; infusion may be followed by a rise in plasma levels of antibody to both human and porcine factor VIII:C; inhibitor levels should be monitored both during and after treatment

Adverse Reactions Reactions tend to lessen in frequency and severity as further infusions are given; hydrocortisone and/or antihistamines may help to prevent or alleviate side effects and may be prescribed as precautionary measures

1% to 10%:

Central nervous system: Fever, headache, chills

Dermatologic: Skin rashes

Gastrointestinal: Nausea, vomiting

Stability Store at temperature of -15°C to <20°C; use before expiration date; reconstituted Hyate®:C must not be stored, stable for 24 hours at room temperature

Mechanism of Action Factor VIII:C is the coagulation portion of the factor VIII complex in plasma. Factor VIII:C acts as a cofactor for factor IX to activate factor X in the intrinsic pathway of blood coagulation.

Usual Dosage Clinical response should be used to assess efficacy rather than relying upon a particular laboratory value for recovery of factor VIII:C.

Initial dose:

Antibody level to human factor VIII:C <50 Bethesda units/mL: 100-150 porcine units/kg (body weight) is recommended

Antibody level to human factor VIII:C >50 Bethesda units/mL: Activity of the antibody to porcine factor VIII:C should be determined; **an antiporcine antibody level** >20 Bethesda units/mL indicates that the patient is unlikely to benefit from treatment; for lower titers, a dose of 100-150 porcine units/kg is recommended

If a patient has previously been treated with Hyate®:C, this may provide a guide to his likely response and, therefore, assist in estimation of the preliminary dose

Subsequent doses: Following administration of the initial dose, if the recovery of factor VIII:C in the patient's plasma is not sufficient, a further higher dose should be administered; if recovery after the second dose is still insufficient, a third and higher dose may prove effective

Administration Administer by I.V. route only; infusion rate should be <10 mL/minute

Reference Range Treatment is not normally indicated in patients with an antibody titer <5 Bethesda units/mL (BU/mL) against human factor VIII:C and is likely to be ineffective in patients with an antibody titer >50 Bethesda units/mL against human factor VIII:C

If a patient has an antibody titer >50 Bethesda units/mL against human factor VIII:C, the activity of the antibody against porcine factor VIII should be determined

An antibody titer <15-20 Bethesda units/mL against porcine factor VIII:C indicates suitability for treatment with antihemophilic factor (Porcine)-Hyate®:C

Factor VIII levels: 50% to 150%, draw 6-8 hours after dose administration

Additional Information Sodium ion concentration is not more than 200 mmol/L; the assayed amount of activity is stated on the label, but may vary depending on the type of assay and hemophilic substrate plasma used

Dosage Forms Powder for injection, lyophilized: 400-700 porcine units to be reconstituted with 20 mL sterile water

Anti-Inhibitor Coagulant Complex (antee-in hi' bi tor coe ag' yu lant com' plecks)

Brand Names Autoplex T®; Feiba VH Immuno®

Use Patients with factor VIII inhibitors who are to undergo surgery or those who are bleeding

Pregnancy Risk Factor C

Contraindications Disseminated intravascular coagulation; patients with normal coagulation mechanism

Warnings/Precautions Products are prepared from pooled human plasma; such plasma may contain the causative agents of viral diseases. Tests used to control efficacy such as APTT, WBCT, and TEG do not correlate with clinical efficacy. Dosing to normalize these values may result in DIC. Identification of the clotting deficiency as caused by factor VIII inhibitors is essential prior to starting therapy. Use with extreme caution in patients with impaired hepatic function.

Adverse Reactions
<1%:
Cardiovascular: Hypotension, flushing, disseminated intravascular coagulation
Central nervous system: Fever, headache, chills
Dermatologic: Rash, urticaria
Miscellaneous: Anaphylaxis, indications of protein sensitivity

Overdosage/Toxicology Rapid infusion may cause hypotension, excessive administration can cause DIC

Stability Store at 2°C to 8°C (36°F to 46°F); use within 1-3 hours after reconstitution

Usual Dosage Dosage range: 25-100 factor VIII correctional units per kg depending on the severity of hemorrhage

Test Interactions ↑ ↓ PT, ↑ ↓ PTT, ↓ WBCT, ↓ fibrin, ↓ platelets, ↑ fibrin split products

Nursing Implications Monitor for hypotension, may reinitiate infusion at a slower rate; have epinephrine ready to treat hypersensitivity reactions

Dosage Forms Injection:
Autoplex T®, with heparin 2 units: Each bottle is labeled with correctional units of Factor VIII
Feiba VH Immuno®, heparin free: Each bottle is labeled with correctional units of Factor VIII

Antilirium® see Physostigmine on page 881

Antimicrobial Drugs of Choice see page 1298

Antiminth® [OTC] see Pyrantel Pamoate on page 957

Antipsychotic Agents Comparison see page 1255

Antispas® see Dicyclomine Hydrochloride on page 330

Antithrombin III (antee throm' bin)

Brand Names ATnativ®; Thrombate III™

Use Agent for hereditary antithrombin III deficiency
Unlabeled use: Has been used effectively for acquired antithrombin III deficiencies related to DIC, pre-eclampsia, liver disease, shock and surgery complicated by DIC

Pregnancy Risk Factor C

Contraindications Hypersensitivity to any component

Warnings/Precautions Test methods and treatment methods may not totally eradicate HBAg and HIV from pooled plasma used in processing of this product

Adverse Reactions
<1%:
Central nervous system: Dizziness, lightheadedness, fever
Cardiovascular: Chest tightness, chest pain, diuretic and vasodilatory effects, edema, fluid overload

(Continued)

Antithrombin III *(Continued)*

Dermatologic: Hives

Gastrointestinal: Nausea, foul taste in mouth, cramps, bowel fullness

Hematologic: Hematoma formation

Ocular: Film over eye

Respiratory: Shortness of breath

Overdosage/Toxicology Levels of 150% to 200% have been documented in patients with no signs or symptoms of complications

Drug Interactions Increased toxicity: Anticoagulation effect of heparin is enhanced

Stability Reconstitute with 10 mL sterile water for injection, normal saline or D_5W; **do not shake**; stability of I.V. admixture: 24 hours at room temperature; do not refrigerate

Mechanism of Action Antithrombin III is the primary physiologic inhibitor of *in vivo* coagulation. It is an alpha₂-globulin. Its principal actions are the inactivation of thrombin, plasmin, and other active serine proteases of coagulation, including factors IXa, Xa, XIa, XIIa, and VIIa. The inactivation of proteases is a major step in the normal clotting process. The strong activation of clotting enzymes at the site of every bleeding injury facilitates fibrin formation and maintains normal hemostasis. Thrombosis in the circulation would be caused by active serine proteases if they were not inhibited by antithrombin III after the localized clotting process. Patients with congenital deficiency are in a prethrombotic state, even if asymptomatic, as evidenced by elevated plasma levels of prothrombin activation fragment, which are normalized following infusions of antithrombin III concentrate.

Usual Dosage After first dose of antithrombin III, level should increase to 120% of normal; thereafter maintain at levels >80%. Generally, achieved by administration of maintenance doses once every 24 hours; initially and until patient is stabilized, measure antithrombin III level at least twice daily, thereafter once daily and always immediately before next infusion. 1 unit = quantity of antithrombin III in 1 mL of normal pooled human plasma; administration of 1 unit/1 kg raises AT-III level by 1% to 2%; assume plasma volume of 40 mL/kg

Initial dosage (units) = [desired AT-III level % - baseline AT-III level %] x body weight (kg) divided by 1%/units/kg, eg, if a 70 kg adult patient had a baseline AT-III level of 57%, the initial dose would be (120% - 57%) x 70/1%/IU/kg = 4,410 IU

Measure antithrombin III preceding and 30 minutes after dose to calculate *in vivo* recovery rate; maintain level within normal range for 2-8 days depending on type of surgery or procedure

Administration Infuse over 5-10 minutes; rate of infusion is 50 units/minute (1 mL/minute) not to exceed 100 units/minute (2 mL/minute)

Monitoring Parameters Monitor antithrombin III levels during treatment period

Reference Range Maintain antithrombin III level in plasma >80%

Dosage Forms Powder for injection: 500 units (50 mL)

Antithymocyte Globulin (Equine) *see* Lymphocyte Immune Globulin *on page 655*

Antithymocyte Immunoglobulin *see* Lymphocyte Immune Globulin *on page 655*

Anti-Tuss® Expectorant [OTC] *see* Guaifenesin *on page 515*

Antivert® *see* Meclizine Hydrochloride *on page 674*

Antrizine® *see* Meclizine Hydrochloride *on page 674*

Anturane® *see* Sulfinpyrazone *on page 1045*

Anucort-HC® *see* Hydrocortisone *on page 546*

Anumed HC™ *see* Hydrocortisone *on page 546*

Anusol-HC® [OTC] *see* Hydrocortisone *on page 546*

Anxanil® *see* Hydroxyzine *on page 556*

Apacet® [OTC] *see* Acetaminophen *on page 17*

APAP *see* Acetaminophen *on page 17*

A.P.L.® *see* Chorionic Gonadotropin *on page 242*

Aplisol® *see* Tuberculin Purified Protein Derivative *on page 1135*

APPG *see* Penicillin G Procaine *on page 853*

Apraclonidine Hydrochloride (a pra kloe' ni deen)
Brand Names Iopidine®
Use Prevention and treatment of postsurgical intraocular pressure elevation
Pregnancy Risk Factor C
Contraindications Known hypersensitivity to apraclonidine or clonidine
Warnings/Precautions Use with caution in patients with cardiovascular disease and in patients with a history of vasovagal reactions
Adverse Reactions
1% to 10%:
  Central nervous system: Lethargy
  Ocular: Upper lid elevation, conjunctival blanching, mydriasis, burning, discomfort, itching, conjunctival microhemorrhage, blurred vision
  Miscellaneous: Dry mouth or nose
<1%:
  Sensitivity reactions: Allergic response
  Miscellaneous: Some systemic effects have also been reported including GI, CNS, and cardiovascular symptoms (arrhythmias)
Drug Interactions Increased effect: Topical beta-blockers, pilocarpine → additive ↓ intraocular pressure
Stability Store in tight, light-resistant containers
Mechanism of Action Apraclonidine is a potent alpha-adrenergic agent similar to clonidine; relatively selective for $alpha_2$-receptors but does retain some binding to $alpha_1$-receptors; appears to result in reduction of aqueous humor formation; its penetration through the blood-brain barrier is more polar than clonidine which reduces its penetration through the blood-brain barrier and suggests that its pharmacological profile is characterized by peripheral rather than central effects.
Pharmacodynamics/Kinetics
Onset of action: 1 hour
Maximum IOP: 3-5 hours
Usual Dosage Adults: Ophthalmic: Instill 1 drop in operative eye 1 hour prior to laser surgery, second drop in eye upon completion of procedure
Monitoring Parameters Closely monitor patients who develop exaggerated reductions in intraocular pressure
Dosage Forms Solution: 1% with benzalkonium chloride 0.01% (0.25 mL)

Apresoline® *see* Hydralazine Hydrochloride *on page 541*

Aprodine® [OTC] *see* Triprolidine and Pseudoephedrine *on page 1131*

Aprotinin ay proe ten' in
Brand Names Trasylol®
Use Reduction or prevention of blood loss in patients undergoing coronary artery bypass surgery when a high risk of excessive bleeding exists; this includes open heart reoperation, pre-existing coagulopathies, operations on the great vessels, and when a patient's beliefs prohibit blood transfusions
Pregnancy Risk Factor C
Contraindications Hypersensitivity to aprotinin or any component, patients with thromboembolic disease requiring anticoagulants or blood factor administration
Warnings/Precautions Patients with a previous exposure to aprotinin are at an increased risk of hypersensitivity reactions
Adverse Reactions
1% to 10%
  Cardiovascular: Atrial fibrillation, myocardial infarction, heart failure, atrial flutter, ventricular tachycardia, hypotension
  Central nervous system: Fever, mental confusion
  Local: Phlebitis
  Renal: Increased potential for postoperative renal dysfunction
  Respiratory: Dyspnea, bronchoconstriction
<1%:
  Cardiovascular: Cerebral embolism, cerebrovascular events
  Central nervous system: Convulsions
  Hematologic: Hemolysis
  Hepatic: Liver damage
  Respiratory: Pulmonary edema
  Miscellaneous: Anaphylactic reactions have been reported in <0.5% of recipients, such reactions are more likely with repeated administration
Overdosage/Toxicology Maximum amount of aprotinin that can safely be given has not yet been determined. One case report of aprotinin overdose was associated with the development of hepatic and renal failure and eventually death. Autopsy demonstrated severe hepatic necrosis and extensive renal tubular and glomerular necrosis. The relationship with these findings and aprotinin remains unclear.
(Continued)

Aprotinin *(Continued)*

Drug Interactions
Decreased effect: Fibrinolytic effects of streptokinase or anistreplase decrease effects of captopril

Increased effect: Heparin's whole blood clotting time may be prolonged; use with succinylcholine can produce prolonged or recurring apnea

Stability Vials should be stored between 2°C and 25°C and protected from freezing; it is **incompatible** with corticosteroids, heparin, tetracyclines, amino acid solutions, and fat emulsion

Mechanism of Action Serine protease inhibitor; inhibits plasmin, kallikrein, and platelet activation producing antifibrinolytic effects; a weak inhibitor of plasma pseudocholinesterase. It also inhibits the contact phase activation of coagulation and preserves adhesive platelet glycoproteins making them resistant to damage from increased circulating plasmin or mechanical injury occurring during bypass

Pharmacodynamics/Kinetics
Half-life: 150 minutes
Elimination: By the kidney

Usual Dosage
Test dose: **All** patients should receive a 1 mL I.V. test dose at least 10 minutes prior to the loading dose to assess the potential for allergic reactions

Regimen A (standard dose):
2 million units (280 mg) loading dose I.V. over 20-30 minutes
2 million units (280 mg) into pump prime volume
500,000 units/hour (70 mg/hour) I.V. during operation

Regimen B (low dose):
1 million units (140 mg) loading dose I.V. over 20-30 minutes
1 million units (140 mg) into pump prime volume
250,000 units/hour (35 mg/hour) I.V. during operation

Administration All intravenous doses should be administered through a central line

Monitoring Parameters Bleeding times, prothrombin time, activated clotting time, platelet count, red blood cell counts, hematocrit, hemoglobin and fibrinogen degradation products; for toxicity also include renal function tests and blood pressure

Reference Range Antiplasmin effects occur when plasma aprotinin concentrations are 125 KIU/mL and antikallikrein effects occur when plasma levels are 250-500 KIU/mL; it remains unknown if these plasma concentrations are required for clinical benefits to occur during cardiopulmonary bypass

Test Interactions Aprotinin prolongs whole blood clotting time of heparinized blood as determined by the Hemochrom® method or similar surface activation methods. Patients may require additional heparin even in the presence of activated clotting time levels that appear to represent adequate anticoagulation.

Dosage Forms Injection: 1.4 mg/mL [10,000 units/mL] (100 mL, 200 mL)

APSAC *see* Anistreplase *on page 79*

Aquacare® [OTC] *see* Urea *on page 1139*

Aquachloral® Supprettes® *see* Chloral Hydrate *on page 217*

AquaMEPHYTON® *see* Phytonadione *on page 882*

Aquaphyllin® *see* Theophylline/Aminophylline *on page 1072*

Aquasol A® [OTC] *see* Vitamin A *on page 1163*

Aquasol E® [OTC] *see* Vitamin E *on page 1164*

Aquatag® *see* Benzthiazide *on page 123*

Aquatensen® *see* Methyclothiazide *on page 718*

Aqueous Procaine Penicillin G *see* Penicillin G Procaine *on page 853*

Aqueous Testosterone *see* Testosterone *on page 1063*

Ara-A *see* Vidarabine *on page 1156*

Arabinofuranosyladenine *see* Vidarabine *on page 1156*

Arabinosylcytosine *see* Cytarabine Hydrochloride *on page 294*

Ara-C *see* Cytarabine Hydrochloride *on page 294*

Aralen® Phosphate *see* Chloroquine Phosphate *on page 225*

Aralen® Phosphate With Primaquine Phosphate *see* Chloroquine and Primaquine *on page 224*

Aramine® *see* Metaraminol Bitartrate *on page 699*

Arduan® *see* Pipecuronium Bromide *on page 887*

Aredia™ *see* Pamidronate Disodium *on page 835*

Arfonad® *see* Trimethaphan Camsylate *on page 1125*

Argesic®**-SA** *see* Salsalate *on page 993*

Arginine Hydrochloride (ar' ji neen)

Brand Names R-Gene®

Use Pituitary function test (growth hormone); management of severe, uncompensated, metabolic alkalosis (pH ≥7.55) **after** optimizing therapy with sodium and potassium supplements

Pregnancy Risk Factor C

Contraindications Known hypersensitivity to arginine; renal or hepatic failure

Warnings/Precautions Arginine may elevate blood urea nitrogen and cause severe hyperkalemia (due to rapid intracellular potassium displacement) in patients with renal dysfunction; serum potassium concentrations must be monitored during arginine administration. Arginine hydrochloride can be metabolized to nitrogen containing products for excretion; temporary effect of a high nitrogen load on the kidneys should be evaluated. Administer with caution due to high chloride (0.475 mEq/mL) content; have agents available (antihistamines) in the event of an allergic reaction; rapid I.V. infusion may produce local irritation, flushing, nausea or vomiting.

Adverse Reactions
1% to 10%: Rapid I.V. infusion may produce flushing, local irritation, nausea & vomiting
  Central nervous system: Headache, numbness
  Gastrointestinal: Nausea, vomiting
  Local: Venous irritation
<1%:
  Endocrine & metabolic: Hyperglycemia, hyperkalemia, increased serum gastrin concentration, hyperchloremia
  Gastrointestinal: Abdominal pain, bloating

Drug Interactions
Increased toxicity: Estrogen-progesterone combinations (increases growth hormone response and decreases glucagon and insulin effects); spironolactone (potentially fatal hyperkalemia has been reported)

Stability Store at room temperature

Mechanism of Action
Stimulates pituitary release of growth hormone and prolactin through origins in the hypothalamus; patients with impaired pituitary function have lower or no increase in plasma concentrations of growth hormone after administration of arginine. Arginine hydrochloride has been used for severe metabolic alkalosis due to its high chloride content.
Arginine hydrochloride has been used investigationally to treat metabolic alkalosis. Arginine contains 475 mEq of hydrogen ions and 475 mEq of chloride ions/L. Arginine is metabolized by the liver to produce hydrogen ions. It may be used in patients with relative hepatic insufficiency because arginine combines with ammonia in the body to produce urea.

Pharmacodynamics/Kinetics
Absorption: Oral: Well absorbed
Time to peak serum concentration: Within 2 hours

Usual Dosage I.V.:
Growth hormone (pituitary function) reserve test:
  Children: 500 mg (5 mL) kg/dose administered over 30 minutes
  Adults: 30 g (300 mL) administered over 30 minutes
Metabolic alkalosis: Children and Adults: Usual dose: 10 g/hour
  Acid required (mEq) =
    [1] 0.2 (L/kg) x wt (kg) x [103 - serum chloride] (mEq/L) **or**
    [2] 0.3 (L/kg) x wt (kg) x base excess (mEq/L) **or**
    [3] 0.5 (L/kg) x wt (kg) x [serum HCO_3 - 24] (mEq/L)
  Give 1/2 to 2/3 of calculated dose and re-evaluate

Note: Arginine hydrochloride should never be used as an alternative to chloride supplementation but used in the patient who is unresponsive to sodium chloride or potassium chloride supplementation

Administration Administer by central line only

Monitoring Parameters Acid-base status (arterial or capillary blood gases), serum electrolytes (sodium, potassium, chloride, HCO_3), BUN, glucose. Arginine may elevate blood urea nitrogen and cause severe hyperkalemia (due to rapid intracellular potassium displacement) in patients with renal dysfunction. Serum potassium concentrations must be monitored during arginine administration.

Nursing Implications Leakage of I.V. arginine may cause necrosis and phlebitis

(Continued)

87

Arginine Hydrochloride *(Continued)*

Additional Information Chloride content: 47.5 mEq/100 mL; 950 mOsmol/L

Dosage Forms Injection: 10% [100 mg/mL = 950 mOsm/L] (500 mL)

8-Arginine Vasopressin *see* Vasopressin *on page 1149*

Aristocort® Forte *see* Triamcinolone *on page 1112*

Aristocort® Intralesional Suspension *see* Triamcinolone *on page 1112*

Aristocort® Tablet *see* Triamcinolone *on page 1112*

Aristospan® *see* Triamcinolone *on page 1112*

Arlidin® *see* Nylidrin Hydrochloride *on page 810*

Arm-a-Med® Isoetharine *see* Isoetharine *on page 593*

Arm-a-Med® Isoproterenol *see* Isoproterenol *on page 597*

Arm-a-Med® Metaproterenol *see* Metaproterenol Sulfate *on page 697*

Armour® Thyroid *see* Thyroid *on page 1088*

Arrestin® *see* Trimethobenzamide Hydrochloride *on page 1126*

Artane® *see* Trihexyphenidyl Hydrochloride *on page 1123*

Artha-G® *see* Salsalate *on page 993*

Arthropan® [OTC] *see* Choline Salicylate *on page 240*

Articulose-50® *see* Prednisolone *on page 919*

ASA *see* Aspirin *on page 92*

A.S.A. [OTC] *see* Aspirin *on page 92*

5-ASA *see* Mesalamine *on page 691*

Asacol® *see* Mesalamine *on page 691*

Ascorbic Acid *(a skor′ bik)*

Brand Names Ascorbicap® [OTC]; Cecon® [OTC]; Cee-1000® T.D. [OTC]; Cetane® [OTC]; Cevalin®; Ce-Vi-Sol® [OTC]; Cevita® [OTC]; C-Span® [OTC]; Flavorcee® [OTC]; Vita-C® [OTC]

Synonyms Vitamin C

Use Prevention and treatment of scurvy and to acidify the urine

Investigational use: In large doses to decrease the severity of "colds"; dietary supplementation

Pregnancy Risk Factor A (C if used in doses above RDA recommendation)

Contraindications Large doses during pregnancy

Warnings/Precautions Diabetics and patients prone to recurrent renal calculi (eg, dialysis patients) should not take excessive doses for extended periods of time

Adverse Reactions

1% to 10%: Renal: Hyperoxaluria

<1%:

Cardiovascular: Flushing

Central nervous system: Faintness, dizziness, headache, fatigue, flank pain

Gastrointestinal: Nausea, vomiting, heartburn, diarrhea

Overdosage/Toxicology Symptoms of overdose include renal calculi, nausea, gastritis, diarrhea; diuresis with forced fluids may be useful following a massive ingestion

Drug Interactions

Decreased effect:

Aspirin decreases ascorbate levels, increases aspirin

Fluphenazine decreases fluphenazine levels

Warfarin decreases effect

Increased effect: Iron enhances absorption; oral contraceptives increase contraceptive effect

Stability Injectable form should be stored under refrigeration (2°C to 8°C); protect oral dosage forms from light; is rapidly oxidized when in solution in air and alkaline media

Mechanism of Action Not fully understood; necessary for collagen formation and tissue repair; involved in some oxidation-reduction reactions as well as other metabolic pathways, such as synthesis of carnitine, steroids, and catecholamines and conversion of folic acid to folinic acid

Pharmacodynamics/Kinetics

Absorption: Oral: Readily absorbed; an active process and is thought to be dose-dependent

Distribution: Widely distributed

Metabolism: In the liver by oxidation and sulfation

Elimination: In urine; there is an individual specific renal threshold for ascorbic acid; when blood levels are high, ascorbic acid is excreted in the urine; whereas when the levels are subthreshold, very little if any ascorbic acid is cleared into the urine

Usual Dosage Oral, I.M., I.V., S.C.:

Recommended daily allowance (RDA):

<6 months: 30 mg
6 months to 1 year: 35 mg
1-3 years: 40 mg
4-10 years: 45 mg
11-14 years: 50 mg
>14 years and Adults: 60 mg

Children:

Scurvy: 100-300 mg/day in divided doses for at least 2 weeks
Urinary acidification: 500 mg every 6-8 hours
Dietary supplement: 35-100 mg/day

Adults:

Scurvy: 100-250 mg 1-2 times/day for at least 2 weeks
Urinary acidification: 4-12 g/day in 3-4 divided doses
Prevention and treatment of colds: 1-3 g/day
Dietary supplement: 50-200 mg/day

Administration Avoid rapid I.V. injection

Monitoring Parameters Monitor pH of urine when using as an acidifying agent

Test Interactions False-positive urinary glucose with cupric sulfate reagent, false-negative urinary glucose with glucose oxidase method; false-negative stool occult blood 48-72 hours after ascorbic acid ingestion

Patient Information Do not take more than the recommended dose; take with plenty of water; report any pain on urination

Additional Information Sodium content of 1 g: ~5 mEq

Dosage Forms

Capsule, timed release: 500 mg
Crystals: 4 g/teaspoonful (1000 g)
Drops: 100 mg/mL (50 mL)
Injection: 250 mg/mL (2 mL, 30 mL); 500 mg/mL (1 mL, 2 mL, 50 mL)
Liquid: 35 mg/0.6 mL (50 mL)
Powder: 4 g/teaspoonful (1000 g)
Syrup: 500 mg/5 mL (5 mL, 10 mL, 120 mL, 480 mL)
Tablet: 25 mg, 50 mg, 100 mg, 250 mg, 500 mg, 1000 mg
Tablet:
  Chewable: 100 mg, 250 mg, 500 mg
  Timed release: 500 mg, 1500 mg, 1 g

Ascorbicap® [OTC] *see* Ascorbic Acid *on previous page*

Ascriptin® [OTC] *see* Aspirin *on page 92*

Asendin® *see* Amoxapine *on page 65*

Asmalix® *see* Theophylline/Aminophylline *on page 1072*

Asparaginase (a spare' a ji nase)

Related Information

Cancer Chemotherapy Regimens *on page 1218-1241*

Brand Names Elspar®; Erwiniar®

Synonyms L-asparaginase

Use Treatment of acute lymphocytic leukemia, lymphoma; used for induction therapy

Pregnancy Risk Factor C

Pregnancy/Breast Feeding Implications Based on limited reports in humans, the use of asparaginase does not seem to pose a major risk to the fetus when used in the 2nd and 3rd trimesters, or when exposure occurs prior to conception in either females or males. Because of the teratogenicity observed in animals and the lack of human data after 1st trimester exposure, asparaginase should be used cautiously, if at all, during this period.

Contraindications Pancreatitis, hypersensitivity to asparaginase or any component; if a reaction occurs to Elspar®, obtain **Erwinia L-asparaginase (must be special ordered from manufacturer)** and use with caution

Warnings/Precautions The U.S. Food and Drug Administration (FDA) currently recommends that procedures for proper handling and disposal of antineoplastic agents be considered. Monitor for severe allergic reactions; risk for hypersensitivity increases with successive doses.

(Continued)

Asparaginase *(Continued)*

The following precautions should be taken when administering:
Only administer in hospital setting
Monitor blood pressure every 15 minutes for 1 hour
Give a small test dose first; the intradermal skin test is commonly given prior to the initial injection, using a dose of 0.1 mL of 20 units/mL solution (~2 units). The skin test site should be observed for at least 1 hour for a wheal or erythema. Note that a negative skin test does not preclude the possibility of an allergic reaction. Desensitization should be performed in patients who have been found to be hypersensitive by the intradermal skin test or who have received previous courses of therapy with the drug.
Have epinephrine, diphenhydramine, and hydrocortisone at the bedside
Have a running I.V. in place
A physician should be readily accessible
Avoid administering at night

Adverse Reactions
>10%:
Immediate effects: Fever, chills, nausea, and vomiting occur in 50% to 60% of patients
Emetic potential: Moderate (30% to 60%)
Hypersensitivity effects: Hypersensitivity and anaphylactic reactions occur in ~10% to 40% of patients and can be fatal. This reaction is more common in patients receiving asparaginase alone or by I.V. administration. Hypersensitivity appears rarely with the first dose and more commonly after the second or third treatment. Hypersensitivity may be treated with antihistamines and/or steroids. If an anaphylactic reaction occurs, a change in treatment to the *Erwinia* preparation may be made, since this preparation does not share antigenic cross-reactivity with the *E. coli* preparation. Note that allergic reactions to the *Erwinia* preparation may also occur and ultimately develop in 5% to 20% of patients.
Pancreatitis: Occur in <15% of patients but may progress to severe hemorrhagic pancreatitis
1% to 10%:
Endocrine & metabolic: Hyperuricemia
Miscellaneous: Mouth sores
<1%:
Central nervous system: Disorientation, drowsiness, seizures, and coma which may be due to elevated NH_4 levels, hyperthermia, fever, malaise
Endocrine & metabolic: Transient diabetes mellitus
Gastrointestinal: Weight loss
Hematologic: Inhibition of protein synthesis will cause a decrease in production of albumin, insulin (resulting in hyperglycemia), serum lipoprotein, antithrombin III, and clotting factors II, V, VII, VIII, IX, and X. The loss of the later two proteins may result in either thrombotic or hemorrhagic events. These protein losses occur in 100% of patients. Leg vein thrombosis.
Myelosuppressive effects: Myelosuppression is uncommon
WBC: Mild
Platelets: Mild
Onset (days): 7
Nadir (days): 14
Recovery (days): 21
Hepatic: Increases in serum bilirubin, ST, alkaline phosphatase, and possible decrease in mobilization of lipids
Hypersensitivity reactions: Hypotension, rash, pruritus, urticaria, laryngeal spasm, chills
Renal: Azotemia
Respiratory: Coughing

Overdosage/Toxicology Symptoms of overdose include nausea, diarrhea
Drug Interactions
Decreased effect: Methotrexate: Asparaginase terminates methotrexate action by inhibition of protein synthesis and prevention of cell entry into the S phase
Increased toxicity:
Vincristine and prednisone: An increased toxicity has been noticed when asparaginase is administered with VCR and prednisone
Cyclophosphamide (decreased metabolism)
Mercaptopurine (increased hepatotoxicity)
Vincristine (increased neuropathy)
Prednisone (increased hyperglycemia)
Stability Powder should be refrigerated (<8°C); lyophilized powder should be reconstituted with sterile water for I.V. administration or NS for I.M. use, reconstituted solutions and those further diluted for I.V. infusion should be stored at 2°C to 8°C and should be discarded after 24 hours; shake well but not too vigorously;

use of a 5 micron in-line filter is recommended to remove fiber-like particles in the solution (not 0.2 micron)

Mechanism of Action Some malignant cells (ie, lymphoblastic leukemia cells and those of lymphocyte derivation) must acquire the amino acid asparagine from surrounding fluid such as blood, whereas normal cells can synthesize their own asparagine. asparaginase is an enzyme that deaminates asparagine to aspartic acid and ammonia in the plasma and extracellular fluid and therefore deprives tumor cells of the amino acid for protein synthesis.

There are two purified preparations of the enzyme, one from *Escherichia coli* and one from *Erwinia carotovora*. These two preparations vary slightly in the gene sequencing and have slight differences in enzyme characteristics. Both are highly specific for asparagine and have less than 10% activity for the D-isomer. The preparation from *E. coli* has had the most use in clinical and research practice.

Pharmacodynamics/Kinetics

Absorption: Not absorbed from GI tract, therefore, requires parenteral administration; I.M. administration produces peak blood levels 50% lower than those from I.V. administration (I.M. may be less immunogenic)

Distribution: V_d: 4-5 L/kg; 70% to 80% of plasma volume; does not penetrate the CSF

Metabolism: Systemically degraded, only trace amounts are found in the urine

Half-life: 8-30 hours

Elimination: Clearance unaffected by age, renal function, or hepatic function

Usual Dosage

Dose must be individualized based upon clinical response and tolerance of the patient (refer to individual protocols)

I.M. administration is **preferred** over I.V. administration; I.M. administration may decrease the risk of anaphylaxis

Asparaginase is available from 2 different microbiological sources: One is from *Escherichia coli* and the other is from *Erwinia carotovora*. The *Erwinia* is restricted to patients who have sustained anaphylaxis to the *E. coli* preparation.

I.M., I.V.: 6000 units/m^2 every other day for 3-4 weeks or daily doses of 10,000 units/m^2 every other day for 10-20 days; other induction regimens have been utilized

Desensitization should be performed before administering the first dose of asparaginase to patients who developed a positive reaction to the intradermal skin test or who are being retreated. One schedule begins with a total of 1 unit given I.V. and doubles the dose every 10 minutes until the total amount given in the planned dose for that day.

Asparaginase Desensitization

Injection No.	Elspar Dose (IU)	Accumulated Total Dose
1	1	1
2	2	3
3	4	7
4	8	15
5	16	31
6	32	63
7	64	127
8	128	255
9	256	511
10	512	1023
11	1024	2047
12	2048	4095
13	4096	8191
14	8192	16383
15	16384	32767
16	32768	65535
17	65536	131071
18	131072	262143

For example, if a patient was to receive a total dose of 4000 units, he/she would receive injections 1 through 12 during the desensitization

Administration Should only be given as a deep intramuscular injection into a large muscle; use two injection sites for I.M. doses >2 mL; do not filter solution; (Continued)

Asparaginase *(Continued)*

may be administered I.V. infusion in 50 mL of D_5W or NS over more than 30 minutes; a small test dose (0.1 mL of a 20 unit/mL solution) should be given first

Monitoring Parameters Vital signs during administration, CBC, urinalysis, amylase, liver enzymes, prothrombin time, renal function tests, urine dipstick for glucose, blood glucose; monitor for onset of abdominal pain and mental status changes

Test Interactions ↓ thyroxine and thyroxine-binding globulin

Patient Information Drowsiness may occur during therapy; nausea or vomiting may interrupt dosing schedule at first

Nursing Implications Appropriate agents for maintenance of an adequate airway and treatment of a hypersensitivity reaction (antihistamine, epinephrine, oxygen, I.V. corticosteroids) should be readily available. Be prepared to treat anaphylaxis at each administration.

Dosage Forms Injection: 10,000 units/vial (*Erwinia*)

Aspergum® [OTC] *see* Aspirin *on this page*

Aspirin (as′ pir in)

Brand Names Anacin® [OTC]; A.S.A. [OTC]; Ascriptin® [OTC]; Aspergum® [OTC]; Bayer® Aspirin [OTC]; Bufferin® [OTC]; Easprin®; Ecotrin® [OTC]; Empirin® [OTC]; Measurin® [OTC]; Synalgos® [OTC]; ZORprin®

Synonyms Acetylsalicylic Acid; ASA

Use Treatment of mild to moderate pain, inflammation, and fever; may be used as a prophylaxis of myocardial infarction and transient ischemic episodes; management of rheumatoid arthritis, rheumatic fever, osteoarthritis, and gout (high dose)

Pregnancy Risk Factor C (D if full-dose aspirin in 3rd trimester)

Contraindications Bleeding disorders (factor VII or IX deficiencies), hypersensitivity to salicylates or other NSAIDs, tartrazine dye and asthma

Warnings/Precautions Use with caution in patients with platelet and bleeding disorders, renal dysfunction, erosive gastritis, or peptic ulcer disease, previous nonreaction does not guarantee future safe taking of medication; do not use aspirin in children <16 years of age for chickenpox or flu symptoms due to the association with Reye's syndrome

Otic: Discontinue use if dizziness, tinnitus, or impaired hearing occurs; surgical patients: avoid ASA if possible, for 1 week prior to surgery because of the possibility of postoperative bleeding; use with caution in impaired hepatic function

Elderly are a high-risk population for adverse effects from nonsteroidal anti-inflammatory agents. As much as 60% of elderly with GI complications to NSAIDs can develop peptic ulceration and/or hemorrhage asymptomatically. Also, concomitant disease and drug use contribute to the risk for GI adverse effects. Use lowest effective dose for shortest period possible. Consider renal function decline with age. Use of NSAIDs can compromise existing renal function especially when Cl_{cr} is <30 mL/minute. Tinnitus may be a difficult and unreliable indication of toxicity due to age-related hearing loss or eighth cranial nerve damage. CNS adverse effects such as confusion, agitation, and hallucination are generally seen in overdose or high-dose situations, but elderly may demonstrate these adverse effects at lower doses than younger adults.

Adverse Reactions

>10%: Gastrointestinal: Nausea, vomiting, dyspepsia, epigastric discomfort, heartburn, stomach pains

1% to 10%:
  Central nervous system: Weakness, tiredness
  Dermatologic: Rash, urticaria
  Gastrointestinal: Gastrointestinal ulceration
  Hematologic: Hemolytic anemia
  Respiratory: Troubled breathing
  Miscellaneous: Anaphylactic shock

<1%:
  Central nervous system: Insomnia, nervousness, jitters
  Hematologic: Occult bleeding, prolongation of bleeding time, leukopenia, thrombocytopenia, iron deficiency anemia
  Hepatic: Hepatotoxicity
  Renal: Impaired renal function
  Respiratory: Bronchospasm

Overdosage/Toxicology Symptoms of overdose include tinnitus, headache, dizziness, confusion, metabolic acidosis, hyperpyrexia, hypoglycemia, coma. The "Done" nomogram may be helpful for estimating the severity of aspirin poisoning and directing treatment using serum salicylate levels. Treatment can also be based upon symptomatology.

Aspirin

Toxic Symptoms	Treatment
Overdose	Induce emesis with ipecac, and/or lavage with saline, followed with activated charcoal
Dehydration	I.V. fluids with KCl (no D₅W only)
Metabolic acidosis (must be treated)	Sodium bicarbonate
Hyperthermia	Cooling blankets or sponge baths
Coagulopathy/hemorrhage	Vitamin K I.V.
Hypoglycemia (with coma, seizures, or change in mental status)	Dextrose 25 g I.V.
Seizures	Diazepam 5-10 mg I.V.

Drug Interactions
Decreased effect: Possible decreased serum concentration of NSAIDs; aspirin may antagonize effects of probenecid

Increased toxicity: Aspirin may increase methotrexate serum levels and may displace valproic acid from binding sites which can result in toxicity; warfarin and aspirin → ↑ bleeding; NSAIDs and aspirin → ↑ GI adverse effects

Stability Keep suppositories in refrigerator, do not freeze; hydrolysis of aspirin occurs upon exposure to water or moist air, resulting in salicylate and acetate, which possess a vinegar-like odor; do not use if a strong odor is present

Mechanism of Action Inhibits prostaglandin synthesis, acts on the hypothalamus heat-regulating center to reduce fever, blocks prostaglandin synthetase action which prevents formation of the platelet-aggregating substance thromboxane A₂

Pharmacodynamics/Kinetics
Absorption: From stomach and small intestine

Distribution: Readily distributes into most body fluids and tissues

Metabolism: Hydrolyzed to salicylate (active) by esterases in the GI mucosa, red blood cells, synovial fluid and blood; metabolism of salicylate occurs primarily by hepatic microsomal enzymes; metabolic pathways are saturable

Half-life:
Parent drug: 15-20 minutes
Salicylates (dose-dependent): From 3 hours at lower doses (300-600 mg), to 5-6 hours (after 1 g) to 10 hours with higher doses

Time to peak serum concentration: ~1-2 hours

Usual Dosage
Children:
Analgesic and antipyretic: Oral, rectal: 10-15 mg/kg/dose every 4-6 hours, up to a total of 60-80 mg/kg/24 hours

Anti-inflammatory: Oral: Initial: 60-90 mg/kg/day in divided doses; usual maintenance: 80-100 mg/kg/day divided every 6-8 hours, maximum dose: 3.6 g/day; monitor serum concentrations

Kawasaki disease: Oral: 80-100 mg/kg/day divided every 6 hours; after fever resolves: 8-10 mg/kg/day once daily; monitor serum concentrations

Antirheumatic: Oral: 60-100 mg/kg/day in divided doses every 4 hours

Adults:
Analgesic and antipyretic: Oral, rectal: 325-650 mg every 4-6 hours up to 4 g/day

Anti-inflammatory: Oral: Initial: 2.4-3.6 g/day in divided doses; usual maintenance: 3.6-5.4 g/day; monitor serum concentrations

TIA: Oral: 1.3 g/day in 2-4 divided doses

Myocardial infarction prophylaxis: 160-325 mg/day

Dosing adjustment in renal impairment: Cl_cr <10 mL/minute: Avoid use
Dialyzable (50% to 100%)

Dosing adjustment in hepatic disease: Avoid use in severe liver disease

Administration Administer with food or a full glass of water to minimize GI distress

Reference Range Timing of serum samples: Peak levels usually occur 2 hours after ingestion. Salicylate serum concentrations correlate with the pharmacological actions and adverse effects observed. See table.

(Continued)

Aspirin *(Continued)*

Serum Salicylate: Clinical Correlations

Serum Salicylate Concentration (mcg/mL)	Desired Effects	Adverse Effects/ Intoxication
~100	Antiplatelet Antipyresis Analgesia	GI intolerance and bleeding, hypersensitivity, hemostatic defects
150-300	Anti-inflammatory	Mild salicylism
250-400	Treatment of rheumatic fever	Nausea/vomiting, hyperventilation, salicylism, flushing, sweating, thirst, headache, diarrhea, and tachycardia
>400-500		Respiratory alkalosis, hemorrhage, excitement, confusion, asterixis, pulmonary edema, convulsions, tetany, metabolic acidosis, fever, coma, cardiovascular collapse, renal and respiratory failure

Test Interactions False-negative results for glucose oxidase urinary glucose tests (Clinistix®); false-positives using the cupric sulfate method (Clinitest®); also, interferes with Gerhardt test, VMA determination; 5-HIAA, xylose tolerance test and T_3 and T_4

Patient Information Watch for bleeding gums or any signs of GI bleeding; take with food or milk to minimize GI distress, notify physician if ringing in ears or persistent GI pain occurs; avoid other concurrent aspirin or salicylate-containing products

Nursing Implications Do not crush sustained release or enteric coated tablet

Dosage Forms
Suppository, rectal: 120 mg, 200 mg, 300 mg, 600 mg
Tablet: 325 mg, 500 mg
Tablet:
  Buffered: 325 mg with magnesium-aluminum hydroxide 150 mg
  Chewable, children's: 81 mg
  Controlled release: 800 mg
  Enteric coated: 165 mg, 325 mg, 500 mg, 650 mg, 975 mg
  Gum: 227.5 mg (16s, 40s)
  Timed release: 800 mg
  With caffeine: 400 mg with 32 mg caffeine

Aspirin and Codeine *(as′ pir in)*
Brand Names Empirin® With Codeine
Synonyms Codeine and Aspirin
Use Relief of mild to moderate pain
Restrictions C-III
Pregnancy Risk Factor D
Contraindications Hypersensitivity to aspirin, codeine or any component; premature infants or during labor for delivery of a premature infant
Warnings/Precautions Use with caution in patients with impaired renal function, erosive gastritis, or peptic ulcer disease; children and teenagers should not use for chickenpox or flu symptoms before a physician is consulted about Reye's syndrome
Adverse Reactions
>10%:
  Central nervous system: Lightheadedness, dizziness, sedation
  Gastrointestinal: Nausea, heartburn, stomach pains, dyspepsia, epigastric discomfort, vomiting
  Respiratory: Shortness of breath
1% to 10%:
  Central nervous system: Weakness, tiredness, euphoria, dysphoria
  Dermatologic: Skin rash, pruritus
  Gastrointestinal: Gastrointestinal ulceration, constipation
  Hematologic: Hemolytic anemia
  Respiratory: Troubled breathing
  Miscellaneous: Anaphylactic shock
<1%:
  Cardiovascular: Palpitations, hypotension, bradycardia, peripheral vasodilation

Central nervous system: Insomnia, nervousness, jitters, increased intracranial pressure

Endocrine & metabolic: Antidiuretic hormone release

Gastrointestinal: Biliary tract spasm

Genitourinary: Urinary retention

Hematologic: Occult bleeding, prolongation of bleeding time, leukopenia, thrombocytopenia, iron deficiency anemia

Hepatic: Hepatotoxicity

Ocular: Miosis

Renal: Impaired renal function

Respiratory: Bronchospasm, respiratory depression

Miscellaneous: Physical and psychological dependence

Overdosage/Toxicology Antidote is naloxone for codeine. Naloxone 2 mg I.V. (0.01 mg/kg for children) with repeat administration as necessary up to a total of 10 mg; see Aspirin monograph for treatment of aspirin toxicity.

Drug Interactions Refer to individual monographs for Aspirin and Codeine

Mechanism of Action Inhibits prostaglandin synthesis, acts on the hypothalamus heat-regulating center to reduce fever, blocks prostaglandin synthetase action which prevents formation of the platelet-aggregating substance thromboxane A_2; binds to opiate receptors in the CNS, causing inhibition of ascending pain pathways, altering the perception of and response to pain; causes cough supression by direct central action in the medulla; produces generalized CNS depression

Usual Dosage Oral:

Children:
Aspirin: 10 mg/kg/dose every 4 hours
Codeine: 0.5-1 mg/kg/dose every 4 hours
Adults: 1-2 tablets every 4-6 hours as needed for pain

Dosing adjustment in renal impairment:
Cl_{cr} 10-50 mL/minute: Administer 75% of dose
Cl_{cr} <10 mL/minute: Avoid use
Dosing interval in hepatic disease: Avoid use in severe liver disease

Administration Administer with food or a full glass of water to minimize GI distress

Monitoring Parameters Observe patient for excessive sedation, respiratory depression, pain relief, blood pressure, mental status

Test Interactions Urine glucose, urinary 5-HIAA, serum uric acid

Patient Information May cause drowsiness; avoid alcohol; watch for bleeding gums or any signs of GI bleeding; take with food or milk to minimize GI distress, notify physician if ringing in ears or persistent GI pain occurs

Dosage Forms Tablet:
#2: Aspirin 325 mg and codeine phosphate 15 mg
#3: Aspirin 325 mg and codeine phosphate 30 mg
#4: Aspirin 325 mg and codeine phosphate 60 mg

Astemizole (a stem' mi zole)

Brand Names Hismanal®

Use Perennial and seasonal allergic rhinitis and other allergic symptoms including urticaria

Pregnancy Risk Factor C

Contraindications Hypersensitivity to astemizole or any component

Warnings/Precautions Use with caution in patients receiving drugs which prolong QRS or Q-T interval; rare cases of severe cardiovascular events (cardiac arrest, arrhythmias) have been reported in the following situations: overdose (even as low as 20-30 mg/day), significant hepatic dysfunction, when used in combination with erythromycin, ketoconazole, or itraconazole

Adverse Reactions

1% to 10%:
Central nervous system: Drowsiness, headache, fatigue, nervousness, dizziness
Gastrointestinal: Appetite increase, weight increase, nausea, diarrhea, abdominal pain, dry mouth
Neuromuscular & skeletal: Arthralgia
Respiratory: Pharyngitis

<1%:
Cardiovascular: Palpitations, edema
Central nervous system: Depression
Dermatologic: Angioedema, photosensitivity, rash
Hepatic: Hepatitis
Neuromuscular & skeletal: Myalgia, paresthesia
Respiratory: Bronchospasm

(Continued)

95

Astemizole *(Continued)*

Miscellaneous: Thickening of mucous, epistaxis

Overdosage/Toxicology Symptoms of overdose include sedation, apnea, diminished mental alertness, ventricular tachycardia, torsade de pointes. There is not a specific treatment for an antihistamine overdose, however most of its clinical toxicity is due to anticholinergic effects. Anticholinesterase inhibitors including physostigmine, neostigmine, pyridostigmine and edrophonium may be useful for the overdose with severe life-threatening symptoms. Physostigmine 1-2 mg (0.5 or 0.02 mg/kg for children) I.V., slowly may be given to reverse the anticholinergic effects. Cases of ventricular arrhythmias following dosages >200 mg have been reported, however, overdoses of up to 500 mg have been reported without ill effect. Patients should be carefully observed with EKG monitoring in cases of suspected overdose. Magnesium may be helpful for torsade de pointes or a lidocaine bolus followed by a titrated infusion.

Drug Interactions Increased toxicity: CNS depressants (sedation), triazole antifungals (torsade de pointes and other cardiotoxicities have been reported), macrolide antibiotics (cardiotoxicity)

Mechanism of Action Competes with histamine for H_1-receptor sites on effector cells in the gastrointestinal tract, blood vessels, and respiratory tract; binds to lung receptors significantly greater than it binds to cerebellar receptors, resulting in a reduced sedative potential

Pharmacodynamics/Kinetics Long-acting, with steady-state plasma levels seen within 4-8 weeks following initiation of chronic therapy

Distribution: Nonsedating action reportedly due to the drug's low lipid solubility and poor penetration through the blood-brain barrier

Protein binding: 97%

Metabolism: Undergoes exclusive first-pass metabolism

Half-life: 20 hours

Time to peak serum concentration: Oral: Long-acting, with steady-state plasma levels of parent compound and metabolites seen within 4-8 weeks following initiation of chronic therapy; peak plasma levels appear in 1-4 hours following administration

Elimination: By metabolism in the liver to active and inactive metabolites, which are thereby excreted in feces and to a lesser degree in urine

Usual Dosage Oral:

Children:

<6 years: 0.2 mg/kg/day

6-12 years: 5 mg/day

Children >12 years and Adults: 10-30 mg/day; give 30 mg on first day, 20 mg on second day, then 10 mg/day in a single dose

Patient Information Take on an empty stomach at least 2 hours after a meal or 1 hour before a meal; may cause drowsiness; do not exceed recommended dose; notify physician or pharmacist if taking any heart medications. Because of its delayed onset, astemizole is useful for prophylaxis of allergic symptoms, rather than for acute relief.

Nursing Implications Raise bed rails at night; may need assistance with ambulation; Give on an empty stomach

Dosage Forms Tablet: 10 mg

AsthmaHaler® *see* Epinephrine *on page 389*

AsthmaNefrin® [OTC] *see* Epinephrine *on page 389*

Astramorph™ PF *see* Morphine Sulfate *on page 756*

Atarax® *see* Hydroxyzine *on page 556*

Atenolol *(a ten' oh lole)*

Related Information

Beta-Blockers Comparison *on page 1257-1259*

Brand Names Tenormin®

Use Treatment of hypertension, alone or in combination with other agents; management of angina pectoris, postmyocardial infarction patients

Unlabeled use: Acute alcohol withdrawal, supraventricular and ventricular arrhythmias, and migraine headache prophylaxis

Pregnancy Risk Factor C

Pregnancy/Breast Feeding Implications Do not use in pregnant or nursing women

Contraindications Hypersensitivity to beta-blocking agents, pulmonary edema, cardiogenic shock, bradycardia, heart block without a pacemaker, uncompensated congestive heart failure, sinus node dysfunction, A-V conduction abnormalities, diabetes mellitus

Warnings/Precautions Safety and efficacy in children have not been established; administer with caution to patients (especially the elderly) with bronchospastic disease, CHF, renal dysfunction, severe peripheral vascular disease, myasthenia gravis, diabetes mellitus, hyperthyroidism. **Abrupt withdrawal of the drug should be avoided**, drug should be discontinued over 1-2 weeks; may potentiate hypoglycemia in a diabetic patient and mask signs and symptoms; modify dosage in patients with renal impairment.

Adverse Reactions

1% to 10%:

Cardiovascular: Persistent bradycardia, hypotension, chest pain, edema, heart failure, second or third degree A-V block, Raynaud's phenomena

Central nervous system: Dizziness, fatigue, insomnia, lethargy, confusion, mental impairment, depression, headache, nightmares

Gastrointestinal: Constipation, diarrhea, nausea

Genitourinary: Impotence

<1%:

Respiratory: Dyspnea (especially with large doses), wheezing

Miscellaneous: Cold extremities

Overdosage/Toxicology Symptoms of intoxication include cardiac disturbances, CNS toxicity, bronchospasm, hypoglycemia and hyperkalemia. The most common cardiac symptoms include hypotension and bradycardia; atrioventricular block, intraventricular conduction disturbances, cardiogenic shock, and systole may occur with severe overdose, especially with membrane-depressant drugs (eg, propranolol); CNS effects include convulsions, coma, and respiratory arrest (commonly seen with propranolol and other membrane-depressant and lipid-soluble drugs).

Treatment includes symptomatic treatment of seizures, hypotension, hyperkalemia, and hypoglycemia; bradycardia and hypotension resistant to atropine, isoproterenol, or pacing may respond to glucagon; wide QRS defects caused by the membrane-depressant poisoning may respond to hypertonic sodium bicarbonate; repeat-dose charcoal, hemoperfusion, or hemodialysis may be helpful in removal of only those beta-blockers with a small V_d, long half-life, or low intrinsic clearance (acebutolol, atenolol, nadolol, sotalol)

Drug Interactions

Decreased effect of beta-blockers with aluminum salts, barbiturates, calcium salts, cholestyramine, colestipol, NSAIDs, penicillins (ampicillin), rifampin, salicylates, and sulfinpyrazone due to decreased bioavailability and plasma levels

Beta-blockers may decrease the effect of sulfonylureas

Increased effect/toxicity of beta-blockers with calcium blockers (diltiazem, felodipine, nicardipine), contraceptives, flecainide, haloperidol (propranolol, hypotensive effects), H_2 antagonists (metoprolol, propranolol only by cimetidine, possibly ranitidine), hydralazine (metoprolol, propranolol), MAO inhibitors (metoprolol, nadolol, bradycardia), phenothiazines (propranolol), propafenone (metoprolol, propranolol), quinidine (in extensive metabolizers), ciprofloxacin, thyroid hormones (metoprolol, propranolol, when hypothyroid patient is converted to euthyroid state)

Beta-blockers may increase the effect/toxicity of flecainide, haloperidol (hypotensive effects), hydralazine, phenothiazines, acetaminophen, anticoagulants (propranolol, warfarin), benzodiazepines (not atenolol), clonidine (hypertensive crisis after or during withdrawal of either agent), epinephrine (initial hypertensive episode followed by bradycardia), nifedipine and verapamil lidocaine, ergots (peripheral ischemia), prazosin (postural hypotension)

Beta-blockers may affect the action or levels of ethanol, disopyramide, nondepolarizing muscle relaxants and theophylline although the effects are difficult to predict

Mechanism of Action Competitively blocks response to beta-adrenergic stimulation, selectively blocks beta$_1$-receptors with little or no effect on beta$_2$-receptors except at high doses

Pharmacodynamics/Kinetics

Absorption: Incomplete from GI tract

Distribution: Low lipophilicity; does **not** cross the blood-brain barrier

Protein binding: Low at 3% to 15%

Metabolism: Partial hepatic

Half-life, beta:

Neonates: Mean: 16 hours, up to 35 hours

Children: 4.6 hours; children >10 years of age may have longer half-life (>5 hours) compared to children 5-10 years of age (<5 hours)

Adults:

Normal renal function: 6-9 hours, longer in those with renal impairment

End stage renal disease: 15-35 hours

Time to peak: Oral: Within 2-4 hours

Elimination: 40% excreted as unchanged drug in urine, 50% in feces

(Continued)

Atenolol *(Continued)*

Usual Dosage

Oral:

Children: 1-2 mg/kg/dose given daily

Adults:

Hypertension: 50 mg once daily, may increase to 100 mg/day; doses >100 mg are unlikely to produce any further benefit

Angina pectoris: 50 mg once daily, may increase to 100 mg/day; some patients may require 200 mg/day

Postmyocardial infarction: Follow I.V. dose with 100 mg/day or 50 mg twice daily for 6-9 days postmyocardial infarction

I.V.: Postmyocardial infarction: Early treatment: 5 mg slow I.V. over 5 minutes; may repeat in 10 minutes; if both doses are tolerated, may start oral atenolol 50 mg every 12 hours or 100 mg/day for 6-9 days postmyocardial infarction

Dosing interval in renal impairment:

Cl_{cr} 15-35 mL/minute: Administer 50 mg/day maximum

Cl_{cr} <15 mL/minute: Administer 50 mg every other day maximum

Moderately dialyzable (20% to 50%) via hemodialysis; administer dose postdialysis or administer 25-50 mg supplemental dose; elimination is not enhanced with peritoneal dialysis; supplemental dose is not necessary

Administration Administer I.V. at 1 mg/minute; intravenous administration requires a cardiac monitor and blood pressure monitor

Monitoring Parameters Monitor blood pressure, apical and radial pulses, fluid I & O, daily weight, respirations, and circulation in extremities before and during therapy

Test Interactions ↑ glucose; ↓ HDL

Patient Information Adhere to dosage regimen; watch for postural hypotension; abrupt withdrawal of the drug should be avoided; take at the same time each day; may mask diabetes symptoms; notify physician if any adverse effects occur; use with caution while driving or performing tasks requiring alertness; may be taken without regard to meals

Dosage Forms

Injection: 0.5 mg/mL (10 mL)

Tablet: 25 mg, 50 mg, 100 mg

ATG *see* Lymphocyte Immune Globulin *on page 655*

Atgam® *see* Lymphocyte Immune Globulin *on page 655*

Ativan® *see* Lorazepam *on page 650*

ATnativ® *see* Antithrombin III *on page 83*

Atolone® *see* Triamcinolone *on page 1112*

Atovaquone *(a toe' va kwone)*

Brand Names Mepron™

Use Acute oral treatment of mild to moderate *Pneumocystis carinii* pneumonia (PCP) in patients who are intolerant to co-trimoxazole

Pregnancy Risk Factor C

Contraindications Life-threatening allergic reaction to the drug or formulation

Warnings/Precautions Has only been used in mild to moderate PCP; use with caution in elderly patients due to potentially impaired renal, hepatic, and cardiac function

Adverse Reactions

>10%:

Central nervous system: Headache, fever, insomnia, anxiety

Dermatologic: Rash

Gastrointestinal: Nausea, diarrhea, vomiting

Respiratory: Cough

1% to 10%:

Central nervous system: Asthenia, dizziness

Dermatologic: Pruritus

Endocrine & metabolic: Hypoglycemia, hyponatremia

Gastrointestinal: Abdominal pain, constipation, anorexia, dyspepsia

Hematologic: Anemia, neutropenia, leukopenia

Renal: Elevated creatinine and BUN

Respiratory: Cough

Miscellaneous: Elevated amylase and liver enzymes, oral *Monilia*

Drug Interactions Possible increased toxicity with other highly protein bound drugs

Mechanism of Action Has not been fully elucidated; may inhibit electron transport in mitochondria inhibiting metabolic enzymes

Pharmacodynamics/Kinetics
  Absorption: Decreased significantly in single doses >750 mg; increased threefold when administered with a high fat meal
  Distribution: Enterohepatically recirculated
  Protein binding: >99.9%
  Bioavailability: ~30%
  Half-life: 2.9 days
  Elimination: In feces

Usual Dosage Adults: Oral: 750 mg 3 times/day with food for 21 days

Patient Information Take only prescribed dose; take each dose with a meal, preferably one with high fat content

Dosage Forms Tablet, film coated: 250 mg

Atozine® *see* Hydroxyzine *on page 556*

Atracurium Besylate (a tra kyoo' ree um)

Related Information
  Neuromuscular Blocking Agents Comparison Charts *on page 1276-1278*

Brand Names Tracrium®

Use Drug of choice for neuromuscular blockade in patients with renal and/or hepatic failure; eases endotracheal intubation as an adjunct to general anesthesia and relaxes skeletal muscle during surgery or mechanical ventilation; does not relieve pain

Pregnancy Risk Factor C

Contraindications Hypersensitivity to atracurium besylate or any component

Warnings/Precautions Reduce initial dosage in patients in whom substantial histamine release would be potentially hazardous (eg, patients with clinically important cardiovascular disease); maintenance of an adequate airway and respiratory support is critical

Adverse Reactions Mild, rare, and generally suggestive of histamine release
  1% to 10%: Flushing
  <1%:
    Cardiovascular: Effects are minimal and transient
    Dermatologic: Erythema, itching, hives
    Respiratory: Wheezing, bronchial secretions

  Causes of prolonged neuromuscular blockade:
    Excessive drug administration
    Cumulative drug effect, decreased metabolism/excretion (hepatic and/or renal impairment)
    Accumulation of active metabolites
    Electrolyte imbalance (hypokalemia, hypocalcemia, hypermagnesemia, hypernatremia)
    Hypothermia
    Drug interactions
    Increased sensitivity to muscle relaxants (eg, neuromuscular disorders such as myasthenia gravis or polymyositis)

Overdosage/Toxicology Symptoms of overdose include respiratory depression, cardiovascular collapse. Neostigmine 1-3 mg slow I.V. push in adults (0.5 mg in children) antagonizes the neuromuscular blockade, and should be administered with or immediately after atropine 1-1.5 mg I.V. push (adults). This may be especially useful in the presence of bradycardia.

Drug Interactions Prolonged neuromuscular blockade:
  Inhaled anesthetics:
    Halothane has only a marginal effect, enflurane and isoflurane ↑ the potency and prolong duration of neuromuscular blockade induced by atracurium by 35% to 50%
    Dosage should be reduced by 33% in patients receiving isoflurane or enflurane and by 20% in patients receiving halothane
    Local anesthetics
    Calcium channel blockers
    Corticosteroids
    Antiarrhythmics (eg, quinidine or procainamide)
    Antibiotics (eg, aminoglycosides, tetracyclines, vancomycin, clindamycin)
    Immunosuppressants (eg, cyclosporine)

Stability Refrigerate; unstable in alkaline solutions; **compatible** with D_5W, D_5NS, and NS; do not dilute in LR

Mechanism of Action Blocks neural transmission at the myoneural junction by binding with cholinergic receptor sites

Pharmacodynamics/Kinetics
  Onset of action: I.V.: 2 minutes
  Peak effect: Within 3-5 minutes
  (Continued)

Atracurium Besylate *(Continued)*

Duration: Recovery begins in 20-35 minutes when anesthesia is balanced

Metabolism: Some metabolites are active; undergoes rapid nonenzymatic degradation in the blood stream, additional metabolism occurs via ester hydrolysis

Half-life, biphasic: Adults:

Initial: 2 minutes

Terminal: 20 minutes

Usual Dosage I.V. (not to be used I.M.):

Children 1 month to 2 years: 0.3-0.4 mg/kg initially followed by maintenance doses of 0.3-0.4 mg/kg as needed to maintain neuromuscular blockade

Atracurium Besylate Infusion Chart

Drug Delivery Rate (mcg/kg/min)	Infusion Rate (mL/kg/min) 0.2 mg/mL (20 mg/100 mL)	Infusion Rate (mL/kg/min) 0.5 mg/mL (50 mg/100 mL)
5	0.025	0.01
6	0.03	0.012
7	0.035	0.014
8	0.04	0.016
9	0.045	0.018
10	0.05	0.02

Children >2 years to Adults: 0.4-0.5 mg/kg then 0.08-0.1 mg/kg 20-45 minutes after initial dose to maintain neuromuscular block

Infusions (requires use of an infusion pump): 0.2 mg/mL or 0.5 mg/mL in D$_5$W or NS, see table.

Continuous infusion: Initial: 9-10 mcg/kg/minute followed by 5-9 mcg/kg/minute maintenance

Dosage adjustment for hepatic or renal impairment is not necessary

Administration Give undiluted as a bolus injection; not for I.M. inject, too much tissue irritation; administration requires the use of an infusion pump

Monitoring Parameters Vital signs (heart rate, blood pressure, respiratory rate)

Patient Information May be difficult to talk because of head and neck muscle blockade

Dosage Forms

Injection: 10 mg/mL (5 mL, 10 mL)

Injection, preservative-free: 10 mg/mL (5 mL)

Atrofen™ *see* Baclofen *on page 114*

Atromid-S® *see* Clofibrate *on page 258*

Atropair® *see* Atropine Sulfate *on this page*

Atropine and Diphenoxylate *see* Diphenoxylate and Atropine *on page 352*

Atropine-Care® *see* Atropine Sulfate *on this page*

Atropine Sulfate (a' troe peen)

Related Information

Cycloplegic Mydriatics Comparison *on page 1269*

Brand Names Atropair®; Atropine-Care®; Atropisol®; Isopto® Atropine; I-Tropine®; Ocu-Tropine®

Use Preoperative medication to inhibit salivation and secretions; treatment of sinus bradycardia; management of peptic ulcer; treat exercise-induced bronchospasm; antidote for organophosphate pesticide poisoning; produce mydriasis and cycloplegia for examination of the retina and optic disc and accurate measurement of refractive errors; uveitis

Pregnancy Risk Factor C

Contraindications Hypersensitivity to atropine sulfate or any component; narrow-angle glaucoma; tachycardia; thyrotoxicosis; obstructive disease of the GI tract; obstructive uropathy

Warnings/Precautions Use with caution in children with spastic paralysis; use with caution in elderly patients. Low doses cause a paradoxical decrease in heart rates. Some commercial products contain sodium metabisulfite, which can cause allergic-type reactions. May accumulate with multiple inhalational administration, particularly in the elderly. Heat prostration may occur in hot weather. Use with caution in patients with autonomic neuropathy, prostatic hypertrophy, hyperthyroidism, congestive heart failure, cardiac arrhythmias, chronic lung disease, biliary tract disease; anticholinergic agents are generally not well tolerated in the elderly and their use should be avoided when possible; atropine is rarely used except as a preoperative agent or in the acute treatment of bradyarrhythmias.

Adverse Reactions

>10%:
Dermatologic: Dry, hot skin
Gastrointestinal: Impaired GI motility, constipation
Local: Irritation at injection site
Miscellaneous: Decreased sweating; dry mouth, nose, throat
1% to 10%: Decreased flow of breast milk, difficulty in swallowing, increased sensitivity to light
<1%:
Cardiovascular: Orthostatic hypotension, tachycardia, palpitations, ventricular fibrillation
Central nervous system: Confusion, drowsiness, ataxia, weakness, fatigue, delirium, headache, loss of memory, restlessness; the elderly may be at increased risk for confusion and hallucinations
Dermatologic: Skin rash
Gastrointestinal: Bloated feeling, nausea, vomiting
Genitourinary: Difficult urination
Neuromuscular & skeletal: Tremor
Ocular: Increased intraocular pain, blurred vision, mydriasis

Overdosage/Toxicology Symptoms of overdose include dilated, unreactive pupils; blurred vision; hot, dry flushed skin; dryness of mucous membranes; difficulty in swallowing, foul breath, diminished or absent bowel sounds, urinary retention, tachycardia, hyperthermia, hypertension, increased respiratory rate.

Anticholinergic toxicity is caused by strong binding of the drug to cholinergic receptors. Anticholinesterase inhibitors reduce acetylcholinesterase, the enzyme that breaks down acetylcholine and thereby allows acetylcholine to accumulate and compete for receptor binding with the offending anticholinergic. For anticholinergic overdose with severe life-threatening symptoms, physostigmine 1-2 mg (0.5 or 0.02 mg/kg for children) S.C. or I.V., slowly may be given to reverse these effects.

Drug Interactions

Decreased effect: Phenothiazines, levodopa, antihistamines with cholinergic mechanisms decrease anticholinergic effects of atropine
Increased toxicity: Amantadine increases anticholinergic effects, thiazides increase effect

Stability Store injection at <40°C, avoid freezing

Mechanism of Action Blocks the action of acetylcholine at parasympathetic sites in smooth muscle, secretory glands and the CNS; increases cardiac output, dries secretions, antagonizes histamine and serotonin

Pharmacodynamics/Kinetics

Absorption: Well absorbed from all dosage forms
Distribution: Widely distributes throughout the body; crosses the placenta; trace amounts appear in breast milk; crosses the blood-brain barrier
Metabolism: In the liver
Half-life: 2-3 hours
Elimination: Both metabolites and unchanged drug (30% to 50%) are excreted into urine

Usual Dosage

Children:
Preanesthetic: I.M., I.V., S.C.:
≤5 kg: 0.02 mg/kg/dose 30-60 minutes preop then every 4-6 hours as needed
>5 kg: 0.01-0.02 mg/kg/dose to a maximum 0.4 mg 30-60 minutes preop; minimum dose: 0.1 mg
Bradycardia: I.V., intratracheal: 0.02 mg/kg every 5 minutes
Minimum dose: 0.1 mg (if administered via endotracheal tube, dilute to 1-2 mL with normal saline prior to endotracheal administration)
Maximum single dose: 0.5 mg (adolescents: 1 mg)
Total maximum dose: 1 mg (adolescents: 2 mg)
When using to treat bradycardia in neonates, reserve use for those patients unresponsive to improved oxygenation
Organophosphate or carbamate poisoning: I.V.: 0.02-0.05 mg/kg every 10-20 minutes until atropine effect (dry flushed skin, tachycardia, mydriasis, fever) is observed then every 1-4 hours for at least 24 hours
Bronchospasm: Inhalation: 0.03-0.05 mg/kg/dose 3-4 times/day; maximum: 1 mg
Ophthalmic, 0.5% solution: Instill 1-2 drops twice daily for 1-3 days before the procedure
(Continued)

Atropine Sulfate *(Continued)*

Adults (doses <0.5 mg have been associated with paradoxical bradycardia):

Asystole: I.V.: 1 mg; may repeat every 3-5 minutes as needed; may give intratracheal in 1 mg/10 mL dilution only, intratracheal dose should be 2-2.5 times the I.V. dose

Preanesthetic: I.M., I.V., S.C.: 0.4-0.6 mg 30-60 minutes preop and repeat every 4-6 hours as needed

Bradycardia: I.V.: 0.5-1 mg every 5 minutes, not to exceed a total of 3 mg or 0.04 mg/kg; may give intratracheal in 1 mg/10 mL dilution only, intratracheal dose should be 2-2.5 times the I.V. dose

Neuromuscular blockade reversal: I.V.: 25-30 mcg/kg 30 seconds before neostigmine or 10 mcg/kg 30 seconds before edrophonium

Organophosphate or carbamate poisoning: I.V.: 1-2 mg/dose every 10-20 minutes until atropine effect (dry flushed skin, tachycardia, mydriasis, fever) is observed, then every 1-4 hours for at least 24 hours; up to 50 mg in first 24 hours and 2 g over several days may be given in cases of severe intoxication

Bronchospasm: Inhalation: 0.025-0.05 mg/kg/dose every 4-6 hours as needed (maximum: 5 mg/dose)

Ophthalmic solution: 1%: Instill 1-2 drops 1 hour before the procedure

Uveitis: Instill 1-2 drops 4 times/day

Ophthalmic ointment: Apply a small amount in the conjunctival sac up to 3 times/day; compress the lacrimal sac by digital pressure for 1-3 minutes after instillation

Monitoring Parameters Heart rate, blood pressure, pulse, mental status; intravenous administration requires a cardiac monitor

Patient Information Maintain good oral hygiene habits because lack of saliva may increase chance of cavities. Observe caution while driving or performing other tasks requiring alertness, as drug may cause drowsiness, dizziness, or blurred vision. Notify physician if skin rash, flushing, or eye pain occurs, or if difficulty in urinating, constipation, or sensitivity to light becomes severe or persists. Do not allow dropper bottle or tube to touch eye during administration.

Nursing Implications Observe for tachycardia if patient has cardiac problems

Dosage Forms

Injection: 0.1 mg/mL (5 mL, 10 mL); 0.3 mg/mL (1 mL, 30 mL); 0.4 mg/mL (1 mL, 20 mL, 30 mL); 0.5 mg/mL (1 mL, 5 mL, 30 mL); 0.8 mg/mL (0.5 mL, 1 mL); 1 mg/mL (1 mL, 10 mL)

Ointment, ophthalmic: 0.5%, 1% (3.5 g)

Solution, ophthalmic: 0.5% (1 mL, 5 mL); 1% (1 mL, 2 mL, 5 mL, 15 mL); 2% (1 mL, 2 mL); 3% (5 mL)

Tablet: 0.4 mg

Tablet, soluble: 0.4 mg, 0.6 mg

Atropisol® *see* Atropine Sulfate *on page 100*

Atrovent® *see* Ipratropium Bromide *on page 590*

Attapulgite *(at a pull' gite)*

Brand Names Children's Kaopectate® [OTC]; Diasorb® [OTC]; Kaopectate® Advanced Formula [OTC]; Kaopectate® Maximum Strength Caplets; Rheaban® [OTC]

Use Symptomatic treatment of diarrhea

Contraindications Hypersensitivity to any component

Warnings/Precautions Use with caution in patients <3 years or >60 years of age or in presence of high fever

Adverse Reactions The powder, if chronically inhaled, can cause pneumoconiosis, since it contains large amounts of silica

1% to 10%: Constipation (dose related)

<1%: Fecal impaction

Overdosage/Toxicology Attapulgite is physiologically inert; upon oral ingestion it swells into a mass that can be up to 12 times the volume of the dry powder, which may cause intestinal obstruction. With an oral ingestion of the dry powder, dilution with 4-8 oz of water for adults (no more than 15 mL/kg in children) along with saline catharsis (magnesium citrate 4 mL/kg) usually prevents any powder-induced intestinal obstruction.

Drug Interactions Decreased GI absorption of orally administered clindamycin, tetracyclines, penicillamine, digoxin

Mechanism of Action Controls diarrhea because of its absorbent action

Pharmacodynamics/Kinetics Absorption: Not absorbed from GI tract

Usual Dosage Oral:

Children:

<3 years: Not recommended

3-6 years: 750 mg/dose up to 2250 mg/24 hours

6-12 years: 1200-1500 mg/dose up to 4500 mg/24 hours

Adults: 1200-1500 mg after each loose bowel movement or every 2 hours; 15-30 mL up to 8 times/day, up to 9000 mg/24 hours

Patient Information If diarrhea is not controlled in 48 hours, contact a physician

Nursing Implications Shake well before giving, dilute accordingly

Dosage Forms

Liquid, oral concentrate: 600 mg/15 mL (180 mL, 240 mL, 360 mL, 480 mL); 750 mg/15 mL (120 mL)

Tablet: 750 mg

Tablet, chewable: 300 mg, 600 mg

Attenuvax® see Measles Virus Vaccine, Live on page 670

Augmentin® see Amoxicillin and Clavulanic Acid on page 67

Auranofin (au rane' oh fin)

Brand Names Ridaura®

Use Management of active stage of classic or definite rheumatoid arthritis in patients that do not respond to or tolerate other agents; psoriatic arthritis; adjunctive or alternative therapy for pemphigus

Pregnancy Risk Factor C

Contraindications Renal disease, history of blood dyscrasias, congestive heart failure, exfoliative dermatitis, necrotizing enterocolitis, history of anaphylactic reactions

Warnings/Precautions NSAIDs and corticosteroids may be discontinued after starting gold therapy; therapy should be discontinued if platelet count falls to <100,000/mm^3; WBC <4000, granulocytes <1500/mm^3, explain possibility of adverse effects and their manifestations; use with caution in patients with renal or hepatic impairment

Adverse Reactions

>10%:

Dermatologic: Itching, skin rash

Gastrointestinal: Stomatitis

Ocular: Conjunctivitis

Renal: Proteinuria

1% to 10%:

Dermatologic: Hives, alopecia

Gastrointestinal: Glossitis

Hematologic: Eosinophilia, leukopenia, thrombocytopenia, hematuria

<1%:

Dermatologic: Angioedema

Gastrointestinal: Ulcerative enterocolitis, GI hemorrhage, gingivitis, metallic taste

Hematologic: Agranulocytosis, anemia, aplastic anemia

Hepatic: Hepatotoxicity

Neuromuscular & skeletal: Peripheral neuropathy

Respiratory: Interstitial pneumonitis

Miscellaneous: Difficulty in swallowing

Overdosage/Toxicology Symptoms of overdose include hematuria, proteinuria, fever, nausea, vomiting, diarrhea; signs of gold toxicity include decrease in hemoglobin, leukopenia, granulocytes and platelets, proteinuria, hematuria, pruritus, stomatitis or persistent diarrhea; advise patients to report any symptoms of toxicity; metallic taste may indicate stomatitis

Mild gold poisoning: Dimercaprol 2.5 mg/kg 4 times/day for 2 days or for more severe forms of gold intoxication, dimercaprol 3 mg/kg every 4 hours for 2 days, should be initiated; after 2 days the initial dose should be repeated twice daily on the third day and once daily thereafter for 10 days; other chelating agents have been used with some success

Drug Interactions Increased toxicity: Penicillamine, antimalarials, hydroxychloroquine, cytotoxic agents, immunosuppressants

Stability Store in tight, light-resistant containers at 15°C to 30°C

Mechanism of Action The exact mechanism of action of gold is unknown; gold is taken up by macrophages which results in inhibition of phagocytosis and lysosomal membrane stabilization; other actions observed are decreased serum rheumatoid factor and alterations in immunoglobulins. Additionally, complement activation is decreased, prostaglandin synthesis is inhibited, and lysosomal enzyme activity is decreased.

Usual Dosage Oral:

Children: Initial: 0.1 mg/kg/day divided daily; usual maintenance: 0.15 mg/kg/day in 1-2 divided doses; maximum: 0.2 mg/kg/day in 1-2 divided doses

(Continued)

Auranofin *(Continued)*

Adults: 6 mg/day in 1-2 divided doses; after 3 months may be increased to 9 mg/day in 3 divided doses; if still no response after 3 months at 9 mg/day, discontinue drug

Dosing adjustment in renal impairment:
Cl_{cr} 50-80 mL/minute: Reduce dose to 50%
Cl_{cr} <50 mL/minute: Avoid use

Monitoring Parameters Monitor urine for protein; CBC and platelets; monitor for mouth ulcers and skin reactions; may monitor auranofin serum levels

Reference Range Gold: Normal: 0-0.1 µg/mL (SI: 0-0.0064 µmol/L); Therapeutic: 1-3 µg/mL (SI: 0.06-0.18 µmol/L); Urine: <0.1 µg/24 hours

Test Interactions May enhance the response to a tuberculin skin test

Patient Information Minimize exposure to sunlight; benefits from drug therapy may take as long as 3 months to appear; notify physician of pruritus, rash, sore mouth; metallic taste may occur; take shortly after a meal or light snack, can be given as bedtime dose if drowsiness occurs; optimum effect may take 2-4 weeks to be achieved; avoid alcohol; be aware of possible photosensitivity reaction; may cause painful erections; avoid sudden changes in position

Nursing Implications Discontinue therapy if platelet count falls <100,000/mm³

Dosage Forms Capsule: 3 mg [29% gold]

Aureomycin® *see* Chlortetracyline Hydrochloride *on page 234*

Auro® Ear Drops [OTC] *see* Carbamide Peroxide *on page 179*

Aurothioglucose *(aur oh thye oh gloo' kose)*

Brand Names Solganal®

Use Adjunctive treatment in adult and juvenile active rheumatoid arthritis; alternative or adjunct in treatment of pemphigus; psoriatic patients who do not respond to NSAIDs

Pregnancy Risk Factor C

Contraindications Renal disease, history of blood dyscrasias, congestive heart failure, exfoliative dermatitis, hepatic disease, SLE, history of hypersensitivity

Warnings/Precautions Use with caution in patients with impaired renal or hepatic function; NSAIDs and corticosteroids may be discontinued over time after initiating gold therapy; explain the possibility of adverse reactions before initiating therapy; pregnancy should be ruled out before therapy is started; therapy should be discontinued if platelet counts fall to <100,000/mm³, WBC <4000, granulocytes <1500/mm³

Adverse Reactions

>10%:
Dermatologic: Itching, skin rash, exfoliative dermatitis, reddened skin
Gastrointestinal: Gingivitis, glossitis, metallic taste, stomatitis

1% to 10%: Renal: Proteinuria

<1%:
Central nervous system: Encephalitis, EKG abnormalities, fever
Dermatologic: Alopecia
Gastrointestinal: Ulcerative enterocolitis
Genitourinary: Vaginitis
Hematologic: Agranulocytosis, aplastic anemia, eosinophilia, leukopenia, thrombocytopenia
Hepatic: Hepatotoxicity
Respiratory: Pharyngitis, bronchitis, pulmonary fibrosis, interstitial pneumonitis
Neuromuscular & skeletal: Peripheral neuropathy
Ocular: Conjunctivitis, corneal ulcers, iritis
Renal: Glomerulitis, hematuria, nephrotic syndrome
Miscellaneous: Anaphylactic shock, allergic reaction (severe)

Overdosage/Toxicology Symptoms of overdose include hematuria, proteinuria, fever, nausea, vomiting, diarrhea; signs of gold toxicity include decrease in hemoglobin, leukopenia, granulocytes and platelets; proteinuria, hematuria, pruritus, stomatitis, persistent diarrhea, rash, or metallic taste; advise patients to report any symptoms of toxicity.

For mild gold poisoning, dimercaprol 2.5 mg/kg 4 times/day for 2 days or for more severe forms of gold intoxication, dimercaprol 3-5 mg/kg every 4 hours for 2 days, should be initiated; then after 2 days the initial dose should be repeated twice daily on the third day, and once daily thereafter for 10 days; other chelating agents have been used with some success

Drug Interactions Increased toxicity: Penicillamine, antimalarials, hydroxychloroquine, cytotoxic agents, immunosuppressants

Stability Protect from light and store at 15°C to 30°C

Mechanism of Action Unknown, may decrease prostaglandin synthesis or may alter cellular mechanisms by inhibiting sulfhydryl systems

Pharmacodynamics/Kinetics
Absorption: I.M.: Erratic and slow
Distribution: Crosses placenta; appears in breast milk
Protein binding: 95% to 99%
Half-life: 3-27 days (half-life dependent upon single or multiple dosing)
Time to peak serum concentration: Within 4-6 hours
Elimination: 70% renal excretion; 30% fecal

Usual Dosage I.M.: Doses should initially be given at weekly intervals
Children 6-12 years: Initial: 0.25 mg/kg/dose first week; increment at 0.25 mg/kg/dose increasing with each weekly dose; maintenance: 0.75-1 mg/kg/dose weekly not to exceed 25 mg/dose to a total of 20 doses, then every 2-4 weeks

Adults: 10 mg first week; 25 mg second and third week; then 50 mg/week until 800 mg to 1 g cumulative dose has been given; if improvement occurs without adverse reactions, give 25-50 mg every 2-3 weeks, then every 3-4 weeks

Administration Administer by deep I.M. injection into the upper outer quadrant of the gluteal region

Monitoring Parameters CBC with differential, platelet count, urinalysis, baseline renal and liver function tests

Reference Range Gold: Normal: 0-0.1 µg/mL (SI: 0-0.0064 µmol/L); Therapeutic: 1-3 µg/mL (SI: 0.06-0.18 µmol/L); Urine: <0.1 µg/24 hours

Patient Information Minimize exposure to sunlight; benefits from drug therapy may take as long as 3 months to appear; notify physician of pruritus, rash, sore mouth; metallic taste may occur

Nursing Implications Therapy should be discontinued if platelet count falls <100,000/mm³; vial should be thoroughly shaken before withdrawing a dose; explain the possibility of adverse reactions before initiating therapy; advise patients to report any symptoms of toxicity

Dosage Forms Suspension, sterile: 50 mg/mL [gold 50%] (10 mL)

Autoplex T® *see* Anti-Inhibitor Coagulant Complex *on page 83*

AVC™ Cream *see* Sulfanilamide *on page 1043*

AVC™ Suppository *see* Sulfanilamide *on page 1043*

Aventyl® Hydrochloride *see* Nortriptyline Hydrochloride *on page 808*

Avitene® *see* Microfibrillar Collagen Hemostat *on page 739*

Avlosulfon® *see* Dapsone *on page 303*

Axid® *see* Nizatidine *on page 803*

Axotal® *see* Butalbital Compound *on page 153*

Aygestin® *see* Norethindrone *on page 805*

Ayr® [OTC] *see* Sodium Chloride *on page 1012*

Azactam® *see* Aztreonam *on page 108*

Azatadine Maleate (a za' ta deen)

Brand Names Optimine®
Use Treatment of perennial and seasonal allergic rhinitis and chronic urticaria
Pregnancy Risk Factor B
Contraindications Hypersensitivity to azatadine or to other related antihistamines including cyproheptadine; patients taking monoamine oxidase inhibitors should not use azatadine
Warnings/Precautions Sedation and somnolence are the most commonly reported adverse effects
Adverse Reactions
>10%:
Central nervous system: Slight to moderate drowsiness
Miscellaneous: Thickening of bronchial secretions
1% to 10%:
Central nervous system: Headache, fatigue, nervousness, dizziness
Gastrointestinal: Appetite increase, weight increase nausea, diarrhea, abdominal pain, dry mouth
Neuromuscular & skeletal: Arthralgia
Respiratory: Pharyngitis
<1%:
Cardiovascular: Palpitations, edema
Central nervous system: Depression
Dermatologic: Angioedema, photosensitivity, rash
(Continued)

105

Azatadine Maleate *(Continued)*

Hepatic: Hepatitis
Neuromuscular & skeletal: Myalgia, paresthesia
Respiratory: Bronchospasm
Miscellaneous: Epistaxis

Overdosage/Toxicology Symptoms of overdose include CNS depression or stimulation, dry mouth, flushed skin, fixed and dilated pupils, apnea.

There is no specific treatment for an antihistamine overdose, however, most of its clinical toxicity is due to anticholinergic effects. Anticholinesterase inhibitors may be useful by reducing acetylcholinesterase; anticholinesterase inhibitors include physostigmine, neostigmine, pyridostigmine, and edrophonium. For anticholinergic overdose with severe life-threatening symptoms, physostigmine 1-2 mg (0.5 or 0.02 mg/kg for children) I.V., slowly may be given to reverse these effects.

Drug Interactions Increased effect/toxicity: Procarbazine, CNS depressants, tricyclic antidepressants, alcohol

Mechanism of Action Azatadine is a piperidine-derivative antihistamine; has both anticholinergic and antiserotonin activity; has been demonstrated to inhibit mediator release from human mast cells *in vitro*; mechanism of this action is suggested to prevent calcium entry into the mast cell through voltage-dependent calcium channels

Pharmacodynamics/Kinetics

Absorption: Oral: Rapid and extensive
Half-life, elimination: ~8.7 hours
Elimination: ~20% of dose excreted unchanged in urine over 48 hours

Usual Dosage Children >12 years and Adults: Oral: 1-2 mg twice daily

Patient Information May cause drowsiness; avoid alcohol; can impair coordination and judgment

Nursing Implications Assist with ambulation

Dosage Forms Tablet: 1 mg

Azathioprine *(ay za thye' oh preen)*

Brand Names Imuran®

Use Adjunct with other agents in prevention of rejection of solid organ transplants; also used in severe active rheumatoid arthritis unresponsive to other agents; **azathioprine is an imidazolyl derivative of 6-mercaptopurine**

Pregnancy Risk Factor D

Contraindications Hypersensitivity to azathioprine or any component; pregnancy and lactation

Warnings/Precautions Chronic immunosuppression increases the risk of neoplasia; has mutagenic potential to both men and women and with possible hematologic toxicities; use with caution in patients with liver disease, renal impairment; monitor hematologic function closely

Adverse Reactions Dose reduction or temporary withdrawal allows reversal
>10%:
Central nervous system: Fever, chills
Gastrointestinal: Nausea, vomiting, anorexia, diarrhea
Hematologic: Thrombocytopenia, leukopenia, secondary infection, anemia
1% to 10%:
Dermatologic: Skin rash
Hematologic: Pancytopenia
Hepatic: Hepatotoxicity
<1%:
Cardiovascular: Hypotension
Dermatologic: Alopecia, rash, maculopapular rash, Aphthous stomatitis
Neuromuscular & skeletal: Arthralgias, which include myalgias, rigors
Ocular: Retinopathy
Respiratory: Dyspnea
Miscellaneous: Rare hypersensitivity reactions

Overdosage/Toxicology Symptoms of overdose include nausea, vomiting, diarrhea, hematologic toxicity. Following initiation of essential overdose management, symptomatic and supportive treatment should be instituted. Dialysis has been reported to remove significant amounts of the drug and its metabolites, and should be considered as a treatment option in those patients who deteriorate despite established forms of therapy.

Drug Interactions Increased toxicity: Allopurinol (reduce azathioprine dose to 1/3 to 1/4 of normal dose)

Stability

Stability of parenteral admixture at room temperature (25°C): 24 hours; at refrigeration (4°C): 16 days

Stable in neutral or acid solutions, but is hydrolyzed to mercaptopurine in alkaline solutions

Mechanism of Action Antagonizes purine metabolism and may inhibit synthesis of DNA, RNA, and proteins; may also interfere with cellular metabolism and inhibit mitosis

Pharmacodynamics/Kinetics
Distribution: Crosses the placenta
Protein binding: ~30%
Metabolism: Extensively by hepatic xanthine oxidase to 6-mercaptopurine (active)
Half-life:
Parent drug: 12 minutes
6-mercaptopurine: 0.7-3 hours
End stage renal disease: Slightly prolonged
Elimination: Small amounts eliminated as unchanged drug; metabolites eliminated eventually in urine

Usual Dosage I.V. dose is equivalent to oral dose
Children and Adults: Renal transplantation: Oral, I.V.: 3-5 mg/kg/day to start, then 1-3 mg/kg/day maintenance

Adults: Rheumatoid arthritis: Oral: 1 mg/kg/day for 6-8 weeks; increase by 0.5 mg/kg every 4 weeks until response or up to 2.5 mg/kg/day

Dosing adjustment in renal impairment:
Cl_{cr} 10-50 mL/minute: Administer 75% of normal dose
Cl_{cr} <10 mL/minute: Administer 50% of normal dose
Slightly dialyzable (5% to 20%); administer dose posthemodialysis

Administration Can be administered IVP over 5 minutes at a concentration not to exceed 10 mg/mL **or** azathioprine can be further diluted with normal saline or D_5W and administered by intermittent infusion over 15-60 minutes

Monitoring Parameters CBC, platelet counts, total bilirubin, alkaline phosphatase

Patient Information Response in rheumatoid arthritis may not occur for up to 3 months; do not stop taking without the physician's approval, do not have any vaccinations before checking with your physician; check with your physician if you have a persistent sore throat, unusual bleeding or bruising, or fatigue

Dosage Forms
Injection, as sodium: 100 mg (20 mL)
Tablet (scored): 50 mg

Extemporaneous Preparations A 50 mg/mL suspension compounded from twenty (20) 50 mg tablets, distilled water, Cologel® 5 mL, and then adding 2:1 simple syrup/cherry syrup mixture to a total volume of 20 mL, was stable for 8 weeks when stored in the refrigerator
Handbook on Extemporaneous Formulations, Bethesda MD: American Society of Hospital Pharmacists, 1987.

Azdone® *see* Hydrocodone and Aspirin *on page 544*

Azidothymidine *see* Zidovudine *on page 1173*

Azithromycin (az ith roe mye′ sin)
Brand Names Zithromax™
Use Treatment of mild to moderate upper and lower respiratory tract infections, infections of the skin and skin structure, and sexually transmitted diseases due to susceptible strains of *C. trachomatis, M. catarrhalis, H. influenzae, S. aureus, S. pneumoniae, Mycoplasma pneumoniae*, and *C. psittaci*
Pregnancy Risk Factor C
Contraindications Hepatic impairment, known hypersensitivity to azithromycin, other macrolide antibiotics, or any Zithromax™ components
Warnings/Precautions Use with caution in patients with hepatic dysfunction; hepatic impairment with or without jaundice has occurred chiefly in older children and adults; it may be accompanied by malaise, nausea, vomiting, abdominal colic, and fever; discontinue use if these occur; may mask or delay symptoms of incubating gonorrhea or syphilis, so appropriate culture and susceptibility tests should be performed prior to initiating azithromycin; pseudomembranous colitis has been reported with use of macrolide antibiotics
Adverse Reactions
1% to 10%: Gastrointestinal: Diarrhea, nausea, abdominal pain, cramping, vomiting
<1%:
Cardiovascular: Ventricular arrhythmias
Central nervous system: Fever headache, dizziness
Dermatologic: Rash, eosinophilia, angioedema
(Continued)
107

Azithromycin *(Continued)*

Genitourinary: Vaginitis
Hepatic: Elevated LFTs, cholestatic jaundice
Local: Thrombophlebitis
Otic: Ototoxicity
Renal: Nephritis
Miscellaneous: Hypertrophic pyloric stenosis, allergic reactions

Overdosage/Toxicology Symptoms of overdose include nausea, vomiting, diarrhea, prostration; treatment is supportive and symptomatic

Drug Interactions
Decreased peak serum levels: Aluminum- and magnesium-containing antacids by 24% but not total absorption
Increased effect/toxicity: Azithromycin increases levels of alfentanil, anticoagulants, astemizole, terfenadine, loratadine, bromocriptine, carbamazepine, cyclosporine, digoxin, disopyramide, theophylline, and triazolam

Mechanism of Action Inhibits RNA-dependent protein synthesis at the chain elongation step; binds to the 50S ribosomal subunit resulting in blockage of transpeptidation

Pharmacodynamics/Kinetics
Absorption: Rapid from the GI tract
Distribution: Extensive tissue distribution
Protein binding: 7% to 50% (concentration-dependent)
Metabolism: In the liver
Bioavailability: 37%, decreased by food
Half-life, terminal: 68 hours
Peak serum concentration: 2.3-4 hours
Elimination: 4.5% to 12% of dose is excreted in urine; 50% of dose is excreted unchanged in bile

Usual Dosage Oral:
Children: Not currently FDA approved for use in children; dosages of 10 mg/kg on day 1 followed by 5 mg/kg/day once daily on days 2-5 have been used in clinical trials
Adolescents ≥16 years and Adults:
Respiratory tract, skin, and soft tissue infections: 500 mg on day 1 (in two divided doses), 250 mg/day on days 2-5
Uncomplicated chlamydial urethritis or cervicitis: Single 1 g dose

Monitoring Parameters Liver function tests, CBC with differential

Patient Information Cream is for topical application to the skin only; avoid contact with the eye; avoid taking antacids at the same time as ketoconazole; may take with food; may cause drowsiness, impair judgment or coordination. Notify physician of unusual fatigue, anorexia, vomiting, dark urine, or pale stools; removal of the curl from permanently waved hair may occur.

Dosage Forms Capsule, as dihydrate: 250 mg

Azmacort™ *see* Triamcinolone *on page 1112*

Azo Gantrisin® *see* Sulfisoxazole and Phenazopyridine *on page 1047*

Azo-Standard® *see* Phenazopyridine Hydrochloride *on page 866*

AZT *see* Zidovudine *on page 1173*

Azthreonam *see* Aztreonam *on this page*

Aztreonam *(az' tree oh nam)*

Related Information
Antimicrobial Drugs of Choice *on page 1298-1302*

Brand Names Azactam®

Synonyms Azthreonam

Use Treatment of patients with documented aerobic gram-negative bacillary infection in which beta-lactam therapy is contraindicated (eg, penicillin or cephalosporin allergy); used for urinary tract infections, lower respiratory tract infections, septicemia, skin/skin structure infections, intra-abdominal infections, and gynecological infections; as part of a multiple-drug regimen for the empirical treatment of neutropenic fever in persons with a history of beta-lactam allergy or with known multidrug-resistant organisms

Pregnancy Risk Factor B

Contraindications Hypersensitivity to aztreonam or any component

Warnings/Precautions Check hypersensitivity to other beta-lactams; may have cross-allergenicity to penicillins and cephalosporins; requires dosage reduction in renal impairment

Adverse Reactions
1% to 10%:
Dermatologic: Rash vomiting

Gastrointestinal: Diarrhea, nausea

Local: Thrombophlebitis, pain at injection site

<1%:

Cardiovascular: Hypotension

Central nervous system: Seizures, confusion, headache, vertigo, insomnia, dizziness, numb tongue, weakness, fever

Endocrine & metabolic: Breast tenderness

Gastrointestinal: Pseudomembranous colitis

Genitourinary: Vaginitis

Hepatic: Hepatitis, jaundice, elevation of liver enzymes

Hematologic: Thrombocytopenia, eosinophilia, leukopenia, neutropenia

Neuromuscular & skeletal: Muscular aches

Ocular: Diplopia

Otic: Tinnitus

Respiratory: Sneezing

Miscellaneous: Anaphylaxis, aphthous ulcer, altered taste, halitosis

Overdosage/Toxicology Symptoms of overdose include seizures; if necessary, dialysis can reduce the drug concentration in the blood

Stability

Reconstituted solutions are colorless to light yellow straw and may turn pink upon standing without affecting potency; use reconstituted solutions and I.V. solutions (in NS and D_5W) within 48 hours if kept at room temperature or 7 days if kept in refrigerator

Stability of I.V. infusion solution is 48 hours at room temperature (25°C) and 7 days at refrigeration (4°C)

Mechanism of Action Monobactam which is active only against gram-negative bacilli (unlikely cross-allergenicity with other beta-lactams); inhibits bacterial cell wall synthesis during active multiplication, causing cell wall destruction

Pharmacodynamics/Kinetics

Absorption: I.M.: Well absorbed; I.M. and I.V. doses produce comparable serum concentrations

Distribution: Relative diffusion of antimicrobial agents from blood into cerebrospinal fluid (CSF): Good only with inflammation (exceeds usual MICs)

V_d:

Neonates: 0.26-0.36 L/kg

Children: 0.2-0.29 L/kg

Adults: 0.2 L/kg

Ratio of CSF to blood level (%):

Inflamed meninges: 8-40

Normal meninges: ~1

Protein binding: 56%

Metabolism: Partial

Half-life:

Neonates:

<7 days, ≤2.5 kg: 5.5-9.9 hours

<7 days, >2.5 kg: 2.6 hours

1 week to 1 month: 2.4 hours

Children 2 months to 12 years: 1.7 hours

Normal renal function: 1.7-2.9 hours

End stage renal disease: 6-8 hours

Time to peak: Within 60 minutes (I.M., I.V. push) and 90 minutes (I.V. infusion)

Elimination: 60% to 70% excreted unchanged in urine and partially in feces

Usual Dosage

Neonates: I.M., I.V.:

Postnatal age ≤7 days:

<2000 g: 30 mg/kg/dose every 12 hours

>2000 g: 30 mg/kg/dose every 8 hours

Postnatal age >7 days:

<1200 g: 30 mg/kg/dose every 12 hours

1200-2000 g: 30 mg/kg/dose every 8 hours

>2000 g: 30 mg/kg/dose every 6 hours

Children >1 month: I.M., I.V.: 90-120 mg/kg/day divided every 6-8 hours

Cystic fibrosis: 50 mg/kg/dose every 6-8 hours (ie, up to 200 mg/kg/day); maximum: 6-8 g/day

Adults:

Urinary tract infection: I.M., I.V.: 500 mg to 1 g every 8-12 hours

Moderately severe systemic infections: 1 g I.V. or I.M. or 2 g I.V. every 8-12 hours

Severe systemic or life-threatening infections (especially caused by *Pseudomonas aeruginosa*): I.V.: 2 g every 6-8 hours; maximum: 8 g/day

Dosing adjustment in renal impairment:

Cl_{cr} 30-50 mL/minute: Administer every 12 hours

Cl_{cr} 10-30 mL/minute: Administer every 24 hours

(Continued)

Aztreonam *(Continued)*

Cl$_{cr}$ <10 mL/minute: Administer every 48 hours

Hemodialysis: Moderately dialyzable (20% to 50%); administer dose postdialysis or supplemental dose of 500 mg after dialysis

Peritoneal dialysis: Administer as for Cl$_{cr}$ <10 mL/minute

Continuous arterio-venous or veno-venous hemofiltration (CAVH/CAVHD): Removes 50 mg of aztreonam per liter of filtrate per day

Administration Administer by IVP over 3-5 minutes or by intermittent infusion over 20-60 minutes at a final concentration not to exceed 20 mg/mL; administer around-the-clock rather than 3 times/day to promote less variation in peak and trough serum levels

Monitoring Parameters Periodic liver function test

Test Interactions Urine glucose (Clinitest®)

Nursing Implications Obtain specimens for culture and sensitivity before the first dose

Dosage Forms Powder for injection: 500 mg (15 mL, 100 mL); 1 g (15 mL, 100 mL); 2 g (15 mL, 100 mL)

Azulfidine® *see* Sulfasalazine *on page 1043*

Azulfidine® EN-tabs® *see* Sulfasalazine *on page 1043*

Babee Teething® [OTC] *see* Benzocaine *on page 121*

B-A-C® *see* Butalbital Compound *on page 153*

Bacid® [OTC] *see Lactobacillus acidophilus* and *Lactobacillus bulgaricus on page 617*

Baciguent® [OTC] *see* Bacitracin *on next page*

Baci-IM® *see* Bacitracin *on next page*

Bacillus Calmette-Guérin (ba cill´ us kall met´ gwair en´)

Related Information

Vaccines *on page 1386-1388*

Brand Names TheraCys™; TICE® BCG

Synonyms BCG

Use Immunization against tuberculosis and immunotherapy for cancer; treatment of bladder cancer

BCG vaccine is not routinely recommended for use in the U.S. for prevention of tuberculosis

BCG vaccine is strongly recommended for infants and children with negative tuberculin skin tests who:

are at high risk of intimate and prolonged exposure to persistently untreated or ineffectively treated patients with infectious pulmonary tuberculosis, and

cannot be removed from the source of exposure, and

cannot be placed on long-term preventive therapy

are continuously exposed with tuberculosis who have bacilli resistant to isoniazid and rifampin

BCG is also recommended for tuberculin-negative infants and children in groups in which the rate of new infections exceeds 1% per year and for whom the usual surveillance and treatment programs have been attempted but are not operationally feasible

BCG should be administered with caution to persons in groups at high risk for HIV infection or persons known to be severely immunocompromised. Although limited data suggest that the vaccine may be safe for use in asymptomatic children infected with HIV, BCG vaccination is not recommended for HIV infected adults or for persons with symptomatic disease. Until further research can clearly define the risks and benefits of BCG vaccination for this population, vaccination should be restricted to persons at exceptionally high risk for tuberculosis infection. HIV infected persons thought to be infected with *Mycobacterium tuberculosis* should be strongly recommended for tuberculosis preventive therapy.

Pregnancy Risk Factor C

Contraindications Tuberculin-positive individual, hypersensitivity to BCG vaccine or any component, immunocompromized and burn patients; pregnancy, unless this is unavoidable exposure to infectious tuberculosis

Warnings/Precautions Protection against tuberculosis is only relative, not permanent, nor entirely predictable; for live bacteria vaccine, proper aseptic technique and disposal of all equipment in contact with BCG vaccine as a biohazardous material is recommended; systemic reactions have been reported in patients treated as immunotherapy for bladder cancer

Adverse Reactions

1% to 10%:

Genitourinary: Bladder infection, dysuria, urinary frequency, prostatitis

Miscellaneous: Flu-like syndrome

<1%:

Dermatologic: Skin ulceration, abscesses

Hematologic: Hematuria

Miscellaneous: Rarely anaphylactic shock in infants, lymphadenitis, tuberculosis in immunosuppressed patients

Drug Interactions Decreased effect: Antimicrobial or immunosuppressive drugs may impair response to BCG or increase risk of infection; antituberculosis drugs

Stability Refrigerate, protect from light, use within 2 (TICE® BCG) hours of mixing

Mechanism of Action BCG live is an attenuated strain of Bacillus Calmette-Guérin used as a biological response modifier; BCG live, when used intravesicular for treatment of bladder carcinoma *in situ*, is thought to cause a local, chronic inflammatory response involving macrophage and leukocyte infiltration of the bladder. By a mechanism not fully understood, this local inflammatory response leads to destruction of superficial tumor cells of the urothelium. Evidence of systemic immune response is also commonly seen, manifested by a positive PPD tuberculin skin test reaction, however, its relationship to clinical efficacy is not well-established. BCG is active immunotherapy which stimulates the host's immune mechanism to reject the tumor.

Usual Dosage Children >1 month and Adults:

Immunization against tuberculosis: 0.2-0.3 mL percutaneous; initial lesion usually appears after 10-14 days consisting of small red papule at injection site and reaches maximum diameter of 3 mm in 4-6 weeks; conduct postvaccinal tuberculin test in 2-3 months; if test is negative, repeat vaccination

Immunotherapy for bladder cancer: TICE® BCG vaccine 6 x 10^8 viable organisms in 50 mL NS (preservative free) instilled into bladder and retained for 2 hours weekly for 6 weeks

Administration Should only be given intravesicularly or percutaneously; **do not give I.V., S.C., or intradermally;** can be used for bladder irrigation

Test Interactions PPD intradermal test

Patient Information Notify physician of persistent pain on urination or blood in urine

Dosage Forms Freeze-dried suspension for reconstitution

Injection: 50 mg (2 mL)

Injection, intravesical: 27 mg (3 vials)

Bacitracin (bass i tray' sin)

Related Information

Antimicrobial Drugs of Choice *on page 1298-1302*

Brand Names AK-Tracin®; Baciguent® [OTC]; Baci-IM®

Use Treatment of susceptible bacterial infections (staphylococcal pneumonia and empyema); due to toxicity risks, systemic and irrigant uses of bacitracin should be limited to situations where less toxic alternatives would not be effective; oral administration has been successful in antibiotic-associated colitis

Pregnancy Risk Factor C

Contraindications Hypersensitivity to bacitracin or any component; I.M. use is contraindicated in patients with renal impairment

Warnings/Precautions Prolonged use may result in overgrowth of nonsusceptible organisms; I.M. use may cause renal failure due to tubular and glomerular necrosis; **do not administer intravenously** because severe thrombophlebitis occurs

Adverse Reactions

1% to 10%:

Cardiovascular: Sweating, hypotension

Dermatologic: Rash, itching

Gastrointestinal: Anorexia, nausea, vomiting, diarrhea

Hematologic: Blood dyscrasias

Respiratory: Tightness of chest

Miscellaneous: Swelling of lips and face, rectal itching and burning, pain

Overdosage/Toxicology Symptoms of overdose include nephrotoxicity (parenteral), nausea, vomiting (oral)

Drug Interactions Increased toxicity: Nephrotoxic drugs, neuromuscular blocking agents, and anesthetics (increased neuromuscular blockade)

Stability Sterile powder should be stored in the refrigerator; do not use diluents containing parabens. For I.M. use; bacitracin sterile powder should be dissolved in 0.9% sodium chloride injection containing 2% procaine hydrochloride; once reconstituted, bacitracin is stable for 1 week under refrigeration (2°C to 8°C).

(Continued)

111

Bacitracin *(Continued)*

Mechanism of Action Inhibits bacterial cell wall synthesis by preventing transfer of mucopeptides into the growing cell wall

Pharmacodynamics/Kinetics

Duration of action: 6-8 hours

Absorption: Poor from mucous membranes and intact or denuded skin; rapidly absorbed following I.M. administration; not absorbed by bladder irrigation, but absorption can occur from peritoneal or mediastinal lavage

Distribution: Relative diffusion of antimicrobial agents from blood into cerebrospinal fluid (CSF): Nil even with inflammation

Protein binding: Minimally bound to plasma proteins

Time to peak serum concentration: I.M.: Within 1-2 hours

Elimination: Slow elimination into urine with 10% to 40% of dose excreted within 24 hours

Usual Dosage Do not administer I.V.:

Infants: I.M.:

<2.5 kg: 900 units/kg/day in 2-3 divided doses

≥2.5 kg: 1000 units/kg/day in 2-3 divided doses

Children: I.M.: 800-1200 units/kg/day divided every 8 hours

Adults: Not recommended

Antibiotic-associated colitis: Adults: Oral: 25,000 units 4 times/day for 7-10 days

Topical: Apply 1-4 times/day to infected area

Ophthalmic ointment: Instill ¼" to ½" ribbon every 3-4 hours into conjunctival sac for acute infections or 2-3 times/day for mild to moderate infections for 7-10 days

Irrigation, solution: 50-100 units/mL in normal saline, lactated Ringer's, or sterile water for irrigation; soak sponges in solution for topical compresses 1-5 times/day or as needed during surgical procedures

Administration For I.M. administration, confirm any orders for parenteral use; pH of urine should be kept >6 by using sodium bicarbonate; bacitracin sterile powder should be dissolved in 0.9% sodium chloride injection containing 2% procaine hydrochloride; do not use diluents containing parabens

Monitoring Parameters I.M.: Urinalysis, renal function tests

Patient Information

Ophthalmic ointment may cause blurred vision; do not share eye medications with others

Ophthalmic administration: Tilt head back, place medication in conjunctival sac and close eyes; apply light finger pressure on lacrimal sac for 1 minute following instillation

Topical bacitracin should not be used for longer than 1 week unless directed by a physician

Additional Information 1 unit is equivalent to 0.026 mg

Dosage Forms

Injection: 50,000 units

Ointment:

Ophthalmic: 500 units/g (1 g, 3.5 g, 3.75 g)

Topical: 500 units/g (0.94 g, 15 g, 30 g, 454 g)

Bacitracin and Polymyxin B *(bass i tray' sin)*

Brand Names AK-Poly-Bac®; Polysporin®

Use Treatment of superficial infections caused by susceptible organisms

Pregnancy Risk Factor C

Contraindications Hypersensitivity to polymyxin, bacitracin, or any component; epithelial herpes simplex keratitis, mycobacterial or fungal infections; topical ointments for external use only

Warnings/Precautions Prolonged use may result in overgrowth of nonsusceptible organisms

Adverse Reactions 1% to 10%: Local: Rash, itching, burning, anaphylactoid reactions, swelling and conjunctival erythema

Mechanism of Action Refer to individual monographs for Bacitracin and Polymyxin B

Usual Dosage Children and Adults:

Ophthalmic ointment: Instill ½" ribbon in the affected eye(s) every 3-4 hours for acute infections or 2-3 times/day for mild to moderate infections for 7-10 days

Topical ointment/powder: Apply to affected area 1-4 times/day; may cover with sterile bandage if needed

Patient Information Ophthalmic ointment may cause blurred vision; do not share eye medications with others. Ophthalmic administration: Tilt head back, place medication in conjunctival sac and close eyes; apply light finger pressure on lacrimal sac for 1 minute following instillation.

Dosage Forms Ointment:
  Ophthalmic: Bacitracin 500 units and polymyxin B sulfate 10,000 units per g (3.5 g)
  Topical: Bacitracin 500 units and polymyxin B sulfate 10,000 units per g in white petrolatum (0.94 g, 10 g, 15 g, 30 g)

Bacitracin, Neomycin, and Polymyxin B (bass i tray' sin)

Brand Names Medi-Quick® Ointment [OTC]; Mycitracin® [OTC]; Neomixin®; Neosporin® Ophthalmic Ointment; Neosporin® Topical Ointment [OTC]; Ocutricin® Topical Ointment; Septa® Ointment [OTC]; Triple Antibiotic®

Use Helps prevent infection in minor cuts, scrapes and burns; short-term treatment of superficial external ocular infections caused by susceptible organisms

Pregnancy Risk Factor C

Contraindications Known hypersensitivity to neomycin, polymyxin B, or zinc bacitracin; epithelial herpes simplex keratitis, mycobacterial or fungal infections; topical ointments for external use only

Warnings/Precautions Symptoms of neomycin sensitization include itching, reddening, edema, failure to heal; do not use topical formulation in eyes or in external ear canal if ear drum is perforated. Prolonged use may result in overgrowth of nonsusceptible organisms. Use neomycin with care in treating extensive burns (>20% body surface area) as absorption is possible which may result in nephrotoxicity and ototoxicity. Ophthalmic ointments may retard corneal healing; do not use topical ointment in or near the eyes.

Adverse Reactions 1% to 10%:
  Local: Itching, reddening, edema, failure to heal
  Sensitivity reactions: Allergic contact dermatitis

Mechanism of Action Refer to individual monographs for Bacitracin, Neomycin Sulfate, and Polymyxin B Sulfate

Usual Dosage Children and Adults:
  Ophthalmic ointment: Instill ½" ribbon into the conjunctival sac every 3-4 hours for acute infections or 2-3 times/day for mild to moderate infections for 7-10 days
  Topical: Apply 1-4 times/day to affected areas and cover with sterile bandage if necessary

Patient Information Ophthalmic ointment may cause blurred vision; do not share eye medications with others
  Ophthalmic administration: Tilt head back, place medication in conjunctival sac and close eyes; apply light finger pressure on lacrimal sac for 1 minute following instillation

Dosage Forms Ointment:
  Ophthalmic: Bacitracin 400 units, neomycin sulfate 3.5 mg, and polymyxin b sulfate 10,000 units and per g
  Topical: Bacitracin 400 units, neomycin sulfate 3.5 mg, and polymyxin b sulfate 5000 units per g

Bacitracin, Neomycin, Polymyxin B, and Hydrocortisone (bass i tray' sin)

Brand Names Cortisporin® Ophthalmic Ointment; Cortisporin® Topical Ointment

Use Prevention and treatment of susceptible superficial topical infections

Pregnancy Risk Factor C

Contraindications Hypersensitivity to polymyxin B, bacitracin, neomycin, hydrocortisone or any component

Warnings/Precautions Prolonged use may result in overgrowth of nonsusceptible organisms

Adverse Reactions
  1% to 10%:
    Dermatologic: Rash, generalized itching
    Respiratory: Apnea

Mechanism of Action Refer to individual monographs for Bacitracin, Neomycin, Polymyxin B, and Hydrocortisone

Usual Dosage Children and Adults:
  Ophthalmic:
    Ointment: Instill ½" ribbon to inside of lower lid every 3-4 hours until improvement occurs
    Suspension: Instill 1-2 drops every 15-30 minutes initially, reducing frequency of instillation as infection improves to 4-6 times/day for moderate infections
  Topical: Apply sparingly 2-4 times/day

Patient Information Ophthalmic ointment may cause blurred vision; do not share eye medications with others
(Continued)

Bacitracin, Neomycin, Polymyxin B, and Hydrocortisone *(Continued)*

Ophthalmic administration: Tilt head back, place medication in conjunctival sac and close eyes; apply light finger pressure on lacrimal sac for 1 minute following instillation

Dosage Forms Ointment:

Ophthalmic: Bacitracin 400 units, neomycin sulfate 3.5 mg, polymyxin b sulfate 10,000 units, and hydrocortisone 10 mg per g (3.5 g)

Topical: Bacitracin 400 units, neomycin sulfate 3.5 mg, polymyxin b sulfate 10,000 units, and hydrocortisone 10 mg per g (15 g)

Baclofen (bak′ loe fen)

Brand Names Atrofen™; Lioresal®

Use Treatment of reversible spasticity associated with multiple sclerosis or spinal cord lesions

There are a number of unlabeled uses for baclofen including, intractable hiccups, intractable pain relief, and bladder spasticity

Pregnancy Risk Factor C

Contraindications Hypersensitivity to baclofen or any component

Warnings/Precautions Use with caution in patients with seizure disorder, impaired renal function; avoid abrupt withdrawal of the drug; elderly are more sensitive to the effects of baclofen and are more likely to experience adverse CNS effects at higher doses.

Adverse Reactions

>10%: Central nervous system: Drowsiness, vertigo, dizziness, psychiatric disturbances, insomnia, slurred speech, weakness, ataxia, hypotonia

1% to 10%:

Cardiovascular: Hypotension

Central nervous system: Fatigue, confusion, headache, insomnia

Dermatologic: Rash

Gastrointestinal: Nausea, constipation

Genitourinary: Urinary frequency

<1%:

Cardiovascular: Palpitations, chest pain, syncope

Central nervous system: Euphoria, excitement, depression, hallucinations

Gastrointestinal: Dry mouth, anorexia, taste disorder, abdominal pain, vomiting, diarrhea

Genitourinary: Enuresis, urinary retention, dysuria, impotence, inability to ejaculate, nocturia

Neuromuscular & skeletal: Paresthesia

Renal: Hematuria

Respiratory: Dyspnea

Overdosage/Toxicology Symptoms of overdose include vomiting, muscle hypotonia, salivation, drowsiness, coma, seizures, respiratory depression. Atropine has been used to improve ventilation, heart rate, blood pressure, and core body temperature. Following initiation of essential overdose management, symptomatic and supportive treatment should be instituted.

Drug Interactions

Decreased effect: Lithium

Increased effect: Opiate analgesics, benzodiazepines, hypertensive agents

Increased toxicity: CNS depressants and alcohol (sedation), tricyclic antidepressants (short-term memory loss), clindamycin (neuromuscular blockade), guanabenz (sedation), MAO inhibitors (↓ blood pressure, CNS, and respiratory effects)

Mechanism of Action Inhibits the transmission of both monosynaptic and polysynaptic reflexes at the spinal cord level, possibly by hyperpolarization of primary afferent fiber terminals, with resultant relief of muscle spasticity

Pharmacodynamics/Kinetics

Onset of action: Muscle relaxation effect requires 3-4 days

Peak effect: Maximal clinical effect is not seen for 5-10 days

Absorption: Oral: Rapid; absorption from GI tract is thought to be dose dependent

Protein binding: 30%

Metabolism: Minimally in the liver

Half-life: 3.5 hours

Time to peak serum concentration: Oral: Within 2-3 hours

Elimination: 85% of oral dose excreted in urine and feces as unchanged drug

Usual Dosage
Oral:
Children:
2-7 years: Initial: 10-15 mg/24 hours divided every 8 hours; titrate dose every 3 days in increments of 5-15 mg/day to a maximum of 40 mg/day
≥8 years: Maximum: 60 mg/day in 3 divided doses
Adults: 5 mg 3 times/day, may increase 5 mg/dose every 3 days to a maximum of 80 mg/day
Intrathecal:
Test dose: 50-100 mcg, doses >50 mcg should be given in 25 mcg increments, separated by 24 hours
Maintenance: After positive response to test dose, a maintenance intrathecal infusion can be administered via an implanted intrathecal pump. Initial dose via pump: Infusion at a 24-hourly rate dosed at twice the test dose.

Dosing adjustment in renal impairment: May be necessary to reduce dosage
Test Interactions ↑ alkaline phosphatase, AST, glucose, ammonia (B); ↓ bilirubin (S)
Patient Information Take with food or milk; abrupt withdrawal after prolonged use may cause anxiety, hallucinations, tachycardia or spasticity; may cause drowsiness and impair coordination and judgment
Nursing Implications Epileptic patients should be closely monitored; supervise ambulation; avoid abrupt withdrawal of the drug
Dosage Forms
Injection, intrathecal: 0.5 mg/mL, 2 mg/mL
Tablet: 10 mg, 20 mg

Bacticort® *see* Neomycin, Polymyxin B, and Hydrocortisone *on page 781*

Bactocill® *see* Oxacillin Sodium *on page 821*

Bactrim™ *see* Co-trimoxazole *on page 278*

Bactrim™ **DS** *see* Co-trimoxazole *on page 278*

Bactroban® *see* Mupirocin *on page 760*

Baking Soda *see* Sodium Bicarbonate *on page 1010*

BAL *see* Dimercaprol *on page 349*

Baldex® *see* Dexamethasone *on page 314*

BAL in Oil® *see* Dimercaprol *on page 349*

Bancap® *see* Butalbital Compound *on page 153*

Bancap HC® *see* Hydrocodone and Acetaminophen *on page 543*

Banesin® **[OTC]** *see* Acetaminophen *on page 17*

Banophen® **[OTC]** *see* Diphenhydramine Hydrochloride *on page 351*

Barbidonna® *see* Hyoscyamine, Atropine, Scopolamine, and Phenobarbital *on page 557*

Barbita® *see* Phenobarbital *on page 869*

Barc™ **[OTC]** *see* Pyrethrins *on page 959*

Baridium® *see* Phenazopyridine Hydrochloride *on page 866*

Barophen® *see* Hyoscyamine, Atropine, Scopolamine, and Phenobarbital *on page 557*

Base Ointment *see* Zinc Oxide *on page 1175*

Bayer® **Aspirin [OTC]** *see* Aspirin *on page 92*

BCG *see* Bacillus Calmette-Guérin *on page 110*

BCNU *see* Carmustine *on page 186*

B Complex *see* Vitamin, Multiple *on page 1166*

B Complex With C *see* Vitamin, Multiple *on page 1166*

Beclomethasone Dipropionate (be kloe meth' a sone)
Related Information
Corticosteroids Comparisons *on page 1266-1268*
Brand Names Beclovent®; Beconase®; Beconase AQ®; Vancenase®; Vancenase® AQ; Vanceril®
Use
Oral inhalation: Treatment of bronchial asthma in patients who require chronic administration of corticosteroids
(Continued)

Beclomethasone Dipropionate *(Continued)*

Nasal aerosol: Symptomatic treatment of seasonal or perennial rhinitis and nasal polyposis

Pregnancy Risk Factor C

Pregnancy/Breast Feeding Implications Data does not support an association between drug and congenital defects in humans

Contraindications Status asthmaticus; hypersensitivity to the drug or fluorocarbons, oleic acid in the formulation, systemic fungal infections

Warnings/Precautions Not to be used in status asthmaticus; safety and efficacy in children <6 years of age have not been established; avoid using higher than recommended dosages since suppression of hypothalamic, pituitary, or adrenal function may occur

Adverse Reactions

>10%:

Local: Growth of *Candida* in the mouth, irritation and burning of the nasal mucosa

Respiratory: Cough, hoarseness

1% to 10%:

Gastrointestinal: Dry mouth

Local: Epistaxis, nasal ulceration

<1%:

Central nervous system: Headache

Dermatologic: Skin rash

Respiratory: Bronchospasm, rhinorrhea, nasal stuffiness, sneezing, nasal septal perforations

Miscellaneous: Difficulty in swallowing

Overdosage/Toxicology Nasal symptoms include irritation and burning of the nasal mucosa, sneezing, intranasal and pharyngeal *Candida* infections, nasal ulceration, epistaxis, rhinorrhea, nasal stuffiness, headache. When consumed in excessive quantities for prolonged periods, systemic hypercorticism and adrenal suppression may occur; in those cases discontinuation and withdrawal of the corticosteroid should be done judiciously.

Stability Do not store near heat or open flame

Mechanism of Action Controls the rate of protein synthesis, depresses the migration of polymorphonuclear leukocytes, fibroblasts, reverses capillary permeability, and lysosomal stabilization at the cellular level to prevent or control inflammation

Pharmacodynamics/Kinetics

Therapeutic effect: Within 1-4 weeks of use

Inhalation:

Absorption: Readily absorbed; quickly hydrolyzed by pulmonary esterases prior to absorption

Distribution: 10% to 25% of dose reaches respiratory tract

Oral:

Absorption: 90%

Distribution: Secreted into breast milk

Protein binding: 87%

Metabolism: Hepatic

Half-life:

Initial: 3 hours

Terminal: 15 hours

Elimination: Renal

Usual Dosage Nasal inhalation and oral inhalation dosage forms are not to be used interchangeably

Nasal:

Children 6-12 years: 1 spray in each nostril 3 times/day

Adults: 1 spray in each nostril 2-4 times/day

Oral inhalation:

Children 6-12 years: 1-2 inhalations 3-4 times/day; alternatively 2-4 inhalations twice daily; do not exceed 10 inhalations/day

Adults: 2 inhalations 3-4 times/day; alternatively 2-4 inhalations twice daily; do not exceed 20 inhalations/day

Patient Information Shake thoroughly before using; inhaled beclomethasone makes many asthmatics cough, to reduce chance, inhale drug slowly or use prescribed inhaled bronchodilator 5 minutes before beclomethasone is used; keep inhaler clean and unobstructed, wash in warm water and dry thoroughly, rinse mouth and throat after use to prevent *Candida* infection, report sore throat or mouth lesions to physician

Nursing Implications Take drug history of patients with perennial rhinitis, may be drug related; check mucous membranes for signs of fungal infection

Dosage Forms
Nasal:
Inhalation: (Beconase®, Vancenase®): 42 mcg/inhalation [200 metered doses] (16.8 g)
Spray, aqueous, nasal (Beconase AQ®, Vancenase® AQ): 42 mcg/inhalation [≥200 metered doses] (25 g)
Oral: Inhalation: (Beclovent®, Vanceril®): 42 mcg/inhalation [200 metered doses] (16.8 g)

Beclovent® *see* Beclomethasone Dipropionate *on page 115*

Beconase® *see* Beclomethasone Dipropionate *on page 115*

Beconase AQ® *see* Beclomethasone Dipropionate *on page 115*

Becotin® Pulvules® *see* Vitamin, Multiple *on page 1166*

Beepen-VK® *see* Penicillin V Potassium *on page 854*

Beesix® *see* Pyridoxine Hydrochloride *on page 961*

Beldin® [OTC] *see* Diphenhydramine Hydrochloride *on page 351*

Belix® [OTC] *see* Diphenhydramine Hydrochloride *on page 351*

Belladonna and Opium (bell a don' a)
Brand Names B&O Supprettes®
Synonyms Opium and Belladonna
Use Relief of moderate to severe pain associated with rectal or bladder tenesmus that may occur in postoperative states and neoplastic situations; pain associated with ureteral spasms not responsive to non-narcotic analgesics and to space intervals between injections of opiates
Restrictions C-II
Pregnancy Risk Factor C
Contraindications Glaucoma, severe renal or hepatic disease, bronchial asthma, respiratory depression, convulsive disorders, acute alcoholism, premature labor
Warnings/Precautions Usual precautions of opiate agonist therapy should be observed; infants <3 months of age are more susceptible to respiratory depression, use with caution and generally in reduced doses in this age group
Adverse Reactions
>10%:
Gastrointestinal: Constipation
Local: Irritation at injection site
Miscellaneous: Decreased sweating; dry mouth, nose, throat, or skin
1% to 10%: Decreased flow of breast milk, difficulty in swallowing, increased sensitivity to light
<1%:
Cardiovascular: Orthostatic hypotension, ventricular fibrillation, tachycardia, palpitations
Central nervous system: Confusion, drowsiness, headache, loss of memory, weakness, tiredness, ataxia, CNS depression
Dermatologic: Skin rash
Endocrine & metabolic: Antidiuretic hormone release
Gastrointestinal: Bloated feeling, nausea, vomiting, constipation
Genitourinary: Difficult urination, urinary retention
Ocular: Increased intraocular pain, blurred vision
Respiratory: Respiratory depression
Miscellaneous: Biliary or urinary tract spasm, histamine release, physical and psychological dependence, sweating
Overdosage/Toxicology Primary attention should be directed to ensuring adequate respiratory exchange; opiate agonist-induced respiratory depression may be reversed with parenteral naloxone hydrochloride
Anticholinergic toxicity may be caused by strong binding of a belladonna alkaloid to cholinergic receptors
Anticholinesterase inhibitors reduce acetylcholinesterase, the enzyme that breaks down acetylcholine and thereby allows acetylcholine to accumulate and compete for receptor binding with the offending anticholinergic
For an overdose with severe life-threatening symptoms, physostigmine 1-2 mg (0.5 or 0.02 mg/kg for children) S.C. or I.V., slowly may be given to reverse these effects
Drug Interactions
Decreased effect: Phenothiazines
Increased effect/toxicity: CNS depressants, tricyclic antidepressants
Stability Store at 15°C to 30°C (avoid freezing)
(Continued)

Belladonna and Opium *(Continued)*

Mechanism of Action Anticholinergic alkaloids act primarily by competitive inhibition of the muscarinic actions of acetylcholine on structures innervated by postganglionic cholinergic neurons and on smooth muscle; resulting effects include antisecretory activity on exocrine glands and intestinal mucosa and smooth muscle relaxation. Contains many narcotic alkaloids including morphine; its mechanism for gastric motility inhibition is primarily due to this morphine content; it results in a decrease in digestive secretions, an increase in GI muscle tone, and therefore a reduction in GI propulsion.

Pharmacodynamics/Kinetics

Onset of action:

Belladonna: 1-2 hours

Opium: Within 30 minutes

Metabolism: Opium metabolized in the liver with formation of glucuronide metabolites

Elimination: Belladonna is excreted unchanged in urine

Usual Dosage Adults: Rectal: 1 suppository 1-2 times/day, up to 4 doses/day

Test Interactions ↑ aminotransferase [ALT (SGPT)/AST (SGOT)] (S)

Patient Information May cause drowsiness and blurred vision

Nursing Implications Prior to rectal insertion, the finger and suppository should be moistened; assist with ambulation, monitor for CNS depression

Dosage Forms Suppository:

#15 A: Belladonna extract 15 mg and opium 30 mg

#16 A: Belladonna extract 15 mg and opium 60 mg

Bellergal-S® *see* Ergotamine *on page 399*

Bemote® *see* Dicyclomine Hydrochloride *on page 330*

Benadryl® [OTC] *see* Diphenhydramine Hydrochloride *on page 351*

Benazepril Hydrochloride *(ben ay′ ze prill)*

Related Information

Angiotensin-Converting Enzyme Inhibitors, Comparative Pharmacokinetics *on page 1244*

Angiotensin-Converting Enzyme Inhibitors, Comparisons of Indications and Adult Dosages *on page 1243*

Brand Names Lotensin®

Use Treatment of hypertension, either alone or in combination with other antihypertensive agents

Pregnancy Risk Factor D

Contraindications Hypersensitivity to benazepril or any component or other ACE inhibitors

Warnings/Precautions Use with caution in patients with collagen vascular disease, hypovolemia, valvular stenosis, hyperkalemia, recent anesthesia; modify dosage in patients with renal impairment (especially renal artery stenosis), severe congestive heart failure, or with coadministered diuretic therapy; experience in children is limited; severe hypotension may occur in patients who are sodium and/or volume depleted; initiate lower doses and monitor closely when starting therapy in these patients

Adverse Reactions

1% to 10%:

Central nervous system: Headache, dizziness, fatigue, somnolence, postural dizziness

Gastrointestinal: Nausea

Respiratory: Transient cough

<1%:

Cardiovascular: Hypotension, tachycardia

Central nervous system: Anxiety, insomnia, nervousness, asthenia

Dermatologic: Rash, photosensitivity, angioedema

Endocrine & metabolic: Hyperkalemia

Gastrointestinal: Constipation, gastritis, vomiting, melena

Genitourinary: Impotence, urinary tract infection

Neuromuscular & skeletal: Hypertonia, paresthesia, arthralgia, arthritis, myalgia

Respiratory: Asthma, bronchitis, dyspnea, sinusitis

Miscellaneous: Sweating

Overdosage/Toxicology Mild hypotension has been the only toxic effect seen with acute overdose. Bradycardia may also occur; hyperkalemia occurs even with therapeutic doses, especially in patients with renal insufficiency and those taking NSAIDs. Following initiation of essential overdose management, toxic symptom treatment and supportive treatment should be initiated. Hypotension usually responds to I.V. fluids or Trendelenburg positioning.

Drug Interactions See table.

Drug-Drug Interactions With ACEIs

Precipitant Drug	Drug (Category) and Effect	Description
Antacids	ACE Inhibitors: decreased	Decreased bioavailability of ACEIs. May be more likely with captopril. Separate administration times by 1-2 hours.
NSAIDs (indomethacin)	ACEIs: decreased	Reduced hypotensive effects of ACEIs. More prominent in low renin or volume dependent hypertensive patients.
Phenothiazines	ACEIs: increased	Pharmacologic effects of ACEIs may be increased.
ACEIs	Allopurinol: increased	Higher risk of hypersensitivity reaction possible when given concurrently. Three case reports of Stevens-Johnson syndrome with captopril.
ACEIs	Digoxin: increased	Increased plasma digoxin levels.
ACEIs	Lithium: increased	Increased serum lithium levels and symptoms of toxicity may occur.
ACEIs	Potassium preps/potassium sparing diuretics increased	Coadministration may result in elevated potassium levels.

Mechanism of Action Competitive inhibition of angiotensin I being converted to angiotensin II, a potent vasoconstrictor, through the angiotensin I-converting enzyme (ACE) activity, with resultant lower levels of angiotensin II which causes an increase in plasma renin activity and a reduction in aldosterone secretion

Pharmacodynamics/Kinetics
Reduction in plasma angiotensin-converting enzyme activity: Oral:
Peak effect: 1-2 hours after administration of 2-20 mg dose
Duration of action: >90% inhibition for 24 hours has been observed after 5-20 mg dose
Reduction in blood pressure:
Peak effect after single oral dose: 2-6 hours
Maximum response With continuous therapy: 2 weeks
Absorption: Rapid (37% of each oral dose); food does not alter significantly; metabolite (benazeprilat) itself unsuitable for oral administration due to poor absorption
Distribution: V_d: ~8.7 L
Metabolism: Rapid and extensive in the liver to its active metabolite, benazeprilat, via enzymatic hydrolysis; undergoes significant first-pass metabolism and is completely eliminated from plasma in 4 hours
Half-life:
Parent drug: 0.6 hour
Metabolite elimination: 22 hours (from 24 hours after dosing onward)
Metabolite: 1.5-2 hours after fasting or 2-4 hours after a meal
Time to peak: 1-1.5 hours (unchanged parent drug)
Elimination: Nonrenal clearance (ie, biliary, metabolic) appears to contribute to the elimination of benazeprilat (11% to 12%), particularly in patients with severe renal impairment; hepatic clearance is the main elimination route of unchanged benazepril
Dialysis: ~6% of metabolite was removed by 4 hours of dialysis following 10 mg of benazepril administered 2 hours prior to procedure; parent compound was not found in the dialysate

Usual Dosage Adults: Oral: 20-40 mg/day as a single dose or 2 divided doses; maximum daily dose: 80 mg

Dosing interval in renal impairment: Cl_{cr} <30 mL/minute: Administer 5 mg/day initially; maximum daily dose: 40 mg
Hemodialysis: Moderately dialyzable (20% to 50%); Administer dose postdialysis or administer 25% to 35% supplemental dose
Peritoneal dialysis: Supplemental dose is not necessary

Patient Information May be taken in disregard to meals; notify physician of persistent cough or other side effects; do not stop therapy except under prescriber advice; may cause dizziness, fainting, and lightheadedness, especially in first week of therapy; sit and stand up slowly; may cause changes in taste or rash; do not add a salt substitute (potassium) without advice of physician
(Continued)

Benazepril Hydrochloride *(Continued)*

Nursing Implications Watch for hypotensive effect within 1-3 hours of first dose or new higher dose; discontinue therapy immediately if angioedema of the face, extremities, lips, tongue, or glottis occurs

Dosage Forms Tablet: 5 mg, 10 mg, 20 mg, 40 mg

Benemid® *see* Probenecid *on page 926*

Benoxyl® *see* Benzoyl Peroxide *on page 122*

Bentiromide *(ben teer' oh mide)*

Brand Names Chymex®

Synonyms BTPABA

Use Screening test for pancreatic exocrine insufficiency

Pregnancy Risk Factor B

Contraindications Known hypersensitivity to bentiromide or PABA

Warnings/Precautions Use in renal or hepatic impairment may alter results; GI absorption defects or concurrent GI testing may alter results; repeat dosing should be done no more frequently than every 7 days; epinephrine 1:1000 should be immediately available in case of hypersensitivity reaction

Adverse Reactions

1% to 10%:
    Central nervous system: Headache
    Gastrointestinal: Diarrhea
<1%:
    Central nervous system: Weakness, drowsiness
    Gastrointestinal: Flatulence, nausea, vomiting, heartburn
    Hepatic: Elevations in liver function tests

Drug Interactions

Decreased effect: Sulfonamides (decreased efficacy)
Increased toxicity:
    Methotrexate increases free MTX levels
    Salicylates increase therapeutic and toxic effects

Stability Store at room temperature

Mechanism of Action Cleaved by the pancreatic enzyme chymotrypsin causing a release of para-aminobenzoic acid (PABA), percentage of PABA metabolites recovered in urine reflects enzymatic activity of chymotrypsin providing a way of determining pancreatic function

Pharmacodynamics/Kinetics

Metabolism: Rapidly hydrolyzed in the small intestine to free para-aminobenzoic acid (PABA)
Time to peak serum concentration: Oral: Within 2-3 hours
Elimination: 40% to 50% of dose excreted in urine within 6 hours, primarily as conjugated PABA metabolites

Usual Dosage Oral:

Children 6-12 years: 14 mg/kg (maximum dose: 500 mg) followed with 8 oz of water immediately and 2 hours post-dosing and an additional 16 oz of water during hours 2-6 post-dosing
Children >12 years and Adults: Administer following an overnight fast and morning void, single 500 mg dose and follow with 8 oz of water immediately and 2 hours post-dosing and an additional 16 oz of water during hours 2-6 post-dosing

Patient Information Urinate before taking the drug; fast after midnight before taking; stop pancreatic supplements 5 days before the test; insulin requirements in diabetics may need to be altered because of fasting

Nursing Implications Obtain a urine sample 0-6 hours post-dosing. Measure the volume of the collection and retain a 10 mL sample for analysis. If retesting is necessary, separate subsequent administrations by at least 7 day intervals to avoid interference of test results.

Dosage Forms Solution: 500 mg [PABA 170 mg] in propylene glycol 40% (7.5 mL)

Bentyl® Hydrochloride *see* Dicyclomine Hydrochloride *on page 330*

Benylin® DM [OTC] *see* Dextromethorphan *on page 321*

Benylin® Cough Syrup [OTC] *see* Diphenhydramine Hydrochloride *on page 351*

Benylin® Expectorant [OTC] *see* Guaifenesin and Dextromethorphan *on page 517*

Benzac AC Wash® *see* Benzoyl Peroxide *on page 122*

Benzac W Wash® *see* Benzoyl Peroxide *on page 122*

Benzathine Benzylpenicillin see Penicillin G Benzathine, Parenteral on page 849

Benzathine Penicillin G see Penicillin G Benzathine, Parenteral on page 849

Benzazoline Hydrochloride see Tolazoline Hydrochloride on page 1102

Benzene Hexachloride see Lindane on page 636

Benzhexol Hydrochloride see Trihexyphenidyl Hydrochloride on page 1123

Benzmethyzin see Procarbazine Hydrochloride on page 931

Benzocaine (ben' zoe kane)

Brand Names Americaine® [OTC]; Anbesol® [OTC]; Anbesol® Maximum Strength [OTC]; Babee Teething® [OTC]; Benzocol® [OTC]; Benzodent® [OTC]; Chigger-Tox® [OTC]; Cylex® [OTC]; Dermoplast® [OTC]; Foille Medicated First Aid® [OTC]; Foille® [OTC]; Hurricaine®; Lanacane® [OTC]; Maximum Strength Anbesol® [OTC]; Maximum Strength Orajel® [OTC]; Mycinettes® [OTC]; Numzitdent® [OTC]; Numzit Teething® [OTC]; Orabase®-B [OTC]; Orabase®-O [OTC]; Orajel® Brace-Aid Oral Anesthetic [OTC]; Orajel® Mouth-Aid [OTC]; Orajel® Maximum Strength [OTC]; Orasept® [OTC]; Orasol® [OTC]; Oratect® [OTC]; Rhulicaine® [OTC]; Rid-A-Pain® [OTC]; Slim-Mint® [OTC]; Solarcaine® [OTC]; Spec-T® [OTC]; Tanac® [OTC]; Unguentine® [OTC]; Vicks Children's Chloraseptic® [OTC]; Vicks Chloraseptic® Sore Throat [OTC]; ZilaDent® [OTC]

Synonyms Ethyl Aminobenzoate

Use Local anesthetic (ester derivative); temporary relief of pain associated with local anesthetic for pruritic dermatosis, pruritus, minor burns, acute congestive and serious otitis media, swimmer's ear, otitis externa, toothache, minor sore throat pain, canker sores, hemorrhoids, rectal fissures, anesthetic lubricant for passage of catheters and endoscopic tubes; nonprescription diet aid

Pregnancy Risk Factor C

Contraindications Known hypersensitivity to benzocaine, other ester-type local anesthetics, or other components in the formulation; ophthalmic use

Warnings/Precautions Not intended for use when infections are present

Adverse Reactions Dose-related and may result in high plasma levels

1% to 10%:
  Dermatologic: Angioedema
  Local: Contact dermatitis, burning, stinging
<1%:
  Cardiovascular: Edema
  Dermatologic: Tenderness, urticaria
  Genitourinary: Urethritis
  Hematologic: Methemoglobinemia in infants

Overdosage/Toxicology Treatment is primarily symptomatic and supportive; termination of anesthesia by pneumatic tourniquet inflation should be attempted when the agent is administered by infiltration or regional injection. Seizures commonly respond to diazepam, while hypotension responds to I.V. fluids and Trendelenburg positioning. Bradyarrhythmias (when the heart rate is <60) can be treated with I.V., I.M., or S.C. atropine 15 mcg/kg. With the development of metabolic acidosis, I.V. sodium bicarbonate 0.5-2 mEq/kg and ventilatory assistance should be instituted.

Mechanism of Action Benzocaine blocks both the initiation and conduction of nerve impulses by decreasing the neuronal membrane's permeability to sodium ions, which results in inhibition of depolarization with resultant blockade of conduction. As a diet aide, the anesthetic effect appears to decrease the ability to detect degrees of sweetness by taste perception.

Pharmacodynamics/Kinetics
  Absorption: Topical: Poorly absorbed after administration to intact skin, but well absorbed from mucous membranes and traumatized skin
  Metabolism: Hydrolyzed in the plasma and, to a lesser extent, the liver by cholinesterase
  Elimination: Metabolites excreted in urine

Usual Dosage
  Children and Adults:
    Mucous membranes: Dosage varies depending on area to be anesthetized and vascularity of tissues
    Oral mouth/throat preparations: Do not administer for >2 days or in children <2 years of age, unless directed by a physician; refer to specific package labeling
    Topical: Apply to affected area as needed
(Continued)

121

Benzocaine *(Continued)*

Adults: Nonprescription diet aid: 6-15 mg just prior to food consumption, not to exceed 45 mg/day

Patient Information Do not eat for 1 hour after application to oral mucosa; chemical burns should be neutralized before application of benzocaine; avoid application to large areas of broken skin, especially in children

Dosage Forms
Topical for mucous membranes:
Gel: 6% (7.5 g); 20% (2.5 g, 3.75 g, 7.5 g, 30 g)
Liquid: 20% (3.75 mL, 9 mL, 13.3 mL, 30 mL)
Topical for skin disorders:
Aerosol, external use: 5% (92 mL, 105 g); 20% (82.5 mL, 90 mL, 92 mL, 150 mL)
Cream: (30 g, 60 g); 5% (30 g, 1 lb); 6% (28.4 g)
Lotion: (120 mL); 8% (90 mL)
Ointment: 5% (3.5 g, 28 g)
Spray: 5% (97.5 mL); 20% (20 g, 60 g, 120 g, 13.3 mL, 120 mL)
Mouth/throat preparations:
Cream: 5% (10 g)
Gel: 6.3% (7.5 g); 7.5% (7.2 g, 9.45 g, 14.1 g); 10% (6 g, 9.45 g, 10 g, 15 g); 15% (10.5 g); 20% (9.45 g, 14.1 g)
Liquid: (3.7 mL); 5% (8.8 mL); 6.3% (9 mL, 22 mL, 14.79 mL); 10% (13 mL); 20% (13.3 mL)
Lotion: 0.2% (15 mL); 2.5% (15 mL)
Lozenges: 5 mg, 6 mg, 10 mg, 15 mg
Ointment: 20% (30 g)
Paste: 20% (5 g, 15 g)
Nonprescription diet aid:
Candy: 6 mg
Gum: 6 mg

Benzocol® [OTC] *see* Benzocaine *on previous page*

Benzodent® [OTC] *see* Benzocaine *on previous page*

Benzodiazepines Comparison *see page 1256*

Benzonatate *(ben zoe' na tate)*

Brand Names Tessalon® Perles

Use Symptomatic relief of nonproductive cough

Pregnancy Risk Factor C

Contraindications Known hypersensitivity to benzonatate or related compounds (such as tetracaine)

Adverse Reactions
1% to 10%:
Central nervous system: Sedation, headache, dizziness
Dermatologic: Skin rash
Gastrointestinal: GI upset
Neuromuscular & skeletal: Numbness in chest
Ocular: Burning sensation in eyes
Respiratory: Nasal congestion

Overdosage/Toxicology Symptoms of overdose include restlessness, tremor, CNS stimulation. The drug's local anesthetic activity can reduce the patient's gag reflex and, therefore, may contradict the use of ipecac following ingestion, this is especially true when the capsules are chewed. Gastric lavage may be indicated if initiated early on following an acute ingestion or in comatose patients. The remaining treatment is supportive and symptomatic.

Mechanism of Action Tetracaine congener with antitussive properties; suppresses cough by topical anesthetic action on the respiratory stretch receptors

Pharmacodynamics/Kinetics
Onset of action: Therapeutic: Within 15-20 minutes
Duration: 3-8 hours

Usual Dosage Children >10 years and Adults: Oral: 100 mg 3 times/day or every 4 hours up to 600 mg/day

Monitoring Parameters Monitor patient's chest sounds and respiratory pattern

Patient Information Swallow capsule whole (do not break or chew capsule); use of hard candy may increase saliva flow to aid in protecting pharyngeal mucosa

Nursing Implications Change patient position every 2 hours to prevent pooling of secretions in lung; capsules are not to be crushed

Dosage Forms Capsule: 100 mg

Benzoyl Peroxide (ben′ zoe ill)

Brand Names Benoxyl®; Benzac AC Wash®; Benzac W Wash®; BlemErase® [OTC]; Clearsil® [OTC]; Dermoxyl® [OTC]; Desquam-E®; Desquam-X®; Dryox® [OTC]; Fostex® [OTC]; Loroxide® [OTC]; Neutrogena® [OTC]; Oxy-5® [OTC]; Oxy-10® [OTC]; PanOxyl-AQ; PanOxyl® [OTC]; Perfectoderm® [OTC]; Persa-Gel®; Vanoxide® [OTC]

Use Adjunctive treatment of mild to moderate acne vulgaris and acne rosacea

Pregnancy Risk Factor C

Pregnancy/Breast Feeding Implications It is not known whether benzoyl peroxide can cause fetal harm when administered to pregnant women; topical application is generally considered safe for use in pregnancy

Contraindications Known hypersensitivity to benzoyl peroxide, benzoic acid, or any of its components

Warnings/Precautions For external use only; may bleach colored fabrics; avoid contact with eyes, eyelids, lips, and mucous membranes, and highly inflamed or denuded skin; discontinue if burning, swelling, or undue dryness occurs

Adverse Reactions 1% to 10%: Dermatologic: Irritation, contact dermatitis, dryness, erythema, peeling, stinging

Overdosage/Toxicology Symptoms include excessive scaling, erythema, or edema; for treatment, discontinue use; to hasten resolution of adverse effects, use emollients, cool compresses or topical corticosteroids

Drug Interactions Increased toxicity: Benzoyl peroxide potentiates adverse reactions seen with tretinoin

Mechanism of Action Releases free-radical oxygen which oxidizes bacterial proteins in the sebaceous follicles decreasing the number of anaerobic bacteria and irritating free fatty acids

Pharmacodynamics/Kinetics

Absorption: ~5% through the skin; gels are more penetrating than creams

Elimination: Major metabolite, benzoic acid, excreted in urine as benzoate

Usual Dosage Children and Adults:

Cleansers: Wash once or twice daily. control amount of drying or peeling by modifying dose frequency or concentration.

Topical: Apply sparingly once daily. Gradually increase to 2-3 times daily if needed. If excessive dryness or peeling occurs, reduce dose frequency or concentration. If excessive stinging or burning occurs, remove with mild soap and water; resume use the next day.

Patient Information Shake lotion before using; cleanse and make sure skin is dry before applying; may bleach color from fabrics; may be worn under water-based makeup. Improvement should occur within 2 weeks; keep away from eyes, mouth, mucous membranes; expect dryness and peeling; if excessive redness or irritation occurs, discontinue use. Avoid excessive sunlight, sun lamps, or other topical medication unless directed by a physician.

Nursing Implications Watch for signs of systemic infection; granulation may indicate effectiveness

Dosage Forms

Bar: 5% (113 g); 10% (106 g, 113 g)

Cream: 5% (18 g, 113.4 g); 10% (18 g, 28 g, 113.4 g)

Gel: 2.5% (30 g, 42.5 g, 45 g, 57 g, 60 g, 90 g, 113 g); 5% (42.5 g, 45 g, 60 g, 80 g, 90 g, 113.4 g); 10% (30 g, 42.5 g, 45 g, 56.7 g, 60 g, 90 g, 113.4 g, 120 g); 20% (30 g, 60 g)

Liquid: 5% (120 mL, 150 mL, 240 mL); 10% (120 mL, 150 mL, 240 mL)

Lotion: 5% (25 mL, 30 mL); 5.5% (25 mL); 10% (12 mL, 29 mL, 30 mL, 60 mL)

Mask: 5% (30 mL, 60 mL, 60 g)

Benzthiazide (benz thye′ a zide)

Brand Names Aquatag®; Exna®; Hydrex®; Marazide®; Proaqua®

Use Management of mild to moderate hypertension; treatment of edema in congestive heart failure and nephrotic syndrome

Pregnancy Risk Factor D

Contraindications Anuria, renal decompensation, hypersensitivity to benzthiazide or any component, cross-sensitivity with other thiazides and sulfonamide derivatives

Warnings/Precautions Hypokalemia, renal disease, hepatic disease, gout, lupus erythematosus, diabetes mellitus; use with caution in severe renal diseases

Adverse Reactions

1% to 10%:

Cardiovascular: Orthostatic hypotension

Endocrine & metabolic: Hyponatremia, hypokalemia

Gastrointestinal: Anorexia, upset stomach, diarrhea

(Continued)

123

Benzthiazide *(Continued)*

<1%:
- Central nervous system: Drowsiness
- Endocrine & metabolic: Hyperuricemia
- Gastrointestinal: Nausea, vomiting
- Genitourinary: Uremia
- Hematologic: Aplastic anemia, hemolytic anemia, leukopenia, agranulocytosis, thrombocytopenia
- Hepatic: Hepatitis, hepatic function impairment
- Neuromuscular & skeletal: Paresthesia
- Renal: Polyuria
- Miscellaneous: Allergic reactions

Overdosage/Toxicology Symptoms of overdose include hypermotility, diuresis, lethargy, confusion, muscle weakness; following GI decontamination, therapy is supportive with I.V. fluids, electrolytes, and I.V. pressors if needed

Drug Interactions
Decreased effect of oral hypoglycemics; decreased absorption with cholestyramine and colestipol
Increased effect with furosemide and other loop diuretics
Increased toxicity/levels of lithium

Pharmacodynamics/Kinetics
Onset of action: Within 2 hours
Duration: 12 hours

Usual Dosage Oral:
Children: 1-4 mg/kg/day in 3 divided doses
Adults: 50-200 mg/day

Monitoring Parameters Assess weight, I & O reports daily to determine fluid loss; blood pressure, serum electrolytes, BUN, creatinine

Patient Information May be taken with food or milk; take early in day to avoid nocturia; take the last dose of multiple doses no later than 6 PM unless instructed otherwise. A few people who take this medication become more sensitive to sunlight and may experience skin rash, redness, itching, or severe sunburn, especially if sun block SPF ≥15 is not used on exposed skin areas.

Nursing Implications Take blood pressure with patient lying down and standing

Dosage Forms Tablet: 50 mg

Benztropine Mesylate *(benz' troe peen)*

Brand Names Cogentin®

Use Adjunctive treatment of Parkinson's disease; also used in treatment of drug-induced extrapyramidal effects (except tardive dyskinesia) and acute dystonic reactions

Pregnancy Risk Factor C

Contraindications Children <3 years of age, use with caution in older children (dosage not established); patients with narrow-angle glaucoma; hypersensitivity to any component; pyloric or duodenal obstruction, stenosing peptic ulcers; bladder neck obstructions; achalasia; myasthenia gravis

Warnings/Precautions Use with caution in hot weather or during exercise. Elderly patients frequently develop increased sensitivity and require strict dosage regulation - side effects may be more severe in elderly patients with atherosclerotic changes. Use with caution in patients with tachycardia, cardiac arrhythmias, hypertension, hypotension, prostatic hypertrophy (especially in the elderly) or any tendency toward urinary retention, liver or kidney disorders and obstructive disease of the GI or GU tract. When given in large doses or to susceptible patients, may cause weakness and inability to move particular muscle groups.

Adverse Reactions
>10%:
- Gastrointestinal: Constipation
- Miscellaneous: Decreased sweating; dry mouth, nose, throat, or skin
1% to 10%: Decreased flow of breast milk, difficulty in swallowing, increased sensitivity to light
<1%:
- Cardiovascular: Coma, tachycardia, orthostatic hypotension, ventricular fibrillation, palpitations, ataxia
- Central nervous system: Drowsiness, nervousness, hallucinations; the elderly may be at increased risk for confusion and hallucinations, headache, loss of memory, weakness, tiredness
- Dermatologic: Skin rash
- Gastrointestinal: Nausea, vomiting, bloated feeling
- Genitourinary: Difficult urination
- Ocular: Blurred vision, mydriasis, increased intraocular pain

Overdosage/Toxicology Symptoms of overdose include CNS depression, confusion, nervousness, hallucinations, dizziness, blurred vision, nausea, vomiting, hyperthermia

For anticholinergic overdose with severe life-threatening symptoms, physostigmine 1-2 mg (0.5 or 0.02 mg/kg for children) S.C. or I.V., slowly may be given to reverse these effects. Anticholinergic toxicity is caused by strong binding of the drug to cholinergic receptors. Anticholinesterase inhibitors reduce acetylcholinesterase, the enzyme that breaks down acetylcholine and thereby allows acetylcholine to accumulate and compete for receptor binding with the offending anticholinergic.

Drug Interactions
Decreased effect: May increase gastric degradation of levodopa and decrease the amount of levodopa absorbed by delaying gastric emptying - the opposite may be true for digoxin
Increased toxicity: Central anticholinergic syndrome can occur when administered with narcotic analgesics, phenothiazines and other antipsychotics, tricyclic antidepressants, quinidine and some other antiarrhythmics, and antihistamines

Mechanism of Action Thought to partially block striatal cholinergic receptors to help balance cholinergic and dopaminergic activity

Pharmacodynamics/Kinetics
Onset of action:
Oral: Within 1 hour
Parenteral: Within 15 minutes
Duration of action: 6-48 hours (wide range)

Usual Dosage Use in children <3 years of age should be reserved for life-threatening emergencies
Drug-induced extrapyramidal reaction: Oral, I.M., I.V.:
Children >3 years: 0.02-0.05 mg/kg/dose 1-2 times/day
Adults: 1-4 mg/dose 1-2 times/day

Acute dystonia: Adults: I.M., I.V.: 1-2 mg
Parkinsonism: Oral:
Adults: 0.5-6 mg/day in 1-2 divided doses; if one dose is greater, give at bedtime; titrate dose in 0.5 mg increments at 5- to 6-day intervals
Elderly: Initial: 0.5 mg once or twice daily; increase by 0.5 mg as needed at 5-6 days; maximum: 6 mg/day

Patient Information Take after meals or with food if GI upset occurs; do not discontinue drug abruptly; notify physician if adverse GI effects, rapid or pounding heartbeat, confusion, eye pain, rash, fever, or heat intolerance occurs. Observe caution when performing hazardous tasks or those that require alertness such as driving, as may cause drowsiness. Avoid alcohol and other CNS depressants. May cause dry mouth - adequate fluid intake or hard sugar-free candy may relieve. Difficult urination or constipation may occur - notify physician if effects persist; may increase susceptibility to heat stroke.

Nursing Implications No significant difference in onset of I.M. or I.V. injection, therefore, there is usually no need to use the I.V. route. Improvement is sometimes noticeable a few minutes after injection.

Dosage Forms
Injection: 1 mg/mL (2 mL)
Tablet: 0.5 mg, 1 mg, 2 mg

Benzylpenicillin Benzathine see Penicillin G Benzathine, Parenteral on page 849

Benzylpenicillin Potassium see Penicillin G, Parenteral, Aqueous on page 850

Benzylpenicillin Sodium see Penicillin G, Parenteral, Aqueous on page 850

Benzylpenicilloyl-polylysine (ben' zil pen i sill' oil polly lie' seen)
Brand Names Pre-Pen®
Synonyms Penicilloyl-polylysine; PPL
Use Adjunct in assessing the risk of administering penicillin (penicillin or benzylpenicillin) in adults with a history of clinical penicillin hypersensitivity
Pregnancy Risk Factor C
Contraindications Patients known to be extremely hypersensitive to penicillin; systemic or marked local reaction to previous administration
Warnings/Precautions PPL test alone does not identify those patients who react to a minor antigenic determinant and does not appear to predict reliably the occurrence of late reactions. A negative skin test is associated with an incidence of allergic reactions <5% after penicillin administration and a positive skin test is (Continued)

Benzylpenicilloyl-polylysine *(Continued)*

associated with a >20% incidence of allergic reaction after penicillin administration; have epinephrine 1:1000 available.

Adverse Reactions
1% to 10%: Local: Intense local inflammatory response at skin test site
<1%:
Local: Pruritus, erythema, wheal, urticaria, edema
Sensitivity reactions: Systemic allergic reactions occur rarely

Drug Interactions Decreased effect: Corticosteroids and other immunosuppressive agents may inhibit the immune response to the skin test

Stability Refrigerate; discard if left at room temperature for longer than one day

Mechanism of Action Elicits IgE antibodies which produce type I accelerate urticarial reactions to penicillins

Usual Dosage PPL is administered by a scratch technique or by intradermal injection. For initial testing, PPL should always be applied via the scratch technique. **Do not give intradermally to patients who have positive reactions to a scratch test.** PPL test alone does not identify those patients who react to a minor antigenic determinant and does not appear to predict reliably the occurrence of late reactions.

Scratch test: Use scratch technique with a 20-gauge needle to make 3-5 mm nonbleeding scratch on epidermis, apply a small drop of solution to scratch, rub in gently with applicator or toothpick. A positive reaction consists of a pale wheal surrounding the scratch site which develops within 10 minutes and ranges from 5-15 mm or more in diameter.

Intradermal test: Use intradermal test with a tuberculin syringe with a 26- to 30-gauge short bevel needle; a dose of 0.01-0.02 mL is injected intradermally. A control of 0.9% sodium chloride should be injected at least 1.5" from the PPL test site. Most skin responses to the intradermal test will develop within 5-15 minutes.

Interpretation:
(-) Negative: No reaction
(±) Ambiguous: Wheal only slightly larger than original bleb with or without erythematous flare and larger than control site
(+) Positive: Itching and marked increase in size of original bleb
Control site should be reactionless

Nursing Implications Always use scratch test for initial testing

Dosage Forms Solution: 0.25 mL

Bepridil Hydrochloride (be' pri dil)

Related Information
Calcium Channel Blockers Cardiovascular Adverse Reactions *on page 1262*
Calcium Channel Blockers Central Nervous System Adverse Reactions *on page 1264*
Calcium Channel Blockers Comparative Actions *on page 1260*
Calcium Channel Blockers Comparative Pharmacokinetics *on page 1261*
Calcium Channel Blockers FDA-Approved Indications *on page 1263*
Calcium Channel Blockers Gastrointestinal and Miscellaneous Adverse Reactions *on page 1265*

Brand Names Vascor®

Use Treatment of chronic stable angina; due to side effect profile, reserve for patients who have been intolerant of other antianginal therapy; bepridil may be used alone or in combination with nitrates or beta-blockers

Pregnancy Risk Factor C

Contraindications History of serious ventricular or atrial arrhythmias (especially tachycardia or those associated with accessory conduction pathways), sick-sinus syndrome, or second or third degree A-V block (without a functioning pacemaker), cardiogenic shock, hypotension, uncompensated cardiac insufficiency, congenital Q-T interval prolongation, patients taking other drugs that prolong the Q-T interval, history of hypersensitivity to bepridil or any component, calcium channel blockers, or adenosine

Warnings/Precautions Use with great caution in patients with history of serious ventricular arrhythmias, IHSS, congenital Q-T interval prolongation, or other drugs that prolong Q-T interval; reserve for patients in whom other antianginals have failed. Carefully titrate dosages for patients with impaired renal or hepatic function; use caution when treating patients with congestive heart failure, sick-sinus syndrome, severe left ventricular dysfunction, hypertrophic cardiomyopathy (especially obstructive), concomitant therapy with beta-blockers or digoxin, edema, or increased intracranial pressure with cranial tumors; do not abruptly withdraw (may cause chest pain); elderly may experience hypotension and constipation more readily.

Adverse Reactions
>10%:
Central nervous system: Dizziness, asthenia, headache
Gastrointestinal: Nausea, dyspepsia, abdominal pain, GI distress
1% to 10%:
Cardiovascular: Bradycardia, palpitations
Central nervous system: Nervousness
Gastrointestinal: Diarrhea, anorexia
Miscellaneous: Flu syndrome, dry mouth
<1%:
Cardiovascular: Ventricular premature contractions, hypertension, torsade de pointes, edema, syncope, prolonged Q-T intervals
Central nervous system: Fever, psychotic behavior, akathisia
Dermatologic: Rash
Genitourinary: Sexual difficulties
Hematologic: Agranulocytosis
Neuromuscular & skeletal: Tremor, myalgia, arthritis
Ocular: Blurred vision
Respiratory: Nasal congestion, cough, pharyngitis
Miscellaneous: Sweating, taste change

Overdosage/Toxicology The primary cardiac symptoms of calcium blocker overdose includes hypotension and bradycardia. The hypotension is caused by peripheral vasodilation, myocardial depression, and bradycardia. Bradycardia results from sinus bradycardia, second- or third-degree atrioventricular block, or sinus arrest with junctional rhythm. Intraventricular conduction is usually not affected so QRS duration is normal (verapamil does prolong the P-R interval and bepridil prolongs the Q-T and may cause ventricular arrhythmias, including torsade de pointes).

The noncardiac symptoms include confusion, stupor, nausea, vomiting, metabolic acidosis and hyperglycemia. Following initial gastric decontamination, if possible, repeated calcium administration may promptly reverse the depressed cardiac contractility (but not sinus node depression or peripheral vasodilation); glucagon, epinephrine, and amrinone may treat refractory hypotension; glucagon and epinephrine also increase the heart rate (outside the U.S., 4-aminopyridine may be available as an antidote); dialysis and hemoperfusion are not effective in enhancing elimination although repeat-dose activated charcoal may serve as an adjunct with sustained-release preparations.

Drug Interactions
Increased toxicity/effect/levels:
H_2 blockers → ↑ bioavailability of bepridil
Beta-blockers → ↑ cardiac depressant effects on A-V conduction
Carbamazepine → ↑ carbamazepine levels
Cyclosporine → ↑ cyclosporine levels
Fentanyl → ↑ hypotension
Digitalis → ↑ digitalis levels
Quinidine → ↑ quinidine levels (hypotension, bradycardia)
Theophylline → ↑ pharmacologic actions of theophylline

Mechanism of Action Bepridil, a type 4 calcium antagonist, possesses characteristics of the traditional calcium antagonists, inhibiting calcium ion from entering the "slow channels" or select voltage-sensitive areas of vascular smooth muscle and myocardium during depolarization and producing a relaxation of coronary vascular smooth muscle and coronary vasodilation. However, bepridil may also inhibit fast sodium channels (inward), which may account for some of its side effects (eg, arrhythmias); a direct bradycardia effect of bepridil has been postulated via direct action on the S-A node.

Pharmacodynamics/Kinetics
Onset of action: 1 hour
Absorption: Oral: 100%
Distribution: Protein binding: >99%
Metabolism: Hepatic
Bioavailability: 60%
Half-life: 24 hours
Time to peak: 2-3 hours
Elimination: Metabolites renally excreted

Usual Dosage Adults: Oral: Initial: 200 mg/day, then adjust dose at 10-day intervals until optimal response is achieved; maximum daily dose: 400 mg

Monitoring Parameters EKG and serum electrolytes, blood pressure, signs and symptoms of congestive heart failure; elderly may need very close monitoring due to underlying cardiac and organ system defects

Reference Range 1-2 ng/mL

Test Interactions ↑ aminotransferases, ↑ CPK, LDH
(Continued)

127

Bepridil Hydrochloride *(Continued)*

Patient Information May cause cardiac arrhythmias if potassium is low; can be taken with food or meals, maintain potassium supplementation as directed, routine EKGs will be necessary during start of therapy or dosage changes; notify physician if the following occur: irregular heartbeat, shortness of breath, pronounced dizziness, constipation, or hypotension

Nursing Implications EKG required; patient should be hospitalized during initiation or escalation of therapy

Dosage Forms Tablet: 200 mg, 300 mg, 400 mg

Beractant *(ber akt' ant)*

Brand Names Survanta®

Synonyms Bovine Lung Surfactant; Natural Lung Surfactant

Use Prevention and treatment of respiratory distress syndrome (RDS) in premature infants

Prophylactic therapy: Body weight <1250 g in infants at risk for developing or with evidence of surfactant deficiency

Rescue therapy: Treatment of infants with RDS confirmed by x-ray and requiring mechanical ventilation (administer as soon as possible - within 8 hours of age)

Warnings/Precautions Rapidly affects oxygenation and lung compliance and should be restricted to a highly supervised use in a clinical setting with immediate availability of clinicians experienced with intubation and ventilatory management of premature infants. If transient episodes of bradycardia and decreased oxygen saturation occur, discontinue the dosing procedure and initiate measures to alleviate the condition.

Adverse Reactions During the dosing procedure:

Cardiovascular: Transient bradycardia, vasoconstriction, hypotension, hypertension, pallor

Respiratory: Oxygen desaturation, endotracheal tube blockage, hypocarbia, hypercarbia, apnea, pulmonary air leaks, pulmonary interstitial emphysema

Miscellaneous: Increased probability of post-treatment nosocomial sepsis

Stability Refrigerate; protect from light, prior to administration warm by standing at room temperature for 20 minutes or held in hand for 8 minutes; **artificial warming methods should not be used**; unused, unopened vials warmed to room temperature may be returned to the refrigerator within 8 hours of warming only once

Mechanism of Action Replaces deficient or ineffective endogenous lung surfactant in neonates with respiratory distress syndrome (RDS) or in neonates at risk of developing RDS. Surfactant prevents the alveoli from collapsing during expiration by lowering surface tension between air and alveolar surfaces.

Pharmacodynamics/Kinetics Alveolar clearance is rapid

Usual Dosage

Prophylactic treatment: Give 100 mg phospholipids (4 mL/kg) intratracheally as soon as possible; as many as 4 doses may be administered during the first 48 hours of life, no more frequently than 6 hours apart. The need for additional doses is determined by evidence of continuing respiratory distress; if the infant is still intubated and requiring at least 30% inspired oxygen to maintain a PaO_2 ≤80 torr.

Rescue treatment: Give 100 mg phospholipids (4 mL/kg) as soon as the diagnosis of RDS is made

Administration

For intratracheal administration only

Suction infant prior to administration; inspect solution to verify complete mixing of the suspension

Administer intratracheally by instillation through a 5-French end-hole catheter inserted into the infant's endotracheal tube

Administer the dose in four 1 mL/kg aliquots. Each quarter-dose is instilled over 2-3 seconds; each quarter-dose is administered with the infant in a different position; slightly downward inclination with head turned to the right, then repeat with head turned to the left; then slightly upward inclination with head turned to the right, then repeat with head turned to the left.

Monitoring Parameters Continuous EKG and transcutaneous O_2 saturation should be monitored during administration; frequent arterial blood gases are necessary to prevent postdosing hyperoxia and hypocarbia

Nursing Implications Do not shake; if settling occurs during storage, swirl gently

Additional Information

Each mL contains 25 mg phospholipids suspended in 0.9% sodium chloride solution

Contents of 1 mL: 0.5-1.75 mg triglycerides, 1.4-3.5 mg free fatty acids, and <1 mg protein

Dosage Forms Suspension: 200 mg (8 mL)

Berocca® *see* Vitamin, Multiple *on page 1166*

Berubigen® *see* Cyanocobalamin *on page 282*

Beta-2® *see* Isoetharine *on page 593*

Beta-Blockers Comparison *see page 1257*

Beta-Carotene (kare′ oh teen)

Brand Names Max-Caro® [OTC]; Provatene® [OTC]; Solatene®

Use Reduces severity of photosensitivity reactions in patients with erythropoietic protoporphyria (EPP)

Pregnancy Risk Factor C

Contraindications Hypersensitivity to beta-carotene

Warnings/Precautions Use with caution in patients with renal or hepatic impairment; not proven effective as a sunscreen

Adverse Reactions
> >10%: Dermatologic: Carotenodermia (yellowing of palms, hands, or soles of feet, and to a lesser extent the face)

> <1%:
> Central nervous system: Dizziness
> Dermatologic: Ecchymoses
> Gastrointestinal: Diarrhea
> Neuromuscular & skeletal: Arthralgia

Drug Interactions Fulfills vitamin A requirements, do not prescribe additional vitamin A

Mechanism of Action The exact mechanism of action in erythropoietic protoporphyria has not as yet been elucidated; although patient must become carotenemic before effects are observed, there appears to be more than a simple internal light screen responsible for the drug's action. A protective effect was achieved when beta-carotene was added to blood samples. The concentrations of solutions used were similar to those achieved in treated patients. Topically applied beta-carotene is considerably less effective than systemic therapy.

Pharmacodynamics/Kinetics
> Metabolism: Prior to absorption, converted to vitamin A in the wall of the small intestine and then further oxidized to retinoic acid and retinol in the presence of fat and bile acids; small amounts are then stored in the liver; retinol (active) is conjugated with glucuronic acid
> Elimination: In urine and feces

Usual Dosage Oral:
> Children <14 years: 30-150 mg/day
> Adults: 30-300 mg/day

Patient Information Take with meals; skin may appear slightly yellow-orange; not a proven sunscreen

Dosage Forms Capsule: 15 mg, 30 mg

Betachron E-R® *see* Propranolol Hydrochloride *on page 947*

Betadine® [OTC] *see* Povidone-Iodine *on page 913*

9-Beta-D-ribofuranosyladenine *see* Adenosine *on page 30*

Betagan® *see* Levobunolol Hydrochloride *on page 623*

Betalin®S *see* Thiamine Hydrochloride *on page 1079*

Betamethasone (bay ta meth′ a sone)

Related Information
> Corticosteroids Comparisons *on page 1266-1268*

Brand Names Alphatrex®; Betatrex®; Beta-Val®; Celestone®; Cel-U-Jec®; Diprolene®; Diprolene® AF; Diprosone®; Maxivate®; Selestoject®; Teladar®; Urticort®; Valisone®

Synonyms Flubenisolone

Use Inflammatory dermatoses such as seborrheic or atopic dermatitis, neurodermatitis, anogenital pruritus, psoriasis, inflammatory phase of xerosis

Pregnancy Risk Factor C

Pregnancy/Breast Feeding Implications There are no reports linking the use of betamethasone with congenital defects in the literature; betamethasone is often used in patients with premature labor [26-34 weeks gestation] to stimulate fetal lung maturation

Contraindications Systemic fungal infections; hypersensitivity to betamethasone or any component

Warnings/Precautions Use with caution in patients with hypothyroidism, cirrhosis, ulcerative colitis; do not use occlusive dressings on weeping or exudative lesions and general caution with occlusive dressings should be observed;
(Continued)

Betamethasone *(Continued)*

discontinue if skin irritation or contact dermatitis should occur; do not use in patients with decreased skin circulation.

Adverse Reactions

>10%:
Central nervous system: Insomnia
Gastrointestinal: Increased appetite, indigestion
Ocular: Temporary mild blurred vision

1% to 10%:
Endocrine & metabolic: Diabetes mellitus
Local: Erythema, dryness, irritation, papular rashes, burning, itching
Ocular: Cataracts

<1%:
Cardiovascular: Hypertension
Central nervous system: Convulsions, vertigo, confusion, headache
Dermatologic: Thin fragile skin, sterile abscess, hyperpigmentation or hypertrichosis, hypopigmentation, impaired wound healing, acneiform eruptions, perioral dermatitis, maceration of skin, skin atrophy, striae, miliaria
Endocrine & metabolic: Cushingoid state
Gastrointestinal: Peptic ulcer
Genitourinary: Sodium retention
Neuromuscular & skeletal: Muscle weakness, osteoporosis
Ocular: Glaucoma, sudden blindness

Overdosage/Toxicology When consumed in excessive quantities for prolonged periods, systemic hypercorticism and adrenal suppression may occur; in those cases, discontinuation and withdrawal of the corticosteroid should be done judiciously

Drug Interactions Decreased effect (corticosteroid) by barbiturates, phenytoin, rifampin

Mechanism of Action Controls the rate of protein synthesis, depresses the migration of polymorphonuclear leukocytes, fibroblasts, reverses capillary permeability, and lysosomal stabilization at the cellular level to prevent or control inflammation

Pharmacodynamics/Kinetics

Protein binding: 64%
Metabolism: Extensively in the liver
Half-life: 6.5 hours
Time to peak serum concentration: I.V.: Within 10-36 minutes
Elimination: <5% of dose excreted renally as unchanged drug

Usual Dosage

Children:
Oral: 0.0175-0.25 mg/kg/day divided every 6-8 hours **or** 0.5-7.5 mg/m²/day divided every 6-8 hours
I.M.: 0.0175-0.125 mg base/kg/day divided every 6-12 hours **or** 0.5-7.5 mg base/m²/day divided every 6-12 hours

Adults:
Oral: 0.6-7.2 mg/day in 2-4 doses
I.M., I.V.: Betamethasone sodium phosphate: 0.6-9 mg/day divided every 12-24 hours

Betamethasone sodium phosphate/acetate suspension: **not for I.V. use**
I.M.: 0.5-9 mg/day (⅓ to ½ of oral dose administered every 12 hours)
Intrabursal, intra-articular, intradermal, intralesional: 0.25-2 mL
Intralesional: Rheumatoid arthritis/osteoarthritis:
Very large joints: 1-2 mL
Large joints: 1 mL
Medium joints: 0.5-1 mL
Small joints: 0.25-0.5 mL
Topical: Apply thin film 2-4 times/day

Patient Information Take oral with food or milk; apply topical sparingly to areas and gently rub in until it disappears, not for use on broken skin or in areas of infection; do not apply to face or inguinal areas

Nursing Implications

Apply topical sparingly to areas; not for use on broken skin or in areas of infection; do not apply to wet skin unless directed; do not apply to face or inguinal area
Not for alternate day therapy; once daily doses should be given in the morning; do not give injectable sodium phosphate/acetate suspension I.V.

Dosage Forms

Base (Celestone®), Oral:
Syrup: 0.6 mg/5 mL (118 mL)
Tablet: 0.6 mg
Benzoate salt (Uticort®)
Cream: 0.025% (60 g)

Gel: 0.025% (15 g, 60 g)
Lotion: 0.025% (60 mL)
Dipropionate salt (Diprosone®)
Aerosol: 0.1% (85 g)
Cream: 0.05% (15 g, 45 g)
Lotion: 0.05% (20 mL, 30 mL, 60 mL)
Ointment: 0.05% (15 g, 45 g)
Dipropionate salt, augmented (Diprolene®)
Cream: 0.05% (15 g, 45 g)
Gel: 0.05% (15 g, 45 g)
Lotion: 0.05% (30 mL, 60 mL)
Ointment, topical: 0.05% (15 g, 45 g)
Valerate salt (Betatrex®, Beta-Val®, Valisone®)
Cream: 0.01% (15 g, 60 g); 0.1% (15 g, 45 g, 110 g, 430 g)
Lotion: 0.1% (20 mL, 60 mL)
Ointment: 0.1% (15 g, 45 g)
Injection: Sodium phosphate salt (Celestone Phosphate®, Cel-U-®, Seles-toject®): 4 mg betamethasone phosphate/mL (equivalent to 3 mg betamethasone/mL) (5 mL)
Injection, suspension: Sodium phosphate and acetate salt (Celestone® Soluspan®): 6 mg/mL (3 mg of betamethasone sodium phosphate and 3 mg of betamethasone acetate per mL) (5 mL)

Betapace® see Sotalol Hydrochloride on page 1022

Betapen®-VK see Penicillin V Potassium on page 854

Betaseron® see Interferon Beta-1b on page 586

Betatrex® see Betamethasone on page 129

Beta-Val® see Betamethasone on page 129

Betaxolol Hydrochloride (be tax' oh lol)
Related Information
Beta-Blockers Comparison on page 1257-1259
Glaucoma Drug Therapy Comparison on page 1270
Brand Names Betoptic®; Betoptic® S; Kerlone®
Use Treatment of chronic open-angle glaucoma and ocular hypertension; management of hypertension
Pregnancy Risk Factor C
Contraindications Bronchial asthma, sinus bradycardia, second and third degree A-V block, cardiac failure (unless a functioning pacemaker present), cardiogenic shock, hypersensitivity to betaxolol or any component
Warnings/Precautions Some products contain sulfites which can cause allergic reactions; diminished response occurs over time; use with caution in patients with decreased renal or hepatic function (dosage adjustment required); patients with a history of asthma, congestive heart failure, diabetes mellitus, or bradycardia appear to be at a higher risk for adverse effects
Adverse Reactions
1% to 10%:
Cardiovascular: Bradycardia, palpitations, edema, congestive heart failure
Central nervous system: Dizziness, fatigue, lethargy, headache
Dermatologic: Erythema, itching
Ocular: Mild ocular stinging and discomfort, tearing, photophobia, decreased corneal sensitivity, keratitis
Miscellaneous: Cold extremities
<1%:
Cardiovascular: Chest pain
Central nervous system: Nervousness, depression, hallucinations
Hematologic: Thrombocytopenia
Overdosage/Toxicology Symptoms of significant overdose include bradycardia, hypotension, A-V block, CHF, bronchospasm, hypoglycemia. Sympathomimetics (eg, epinephrine or dopamine), glucagon, or a pacemaker can be used to treat the toxic bradycardia, asystole, and/or hypotension; initially, fluids may be the best treatment for toxic hypotension.
Drug Interactions
Decreased effect of beta-blockers with aluminum salts, barbiturates, calcium salts, cholestyramine, colestipol, NSAIDs, penicillins (ampicillin), rifampin, salicylates and sulfinpyrazone due to decreased bioavailability and plasma levels
Beta-blockers may decrease the effect of sulfonylureas
Increased effect/toxicity of beta-blockers with calcium blockers (diltiazem, felodipine, nicardipine), contraceptives, flecainide, haloperidol (propranolol, hypotensive effects), H_2 antagonists (metoprolol, propranolol only by cimetidine,
(Continued)
131

Betaxolol Hydrochloride *(Continued)*

possibly ranitidine), hydralazine (metoprolol, propranolol), loop diuretics (propranolol, not atenolol), MAO inhibitors (metoprolol, nadolol, bradycardia), phenothiazines (propranolol), propafenone (metoprolol, propranolol), quinidine (in extensive metabolizers), ciprofloxacin, thyroid hormones (metoprolol, propranolol, when hypothyroid patient is converted to euthyroid state)

Beta-blockers may increase the effect/toxicity of flecainide, haloperidol (hypotensive effects), hydralazine, phenothiazines, acetaminophen, anticoagulants (propranolol, warfarin), benzodiazepines (not atenolol), clonidine (hypertensive crisis after or during withdrawal of either agent), epinephrine (initial hypertensive episode followed by bradycardia), nifedipine and verapamil lidocaine, ergots (peripheral ischemia), prazosin (postural hypotension)

Beta-blockers may affect the action or levels of ethanol, disopyramide, nondepolarizing muscle relaxants and theophylline although the effects are difficult to predict

Stability Avoid freezing

Mechanism of Action Competitively blocks $beta_1$-receptors, with little or no effect on $beta_2$-receptors; ophthalmic reduces intraocular pressure by reducing the production of aqueous humor

Pharmacodynamics/Kinetics

Onset of action: 1-1.5 hours

Duration: ≥12 hours

Absorption: Systemically absorbed

Metabolism: Hepatic (multiple metabolites)

Half-life: 12-22 hours

Time to peak: Within 2 hours

Elimination: Renal

Usual Dosage Adults:

Ophthalmic: Instill 1 drop twice daily

Oral: 10 mg/day; may increase dose to 20 mg/day after 7-14 days if desired response is not achieved; initial dose in elderly patients: 5 mg/day

Monitoring Parameters Ophthalmic: Intraocular pressure. Systemic: Blood pressure, pulse

Patient Information Intended for twice daily dosing; keep eye open and do not blink for 30 seconds after instillation; wear sunglasses to avoid photophobic discomfort; apply gentle pressure to lacrimal sac during and immediately following instillation (1 minute)

Nursing Implications Monitor for systemic effect of beta blockade

Dosage Forms

Solution, ophthalmic (Betoptic®): 0.5% (2.5 mL, 5 mL, 10 mL)

Suspension, ophthalmic (Betoptic® S): 0.25% (2.5 mL, 10 mL, 15 mL)

Tablet (Kerlone®): 10 mg, 20 mg

Bethanechol Chloride *(be than' e kole)*

Brand Names Duvoid®; Myotonachol™; Urabeth®; Urecholine®

Use Nonobstructive urinary retention and retention due to neurogenic bladder; treatment and prevention of bladder dysfunction caused by phenothiazines; diagnosis of flaccid or atonic neurogenic bladder; gastroesophageal reflux

Pregnancy Risk Factor C

Contraindications Hypersensitivity to bethanechol; do not use in patients with mechanical obstruction of the GI or GU tract or when the strength or integrity of the GI or bladder wall is in question. It is also contraindicated in patients with hyperthyroidism, peptic ulcer disease, epilepsy, obstructive pulmonary disease, bradycardia, vasomotor instability, atrioventricular conduction defects, hypotension, or parkinsonism; **contraindicated for I.M. or I.V. use due to a likely severe cholinergic reaction**

Warnings/Precautions Potential for reflux infection if the sphincter fails to relax as bethanechol contracts the bladder; use with caution when administering to nursing women, as it is unknown if the drug is excreted in breast milk; safety and efficacy in children <5 years of age have not been established; syringe containing atropine should be readily available for treatment of serious side effects; for S.C. injection only; do not give I.M. or I.V.

Adverse Reactions

Oral: <1%:

Cardiovascular: Hypotension, cardiac arrest, flushed skin

Gastrointestinal: Abdominal cramps, diarrhea, nausea, vomiting

Respiratory: Bronchial constriction

Miscellaneous: Sweating, salivation, vasomotor response

Subcutaneous: 1% to 10%:

Cardiovascular: Hypotension, cardiac arrest, flushed skin

Gastrointestinal: Abdominal cramps, diarrhea, nausea, vomiting

Respiratory: Bronchial constriction

Miscellaneous: Sweating, salivation, vasomotor response

Overdosage/Toxicology Symptoms of overdose include nausea, vomiting, abdominal cramps, diarrhea, involuntary defecation, flushed skin, hypotension, bronchospasm

Atropine is the treatment of choice for intoxications manifesting with significant muscarinic symptoms; atropine I.V. 0.6 mg every 3-60 minutes (or 0.01 mg/kg I.V. every 2 hours if needed for children) should be repeated to control symptoms and then continued as needed for 1-2 days following the acute ingestion. Epinephrine 0.1-1 mg S.C. may be useful in reversing severe cardiovascular or pulmonary sequel.

Drug Interactions

Decreased effect: Procainamide, quinidine

Increased toxicity: Bethanechol and ganglionic blockers → critical fall in blood pressure; cholinergic drugs or anticholinesterase agents

Mechanism of Action Stimulates cholinergic receptors in the smooth muscle of the urinary bladder and gastrointestinal tract resulting in increased peristalsis, increased GI and pancreatic secretions, bladder muscle contraction, and increased ureteral peristaltic waves

Pharmacodynamics/Kinetics

Onset of action:

Oral: 30-90 minutes

S.C.: 5-15 minutes

Duration of action:

Oral: Up to 6 hours

S.C.: 2 hours

Absorption: Oral: Variable

Metabolism and elimination have not been determined

Usual Dosage

Children:

Oral:

Abdominal distention or urinary retention: 0.6 mg/kg/day divided 3-4 times/day

Gastroesophageal reflux: 0.1-0.2 mg/kg/dose given 30 minutes to 1 hour before each meal to a maximum of 4 times/day

S.C.: 0.15-0.2 mg/kg/day divided 3-4 times/day

Adults:

Oral: 10-50 mg 2-4 times/day

S.C.: 2.5-5 mg 3-4 times/day, up to 7.5-10 mg every 4 hours for neurogenic bladder

Administration Do **not** administer I.V. or I.M., a severe cholinergic reaction may occur

Monitoring Parameters Observe closely for side effects

Test Interactions ↑ lipase, AST, amylase (S), bilirubin, aminotransferase [ALT (SGPT)/AST (SGOT)] (S)

Patient Information Oral should be taken 1 hour before meals or 2 hours after meals to avoid nausea or vomiting; may cause abdominal discomfort, salivation, sweating or flushing - notify physician if these symptoms become pronounced; rise slowly from sitting/lying down

Nursing Implications Have bedpan readily available, if administered for urinary retention

Dosage Forms

Injection: 5 mg/mL (1 mL)

Tablet: 5 mg, 10 mg, 25 mg, 50 mg

Betoptic® see Betaxolol Hydrochloride on page 131

Betoptic® S see Betaxolol Hydrochloride on page 131

Biamine® see Thiamine Hydrochloride on page 1079

Biavax®ᵢᵢ see Rubella and Mumps Vaccines, Combined on page 989

Biaxin™ Filmtabs® see Clarithromycin on page 252

Bicillin® L-A see Penicillin G Benzathine, Parenteral on page 849

Bicitra® see Sodium Citrate and Citric Acid on page 1013

BiCNU® see Carmustine on page 186

Biltricide® see Praziquantel on page 917

Biocal® [OTC] see Calcium Carbonate on page 161

Biphenabid see Probucol on page 927

Bisac-Evac® [OTC] see Bisacodyl on this page

Bisacodyl (bis a koe' dill)

Related Information
Laxatives, Classification and Properties *on page 1272*

Brand Names
Bisac-Evac® [OTC]; Bisacodyl Uniserts®; Bisco-Lax® [OTC]; Carter's Little Pills® [OTC]; Clysodrast®; Dacodyl® [OTC]; Deficol® [OTC]; Dulcolax® [OTC]; Fleet® Laxative [OTC]; Theralax® [OTC]

Use
Treatment of constipation; colonic evacuation prior to procedures or examination

Pregnancy Risk Factor
C

Contraindications
Do not use in patients with abdominal pain, obstruction, nausea or vomiting; do not administer bisacodyl tannex enema to children <10 years of age

Warnings/Precautions
Bisacodyl tannex should be used with caution in patients with ulceration of the colon and during pregnancy or lactation; safety of bisacodyl tannex usage in children <10 years of age has not been established

Adverse Reactions
<1%:
Central nervous system: Vertigo
Endocrine & metabolic: Electrolyte and fluid imbalance (metabolic acidosis or alkalosis, hypocalcemia)
Gastrointestinal: Mild abdominal cramps, nausea, vomiting, rectal burning

Overdosage/Toxicology
Diarrhea, abdominal pain, electrolyte disturbances

Drug Interactions
Decreased effect: Milk, antacids; decreased effect of warfarin

Mechanism of Action
Stimulates peristalsis by directly irritating the smooth muscle of the intestine, possibly the colonic intramural plexus; alters water and electrolyte secretion producing net intestinal fluid accumulation and laxation

Pharmacodynamics/Kinetics
Onset of action:
Oral: 6-10 hours
Rectal: 0.25-1 hour
Absorption: Oral, rectal: <5% absorbed systemically
Metabolism: In the liver
Elimination: Conjugated metabolites excreted in milk, bile, and urine

Usual Dosage
Children:
Oral: >6 years: 5-10 mg (0.3 mg/kg) at bedtime or before breakfast
Rectal suppository:
<2 years: 5 mg as a single dose
>2 years: 10 mg
Adults:
Oral: 5-15 mg as single dose (up to 30 mg when complete evacuation of bowel is required)
Rectal suppository: 10 mg as single dose
Tannex:
Enema: 2.5 g in 1000 mL warm water
Barium enema: 2.5-5 g in 1000 mL barium suspension
Do not give >10 g within 72-hour period

Administration
Administer tablets 2 hours prior to, or 4 hours after antacids

Patient Information
Swallow tablets whole, do **not** crush or chew; do not take antacid or milk within 1 hour of taking drug

Nursing Implications
Increased pH may dissolve the enteric coating leading to GI distress; do not crush enteric coated drug product

Dosage Forms
Powder, as tannex: 2.5 g packets (50 packet/box)
Suppository, rectal: 5 mg, 10 mg
Tablet, enteric coated: 5 mg

Bisacodyl Uniserts® *see Bisacodyl on this page*

Bisco-Lax® [OTC] *see Bisacodyl on this page*

Bismatrol® [OTC] *see Bismuth on this page*

Bismuth (bis' muth)

Brand Names
Bismatrol® [OTC]; Devrom® [OTC]; Pepto-Bismol® [OTC]; Pink Bismuth® [OTC]

Synonyms
Bismuth Subgallate; Bismuth Subsalicylate

Use
Symptomatic treatment of mild, nonspecific diarrhea; indigestion, nausea, control of traveler's diarrhea (enterotoxigenic *Escherichia coli*); as an adjunct in the treatment of *Helicobacter pylori*-associated peptic ulcer disease

Pregnancy Risk Factor
C (D in 3rd trimester)

Contraindications Do not use subsalicylate in patients with influenza or chickenpox because of risk of Reye's syndrome; do not use in patients with known hypersensitivity to salicylates; history of severe GI bleeding; history of coagulopathy

Warnings/Precautions Subsalicylate should be used with caution if patient is taking aspirin, additive toxicity; use with caution in children <3 years of age; beware of salicylate content when prescribing for use in children

Adverse Reactions
>10%: Discoloration of the tongue (darkening), grayish black stools
<1%:
Central nervous system: Anxiety, confusion, slurred speech, headache, mental depression, weakness
Gastrointestinal: Impaction may occur in infants and debilitated patients
Neuromuscular & skeletal: Muscle spasms
Otic: Loss of hearing, buzzing in ears

Overdosage/Toxicology Symptoms of overdose include tinnitus (subsalicylate), fever. Unusual to develop toxicity from short-term administrations of bismuth salts, and most toxic symptoms occur following subacute or chronic intoxications. Chelation with dimercaprol in doses of 3 mg/kg or penicillamine 100 mg/kg/day for 5 days can hasten recovery from bismuth-induced encephalopathy. When associated with methemoglobinemia, bismuth intoxications should be treated with methylene blue 1-2 mg/kg in a 1% sterile aqueous solution I.V. push over 4-6 minutes. This may be repeated within 60 minutes if necessary, up to a total dose of 7 mg/kg. Seizures usually respond to I.V. diazepam.

Drug Interactions
Decreased effect: Tetracyclines and uricosurics
Increased toxicity: Aspirin, warfarin, hypoglycemics

Mechanism of Action Bismuth subsalicylate exhibits both antisecretory and antimicrobial action. This agent may provide some anti-inflammatory action as well. The salicylate moiety provides antisecretory effect and the bismuth exhibits antimicrobial directly against bacterial and viral gastrointestinal pathogens. Bismuth has some antacid properties.

Pharmacodynamics/Kinetics
Absorption: Minimally absorbed across the GI tract while the salt (eg, salicylate) may be readily absorbed
Metabolism: Undergoes chemical dissociation to various bismuth salts after oral administration

Usual Dosage Oral:
Nonspecific diarrhea: Subsalicylate:
Children: Up to 8 doses/24 hours:
3-6 years: 1/3 tablet or 5 mL every 30 minutes to 1 hour as needed
6-9 years: 2/3 tablet or 10 mL every 30 minutes to 1 hour as needed
9-12 years: 1 tablet or 15 mL every 30 minutes to 1 hour as needed
Adults: 2 tablets or 30 mL every 30 minutes to 1 hour as needed up to 8 doses/24 hours
Prevention of traveler's diarrhea: 2.1 g/day or 2 tablets 4 times/day before meals and at bedtime
Subgallate: 1-2 tablets 3 times/day with meals

Dosing adjustment in renal impairment: Should probably be avoided in patients with renal failure

Test Interactions ↑ uric acid, ↑ AST

Patient Information Chew tablet well or shake suspension well before using; may darken stools; if diarrhea persists for more than 2 days, consult a physician; can turn tongue black, tinnitus may indicate toxicity and use should be discontinued

Nursing Implications Seek causes for diarrhea; monitor for tinnitus; may aggravate or cause gout attack; may enhance bleeding if used with anticoagulants

Dosage Forms
Liquid, as subsalicylate (Pepto-Bismol®, Bismatrol®): 262 mg/15 mL (120 mL, 240 mL, 360 mL, 480 mL); 524 mg/15 mL (120 mL, 240 mL, 360 mL)
Tablet:
Chewable, as subsalicylate (Pepto-Bismol®, Bismatrol®): 262 mg
Chewable, as subgallate (Devrom®): 200 mg

Bismuth Subgallate *see* Bismuth *on previous page*

Bismuth Subsalicylate *see* Bismuth *on previous page*

Bisoprolol Fumarate (bis oh' proe lol)
Related Information
Beta-Blockers Comparison *on page 1257-1259*
Brand Names Zebeta®
(Continued)

Bisoprolol Fumarate *(Continued)*

Use Treatment of hypertension, alone or in combination with other agents
  Unlabeled use: Angina pectoris, supraventricular arrhythmias, PVCs

Contraindications Hypersensitivity to beta-blocking agents, uncompensated congestive heart failure; cardiogenic shock; bradycardia or heart block; sinus node dysfunction; A-V conduction abnormalities. Although bisoprolol primarily blocks beta$_1$-receptors, high doses can result in beta$_2$-receptor blockage. Therefore, use with caution in patients (especially elderly) with bronchospastic lung disease and renal dysfunction.

Warnings/Precautions Use with caution in patients with inadequate myocardial function, bronchospastic disease, hyperthyroidism, undergoing anesthesia; and in those with impaired hepatic function; acute withdrawal may exacerbate symptoms (gradually taper over a 2-week period)

Adverse Reactions
  >10%: Central nervous system: Fatigue, lethargy
  1% to 10%:
    Central nervous system: Headache, dizziness, insomnia, confusion, depression, abnormal dreams
    Cardiovascular: Hypotension, chest pain, heart failure, Raynaud's phenomena, heart block, edema, bradycardia
    Dermatologic: Rash
    Gastrointestinal: Constipation, diarrhea, dyspepsia, nausea, flatulence, anorexia
    Genitourinary: Micturition (frequency), impotence, urinary retention
    Neuromuscular & skeletal: Arthralgia, myalgia
    Ocular: Abnormal vision
    Respiratory: Dyspnea, rhinitis, cough

Overdosage/Toxicology Symptoms of overdose include severe hypotension, bradycardia, heart failure, and bronchospasm, hypoglycemia. Sympathomimetics (eg, epinephrine or dopamine), glucagon, or a pacemaker can be used to treat the toxic bradycardia, asystole, and/or hypotension (I.V. fluids-initial treatment); may be removed by hemodialysis; other treatment is symptomatic and supportive.

Drug Interactions
  Decreased effect/levels with barbiturates, rifampin, sulfinpyrazone
  Increased effect/toxicity/levels of flecainide

Mechanism of Action Selective inhibitor of beta$_1$-adrenergic receptors; competitively blocks beta$_1$-receptors, with little or no effect on beta$_2$-receptors at doses <10 mg

Pharmacodynamics/Kinetics
  Absorption: Rapid and almost complete from GI tract
  Distribution: Distributed widely to body tissues; highest concentrations in heart, liver, lungs, and saliva; crosses the blood-brain barrier; distributes into breast milk
  Protein binding: 26% to 33%
  Metabolism: Significant first-pass metabolism; extensively metabolized in the liver
  Half-life: 9-12 hours
  Time to peak: 1.7-3 hours
  Elimination: In urine (3% to 10% as unchanged drug); <2% excreted in feces

Usual Dosage Oral:
  Adults: 5 mg once daily, may be increased to 10 mg, and then up to 20 mg once daily, if necessary
  Elderly: Initial dose: 2.5 mg/day; may be increased by 2.5-5 mg/day; maximum recommended dose: 20 mg/day

  Dosing adjustment in renal/hepatic impairment: Cl$_{cr}$ <40 mL/minute: Initial: 2.5 mg/day; increase cautiously
  Not dialyzable

Monitoring Parameters Blood pressure, EKG, neurologic status

Test Interactions ↑ thyroxine (S), cholesterol (S), glucose; ↑ triglycerides, uric acid; ↓ HDL

Patient Information Do not discontinue abruptly (angina may be precipitated); notify physician if CHF symptoms become worse or side effects occur; take at the same time each day; may mask diabetes symptoms; consult pharmacist or physician before taking with other adrenergic drugs (eg, cold medications); use with caution while driving or performing tasks requiring alertness; may be taken without regard to meals

Dosage Forms Tablet: 5 mg, 10 mg

Bistropamide *see* Tropicamide *on page 1134*

Bitolterol Mesylate (bye tole' ter ole)

Brand Names Tornalate®

Use Prevention and treatment of bronchial asthma and bronchospasm

Pregnancy Risk Factor C

Contraindications Known hypersensitivity to bitolterol

Warnings/Precautions Use with caution in patients with unstable vasomotor symptoms, diabetes, hyperthyroidism, prostatic hypertrophy or a history of seizures; also use caution in the elderly and those patients with cardiovascular disorders such as coronary artery disease, arrhythmias, and hypertension; excessive use may result in cardiac arrest and death; do not use concurrently with other sympathomimetic bronchodilators

Adverse Reactions

>10%: Neuromuscular & skeletal: Trembling

1% to 10%:

Cardiovascular: Flushing of face, hypertension, pounding heartbeat

Central nervous system: Dizziness, lightheadedness, nervousness

Gastrointestinal: Dry mouth, nausea, unpleasant taste

Respiratory: Bronchial irritation, coughing

<1%:

Cardiovascular: Chest pain, arrhythmias, tachycardia

Central nervous system: Insomnia

Respiratory: Paradoxical bronchospasm

Overdosage/Toxicology Symptoms of overdose include tremor, dizziness, nervousness, headache, nausea, coughing; treatment is symptomatic/supportive; in cases of severe overdose, supportive therapy should be instituted, and prudent use of a cardioselective beta-adrenergic blocker (eg, atenolol or metoprolol) should be considered, keeping in mind the potential for induction of bronchoconstriction in an asthmatic individual. Dialysis has not been shown to be of value in the treatment of an overdose with this agent.

Drug Interactions

Decreased effect: Beta-adrenergic blockers (eg, propranolol)

Increased effect: Inhaled ipratropium → ↑ duration of bronchodilation, nifedipine → ↑ FEV-1

Increased toxicity: MAO inhibitors, tricyclic antidepressants, sympathomimetic agents (eg, amphetamine, dopamine, dobutamine), inhaled anesthetics (eg, enflurane)

Mechanism of Action Selectively stimulates beta$_2$-adrenergic receptors in the lungs producing bronchial smooth muscle relaxation; minor beta$_1$ activity

Pharmacodynamics/Kinetics

Duration of effect: 4-8 hours

Metabolism: Bitolterol, a prodrug, is hydrolyzed to colterol (active) following inhalation

Half-life: 3 hours

Time to peak serum concentration (colterol): Inhalation: Within 1 hour

Elimination: In urine and feces

Usual Dosage Children >12 years and Adults:

Bronchospasm: 2 inhalations at an interval of at least 1-3 minutes, followed by a third inhalation if needed

Prevention of bronchospasm: 2 inhalations every 8 hours; do not exceed 3 inhalations every 6 hours or 2 inhalations every 4 hours

Administration Administer around-the-clock rather than 3 times/day, to promote less variation in peak and trough serum levels

Monitoring Parameters Assess lung sounds, pulse, and blood pressure before administration and during peak of medication; observe patient for wheezing after administration

Patient Information Do not exceed recommended dosage, excessive use may lead to adverse effects or loss of effectiveness; shake canister well before use; administer pressurized inhalation during the second half of inspiration, as the airways are open, water and the aerosol distribution is more extensive. If more than one inhalation per dose is necessary, wait at least 1 full minute between inhalations - second inhalation is best delivered after 10 minutes. May cause nervousness, restlessness, and insomnia; if these effects continue after dosage reduction, notify physician. Also notify physician if palpitations, tachycardia, chest pain, muscle tremors, dizziness, headache, flushing, or if breathing difficulty persists.

Nursing Implications Before using, the inhaler must be shaken well

Dosage Forms Aerosol, oral: 370 mcg/metered spray

Blanex® see Chlorzoxazone on page 236

BlemErase® [OTC] see Benzoyl Peroxide on page 122

Blenoxane® see Bleomycin Sulfate on this page

Bleomycin Sulfate (blee oh mye' sin)

Related Information
Cancer Chemotherapy Regimens *on page 1218-1241*

Brand Names Blenoxane®

Synonyms BLM; NIM

Use Treatment of squamous cell carcinomas, melanomas, sarcomas, testicular carcinomas, Hodgkin's lymphoma, and non-Hodgkin's lymphoma; may also be used as a sclerosing agent for malignant pleural effusion

Pregnancy Risk Factor D

Contraindications Hypersensitivity to bleomycin sulfate or any component, severe pulmonary disease

Warnings/Precautions The U.S. Food and Drug Administration (FDA) currently recommends that procedures for proper handling and disposal of antineoplastic agents be considered. Occurrence of pulmonary fibrosis is higher in elderly patients and in those receiving >400 units total and in smokers and patients with prior radiation therapy; a severe idiosyncratic reaction consisting of hypotension, mental confusion, fever, chills, and wheezing is possible; check lungs prior to each treatment for crackles.

Adverse Reactions
>10%:
Cardiovascular: Raynaud's phenomenon
Central nervous system: Fever, chills
Dermatologic: Pruritic erythema
Emetic potential: Moderately low (10% to 30%)
Gastrointestinal: Stomatitis, nausea, vomiting, anorexia, weight loss
Integument: Approximately 50% of patients will develop erythema, induration, hyperkeratosis, and peeling of the skin. Hyperpigmentation, alopecia, nailbed changes may occur; this appears to be dose-related and is reversible after cessation of therapy.
Irritant chemotherapy
Local: Pain at tumor site, phlebitis
Miscellaneous: Mild febrile reaction, mucocutaneous toxicity, patients may become febrile after intracavitary administration
1% to 10%:
Idiosyncratic: Similar to anaphylaxis and occurs in 1% of lymphoma patients; may include hypotension, confusion, fever, chills, and wheezing. May be immediate or delayed for several hours; symptomatic treatment includes volume expansion, pressor agents, antihistamines, and steroids.
<1%:
Cardiovascular: Myocardial infarction, cerebrovascular accident
Dermatologic: Skin thickening
Hepatic: Hepatotoxicity
Myelosuppressive:
WBC: Rare
Platelets: Rare
Onset (days): 7
Nadir (days): 14
Recovery (days): 21
Renal: Renal toxicity
Respiratory: Tachypnea, rales; dose-related when total dose is >400 units or with single doses >30 units. Pathogenesis is poorly understood, but may be related to damage of pulmonary, vascular, or connective tissue. Manifested as an acute or chronic interstitial pneumonitis with interstitial fibrosis, hypoxia, and death. Symptoms include cough, dyspnea, and bilateral pulmonary infiltrates noted on CXR. It is controversial whether steroids improve symptoms of bleomycin pulmonary toxicity.

Overdosage/Toxicology Symptoms of overdose include chills, fever, pulmonary fibrosis, hyperpigmentation

Drug Interactions
Decreased effect:
Digitalis glycosides: May decrease plasma levels and renal excretion of digoxin
Phenytoin: Results in decreased phenytoin levels, possibly due to decreased oral absorption
Increased toxicity:
CCNU: Increased severity of leukopenia
Cisplatin: Results in delayed bleomycin elimination due to decrease in creatinine clearance secondary to cisplatin

Stability Refrigerate powder; reconstituted at room temperature is stable for 28 days or in refrigerator for 14 days; stability may decrease in D_5W (10% to 16% in 24 hours) in glass or PVC containers, therefore, NS may be a preferred diluent for bleomycin 24-hour continuous infusions

Incompatible with amino acid solutions, ascorbic acid, cefazolin, furosemide, diazepam, hydrocortisone, mitomycin, nafcillin, penicillin G, aminophylline

Compatible with cyclophosphamide, doxorubicin, mesna, vinblastine, vincristine

Mechanism of Action Inhibits synthesis of DNA; binds to DNA leading to single- and double-strand breaks; isolated from *Streptomyces verticillus*

Pharmacodynamics/Kinetics

Absorption: I.M. and intrapleural administration produces serum concentrations of 30% of I.V. administration; intraperitoneal and S.C. routes produce serum concentrations equal to those of I.V.

Distribution: V_d: 22 L/m²; highest concentrations seen in skin, kidney, lung, heart tissues; low concentrations seen in testes and GI tract; does not cross blood-brain barrier

Protein binding: 1%

Metabolism: By several tissue types, including the liver, GI tract, skin, lungs, kidney, and serum

Half-life (biphasic): Dependent upon renal function:

Normal renal function:

Initial: 1.3 hours

Terminal: 9 hours

End stage renal disease:

Initial: 2 hours

Terminal: 30 hours

Time to peak serum concentration: I.M.: Within 30 minutes

Elimination: 50% to 70% of dose excreted in urine as active drug; not removed by hemodialysis

Usual Dosage Refer to individual protocols; 1 unit = 1 mg

Children and Adults:

Test dose for lymphoma patients: I.M., I.V., S.C.: 1-5 units of bleomycin before the first dose; monitor vital signs every 15 minutes; wait a minimum of 1 hour before administering remainder of dose

I.M., I.V., S.C.: 10-20 units/m² (0.25-0.5 units/kg) 1-2 times/week in combination regimens

I.V. continuous infusion: 15-20 units/m²/day for 4-5 days

Maximum cumulative lifetime dose: 400 units

Dosing adjustment in renal impairment:

Cl_{cr} 10-50 mL/minute: Administer 75% of normal dose

Cl_{cr} <10 mL/minute: Administer 50% of normal dose

Not removed by hemodialysis

Adults: Intracavitary injection for pleural effusion: 60 units have been given in 50-100 mL SWI for malignant pleural effusion

Administration Administer I.V. at ≤1 unit/minute I.M. or S.C. injection may cause pain at injection site

Monitoring Parameters Pulmonary function tests (total lung volume, forced vital capacity, carbon monoxide diffusion), renal function, chest x-ray, temperature initially, CBC with differential and platelet count

Patient Information Hair should reappear after discontinuance of medication; maintain excellent oral hygiene habits; report any coughing, shortness of breath, or wheezing; skin rashes, shaking, chills, or transient high fever may occur following administration

Nursing Implications Patients should be closely monitored for signs of pulmonary toxicity; check body weight at regular intervals

Dosage Forms Injection: 15 units/bottle

Bleph®-10 *see* Sodium Sulfacetamide *on page 1018*

Blephamide® *see* Sodium Sulfacetamide and Prednisolone Acetate *on page 1019*

BLM *see* Bleomycin Sulfate *on previous page*

Blocadren® *see* Timolol Maleate *on page 1094*

Blue® [OTC] *see* Pyrethrins *on page 959*

Bonine® [OTC] *see* Meclizine Hydrochloride *on page 674*

B&O Supprettes® *see* Belladonna and Opium *on page 117*

Botox® *see* Botulinum Toxin Type A *on this page*

Botulinum Toxin Type A (bot' yoo lin num)

Brand Names Botox®

Use

Treatment of strabismus and blepharospasm associated with dystonia (including benign essential blepharospasm or VII nerve disorders in patients ≥12 years of age)

Unlabeled uses: Treatment of hemifacial spasms, spasmodic torticollis (ie, cervical dystonia, clonic twisting of the head), oromandibular dystonia, spasmodic dysphonia (laryngeal dystonia) and other dystonias (ie, writer's cramp, focal task-specific dystonias)

Orphan drug: Treatment of dynamic muscle contracture in pediatric cerebral palsy patients

Pregnancy Risk Factor C

Contraindications

Hypersensitivity to botulinum A toxin

Relative contraindications to botulinum toxin therapy include diseases of neuromuscular transmission and coagulopathy, including anticoagulant therapy; injections into the central area of the upper eyelid (rapid diffusion of toxin into the levator can occur resulting in a marked ptosis).

Warnings/Precautions
Use with caution in patients taking aminoglycosides or any other antibiotic or other drugs that interfere with neuromuscular transmission; do not exceed recommended dose

Adverse Reactions

>10%: Ocular: Dry eyes, lagophthalmos, ptosis, photophobia, vertical deviation

1% to 10%:

Dermatologic: Diffuse skin rash

Ocular: Swelling of eyelid, blepharospasm

<1%: Ocular: Ectropion, keratitis, diplopia, entropion

Overdosage/Toxicology
In the event of an overdosage or injection into the wrong muscle, additional information may be obtained by contacting Allergan Pharmaceuticals at (800)-347-5063 from 8 AM to 4 PM Pacific time, or at (714)-724-5954 at other times

Drug Interactions
Increased effect: Botulinum toxin may be potentiated by aminoglycosides

Stability
Keep in undiluted vials in freezer (at or below -5°C/23°F); administer within 4 hours after the vial is removed from the freezer and reconstituted; store reconstituted solution in refrigerator (2°C to 8°C/36°F to 46°F)

Mechanism of Action
Botulinum A toxin is a neurotoxin produced by *Clostridium botulinum*, spore-forming anaerobic bacillus, which appears to affect only the presynaptic membrane of the neuromuscular junction in humans, where it prevents calcium-dependent release of acetylcholine and produces a state of denervation. Muscle inactivation persists until new fibrils grow from the nerve and form junction plates on new areas of the muscle-cell walls. The antagonist muscle shortens simultaneously ("contracture"), taking up the slack created by agonist paralysis; following several weeks of paralysis, alignment of the eye is measurably changed, despite return of innervation to the injected muscle.

Pharmacodynamics/Kinetics

Strabismus:

Onset of action: 1-2 days after injection

Duration of paralysis: 2-6 weeks

Blepharospasm:

Onset: 3 days after injection

Peak: 1-2 weeks

Duration of paralysis: 3 months

Usual Dosage

Strabismus: 1.25-5 units (0.05-0.15 mL) injected into any one muscle

Subsequent doses for residual/recurrent strabismus: Re-examine patients 7-14 days after each injection to assess the effect of that dose. Subsequent doses for patients experiencing incomplete paralysis of the target may be increased up to two fold the previously administered dose. Maximum recommended dose as a single injection for any one muscle is 25 units.

Blepharospasm: 1.25-2.5 units (0.05-0.10 mL) injected into the orbicularis oculi muscle

Subsequent doses: Each treatment lasts approximately 3 months. At repeat treatment sessions, the dose may be increased up to twofold if the response from the initial treatment is considered insufficient (usually defined as an effect that does not last >2 months). There appears to be little benefit obtainable from injecting >5 units per site. Some tolerance may be found if treatments are given any more frequently than every 3 months.

The cumulative dose should not exceed 200 units in a 30-day period

Administration
Inject using a 27- to 30-gauge needle

Patient Information Patients with blepharospasm may have been extremely sedentary for a long time; caution these patients to resume activity slowly and carefully following administration

Nursing Implications To alleviate spatial disorientation or double vision in strabismic patients, cover the affected eye; have epinephrine ready for hypersensitivity reactions

Dosage Forms Injection: 100 units *Clostridium botulinum* toxin type A

Bovine Lung Surfactant *see* Beractant *on page 128*

Breonesin® [OTC] *see* Guaifenesin *on page 515*

Brethaire® *see* Terbutaline Sulfate *on page 1060*

Brethine® *see* Terbutaline Sulfate *on page 1060*

Bretylium Tosylate (bre til' ee um)
Related Information
Antiarrhythmic Drugs *on page 1246-1248*

Brand Names Bretylol®

Use Treatment of ventricular tachycardia and fibrillation; used in the treatment of other serious ventricular arrhythmias resistant to lidocaine

Pregnancy Risk Factor C

Contraindications Digitalis intoxication-induced arrhythmias, hypersensitivity to bretylium or any component

Warnings/Precautions Hypotension, patients with fixed cardiac output (severe pulmonary hypertension or aortic stenosis) may experience severe hypotension due to decrease in peripheral resistance without ability to increase cardiac output; reduce dose in renal failure patients; may have prolonged half-life with aging

Adverse Reactions
>10%: Cardiovascular: Hypotension (both postural and supine)

1% to 10%: Gastrointestinal: Nausea, vomiting

<1%:
Cardiovascular: Transient initial hypertension, increase in PVCs, bradycardia, angina, flushing, syncope
Central nervous system: Vertigo, confusion, hyperthermia
Dermatologic: Rash
Gastrointestinal: Diarrhea, abdominal pain
Neuromuscular & skeletal: Muscle atrophy and necrosis with repeated I.M. injections at same site
Ocular: Conjunctivitis
Renal: Renal impairment
Respiratory: Respiratory depression, nasal congestion
Miscellaneous: Hiccups

Overdosage/Toxicology Symptoms of overdose include significant hypertension followed by severe hypotension. Administration of short-acting hypotensive agent (Nipride®) should be used for the hypertensive response; hypotension should be treated with fluid administration and dopamine or norepinephrine; dialysis is not useful.

Drug Interactions
Increased toxicity: Other antiarrhythmic agents
Additive toxicity or effect by bretylium, pressor catecholamines, digitalis

Stability Standard diluent: 2 g/250 mL D_5W; the premix infusion should be stored at room temperature and protected from freezing

Mechanism of Action Class II antiarrhythmic; after an initial release of norepinephrine at the peripheral adrenergic nerve terminals, inhibits further release by postganglionic nerve endings in response to sympathetic nerve stimulation

Pharmacodynamics/Kinetics
Onset of antiarrhythmic effect:
I.M.: May require 2 hours
I.V.: Within 6-20 minutes
Peak effect: 6-9 hours
Duration: 6-24 hours
Protein binding: 1% to 6%
Metabolism: Not metabolized
Half-life: 7-11 hours; average: 4-17 hours
End stage renal disease: 16-32 hours
Elimination: 70% to 80% excreted over the first 24 hours; excreted unchanged in the urine

Usual Dosage (Note: Patients should undergo defibrillation/cardioversion before and after bretylium doses as necessary)
(Continued)

Bretylium Tosylate *(Continued)*

Children:
  I.M.: 2-5 mg/kg as a single dose
  I.V.: Initial: 5 mg/kg, then attempt electrical defibrillation; repeat with 10 mg/kg if ventricular fibrillation persists at 15-minute intervals to maximum total of 30 mg/kg
  Maintenance dose: I.M., I.V.: 5 mg/kg every 6-8 hours

Adults:
  Immediate life-threatening ventricular arrhythmias, ventricular fibrillation, unstable ventricular tachycardia: Initial dose: I.V.: 5 mg/kg (undiluted) over 1 minute; if arrhythmia persists, give 10 mg/kg (undiluted) over 1 minute and repeat as necessary (usually at 15- to 30-minute intervals) up to a total dose of 30-35 mg/kg
  Other life-threatening ventricular arrhythmias:
    Initial dose: I.M., I.V.: 5-10 mg/kg, may repeat every 1-2 hours if arrhythmia persist; give I.V. dose (diluted) over 8-10 minutes
    Maintenance dose: I.M.: 5-10 mg/kg every 6-8 hours; I.V. (diluted): 5-10 mg/kg every 6 hours; I.V. infusion (diluted): 1-2 mg/minute (little experience with doses >40 mg/kg/day)
    2 g/250 mL D_5W (infusion pump should be used for I.V. infusion administration)
      Rate of I.V. infusion: 1-4 mg/minute
      1 mg/minute = 7 mL/hour
      2 mg/minute = 15 mL/hour
      3 mg/minute = 22 mL/hour
      4 mg/minute = 30 mL/hour

Dosing adjustment in renal impairment:
  Cl_{cr} 10-50 mL/minute: Administer 25% to 50% of dose
  Cl_{cr} <10 mL/minute: Administer 25% of dose
  Not dialyzable (0% to 5%) via hemo- or peritoneal dialysis; supplemental doses are not needed
Administration I.M. injection in adults should not exceed 5 mL volume in any one site
Monitoring Parameters EKG, heart rate, blood pressure; requires a cardiac monitor
Patient Information Anticipate vomiting
Nursing Implications Monitor EKG and blood pressure throughout therapy; onset of action may be delayed 15-30 minutes; rapid infusion may result in nausea and vomiting
Dosage Forms
  Injection: 50 mg/mL (10 mL, 20 mL)
  Injection, premixed in D_5W: 1 mg/mL (500 mL); 2 mg/mL (250 mL); 4 mg/mL (250 mL, 500 mL)

Bretylol® *see* Bretylium Tosylate *on previous page*

Brevibloc® *see* Esmolol Hydrochloride *on page 404*

Brevicon® *see* Ethinyl Estradiol and Norethindrone *on page 425*

Brevital® Sodium *see* Methohexital Sodium *on page 710*

Bricanyl® *see* Terbutaline Sulfate *on page 1060*

British Anti-Lewisite *see* Dimercaprol *on page 349*

Bromarest® [OTC] *see* Brompheniramine Maleate *on next page*

Brombay® [OTC] *see* Brompheniramine Maleate *on next page*

Bromocriptine Mesylate *(broe moe krip' teen mess' a late)*
Brand Names Parlodel®
Use
  Usually used with levodopa or levodopa/carbidopa to treat Parkinson's disease - treatment of parkinsonism in patients unresponsive or allergic to levodopa
  Prolactin-secreting pituitary adenomas, acromegaly, amenorrhea/galactorrhea secondary to hyperprolactinemia in the absence of primary tumor
  The indication for prevention of postpartum lactation has been withdrawn voluntarily by Sandoz Pharmaceuticals Corporation
Pregnancy Risk Factor C (See Contraindications)
Contraindications Hypersensitivity to bromocriptine or any component, severe ischemic heart disease or peripheral vascular disorders, pregnancy
Warnings/Precautions Use with caution in patients with impaired renal or hepatic function

Adverse Reactions Incidence of adverse effects is high, especially at beginning of treatment and with dosages >20 mg/day

1% to 10%:
  Cardiovascular: Hypotension, Raynaud's phenomenon
  Central nervous system: Mental depression, confusion, hallucinations
  Gastrointestinal: Nausea, constipation, anorexia
  Neuromuscular & skeletal: Leg cramps
  Respiratory: Stuffy nose
<1%:
  Cardiovascular: Hypertension, myocardial infarction, syncope
  Central nervous system: Dizziness, drowsiness, fatigue, insomnia, headache, seizures
  Gastrointestinal: Vomiting, abdominal cramps
Overdosage/Toxicology Symptoms of overdose include nausea, vomiting, hypotension; hypotension, when unresponsive to I.V. fluids or Trendelenburg positioning, often responds to norepinephrine infusions started at 0.1-0.2 mcg/kg/minute followed by a titrated infusion
Drug Interactions
  Decreased effect: Amitriptyline, butyrophenones, imipramine, methyldopa, phenothiazines, reserpine, → ↓ bromocriptine's efficacy at reducing prolactin
  Increased toxicity: Ergot alkaloids (increased cardiovascular toxicity)
Mechanism of Action Semisynthetic ergot alkaloid derivative with dopaminergic properties; inhibits prolactin secretion and can improve symptoms of Parkinson's disease by directly stimulating dopamine receptors in the corpus stratum
Pharmacodynamics/Kinetics
  Protein binding: 90% to 96%
  Metabolism: Majority of drug metabolized in the liver
  Half-life (biphasic):
    Initial: 6-8 hours
    Terminal: 50 hours
  Time to peak serum concentration: Oral: Within 1-2 hours
  Elimination: In bile; only 2% to 6% excreted unchanged in urine
Usual Dosage Adults: Oral:
  Parkinsonism: 1.25 mg 2 times/day, increased by 2.5 mg/day in 2- to 4-week intervals (usual dose range is 30-90 mg/day in 3 divided doses), though elderly patients can usually be managed on lower doses
  Hyperprolactinemia: 2.5 mg 2-3 times/day
  Acromegaly: Initial: 1.25-2.5 mg increasing as necessary every 3-7 days; usual dose: 20-30 mg/day

  Dosing adjustment in hepatic impairment: No guidelines are available, however, may be necessary
Monitoring Parameters Monitor blood pressure closely as well as hepatic, hematopoietic, and cardiovascular function
Patient Information Take with food or milk; drowsiness commonly occurs upon initiation of therapy; limit use of alcohol; avoid exposure to cold; incidence of side effects is high (68%) with nausea the most common; hypotension occurs commonly with initiation of therapy, usually upon rising after prolonged sitting or lying

  Discontinue immediately if pregnant; may restore fertility; women desiring not to become pregnant should use mechanical contraceptive means
Nursing Implications Raise bed rails and institute safety measures; aid patient with ambulation; may cause postural hypotension and drowsiness
Dosage Forms
  Capsule: 5 mg
  Tablet: 2.5 mg

Brompheniramine Maleate (brome fen ir' a meen)
Brand Names Bromarest® [OTC]; Brombay® [OTC]; Bromphen® [OTC]; Brotane® [OTC]; Chlorphed® [OTC]; Codimal-A®; Cophene-B®; Dehist®; Diamine T.D.® [OTC]; Dimetane® [OTC]; Histaject®; Nasahist B®; ND-Stat®; Oraminic® II; Sinusol-B®; Veltane®
Synonyms Parabromdylamine
Use Perennial and seasonal allergic rhinitis and other allergic symptoms including urticaria
Pregnancy Risk Factor C
Contraindications Narrow-angle glaucoma, bladder neck obstruction, symptomatic prostatic hypertrophy, asthmatic attacks, and stenosing peptic ulcer, hypersensitivity to brompheniramine or any component
(Continued)

Brompheniramine Maleate *(Continued)*

Warnings/Precautions Use with caution in patients with heart disease, hypertension, thyroid disease, and asthma; swallow whole, do not crush or chew; antihistamines are more likely to cause dizziness, excessive sedation, syncope, toxic confusional states, and hypotension in the elderly

Adverse Reactions

>10%:

Central nervous system: Slight to moderate drowsiness (compared with other first generation antihistamines, brompheniramine is relatively nonsedating)

Respiratory: Thickening of bronchial secretions

1% to 10%:

Central nervous system: Headache, fatigue, nervousness, dizziness

Gastrointestinal: Appetite increase, weight increase, nausea, diarrhea, abdominal pain, dry mouth

Neuromuscular & skeletal: Arthralgia

Respiratory: Pharyngitis

<1%:

Cardiovascular: Palpitations

Central nervous system: Depression

Dermatologic: Photosensitivity, rash, angioedema

Hepatic: Hepatitis

Neuromuscular & skeletal: Myalgia, paresthesia

Respiratory: Bronchospasm

Miscellaneous: Epistaxis

Overdosage/Toxicology Symptoms of overdose include dry mouth, flushed skin, dilated pupils, CNS depression

There is no specific treatment for an antihistamine overdose, however, most of its clinical toxicity is due to anticholinergic effects; anticholinesterase inhibitors including physostigmine, neostigmine, pyridostigmine, and edrophonium may be useful by reducing acetylcholinesterase; for anticholinergic overdose with severe life-threatening symptoms, physostigmine 1-2 mg (0.5 or 0.02 mg/kg for children) I.V., slowly may be given to reverse these effects

Drug Interactions Increased toxicity: CNS depressants, MAO inhibitors, alcohol, tricyclic antidepressants

Stability Solutions may crystallize if stored at <0°C, crystals will dissolve when warmed

Mechanism of Action Competes with histamine for H_1-receptor sites on effector cells in the gastrointestinal tract, blood vessels, and respiratory tract

Pharmacodynamics/Kinetics

Peak effect: Within 3-9 hours

Time to peak serum concentration: Oral: Within 2-5 hours

Duration of action: Varies with formulation

Metabolism: Extensively by the liver

Half-life: 12-34 hours

Elimination: In urine as inactive metabolites; 2% fecal elimination

Usual Dosage

Oral:

Children:

≤6 years: 0.125 mg/kg/dose given every 6 hours; maximum: 6-8 mg/day

6-12 years: 2-4 mg every 6-8 hours; maximum: 12-16 mg/day

Adults: 4 mg every 4-6 hours or 8 mg of sustained release form every 8-12 hours or 12 mg of sustained release every 12 hours; maximum: 24 mg/day

Elderly: Initial: 4 mg once or twice daily. **Note:** Duration of action may be 36 hours or more, even when serum concentrations are low.

I.M., I.V., S.C.:

Children ≤12 years: 0.5 mg/kg/24 hours divided every 6-8 hours

Adults: 10 mg every 6-12 hours, maximum: 40 mg/24 hours

Patient Information Avoid alcohol; take with food or milk; swallow whole, do not crush or chew extended release products; may cause drowsiness

Nursing Implications Raise bed rails, institute safety measure, aid patient with ambulation

Dosage Forms

Elixir: 2 mg/5 mL with 3% alcohol (120 mL, 480 mL, 4000 mL)

Injection: 10 mg/mL (10 mL)

Tablet: 4 mg, 8 mg, 12 mg

Tablet, sustained release: 8 mg, 12 mg

Bromphen® [OTC] *see* Brompheniramine Maleate *on previous page*

Bronitin® *see* Epinephrine *on page 389*

Bronkaid® Mist [OTC] *see* Epinephrine *on page 389*

Bronkodyl® *see* Theophylline/Aminophylline *on page 1072*

Bronkometer® *see* Isoetharine *on page 593*

Bronkosol® *see* Isoetharine *on page 593*

Brotane® [OTC] *see* Brompheniramine Maleate *on page 143*

BTPABA *see* Bentiromide *on page 120*

Bucladin®-S Softab® *see* Buclizine Hydrochloride *on this page*

Buclizine Hydrochloride (byoo' kli zeen)
Brand Names Bucladin®-S Softab®; Vibazine®
Use Prevention and treatment of motion sickness; symptomatic treatment of vertigo
Pregnancy Risk Factor C
Contraindications Known hypersensitivity to buclizine
Warnings/Precautions Product contains tartrazine; use with caution in patients with angle-closure glaucoma, peptic ulcer, urinary tract obstruction, hyperthyroidism; some preparations contain sodium bisulfite; syrup contains alcohol
Adverse Reactions
>10%: Central nervous system: Drowsiness
<1%:
  Cardiovascular: Hypotension, palpitations
  Central nervous system: Sedation, dizziness, paradoxical excitement, fatigue, insomnia
  Gastrointestinal: Nausea, vomiting
  Genitourinary: Urinary retention
  Neuromuscular & skeletal: Tremor
  Ocular: Blurred vision
Overdosage/Toxicology CNS stimulation or depression; overdose may result in death in infants and children

There is no specific treatment for an antihistamine overdose, however, most of its clinical toxicity is due to anticholinergic effects; anticholinesterase inhibitors including physostigmine, neostigmine, pyridostigmine, and edrophonium may be useful by reducing acetylcholinesterase; for anticholinergic overdose with severe life-threatening symptoms, physostigmine 1-2 mg (0.5 or 0.02 mg/kg for children) I.V., slowly may be given to reverse these effects
Drug Interactions Increased toxicity: CNS depressants, MAO inhibitors, tricyclic antidepressants
Mechanism of Action Buclizine acts centrally to suppress nausea and vomiting. It is a piperazine antihistamine closely related to cyclizine and meclizine. It also has CNS depressant, anticholinergic, antispasmodic, and local anesthetic effects, and suppresses labyrinthine activity and conduction in vestibular-cerebellar nerve pathways.
Usual Dosage Adults: Oral:
  Motion sickness (prophylaxis): 50 mg 30 minutes prior to traveling; may repeat 50 mg after 4-6 hours
  Vertigo: 50 mg twice daily, up to 150 mg/day
Patient Information May cause drowsiness
Nursing Implications Bucladin®-S Softab® may be chewed, swallowed whole, or allowed to dissolve in mouth
Dosage Forms Tablet: 50 mg

Budesonide (byoo des' oh nide)
Brand Names Rhinocort™
Use Management of symptoms of seasonal or perennial rhinitis in adults and nonallergic perennial rhinitis in adults
Adverse Reactions
>10%:
  Cardiovascular: Pounding heartbeat
  Central nervous system: Nervousness, headache, dizziness
  Dermatologic: Itching, skin rash
  Gastrointestinal: GI irritation, bitter taste
  Respiratory: Coughing, upper respiratory tract infection, bronchitis, hoarseness
  Miscellaneous: Oral candidiasis, increased susceptibility to infections, diaphoresis
1% to 10%:
  Central nervous system: Insomnia, psychic changes
  Dermatologic: Acne, hives
  Endocrine & metabolic: Menstrual problems
  Gastrointestinal: Anorexia, increase in appetite
  Ocular: Cataracts
(Continued)

Budesonide *(Continued)*

Miscellaneous: Loss of smell/taste, epistaxis, dry mouth/throat

<1%:

Gastrointestinal: Abdominal fullness

Respiratory: Bronchospasm, shortness of breath

Drug Interactions Although there have been no reported drug interactions to date, one would expect budesonide could potentially interact with drugs known to interact with other corticosteroids

Usual Dosage

Children <6 years of age: Not Recommended

Children ≥6 years and Adults: 256 mcg daily, given as either 2 sprays in each nostril in the morning and evening or as 4 sprays in each nostril in the morning

Patient Information Inhaler should be shaken well immediately prior to use; while activating inhaler, deep breathe for 3-5 seconds, hold breath for ~10 seconds and allow ≥1 minute between inhalations

Dosage Forms Aerosol: 32 mcg per actuation (7 g)

Bufferin® [OTC] *see* Aspirin *on page 92*

Bumetanide *(byoo met' a nide)*

Related Information

Diuretics, Loop Comparison *on page 1269*

Brand Names Bumex®

Use Management of edema secondary to congestive heart failure or hepatic or renal disease including nephrotic syndrome; may be used alone or in combination with antihypertensives in the treatment of hypertension; can be used in furosemide-allergic patients; (1 mg = 40 mg furosemide)

Pregnancy Risk Factor D

Contraindications Hypersensitivity to bumetanide or any component; in anuria or increasing azotemia

Warnings/Precautions Loop diuretics are potent diuretics; excess amounts can lead to profound diuresis with fluid and electrolyte loss; close medical supervision and dose evaluation is required

Adverse Reactions

>10%:

Endocrine & metabolic: Hyperuricemia, hypochloremia, hypokalemia

Genitourinary: Azotemia

1% to 10%:

Central nervous system: Dizziness, encephalopathy, weakness, headache

Endocrine & metabolic: Hyponatremia

Neuromuscular & skeletal: Muscle cramps

<1%:

Cardiovascular: Hypotension

Dermatologic: Rash, pruritus

Endocrine & metabolic: Hyperglycemia, hyperuricemia

Gastrointestinal: Cramps, nausea, vomiting

Hepatic: Alteration of liver function test results

Otic: Hearing loss

Renal: Increased serum creatinine

Overdosage/Toxicology Symptoms of overdose include electrolyte depletion, volume depletion; treatment is primarily symptomatic and supportive

Drug Interactions

Decreased effect: Indomethacin and other NSAIDs, probenecid

Increased effect: Other antihypertensive agents; lithium's excretion may be decreased

Stability I.V. infusion solutions should be used within 24 hours after preparation; light sensitive, → discoloration when exposed to light

Mechanism of Action Inhibits reabsorption of sodium and chloride in the ascending loop of Henle and proximal renal tubule, interfering with the chloride-binding cotransport system, thus causing increased excretion of water, sodium, chloride, magnesium, phosphate and calcium; it does not appear to act on the distal tubule

Pharmacodynamics/Kinetics

Onset of effect:

Oral, I.M.: 0.5-1 hour

I.V.: 2-3 minutes

Duration of action: 6 hours

Distribution: V_d: 13-25 L/kg

Protein binding: 95%

Metabolism: Partial, occurs in the liver

Half-life:
  Infants <6 months: Possibly 2.5 hours
  Children and Adults: 1-1.5 hours
Elimination: Majority of unchanged drug and metabolites excreted in urine

Usual Dosage
  Children:
    <6 months: Dose not established
    >6 months:
      Oral: Initial: 0.015 mg/kg/dose once daily or every other day; maximum
        dose: 0.1 mg/kg/day
      I.M., I.V.: Dose not established
  Adults:
    Oral: 0.5-2 mg/dose 1-2 times/day; maximum: 10 mg/day
    I.M., I.V.: 0.5-1 mg/dose; maximum: 10 mg/day
    Continuous I.V. infusions of 0.9-1 mg/hour may be more effective than bolus
      dosing

Administration Give I.V. slowly, over 1-2 minutes

Monitoring Parameters Blood pressure, serum electrolytes, renal function

Patient Information May be taken with food or milk; rise slowly from a lying or
sitting position to minimize dizziness, lightheadedness or fainting; also use extra
care when exercising, standing for long periods of time, and during hot weather;
take last dose of day early in the evening to prevent nocturia

Nursing Implications Be alert to complaints about hearing difficulty

Dosage Forms
  Injection: 0.25 mg/mL (2 mL, 4 mL, 10 mL)
  Tablet: 0.5 mg, 1 mg, 2 mg

Bumex® see Bumetanide *on previous page*

Buminate® see Albumin, Human *on page 32*

Bupivacaine Hydrochloride (byoo piv′ a kane)

Brand Names Marcaine®; Sensorcaine®

Use Local anesthetic (injectable) for peripheral nerve block, infiltration, sympathetic block, caudal or epidural block, retrobulbar block

Pregnancy Risk Factor C

Contraindications Hypersensitivity to bupivacaine hydrochloride or any component, para-aminobenzoic acid or parabens

Warnings/Precautions Use with caution in patients with liver disease. Some
commercially available formulations contain sodium metabisulfite, which may
cause allergic-type reactions. Pending further data, should not be used in children <12 years of age and the solution for spinal anesthesia should not be used
in children <18 years of age. **Do not use solutions containing preservatives
for caudal or epidural block**; convulsions due to systemic toxicity leading to
cardiac arrest have been reported, presumably following unintentional intravascular injection. 0.75% is **not** recommended for obstetrical anesthesia.

Adverse Reactions
  1% to 10% (dose related):
    Cardiovascular: Cardiac arrest, hypotension, bradycardia, palpitations
    Central nervous system: Seizures, restlessness, anxiety, dizziness, weakness
    Gastrointestinal: Nausea, vomiting
    Ocular: Blurred vision
    Otic: Tinnitus
    Respiratory: Apnea

Overdosage/Toxicology
  Treatment is primarily symptomatic and supportive
  Termination of anesthesia by pneumatic tourniquet inflation should be attempted
    when the agent is administered by infiltration or regional injection
  Seizures commonly respond to diazepam, while hypotension responds to I.V.
    fluids and Trendelenburg positioning
  Bradyarrhythmias (when the heart rate is <60) can be treated with I.V., or S.C.
    atropine 15 mcg/kg
  With the development of metabolic acidosis, I.V. sodium bicarbonate 0.5-2
    mEq/kg and ventilatory assistance should be instituted
  Methemoglobinemia should be treated with methylene blue 1-2 mg/kg in a 1%
    sterile aqueous solution I.V. push over 4-6 minutes repeated up to a total dose
    of 7 mg/kg.

Drug Interactions
  Increased effect: Hyaluronidase
  Increased toxicity: Beta-blockers, ergot-type oxytocics, MAO inhibitors, TCAs,
    phenothiazines, vasopressors

Stability Solutions with epinephrine should be protected from light
(Continued)

Bupivacaine Hydrochloride (Continued)

Mechanism of Action Blocks both the initiation and conduction of nerve impulses by decreasing the neuronal membrane's permeability to sodium ions, which results in inhibition of depolarization with resultant blockade of conduction

Pharmacodynamics/Kinetics

Onset of anesthesia (dependent on route administered): Within 4-10 minutes generally

Duration of action: 1.5-8.5 hours

Metabolism: In the liver

Half-life (age dependent):

Neonates: 8.1 hours

Adults: 1.5-5.5 hours

Elimination: Small amounts (~6%) excreted in urine

Usual Dosage Dose varies with procedure, depth of anesthesia, vascularity of tissues, duration of anesthesia and condition of patient. Metabisulfites (in epinephrine-containing injection); do not use solutions containing preservatives for caudal or epidural block.

Caudal block (with or without epinephrine):

Children: 1-3.7 mg/kg

Adults: 15-30 mL of 0.25% or 0.5%

Epidural block (other than caudal block):

Children: 1.25 mg/kg/dose

Adults: 10-20 mL of 0.25% or 0.5%

Peripheral nerve block: 5 mL dose of 0.25% or 0.5% (12.5-25 mg); maximum: 2.5 mg/kg (plain); 3 mg/kg (with epinephrine); up to a maximum of 400 mg/day

Sympathetic nerve block: 20-50 mL of 0.25% (no epinephrine) solution

Monitoring Parameters Monitor fetal heart rate during paracervical anesthesia

Patient Information Do not chew food in anesthetized region to prevent traumatizing tongue, lip, or buccal mucosa; single dose is usually sufficient in most applications

Dosage Forms

Injection: 0.25% (10 mL, 20 mL, 30 mL, 50 mL); 0.5% (10 mL, 20 mL, 30 mL, 50 mL); 0.75% (2 mL, 10 mL, 20 mL, 30 mL)

Injection, with epinephrine (1:200,000): 0.25% (10 mL, 30 mL, 50 mL); 0.5% (1.8 mL, 3 mL, 5 mL, 10 mL, 30 mL, 50 mL); 0.75% (30 mL)

Buprenex® *see* Buprenorphine Hydrochloride *on this page*

Buprenorphine Hydrochloride (byoo pre nor' feen)

Related Information

Narcotic Agonist Comparison Charts *on page 1274-1275*

Brand Names Buprenex®

Use Management of moderate to severe pain

Restrictions C-V

Pregnancy Risk Factor C

Contraindications Hypersensitivity to buprenorphine or any component

Warnings/Precautions Use with caution in patients with hepatic dysfunction or possible neurologic injury; may precipitate abstinence syndrome in narcotic-dependent patients

Adverse Reactions

>10%: Central nervous system: Drowsiness

1% to 10%:

Cardiovascular: Hypotension

Central nervous system: Respiratory depression, dizziness, headache

Gastrointestinal: Vomiting, nausea

<1%:

Central nervous system: Euphoria, slurred speech, malaise

Dermatologic: Allergic dermatitis

Genitourinary: Urinary retention

Neuromuscular & skeletal: Paresthesia

Ocular: Blurred vision

Overdosage/Toxicology Symptoms of overdose include CNS depression, pinpoint pupils, hypotension, bradycardia; treatment of an overdose includes support of the patient's airway, establishment of an I.V. line, and administration of naloxone 2 mg I.V. (0.01 mg/kg for children) with repeat administration as necessary up to a total of 10 mg

Drug Interactions Increased toxicity: Barbiturates, benzodiazepines (increase CNS and respiratory depression)

Stability Protect from excessive heat (>40°C/104°F) and light
  Compatible with 0.9% sodium chloride, Lactated Ringer's Solution, 5% dextrose in water, scopolamine, haloperidol, glycopyrrolate, droperidol, and hydroxyzine
  Incompatible with diazepam, lorazepam
Mechanism of Action Opiate agonist/antagonist that produces analgesia by binding to kappa and mu opiate receptors in the CNS
Pharmacodynamics/Kinetics
  Onset of analgesia: Within 10-30 minutes
  Absorption: I.M., S.C.: 30% to 40%
  Distribution: V_d: 97-187 L/kg
  Protein binding: High
  Metabolism: Mainly in the liver; undergoes extensive first-pass metabolism
  Half-life: 2.2-3 hours
  Elimination: 70% excreted in feces via bile and 20% in urine as unchanged drug
Usual Dosage I.M., slow I.V.:
  Children ≥13 years and Adults: 0.3-0.6 mg every 6 hours as needed
  Elderly: 0.15 mg every 6 hours; elderly patients are more likely to suffer from confusion and drowsiness compared to younger patients
  Long-term use is not recommended
Monitoring Parameters Pain relief, respiratory and mental status, CNS depression, blood pressure
Patient Information May cause drowsiness
Nursing Implications Gradual withdrawal of drug is necessary to avoid withdrawal symptoms
Additional Information 0.3 mg = 10 mg morphine or 75 mg meperidine, has longer duration of action than either agent
Dosage Forms Injection: 0.324 mg buprenorphine HCl (which is equivalent to 0.3 mg buprenorphine)/mL (1 mL)

Bupropion (byoo proe' pee on)
Related Information
  Antidepressant Agents Comparison *on page 1250-1252*
Brand Names Wellbutrin®
Use Treatment of depression
Pregnancy Risk Factor B
Contraindications Seizure disorder, prior diagnosis of bulimia or anorexia nervosa, known hypersensitivity to bupropion, concurrent use of a monoamine oxidase (MAO) inhibitor
Warnings/Precautions The estimated seizure potential is increased many fold in doses in the 450-600 mg/day range; giving a single dose <150 mg will lessen the seizure potential; use in patients with renal or hepatic impairment increases possible toxic effects
Adverse Reactions
  >10%:
    Central nervous system: Agitation, insomnia, fever, headache, psychosis, confusion, anxiety, restlessness, dizziness, seizures, chills, akathisia
    Gastrointestinal: Nausea, vomiting, dry mouth, constipation, weight loss
    Genitourinary: Impotence
    Neuromuscular & skeletal: Tremor
  1% to 10%:
    Central nervous system: Hallucinations, chills, tiredness
    Dermatologic: Skin rash
    Ocular: Blurred vision
  <1%: Central nervous system: Fainting, drowsiness, seizures
Overdosage/Toxicology Symptoms of overdose include labored breathing, salivation, arched back, ataxia, convulsions

  Hospitalize patient; if still conscious, induce vomiting; administer activated charcoal every 6 hours for two times and obtain baseline labs, obtain EKG and EEG over the next 48 hours; maintain hydration. In patients who are comatose, stuporous, or seizing, perform gastric lavage after adequate airway has been established via intubation. Treat seizures with I.V. benzodiazepines and supportive therapies; dialysis may be of limited value after drug absorption because of slow tissue to plasma diffusion.
Drug Interactions
  Decreased effects: Increased clearance: Carbamazepine, phenytoin, cimetidine, phenobarbital
  Increased effects: Levodopa, MAO inhibitors
Mechanism of Action Antidepressant structurally different from all other previously marketed antidepressants; like other antidepressants the mechanism of
(Continued)

Bupropion *(Continued)*

bupropion's activity is not fully understood; weak blocker of serotonin and norepinephrine re-uptake, inhibits neuronal dopamine re-uptake and is **not** a monoamine oxidase A or B inhibitor

Pharmacodynamics/Kinetics

Absorption: Rapidly absorbed from GI tract

Distribution: V_d: 19-21 L/kg

Protein binding: 82% to 88%

Metabolism: Extensively in the liver to multiple metabolites

Half-life: 14 hours

Time to peak serum concentration: Oral: Within 3 hours

Usual Dosage Oral:

Adults: 100 mg 3 times/day; begin at 100 mg twice daily; may increase to a maximum dose of 450 mg/day

Elderly: 50-100 mg/day, increase by 50-100 mg every 3-4 days as tolerated; there is evidence that the elderly respond at 150 mg/day in divided doses, but some may require a higher dose

Dosing adjustment/comments in renal or hepatic impairment: Patients with renal or hepatic failure should receive a reduced dosage initially and be closely monitored

Monitoring Parameters Monitor body weight

Reference Range Therapeutic levels (trough, 12 hours after last dose): 50-100 ng/mL

Test Interactions Decreased prolactin levels

Patient Information Take in equally divided doses 3-4 times/day to minimize the risk of seizures; avoid alcohol; do not take more than recommended dose or more than 150 mg in a single dose; do not discontinue abruptly, may take 3-4 weeks for full effect; may impair driving or other motor or cognitive skills and judgment

Nursing Implications Be aware that drug may cause seizures; dose should not be increased by more than 50 mg/day once weekly

Dosage Forms Tablet: 75 mg, 100 mg

BuSpar® *see* Buspirone Hydrochloride *on this page*

Buspirone Hydrochloride *(byoo spye' rone)*

Brand Names BuSpar®

Use Management of anxiety; has shown little potential for abuse

Unlabeled use: Panic attacks

Pregnancy Risk Factor B

Contraindications Hypersensitivity to buspirone or any component

Warnings/Precautions Safety and efficacy not established in children <18 years of age; use in hepatic or renal impairment is not recommended; does not prevent or treat withdrawal from benzodiazepines

Adverse Reactions

>10%:

Central nervous system: Dizziness, lightheadedness, headache, restlessness

Gastrointestinal: Nausea

1% to 10%: Central nervous system: Drowsiness

<1%:

Cardiovascular: Chest pain, tachycardia

Central nervous system: Confusion, insomnia, nightmares, sedation, disorientation, excitement, fever, ataxia

Dermatologic: Rash, urticaria

Gastrointestinal: Dry mouth, vomiting, diarrhea, flatulence

Hematologic: Leukopenia, eosinophilia

Neuromuscular & skeletal: Muscle weakness

Ocular: Blurred vision

Otic: Tinnitus

Overdosage/Toxicology Symptoms of overdose include dizziness, drowsiness, pinpoint pupils, nausea, vomiting; there is no known antidote for buspirone, treatment is supportive

Drug Interactions

Increased effects: Cimetidine, food

Increased toxicity: MAO inhibitors, phenothiazines, CNS depressants; increased toxicity of digoxin and haloperidol

Mechanism of Action Selectively antagonizes CNS serotonin $5-HT_1A$ receptors without affecting benzodiazepine-GABA receptors; may down-regulate postsynaptic $5-HT_2$ receptors as do antidepressants

Pharmacodynamics/Kinetics
Protein binding: 95%

Metabolism: In the liver by oxidation and undergoes extensive first-pass metabolism

Half-life: 2-3 hours

Time to peak serum concentration: Oral: Within 40-60 minutes

Usual Dosage Adults: Oral: 15 mg/day (5 mg 3 times/day); may increase in increments of 5 mg/day every 2-4 days to a maximum of 60 mg/day

Dosing adjustment in renal or hepatic impairment: Dosage should be decreased in patients with severe hepatic insufficiency; anuric patients should be dosed at 25% to 50% of the usual dose

Monitoring Parameters Mental status, symptoms of anxiety; monitor for benzodiazepine withdrawal

Test Interactions ↑ AST, ALT, growth hormone(s), prolactin (S)

Patient Information Take with food; report any change in senses (ie, smelling, hearing, vision); cautious use with alcohol is recommended; cannot be substituted for benzodiazepines unless directed by a physician; takes 2-3 weeks to see the full effect of this medication; if you miss a dose, do **not** double your next dose

Dosage Forms Tablet: 5 mg, 10 mg

Busulfan (byoo sul' fan)
Related Information
Cancer Chemotherapy Regimens *on page 1218-1241*

Brand Names Myleran®

Use Chronic myelogenous leukemia and bone marrow disorders, such as polycythemia vera and myeloid metaplasia, conditioning regimens for bone marrow transplantation

Pregnancy Risk Factor D

Contraindications Failure to respond to previous courses; should not be used in pregnancy or lactation; hypersensitivity to busulfan or any component

Warnings/Precautions The U.S. Food and Drug Administration (FDA) currently recommends that procedures for proper handling and disposal of antineoplastic agents be considered. May induce severe bone marrow hypoplasia; reduce or discontinue dosage at first sign, as reflected by an abnormal decrease in any of the formed elements of the blood; use with caution in patients recently given other myelosuppressive drugs or radiation treatment. If white blood count is high, hydration and allopurinol should be employed to prevent hyperuricemia.

Adverse Reactions
Fertility/carcinogenesis: Sterility, ovarian suppression, amenorrhea, azoospermia, and testicular atrophy; malignant tumors have been reported in patients on busulfan therapy

>10%:
Hematologic: Severe pancytopenia, leukopenia, thrombocytopenia, anemia, and bone marrow suppression are common and patients should be monitored closely while on therapy. Since this is a delayed effect (busulfan affects the stem cells), the drug should be discontinued temporarily at the first sign of a large or rapid fall in any blood element. Some patients may develop bone marrow fibrosis or chronic aplasia which is probably due to the busulfan toxicity. In large doses, busulfan is myeloablative and is used for this reason in BMT.

Myelosuppressive:
WBC: Moderate
Platelets: Moderate
Onset (days): 7-10
Nadir (days): 14-21
Recovery (days): 28

1% to 10%:
Cardiovascular: Endocardial fibrosis
Central nervous system: Weakness
Dermatologic: Hyperpigmentation skin (busulfan tan), urticaria, erythema, alopecia
Endocrine & metabolic: Amenorrhea
Gastrointestinal: **Emetic potential:** Low (<10%); nausea, vomiting, diarrhea; drug has little effect on the GI mucosal lining

<1%:
Central nervous system: Generalized or myoclonic seizures and loss of consciousness have been associated with high-dose busulfan (4 mg/kg/day), blurred vision
Endocrine & metabolic: Adrenal suppression, gynecomastia, hyperuricemia
Genitourinary: Isolated cases of hemorrhagic cystitis have been reported
(Continued)

Busulfan *(Continued)*

Hepatic: Hepatic dysfunction

Ocular: Cataracts

Respiratory: After long-term or high-dose therapy, a syndrome known as busulfan lung may occur. This syndrome is manifested by a diffuse interstitial pulmonary fibrosis and persistent cough, fever, rales, and dyspnea. May be relieved by corticosteroids.

Overdosage/Toxicology Symptoms of overdose include leukopenia, thrombocytopenia

Mechanism of Action Reacts with N-7 position of guanosine and interferes with DNA replication and transcription of RNA. Busulfan has a more marked effect on myeloid cells (and is, therefore, useful in the treatment of CML) than on lymphoid cells. The drug is also very toxic to hematopoietic stem cells (thus its usefulness in high doses in BMT preparative regimens). Busulfan exhibits little immunosuppressive activity. Interferes with the normal function of DNA by alkylation and cross-linking the strands of DNA.

Pharmacodynamics/Kinetics

Absorption: Rapidly and completely from the GI tract

Distribution: V_d: ~1 L/kg; distributed into the CSF and saliva with levels similar to plasma

Protein binding: ~14%

Metabolism: Extensive in the liver (may increase with multiple dosing)

Half-life:

After first dose: 3.4 hours

After last dose: 2.3 hours

Time to peak serum concentration:

Oral: Within 4 hours

I.V.: Within 5 minutes

Elimination: 10% to 50% excreted in the urine as metabolites within 24 hours; <2% seen as unchanged drug

Usual Dosage Oral (refer to individual protocols):

Children: 0.06-0.12 mg/kg/day or 1.8-4.6 mg/m^2/day; titrate dosage to maintain leukocyte count about 20,000/mm^3 (dosages >4 mg/day are especially likely to reduce the leukocyte count). Higher doses may be utilized in young children due to different pharmacokinetics.

Adults:

Bone marrow transplantation: 1 mg/kg ideal body weight 4 times/day for 4 days (total dose: 16 mg/kg) or as per protocol

Remission:

Induction of CML: 4-8 mg/day (may be as high as 12 mg/day)

Maintenance doses: Controversial, range from 1-4 mg/day to 2 mg/week; treatment is continued until WBC reaches 10,000-20,000 cells/mm^3 at which time drug is discontinued; when WBC reaches 50,000/mm^3, maintenance dose is resumed

Unapproved uses:

Polycythemia vera: 2-6 mg/day

Thrombocytosis: 4-6 mg/day

Administration Avoid I.M. injection if platelet count falls <100,000/mm^3

Monitoring Parameters CBC with differential and platelet count, hemoglobin, liver function tests

Patient Information Watch for signs of bleeding; excellent oral hygiene is needed to minimize oral discomfort

Dosage Forms Tablet: 2 mg

Butabarbital Sodium *(byoo ta bar′ bi tal)*

Brand Names Butalan®; Buticaps®; Butisol Sodium®

Use Sedative, hypnotic

Restrictions C-III

Pregnancy Risk Factor D

Contraindications Hypersensitivity to butabarbital or any component, presence of acute or chronic pain, latent porphyria, marked liver impairment

Adverse Reactions

>10%: Central nervous system: Dizziness, lightheadedness, drowsiness, "hangover" effect

1% to 10%:

Central nervous system: Confusion, mental depression, unusual excitement, nervousness, faint feeling, headache, insomnia, nightmares

Gastrointestinal: Constipation, nausea, vomiting

<1%:

Cardiovascular: Hypotension

Central nervous system: Hallucinations
Dermatologic: Skin rash, exfoliative dermatitis, Stevens-Johnson syndrome, angioedema
Hematologic: Agranulocytosis, megaloblastic anemia, thrombocytopenia
Local: Thrombophlebitis
Respiratory: Respiratory depression
Miscellaneous: Dependence

Overdosage/Toxicology Symptoms of overdose include slurred speech, confusion, nystagmus, tachycardia, hypotension

If hypotension occurs, administer I.V. fluids and place the patient in the Trendelenburg position; if unresponsive, an I.V. vasopressor (eg, dopamine, epinephrine) may be required. Forced alkaline diuresis is of no value in the treatment of intoxications with short-acting barbiturates. Charcoal hemoperfusion or hemodialysis may be useful in the harder to treat intoxications, especially in the presence of very high serum barbiturate levels.

Drug Interactions
Decreased effect: Phenothiazines, haloperidol, quinidine, cyclosporine, TCAs, corticosteroids, theophylline, ethosuximide, warfarin, oral contraceptives, chloramphenicol, griseofulvin, doxycycline, beta-blockers
Increased effect/toxicity: Propoxyphene, benzodiazepines, CNS depressants, valproic acid, methylphenidate, chloramphenicol

Mechanism of Action Interferes with transmission of impulses from the thalamus to the cortex of the brain resulting in an imbalance in central inhibitory and facilitatory mechanisms

Pharmacodynamics/Kinetics
Distribution: V_d: 0.8 L/kg
Protein binding: 26%
Metabolism: In the liver
Half-life: 40-140 hours
Time to peak serum concentration: Oral: Within 40-60 minutes
Elimination: In urine as metabolites

Usual Dosage Oral:
Children: Preop: 2-6 mg/kg/dose; maximum: 100 mg

Adults:
Sedative: 15-30 mg 3-4 times/day
Hypnotic: 50-100 mg
Preop: 50-100 mg 1-1½ hours before surgery

Reference Range Therapeutic: Not established; Toxic: 28-73 µg/mL

Test Interactions ↑ ammonia (B); ↓ bilirubin (S)

Patient Information May cause drowsiness, avoid alcohol or other CNS depressants, may impair judgment and coordination; may cause physical and psychological dependence with prolonged use; do not exceed recommended dose

Nursing Implications Raise bed rails; initiate safety measures; aid with ambulation; monitor for CNS depression

Dosage Forms
Capsule: 15 mg, 30 mg
Elixir, with alcohol 7%: 30 mg/5 mL (480 mL, 3780 mL); 33.3 mg/5 mL (480 mL, 3780 mL)
Tablet: 15 mg, 30 mg, 50 mg, 100 mg

Butace® see Butalbital Compound on this page

Butalan® see Butabarbital Sodium on previous page

Butalbital Compound (byoo tal' bi tal)
Brand Names Amaphen®; Anoquan®; Axotal®; B-A-C®; Bancap®; Butace®; Endolor®; Esgic®; Femcet®; Fiorgen PF®; Fioricet®; Fiorinal®; G-1®; Isollyl Improved®; Lanorinal®; Marnal®; Medigesic®; Phrenilin®; Phrenilin Forte®; Repan®; Sedapap-10®; Triapin®; Two-Dyne®
Use Relief of symptomatic complex of tension or muscle contraction headache
Restrictions C-III (Fiorinal®)
Pregnancy Risk Factor D
Contraindications Patients with porphyria, known hypersensitivity to butalbital or any component
Warnings/Precautions Children and teenagers should not use for chickenpox or flu symptoms before a physician is consulted about Reye's syndrome (Fiorinal®)
Adverse Reactions
>10%:
Central nervous system: Dizziness, lightheadedness, drowsiness, "hangover" effect
(Continued)

Butalbital Compound *(Continued)*

Gastrointestinal: Nausea, heartburn, stomach pains, dyspepsia, epigastric discomfort

1% to 10%:

Central nervous system: Confusion, mental depression, unusual excitement, nervousness, faint feeling, headache, insomnia, nightmares, weakness, tiredness

Dermatologic: Skin rash

Gastrointestinal: Constipation, vomiting, gastrointestinal ulceration

Hematologic: Hemolytic anemia

Respiratory: Troubled breathing

Miscellaneous: Anaphylactic shock

<1%:

Cardiovascular: Hypotension

Central nervous system: Hallucinations, insomnia, nervousness, jitters

Dermatologic: Skin rash, exfoliative dermatitis, Stevens-Johnson syndrome

Hematologic: Agranulocytosis, megaloblastic anemia, occult bleeding, prolongation of bleeding time, leukopenia, thrombocytopenia, iron deficiency anemia

Hepatic: Hepatotoxicity

Local: Thrombophlebitis

Renal: Impaired renal function

Respiratory: Respiratory depression, bronchospasm

Overdosage/Toxicology Symptoms of overdose include slurred speech, confusion, nystagmus, tachycardia, hypotension, tinnitus, headache, dizziness, confusion, metabolic acidosis, hyperpyrexia, hypoglycemia, coma, hepatic necrosis, blood dyscrasias, respiratory depression

Forced alkaline diuresis is of no value in the treatment of intoxications with short-acting barbiturates. Charcoal hemoperfusion or hemodialysis may be useful in the harder to treat intoxications, especially in the presence of very high serum barbiturate levels; see also Acetaminophen for Fioricet® toxicology or Aspirin for Fiorinal® toxicology.

Drug Interactions

Decreased effect: Phenothiazines, haloperidol, quinidine, cyclosporine, TCAs, corticosteroids, theophylline, ethosuximide, warfarin, oral contraceptives, chloramphenicol, griseofulvin, doxycycline, beta-blockers

Increased effect/toxicity: Propoxyphene, benzodiazepines, CNS depressants, valproic acid, methylphenidate, chloramphenicol

Mechanism of Action Butalbital, like other barbiturates, has a generalized depressant effect on the central nervous system (CNS). Barbiturates have little effect on peripheral nerves or muscle at usual therapeutic doses. However, at toxic doses serious effects on the cardiovascular system and other peripheral systems may be observed. These effects may result in hypotension or skeletal muscle weakness. While all areas of the central nervous system are acted on by barbiturates, the mesencephalic reticular activating system is extremely sensitive to their effects. Barbiturates act at synapses where gamma-aminobenzoic acid is a neurotransmitter, but they may act in other areas as well.

Usual Dosage Adults: Oral: 1-2 tablets or capsules every 4 hours; not to exceed 6/day

Dosing interval in renal or hepatic impairment: Should be reduced

Patient Information Children and teenagers should not use this product; may cause drowsiness, avoid alcohol or other CNS depressants, may impair judgment and coordination; may cause physical and psychological dependence with prolonged use; do not exceed recommended dose

Nursing Implications Raise bed rails; initiate safety measures; aid with ambulation; monitor for CNS depression

Dosage Forms

Capsule, with acetaminophen:

Amaphen®, Anoquan®, Butace®, Endolor®, Esgic®, Femcet®, G-1®, Medigesic®, Repan®, Two-Dyne®: Butalbital 50 mg, caffeine 40 mg, and acetaminophen 325 mg

Bancap®, Triapin®: Butalbital 50 mg and acetaminophen 325 mg

Phrenilin Forte®: Butalbital 50 mg and acetaminophen 650 mg

Capsule, with aspirin: (Fiorgen PF®, Fiorinal®, Isollyl Improved®, Lanorinal®, Marnal®): Butalbital 50 mg, caffeine 40 mg, and aspirin 325 mg

Tablet, with acetaminophen:

Esgic®, Fioricet®, Repan®: Butalbital 50 mg, caffeine 40 mg, and acetaminophen 325 mg

Phrenilin®: Butalbital 50 mg and acetaminophen 325 mg

Sedapap-10®: Butalbital 50 mg and acetaminophen 650 mg

Tablet, with aspirin:
Axotal®: Butalbital 50 mg and aspirin 650 mg
B-A-C®: Butalbital 50 mg, caffeine 40 mg, and aspirin 650 mg
Fiorinal®, Isollyl Improved®, Lanorinal®, Marnal®: Butalbital 50 mg, caffeine 40 mg, and aspirin 325 mg

Buticaps® *see* Butabarbital Sodium *on page 152*

Butisol Sodium® *see* Butabarbital Sodium *on page 152*

Butoconazole Nitrate (byoo toe koe' na zole)
Brand Names Femstat®
Use Local treatment of vulvovaginal candidiasis
Pregnancy Risk Factor C (For use only in 2nd or 3rd trimester)
Contraindications Known hypersensitivity to butoconazole
Warnings/Precautions In pregnancy, use only during second or third trimesters; if irritation or sensitization occurs, discontinue use
Adverse Reactions
1% to 10%: Genitourinary: Vulvar/vaginal burning
<1%: Genitourinary: Vulvar itching, soreness, swelling, or discharge; urinary frequency
Stability Do not store at temperatures >40°C/104°F; avoid freezing
Mechanism of Action Increases cell membrane permeability in susceptible fungi (*Candida*)
Pharmacodynamics/Kinetics
Absorption: Following intravaginal application small amounts of drug are absorbed systemically (25%) within 2-8 hours
Half-life: 21-24 hours
Elimination: Into urine and feces in approximate equal amounts
Usual Dosage Adults:
Nonpregnant: Insert 1 applicatorful (~5 g) intravaginally at bedtime for 3 days, may extend for up to 6 days if necessary
Pregnant: **Use only during second or third trimesters**
Patient Information May cause burning or stinging on application; if symptoms of vaginitis persist, contact physician
Dosage Forms Cream, vaginal: 2% with applicator (28 g)

Butorphanol Tartrate (byoo tor' fa nole)
Related Information
Narcotic Agonist Comparison Charts *on page 1274-1275*
Brand Names Stadol®; Stadol® NS
Use Management of moderate to severe pain
Pregnancy Risk Factor B (D if used for prolonged periods or in high doses at term)
Contraindications Hypersensitivity to butorphanol or any component; avoid use in opiate-dependent patients who have not been detoxified, may precipitate opiate withdrawal
Warnings/Precautions Use with caution in patients with hepatic/renal dysfunction, may elevate CSF pressure, may increase cardiac workload
Adverse Reactions
>10%: Central nervous system: Drowsiness
1% to 10%:
Cardiovascular: Flushing of the face, hypotension
Central nervous system: Dizziness, lightheadedness, headache
Gastrointestinal: Anorexia, nausea, vomiting
Genitourinary: Decreased urination
Miscellaneous: Increased sweating
<1%:
Cardiovascular: Bradycardia or tachycardia, hypertension
Central nervous system: Paradoxical CNS stimulation, confusion, hallucinations, mental depression, false sense of well being, malaise, restlessness, nightmares, weakness, CNS depression
Dermatologic: Skin rash
Gastrointestinal: Stomach cramps, constipation, dry mouth
Genitourinary: Painful urination
Ocular: Blurred vision
Otic: Tinnitus
Respiratory: Shortness of breath, troubled breathing, respiratory depression
Miscellaneous: Dependence with prolonged use
Overdosage/Toxicology Symptoms of overdose include respiratory depression, cardiac and CNS depression; treatment of an overdose includes support of the
(Continued)

Butorphanol Tartrate *(Continued)*

patient's airway, establishment of an I.V. line and administration of naloxone 2 mg I.V. (0.01 mg/kg for children) with repeat administration as necessary up to a total of 10 mg

Drug Interactions Increased toxicity: CNS depressants, phenothiazines, barbiturates, skeletal muscle relaxants, alfentanil, guanabenz, MAO inhibitors

Stability Store at room temperature, protect from freezing; **incompatible** when mixed in the same syringe with diazepam, dimenhydrinate, methohexital, pentobarbital, secobarbital, thiopental

Mechanism of Action Mixed narcotic agonist-antagonist with central analgesic actions; binds to opiate receptors in the CNS, causing inhibition of ascending pain pathways, altering the perception of and response to pain; produces generalized CNS depression

Pharmacodynamics/Kinetics
Peak effect:
I.M.: Within 0.5-1 hour
I.V.: Within 4-5 minutes
Absorption: Rapidly and well absorbed
Protein binding: 80%
Metabolism: In the liver
Half-life: 2.5-4 hours
Elimination: Primarily in urine

Usual Dosage Adults:
I.M.: 1-4 mg every 3-4 hours as needed
I.V.: 0.5-2 mg every 3-4 hours as needed
Nasal spray: Headache: 1 spray in 1 nostril; if adequate pain relief is not achieved within 60-90 minutes, an additional 1 spray in 1 nostril may be given (each spray gives ~1 mg of butorphanol)

Dosing adjustment in renal impairment:
Cl_{cr} 10-50 mL/minute: Administer 75% of dose
Cl_{cr} <10 mL/minute: Administer 50% of dose

Monitoring Parameters Pain relief, respiratory and mental status, blood pressure

Reference Range 0.7-1.5 ng/mL

Patient Information May cause drowsiness; avoid alcohol

Nursing Implications Observe for excessive sedation or confusion, respiratory depression; raise bed rails; aid with ambulation

Dosage Forms
Injection: 1 mg/mL (1 mL); 2 mg/mL (1 mL, 2 mL, 10 mL)
Nasal spray: 10 mg/mL [14-15 doses] (2.5 mL)

BW-430C *see* Lamotrigine *on page 618*

Byclomine® *see* Dicyclomine Hydrochloride *on page 330*

C8-CCK *see* Sincalide *on page 1007*

Cafatine® *see* Ergotamine *on page 399*

Cafatine-PB® *see* Ergotamine *on page 399*

Cafergot® *see* Ergotamine *on page 399*

Cafetrate® *see* Ergotamine *on page 399*

Calan® *see* Verapamil Hydrochloride *on page 1153*

Calci-Chew™ *see* Calcium Carbonate *on page 161*

Calcifediol *(kal si fe dye' ole)*

Brand Names Calderol®

Synonyms 25-HCC; 25-Hydroxycholecalciferol; 25-Hydroxyvitamin D_3

Use Treatment and management of metabolic bone disease associated with chronic renal failure

Pregnancy Risk Factor A (D if used in doses above the recommended daily allowance)

Contraindications Hypercalcemia; known hypersensitivity to calcifediol; malabsorption syndrome; hypervitaminosis D; significantly decreased renal function

Warnings/Precautions Adequate (supplemental) dietary calcium is necessary for clinical response to vitamin D; calcium-phosphate product (serum calcium times phosphorus) must not exceed 70; avoid hypercalcemia

Adverse Reactions
1% to 10%:
Cardiovascular: Hypotension, cardiac arrhythmias, hypertension, irregular heartbeat

Central nervous system: Irritability, headache

Dermatologic: Pruritus

Endocrine & metabolic: Polydipsia, hypermagnesemia

Gastrointestinal: Nausea, vomiting, constipation, anorexia, pancreatitis, metallic taste

Neuromuscular & skeletal: Muscle/bone pain

Ocular: Conjunctivitis, photophobia

Renal: Polyuria

<1%:

Central nervous system: Overt psychosis, seizures

Gastrointestinal: Weight loss

Hepatic: Elevated AST/ALT

Miscellaneous: Calcification

Overdosage/Toxicology Symptoms of overdose include hypercalcemia, hypercalciuria; following withdrawal of the drug, treatment consists of bed rest, liberal intake of fluids, reduced calcium intake, and cathartic administration. Severe hypercalcemia requires I.V. hydration and forced diuresis. Urine output should be monitored and maintained at >3 mL/kg/hour. I.V. saline can quickly and significantly increase excretion of calcium into urine. Calcitonin, cholestyramine, prednisone, sodium EDTA, biphosphonates, and mithramycin have all been used successfully to treat the more resistant cases of vitamin D-induced hypercalcemia.

Drug Interactions

Decreased effect: Cholestyramine, colestipol

Increased effect: Thiazide diuretics

Additive effect: Antacids (magnesium)

Mechanism of Action Vitamin D analog that (along with calcitonin and parathyroid hormone) regulates serum calcium homeostasis by promoting absorption of calcium and phosphorus in the small intestine; promotes renal tubule resorption of phosphate; increases rate of accretion and resorption in bone minerals

Pharmacodynamics/Kinetics

Absorption: Rapid from the small intestines

Distribution: Activated in the kidneys; stored in liver and fat depots

Half-life: 12-22 days

Time to peak: Within 4 hours (oral)

Elimination: In bile and feces

Usual Dosage Oral: Hepatic osteodystrophy:

Infants: 5-7 mcg/kg/day

Children and Adults: 20-100 mcg/day or every other day; titrate to obtain normal serum calcium/phosphate levels; increase dose at 4-week intervals

Test Interactions ↑ calcium (S), cholesterol (S), magnesium, BUN, AST, ALT; ↓ alk phos

Patient Information Compliance with dose, diet, and calcium supplementation is essential; avoid taking magnesium supplements or magnesium-containing antacids; notify physician if weakness, lethargy, headache, and decreased appetite occur

Dosage Forms Capsule: 20 mcg, 50 mcg

Calciferol™ see Ergocalciferol on page 396

Calcijex™ see Calcitriol on page 159

Calcilac® [OTC] see Calcium Carbonate on page 161

Calcimar® see Calcitonin on next page

Calci-Mix™ see Calcium Carbonate on page 161

Calciparine® see Heparin on page 528

Calcipotriene (kal si poe' try een)

Brand Names Dovonex®

Use Treatment of moderate plaque psoriasis

Pregnancy Risk Factor C

Contraindications Hypersensitivity to any components of the preparation; patients with demonstrated hypercalcemia or evidence of vitamin D toxicity; use on the face

Warnings/Precautions Use may cause irritations of lesions and surrounding uninvolved skin. If irritation develops, discontinue use. Transient, rapidly reversible elevation of serum calcium has occurred during use. If elevation in serum calcium occurs above the normal range, discontinue treatment until calcium levels are normal. For external use only: not for ophthalmic, oral or intravaginal use.

(Continued)

Calcipotriene (Continued)

Adverse Reactions
>10%: Topical: Burning, itching, skin irritation, erythema, dry skin, peeling, rash, worsening of psoriasis

1% to 10%: Topical: Dermatitis

<1%:
Endocrine & metabolic: Hypercalcemia
Topical: Skin atrophy, hyperpigmentation, folliculitis

Mechanism of Action Synthetic vitamin D_3 analog which regulates skin cell production and proliferation

Usual Dosage Adults: Topical: Apply in a thin film to the affected skin twice daily and rub in gently and completely

Patient Information For external use only; avoid contact with the face or eyes; wash hands after application

Nursing Implications Wear gloves

Dosage Forms Ointment, topical: 0.005% (30 g, 60 g, 100 g)

Calcitonin (kal si toe' nin)

Brand Names Calcimar®; Cibacalcin®; Miacalcin®

Synonyms Calcitonin (Human); Calcitonin (Salmon)

Use
Calcitonin (salmon): Treatment of Paget's disease of bone and as adjunctive therapy for hypercalcemia; also used in postmenopausal osteoporosis

Calcitonin (human): Treatment of Paget's disease of bone

Pregnancy Risk Factor B

Contraindications Hypersensitivity to salmon protein or gelatin diluent with the salmon product

Warnings/Precautions A skin test should be performed prior to initiating therapy of calcitonin salmon; have epinephrine immediately available for a possible hypersensitivity reaction

Adverse Reactions
>10%:
Cardiovascular: Facial flushing
Gastrointestinal: Nausea, diarrhea, anorexia
Local: Swelling at injection site

1% to 10%: Frequency of urination

<1%:
Central nervous system: Chills, headache, tingling of hands/feet, swelling, dizziness, weakness
Dermatologic: Skin rash, urticaria
Respiratory: Shortness of breath, nasal congestion, stuffy nose

Overdosage/Toxicology Symptoms of overdose include nausea, vomiting, hypocalcemia, hypocalcemic tetany

Stability
Salmon calcitonin: Store under refrigeration at 2°C to 6°C/36°F to 43°F; stable for up to 2 weeks at room temperature; NS has been recommended for the dilution to prepare a skin test

Human calcitonin: Store at <25°C/77°F and protect from light

Mechanism of Action Structurally similar to human calcitonin; it directly inhibits osteoclastic bone resorption; promotes the renal excretion of calcium, phosphate, sodium, magnesium and potassium by decreasing tubular reabsorption; increases the jejunal secretion of water, sodium, potassium, and chloride

Pharmacodynamics/Kinetics
Hypercalcemia:
Onset of reduction in calcium: 2 hours
Duration of effect: 6-8 hours
Distribution: Does not cross into the placenta
Metabolism: Rapidly by the kidneys
Half-life: S.C.: 1.2 hours
Elimination: As inactive metabolites in urine

Usual Dosage Dosage for calcitonin salmon is expressed in international units (IU); dosage of calcitonin human is expressed in mg

Calcitonin salmon:
Skin test: 1 IU/0.1 mL intracutaneously on the inner aspect of the forearm
The skin test is 0.1 mL of 10 IU dilution of calcitonin (must be prepared) injected intradermally; observe injection site for 15 minutes for wheal or significant erythema
Paget's disease: S.C.: 100 IU/day
Postmenopause osteoporosis: I.M., S.C.: 100 IU/day (concomitant therapy with supplemental calcium and vitamin D is recommended)

Hypercalcemia: I.M., S.C.: 4 IU/kg every 12 hours. If response is unsatisfactory, may increase at 2 day intervals to 8 IU/kg every 12 hours then to maximum of 8 IU/kg every 6 hours

Calcitonin human: Paget's disease: S.C.: 0.5 mg/day initially; some patients require as little as 0.25 mg or 0.5 mg 2-3 times/week; some patients require up to 0.5 mg twice daily

Monitoring Parameters Serum calcium and electrolytes

Reference Range Therapeutic: <19 pg/mL (SI: 19 ng/L) basal, depending on the assay

Patient Information Keep salmon calcitonin in refrigerator

Nursing Implications Skin test should be performed prior to administration of salmon calcitonin; refrigerate; I.M. administration is preferred if the volume to injection exceeds 2 mL

Dosage Forms Injection:
Human (Cibacalcin®): 0.5 mg/vial
Salmon:
Calcimar®: 200 units/mL (2 mL)
Miacalcin®: 100 units/mL (1 mL)

Calcitonin (Human) *see* Calcitonin *on previous page*

Calcitonin (Salmon) *see* Calcitonin *on previous page*

Calcitriol (kal si trye' ole)

Brand Names Calcijex™; Rocaltrol®

Synonyms 1,25 Dihydroxycholecalciferol

Use Management of hypocalcemia in patients on chronic renal dialysis; reduce elevated parathyroid hormone levels; decrease severity of psoriatic lesions in psoriatic vulgaris

Pregnancy Risk Factor A (D if used in doses above the recommended daily allowance)

Contraindications Hypercalcemia; vitamin D toxicity; abnormal sensitivity to the effects of vitamin D; malabsorption syndrome

Warnings/Precautions Adequate dietary (supplemental) calcium is necessary for clinical response to vitamin D; maintain adequate fluid intake; calcium-phosphate product (serum calcium times phosphorus) must not exceed 70; avoid hypercalcemia or use with renal function impairment and secondary hyperparathyroidism

Adverse Reactions
1% to 10%:
Cardiovascular: Hypotension, cardiac arrhythmias, hypertension, irregular heartbeat
Central nervous system: Irritability, headache
Dermatologic: Pruritus
Endocrine & metabolic: Polydipsia
Gastrointestinal: Nausea, vomiting, constipation, anorexia, pancreatitis, metallic taste
Neuromuscular & skeletal: Muscle/bone pain
Ocular: Conjunctivitis, photophobia
Renal: Polyuria
<1%:
Central nervous system: Overt psychosis, hyperthermia
Endocrine & metabolic: Hypercalcemia
Gastrointestinal: Weight loss
Hepatic: Increased LFTs
Respiratory: Rhinorrhea
Miscellaneous: Hypercholesterolemia

Overdosage/Toxicology Symptoms of overdose include hypercalcemia, hypercalciuria; following withdrawal of the drug, treatment consists of bed rest, liberal intake of fluids, reduced calcium intake, and cathartic administration. Severe hypercalcemia requires I.V. hydration and forced diuresis. Urine output should be monitored and maintained at >3 mL/kg/hour. I.V. saline can quickly and significantly increase excretion of calcium into urine. Calcitonin, cholestyramine, prednisone, sodium EDTA, biphosphonates, and mithramycin have all been used successfully to treat the more resistant cases of vitamin D-induced hypercalcemia.

Drug Interactions
Decreased effect/absorption: Cholestyramine, colestipol
Increased effect: Thiazide diuretics
Additive effect: Magnesium-containing antacids

Stability Store in tight, light-resistant container; calcitriol degrades upon prolonged exposure to light
(Continued)

Calcitriol *(Continued)*

Mechanism of Action Promotes absorption of calcium in the intestines and retention at the kidneys thereby increasing calcium levels in the serum; decreases excessive serum phosphatase levels, parathyroid hormone levels, and decreases bone resorption; increases renal tubule phosphate resorption

Pharmacodynamics/Kinetics

Onset of action: ~2-6 hours

Duration: 3-5 days

Absorption: Oral: Rapid

Metabolism: Primarily to 1,24,25-trihydroxycholecalciferol and 1,24,25-trihydroxy ergocalciferol

Half-life: 3-8 hours

Elimination: Principally in bile and feces with 4% to 6% excreted in urine

Usual Dosage Individualize dosage to maintain calcium levels of 9-10 mg/dL

Renal failure:

Oral:

Children: Initial: 15 ng/kg/day; maintenance: 5-40 ng/kg/day

Adults: 0.25 mcg/day or every other day (may require 0.5-1 mcg/day)

I.V.: Adults: 0.5 mcg (0.01 mcg/kg) 3 times/week; most doses in the range of 0.5-3 mcg (0.01-0.05 mcg/kg) 3 times/week

Hypoparathyroidism/pseudohypoparathyroidism: Oral:

Children:

<1 year: 0.04-0.08 mcg/kg/day

1-6 years: Initial: 0.25 mcg/day, increase at 2- to 4-week intervals

Children >6 years and Adults: 0.5-2 mcg/day

Vitamin D-resistant rickets (familial hypophosphatemia): Oral: 2 mcg/day; initial: 15-20 ng/kg/day; maintenance: 30-60 ng/kg/day

Monitoring Parameters Monitor symptoms of hypercalcemia (weakness, fatigue, somnolence, headache, anorexia, dry mouth, metallic taste, nausea, vomiting, cramps, diarrhea, muscle pain, bone pain and irritability)

Reference Range Calcium (serum) 9-10 mg/dL (4.5-5 mEq/L) but do not include the I.V. dosages; phosphate: 2.5-5 mg/dL

Test Interactions ↑ calcium, cholesterol, magnesium, BUN, AST, ALT, calcium (S), cholesterol (S); ↓ alkaline phosphatase

Patient Information Compliance with dose, diet, and calcium supplementation is essential; notify physician if weakness, lethargy, headache, and decreased appetite occur; avoid taking magnesium supplements or magnesium-containing antacids

Dosage Forms

Capsule: 0.25 mcg, 0.5 mcg

Injection: 1 mcg/mL (1 mL); 2 mcg/mL (1 mL)

Calcium Acetate *(kal' see um as' e tate)*

Brand Names Phos-Ex®; PhosLo®

Use Control of hyperphosphatemia in end stage renal failure; calcium acetate binds phosphorus in the GI tract better than other calcium salts due to its lower solubility and subsequent reduced absorption and increased formation of calcium phosphate; calcium acetate does not promote aluminum absorption

Pregnancy Risk Factor C

Contraindications Hypercalcemia

Warnings/Precautions Use with caution in patients on digitalis, with CHF or renal failure. No other calcium supplements should be given concurrently; therapy should be initiated at a low dose and increase only with careful monitoring (2 times/week); chronic hypercalcemia may lead to vascular calcification, and other soft tissue calcification; the serum calcium times phosphate product should not be allowed to exceed 66.

Adverse Reactions

Mild hypercalcemia (calcium: >10.5 mg/dL) may be asymptomatic or manifest itself as constipation, anorexia, nausea, and vomiting

More severe hypercalcemia (calcium: >12 mg/dL) is associated with confusion, delirium, stupor, and coma

<1%:

Central nervous system: Headache

Endocrine & metabolic: Hypophosphatemia, hypercalcemia

Gastrointestinal: Nausea, anorexia, vomiting, abdominal pain, constipation

Miscellaneous: Thirst

Overdosage/Toxicology Symptoms of overdose include hypercalcemia, lethargy, nausea, vomiting, coma; following withdrawal of the drug, treatment consists of bed rest, liberal intake of fluids, reduced calcium intake, and cathartic

ALPHABETICAL LISTING OF DRUGS

administration. Severe hypercalcemia requires I.V. hydration and forced diuresis. Urine output should be monitored and maintained at >3 mL/kg/hour. I.V. saline can quickly and significantly increase excretion of calcium into urine.

Drug Interactions
Decreased effect:
  Calcium may antagonize the effects of calcium channel blockers
  May decrease the bioavailability of tetracyclines
  Renders tetracycline antibiotics inactive
Increased toxicity: Administer cautiously to a digitalized patient, may precipitate arrhythmias

Mechanism of Action Moderates nerve and muscle performance via action potential excitation threshold regulation; combines with dietary phosphate to form insoluble calcium phosphate which is excreted in feces

Pharmacodynamics/Kinetics
Absorption: Absorption from the GI tract requires vitamin D
Distribution: Crosses the placenta; appears in breast milk
Elimination: Mainly in feces as unabsorbed calcium with 20% eliminated by the kidneys

Usual Dosage Adults: Oral: 2 tablets with each meal; dosage may be increased to bring serum phosphate value to <6 mg/dL; most patients require 3-4 tablets with each meal

Reference Range
Serum calcium: 8.4-10.2 mg/dL
Due to a poor correlation between the serum ionized calcium (free) and total serum calcium, particularly in states of low albumin or acid/base imbalances, direct measurement of ionized calcium is recommended
In low albumin states, the corrected **total** serum calcium may be estimated by this equation (assuming a normal albumin of 4 g/dL)
Corrected total calcium = total serum calcium + 0.8 (4.0 - measured serum albumin)
or
Corrected calcium = measured calcium - measured albumin + 4.0

Test Interactions ↑ calcium (S); ↓ magnesium

Patient Information Can take with food; do not take calcium supplements within 1-2 hours of taking other medicine by mouth or eating large amounts of fiber-rich foods; do not use nonprescription antacids or drink large amounts of alcohol, caffeine-containing beverages, or use tobacco

Additional Information 12.7 mEq/g; 250 mg/g elemental calcium (25% elemental calcium); see table.

Elemental Calcium Content of Calcium Salts

Calcium Salt	% Calcium	mEq Ca⁺⁺/g
Calcium acetate	25	12.6
Calcium carbonate	40	20
Calcium chloride	27.2	13.6
Calcium gluconate	9	4.5

Dosage Forms
Capsule: 500 mg
Tablet: 250 mg, 667 mg, 1000 mg

Calcium Carbonate (kal' see um kar' bon ate)
Brand Names Alka-Mints® [OTC]; Amitone® [OTC]; Biocal® [OTC]; Calci-Chew™; Calcilac® [OTC]; Calci-Mix™; CalSup® [OTC]; Caltrate® [OTC]; Chooz® [OTC]; Dicarbosil® [OTC]; Glycate® [OTC]; Os-Cal® 250 [OTC]; Os-Cal® 500 [OTC]; Rolaids® Calcium Rich [OTC]; Suplical® [OTC]; Titralac® [OTC]; Tums® [OTC]

Use Adjunct in prevention of postmenopausal osteoporosis, antacid, treatment and prevention of calcium depletion (osteoporosis, osteomalacia, etc); control of hyperphosphatemia in end stage renal disease

Pregnancy Risk Factor C

Contraindications Hypercalcemia, renal calculi, hypophosphatemia, ventricular fibrillation; patients with risk of digitalis toxicity, renal or cardiac disease

Warnings/Precautions Use with caution in patients on digitalis, with CHF or renal failure. No other calcium supplements should be given concurrently; no more than 300-350 mg of elemental calcium should be given at a time; therapy should be initiated at a low dose and increase only with careful monitoring (2 times/week); calcium carbonate absorption is impaired in achlorhydria (common in elderly - use alternate salt, administer with food); chronic hypercalcemia may
(Continued)

Calcium Carbonate *(Continued)*

lead to vascular calcification, and other soft tissue calcification; the serum calcium times phosphate product should not be allowed to exceed 66. Calcium carbonate administration is followed by increased gastric acid secretion within 2 hours of administration.

Adverse Reactions

1% to 10%: Gastrointestinal: Constipation, flatulence

<1%:

Cardiovascular: Hypotension, bradycardia, cardiac arrhythmias

Central nervous system: Mood and mental changes, lethargy

Dermatologic: Erythema

Endocrine & metabolic: Hypercalcemia (with prolonged use), metastatic calcinosis, hypomagnesemia, hypophosphatemia, milk-alkali syndrome

Gastrointestinal: Laxative effect, acid rebound, nausea, vomiting, GI hemorrhage, fecal impaction

Hematologic: Elevated serum amylase

Neuromuscular & skeletal: Myalgia

Renal: Polyuria, renal calculi, renal dysfunction, hypercalciuria

Overdosage/Toxicology

Symptoms of overdose include hypercalcemia, lethargy, nausea, vomiting, coma; following withdrawal of the drug, treatment consists of bed rest, liberal intake of fluids, reduced calcium intake, and cathartic administration. Severe hypercalcemia requires I.V. hydration and forced diuresis. Urine output should be monitored and maintained at >3 mL/kg/hour. I.V. saline can quickly and significantly increase excretion of calcium into urine. Calcitonin, cholestyramine, prednisone, sodium EDTA, biphosphonates, and mithramycin have all been used successfully to treat the more resistant cases of vitamin D-induced hypercalcemia.

Drug Interactions

Decreased effect:

Calcium may antagonize the effects of calcium channel blockers

May decrease the bioavailability of tetracyclines

Renders tetracycline antibiotics inactive

Increased toxicity: Administer cautiously to a digitalized patient, may precipitate arrhythmias

Stability

Admixture **incompatibilities** include carbonates, phosphates, sulfates, tartrates

Mechanism of Action

Moderates nerve and muscle performance via action potential excitation threshold regulation; combines with dietary phosphate to form insoluble calcium phosphate which is excreted in feces; may prevent negative calcium balance when used as a dietary supplement, or for calcium balance when used as a dietary supplement, or as treatment for osteoporosis

Pharmacodynamics/Kinetics

Absorption: From the GI tract requires vitamin D; calcium is absorbed in soluble, ionized form; solubility of calcium is increased in an acid environment

Distribution: Crosses the placenta; appears in breast milk

Elimination: Mainly in feces as unabsorbed calcium with 20% eliminated by the kidneys

Usual Dosage

Oral (dosage is in terms of elemental calcium):

Recommended daily allowance (RDA):

<6 months: 360 mg/day

6-12 months: 540 mg/day

1-10 years: 800 mg/day

10-18 years: 1200 mg/day

Adults: 800 mg/day

Hypocalcemia (dose depends on clinical condition and serum calcium level):

Neonates: 50-150 mg/kg/day in 4-6 divided doses; not to exceed 1 g/day

Children: 45-65 mg/kg/day in 4 divided doses

Adults: 1-2 g or more/day

Adults:

Dietary supplementation: 500 mg to 2 g divided 2-4 times/day

To reduce bone loss with aging/osteoporosis: 1000-1500 mg/day

Antacid: 2 tablets or 10 mL every 2 hours, up to 12 times/day

Reference Range

Serum calcium: 8.4-10.2 mg/dL

Due to a poor correlation between the serum ionized calcium (free) and total serum calcium, particularly in states of low albumin or acid/base imbalances, direct measurement of ionized calcium is recommended

In low albumin states, the corrected **total** serum calcium may be estimated by this equation (assuming a normal albumin of 4 g/dL)

Corrected total calcium = total serum calcium + 0.8 (4.0 - measured serum albumin)

or

Corrected calcium = measured calcium - measured albumin + 4.0

Test Interactions ↑ calcium (S); ↓ magnesium

Patient Information Shake suspension well; take with large quantities of water or juice; do not take calcium supplements within 1-2 hours of taking other medicine by mouth or eating large amounts of fiber-rich foods; do not take other antacids or calcium supplements or drink large amounts of alcohol or caffeine-containing beverages

Additional Information 20 mEq calcium/g; 400 mg calcium/g calcium carbonate (40% elemental calcium); see table.

Elemental Calcium Content of Calcium Salts

Calcium Salt	% Calcium	mEq Ca⁺⁺/g
Calcium acetate	25	12.6
Calcium carbonate	40	20
Calcium chloride	27.2	13.6
Calcium gluconate	9	4.5

Dosage Forms

Capsule:
Calci-Mix™: 1250 mg
Florical®: 364 mg with sodium fluoride 8.3 mg
Liquid (Tums® Extra Strength): 1000 mg/5 mL (360 mL)
Powder (Cal Carb-HD®): 6.5 g/packet
Suspension, oral: 1.25 g/5 mL
Tablet:
650 mg
Calciday-667®: 667 mg
Os-Cal® 500, Oyst-Cal® 500, Oystercal® 500: 1.25 g
Cal-Plus®, Caltrate® 600, Gencalc® 600, Nephro-Calci®: 1.5 g
Chewable:
Alka-Mints®: 850 mg
Amitone®: 350 mg
Caltrate, Jr.®: 750 mg
Calci-Chew™, Os-Cal®: 750 mg
Chooz®, Dicarbosil®, Equilet®, Tums®: 500 mg
Mallamint®: 420 mg
Rolaids® Calcium Rich: 550 mg
Tums® E-X Extra Strength: 750 mg
Florical®: 364 mg with sodium fluoride 8.3 mg

Calcium Channel Blockers Cardiovascular Adverse Reactions *see page 1262*

Calcium Channel Blockers Central Nervous System Adverse Reactions *see page 1264*

Calcium Channel Blockers Comparative Actions *see page 1260*

Calcium Channel Blockers Comparative Pharmacokinetics *see page 1261*

Calcium Channel Blockers FDA-Approved Indications *see page 1263*

Calcium Channel Blockers Gastrointestinal and Miscellaneous Adverse Reactions *see page 1265*

Calcium Chloride (kal' see um klor' ide)

Related Information
Extravasation Treatment of Other Drugs *on page 1209*

Brand Names Cal Plus®

Use Cardiac resuscitation when epinephrine fails to improve myocardial contractions, cardiac disturbances of hyperkalemia, hypocalcemia, or calcium channel blocking agent toxicity; emergent treatment of hypocalcemic tetany, treatment of hypermagnesemia

Pregnancy Risk Factor C

Contraindications In ventricular fibrillation during cardiac resuscitation, hypercalcemia, and in patients with risk of digitalis toxicity, renal or cardiac disease

Warnings/Precautions Avoid too rapid I.V. administration (<1 mL/minute) and extravasation; use with caution in digitalized patients, respiratory failure, or acidosis; hypercalcemia may occur in patients with renal failure, and frequent

(Continued)

163

Calcium Chloride *(Continued)*

determination of serum calcium is necessary; avoid metabolic acidosis (ie, give only 2-3 days then change to another calcium salt)

Adverse Reactions

<1%:

Cardiovascular: Vasodilation, hypotension, bradycardia, cardiac arrhythmias, ventricular fibrillation, syncope

Central nervous system: Lethargy, coma, mania

Dermatologic: Erythema

Endocrine & metabolic: Decreased serum magnesium, hypercalcemia

Hematologic: Elevated serum amylase

Local: Tissue necrosis

Neuromuscular & skeletal: Muscle weakness

Renal: Hypercalciuria

Overdosage/Toxicology Symptoms of overdose include lethargy, nausea, vomiting, coma; following withdrawal of the drug, treatment consists of bed rest, liberal intake of fluids, reduced calcium intake, and cathartic administration. Severe hypercalcemia requires I.V. hydration and forced diuresis. Urine output should be monitored and maintained at >3 mL/kg/hour. I.V. saline can quickly and significantly increase excretion of calcium into urine.

Drug Interactions

Decreased effect: Calcium may antagonize the effects of calcium channel blockers; concomitant administration with tetracyclines decreases tetracycline bioavailability

Increased toxicity: Administer cautiously to a digitalized patient, may precipitate arrhythmias

Stability

Do not refrigerate solutions; IVPB solutions/I.V. infusion solutions are stable for 24 hours at room temperature

Maximum concentration in parenteral nutrition solutions: 15 mEq/L of calcium and 30 mmol/L of phosphate

Incompatibilities include sodium bicarbonate, carbonates, phosphates, sulfates, and tartrates

Mechanism of Action Moderates nerve and muscle performance via action potential excitation threshold regulation

Pharmacodynamics/Kinetics

Absorption: I.V. calcium salts are absorbed directly into the bloodstream

Distribution: Crosses the placenta; appears in breast milk

Elimination: Mainly in feces as unabsorbed calcium with 20% eliminated by the kidneys

Usual Dosage Note: Calcium chloride is 3 times as potent as calcium gluconate

Cardiac arrest in the presence of hyperkalemia or hypocalcemia, magnesium toxicity, or calcium antagonist toxicity: I.V.:

Infants and Children: 20 mg/kg; may repeat in 10 minutes if necessary

Adults: 2-4 mg/kg (10% solution), repeated every 10 minutes

Hypocalcemia: I.V.:

Infants and Children: 10-20 mg/kg/dose (infants: <1 mEq; children: 1-7 mEq), repeat every 4-6 hours if needed; doses may be repeated every 1-3 days if needed

Adults: 500 mg to 1 g (7-14 mEq), repeated at 1- to 3-day intervals if necessary

Hypocalcemic tetany: I.V.:

Neonates: Divided doses totalling about 2.4 mEq/kg/day

Infants and Children: 10 mg/kg (0.5-0.7 mEq/kg) over 5-10 minutes; may repeat after 6-8 hours or follow with an infusion with a maximum dose of 200 mg/kg/day

Adults: 4.5-16 mEq may be administered until response occurs

Hypocalcemia secondary to citrated blood transfusion give 0.45 mEq **elemental** calcium for each 100 mL citrated blood infused

Reference Range

Serum calcium: 8.4-10.2 mg/dL

Due to a poor correlation between the serum ionized calcium (free) and total serum calcium, particularly in states of low albumin or acid/base imbalances, direct measurement of ionized calcium is recommended

In low albumin states, the corrected **total** serum calcium may be estimated by this equation (assuming a normal albumin of 4 g/dL)

Corrected total calcium = total serum calcium + 0.8 (4.0 - measured serum albumin)

or

Corrected calcium = measured calcium - measured albumin + 4.0

Serum/plasma chloride: 95-108 mEq/L

Test Interactions ↑ calcium (S); ↓ magnesium

Nursing Implications Do not inject calcium chloride I.M. or administer S.C. or use scalp, small hand or foot veins for I.V. administration since severe necrosis and sloughing may occur. Monitor EKG if calcium is infused faster than 2.5 mEq/minute; usual: 0.7-1.5 mEq/minute (0.5-1 mL/minute); **stop the infusion if the patient complains of pain or discomfort.** Warm to body temperature; administer slowly, do not exceed 1 mL/minute (inject into ventricular cavity - not myocardium); **do not infuse calcium chloride in the same I.V. line as phosphate-containing solutions.**

Extravasation treatment:
Hyaluronidase: Add 1 mL NS to 150 unit vial to make 150 units/mL of concentration; mix 0.1 mL of above with 0.9 mL NS in 1 mL syringe to make final concentration = 15 units/mL
Phentolamine: Mix 5 mg with 9 mL NS; inject small amount of this dilution into extravasated area. Blanching should reverse immediately; monitor site; if blanching should recur, additional injections of phentolamine may be needed.

Additional Information 14 mEq/g/10 mL; 270 mg elemental calcium/g (27% elemental calcium); see table.

Elemental Calcium Content of Calcium Salts

Calcium Salt	% Calcium	mEq Ca^{++}/g
Calcium acetate	25	12.6
Calcium carbonate	40	20
Calcium chloride	27.2	13.6
Calcium gluconate	9	4.5

Dosage Forms Injection: 10% [100 mg/mL] (10 mL)

Calcium Citrate (kal′ see um si′ trate)
Brand Names Citracal® [OTC]
Use Adjunct in prevention of postmenopausal osteoporosis; treatment and prevention of calcium depletion
Pregnancy Risk Factor C
Contraindications Hypercalcemia, renal calculi, ventricular fibrillation
Warnings/Precautions Use with caution in patients on digitalis, because hypercalcemia may precipitate cardiac arrhythmias. Always start at low dose and do not increase without careful monitoring of serum calcium; estimate of daily dietary calcium intake should be made initially and the intake adjusted as needed. Use with caution in patients with CHF, renal failure. No other calcium supplements should be given concurrently; progressive hypercalcemia due to overdose may be severe as to require emergency measures; chronic hypercalcemia may lead to vascular calcification, and other soft tissue calcification. The serum calcium level should be monitored twice weekly during the early dose adjustment period.
Adverse Reactions
<1%:
Central nervous system: Mental confusion, headache
Endocrine & metabolic: Hypercalcemia, milk-alkali syndrome, hypophosphatemia
Gastrointestinal: Constipation, vomiting, nausea
Overdosage/Toxicology Lethargy, nausea, vomiting, coma
Drug Interactions Administer cautiously to a digitalized patient, may precipitate arrhythmias; calcium may antagonize the effects of calcium channel blockers; concomitant administration renders tetracycline antibiotics inactive by blocking absorption
Mechanism of Action Moderates nerve and muscle performance via action potential excitation threshold regulation
Pharmacodynamics/Kinetics
Absorption: Absorption from the GI tract requires vitamin D
Distribution: Crosses the placenta; appears in breast milk
Elimination: Mainly in feces as unabsorbed calcium with 20% eliminated by the kidneys
Usual Dosage Dosage is in terms of elemental calcium
Recommended daily allowance (RDA):
<6 months: 360 mg/day
6-12 months: 540 mg/day
1-10 years: 800 mg/day
10-18 years: 1200 mg/day
(Continued)

Calcium Citrate *(Continued)*

Adults: 800 mg/day
Adults: Oral: 1-2 g/day

Reference Range Serum: 8.4-10.2 mg/dL; due to a poor correlation between the serum ionized calcium (free) and total serum calcium, particularly in states of low albumin or acid/base imbalances, direct measurement of ionized calcium is recommended. In low albumin states, the corrected **total** serum calcium may be estimated by this equation (assuming a normal albumin of 4 g/dL); corrected total calcium = total serum calcium + 0.8 (4- measured serum albumin)

Test Interactions ↑ calcium (S); ↓ magnesium

Patient Information Chew tablets well, followed by water; do not take calcium supplements within 1-2 hours of taking other medicine by mouth or eating large amounts of fiber-rich foods; do not drink large amounts of alcohol or caffeine-containing beverages or use tobacco

Additional Information 10.6 mEq/g; 211 mg elemental calcium/g (21% elemental calcium)

Dosage Forms
Tablet: 950 mg
Tablet, effervescent: 2376 mg

Calcium Disodium Versenate® *see* Edetate Calcium Disodium *on page 379*

Calcium EDTA *see* Edetate Calcium Disodium *on page 379*

Calcium Glubionate *(gloo bye' oh nate)*

Brand Names Neo-Calglucon® [OTC]

Use Adjunct in prevention of postmenopausal osteoporosis; treatment and prevention of calcium depletion

Pregnancy Risk Factor C

Contraindications Hypercalcemia, renal calculi, ventricular fibrillation

Warnings/Precautions Use cautiously in patients with sarcoidosis, CHF, renal insufficiency, cardiac disease, receiving digitalis, because hypercalcemia may precipitate cardiac arrhythmias. Always start at low dose and do not increase without careful monitoring of serum calcium (twice weekly); avoid other calcium supplements given concurrently; chronic hypercalcemia may lead to vascular calcification, and other soft tissue calcification.

Adverse Reactions
<1%:
Central nervous system: Dizziness, headache, mental confusion
Endocrine & metabolic: Hypercalcemia, hypomagnesemia, hypophosphatemia, milk-alkali syndrome
Gastrointestinal: GI irritation, diarrhea, constipation, dry mouth
Renal: Hypercalciuria

Overdosage/Toxicology Symptoms of overdose include lethargy, nausea, vomiting, coma; following withdrawal of the drug, treatment consists of bed rest, liberal intake of fluids, reduced calcium intake, and cathartic administration. Severe hypercalcemia requires I.V. hydration and forced diuresis. Urine output should be monitored and maintained at >3 mL/kg/hour. I.V. saline can quickly and significantly increase excretion of calcium into urine.

Drug Interactions
Decreased effect: Calcium may antagonize the effects of calcium channel blockers; concomitant administration renders tetracycline antibiotics inactive
Increased toxicity: Administer cautiously to a digitalized patient, may precipitate arrhythmias

Mechanism of Action Moderates nerve and muscle performance via action potential excitation threshold regulation

Pharmacodynamics/Kinetics
Absorption: Absorption from the GI tract requires vitamin D
Distribution: Crosses the placenta; appears in breast milk
Elimination: Mainly in feces as unabsorbed calcium with 20% eliminated by the kidneys

Usual Dosage Oral:
Recommended daily allowance (RDA) (in terms of elemental calcium):
<6 months: 360 mg/day
6-12 months: 540 mg/day
1-10 years: 800 mg/day
10-18 years: 1200 mg/day
Adults: 800 mg/day

Syrup is a hyperosmolar solution; dosage is in terms of calcium glubionate
Neonatal hypocalcemia: 1200 mg/kg/day in 4-6 divided doses

Maintenance: Infants and Children: 600-2000 mg/kg/day in 4 divided doses up to a maximum of 9 g/day

Adults: 6-18 g/day in divided doses

Reference Range
Serum calcium: 8.4-10.2 mg/dL
Due to a poor correlation between the serum ionized calcium (free) and total serum calcium, particularly in states of low albumin or acid/base imbalances, direct measurement of ionized calcium is recommended
In low albumin states, the corrected **total** serum calcium may be estimated by this equation (assuming a normal albumin of 4 g/dL)
Corrected total calcium = total serum calcium + 0.8 (4.0 - measured serum albumin)
or
Corrected calcium = measured calcium - measured albumin + 4.0

Test Interactions $\uparrow$ calcium (S); $\downarrow$ magnesium

Patient Information Do not take calcium supplements within 1-2 hours of taking other medicine by mouth or eating large amounts of fiber-rich foods; do not take other calcium-containing products or antacids, drink large amounts of alcohol or caffeine-containing beverages

Additional Information 3.3 mEq/g; 64 mg elemental calcium/g (6% elemental calcium)

Dosage Forms Syrup: 1.8 g/5 mL (480 mL)

Calcium Gluceptate (gloo sep' tate)

Use Treatment of cardiac disturbances of hyperkalemia, hypocalcemia, or calcium channel blocker toxicity; cardiac resuscitation when epinephrine fails to improve myocardial contractions; treatment of hypermagnesemia and hypocalcemia

Pregnancy Risk Factor C

Contraindications In ventricular fibrillation during cardiac resuscitation; patients with risk of digitalis toxicity, renal or cardiac disease; hypercalcemia

Warnings/Precautions Avoid too rapid I.V. administration; avoid extravasation; use with caution in digitalized patients, respiratory failure or acidosis; metabolic acidosis (give only 2-3 days then change to another calcium salt)

Adverse Reactions
<1%:
Cardiovascular: Vasodilation, hypotension, bradycardia, cardiac arrhythmias, ventricular fibrillation, syncope, coma
Central nervous system: Lethargy, mania
Dermatologic: Erythema
Endocrine & metabolic: Hypomagnesemia, hypercalcemia
Hematologic: Elevated serum amylase
Local: Tissue necrosis
Neuromuscular & skeletal: Muscle weakness
Renal: Hypercalciuria

Overdosage/Toxicology Symptoms of overdose include lethargy, nausea, vomiting, coma; following withdrawal of the drug, treatment consists of bed rest, liberal intake of fluids, reduced calcium intake, and cathartic administration. Severe hypercalcemia requires I.V. hydration and forced diuresis with I.V. furosemide (20-40 mg I.V. every 4-6 hours for adults). Urine output should be monitored and maintained at >3 mL/kg/hour. I.V. saline can quickly and significantly increase excretion of calcium into urine. Calcitonin, cholestyramine, prednisone, sodium EDTA, biphosphonates, and mithramycin have all been used successfully to treat the more resistant cases of vitamin D-induced hypercalcemia.

Drug Interactions Administer cautiously to digitalized patients, may precipitate arrhythmias; calcium may antagonize effects of calcium channel blockers

Stability Admixture **incompatibilities** include carbonates, phosphates, sulfates, tartrates

Mechanism of Action Moderates nerve and muscle performance via action potential excitation threshold regulation

Pharmacodynamics/Kinetics
Absorption: I.M. and I.V. calcium salts are absorbed directly into the bloodstream
Distribution: Crosses the placenta; appears in breast milk
Elimination: Mainly in feces as unabsorbed calcium with 20% eliminated by the kidneys

Usual Dosage I.V. (dose expressed in mg of calcium gluceptate):
Cardiac resuscitation in the presence of hypocalcemia, hyperkalemia, magnesium toxicity, or calcium channel blocker toxicity:
Children: 110 mg/kg/dose
Adults: 1.1-1.5 g (5-7 mL)
Hypocalcemia:
Children: 200-500 mg/kg/day divided every 6 hours
(Continued)

Calcium Gluceptate *(Continued)*

Adults: 500 mg to 1.1 g/dose as needed

After citrated blood administration: Children and Adults: 0.4 mEq/100 mL blood infused

Reference Range

Serum calcium: 8.4-10.2 mg/dL

Due to a poor correlation between the serum ionized calcium (free) and total serum calcium, particularly in states of low albumin or acid/base imbalances, direct measurement of ionized calcium is recommended

In low albumin states, the corrected **total** serum calcium may be estimated by this equation (assuming a normal albumin of 4 g/dL)

Corrected total calcium = total serum calcium + 0.8 (4.0 - measured serum albumin)

or

Corrected calcium = measured calcium - measured albumin + 4.0

Test Interactions ↑ calcium (S); ↓ magnesium

Nursing Implications Warm to body temperature; administer slowly, do not exceed 1 mL/minute (inject into ventricular cavity - not myocardium)

Additional Information 4.1 mEq/g; 82 mg elemental calcium/g (8% elemental calcium)

Dosage Forms Elemental calcium listed in brackets

Injection: 220 mg/mL [18 mg/mL] (5 mL, 50 mL)

Calcium Gluconate (gloo' koe nate)

Brand Names Kalcinate®

Use Treatment and prevention of hypocalcemia; treatment of tetany, cardiac disturbances of hyperkalemia, cardiac resuscitation when epinephrine fails to improve myocardial contractions, hypocalcemia, or calcium channel blocker toxicity; calcium supplementation

Pregnancy Risk Factor C

Contraindications In ventricular fibrillation during cardiac resuscitation; patients with risk of digitalis toxicity, renal or cardiac disease, hypercalcemia, renal calculi, hypophosphatemia

Warnings/Precautions Avoid too rapid I.V. administration (1.5-3.3 mL/minute); use with caution in digitalized patients, severe hyperphosphatemia, respiratory failure or acidosis; avoid extravasation; may produce cardiac arrest; hypercalcemia may occur in patients with renal failure and frequent determination of serum calcium is necessary; avoid injection into myocardium; the serum calcium level should be monitored twice weekly during the early dose adjustment period; no more than 300-350 mg of elemental calcium should be given at a time

Adverse Reactions

<1%:

Cardiovascular: Vasodilation, hypotension, bradycardia, cardiac arrhythmias, ventricular fibrillation, syncope, coma

Central nervous system: Lethargy, mania

Endocrine & metabolic: Decrease serum magnesium, hypercalcemia

Hematologic: Erythema, elevated serum amylase

Local: Tissue necrosis

Neuromuscular & skeletal: Muscle weakness

Renal: Hypercalciuria

Overdosage/Toxicology Symptoms of overdose include lethargy, nausea, vomiting, delirium, coma; following withdrawal of the drug, treatment consists of bed rest, liberal intake of fluids, reduced calcium intake, and cathartic administration. Severe hypercalcemia requires I.V. hydration. Urine output should be monitored and maintained at >3 mL/kg/hour. I.V. saline can quickly and significantly increase excretion of calcium into urine.

Drug Interactions

Decreased effect: Calcium may antagonize the effects of verapamil; concomitant oral administration renders tetracycline antibiotics inactive

Increased toxicity: Administer cautiously to a digitalized patient, may precipitate arrhythmias

Stability

Do not refrigerate solutions; IVPB solutions/I.V. infusion solutions are stable for 24 hours at room temperature

Standard diluent: 1 g/100 mL D_5W or NS; 2 g/100 mL D_5W or NS

Maximum concentration in parenteral nutrition solutions is 15 mEq/L of calcium and 30 mmol/L of phosphate

Incompatibilities include sodium bicarbonate, carbonates, phosphates, sulfates, and tartrates

Mechanism of Action Moderates nerve and muscle performance via action potential excitation threshold regulation

Pharmacodynamics/Kinetics

Absorption: I.M. and I.V. calcium salts are absorbed directly into the bloodstream; absorption from the GI tract requires vitamin D; calcium is absorbed in soluble, ionized form; solubility of calcium is increased in an acid environment (except calcium lactate)

Distribution: Crosses the placenta; appears in breast milk

Elimination: Mainly in feces as unabsorbed calcium with 20% eliminated by the kidneys

Usual Dosage Dosage is in terms of elemental calcium

Recommended daily allowance (RDA):
<6 months: 400 mg/day
6-12 months: 600 mg/day
1-10 years: 800 mg/day
10-18 years: 1200 mg/day
Adults: 800 mg/day

Calcium gluconate electrolyte requirement in newborn period:
Premature: 200-1000 mg/kg/24 hours
Term:
0-24 hours: 0-500 mg/kg/24 hours
24-48 hours: 200-500 mg/kg/24 hours
48-72 hours: 200-600 mg/kg/24 hours
>3 days: 200-800 mg/kg/24 hours

Hypocalcemia:
Oral:
Children: 200-500 mg/kg/day divided every 6 hours
Adults: 500 mg to 2 g 2-4 times/day
I.V.:
Neonates: 200-800 mg/kg/day as a continuous infusion or in 4 divided doses
Infants and Children: 200-500 mg/kg/day (infants <1 mEq/day; children 1-7 mEq/day) as a continuous infusion or in 4 divided doses; doses may be repeated every 1-3 days if necessary
Adults: 2-15 g/24 hours as a continuous infusion or in divided doses, which may be repeated every 1-3 days if necessary

Hypocalcemic tetany: I.V.:
Neonates: 100-200 mg/kg/dose, may follow with 500 mg/kg/day in 3-4 divided doses or as an infusion up to 2.4 mEq/kg/day
Infants and Children: 100-200 mg/kg/dose (0.5-0.7 mEq/kg/dose) over 5-10 minutes; may repeat every 6-8 hours or follow with an infusion of 500 mg/kg/day
Adults: 1-3 g (4.5-16 mEq) may be administered until therapeutic response occurs

Osteoporosis/bone loss: Oral: 1000-1500 mg in divided doses/day

Calcium antagonist toxicity, magnesium intoxication, or cardiac arrest in the presence of hyperkalemia or hypocalcemia: I.V.:
Infants and Children: Calcium chloride is recommended: Calcium salt; refer to calcium chloride monograph
Adults: 5-8 mL/dose and repeated as necessary at 10-minute intervals, however, calcium chloride is recommended calcium salt; refer to Calcium Chloride monograph

Hypocalcemia secondary to citrated blood infusion: I.V.: Give 0.45 mEq elemental calcium for each 100 mL citrated blood infused

Exchange transfusion:
Neonates: 100 mg/100 mL of citrated blood exchanged
Adults: 300 mg/100 mL of citrated blood exchanged

Maintenance electrolyte requirements for total parenteral nutrition: I.V.: Daily requirements: Adults: 8-16 mEq/1000 kcals/24 hours

Administration I.M. injections should be administered in the gluteal region in adults, usually in volumes <2 mL; avoid I.M. injections in children and adults with muscle mass wasting; do not use scalp veins or small hand or foot veins for I.V. administration; generally, I.V. infusion rates should not exceed 0.7-1.5 mEq/minute (1.5-3.3 mL/minute); stop the infusion if the patient complains of pain or discomfort. Warm to body temperature; do not inject into the myocardium when using calcium during advanced cardiac life support.

Reference Range

Serum calcium: 8.4-10.2 mg/dL

Due to a poor correlation between the serum ionized calcium (free) and total serum calcium, particularly in states of low albumin or acid/base imbalances, direct measurement of ionized calcium is recommended

In low albumin states, the corrected total serum calcium may be estimated by this equation (assuming a normal albumin of 4 g/dL)

Corrected total calcium = total serum calcium + 0.8 (4.0 - measured serum albumin)

or

(Continued)

Calcium Gluconate (Continued)

Corrected calcium = measured calcium - measured albumin + 4.0

Test Interactions ↑ calcium (S); ↓ magnesium

Patient Information Do not take calcium supplements within 1-2 hours of taking other medicine by mouth or eating large amounts of fiber-rich foods; do not drink large amounts of alcohol or caffeine-containing beverages; take with food

Nursing Implications

Extravasation treatment:

Hyaluronidase: Add 1 mL NS to 150 unit vial to make 150 units/mL of concentration; mix 0.1 mL of above with 0.9 mL NS in 1 mL syringe to make final concentration = 15 units/mL

Phentolamine: Mix 5 mg with 9 mL NS; inject small amount of this dilution into extravasated area. Blanching should reverse immediately; monitor site; if blanching should recur, additional injections of phentolamine may be needed.

Do not infuse calcium gluconate solutions in the same I.V. line as phosphate-containing solutions (eg, TPN)

Additional Information 4.5 mEq/g; 90 mg elemental calcium/g (9% elemental calcium); see table.

Elemental Calcium Content of Calcium Salts

Calcium Salt	% Calcium	mEq Ca⁺⁺/g
Calcium acetate	25	12.6
Calcium carbonate	40	20
Calcium chloride	27.2	13.6
Calcium gluconate	9	4.5

Dosage Forms

Injection: 10% [100 mg/mL] (10 mL, 50 mL, 100 mL, 200 mL)

Tablet: 500 mg, 650 mg, 975 mg, 1 g

Calcium Lactate (lak' tate)

Use Adjunct in prevention of postmenopausal osteoporosis; treatment and prevention of calcium depletion

Pregnancy Risk Factor C

Contraindications Hypercalcemia, renal calculi, ventricular fibrillation

Warnings/Precautions Use with caution in patients on digitalis, because hypercalcemia may precipitate cardiac arrhythmias, CHF, hyperphosphatemia, respiratory failure or acidosis, renal failure. Always start at low dose and do not increase without careful monitoring of serum calcium (twice weekly); estimate of daily dietary calcium intake should be made initially and the intake adjusted as needed. No other calcium supplements should be given concurrently; chronic hypercalcemia may lead to vascular calcification and other soft tissue calcification; avoid extravasation; no more than 300-350 mg of elemental calcium should be given at a time.

Adverse Reactions

<1%:

Central nervous system: Headache, mental confusion, dizziness

Endocrine & metabolic: Hypercalcemia, hypophosphatemia, hypomagnesemia, milk-alkali syndrome

Gastrointestinal: Constipation, nausea, dry mouth, vomiting

Renal: Hypercalciuria

Overdosage/Toxicology Symptoms of overdose include lethargy, nausea, vomiting, coma; following withdrawal of the drug, treatment consists of bed rest, liberal intake of fluids, reduced calcium intake, and cathartic administration. Severe hypercalcemia requires I.V. hydration and forced diuresis. Urine output should be monitored and maintained at >3 mL/kg/hour. I.V. saline can quickly and significantly increase excretion of calcium into urine. D-induced hypercalcemia.

Drug Interactions

Decreased effect: Calcium may antagonize the effects of calcium channel blockers; concomitant oral administration renders tetracycline antibiotics inactive

Increased toxicity: Administer cautiously to a digitalized patient, may precipitate arrhythmias

Mechanism of Action Moderates nerve and muscle performance via action potential excitation threshold regulation

Pharmacodynamics/Kinetics
  Absorption: Absorption from the GI tract requires vitamin D
  Distribution: Crosses the placenta; appears in breast milk
  Elimination: Mainly in feces as unabsorbed calcium with 20% eliminated by the kidneys

Usual Dosage Oral (in terms of calcium lactate)
  Recommended daily allowance (RDA) (in terms of elemental calcium):
    <6 months: 360 mg/day
    6-12 months: 540 mg/day
    1-10 years: 800 mg/day
    10-18 years: 1200 mg/day
    Adults: 800 mg/day

  Infants: 400-500 mg/kg/day divided every 4-6 hours
  Children: 500 mg/kg/day divided every 6-8 hours
    Maximum daily dose: 9 g
  Adults: 1.5-3 g divided every 8 hours

Reference Range
  Serum calcium: 8.4-10.2 mg/dL
  Due to a poor correlation between the serum ionized calcium (free) and total serum calcium, particularly in states of low albumin or acid/base imbalances, direct measurement of ionized calcium is recommended
  In low albumin states, the corrected **total** serum calcium may be estimated by this equation (assuming a normal albumin of 4 g/dL)
  Corrected total calcium = total serum calcium + 0.8 (4.0 - measured serum albumin)
    or
  Corrected calcium = measured calcium - measured albumin + 4.0

Test Interactions ↑ calcium (S); ↓ magnesium

Patient Information Do not take calcium supplements within 1-2 hours of taking other medicine by mouth or eating large amounts of fiber-rich foods; do not drink large amounts of alcohol or caffeine-containing beverages

Additional Information 6.5 mEq/g; 130 mg elemental calcium/g (13% elemental calcium)

Dosage Forms Elemental calcium listed in brackets
  Tablet: 325 mg [42.25 mg], 650 mg [84.5 mg]

Calcium Leucovorin see Leucovorin Calcium on page 619

Calcium Phosphate, Tribasic (kal' see um fos' fate tri ba' sik)
Brand Names Posture® [OTC]
Synonyms Dicalcium Phosphate
Use Adjunct in prevention of postmenopausal osteoporosis; treatment and prevention of calcium depletion
Pregnancy Risk Factor C
Contraindications Hypercalcemia, renal calculi, ventricular fibrillation
Warnings/Precautions Calcium, CBC, serum amylase, triglycerides, baseline and periodic total blood chemistries
Adverse Reactions
  <1%:
    Endocrine & metabolic: Hypercalcemia, milk-alkali syndrome, hypophosphatemia
    Gastrointestinal: Constipation, nausea, dry mouth
Overdosage/Toxicology Symptoms of overdose include lethargy, nausea, vomiting, coma; following withdrawal of the drug, treatment consists of bed rest, liberal intake of fluids, reduced calcium intake, and cathartic administration. Severe hypercalcemia requires I.V. hydration and forced diuresis with I.V. furosemide (20-40 mg I.V. every 4-6 hours for adults). Urine output should be monitored and maintained at >3 mL/kg/hour. I.V. saline can quickly and significantly increase excretion of calcium into urine.
Drug Interactions
  Decreased effect: Calcium may antagonize the effects of calcium channel blockers; concomitant oral administration renders tetracycline antibiotics inactive
  Increased toxicity: Administer cautiously to a digitalized patient, may precipitate arrhythmias
Mechanism of Action Moderates nerve and muscle performance via action potential excitation threshold regulation
Usual Dosage Oral (all doses in terms of elemental calcium):
  Recommended daily allowance (RDA) (elemental calcium):
    <6 months: 360 mg/day
    6-12 months: 540 mg/day
(Continued)

Calcium Phosphate, Tribasic (Continued)

    1-10 years: 800 mg/day
    10-18 years: 1200 mg/day
    Adults: 800 mg/day

    Children: 45-65 mg/kg/day
    Adults: 1-2 g/day

Reference Range
Serum calcium: 8.4-10.2 mg/dL
Due to a poor correlation between the serum ionized calcium (free) and total serum calcium, particularly in states of low albumin or acid/base imbalances, direct measurement of ionized calcium is recommended
In low albumin states, the corrected **total** serum calcium may be estimated by this equation (assuming a normal albumin of 4 g/dL)
Corrected total **calcium** = total serum calcium + 0.8 (4.0 - measured serum albumin)
    or
Corrected calcium = measured calcium - measured albumin + 4.0

Test Interactions ↑ calcium (S); ↓ magnesium

Patient Information Do not take calcium supplements within 1-2 hours of taking other medicine by mouth or eating large amounts of fiber-rich foods; do not drink large amounts of alcohol or caffeine-containing beverages

Additional Information 19.3 mEq/g; 390 mg elemental calcium/g (39% elemental calcium)

Dosage Forms Tablet, sugar free: 1565.2 mg

Calcium Polycarbophil (pol ee kar' boe fil)

Brand Names Equalactin® Chewable Tablet [OTC]; Fiberall® Chewable Tablet [OTC]; FiberCon® Tablet [OTC]; Fiber-Lax® Tablet [OTC]; Mitrolan® Chewable Tablet [OTC]

Use Treatment of constipation or diarrhea by restoring a more normal moisture level and providing bulk in the patient's intestinal tract; calcium polycarbophil is supplied as the approved substitute whenever a bulk-forming laxative is ordered in a tablet, capsule, wafer, or other oral solid dosage form

Pregnancy Risk Factor C

Adverse Reactions 1% to 10%: Abdominal fullness

Drug Interactions Decreased absorption of oral anticoagulants, digoxin, potassium-sparing diuretics, salicylates, tetracyclines

Usual Dosage Oral:
Children:
    2-6 years: 500 mg (1 tablet) 1-2 times/day, up to 1.5 g/day
    6-12 years: 500 mg (1 tablet) 1-3 times/day, up to 3 g/day
Adults: 1 g 4 times/day, up to 6 g/day

Test Interactions ↓ potassium (S)

Patient Information When used as an antacid or for constipation, drink 8 oz of water or other liquid with each dose; diarrhea dose may be repeated every 30 minutes until total dose in achieved

Dosage Forms Tablet:
Sodium free:
    Fiber-Lax®: 625 mg
    FiberCon®: 500 mg
Chewable:
    Equalactin®, Mitrolan®: 500 mg
    Fiberall®: 1250 mg

Caldecort® Anti-Itch Spray [OTC] see Hydrocortisone on page 546

Caldecort® [OTC] see Hydrocortisone on page 546

Calderol® see Calcifediol on page 156

Calm-X® [OTC] see Dimenhydrinate on page 347

Cal Plus® see Calcium Chloride on page 163

CalSup® [OTC] see Calcium Carbonate on page 161

Caltrate® [OTC] see Calcium Carbonate on page 161

Camphorated Tincture of Opium see Paregoric on page 840

Cancer Chemotherapy Regimens see page 1218

Cankaid® [OTC] see Carbamide Peroxide on page 179

Capastat® Sulfate see Capreomycin Sulfate on next page

Capital® and Codeine see Acetaminophen and Codeine on page 19

Capoten® *see* Captopril *on next page*

Capozide® *see* Captopril *on next page*

Capreomycin Sulfate (kap ree oh mye' sin)
Related Information
Antimicrobial Drugs of Choice *on page 1298-1302*
Brand Names Capastat® Sulfate
Use Treatment of tuberculosis in conjunction with at least one other anti-tuberculosis agent
Pregnancy Risk Factor C
Contraindications Known hypersensitivity to capreomycin sulfate
Warnings/Precautions The use of capreomycin in patients with renal insufficiency, pre-existing auditory impairment, and other oto- and nephrotoxic drug (especially other parenteral antituberculous agents) must be undertaken with great caution, and the risk of additional eighth nerve impairment or renal injury should be weighed against the benefits to be derived from therapy
Adverse Reactions
>10%:
Otic: Ototoxicity
Renal: Nephrotoxicity
1% to 10%: Hematologic: Eosinophilia
<1%:
Central nervous system: Vertigo, fever, rash
Hematologic: Leukocytosis, thrombocytopenia
Local: Pain, induration, bleeding at injection site
Otic: Tinnitus
Overdosage/Toxicology Symptoms of overdose include renal failure, ototoxicity, thrombocytopenia; treatment is supportive
Drug Interactions
Increased effect/duration of nondepolarizing neuromuscular blocking agents
Additive toxicity (nephro- and ototoxicity, respiratory paralysis): Aminoglycosides (eg, streptomycin)
Mechanism of Action Capreomycin is a cyclic polypeptide antimicrobial. It is administered as a mixture of capreomycin IA and capreomycin IB. The mechanism of action of capreomycin is not well understood. Mycobacterial species that have become resistant to other agents are usually still sensitive to the action of capreomycin. However, significant cross-resistance with viomycin, kanamycin, and neomycin occurs.
Pharmacodynamics/Kinetics
Absorption: Oral: Poor absorption necessitates parenteral administration
Half-life: Dependent upon renal function and varies with creatinine clearance; 4-6 hours
Time to peak serum concentration: I.M.: Within 1 hour
Elimination: Essentially excreted unchanged in the urine; no significant accumulation after ≥30 day of 1 g/day dosing in patients with normal renal function
Usual Dosage I.M.:
Infants and Children: 15-20 mg/kg/day, up to 1 g/day maximum
Adults: 15-30 mg/kg/day up to 1 g/day for 60-120 days, followed by 1 g 2-3 times/week

Dosing interval in renal impairment: Cl_{cr} <10 mL/minute: Decrease dose to ~33% of usual and administer every 48 hours; consult manufacturer's guidelines for specific dosing recommendations
Test Interactions ↓ potassium (S), ↑ BUN, leukocytosis ↓ platelets
Patient Information Report any hearing loss to physician immediately; do not discontinue without notifying physician
Nursing Implications The solution for injection may acquire a pale straw color and darken with time; this is not associated with a loss of potency or development of toxicity
Dosage Forms Injection: 100 mg/mL (10 mL)

Capsaicin (kap say' sin)
Brand Names Zostrix®-HP [OTC]; Zostrix® [OTC]
Use FDA approved for the topical treatment of pain associated with postherpetic neuralgia, rheumatoid arthritis, osteoarthritis, diabetic neuropathy, and post-surgical pain.
Unlabeled uses: Treatment of pain associated with psoriasis, chronic neuralgias unresponsive to other forms of therapy, and intractable pruritus
Pregnancy Risk Factor C
Contraindications Hypersensitivity to capsaicin or components
(Continued)

Capsaicin (Continued)

Warnings/Precautions Avoid contact with eyes, mucous membrane, or with damaged or irritated skin

Adverse Reactions

>10%: Local: ≥30%: Transient burning on application which usually diminishes with repeated use

1% to 10%:

Local: Itching, stinging sensation, erythema

Respiratory: Cough

Mechanism of Action Induces release of substance P, the principal chemomediator of pain impulses from the periphery to the CNS, from peripheral sensory neurons; after repeated application, capsaicin depletes the neuron of substance P and prevents reaccumulation

Pharmacodynamics/Kinetics Data following the use of topical capsaicin in humans are lacking

Onset of action: Pain relief is usually seen within 14-28 days of regular topical application; maximal response may require 4-6 weeks of continuous therapy

Duration: Several hours

Usual Dosage Children ≥2 years and Adults: Topical: Apply to affected area at least 3-4 times/day; application frequency less than 3-4 times/day prevents the total depletion, inhibition of synthesis, and transport of substance P resulting in decreased clinical efficacy and increased local discomfort

Patient Information For external use only. Avoid washing treated areas for 30 minutes after application; should not be applied to wounds or damaged skin; avoid eye and mucous membrane exposure; discontinue if severe burning or itching occurs; if symptoms persist longer than 14-28 days, contact physician

Dosage Forms Cream: 0.025% (45 g, 90 g); 0.075% (30 g, 60 g)

Captopril (kap' toe pril)

Related Information

Angiotensin-Converting Enzyme Inhibitors, Comparative Pharmacokinetics on page 1244

Angiotensin-Converting Enzyme Inhibitors, Comparisons of Indications and Adult Dosages on page 1243

Brand Names Capoten®; Capozide®

Synonyms ACE; Captopril and Hydrochlorothiazide

Use Management of hypertension and treatment of congestive heart failure

Unlabeled use: Hypertensive crisis, diabetic nephropathy, rheumatoid arthritis, diagnosis of anatomic renal artery stenosis, hypertension secondary to scleroderma renal crisis, diagnosis of aldosteronism, idiopathic edema, Bartter's syndrome, postmyocardial infarction for prevention of ventricular failure; increase circulation in Raynaud's phenomenon

Pregnancy Risk Factor D

Contraindications Hypersensitivity to captopril, other ACE inhibitors, or any component

Warnings/Precautions Use with caution and modify dosage in patients with renal impairment (decrease dosage) (especially renal artery stenosis), severe congestive heart failure, or with coadministered diuretic therapy; experience in children is limited. Severe hypotension may occur in patients who are sodium and/or volume depleted, initiate lower doses and monitor closely when starting therapy in these patients; ACE inhibitors may be preferred agents in elderly patients with congestive heart failure and diabetes mellitus (diabetic proteinuria is reduced, minimal CNS effects, and enhanced insulin sensitivity); however due to decreased renal function, tolerance must be carefully monitored.

Adverse Reactions

1% to 10%:

Cardiovascular: Tachycardia, chest pain, palpitations

Central nervous system: Insomnia, headache, dizziness, fatigue, malaise

Dermatologic: Rash, pruritus, alopecia

Gastrointestinal: Abdominal pain, vomiting, nausea, diarrhea, anorexia, constipation, dysgeusia

Neuromuscular & skeletal: Paresthesias

Renal: Oliguria

Respiratory: Transient cough

<1%:

Cardiovascular: Hypotension

Dermatologic: Angioedema

Endocrine & metabolic: Hyperkalemia

Hematologic: Neutropenia, agranulocytosis

Renal: Proteinuria, increased BUN, serum creatinine

Miscellaneous: Loss of taste perception

Overdosage/Toxicology Mild hypotension has been the only toxic effect seen with acute overdose. Bradycardia may also occur; hyperkalemia occurs even with therapeutic doses, especially in patients with renal insufficiency and those taking NSAIDs. Following initiation of essential overdose management, toxic symptom treatment and supportive treatment should be initiated. Hypotension usually responds to I.V. fluids or Trendelenburg positioning.

Drug Interactions

Increased toxicity:

Probenecid increases blood levels of captopril

Captopril and diuretics have additive hypotensive effects; see table.

Drug-Drug Interactions With ACEIs

Precipitant Drug	Drug (Category) and Effect	Description
Antacids	ACEIs: decreased	Decreased bioavailability of ACEIs. May be more likely with captopril. Separate administration times by 1-2 hours.
NSAIDs (indomethacin)	ACEIs: decreased	Reduced hypotensive effects of ACEIs. More prominent in low renin or volume dependent hypertensive patients.
Phenothiazines	ACEIs: increased	Pharmacologic effects of ACEIs may be increased.
ACEIs	Allopurinol: increased	Higher risk of hypersensitivity reaction possible when given concurrently. Three case reports of Stevens-Johnson syndrome with captopril.
ACEIs	Digoxin: increased	Increased plasma digoxin levels.
ACEIs	Lithium: increased	Increased serum lithium levels and symptoms of toxicity may occur.
ACEIs	Potassium preps/potassium-sparing diuretics increased	Coadministration may result in elevated potassium levels.

Stability Unstable in aqueous solutions; to prepare solution for oral administration, mix prior to administration and use within 10 minutes

Mechanism of Action Competitive inhibitor of angiotensin-converting enzyme (ACE); prevents conversion of angiotensin I to angiotensin II, a potent vasoconstrictor; results in lower levels of angiotensin II which causes an increase in plasma renin activity and a reduction in aldosterone secretion

Pharmacodynamics/Kinetics

Onset of effect: Maximal decrease in blood pressure 1-1.5 hours after dose

Duration: Dose related, may require several weeks of therapy before full hypotensive effect is seen

Absorption: Oral: 60% to 75%

Protein binding: 25% to 30%

Metabolism: 50%

Half-life (dependent upon renal and cardiac function):

Adults, normal: 1.9 hours

Congestive heart failure: 2.06 hours

Anuria: 20-40 hours

Time to peak: Within 1-2 hours

Elimination: 95% excreted in urine in 24 hours

Usual Dosage Note: Dosage must be titrated according to patient's response; use lowest effective dose. Oral:

Neonates: Initial: 0.05-0.1 mg/kg/dose every 8-24 hours; titrate dose up to 0.5 mg/kg/dose given every 6-24 hours

Infants: Initial: 0.15-0.3 mg/kg/dose; titrate dose upward to maximum of 6 mg/kg/day in 1-4 divided doses; usual required dose: 2.5-6 mg/kg/day

Children: Initial: 0.5 mg/kg/dose; titrate upward to maximum of 6 mg/kg/day in 2-4 divided doses

Older Children: Initial: 6.25-12.5 mg/dose every 12-24 hours; titrate upward to maximum of 6 mg/kg/day

Adolescents: Initial: 12.5-25 mg/dose given every 8-12 hours; increase by 25 mg/dose to maximum of 450 mg/day

Adults:

Hypertension:

Initial dose: 12.5-25 mg 2-3 times/day; may increase by 12.5-25 mg/dose at 1- to 2-week intervals up to 50 mg 3 times/day; add diuretic before further dosage increases

(Continued)

Captopril *(Continued)*

Maximum dose: 150 mg 3 times/day

Congestive heart failure:

Initial dose: 6.25-12.5 mg 3 times/day in conjunction with cardiac glycoside and diuretic therapy; initial dose depends upon patient's fluid/electrolyte status

Target dose: 50 mg 3 times/day

Maximum dose: 100 mg 3 times/day

Dosing adjustment in renal impairment:

Cl_{cr} 10-50 mL/minute: Administer at 75% of normal dose

Cl_{cr} <10 mL/minute: Administer at 50% of normal dose

Note: Smaller dosages given every 8-12 hours are indicated in patients with renal dysfunction; renal function and leukocyte count should be carefully monitored during therapy

Hemodialysis: Moderately dialyzable (20% to 50%); administer dose postdialysis or administer 25% to 35% supplemental dose

Peritoneal dialysis: Supplemental dose is not necessary

Monitoring Parameters BUN, serum creatinine, urine dipstick for protein, complete leukocyte count, and blood pressure

Test Interactions ↑ BUN, creatinine, potassium, positive Coombs' [direct]; ↓ cholesterol (S); may cause false-positive results in urine acetone determinations using sodium nitroprusside reagent

Patient Information Take 1 hour before meals; do not stop therapy except under prescriber advice; notify physician if you develop sore throat, fever, swelling, rash, difficult breathing, irregular heartbeats, chest pains, or cough. May cause dizziness, fainting, and lightheadedness, especially in first week of therapy; sit and stand up slowly; do not add a salt substitute (potassium) without advice of physician.

Nursing Implications Watch for hypotensive effect within 1-3 hours of first dose or new higher dose; food decreases absorption of captopril 30% to 40%

Dosage Forms Tablet:

Capoten®: 12.5 mg, 25 mg, 50 mg, 100 mg

Capozide®:

25/15: Captopril 25 mg and hydrochlorothiazide 15 mg

25/25: Captopril 25 mg and hydrochlorothiazide 25 mg

50/15: Captopril 50 mg and hydrochlorothiazide 15 mg

50/25: Captopril 50 mg and hydrochlorothiazide 25 mg

Captopril and Hydrochlorothiazide *see* Captopril *on page 174*

Carafate® *see* Sucralfate *on page 1036*

Carbachol *(kar′ ba kole)*

Related Information

Glaucoma Drug Therapy Comparison *on page 1270*

Brand Names Isopto® Carbachol; Miostat®

Synonyms Carbacholine; Carbamylcholine Chloride

Use Lowers intraocular pressure in the treatment of glaucoma; cause miosis during surgery

Pregnancy Risk Factor C

Contraindications Acute iritis, acute inflammatory disease of the anterior chamber, hypersensitivity to carbachol or any component

Warnings/Precautions Use with caution in patients undergoing general anesthesia and in presence of corneal abrasion

Adverse Reactions

1% to 10%: Ocular: Blurred vision, eye pain

<1%:

Cardiovascular: Transient fall in blood pressure

Central nervous system: Headache

Gastrointestinal: Stomach cramps, diarrhea

Local: Ciliary spasm with temporary decrease of visual acuity

Ocular: Corneal clouding, persistent bullous keratopathy, postoperative keratitis, retinal detachment, transient ciliary and conjunctival injection

Respiratory: Asthma

Miscellaneous: Increased peristalsis

Overdosage/Toxicology Symptoms of overdose include miosis, flushing, vomiting, bradycardia, bronchospasm, involuntary urination. Atropine is the treatment of choice for intoxications manifesting with significant muscarinic symptoms. Atropine I.V. 2-4 mg every 3-60 minutes (or 0.04-0.08 mg I.V. every 5-60 minutes if needed for children) should be repeated to control symptoms and then continued as needed for 1-2 days following the acute ingestion. Epinephrine 0.1-

1 mg S.C. may be useful in reversing severe cardiovascular or pulmonary sequel.

Stability

Intraocular: Store at room temperature of 15°C to 30°C/59°F to 86°F

Topical: Store at 8°C to 27°C/46°F to 80°F

Mechanism of Action Synthetic direct-acting cholinergic agent that causes miosis by stimulating muscarinic receptors in the eye

Pharmacodynamics/Kinetics

Ophthalmic instillation:

Onset of miosis: 10-20 minutes

Duration of reduction in intraocular pressure: 4-8 hours

Intraocular administration:

Onset of miosis: Within 2-5 minutes

Duration: 24 hours

Usual Dosage Adults:

Ophthalmic: Instill 1-2 drops up to 3 times/day

Intraocular: 0.5 mL instilled into anterior chamber before or after securing sutures

Patient Information May sting on instillation; may cause headache, altered distance vision, and decreased night vision

Nursing Implications Finger pressure should be applied on the lacrimal sac for 1-2 minutes following topical instillation; remove excess around the eye with a tissue. Instillation for miosis prior to eye surgery should be gentle and parallel to the iris face and tangential to the pupil border; discard unused portion.

Dosage Forms Solution:

Intraocular (Miostat®): 0.01% (1.5 mL)

Topical, ophthalmic (Isopto® Carbachol): 0.75% (15 mL, 30 mL); 1.5% (15 mL, 30 mL); 2.25% (15 mL); 3% (15 mL, 30 mL)

Carbacholine *see Carbachol on previous page*

Carbamazepine (kar ba maz' e peen)

Brand Names Epitol®; Tegretol®

Use Prophylaxis of generalized tonic-clonic, partial (especially complex partial), and mixed partial or generalized seizure disorder

Unlabeled use: Treat bipolar disorders and other affective disorders; resistant schizophrenia, alcohol withdrawal, restless leg syndrome, and psychotic behavior associated with dementia; may be used to relieve pain in trigeminal neuralgia or diabetic neuropathy

Pregnancy Risk Factor C

Contraindications Hypersensitivity to carbamazepine or any component; **may have cross-sensitivity with tricyclic antidepressants**; should not be used in any patient with bone marrow depression, MAO inhibitor use

Warnings/Precautions MAO inhibitors should be discontinued for a minimum of 14 days before carbamazepine is begun; administer with caution to patients with history of cardiac damage or hepatic disease; potentially fatal blood cell abnormalities have been reported following treatment; early detection of hematologic change is important; advise patients of early signs and symptoms including fever, sore throat, mouth ulcers, infections, easy bruising, petechial or purpuric hemorrhage; carbamazepine is not effective in absence, myoclonic or akinetic seizures; exacerbation of certain seizure types have been seen after initiation of carbamazepine therapy in children with mixed seizure disorders. Elderly may have increased risk of SIADH-like syndrome.

Adverse Reactions

Dermatologic: Rash; but does not necessarily mean the drug should not be stopped

>10%:

Central nervous system: Sedation, dizziness, fatigue, slurred speech, ataxia, clumsiness, confusion

Gastrointestinal: Nausea, vomiting

Ocular: Blurred vision, nystagmus

1% to 10%:

Dermatologic: Stevens-Johnson syndrome, toxic epidermal necrolysis

Endocrine & metabolic: Hyponatremia, SIADH

Gastrointestinal: Diarrhea

Miscellaneous: Diaphoresis

<1%:

Cardiovascular: Edema, congestive heart failure, syncope, bradycardia, hypertension or hypotension, A-V block, arrhythmias

Central nervous system: Slurred speech, mental depression, peripheral neuritis

Endocrine & metabolic: Hypocalcemia

Genitourinary: Hyponatremia, urinary retention, sexual problems in males

(Continued)

Carbamazepine *(Continued)*

Hematologic: Neutropenia (can be transient), aplastic anemia, agranulocytosis, eosinophilia, leukopenia, pancytopenia, thrombocytopenia, bone marrow depression

Hepatic: Hepatitis

Ocular: Nystagmus, diplopia

Miscellaneous: Swollen glands, hypersensitivity

Overdosage/Toxicology Symptoms of overdose include dizziness ataxia, drowsiness, nausea, vomiting, tremor, agitation, nystagmus, urinary retention, dysrhythmias, coma, seizures, twitches, respiratory depression, neuromuscular disturbances; provide general supportive care. Activated charcoal is effective at binding certain chemicals and this is especially true for carbamazepine; other treatment is supportive/symptomatic. Treatment consists of inducing emesis or gastric lavage. EKG should also be monitored to detect cardiac dysfunction. Monitor blood pressure, body temperature, pupillary reflexes, bladder function for several days following ingestion.

Drug Interactions

Decreased effect: Carbamazepine may induce the metabolism of warfarin, cyclosporine, doxycycline, oral contraceptives, phenytoin, theophylline, benzodiazepines, ethosuximide, valproic acid, corticosteroids, and thyroid hormones

Increased toxicity: Erythromycin, isoniazid, propoxyphene, verapamil, danazol, isoniazid, diltiazem, and cimetidine may inhibit hepatic metabolism of carbamazepine with resultant increase of carbamazepine serum concentrations and toxicity

Mechanism of Action In addition to anticonvulsant effects, carbamazepine has anticholinergic, antineuralgic, antidiuretic, muscle relaxant and antiarrhythmic properties; may depress activity in the nucleus ventralis of the thalamus or decrease synaptic transmission or decrease summation of temporal stimulation leading to neural discharge by limiting influx of sodium ions across cell membrane or other unknown mechanisms; stimulates the release of ADH and potentiates its action in promoting reabsorption of water; chemically related to tricyclic antidepressants

Pharmacodynamics/Kinetics

Absorption: Slowly absorbed from GI tract

Distribution: V_d:

Neonates: 1.5 L/kg

Children: 1.9 L/kg

Adults: 0.59-2 L/kg

Protein binding: 75% to 90%; may be decreased in newborns

Metabolism: In the liver to active epoxide metabolite; induces liver enzymes to increase metabolism and shorten half-life over time

Bioavailability, oral: 85%

Half-life:

Initial: 18-55 hours

Multiple dosing:

Children: 8-14 hours

Adults: 12-17 hours

Time to peak serum concentration: Unpredictable, within 4-8 hours

Elimination: 1% to 3% excreted unchanged in urine

Usual Dosage Oral (dosage must be adjusted according to patient's response and serum concentrations):

Children:

<6 years: Initial: 5 mg/kg/day; dosage may be increased every 5-7 days to 10 mg/kg/day; then up to 20 mg/kg/day if necessary; administer in 2-4 divided doses/day

6-12 years: Initial: 100 mg twice daily or 10 mg/kg/day in 2 divided doses; increase by 100 mg/day at weekly intervals depending upon response; usual maintenance: 20-30 mg/kg/day in 2-4 divided doses/day; maximum dose: 1000 mg/day

Children >12 years and Adults: 200 mg twice daily to start, increase by 200 mg/day at weekly intervals until therapeutic levels achieved; usual dose: 800-1200 mg/day in 3-4 divided doses; some patients have required up to 1.6-2.4 g/day

Dosing adjustment in renal impairment: Cl_{cr} <10 mL/minute: Administer 75% of dose

Reference Range

Timing of serum samples: Absorption is slow, peak levels occur 6-8 hours after ingestion of the first dose; the half-life ranges from 8-60 hours, therefore, steady-state is achieved in 2-5 days

Therapeutic levels: 6-12 µg/mL (SI: 25-51 µmol/L)

Toxic concentration: >15 µg/mL; patients who require higher levels of 8-12 µg/mL (SI: 34-51 µmol/L) should be watched closely. Side effects including CNS effects occur commonly at higher dosage levels. If other anticonvulsants are given therapeutic range is 4-8 µg/mL.

Test Interactions ↑ BUN, AST, ALT, bilirubin, alkaline phosphatase (S); ↓ calcium, T_3, T_4, sodium (S)

Patient Information Take with food, may cause drowsiness, periodic blood test monitoring required; notify physician if you observe bleeding, bruising, jaundice, abdominal pain, pale stools, mental disturbances, fever, chills, sore throat, or mouth ulcers

Nursing Implications Observe patient for excessive sedation; suspension dosage form must be given on a 3-4 times/day schedule versus tablets which can be given 2-4 times/day

Dosage Forms
Suspension, oral (citrus-vanilla flavor): 100 mg/5 mL (450 mL)
Tablet: 200 mg
Tablet, chewable: 100 mg

Extemporaneous Preparations A more concentrated oral suspension can be prepared with 24-hour carbamazepine 200 mg tablets to provide a final concentration of 200 mg/5 mL when mixed with 120 mL of simple syrup. The resultant suspension is stable for 90 days when refrigerated; "shake well" label and "refrigerate" label should be included.

Carbamide see Urea on page 1139

Carbamide Peroxide (kar' ba mide per ox' ide)

Brand Names Auro® Ear Drops [OTC]; Cankaid® [OTC]; Debrox® [OTC]; ERO Ear® [OTC]; Gly-Oxide® [OTC]; Murine® Ear Drops [OTC]; Orajel® Brace-Aid Rinse [OTC]; Proxigel® [OTC]

Synonyms Urea Peroxide

Use Relief of minor inflammation of gums, oral mucosal surfaces and lips including canker sores and dental irritation; emulsify and disperse ear wax

Pregnancy Risk Factor C

Contraindications Otic preparation should not be used in patients with a perforated tympanic membrane; ear drainage, ear pain or rash in the ear; do not use in the eye; do not use otic preparation longer than 4 days; oral preparation should not be used in children <3 years

Warnings/Precautions
Oral: With prolonged use of oral carbamide peroxide, there is a potential for overgrowth of opportunistic organisms; damage to periodontal tissues; delayed wound healing; should not be used for longer than 7 days
Otic: Do not use if ear drainage or discharge, ear pain, irritation, or rash in ear; should not be used for longer than 4 days

Adverse Reactions 1% to 10%: Local: Rash, irritation, superinfections, redness

Stability Store in tight, light-resistant containers; oral gel should be stored under refrigeration

Mechanism of Action Carbamide peroxide releases hydrogen peroxide which serves as a source of nascent oxygen upon contact with catalase; deodorant action is probably due to inhibition of odor-causing bacteria; softens impacted cerumen due to its foaming action

Usual Dosage Children and Adults:
Gel: Gently massage on affected area 4 times/day; do not drink or rinse mouth for 5 minutes after use
Oral solution (should not be used for >7 days): Oral preparation should not be used in children <3 years of age; apply several drops undiluted on affected area 4 times/day after meals and at bedtime; expectorate after 2-3 minutes or place 10 drops onto tongue, mix with saliva, swish for several minutes, expectorate
Otic solution (should not be used for >4 days): Tilt head sideways and instill 5-10 drops twice daily up to 4 days, tip of applicator should not enter ear canal; keep drops in ear for several minutes by keeping head tilted and placing cotton in ear

Patient Information Contact physician if dizziness or otic redness, rash, irritation, tenderness, pain, drainage, or discharge develop; do not drink or rinse mouth for 5 minutes after oral use of gel

Nursing Implications Patient may complain of foaming

Dosage Forms
Gel, oral (Proxigel®): 10% (34 g)
Solution:
Oral :10% in glycerol (15 mL, 60 mL); 15% in glycerin (13.3 mL)
(Continued)

Carbamide Peroxide *(Continued)*

Otic (Auro® Ear Drops, Debrox®, Murine® Ear Drops): 6.5% in glycerin (15 mL, 30 mL)

Carbamylcholine Chloride *see* Carbachol *on page 176*

Carbenicillin *(kar ben i sill' in)*

Related Information

Antimicrobial Drugs of Choice *on page 1298-1302*

Brand Names Geocillin®

Synonyms Carindacillin; Indanyl Sodium

Use Treatment of serious urinary tract infections and prostatitis caused by susceptible gram-negative aerobic bacilli or mixed aerobic-anaerobic bacterial infections excluding those secondary to *Klebsiella* sp and *Serratia marcescens*

Pregnancy Risk Factor B

Contraindications Hypersensitivity to carbenicillin or any component or penicillins

Warnings/Precautions Avoid use in patients with severe renal impairment (Cl_{cr} <10 mL/minute); dosage modification required in patients with impaired renal and/or hepatic function; use with caution in patients with history of hypersensitivity to cephalosporins

Adverse Reactions

>10%: Gastrointestinal: Diarrhea

1% to 10%: Gastrointestinal: Nausea, bad taste, vomiting, flatulence, glossitis

<1%:

Central nervous system: Headache, hyperthermia

Dermatologic: Skin rash, urticaria

Endocrine & metabolic: Hypokalemia

Genitourinary: Vaginitis

Hematologic: Anemia, thrombocytopenia, leukopenia, neutropenia, eosinophilia

Hepatic: Elevated LFTs

Local: Thrombophlebitis

Ocular: Itchy eyes

Renal: Hematuria

Miscellaneous: Furry tongue

Overdosage/Toxicology Symptoms of overdose include neuromuscular hypersensitivity, convulsions. Hemodialysis may be helpful to aid in the removal of the drug from the blood, otherwise most treatment is supportive or symptom directed.

Drug Interactions

Decreased effect with administration of aminoglycosides within 1 hour; may inactivate both drugs

Increased duration of half-life with probenecid

Mechanism of Action Interferes with bacterial cell wall synthesis during active multiplication

Pharmacodynamics/Kinetics

Absorption: Oral: 30% to 40%

Distribution: Crosses the placenta; small amounts appear in breast milk; distributes into bile, low concentrations attained in CSF

Protein binding: 50%

Half-life:

Children: 0.8-1.8 hours

Adults: 1-1.5 hours, prolonged to 10-20 hours with renal insufficiency

Time to peak serum concentration: Within 0.5-2 hours in patients with normal renal function; serum concentrations following oral absorption are inadequate for treatment of systemic infections

Elimination: ~80% to 99% of dose is excreted unchanged in urine

Usual Dosage Oral:

Children: 30-50 mg/kg/day divided every 6 hours; maximum dose: 2-3 g/day

Adults: 1-2 tablets every 6 hours for urinary tract infections or 2 tablets every 6 hours for prostatitis

Dosing interval in renal impairment:

Cl_{cr} 10-50 mL/minute: Administer every 12-24 hours

Cl_{cr} <10 mL/minute: Administer every 24-48 hours

Moderately dialyzable (20% to 50%)

Administration Administer around-the-clock to promote less variation in peak and trough serum levels

Monitoring Parameters Monitor for increased edema, rales, or signs of congestion, bruising, or bleeding

Reference Range Therapeutic: Not established; Toxic: >250 µg/mL (SI: >660 µmol/L)

Test Interactions False-positive urine or serum proteins; false-positive urine glucose (Clinitest®)

Patient Information Tablets have a bitter taste; take with a full glass of water; take all medication for 7-14 days, do not skip doses; may interfere with oral contraceptives; notify physician of edema, difficulty breathing, bruising, or bleeding

Nursing Implications Give at least 1 hour before aminoglycosides

Dosage Forms Tablet, film coated: 382 mg

Carbidopa (kar bi doe' pa)

Brand Names Lodosyn®

Use

Given with levodopa in the treatment of parkinsonism to enable a lower dosage of levodopa to be used and a more rapid response to be obtained and to decrease side-effects; for details of administration and dosage, see Levodopa

Has no effect without levodopa

Pregnancy Risk Factor C

Contraindications Hypersensitivity to carbidopa or levodopa

Adverse Reactions Adverse reactions are associated with concomitant administration with levodopa

>10%: Central nervous system: Anxiety, confusion, nervousness, mental depression

1% to 10%:
Cardiovascular: Orthostatic hypotension, palpitations, cardiac arrhythmias
Central nervous system: Memory loss, nervousness, insomnia, fatigue, hallucinations, ataxia, dystonic movements
Gastrointestinal: Nausea, vomiting, GI bleeding
Ocular: Blurred vision

<1%:
Cardiovascular: Hypertension
Gastrointestinal: Duodenal ulcer
Hematologic: Hemolytic anemia

Drug Interactions Increased toxicity: Tricyclic antidepressant → hypertensive reactions and dyskinesia

Mechanism of Action Carbidopa is a peripheral decarboxylase inhibitor with little or no pharmacological activity when given alone in usual doses. It inhibits the peripheral decarboxylation of levodopa to dopamine; and as it does not cross the blood-brain barrier, unlike levodopa, effective brain concentrations of dopamine are produced with lower doses of levodopa. At the same time reduced peripheral formation of dopamine reduces peripheral side-effects, notably nausea and vomiting, and cardiac arrhythmias, although the dyskinesias and adverse mental effects associated with levodopa therapy tend to develop earlier.

Pharmacodynamics/Kinetics

Absorption: Rapid but incomplete from GI tract
Distribution: Does not cross the blood-brain barrier; in rats, it has been reported to cross the placenta and to be excreted in milk
Elimination: Rapidly excreted in urine both unchanged and in the form of metabolites

Usual Dosage Adults: Oral: 70-100 mg/day; maximum daily dose: 200 mg

Patient Information Can take with food to prevent GI upset, do not stop taking this drug even if you do not think it is working; dizziness, lightheadedness, fainting may occur when getting up from a sitting or lying position

Nursing Implications Give with meals to decrease GI upset

Dosage Forms Tablet: 25 mg

Carbidopa and Levodopa see Levodopa and Carbidopa *on page 625*

Carbinoxamine and Pseudoephedrine (kar bi nox' a meen)

Related Information

Pseudoephedrine *on page 955*

Brand Names Carbiset® Tablet; Carbiset-TR® Tablet; Carbodec® Syrup; Carbodec® Tablet; Carbodec TR® Tablet; Cardec-S® Syrup; Rondec® Drops; Rondec® Filmtab®; Rondec® Syrup; Rondec-TR®

Use Temporary relief of nasal congestion, running nose, sneezing, itching of nose or throat, and itchy, watery eyes due to the common cold, hay fever, or other respiratory allergies

Pregnancy Risk Factor C

(Continued)

181

Carbinoxamine and Pseudoephedrine *(Continued)*

Contraindications Hypersensitivity to carbinoxamine or pseudoephedrine or any component; severe hypertension or coronary artery disease, MAO inhibitor therapy, GI or GU obstruction, narrow-angle glaucoma; avoid use in premature or term infants due to a possible association with SIDS

Warnings/Precautions Narrow-angle glaucoma, bladder neck obstruction, symptomatic prostatic hypertrophy, asthmatic attack, and stenosing peptic ulcer

Adverse Reactions

>10%:

Central nervous system: Slight to moderate drowsiness

Miscellaneous: Thickening of bronchial secretions

1% to 10%:

Central nervous system: Headache, fatigue, nervousness, dizziness

Gastrointestinal: Appetite increase, weight increase, nausea, diarrhea, abdominal pain, dry mouth

Neuromuscular & skeletal: Arthralgia

Respiratory: Pharyngitis

<1%:

Cardiovascular: Edema, palpitations

Central nervous system: Depression

Dermatologic: Angioedema, photosensitivity, rash

Hepatic: Hepatitis

Neuromuscular & skeletal: Myalgia, paresthesia

Respiratory: Bronchospasm

Miscellaneous: Epistaxis

Overdosage/Toxicology Symptoms of overdose include dry mouth, flushed skin, dilated pupils, CNS depression

There is no specific treatment for an antihistamine overdose, however, most of its clinical toxicity is due to anticholinergic effects. Anticholinesterase inhibitors including physostigmine, neostigmine, pyridostigmine, and edrophonium may be useful by reducing acetylcholinesterase; for anticholinergic overdose with severe life-threatening symptoms, physostigmine 1-2 mg (0.5 or 0.02 mg/kg for children) I.V., slowly may be given to reverse these effects.

Drug Interactions Increased toxicity: Barbiturates, TCAs, MAO inhibitors, ethanolamine antihistamines

Mechanism of Action Carbinoxamine competes with histamine for H_1-receptor sites on effector cells in the gastrointestinal tract, blood vessels, and respiratory tract

Usual Dosage Oral:

Children:

Drops: 1-18 months: 0.25-1 mL 4 times/day

Syrup:

18 months to 6 years: 2.5 mL 3-4 times/day

>6 years: 5 mL 2-4 times/day

Adults:

Liquid: 5 mL 4 times/day

Tablets: 1 tablet 4 times/day

Patient Information May cause drowsiness, impaired coordination, or judgment; may cause blurred vision; may also cause CNS excitation and difficulty sleeping

Nursing Implications Raise bed rails; institute safety measures; assist with ambulation

Dosage Forms

Drops: Carbinoxamine maleate 2 mg and pseudoephedrine hydrochloride 25 mg per mL (30 mL with dropper)

Syrup: Carbinoxamine maleate 4 mg and pseudoephedrine hydrochloride 60 mg per 5 mL (120 mL, 480 mL)

Tablet:

Film-coated: Carbinoxamine maleate 4 mg and pseudoephedrine hydrochloride 60 mg

Sustained release: Carbinoxamine maleate 8 mg and pseudoephedrine hydrochloride 120 mg

Carbiset® Tablet *see* Carbinoxamine and Pseudoephedrine *on previous page*

Carbiset-TR® Tablet *see* Carbinoxamine and Pseudoephedrine *on previous page*

Carbocaine® *see* Mepivacaine Hydrochloride *on page 688*

Carbodec® Syrup *see* Carbinoxamine and Pseudoephedrine *on previous page*

Carbodec® Tablet *see* Carbinoxamine and Pseudoephedrine *on page 181*

Carbodec TR® Tablet *see* Carbinoxamine and Pseudoephedrine *on page 181*

Carboplatin (kar' boe pla tin)
Related Information
Antiemetics for Chemotherapy Induced Nausea and Vomiting *on page 1202*
Cancer Chemotherapy Regimens *on page 1218-1241*
Brand Names Paraplatin®
Synonyms CBDCA
Use Ovarian carcinoma, cervical, small cell lung carcinoma, esophageal cancer, testicular, bladder cancer, mesothelioma, pediatric brain tumors, sarcoma, neuroblastoma
Pregnancy Risk Factor D
Contraindications Hypersensitivity to carboplatin or any component (anaphylactic-like reactions may occur), severe bone marrow depression, or excessive bleeding
Warnings/Precautions The U.S. Food and Drug Administration (FDA) currently recommends that procedures for proper handling and disposal of antineoplastic agents be considered. High doses have resulted in severe abnormalities of liver function tests. Bone marrow depression, which may be severe, and vomiting are dose related; reduce dosage in patients with bone marrow suppression and impaired renal function.
Adverse Reactions
>10%:
  Endocrine & metabolic: Electrolyte abnormalities such as hypocalcemia and hypomagnesemia, hyponatremia, hypokalemia
  Gastrointestinal: **Emetic potential: Moderate**
  Hematologic: Neutropenia, leukopenia, thrombocytopenia, anemia
  Local: Asthenia, pain at injection site
  Myelosuppressive: Dose-limiting toxicity
    WBC: Severe (dose-dependent)
    Platelets: Severe
    Nadir: 21-24 days
    Recovery: 5-6 weeks
  Hepatic: Abnormal liver function tests
1% to 10%:
  Dermatologic: Alopecia
  Gastrointestinal: Diarrhea, anorexia
  Hematologic: Hemorrhagic complications
  Neuromuscular & skeletal: Peripheral neuropathy
  Otic: Ototoxicity in 1% of patients
<1%:
  Central nervous system: Neurotoxicity has only been noted in patients previously treated with cisplatin
  Dermatologic: Urticaria, rash
  Gastrointestinal: Nausea, vomiting, stomatitis
  Ocular: Blurred vision
  Renal: Nephrotoxicity (uncommon)
Overdosage/Toxicology Symptoms of overdose include bone marrow depression, hepatic toxicity
Drug Interactions Increased toxicity: Nephrotoxic drugs; aminoglycosides increase risk of ototoxicity
Stability
Store unopened vials at room temperature (15°C to 30°C/59°F to 86°F)
After preparation, solutions are stable for 8 hours at room temperature (25°C/77°F); dilute dose to concentrations as low as 0.5-2 mg/mL in D_5W or NS; aluminum needles should not be used for administration due to binding with the platinum ion; protect from light
Compatible with etoposide
Mechanism of Action Analogue of cisplatin which covalently binds to DNA; possible cross-linking and interference with the function of DNA
Pharmacodynamics/Kinetics
Distribution: V_d: 16 L/kg; distributes into liver, kidney, skin, and tumor tissue
Protein binding: 0%; however, platinum is 30% protein bound
Metabolism: To aquated and hydroxylated compounds
Half-life, terminal: 22-40 hours; 2.5-5.9 hours in patients with Cl_{cr} >60 mL/minute
Elimination: ~60% to 90% excreted renally in the first 24 hours
Usual Dosage IVPB/I.V. infusion (refer to individual protocols):
(Continued)

Carboplatin *(Continued)*

Children:

Solid tumor: 560 mg/m² once every 4 weeks

Brain tumor: 175 mg/m² once weekly for 4 weeks with a 2-week recovery period between courses; dose is then adjusted on platelet count and neutrophil count values

Adults:

Ovarian cancer: Usual doses range from 360 mg/m² I.V. every 4 weeks to 400 mg/m² as a 24-hour infusion for 2 consecutive days

Carboplatin in doses of 200-500 mg/m² in 2 L of dialysis fluid have been administered into the peritoneum of ovarian cancer patients.

Head and neck cancer and small cell lung cancer: 300-400 mg/m² every 4 weeks or 60-80 mg/m²/day IVP for 5 days have been utilized.

In general, however, **single intermittent courses of carboplatin should not be repeated until the neutrophil count is at least 2000 and the platelet count is at least 100,000.**

The dose adjustments in the table are modified from a controlled trial in previously treated patients with ovarian carcinoma. Blood counts were done weekly and the recommendations are based on the lowest post-treatment platelet or neutrophil value.

Carboplatin

Platelets (cells/mm³)	Neutrophils (cells/mm³)	Adjusted Dose (From Prior Course)
>100,000	>2000	125%
50-100,000	500-2000	No adjustment
<50,000	<500	75%

Dosing adjustment in renal impairment:

Cl$_{cr}$ <60 mL/minute are at increased risk of severe bone marrow suppression. In renally impaired patients who received single agent carboplatin therapy, the incidence of severe leukopenia, neutropenia, or thrombocytopenia has been about 25% when the following dosage modifications have been used:

Cl$_{cr}$ 41-59 mL/minute: Recommended dose on day 1 is 250 mg/m²

Cl$_{cr}$ 16-40 mL/minute: Recommended dose on day 1 is 200 mg/m²

The data available for patients with severely impaired kidney function (Cl$_{cr}$ <15 mL/minute) are too limited to permit a recommendation for treatment

These dosing recommendations apply to the initial course of treatment. Subsequent dosages should be adjusted according to the patient's tolerance based on the degree of bone marrow suppression.

Administration Do not use needles or I.V. administration sets containing aluminum parts that may come in contact with carboplatin (aluminum can react causing precipitate formation and loss of potency); administer dose over at least 30 minutes

Monitoring Parameters CBC with differential and platelet count, serum electrolytes, urinalysis, creatinine clearance, liver function tests

Patient Information Delayed nausea and vomiting can occur 2-5 days after receiving the drug; report any loss of hearing, numbness, or tingling in the extremities to the physician

Dosage Forms Powder for injection, lyophilized: 50 mg, 150 mg, 450 mg

Carboprost Tromethamine *(kar' boe prost tro meth' a meen)*

Brand Names Hemabate™

Use Termination of pregnancy and refractory postpartum uterine bleeding

Investigational use: Hemorrhagic cystitis

Pregnancy Risk Factor X

Contraindications Hypersensitivity to carboprost tromethamine or any component; acute pelvic inflammatory disease

Warnings/Precautions Use with caution in patients with history of asthma, hypotension or hypertension, cardiovascular, adrenal, renal or hepatic disease, anemia, jaundice, diabetes, epilepsy or compromised uteri

Adverse Reactions

>10%: Gastrointestinal: Nausea

1% to 10%: Cardiovascular: Flushing

<1%:

Cardiovascular: Hypertension, hypotension

Central nervous system: Drowsiness, vertigo, nervousness, fever, headache, dystonia, vasovagal syndrome

Endocrine & metabolic: Breast tenderness
Gastrointestinal: Dry mouth, vomiting, diarrhea, hematemesis
Genitourinary: Bladder spasms
Neuromuscular & skeletal: Muscle pain
Ocular: Blurred vision
Respiratory: Coughing, asthma, respiratory distress
Miscellaneous: Taste alterations, septic shock, hiccups

Drug Interactions Increased toxicity: Oxytocic agents

Stability Refrigerate ampuls

Bladder irrigation: Dilute immediately prior to administration in NS; stability unknown

Mechanism of Action Carboprost tromethamine is a prostaglandin similar to prostaglandin F_2 alpha (dinoprost) except for the addition of a methyl group at the C-15 position. This substitution produces longer duration of activity than dinoprost; carboprost stimulates uterine contractility which usually results in expulsion of the products of conception and is used to induce abortion between 13-20 weeks of pregnancy. Hemostasis at the placentation site is achieved through the myometrial contractions produced by carboprost.

Usual Dosage Adults: I.M.:

Abortion: 250 mcg to start, 250 mcg at $1^1/_2$-hour to $3^1/_2$-hour intervals depending on uterine response; a 500 mcg dose may be given if uterine response is not adequate after several 250 mcg doses; do not exceed 12 mg total dose

Refractory postpartum uterine bleeding: Initial: 250 mcg; may repeat at 15- to 90-minute intervals to a total dose of 2 mg

Bladder irrigation for hemorrhagic cystitis (refer to individual protocols): [0.4-1.0 mg/dL as solution] 50 mL instilled into bladder 4 times/day for 1 hour

Administration Do not inject I.V.; may result in bronchospasm, hypertension, vomiting, and anaphylaxis

Dosage Forms Injection: Carboprost 250 mcg and tromethamine 83 mcg per mL (1 mL)

Cardec-S® Syrup see Carbinoxamine and Pseudoephedrine on page 181

Cardene® see Nicardipine Hydrochloride on page 790

Cardene® SR see Nicardipine Hydrochloride on page 790

Cardilate® see Erythrityl Tetranitrate on page 400

Cardioquin® see Quinidine on page 968

Cardizem® CD see Diltiazem on page 345

Cardizem® Injectable see Diltiazem on page 345

Cardizem® SR see Diltiazem on page 345

Cardizem® Tablet see Diltiazem on page 345

Cardura® see Doxazosin on page 368

Carindacillin see Carbenicillin on page 180

Carisoprodate see Carisoprodol on this page

Carisoprodol (kar eye soe proe' dole)

Brand Names Rela®; Sodol®; Soma®; Soma® Compound; Soprodol®; Soridol®

Synonyms Carisoprodate; Isobamate

Use Skeletal muscle relaxant

Pregnancy Risk Factor C

Contraindications Acute intermittent porphyria, hypersensitivity to carisoprodol, meprobamate or any component

Warnings/Precautions Use with caution in renal and hepatic dysfunction

Adverse Reactions

>10%: Central nervous system: Drowsiness

1% to 10%:

Cardiovascular: Tachycardia, tightness in chest, flushing of face
Central nervous system: Fainting, mental depression, allergic fever, dizziness, lightheadedness, headache, paradoxical stimulation
Dermatologic: Angioedema
Gastrointestinal: Nausea, vomiting, stomach cramps
Neuromuscular & skeletal: Trembling
Ocular: Burning of eyes
Respiratory: Shortness of breath
Miscellaneous: Hiccups

<1%:

Central nervous system: Clumsiness

(Continued)

Carisoprodol *(Continued)*

Dermatologic: Skin rash, hives erythema multiforme
Hematologic: Aplastic anemia, leukopenia, eosinophilia
Ocular: Blurred vision

Overdosage/Toxicology Symptoms of overdose include CNS depression, stupor, coma, shock, respiratory depression; treatment is supportive following attempts to enhance drug elimination. Hypotension should be treated with I.V. fluids and/or Trendelenburg positioning.

Drug Interactions Increased toxicity: Alcohol, CNS depressants, phenothiazines, clindamycin, MAO inhibitors

Mechanism of Action Precise mechanism is not yet clear, but many effects have been ascribed to its central depressant actions

Pharmacodynamics/Kinetics
Onset of action: Within 30 minutes
Duration: 4-6 hours
Distribution: Crosses the placenta; appears in high concentrations in breast milk
Metabolism: By the liver
Half-life: 8 hours
Elimination: By the kidneys

Usual Dosage Adults: Oral: 350 mg 3-4 times/day; take last dose at bedtime; compound: 1-2 tablets 4 times/day

Monitoring Parameters Look for relief of pain and/or muscle spasm and avoid excessive drowsiness

Patient Information May cause drowsiness or dizziness; avoid alcohol and other CNS depressants

Nursing Implications Raise bed rails; institute safety measures; assist with ambulation

Dosage Forms Tablet:
Rela®, Sodol®, Soma®, Soprodol®, Soridol®: 350 mg
Soma® Compound: Carisoprodol 200 mg and aspirin 325 mg

Extemporaneous Preparations A suspension can be prepared by triturating 60 carisoprodol 350 mg tablets, a small amount of water or glycerin, then mixing with a sufficient quantity of cherry syrup to bring the final volume to 60 mL; when refrigerated, the suspension is stable for 14 days; shake well before administration

Carmol® [OTC] *see Urea on page 1139*

Carmustine *(kar mus' teen)*

Related Information
Antiemetics for Chemotherapy Induced Nausea and Vomiting *on page 1202*
Cancer Chemotherapy Regimens *on page 1218-1241*

Brand Names BiCNU®

Synonyms BCNU

Use Treatment of brain tumors, multiple myeloma, Hodgkin's disease and non-Hodgkin's lymphomas, melanoma, lung cancer, colon cancer

Pregnancy Risk Factor D

Contraindications Hypersensitivity to carmustine or any component, myelosuppression from previous chemotherapy or other causes

Warnings/Precautions The U.S. Food and Drug Administration (FDA) currently recommends that procedures for proper handling and disposal of antineoplastic agents be considered. Administer with caution to patients with depressed platelet, leukocyte or erythrocyte counts, renal or hepatic impairment. Bone marrow depression, notably thrombocytopenia and leukopenia, may lead to bleeding and overwhelming infections in an already compromised patient; will last for at least 6 weeks after a dose, do not give courses more frequently than every 6 weeks because the toxicity is cumulative.

Adverse Reactions
>10%:
Central nervous system: Dizziness and ataxia
Dermatologic: Hyperpigmentation of skin
Gastrointestinal: Nausea and vomiting occur within 2-4 hours after drug injection and are dose-related
Emetic potential:
<200 mg: Moderately high (60% to 90%)
≥200 mg: High (>90%)
Local: Irritant, pain at injection site
Myelosuppressive: Delayed, occurs 4-6 weeks after administration and is dose-related; usually persists for 1-2 weeks; thrombocytopenia is usually more severe than leukopenia. Myelofibrosis and preleukemic syndromes are being reported.

WBC: Moderate

Platelets: Severe

Onset (days): 14

Nadir (days): 21-35

Recovery (days): 42-50

Ocular: Ocular toxicity, and retinal hemorrhages

1% to 10%:

Dermatologic: Facial flushing is probably due to the ethanol used in reconstitution, alopecia

Gastrointestinal: Diarrhea, anorexia, stomatitis

Hematologic: Anemia

<1%:

Dermatologic: Dermatitis

Hepatic: Reversible toxicity, increased LFTs in 20%

Renal: Azotemia, decrease in kidney size

Respiratory: Pulmonary fibrosis occurs mostly in patients treated with prolonged total doses >1400 mg/m² or with bone marrow transplantation doses. Risk factors include a history of lung disease, concomitant bleomycin, or radiation therapy. PFTs should be conducted prior to therapy and monitored. Patients with predicted FVC or DL_{co} <70% are at a higher risk.

Overdosage/Toxicology Symptoms of overdose include nausea, vomiting, thrombocytopenia, leukopenia; there are no known antidotes; treatment is primarily symptomatic and supportive

Drug Interactions Increased toxicity:

Cimetidine: Reported to cause bone marrow depression

Etoposide: Reported to cause severe hepatic dysfunction with hyperbilirubinemia, ascites, and thrombocytopenia

Stability

Store unreconstituted powder in vials in refrigerator (2°C to 8°C/36°F to 46°F), protect from light

Reconstituted solution in vials are stable for 8 hours at room temperature and 24 hours under refrigeration

After further dilution in D_5W or NS in glass bottle or Excell™ bag to a concentration of 0.2 mg/mL, solution is stable for 8 hours at room temperature and 48 hours at room temperature

Incompatible with sodium bicarbonate

Compatible with cisplatin

Mechanism of Action Interferes with the normal function of DNA by alkylation and cross-linking the strands of DNA, and by possible protein modification

Pharmacodynamics/Kinetics

Absorption: Highly lipid soluble

Distribution: Readily crosses the blood-brain barrier producing CSF levels equal to 15% to 70% of blood plasma levels; distributes into breast milk

Metabolism: Rapid

Half-life (biphasic):

Initial: 1.4 minutes

Secondary: 20 minutes (active metabolites may persist for days and have a plasma half-life of 67 hours)

Elimination: ~60% to 70% excreted in the urine within 96 hours and 6% to 10% excreted as CO_2 by the lungs

Usual Dosage I.V. infusion (refer to individual protocols):

Children: 200-250 mg/m² every 4-6 weeks as a single dose

Adults: 150-200 mg/m² every 6 weeks as a single dose or divided into daily injections on 2 successive days; next dose is to be determined based on hematologic response to the previous dose; see table.

Suggested Carmustine Dose Following Initial Dose

Nadir After Prior Dose		% of Prior Dose to Be Given
Leukocytes/mm³	Platelets/mm³	
>4000	>100,000	100
3000-3999	75,000-99,999	100
2000-2999	25,000-74,999	70
<2000	<25,000	50

Dosing adjustment in hepatic impairment: Adjustments may be necessary; however, no specific guidelines are available.

Administration Do not mix with solutions containing sodium bicarbonate; must administer in non-PVC containers; pain during infusion may be reduced by slowing infusion rate; may be irritating to veins and cause burning

(Continued)

Carmustine *(Continued)*

Monitoring Parameters CBC with differential and platelet count, pulmonary function, liver function, and renal function tests; monitor blood pressure during administration

Patient Information Contraceptive measures are recommended during therapy

Dosage Forms Powder for injection: 100 mg/vial packaged with 3 mL of absolute alcohol for use as a sterile diluent

Carteolol Hydrochloride *(kar' tee oh lole)*

Brand Names Cartrol®; Ocupress®

Use Management of hypertension; treatment of chronic open-angle glaucoma and intraocular hypertension

Pregnancy Risk Factor C

Contraindications Bronchial asthma, sinus bradycardia, second and third degree A-V block, cardiac failure (unless a functioning pacemaker present), cardiogenic shock, hypersensitivity to betaxolol or any component

Warnings/Precautions Some products contain sulfites which can cause allergic reactions; diminished response over time; may increase muscle weaknesses; use with a miotic in angle-closure glaucoma; use with caution in patients with decreased renal or hepatic function (dosage adjustment required) or patients with a history of asthma, congestive heart failure, or bradycardia; severe CNS, cardiovascular, and respiratory adverse effects have been seen following ophthalmic use

Adverse Reactions

1% to 10%:
Cardiovascular: Congestive heart failure, irregular heartbeat
Central nervous system: Mental depression, headache, dizziness
Neuromuscular & skeletal: Back pain, joint pain

<1%:
Cardiovascular: Bradycardia, chest pain, mesenteric arterial thrombosis, A-V block, persistent bradycardia, hypotension, edema, Raynaud's phenomena
Central nervous system: Fatigue, dizziness, headache, insomnia, lethargy, nightmares, depression, confusion
Dermatologic: Purpura
Endocrine & metabolic: Hyperglycemia
Gastrointestinal: Ischemic colitis, constipation, nausea, diarrhea
Genitourinary: Impotence
Hematologic: Thrombocytopenia
Respiratory: Bronchospasm
Miscellaneous: Cold extremities

Overdosage/Toxicology Symptoms of intoxication include cardiac disturbances, CNS toxicity, bronchospasm, hypoglycemia, and hyperkalemia. The most common cardiac symptoms include hypotension and bradycardia; atrioventricular block, intraventricular conduction disturbances, cardiogenic shock, and systole may occur with severe overdose, especially with membrane-depressant drugs (eg, propranolol); CNS effects include convulsions, coma, and respiratory arrest (commonly seen with propranolol and other membrane-depressant and lipid-soluble drugs)

Treatment includes symptomatic treatment of seizures, hypotension, hyperkalemia, and hypoglycemia; bradycardia and hypotension resistant to atropine, isoproterenol, or pacing may respond to glucagon; wide QRS defects caused by the membrane-depressant poisoning may respond to hypertonic sodium bicarbonate; repeat-dose charcoal, hemoperfusion, or hemodialysis may be helpful in removal of only those beta-blockers with a small V_d, long half-life, or low intrinsic clearance (acebutolol, atenolol, nadolol, sotalol).

Drug Interactions

Decreased effect of beta-blockers with aluminum salts, barbiturates, calcium salts, cholestyramine, colestipol, NSAIDs, penicillins (ampicillin), rifampin, salicylates, and sulfinpyrazone due to decreased bioavailability and plasma levels

Beta-blockers may decrease the effect of sulfonylureas

Increased effect/toxicity of beta-blockers with calcium blockers (diltiazem, felodipine, nicardipine), contraceptives, flecainide, haloperidol (propranolol, hypotensive effects), H_2 antagonists (metoprolol, propranolol only by cimetidine, possibly ranitidine), hydralazine (metoprolol, propranolol), loop diuretics (propranolol, not atenolol), MAO inhibitors (metoprolol, nadolol, bradycardia), phenothiazines (propranolol), propafenone (metoprolol, propranolol), quinidine (in extensive metabolizers), ciprofloxacin, thyroid hormones (metoprolol, propranolol, when hypothyroid patient is converted to euthyroid state)

Beta-blockers may increase the effect/toxicity of flecainide, haloperidol (hypotensive effects), hydralazine, phenothiazines, acetaminophen, anticoagulants (propranolol, warfarin), benzodiazepines (not atenolol), clonidine (hypertensive crisis after or during withdrawal of either agent), epinephrine (initial hypertensive episode followed by bradycardia), nifedipine and verapamil lidocaine, ergots (peripheral ischemia), prazosin (postural hypotension)

Beta-blockers may affect the action or levels of ethanol, disopyramide, nondepolarizing muscle relaxants and theophylline although the effects are difficult to predict

Mechanism of Action Blocks both beta$_1$- and beta$_2$-receptors and has mild intrinsic sympathomimetic activity; has negative inotropic and chronotropic effects and can significantly slow A-V nodal conduction

Pharmacodynamics/Kinetics
Onset of effect: Oral: 1-1.5 hours
Peak effect: 2 hours
Duration: 12 hours
Absorption: Oral: 80%
Protein binding: 23% to 30%
Metabolism: 30% to 50%
Half-life: 6 hours
Elimination: Renally excreted metabolites

Usual Dosage Adults:
Oral: 2.5 mg as a single daily dose, with a maintenance dose normally 2.5-5 mg once daily; maximum daily dose: 10 mg; doses >10 mg do not increase response and may in fact decrease effect
Ophthalmic: Instill 1 drop in affected eye(s) twice daily; see Additional Information

Dosing interval in renal impairment:
Cl_{cr} >60 (mL/min/1.73 m^2): Administer every 24 hours
Cl_{cr} 20-60 (mL/min/1.73 m^2): Administer every 48 hours
Cl_{cr} <20 (mL/min/1.73 m^2): Administer every 72 hours

Monitoring Parameters Ophthalmic: Intraocular pressure; Systemic: Blood pressure, pulse, CNS status

Patient Information Intended for twice daily dosing; keep eye open and do not blink for 30 seconds after instillation; wear sunglasses to avoid photophobic discomfort; apply gentle pressure to lacrimal sac during and immediately following instillation (1 minute); do not discontinue medication abruptly, sudden stopping of medication may precipitate or cause angina; consult pharmacist or physician before taking with other adrenergic drugs (eg, cold medications); notify physician if any systemic side effects occur; use with caution while driving or performing tasks requiring alertness; may mask signs of hypoglycemia in diabetics; may be taken without regard to meals

Nursing Implications Advise against abrupt withdrawal; monitor orthostatic blood pressures, apical and peripheral pulse, and mental status changes (ie, confusion, depression)

Dosage Forms
Solution, ophthalmic (Ocupress®): 1% (5 mL, 10 mL)
Tablet (Cartrol®): 2.5 mg, 5 mg

Carter's Little Pills® [OTC] *see* Bisacodyl *on page 134*

Cartrol® *see* Carteolol Hydrochloride *on previous page*

Cascara Sagrada (kas kar' a)
Related Information
Laxatives, Classification and Properties *on page 1272*

Use Temporary relief of constipation; sometimes used with milk of magnesia ("black and white" mixture)

Pregnancy Risk Factor C

Contraindications Nausea, vomiting, abdominal pain, fecal impaction, intestinal obstruction, GI bleeding, appendicitis, congestive heart failure

Warnings/Precautions Excessive use can lead to electrolyte imbalance, fluid imbalance, vitamin deficiency, steatorrhea, osteomalacia, cathartic colon, and dependence; should be avoided during nursing because it may have a laxative effect on the infant

Adverse Reactions
1% to 10%:
Central nervous system: Faintness
Endocrine & metabolic: Electrolyte and fluid imbalance
Gastrointestinal: Abdominal cramps, nausea, diarrhea
Miscellaneous: Discolors urine reddish pink or brown

Drug Interactions Decreased effect of oral anticoagulants

Stability Protect from light and heat

(Continued)

Cascara Sagrada *(Continued)*

Mechanism of Action Direct chemical irritation of the intestinal mucosa resulting in an increased rate of colonic motility and change in fluid and electrolyte secretion

Pharmacodynamics/Kinetics
Onset of action: 6-10 hours
Absorption: Oral: Small amount absorbed from small intestine
Metabolism: In the liver

Usual Dosage Note: Cascara sagrada fluid extract is 5 times more potent than cascara sagrada aromatic fluid extract.

Oral (aromatic fluid extract):
Infants: 1.25 mL/day (range: 0.5-1.5 mL) as needed
Children 2-11 years: 2.5 mL/day (range: 1-3 mL) as needed
Children ≥12 years and Adults: 5 mL/day (range: 2-6 mL) as needed at bedtime (1 tablet as needed at bedtime)

Test Interactions ↓ calcium (S), ↓ potassium (S)

Patient Information Should not be used regularly for more than 1 week

Dosage Forms
Aromatic fluid extract: 120 mL, 473 mL
Tablet: 325 mg

Castor Oil (kas′ tor)

Related Information
Laxatives, Classification and Properties *on page 1272*

Brand Names Alphamul® [OTC]; Emulsoil® [OTC]; Fleet® Flavored Castor Oil [OTC]; Neoloid® [OTC]; Purge® [OTC]

Synonyms Oleum Ricini

Use Preparation for rectal or bowel examination or surgery; rarely used to relieve constipation; also applied to skin as emollient and protectant

Pregnancy Risk Factor X

Contraindications Known hypersensitivity to castor oil; nausea, vomiting, abdominal pain, fecal impaction, GI bleeding, appendicitis, congestive heart failure, menstruation, dehydration

Warnings/Precautions Use only when a prompt and thorough catharsis is desired; use with caution during menstruation

Adverse Reactions
1% to 10%:
Central nervous system: Dizziness
Endocrine & metabolic: Electrolyte disturbance
Gastrointestinal: Abdominal cramps, nausea, diarrhea
<1%: Pelvic congestion

Stability Protect from heat (castor oil emulsion should be protected from freezing)

Mechanism of Action Acts primarily in the small intestine; hydrolyzed to ricinoleic acid which reduces net absorption of fluid and electrolytes and stimulates peristalsis

Pharmacodynamics/Kinetics Onset of action: Oral: 2-6 hours

Usual Dosage Oral:
Liquid:
Infants <2 years: 1-5 mL or 15 mL/m²/dose as a single dose
Children 2-11 years: 5-15 mL as a single dose
Children ≥12 years and Adults: 15-60 mL as a single dose

Emulsified:
36.4%:
Infants: 2.5-7.5 mL/dose
Children <2 years: 5-15 mL/dose
Children 2-11 years: 7.5-30 mL/dose
Children ≥12 years and Adults: 30-60 mL/dose
60% to 67%:
Children <2 years: 1.25-5 mL
Children 2-12 years: 5-15 mL
Adults: 15-45 mL
95%, mix with ½ to 1 full glass liquid:
Children: 5-10 mL
Adults: 15-60 mL

Administration Do not administer at bedtime because of rapid onset of action

Patient Information Chill or take with juice or carbonated beverage to improve taste

Dosage Forms
Emulsion, oral:
Alphamul®: 60% (90 mL, 3780 mL)
Emulsoil®: 95% (63 mL)
Fleet® Flavored Castor Oil: 67% (45 mL, 90 mL)
Neoloid®: 36.4% (118 mL)
Liquid, oral:
100% (60 mL, 120 mL, 480 mL)
Purge®: 95% (30 mL, 60 mL)

Cataflam® see Diclofenac on page 327

Catapres® see Clonidine on page 262

Catapres-TTS® see Clonidine on page 262

Catarase® see Chymotrypsin, Alpha on page 243

CBDCA see Carboplatin on page 183

CCNU see Lomustine on page 646

2-CdA see Cladribine on page 251

CDDP see Cisplatin on page 248

Ceclor® see Cefaclor on this page

Cecon® [OTC] see Ascorbic Acid on page 88

Cee-1000® T.D. [OTC] see Ascorbic Acid on page 88

CeeNU® see Lomustine on page 646

Cefaclor (sef′ a klor)

Brand Names Ceclor®
Use Infections caused by susceptible organisms including *Staphylococcus aureus* and *H. influenzae*; treatment of otitis media, sinusitis, and infections involving the respiratory tract, skin and skin structure, bone and joint, and urinary tract
Pregnancy Risk Factor B
Contraindications Hypersensitivity to cefaclor, any component, or cephalosporins
Warnings/Precautions Modify dosage in patients with severe renal impairment; prolonged use may result in superinfection; a low incidence of cross-hypersensitivity to penicillins exists
Adverse Reactions
1% to 10%: Pseudomembranous colitis, diarrhea
<1%: Rash, urticaria, pruritus, nausea, eosinophilia, cholestatic jaundice, arthralgia, Stevens-Johnson syndrome, vomiting, slight elevation of AST, ALT, hemolytic anemia, neutropenia, positive Coombs' test
Overdosage/Toxicology Symptoms of overdose include neuromuscular hypersensitivity, convulsions; hemodialysis may be helpful to aid in the removal of the drug from the blood, otherwise most treatment is supportive or symptom directed
Drug Interactions
Increased effect: Probenecid may decrease cephalosporin elimination
Increased toxicity: Furosemide, aminoglycosides may be a possible additive to nephrotoxicity
Stability Refrigerate suspension after reconstitution; discard after 14 days; do not freeze
Mechanism of Action Inhibits bacterial cell wall synthesis by binding to one or more of the penicillin-binding proteins (PBPs) which in turn inhibits the final transpeptidation step of peptidoglycan synthesis in bacterial cell walls, thus inhibiting cell wall biosynthesis. Bacteria eventually lyse due to ongoing activity of cell wall autolytic enzymes (autolysins and murein hydrolases) while cell wall assembly is arrested.
Pharmacodynamics/Kinetics
Peak serum levels:
Capsule: 60 minutes
Suspension: 45 minutes
Absorption: Oral: Well absorbed, acid stable
Distribution: Crosses the placenta; appears in breast milk
Protein binding: 25%
Metabolism: Partially
Half-life: 0.5-1 hour, prolonged with renal impairment
Elimination: 80% excreted unchanged in urine
Usual Dosage Oral:
Children >1 month: 20-40 mg/kg/day divided every 8-12 hours; maximum dose: 2 g/day (twice daily option is for treatment of otitis media or pharyngitis)
Adults: 250-500 mg every 8 hours or daily dose can be given in 2 divided doses
(Continued)
191

Cefaclor *(Continued)*

Dosing adjustment in renal impairment: Cl$_{cr}$ <50 mL/minute: Administer 50% of dose

Moderately dialyzable (20% to 50%)

Administration Administer around-the-clock rather than 3 times/day to promote less variation in peak and trough serum levels

Monitoring Parameters Assess patient at beginning and throughout therapy for infection

Test Interactions Positive Coombs' [direct], false-positive urine glucose (Clinitest®)

Patient Information Chilling of the oral suspension improves flavor (do not freeze); report persistent diarrhea; entire course of medication (10-14 days) should be taken to ensure eradication of organism; should be taken in equal intervals around-the-clock to maintain adequate blood levels; may interfere with oral contraceptives; females should report symptoms of vaginitis

Dosage Forms

Capsule: 250 mg, 500 mg

Powder for oral suspension (strawberry flavor): 125 mg/5 mL (75 mL, 150 mL); 187 mg/5 mL (50 mL, 100 mL); 250 mg/5 mL (75 mL, 150 mL); 375 mg/5 mL (50 mL, 100 mL)

Cefadroxil Monohydrate *(sef a drox' ill)*

Brand Names Duricef®; Ultracef®

Use Treatment of susceptible bacterial infections, including those caused by group A beta-hemolytic *Streptococcus*

Pregnancy Risk Factor B

Contraindications Hypersensitivity to cefadroxil or other cephalosporins

Warnings/Precautions Modify dosage in patients with severe renal impairment; prolonged use may result in superinfection; a low incidence of cross-hypersensitivity to penicillins exists

Adverse Reactions

1% to 10%: Gastrointestinal: Diarrhea

<1%:

Central nervous system: Fatigue, chills

Dermatologic: Maculopapular and erythematous rash

Gastrointestinal: Dyspepsia, pseudomembranous colitis, nausea, vomiting, heartburn, gastritis, bloating

Hematologic: Neutropenia

Miscellaneous: Superinfections

Overdosage/Toxicology Symptoms of overdose include neuromuscular hypersensitivity, convulsions; hemodialysis may be helpful to aid in the removal of the drug from the blood, otherwise most treatment is supportive or symptom directed

Drug Interactions

Increased effect: Probenecid may decrease cephalosporin elimination

Increased toxicity: Furosemide, aminoglycosides may be a possible additive to nephrotoxicity

Stability Refrigerate suspension after reconstitution; discard after 14 days

Mechanism of Action Inhibits bacterial cell wall synthesis by binding to one or more of the penicillin-binding proteins (PBPs) which in turn inhibits the final transpeptidation step of peptidoglycan synthesis in bacterial cell walls, thus inhibiting cell wall biosynthesis. Bacteria eventually lyse due to ongoing activity of cell wall autolytic enzymes (autolysins and murein hydrolases) while cell wall assembly is arrested.

Pharmacodynamics/Kinetics

Absorption: Oral: Rapid and well absorbed from GI tract

Distribution: V$_d$: 0.31 L/kg; crosses the placenta; appears in breast milk

Protein binding: 20%

Half-life: 1-2 hours; 20-24 hours in renal failure

Time to peak serum concentration: Within 70-90 minutes

Elimination: >90% of dose excreted unchanged in urine within 8 hours

Usual Dosage Oral:

Children: 30 mg/kg/day divided twice daily up to a maximum of 2 g/day

Adults: 1-2 g/day in 2 divided doses

Dosing interval in renal impairment:

Cl$_{cr}$ 10-25 mL/minute: Administer every 24 hours

Cl$_{cr}$ <10 mL/minute: Administer every 36 hours

Administration Administer around-the-clock to promote less variation in peak and trough serum levels

Test Interactions Positive Coombs' [direct], glucose, protein; ↓ glucose

Patient Information Report persistent diarrhea; entire course of medication (10-14 days) should be taken to ensure eradication of organism; should be taken in equal intervals around-the-clock to maintain adequate blood levels; may interfere with oral contraceptives; females should report symptoms of vaginitis

Dosage Forms
Capsule: 500 mg
Suspension, oral: 125 mg/5 mL, 250 mg/5 mL, 500 mg/5 mL (50 mL, 100 mL)
Tablet: 1 g

Cefadyl® see Cephapirin Sodium on page 212

Cefamandole Nafate (sef a man' dole)

Brand Names Mandol®

Use Treatment of susceptible bacterial infection; mainly respiratory tract, skin and skin structure, bone and joint, urinary tract and gynecologic, as well as, septicemia

Pregnancy Risk Factor B

Contraindications Hypersensitivity to cefamandole nafate, any component, or cephalosporins

Warnings/Precautions Modify dosage in patients with severe renal impairment; prolonged use may result in superinfection; a low incidence of cross-hypersensitivity to penicillins exists

Adverse Reactions
1% to 10%: Gastrointestinal: Diarrhea
<1%:
Central nervous system: CNS irritation, seizures, fever
Dermatologic: Rash, urticaria
Gastrointestinal: Abdominal cramps, pseudomembraneous colitis
Hematologic: Eosinophilia, hypoprothrombinemia, leukopenia, thrombocytopenia
Hepatic: Transient elevation of liver enzymes, cholestatic jaundice
Local: Pain at injection site
Miscellaneous: Superinfections

Overdosage/Toxicology Symptoms of overdose include neuromuscular hypersensitivity, convulsions; hemodialysis may be helpful to aid in the removal of the drug from the blood, otherwise most treatment is supportive or symptom directed

Drug Interactions
Disulfiram-like reaction has been reported when taken within 72 hours of alcohol consumption
Increased cefamandole plasma levels: Probenecid
Increased nephrotoxicity: Aminoglycosides, furosemide
Hypoprothrombinemic effect increased: Warfarin and heparin

Stability After reconstitution, CO_2 gas is liberated which allows solution to be withdrawn without injecting air; solution is stable for 24 hours at room temperature and 96 hours when refrigerated; for I.V., infusion in NS and D_5W is stable for 24 hours at room temperature, 1 week when refrigerated, or 26 weeks when frozen

Mechanism of Action Inhibits bacterial cell wall synthesis by binding to one or more of the penicillin-binding proteins (PBPs) which in turn inhibits the final transpeptidation step of peptidoglycan synthesis in bacterial cell walls, thus inhibiting cell wall biosynthesis. Bacteria eventually lyse due to ongoing activity of cell wall autolytic enzymes (autolysins and murein hydrolases) while cell wall assembly is arrested.

Pharmacodynamics/Kinetics
Time to peak serum concentration:
I.M.: Within 1-2 hours
I.V.: Within 10 minutes
Distribution: Distributes well throughout body, except CSF; poor penetration even with inflamed meninges; extensive enterohepatic circulation; high concentrations in the bile
Protein binding: 56% to 78%
Half-life: 30-60 minutes
Elimination: Extensive enterohepatic circulation; high concentrations in bile; majority of drug excreted unchanged in urine

Usual Dosage I.M., I.V.:
Children: 100-150 mg/kg/day in divided doses every 4-6 hours

Adults: 4-12 g/24 hours divided every 4-6 hours or 500-1000 mg every 4-8 hours; maximum: 2 g/dose

Dosing interval in renal impairment:
Cl_{cr} 25-50 mL/minute: 1-2 g every 8 hours
(Continued)

Cefamandole Nafate *(Continued)*

    Cl_{cr} 10-25 mL/minute: 1 g every 8 hours
    Cl_{cr} <10 mL/minute: 1 g every 12 hours
   Moderately dialyzable (20% to 50%)

Administration Administer around-the-clock to promote less variation in peak and trough serum levels

Monitoring Parameters Monitor for signs of bruising or bleeding

Test Interactions ↑ alkaline phosphatase, AST, ALT, BUN, creatinine, prothrombin time (S), glucose, protein; ↓ glucose; positive Coombs' [direct]

Additional Information Sodium content of 1 g: 3.3 mEq

Dosage Forms Powder for injection: 500 mg (10 mL); 1 g (10 mL, 100 mL); 2 g (20 mL, 100 mL); 10 g (100 mL)

Cefanex® *see* Cephalexin Monohydrate *on page 210*

Cefazolin Sodium *(sef a′ zoe lin)*

Brand Names Ancef®; Kefzol®; Zolicef®

Use Treatment of gram-positive bacilli and cocci (except enterococcus); some gram-negative bacilli including *E. coli*, *Proteus*, and *Klebsiella* may be susceptible

Pregnancy Risk Factor B

Contraindications Hypersensitivity to cefazolin sodium, any component, or cephalosporins

Warnings/Precautions Modify dosage in patients with severe renal impairment; prolonged use may result in superinfection; a low incidence of cross-hypersensitivity to penicillins exists

Adverse Reactions
  1% to 10%: Gastrointestinal: Diarrhea
  <1%:
    Central nervous system: CNS irritation, seizures, confusion, fever
    Dermatologic: Rash, urticaria
    Hematologic: Leukopenia, thrombocytopenia, neutropenia
    Hepatic: Transient elevation of liver enzymes, cholestatic jaundice
    Miscellaneous: Superinfections

Overdosage/Toxicology Symptoms of overdose include neuromuscular hypersensitivity, convulsions; many beta-lactam containing antibiotics have the potential to cause neuromuscular hyperirritability or convulsive seizures. Hemodialysis may be helpful to aid in the removal of the drug from the blood, otherwise most treatment is supportive or symptom directed.

Drug Interactions
  Increased effect: High-dose probenecid decreases clearance
  Increased toxicity: Aminoglycosides increase nephrotoxic potential

Stability
  Store intact vials at room temperature and protect from temperatures exceeding 40°C
  Reconstituted solutions of cefazolin are light yellow to yellow
  Protection from light is recommended for the powder and for the reconstituted solutions
  Reconstituted solutions are stable for 24 hours at room temperature and 10 days under refrigeration
  Stability of parenteral admixture at room temperature (25°C): 48 hours
  Stability of parenteral admixture at refrigeration temperature (4°C): 14 days
  Standard diluent: 1 g/50 mL D_5W; 2 g/50 mL D_5W

Mechanism of Action Inhibits bacterial cell wall synthesis by binding to one or more of the penicillin-binding proteins (PBPs) which in turn inhibits the final transpeptidation step of peptidoglycan synthesis in bacterial cell walls, thus inhibiting cell wall biosynthesis. Bacteria eventually lyse due to ongoing activity of cell wall autolytic enzymes (autolysins and murein hydrolases) while cell wall assembly is arrested.

Pharmacodynamics/Kinetics
  Time to peak serum concentration:
    I.M.: Within 0.5-2 hours
    I.V.: Within 5 minutes
  Distribution: Crosses the placenta; small amounts appear in breast milk; CSF penetration is poor
  Protein binding: 74% to 86%
  Metabolism: Hepatic is minimal
  Half-life: 90-150 minutes (prolonged with renal impairment)
    End stage renal disease: 40-70 hours
  Elimination: 80% to 100% is excreted unchanged in urine

Usual Dosage I.M., I.V.:

Neonates:

Postnatal age ≤7 days: 20 mg/kg/dose every 12 hours

Postnatal age >7 days:

≤2000 g: 20 mg/kg/dose every 12 hours

>2000 g: 20 mg/kg/dose every 8 hours

Children >1 month: 50-100 mg/kg/day divided every 8 hours; maximum: 6 g/day

Adults: 1-2 g every 8 hours, depending on severity of infection; maximum dose: 12 g/day

Dosing adjustment in renal impairment:

Cl_{cr} 10-30 mL/minute: Administer every 12 hours

Cl_{cr} <10 mL/minute: Administer every 24 hours

Moderately dialyzable (20% to 50%); administer dose postdialysis or administer supplemental dose of 0.5-1 g after dialysis

Peritoneal dialysis: Administer 0.5 g every 12 hours

Continuous arterio-venous or veno-venous hemofiltration (CAVH/CAVHD): Removes 30 mg of cefazolin per liter of filtrate per day

Administration Administer around-the-clock rather than 3 times/day to promote less variation in peak and trough serum levels

Monitoring Parameters Renal function periodically when used in combination with other nephrotoxic drugs, hepatic function tests, CBC

Test Interactions False-positive urine glucose using Clinitest®, positive Coombs' [direct], false increase serum or urine creatinine

Additional Information Sodium content of 1 g: 47 mg (2 mEq)

Dosage Forms

Infusion, premixed, in D_5W (frozen) (Ancef®): 500 mg (50 mL); 1 g (50 mL)

Injection (Kefzol®): 500 mg, 1 g

Powder for injection (Ancef®, Zolicef®): 250 mg, 500 mg, 1 g, 5 g, 10 g, 20 g

Cefixime (sef ix' eem)

Related Information

Antimicrobial Drugs of Choice on page 1298-1302

Brand Names Suprax®

Use Treatment of urinary tract infections, otitis media, respiratory infections due to susceptible organisms including S. pneumoniae and S. pyogenes, H. influenzae and many Enterobacteriaceae; documented poor compliance with other oral antimicrobials; outpatient therapy of serious soft tissue or skeletal infections due to susceptible organisms; single-dose oral treatment of uncomplicated cervical/urethral gonorrhea due to N. gonorrhoeae

Pregnancy Risk Factor B

Contraindications Hypersensitivity to cefixime or cephalosporins

Warnings/Precautions Modify dosage in patients with severe renal impairment; prolonged use may result in superinfection; a low incidence of cross-hypersensitivity to penicillins exists

Adverse Reactions

1% to 10%: Gastrointestinal: Diarrhea (up to 15% of children), abdominal pain, nausea, dyspepsia, flatulence, pseudomembranous colitis

<1%:

Central nervous system: Headache, dizziness, fever

Dermatologic: Rash, urticaria, pruritus

Genitourinary: Vaginitis

Hematologic: Thrombocytopenia, leukopenia, eosinophilia

Miscellaneous: Transient elevation of BUN or creatinine and LFTs

Overdosage/Toxicology Symptoms of overdose include neuromuscular hypersensitivity, convulsions; hemodialysis may be helpful to aid in the removal of the drug from the blood, otherwise most treatment is supportive or symptom directed

Drug Interactions

Increased effect: Probenecid may decrease cephalosporin elimination

Increased toxicity: Furosemide, aminoglycosides may be a possible additive to nephrotoxicity

Stability After mixing, suspension may be kept for 14 days at room temperature

Mechanism of Action Inhibits bacterial cell wall synthesis by binding to one or more of the penicillin-binding proteins (PBPs) which in turn inhibits the final transpeptidation step of peptidoglycan synthesis in bacterial cell walls, thus inhibiting cell wall biosynthesis. Bacteria eventually lyse due to ongoing activity of cell wall autolytic enzymes (autolysins and murein hydrolases) while cell wall assembly is arrested.

Pharmacodynamics/Kinetics

Absorption: Oral: 40% to 50%

Protein binding: 65%

(Continued)

195

Cefixime *(Continued)*

Half-life:
  Normal renal function: 3-4 hours
  Renal failure: Up to 11.5 hours
Peak serum levels: Within 2-6 hours; peak serum concentrations are 15% to 50% higher for the oral suspension versus tablets
Elimination: 50% of absorbed dose excreted as active drug in urine and 10% in bile

Usual Dosage Oral:
Children: 8 mg/kg/day in 1-2 divided doses; maximum dose: 400 mg/day

Children >50 kg or >12 years and Adults: 400 mg/day in 1-2 divided doses
  Uncomplicated cervical/urethral gonorrhea due to *N. gonorrhoeae*: 400 mg as a single dose

Dosing adjustment in renal impairment:
  Cl_{cr} 21-60 mL/minute: Administer 75% of the standard dose
  Cl_{cr} ≤20 mL/minute: Administer 50% of the standard dose
  Moderately dialyzable (10%)

Administration Administer at regular intervals, around-the-clock to maintain adequate levels

Monitoring Parameters Renal and hepatic function periodically, with prolonged therapy

Test Interactions False-positive reaction for urine glucose using Clinitest®

Patient Information Report persistent diarrhea; entire course of medication (10-14 days) should be taken to ensure eradication of organism; should be taken in equal intervals around-the-clock to maintain adequate blood levels; may interfere with oral contraceptives; females should report symptoms of vaginitis; take with food to decrease GI distress

Dosage Forms
Powder for oral suspension (strawberry flavor): 100 mg/5 mL (50 mL, 100 mL)
Tablet, film coated: 200 mg, 400 mg

Cefizox® see Ceftizoxime on page 206

Cefmetazole Sodium *(sef met' a zole)*

Brand Names Zefazone®

Use Second generation cephalosporin with an antibacterial spectrum similar to cefoxitin, useful on many aerobic and anaerobic gram-positive and gram-negative bacteria

Pregnancy Risk Factor B

Contraindications Hypersensitivity to cefmetazole or any component or cephalosporins

Warnings/Precautions Modify dosage in patients with severe renal impairment; prolonged use may result in superinfection; a low incidence of cross-hypersensitivity to penicillins exists

Adverse Reactions
1% to 10%:
  Dermatologic: Rash
  Gastrointestinal: Diarrhea, nausea
<1%:
  Cardiovascular: Shock, hypotension
  Central nervous system: Headache, fever
  Endocrine & metabolic: Hot flashes
  Gastrointestinal: Epigastric pain, pseudomembraneous colitis
  Genitourinary: Vaginitis
  Hematologic: Hypoprothrombinemia, anemia
  Local: Pain at injection site, phlebitis
  Respiratory: Respiratory distress, dyspnea
  Miscellaneous: Epistaxis, alteration of color, candidiasis

Overdosage/Toxicology Symptoms of overdose include neuromuscular hypersensitivity, convulsions; many beta-lactam containing antibiotics have the potential to cause neuromuscular hyperirritability or convulsive seizures. Hemodialysis may be helpful to aid in the removal of the drug from the blood, otherwise most treatment is supportive or symptom directed.

Drug Interactions
Increased effect: Probenecid may decrease cephalosporin elimination
Increased toxicity: Furosemide, aminoglycosides may be a possible additive to nephrotoxicity

Stability Reconstituted solution and I.V. infusion in NS or D_5W solution are stable for 24 hours at room temperature, 7 days when refrigerated, or 6 weeks when frozen; after freezing, thawed solution is stable for 24 hours at room temperature or 7 days when refrigerated

Mechanism of Action Inhibits bacterial cell wall synthesis by binding to one or more of the penicillin-binding proteins (PBPs) which in turn inhibits the final transpeptidation step of peptidoglycan synthesis in bacterial cell walls, thus inhibiting cell wall biosynthesis. Bacteria eventually lyse due to ongoing activity of cell wall autolytic enzymes (autolysins and murein hydrolases) while cell wall assembly is arrested.

Pharmacodynamics/Kinetics

Protein binding: 65%
Metabolism: <15%
Half-life: 72 minutes
Elimination: Renal

Usual Dosage Adults: I.V.:

Infections: 2 g every 6-12 hours for 5-14 days

Prophylaxis: 2 g 30-90 minutes before surgery **or** 1 g 30-90 minutes before surgery; repeat 8 and 16 hours later

Dosing interval in renal impairment:
Cl_{cr} 50-90 mL/minute: Administer every 12 hours
Cl_{cr} 10-50 mL/minute: Administer every 16-24 hours
Cl_{cr} <10 mL/minute: Administer every 48 hours

Administration Administer around-the-clock rather than 2 times/day to promote less variation in peak and trough serum levels

Monitoring Parameters Monitor prothrombin times

Patient Information Do not drink alcohol for at least 24 hours after receiving dose; report persistent diarrhea; may interfere with oral contraceptives, females should report symptoms of vaginitis

Nursing Implications Do not admix with aminoglycosides in same bottle/bag

Additional Information Sodium content of 1 g: 2 mEq

Dosage Forms Powder for injection: 1 g, 2 g

Cefobid® *see* Cefoperazone Sodium *on next page*

Cefol® Filmtab® *see* Vitamin, Multiple *on page 1166*

Cefonicid Sodium (se fon' i sid)

Brand Names Monocid®

Use Treatment of susceptible bacterial infection; mainly respiratory tract, skin and skin structure, bone and joint, urinary tract and gynecologic, as well as, septicemia; second generation cephalosporin

Pregnancy Risk Factor B

Contraindications Hypersensitivity to cefonicid sodium, any component, or cephalosporins

Warnings/Precautions Modify dosage in patients with severe renal impairment; prolonged use may result in superinfection; a low incidence of cross-hypersensitivity to penicillins exists

Adverse Reactions

1% to 10%:
Local: Pain at injection site
Hematologic: Increased platelets and eosinophils
Hepatic: Liver function alterations

<1%:
Central nervous system: Fever, headache
Dermatologic: Skin rash
Gastrointestinal: Nausea, diarrhea, abdominal pain, pseudomembranous colitis
Hematologic: Increased platelets and eosinophils
Miscellaneous: Transient elevations in liver enzymes, BUN, or creatinine

Overdosage/Toxicology Symptoms of overdose include neuromuscular hypersensitivity, convulsions; hemodialysis may be helpful to aid in the removal of the drug from the blood, otherwise most treatment is supportive or symptom directed

Drug Interactions

Increased effect: Probenecid may decrease cephalosporin elimination
Increased toxicity: Furosemide, aminoglycosides may be a possible additive to nephrotoxicity

Stability Reconstituted solution and I.V. infusion in NS or D_5W solution are stable for 24 hours at room temperature or 72 hours if refrigerated

Mechanism of Action Inhibits bacterial cell wall synthesis by binding to one or more of the penicillin-binding proteins (PBPs) which in turn inhibits the final transpeptidation step of peptidoglycan synthesis in bacterial cell walls, thus inhibiting cell wall biosynthesis. Bacteria eventually lyse due to ongoing activity of cell

(Continued)

Cefonicid Sodium *(Continued)*

wall autolytic enzymes (autolysins and murein hydrolases) while cell wall assembly is arrested.

Pharmacodynamics/Kinetics
Protein binding: 98%
Metabolism: None
Half-life: 6-7 hours
Elimination: Renal

Usual Dosage Adults: I.M., I.V.: 0.5-2 g every 24 hours
Prophylaxis: Preop: 1 g/hour

Dosing interval in renal impairment: See table.

Cefonicid Sodium

Cl$_{cr}$ (mL/min/1.73 m^2)	Dose (mg/kg) for each dosing interval
60-79	10-24 q24h
40-59	8-20 q24h
20-39	4-15 q24h
10-19	4-15 q48h
5-9	4-15 q3-5d
<5	3-4 q3-5d

Administration Administer around-the-clock rather than 3 times/day to promote less variation in peak and trough serum levels
Additional Information Sodium content of 1 g: 3.7 mEq
Dosage Forms Powder for injection: 500 mg, 1 g, 10 g

Cefoperazone Sodium (sef oh per′ a zone)

Brand Names Cefobid®
Use Treatment of susceptible bacterial infection; mainly respiratory tract, skin and skin structure, bone and joint, urinary tract and gynecologic, as well as, septicemia
Pregnancy Risk Factor B
Contraindications Hypersensitivity to cefoperazone or any component or cephalosporins
Warnings/Precautions Modify dosage in patients with severe renal impairment; prolonged use may result in superinfection; a low incidence of cross-hypersensitivity to penicillins exists
Adverse Reactions
1% to 10%: Gastrointestinal: Diarrhea
<1%:
Dermatologic: Maculopapular and erythematous rash
Gastrointestinal: Dyspepsia, pseudomembranous colitis, nausea, vomiting
Hematologic: Hypoprothrombinemia
Local: Pain and induration at injection site
Overdosage/Toxicology Symptoms of overdose include neuromuscular hypersensitivity, convulsions; hemodialysis may be helpful to aid in the removal of the drug from the blood, otherwise most treatment is supportive or symptom directed
Stability Reconstituted solution and I.V. infusion in NS or D$_5$W solution are stable for 24 hours at room temperature, 5 days when refrigerated or 3 weeks, when frozen; after freezing, thawed solution is stable for 48 hours at room temperature or 10 days when refrigerated
Mechanism of Action Inhibits bacterial cell wall synthesis by binding to one or more of the penicillin-binding proteins (PBPs) which in turn inhibits the final transpeptidation step of peptidoglycan synthesis in bacterial cell walls, thus inhibiting cell wall biosynthesis. Bacteria eventually lyse due to ongoing activity of cell wall autolytic enzymes (autolysins and murein hydrolases) while cell wall assembly is arrested.
Pharmacodynamics/Kinetics
Distribution: Widely distributed in most body tissues and fluids; highest concentrations in bile; low penetration in CSF; variable when meninges are inflamed; crosses placenta; small amounts into breast milk
Half-life: 2 hours, higher with hepatic disease or biliary obstruction
Time to peak serum concentration:
I.M.: Within 1-2 hours
I.V.: Within 15-20 minutes (serum levels 2-3 times the serum levels following I.M. administration)

Elimination: Principally in bile (70% to 75%); 20% to 30% recovered unchanged in urine within 6-12 hours

Usual Dosage I.M., I.V.:
Neonates: 50 mg/kg/dose every 12 hours
Children: 100-150 mg/kg/day divided every 8-12 hours; up to 12 g/day
Adults: 2-4 g/day in divided doses every 12 hours; up to 12 g/day

Dosing adjustment in hepatic impairment: Reduce dose 50% in patients with advanced liver cirrhosis; maximum daily dose: 4 g

Administration Administer around-the-clock to promote less variation in peak and trough serum levels

Monitoring Parameters Monitor for coagulation abnormalities and diarrhea; observe for signs and symptoms of anaphylaxis during first dose

Test Interactions Prothrombin time (S), glucose, protein; ↓ positive Coombs' [direct]

Nursing Implications Do not admix with aminoglycosides in same bottle/bag

Additional Information Sodium content of 1 g: 34.5 mg (1.5 mEq); contains the n-methylthiotetrazole side chain

Dosage Forms
Injection, premixed (frozen): 1 g (50 mL); 2 g (50 mL)
Powder for injection: 1 g, 2 g

Cefotan® see Cefotetan Disodium on next page

Cefotaxime Sodium (sef oh taks' eem)

Related Information
Antimicrobial Drugs of Choice on page 1298-1302

Brand Names Claforan®

Use Treatment of susceptible infection in respiratory tract, skin and skin structure, bone and joint, urinary tract, gynecologic as well as septicemia, and documented or suspected meningitis

Pregnancy Risk Factor B

Contraindications Hypersensitivity to cefotaxime, any component, or cephalosporins

Warnings/Precautions Modify dosage in patients with severe renal impairment; prolonged use may result in superinfection; a low incidence of cross-hypersensitivity to penicillins exists

Adverse Reactions
1% to 10%:
Central nervous system: Fever
Dermatologic: Rash, pruritus
Gastrointestinal: Colitis, diarrhea, nausea, vomiting
Hematologic: Eosinophilia
Local: Pain at injection site
<1%:
Central nervous system: Headache
Gastrointestinal: Pseudomembranous colitis
Hematologic: Transient neutropenia, thrombocytopenia
Local: Phlebitis
Miscellaneous: Transient elevation of BUN, creatinine and liver enzymes

Overdosage/Toxicology Symptoms of overdose include neuromuscular hypersensitivity, convulsions; hemodialysis may be helpful to aid in the removal of the drug from the blood, otherwise most treatment is supportive or symptom directed

Drug Interactions
Increased effect: Probenecid may decrease cephalosporin elimination
Increased toxicity: Furosemide, aminoglycosides may be a possible additive to nephrotoxicity

Stability Reconstituted solution is stable for 24 hours at room temperature and 10 days when refrigerated; for I.V. infusion in NS or D_5W solution is stable for 24 hours at room temperature, 5 days when refrigerated, or 13 weeks when frozen; after freezing, thawed solution is stable for 24 hours at room temperature or 10 days when refrigerated

Mechanism of Action Inhibits bacterial cell wall synthesis by binding to one or more of the penicillin-binding proteins (PBPs) which in turn inhibits the final transpeptidation step of peptidoglycan synthesis in bacterial cell walls, thus inhibiting cell wall biosynthesis. Bacteria eventually lyse due to ongoing activity of cell wall autolytic enzymes (autolysins and murein hydrolases) while cell wall assembly is arrested.

Pharmacodynamics/Kinetics
Distribution: Widely distributed to body tissues and fluids including aqueous humor, ascitic and prostatic fluids, and bone; penetrates CSF when meninges are inflamed; crosses the placenta and appears in breast milk
(Continued)

199

Cefotaxime Sodium *(Continued)*

Metabolism: Partially in the liver to active metabolite, desacetylcefotaxime

Half-life:

Cefotaxime:

Premature neonates <1 week: 5-6 hours

Full-term neonates <1 week: 2-3.4 hours

Adults: 1-1.5 hours (prolonged with renal and/or hepatic impairment)

Desacetylcefotaxime: 1.5-1.9 hours (prolonged with renal impairment)

Time to peak serum concentration: I.M.: Within 30 minutes

Elimination: Renal excretion of parent drug and metabolites

Usual Dosage I.M., I.V.:

Neonates: Postnatal age:

<7 days: 50 mg/kg/dose every 12 hours

>7 days: 50 mg/kg/dose every 8 hours

Infants and Children 1 month to 12 years:

<50 kg: 100-150 mg/kg/day in divided doses every 6-8 hours

Meningitis: 200 mg/kg/day in divided doses every 6 hours

>50 kg: Moderate to severe infection: 1-2 g every 6-8 hours; life-threatening infection: 2 g/dose every 4 hours; maximum dose: 12 g/day

Children >12 years and Adults: 1-2 g every 6-8 hours (up to 12 g/day)

Dosing interval in renal impairment:

Cl_{cr} 10-50 mL/minute: Administer every 8-12 hours

Cl_{cr} <10 mL/minute: Administer every 24 hours

Moderately dialyzable (20% to 50%)

Dosing adjustment in hepatic impairment: Moderate dosage reduction is recommended in severe liver disease

Administration Can be administered IVP over 3-5 minutes or I.V. retrograde or I.V. intermittent infusion over 15-30 minutes; do not admix with aminoglycosides in same bottle/bag

Monitoring Parameters Observe for signs and symptoms of anaphylaxis during first dose

Test Interactions False-positive Coombs' test, false-positive reaction for urine glucose tests using Clinitest® or Benedict's solution, false elevation of creatinine using Jaffé test

Additional Information Sodium content of 1 g: 2.2 mEq

Dosage Forms

Infusion, premixed, in D_5W (frozen): 1 g (50 mL); 2 g (50 mL)

Powder for injection: 1 g, 2 g, 10 g

Cefotetan Disodium (sef' oh tee tan)

Brand Names Cefotan®

Use Treatment of susceptible bacterial infection; mainly respiratory tract, skin and skin structure, bone and joint, urinary tract and gynecologic, as well as, septicemia, similar spectrum to cefoxitin

Pregnancy Risk Factor B

Contraindications Hypersensitivity to cefotetan, any component, or cephalosporins

Warnings/Precautions Modify dosage in patients with severe renal impairment; prolonged use may result in superinfection; a low incidence of cross-hypersensitivity to penicillins exists

Adverse Reactions

1% to 10%:

Gastrointestinal: Diarrhea

Hepatic: Hepatic enzyme elevation

Miscellaneous: Hypersensitivity reactions

<1%:

Central nervous system: Fever

Dermatologic: Rash, pruritus

Gastrointestinal: Nausea, vomiting, antibiotic-associated colitis

Hematologic: Prolongation of bleeding time or prothrombin time, neutropenia, thrombocytopenia

Local: Phlebitis

Overdosage/Toxicology Symptoms of overdose include neuromuscular hypersensitivity, convulsions; hemodialysis may be helpful to aid in the removal of the drug from the blood, otherwise most treatment is supportive or symptom directed

Drug Interactions

Increased effect: Probenecid may decrease cephalosporin elimination

Increased toxicity: Furosemide, aminoglycosides may be a possible additive to nephrotoxicity

May cause disulfiram-like reaction with concomitant alcohol use

Stability Reconstituted solution is stable for 24 hours at room temperature and 96 hours when refrigerated; for I.V. infusion in NS or D_5W solution and after freezing, thawed solution is stable for 24 hours at room temperature or 96 hours when refrigerated; frozen solution is stable for 12 weeks

Mechanism of Action Inhibits bacterial cell wall synthesis by binding to one or more of the penicillin-binding proteins (PBPs) which in turn inhibits the final transpeptidation step of peptidoglycan synthesis in bacterial cell walls, thus inhibiting cell wall biosynthesis. Bacteria eventually lyse due to ongoing activity of cell wall autolytic enzymes (autolysins and murein hydrolases) while cell wall assembly is arrested.

Pharmacodynamics/Kinetics

Distribution: Widely distributed to body tissues and fluids including bile, sputum, prostatic and peritoneal fluids; low concentrations enter CSF; crosses the placenta and appears in breast milk

Protein binding: 76% to 90%

Half-life: 1.5-3 hours

Time to peak serum concentration: I.M.: Within 1.5-3 hours

Elimination: Primarily excreted unchanged in urine with 20% excreted in bile

Usual Dosage I.M., I.V.:

Children: 20-40 mg/kg/dose every 12 hours

Adults: 1-6 g/day in divided doses every 12 hours, 1-2 g may be given every 24 hours for urinary tract infection

Dosing interval in renal impairment:

Cl_{cr} 10-30 mL/minute: Administer every 24 hours

Cl_{cr} <10 mL/minute: Administer every 48 hours

Slightly dialyzable (5% to 20%)

Administration Administer around-the-clock to promote less variation in peak and trough serum levels

Monitoring Parameters Monitor for unusual bleeding or bruising; observe for signs and symptoms of anaphylaxis during first dose

Test Interactions ↑ alkaline phosphatase, AST, ALT, BUN, creatinine, glucose, protein; decreased glucose; positive Coombs' test

Nursing Implications Do not admix with aminoglycosides in same bottle/bag

Additional Information Sodium content of 1 g: 34.5 mg (1.5 mEq); contains the n-methylthiotetrazole side chain

Dosage Forms Powder for injection: 1 g (10 mL, 100 mL); 2 g (20 mL, 100 mL); 10 g (100 mL)

Cefoxitin Sodium (se fox' i tin)

Related Information

Antimicrobial Drugs of Choice on page 1298-1302

Brand Names Mefoxin®

Use Less active against staphylococci and streptococci than first generation cephalosporins, but active against anaerobes including *Bacteroides fragilis*; active against gram-negative enteric bacilli including *E. coli*, *Klebsiella*, and *Proteus*; used predominantly for respiratory tract, skin and skin structure, bone and joint, urinary tract and gynecologic as well as septicemia; surgical prophylaxis; intra-abdominal infections and other mixed infections

Pregnancy Risk Factor B

Contraindications Hypersensitivity to cefoxitin, any component, or cephalosporins

Warnings/Precautions Use with caution in patients with history of colitis; cefoxitin may increase resistance of organisms by inducing beta-lactamase; modify dosage in patients with severe renal impairment; prolonged use may result in superinfection; a low incidence of cross-hypersensitivity to penicillins exists

Adverse Reactions

1% to 10%: Gastrointestinal: Diarrhea

<1%:

Cardiovascular: Hypotension

Central nervous system: Fever

Dermatologic: Rash, exfoliative dermatitis

Gastrointestinal: Nausea, vomiting, pseudomembranous colitis

Hematologic: Transient leukopenia, thrombocytopenia, anemia, eosinophilia

Hepatic: Elevation in serum AST concentration

Local: Thrombophlebitis

Respiratory: Dyspnea

Miscellaneous: Elevations in serum creatinine and/or BUN

(Continued)

Cefoxitin Sodium *(Continued)*

Overdosage/Toxicology Symptoms of overdose include neuromuscular hypersensitivity, convulsions; hemodialysis may be helpful to aid in the removal of the drug from the blood, otherwise most treatment is supportive or symptom directed

Drug Interactions

Increased effect: Probenecid may decrease cephalosporin elimination

Increased toxicity: Furosemide, aminoglycosides may be a possible additive to nephrotoxicity

Stability Reconstituted solution is stable for 24 hours at room temperature and 48 hours when refrigerated; I.V. infusion in NS or D_5W solution is stable for 24 hours at room temperature, 1 week when refrigerated, or 26 weeks when frozen; after freezing, thawed solution is stable for 24 hours at room temperature or 5 days when refrigerated

Mechanism of Action Inhibits bacterial cell wall synthesis by binding to one or more of the penicillin-binding proteins (PBPs) which in turn inhibits the final transpeptidation step of peptidoglycan synthesis in bacterial cell walls, thus inhibiting cell wall biosynthesis. Bacteria eventually lyse due to ongoing activity of cell wall autolytic enzymes (autolysins and murein hydrolases) while cell wall assembly is arrested.

Pharmacodynamics/Kinetics

Distribution: Widely distributed to body tissues and fluids including pleural, synovial, ascitic fluid, and bile; poorly penetrates into CSF even with inflammation of the meninges; crosses the placenta and small amounts appear in breast milk

Protein binding: 65% to 79%

Half-life: 45-60 minutes, increases significantly with renal insufficiency

Time to peak serum concentration:

I.M.: Within 20-30 minutes

I.V.: Within 5 minutes

Elimination: Rapidly excreted as unchanged drug (85%) in urine

Usual Dosage I.M., I.V.:

Infants >3 months and Children:

Mild-moderate infection: 80-100 mg/kg/day in divided doses every 4-6 hours

Severe infection: 100-160 mg/kg/day in divided doses every 4-6 hours

Maximum dose: 12 g/day

Adults: 1-2 g every 6-8 hours (I.M. injection is painful); up to 12 g/day

Dosing interval in renal impairment:

Cl_{cr} 30-50 mL/minute: Administer every 8-12 hours

Cl_{cr} 10-30 mL/minute: Administer every 12-24 hours

Cl_{cr} <10 mL/minute: Administer every 24-48 hours

Moderately dialyzable (20% to 50%)

Administration Administer around-the-clock rather than 4 times/day to promote less variation in peak and trough serum levels

Monitoring Parameters Monitor renal function periodically when used in combination with other nephrotoxic drugs

Test Interactions Positive Coombs' [direct]; false-positive urine glucose (Clinitest®), false increase in serum or urine creatinine with the Jaffé method

Additional Information Sodium content of 1 g: 53 mg (2.3 mEq)

Dosage Forms

Infusion, premixed, in D_5W (frozen): 1 g (50 mL); 2 g (50 mL)

Powder for injection: 1 g, 2 g, 10 g

Cefpodoxime Proxetil *(sef pode ox' eem)*

Brand Names Vantin®

Use Treatment of susceptible acute, community-acquired pneumonia caused by *S. pneumoniae* or nonbeta-lactamase producing *H. influenzae*; acute uncomplicated gonorrhea caused by *N. gonorrhoeae*; uncomplicated skin and skin structure infections caused by *S. aureus* or *S. pyogenes*; acute otitis media caused by *S. pneumoniae*, *H. influenzae*, or *M. catarrhalis*; pharyngitis or tonsillitis; and uncomplicated urinary tract infections caused by *E. coli*, *Klebsiella*, and *Proteus*

Pregnancy Risk Factor B

Contraindications Hypersensitivity to cefpodoxime or cephalosporins

Warnings/Precautions Modify dosage in patients with severe renal impairment; prolonged use may result in superinfection; a low incidence of cross-hypersensitivity to penicillins exists

Adverse Reactions

1% to 10%: Gastrointestinal: Diarrhea

<1%:

Central nervous system: Headache

Dermatologic: Diaper rash

Gastrointestinal: Nausea, vomiting, abdominal pain, pseudomembranous colitis

Genitourinary: Vaginal fungal infections

Overdosage/Toxicology Symptoms of overdose include neuromuscular hypersensitivity, convulsions; hemodialysis may be helpful to aid in the removal of the drug from the blood, otherwise most treatment is supportive or symptom directed

Drug Interactions

Decreased effect: Antacids and H_2-receptor antagonists (reduce absorption and serum concentration of cefpodoxime)

Increased effect: Probenecid may decrease cephalosporin elimination

Increased toxicity: Furosemide, aminoglycosides may be a possible additive to nephrotoxicity

Stability After mixing, keep suspension in refrigerator, shake well before using; discard unused portion after 14 days

Mechanism of Action Inhibits bacterial cell wall synthesis by binding to one or more of the penicillin-binding proteins (PBPs) which in turn inhibits the final transpeptidation step of peptidoglycan synthesis in bacterial cell walls, thus inhibiting cell wall biosynthesis. Bacteria eventually lyse due to ongoing activity of cell wall autolytic enzymes (autolysins and murein hydrolases) while cell wall assembly is arrested.

Pharmacodynamics/Kinetics

Absorption: Oral: Rapidly and well absorbed (50%), acid stable; enhanced in the presence of food or low gastric pH

Distribution: Good tissue penetration, including lung and tonsils; penetrates into pleural fluid

Protein binding: 18% to 23%

Metabolism: Oral: De-esterified in the GI tract to the active metabolite, cefpodoxime

Half-life: 2.2 hours (prolonged with renal impairment)

Time to peak: Within 1 hour (oral)

Elimination: Plasma clearance: ~200-300 mL/minute; primarily eliminated by the kidney with 80% of dose excreted unchanged in urine in 24 hours

Usual Dosage Oral:

Children >6 months to 12 years: 10 mg/kg/day divided every 12 hours

Children ≥13 years and Adults: 100-400 mg every 12 hours
Uncomplicated gonorrhea: 200 mg as a single dose

Dosing adjustment in renal impairment: Cl_{cr} <30 mL/minute: Administer every 24 hours

Administration Administer around-the-clock to promote less variation in peak and trough serum levels

Monitoring Parameters Assess patient at beginning and throughout therapy for infection

Test Interactions Positive Coombs' [direct]

Patient Information Take with food; chilling improves flavor (do not freeze); report persistent diarrhea; entire course of medication (10-14 days) should be taken to ensure eradication of organism; should be taken in equal intervals around-the-clock to maintain adequate blood levels; may interfere with oral contraceptives; females should report symptoms of vaginitis

Additional Information Dose adjustment is not necessary in patients with cirrhosis

Dosage Forms

Granules for oral suspension (lemon creme flavor): 50 mg/5 mL (100 mL); 100 mg/5 mL (100 mL)

Tablet, film coated: 100 mg, 200 mg

Cefprozil (sef proe' zil)

Brand Names Cefzil®

Use Infections causes by susceptible organisms including *S. pneumoniae*, *S. aureus*, *S. pyogenes*; treatment of otitis media and infections involving the respiratory tract and skin and skin structure

Pregnancy Risk Factor B

Contraindications Hypersensitivity to cefprozil or any component or cephalosporins

Warnings/Precautions Modify dosage in patients with severe renal impairment; prolonged use may result in superinfection; a low incidence of cross-hypersensitivity to penicillins exists

Adverse Reactions

1% to 10%:

Central nervous system: Dizziness

Dermatologic: Diaper rash and superinfection, genital pruritus

(Continued)

Cefprozil *(Continued)*

    Gastrointestinal: Diarrhea, nausea, vomiting, abdominal pain
    Genitourinary: Vaginitis
    Hematologic: Eosinophilia
    Hepatic: Elevation of AST and ALT, elevation of alkaline phosphatase
    <1%:
    Central nervous system: Headache, insomnia, confusion
    Dermatologic: Rash, urticaria
    Hematologic: Prolonged PT
    Hepatic: Cholestatic jaundice
    Neuromuscular & skeletal: Arthralgia
    Renal: Elevated BUN and serum creatinine

Overdosage/Toxicology Symptoms of overdose include neuromuscular hypersensitivity, convulsions; hemodialysis may be helpful to aid in the removal of the drug from the blood, otherwise most treatment is supportive or symptom directed

Drug Interactions
    Increased effect: Probenecid may decrease cephalosporin elimination
    Increased toxicity: Furosemide, aminoglycosides may be a possible additive to nephrotoxicity

Mechanism of Action Inhibits bacterial cell wall synthesis by binding to one or more of the penicillin-binding proteins (PBPs) which in turn inhibits the final transpeptidation step of peptidoglycan synthesis in bacterial cell walls, thus inhibiting cell wall biosynthesis. Bacteria eventually lyse due to ongoing activity of cell wall autolytic enzymes (autolysins and murein hydrolases) while cell wall assembly is arrested.

Pharmacodynamics/Kinetics
    Absorption: Oral: Well absorbed (94%)
    Distribution: Low distribution into breast milk
    Protein binding: 35% to 45%
    Half-life, elimination: 1.3 hours (normal renal function)
    Peak serum levels: 1.5 hours (fasting state)
    Elimination: 61% excreted unchanged in urine

Usual Dosage Oral:
    Infants and Children >6 months to 12 years: 7.5-15 mg/kg every 12 hours for 10 days
    Pharyngitis/tonsillitis:
    Children 2-12 years: 15 mg/kg/day divided every 12 hours; maximum: 1 g/day
    Children >13 years and Adults: 250-500 mg every 12-24 hours for 10-14 days

    Dosing adjustment in renal impairment: Cl_{cr} <30 mL/minute: Reduce dose by 50%
    55% reduced by hemodialysis

Administration Administer around-the-clock to promote less variation in peak and trough serum levels

Monitoring Parameters Assess patient at beginning and throughout therapy for infection

Test Interactions Positive Coombs' [direct]; may produce false-positive reaction for urine glucose with Clinitest®

Patient Information Chilling improves flavor (do not freeze); report persistent diarrhea; entire course of medication (10-14 days) should be taken to ensure eradication of organism; should be taken in equal intervals around-the-clock to maintain adequate blood levels; may interfere with oral contraceptives; females should report symptoms of vaginitis

Dosage Forms
    Powder for oral suspension, as anhydrous: 125 mg/5 mL (50 mL, 75 mL, 100 mL); 250 mg/5 mL (50 mL, 75 mL, 100 mL)
    Tablet, as anhydrous: 250 mg, 500 mg

Ceftazidime *(sef′ tay zi deem)*

Related Information
    Antimicrobial Drugs of Choice *on page 1298-1302*

Brand Names Fortaz®; Tazicef®; Tazidime®

Use Treatment of documented susceptible *Pseudomonas aeruginosa* infection; *Pseudomonas* infection in patients at risk of developing aminoglycoside-induced nephrotoxicity and/or ototoxicity; empiric therapy of febrile, granulocytopenic patients

Pregnancy Risk Factor B

Contraindications Hypersensitivity to ceftazidime, any component, or cephalosporins

Warnings/Precautions Modify dosage in patients with severe renal impairment; prolonged use may result in superinfection; a low incidence of cross-hypersensitivity to penicillins exists

Adverse Reactions

1% to 10%:
  Gastrointestinal: Diarrhea
  Local: Pain at injection site

<1%:
  Central nervous system: Fever, headache, dizziness
  Dermatologic: Rash, angioedema
  Gastrointestinal: Nausea, vomiting, pseudomembranous colitis
  Hematologic: Eosinophilia, thrombocytosis, transient leukopenia, hemolytic anemia
  Local: Phlebitis
  Neuromuscular & skeletal: Paresthesia
  Miscellaneous: Transient elevation in liver enzymes, BUN and creatinine, candidiasis

Overdosage/Toxicology Symptoms of overdose include neuromuscular hypersensitivity, convulsions; hemodialysis may be helpful to aid in the removal of the drug from the blood, otherwise most treatment is supportive or symptom directed

Drug Interactions
  Increased effect: Probenecid may decrease cephalosporin elimination; aminoglycosides: *in vitro* studies indicate additive or synergistic effect against some strains of Enterobacteriaceae and *Pseudomonas aeruginosa*
  Increased toxicity: Furosemide, aminoglycosides may be a possible additive to nephrotoxicity

Stability Reconstituted solution and I.V. infusion in NS or D_5W solution are stable for 24 hours at room temperature, 10 days when refrigerated, or 12 weeks when frozen; after freezing, thawed solution is stable for 24 hours at room temperature or 4 days when refrigerated; 96 hours under refrigeration, after mixing

Mechanism of Action Inhibits bacterial cell wall synthesis by binding to one or more of the penicillin-binding proteins (PBPs) which in turn inhibits the final transpeptidation step of peptidoglycan synthesis in bacterial cell walls, thus inhibiting cell wall biosynthesis. Bacteria eventually lyse due to ongoing activity of cell wall autolytic enzymes (autolysins and murein hydrolases) while cell wall assembly is arrested.

Pharmacodynamics/Kinetics
  Distribution: Widely distributes throughout the body including bone, bile, skin, CSF (diffuses into CSF with higher concentrations when the meninges are inflamed), endometrium, heart, pleural and lymphatic fluids
  Protein binding: 17%
  Half-life: 1-2 hours (prolonged with renal impairment)
    Neonates <23 days: 2.2-4.7 hours
  Time to peak serum concentration: I.M.: Within 1 hour
  Elimination: By glomerular filtration with 80% to 90% of the dose excreted as unchanged drug within 24 hours

Usual Dosage I.M., I.V.:
  Neonates:
    Postnatal age <7 days:
      ≤2000 g: 30 mg/kg/dose every 12 hours
      >2000 g: 30 mg/kg/dose every 8 hours
    Postnatal age >7 days:
      <1200 g: 50 mg/kg/dose every 12 hours
      ≥1200 g: 50 mg/kg/dose every 8 hours
  Infants and Children 1 month to 12 years: 30-50 mg/kg/dose every 8 hours; maximum dose: 6 g/day
  Adults: 1-2 g every 8-12 hours
    Urinary tract infections: 250-500 mg every 12 hours

  Dosing interval in renal impairment:
    Cl_{cr} 30-50 mL/minute: Administer every 12 hours
    Cl_{cr} 10-30 mL/minute: Administer every 24 hours
    Cl_{cr} <10 mL/minute: Administer every 48-72 hours
  Dialyzable (50% to 100%)

Administration Any carbon dioxide bubbles that may be present in the withdrawn solution should be expelled prior to injection; administer around-the-clock to promote less variation in peak and trough serum levels; ceftazidime can be administered IVP over 3-5 minutes, or I.V. retrograde or I.V. intermittent infusion over 15-30 minutes; do not admix with aminoglycosides in same bottle/bag; final concentration for I.V. administration should not exceed 100 mg/mL

Monitoring Parameters Observe for signs and symptoms of anaphylaxis during first dose

(Continued)

Ceftazidime *(Continued)*

Test Interactions Positive Coombs' [direct], false-positive urine glucose (Clinitest®)

Additional Information Sodium content of 1 g: 2.3 mEq

Dosage Forms

Infusion, premixed (frozen):
In D_5W: 500 mg (50 mL)
In $D_{1.4}W$: 1 g (50 mL)
In $D_{3.2}W$: 2 g (50 mL)
In NS: 1 g (50 mL); 2 g (100 mL)
Powder for injection: 500 mg, 1 g, 2 g, 6 g

Ceftin® *see* Cefuroxime *on page 208*

Ceftizoxime *(sef ti zox' eem)*

Related Information

Antimicrobial Drugs of Choice *on page 1298-1302*

Brand Names Cefizox®

Use Treatment of susceptible nonpseudomonal gram-negative rod infections or mixed gram-negative and anaerobic infections; predominantly respiratory tract, skin and skin structure, bone and joint, urinary tract and gynecologic, as well as septicemia

Pregnancy Risk Factor B

Contraindications Hypersensitivity to ceftizoxime, any component, or cephalosporins

Warnings/Precautions Modify dosage in patients with severe renal impairment; prolonged use may result in superinfection; a low incidence of cross-hypersensitivity to penicillins exists

Adverse Reactions

1% to 10%:
Central nervous system: Fever
Dermatologic: Rash, pruritus
Hematologic: Eosinophilia, thrombocytosis
Local: Pain, burning at injection site
Miscellaneous: Transient elevation of AST, ALT, and alkaline phosphatase
<1%:
Central nervous system: Numbness
Genitourinary: Vaginitis
Hematologic: Anemia, leukopenia, neutropenia, thrombocytopenia
Hepatic: Elevation of bilirubin
Renal: Transient elevations of BUN and creatinine

Overdosage/Toxicology Symptoms of overdose include neuromuscular hypersensitivity, convulsions; hemodialysis may be helpful to aid in the removal of the drug from the blood, otherwise most treatment is supportive or symptom directed

Drug Interactions

Increased effect: Probenecid may decrease cephalosporin elimination
Increased toxicity: Furosemide, aminoglycosides may be a possible additive to nephrotoxicity

Stability Reconstituted solution is stable for 24 hours at room temperature and 96 hours when refrigerated; for I.V. infusion in NS or D_5W solution is stable for 24 hours at room temperature, 96 hours when refrigerated or 12 weeks when frozen; after freezing, thawed solution is stable for 24 hours at room temperature or 10 days when refrigerated

Mechanism of Action Inhibits bacterial cell wall synthesis by binding to one or more of the penicillin-binding proteins (PBPs) which in turn inhibits the final transpeptidation step of peptidoglycan synthesis in bacterial cell walls, thus inhibiting cell wall biosynthesis. Bacteria eventually lyse due to ongoing activity of cell wall autolytic enzymes (autolysins and murein hydrolases) while cell wall assembly is arrested.

Pharmacodynamics/Kinetics

Distribution: V_d: 0.35-0.5 L/kg; widely distributed into most body tissues and fluids including gallbladder, liver, kidneys, bone, sputum, bile, and pleural and synovial fluids; has good CSF penetration; crosses placenta; small amounts excreted in breast milk
Protein binding: 30%
Half-life: 1.6 hours, increases to 25 hours when Cl_{cr} falls to <10 mL/minute
Time to peak serum concentration: I.M.: Within 0.5-1 hour
Elimination: Excreted unchanged in urine

Usual Dosage I.M., I.V.:

Children ≥6 months: 150-200 mg/kg/day divided every 6-8 hours (maximum of 12 g/24 hours)

Adults: 1-2 g every 8-12 hours, up to 2 g every 4 hours or 4 g every 8 hours for life-threatening infections

Dosing interval in renal impairment:
Cl$_{cr}$ 10-50 mL/minute: Administer every 24-48 hours
Cl$_{cr}$ <10 mL/minute: Administer every 48-72 hours
Moderately dialyzable (20% to 50%)

Monitoring Parameters Observe for signs and symptoms of anaphylaxis during first dose

Test Interactions False-positive Coombs' test, may falsely elevate creatinine values when Jaffé reaction is used, may cause false-positive results in urine glucose tests using cupric sulfate (Benedict's solution, Clinitest®)

Nursing Implications Do not admix with aminoglycosides in same bottle/bag

Additional Information Sodium content of 1 g: 60 mg (2.6 mEq)

Dosage Forms
Injection, in D$_5$W (frozen): 1 g (50 mL); 2 g (50 mL)
Powder for injection: 500 mg, 1 g, 2 g, 10 g

Ceftriaxone Sodium (sef try ax' one)

Related Information
Antimicrobial Drugs of Choice on page 1298-1302

Brand Names Rocephin®

Use Treatment of lower respiratory tract infections, skin and skin structure infections, bone and joint infections, intra-abdominal and urinary tract infections, sepsis and meningitis due to susceptible organisms; documented or suspected infection due to susceptible organisms in home care patients and patients without I.V. line access; treatment of documented or suspected gonococcal infection or chancroid; emergency room management of patients at high risk for bacteremia, periorbital or buccal cellulitis, salmonellosis or shigellosis, and pneumonia of unestablished etiology (<5 years of age)

Pregnancy Risk Factor B

Contraindications Hypersensitivity to ceftriaxone sodium, any component, or cephalosporins; **do not use in hyperbilirubinemic neonates,** particularly those who are premature since ceftriaxone is reported to displace bilirubin from albumin binding sites

Warnings/Precautions Modify dosage in patients with severe renal impairment; prolonged use may result in superinfection with yeasts, enterococci, B. fragilis, or P. aeruginosa; a low incidence of cross-hypersensitivity to penicillins exists

Adverse Reactions
1% to 10%:
Dermatologic: Rash
Gastrointestinal: Diarrhea
Hematologic: Eosinophilia, thrombocytosis, leukopenia
Hepatic: Elevations of SGOT [AST], SGPT [ALT]
Local: Pain at injection site
Renal: Elevations of BUN
<1%:
Cardiovascular: Flushing
Central nervous system: Fever, chills, headache, dizziness
Dermatologic: Pruritus
Gastrointestinal: Nausea, vomiting, dysgeusia
Genitourinary: Presence of casts in urine, vaginitis
Hematologic: Anemia, hemolytic anemia, neutropenia, lymphopenia, thrombocytopenia
Local: Phlebitis
Renal: Elevation of creatinine
Miscellaneous: Elevations of alkaline phosphatase and bilirubin, moniliasis, diaphoresis

Overdosage/Toxicology Symptoms of overdose include neuromuscular hypersensitivity, convulsions; hemodialysis may be helpful to aid in the removal of the drug from the blood, otherwise most treatment is supportive or symptom directed

Drug Interactions
Increased effect:
Aminoglycosides may result in synergistic antibacterial activity
High-dose probenecid decreases clearance
Increased toxicity: Aminoglycosides increase nephrotoxic potential

Stability Reconstituted solution (100 mg/mL) is stable for 3 days at room temperature and 3 days when refrigerated; for I.V. infusion in NS or D$_5$W solution is stable for 3 days at room temperature, 10 days when refrigerated, or 26 weeks when frozen; after freezing, thawed solution is stable for 3 days at room temperature or 10 days when refrigerated

(Continued)

Ceftriaxone Sodium (Continued)

Mechanism of Action Inhibits bacterial cell wall synthesis by binding to one or more of the penicillin-binding proteins (PBPs) which in turn inhibits the final transpeptidation step of peptidoglycan synthesis in bacterial cell walls, thus inhibiting cell wall biosynthesis. Bacteria eventually lyse due to ongoing activity of cell wall autolytic enzymes (autolysins and murein hydrolases) while cell wall assembly is arrested.

Pharmacodynamics/Kinetics

Distribution: Widely distributes throughout the body including gallbladder, lungs, bone, bile, CSF (diffuses into the CSF at higher concentrations when the meninges are inflamed)

Protein binding: 85% to 95%

Half-life: Normal renal and hepatic function: 5-9 hours

Neonates: Postnatal:

1-4 days: 16 hours

9-30 days: 9 hours

Time to peak serum concentration:

I.M.: Within 1-2 hours

I.V.: Within minutes

Elimination: Excreted unchanged in urine (33% to 65%) by glomerular filtration and in feces

Usual Dosage

Neonates: I.M., I.V.:

Postnatal age <7 days: 50 mg/kg/day given every 24 hours

Postnatal age >7 days:

<2000 g: 50 mg/kg/day given every 24 hours

>2000 g: 75 mg/kg/day given every 24 hours

Gonococcal prophylaxis: I.M.:

LBW neonates: 25-50 mg/kg as a single dose (dose not to exceed 125 mg)

Neonates: 125 mg as a single dose

Neonatal gonococcal ophthalmia: I.M.: 25-50 mg/kg/day given every 24 hours

Infants and Children: 50-100 mg/kg/day in 1-2 divided doses

Meningitis: Loading dose: 75 mg/kg may be administered at the start of therapy; then 100 mg/kg/day divided every 12 hours; maximum: 4 g/day

Chancroid, uncomplicated gonorrhea: I.M.:

<45 kg: 125 mg as a single dose

>45 kg: 250 mg as a single dose

Adults: 1-2 g every 12-24 hours depending on the type and severity of the infection; maximum dose: 4 g/day

A single I.M. dose of 250 mg of ceftriaxone is the treatment of choice for gonorrhea

Not dialyzable (0% to 5%)

Monitoring Parameters Assess patient at beginning and throughout therapy for infection; observe for signs and symptoms of anaphylaxis

Test Interactions False-positive urine glucose with Clinitest®

Nursing Implications Obtain specimens for culture and sensitivity before the first dose

Additional Information Sodium content of 1 g: 2.6 mEq

Dosage Forms

Infusion, premixed (frozen): 1 g in $D_{3.8}W$ (50 mL); 2 g in $D_{2.4}W$ (50 mL)

Powder for injection: 250 mg, 500 mg, 1 g, 2 g, 10 g

Cefuroxime (se fyoor ox′ eem)

Related Information

Antimicrobial Drugs of Choice on page 1298-1302

Brand Names Ceftin®; Kefurox®; Zinacef®

Use Treatment of infections caused by staphylococci, group B streptococci, *H. influenzae* (type A and B), *E. coli*, *Enterobacter*, *Salmonella*, and *Klebsiella*; treatment of susceptible infections of the lower respiratory tract, otitis media, urinary tract, skin and soft tissue, bone and joint, sepsis and gonorrhea

Pregnancy Risk Factor B

Contraindications Hypersensitivity to cefuroxime, any component, or cephalosporins

Warnings/Precautions Modify dosage in patients with severe renal impairment; prolonged use may result in superinfection; a low incidence of cross-hypersensitivity to penicillins exists

Adverse Reactions

1% to 10%:

Hematologic: Decreased hemoglobin and hematocrit, eosinophilia

Local: Thrombophlebitis

Miscellaneous: Transient rise in SGOT [AST]/SGPT [ALT] and alkaline phosphatase

<1%:

Central nervous system: Dizziness, fever, headache

Dermatologic: Rash

Gastrointestinal: Nausea, vomiting, diarrhea, stomach cramps, colitis, GI bleeding

Genitourinary: Vaginitis

Hematologic: Transient neutropenia and leukopenia

Hepatic: Transient increase in liver enzymes

Local: Pain at the injection site

Renal: Increase in creatinine and/or BUN

Overdosage/Toxicology Symptoms of overdose include neuromuscular hypersensitivity, convulsions; hemodialysis may be helpful to aid in the removal of the drug from the blood, otherwise most treatment is supportive or symptom directed

Drug Interactions

Increased effect: High-dose probenecid decreases clearance

Increased toxicity: Aminoglycosides increase nephrotoxic potential

Stability Reconstituted solution is stable for 24 hours at room temperature and 48 hours when refrigerated; I.V. infusion in NS or D_5W solution is stable for 24 hours at room temperature, 7 days when refrigerated, or 26 weeks when frozen; after freezing, thawed solution is stable for 24 hours at room temperature or 21 days when refrigerated

Mechanism of Action Inhibits bacterial cell wall synthesis by binding to one or more of the penicillin-binding proteins (PBPs) which in turn inhibits the final transpeptidation step of peptidoglycan synthesis in bacterial cell walls, thus inhibiting cell wall biosynthesis. Bacteria eventually lyse due to ongoing activity of cell wall autolytic enzymes (autolysins and murein hydrolases) while cell wall assembly is arrested.

Pharmacodynamics/Kinetics

Absorption: Increased when given with or shortly after food or infant formula

Distribution: Widely distributed to body tissues and fluids; crosses blood-brain barrier; therapeutic concentrations achieved in CSF even when meninges are not inflamed; crosses placenta and reaches breast milk

Protein binding: 33% to 50%

Bioavailability, axetil: Oral: 37% to 52%

Half-life:

Neonates:

≤3 days: 5.1-5.8 hours

6-14 days: 2-4.2 hours

3-4 weeks: 1-1.5 hours

Adults: 1-2 hours (prolonged in renal impairment)

I.M.: Within 15-60 minutes

I.V.: 2-3 minutes

Elimination: Primarily excreted 66% to 100% as unchanged drug in urine by both glomerular filtration and tubular secretion

Usual Dosage

Neonates: 10-25 mg/kg/dose every 12 hours

Children:

Oral:

<12 years: 125 mg twice daily

>12 years: 250 mg twice daily

I.M., I.V.: 75-150 mg/kg/day divided every 8 hours; maximum dose: 9 g/day

Adults:

Oral: 125-500 mg twice daily, depending on severity of infection

I.M., I.V.: 100-150 mg/kg/day in divided doses every 6-8 hours; maximum: 6 g/24 hours

Dosing adjustment in renal impairment:

Cl_{cr} 10-20 mL/minute: Administer every 12 hours

Cl_{cr} <10 mL/minute: Administer every 24 hours

Dialyzable (25%)

Administration Administer around-the-clock to promote less variation in peak and trough serum levels

Monitoring Parameters Observe for signs and symptoms of anaphylaxis during first dose; with prolonged therapy, monitor renal, hepatic, and hematologic function periodically

(Continued)

209

Cefuroxime *(Continued)*

Test Interactions False-positive Coombs' test; may falsely elevate creatinine values when Jaffé reaction is used; may cause false-positive results in urine glucose tests using cupric sulfate (Benedict's solution, Clinitest®)

Patient Information Report prolonged diarrhea; entire course of medication (10-14 days) should be taken to ensure eradication of organism; should be taken in equal intervals around-the-clock to maintain adequate blood levels; may interfere with oral contraceptives; females should report symptoms of vaginitis

Nursing Implications Do not admix with aminoglycosides in same bottle/bag; obtain specimens for culture and sensitivity prior to the first dose

Additional Information Sodium content of 1 g: 54.2 mg (2.4 mEq)

Dosage Forms

Infusion, premixed (frozen) (Zinacef®): 750 mg (50 mL); 1.5 g (50 mL)
Powder for injection, as sodium (Kefurox®, Zinacef®): 750 mg, 1.5 g, 7.5 g
Tablet, as axetil (Ceftin®): 125 mg, 250 mg, 500 mg

Cefzil® *see* Cefprozil *on page 203*

Celestone® *see* Betamethasone *on page 129*

Celontin® *see* Methsuximide *on page 718*

Cel-U-Jec® *see* Betamethasone *on page 129*

Cenafed® [OTC] *see* Pseudoephedrine *on page 955*

Cenafed® Plus [OTC] *see* Triprolidine and Pseudoephedrine *on page 1131*

Cena-K® *see* Potassium Chloride *on page 906*

Cenocort® *see* Triamcinolone *on page 1112*

Cenocort® Forte *see* Triamcinolone *on page 1112*

Cenolate® *see* Sodium Ascorbate *on page 1009*

Centrax® *see* Prazepam *on page 916*

Cephalexin Monohydrate *(sef a lex' in)*

Brand Names Cefanex®; C-Lexin®; Entacef®; Keflet®; Keflex®; Keftab®

Use Treatment of susceptible bacterial infections, including those caused by group A beta-hemolytic *Streptococcus, Staphylococcus, Klebsiella pneumoniae, E. coli, Proteus mirabilis,* and *Shigella;* predominantly used for lower respiratory tract, urinary tract, skin and soft tissue, and bone and joint

Pregnancy Risk Factor B

Contraindications Hypersensitivity to cephalexin, any component, or cephalosporins

Warnings/Precautions Modify dosage in patients with severe renal impairment; prolonged use may result in superinfection; a low incidence of cross-hypersensitivity to penicillins exists

Adverse Reactions

1% to 10%: Gastrointestinal: Diarrhea

<1%:

Central nervous system: Dizziness, fatigue, headache
Dermatologic: Rash
Gastrointestinal: Nausea, vomiting, pseudomembranous colitis
Hematologic: Transient neutropenia, anemia
Hepatic: Transient elevation in liver enzymes

Overdosage/Toxicology Symptoms of overdose include neuromuscular hypersensitivity, convulsions; hemodialysis may be helpful to aid in the removal of the drug from the blood, otherwise most treatment is supportive or symptom directed

Drug Interactions

Increased effect: High-dose probenecid increases clearance
Increased toxicity: Aminoglycosides increase nephrotoxic potential

Stability Refrigerate suspension after reconstitution; discard after 14 days

Mechanism of Action Inhibits bacterial cell wall synthesis by binding to one or more of the penicillin-binding proteins (PBPs) which in turn inhibits the final transpeptidation step of peptidoglycan synthesis in bacterial cell walls, thus inhibiting cell wall biosynthesis. Bacteria eventually lyse due to ongoing activity of cell wall autolytic enzymes (autolysins and murein hydrolases) while cell wall assembly is arrested.

Pharmacodynamics/Kinetics

Absorption: Delayed in young children; may be decreased up to 50% in neonates
Distribution: Widely distributed into most body tissues and fluids, including gallbladder, liver, kidneys, bone, sputum, bile, and pleural and synovial fluids; CSF penetration is poor; crosses placenta; appears in breast milk

Protein binding: 6% to 15%

Half-life:

Neonates: 5 hours

Children 3-12 months: 2.5 hours

Adults: 0.5-1.2 hours (prolonged with renal impairment)

Time to peak serum concentration: Oral: Within 1 hour

Elimination: 80% to 100% of dose excreted as unchanged drug in urine within 8 hours

Usual Dosage Oral:

Children: 25-50 mg/kg/day every 6 hours; severe infections: 50-100 mg/kg/day in divided doses every 6 hours; maximum: 3 g/24 hours

Adults: 250-1000 mg every 6 hours; maximum: 4 g/day

Dosing interval in renal impairment: Cl_{cr} <10 mL/minute: Administer every 8-12 hours

Moderately dialyzable (20% to 50%)

Administration Administer on an empty stomach (ie, 1 hour prior to, or 2 hours after meals) to increase total absorption; give around-the-clock rather than 4 times/day to promote less variation in peak and trough serum levels

Monitoring Parameters With prolonged therapy monitor renal, hepatic, and hematologic function periodically

Test Interactions False-positive Coombs' test, may falsely elevate creatinine values when Jaffé reaction is used, may cause false-positive results in urine glucose tests using cupric sulfate (Benedict's solution, Clinitest®), false-positive urinary proteins and steroids

Patient Information Report prolonged diarrhea; entire course of medication (10-14 days) should be taken to ensure eradication of organism; should be taken in equal intervals around-the-clock to maintain adequate blood levels; may interfere with oral contraceptives; females should report symptoms of vaginitis

Nursing Implications Obtain specimens for culture and sensitivity prior to the first dose

Dosage Forms

Capsule: 250 mg, 500 mg

Drops, pediatric: 100 mg/mL (10 mL)

Suspension: 125 mg/5 mL (5 mL unit dose, 60 mL, 100 mL, 200 mL); 250 mg/5 mL (5 mL unit dose, 100 mL, 200 mL)

Tablet: 250 mg, 500 mg, 1 g

Tablet, as hydrochloride (Keftab®): 250 mg, 500 mg

Cephalothin Sodium (sef a′ loe thin)

Brand Names Keflin®

Use Treatment of susceptible bacterial infections, including those caused by group A beta-hemolytic *Streptococcus*; respiratory, genitourinary, gastrointestinal, skin and soft tissue, bone and joint infections; septicemia; cephalexin is the oral equivalent

Pregnancy Risk Factor B

Contraindications Hypersensitivity to cephalothin or cephalosporins

Warnings/Precautions Modify dosage in patients with severe renal impairment; prolonged use may result in superinfection; a low incidence of cross-hypersensitivity to penicillins exists

Adverse Reactions

1% to 10%: Gastrointestinal: Nausea, vomiting, diarrhea

<1%:

Dermatologic: Maculopapular and erythematous rash

Gastrointestinal: Dyspepsia, pseudomembranous colitis

Hematologic: Bleeding, thrombocytopenia

Local: Pain and induration at injection site

Overdosage/Toxicology Symptoms of overdose include neuromuscular hypersensitivity, convulsions; hemodialysis may be helpful to aid in the removal of the drug from the blood, otherwise most treatment is supportive or symptom directed

Stability Reconstituted solution is stable for 12-24 hours at room temperature and 96 hours when refrigerated; for I.V. infusion in NS or D_5W solution is stable for 24 hours at room temperature, 96 hours when refrigerated or 12 weeks when frozen; after freezing, thawed solution is stable for 24 hours at room temperature or 96 hours when refrigerated

Mechanism of Action Inhibits bacterial cell wall synthesis by binding to one or more of the penicillin-binding proteins (PBPs) which in turn inhibits the final transpeptidation step of peptidoglycan synthesis in bacterial cell walls, thus inhibiting cell wall biosynthesis. Bacteria eventually lyse due to ongoing activity of cell wall autolytic enzymes (autolysins and murein hydrolases) while cell wall assembly is arrested.

(Continued)

segmenterALPHABETICAL LISTING OF DRUGS

Cephalothin Sodium *(Continued)*

Pharmacodynamics/Kinetics

Distribution: Does not penetrate the CSF unless the meninges are inflamed; crosses the placenta; small amounts appear in breast milk

Protein binding: 65% to 80%

Metabolism: Partially deacetylated in the liver and kidney

Half-life: 30-60 minutes

Time to peak serum concentration:
- I.M.: Within 30 minutes
- I.V.: Within 15 minutes

Elimination: 50% to 75% of a dose appearing as unchanged drug in urine

Usual Dosage

Neonates: I.V.:

<7 days:
- <2000 g: 20 mg/kg/dose every 12 hours
- >2000 g: 20 mg/kg/dose every 8 hours

>7 days:
- <2000 g: 20 mg/kg/dose every 8 hours
- >2000 g: 20 mg/kg/dose every 6 hours

Children: I.M., I.V.: 75-125 mg/kg/day divided every 4-6 hours; maximum dose: 10 g in a 24-hour period

Adults: I.M., I.V.: 500 mg to 2 g every 4-6 hours

Dosing interval in renal impairment:

Cl_{cr} 10-50 mL/minute: Administer every 6-8 hours

Cl_{cr} <10 mL/minute: Administer every 12 hours

Administration Administer around-the-clock to promote less variation in peak and trough serum levels

Monitoring Parameters Observe for signs and symptoms of anaphylaxis during first dose; obtain specimen for culture and sensitivity prior to the first dose

Test Interactions False-positive Coombs' test, may falsely elevate creatinine values when Jaffé reaction is used; may cause false-positive results in urine glucose test using cupric sulfate (Benedict's solution, Clinitest®), false-positive urinary proteins and steroids

Nursing Implications Do not admix with aminoglycosides in same bottle/bag

Additional Information Sodium content of 1 g: 2.8 mEq

Dosage Forms

Infusion, in D_5W (frozen): 1 g (50 mL); 2 g (50 mL)

Powder for injection: 1 g, 2 g, 20 g

Cephapirin Sodium *(sef a pye' rin)*

Brand Names Cefadyl®

Use Treatment of infections when caused by susceptible strains including group A beta-hemolytic *Streptococcus*; used in serious respiratory, genitourinary, gastrointestinal, skin and soft tissue, bone and joint infections; septicemia; endocarditis; identical to cephalothin

Pregnancy Risk Factor B

Contraindications Hypersensitivity to cephapirin sodium, any component, or cephalosporins

Warnings/Precautions Modify dosage in patients with severe renal impairment; prolonged use may result in superinfection; a low incidence of cross-hypersensitivity to penicillins exists

Adverse Reactions

1% to 10%: Gastrointestinal: Diarrhea

<1%:
- Central nervous system: CNS irritation, seizures, fever
- Dermatologic: Rash, urticaria
- Hematologic: Leukopenia, thrombocytopenia
- Hepatic: Transient elevation of liver enzymes

Overdosage/Toxicology Symptoms of overdose include neuromuscular hypersensitivity, convulsions; hemodialysis may be helpful to aid in the removal of the drug from the blood, otherwise most treatment is supportive or symptom directed

Drug Interactions

Increased effect: High-dose probenecid decreases clearance

Increased toxicity: Aminoglycosides increase nephrotoxic potential

Stability Reconstituted solution is stable for 24 hours at room temperature and 10 days when refrigerated; for I.V. infusion in NS or D_5W solution is stable for 24 hours at room temperature, 10 days when refrigerated or 14 days when frozen; after freezing, thawed solution is stable for 12 hours at room temperature or 10 days when refrigerated

212

Mechanism of Action Inhibits bacterial cell wall synthesis by binding to one or more of the penicillin-binding proteins (PBPs) which in turn inhibits the final transpeptidation step of peptidoglycan synthesis in bacterial cell walls, thus inhibiting cell wall biosynthesis. Bacteria eventually lyse due to ongoing activity of cell wall autolytic enzymes (autolysins and murein hydrolases) while cell wall assembly is arrested.

Pharmacodynamics/Kinetics
Distribution: Widely distributed into most body tissues and fluids including gallbladder, liver, kidneys, bone, sputum, bile, and pleural and synovial fluids; CSF penetration is poor; crosses the placenta and small amounts appear in breast milk

Protein binding: 22% to 25%

Metabolism: Partially in the liver, kidney, and plasma to metabolites (50% active)

Half-life: 36-60 minutes

Time to peak serum concentration:
I.M.: Within 30 minutes
I.V.: Within 5 minutes

Elimination: 60% to 85% excreted as unchanged drug in urine

Usual Dosage I.M., I.V.:
Children: 10-20 mg/kg/dose every 6 hours up to 4 g/24 hours
Adults: 500 mg to 1 g every 6 hours up to 12 g/day

Dosing interval in renal impairment:
Cl_{cr} 10-50 mL/minute: Administer every 6-8 hours
Cl_{cr} <10 mL/minute: Administer every 12 hours

Administration Administer around-the-clock rather than 4 times/day to promote less variation in peak and trough serum levels

Monitoring Parameters Observe for signs and symptoms of anaphylaxis during first dose

Test Interactions False-positive Coombs' test, may falsely elevate creatinine values when Jaffé reaction is used, may cause false-positive results in urine glucose tests using cupric sulfate (Benedict's solution, Clinitest®), false-positive urinary proteins and steroids

Nursing Implications Do not admix with aminoglycosides in same bottle/bag; obtain specimens for culture and sensitivity prior to administration of first dose

Additional Information Sodium content of 1 g: 2.4 mEq

Dosage Forms Powder for injection: 500 mg, 1 g, 2 g, 4 g, 20 g

Cephradine (sef' ra deen)
Brand Names Velosef®

Use Treatment of susceptible bacterial infections, including those caused by group A beta-hemolytic *Streptococcus*; used in in respiratory, genitourinary, gastrointestinal, skin and soft tissue, bone and joint infections

Pregnancy Risk Factor B

Contraindications Hypersensitivity to cephradine, any component, or cephalosporins

Warnings/Precautions Prolonged use may result in superinfection; use with caution in patients with a history of colitis; reduce dose in patients with renal dysfunction; a low incidence of cross-hypersensitivity with penicillins exists

Adverse Reactions
1% to 10%: Gastrointestinal: Diarrhea
<1%:
Dermatologic: Rash
Gastrointestinal: Nausea, vomiting, pseudomembranous colitis
Renal: Increased BUN and creatinine

Overdosage/Toxicology Symptoms of overdose include neuromuscular hypersensitivity, convulsions; hemodialysis may be helpful to aid in the removal of the drug from the blood, otherwise most treatment is supportive or symptom directed

Stability Reconstituted solution is stable for 2 hours at room temperature and 24 hours when refrigerated; for I.V. infusion in NS or D_5W solution is stable for 10 hours at room temperature, 48 hours when refrigerated or 6 weeks when frozen; after freezing, thawed solution is stable for 10 hours at room temperature or 48 hours when refrigerated

Mechanism of Action Inhibits bacterial cell wall synthesis by binding to one or more of the penicillin-binding proteins (PBPs) which in turn inhibits the final transpeptidation step of peptidoglycan synthesis in bacterial cell walls, thus inhibiting cell wall biosynthesis. Bacteria eventually lyse due to ongoing activity of cell wall autolytic enzymes (autolysins and murein hydrolases) while cell wall assembly is arrested.

Pharmacodynamics/Kinetics
Absorption: Oral is faster than I.M., but well absorbed from all routes
(Continued)

Cephradine *(Continued)*

Distribution: Widely distributed into most body tissues and fluids including gall-bladder, liver, kidneys, bone, sputum, bile, and pleural and synovial fluids; CSF penetration is poor; crosses the placenta and appears in breast milk

Protein binding: 18% to 20%

Half-life: 1-2 hours

Time to peak serum concentration: Oral, I.M.: Within 1-2 hours

Elimination: ~80% to 90% unchanged drug is recovered in urine within 6 hours

Usual Dosage

Children ≥9 months:

Oral: 25-50 mg/kg/day in divided doses every 6 hours

I.M., I.V.: 50-100 mg/kg/day in equally divided doses every 6 hours up to 4 g/day

Adults:

Oral: 250-500 mg every 6-12 hours

I.M., I.V.: 1 g every 6 hours

Dosing adjustment in renal impairment:

Cl_{cr} 10-50 mL/minute: Administer 50% of dose

Cl_{cr} <10 mL/minute: Administer 25% of dose

or

Cl_{cr} 25-50 mL/minute: Administer every 12 hours

Cl_{cr} 10-25 mL/minute: Administer every 24 hours

Cl_{cr} <10 mL/minute: Administer every 36 hours

Administration Administer around-the-clock to promote less variation in peak and trough serum levels

Monitoring Parameters Observe for signs and symptoms of anaphylaxis during first dose

Test Interactions False-positive Coombs' test, may falsely elevate creatinine values when Jaffé reaction is used, may cause false-positive results in urine glucose tests using cupric sulfate (Benedict's solution, Clinitest®), false-positive urinary proteins and steroids

Patient Information Take until gone, do not miss doses; report diarrhea promptly; entire course of medication (10-14 days) should be taken to ensure eradication of organism; should be taken in equal intervals around-the-clock to maintain adequate blood levels; may interfere with oral contraceptives; females should report symptoms of vaginitis

Nursing Implications Do not admix with aminoglycosides in same bottle/bag; obtain specimen for culture and sensitivity prior to the first dose

Dosage Forms

Capsule: 250 mg, 500 mg

Powder for injection: 250 mg, 500 mg, 1 g, 2 g

Powder for oral suspension: 125 mg/5 mL (5 mL, 100 mL, 200 mL); 250 mg/5 mL (5 mL, 100 mL, 200 mL)

Charcoal (char′ kole)

Brand Names Actidose-Aqua® [OTC]; Actidose® With Sorbitol [OTC]; Charcoaid® [OTC]; Charcocaps® [OTC]; Insta-Char® [OTC]; Liqui-Char® [OTC]; SuperChar® [OTC]

Synonyms Activated Carbon; Activated Charcoal; Adsorbent Charcoal; Liquid Antidote; Medicinal Carbon; Medicinal Charcoal

Use Emergency treatment in poisoning by drugs and chemicals; repetitive doses for gastric dialysis in uremia to adsorb various waste products, and repetitive doses have proven useful to enhance the elimination of certain drugs (eg, theophylline, phenobarbital, and aspirin)

Pregnancy Risk Factor C

Contraindications Not effective for cyanide, mineral acids, caustic alkalis, organic solvents, iron, ethanol, methanol poisoning, lithium; do not use charcoal with sorbitol in patients with fructose intolerance; charcoal with sorbitol is not recommended in children <1 year.

Warnings/Precautions When using ipecac with charcoal, induce vomiting with ipecac before administering activated charcoal since charcoal adsorbs ipecac syrup; charcoal may cause vomiting which is hazardous in petroleum distillate and caustic ingestions; if charcoal in sorbitol is administered, doses should be limited to prevent excessive fluid and electrolyte losses; do not mix charcoal with milk, ice cream, or sherbet

Adverse Reactions

>10%:

    Gastrointestinal: Emesis, vomiting, diarrhea with sorbitol, constipation

    Miscellaneous: Stools will turn black

<1%: Swelling of abdomen

Drug Interactions Do not administer concomitantly with syrup of ipecac; do not mix with milk, ice cream, or sherbet

Stability Adsorbs gases from air, store in closed container

Mechanism of Action Adsorbs toxic substances or irritants, thus inhibiting GI absorption; adsorbs intestinal gas; the addition of sorbitol results in hyperosmotic laxative action causing catharsis

Pharmacodynamics/Kinetics

Absorption: Not absorbed from GI tract

Metabolism: Not metabolized

Elimination: As charcoal in feces

Usual Dosage Oral:

Acute poisoning:

Charcoal with sorbitol: Single-dose:

    Children 1-12 years: 1-2 g/kg/dose or 15-30 g or approximately 5-10 times the weight of the ingested poison; 1 g absorbs 100-1000 mg of poison; the use of repeat oral charcoal with sorbitol doses is not recommended. In young children, sorbitol should be repeated no more than 1-2 times/day.

    Adults: 30-100 g

Charcoal in water:

    Single-dose:

        Infants <1 year: 1 g/kg

        Children 1-12 years: 15-30 g or 1-2 g/kg

        Adults: 30-100 g or 1-2 g/kg

    Multiple-dose:

        Infants <1 year: 0.5 g/kg every 4-6 hours

        Children 1-12 years: 20-60 g or 0.5-1 g/kg every 2-6 hours until clinical observations, serum drug concentration have returned to a subtherapeutic range, or charcoal stool apparent

        Adults: 20-60 g or 0.5-1 g/kg every 2-6 hours

Gastric dialysis: Adults: 20-50 g every 6 hours for 1-2 days

Intestinal gas, diarrhea, GI distress: Adults: 520-975 mg after meals or at first sign of discomfort; repeat as needed to a maximum dose of 4.16 g/day

Administration Flavoring agents (eg, chocolate) and sorbitol can enhance charcoal's palatability; marmalade, milk, ice cream, and sherbet should be avoided since they can reduce charcoal's effectiveness

Patient Information Charcoal causes the stools to turn black; should not be used prior to calling a poison control center or a physician

Nursing Implications Too concentrated of slurries may clog airway; often given with a laxative or cathartic; check for presence of bowel sounds before administration

Dosage Forms

Capsule (Charcocaps®): 260 mg

Liquid, activated:

    Actidose-Aqua®: 12.5 g (60 mL); 25 g (120 mL)

(Continued)

Charcoal *(Continued)*

    Liqui-Char®: 12.5 g (60 mL); 15 g (75 mL); 25 g (120 mL); 30 g (120 mL); 50 g (240 mL)

    SuperChar®: 30 g (240 mL)

  Liquid, activated, with propylene glycol: 12.5 g (60 mL); 25 g (120 mL)

  Liquid, activated, with sorbitol:

    Actidose® With Sorbitol: 25 g (120 mL); 50 g (240 mL)

    Charcoaid®: 30 g (150 mL)

    SuperChar®: 30 g (240 mL)

  Powder for suspension, activated:

    15 g, 30 g, 40 g, 120 g, 240 g

    SuperChar®: 30 g

Charcocaps® [OTC] *see* Charcoal *on page 214*

Chealamide® *see* Edetate Disodium *on page 381*

Chelated Manganese® [OTC] *see* Manganese *on page 663*

Chemet® *see* Succimer *on page 1034*

Chenix® *see* Chenodiol *on this page*

Chenodeoxycholic Acid *see* Chenodiol *on this page*

Chenodiol *(kee noe dye' ole)*

Brand Names Chenix®

Synonyms Chenodeoxycholic Acid

Use Oral dissolution of cholesterol gallstones in selected patients

Pregnancy Risk Factor X

Contraindications Presence of known hepatocyte dysfunction or bile ductal abnormalities; a gallbladder confirmed as nonvisualizing after two consecutive single doses of dye; radiopaque stones; gallstone complications or compelling reasons for gallbladder surgery; inflammatory bowel disease or active gastric or duodenal ulcer; pregnancy

Warnings/Precautions Chenodiol is hepatotoxic in animal models including subhuman Primates; chenodiol should be discontinued if aminotransferases exceed 3 times the upper normal limit; chenodiol may contribute to colon cancer in otherwise susceptible individuals

Adverse Reactions

>10%:

  Gastrointestinal: Diarrhea (mild), biliary pain

  Miscellaneous: Aminotransferase increases

1% to 10%:

  Endocrine & metabolic: Increases in cholesterol and LDL cholesterol

  Gastrointestinal: Dyspepsia

<1%:

  Gastrointestinal: Diarrhea (severe), cramps, nausea, vomiting, flatulence, constipation

  Hematologic: Leukopenia

  Hepatic: Intrahepatic cholestasis, higher cholecystectomy rates

Overdosage/Toxicology Symptoms of overdose include diarrhea and a rise in liver function tests have been observed; no specific antidote, institute supportive therapy

Drug Interactions Decreased effect: Antacids, cholestyramine, colestipol, oral contraceptives

Mechanism of Action Chenodiol is a primary acid excreted into bile, normally constituting one-third of the total biliary bile acids. Synthesis of chenodiol is regulated by the relative composition and flux of cholesterol and bile acids through the hepatocyte by a negative feedback effect on the rate-limiting enzymes for synthesis of cholesterol (HMGCoA reductase) and bile acids (cholesterol 7 alpha-hydroxyl).

Usual Dosage Adults: Oral: 13-16 mg/kg/day in 2 divided doses, starting with 250 mg twice daily the first 2 weeks and increasing by 250 mg/day each week thereafter until the recommended or maximum tolerated dose is achieved

  Dosing comments in hepatic impairment: Contraindicated for use in presence of known hepatocyte dysfunction or bile ductal abnormalities

Monitoring Parameters Oral cholecystograms and/or ultrasonograms should be used to monitor response; dissolutions of stones should be confirmed 1-3 months later

Test Interactions ↑ aminotransferases, ↑ cholesterol, ↑ LDL cholesterol, ↓ triglycerides, ↑ bilirubin (I)

Patient Information Periodic liver function tests and oral cholecystograms are required to monitor therapy; contact the physician immediately if nonspecific abdominal pain, right upper quadrant pain, nausea, and vomiting are severe
Dosage Forms Tablet, film coated: 250 mg

Cheracol® *see* Guaifenesin and Codeine *on page 516*

Cheracol D® [OTC] *see* Guaifenesin and Dextromethorphan *on page 517*

Chibroxin™ *see* Norfloxacin *on page 806*

Chicken Pox Vaccine *see* Varicella Virus Vaccine *on page 1147*

Chigger-Tox® [OTC] *see* Benzocaine *on page 121*

Children's Hold® [OTC] *see* Dextromethorphan *on page 321*

Children's Kaopectate® [OTC] *see* Attapulgite *on page 102*

Children's Vitamins *see* Vitamin, Multiple *on page 1166*

Chlo-Amine® [OTC] *see* Chlorpheniramine Maleate *on page 229*

Chloral *see* Chloral Hydrate *on this page*

Chloral Hydrate (klor al hye' drate)
Brand Names Aquachloral® Supprettes®; Noctec®; Somnos®
Synonyms Chloral; Hydrated Chloral; Trichloroacetaldehyde Monohydrate
Use Short-term sedative and hypnotic (<2 weeks), sedative/hypnotic for dental and diagnostic procedures; sedative prior to EEG evaluations
Restrictions C-IV
Pregnancy Risk Factor C
Contraindications Hypersensitivity to chloral hydrate or any component; hepatic or renal impairment; gastritis or ulcers; severe cardiac disease
Warnings/Precautions Use with caution in patients with porphyria; use with caution in neonates, drug may accumulate with repeated use, prolonged use in neonates associated with hyperbilirubinemia; tolerance to hypnotic effect develops, therefore, not recommended for use >2 weeks; taper dosage to avoid withdrawal with prolonged use; trichloroethanol (TCE), a metabolite of chloral hydrate, is a carcinogen in mice; there is no data in humans. Chloral hydrate is considered a second line hypnotic agent in the elderly. Recent interpretive guidelines from the Health Care Financing Administration (HCFA) discourage the use of chloral hydrate in residents of long-term care facilities.
Adverse Reactions
>10%: Gastrointestinal: Gastric irritation, nausea, vomiting, diarrhea
1% to 10%:
Central nervous system: Clumsiness, hallucinations, drowsiness, "hangover" effect
Dermatologic: Rash, urticaria
<1%:
Central nervous system: Disorientation, sedation, ataxia, excitement (paradoxical), dizziness, fever, headache, confusion
Gastrointestinal: Gastric irritation, flatulence
Hematologic: Leukopenia, eosinophilia
Miscellaneous: Physical and psychological dependence may occur with prolonged use of large doses
Overdosage/Toxicology Symptoms of overdose include hypotension, respiratory depression, coma, hypothermia, cardiac arrhythmias; treatment is supportive and symptomatic; lidocaine or propranolol may be used for ventricular dysrhythmias, while isoproterenol or atropine may be required for torsade de pointes; activated charcoal may prevent drug absorption
Drug Interactions Increased toxicity: May potentiate effects of warfarin, central nervous system depressants, alcohol; vasodilation reaction (flushing, tachycardia, etc) may occur with concurrent use of alcohol; concomitant use of furosemide (I.V.) may result in flushing, diaphoresis, and blood pressure changes
Stability Sensitive to light; exposure to air causes volatilization; store in light-resistant, airtight container
Mechanism of Action Central nervous system depressant effects are due to its active metabolite trichloroethanol, mechanism unknown
Pharmacodynamics/Kinetics
Peak effect: Within 0.5-1 hour
Duration: 4-8 hours
Absorption: Oral, rectal: Well absorbed
Distribution: Crosses the placenta; negligible amounts appear in breast milk
Metabolism: Rapidly to trichloroethanol (active metabolite); variable amounts metabolized in liver and kidney to trichloroacetic acid (inactive)
Half-life: Active metabolite: 8-11 hours
(Continued)

Chloral Hydrate *(Continued)*

Elimination: Metabolites excreted in urine, small amounts excreted in feces via bile

Usual Dosage

Neonates: Oral, rectal: 25 mg/kg/dose for sedation prior to a procedure or 50 mg/kg as hypnotic

Children:

Sedation, anxiety: Oral, rectal: 5-15 mg/kg/dose every 8 hours, maximum: 500 mg/dose

Prior to EEG: Oral, rectal: 20-25 mg/kg/dose, 30-60 minutes prior to EEG; may repeat in 30 minutes to maximum of 100 mg/kg or 2 g total

Hypnotic: Oral, rectal: 20-40 mg/kg/dose up to a maximum of 50 mg/kg/24 hours or 1 g/dose or 2 g/24 hours

Sedation, nonpainful procedure: Oral: 50-75 mg/kg/dose 30-60 minutes prior to procedure; may repeat 30 minutes after initial dose if needed, to a total maximum dose of 120 mg/kg or 1 g total

Adults: Oral, rectal:

Sedation, anxiety: 250 mg 3 times/day

Hypnotic: 500-1000 mg at bedtime or 30 minutes prior to procedure, not to exceed 2 g/24 hours

Dosing adjustment/comments in renal impairment: Cl_{cr} <50 mL/minute: Avoid use

Hemodialysis effects: Supplemental dose is not necessary; dialyzable (50% to 100%)

Dosing adjustment/comments in hepatic impairment: Avoid use in patients with severe hepatic impairment

Administration Do not crush capsule, contains drug in liquid form

Monitoring Parameters Vital signs, O_2 saturation and blood pressure with doses used for conscious sedation

Test Interactions False-positive urine glucose using Clinitest® method; may interfere with fluorometric urine catecholamine and urinary 17-hydroxycorticosteroid tests

Patient Information Take a capsule with a full glass of water or fruit juice; swallow capsules whole, do not chew; avoid alcohol and other CNS depressants; avoid activities needing good psychomotor coordination until CNS effects are known; drug may cause physical or psychological dependence; avoid abrupt discontinuation after prolonged use; if taking at home prior to a diagnostic procedure, have someone else transport

Nursing Implications Gastric irritation may be minimized by diluting dose in water or other oral liquid

Dosage Forms

Capsule: 250 mg, 500 mg

Suppository, rectal: 324 mg, 500 mg, 648 mg

Syrup: 250 mg/5 mL (10 mL); 500 mg/5 mL (5 mL, 10 mL, 480 mL)

Chlorambucil *(klor am′ byoo sil)*

Related Information

Cancer Chemotherapy Regimens on page 1218-1241

Brand Names Leukeran®

Use Management of chronic lymphocytic leukemia, Hodgkin's and non-Hodgkin's lymphoma; breast and ovarian carcinoma; Waldenström's macroglobulinemia, testicular carcinoma, thrombocythemia, choriocarcinoma

Pregnancy Risk Factor D

Pregnancy/Breast Feeding Implications Carcinogenic and mutagenic in humans

Contraindications Previous resistance; hypersensitivity to chlorambucil or any component or other alkylating agents

Warnings/Precautions The U.S. Food and Drug Administration (FDA) currently recommends that procedures for proper handling and disposal of antineoplastic agents be considered. Use with caution in patients with seizure disorder and bone marrow suppression; reduce initial dosage if patient has received radiation therapy, myelosuppressive drugs or has a depressed baseline leukocyte or platelet count within the previous 4 weeks. Can severely suppress bone marrow function; affects human fertility; carcinogenic in humans and probably mutagenic and teratogenic as well; chromosomal damage has been documented; secondary AML may be associated with chronic therapy.

Adverse Reactions

>10%: Myelosuppressive: Use with caution when receiving radiation; bone marrow suppression frequently occurs and occasionally bone marrow failure

has occurred; blood counts should be monitored closely while undergoing treatment; leukopenia, thrombocytopenia, anemia

WBC: Moderate

Platelets: Moderate

Onset (days): 7

Nadir (days): 10-14

Recovery (days): 28

1% to 10%:

Dermatologic: Skin rashes

Emetic potential: Low (<10%)

Endocrinological: Menstrual changes, hyperuricemia

Gastrointestinal: Nausea, vomiting, diarrhea, oral ulceration are all infrequent

<1%:

Central nervous system: Confusion, agitation, ataxia, hallucination; rarely generalized or focal seizures, weakness

Dermatologic: Rash, skin hypersensitivity, keratitis

Fertility impairment: Has caused chromosomal damage in man, oligospermia, both reversible and permanent sterility have occurred in both sexes; can produce amenorrhea in females and oligospermia in males

Gastrointestinal: Oral ulceration, hepatic necrosis

Hematologic: Leukopenia, thrombocytopenia

Neuromuscular & skeletal: Tremor, muscle twitching, peripheral neuropathy

Respiratory: Pulmonary fibrosis

Secondary malignancies: Increased incidence of AML

Miscellaneous: Drug fever

Overdosage/Toxicology Symptoms of overdose include vomiting, ataxia, coma, seizures, pancytopenia; there are no known antidotes for chlorambucil intoxication; treatment is mainly supportive, directed at decontaminating the GI tract and controlling symptoms; blood products may be used to treat the hematologic toxicity

Stability Protect from light

Mechanism of Action Interferes with DNA replication and RNA transcription by alkylation and cross-linking the strands of DNA

Pharmacodynamics/Kinetics

Absorption/bioavailability: 70% to 80%; **food will interfere with absorption** resulting in a 10% to 20% decrease in bioavailability

Distribution: V_d: 0.14-0.24 L/kg

Protein binding: ~99% bound to albumin; extensive binding to tissues and plasma proteins

Metabolism: In the liver to an active metabolite

Half-life: 90 minutes to 2 hours

Elimination: 60% excreted in urine within 24 hours, principally as metabolites

Usual Dosage Oral (refer to individual protocols):

Nephrotic syndrome: 0.1-0.2 mg/kg/day every day for 5-15 weeks with low-dose prednisone

Children: 0.1-0.2 mg/kg/day or 4-8 mg/m^2/day for 3-6 weeks for remission induction; maintenance therapy: 0.03-0.1 mg/kg/day

Adults: 0.1-0.2 mg/kg/day (4-8 mg/m^2/day) for 3-6 weeks, then adjust dose on basis of blood counts. Pulse dosing has been used in CLL as intermittent, biweekly, or monthly doses of 0.4 mg/kg and increased by 0.1 mg/kg until the disease is under control or toxicity ensues. An alternate regimen is 14 mg/m^2/day for 5 days, repeated every 21-28 days.

Probably not dialyzable

Monitoring Parameters Liver function tests, CBC, platelet count, serum uric acid

Patient Information Notify physician immediately if sore throat or bleeding occurs, contraceptive measures are recommended during therapy

Dosage Forms Tablet, sugar coated: 2 mg

Chloramphenicol (klor am fen' i kole)

Related Information

Antimicrobial Drugs of Choice *on page 1298-1302*

Brand Names AK-Chlor®; Chloromycetin®; Chloroptic®; Ophthochlor®

Use Treatment of serious infections due to organisms resistant to other less toxic antibiotics or when its penetrability into the site of infection is clinically superior to other antibiotics to which the organism is sensitive; useful in infections caused by *Bacteroides, H. influenzae, Neisseria meningitidis, Salmonella,* and *Rickettsia*

Pregnancy Risk Factor C

Contraindications Hypersensitivity to chloramphenicol or any component

Warnings/Precautions Use with caution in patients with impaired renal or hepatic function and in neonates; reduce dose with impaired liver function; use

(Continued)

219

Chloramphenicol *(Continued)*

with care in patients with glucose 6-phosphate dehydrogenase deficiency. Serious and fatal blood dyscrasias have occurred after both short-term and prolonged therapy; should not be used when less potentially toxic agents are effective; prolonged use may result in superinfection.

Adverse Reactions

<1%:

Central nervous system: Nightmares, headache

Dermatologic: Rash

Gastrointestinal: Diarrhea, stomatitis, enterocolitis, nausea, vomiting

Hematologic: Bone marrow depression, aplastic anemia

Neuromuscular & skeletal: Peripheral neuropathy

Ocular: Optic neuritis

Miscellaneous: Gray baby syndrome

Three (3) major toxicities associated with chloramphenicol include:

Aplastic anemia, an idiosyncratic reaction which can occur with any route of administration; usually occurs 3 weeks to 12 months after initial exposure to chloramphenicol

Bone marrow suppression is thought to be dose-related with serum concentrations >25 mcg/mL and reversible once chloramphenicol is discontinued; anemia and neutropenia may occur during the first week of therapy

Gray baby syndrome is characterized by circulatory collapse, cyanosis, acidosis, abdominal distention, myocardial depression, coma, and death; reaction appears to be associated with serum levels ≥50 mcg/mL; may result from drug accumulation in patients with impaired hepatic or renal function

Overdosage/Toxicology Symptoms of overdose include anemia, metabolic acidosis, hypotension, hypothermia; treatment is supportive following GI decontamination

Drug Interactions

Decreased effect: Phenobarbital and rifampin may decrease concentration of chloramphenicol

Increased toxicity: Chloramphenicol inhibits the metabolism of chlorpropamide, phenytoin, oral anticoagulants

Stability Refrigerate ophthalmic solution; constituted solutions remain stable for 30 days; use only clear solutions; frozen solutions remain stable for 6 months

Mechanism of Action Reversibly binds to 50S ribosomal subunits of susceptible organisms preventing amino acids from being transferred to growing peptide chains thus inhibiting protein synthesis

Pharmacodynamics/Kinetics

Absorption: Oral: 75% to 100%; in neonates, GI absorption of chloramphenicol palmitate is slow and erratic

Distribution: Readily crosses placenta; appears in breast milk; distributes to most tissues and body fluids

Relative diffusion of antimicrobial agents from blood into cerebrospinal fluid (CSF): Adequate with or without inflammation (exceeds usual MICs)

Ratio of CSF to blood level (%):

Normal meninges: 66

Inflamed meninges: 66+

Protein binding: 60%

Metabolism: Extensive in the liver (90%) to inactive metabolites, principally by glucuronidation, chloramphenicol palmitate is hydrolyzed by lipases in the GI tract to the active base; chloramphenicol sodium succinate is hydrolyzed by esterases to active base

Half-life: (Prolonged with markedly reduced liver function or combined liver/kidney dysfunction):

Normal renal function: 1.6-3.3 hours

End stage renal disease: 3-7 hours

Cirrhosis: 10-12 hours

Neonates: Postnatal:

1-2 days: 24 hours

10-16 days: 10 hours

Time to peak serum concentration: Oral: Within 0.5-3 hours

Elimination: 5% to 15% excreted as unchanged drug in the urine, 4% excreted in bile; in neonates, 6% to 80% may be excreted unchanged in urine

Usual Dosage

Neonates: Initial loading dose: Oral, I.V. (I.M. administration is not recommended):

Postnatal age 0-4 weeks:

<2000 g: 25 mg/kg/day every 24 hours

<7 days, >2000 g: 25 mg/kg/day every 24 hours

7-28 days, >2000 g: 25 mg/kg/dose every 12 hours

Meningitis: Oral, I.V.: Infants >30 days and Children: 75-100 mg/kg/day divided every 6 hours

Other infections: Oral, I.V.:

Infants and Children: 50-75 mg/kg/day divided every 6 hours; maximum daily dose: 4 g/day

Adults: 50-100 mg/kg/day in divided doses every 6 hours; maximum daily dose: 4 g/day

Ophthalmic: Children and Adults: Instill 1-2 drops or 1.25 cm (½" of ointment every 3-4 hours); increase interval between applications after 48 hours to 2-3 times/day

Otic solution: Instill 2-3 drops into ear 3 times/day

Topical: Gently rub into the affected area 1-4 times/day

Dosing adjustment/comments in hepatic impairment: Avoid use in severe liver impairment as increased toxicity may occur

Slightly dialyzable (5% to 20%) via hemo- and peritoneal dialysis; no supplemental doses needed in dialysis or continuous arterio-venous or veno-venous hemofiltration (CAVH/CAVHD)

Administration Administer around-the-clock rather than 4 times/day to promote less variation in peak and trough serum levels

Monitoring Parameters CBC with reticulocyte and platelet counts, periodic liver and renal function tests, serum drug concentration

Reference Range

Therapeutic levels: 15-20 µg/mL; Toxic concentration: >40 µg/mL; Trough: 5-10 µg/mL

Timing of serum samples: Draw levels 1.5 hours and 3 hours after completion of I.V. or oral dose; trough levels may be preferred; should be drawn ≤1 hour prior to dose

Test Interactions ↑ iron (B), prothrombin time (S); ↓ urea nitrogen (B)

Patient Information Take on empty stomach; take with food if GI upset occurs, at evenly spaced intervals (every 6 hours around-the-clock); notify physician if persistent sore throat, tiredness, or unusual bleeding or bruising

Additional Information Sodium content of 1 g (injection): 51.8 mg (2.25 mEq)

Dosage Forms

Capsule: 250 mg

Cream (Chloromycetin®): 1% (30 g)

Ointment, ophthalmic (AK-Chlor®, Chloromycetin®, Chloroptic®): 1% [10 mg/g] (3.5 g)

Powder for injection, as sodium succinate: 1 g

Powder for ophthalmic solution (Chloromycetin®): 25 mg/vial

Solution:

Ophthalmic (AK-Chlor®, Chloroptic®, Ophthochlor®): 0.5% [5 mg/mL] (2.5 mL, 7.5 mL, 15 mL)

Otic (Chloromycetin®): 0.5% (15 mL)

Chlorate® [OTC] *see* Chlorpheniramine Maleate *on page 229*

Chlordiazepoxide (klor dye az e pox' ide)

Related Information

Benzodiazepines Comparison *on page 1256*

Brand Names Libritabs®; Librium®; Mitran®; Reposans-10®

Synonyms Methaminodiazepoxide Hydrochloride

Use Approved for anxiety, may be useful for acute alcohol withdrawal symptoms

Restrictions C-IV

Pregnancy Risk Factor D

Contraindications Hypersensitivity to chlordiazepoxide or any component, preexisting CNS depression, severe uncontrolled pain

Warnings/Precautions Use with caution in patients with respiratory depression, CNS impairment, liver dysfunction, or a history of drug dependence

Adverse Reactions

>10%:

Cardiovascular: Chest pain

Central nervous system: Drowsiness, fatigue, impaired coordination, lightheadedness, memory impairment, insomnia, anxiety, depression, headache

Dermatologic: Skin eruptions, rash

Endocrine & metabolic: Decreased libido

Gastrointestinal: Nausea, constipation, vomiting, diarrhea, dry mouth, increased or decreased appetite

Neuromuscular & skeletal: Dysarthria

Ocular: Blurred vision

Miscellaneous: Decreased salivation, sweating

(Continued)

221

Chlordiazepoxide *(Continued)*

1% to 10%:
Cardiovascular: Hypotension, tachycardia, edema, syncope
Central nervous system: Drowsiness, ataxia, confusion, mental impairment, nervousness, dizziness, akathisia
Dermatologic: Dermatitis
Gastrointestinal: Nausea, vomiting, weight gain or loss
Neuromuscular & skeletal: Rigidity, tremor, muscle cramps
Ocular: Blurred vision
Otic: Tinnitus
Respiratory: Nasal congestion, hyperventilation
Miscellaneous: Increased salivation
<1%:
Endocrine & metabolic: Menstrual irregularities
Hematologic: Blood dyscrasias
Neuromuscular & skeletal: Depressed reflexes
Miscellaneous: Drug dependence

Overdosage/Toxicology Symptoms of overdose include hypotension, respiratory depression, coma, hypothermia, cardiac arrhythmias

Treatment for benzodiazepine overdose is supportive; rarely is mechanical ventilation required; flumazenil has been shown to selectively block the binding of benzodiazepines to CNS receptors, resulting in a reversal of benzodiazepine-induced CNS depression. Respiratory depression may not be reversed.

Drug Interactions Increased toxicity (CNS depression): Oral anticoagulants, alcohol, tricyclic antidepressants, sedative-hypnotics, MAO inhibitors

Stability Refrigerate injection; protect from light; **incompatible** when mixed with Ringer's solution, normal saline, ascorbic acid, benzquinamide, heparin, phenytoin, promethazine, secobarbital

Pharmacodynamics/Kinetics

Distribution: V_d: 3.3 L/kg; crosses the placenta; appears in breast milk
Protein binding: 90% to 98%
Metabolism: Extensive in the liver to desmethyldiazepam (active and long-acting)
Half-life: 6.6-25 hours
End stage renal disease: 5-30 hours
Cirrhosis: 30-63 hours
Time to peak serum concentration:
Oral: Within 2 hours
I.M.: Results in lower peak plasma levels than oral
Elimination: Very little excretion in urine as unchanged drug

Usual Dosage

Children:
<6 years: Not recommended
>6 years: Anxiety: Oral, I.M.: 0.5 mg/kg/24 hours divided every 6-8 hours

Adults:
Anxiety:
Oral: 15-100 mg divided 3-4 times/day
I.M., I.V.: Initial: 50-100 mg followed by 25-50 mg 3-4 times/day as needed
Preoperative anxiety: I.M.: 50-100 mg prior to surgery
Alcohol withdrawal symptoms: Oral, I.V.: 50-100 mg to start, dose may be repeated in 2-4 hours as necessary to a maximum of 300 mg/24 hours

Dosing adjustment in renal impairment:
Cl_{cr} <10 mL/minute: Administer 50% of dose
Not dialyzable (0% to 5%)

Dosing adjustment/comments in hepatic impairment: Avoid use

Administration Up to 300 mg may be given I.M. or I.V. during a 6-hour period, but not more than this in any 24-hour period; do not use diluent provided with parenteral form for I.V. administration; dissolve with normal saline instead; I.V. form is a powder and should be reconstituted with 5 mL of sterile water or saline prior to administration

Monitoring Parameters Respiratory and cardiovascular status, mental status, check for orthostasis

Reference Range Therapeutic: 0.1-3 µg/mL (SI: 0-10 µmol/L); Toxic: >23 µg/mL (SI: >77 µmol/L)

Test Interactions ↓ HDL, ↑ triglycerides (S)

Patient Information Avoid alcohol and other CNS depressants; avoid activities needing good psychomotor coordination until CNS effects are known; drug may cause physical or psychological dependence; avoid abrupt discontinuation after prolonged use, may cause drowsiness, poor balance

Nursing Implications Raise bed rails; initiate safety measures; aid with ambulation

Dosage Forms
Capsule, as hydrochloride: 5 mg, 10 mg, 25 mg
Powder for injection, as hydrochloride: 100 mg
Tablet: 5 mg, 10 mg, 25 mg

Chlorhexidine Gluconate (klor hex' i deen)

Brand Names Dyna-Hex® [OTC]; Exidine® Scrub [OTC]; Hibiclens® [OTC]; Hibistat® [OTC]; Peridex®

Use Skin cleanser for surgical scrub, cleanser for skin wounds, germicidal hand rinse, and as antibacterial dental rinse. Chlorhexidine is active against gram-positive and gram-negative organisms, facultative anaerobes, aerobes, and yeast.

Pregnancy Risk Factor B

Contraindications Known hypersensitivity to chlorhexidine gluconate

Warnings/Precautions Staining of oral surfaces, teeth, restorations, and dorsum of tongue may occur; keep out of eyes and ears; for topical use only; there have been several case reports of anaphylaxis following disinfection with chlorhexidine

Adverse Reactions
>10%: Increase of tartar on teeth, changes in taste. Staining of oral surfaces (mucosa, teeth, dorsum of tongue) may be visible as soon as 1 week after therapy begins and is more pronounced when there is a heavy accumulation of unremoved plaque and when teeth fillings have rough surfaces. Stain does not have a clinically adverse effect but because removal may not be possible, patient with frontal restoration should be advised of the potential permanency of the stain.

1% to 10%: Tongue irritation, oral irritation

<1%:
Respiratory: Nasal congestion, shortness of breath
Miscellaneous: Swelling of face

Overdosage/Toxicology Symptoms of oral overdose include gastric distress, nausea, or signs of alcohol intoxication

Mechanism of Action The bactericidal effect of chlorhexidine is a result of the binding of this cationic molecule to negatively charged bacterial cell walls and extramicrobial complexes. At low concentrations, this causes an alteration of bacterial cell osmotic equilibrium and leakage of potassium and phosphorous resulting in a bacteriostatic effect. At high concentrations of chlorhexidine, the cytoplasmic contents of the bacterial cell precipitate and result in cell death.

Pharmacodynamics/Kinetics
Absorption: ~30% of chlorhexidine is retained in the oral cavity following rinsing and is slowly released into the oral fluids; chlorhexidine is poorly absorbed from the GI tract
Serum concentrations: Detectable levels are not present in the plasma 12 hours after administration
Elimination: Primarily through the feces (approximately 90%); <1% excreted in the urine

Usual Dosage
Oral rinse (Peridex®):
Precede use of solution by flossing and brushing teeth, completely rinse toothpaste from mouth; swish 15 mL undiluted oral rinse around in mouth for 30 seconds, then expectorate. Caution patient not to swallow the medicine; avoid eating for 2-3 hours after treatment. (The cap on bottle of oral rinse is a measure for 15 mL.)
When used as a treatment of gingivitis, the regimen begins with oral prophylaxis. Patient treats mouth with 15 mL chlorhexidine; swish for 30 seconds, then expectorate. This is repeated twice daily (morning and evening). Patient should have a re-evaluation followed by a dental prophylaxis every 6 months.

Cleanser:
Surgical scrub: Scrub 3 minutes and rinse thoroughly, wash for an additional 3 minutes
Hand wash: Wash for 15 seconds and rinse
Hand rinse: Rub 15 seconds and rinse

Patient Information
Oral rinse: Do not swallow, do not rinse after use; may cause reduced taste perception which is reversible; may cause discoloration of teeth
Topical administration is for external use only

Dosage Forms
Rinse:
Oral (mint flavor) (Peridex®): 0.12% with alcohol 11.6% (480 mL)
(Continued)

223

Chlorhexidine Gluconate *(Continued)*

Topical (Hibistat® Hand Rinse): 0.5% with isopropyl alcohol 70% (120 mL, 240 mL)

Topical, Liquid with isopropyl alcohol 4%:
Skin cleanser (Dyna-Hex®, Exidine®, Hibiclens®): 2% (120 mL, 240 mL, 480 mL, 960 mL, 960 mL); 4% (15 mL, 120 mL, 240 mL, 480 mL, 4000 mL)
Sponge/brush (Hibiclens®): 4% with isopropyl alcohol 4% (22 mL)
Wipes (Hibistat®): 0.5%

2-Chlorodeoxyadenosine *see* Cladribine *on page 251*

Chlorofon-F® *see* Chlorzoxazone *on page 236*

Chloromycetin® *see* Chloramphenicol *on page 219*

Chloroprocaine Hydrochloride *(klor oh proe' kane)*

Brand Names Nesacaine®; Nesacaine®-MPF

Use Infiltration anesthesia and peripheral and epidural anesthesia

Pregnancy Risk Factor C

Contraindications Known hypersensitivity to chloroprocaine, or other ester type anesthetics; myasthenia gravis; concurrent use of bupivacaine; do not use for subarachnoid administration

Warnings/Precautions Use with caution in patients with cardiac disease, renal disease, and hyperthyroidism; convulsions and cardiac arrest have been reported presumably due to intravascular injection

Adverse Reactions

<1%:
Cardiovascular: Myocardial depression, hypotension, bradycardia, cardiovascular collapse, edema
Central nervous system: Anxiety, restlessness, disorientation, confusion, seizures, drowsiness, unconsciousness, chills, shivering
Dermatologic: Urticaria
Gastrointestinal: Nausea, vomiting
Local: Transient stinging or burning at injection site
Neuromuscular & skeletal: Tremor
Ocular: Blurred vision
Otic: Tinnitus
Respiratory: Respiratory arrest
Miscellaneous: Anaphylactoid reactions

Overdosage/Toxicology Treatment is primarily symptomatic and supportive. Termination of anesthesia by pneumatic tourniquet inflation should be attempted when the agent is administered by infiltration or regional injection. Hypotension responds to I.V. fluids and Trendelenburg positioning. Other symptoms (seizures, bradyarrhythmias, metabolic acidosis, methemoglobinemia) respond to conventional treatments.

Mechanism of Action Chloroprocaine HCl is benzoic acid, 4-amino-2-chloro-2-(diethylamino) ethyl ester monohydrochloride. Chloroprocaine is an ester-type local anesthetic, which stabilizes the neuronal membranes and prevents initiation and transmission of nerve impulses thereby affecting local anesthetic actions. Local anesthetics including chloroprocaine, reversibly prevent generation and conduction of electrical impulses in neurons by decreasing the transient increase in permeability to sodium. The differential sensitivity generally depends on the size of the fiber; small fibers are more sensitive than larger fibers and require a longer period for recovery. Sensory pain fibers are usually blocked first, followed by fibers that transmit sensations of temperature, touch, and deep pressure. High concentrations block sympathetic somatic sensory and somatic motor fibers. The spread of anesthesia depends upon the distribution of the solution. This is primarily dependent on the volume of drug injected.

Usual Dosage Dosage varies with anesthetic procedure, the area to be anesthetized, the vascularity of the tissues, depth of anesthesia required, degree of muscle relaxation required, and duration of anesthesia; range: 1.5-25 mL of 2% to 3% solution; single adult dose should not exceed 800 mg
Infiltration and peripheral nerve block: 1% to 2%
Infiltration, peripheral and central nerve block, including caudal and epidural block: 2% to 3%, without preservatives

Administration Before injecting, withdraw syringe plunger to ensure injection is not into vein or artery

Nursing Implications Must have resuscitative equipment available

Dosage Forms Injection:
Preservative free (Nesacaine®-MPF): 2% (30 mL); 3% (30 mL)
With preservative (Nesacaine®): 1% (30 mL); 2% (30 mL)

Chloroptic® *see* Chloramphenicol *on page 219*

Chloroquine and Primaquine (klor' oh kwin)

Brand Names Aralen® Phosphate With Primaquine Phosphate

Synonyms Primaquine and Chloroquine

Use Prophylaxis of malaria, regardless of species, in all areas where the disease is endemic

Pregnancy Risk Factor C

Contraindications Retinal or visual field changes, known hypersensitivity to chloroquine or primaquine

Warnings/Precautions Use with caution in patients with psoriasis, porphyria, hepatic dysfunction, G-6-PD deficiency

Adverse Reactions

1% to 10%: Gastrointestinal: Diarrhea, nausea

<1%:

Cardiovascular: Hypotension, EKG changes

Central nervous system: Fatigue, personality changes, headache

Dermatologic: Pruritus, hair bleaching

Gastrointestinal: Anorexia, vomiting, stomatitis

Hematologic: Blood dyscrasias

Ocular: Retinopathy, blurred vision

Overdosage/Toxicology Symptoms of overdose include headache, visual changes, cardiovascular collapse, seizures, abdominal cramps, vomiting, cyanosis, methemoglobinemia, leukopenia, respiratory and cardiac arrest; following initial measures (immediate GI decontamination), treatment is supportive and symptomatic

Drug Interactions

Decreased absorption if administered concomitantly with kaolin and magnesium trisilicate

Increased toxicity/levels with cimetidine

Mechanism of Action Chloroquine concentrates within parasite acid vesicles and raises internal pH resulting in inhibition of parasite growth; may involve aggregates of ferriprotoporphyrin IX acting as chloroquine receptors causing membrane damage; may also interfere with nucleoprotein synthesis. Primaquine eliminates the primary tissue exoerythrocytic forms of *P. falciparum*; disrupts mitochondria and binds to DNA

Pharmacodynamics/Kinetics

Absorption: Oral: Both drugs are readily absorbed

Distribution: Concentrated in liver, spleen, kidney, heart, and brain

Protein binding: ~55%; binds strongly to melanin

Metabolism: 25% of chloroquine is metabolized

Elimination: Drug may remain in tissue for 3-5 days; up to 70% excreted unchanged

Usual Dosage Oral: Start at least 1 day before entering the endemic area; continue for 8 weeks after leaving the endemic area

Children: For suggested weekly dosage (based on body weight), see table:

Weight		Chloroquine Base (mg)	Primaquine Base (mg)	Dose* (mL)
lb	kg			
10-15	4.5-6.8	20	3	2.5
16-25	7.3-11.4	40	6	5
26-35	11.8-15.9	60	9	7.5
36-45	16.4-20.5	80	12	10
46-55	20.9-25	100	15	12.5
56-100	25.4-45.4	150	22.5	½ tablet
100+	>45.4	300	45	1 tablet

*Dose based on liquid containing approximately 40 mg of chloroquine base and 6 mg primaquine base per 5 mL, prepared from chloroquine phosphate with primaquine phosphate tablets.

Adults: 1 tablet/week on the same day each week

Monitoring Parameters Periodic CBC, examination for muscular weakness, and ophthalmologic examination in patients receiving prolonged therapy

Patient Information Take with meals; report any visual disturbances or difficulty in hearing or ringing in the ears; tablets are bitter tasting; may cause diarrhea, loss of appetite, nausea, stomach pain; notify physician if these become severe

Dosage Forms Tablet: Chloroquine phosphate 500 mg [base 300 mg] and primaquine phosphate 79 mg [base 45 mg]

Chloroquine Phosphate (klor' oh kwin)

Related Information

Prevention of Malaria *on page 1405*

Brand Names Aralen® Phosphate

Use Suppression or chemoprophylaxis of malaria; treatment of uncomplicated or mild-moderate malaria; extraintestinal amebiasis; rheumatoid arthritis; discoid lupus erythematosus, scleroderma, pemphigus

Pregnancy Risk Factor C

Contraindications Retinal or visual field changes; patients with psoriasis; known hypersensitivity to chloroquine

Warnings/Precautions Use with caution in patients with liver disease, G-6-PD deficiency, alcoholism or in conjunction with hepatotoxic drugs, psoriasis, porphyria

Adverse Reactions

1% to 10%: Gastrointestinal: Nausea, diarrhea

<1%:

Cardiovascular: Hypotension, EKG changes

Central nervous system: Fatigue, personality changes, headache

Dermatologic: Pruritus, hair bleaching

Gastrointestinal: Anorexia, vomiting, stomatitis

Hematologic: Blood dyscrasias

Ocular: Retinopathy, blurred vision

Overdosage/Toxicology Symptoms of overdose include headache, visual changes, cardiovascular collapse, seizures, abdominal cramps, vomiting, cyanosis, methemoglobinemia, leukopenia, respiratory and cardiac arrest; following initial measures (immediate GI decontamination), treatment is supportive and symptomatic

Drug Interactions

Decreased absorption if administered concomitantly with kaolin and magnesium trisilicate

Increased toxicity/levels with cimetidine

Mechanism of Action Binds to and inhibits DNA and RNA polymerase; interferes with metabolism and hemoglobin utilization by parasites; inhibits prostaglandin effects; chloroquine concentrates within parasite acid vesicles and raises internal pH resulting in inhibition of parasite growth; may involve aggregates of ferriprotoporphyrin IX acting as chloroquine receptors causing membrane damage; may also interfere with nucleoprotein synthesis

Pharmacodynamics/Kinetics

Absorption: Oral: Rapid (~89%)

Distribution: Widely distributed in body tissues such as eyes, heart, kidneys, liver, and lungs where retention is prolonged; crosses the placenta; appears in breast milk

Metabolism: Partial hepatic metabolism occurs

Half-life: 3-5 days

Time to peak serum concentration: Within 1-2 hours

Elimination: ~70% excreted unchanged in urine; acidification of the urine increases elimination of drug; small amounts of drug may be present in urine months following discontinuation of therapy

Usual Dosage Oral (**dosage expressed in terms of mg of base**):

Suppression or prophylaxis of malaria:

Children: Administer 5 mg base/kg/week on the same day each week (not to exceed 300 mg base/dose); begin 1-2 weeks prior to exposure; continue for 4-6 weeks after leaving endemic area; if suppressive therapy is not begun prior to exposure, double the initial loading dose to 10 mg base/kg and give in 2 divided doses 6 hours apart, followed by the usual dosage regimen

Adults: 300 mg/week (base) on the same day each week; begin 1-2 weeks prior to exposure; continue for 4-6 weeks after leaving endemic area; if suppressive therapy is not begun prior to exposure, double the initial loading dose to 600 mg base and give in 2 divided doses 6 hours apart, followed by the usual dosage regimen

Acute attack:

Children: 10 mg/kg on day 1, followed by 5 mg/kg 6 hours later and 5 mg/kg on days 2 and 3

Adults: 600 mg on day 1, followed by 300 mg 6 hours later, followed by 300 mg on days 2 and 3

Extraintestinal amebiasis:

Children: 10 mg/kg once daily for 2-3 weeks (up to 300 mg base/day)

Adults: 600 mg base/day for 2 days followed by 300 mg base/day for at least 2-3 weeks

Dosing adjustment in renal impairment: Cl_{cr} <10 mL/minute: Administer 50% of dose

Minimally removed by hemodialysis

Monitoring Parameters Periodic CBC, examination for muscular weakness, and ophthalmologic examination in patients receiving prolonged therapy

Patient Information Take with meals; report any visual disturbances or difficulty in hearing or ringing in the ears; tablets are bitter tasting; may cause diarrhea, loss of appetite, nausea, stomach pain; notify physician if these become severe

Dosage Forms Tablet: 250 mg [150 mg base]; 500 mg [300 mg base]

Chlorothiazide (klor oh thye' a zide)

Brand Names Diurigen®; Diuril®

Use Management of mild to moderate hypertension, or edema associated with congestive heart failure, pregnancy, or nephrotic syndrome in patients unable to take oral hydrochlorothiazide, when a thiazide is the diuretic of choice

Pregnancy Risk Factor D

Contraindications Hypersensitivity to chlorothiazide or any component; cross-sensitivity with other thiazides or sulfonamides; do not use in anuric patients.

Warnings/Precautions Injection must not be administered S.C. or I.M.; may cause hyperbilirubinemia, hypokalemia, alkalosis, chlorothiazide is minimally effective in patients with a Cl_{cr} <40 mL/minute; this may limit the usefulness of chlorothiazide in the elderly

Adverse Reactions

1% to 10%: Endocrine & metabolic: Hypokalemia, hyponatremia

<1%:

Cardiovascular: Irregular heartbeat, weak pulse, orthostatic hypotension

Central nervous system: Dizziness, vertigo, headache, fever

Dermatologic: Rash, photosensitivity

Endocrine & metabolic: Hypochloremic alkalosis, hyperglycemia, hyperlipidemia, hyperuricemia

Hematologic: Rarely blood dyscrasias, leukopenia, agranulocytosis, aplastic anemia

Neuromuscular & skeletal: Paresthesias

Renal: Prerenal azotemia

Overdosage/Toxicology Symptoms of overdose include hypermotility, diuresis, lethargy, confusion, muscle weakness, coma; following GI decontamination, therapy is supportive with I.V. fluids, electrolytes, and I.V. pressors if needed

Drug Interactions

Decreased effect: NSAIDs + chlorothiazide → decreased antihypertensive effect; decreased absorption of thiazides with cholestyramine resins; chlorothiazide causes a decreased effect of oral hypoglycemics

Increased toxicity: Digitalis glycosides, lithium (decreased clearance), probenecid

Stability Reconstituted solution is stable for 24 hours at room temperature; precipitation will occur in <24 hours in pH <7.4

Mechanism of Action Inhibits sodium reabsorption in the distal tubules causing increased excretion of sodium and water as well as potassium and hydrogen ions, magnesium, phosphate, calcium

Pharmacodynamics/Kinetics

Absorption: Oral: Poor

Onset of diuresis: Oral: 2 hours

Duration of diuretic action:

Oral: 6-12 hours

I.V.: ~2 hours

Half-life: 1-2 hours

Time to peak serum concentration: Within 4 hours

Usual Dosage I.V. form not recommended for children and should only be used in adults if unable to take oral in emergency situations:

Infants <6 months:

Oral: 20-40 mg/kg/day in 2 divided doses

I.V.: 2-8 mg/kg/day in 2 divided doses

Infants >6 months and Children:

Oral: 20 mg/kg/day in 2 divided doses

I.V.: 4 mg/kg/day

Adults:

Oral: 500 mg to 2 g/day divided in 1-2 doses

I.V.: 100-500 mg/day

Elderly: Oral: 500 mg once daily **or** 1 g 3 times/week

Administration Injection must **not** be administered S.C. or I.M.

Monitoring Parameters Serum electrolytes, renal function, blood pressure; assess weight, I & O reports daily to determine fluid loss

(Continued)

Chlorothiazide *(Continued)*

Test Interactions ↑ creatine phosphokinase [CPK] (S), ammonia (B), amylase (S), calcium (S), chloride (S), cholesterol (S), glucose, ↑ acid (S), ↓ chloride (S), magnesium, potassium (S), sodium (S)

Patient Information Shake well; may be taken with food or milk; take early in day to avoid nocturia; take the last dose of multiple doses no later than 6 PM unless instructed otherwise; to avoid photosensitivity, use sun block SPF ≥15 on exposed skin areas

Nursing Implications Take blood pressure with patient lying down and standing; avoid extravasation of parenteral solution since it is extremely irritating to tissues

Additional Information Sodium content of injection, 500 mg: 57.5 mg (2 mEq)

Dosage Forms
Powder for injection, lyophilized, as sodium: 500 mg
Suspension, oral: 250 mg/5 mL (237 mL)
Tablet: 250 mg, 500 mg

Chlorotrianisene *(klor oh trye an' i seen)*

Brand Names TACE®

Use Treat inoperable prostatic cancer; management of atrophic vaginitis, female hypogonadism, vasomotor symptoms of menopause

Pregnancy Risk Factor X

Contraindications Thrombophlebitis, breast cancer, undiagnosed abnormal vaginal bleeding, known or suspected pregnancy

Warnings/Precautions Estrogens have been reported to increase the risk of endometrial carcinoma; do not use estrogens during pregnancy

Adverse Reactions
>10%:
Endocrine & metabolic: Peripheral edema, enlargement of breasts (female and male), breast tenderness
Gastrointestinal: Nausea, anorexia, bloating
1% to 10%:
Central nervous system: Headache
Endocrine & metabolic: Increased libido (female), decreased libido (male)
Gastrointestinal: Vomiting, diarrhea
<1%:
Cardiovascular: Hypertension, thromboembolism, stroke, myocardial infarction, edema
Central nervous system: Depression, dizziness, anxiety
Dermatologic: Chloasma, melasma, rash
Endocrine & metabolic: Breast tumors, amenorrhea, alterations in frequency and flow of menses, decreased glucose tolerance, increased triglycerides and LDL
Gastrointestinal: Nausea, GI distress
Hepatic: Cholestatic jaundice
Ocular: Intolerance to contact lenses
Miscellaneous: Increased susceptibility to *Candida* infection

Overdosage/Toxicology Serious adverse effects have not been reported following ingestion of large doses of estrogen-containing oral contraceptives; overdosage of estrogen may cause nausea; withdrawal bleeding may occur in females

Mechanism of Action Diethylstilbestrol derivative with similar estrogenic actions

Pharmacodynamics/Kinetics
Onset of therapeutic effect: Commonly occurs within 14 days of therapy
Distribution: Stored in fat tissues and slowly released
Metabolism: In the liver to a more potent estrogen compound

Usual Dosage Adults: Oral:
Atrophic vaginitis: 12-25 mg/day in 28-day cycles (21 days on and 7 days off)
Female hypogonadism: 12-25 mg cyclically for 21 days. May be followed by I.M. progesterone 100 mg or 5 days of oral progestin; next course may begin on day 5 of induced uterine bleeding.
Postpartum breast engorgement: 12 mg 4 times/day for 7 days or 50 mg every 6 hours for 6 doses; give first dose within 8 hours after delivery
Vasomotor symptoms associated with menopause: 12-25 mg cyclically for 30 days; one or more courses may be prescribed
Prostatic cancer (inoperable/progressing): 12-25 mg/day

Patient Information Patients should inform their physicians if signs or symptoms of thromboembolic or thrombotic disorders including sudden severe headache or vomiting, disturbance of vision or speech, loss of vision, numbness or weakness in an extremity, sharp or crushing chest pain, calf pain, shortness of breath, severe abdominal pain or mass, mental depression or unusual bleeding.

Dosage Forms Capsule: 12 mg, 25 mg

Chlorphed®-LA Nasal Solution [OTC] *see* Oxymetazoline Hydrochloride *on page 829*

Chlorphed® [OTC] *see* Brompheniramine Maleate *on page 143*

Chlorpheniramine Maleate (klor fen ir' a meen)

Brand Names Aller-Chlor® [OTC]; AL-R® [OTC]; Chlo-Amine® [OTC]; Chlorate® [OTC]; Chlor-Pro® [OTC]; Chlor-Trimeton® [OTC]; Kloromin® [OTC]; Phenetron®; Telachlor®; Teldrin® [OTC]

Synonyms CTM

Use Perennial and seasonal allergic rhinitis and other allergic symptoms including urticaria

Pregnancy Risk Factor B

Contraindications Hypersensitivity to chlorpheniramine maleate or any component; narrow-angle glaucoma, bladder neck obstruction, symptomatic prostate hypertrophy, during acute asthmatic attacks, stenosing peptic ulcer, pyloroduodenal obstruction. Avoid use in premature and term newborns due to possible association with SIDS.

Warnings/Precautions Do not administer to premature or full-term neonates; young children may be more susceptible to side effects and CNS stimulation; bladder neck obstruction, symptomatic prostate hypertrophy, asthmatic attacks, and stenosing peptic ulcer; swallow whole, do not crush or chew sustained release tablets. Anticholinergic action may cause significant confusional symptoms.

Adverse Reactions
Genitourinary: Polyuria, urinary retention
Ocular: Diplopia

>10%:
Central nervous system: Slight to moderate drowsiness
Respiratory: Thickening of bronchial secretions
1% to 10%:
Central nervous system: Weakness, headache, excitability, fatigue, nervousness, dizziness
Gastrointestinal: Nausea, dry mouth, diarrhea, abdominal pain, appetite increase, weight increase
Neuromuscular & skeletal: Arthralgia
Respiratory: Pharyngitis
<1%:
Cardiovascular: Palpitations
Central nervous system: Depression
Dermatologic: Dermatitis, photosensitivity, angioedema
Hepatic: Hepatitis
Neuromuscular & skeletal: Myalgia, paresthesia
Respiratory: Bronchospasm
Miscellaneous: Epistaxis

Overdosage/Toxicology Symptoms of overdose include dry mouth, flushed skin, dilated pupils, CNS depression

There is no specific treatment for an antihistamine overdose, however, most of its clinical toxicity is due to anticholinergic effects. For anticholinergic overdose with severe life-threatening symptoms, physostigmine 1-2 mg (0.5 or 0.02 mg/kg for children) I.V., slowly may be given to reverse these effects.

Drug Interactions Increased toxicity (CNS depression): CNS depressants, MAO inhibitors, tricyclic antidepressants, phenothiazines

Stability Injectable form should be protected from light; **incompatible** when mixed in same syringe with calcium chloride, kanamycin, norepinephrine, pentobarbital

Mechanism of Action Competes with histamine for H_1-receptor sites on effector cells in the gastrointestinal tract, blood vessels, and respiratory tract

Pharmacodynamics/Kinetics
Protein binding: 69% to 72%
Metabolism: In the liver
Half-life: 20-24 hours
Elimination: Metabolites and parent drug (3% to 4%) excreted in urine, 35% of total within 48 hours

Usual Dosage
Children: Oral: 0.35 mg/kg/day in divided doses every 4-6 hours
2-6 years: 1 mg every 4-6 hours, not to exceed 6 mg in 24 hours
6-12 years: 2 mg every 4-6 hours, not to exceed 12 mg/day or sustained release 8 mg at bedtime
(Continued)

229

Chlorpheniramine Maleate *(Continued)*

Children >12 years and Adults: Oral: 4 mg every 4-6 hours, not to exceed 24 mg/day or sustained release 8-12 mg every 8-12 hours, not to exceed 24 mg/day

Adults: Allergic reactions: I.M., I.V., S.C.: 10-20 mg as a single dose; maximum recommended dose: 40 mg/24 hours

Elderly: 4 mg once or twice daily. **Note:** Duration of action may be 36 hours or more when serum concentrations are low.

Hemodialysis effects: Supplemental dose is not necessary

Patient Information May cause drowsiness; swallow whole, do not crush or chew sustained release product; avoid alcohol, may impair coordination and judgment

Nursing Implications Do not crush sustained release drug product; raise bed rails, institute safety measures, assist with ambulation

Dosage Forms

Capsule: 12 mg

Capsule, timed release: 8 mg, 12 mg

Injection: 10 mg/mL (1 mL, 30 mL); 100 mg/mL (2 mL)

Syrup: 2 mg/5 mL (120 mL, 473 mL)

Tablet: 4 mg, 8 mg, 12 mg

Tablet:

Chewable: 2 mg

Timed release: 8 mg, 12 mg

Chlorpromazine Hydrochloride *(klor proe' ma zeen)*

Related Information

Antipsychotic Agents Comparison *on page 1255*

Brand Names Ormazine; Thorazine®

Use Treatment of nausea and vomiting; psychoses; Tourette's syndrome; mania; intractable hiccups (adults); behavioral problems (children)

Pregnancy Risk Factor C

Contraindications Hypersensitivity to chlorpromazine hydrochloride or any component; cross-sensitivity with other phenothiazines may exist; avoid use in patients with narrow-angle glaucoma

Warnings/Precautions Safety in children <6 months of age has not been established; use with caution in patients with seizures, bone marrow depression, or severe liver disease

Significant hypotension may occur, especially when the drug is administered parenterally; injection contains benzyl alcohol; injection also contains sulfites which may cause allergic reaction

Tardive dyskinesia: Prevalence rate may be 40% in elderly; development of the syndrome and the irreversible nature are proportional to duration and total cumulative dose over time. May be reversible if diagnosed early in therapy.

Extrapyramidal reactions are more common in elderly with up to 50% developing these reactions after 60 years of age. Drug-induced **Parkinson's syndrome** occurs often. **Akathisia** is the most common extrapyramidal reaction in elderly.

Increased confusion, memory loss, psychotic behavior, and agitation frequently occur as a consequence of anticholinergic effects

Orthostatic hypotension is due to alpha-receptor blockade, the elderly are at greater risk for orthostatic hypotension

Antipsychotic associated sedation in nonpsychotic patients is extremely unpleasant due to feelings of depersonalization, derealization, and dysphoria

Life-threatening arrhythmias have occurred at therapeutic doses of antipsychotics

Adverse Reactions

>10%:

Cardiovascular: Hypotension (especially with I.V. use), tachycardia, arrhythmias, orthostatic hypotension

Central nervous system: Pseudoparkinsonism, akathisia, dystonias, tardive dyskinesia (persistent), dizziness,

Gastrointestinal: Constipation

Ocular: Pigmentary retinopathy

Respiratory: Nasal congestion

Miscellaneous: Decreased sweating

1% to 10%:

Central nervous system: Dizziness, trembling of fingers

Dermatologic: Pruritus, rash, increased sensitivity to sun

Endocrine & metabolic: Amenorrhea, galactorrhea, gynecomastia, changes in libido

Gastrointestinal: GI upset, nausea, vomiting, stomach pain, weight gain, dry mouth, constipation

Genitourinary: Difficulty in urination, ejaculatory disturbances, urinary retention
Ocular: Blurred vision
Miscellaneous: Pain in breasts
<1%:
Central nervous system: Sedation, drowsiness, restlessness, anxiety, extrapyramidal reactions, seizures, altered central temperature regulation, lowering of seizures threshold, neuroleptic malignant syndrome (NMS)
Dermatologic: Discoloration of skin (blue-gray), photosensitivity
Endocrine & metabolic: Galactorrhea
Genitourinary: Priapism
Hematologic: Agranulocytosis (more often in women between 4th and 10th weeks of therapy), leukopenia (usually in patients with large doses for prolonged periods)
Hepatic: Cholestatic jaundice, hepatotoxicity
Ocular: Cornea and lens changes, pigmentary retinopathy
Miscellaneous: Anaphylactoid reactions

Overdosage/Toxicology Symptoms of overdose include deep sleep, coma, extrapyramidal symptoms, abnormal involuntary muscle movements, hypotension

Following initiation of essential overdose management, toxic symptom treatment and supportive treatment should be initiated. Hypotension usually responds to I.V. fluids or Trendelenburg positioning. If unresponsive to these measures, the use of a parenteral inotrope may be required. Seizures commonly respond to diazepam (I.V. 5-10 mg bolus in adults every 15 minutes if needed up to a total of 30 mg; I.V. 0.25-0.4 mg/kg/dose up to a total of 10 mg in children) or to phenytoin or phenobarbital; critical cardiac arrhythmias often respond to I.V. phenytoin (15 mg/kg up to 1 g), while other antiarrhythmics can be used. Neuroleptics often cause extrapyramidal symptoms (eg, dystonic reactions) requiring management with benztropine mesylate I.V. 1-2 mg (adults) may be effective. These agents are generally effective within 2-5 minutes.

Drug Interactions Increased toxicity: Additive effects with other CNS-depressants; epinephrine (hypotension); may increase valproic acid serum concentrations

Stability Protect from light; a slightly yellowed solution does not indicate potency loss, but a markedly discolored solution should be discarded; diluted injection (1 mg/mL) with NS and stored in 5 mL vials remains stable for 30 days

Mechanism of Action Blocks postsynaptic mesolimbic dopaminergic receptors in the brain; exhibits a strong alpha-adrenergic blocking effect and depresses the release of hypothalamic and hypophyseal hormones; believed to depress the reticular-activating system, thus affecting basal metabolism, body temperature, wakefulness, vasomotor tone, and emesis

Pharmacodynamics/Kinetics
Distribution: Crosses the placenta; appears in breast milk
Metabolism: Extensively in the liver to active and inactive metabolites
Half-life, biphasic:
Initial: 2 hours
Terminal: 30 hours
Elimination: <1% excreted in urine as unchanged drug within 24 hours

Usual Dosage
Children >6 months:
Psychosis:
Oral: 0.5-1 mg/kg/dose every 4-6 hours; older children may require 200 mg/day or higher
I.M., I.V.: 0.5-1 mg/kg/dose every 6-8 hours; maximum dose for <5 years (22.7 kg): 40 mg/day; maximum for 5-12 years (22.7-45.5 kg): 75 mg/day
Nausea and vomiting:
Oral: 0.5-1 mg/kg/dose every 4-6 hours as needed
I.M., I.V.: 0.5-1 mg/kg/dose every 6-8 hours; maximum dose for <5 years (22.7 kg): 40 mg/day; maximum for 5-12 years (22.7-45.5 kg): 75 mg/day
Rectal: 1 mg/kg/dose every 6-8 hours as needed
Adults:
Psychosis:
Oral: Range: 30-800 mg/day in 1-4 divided doses, initiate at lower doses and titrate as needed; usual dose: 200 mg/day; some patients may require 1-2 g/day
I.M., I.V.: Initial: 25 mg, may repeat (25-50 mg) in 1-4 hours, gradually increase to a maximum of 400 mg/dose every 4-6 hours until patient is controlled; usual dose: 300-800 mg/day
Intractable hiccups: Oral, I.M.: 25-50 mg 3-4 times/day
Nausea and vomiting:
Oral: 10-25 mg every 4-6 hours
I.M., I.V.: 25-50 mg every 4-6 hours
Rectal: 50-100 mg every 6-8 hours
(Continued)

ALPHABETICAL LISTING OF DRUGS

Chlorpromazine Hydrochloride *(Continued)*

Elderly (nonpsychotic patient; dementia behavior): Initial: 10-25 mg 1-2 times/day; increase at 4- to 7-day intervals by 10-25 mg/day. Increase dose intervals (bid, tid, etc) as necessary to control behavior response or side effects; maximum daily dose: 800 mg; gradual increases (titration) may prevent some side effects or decrease their severity.

Not dialyzable (0% to 5%)

Dosing adjustment/comments in hepatic impairment: Avoid use in severe hepatic dysfunction

Administration Dilute oral concentrate solution in juice before administration

Monitoring Parameters Orthostatic blood pressures; tremors, gait changes, abnormal movement in trunk, neck, buccal area, or extremities; monitor target behaviors for which the agent is given; watch for hypotension when administering I.M. or I.V.

Reference Range
Therapeutic: 50-300 ng/mL (SI: 157-942 nmol/L)
Toxic: >750 ng/mL (SI: >2355 nmol/L); serum concentrations poorly correlate with expected response

Test Interactions False-positives for phenylketonuria, amylase, uroporphyrins, urobilinogen; may cause photosensitivity; avoid excessive sunlight; do not stop taking without consulting physician

Patient Information Do not stop taking unless informed by your physician; oral concentrate may be diluted in 2-4 oz of liquid (water, fruit juice, carbonated drinks, milk, or pudding); do not take antacid within 1 hour of taking drug; avoid alcohol; avoid excess sun exposure (use sun block); may cause drowsiness, rise slowly from recumbent position; use of supportive stockings may help prevent orthostatic hypotension

Nursing Implications Avoid contact of oral solution or injection with skin (contact dermatitis)

Dosage Forms
Capsule, sustained action: 30 mg, 75 mg, 150 mg, 200 mg, 300 mg
Concentrate, oral: 30 mg/mL (120 mL); 100 mg/mL (60 mL, 240 mL)
Injection: 25 mg/mL (1 mL, 2 mL, 10 mL)
Suppository, rectal, as base: 25 mg, 100 mg
Syrup: 10 mg/5 mL (120 mL)
Tablet: 10 mg, 25 mg, 50 mg, 100 mg, 200 mg

Chlorpropamide *(klor proe' pa mide)*

Related Information
Hypoglycemic Agents Comparison *on page 1271*

Brand Names Diabinese®

Use Control blood sugar in adult onset, noninsulin-dependent diabetes (type II)
Unlabeled use: Nephrogenic diabetes insipidus

Pregnancy Risk Factor C

Contraindications Cross-sensitivity may exist with other hypoglycemics or sulfonamides; do not use with type I diabetes, or with severe renal, hepatic, thyroid, or other endocrine disease, diabetes complicated by ketoacidosis; patients with reduced renal function, dietary noncompliance or irregular meals, alcohol abusers

Warnings/Precautions Patients should be properly instructed in the early detection and treatment of hypoglycemia; long half-life may complicate recovery from excess effects. Because of chlorpropamide's long half-life, duration of action, and the increased risk for hypoglycemia, it is not considered a hypoglycemic agent of choice in the elderly; see Pharmacodynamics/Kinetics

Adverse Reactions
>10%:
Central nervous system: Headache, dizziness
Gastrointestinal: Anorexia, constipation, heartburn, epigastric fullness, nausea, vomiting, diarrhea
1% to 10%: Dermatologic: Skin rash, hives, photosensitivity
<1%:
Cardiovascular: Edema
Endocrine & metabolic: Hypoglycemia, hyponatremia, SIADH
Hematologic: Blood dyscrasias, aplastic anemia, hemolytic anemia, bone marrow depression, thrombocytopenia, agranulocytosis
Hepatic: Cholestatic jaundice

Overdosage/Toxicology Symptoms of overdose include low blood glucose levels, tingling of lips and tongue, tachycardia, convulsions, stupor, coma. Antidote is glucose. Intoxications with sulfonylureas can cause hypoglycemia and are

232

best managed with glucose administration (oral for milder hypoglycemia or by injection in more severe forms); prolonged effects lasting up to 1 week may occur with this agent.

Drug Interactions

Decreased effect: Thiazides and hydantoins (eg, phenytoin) decrease chlorpropamide effectiveness → ↑ blood glucose

Increased toxicity:

Increased alcohol associated disulfiram reactions

Increased oral anticoagulant effects

Salicylates → ↑ chlorpropamide effects → ↓ blood glucose

Sulfonamides → ↓ sulfonylureas clearance

Mechanism of Action Stimulates insulin release from the pancreatic beta cells; reduces glucose output from the liver; insulin sensitivity is increased at peripheral target sites

Pharmacodynamics/Kinetics

Peak effect: Oral: Within 6-8 hours

Distribution: V_d: 0.13-0.23 L/kg; appears in breast milk

Protein binding: 60% to 90%

Metabolism: Extensive (~80%) in the liver; clearance decreased in older patients with diabetes

Half-life: 30-42 hours; prolonged in the elderly or with renal disease

End stage renal disease: 50-200 hours

Time to peak serum concentration: Within 3-4 hours

Elimination: 10% to 30% excreted in the urine as unchanged drug

Usual Dosage Oral: The dosage of chlorpropamide is variable and should be individualized based upon the patient's response

Initial dose:

Adults: 250 mg/day in mild to moderate diabetes in middle-aged, stable diabetic

Elderly: 100-125 mg/day in older patients

Maintenance dose: 100-250 mg/day; severe diabetics may require 500 mg/day; avoid doses >750 mg/day

Dosing adjustment/comments in renal impairment: Cl_{cr} <50 mL/minute: Avoid use

Peritoneal dialysis effects: Supplemental dose is not necessary

Dosing adjustment in hepatic impairment: Dosage reduction is recommended

Monitoring Parameters Fasting blood glucose, normal Hgb A_{1c} or fructosamine levels; monitor for signs and symptoms of hypoglycemia, (fatigue, sweating, numbness of extremities); monitor urine for glucose and ketones

Reference Range Fasting glucose:

Adults: 60-110 mg/dL

Elderly: 100-180 mg/dL

Patient Information Avoid alcohol; take at the same time each day; avoid hypoglycemia, eat regularly, do not skip meals; carry a quick source of sugar

Dosage Forms Tablet: 100 mg, 250 mg

Chlor-Pro® [OTC] *see* Chlorpheniramine Maleate *on page 229*

Chlorprothixene (klor proe thix' een)

Brand Names Taractan®

Use Management of psychotic disorders

Pregnancy Risk Factor C

Contraindications Circulatory collapse, hypersensitivity to chlorprothixene or any component, comatose states due to central depressant drugs

Warnings/Precautions Safety in children <6 months of age has not been established; use with caution in patients with cardiovascular disease or seizures; bone marrow depression, severe liver or cardiac disease; significant hypotension may occur, especially when the drug is administered parenterally; extended release capsules and injection contain benzyl alcohol; injection also contains sulfites which may cause allergic reaction

Adverse Reactions

>10%:

Cardiovascular: Hypotension, orthostatic hypotension

Central nervous system: Pseudoparkinsonism, akathisia, dystonias, tardive dyskinesia (persistent), dizziness

Gastrointestinal: Constipation

Ocular: Pigmentary retinopathy

Respiratory: Nasal congestion

Miscellaneous: Decreased sweating

(Continued)

Chlorprothixene *(Continued)*

1% to 10%:
Dermatologic: Increased sensitivity to sun, skin rash
Endocrine & metabolic: Changes in menstrual cycle, ejaculatory disturbances, changes in libido, pain in breasts
Gastrointestinal: Weight gain, nausea, vomiting, stomach pain
Genitourinary: Difficulty in urination
Neuromuscular & skeletal: Trembling of fingers

<1%:
Central nervous system: Neuroleptic malignant syndrome (NMS)
Dermatologic: discoloration of skin (blue-gray)
Endocrine & metabolic: Galactorrhea
Genitourinary: Priapism
Hematologic: Agranulocytosis, leukopenia
Hepatic: Cholestatic jaundice, hepatotoxicity
Ocular: Cornea and lens changes, pigmentary retinopathy
Miscellaneous: Impairment of temperature regulation lowering of seizures threshold

Overdosage/Toxicology Symptoms of overdose include deep sleep, coma, extrapyramidal symptoms, abnormal involuntary muscle movements, hypotension

Following initiation of essential overdose management, toxic symptom treatment and supportive treatment should be initiated. Hypotension usually responds to I.V. fluids or Trendelenburg positioning. If unresponsive to these measures, the use of a parenteral inotrope may be required. Seizures commonly respond to diazepam (I.V. 5-10 mg bolus in adults every 15 minutes if needed up to a total of 30 mg; I.V. 0.25-0.4 mg/kg/dose up to a total of 10 mg in children) or to phenytoin or phenobarbital; critical cardiac arrhythmias often respond to I.V. phenytoin (15 mg/kg up to 1 g), while other antiarrhythmics can be used. Neuroleptics often cause extrapyramidal symptoms (eg, dystonic reactions) requiring management with benztropine mesylate I.V. 1-2 mg (adults) may be effective. These agents are generally effective within 2-5 minutes.

Drug Interactions
Decreased effect of guanethidine
Increased effect/toxicity: Alcohol, CNS depressants

Mechanism of Action The mechanism of action for chlorprothixene, like other thioxanthenes and phenothiazines, is not fully understood. The sites of action appear to be the reticular activating system of the midbrain, the limbic system, the hypothalamus, and the globus pallidus and corpus striatum. The mechanism appears to be one or more of a combination of postsynaptic blockade of adrenergic, dopaminergic, or serotoninergic receptor sites, metabolic inhibition of oxidative phosphorylation, or decrease in the excitability of neuronal membranes.

Usual Dosage
Children >6 years: Oral: 10-25 mg 3-4 times/day

Adults:
Oral: 25-50 mg 3-4 times/day, to be increased as needed; doses exceeding 600 mg/day are rarely required
I.M.: 25-50 mg up to 3-4 times/day

Not dialyzable (0% to 5%)

Monitoring Parameters Monitor for reduction of psychotic symptoms
Test Interactions ↑ cholesterol (S), glucose; ↓ uric acid (S)
Patient Information May cause drowsiness; avoid alcohol
Dosage Forms
Concentrate, oral, as lactate and hydrochloride (fruit flavor): 100 mg/5 mL (480 mL)
Injection, as hydrochloride: 12.5 mg/mL (2 mL)
Tablet: 10 mg, 25 mg, 50 mg, 100 mg

Chlortetracycline Hydrochloride *(klor te tra sye' kleen)*

Brand Names Aureomycin®
Use
Ophthalmic: Treatment of superficial ocular infections involving the conjunctiva or cornea due to strains of susceptible microorganisms
Topical: Treatment of superficial infections of the skin due to susceptible organisms, also infection prophylaxis in minor skin abrasions

Pregnancy Risk Factor D
Contraindications Hypersensitivity to tetracycline or any component; do not use topical formulation in eyes

Warnings/Precautions Prolonged use may cause superinfection; ophthalmic ointments may retard corneal epithelial healing

Adverse Reactions
1% to 10%: Dermatologic: Faint yellowing of skin
<1%: Dermatologic: Redness, swelling, irritation, photosensitivity

Mechanism of Action Inhibits bacterial protein synthesis by binding with the 30S and possibly the 50S ribosomal subunit(s) of susceptible bacteria; may also cause alterations in the cytoplasmic membrane; usually bacteriostatic, may be bactericidal

Usual Dosage
Ophthalmic:
Acute infections: Instill ½" (1.25 cm) every 3-4 hours until improvement
Mild to moderate infections: Instill ½" (1.25 cm) 2-3 times/day

Topical: Apply 1-4 times/day, cover with sterile bandage if needed

Patient Information
For ophthalmic use, tilt head back, place medication in conjunctival sac and close eye, apply light finger pressure on lacrimal sac following instillation
Topical is for external use only, contact physician if rash or irritation develops, may stain clothing

Nursing Implications Cleanse affected area of skin prior to application unless otherwise directed

Dosage Forms Ointment:
Ophthalmic: 1% [10 mg/g] (3.5 g)
Topical: 3% (14.2 g, 30 g)

Chlorthalidone (klor thal' i done)

Brand Names Hygroton®; Thalitone®

Use Management of mild to moderate hypertension, used alone or in combination with other agents; treatment of edema associated with congestive heart failure, nephrotic syndrome, or pregnancy. Recent studies have found chlorthalidone effective in the treatment of isolated systolic hypertension in the elderly.

Pregnancy Risk Factor D

Contraindications Hypersensitivity to chlorthalidone or any component, cross-sensitivity with other thiazides or sulfonamides; do not use in anuric patients

Warnings/Precautions Use with caution in patients with hypokalemia, renal disease, hepatic disease, gout, lupus erythematosus, diabetes mellitus; use with caution in severe renal diseases

Adverse Reactions
1% to 10%: Endocrine & metabolic: Hypokalemia
<1%:
Cardiovascular: Hypotension
Dermatologic: Photosensitivity
Endocrine & metabolic: Fluid and electrolyte imbalances (hypocalcemia, hypomagnesemia, hyponatremia), hyperglycemia
Hematologic: Rarely blood dyscrasias
Renal: Prerenal azotemia

Overdosage/Toxicology Symptoms of overdose include hypermotility, diuresis, lethargy, confusion, muscle weakness, coma; following GI decontamination, therapy is supportive with I.V. fluids, electrolytes, and I.V. pressors if needed

Drug Interactions
Decreased effect: NSAIDs + chlorothiazide → decreased antihypertensive effect; decreased absorption of thiazides with cholestyramine resins; chlorothiazide causes a decreased effect of oral hypoglycemics
Increased toxicity: Digitalis glycosides, lithium (decreased clearance), probenecid
Increased effect: Furosemide and other loop diuretics

Mechanism of Action Sulfonamide-derived diuretic that inhibits sodium and chloride reabsorption in the cortical-diluting segment of the ascending loop of Henle

Pharmacodynamics/Kinetics
Peak effect: 2-6 hours
Absorption: Oral: 65%
Distribution: Crosses placenta; appears in breast milk
Metabolism: In the liver
Half-life: 35-55 hours; may be prolonged with renal impairment, with anuria: 81 hours
Elimination: ~50% to 65% excreted unchanged in urine

Usual Dosage Oral:
Children: 2 mg/kg/dose 3 times/week or 1-2 mg/kg/day
Adults: 25-100 mg/day or 100 mg 3 times/week
(Continued)

Chlorthalidone *(Continued)*

Elderly: Initial: 12.5-25 mg/day or every other day; there is little advantage to using doses >25 mg/day

Dosing interval in renal impairment: Cl$_{cr}$ <10 mL/minute: Administer every 48 hours

Monitoring Parameters Assess weight, I & O records daily to determine fluid loss; blood pressure, serum electrolytes, renal function

Test Interactions ↑ creatine phosphokinase [CPK] (S), ammonia (B), amylase (S), calcium (S), chloride (S), cholesterol (S), glucose, ↑ acid (S), ↓ chloride (S), magnesium, potassium (S), sodium (S)

Patient Information May be taken with food or milk; take early in day to avoid nocturia; take the last dose of multiple doses no later than 6 PM unless instructed otherwise; to avoid photosensitivity, use sun block SPF ≥15 on exposed skin areas

Nursing Implications Take blood pressure with patient lying down and standing

Dosage Forms
Tablet:
Hygroton®: 25 mg, 50 mg, 100 mg
Thalitone®: 15 mg, 25 mg

Chlor-Trimeton® [OTC] *see* Chlorpheniramine Maleate *on page 229*

Chlorzoxazone *(klor zox′ a zone)*

Brand Names Blanex®; Chlorofon-F®; Flexaphen®; Lobac®; Miflex®; Mus-Lac®; Paraflex®; Parafon Forte™ DSC; Pargen Fortified®; Polyflex®; Skelex®

Use Symptomatic treatment of muscle spasm and pain associated with acute musculoskeletal conditions

Pregnancy Risk Factor C

Contraindications Known hypersensitivity to chlorzoxazone; impaired liver function

Adverse Reactions
>10%: Central nervous system: Drowsiness
1% to 10%:
Cardiovascular: Tachycardia, tightness in chest, flushing of face
Central nervous system: Fainting, mental depression, allergic fever, dizziness, lightheadedness, headache, paradoxical stimulation
Dermatologic: Angioedema
Gastrointestinal: Nausea, vomiting, stomach cramps
Neuromuscular & skeletal: Trembling
Ocular: Burning of eyes
Respiratory: Shortness of breath
Miscellaneous: Hiccups
<1%:
Central nervous system: Clumsiness
Dermatologic: Skin rash, hives, erythema multiforme
Hematologic: Aplastic anemia, leukopenia, eosinophilia
Ocular: Blurred vision

Overdosage/Toxicology Symptoms of overdose include nausea, vomiting, diarrhea, drowsiness, dizziness, headache, absent tendon reflexes, hypotension

Treatment is supportive following attempts to enhance drug elimination. Hypotension should be treated with I.V. fluids and/or Trendelenburg positioning. Dialysis and hemoperfusion and osmotic diuresis have all been useful in reducing serum drug concentrations; patient should be observed for possible relapses due to incomplete gastric emptying.

Drug Interactions Increased effect/toxicity: Alcohol, CNS depressants

Mechanism of Action Acts on the spinal cord and subcortical levels by depressing polysynaptic reflexes

Pharmacodynamics/Kinetics
Onset of action: Within 1 hour
Absorption: Oral: Readily absorbed
Metabolism: Extensively in the liver by glucuronidation
Elimination: Excretion in urine as conjugates

Usual Dosage Oral:
Children: 20 mg/kg/day or 600 mg/m²/day in 3-4 divided doses
Adults: 250-500 mg 3-4 times/day up to 750 mg 3-4 times/day

Monitoring Parameters Periodic liver functions tests

Patient Information May cause drowsiness or dizziness; avoid alcohol and other CNS depressants

Nursing Implications Raise bed rails; institute safety measures; assist with ambulation

Dosage Forms

Caplet (Parafon Forte™ DSC): 500 mg

Capsule (Blanex®, Lobac®, Miflex®, Mus-Lac®, Skelex®): 250 mg with acetaminophen 300 mg

Tablet:

Paraflex®: 250 mg

Chlorofon-F®, Pargen® Fortified, Polyflex: 250 mg with acetaminophen 300 mg

Cholac® see Lactulose on page 617

Choledyl® see Theophylline/Aminophylline on page 1072

Cholera Vaccine (kol' er a)

Related Information

Vaccines on page 1386-1388

Use The World Health Organization no longer recommends cholera vaccination for travel to or from cholera-endemic areas. Some countries may still require evidence of a complete primary series or a booster dose given within 6 months of arrival. Vaccination should not be considered as an alternative to continued careful selection of foods and water. Ideally, cholera and yellow fever vaccines should be administered at least 3 weeks apart.

Pregnancy Risk Factor C

Contraindications Presence of any acute illness, history of severe systemic reaction, or allergic response following a prior dose of cholera vaccine

Warnings/Precautions There is no data on the safety of cholera vaccination during pregnancy. Use in pregnancy should reflect actual increased risk. Persons who have had severe local or systemic reactions to a previous dose should not be revaccinated. Have epinephrine (1:1000) available for immediate use.

Adverse Reactions

>10%:

Central nervous system: Malaise, fever, headache

Local: Pain, swelling, tenderness, erythema, and induration at injection site

Drug Interactions Decreased effect with yellow fever vaccine; data suggests that giving both vaccines within 3 weeks of each other may decrease the response to both

Stability Refrigerate, avoid freezing

Mechanism of Action Inactivated vaccine producing active immunization

Usual Dosage

Children:

6 months to 4 years: Two 0.2 mL doses I.M./S.C. 1 week to 1 month apart; booster doses (0.2 mL I.M./S.C.) every 6 months

5-10 years: Two 0.3 mL doses I.M./S.C. or two 0.2 mL intradermal doses 1 week to 1 month apart; booster doses (0.3 mL I.M./S.C. or 0.2 mL I.D.) every 6 months

Children ≥10 years and Adults: Two 0.5 mL doses given I.M./S.C. or two 0.2 mL doses I.D. 1 week to 1 month apart; booster doses (0.5 mL I.M. or S.C. or 0.2 mL I.D.) every 6 months

Administration Do not give I.V.

Patient Information Local reactions can occur up to 7 days after injection

Nursing Implications Defer immunization in individuals with moderate or severe febrile illness

Additional Information Inactivated bacteria vaccine

Dosage Forms Injection: Suspension of killed Vibrio cholerae (Inaba and Ogawa types) 8 units of each serotype per mL (1.5 mL, 20 mL)

Cholestyramine Resin (koe less' tir a meen)

Related Information

Lipid-Lowering Agents on page 1273

Brand Names Questran®; Questran® Light

Use Adjunct in the management of primary hypercholesterolemia; pruritus associated with elevated levels of bile acids; diarrhea associated with excess fecal bile acids; binding toxicologic agents; pseudomembraneous colitis

Pregnancy Risk Factor C

Contraindications Avoid using in complete biliary obstruction; hypersensitive to cholestyramine or any component; hypolipoproteinemia types III, IV, V

(Continued)

Cholestyramine Resin *(Continued)*

Warnings/Precautions Use with caution in patients with constipation (GI dysfunction); caution patients with phenylketonuria (Questran® Light contains aspartame); overdose may result in GI obstruction

Adverse Reactions

1% to 10%: Gastrointestinal: Constipation

<1%:

Dermatologic: Rash, irritation of perianal area, skin, or tongue

Endocrine & metabolic: Hyperchloremic acidosis

Gastrointestinal: Nausea, vomiting, abdominal distention and pain, malabsorption of fat-soluble vitamins, intestinal obstruction, steatorrhea

Hematologic: Hypoprothrombinemia (secondary to vitamin K deficiency)

Renal: Increased urinary calcium excretion

Overdosage/Toxicology Symptoms of overdose include GI obstruction; treatment is supportive

Drug Interactions Decreased effect: Decreased absorption (oral) of digitalis glycosides, warfarin, thyroid hormones, thiazide diuretics, propranolol, phenobarbital, amiodarone, methotrexate, NSAIDs, and other drugs by binding to the drug in the intestine

Mechanism of Action Forms a nonabsorbable complex with bile acids in the intestine, releasing chloride ions in the process; inhibits enterohepatic reuptake of intestinal bile salts and thereby increases the fecal loss of bile salt-bound low density lipoprotein cholesterol

Pharmacodynamics/Kinetics

Peak effect: 21 days

Absorption: Not absorbed from the GI tract

Elimination: In feces as an insoluble complex with bile acids

Usual Dosage Oral (dosages are expressed in terms of anhydrous resin):

Powder:

Children: 240 mg/kg/day in 3 divided doses; need to titrate dose depending on indication

Adults: 4 g 1-6 times/day to a maximum of 16-32 g/day

Tablet: Adults: Initial: 4 g once or twice daily; maintenance: 8-16 g/day in 2 divided doses

Not removed by hemo- or peritoneal dialysis; supplemental doses not necessary with dialysis or continuous arterio-venous or veno-venous hemofiltration effects

Test Interactions ↑ prothrombin time (S); ↓ cholesterol (S), iron (B)

Patient Information Do not administer the powder in its dry form, mix with fluid or with applesauce; chew bars thoroughly; drink plenty of fluids; take other medications 1 hour before or 4-6 hours after binding resin; GI adverse reactions may decrease over time with continued use; do not take with meals; adhere to prescribed diet

Nursing Implications Administer warfarin and other drugs at least 1-2 hours prior to, or 6 hours after cholestyramine because cholestyramine may bind to them, decreasing their total absorption. (**Note:** Cholestyramine itself may cause hypoprothrombinemia in patients with impaired enterohepatic circulation.)

Dosage Forms

Powder: 4 g of resin/9 g of powder (9 g, 378 g)

Powder, for oral suspension, with aspartame: 4 g of resin/5 g of powder (5 g, 210 g)

Tablet: 1 g

Choline Magnesium Salicylate *(koe' leen)*

Brand Names Trilisate®

Use Management of osteoarthritis, rheumatoid arthritis, and other arthritis; salicylate salts may not inhibit platelet aggregation and, therefore, should not be substituted for aspirin in the prophylaxis of thrombosis

Pregnancy Risk Factor C

Contraindications Bleeding disorders; hypersensitivity to salicylates or other nonacetylated salicylates or other NSAIDs; tartrazine dye hypersensitivity, asthma

Warnings/Precautions Use with caution in patients with impaired renal function, erosive gastritis, or peptic ulcer; avoid use in patients with suspected varicella or influenza (salicylates have been associated with Reye's syndrome in children <16 years of age when used to treat symptoms of chickenpox or the flu). Tinnitus or impaired hearing may indicate toxicity; discontinue use 1 week prior to surgical procedures.

Elderly are a high-risk population for adverse effects from nonsteroidal anti-inflammatory agents. As much as 60% of elderly can develop peptic ulceration and/or hemorrhage asymptomatically. Use lowest effective dose for shortest period possible. Tinnitus may be a difficult and unreliable indication of toxicity due to age-related hearing loss or eighth cranial nerve damage. CNS adverse effects may be observed in the elderly at lower doses than younger adults.

Adverse Reactions
>10%: Gastrointestinal: Nausea, heartburn, stomach pains, dyspepsia, epigastric discomfort

1% to 10%:
Central nervous system: Weakness, tiredness
Dermatologic: Skin rash
Gastrointestinal: Gastrointestinal ulceration
Hematologic: Hemolytic anemia
Respiratory: Troubled breathing
Miscellaneous: Anaphylactic shock

<1%:
Central nervous system: Insomnia, nervousness, jitters
Hematologic: Occult bleeding, prolongation of bleeding time, leukopenia, thrombocytopenia, iron deficiency anemia
Hepatic: Hepatotoxicity
Renal: Impaired renal function
Respiratory: Bronchospasm

Overdosage/Toxicology Symptoms of overdose include tinnitus, vomiting, acute renal failure, hyperthermia, irritability, seizures, coma, metabolic acidosis; for acute ingestions, determine serum salicylate levels 6 hours after ingestion; the "Done" nomogram may be helpful for estimating the severity of aspirin poisoning and directing treatment using serum salicylate levels. Treatment can also be based upon symptomatology.

Salicylates

Toxic Symptoms	Treatment
Overdose	Induce emesis with ipecac, and/or lavage with saline, followed with activated charcoal
Dehydration	I.V. fluids with KCl (no D_5W only)
Metabolic acidosis (must be treated)	Sodium bicarbonate
Hyperthermia	Cooling blankets or sponge baths
Coagulopathy/hemorrhage	Vitamin K I.V.
Hypoglycemia (with coma, seizures, or change in mental status)	Dextrose 25 g I.V.
Seizures	Diazepam 5-10 mg I.V.

Drug Interactions
Decreased effect: Antacids + Trilisate® → decreased salicylate concentration
Increased toxicity: Warfarin + Trilisate® → possible increased hypoprothrombinemic effect

Mechanism of Action Inhibits prostaglandin synthesis; acts on the hypothalamus heat-regulating center to reduce fever; blocks the generation of pain impulses

Pharmacodynamics/Kinetics
Absorption: Absorbed from the stomach and small intestine
Distribution: Readily distributes into most body fluids and tissues; crosses the placenta; appears in breast milk
Half-life: Dose-dependent ranging from 2-3 hours at low doses to 30 hours at high doses
Time to peak serum concentration: ~2 hours

Usual Dosage Oral (based on total salicylate content):
Children <37 kg: 50 mg/kg/day given in 2 divided doses
Adults: 500 mg to 1.5 g 2-3 times/day; usual maintenance dose: 1-4.5 g/day

Dosing adjustment/comments in renal impairment: Avoid use in severe renal impairment

Monitoring Parameters Serum magnesium with high dose therapy or in patients with impaired renal function; serum salicylate levels, renal function, hearing changes or tinnitus, abnormal bruising, weight gain and response (ie, pain)

Reference Range Salicylate blood levels for anti-inflammatory effect: 150-300 µg/mL; analgesia and antipyretic effect: 30-50 µg/mL

Test Interactions False-negative results for glucose oxidase urinary glucose tests (Clinistix®); false-positives using the cupric sulfate method (Clinitest®); also, interferes with Gerhardt test (urinary ketone analysis), VMA determination; 5-HIAA, xylose tolerance test, and T_3 and T_4; increased PBI; increased uric acid
(Continued)

Choline Magnesium Salicylate *(Continued)*

Patient Information Take with food; do not take with antacids; watch for bleeding gums or any signs of GI bleeding; take with food or milk to minimize GI distress; notify physician if ringing in ears or persistent GI pain occurs

Nursing Implications Liquid may be mixed with fruit juice just before drinking; do not administer with antacids

Dosage Forms See table.

Choline Magnesium Trisalicylate

Brand Name	Dosage Form	Total Salicylate	Choline Salicylate	Magnesium Salicylate
Trilisate®	Liquid	500 mg/5 mL	293 mg/5 mL	362 mg/5 mL
Trilisate 500®	Tablet	500 mg	293 mg	362 mg
Trilisate 750®	Tablet	750 mg	440 mg	544 mg
Trilisate 1000®	Tablet	1000 mg	587 mg	725 mg

Choline Salicylate (ko' leen sal' i sil ate)

Brand Names Arthropan® [OTC]

Use Temporary relief of pain of rheumatoid arthritis, rheumatic fever, osteoarthritis, and other conditions for which oral salicylates are recommended; useful in patients in which there is difficulty in administering doses in a tablet or capsule dosage form, because of the liquid dosage form

Pregnancy Risk Factor C

Contraindications Hypersensitivity to salicylates or any component or other nonacetylated salicylates

Warnings/Precautions Use with caution in patients with impaired renal function, erosive gastritis, or peptic ulcer; avoid use in patients with suspected varicella or influenza (salicylates have been associated with Reye's syndrome in children <16 years of age when used to treat symptoms of chickenpox or the flu)

Adverse Reactions

>10%: Gastrointestinal: Nausea, heartburn, stomach pains, dyspepsia, epigastric discomfort

1% to 10%:
  Central nervous system: Weakness, tiredness
  Dermatologic: Skin rash
  Gastrointestinal: Gastrointestinal ulceration
  Hematologic: Hemolytic anemia
  Respiratory: Troubled breathing
  Miscellaneous: Anaphylactic shock

<1%:
  Central nervous system: Insomnia, nervousness, jitters
  Hematologic: Occult bleeding, prolongation of bleeding time, leukopenia, thrombocytopenia, iron deficiency anemia
  Hepatic: Hepatotoxicity
  Renal: Impaired renal function
  Respiratory: Bronchospasm

Overdosage/Toxicology Symptoms of overdose include tinnitus, vomiting, acute renal failure, hyperthermia, irritability, seizures, coma, metabolic acidosis; for acute ingestions, determine serum salicylate levels 6 hours after ingestion; the "Done" nomogram may be helpful for estimating the severity of aspirin poisoning and directing treatment using serum salicylate levels. Treatment can also be based upon symptomatology.

Drug Interactions

Decreased effect with antacids

Increased effect of warfarin

Mechanism of Action Inhibits prostaglandin synthesis; acts on the hypothalamus heat-regulating center to reduce fever; blocks the generation of pain impulses

Pharmacodynamics/Kinetics

Absorption: From the stomach and small intestine within ~2 hours

Distribution: Readily distributes into most body fluids and tissues; crosses the placenta; appears in breast milk

Protein binding: 75% to 90%

Metabolism: Hydrolyzed to salicylate in the liver

Half-life: Dose-dependent ranging from 2-3 hours at low doses to 30 hours at high doses

Time to peak serum concentration: 1-2 hours

Elimination: In urine

Salicylates

Toxic Symptoms	Treatment
Overdose	Induce emesis with ipecac, and/or lavage with saline, followed with activated charcoal
Dehydration	I.V. fluids with KCl (no D_5W only)
Metabolic acidosis (must be treated)	Sodium bicarbonate
Hyperthermia	Cooling blankets or sponge baths
Coagulopathy/hemorrhage	Vitamin K I.V.
Hypoglycemia (with coma, seizures, or change in mental status)	Dextrose 25 g I.V.
Seizures	Diazepam 5-10 mg I.V.

Usual Dosage
 Children >12 years and Adults: Oral: 5 mL (870 mg) every 3-4 hours, if necessary, but not more than 6 doses in 24 hours
 Rheumatoid arthritis: 870-1740 mg (5-10 mL) up to 4 times/day

 Dosing adjustment/comments in renal impairment: Avoid use in severe renal impairment
Test Interactions False-negative results for Clinistix® urine test; false-positive results with Clinitest®; ↑ bleeding time
Patient Information Take with food; do not take with antacids; watch for bleeding gums or any signs of GI bleeding; take with food or milk to minimize GI distress, notify physician if ringing in ears or persistent GI pain occurs
Nursing Implications Liquid may be mixed with fruit juice just before drinking; do not administer with antacids
Dosage Forms Liquid (mint flavor): 870 mg/5 mL (240 mL, 480 mL)

Choline Theophyllinate see Theophylline/Aminophylline on page 1072

Choloxin® see Dextrothyroxine Sodium on page 322

Chondroitin Sulfate-Sodium Hyaluronate (kon droy' tin sul' fate-so' de um hi a lu ron' ate)
Brand Names Viscoat®
Synonyms Sodium Hyaluronate-Chrondroitin Sulfate
Use Surgical aid in anterior segment procedures, protects corneal endothelium and coats intraocular lens thus protecting it
Pregnancy Risk Factor C
Contraindications Hypersensitivity to hyaluronate
Warnings/Precautions Product is extracted from avian tissues and contains minute amounts of protein, potential risks of hypersensitivity may exist. Intraocular pressure may be elevated as a result of pre-existing glaucoma, compromised outflow and by operative procedures and sequelae, including coma, compromised outflow and by operative procedures and sequelae, including enzymatic zonulysis, absence of an iridectomy, trauma to filtration structures and by blood and lenticular remnants in the anterior chamber. Monitor IOP, especially during the immediate postoperative period.
Adverse Reactions 1% to 10%: Increased intraocular pressure
Stability Store at 2°C to 8°C/36°F to 46°F; do not freeze
Mechanism of Action Functions as a tissue lubricant and is thought to play an important role in modulating the interactions between adjacent tissues
Pharmacodynamics/Kinetics
 Absorption: Following intravitreous injection, diffusion occurs slowly
 Elimination: By way of the Canal of Schlemm
Usual Dosage Carefully introduce (using a 27-gauge needle or cannula) into anterior chamber after thoroughly cleaning the chamber with a balanced salt solution
Administration May inject prior to or following delivery of the crystalline lens. Instillation prior to lens delivery provides additional protection to corneal endothelium, protecting it from possible damage arising from surgical instrumentation. May also be used to coat intraocular lens and tips of surgical instruments prior to implantation surgery. May inject additional solution during anterior segment surgery to fully maintain the solution lost during surgery. At the end of surgery, remove solution by thoroughly irrigating with a balanced salt solution.
Test Interactions False-negative results for Clinistix® urine test; false-positive results with Clinitest®
(Continued)

Chondroitin Sulfate-Sodium Hyaluronate *(Continued)*
Dosage Forms Solution: Sodium chondroitin 40 mg and sodium hyaluronate 30 mg (0.25 mL, 0.5 mL)

Chooz® [OTC] *see* Calcium Carbonate *on page 161*

Chorex® *see* Chorionic Gonadotropin *on this page*

Chorionic Gonadotropin (kor re on' ik goe nad' oh troe pin)
Brand Names A.P.L.®; Chorex®; Choron®; Corgonject®; Follutein®; Glukor®; Gonic®; Pregnyl®; Profasi® HP
Synonyms CG; hCG
Use Induces ovulation and pregnancy in anovulatory, infertile females; treatment of hypogonadotropic hypogonadism, prepubertal cryptorchidism
Pregnancy Risk Factor C
Contraindications Hypersensitivity to chorionic gonadotropin or any component; precocious puberty, prostatic carcinoma or similar neoplasms
Warnings/Precautions Use with caution in asthma, seizure disorders, migraine, cardiac or renal disease; **not** effective in the treatment of obesity
Adverse Reactions
1% to 10%:
Central nervous system: Mental depression, tiredness
Endocrine & metabolic: Pelvic pain, ovarian cysts, enlargement of breasts, precocious puberty
Local: Pain at the injection site
Neuromuscular & skeletal: Premature closure of epiphyses
<1%:
Cardiovascular: Peripheral edema
Central nervous system: Irritability, restlessness, fatigue, headache
Endocrine & metabolic: Ovarian hyperstimulation syndrome, gynecomastia
Stability Following reconstitution with the provided diluent, solutions are stable for 30-90 days, depending on the specific preparation, when stored at 2°C to 15°C
Mechanism of Action Stimulates production of gonadal steroid hormones by causing production of androgen by the testis; as a substitute for luteinizing hormone (LH) to stimulate ovulation
Pharmacodynamics/Kinetics
Half-life, biphasic:
Initial: 11 hours
Terminal: 23 hours
Elimination: Excreted unchanged in urine within 3-4 days
Usual Dosage I.M.:
Children:
Prepubertal cryptorchidism (not due to anatomical obstruction): 4000 units 3 times/week for 3 weeks
or
5000 units every other day for 4 injections
or
15 injections of 500-1000 units over a period of 6 weeks
or
500 units 3 times per week for 4-6 weeks. If unsuccessful, start another course 1 month later, giving 1000 units/injection.
Hypogonadotropic hypogonadism in males: 500-1000 units 3 times/week for 3 weeks, followed by the same dose twice weekly for 3 weeks
or
1000-2000 units 3 times/week
or
4000 units 3 times/week for 6-9 months; reduce dose to 2000 units 3 times/week for an additional 3 months

Adults:
Use with menotropins to stimulate spermatogenesis: 5000 units 3 times/week for 4-6 months. With the beginning of menotropins therapy, hCG dose is continued at 2000 2 times/week.
Induction of ovulation and pregnancy: 5000-10,000 units one day following last dose of menotropins
Administration I.M. administration only
Reference Range Depends on application and methodology; <3 mIU/mL (SI: <3 units/L) usually normal (nonpregnant)
Patient Information Discontinue immediately if possibility of pregnancy
Dosage Forms Powder for injection (human origin): 200 units/mL (10 mL, 25 mL); 500 units/mL (10 mL); 1000 units/mL (10 mL); 2000 units/mL (10 mL)

Choron® *see* Chorionic Gonadotropin *on previous page*

Chromagen® OB [OTC] *see* Vitamin, Multiple *on page 1166*

Chronulac® *see* Lactulose *on page 617*

Chymex® *see* Bentiromide *on page 120*

Chymodiactin® *see* Chymopapain *on this page*

Chymopapain (kye' moe pa pane)

Brand Names Chymodiactin®; Discase®

Use Alternative to surgery in patients with herniated lumbar intervertebral discs

Pregnancy Risk Factor C

Contraindications Known hypersensitivity to chymopapain, papaya or its derivatives, neurologic impairment, use in spondylolisthesis or cauda equina lesion

Warnings/Precautions Prophylaxis (for anaphylactic reaction) with a histamine H_1- or H_2-receptor antagonist and/or a corticosteroid is recommended prior to chymopapain administration; anaphylaxis occurs in approximately 0.5% of patients; it can be fatal; paraplegia or paraparesis, central nervous system hemorrhage and other serious neurologic adverse effects have been observed within hours or days after the injection; extremely toxic when injected intrathecally

Adverse Reactions

>10%: Back pain

1% to 10%:

Central nervous system: Dizziness, headache

Gastrointestinal: Nausea

Neuromuscular & skeletal: Weakness in legs

<1%:

Central nervous system: CNS hemorrhage

Central nervous system: Seizures

Dermatologic: Allergic dermatitis

Gastrointestinal: Paralytic ileus

Local: Thrombophlebitis

Ocular: Conjunctivitis

Respiratory: Runny nose, shortness of breath

Miscellaneous: Anaphylaxis

Drug Interactions Avoid discography (with intradiscal radiographic contrast media)

Stability Store at 2°C to 8°C (36°F to 46°F); use within 2 hours of reconstitution

Mechanism of Action Chymopapain, when injected into the disc center, causes hydrolysis of the mucal mucopolysaccharide protein complex into acid polysaccharide, polypeptides, and amino acids. Subsequently, the water trapping properties of the nucleus pulposus are destroyed which permanently diminishes the pressure within the disc. The adjacent structures including the annulus fibrosus are not affected by chymopapain.

Usual Dosage Adults: 2000-4000 units/disc with a maximum cumulative dose not to exceed 8000 units for patients with multiple disc herniations

Patient Information The risk of serious adverse reactions must be discussed with the patient

Nursing Implications Patients should be well hydrated prior to chymopapain administration; anaphylactic reactions may occur up to 1 hour after injection; observe the patient closely

Dosage Forms Injection: 4000 units [4 nKat]; 10,000 units [10 nKat]

Chymotrypsin, Alpha (kye moe trip' sin)

Brand Names Catarase®; Zolyse®

Synonyms Alpha Chymotrypsin

Use Enzymatic zonulysis for intracapsular lens extraction in cataract surgery

Pregnancy Risk Factor C

Contraindications Known hypersensitivity to alpha chymotrypsin, high vitreous pressure, congenital cataracts

Warnings/Precautions Chymotrypsin may produce an acute rise in intraocular pressure following surgery, especially in patients with poor facility of outflow. The enzyme will not lyse the synechiae that may exist between the lens and other eye structures. Use of chymotrypsin in cataract surgery is not recommended in patients <20 years of age.

Adverse Reactions <1%: Ocular: Moderate uveitis, transient increases in intraocular pressure, corneal edema, striation

Drug Interactions Epinephrine 1:100 will inactivate chymotrypsin in approximately 1 hour; isoflurophate and chloramphenicol inhibit chymotrypsin

(Continued)

Chymotrypsin, Alpha *(Continued)*

Stability Reconstitute immediately prior to use

Usual Dosage Adults: Irrigate area (posterior chamber under iris) with 1-2 mL of chymotrypsin solution

Administration Dilute powder with 5 mL of diluent to give 150 units/mL solution; reconstitute immediately prior to use with 5-10 mL diluent

Dosage Forms Powder for ophthalmic solution:

Catarase®: 150 units [1:10,000] (with 2 mL diluent); 300 units [1:5000] (with 2 mL diluent)

Zolyse®: 750 units (with 9 mL diluent)

Cibacalcin® *see* Calcitonin *on page 158*

Cibalith-S® *see* Lithium *on page 643*

Ciclopirox Olamine (sye kloe peer' ox)

Brand Names Loprox®

Use Treatment of tinea pedis (athlete's foot), tinea cruris (jock itch), tinea corporis (ringworm), cutaneous candidiasis, and tinea versicolor (pityriasis)

Pregnancy Risk Factor B

Contraindications Known hypersensitivity to ciclopirox

Warnings/Precautions For external use only; avoid contact with eyes

Adverse Reactions 1% to 10%: Local: Irritation, redness, pain or burning; worsening of clinical condition

Mechanism of Action Inhibiting transport of essential elements in the fungal cell causing problems in synthesis of DNA, RNA, and protein

Pharmacodynamics/Kinetics

Absorption: <2% absorbed through intact skin

Protein binding: 94% to 98%

Half-life: 1.7 hours

Elimination: Of the small amounts of systemically absorbed drug, majority excreted by the kidney with small amounts excreted in feces

Usual Dosage Children >10 years and Adults: Apply twice daily, gently massage into affected areas; if no improvement after 4 weeks of treatment, re-evaluate the diagnosis

Patient Information Avoid contact with eyes; if sensitivity or irritation occurs, discontinue use

Dosage Forms

Cream, topical: 1% (15 g, 30 g, 90 g)

Lotion: 1% (30 mL)

Ciloxan™ Ophthalmic *see* Ciprofloxacin Hydrochloride *on page 246*

Cimetidine (sye met' i deen)

Brand Names Tagamet®

Use Short-term treatment of active duodenal ulcers and benign gastric ulcers; long-term prophylaxis of duodenal ulcer; gastric hypersecretory states; gastroesophageal reflux; prevention of upper GI bleeding in critically ill patients.

Pregnancy Risk Factor B

Contraindications Hypersensitivity to cimetidine, other component, or other H_2 antagonists

Warnings/Precautions Adjust dosages in renal/hepatic impairment or patients receiving drugs metabolized through the P-450 system

Adverse Reactions

1% to 10%:

Central nervous system: Dizziness, agitation, headache, drowsiness

Gastrointestinal: Diarrhea, nausea, vomiting

<1%:

Cardiovascular: Bradycardia, hypotension, tachycardia

Central nervous system: Confusion, fever

Dermatologic: Rash

Endocrine & metabolic: Gynecomastia, swelling of breasts

Genitourinary: Decreased sexual ability

Hematologic: Neutropenia, agranulocytosis, thrombocytopenia

Hepatic: Elevated creatinine, elevated AST and ALT

Neuromuscular & skeletal: Myalgia

Overdosage/Toxicology Treatment is primarily symptomatic and supportive. No experience with intentional overdose; reported ingestions of 20 g have had transient side effects seen with recommended doses; animal data have shown respiratory failure, tachycardia, muscle tremors, vomiting, restlessness, hypotension, salivation, emesis, and diarrhea.

Drug Interactions
Increased toxicity: Decreased elimination of lidocaine, theophylline, phenytoin, metronidazole, triamterene, procainamide, quinidine, and propranolol
Inhibition of warfarin metabolism, tricyclic antidepressant metabolism, diazepam elimination and cyclosporine elimination

Stability
Intact vials of cimetidine should be stored at room temperature and protected from light; cimetidine may precipitate from solution upon exposure to cold but can be redissolved by warming without degradation
Stability at room temperature:
Prepared bags: 7 days
Premixed bags: Manufacturer expiration dating and out of overwrap stability: 15 days
Stable in parenteral nutrition solutions for up to 7 days when protected from light
Physically incompatible with barbiturates, amphotericin B, and cephalosporins

Mechanism of Action Competitive inhibition of histamine at H_2-receptors of the gastric parietal cells resulting in reduced gastric acid secretion, gastric volume and hydrogen ion concentration reduced

Pharmacodynamics/Kinetics
Distribution: Crosses the placenta; appears in breast milk
Protein binding: 20%
Bioavailability: 60% to 70%
Half-life:
Neonates: 3.6 hours
Children: 1.4 hours
Adults (with normal renal function): 2 hours
Time to peak serum concentration: Oral: Within 1-2 hours
Elimination: Principally as unchanged drug by the kidney; some excretion in bile and feces

Usual Dosage
Neonates: Oral, I.M., I.V.: 10-20 mg/kg/day divided every 4-6 hours
Children: Oral, I.M., I.V.: 20-40 mg/kg/day in divided doses every 4 hours
Adults: Short-term treatment of active ulcers:
Oral: 300 mg 4 times/day or 800 mg at bedtime or 400 mg twice daily for up to 8 weeks
I.M., I.V.: 300 mg every 6 hours or 37.5 mg/hour by continuous infusion; I.V. dosage should be adjusted to maintain an intragastric pH ≥5

Patients with an active bleed: Give cimetidine as a continuous infusion (see above)
Duodenal ulcer prophylaxis: Oral: 400-800 mg at bedtime
Gastric hypersecretory conditions: Oral, I.M., I.V.: 300-600 mg every 6 hours; dosage not to exceed 2.4 g/day

Dosing adjustment/interval in renal impairment: Children and Adults:
Cl_{cr} 20-40 mL/minute: Administer every 8 hours or 75% of normal dose
Cl_{cr} 0-20 mL/minute: Administer every 12 hours or 50% of normal dose
Slightly dialyzable (5% to 20%)

Dosing adjustment/comments in hepatic impairment: Usual dose is safe in mild liver disease but use with caution and in reduced dosage in severe liver disease; increased risk of CNS toxicity in cirrhosis suggested by enhanced penetration of CNS

Monitoring Parameters Blood pressure with I.V. push administration, CBC, gastric pH, signs and symptoms of peptic ulcer disease, occult blood with GI bleeding, monitor renal function to correct dose; monitor for side effects

Test Interactions ↑ creatinine, AST, ALT, creatinine (S)

Patient Information Take with or immediately after meals; take 1 hour before or 2 hours after antacids; may cause drowsiness, impaired judgment, or coordination; avoid excessive alcohol

Nursing Implications Give with meals so that the drug's peak effect occurs at the proper time (peak inhibition of gastric acid secretion occurs at 1 and 3 hours after dosing in fasting subjects and approximately 2 hours in nonfasting subjects; this correlates well with the time food is no longer in the stomach offering a buffering effect)

Dosage Forms
Infusion, as hydrochloride, in NS: 300 mg (50 mL)
Injection, as hydrochloride: 150 mg/mL (2 mL, 8 mL)
Liquid, oral, as hydrochloride (mint-peach flavor): 300 mg/5 mL with alcohol 2.8% (5 mL, 240 mL)
Tablet: 200 mg, 300 mg, 400 mg, 800 mg

Cinobac® Pulvules® *see* Cinoxacin *on this page*

Cinoxacin (sin ox' a sin)

Brand Names Cinobac® Pulvules®

Use Treatment of urinary tract infections

Pregnancy Risk Factor B

Contraindications History of convulsive disorders, hypersensitivity to cinoxacin or any component or other quinolones

Warnings/Precautions CNS stimulation may occur (tremor, restlessness, confusion, and very rarely hallucinations or seizures). Use with caution in patients with known or suspected CNS disorders or renal impairment. Not recommended in children <18 years of age, ciprofloxacin (a related compound), has caused a transient arthropathy in children; prolonged use may result in superinfection; modify dosage in patients with renal impairment.

Adverse Reactions

1% to 10%:

Central nervous system: Headache, dizziness

Gastrointestinal: Heartburn, abdominal pain, GI bleeding, belching, flatulence, anorexia, nausea

<1%:

Central nervous system: Insomnia, confusion

Gastrointestinal: Diarrhea

Hematologic: Thrombocytopenia

Ocular: Photophobia

Otic: Tinnitus

Overdosage/Toxicology Symptoms of overdose include acute renal failure, seizures; GI decontamination and supportive care; not removed by peritoneal or hemodialysis

Drug Interactions

Decreased effect: Decreased urine levels with probenecid; decreased absorption with aluminum-, magnesium-, calcium-containing antacids

Increased serum levels: Probenecid

Mechanism of Action Inhibits microbial synthesis of DNA with resultant inhibition of protein synthesis

Pharmacodynamics/Kinetics

Absorption: Oral: Rapid and complete; food decreases peak levels by 30% but not total amount absorbed

Distribution: Crosses the placenta; concentrates in prostate tissue

Protein binding: 60% to 80%

Half-life: 1.5 hours, prolonged in renal impairment

Time to peak serum concentration: Oral: Within 2-3 hours

Elimination: ~60% excreted as unchanged drug in urine

Usual Dosage Children >12 years and Adults: 1 g/day in 2-4 doses for 7-14 days

Dosing interval in renal impairment:

Cl_{cr} 20-50 mL/minute: 250 mg twice daily

Cl_{cr} <20 mL/minute: 250 mg/day

Administration Administer around-the-clock to promote less variation in peak and trough serum levels

Patient Information May be taken with food to minimize upset stomach; avoid antacid use; drink fluid liberally; may cause dizziness; use caution when driving or performing other tasks requiring alertness

Nursing Implications Hold antacids for 3-4 hours after giving

Dosage Forms Capsule: 250 mg, 500 mg

Cipro™ *see* Ciprofloxacin Hydrochloride *on this page*

Ciprofloxacin Hydrochloride (sip roe flox' a sin)

Related Information

Antimicrobial Drugs of Choice *on page 1298-1302*

Brand Names Ciloxan™ Ophthalmic; Cipro™

Use Treatment of documented or suspected pseudomonal infection (eg, home care patients); documented multi-drug resistant gram-negative organisms; documented infectious diarrhea due to *Campylobacter jejuni*, *Shigella*, or *Salmonella*; osteomyelitis caused by susceptible organisms in which parenteral therapy is not feasible; used ophthalmically for superficial ocular infections (corneal ulcers, conjunctivitis) due to strains of microorganisms susceptible to ciprofloxacin

Pregnancy Risk Factor C

Contraindications Hypersensitivity to ciprofloxacin, any component or other quinolones

Warnings/Precautions Not recommended in children <18 years of age; has caused transient arthropathy in children; CNS stimulation may occur (tremor, restlessness, confusion, and very rarely hallucinations or seizures). Use with caution in patients with known or suspected CNS disorders.

Adverse Reactions
1% to 10%:
  Central nervous system: Headache, restlessness
  Gastrointestinal: Nausea, diarrhea, vomiting, abdominal pain
  Dermatologic: Rash
<1%:
  Central nervous system: Dizziness, confusion, seizures
  Hematologic: Anemia
  Hepatic: Increased liver enzymes
  Neuromuscular & skeletal: Tremor, arthralgia
  Renal: Acute renal failure

Overdosage/Toxicology Symptoms of overdose include acute renal failure, seizures; GI decontamination and supportive care; not removed by peritoneal or hemodialysis

Drug Interactions
Decreased effect: Decreased absorption with antacids containing aluminum, magnesium, and/or calcium (by up to 98% if given at the same time)
Increased toxicity/serum levels: Quinolones cause increased levels of caffeine, warfarin, cyclosporine, and theophylline; azlocillin, cimetidine, probenecid increase quinolone levels

Stability Refrigeration and room temperature: Prepared bags: 14 days; Premixed bags: Manufacturer expiration dating

Mechanism of Action Inhibits DNA-gyrase in susceptible organisms; inhibits relaxation of supercoiled DNA and promotes breakage of double-stranded DNA

Pharmacodynamics/Kinetics
Absorption: Oral: Rapid from GI tract (~85%)
Distribution: Crosses the placenta; appears in breast milk; distributes widely throughout body; tissue concentrations often exceed serum concentrations especially in the kidneys, gallbladder, liver, lungs, gynecological tissue, and prostatic tissue; distributes to saliva, nasal secretions, aqueous humor, sputum, skin blister fluid, lymph, peritoneal fluid, bile, and prostatic secretions; also to skin, fat, muscle, bone, and cartilage; CSF concentrations reach 10% with noninflamed meninges and 14% to 37% with inflamed meninges
Metabolism: Partially metabolized in the liver
Half-life: 3-5 hours in patients with normal renal function
Time to peak serum concentration: Oral: Within 0.5-2 hours
Elimination: 30% to 50% excreted as unchanged drug in urine; 20% to 40% of dose excreted in feces primarily from biliary excretion

Usual Dosage
Children >18 years: Oral: 20-30 mg/kg/day in 2 divided doses; maximum dose: 1.5 g/day
Adults:
  Oral: 250-750 mg every 12 hours, depending on severity of infection and susceptibility
  I.V.: 200-400 mg every 12 hours depending on severity of infection
  Ophthalmic: Instill 1-2 drops in eye(s) every 2 hours while awake for 2 days and 1-2 drops every 4 hours while awake for the next 5 days

Dosing adjustment in renal impairment: Cl_{cr} <30 mL/minute: Administer every 24 hours
Only small amounts of ciprofloxacin are removed by dialysis (<10%)

Administration Administer around-the-clock to promote less variation in peak and trough serum levels

Monitoring Parameters Patients receiving concurrent ciprofloxacin, theophylline, or cyclosporine should have serum levels monitored

Reference Range Therapeutic: 2.6-3 µg/mL; Toxic: >5 µg/mL

Patient Information May be taken with food to minimize upset stomach; avoid antacids containing magnesium or aluminum, or products containing zinc or iron within 4 hours before or 2 hours after dosing; may cause dizziness or drowsiness; drink fluid liberally

Nursing Implications Hold antacids for 2 hours after giving

Dosage Forms
Infusion, in D_5W: 400 mg (200 mL)
Infusion, in NS or D_5W: 200 mg (100 mL)
Injection: 200 mg (20 mL); 400 mg (40 mL)
Solution, ophthalmic: 3.5 mg/mL (2.5 mL, 5 mL)
Tablet: 250 mg, 500 mg, 750 mg

Cisapride (sis' a pride)

Brand Names Propulsid®

Use Treatment of nocturnal symptoms of gastroesophageal reflux disease (GERD), also demonstrated effectiveness for gastroparesis, refractory constipation, and nonulcer dyspepsia

Pregnancy Risk Factor C

Contraindications Hypersensitivity to cisapride or any of its components; GI hemorrhage, mechanical obstruction, GI perforation, or other situations when GI motility stimulation is dangerous

Warnings/Precautions Pregnancy, lactation and when stimulation of GI motility may be dangerous (eg, obstruction, perforation, hemorrhage)

Adverse Reactions

>5%:

Central nervous system: Headache

Dermatologic: Rash

Gastrointestinal: Diarrhea, GI cramping, dyspepsia, flatulence, nausea, dry mouth

Respiratory: Rhinitis

<5%:

Cardiovascular: Tachycardia

Central nervous system: Extrapyramidal effects, somnolence, fatigue, seizures, insomnia, anxiety

Hematologic: Thrombocytopenia, increased LFTs, pancytopenia, leukopenia, granulocytopenia, aplastic anemia

Respiratory: Rhinitis, sinusitis, coughing, upper respiratory tract infection, increased incidence of viral infection

Drug Interactions

Decreased effect: Atropine, digoxin

Increased toxicity: Warfarin, diazepam increased levels, cimetidine, and ranitidine, CNS depressants

Mechanism of Action Enhances the release of acetylcholine at the myenteric plexus. *In vitro* studies have shown cisapride to have serotonin-4 receptor agonistic properties which may increase gastrointestinal motility and cardiac rate; increases lower esophageal sphincter pressure and lower esophageal peristalsis; accelerates gastric emptying of both liquids and solids.

Pharmacodynamics/Kinetics

Onset of effect: 0.5-1 hour

Bioavailability: 35% to 40%

Protein binding: 97.5% to 98%

Metabolism: Extensively to norcisapride, which is eliminated in urine and feces

Half-life: 6-12 hours

Elimination: <10% of dose excreted into feces and urine

Usual Dosage Oral:

Children: 0.15-0.3 mg/kg/dose 3-4 times/day; maximum: 10 mg/dose

Adults: Initial: 10 mg 4 times/day at least 15 minutes before meals and at bedtime; in some patients the dosage will need to be increased to 20 mg to obtain a satisfactory result

Additional Information Safety and effectiveness in children have not been established

Dosage Forms Tablet, scored: 10 mg

Cisplatin (sis' pla tin)

Related Information

Antiemetics for Chemotherapy Induced Nausea and Vomiting *on page 1202*
Cancer Chemotherapy Regimens *on page 1218-1241*

Brand Names Platinol®; Platinol®-AQ

Synonyms CDDP

Use Treatment of head and neck, breast, testicular, and ovarian cancer; Hodgkin's and non-Hodgkin's lymphoma; sarcomas, bladder, gastric, lung, esophageal, cervical, and prostate cancer; myeloma, melanoma, mesothelioma, small cell lung cancer, and osteosarcoma

Pregnancy Risk Factor D

Contraindications Hypersensitivity to cisplatin or any other platinum-containing compounds or any component, anaphylactic-like reactions have been reported; pre-existing renal insufficiency, myelosuppression, hearing impairment

Warnings/Precautions The U.S. Food and Drug Administration (FDA) currently recommends that procedures for proper handling and disposal of antineoplastic agents be considered. All patients should receive adequate hydration prior to and for 24 hours after cisplatin administration, with or without mannitol and/or furosemide, to ensure good urine output and decrease the chance of nephrotoxicity; reduce dosage in renal impairment. Cumulative renal toxicity may be severe;

dose-related toxicities include myelosuppression, nausea, and vomiting; ototoxicity, especially pronounced in children, is manifested by tinnitus or loss of high frequency hearing and occasionally, deafness. **Serum magnesium, as well as other electrolytes, should be monitored both before and within 48 hours after cisplatin therapy.** Patients who are magnesium depleted should receive replacement therapy before the cisplatin is administered.

Adverse Reactions

>10%:

Gastrointestinal: Cisplatin is one of the most emetogenic agents used in cancer chemotherapy; nausea and vomiting occur in 76% to 100% of patients and is dose related. Prophylactic antiemetics should always be prescribed; nausea and vomiting may last up to 1 week after therapy.

Emetic potential:

<75 mg: Moderately high (60% to 90%)

≥75 mg: High (>90%)

Myelosuppressive: Mild with moderate doses, mild to moderate with high-dose therapy

WBC: Mild

Platelets: Mild

Onset (days): 10

Nadir (days): 14-23

Recovery (days): 21-39

Nephrotoxicity: Related to elimination, protein binding, and uptake of cisplatin. Two types of nephrotoxicity: Acute renal failure and chronic renal insufficiency.

Acute renal failure and azotemia is a dose-dependent process and can be minimized with proper administration and prophylaxis. Damage to the proximal tubules by the degradation products of cisplatin is suspected to cause the toxicity. It is manifested as increased BUN and creatinine, oliguria, protein wasting, and potassium, calcium, and magnesium wasting.

Chronic renal dysfunction can develop in patients receiving multiple courses of cisplatin. This occurs with slow release of the platinum ion from tissues, which then accumulates in the distal tubules. Manifestations of this toxicity are varied, and can include sodium and water wasting, nephropathy, hyperuricemia, decreased Cl_{cr}, and magnesium wasting.

Recommendations for minimizing nephrotoxicity include:

Prepare cisplatin in saline-containing vehicles

Vigorous hydration (125-150 mL/hour) before, during, and after cisplatin administration

Simultaneous administration of either mannitol or furosemide

Avoid other nephrotoxic agents (aminoglycosides, amphotericin, etc)

Neurotoxicity: Peripheral neuropathy is dose- and duration-dependent. The mechanism is through axonal degeneration with subsequent damage to the long sensory nerves. Toxicity can first be noted at doses of 200 mg/m², with measurable toxicity at doses >350 mg/m². This process is irreversible and progressive with continued therapy.

Ototoxicity: Ototoxicity occurs in 10% to 30%, and is manifested as high frequency hearing loss. Baseline audiography should be performed. Ototoxicity is especially pronounced in children.

Miscellaneous: Elevation of liver enzymes, mild alopecia

1% to 10%:

Extravasation: May cause thrombophlebitis and tissue damage if infiltrated; may use sodium thiosulfate as antidote, but consult hospital policy for guidelines

Irritant chemotherapy

<1%:

Anaphylactic reaction occurs within minutes after administration and can be controlled with epinephrine, antihistamines, and steroids

Cardiovascular: Bradycardia, arrhythmias

Dermatologic: Mild alopecia

Endocrine & metabolic: SIADH

Local: Phlebitis

Ocular: Optic neuritis, blurred vision, papilledema

Miscellaneous: Mouth sores

Overdosage/Toxicology Symptoms of overdose include leukopenia, thrombocytopenia, nausea, vomiting; antidote is sodium thiosulfate

Drug Interactions

Decreased toxicity: Sodium thiosulfate theoretically inactivates drug systemically; has been used clinically to reduce systemic toxicity with intraperitoneal administration of cisplatin

(Continued)

Cisplatin *(Continued)*

Increased toxicity: Ethacrynic acid has resulted in severe ototoxicity in animals; loop diuretics increase ototoxicity of cisplatin; cisplatin has resulted in delayed bleomycin elimination

Stability

Do not infuse in solutions containing <0.2% sodium chloride; do not refrigerate reconstituted solutions since precipitation may occur; protect from light; aluminum needles should not be used to administer the drug due to binding with the platinum

Incompatible with sodium bicarbonate

Mechanism of Action Inhibits DNA synthesis by the formation of DNA cross-links; denatures the double helix; covalently binds to DNA bases and disrupts DNA function; may also bind to proteins; the *cis*-isomer is 14 times more cytotoxic than the *trans*-isomer; both forms cross-link but cis-platinum is less easily recognized by cell enzymes and, therefore, not repaired. Cisplatin can also bind two adjacent guanines on the same strand of DNA producing intrastrand cross-linking and breakage

Pharmacodynamics/Kinetics

Distribution: I.V.: Rapidly distributes into tissue following administration; found in high concentrations in the kidneys, liver, ovaries, uterus, and lungs

Protein binding: >90%

Half-life:

Initial: 20-30 minutes

Beta: 1 hour

Terminal: ~24 hours

Secondary half-life: 44-73 hours

Metabolism: Undergoes nonenzymatic metabolism; the drug is inactivated (in both the cell and the bloodstream) by sulfhydryl groups; cisplatin covalently binds to glutathione and to thiosulfate

Elimination: >90% in urine and 10% in bile

Usual Dosage I.V. (refer to individual protocols):

An estimated Cl_{cr} should be on all cisplatin chemotherapy orders along with other patient parameters (ie, patient's height, weight, and body surface area). Pharmacy and nursing staff should check the Cl_{cr} on the order and determine the appropriateness of cisplatin dosing.

It is recommended that a 24-hour urine creatinine clearance be checked prior to a patient's first dose of cisplatin and periodically thereafter (ie, after every 2-3 cycles of cisplatin)

If the dose prescribed is a reduced dose, then this should be indicated on the chemotherapy order

Children: Various dosage schedules range from 30-100 mg/m² once every 2-3 weeks; may also dose similar to adult dosing

Adults:

Head and neck cancer: 100-150 mg/m² every 3-4 weeks

Testicular cancer: 10-20 mg/m²/day for 5 days repeated every 3-4 weeks

Metastatic ovarian cancer: 50 mg/m² every 3 weeks

Rate of infusion varies from 30 minutes to 24-hour continuous infusion; cisplatin has been administered intraperitoneal with systemic sodium thiosulfate for ovarian cancer; doses up to 90-270 mg/m² have been administered and retained for 4 hours before draining

Dosing adjustment in renal impairment:

Cl_{cr} 10-50 mL/minute: Administer 50% to 75% of normal dose

Cl_{cr} <10 mL/minute: Administer 25% to 50% of normal dose

Partially cleared by hemodialysis

Administer dose posthemodialysis

Administration I.V.: Rate of administration has varied from a 15- to 20-minute infusion, 1 mg/minute infusion, 6- to 8-hour infusion, 24-hour infusion, or per protocol; needles, syringes, catheters, or I.V. administration sets that contain aluminum parts should not be used for administration of drug

Monitoring Parameters Renal function tests (serum creatinine, BUN, Cl_{cr}), electrolytes (particularly magnesium, calcium, potassium); hearing test, neurologic exam (with high dose), liver function tests periodically, CBC with differential and platelet count; urine output, urinalysis

Patient Information Drink plenty of fluids to maintain urine output, be prepared for severe nausea and vomiting following drug administration which can be delayed up to 48 hours; notify physician of numbness or tingling in extremities or hearing loss

Nursing Implications Perform pretreatment hydration with 1-2 L of fluid infused for 8-12 hours prior to dose; monitor for possible anaphylactoid reaction; monitor renal, hematologic, otic, and neurologic function frequently

Management of extravasation: Large extravasations of concentrated solutions produce tissue necrosis; **treatment is not recommended unless a large amount of highly concentrated solution is extravasated;** mix 4 mL of 10% sodium thiosulfate with 6 mL sterile water for injection: Inject 1-4 mL through existing I.V. line cannula; administer 1 mL for each mL extravasated; inject S.C. if needle is removed

Additional Information Sodium content (10 mg): 35.4 mg (1.54 mEq)

Dosage Forms
Injection, aqueous: 1 mg/mL (50 mL, 100 mL)
Powder for injection: 10 mg, 50 mg

13-*cis*-Retinoic Acid *see* Isotretinoin *on page 602*

Citracal® [OTC] *see* Calcium Citrate *on page 165*

Citrate of Magnesia *see* Magnesium Citrate *on page 657*

Citroma® [OTC] *see* Magnesium Citrate *on page 657*

Citro-Nesia™ [OTC] *see* Magnesium Citrate *on page 657*

Citrovorum Factor *see* Leucovorin Calcium *on page 619*

CI-719 *see* Gemfibrozil *on page 498*

Cla *see* Clarithromycin *on next page*

Cladribine (kla′ dri been)

Related Information
Cancer Chemotherapy Regimens *on page 1218-1241*

Brand Names Leustatin™

Synonyms 2-CdA; 2-Chlorodeoxyadenosine

Use Treatment of hairy cell and chronic lymphocytic leukemias

Pregnancy Risk Factor D

Contraindications Patients with a prior history of hypersensitivity to cladribine

Warnings/Precautions The U.S. Food and Drug Administration (FDA) currently recommends that procedures for proper handling and disposal of antineoplastic agents be considered. Because of its myelosuppressive properties, cladribine should be used with caution in patients with pre-existing hematologic or immunologic abnormalities; prophylactic administration of allopurinol should be considered in patients receiving cladribine because of the potential for hyperuricemia secondary to tumor lysis; appropriate antibiotic therapy should be administered promptly in patients exhibiting signs and symptoms of neutropenia and infection.

Adverse Reactions
>10%:
Bone marrow suppression: Commonly observed in patients treated with cladribine, especially at high doses; at the initiation of treatment, however, most patients in clinical studies had hematologic impairment as a result of HCL. During the first 2 weeks after treatment initiation, mean platelet counts decline and subsequently increased with normalization of mean counts by day 12. Absolute neutrophil counts and hemoglobin declined and subsequently increased with normalization of mean counts by week 5 and week 6.
Fever: Temperature ≥101°F has been associated with the use of cladribine in approximately 66% of patients in the first month of therapy. Although 69% of patients developed fevers, less than 33% of febrile events were associated with documented infection.
Gastrointestinal: Nausea and vomiting are not severe with cladribine at any dose level. Most cases of nausea were mild, not accompanied by vomiting and did not require treatment with antiemetics. In patients requiring antiemetics, nausea was easily controlled most often by chlorpromazine.
Local: Injection site reactions
Miscellaneous: Fatigue, rash, headache
1% to 10%:
Cardiovascular: Edema, tachycardia
Central nervous system: Dizziness, insomnia, chills, asthenia, malaise
Dermatologic: Pruritus, erythema
Gastrointestinal: Constipation, abdominal pain
Neuromuscular & skeletal: Arthralgia, myalgia
Miscellaneous: Pain, diaphoresis, trunk pain

Stability Refrigerate unopened vials (2°C to 8°C/36°F to 46°F); protect from light. Solutions should be administered immediately after the initial dilution or stored in the refrigerator (2°C to 8°C) for ≤8 hours. **The use of dextrose 5% in water as a diluent is not recommended due to increased degradation of cladribine;** should not be mixed with other intravenous drugs or additive or infused simultaneously via a common intravenous line. Admixtures for single daily infusion are
(Continued)

Cladribine *(Continued)*

stable for at least 24 hours at room temperature under normal room light in polyvinyl chloride infusion containers. Admixtures for 7-day infusion are stable (chemically and physically) for at least 7 days in the Pharmacia Deltec™ medication cassettes.

Mechanism of Action A purine nucleoside analogue; prodrug which is activated via phosphorylation by deoxycytidine kinase to a 5'-triphosphate derivative. This active form incorporates into susceptible cells and into DNA to result in the breakage of DNA strand and shutdown of DNA synthesis and also results in a depletion of nicotinamide adenine dinucleotide and adenosine triphosphate (ATP). The induction of strand breaks results in a drop in the cofactor nicotinamide adenine dinucleotide and disruption of cell metabolism. ATP is depleted to deprive cells of an important source of energy. Cladribine is able to kill resting as well as dividing cells, unlike most other cytotoxic drugs.

Pharmacodynamics/Kinetics

Distribution: V_d: 4.52±2.82 L/kg

Protein binding: 20% to plasma proteins

Half-life: Biphasic:

Alpha: 25 minutes

Beta: 6.7 hours

Terminal, mean (normal renal function): 5.4 hours

Elimination: Mean: 978±422 mL/hour/kg; estimated systemic clearance: 640 mL/hour/kg

Usual Dosage I.V.:

Children: Safety and effectiveness have not been established; in a phase I study involving patients 1-21 years of age with relapsed acute leukemia, cladribine was administered by continuous infusion at doses ranging from 3-10.7 mg/m²/day for 5 days (0.5-2 times the dose recommended in HCL). Investigators reported beneficial responses in this study; the dose-limiting toxicity was severe myelosuppression with profound neutropenia and thrombocytopenia.

Adults: 0.09-0.1 mg/kg/day continuous infusion for 7 consecutive days

Administration

Single daily infusion: Administer diluted in an infusion bag containing 500 mL of 0.9% sodium chloride and repeated for a total of 7 consecutive days

7-day infusion: Prepare with bacteriostatic 0.9% sodium chloride. Both cladribine and diluent should be passed through a sterile 0.22 micron hydrophilic filter as it is being introduced into the infusion reservoir. The calculated dose of cladribine (7 days x 0.09 mg/kg) should first be added to the infusion reservoir through a filter then the bacteriostatic 0.9% sodium chloride should be added to the reservoir to obtain a total volume of 100 mL.

Dosage Forms Injection, preservative free: 1 mg/mL (10 mL)

Claforan® *see* Cefotaxime Sodium *on page 199*

Clarithromycin *(kla rith' roe mye sin)*

Brand Names Biaxin™ Filmtabs®

Synonyms Cla

Use Treatment against most respiratory pathogens (eg, *S. pyogenes, S. pneumoniae, S. agalactiae,* viridans *Streptococcus, M. catarrhalis, C. trachomatis, Legionella* sp, *Mycoplasma pneumoniae, S. aureus*). Clarithromycin is highly active (MICs ≤0.25 mcg/mL) against *H. influenzae,* the combination of clarithromycin and its metabolite demonstrate an additive effect. Additionally, clarithromycin has shown activity against *C. pneumoniae* (including strain TWAR) and *M. avium* infection.

Pregnancy Risk Factor C

Contraindications Hypersensitivity to clarithromycin, erythromycin, or any macrolide antibiotic

Warnings/Precautions In presence of severe renal impairment with or without coexisting hepatic impairment, decreased dosage or prolonged dosing interval may be appropriate; antibiotic associated colitis has been reported with use of clarithromycin; elderly patients have experienced increased incidents of adverse effects due to known age-related decreases in renal function

Adverse Reactions

1% to 10%:

Central nervous system: Headache

Gastrointestinal: Diarrhea, nausea, abnormal taste, dyspepsia, abdominal pain

<1%:

Cardiovascular: Ventricular tachycardia, torsade de pointes

Hematologic: Decreased white blood count

Miscellaneous: Elevated AST, alkaline phosphatase, and bilirubin, elevated BUN and serum creatinine, elevated prothrombin time

Overdosage/Toxicology Symptoms of overdose include nausea, vomiting, diarrhea, prostration, reversible pancreatitis, hearing loss with or without tinnitus or vertigo; treatment includes symptomatic and supportive care

Drug Interactions Increased levels: Clarithromycin increases serum theophylline levels by as much as 20% and significantly increases carbamazepine levels

Note: While other drug interactions (digoxin, anticoagulants, ergotamine, triazolam) known to occur with erythromycin have not been reported in clinical trials with clarithromycin, concurrent use of these drugs should be monitored closely

Mechanism of Action Exerts its antibacterial action by binding to 50S ribosomal subunit resulting in inhibition of protein synthesis. The 14-OH metabolite of clarithromycin is twice as active as the parent compound.

Pharmacodynamics/Kinetics

Absorption: Highly stable in the presence of gastric acid (unlike erythromycin)

Distribution: Widely distributes into most body tissues with the exception of the CNS

Metabolism: Partially converted to the microbiologically active metabolite, 14-OH clarithromycin

Bioavailability: 50% (250 mg tablet)

Half-life, elimination: 3-4 hours with a 250 mg dose; 5-7 hours with a 500 mg dose

Time to peak serum concentration: Oral: 2-4 hours

Elimination: Following 250 mg or 500 mg doses every 12 hours, ~20% to 30% of unchanged parent drug is excreted in urine

Usual Dosage Safe use in children has not been established. Adults: Oral: Usual dose: 250-500 mg every 12 hours for 7-14 days

Upper respiratory tract: 250-500 mg every 12 hours for 10-14 days
Pharyngitis/tonsillitis: 250 mg every 12 hours for 10 days
Acute maxillary sinusitis: 500 mg every 12 hours for 14 days

Lower respiratory tract: 250-500 mg every 12 hours for 7-14 days
Acute exacerbation of chronic bronchitis due to:
M. catarrhalis and S. pneumoniae: 250 mg every 12 hours for 7-14 days
H. influenzae: 500 mg every 12 hours for 7-14 days
Pneumonia due to M. pneumoniae and S. pneumoniae: 250 mg every 12 hours for 7-14 days

Uncomplicated skin and skin structure: 250 mg every 12 hours for 7-14 days

Helicobacter pylori: Combination regimen with bismuth subsalicylate, tetracycline, clarithromycin, and an H_2 receptor antagonist; or combination of omeprazole and clarithromycin. Adult dosage: Oral: 250 mg twice daily to 500 mg 3 times/day

Dosing adjustment in severe renal impairment: Decreased doses or prolonged dosing intervals are recommended

Patient Information May be taken with meals; finish all medication; do not skip doses

Nursing Implications Clarithromycin may be given with or without meals; give every 12 hours rather than twice daily to avoid peak and trough variation

Dosage Forms Tablet, film coated: 250 mg, 500 mg

Claritin® see Loratadine on page 649

ClearAway® see Salicylic Acid on page 991

Clear Eyes® [OTC] see Naphazoline Hydrochloride on page 775

Clearsil® [OTC] see Benzoyl Peroxide on page 122

Clemastine Fumarate (klem' as teen fume' a rate)

Brand Names Tavist®

Use Perennial and seasonal allergic rhinitis and other allergic symptoms including urticaria

Pregnancy Risk Factor C

Contraindications Narrow-angle glaucoma, hypersensitivity to clemastine or any component

Warnings/Precautions Safety and efficacy have not been established in children <6 years of age; bladder neck obstruction, symptomatic prostate hypertrophy, asthmatic attacks, and stenosing peptic ulcer

Adverse Reactions

>10%:

Central nervous system: Slight to moderate drowsiness

Miscellaneous: Thickening of bronchial secretions

(Continued)

253

Clemastine Fumarate *(Continued)*

1% to 10%:
  Central nervous system: Headache, fatigue, nervousness, increased dizziness
  Gastrointestinal: Appetite increase, weight nausea, diarrhea, abdominal pain, dry mouth
  Neuromuscular & skeletal: Arthralgia
  Respiratory: Pharyngitis
<1%:
  Cardiovascular: Edema, palpitations
  Central nervous system: Depression
  Dermatologic: Angioedema, photosensitivity, rash
  Hepatic: Hepatitis
  Neuromuscular & skeletal: Myalgia, paresthesia
  Respiratory: Bronchospasm
  Miscellaneous: Epistaxis

Overdosage/Toxicology Symptoms of overdose include anemia, metabolic acidosis, hypotension, hypothermia; there is no specific treatment for an antihistamine overdose, however, most of its clinical toxicity is due to anticholinergic effects. For anticholinergic overdose with severe life-threatening symptoms, physostigmine 1-2 mg (0.5 or 0.02 mg/kg for children) I.V., slowly may be given to reverse these effects.

Drug Interactions Increased toxicity (CNS depression): CNS depressants, MAO inhibitors, tricyclic antidepressants, phenothiazines

Mechanism of Action Competes with histamine for H_1-receptor sites on effector cells in the gastrointestinal tract, blood vessels, and respiratory tract

Pharmacodynamics/Kinetics
  Peak therapeutic effect: Within 5-7 hours
  Absorption: Almost 100% from GI tract
  Metabolism: In the liver
  Elimination: In urine

Usual Dosage Oral:
  Children: <12 years: 0.4-1 mg twice daily

  Children >12 years and Adults: 1.34 mg twice daily to 2.68 mg 3 times/day; do not exceed 8.04 mg/day; lower doses should be considered in patients >60 years

Monitoring Parameters Look for a reduction of rhinitis, urticaria, eczema, pruritus, or other allergic symptoms

Patient Information Avoid alcohol; may cause drowsiness, may impair coordination or judgment

Nursing Implications Raise bed rails, institute safety measures, assist with ambulation

Dosage Forms
  Syrup (citrus flavor): 0.67 mg/5 mL with alcohol 5.5% (120 mL)
  Tablet: 1.34 mg, 2.68 mg

Cleocin HCl® *see* Clindamycin *on this page*

Cleocin Pediatric® *see* Clindamycin *on this page*

Cleocin Phosphate® *see* Clindamycin *on this page*

Cleocin T® *see* Clindamycin *on this page*

C-Lexin® *see* Cephalexin Monohydrate *on page 210*

Clindamycin *(klin da mye' sin)*

Related Information
  Antimicrobial Drugs of Choice *on page 1298-1302*
  Prevention of Bacterial Endocarditis *on page 1285-1288*

Brand Names Cleocin HCl®; Cleocin Pediatric®; Cleocin Phosphate®; Cleocin T®

Use Treatment against aerobic and anaerobic streptococci (except enterococci), most staphylococci, *Bacteroides* sp and *Actinomyces*; used topically in treatment of severe acne, vaginally for *Gardnerella vaginalis*, alternate treatment for toxoplasmosis, PCP

Pregnancy Risk Factor B

Contraindications Hypersensitivity to clindamycin or any component; previous pseudomembranous colitis, hepatic impairment

Warnings/Precautions Dosage adjustment may be necessary in patients with severe hepatic dysfunction; no change necessary with renal insufficiency; can cause severe and possibly fatal colitis; use with caution in patients with a history of pseudomembranous colitis; discontinue drug if significant diarrhea, abdominal cramps, or passage of blood and mucus occurs

Adverse Reactions
>10%: Gastrointestinal: Diarrhea
1% to 10%:
  Dermatologic: Skin rashes
  Gastrointestinal: Pseudomembranous colitis, nausea, vomiting
<1%:
  Cardiovascular: Hypotension
  Dermatologic: Urticaria, Stevens-Johnson syndrome
  Hematologic: Eosinophilia, neutropenia, granulocytopenia, thrombocytopenia
  Hepatic: Elevation of liver enzymes
  Local: Thrombophlebitis, sterile abscess at I.M. injection site
  Neuromuscular & skeletal: Polyarthritis
  Renal: Rare renal dysfunction

Overdosage/Toxicology Symptoms of overdose include diarrhea, nausea, vomiting; following GI decontamination, treatment is supportive

Drug Interactions Increased duration of neuromuscular blockade from tubocurarine, pancuronium

Stability Do **not** refrigerate reconstituted oral solution because it will thicken; oral solution is stable for 2 weeks at room temperature following reconstitution; I.V. infusion solution in NS or D_5W solution is stable for 24 hours at room temperature

Mechanism of Action Reversibly binds to 50S ribosomal subunits preventing peptide bond formation thus inhibiting bacterial protein synthesis; bacteriostatic or bactericidal depending on drug concentration, infection site, and organism

Pharmacodynamics/Kinetics
Absorption: ~10% of topically applied drug is absorbed systemically; 90% absorbed rapidly from GI tract following oral administration
Distribution: No significant levels are seen in CSF, even with inflamed meninges; crosses the placenta; distributes into breast milk; high concentrations in bone, bile, and urine
Metabolism: Hepatic
Half-life:
  Neonates:
    Premature: 8.7 hours
    Full-term: 3.6 hours
  Adults: 1.6-5.3 hours, average: 2-3 hours
Time to peak serum concentration:
  Oral: Within 60 minutes
  I.M.: Within 1-3 hours
Elimination: Most of drug eliminated by hepatic metabolism

Usual Dosage Avoid in neonates (contains benzyl alcohol)
Neonates: I.M., I.V.:
  Postnatal age <7 days:
    ≤2000 g: 10 mg/kg/day in 2 equally divided doses
    >2000 g: 15 mg/kg/day in 3 divided doses
  Postnatal age >7 days:
    <1200 g: 10 mg/kg/day in 2 equally divided doses
    1200-2000 g: 15 mg/kg/day in 3 divided doses
    >2000 g: 20 mg/kg/day in 3-4 divided doses
Infants and Children:
  Oral: 10-30 mg/kg/day in 3-4 divided doses
  I.M., I.V.: 25-40 mg/kg/day in 3-4 divided doses
Children and Adults: Topical: Apply twice daily
Adults:
  Oral: 150-450 mg/dose every 6-8 hours; maximum dose: 1.8 g/day
  I.M., I.V.: 1.2-1.8 g/day in 2-4 divided doses; maximum dose: 4.8 g/day
Pneumocystis carinii pneumonia:
  Oral: 300-450 mg 4 times/day with primaquine
  I.M., I.V.: 1200-2400 mg/day with pyrimethamine
  I.V.: 600 mg 4 times/day with primaquine
Vaginal: One full applicator (100 mg) inserted intravaginally once daily before bedtime for seven consecutive days
Topical: Apply a thin film twice daily

Dosing adjustment in hepatic impairment: Adjustment recommended in patients with severe hepatic disease

Administration Administer oral dosage form with a full glass of water to minimize esophageal ulceration; give around-the-clock to promote less variation in peak and trough serum levels

Monitoring Parameters Observe for changes in bowel frequency, monitor for colitis and resolution of symptoms; during prolonged therapy monitor CBC, liver and renal function tests periodically

Patient Information Report any severe diarrhea immediately and do not take antidiarrheal medication; take each oral dose with a full glass of water; finish all
(Continued)
255

Clindamycin *(Continued)*

medication; do not skip doses; should not engage in sexual intercourse during treatment with vaginal product; avoid contact of topical gel/solution with eyes, abraded skin, or mucous membranes

Dosage Forms

Capsule, as hydrochloride: 75 mg, 150 mg, 300 mg

Cream, vaginal: 2% (40 g)

Gel, topical, as phosphate: 1% [10 mg/g] (7.5 g, 30 g)

Granules for oral solution, as palmitate: 75 mg/5 mL (100 mL)

Infusion, as phosphate, in D_5W: 300 mg (50 mL); 600 mg (50 mL)

Injection, as phosphate: 150 mg/mL (2 mL, 4 mL, 6 mL, 50 mL, 60 mL)

Solution, topical, as phosphate: 1% [10 mg/mL] (30 mL, 60 mL, 480 mL)

Clinoril® *see* Sulindac *on page 1048*

Clioquinol *see* Iodochlorhydroxyquin *on page 588*

Clobetasol Propionate *(kloe bay' ta sol dye pro pee oh' nate)*

Related Information

Corticosteroids Comparisons *on page 1266-1268*

Brand Names Temovate®

Use Short-term relief of inflammation of moderate to severe corticosteroid-responsive dermatosis (very high potency topical corticosteroid)

Pregnancy Risk Factor C

Contraindications Known hypersensitivity to clobetasol; viral, fungal, or tubercular skin lesions

Warnings/Precautions Adrenal suppression can occur if used for >14 days

Adverse Reactions

1% to 10%: Local: Itching, burning, erythema, dryness, irritation, papular rashes

<1%: Local: Hypertrichosis, acneiform eruptions, hypopigmentation, perioral dermatitis, maceration of skin, skin atrophy, striae, miliaria

Mechanism of Action Stimulates the synthesis of enzymes needed to decrease inflammation, suppress mitotic activity, and cause vasoconstriction

Pharmacodynamics/Kinetics

Absorption: Percutaneous absorption variable and dependent upon many factors including vehicle used, integrity of epidermis, dose, and use of occlusive dressings

Metabolism: Remains to be defined

Elimination: In urine and bile

Usual Dosage Adults: Topical: Apply twice daily for up to 2 weeks with no more than 50 g/week

Patient Information A thin film of cream or ointment is effective; do not overuse; do not use tight-fitting diapers or plastic pants on children being treated in the diaper area; use only as prescribed and for no longer than the period prescribed; apply sparingly in light film; rub in lightly; avoid contact with eyes; notify physician if condition being treated persists or worsens

Nursing Implications For external use only; do not use on open wounds; apply sparingly to occlusive dressings; should not be used in the presence of open or weeping lesions

Dosage Forms

Cream, topical: 0.05% (15 g, 30 g, 45 g)

Ointment, topical: 0.05% (15 g, 30 g, 45 g)

Scalp application: 0.05% (25 mL, 50 mL)

Clocort® Maximum Strength *see* Hydrocortisone *on page 546*

Clocortolone Pivalate *(kloe kor' toe lone)*

Related Information

Corticosteroids Comparisons *on page 1266-1268*

Brand Names Cloderm®

Use Inflammation of corticosteroid-responsive dermatoses (medium potency topical corticosteroid)

Pregnancy Risk Factor C

Contraindications Known hypersensitivity to clocortolone; viral, fungal, or tubercular skin lesions

Warnings/Precautions Adrenal suppression can occur if used for >14 days

Adverse Reactions

1% to 10%: Local: Itching, burning, erythema, dryness, irritation, papular rashes

<1%: Local: Hypertrichosis, acneiform eruptions, hypopigmentation, perioral dermatitis, maceration of skin, skin atrophy, striae, miliaria

Mechanism of Action Stimulates the synthesis of enzymes needed to decrease inflammation, suppress mitotic activity, and cause vasoconstriction

Pharmacodynamics/Kinetics

Absorption: Percutaneous absorption is variable and dependent upon many factors including vehicle used, integrity of epidermis, dose, and use of occlusive dressings;

Distribution: Small amounts enter systemic circulation mostly throughout skin

Metabolism: Remains to be defined (largely in liver)

Elimination: In urine and bile

Usual Dosage Adults: Apply sparingly and gently; rub into affected area from 1-4 times/day

Patient Information A thin film of cream or ointment is effective; do not overuse; do not use tight-fitting diapers or plastic pants on children being treated in the diaper area; use only as prescribed, and for no longer than the period prescribed; apply sparingly in light film; rub in lightly; avoid contact with eyes; notify physician if condition being treated persists or worsens

Nursing Implications For external use only; do not use on open wounds; apply sparingly to occlusive dressings; should not be used in the presence of open or weeping lesions

Dosage Forms Cream: 0.1% (15 g, 45 g)

Cloderm® *see* Clocortolone Pivalate *on previous page*

Clofazimine Palmitate (kloe fa′ zi meen)

Brand Names Lamprene®

Use Treatment of dapsone-resistant leprosy; multibacillary dapsone-sensitive leprosy; erythema nodosum leprosum; *Mycobacterium avium-intracellulare* (MAI) infections

Pregnancy Risk Factor C

Contraindications Hypersensitivity to clofazimine or any component

Warnings/Precautions Use with caution in patients with GI problems; dosages >100 mg/day should be used for as short a duration as possible; skin discoloration may lead to depression

Adverse Reactions

>10%:

Dermatologic: Dry skin

Gastrointestinal: Abdominal pain, nausea, vomiting, diarrhea

Miscellaneous: Pink to brownish-black discoloration of the skin and conjunctiva

1% to 10%:

Dermatologic: Rash, pruritus

Endocrine & metabolic: Elevated blood sugar

Ocular: Irritation of the eyes

Miscellaneous: Discoloration of urine, feces, sputum, sweat

<1%:

Cardiovascular: Edema, vascular pain

Central nervous system: Dizziness, drowsiness, fatigue, headache, giddiness, neuralgia, taste disorder, fever

Dermatologic: Erythroderma, acneiform eruptions, monilial cheilosis, phototoxicity

Endocrine & metabolic: Hypokalemia

Gastrointestinal: Bowel obstruction, GI bleeding, anorexia, constipation, weight loss, eosinophilic enteritis

Genitourinary: Cystitis

Hematologic: Eosinophilia, anemia

Hepatic: Hepatitis, jaundice, enlarged liver, elevated albumin, serum bilirubin and AST

Neuromuscular & skeletal: Bone pain

Ocular: Diminished vision

Miscellaneous: Lymphadenopathy

Overdosage/Toxicology Following GI decontamination, treatment is supportive

Drug Interactions Decreased effect with dapsone (unconfirmed)

Mechanism of Action Binds preferentially to mycobacterial DNA to inhibit mycobacterial growth; also has some anti-inflammatory activity through an unknown mechanism

Pharmacodynamics/Kinetics

Absorption: Oral: 45% to 70% absorbed slowly

Distribution: Remains in tissues for prolonged periods; appears in breast milk; highly lipophilic; deposited primarily in fatty tissue and cells of the reticuloendothelial system; taken up by macrophages throughout the body; also distributed to breast milk, mesenteric lymph nodes, adrenal glands, subcutaneous fat, liver, bile, gallbladder, spleen, small intestine, muscles, bones, and skin; does not appear to cross blood-brain barrier

(Continued)

Clofazimine Palmitate *(Continued)*

Metabolism: Partially in the liver to two metabolites

Half-life:

Terminal: 8 days

Tissue: 70 days

Time to peak serum concentration: 1-6 hours with chronic therapy

Elimination: Mainly in feces; negligible amounts excreted unchanged in urine; small amounts excreted in sputum, saliva, and sweat

Usual Dosage Oral:

Children: Leprosy: 1 mg/kg/day every 24 hours in combination with dapsone and rifampin

Adults:

Dapsone-resistant leprosy: 100 mg/day in combination with one or more antileprosy drugs for 3 years; then alone 100 mg/day

Dapsone-sensitive multibacillary leprosy: 100 mg/day in combination with two or more antileprosy drugs for at least 2 years and continue until negative skin smears are obtained, then institute single drug therapy with appropriate agent

Erythema nodosum leprosum: 100-200 mg/day for up to 3 months or longer then taper dose to 100 mg/day when possible

Pyoderma gangrenosum: 300-400 mg/day for up to 12 months

Dosing adjustment in hepatic impairment: Should be considered in severe hepatic dysfunction

Monitoring Parameters GI complaints

Test Interactions ↑ ESR, ↑ glucose (S), ↑ albumin, ↑ bilirubin, ↑ AST

Patient Information Drug may cause a pink to brownish-black discoloration of the skin, conjunctiva, tears, sweat, urine, feces, and nasal secretions; although reversible, may take months to years to disappear after therapy is complete; take with meals

Dosage Forms Capsule: 50 mg, 100 mg

Clofibrate *(kloe fye' brate)*

Related Information

Lipid-Lowering Agents *on page 1273*

Brand Names Atromid-S®

Use Adjunct to dietary therapy in the management of hyperlipidemias associated with high triglyceride levels (types III, IV, V); primarily lowers triglycerides and very low density lipoprotein

Pregnancy Risk Factor C

Contraindications Hypersensitivity to clofibrate or any component, severe hepatic or renal impairment, primary biliary cirrhosis

Warnings/Precautions Clofibrate has been shown to be tumorigenic in animal studies; increased risk of cholelithiasis, cholecystitis; discontinue if lipid response is not obtained; no evidence substantiates a beneficial effect on cardiovascular mortality

Adverse Reactions

>10%: Gastrointestinal: Nausea

1% to 10%: Gastrointestinal: Diarrhea, vomiting, dyspepsia, flatulence, abdominal distress

<1%:

Cardiovascular: Angina, cardiac arrhythmias

Central nervous system: Headache, dizziness, fatigue

Dermatologic: Skin rash, urticaria, pruritus, alopecia

Gastrointestinal: Gallstones

Genitourinary: Impotence

Hematologic: Leukopenia, anemia, eosinophilia, agranulocytosis

Hepatic: Increased liver function test

Neuromuscular & skeletal: Muscle cramping, aching, weakness, myalgia

Renal: Renal toxicity, rhabdomyolysis-induced renal failure

Miscellaneous: Dry, brittle hair

Overdosage/Toxicology Symptoms of overdose include nausea, vomiting, diarrhea, GI distress; following GI decontamination, treatment is supportive

Drug Interactions

Increased effect: Effects of warfarin, insulin, and sulfonylureas may be increased

Increased toxicity/levels: Clofibrate's levels may be increased with probenecid

Mechanism of Action Mechanism is unclear but thought to reduce cholesterol synthesis and triglyceride hepatic-vascular transference

Pharmacodynamics/Kinetics

Absorption: Occurs completely; intestinal transformation is required to activate the drug

Distribution: V_d: 5.5 L/kg; crosses the placenta

Protein binding: 95%

Metabolism: In the liver to an inactive glucuronide ester

Half-life: 6-24 hours, increases significantly with reduced renal function; with anuria: 110 hours

Time to peak serum concentration: Within 3-6 hours

Elimination: 40% to 70% excreted in urine

Usual Dosage Adults: Oral: 500 mg 4 times/day; some patients may respond to lower doses

Dosing interval in renal impairment:

Cl_{cr} >50 mL/minute: Administer every 6-12 hours

Cl_{cr} 10-50 mL/minute: Administer every 12-18 hours

Cl_{cr} <10 mL/minute: Avoid use

Elimination is not enhanced via hemodialysis; supplemental dose is not necessary

Monitoring Parameters Serum lipids, cholesterol and triglycerides, LFTs, CBC

Test Interactions ↑ creatine phosphokinase [CPK] (S); ↓ alkaline phosphatase (S), cholesterol (S), glucose, uric acid (S)

Patient Information If GI upset occurs, may be taken with food; notify physician of chest pain, shortness of breath, irregular heartbeat, severe stomach pain with nausea and vomiting, persistent fever, sore throat, or unusual bleeding or bruising; adhere to prescribed diet

Dosage Forms Capsule: 500 mg

Clomid® see Clomiphene Citrate on this page

Clomiphene Citrate (kloe′ mi feen)

Brand Names Clomid®; Serophene®

Use Treatment of ovulatory failure in patients desiring pregnancy

Unlabeled use: Male infertility

Pregnancy Risk Factor X

Contraindications Liver disease, abnormal uterine bleeding, suspected pregnancy, enlargement or development of ovarian cyst, uncontrolled thyroid or adrenal dysfunction

Warnings/Precautions Patients unusually sensitive to pituitary gonadotropins (eg, polycystic ovary disease); multiple pregnancies, blurring or other visual symptoms can occur

Adverse Reactions

>10%: Endocrine & metabolic: Hot flashes, ovarian enlargement

1% to 10%:

Cardiovascular: Thromboembolism

Central nervous system: Mental depression, headache

Endocrine & metabolic: Breast enlargement (males), abnormal menstrual flow

Gastrointestinal: Distention, bloating, nausea, vomiting, hepatotoxicity

Ocular: Blurring of vision, diplopia, floaters, after-images, phosphenes, photophobia

<1%:

Central nervous system: Insomnia, fatigue

Dermatologic: Alopecia (reversible)

Gastrointestinal: Weight gain

Genitourinary: Increased urination

Stability Protect from light

Mechanism of Action Induces ovulation by stimulating the release of pituitary gonadotropins

Pharmacodynamics/Kinetics

Half-life: 5-7 days

Elimination: Enterohepatically circulated; excreted primarily in feces with small amounts appearing in urine

Usual Dosage Adults: Oral:

Males (infertility): 25 mg/day for 25 days with 5 days rest, or 100 mg every Monday, Wednesday, Friday

Females (ovulatory failure): Oral: 50 mg/day for 5 days (first course); start the regimen on or about the fifth day of cycle; if ovulation occurs do not increase dosage; if not, increase next course to 100 mg/day for 5 days. Three courses of therapy are an adequate therapeutic trial. Further treatment is not recommended in patients who do not exhibit ovulation.

(Continued)

Clomiphene Citrate *(Continued)*

Reference Range FSH and LH are expected to peak 5-9 days after completing clomiphene; ovulation assessed by basal body temperature or serum progesterone 2 weeks after last clomiphene dose

Test Interactions Clomiphene may increase levels of serum thyroxine and thyroxine-binding globulin (TBG)

Patient Information May cause visual disturbances, dizziness, lightheadedness; if possibility of pregnancy, stop the drug and consult your physician

Dosage Forms Tablet: 50 mg

Clomipramine Hydrochloride (kloe mi' pra meen)

Related Information

Antidepressant Agents Comparison *on page 1250-1252*

Brand Names Anafranil®

Use Treatment of obsessive-compulsive disorder (OCD); may also relieve depression, panic attacks, and chronic pain

Pregnancy Risk Factor C

Contraindications Patients in acute recovery stage of recent myocardial infarction; not to be used within 14 days of MAO inhibitors

Warnings/Precautions Seizures are likely and are dose-related; can be additive when coadministered with other drugs that can lower the seizure threshold; use with caution in patients with asthma, bladder outlet destruction, narrow-angle glaucoma

Adverse Reactions

>10%:

Central nervous system: Dizziness, drowsiness, headache

Gastrointestinal: Dry mouth, constipation, increased appetite, nausea, weakness, unpleasant taste, weight gain

1% to 10%:

Cardiovascular: Arrhythmias, hypotension

Central nervous system: Confusion, delirium, hallucinations, nervousness, restlessness, parkinsonian syndrome, insomnia

Gastrointestinal: Diarrhea, heartburn

Genitourinary: Difficult urination, sexual function impairment

Neuromuscular & skeletal: Fine muscle tremors

Ocular: Blurred vision, eye pain

Miscellaneous: Excessive sweating

<1%:

Central nervous system: Anxiety, seizures

Dermatologic: Alopecia, photosensitivity

Endocrine & metabolic: Breast enlargement, galactorrhea, SIADH

Genitourinary: Testicular swelling

Hematologic: Agranulocytosis, leukopenia, eosinophilia

Hepatic: Cholestatic jaundice, increased liver enzymes

Ocular: Increased intraocular pressure

Otic: Tinnitus

Miscellaneous: Trouble with gums, decreased lower esophageal sphincter tone may cause GE reflux, allergic reactions

Overdosage/Toxicology Symptoms of overdose include agitation, confusion, hallucinations, urinary retention, hypothermia, hypotension, tachycardia, ventricular tachycardia, seizures, coma

Following initiation of essential overdose management, toxic symptoms should be treated. Ventricular arrhythmias and EKG abnormalities (eg, QRS widening) often respond to systemic alkalinization (sodium bicarbonate 0.5-2 mEq/kg I.V.) and/or phenytoin 15-20 mg/kg (adults). Arrhythmias unresponsive to this therapy may respond to lidocaine 1 mg/kg I.V. followed by a titrated infusion. Physostigmine (1-2 mg I.V. slowly for adults or 0.5 mg I.V. slowly for children) may be indicated in reversing cardiac arrhythmias that are life-threatening. Seizures usually respond to diazepam I.V. boluses (5-10 mg for adults up to 30 mg or 0.25-0.4 mg/kg/dose for children up to 10 mg/dose). If seizures are unresponsive or recur, phenytoin or phenobarbital may be required.

Drug Interactions

Decreased effect with barbiturates, carbamazepine, phenytoin

Increased effect of alcohol, CNS depressants, anticholinergics, sympathomimetics

Increased toxicity: MAO inhibitors ($\uparrow$ temperature, seizures, coma, and death)

Mechanism of Action Clomipramine appears to affect serotonin uptake while its active metabolite, desmethylclomipramine, affects norepinephrine uptake

Pharmacodynamics/Kinetics

Absorption: Oral: Rapid

Metabolism: Extensive first-pass metabolism; metabolized to desmethyl-clomipramine (active) in the liver

Half-life: 20-30 hours

Usual Dosage Oral: Initial:

Children: 25 mg/day and gradually increase, as tolerated, to a maximum of 3 mg/kg/day or 200 mg/day, whichever is smaller

Adults: 25 mg/day and gradually increase, as tolerated, to 100 mg/day the first 2 weeks, may then be increased to a total of 250 mg/day maximum

Test Interactions ↑ glucose

Patient Information May cause seizures; caution should be used in activities that require alertness like driving, operating machinery, or swimming; effect of drug may take several weeks to appear

Dosage Forms Capsule: 25 mg, 50 mg, 75 mg

Clonazepam (kloe na′ ze pam)

Related Information

Benzodiazepines Comparison on page 1256

Brand Names Klonopin™

Use Prophylaxis of petit mal, petit mal variant (Lennox-Gastaut), akinetic, and myoclonic seizures

Unlabeled use: Restless legs syndrome, neuralgia, multifocal tic disorder, parkinsonian dysarthria, acute manic episodes, and adjunct therapy for schizophrenia

Restrictions C-IV

Pregnancy Risk Factor C

Contraindications Hypersensitivity to clonazepam, any component, or other benzodiazepines; severe liver disease, acute narrow-angle glaucoma

Warnings/Precautions Use with caution in patients with chronic respiratory disease or impaired renal function; abrupt discontinuance may precipitate withdrawal symptoms, status epilepticus or seizures, in patients with a history of substance abuse; clonazepam-induced behavioral disturbances may be more frequent in mentally handicapped patients

Adverse Reactions

>10%:

Cardiovascular: Tachycardia, chest pain

Central nervous system: Drowsiness, fatigue, impaired coordination, lightheadedness, memory impairment, insomnia, anxiety, depression, headache

Dermatologic: Rash

Endocrine & metabolic: Decreased libido

Gastrointestinal: Dry mouth, constipation, diarrhea, nausea, increased or decreased appetite, vomiting

Neuromuscular & skeletal: Dysarthria

Ocular: Blurred vision

Miscellaneous: Decreased salivation sweating

1% to 10%:

Cardiovascular: Syncope, hypotension

Central nervous system: Confusion, nervousness, dizziness, akathisia

Dermatologic: Dermatitis

Gastrointestinal: Weight gain or loss

Neuromuscular & skeletal: Rigidity, tremor, muscle cramps

Otic: Tinnitus

Respiratory: Nasal congestion, hyperventilation

Miscellaneous: Increased salivation

<1%:

Central nervous system: Reflex slowing

Endocrine & metabolic: Menstrual irregularities

Hematologic: Blood dyscrasias

Miscellaneous: Drug dependence

Overdosage/Toxicology May produce somnolence, confusion, ataxia, diminished reflexes, or coma

Treatment for benzodiazepine overdose is supportive. Rarely is mechanical ventilation required.

Flumazenil has been shown to selectively block the binding of benzodiazepines to CNS receptors, resulting in a reversal of benzodiazepine-induced CNS depression, but not respiratory depression

Drug Interactions

Decreased effect: Phenytoin, barbiturates → ↑ clonazepam clearance

Increased toxicity: CNS depressants → ↑ sedation

Mechanism of Action Suppresses the spike-and-wave discharge in absence seizures by depressing nerve transmission in the motor cortex

Pharmacodynamics/Kinetics

Onset of effect: 20-60 minutes

(Continued)

Clonazepam (Continued)

Duration: Up to 6-8 hours in infants and young children, up to 12 hours in adults

Absorption: Oral: Well absorbed

Distribution: Adults: V_d: 1.5-4.4 L/kg

Protein binding: 85%

Metabolism: Extensive; glucuronide and sulfate conjugation

Half-life:

Children: 22-33 hours

Adults: 19-50 hours

Time to peak serum concentration: Oral: 1-3 hours

Steady-state: 5-7 days

Elimination: <2% excreted unchanged in urine; metabolites excreted as glucuronide or sulfate conjugates

Usual Dosage Oral:

Children <10 years or 30 kg:

Initial daily dose: 0.01-0.03 mg/kg/day (maximum: 0.05 mg/kg/day) given in 2-3 divided doses; increase by no more than 0.5 mg every third day until seizures are controlled or adverse effects seen

Usual maintenance dose: 0.1-0.2 mg/kg/day divided 3 times/day; not to exceed 0.2 mg/kg/day

Adults:

Initial daily dose not to exceed 1.5 mg given in 3 divided doses; may increase by 0.5-1 mg every third day until seizures are controlled or adverse effects seen

Usual maintenance dose: 0.05-0.2 mg/kg; do not exceed 20 mg/day

Hemodialysis effects: Supplemental dose is not necessary

Reference Range Relationship between serum concentration and seizure control is not well established

Timing of serum samples: Peak serum levels occur 1-3 hours after oral ingestion; the half-life is 20-40 hours; therefore, steady-state occurs in 5-7 days

Therapeutic levels: 20-80 ng/mL; Toxic concentration: >80 ng/mL

Patient Information Avoid alcohol and other CNS depressants; avoid activities needing good psychomotor coordination until CNS effects are known; drug may cause physical or psychological dependence; avoid abrupt discontinuation after prolonged use

Nursing Implications Observe patient for excess sedation, respiratory depression; raise bed rails, initiate safety measures, assist with ambulation

Dosage Forms Tablet: 0.5 mg, 1 mg, 2 mg

Clonidine (kloe' ni deen)

Brand Names Catapres®; Catapres-TTS®

Use Management of mild to moderate hypertension; either used alone or in combination with other antihypertensives; not recommended for first-line therapy for hypertension; also used for heroin withdrawal and in smoking cessation therapy; other uses may include prophylaxis of migraines, glaucoma, paralytic ileus, and diabetes-associated diarrhea

Pregnancy Risk Factor C

Contraindications Hypersensitivity to clonidine hydrochloride or any component

Warnings/Precautions Use with caution in cerebrovascular disease, coronary insufficiency, renal impairment, sinus node dysfunction; do not abruptly discontinue (rapid increase in blood pressure, and symptoms of sympathetic overactivity, ie, increased heart rate, tremor, agitation, anxiety, insomnia, sweating, palpitations) may occur; **if need to discontinue, taper dose gradually over more than 1 week**; adjust dosage in patients with renal dysfunction (especially the elderly)

Adverse Reactions

>10%:

Central nervous system: Drowsiness, dizziness

Gastrointestinal: Dry mouth, constipation

1% to 10%:

Cardiovascular: Orthostatic hypotension

Central nervous system: Nervousness, agitation, mental depression, headache, weakness, fatigue

Dermatologic: Rash

Endocrine & metabolic: Decreased sexual activity, impotence, loss of libido

Gastrointestinal: Nausea, vomiting

Genitourinary: Nocturia

Hepatic: Abnormal liver function tests

<1%:

Cardiovascular: Palpitations, tachycardia, bradycardia, Raynaud's phenomenon, congestive heart failure

Central nervous system: Insomnia, vivid dreams, delirium, fever

Dermatologic: Pruritus, hives, urticaria, alopecia

Endocrine & metabolic: Gynecomastia

Gastrointestinal: Weight gain

Genitourinary: Difficulty in micturition, urinary retention

Ocular: Burning of the eyes, blurred vision

Overdosage/Toxicology Symptoms of overdose include bradycardia, CNS depression, hypothermia, diarrhea, respiratory depression, apnea; treatment is primarily supportive and symptomatic. Hypotension usually responds to I.V. fluids or Trendelenburg positioning. Naloxone may be utilized in treating the CNS depression and/or apnea and should be given I.V. 0.4-2 mg, with repeated doses as needed.

Drug Interactions

Decreased effect: Tricyclic antidepressants antagonize hypotensive effects of clonidine

Increased toxicity: Beta-blockers may potentiate bradycardia in patients receiving clonidine and may increase the rebound hypertension of withdrawal; discontinue beta-blocker several days before clonidine is tapered

Mechanism of Action Stimulates alpha$_2$-adrenoreceptors in the brain stem, thus activating an inhibitory neuron, resulting in reduced sympathetic outflow, producing a decrease in vasomotor tone and heart rate

Pharmacodynamics/Kinetics

Onset of effect: Oral: 0.5-1 hour

Peak effect: Within 2-4 hours

Duration: 6-10 hours

Distribution: V$_d$: 2.1 L/kg (adults)

Metabolism: Hepatic (enterohepatic recirculation); metabolized to inactive metabolites

Bioavailability: 75% to 95%

Half-life: Adults:

Normal renal function: 6-20 hours

Renal impairment: 18-41 hours

Elimination: 65% excreted in urine, 32% unchanged, and 22% excreted in feces

Usual Dosage

Oral:

Children: Initial: 5-10 mcg/kg/day in divided doses every 8-12 hours; increase gradually at 5- to 7-day intervals to 25 mcg/kg/day in divided doses every 6 hours; maximum: 0.9 mg/day

Clonidine tolerance test (test of growth hormone release from pituitary): 0.15 mg/m^2 or 4 mcg/kg as single dose

Adults: Initial dose: 0.1 mg twice daily, usual maintenance dose: 0.2-1.2 mg/day in 2-4 divided doses; maximum recommended dose: 2.4 mg/day

Elderly: Initial: 0.1 mg once daily at bedtime, increase gradually as needed

Transdermal: Apply once every 7 days; for initial therapy start with 0.1 mg and increase by 0.1 mg at 1- to 2-week intervals; dosages >0.6 mg do not improve efficacy

Dosing adjustment in renal impairment: Cl$_{cr}$ <10 mL/minute: Administer 50% to 75% of normal dose initially

Not dialyzable (0% to 5%) via hemo- or peritoneal dialysis; supplemental dose not necessary

Monitoring Parameters Blood pressure, standing and sitting/supine, mental status, heart rate

Reference Range Therapeutic: 1-2 ng/mL (SI: 4.4-8.7 nmol/L)

Test Interactions ↑ sodium (S); ↓ catecholamines (U)

Patient Information Do not discontinue drug except on instruction of physician; check daily to be sure patch is present; may cause drowsiness, impaired coordination, and judgment

Nursing Implications Patches should be applied weekly at bedtime to a clean, hairless area of the upper outer arm or chest; rotate patch sites weekly; redness under patch may be reduced if a topical corticosteroid spray is applied to the area before placement of the patch; if needed, gradually reduce dose over 2-4 days to avoid rebound hypertension

Dosage Forms

Patch, transdermal: 1, 2, and 3 (0.1 mg, 0.2 mg, 0.3 mg/day to 7-day duration)

Tablet, as hydrochloride: 0.1 mg, 0.2 mg, 0.3 mg

Clopra® see Metoclopramide on page 728

Clorazepate Dipotassium (klor az' e pate)

Related Information

Benzodiazepines Comparison *on page 1256*

Brand Names Gen-XENE®; Tranxene®

Use Treatment of generalized anxiety and panic disorders; management of alcohol withdrawal; adjunct anticonvulsant in management of partial seizures

Restrictions C-IV

Pregnancy Risk Factor D

Contraindications Hypersensitivity to clorazepate dipotassium or any component; cross-sensitivity with other benzodiazepines may exist; avoid using in patients with pre-existing CNS depression, severe uncontrolled pain, or narrow-angle glaucoma

Warnings/Precautions Use with caution in patients with hepatic or renal disease; abrupt discontinuation may cause withdrawal symptoms or seizures

Adverse Reactions

>10%:

Cardiovascular: Tachycardia, chest pain

Central nervous system: Drowsiness, fatigue, impaired coordination, lightheadedness, memory impairment, insomnia, anxiety, headache, depression

Dermatologic: Rash

Endocrine & metabolic: Decreased libido

Gastrointestinal: Dry mouth, constipation, diarrhea, decreased salivation, nausea, vomiting, increased or decreased appetite

Neuromuscular & skeletal: Dysarthria

Ocular: Blurred vision

Miscellaneous: Sweating

1% to 10%:

Cardiovascular: Syncope, hypotension

Central nervous system: Confusion, nervousness, dizziness, akathisia

Dermatologic: Dermatitis

Gastrointestinal: Nausea, increased salivation, weight gain or loss

Neuromuscular & skeletal: Rigidity, tremor, muscle cramps

Otic: Tinnitus

Respiratory: Nasal congestion, hyperventilation

<1%:

Central nervous system: Reflex slowing

Endocrine & metabolic: Menstrual irregularities

Hematologic: Blood dyscrasias

Miscellaneous: Drug dependence, long-term use may also be associated with renal or hepatic injury and reduced hematocrit

Overdosage/Toxicology May produce somnolence, confusion, ataxia, diminished reflexes, coma. Treatment for benzodiazepine overdose is supportive; rarely is mechanical ventilation required; flumazenil has been shown to selectively block the binding of benzodiazepines to CNS receptors, resulting in a reversal of benzodiazepine-induced CNS depression, but not respiratory depression.

Drug Interactions Increased effect: Cimetidine, CNS depressants, alcohol

Stability Unstable in water

Mechanism of Action Facilitates gamma aminobutyric acid (GABA)-mediated transmission inhibitory neurotransmitter action, depresses subcortical levels of CNS

Pharmacodynamics/Kinetics

Distribution: Crosses the placenta; appears in urine

Metabolism: Rapidly decarboxylated to desmethyldiazepam (active) in acidic stomach prior to absorption; metabolized in the liver to oxazepam (active)

Half-life: Adults:

Desmethyldiazepam: 48-96 hours

Oxazepam: 6-8 hours

Time to peak serum concentration: Oral: Within 1 hour

Elimination: Primarily in urine

Usual Dosage Oral:

Children 9-12 years: Anticonvulsant: Initial: 3.75-7.5 mg/dose twice daily; increase dose by 3.75 mg at weekly intervals, not to exceed 60 mg/day in 2-3 divided doses

Children >12 years and Adults: Anticonvulsant: Initial: Up to 7.5 mg/dose 2-3 times/day; increase dose by 7.5 mg at weekly intervals; not to exceed 90 mg/day

Adults:

Anxiety: 7.5-15 mg 2-4 times/day, or given as single dose of 11.25 or 22.5 mg at bedtime

Alcohol withdrawal: Initial: 30 mg, then 15 mg 2-4 times/day on first day; maximum daily dose: 90 mg; gradually decrease dose over subsequent days

Monitoring Parameters Respiratory and cardiovascular status, excess CNS depression

Reference Range Therapeutic: 0.12-1 µg/mL (SI: 0.36-3.01 µmol/L)

Test Interactions ↓ hematocrit, abnormal liver and renal function tests

Patient Information Avoid alcohol and other CNS depressants; avoid activities needing good psychomotor coordination until CNS effects are known; drug may cause physical or psychological dependence; avoid abrupt discontinuation after prolonged use

Nursing Implications Observe patient for excess sedation, respiratory depression; raise bed rails, initiate safety measures, assist with ambulation

Dosage Forms
Capsule: 3.75 mg, 7.5 mg, 15 mg
Tablet: 3.75 mg, 7.5 mg, 15 mg
Tablet, single dose: 11.25 mg, 22.5 mg

Clotrimazole (kloe trim' a zole)

Brand Names Femcare® [OTC]; Gyne-Lotrimin® [OTC]; Lotrimin®; Lotrimin AF® [OTC]; Mycelex®; Mycelex-7® [OTC]; Mycelex®-G; Mycelex OTC® [OTC]; Mycelex Twin Pack®

Use Treatment of susceptible fungal infections, including oropharyngeal candidiasis, dermatophytoses, superficial mycoses, and cutaneous candidiasis, as well as vulvovaginal candidiasis; limited data suggests that the use of clotrimazole troches may be effective for prophylaxis against oropharyngeal candidiasis in neutropenic patients

Pregnancy Risk Factor B/C (oral)

Contraindications Hypersensitivity to clotrimazole or any component

Warnings/Precautions Clotrimazole should not be used for treatment of systemic fungal infection; safety and effectiveness of clotrimazole lozenges (troches) in children <3 years of age have not been established

Adverse Reactions
>10%: Hepatic: Abnormal liver function tests
1% to 10%:
Gastrointestinal: Nausea and vomiting may occur in patients on clotrimazole troches
Local: Mild burning, irritation, stinging to skin or vaginal area

Mechanism of Action Binds to phospholipids in the fungal cell membrane altering cell wall permeability resulting in loss of essential intracellular elements

Pharmacodynamics/Kinetics
Absorption: Topical: Negligible through intact skin
Time to peak serum concentration:
Oral topical administration: Salivary levels occur within 3 hours following 30 minutes of dissolution time in the mouth
Vaginal cream: High vaginal levels occur within 8-24 hours
Vaginal tablet: High vaginal levels occur within 1-2 days
Elimination: As metabolites via bile

Usual Dosage
Children >3 years and Adults:
Oral:
Prophylaxis: 10 mg trough dissolved 3 times/day for the duration of chemotherapy or until steroids are reduced to maintenance levels
Treatment: 10 mg troche dissolved slowly 5 times/day for 14 consecutive days
Topical: Apply twice daily; if no improvement occurs after 4 weeks of therapy, re-evaluate diagnosis
Children >12 years and Adults: Vaginal:
Cream, vaginal:
Intravaginal: Insert 1 applicatorful of 1% vaginal cream daily (preferably at bedtime) for 7 consecutive days
Topical: Apply to affected are twice daily (morning and evening) for 7 consecutive days.
Tablets: Insert 100 mg/day for 7 days or 500 mg single dose

Monitoring Parameters Periodic liver function tests during oral therapy with clotrimazole lozenges

Patient Information May cause irritation to the skin; avoid contact with eyes; lozenge (troche) must be dissolved slowly in the mouth

Dosage Forms
Cream:
Topical : 1% (12 g, 15 g, 30 g, 45 g, 90 g)
Vaginal : 1% (45 g)
(Continued)

Clotrimazole *(Continued)*

Lotion, topical: 1% (30 mL)
Solution, topical : 1% (10 mL, 30 mL)
Tablet, vaginal : 100 mg (7s); 500 mg (1s)
Troche, oral (Mycelex®): 10 mg
Twin pack/Combination pack (Gyne-Lotrimin®, Mycelex®): Tablet 500 mg (1s) and vaginal cream 1% (7 g)

Cloxacillin Sodium *(klox a sill' in)*

Brand Names Cloxapen®; Tegopen®

Use Treatment of susceptible bacterial infections, notably penicillinase-producing staphylococci causing respiratory tract, skin and skin structure, bone and joint, urinary tract infections, endocarditis, septicemia, and meningitis

Pregnancy Risk Factor B

Contraindications Hypersensitivity to cloxacillin or any component, or penicillins

Warnings/Precautions Monitor PT if patient concurrently on warfarin, elimination of drug is slow in renally impaired; use with caution in patients allergic to cephalosporins due to a low incidence of cross-hypersensitivity

Adverse Reactions

1% to 10%: Gastrointestinal: Nausea, diarrhea
<1%:
Central nervous system: Fever
Dermatologic: Rash
Gastrointestinal: Vomiting
Hematologic: Eosinophilia, leukopenia, neutropenia, thrombocytopenia, agranulocytosis
Hepatic: Hepatotoxicity
Renal: Hematuria
Miscellaneous: Serum sickness-like reactions

Overdosage/Toxicology Symptoms of penicillin overdose include neuromuscular hypersensitivity (agitation, hallucinations, asterixis, encephalopathy, confusion, and seizures) and electrolyte imbalance with potassium or sodium salts, especially in renal failure; hemodialysis may be helpful to aid in the removal of the drug from the blood, otherwise most treatment is supportive or symptom directed

Drug Interactions

Decreased effect: Efficacy of oral contraceptives may be reduced
Increased effect: Disulfiram, probenecid → ↑ penicillin levels, increased effect of anticoagulants

Stability Refrigerate oral solution after reconstitution; discard after 14 days; stable for 3 days at room temperature

Mechanism of Action Inhibits bacterial cell wall synthesis by binding to one or more of the penicillin-binding proteins (PBPs) which in turn inhibits the final transpeptidation step of peptidoglycan synthesis in bacterial cell walls, thus inhibiting cell wall biosynthesis. Bacteria eventually lyse due to ongoing activity of cell wall autolytic enzymes (autolysins and murein hydrolases) while cell wall assembly is arrested.

Pharmacodynamics/Kinetics

Absorption: Oral: ~50%
Distribution: Crosses the placenta; appears in breast milk; distributed widely to most body fluids and bone; penetration into cells, into the eye, and across normal meninges is poor; inflammation increased amount that crosses the blood-brain barrier
Protein binding: 90% to 98%
Metabolism: Significant in the liver to active and inactive metabolites
Half-life: 0.5-1.5 hours (prolonged with renal impairment and in neonates)
Time to peak serum concentration: Oral: Within 0.5-2 hours
Elimination: In urine and through bile

Usual Dosage Oral:

Children >1 month (<20 kg): 50-100 mg/kg/day in divided doses every 6 hours; up to a maximum of 4 g/day

Children (>20 kg) and Adults: 250-500 mg every 6 hours

Not dialyzable (0% to 5%)

Administration Administer around-the-clock to lessen peak and tough concentrations

Test Interactions May interfere with urinary glucose tests using cupric sulfate (Benedict's solution, Clinitest®); may inactivate aminoglycosides *in vitro*; false-positive urine and serum proteins; false-positive in uric acid, urinary steroids

Patient Information Take 1 hour before or 2 hours after meals; finish all medication; do not skip doses

Dosage Forms
Capsule: 250 mg, 500 mg
Powder for oral suspension: 125 mg/5 mL (100 mL, 200 mL)

Cloxapen® see Cloxacillin Sodium on previous page

Clozapine (kloe' za peen)

Related Information
Antipsychotic Agents Comparison on page 1255

Brand Names Clozaril®

Use Management of schizophrenic patients

Pregnancy Risk Factor B

Contraindications In patients with WBC ≤3500 cells/mm³ before therapy; if WBC falls to <3000 cells/mm³ during therapy the drug should be withheld until signs and symptoms of infection disappear and WBC rises to >3000 cells/mm³

Warnings/Precautions Medication should not be stopped abruptly; taper off over 1-2 weeks; WBC testing should occur weekly for the duration of therapy; significant risk of agranulocytosis, potentially life-threatening; use with caution in patients receiving other marrow suppressive agents

Adverse Reactions
>10%:
  Cardiovascular: Tachycardia, hypotension, orthostatic hypotension
  Central nervous system: Fever, headache, drowsiness
  Gastrointestinal: Constipation, nausea, vomiting, unusual weight gain
1% to 10%:
  Cardiovascular: EKG changes, hypertension
  Central nervous system: Agitation, akathisia
  Gastrointestinal: Abdominal discomfort, heartburn, dry mouth
  Ocular: Blurred vision
  Miscellaneous: Increased sweating
<1%:
  Central nervous system: Insomnia, seizures, tardive dyskinesia, neuroleptic malignant syndrome
  Genitourinary: Difficult urination, impotence
  Hematologic: Agranulocytosis, eosinophilia, granulocytopenia, leukopenia, thrombocytopenia
  Neuromuscular & skeletal: Rigidity, tremor

Overdosage/Toxicology Symptoms of overdose include altered states of consciousness, tachycardia, hypotension, hypersalivation, respiratory depression

Following initiation of essential overdose management, toxic symptom treatment and supportive treatment should be initiated. Hypotension usually responds to I.V. fluids or Trendelenburg positioning. If unresponsive to these measures, the use of a parenteral inotrope may be required. Seizures commonly respond to diazepam (I.V. 5-10 mg bolus in adults every 15 minutes if needed up to a total of 30 mg; I.V. 0.25-0.4 mg/kg/dose up to a total of 10 mg in children) or to phenytoin or phenobarbital; critical cardiac arrhythmias often respond to I.V. phenytoin (15 mg/kg up to 1 g), while other antiarrhythmics can be used. Neuroleptics often cause extrapyramidal symptoms (eg, dystonic reactions) requiring management with benztropine mesylate I.V. 1-2 mg (adults) may be effective. These agents are generally effective within 2-5 minutes.

Drug Interactions
Decreased effect of epinephrine; decreased effect with phenytoin
Increased effect of CNS depressants, guanabenz, anticholinergics
Increased toxicity with cimetidine, MAO inhibitors, neuroleptics, TCAs

Mechanism of Action Clozapine is a weak dopamine₁ and dopamine₂ receptor blocker; in addition, it blocks the serotonin₂, alpha-adrenergic, and histamine H₁ central nervous system receptors

Pharmacodynamics/Kinetics
Metabolism: Undergoes extensive metabolism primarily to unconjugated forms
Elimination: In urine

Usual Dosage Adults: Oral: 25 mg once or twice daily initially and increased, as tolerated to a target dose of 300-450 mg/day after 2 weeks, but may require doses as high as 600-900 mg/day

Patient Information Report any lethargy, fever, sore throat, flu-like symptoms, or any other signs or symptoms of infection; may cause drowsiness; frequent blood samples must be taken; do not stop taking even if you think it is not working

Nursing Implications Benign, self-limiting temperature elevations sometimes occur during the first 3 weeks of treatment, weekly CBC mandatory
(Continued)

Clozapine *(Continued)*
Dosage Forms Tablet: 25 mg, 100 mg

Clozaril® *see* Clozapine *on previous page*

Clysodrast® *see* Bisacodyl *on page 134*

CMV-IGIV *see* Cytomegalovirus Immune Globulin Intravenous, Human *on page 296*

Cobex® *see* Cyanocobalamin *on page 282*

Cocaine Hydrochloride *(koe' kane)*
Use Topical anesthesia (ester derivative) for mucous membranes
Restrictions C-II
Pregnancy Risk Factor C (X if nonmedicinal use)
Contraindications Systemic use, hypersensitivity to cocaine or any component
Warnings/Precautions Use with caution in patients with hypertension, severe cardiovascular disease, or thyrotoxicosis; use with caution in patients with severely traumatized mucosa and sepsis in the region of intended application. Repeated topical application can result in psychic dependence and tolerance. May cause cornea to become clouded or pitted, therefore, normal saline should be used to irrigate and protect cornea during surgery; not for injection.
Adverse Reactions
>10%:
  Central nervous system: CNS stimulation
  Local: Loss of smell/taste, chronic rhinitis, stuffy nose
1% to 10%:
  Cardiovascular: Decreased heart rate with low doses, increased heart rate with moderate doses, hypertension, tachycardia, cardiac arrhythmias
  Central nervous system: Nervousness, restlessness, euphoria, excitement, hallucination, seizures
  Gastrointestinal: Vomiting
  Neuromuscular & skeletal: Tremors and clonic-tonic reactions
  Ocular: Sloughing of the corneal epithelium, ulceration of the cornea
  Respiratory: Tachypnea, respiratory failure
Overdosage/Toxicology Symptoms of overdose include respiratory depression, restlessness, hallucinations, dilated pupils, vomiting, muscular spasms, sensory aberrations, cardiac arrhythmias. Fatal dose: Oral: 500 mg to 1.2 g. Severe toxic effects have occurred with doses as low as 20 mg. Since no specific antidote for cocaine exists, serious toxic effects are treated symptomatically. Maintain airway and respiration. Attempt delay of absorption (if ingested) with activated charcoal, gastric lavage or emesis. Seizures are treated with diazepam while propranolol or labetalol may be useful for life-threatening arrhythmias, agitation, and/or hypertension.
Drug Interactions Increased toxicity: MAO inhibitors
Stability Store in well closed, light-resistant containers
Mechanism of Action Blocks both the initiation and conduction of nerve impulses by decreasing the neuronal membrane's permeability to sodium ions, which results in inhibition of depolarization with resultant blockade of conduction; interferes with the uptake of norepinephrine by adrenergic nerve terminals producing vasoconstriction
Pharmacodynamics/Kinetics
Following topical administration to mucosa:
  Onset of action: Within 1 minute
  Peak action: Within 5 minutes
  Duration: ≥30 minutes, depending on dosage administered
  Absorption: Limited by drug-induced vasoconstriction; enhanced by inflammation
  Distribution: Appears in breast milk
  Metabolism: In the liver
  Half-life: 75 minutes
  Elimination: Primarily in urine as metabolites and unchanged drug (<10%)
Usual Dosage Dosage depends on the area to be anesthetized, tissue vascularity, technique of anesthesia, and individual patient tolerance; use the lowest dose necessary to produce adequate anesthesia should be used, not to exceed 1 mg/kg. Use reduced dosages for children, elderly, or debilitated patients.

Topical application (ear, nose, throat, bronchoscopy): Concentrations of 1% to 4% are used; concentrations >4% are not recommended because of potential for increased incidence and severity of systemic toxic reactions
Monitoring Parameters Vital signs
Reference Range Therapeutic: 100-500 ng/mL (SI: 330 nmol/L); Toxic: >1000 ng/mL (SI: >3300 nmol/L)

Nursing Implications Use only on mucous membranes of the oral, laryngeal, and nasal cavities, do not use on extensive areas of broken skin

Dosage Forms

Powder: 5 g, 25 g

Solution, topical: 4% [40 mg/mL] (4 mL, 10 mL); 10% [100 mg/mL] (4 mL, 10 mL)

Tablet, soluble, for topical solution: 135 mg

Codeine (koe' deen)

Related Information

Narcotic Agonist Comparison Charts *on page 1274-1275*

Synonyms Codeine Phosphate; Codeine Sulfate; Methylmorphine

Use Treatment of mild to moderate pain; antitussive in lower doses; dextromethorphan has equivalent antitussive activity but has much lower toxicity in accidental overdose

Restrictions C-II

Pregnancy Risk Factor C (D if used for prolonged periods or in high doses at term)

Contraindications Hypersensitivity to codeine or any component

Warnings/Precautions Use with caution in patients with hypersensitivity reactions to other phenanthrene derivative opioid agonists (morphine, hydrocodone, hydromorphone, levorphanol, oxycodone, oxymorphone); respiratory diseases including asthma, emphysema, COPD, or severe liver or renal insufficiency; some preparations contain sulfites which may cause allergic reactions; may be habit-forming

Not recommended for use for cough control in patients with a productive cough; not recommended as an antitussive for children <2 years of age; the elderly may be particularly susceptible to the CNS depressant and confusion as well as constipating effects of narcotics

Adverse Reactions

>10%:

Central nervous system: Drowsiness

Gastrointestinal: Constipation

1% to 10%:

Cardiovascular: Tachycardia or bradycardia, hypotension

Central nervous system: Dizziness, lightheadedness, false feeling of well being, malaise, headache, restlessness, weakness, paradoxical CNS stimulation, confusion

Dermatologic: Skin rash, hives

Gastrointestinal: Dry mouth, anorexia, nausea, vomiting

Genitourinary: Decreased urination, ureteral spasm

Local: Burning at injection site

Ocular: Blurred vision

Respiratory: Shortness of breath, troubled breathing

Miscellaneous: Histamine release

<1%:

Central nervous system: Convulsions, hallucinations, mental depression, nightmares, insomnia

Gastrointestinal: Paralytic ileus, biliary spasm, stomach cramps

Neuromuscular & skeletal: Muscle rigidity, trembling

Overdosage/Toxicology Symptoms of overdose include CNS and respiratory depression, gastrointestinal cramping, constipation; naloxone 2 mg I.V. (0.01 mg/kg for children) with repeat administration as necessary up to a total of 10 mg

Drug Interactions

Decreased effect with cigarette smoking

Increased toxicity: CNS depressants, phenothiazines, TCAs, other narcotic analgesics, guanabenz, MAO inhibitors, neuromuscular blockers

Stability Store injection between 15°C to 30°C, avoid freezing; do not use if injection is discolored or contains a precipitate; protect injection from light

Mechanism of Action Binds to opiate receptors in the CNS, causing inhibition of ascending pain pathways, altering the perception of and response to pain; causes cough supression by direct central action in the medulla; produces generalized CNS depression

Pharmacodynamics/Kinetics

Onset of action:

Oral: 0.5-1 hour

I.M.: 10-30 minutes

Peak action:

Oral: 1-1.5 hours

I.M.: 0.5-1 hour

Duration of action: 4-6 hours

Absorption: Oral: Adequate

(Continued)

Codeine *(Continued)*

Distribution: Crosses the placenta; appears in breast milk

Protein binding: 7%

Metabolism: Hepatic to morphine (active)

Half-life: 2.5-3.5 hours

Elimination: 3% to 16% excreted in urine as unchanged drug, norcodeine, and free and conjugated morphine

Usual Dosage Doses should be titrated to appropriate analgesic effect; when changing routes of administration, note that oral dose is $^2/_3$ as effective as parenteral dose

Analgesic:

Children: Oral, I.M., S.C.: 0.5-1 mg/kg/dose every 4-6 hours as needed; maximum: 60 mg/dose

Adults: Oral, I.M., I.V., S.C.: 30 mg/dose; range: 15-60 mg every 4-6 hours as needed; maximum: 360 mg/24 hours

Antitussive: Oral (for nonproductive cough):

Children: 1-1.5 mg/kg/day in divided doses every 4-6 hours as needed: Alternative dose according to age:

2-6 years: 2.5-5 mg every 4-6 hours as needed; maximum: 30 mg/day

6-12 years: 5-10 mg every 4-6 hours as needed; maximum: 60 mg/day

Adults: 10-20 mg/dose every 4-6 hours as needed; maximum: 120 mg/day

Dosing adjustment in renal impairment:

Cl_{cr} 10-50 mL/minute: Administer 75% of dose

Cl_{cr} <10 mL/minute: Administer 50% of dose

Dosing adjustment in hepatic impairment: Probably necessary in hepatic insufficiency

Monitoring Parameters Pain relief, respiratory and mental status, blood pressure, heart rate

Reference Range Therapeutic: Not established; Toxic: >1.1 µg/mL

Test Interactions ↑ aminotransferase [ALT (SGPT)/AST (SGOT)] (S)

Patient Information Avoid alcohol, may cause drowsiness, impaired judgment or coordination; may cause physical and psychological dependence with prolonged use

Nursing Implications Observe patient for excessive sedation, respiratory depression, implement safety measures, assist with ambulation

Dosage Forms

Injection, as phosphate: 30 mg (1 mL, 2 mL); 60 mg (1 mL, 2 mL)

Solution, oral: 15 mg/5 mL

Tablet, as sulfate: 15 mg, 30 mg, 60 mg

Tablet, as phosphate, soluble: 30 mg, 60 mg

Tablet, as sulfate, soluble: 15 mg, 30 mg, 60 mg

Codeine and Acetaminophen *see* Acetaminophen and Codeine *on page 19*

Codeine and Aspirin *see* Aspirin and Codeine *on page 94*

Codeine and Guaifenesin *see* Guaifenesin and Codeine *on page 516*

Codeine Phosphate *see* Codeine *on previous page*

Codeine Sulfate *see* Codeine *on previous page*

Codimal-A® *see* Brompheniramine Maleate *on page 143*

Codoxy® *see* Oxycodone and Aspirin *on page 828*

Codroxomin® *see* Hydroxocobalamin *on page 552*

Cogentin® *see* Benztropine Mesylate *on page 124*

Co-Gesic® *see* Hydrocodone and Acetaminophen *on page 543*

Cognex® *see* Tacrine Hydrochloride *on page 1052*

Colace® [OTC] *see* Docusate *on page 362*

Colchicine *(kol' chi seen)*

Use Treat acute gouty arthritis attacks and to prevent recurrences of such attacks; management of familial Mediterranean fever

Pregnancy Risk Factor C (oral)/D (parenteral)

Contraindications Hypersensitivity to colchicine or any component; serious renal, gastrointestinal, hepatic, or cardiac disorders; blood dyscrasias

Warnings/Precautions Severe local irritation can occur following S.C. or I.M. administration; use with caution in debilitated patients or elderly patients or patients with severe GI, renal, or liver disease

Adverse Reactions

>10%: Gastrointestinal: Nausea, vomiting, diarrhea, abdominal pain

1% to 10%:

Dermatologic: Alopecia

Gastrointestinal: Anorexia

<1%:

Central nervous system: Myopathy, peripheral neuritis

Dermatologic: Rash

Genitourinary: Azoospermia

Hematologic: Bone marrow suppression, agranulocytosis, aplastic anemia

Hepatic: Hepatotoxicity

Overdosage/Toxicology Symptoms of overdose include nausea, vomiting, abdominal pain, shock, kidney damage, muscle weakness, burning in throat, watery to bloody diarrhea, hypotension, anuria, cardiovascular collapse, delirium, convulsions; treatment includes gastric lavage and measures to prevent shock, hemodialysis or peritoneal dialysis; atropine and morphine may relieve abdominal pain

Drug Interactions

Decreased effect: Vitamin B_{12} absorption may be reduced

Increased toxicity: Sympathomimetic agents; CNS depressant effects are enhanced

Stability Protect tablets from light; I.V. colchicine is **incompatible** with dextrose or I.V. solutions with preservatives

Mechanism of Action Decreases leukocyte motility, decreases phagocytosis in joints and lactic acid production, thereby reducing the deposition of urate crystals that perpetuates the inflammatory response

Pharmacodynamics/Kinetics

Protein binding: 10% to 31%

Metabolism: Partially deacetylated in the liver

Half-life: 12-30 minutes

End stage renal disease: 45 minutes

Time to peak serum concentration: Oral: Within 0.5-2 hours declining for the next 2 hours before increasing again due to enterohepatic recycling

Elimination: Primarily in the feces via bile

Usual Dosage

Prophylaxis of familial Mediterranean fever: Oral:

Children:

≤5 years: 0.5 mg/day

>5 years: 1-1.5 mg/day in 2-3 divided doses

Adults: 1-2 mg/day in 2-3 divided doses

Gouty arthritis, acute attacks: Adults:

Oral: Initial: 0.5-1.2 mg, then 0.5-0.6 mg every 1-2 hours or 1-1.2 mg every 2 hours until relief or GI side effects (nausea, vomiting, or diarrhea) occur to a maximum total dose of 8 mg; wait 3 days before initiating another course of therapy

I.V.: Initial: 2 mg, then 0.5 mg every 6 hours until response, not to exceed 4 mg/day; if pain recurs, it may be necessary to administer a daily dose of 1-2 mg for several days, however, do not give more colchicine by any route for at least 7 days after a full course of I.V. therapy (4 mg), transfer to oral colchicine in a dose similar to that being given I.V.

Gouty arthritis, prophylaxis of recurrent attacks: Adults: Oral: 0.5-0.6 mg/day or every other day

Dosing adjustment in renal impairment:

Cl_{cr} <50 mL/minute: Avoid chronic use or administration

Cl_{cr} <10 mL/minute: Decrease dose by 50% for treatment of acute attacks

Not dialyzable (0% to 5%)

Supplemental dose is not necessary

Administration Injection should be made over 2-5 minutes into tubing of free-flowing I.V. with compatible fluid; do not give I.M. or S.C.

Monitoring Parameters CBC and renal function test

Test Interactions May cause false-positive results in urine tests for erythrocytes or hemoglobin

Patient Information Avoid alcohol; discontinue if nausea or vomiting occurs; if taking for acute attack, discontinue as soon as pain resolves or if nausea, vomiting, or diarrhea occurs

Dosage Forms

Injection: 0.5 mg/mL (2 mL)

Tablet: 0.5 mg, 0.6 mg

Colestid® *see* Colestipol Hydrochloride *on this page*

Colestipol Hydrochloride (koe les' ti pole)
Related Information
Lipid-Lowering Agents *on page 1273*
Brand Names Colestid®
Use Adjunct in management of primary hypercholesterolemia; regression of arteri-olosclerosis; relief of pruritus associated with elevated levels of bile acids; possibly used to decrease plasma half-life of digoxin in toxicity
Pregnancy Risk Factor C
Contraindications Hypersensitivity to colestipol or any component; avoid using in complete biliary obstruction
Warnings/Precautions Avoid in patients with high triglycerides, GI dysfunction (constipation); may be associated with increased bleeding tendency as a result of hypothrombinemia secondary to vitamin K deficiency; may cause depletion of vitamins A, D, E
Adverse Reactions
>10%: Gastrointestinal: Constipation
1% to 10%: Gastrointestinal: Abdominal pain and distention, belching, flatulence, nausea, vomiting, diarrhea
<1%:
Central nervous system: Headache, dizziness, anxiety, vertigo, drowsiness, fatigue
Dermatologic: Dermatitis, urticaria
Gastrointestinal: Peptic ulceration, GI irritation and bleeding, cholecystitis, anorexia
Hepatic: Cholelithiasis
Neuromuscular & skeletal: Joint pain, arthritis, weakness
Respiratory: Shortness of breath
Miscellaneous: Increased serum phosphorous and chloride with decrease of sodium and potassium
Overdosage/Toxicology Symptoms of overdose include GI obstruction, nausea, GI distress; treatment is supportive
Drug Interactions Decreased absorption of tetracycline, penicillin G, vitamins A, D, E and K, digitalis glycosides, warfarin, thyroid hormones, thiazide diuretics, propranolol, phenobarbital, amiodarone, methotrexate, NSAIDs, and other drugs by binding to the drug in the intestine
Mechanism of Action Binds with bile acids to form an insoluble complex that is eliminated in feces; it thereby increases the fecal loss of bile acid-bound low density lipoprotein cholesterol
Pharmacodynamics/Kinetics Absorption: Oral: Not absorbed
Usual Dosage Adults: Oral: 5-30 g/day in divided doses 2-4 times/day
Administration Dry powder should be added to at least 90 mL of liquid and stirred until completely mixed; other drugs should be administered at least 1 hour before or 4 hours after colestipol
Test Interactions ↑ prothrombin time (S); ↓ cholesterol (S)
Patient Information Take in water or fruit juice (~90 mL) or sprinkled on food; other drugs should not be taken at least 1 hour before or 4 hours after colestipol; rinse glass with small amount of liquid to ensure full dose is taken
Dosage Forms Granules: 5 g packet, 300 g, 500 g

Colfosceril Palmitate (kole fos' er il)
Brand Names Exosurf® Neonatal
Synonyms Dipalmitoylphosphatidylcholine; DPPC; Synthetic Lung Surfactant
Use Neonatal respiratory distress syndrome:
Prophylactic therapy: Body weight <1350 g in infants at risk for developing RDS; body weight >1350 g in infants with evidence of pulmonary immaturity
Rescue therapy: Treatment of infants with RDS based on respiratory distress not attributable to any other causes and chest radiographic findings consistent with RDS
Warnings/Precautions This drug may rapidly affect oxygenation and lung compliance. If chest expansion improves substantially the ventilator PIP setting should be reduced immediately. Hyperoxia and hypocarbia (hypocarbia can decrease blood flow to the brain) may occur requiring appropriate ventilator adjustments.
Adverse Reactions 1% to 10%: Respiratory: Pulmonary hemorrhage, apnea, mucous plugging, decrease in transcutaneous O_2 >20%
Stability Reconstituted suspension should be used immediately (within 12 hours after reconstitution) and unused portion discarded; store at room temperature

(8°C to 24°C/46°F to 75°F); protect from excessive heat and light; do not refrigerate or freeze

Mechanism of Action Replaces deficient or ineffective endogenous lung surfactant in neonates with respiratory distress syndrome (RDS) or in neonates at risk of developing RDS; reduces surface tension and stabilizes the alveoli from collapsing

Pharmacodynamics/Kinetics

Absorption: Intratracheal: Absorbed from the alveolus

Metabolism: Catabolized and reutilized for further synthesis and secretion in lung tissue

Usual Dosage For intratracheal use only

Prophylactic treatment: Give 5 mL/kg (as two 2.5 mL/kg half-doses) as soon as possible; the second and third doses should be administered at 12 and 24 hours later to those infants remaining on ventilators

Rescue treatment: Give 5 mL/kg (as two 2.5 mL/kg half-doses) as soon as the diagnosis of RDS is made; the second 5 mL/kg (as two 2.5 mL/kg half-doses) dose should be administered 12 hours later

Administration For intratracheal administration only. Suction infant prior to administration; inspect solution to verify complete mixing of the suspension. Administer via sideport on the special ETT adapter without interrupting mechanical ventilation. Administer the dose in two 2.5 mL/kg aliquots. Each half-dose is instilled slowly over 1-2 minutes in small bursts with each inspiration. After the first 2.5 mL/kg dose, turn the infant's head and torso 45° to the right for 30 seconds, then return to the midline position and administer the second dose as above. Following the second dose, turn the infant's head and torso 45° to the left for 30 seconds and return the infant to the midline position.

Monitoring Parameters Continuous EKG and transcutaneous O_2 saturation should be monitored during administration; frequent arterial blood gas sampling is necessary to prevent post-dosing hyperoxia and hypocarbia

Dosage Forms Suspension, intratracheal: 108 mg (10 mL)

Colistin Sulfate (koe lis' tin)

Brand Names Coly-Mycin® S

Synonyms Polymyxin E

Use Treatment of diarrhea in infants and children caused by susceptible organisms, especially *E. coli* and *Shigella*, however, other agents are preferred; treatment of superficial infections of external ear canal and of mastoidectomy and fenestration cavities

Pregnancy Risk Factor C

Contraindications Known hypersensitivity to colistin

Warnings/Precautions Use with caution in patients with impaired renal function; some systemic absorption may occur; potential for renal toxicity exists; prolonged use may lead to superinfection

Adverse Reactions

<1%:

Gastrointestinal: Nausea, vomiting

Neuromuscular & skeletal: Neuromuscular blockade

Renal: Nephrotoxicity

Respiratory: Respiratory arrest

Miscellaneous: Hypersensitivity reactions, superinfections

Stability Stable for 2 weeks when refrigerated, shake well

Mechanism of Action A polypeptide antibiotic that binds to and damages the bacterial cell membrane

Pharmacodynamics/Kinetics

Absorption: Oral: Slightly absorbed from GI tract (adults); unpredictable absorption occurs in infants, can lead to significant serum levels

Half-life: 2.8-4.8 hours, prolonged in renal insufficiency; with anuria: 48-72 hours

Elimination: ~65% to 75% of dose excreted unchanged in urine

Usual Dosage Diarrhea: Children: Oral: 5-15 mg/kg/day in 3 divided doses given every 8 hours

Patient Information Keep refrigerated, shake well, discard after 14 days

Dosage Forms Powder for oral suspension: 25 mg/5 mL (60 mL)

Collagen see Microfibrillar Collagen Hemostat *on page 739*

Collagenase (kol' la je nase)

Brand Names Santyl®

Use Promotes debridement of necrotic tissue in dermal ulcers and severe burns

Pregnancy Risk Factor C

Contraindications Known hypersensitivity to collagenase

(Continued)

Collagenase *(Continued)*

Warnings/Precautions For external use only; avoid contact with eyes; monitor debilitated patients for systemic bacterial infections because debriding enzymes may increase the risk of bacteremia

Adverse Reactions

1% to 10%: Local: Irritation

<1%: Local: Pain and burning may occur at site of application

Overdosage/Toxicology Action of enzyme may be stopped by applying Burow's solution

Drug Interactions Decreased effect: Enzymatic activity is inhibited by detergents, benzalkonium chloride, hexachlorophene, nitrofurazone, tincture of iodine, and heavy metal ions (silver and mercury)

Mechanism of Action Collagenase is an enzyme derived from the fermentation of *Clostridium histolyticum* and differs from other proteolytic enzymes in that its enzymatic action has a high specificity for native and denatured collagen. Collagenase will not attack collagen in healthy tissue or newly formed granulation tissue. In addition, it does not act on fat, fibrin, keratin, or muscle.

Usual Dosage Topical: Apply once daily

Nursing Implications Do not introduce into major body cavities; monitor debilitated patients for systemic bacterial infections

Dosage Forms Ointment, topical: 250 units/g (15 g, 30 g)

Collyrium Fresh® [OTC] *see* Tetrahydrozoline Hydrochloride *on page 1071*

Colovage® *see* Polyethylene Glycol-Electrolyte Solution *on page 900*

Coly-Mycin® S *see* Colistin Sulfate *on previous page*

CoLyte® *see* Polyethylene Glycol-Electrolyte Solution *on page 900*

Comfort® [OTC] *see* Naphazoline Hydrochloride *on page 775*

Compazine® *see* Prochlorperazine *on page 932*

Compound F *see* Hydrocortisone *on page 546*

Compound S *see* Zidovudine *on page 1173*

Compound W® [OTC] *see* Salicylic Acid *on page 991*

Compoz® [OTC] *see* Diphenhydramine Hydrochloride *on page 351*

Constant-T® *see* Theophylline/Aminophylline *on page 1072*

Constilac® *see* Lactulose *on page 617*

Constulose® *see* Lactulose *on page 617*

Contac® Cough Formula Liquid [OTC] *see* Guaifenesin and Dextromethorphan *on page 517*

Control-L™ [OTC] *see* Pyrethrins *on page 959*

Control® [OTC] *see* Phenylpropanolamine Hydrochloride *on page 876*

Cophene-B® *see* Brompheniramine Maleate *on page 143*

Cordarone® *see* Amiodarone Hydrochloride *on page 58*

Cordran® *see* Flurandrenolide *on page 480*

Cordran® SP *see* Flurandrenolide *on page 480*

Corgard® *see* Nadolol *on page 765*

Corgonject® *see* Chorionic Gonadotropin *on page 242*

CortaGel® [OTC] *see* Hydrocortisone *on page 546*

Cortaid® Maximum Strength [OTC] *see* Hydrocortisone *on page 546*

Cortaid® with Aloe [OTC] *see* Hydrocortisone *on page 546*

Cortatrigen® *see* Neomycin, Polymyxin B, and Hydrocortisone *on page 781*

Cort-Dome® *see* Hydrocortisone *on page 546*

Cortef® *see* Hydrocortisone *on page 546*

Cortef® Feminine Itch [OTC] *see* Hydrocortisone *on page 546*

Cortenema® *see* Hydrocortisone *on page 546*

Corticaine® [OTC] *see* Hydrocortisone *on page 546*

Corticosteroids Comparisons *see page 1266*

Corticotropin (kor ti koe troe' pin)

Brand Names ACTH®; Acthar®; H.P. Acthar® Gel

Synonyms Adrenocorticotropic Hormone; Corticotropin, Repository

Use Acute exacerbations of multiple sclerosis; diagnostic aid in adrenocortical insufficiency, severe muscle weakness in myasthenia gravis

Cosyntropin is preferred over corticotropin for diagnostic test of adrenocortical insufficiency (cosyntropin is less allergenic and test is shorter in duration)

Pregnancy Risk Factor C

Contraindications Scleroderma, osteoporosis, systemic fungal infections, ocular herpes simplex, peptic ulcer, hypersensitivity to corticotropin or any component

Warnings/Precautions May mask signs of infection; do not administer live vaccines; use with caution in patients with hypothyroidism, cirrhosis, thromboembolic disorders, seizure disorders or renal insufficiency, hypertension, congestive heart failure; may mask signs of infection; do not administer live vaccines

Adverse Reactions

>10%:

Central nervous system: Insomnia, nervousness

Gastrointestinal: Increased appetite, indigestion

1% to 10%:

Endocrine & metabolic: Diabetes mellitus

Neuromuscular & skeletal: Joint pain

Ocular: Cataracts

Miscellaneous: Epistaxis

<1%:

Central nervous system: Seizures, mood swings, headache, delirium, hallucinations, euphoria

Dermatologic: Skin atrophy, bruising, hyperpigmentation, acne, hirsutism

Endocrine & metabolic: Amenorrhea, sodium and water retention, Cushing's syndrome, hyperglycemia

Gastrointestinal: Abdominal distention, ulcerative esophagitis, pancreatitis

Neuromuscular & skeletal: Muscle wasting, bone growth suppression

Miscellaneous: Hypersensitivity reactions

Drug Interactions Decreased effect: Spironolactone, hydrocortisone, cortisone; can antagonize the effects of anticholinesterases (eg, neostigmine)

Stability

Reconstituted solution remains stable for 8 hours at room temperature and 24 hours refrigerated

Standard diluent: 25-80 units/500 mL D_5W

Stability of parenteral admixture at room temperature (25°C): 8 hours; refrigeration temperature (4°C): 24 hours

Store repository injection in the refrigerator; warm gel before administration; repository is stable for <72 hours at room temperature

Mechanism of Action Stimulates the adrenal cortex to secrete adrenal steroids (including hydrocortisone, cortisone), androgenic substances, and a small amount of aldosterone

Pharmacodynamics/Kinetics

Time to peak serum concentration:

I.M., I.V. (aqueous): Within 1 hour

I.M., S.C. (gel): Within 7-24 hours

Repository injection: 3-12 hours

Onset of action: 6 hours

Duration of action:

Aqueous: 2-4 hours

Repository: 3 days

Absorption: I.M. (repository): Over 8-16 hours

Half-life: 15 minutes

Elimination: In urine

Usual Dosage Injection has a rapid onset and duration of activity of approximately 2 hours; the repository injection has a slower onset, but may sustain effects for ≤3 days

Children:

Anti-inflammatory/immunosuppressant:

I.M., I.V., S.C. (aqueous): 1.6 units/kg/day or 50 units/m²/day divided every 6-8 hours

I.M. (gel): 0.8 units/kg/day or 25 units/m²/day divided every 12-24 hours

Infantile spasms: Various regimens have been used. Some neurologists recommend low-dose ACTH (5-40 units/day) for short periods (1-6 weeks), while others recommend larger doses of ACTH (40-160 units/day) for long

(Continued)

Corticotropin (Continued)

periods of treatment (3-12 months). Well designed comparative dosing studies are needed. Example of low dose regimen:

Initial: I.M. (gel): 20 units/day for 2 weeks, if patient responds, taper and discontinue; if patient does not respond, increase dose to 30 units/day for 4 weeks then taper and discontinue

I.M. usual dose (gel): 20-40 units/day or 5-8 units/kg/day in 1-2 divided doses; range: 5-160 units/day

Oral prednisone (2 mg/kg/day) was as effective as I.M. ACTH gel (20 units/day) in controlling infantile spasms

Adults: Acute exacerbation of multiple sclerosis: I.M.: 80-120 units/day for 2-3 weeks

Diagnostic purposes: I.V.: 10-25 units in 500 mL 5% dextrose in water infused over 8 hours

Repository injection: I.M., S.C.: 40-80 units every 24-72 hours

Test Interactions Spironolactone, hydrocortisone, cortisone

Patient Information Do not abruptly discontinue the medication; your physician may want you to follow a low salt/potassium rich diet; tell your physician if you are using this drug before having skin tests, before surgery, or emergency treatment if you get a serious infection or injury

Additional Information Repository injection with zinc contains benzyl alcohol

Dosage Forms

Injection, repository: 40 units/mL (1 mL, 5 mL); 80 units/mL (1 mL, 5 mL)

Powder for injection: 25 units, 40 units

Corticotropin, Repository see Corticotropin on page 274

Cortisol see Hydrocortisone on page 546

Cortisone Acetate (kor' ti sone)

Related Information

Corticosteroids Comparisons on page 1266-1268

Brand Names Cortone® Acetate

Use Management of adrenocortical insufficiency

Pregnancy Risk Factor D

Contraindications Serious infections, except septic shock or tuberculous meningitis, idiopathic thrombocytopenia purpura (I.M. use), administration of live virus vaccines

Warnings/Precautions Use with caution in patients with hypothyroidism, cirrhosis, hypertension, congestive heart failure, ulcerative colitis, thromboembolic disorders, osteoporosis, convulsive disorders, peptic ulcer, diabetes mellitus, myasthenia gravis; prolonged therapy (>5 days) of pharmacologic doses of corticosteroids may lead to hypothalamic-pituitary-adrenal suppression, the degree of adrenal suppression varies with the degree and duration of glucocorticoid therapy; this must be taken into consideration when taking patients off steroids

Adverse Reactions

>10%:

Central nervous system: Insomnia, nervousness

Gastrointestinal: Increased appetite, indigestion

1% to 10%:

Endocrine & metabolic: Diabetes mellitus, hirsutism

Gastrointestinal: Peptic ulcer, nausea, vomiting

Neuromuscular & skeletal: Muscle weakness, osteoporosis, fractures, joint pain, epistaxis

Ocular: Cataracts, glaucoma

<1%:

Cardiovascular: Edema, hypertension

Central nervous system: Mood swings, vertigo, seizures, headache, psychoses, pseudotumor cerebri, delirium, hallucinations, euphoria

Dermatologic: Acne, skin atrophy, hyperpigmentation

Endocrine & metabolic: Cushing's syndrome, pituitary-adrenal axis suppression, growth suppression, glucose intolerance, hypokalemia, alkalosis, amenorrhea, sodium and water retention, hyperglycemia

Gastrointestinal: Abdominal distention, ulcerative esophagitis, pancreatitis

Hematologic: Bruising

Neuromuscular & skeletal: Muscle wasting

Miscellaneous: Hypersensitivity reactions

Overdosage/Toxicology When consumed in excessive quantities for prolonged periods, systemic hypercorticism and adrenal suppression may occur; in those cases, discontinuation and withdrawal of the corticosteroid should be done judiciously. Cushingoid changes from continued administration of large doses results in moonface, central obesity, striae, hirsutism, acne, ecchymoses, hypertension, osteoporosis, myopathy, sexual dysfunction, diabetes, hyperlipidemia, peptic ulcer, increased susceptibility to infection and electrolyte and fluid imbalance.

Drug Interactions
Decreased effect:
Barbiturates, phenytoin, rifampin → ↓ cortisone effects
Live virus vaccines, diuretics (potassium depleting)
Anticholinesterase agents → ↓ effect
Cortisone → ↓ warfarin effects
Cortisone → ↓ effects of salicylates
Increased effect: Estrogens (increased cortisone effects)
Increased toxicity:
Cortisone + NSAIDs → ↑ ulcerogenic potential
Cortisone → ↑ potassium deletion due to diuretics

Mechanism of Action Decreases inflammation by suppression of migration of polymorphonuclear leukocytes and reversal of increased capillary permeability

Pharmacodynamics/Kinetics
Peak effect:
Oral: Within 2 hours
I.M.: Within 20-48 hours
Duration of action: 30-36 hours
Absorption: Slow rate of absorption
Distribution: Crosses the placenta; appears in breast milk; distributes to muscles, liver, skin, intestines, and kidneys
Metabolism: In the liver to inactive metabolites
Half-life: 30 minutes to 2 hours
End stage renal disease: 3.5 hours
Elimination: In bile and urine
Note: Insoluble in water; supplemental doses may be warranted during times of stress in the course of withdrawing therapy

Usual Dosage If possible, administer glucocorticoids before 9 AM to minimize adrenocortical suppression; dosing depends upon the condition being treated and the response of the patient. Supplemental doses may be warranted during times of stress in the course of withdrawing therapy.

Children:
Anti-inflammatory or immunosuppressive:
Oral: 2.5-10 mg/kg/day in divided doses every 6-8 hours
I.M.: 1-5 mg/kg/day or 30-150 mg/m^2/day in divided doses every 12-24 hours
Physiologic replacement:
Oral: 0.5-0.75 mg/kg/day or 12-15 mg/m^2/day in divided doses every 8 hours
I.M.: 0.25-0.35 mg/kg/day once daily or 12-15 mg/m^2/day

Adults: Oral, I.M.: 25-300 mg/day in divided doses every 12-24 hours

Hemodialysis effects: Supplemental dose is not necessary

Administration Administer I.M. daily dose before 9 AM to minimize adrenocortical suppression

Patient Information Take with meals or with food or milk; do not discontinue drug or reduce dose without notifying physician

Nursing Implications I.M. use only; shake vial before measuring out dose; withdraw gradually following long-term therapy

Additional Information Insoluble in water

Dosage Forms
Injection: 50 mg/mL (10 mL)
Tablet: 5 mg, 10 mg, 25 mg

Cortisporin® Ophthalmic Ointment see Bacitracin, Neomycin, Polymyxin B, and Hydrocortisone on page 113

Cortisporin® Ophthalmic Suspension see Neomycin, Polymyxin B, and Hydrocortisone on page 781

Cortisporin® Otic see Neomycin, Polymyxin B, and Hydrocortisone on page 781

Cortisporin® Topical Cream see Neomycin, Polymyxin B, and Hydrocortisone on page 781

Cortisporin® Topical Ointment see Bacitracin, Neomycin, Polymyxin B, and Hydrocortisone on page 113

Cortizone®-5 [OTC] see Hydrocortisone on page 546

Cortizone®-10 [OTC] *see* Hydrocortisone *on page 546*

Cortone® Acetate *see* Cortisone Acetate *on page 276*

Cortrosyn® *see* Cosyntropin *on this page*

Cosmegen® *see* Dactinomycin *on page 298*

Cosyntropin (koe sin troe' pin)
Brand Names Cortrosyn®
Synonyms Synacthen; Tetracosactide
Use Diagnostic test to differentiate primary adrenal from secondary (pituitary) adrenocortical insufficiency
Pregnancy Risk Factor C
Contraindications Known hypersensitivity to cosyntropin
Warnings/Precautions Use with caution in patients with pre-existing allergic disease or a history of allergic reactions to corticotropin
Adverse Reactions
  1% to 10%:
    Cardiovascular: Flushing
    Central nervous system: Mild fever
    Dermatologic: Pruritus
    Gastrointestinal: Chronic pancreatitis
  <1%: Hypersensitivity reactions
Stability Reconstitute with NS
  Stability of parenteral admixture at room temperature (25°C): 24 hours
  Stability of parenteral admixture at refrigeration temperature (4°C): 21 days
  I.V. infusion in NS or D_5W is stable 12 hours at room temperature
Mechanism of Action Stimulates the adrenal cortex to secrete adrenal steroids (including hydrocortisone, cortisone), androgenic substances, and a small amount of aldosterone
Pharmacodynamics/Kinetics
  Distribution: Crosses the placenta
  Metabolism: Unknown
  Time to peak serum concentration: Within 1 hour (plasma cortisol levels rise in healthy individuals within 5 minutes of administration I.M. or I.V. push)
Usual Dosage
  Adrenocortical insufficiency: I.M., I.V. (over 2 minutes):
    Neonates: 0.015 mg/kg/dose
    Children <2 years: 0.125 mg
    Children >2 years and Adults: 0.25 mg
  When greater cortisol stimulation is needed, an I.V. infusion may be used: I.V. infusion: 0.25 mg administered at 0.04 mg/hour over 6 hours
  Peak plasma cortisol concentrations usually occur 45-60 minutes after cosyntropin administration
Reference Range Normal baseline cortisol >5 µg/dL (SI: >138 nmol/L); increase in serum cortisol after cosyntropin injection >7 µg/dL (SI: >193 nmol/L) or peak response >18 µg/dL (SI: >497 nmol/L). Plasma cortisol concentrations should be measured immediately before and exactly 30 minutes after a dose.
Test Interactions Decreased effect: Spironolactone, hydrocortisone, cortisone
Nursing Implications Patient should not receive corticosteroids or spironolactone the day prior and the day of the test
Additional Information Each 0.25 mg of cosyntropin is equivalent to 25 units of corticotropin
Dosage Forms Powder for injection: 0.25 mg

Cotazym® *see* Pancrelipase *on page 837*

Cotazym-S® *see* Pancrelipase *on page 837*

Cotrim® *see* Co-trimoxazole *on this page*

Cotrim® DS *see* Co-trimoxazole *on this page*

Co-trimoxazole (koe-trye mox' a zole)
Related Information
  Antimicrobial Drugs of Choice *on page 1298-1302*
Brand Names Bactrim™; Bactrim™ DS; Cotrim®; Cotrim® DS; Septra®; Septra® DS; Sulfamethoprim®; Sulfatrim®; Sulfatrim® DS; Sulfoxaprim®; Sulfoxaprim® DS; Trisulfam®; Uroplus® DS; Uroplus® SS
Synonyms SMX-TMP; Sulfamethoxazole and Trimethoprim; TMP-SMX; Trimethoprim and Sulfamethoxazole

Use
Oral treatment of urinary tract infections; acute otitis media in children; acute exacerbations of chronic bronchitis in adults; prophylaxis of *Pneumocystis carinii* pneumonitis (PCP)

I.V. treatment of documented PCP, empiric treatment of PCP in immune compromised patients; treatment of documented or suspected shigellosis, typhoid fever, *Nocardia asteroides* infection, or other infections caused by susceptible bacterial

Pregnancy Risk Factor C

Contraindications Hypersensitivity to any sulfa drug or any component; porphyria; megaloblastic anemia due to folate deficiency; infants <2 months of age

Warnings/Precautions Use with caution in patients with G-6-PD deficiency, impaired renal or hepatic function; adjust dosage in patients with renal impairment; injection vehicle contains benzyl alcohol and sodium metabisulfite; fatalities associated with severe reactions including Stevens-Johnson syndrome, toxic epidermal necrolysis, hepatic necrosis, agranulocytosis, aplastic anemia and other blood dyscrasias; discontinue use at first sign of rash; elderly patients appear at greater risk for more severe adverse reactions

Adverse Reactions
>10%:
  Dermatologic: Allergic skin reactions including rashes and urticaria, photosensitivity
  Gastrointestinal: Nausea, vomiting, anorexia
1% to 10%:
  Dermatologic: Stevens-Johnson syndrome, toxic epidermal necrolysis
  Hematologic: Blood dyscrasias
  Hepatic: Hepatitis
<1%:
  Central nervous system: Confusion, depression, hallucinations, seizures, fever, ataxia
  Dermatologic: Erythema multiforme
  Gastrointestinal: Stomatitis, diarrhea, pseudomembranous colitis
  Hematologic: Thrombocytopenia, megaloblastic anemia, granulocytopenia, aplastic anemia, hemolysis (with G-6-PD deficiency)
  Hepatic: Hepatitis, kernicterus in neonates
  Renal: Interstitial nephritis
  Miscellaneous: Serum sickness

Overdosage/Toxicology Symptoms of overdose include nausea, vomiting, GI distress, hematuria, crystalluria; following GI decontamination, treatment is supportive; adequate fluid intake is essential; peritoneal dialysis is not effective and hemodialysis only moderately effective in removing co-trimoxazole

Drug Interactions Co-trimoxazole causes:
Decreased effect: Cyclosporines
Increased effect: Sulfonylureas and oral anticoagulants
Increased toxicity: Phenytoin, cyclosporines (nephrotoxicity), methotrexate (displaced from binding sites)

Stability Do not refrigerate injection; is less soluble in more alkaline pH; protect from light; do not use NS as a diluent; injection vehicle contains benzyl alcohol and sodium metabisulfite
Stability of parenteral admixture at room temperature (25°C):
  5 mL/125 mL D_5W = 6 hours
  5 mL/100 mL D_5W = 4 hours
  5 mL/75 mL D_5W = 2 hours

Mechanism of Action Sulfamethoxazole interferes with bacterial folic acid synthesis and growth via inhibition of dihydrofolic acid formation from para-aminobenzoic acid; trimethoprim inhibits dihydrofolic acid reduction to tetrahydrofolate resulting in sequential inhibition of enzymes of the folic acid pathway

Pharmacodynamics/Kinetics
Absorption: Oral: 90% to 100%
Distribution: Crosses the placenta; distributes into breast milk
Protein binding:
  SMX: 68%
  TMP: 68%
Metabolism:
  SMX is N-acetylated and glucuronidated
  TMP is metabolized to oxide and hydroxylated metabolites
Half-life:
  SMX: 9 hours
  TMP: 6-17 hours, both are prolonged in renal failure
Time to peak serum concentration: Within 1-4 hours
Elimination: In urine as metabolites and unchanged drug
(Continued)

Co-trimoxazole (Continued)

Usual Dosage Dosage recommendations are based on the trimethoprim component

Children >2 months:
  Mild to moderate infections: Oral, I.V.: 8 mg TMP/kg/day in divided doses every 12 hours
  Serious infection/*Pneumocystis*: I.V.: 20 mg TMP/kg/day in divided doses every 6 hours
  Urinary tract infection prophylaxis: Oral: 2 mg TMP/kg/dose daily
  Prophylaxis of *Pneumocystis*: Oral, I.V.: 10 mg TMP/kg/day or 150 mg TMP/m²/day in divided doses every 12 hours for 3 days/week; dose should not exceed 320 mg trimethoprim and 1600 mg sulfamethoxazole 3 days/week

Adults:
  Urinary tract infection/chronic bronchitis: Oral: 1 double strength tablet every 12 hours for 10-14 days
  Sepsis: I.V.: 20 TMP/kg/day divided every 6 hours
  Pneumocystis carinii:
    Prophylaxis: Oral, I.V.: 10 mg TMP/kg/day divided every 12 hours for 3 days/week
    Treatment: I.V.: 20 mg TMP/kg/day divided every 6 hours

Dosing interval/adjustment in renal impairment:
  Cl_{cr} 30-50 mL/minute: Administer every 12-18 hours or reduce dose by 25%
  Cl_{cr} 15-30 mL/minute: Administer every 18-24 hours or reduce dose by 50%
  Cl_{cr} <15 mL/minute: Not recommended

Administration Infuse over 60-90 minutes, must dilute well before giving; may be given less diluted in a central line; not for I.M. injection; maintain adequate fluid intake to prevent crystalluria; administer around-the-clock every 6-12 hours

Test Interactions ↑ creatinine (Jaffé alkaline picrate reaction); increased serum methotrexate by dihydrofolate reductase method; does not interfere with RAI method

Patient Information Take oral medication with 8 oz of water on an empty stomach (1 hour before or 2 hours after meals) for best absorption; report any skin rashes immediately; finish all medication, do not skip doses

Dosage Forms The 5:1 ratio (SMX to TMP) remains constant in all dosage forms:
  Injection: Sulfamethoxazole 80 mg and trimethoprim 16 mg per mL (5 mL, 10 mL, 20 mL, 30 mL, 50 mL)
  Suspension, oral: Sulfamethoxazole 200 mg and trimethoprim 40 mg per 5 mL (20 mL, 100 mL, 150 mL, 200 mL, 480 mL)
  Tablet: Sulfamethoxazole 400 mg and trimethoprim 80 mg
  Tablet, double strength: Sulfamethoxazole 800 mg and trimethoprim 160 mg

Coumadin® see Warfarin Sodium *on page 1168*

CPM see Cyclophosphamide *on page 286*

Creon® see Pancrelipase *on page 837*

Creon® 25 see Pancrelipase *on page 837*

Crolom® Ophthalmic Solution see Cromolyn Sodium *on this page*

Cromoglycic Acid see Cromolyn Sodium *on this page*

Cromolyn Sodium (kroe' moe lin)

Brand Names Crolom® Ophthalmic Solution; Gastrocrom® Oral; Intal® Inhalation Capsule; Intal® Nebulizer Solution; Intal® Oral Inhaler; Nasalcrom® Nasal Solution

Synonyms Cromoglycic Acid; Disodium Cromoglycate; DSCG

Use Adjunct in the prophylaxis of allergic disorders, including rhinitis, giant papillary conjunctivitis, and asthma; inhalation product may be used for prevention of exercise-induced bronchospasm; systemic mastocytosis, food allergy, and treatment of inflammatory bowel disease; **cromolyn is a prophylactic drug with no benefit for acute situations**

Pregnancy Risk Factor B

Contraindications Hypersensitivity to cromolyn or any component; acute asthma attacks

Warnings/Precautions Severe anaphylactic reactions may occur rarely; cromolyn is a prophylactic drug with no benefit for acute situations; do not use in patients with severe renal or hepatic impairment; caution should be used when withdrawing the drug or tapering the dose as symptoms may reoccur; use with caution in patients with a history of cardiac arrhythmias

Adverse Reactions
>10%: Local: Hoarseness, coughing, unpleasant taste (inhalation aerosol)
1% to 10%:
Dermatologic: Angioedema
Local: Dry mouth, sneezing, stuffy nose
Renal: Dysuria
<1%:
Central nervous system: Dizziness, headache
Dermatologic: Rash, urticaria
Gastrointestinal: Nausea, vomiting, diarrhea
Hypersensitivity: Anaphylactic reactions
Local: Nasal burning
Neuromuscular & skeletal: Joint pain
Ocular: Ocular stinging, lacrimation
Respiratory: Wheezing, throat irritation, eosinophilic pneumonia, pulmonary infiltrates

Overdosage/Toxicology Symptoms of overdose include bronchospasm, laryngeal edema, dysuria

Stability Nebulizer solution is **compatible** with metaproterenol sulfate, isoproterenol hydrochloride, 0.25% isoetharine hydrochloride, epinephrine hydrochloride, terbutaline sulfate, and 20% acetylcysteine solution for at least 1 hour after their admixture; store nebulizer solution protected from direct light

Mechanism of Action Prevents the mast cell release of histamine, leukotrienes and slow-reacting substance of anaphylaxis by inhibiting degranulation after contact with antigens

Pharmacodynamics/Kinetics
Absorption:
Inhalation: ~8% of dose reaches the lungs upon inhalation of the powder and is well absorbed
Oral: Only 0.5% to 2% of dose absorbed
Half-life: 80-90 minutes
Time to peak serum concentration: Inhalation: Within 15 minutes
Elimination: Absorbed cromolyn is equally excreted unchanged in the urine and the feces (via bile); small amounts are exhaled

Usual Dosage
Children and Adults:
Inhalation (taper frequency to lowest effective dose):
>2 years: 20 mg 4 times/day by nebulization solution
>5 years: 2 inhalations 4 times/day by metered spray or 20 mg 4 times/day (Spinhaler®)
For prevention of exercise-induced bronchospasm: Single dose of 2 inhalations (aerosol) or 20 mg (powder inhalation) just prior to exercise (no more than 1 hour)
Nasal: >6 years: Instill 1 spray in each nostril 3-4 times/day
Ophthalmic: Instill 1-2 drops 4-6 times/day into each eye
Oral:
Infants ≤2 years: 20 mg/kg/day in 4 divided doses, not to exceed 30 mg/kg/day
Children 2-12 years: 100 mg 4 times/day 15-20 minutes before meals, not to exceed 40 mg/kg/day
Children >12 years and Adults: 200 mg 4 times/day 15-20 minutes before meal, up to 400 mg 4 times/day

Monitoring Parameters Periodic pulmonary function tests

Patient Information Do not discontinue abruptly; not effective for acute relief of symptoms; must be taken on a regularly scheduled basis; do not mix oral capsule with fruit juice, milk, or foods

Nursing Implications Advise patient to clear as much mucus as possible before inhalation treatments

Dosage Forms
Capsule:
Oral (Gastrocrom®): 100 mg
Oral inhalation (Intal®): 20 mg [to be used with Spinhaler® turbo-inhaler]
Inhalation, oral (Intal®): 800 mcg/spray (8.1 g)
Solution, for nebulization (Intal®): 10 mg/mL (2 mL)
Solution, nasal (Nasalcrom®): 40 mg/mL (13 mL)
Solution, ophthalmic (Crolom®): 4% [40 mg/mL] (2.5 mL, 10 mL)

Crotamiton (kroe tam' i tonn)
Brand Names Eurax®
Use Treatment of scabies and symptomatic treatment of pruritus
Pregnancy Risk Factor C
(Continued)

Crotamiton *(Continued)*

Contraindications Hypersensitivity to crotamiton or other components; patients who manifest a primary irritation response to topical medications

Warnings/Precautions Avoid contact with face, eyes, mucous membranes, and urethral meatus; do not apply to acutely inflamed or raw skin; for external use only

Adverse Reactions <1%: Local: Pruritus, irritation, contact dermatitis, warm sensation

Overdosage/Toxicology Symptoms of ingestion include burning sensation in mouth, irritation of the buccal, esophageal and gastric mucosa, nausea, vomiting and abdominal pain; there is no specific antidote; general measures to eliminate the drug and reduce its absorption, combined with symptomatic treatment, are recommended

Mechanism of Action Crotamiton has scabicidal activity against *Sarcoptes scabiei*; mechanism of action unknown

Usual Dosage Topical:

Scabicide: Children and Adults: Wash thoroughly and scrub away loose scales, then towel dry; apply a thin layer and massage drug onto skin of the entire body from the neck to the toes (with special attention to skin folds, creases, and interdigital spaces). Repeat application in 24 hours. Take a cleansing bath 48 hours after the final application. Treatment may be repeated after 7-10 days if live mites are still present.

Pruritus: Massage into affected areas until medication is completely absorbed; repeat as necessary

Patient Information For topical use only; all contaminated clothing and bed linen should be washed to avoid reinfestation

Nursing Implications Lotion: Shake well before using; avoid contact with face, eyes, mucous membranes, and urethral meatus

Dosage Forms
Cream: 10% (60 g)
Lotion: 10% (60 mL, 454 mL)

Crystalline Penicillin *see* Penicillin G, Parenteral, Aqueous *on page 850*

Crystal Violet *see* Gentian Violet *on page 503*

Crystamine® *see* Cyanocobalamin *on this page*

Crysticillin® A.S. *see* Penicillin G Procaine *on page 853*

Crystodigin® *see* Digitoxin *on page 337*

CSA *see* Cyclosporine *on page 290*

C-Span® [OTC] *see* Ascorbic Acid *on page 88*

CTM *see* Chlorpheniramine Maleate *on page 229*

CTX *see* Cyclophosphamide *on page 286*

Cuprid® *see* Trientine Hydrochloride *on page 1120*

Cuprimine® *see* Penicillamine *on page 847*

Curretab® *see* Medroxyprogesterone Acetate *on page 677*

Cutivate™ *see* Fluticasone Propionate *on page 484*

CyA *see* Cyclosporine *on page 290*

Cyanocobalamin *(sye an oh koe bal' a min)*

Brand Names Berubigen®; Cobex®; Crystamine®; Cyanoject®; Cyomin®; Ener-B® [OTC]; Kaybovite-1000®; Redisol®; Rubramin-PC®; Sytobex®

Synonyms Vitamin B_{12}

Use Treatment of pernicious anemia; vitamin B_{12} deficiency; increased B_{12} requirements due to pregnancy, thyrotoxicosis, hemorrhage, malignancy, liver or kidney disease

Pregnancy Risk Factor A (C if dose exceeds RDA recommendation)

Contraindications Hypersensitivity to cyanocobalamin or any component, cobalt; patients with hereditary optic nerve atrophy

Warnings/Precautions I.M. route used to treat pernicious anemia; vitamin B_{12} deficiency for >3 months results in irreversible degenerative CNS lesions; treatment of vitamin B_{12} megaloblastic anemia may result in severe hypokalemia, sometimes, fatal, when anemia corrects due to cellular potassium requirements. B_{12} deficiency masks signs of polycythemia vera; vegetarian diets may result in B_{12} deficiency; pernicious anemia occurs more often in gastric carcinoma than in general population.

Adverse Reactions
1% to 10%:
Dermatologic: Itching
Gastrointestinal: Diarrhea
<1%:
Cardiovascular: Peripheral vascular thrombosis
Dermatologic: Urticaria
Miscellaneous: Anaphylaxis

Stability Clear pink to red solutions are stable at room temperature; protect from light; **incompatible** with chlorpromazine, phytonadione, prochlorperazine, warfarin, ascorbic acid, dextrose, heavy metals, oxidizing or reducing agents

Mechanism of Action Coenzyme for various metabolic functions, including fat and carbohydrate metabolism and protein synthesis, used in cell replication and hematopoiesis

Pharmacodynamics/Kinetics
Absorption: Absorbed from the terminal ileum in the presence of calcium; for absorption to occur gastric "intrinsic factor" must be present to transfer the compound across the intestinal mucosa
Distribution: Principally stored in the liver, also stored in the kidneys and adrenals
Protein binding: Bound to transcobalamin II
Metabolism: Converted in the tissues to active coenzymes methylcobalamin and deoxyadenosylcobalamin

Usual Dosage I.M. or deep S.C. (oral is not generally recommended due to poor absorption and I.V. is not recommended due to more rapid elimination):

Recommended daily allowance (RDA):
Children: 0.3-2 mcg
Adults: 2 mcg
Pernicious anemia, congenital (if evidence of neurologic involvement): 1000 mcg/day for at least 2 weeks; maintenance: 50 mcg/month
Children: 30-50 mcg/day for 2 or more weeks (to a total dose of 1000-5000 mcg), then follow with 100 mcg month as maintenance dosage
Adults: 100 mcg/day for 6-7 days; if improvement, give same dose on alternate days for 7 doses; then every 3-4 days for 2-3 weeks; once hematologic values have returned to normal, maintenance dosage: 100 mcg/month.
Note: Use only parenteral therapy as oral therapy is not dependable.
Vitamin B$_{12}$ deficiency:
Children: 100 mcg/day for 10-15 days (total dose of 1-1.5 mg), then once or twice weekly for several months; may taper to 60 mcg every month
Adults: Initial: 30 mcg/day for 5-10 days; maintenance: 100-200 mcg/month

Administration I.M. or deep S.C. are preferred routes of administration

Monitoring Parameters Serum potassium, erythrocyte and reticulocyte count, hemoglobin, hematocrit

Reference Range Normal range of serum B$_{12}$ is 150-750 pg/mL; this represents 0.1% of total body content. Metabolic requirements are 2-5 µg/day; years of deficiency required before hematologic and neurologic signs and symptoms are seen. Occasional patients with significant neuropsychiatric abnormalities may have no hematologic abnormalities and normal serum cobalamin levels, 200 pg/mL (SI: >150 pmol/L), or more commonly between 100-200 pg/mL (SI: 75-150 pmol/L). There exists evidence that people, particularly elderly whose serum cobalamin concentrations <300 pg/mL, should receive replacement parenteral therapy; this recommendation is based upon neuropsychiatric disorders and cardiovascular disorders associated with lower sodium cobalamin concentrations.

Test Interactions Methotrexate, pyrimethamine, and most antibiotics invalidate folic acid and vitamin B$_{12}$ diagnostic microbiological blood assays

Patient Information Pernicious anemia will require monthly injections for life

Nursing Implications Oral therapy is markedly inferior to parenteral therapy; monitor potassium concentrations during early therapy

Dosage Forms
Gel, nasal (Ener-B®): 400 mcg/0.1 mL
Injection: 30 mcg/mL (30 mL); 100 mcg/mL (1 mL, 10 mL, 30 mL); 1000 mcg/mL (1 mL, 10 mL, 30 mL)
Tablet [OTC]: 25 mcg, 50 mcg, 100 mcg, 250 mcg, 500 mcg, 1000 mcg

Cyanoject® see Cyanocobalamin *on previous page*

Cyclan® see Cyclandelate *on this page*

Cyclandelate (sye klan' de late)
Brand Names Cyclan®; Cyclospasmol®
Use Considered as "possibly effective" for adjunctive therapy in peripheral vascular disease and possibly senility due to cerebrovascular disease or multi-
(Continued)

Cyclandelate *(Continued)*

infarct dementia; migraine prophylaxis, vertigo, tinnitus, and visual disturbances secondary to cerebrovascular insufficiency and diabetic peripheral polyneuropathy

Pregnancy Risk Factor C

Contraindications Hypersensitivity to cyclandelate or any component

Warnings/Precautions Use with caution in patients with severe obliterative coronary artery or cerebral vascular disease, in patients with active bleeding or a bleeding tendency, and patients with glaucoma

Adverse Reactions

<1%:

Cardiovascular: Flushing of face, tachycardia

Central nervous system: Headache, pain, dizziness; tingling sensation in face, fingers, or toes

Gastrointestinal: Belching, heartburn

Neuromuscular & skeletal: Weakness

Overdosage/Toxicology Symptoms of overdose include drowsiness, weakness, respiratory depression, hypotension; treatment following decontamination is supportive; fluids followed by vasopressors are most helpful

Mechanism of Action Cyclandelate, 3,3,5-trimethylcyclohexyl mandelate is a vasodilator that exerts a direct, papaverine-like action on smooth muscles, particularly that found within the blood vessels. Animal data indicate that cyclandelate also has antispasmodic properties; exhibits no adrenergic stimulation or blocking action; action exceeds that of papaverine; mild calcium channel blocking agent, may benefit in mild hypercalcemia; calcium channel blocking activity may explain some of its pharmacologic effects (enhanced blood flow) and inhibition of platelet aggregation

Usual Dosage Adults: Oral: Initial: 1.2-1.6 g/day in divided doses before meals and at bedtime until response; maintenance therapy: 400-800 mg/day in 2-4 divided doses; start with lowest dose in elderly due to hypotensive potential; decrease dose by 200 mg decrements to achieve minimal maintenance dose; improvement can usually be seen over weeks of therapy and prolonged use; short courses of therapy are usually ineffective and not recommended

Patient Information Take medication with meals or antacids to decrease gastrointestinal side effects. **Note:** Use of antacids not recommended with reduced renal function (Cl$_{cr}$ <30 mL/minute) or when bowel function may be adversely affected (eg, elderly).

Nursing Implications Administer with meals; observe for orthostatic hypotension

Dosage Forms

Capsule: 200 mg, 400 mg

Tablet: 200 mg, 400 mg

Cyclizine *(sye' kli zeen)*

Brand Names Marezine® [OTC]

Use Prevention and treatment of nausea, vomiting, and vertigo associated with motion sickness; control of postoperative nausea and vomiting

Pregnancy Risk Factor B

Contraindications Hypersensitivity to cyclizine or any component

Warnings/Precautions Do not administer to premature or full-term neonates; young children may be more susceptible to side effects and CNS stimulation; bladder neck obstruction, symptomatic prostate hypertrophy, asthmatic attacks, and stenosing peptic ulcer

Adverse Reactions

>10%:

Central nervous system: Drowsiness

Gastrointestinal: Dry mouth

1% to 10%:

Central nervous system: Headache

Dermatologic: Dermatitis

Gastrointestinal: Nausea

Ocular: Diplopia

Renal: Polyuria, urinary retention

Overdosage/Toxicology Symptoms of overdose include dry mouth, flushed skin, dilated pupils, CNS depression; there is no specific treatment for an antihistamine overdose, however, most of its clinical toxicity is due to anticholinergic effects. For anticholinergic overdose with severe life-threatening symptoms, physostigmine 1-2 mg (0.5 or 0.02 mg/kg for children) I.V., slowly may be given to reverse these effects.

Drug Interactions Increased effect/toxicity with CNS depressants, alcohol

Stability I.M. formulation is **incompatible** when mixed in the same syringe with tetracyclines, methohexital, penicillin, pentobarbital, phenobarbital, secobarbital, thiopental

Mechanism of Action Cyclizine is a piperazine derivative with properties of histamines. The precise mechanism of action in inhibiting the symptoms of motion sickness is not known. It may have effects directly on the labyrinthine apparatus and central actions on the labyrinthine apparatus and on the chemoreceptor trigger zone. Cyclizine exerts a central anticholinergic action.

Usual Dosage

Children 6-12 years:
Oral: 25 mg up to 3 times/day
I.M.: Not recommended

Adults:
Oral: 50 mg taken 30 minutes before departure, may repeat in 4-6 hours if needed, up to 200 mg/day
I.M.: 50 mg every 4-6 hours as needed

Monitoring Parameters CNS effects or unusual movements

Patient Information May cause drowsiness, may impair judgment and coordination; avoid alcohol; drink plenty of fluids for dry mouth and to prevent constipation

Nursing Implications Raise bed rails, institute safety measures, assist with ambulation

Dosage Forms

Injection, as lactate: 50 mg/mL (1 mL)
Tablet, as hydrochloride: 50 mg

Cyclobenzaprine Hydrochloride (sye kloe ben' za preen)

Brand Names Cycoflex®; Flexeril®

Use Treatment of muscle spasm associated with acute painful musculoskeletal conditions; supportive therapy in tetanus

Pregnancy Risk Factor B

Contraindications Hypersensitivity to cyclobenzaprine or any component; do not use concomitantly or within 14 days of MAO inhibitors; hyperthyroidism, congestive heart failure, arrhythmias

Warnings/Precautions Cyclobenzaprine shares the toxic potentials of the tricyclic antidepressants and the usual precautions of tricyclic antidepressant therapy should be observed; use with caution in patients with urinary hesitancy or angle-closure glaucoma

Adverse Reactions

>10%:
Central nervous system: Drowsiness, dizziness, lightheadedness
Gastrointestinal: Dry mouth

1% to 10%:
Cardiovascular: Swelling of face, lips, syncope
Gastrointestinal: Bloated feeling
Genitourinary: Problems in urinating, urinary frequency
Hepatic: Hepatitis
Neuromuscular & skeletal: Problems in speaking, muscle weakness
Ocular: Blurred vision
Otic: Tinnitus

<1%:
Cardiovascular: Tachycardia, hypotension, arrhythmia
Central nervous system: Headache, fatigue, asthenia, nervousness, confusion, clumsiness
Dermatologic: Rash, dermatitis
Gastrointestinal: Dyspepsia, nausea, constipation, stomach cramps, unpleasant taste

Overdosage/Toxicology Symptoms of overdose include troubled breathing, drowsiness, syncope, seizures, tachycardia, hallucinations, vomiting. Following initiation of essential overdose management, toxic symptoms should be treated. Ventricular arrhythmias often respond to systemic alkalinization (sodium bicarbonate 0.5-2 mEq/kg I.V.) and/or phenytoin 15-20 mg/kg (adults). Arrhythmias unresponsive to this therapy may respond to lidocaine 1 mg/kg I.V. followed by a titrated infusion. Physostigmine (1-2 mg I.V. slowly for adults or 0.5 mg I.V. slowly for children) may be indicated in reversing cardiac arrhythmias that are life-threatening. Seizures usually respond to diazepam I.V. boluses (5-10 mg for adults up to 30 mg or 0.25-0.4 mg/kg/dose for children up to 10 mg/dose). If seizures are unresponsive or recur, phenytoin or phenobarbital may be required.

Drug Interactions Increased toxicity:
Do not use concomitantly or within 14 days after MAO inhibitors
Because of similarities to the tricyclic antidepressants, may have additive toxicities

(Continued)

Cyclobenzaprine Hydrochloride *(Continued)*

Anticholinergics: Because of cyclobenzaprine's anticholinergic action, use with caution in patients receiving these agents

Alcohol, barbiturates, and other CNS depressants: Effects may be enhanced by cyclobenzaprine

Mechanism of Action Centrally acting skeletal muscle relaxant pharmacologically related to tricyclic antidepressants; reduces tonic somatic motor activity influencing both alpha and gamma motor neurons

Pharmacodynamics/Kinetics

Onset of action: Commonly occurs within 1 hour

Absorption: Oral: Completely

Metabolism: Hepatic; may undergo enterohepatic recycling

Time to peak serum concentration: Within 3-8 hours

Elimination: Renally as inactive metabolites and in feces (via bile) as unchanged drug

Usual Dosage Oral: **Note:** Do not use longer than 2-3 weeks

Children: Dosage has not been established

Adults: 20-40 mg/day in 2-4 divided doses; maximum dose: 60 mg/day

Patient Information Drug may impair ability to perform hazardous activities requiring mental alertness or physical coordination, such as operating machinery or driving a motor vehicle

Nursing Implications Raise bed rails, institute safety measures, assist with ambulation

Dosage Forms Tablet: 10 mg

Cyclocort® *see* Amcinonide *on page 51*

Cyclogyl® *see* Cyclopentolate Hydrochloride *on this page*

Cyclopentolate Hydrochloride (sye kloe pen' toe late)

Related Information

Cycloplegic Mydriatics Comparison *on page 1269*

Brand Names AK-Pentolate®; Cyclogyl®; I-Pentolate®; Ocu-Pentolate®

Use Diagnostic procedures requiring mydriasis and cycloplegia

Pregnancy Risk Factor C

Contraindications Narrow-angle glaucoma, known hypersensitivity to drug

Warnings/Precautions 2% solution may result in psychotic reactions and behavioral disturbances in children, usually occurring approximately 30-45 minutes after instillation; use with caution in elderly patients and other patients who may be predisposed to increased intraocular pressure

Adverse Reactions

1% to 10%:

Cardiovascular: Tachycardia

Central nervous system: Restlessness, hallucinations, psychosis, hyperactivity, seizures, incoherent speech, ataxia, burning sensation

Ocular: Increase in intraocular pressure, loss of visual accommodation

Miscellaneous: Allergic reaction

Overdosage/Toxicology Antidote, if needed, is pilocarpine

Drug Interactions Decreased effect of carbachol, cholinesterase inhibitors

Stability Store in tight containers

Mechanism of Action Prevents the muscle of the ciliary body and the sphincter muscle of the iris from responding to cholinergic stimulation, causing mydriasis and cycloplegia

Pharmacodynamics/Kinetics

Peak effect:

Cycloplegia: 25-75 minutes

Mydriasis: 30-60 minutes

Duration: Recovery takes up to 24 hours

Usual Dosage

Infants: Instill 1 drop of 0.5% into each eye 5-10 minutes before examination

Children: Instill 1 drop of 0.5%, 1%, or 2% in eye followed by 1 drop of 0.5% or 1% in 5 minutes, if necessary

Adults: Instill 1 drop of 1% followed by another drop in 5 minutes; 2% solution in heavily pigmented iris

Patient Information May cause blurred vision and increased sensitivity to light

Nursing Implications Finger pressure should be applied to lacrimal sac for 1-2 minutes after instillation to decrease risk of absorption and systemic reactions

Dosage Forms Solution, ophthalmic: 0.5% (2 mL, 5 mL, 15 mL); 1% (2 mL, 5 mL, 15 mL); 2% (2 mL, 5 mL, 15 mL)

Cyclophosphamide (sye kloe foss' fa mide)

Related Information

Antiemetics for Chemotherapy Induced Nausea and Vomiting *on page 1202*

Cancer Chemotherapy Regimens *on page 1218-1241*

Brand Names Cytoxan®; Neosar®

Synonyms CPM; CTX; CYT

Use Treatment of Hodgkin's and non-Hodgkin's lymphoma, Burkitt's lymphoma, chronic lymphocytic leukemia, chronic granulocytic leukemia, AML, ALL, mycosis fungoides, breast cancer, multiple myeloma, neuroblastoma, retinoblastoma, rhabdomyosarcoma, Ewing's sarcoma; testicular, endometrium and ovarian, and lung cancer, and as a conditioning regimen for BMT; prophylaxis of rejection for kidney, heart, liver, and BMT transplants, severe rheumatoid disorders, nephrotic syndrome, Wegener's granulomatosis, idiopathic pulmonary hemosideroses, myasthenia gravis, multiple sclerosis, systemic lupus erythematosus, lupus nephritis, autoimmune hemolytic anemia, idiopathic thrombocytic purpura, macroglobulinemia, and antibody-induced pure red cell aplasia

Pregnancy Risk Factor D

Contraindications Hypersensitivity to cyclophosphamide or any component

Warnings/Precautions The U.S. Food and Drug Administration (FDA) currently recommends that procedures for proper handling and disposal of antineoplastic agents be considered. Dosage adjustment needed for renal or hepatic failure; use with caution in patients with bone marrow depression.

Adverse Reactions

>10%:

Dermatologic: Alopecia is frequent, but hair will regrow although it may be of a different color or texture; hair loss usually occurs 3 weeks after therapy

Fertility: May cause sterility; interferes with oogenesis and spermatogenesis; may be irreversible in some patients; gonadal suppression (amenorrhea)

Gastrointestinal: Nausea and vomiting occur more frequently with larger doses, usually beginning 6-10 hours after administration; also seen are anorexia, diarrhea, stomatitis; mucositis

Emetic potential:

Oral: Low (<10%)

<1 g: Moderate (30% to 60%)

≥1 g: High (>90%)

Hepatic: Jaundice seen occasionally

1% to 10%:

Central nervous system: Headache

Dermatologic: Skin rash, facial flushing

Myelosuppressive: Thrombocytopenia occurs less frequently than with mechlorethamine, anemia

WBC: Moderate

Platelets: Moderate

Onset (days): 7

Nadir (days): 10-14

Recovery (days): 21

<1%:

Cardiovascular: High-dose therapy may cause cardiac dysfunction manifested as congestive heart failure; cardiac necrosis or hemorrhagic myocarditis has occurred rarely, but is fatal. Cyclophosphamide may also potentiate the cardiac toxicity of anthracyclines.

Central nervous system: Dizziness

Dermatologic: Darkening of skin/fingernails

Endocrine & metabolic: Hyperglycemia, hypokalemia, distortion, hyperuricemia

Gastrointestinal: Stomatitis

Genitourinary: Acute hemorrhagic cystitis is believed to be a result of chemical irritation of the bladder by acrolein, a cyclophosphamide metabolite. Acute hemorrhagic cystitis occurs in 7% to 12% of patients, and has been reported in up to 40% of patients. Hemorrhagic cystitis can be severe and even fatal. Patients should be encouraged to drink plenty of fluids (3-4 L/day) during therapy, void frequently, and avoid taking the drug at nighttime. If large I.V. doses are being administered, I.V. hydration should be given during therapy. The administration of mesna or continuous bladder irrigation may also be warranted.

Hepatic: Hepatic toxicity

Respiratory: Nasal stuffiness: Occurs when given in large I.V. doses; patients experience runny eyes, rhinorrhea, sinus congestion, and sneezing during or immediately after the infusion; interstitial pulmonary fibrosis with prolonged high dosage has occurred

Renal: SIADH has occurred with I.V. doses >50 mg/kg; renal tubular necrosis has also occurred, but usually resolves after the discontinuation of therapy

(Continued)

Cyclophosphamide *(Continued)*

Secondary malignancy: Has developed with cyclophosphamide alone or in combination with other antineoplastics; both bladder carcinoma and acute leukemia are well documented

Overdosage/Toxicology Symptoms of overdose include myelosuppression, alopecia, nausea, vomiting; treatment is supportive

Drug Interactions

Decreased effect: Digoxin: Cyclophosphamide may reduce digoxin serum levels

Increased toxicity:

Allopurinol may cause an increase in bone marrow depression and may result in significant elevations of cyclophosphamide cytotoxic metabolites

Anesthetic agents: Cyclophosphamide reduces serum pseudocholinesterase concentrations and may prolong the neuromuscular blocking activity of succinylcholine; use with caution with halothane, nitrous oxide, and succinylcholine

Chloramphenicol results in prolonged cyclophosphamide half-life to increase toxicity

Cimetidine inhibits hepatic metabolism of drugs and may reduce the activation of cyclophosphamide

Doxorubicin: Cyclophosphamide may enhance cardiac toxicity of anthracyclines

Phenobarbital and phenytoin induce hepatic enzymes and cause a more rapid production of cyclophosphamide metabolites with a concurrent decrease in the serum half-life of the parent compound

Tetrahydrocannabinol results in enhanced immunosuppression in animal studies

Thiazide diuretics: Leukopenia may be prolonged

Stability I.V. solution is usually reconstituted in 20 mg/mL concentrations; solutions may be administered I.V., I.M., intraperitoneally, or intrapleurally; they may be infused I.V. in D_5W, 0.9% sodium chloride, D_5LR, lactated Ringer's, or 0.45% sodium chloride; prepared solutions should be used within 24 hours or may be stored up to 6 days under refrigeration; oral elixir may be prepared from the injectable preparation and is stable for 14 days if refrigerated

Mechanism of Action Interferes with the normal function of DNA by alkylation and cross-linking the strands of DNA, and by possible protein modification; cyclophosphamide also possesses potent immunosuppressive activity; note that cyclophosphamide must be metabolized to its active form in the liver

Pharmacodynamics/Kinetics

Absorption: Complete from GI tract (>75%)

Distribution: V_d: 0.48-0.71 L/kg; well distributed; crosses the placenta; appears in breast milk; does cross into the CSF, but not in concentrations high enough to treat meningeal leukemia

Protein binding: 10% to 56%

Metabolism: In the liver into its active components, one of which is 4-HC

Bioavailability: >75%

Half-life: 4-6.5 hours

Time to peak serum concentration: Oral: Within 1 hour

Elimination: In urine as unchanged drug (<30%) and as metabolites (85% to 90%)

Usual Dosage Patients with compromised bone marrow function may require a 33% to 50% reduction in initial loading dose; I.V. infusions may be administered over 1-2 hours

Doses >500 mg to approximately 1 g may be administered over 20-30 minutes; may also be administered slow IVP in lower doses

Children: Neuroblastomas/sarcomas: I.V.: 3 g/m^2/day for 2 days or 2 g/m^2/day for 3 days

Children and Adults:

Oral: 50-100 mg/m^2/day as continuous therapy or 400-1000 mg/m^2 in divided doses over 4-5 days as intermittent therapy

I.V.: 400-1500 mg/m^2 every 21-28 days

BMT-conditioning regimen: I.V.: 50 mg/kg/dose once daily for 3-4 days or 60 mg/kg/dose for 2 days

Nephrotic syndrome: Oral: 2-3 mg/kg/day every day for up to 12 weeks when corticosteroids are unsuccessful

Dosing adjustment in renal impairment:

Cl_{cr} 25-50 mL/minute: Administer 75% of normal dose

Cl_{cr} <25 mL/minute: Administer 50% of normal dose

Moderately dialyzable (20% to 50%)

Administer dose posthemodialysis or administer supplemental 50% dose

Dosing adjustment in hepatic impairment:
Bilirubin 3.5-5 mg/dL or AST >180 units: Administer 75% of normal dose
Bilirubin >5 mg/dL: Omit dose

Administration I.V. infusions may be administered over 1-2 hours; doses >500 mg to approximately 1 g may be administered over 20-30 minutes; may also be administered slow IVP in lower doses

Monitoring Parameters CBC with differential and platelet count, ESR, BUN, UA, serum electrolytes, serum creatinine

Patient Information Drink plenty of fluids before and after doses; report any blood in urine

Nursing Implications Encourage adequate hydration and frequent voiding to help prevent hemorrhagic cystitis

Dosage Forms
Powder for injection: 100 mg, 200 mg, 500 mg, 1 g, 2 g
Powder for injection, lyophilized: 100 mg, 200 mg, 500 mg, 1 g, 2 g
Tablet: 25 mg, 50 mg

Cycloplegic Mydriatics Comparison *see page 1269*

Cycloserine (sye kloe ser' een)
Related Information
Antimicrobial Drugs of Choice *on page 1298-1302*
Brand Names Seromycin® Pulvules®
Use Adjunctive treatment in pulmonary or extrapulmonary tuberculosis; treatment of acute urinary tract infections caused by *E. coli* or *Enterobacter* sp when less toxic conventional therapy has failed or is contraindicated
Pregnancy Risk Factor C
Contraindications Known hypersensitivity to cycloserine
Warnings/Precautions Epilepsy, depression, severe anxiety, psychosis, severe renal insufficiency, chronic alcoholism
Adverse Reactions
1% to 10%: Central nervous system: Drowsiness, headache
<1%:
Cardiovascular: Cardiac arrhythmias, coma
Central nervous system: Dizziness, vertigo, seizures, confusion, psychosis, paresis
Dermatologic: Rash
Hepatic: Elevated liver enzymes
Neuromuscular & skeletal: Tremor
Miscellaneous: Vitamin B_{12} deficiency, folate deficiency
Overdosage/Toxicology Symptoms of overdose include confusion, CNS depression, psychosis, coma, seizures; decontaminate with activated charcoal; can be hemodialyzed; management is supportive; administer 100-300 mg/day of pyridoxine to reduce neurotoxic effects; acute toxicity can occur with ingestions >1 g
Drug Interactions Increased toxicity: Alcohol, isoniazid, ethionamide increase toxicity of cycloserine; cycloserine inhibits the hepatic metabolism of phenytoin
Mechanism of Action Inhibits bacterial cell wall synthesis by competing with amino acid (D-alanine) for incorporation into the bacterial cell wall; bacteriostatic or bactericidal
Pharmacodynamics/Kinetics
Absorption: Oral: ~70% to 90% from the GI tract
Distribution: Crosses the placenta; appears in breast milk; distributed widely to most body fluids and tissues including CSF, breast milk, bile, sputum, lymph tissue, lungs, and ascitic, pleural, and synovial fluids
Half-life: 10 hours in patients with normal renal function
Metabolism: Extensive in liver
Time to peak serum concentration: Oral: Within 3-4 hours
Elimination: 60% to 70% of oral dose excreted unchanged in urine by glomerular filtration within 72 hours, small amounts excreted in feces, remainder is metabolized
Usual Dosage Some of the neurotoxic effects may be relieved or prevented by the concomitant administration of pyridoxine

Tuberculosis: Oral:
Children: 10-20 mg/kg/day in 2 divided doses up to 1000 mg/day for 18-24 months
Adults: Initial: 250 mg every 12 hours for 14 days, then give 500 mg to 1 g/day in 2 divided doses for 18-24 months (maximum daily dose: 1 g)

Dosing interval in renal impairment:
Cl_{cr} 10-50 mL/minute: Administer every 12-24 hours
(Continued)

Cycloserine *(Continued)*

Cl$_{cr}$ <10 mL/minute: Administer every 24 hours

Monitoring Parameters Periodic renal, hepatic, hematological tests, and plasma cycloserine concentrations

Reference Range Toxicity is greatly increased at levels >30 µg/mL

Patient Information May cause drowsiness; notify physician if skin rash, mental confusion, dizziness, headache, or tremors occur; do not skip doses; do not drink excessive amounts of alcoholic beverages

Dosage Forms Capsule: 250 mg

Cyclospasmol® *see* Cyclandelate *on page 283*

Cyclosporin A *see* Cyclosporine *on this page*

Cyclosporine *(sye' kloe spor een)*

Brand Names Sandimmune®

Synonyms CSA; CyA; Cyclosporin A

Use Immunosuppressant which may be used with azathioprine and/or corticosteroids to prolong organ and patient survival in kidney, liver, heart, and bone marrow transplants

Pregnancy Risk Factor C

Pregnancy/Breast Feeding Implications Based on small numbers of patients, the use of cyclosporine during pregnancy apparently does not pose a major risk to the fetus

Contraindications Hypersensitivity to cyclosporine or Cremephor EL (I.V. solution) or any component

Warnings/Precautions Infection and possible development of lymphoma may result. Make dose adjustments to avoid toxicity or possible organ rejection using cyclosporine blood levels because absorption is erratic and elimination is highly variable; administer with adrenal corticosteroids but not with other immunosuppressive agents. Adjustment of dose should only be made under the direct supervision of an experienced physician; reserve the use of I.V. for use only in patients who cannot take oral; adequate airway and other supportive measures and agents for treating anaphylaxis should be present when I.V. drug is given. Nephrotoxic, if possible avoid concomitant use of other potentially nephrotoxic drugs (eg, acyclovir, aminoglycoside antibiotics, amphotericin B, ciprofloxacin).

Adverse Reactions

>10%:

Cardiovascular: Hypertension

Dermatologic: Hirsutism

Neuromuscular & skeletal: Tremor

Renal: Nephrotoxicity

Miscellaneous: Gingival hypertrophy

1% to 10%:

Central nervous system: Seizure, headache

Dermatologic: Acne

Gastrointestinal: Abdominal discomfort, nausea, vomiting

Neuromuscular & skeletal: Leg cramps

<1%:

Cardiovascular: Hypotension, tachycardia, warmth, flushing

Endocrine & metabolic: Hyperkalemia, hypomagnesemia, hyperuricemia

Hepatic: Hepatotoxicity

Neuromuscular & skeletal: Myositis, paresthesias

Respiratory: Respiratory distress, sinusitis

Miscellaneous: Anaphylaxis, pancreatitis, increased susceptibility to infection, and sensitivity to temperature extremes

Overdosage/Toxicology Hepatotoxicity, nephrotoxicity, nausea, vomiting, tremor, seizures; CNS secondary to direct action of the drug may not be reflected in serum concentrations, may be more predictable by renal magnesium loss

Drug Interactions

Decreased effect: Rifampin, phenytoin, phenobarbital decreases plasma concentration of cyclosporine

Increased toxicity: Ketoconazole, fluconazole, and itraconazole increase plasma concentration of cyclosporine

Stability

Cyclosporine injection is a clear, faintly brown-yellow solution which should be stored at <30°C and protected from light

Cyclosporine concentrate for injection should be further diluted [1 mL (50 mg)] of concentrate in 20-100 mL of D$_5$W or or NS] for administration by intravenous infusion. Light protection is not required for intravenous admixtures of cyclosporine.

Stability of injection of parenteral admixture at room temperature (25°C): 6 hours in PVC; 24 hours in Excel, PAB containers, or glass

Polyoxyethylated castor oil (Cremophor EL®) surfactant in cyclosporin injection may leach phthalate from PVC containers such as bags and tubing. The actual amount of diethylhexyl phthalate (DEHP) plasticizer leached from PVC containers and administration sets may vary in clinical situations, depending on surfactant concentration, bag size, and contact time.

Doses <250 mg should be prepared in 100 mL of D_5W or NS

Doses >250 mg should be prepared in 250 mL of D_5W or NS

Minimum volume: 100 mL D_5W or NS

Do not refrigerate oral or I.V. solution

Oral solution: Use the contents of the oral solution within two months after opening; should be mixed in glass containers

Mechanism of Action Inhibition of production and release of interleukin II and inhibits interleukin II-induced activation of resting T-lymphocytes

Pharmacodynamics/Kinetics

Absorption: Oral: Incomplete and erratic

Distribution: Distributes into breast milk

Protein binding: 90%

Metabolism: By mixed function oxidase enzymes in the liver

Bioavailability: 31% in pediatric renal transplant patients; gut dysfunction, commonly seen in BMT recipients, reduces oral bioavailability further

Half-life (normal renal function and end stage renal disease): Adults: 19-40 hours

Time to peak serum concentration: 3-4 hours

Elimination: Primarily in bile; clearance is more rapid in pediatric patients than in adults; clearance is decreased in patients with liver disease

Usual Dosage Children and Adults (oral dosage is ~3 times the I.V. dosage):

Oral: Initial: 14-18 mg/kg/day, beginning 4-12 hours prior to organ transplantation; maintenance: 3-15 mg/kg/day divided every 12-24 hours

I.V.: Initial: 5-6 mg/kg/day beginning 4-12 hours prior to organ transplantation; patients should be switched to oral cyclosporine as soon as possible; dose should be in fused over 2-24 hours

Dosing considerations of cyclosporine, see table.

Cyclosporine

Condition	Cyclosporine
Switch from I.V. to oral therapy	Threefold increase in dose
T-tube clamping	Decrease dose; increase availability of bile facilitates absorption of CsA
Pediatric patients	About 2-3 times higher dose compared to adults
Liver dysfunction	Decrease I.V. dose; increase oral dose
Renal dysfunction	Decrease dose to decrease levels if renal dysfunction is related to the drug
Dialysis	Not removed
Inhibitors of hepatic metabolism	Decrease dose
Inducers of hepatic metabolism	Monitor drug level; may need to increase dose

Hemodialysis effects: Supplemental dose is not necessary

Peritoneal dialysis effects: Supplemental dose is not necessary

Dosing adjustment in hepatic impairment: Probably necessary, monitor levels closely

Monitoring Parameters Cyclosporine levels, serum electrolytes, renal function, hepatic function, blood pressure, pulse

Reference Range

Method-dependent and specimen-dependent

Trough levels should be obtained:

Oral: 12-18 hours after dose (chronic usage)

I.V.: 12 hours after dose **or** immediately prior to next dose

Therapeutic range: Not absolutely defined, dependent on organ transplanted, time after transplant, organ function and CSA toxicity

Kidney: 100-200 ng/mL (whole blood HPLC)

Heart: 200-400 ng/mL (whole blood HPLC)

Bone marrow transplant: 100-400 ng/mL (whole blood HPLC)

Liver: 100-300 ng/mL (whole blood HPLC)

Toxic level: Not well defined, nephrotoxicity may occur at any level

(Continued)

Cyclosporine *(Continued)*

Test Interactions Specific whole blood, HPLC assay for cyclosporine may be falsely elevated if sample is drawn from the same line through which dose was administered (even if flush has been administered and/or dose was given hours before)

Patient Information Use glass droppers or glass to hold dose; rinse container to get full dose; mix with milk, chocolate milk, or orange juice preferably at room temperature, improves palatability; stir well and drink at once

Nursing Implications Do not administer liquid from plastic or styrofoam cup; mixing with milk, chocolate milk, or orange juice preferably at room temperature, improves palatability; stir well; do not allow to stand before drinking; rinse with more diluent to ensure that the total dose is taken; after use, dry outside of pipette; do not rinse with water or other cleaning agents; may cause inflamed gums

Dosage Forms
Capsule: 25 mg, 100 mg
Injection: 50 mg/mL (5 mL)
Solution, oral: 100 mg/mL (50 mL)

Cycoflex® *see* Cyclobenzaprine Hydrochloride *on page 285*

Cycrin® *see* Medroxyprogesterone Acetate *on page 677*

Cyklokapron® *see* Tranexamic Acid *on page 1109*

Cylert® *see* Pemoline *on page 846*

Cylex® [OTC] *see* Benzocaine *on page 121*

Cyomin® *see* Cyanocobalamin *on page 282*

Cyproheptadine Hydrochloride (si proe hep′ ta deen)

Brand Names Periactin®

Use Perennial and seasonal allergic rhinitis and other allergic symptoms including urticaria; its off-labeled uses have included appetite stimulation, blepharospasm, cluster headaches, migraine headaches, Nelson's syndrome, pruritus, schizophrenia, spinal cord damage associated spasticity, and tardive dyskinesia

Pregnancy Risk Factor B

Contraindications Hypersensitivity to cyproheptadine or any component; narrow-angle glaucoma, bladder neck obstruction, acute asthmatic attack, stenosing peptic ulcer, GI tract obstruction, those on MAO inhibitors; avoid use in premature and term newborns due to potential association with SIDS

Warnings/Precautions Do not use in neonates, safety and efficacy have not been established in children <2 years of age; symptomatic prostate hypertrophy; antihistamines are more likely to cause dizziness, excessive sedation, syncope, toxic confusion states, and hypotension in the elderly. In case reports, cyproheptadine has promoted weight gain in anorexic adults, though it has not been specifically studied in the elderly. All cases of weight loss or decreased appetite should be adequately assessed.

Adverse Reactions
>10%:
Central nervous system: Slight to moderate drowsiness
Respiratory: Thickening of bronchial secretions
1% to 10%:
Central nervous system: Headache, fatigue, nervousness, dizziness
Gastrointestinal: Appetite stimulation, nausea, diarrhea, abdominal pain, dry mouth
Neuromuscular & skeletal: Arthralgia
Respiratory: Pharyngitis
<1%:
Cardiovascular: Tachycardia, palpitations, edema
Central nervous system: Sedation, CNS stimulation, seizures, depression
Dermatologic: Photosensitivity, rash, angioedema
Hematologic: Hemolytic anemia, leukopenia, thrombocytopenia
Hepatic: Hepatitis
Neuromuscular & skeletal: Myalgia, paresthesia
Respiratory: Bronchospasm
Miscellaneous: Epistaxis, allergic reactions

Overdosage/Toxicology Symptoms of overdose include CNS depression or stimulation, dry mouth, flushed skin, fixed and dilated pupils, apnea. There is no specific treatment for an antihistamine overdose, however, most of its clinical toxicity is due to anticholinergic effects. Anticholinesterase inhibitors may be useful by reducing acetylcholinesterase. Anticholinesterase inhibitors include physostigmine, neostigmine, pyridostigmine, and edrophonium. For anticholinergic overdose with severe life-threatening symptoms, physostigmine 1-2 mg (0.5 or 0.02 mg/kg for children) I.V., slowly may be given to reverse these effects.

Drug Interactions Increased toxicity: MAO inhibitors → hallucinations

Mechanism of Action A potent antihistamine and serotonin antagonist, competes with histamine for H_1-receptor sites on effector cells in the gastrointestinal tract, blood vessels, and respiratory tract

Pharmacodynamics/Kinetics
Metabolism: Almost completely
Elimination: >50% excreted in urine (primarily as metabolites); ~25% excreted in feces

Usual Dosage Oral:
Children: 0.25 mg/kg/day in 2-3 divided doses or 8 mg/m²/day in 2-3 divided doses
2-6 years: 2 mg every 8-12 hours (not to exceed 12 mg/day)
7-14 years: 4 mg every 8-12 hours (not to exceed 16 mg/day)
Adults: 4-20 mg/day divided every 8 hours (not to exceed 0.5 mg/kg/day)

Dosing adjustment in hepatic impairment: Dosage should be reduced in patients with significant hepatic dysfunction

Test Interactions Diagnostic antigen skin tests, ↑ amylases (S), ↓ fasting glucose (S)

Patient Information May cause drowsiness; may stimulate appetite, avoid alcohol and other CNS depressants; may impair judgment and coordination

Nursing Implications Raise bed rails, institute safety measures, assist with ambulation

Dosage Forms
Syrup: 2 mg/5 mL with alcohol 5% (473 mL)
Tablet: 4 mg

Cystagon® *see* Cysteamine *on this page*

Cysteamine (sis tee' a meen)

Brand Names Cystagon®

Use Management of nephropathic cystinosis; approved as orphan drug 8/15/94

Pregnancy Risk Factor C

Pregnancy/Breast Feeding Implications Use only when the potential benefits outweigh the potential hazards to the fetus; in animal studies, cysteamine reduced the fertility of rats and offspring survival at very large doses; it is unknown whether cysteamine is excreted in breast milk; discontinue nursing or discontinue drug during lactation

Contraindications Hypersensitivity to cysteamine or penicillamine

Warnings/Precautions Withhold cysteamine if a mild rash develops; restart at a lower dose and titrate to therapeutic dose; adjust cysteamine dose if CNS symptoms due to the drug, rather than the disease, develop

Adverse Reactions
5% to 10%:
Gastrointestinal: Vomiting, anorexia, diarrhea
Central nervous system: Fever, lethargy
Dermatologic: Rash
<5%:
Cardiovascular: Hypertension
Central nervous system: Somnolence, encephalopathy, headache, seizures, ataxia, confusion, dizziness, jitteriness, nervousness, impaired cognition, emotional changes, hallucinations, nightmares
Dermatologic: Urticaria
Endocrine & metabolic: Dehydration
Gastrointestinal: Bad breath, abdominal pain, dyspepsia, constipation, gastroenteritis, duodenitis, duodenal ulceration
Hematologic: Anemia, leukopenia
Hepatic: Abnormal LFTs
Neuromuscular & skeletal: Tremor, hyperkinesia
Otic: Decreased hearing

Overdosage/Toxicology Symptoms may include vomiting, reduction of motor activity, GI or renal hemorrhage; treatment is generally supportive; hemodialysis may be appropriate

Mechanism of Action Reacts with cystine in the lysosome to convert it to cysteine and to a cysteine-cysteamine mixed disulfide, both of which can then exit the lysosome in patients with cystinosis, an inherited defect of lysosomal transport

Usual Dosage Initiate therapy with ¼ to ⅛ of maintenance dose; titrate slowly upward over 4-6 weeks
(Continued)

Cysteamine *(Continued)*

Children <12 years: Oral: Maintenance: 1.3 g/m²/day divided into 4 doses
Children >12 years and Adults (>110 lbs): 2 g/day in 4 divided doses; dosage may in increased to 1.95 g/m²/day if cystine levels are <1 nmol/½ cystine/mg protein, although intolerance and incidence of adverse events may be increased

Administration Sprinkle capsule contents over food for children <6 years of age

Monitoring Parameters Blood counts and LFTs during therapy; monitor leukocyte cystine measurements every 3 months to determine adequate dosage and compliance (measure 5-6 hours after administration); monitor more frequently when switching salt forms

Reference Range Leukocyte cystine: <1 nmol/½ cystine/mg protein

Patient Information Following initiation of therapy, do not engage in hazardous tasks until the effects of the drug on mental performance are known

Cystospaz® *see* Hyoscyamine Sulfate *on page 559*

Cystospaz-M® *see* Hyoscyamine Sulfate *on page 559*

CYT *see* Cyclophosphamide *on page 286*

Cytadren® *see* Aminoglutethimide *on page 56*

Cytarabine Hydrochloride (sye tare' a been)

Related Information

Antiemetics for Chemotherapy Induced Nausea and Vomiting *on page 1202*
Cancer Chemotherapy Regimens *on page 1218-1241*

Brand Names Cytosar-U®

Synonyms Arabinosylcytosine; Ara-C; Cytosine Arabinosine Hydrochloride

Use Ara-C is one of the most active agents in leukemia; also active against lymphoma, meningeal leukemia, and meningeal lymphoma; has little use in the treatment of solid tumors

Pregnancy Risk Factor D

Contraindications Hypersensitivity to cytarabine or any component

Warnings/Precautions The U.S. Food and Drug Administration (FDA) currently recommends that procedures for proper handling and disposal of antineoplastic agents be considered. Use with caution in pregnant women or women of childbearing age and in infants; must monitor drug tolerance, protect and maintain a patient compromised by drug toxicity that includes bone marrow depression with leukopenia, thrombocytopenia and anemia along with nausea, vomiting, diarrhea, abdominal pain, oral ulceration and hepatic impairment; marked bone marrow depression necessitates dosage reduction in the number of days of administration.

Adverse Reactions

Central nervous system: Has produced seizures when given I.T.; cerebellar syndrome (or cerebellar toxicity), manifested as ataxia, dysarthria, and dysdiadochokinesia, has been reported to be dose-related. This may or may not be reversible.

High-dose therapy toxicities: Cerebellar toxicity, conjunctivitis (make sure the patient is on steroid eye drops during therapy), corneal keratitis, hyperbilirubinemia, pulmonary edema, pericarditis, and tamponade

>10%:

Central nervous system: Fever, rash

Dermatologic: Oral/anal ulceration

Gastrointestinal: Nausea, vomiting, diarrhea, and mucositis which subside quickly after discontinuing the drug; GI effects may be more pronounced with divided I.V. bolus doses than with continuous infusion

Emetic potential:

≤20 mg: Moderately low (10% to 30%)
250 mg to 1 g: Moderately high (60% to 90%)
>1 g: High (>90%)

Hematologic: Bleeding

Hepatic: Hepatic dysfunction, mild jaundice and acute increase in transaminases can be produced

Local: Thrombophlebitis

Myelosuppressive: Occurs within the first week of treatment and lasts for 10-14 days; primarily manifested as granulocytopenia, but anemia can also occur
WBC: Severe
Platelets: Severe
Onset (days): 4-7
Nadir (days): 14-18
Recovery (days): 21-28

1% to 10%:

Cardiovascular: Cardiomegaly

Central nervous system: Dizziness, headache, somnolence, confusion, neuritis, malaise

Dermatologic: Skin freckling, itching, alopecia, cellulitis at injection site

Genitourinary: Urinary retention

Neuromuscular & skeletal: Myalgia, bone pain, peripheral neuropathy

Respiratory: Syndrome of sudden respiratory distress progressing to pulmonary edema, pneumonia

Miscellaneous: Sepsis

Overdosage/Toxicology Symptoms of overdose include myelosuppression, megaloblastosis, nausea, vomiting, respiratory distress, pulmonary edema. A syndrome of sudden respiratory distress progressing to pulmonary edema and cardiomegaly has been reported following high doses.

Drug Interactions

Decreased effect of gentamicin, flucytosine; decreased digoxin oral tablet absorption

Increased toxicity: Alkylating agents and radiation; purine analogs; methotrexate

Stability Keep in refrigerator until reconstituted; after reconstitution, solutions remain stable for 48 hours at room temperature; discard hazy solutions; I.V. infusion solution in NS or D_5W solution is stable for 192 hours at room temperature

I.T. Ara-C is **compatible** with methotrexate and hydrocortisone mixed in the same syringe

Compatible with vincristine, potassium chloride, calcium, magnesium, and idarubicin

Incompatible with 5-FU, gentamicin, heparin, insulin, methylprednisolone, nafcillin, oxacillin, penicillin G sodium

Mechanism of Action Inhibition of DNA synthesis; cell cycle-specific for the S phase of cell division; cytosine gains entry into cells by a carrier process, and then must be converted to its active compound; cytosine acts as an analog and is incorporated into DNA; however, the primary action is inhibition of DNA polymerase resulting in decreased DNA synthesis and repair; degree of its cytotoxicity correlates linearly with its incorporation into DNA; therefore, incorporation into the DNA is responsible for drug activity and toxicity

Pharmacodynamics/Kinetics

Absorption: Because high concentrations of cytidine deaminase are in the GI mucosa and liver, three- to tenfold higher doses than I.V. would need to be given orally; therefore, the oral route is not used

Distribution: V_d: Total body water; widely and rapidly distributed since it enters the cells readily; crosses the blood-brain barrier, and CSF levels of 40% to 50% of the plasma level are reached

Metabolism: Primarily in the liver; Ara-C must be metabolized to Ara-CTP to be active

Half-life:

Initial: 7-20 minutes

Terminal: 0.5-2.6 hours

Elimination: ~80% of dose excreted in the urine as metabolites within 36 hours

Usual Dosage Bolus doses are relatively well tolerated since the drug is rapidly metabolized; continuous infusion uniformly results in myelosuppression. Children and Adults (refer to individual protocols):

Induction remission:

I.V.: 200 mg/m²/day for 5 days at 2-week intervals; 100-200 mg/m²/day for 5- to 10-day therapy course or every day until remission

Give I.V. continuous drip, or in 2-3 divided doses

I.T.: 5-75 mg/m² every 2-7 days until CNS findings normalize

or

<1 year: 20 mg

1-2 years: 30 mg

2-3 years: 50 mg

>3 years: 70 mg

Maintenance remission:

I.V.: 70-200 mg/m²/day for 2-5 days at monthly intervals

I.M., S.C.: 1-1.5 mg/kg single dose for maintenance at 1- to 4-week intervals

High-dose therapies:

Doses as high as 1-3 g/m² have been used for refractory or secondary leukemias or refractory non-Hodgkin's lymphoma

Doses of 3 g/m² every 12 hours for up to 12 doses have been used

Bone marrow transplant: 1.5 g/m² continuous infusion over 48 hours

Dose may need to be adjusted in patients with liver failure since cytarabine is partially detoxified in the liver

Administration Administer corticosteroid eye drops around-the-clock prior to, during, and after high-dose Ara-C for prophylaxis of conjunctivitis; pyridoxine has

(Continued)

Cytarabine Hydrochloride *(Continued)*

been administered on days of high-dose Ara-C therapy for prophylaxis of CNS toxicity. Can be administered I.M., IVP, I.V. infusion, or S.C. at a concentration not to exceed 100 mg/mL; high-dose regimens are usually administered by I.V. infusion over 1-3 hours or as I.V. continuous infusion; for I.T. use, reconstitute with preservative-free saline or preservative-free lactated Ringer's solution; add hydrocortisone to intrathecal doses.

Monitoring Parameters Liver function tests, CBC with differential and platelet count, serum creatinine, BUN, serum uric acid

Patient Information Notify physician of any fever, sore throat, bleeding, or bruising

Additional Information Supplied with diluent containing benzyl alcohol, which should not be used when preparing either high-dose or I.T. doses

Dosage Forms Powder for injection: 100 mg, 500 mg, 1 g, 2 g

CytoGam™ *see* Cytomegalovirus Immune Globulin Intravenous, Human *on this page*

Cytomegalovirus Immune Globulin Intravenous, Human

(sye toe meg a low vi′ rus)

Brand Names CytoGam™

Synonyms CMV-IGIV

Use Attenuation of primary CMV disease associated with kidney transplantation

Contraindications Hypersensitivity to any component, patients with selective immunoglobulin A deficiency (↑ potential for anaphylaxis)

Warnings/Precautions Studies indicate that product carries little or no risk for transmission of HIV

Adverse Reactions

1% to 10%:
   Cardiovascular: Flushing of the face
   Gastrointestinal: Nausea, vomiting
   Neuromuscular & skeletal: Muscle cramps, back pain
   Respiratory: Wheezing
   Miscellaneous: Diaphoresis
<1%:
   Cardiovascular: Tightness in the chest
   Central nervous system: Dizziness, fever, headache, chills
   Miscellaneous: Hypersensitivity reactions

Drug Interactions May inactivate live virus vaccines (eg, measles, mumps, rubella)

Stability Use reconstituted product within 6 hours

Mechanism of Action CMV-IGIV is a preparation of immunoglobulin G derived from pooled healthy blood donors with a high titer of CMV antibodies; administration provides a passive source of antibodies against cytomegalovirus

Usual Dosage I.V.:
   Dosing schedule:
      Initial dose (within 72 hours after transplant): 150 mg/kg/dose
      2 weeks after transplant: 100 mg/kg/dose
      4, 6, 8 weeks after transplant: 100 mg/kg/dose
      12 and 16 weeks after transplant: 50 mg/kg/dose

   Administration rate: Administer at 15 mg/kg/hour initially, then increase to 30 mg/kg/hour after 30 minutes if no untoward reactions, then increase to 60 mg/kg/hour after another 30 minutes; volume not to exceed 75 mL/hour

Administration I.V. use only; administer as separate infusion; infuse beginning at 15 mg/kg/hour; may titrate up to 60 mg/kg/hour; do not administer faster than 75 mL/hour

Dosage Forms Powder for injection, lyophilized: 2500±250 mg (50 mL)

Cytomel® *see* Liothyronine Sodium *on page 637*

Cytosar-U® *see* Cytarabine Hydrochloride *on page 294*

Cytosine Arabinosine Hydrochloride *see* Cytarabine Hydrochloride *on page 294*

Cytotec® *see* Misoprostol *on page 746*

Cytovene® *see* Ganciclovir *on page 496*

Cytoxan® *see* Cyclophosphamide *on page 286*

D-3-Mercaptovaline *see* Penicillamine *on page 847*

d4T *see* Stavudine *on page 1028*

Dacarbazine (da kar' ba zeen)

Related Information
Antiemetics for Chemotherapy Induced Nausea and Vomiting *on page 1202*
Cancer Chemotherapy Regimens *on page 1218-1241*

Brand Names DTIC-Dome®

Synonyms DIC; Dimethyl Triazeno Imidazol Carboxamide; DTIC; Imidazole Carboxamide

Use Treatment of malignant melanoma, Hodgkin's disease, soft-tissue sarcomas, fibrosarcomas, rhabdomyosarcoma, islet cell carcinoma, medullary carcinoma of the thyroid, and neuroblastoma

Pregnancy Risk Factor C

Contraindications Hypersensitivity to dacarbazine or any component

Warnings/Precautions The U.S. Food and Drug Administration (FDA) currently recommends that procedures for proper handling and disposal of antineoplastic agents be considered. Use with caution in patients with bone marrow depression; in patients with renal and/or hepatic impairment since dosage reduction may be necessary; avoid extravasation of the drug.

Adverse Reactions
>10%: Pain and burning at infusion site
  Extravasation: Dacarbazine is an irritant; may cause tissue necrosis after extravasation; apply ice and consult extravasation policy if this occurs
  Irritant chemotherapy:
    Gastrointestinal: Moderate to severe nausea and vomiting in 90% of patients and lasting up to 12 hours after administration; nausea and vomiting are dose-related and occur more frequently when given as a one-time dose, as opposed to a less intensive 5-day course; diarrhea may also occur
  Emetic potential:
    <500 mg: Moderately high (60% to 90%)
    ≥500 mg: High (>90%)
1% to 10%:
  Cardiovascular: Facial flushing
  Central nervous system: Headache
  Dermatologic: Alopecia, rash
  Flu-like effects: Fever, malaise, headache, myalgia, and sinus congestion may last up to several days after administration
  Gastrointestinal: Anorexia, metallic taste
  Myelosuppressive: Mild to moderate is common and dose-related; leukopenia and thrombocytopenia may be delayed 2-3 weeks and may be the dose-limiting toxicity
    WBC: Mild (primarily leukocytes)
      Platelets: Mild
      Onset (days): 7
      Nadir (days): 10-14
      Recovery (days): 21-28
  Neuromuscular & skeletal: Paresthesias
  Respiratory: Sinus congestion
  Miscellaneous: Anaphylactic reactions
<1%:
  Cardiovascular: Orthostatic hypotension
  Central nervous system: Weakness, polyneuropathy, blurred vision, headache, and seizures have been reported
  Dermatologic: Photosensitivity reactions, alopecia
  Gastrointestinal: Stomatitis, diarrhea
  Hepatic: Elevated LFTs
  Miscellaneous: Anaphylaxis

Overdosage/Toxicology Symptoms of overdose include myelosuppression, diarrhea; there are no known antidotes; treatment is primarily symptomatic and supportive

Stability Vials require refrigeration and are stable for up to 72 hours under refrigeration and up to 8 hours at room temperature once reconstituted. DTIC-Dome® should be protected from light. Solutions further diluted in D_5W or NS are stable under refrigeration for up to 24 hours.

Mechanism of Action Alkylating agent which forms methylcarbonium ions that attack nucleophilic groups in DNA; cross-links strands of DNA resulting in the inhibition of DNA, RNA, and protein synthesis, but the exact mechanism of action is still unclear; originally developed as a purine antimetabolite, but it does not interfere with purine synthesis; metabolism by the host is necessary for activation of dacarbazine, then the methylated species acts by alkylation of nucleic acids; dacarbazine is active in all phases of the cell cycle

Pharmacodynamics/Kinetics
Onset of action: I.V.: 18-24 days
(Continued)

Dacarbazine *(Continued)*

Absorption: Oral administration demonstrates slow and variable absorption; preferable to administer by I.V. route

Distribution: V_d: 0.6 L/kg, exceeding total body water and suggesting binding to some tissue (probably the liver)

Protein binding: Minimal (5%)

Metabolism: Extensive in the liver, and hepatobiliary excretion is probably of some importance; metabolites may also have an antineoplastic effect

Half-life (biphasic):
Initial: 20-40 minutes
Terminal: 5 hours

Elimination: Hepatobiliary; ~30% to 50% of dose excreted unchanged in the urine by tubular secretion

Usual Dosage I.V. (refer to individual protocols):

Children and Adults: As a single dose, has been administered 800-900 mg/m² every 3-4 weeks

Adults:
Malignant melanoma: 2-4.5 mg/kg/day for 10 days, repeat in 4 weeks or may use 250 mg/m²/day for 5 days, repeat in 3 weeks

Hodgkin's disease: 150 mg/m²/day for 5 days, repeat every 4 weeks or 375 mg/m² on day 1, repeat in 15 days of each 28-day cycle in combination with other agents

Dosing adjustment in renal impairment: Adjustment is warranted

Dosing adjustment/comments in hepatic impairment: Monitor closely for signs of toxicity

Monitoring Parameters CBC with differential, platelet count, liver function tests

Patient Information Report any persistent fever, sore throat, or malaise or fatigue

Nursing Implications Extravasation management: Local pain, burning sensation, and irritation at the injection site may be relieved by local application of hot packs; if extravasation occurs, apply cold packs; protect exposed tissue from light following extravasation

Dosage Forms Injection: 100 mg, 200 mg, 500 mg

Dacodyl® [OTC] *see* Bisacodyl *on page 134*

Dactinomycin *(dak ti noe mye' sin)*

Related Information

Antiemetics for Chemotherapy Induced Nausea and Vomiting *on page 1202*
Cancer Chemotherapy Regimens *on page 1218-1241*

Brand Names Cosmegen®

Synonyms ACT; Actinomycin D

Use Treatment of testicular tumors, melanoma, choriocarcinoma, Wilms tumor, neuroblastoma, retinoblastoma, rhabdomyosarcoma, uterine sarcomas, Ewing's sarcoma, Kaposi's sarcoma, and soft tissue sarcoma

Pregnancy Risk Factor C

Contraindications Hypersensitivity to dactinomycin or any component; patients with chickenpox or herpes zoster; avoid in infants <6 months of age

Warnings/Precautions The U.S. Food and Drug Administration (FDA) currently recommends that procedures for proper handling and disposal of antineoplastic agents be considered. Drug is extremely irritating to tissues and must be administered I.V.; if extravasation occurs during I.V. use, severe damage to soft tissues will occur; use with caution in patients who have received radiation therapy or in the presence of hepatobiliary dysfunction; reduce dosage in patients who are receiving radiation therapy simultaneously.

Adverse Reactions

Extravasation: An irritant and should be administered through a rapidly running I.V. line; extravasation can lead to tissue necrosis, pain, and ulceration

Vesicant chemotherapy

Myelosuppressive: Dose-limiting toxicity; anemia, aplastic anemia, agranulocytosis, pancytopenia
WBC: Moderate
Platelets: Moderate
Onset (days): 7
Nadir (days): 14-21
Recovery (days): 21-28

>10%:
Central nervous system: Unusual tiredness, malaise, fatigue, fever
Dermatologic: Alopecia (reversible), skin eruptions, acne, increased pigmentation of previously irradiated skin

Endocrine & metabolic: Hypocalcemia

Gastrointestinal: **Highly emetogenic**

Severe nausea and vomiting occurs in most patients and persists for up to 24 hours; stomatitis, anorexia, abdominal pain, esophagitis, diarrhea

1% to 10%: Gastrointestinal: Diarrhea, mucositis

<1%:

Endocrine & metabolic: Hyperuricemia

Hepatic: Hepatitis, liver function tests abnormalities

Miscellaneous: Anaphylactoid reaction

Overdosage/Toxicology Symptoms of overdose include myelosuppression, nausea, vomiting, glossitis, oral ulceration; there are no known antidotes and treatment is primarily symptomatic and supportive

Drug Interactions Increased toxicity:

Dactinomycin potentiates the effects of radiation therapy

Radiation may cause skin erythema which may become severe

Also associated with incidence of GI toxicity

Stability Although chemically stable after reconstitution, there is no preservatives present, discard any used portion; use of a diluent containing preservatives to reconstitute will result in a precipitate. Reconstituted solutions should be discarded within a few hours; may exhibit considerable binding to Millex or Millex GV filters; binds to cellulose filters, so avoid in-line filtration; adsorbs to glass and plastic so dactinomycin should not be given by continuous or intermittent infusion.

Mechanism of Action Binds to the guanine portion of DNA intercalating between guanine and cytosine base pairs inhibiting DNA and RNA synthesis and protein synthesis; product of *Streptomyces parvullus* (a yeast species)

Pharmacodynamics/Kinetics

Distribution: Poor penetration into CSF; crosses placenta; high concentrations found in bone marrow and tumor cells, submaxillary gland, liver, and kidney

Metabolism: Minimal

Half-life: 36 hours

Time to peak serum concentration: I.V.: Within 2-5 minutes

Elimination: ~10% of dose excreted as unchanged drug in the urine, 14% excreted in feces, while 50% appears in the bile

Usual Dosage Dosage should be based on body surface area in obese or edematous patients (refer to individual protocols)

Children >6 months and Adults: I.V.:

15 mcg/kg/day or 400-600 mcg/m^2/day for 5 days, may repeat every 3-6 weeks; or

2.5 mg/m^2 given in divided doses over 1 week

0.75-2 mg/m^2 as a single dose given at intervals of 1-4 weeks have been used

Dosing in renal impairment: No adjustment necessary

Administration Do not give I.M. or S.C.

Monitoring Parameters CBC with differential and platelet count, liver function tests, and renal function tests

Patient Information Notify physician if fever, persistent sore throat, bleeding, bruising, fatigue, or malaise occurs

Nursing Implications Care should be taken to avoid extravasation of the drug; an in-line cellulose membrane filter should not be used during administration of dactinomycin solutions

Dosage Forms Powder for injection, lyophilized: 0.5 mg

Dakin's Solution *see* Sodium Hypochlorite Solution *on page 1015*

Dalalone L.A.® *see* Dexamethasone *on page 314*

Dalcaine® *see* Lidocaine Hydrochloride *on page 633*

Dalgan® *see* Dezocine *on page 322*

Dalmane® *see* Flurazepam Hydrochloride *on page 481*

d-Alpha Tocopherol *see* Vitamin E *on page 1164*

Dalteparin (dal te' pa rin)

Brand Names Fragmin®

Use Prevention of deep vein thrombosis which may lead to pulmonary embolism, in patients requiring abdominal surgery who are at risk for thromboembolism complications (ie, patients >40 years of age, obese, patients with malignancy, history of deep vein thrombosis or pulmonary embolism, and surgical procedures requiring general anesthesia and lasting longer than 30 minutes)

(Continued)

Dalteparin *(Continued)*

Contraindications Hypersensitivity to dalteparin or other low-molecular weight heparins; cerebrovascular disease or other active hemorrhage; cerebral aneurysm; severe uncontrolled hypertension

Warnings/Precautions Use with caution in patients with pre-existing thrombocytopenia, recent childbirth, subacute bacterial endocarditis, peptic ulcer disease, pericarditis or pericardial effusion, liver or renal function impairment, recent lumbar puncture, vasculitis, concurrent use of aspirin (increased bleeding risk), previous hypersensitivity to heparin, heparin-associated thrombocytopenia

Adverse Reactions

1% to 10%:

Dermatologic: Allergic reactions (eg, pruritus, rash, fever, injection site reaction, bullous eruption), anaphylactoid reactions and skin necrosis

Hematologic: Bleeding, wound hematoma, injection site hematoma, thrombocytopenia

Local: Pain at injection site

Drug Interactions Increased toxicity: Caution should be used when using aspirin, other platelet inhibitors, and oral anticoagulants in combination with dalteparin due to an increased risk of bleeding

Stability Store at temperatures ≤25°C

Mechanism of Action Low molecular weight heparin analog with a molecular weight of 4000-6000 daltons; the commercial product contains 3% to 15% heparin with a molecular weight <3000 daltons, 65% to 78% with a molecular weight of 3000-8000 daltons and 14% to 26% with a molecular weight >8000 daltons; while dalteparin has been shown to inhibit both factor Xa and factor IIa (thrombin), the antithrombotic effect of dalteparin is characterized by a higher ratio of antifactor Xa to antifactor IIa activity (ratio = 4)

Usual Dosage Adults: S.C.: 2500 units 1-2 hours prior to surgery, then once daily for 5-10 days postoperatively

Monitoring Parameters Periodic CBC including platelet count; stool occult blood tests; monitoring of PT and PTT is not necessary

Dosage Forms Injection: Prefilled syringe: 2500 units (16 mg) in 0.2 mL

Damason-P® *see* Hydrocodone and Aspirin *on page 544*

Danazol *(da′ na zole)*

Brand Names Danocrine®

Use Treatment of endometriosis, fibrocystic breast disease, and hereditary angioedema

Pregnancy Risk Factor X

Contraindications Undiagnosed genital bleeding, hypersensitivity to danazol or any component, significant renal, hepatic, or cardiac impairment; pregnancy and lactation

Warnings/Precautions Use with caution in patients with seizure disorders, migraine, impaired hepatic, renal, or cardiac disease

Adverse Reactions

>10%:

Androgenic: Weight gain, oily skin, acne, hirsutism, voice deepening, breakthrough bleeding, irregular menstrual periods, decreased breast size

Cardiovascular: Fluid retention, edema

Hepatic: Hepatic impairment

1% to 10%:

Central nervous system: Weakness

Endocrine & metabolic: Virilization, androgenic effects, amenorrhea, hypoestrogenism

<1%:

Central nervous system: Dizziness, headache

Dermatologic: Skin rashes, photosensitivity

Genitourinary: Monilial vaginitism testicular atrophy, enlarged clitoris

Hepatic: Cholestatic jaundice

Miscellaneous: Bleeding gums, carpal tunnel syndrome, benign intracranial hypertension, pancreatitis

Drug Interactions Increased toxicity: Decreased insulin requirements; warfarin → ↑ anticoagulant effects

Mechanism of Action Suppresses pituitary output of follicle-stimulating hormone and luteinizing hormone that causes regression and atrophy of normal and ectopic endometrial tissue; decreases rate of growth of abnormal breast tissue; reduces attacks associated with hereditary angioedema by increasing levels of C4 component of complement

Pharmacodynamics/Kinetics

Onset of therapeutic effect: Within 4 weeks following daily doses

Metabolism: Extensive hepatic metabolism, primarily to 2-hydroxymethylethis-
terone

Half-life: 4.5 hours (variable)

Time to peak serum concentration: Within 2 hours

Elimination: In urine

Usual Dosage Adults: Oral:

Endometriosis: 100-400 mg twice daily for 3-6 months (may extend to 9 months)

Fibrocystic breast disease: 50-200 mg twice daily for 2-6 months

Hereditary angioedema: 400-600 mg/day in 2-3 divided doses

Patient Information Notify physician if masculinity effects occur; virilization may
occur in female patients; report menstrual irregularities; male patients report
persistent penile erections; all patients should report persistent GI distress, diarrhea, or jaundice

Dosage Forms Capsule: 50 mg, 100 mg, 200 mg

Danocrine® see Danazol on previous page

Dantrium® see Dantrolene Sodium on this page

Dantrolene Sodium (dan' troe leen)

Brand Names Dantrium®

Use Treatment of spasticity associated with spinal cord injury, stroke, cerebral
palsy, or multiple sclerosis; also used as treatment of malignant hyperthermia

Pregnancy Risk Factor C

Contraindications Active hepatic disease; should not be used where spasticity is
used to maintain posture or balance

Warnings/Precautions Use with caution in patients with impaired cardiac function or impaired pulmonary function; has potential for hepatotoxicity; overt hepatitis has been most frequently observed between the third and twelfth month of
therapy; hepatic injury appears to be greater in females and in patients >35 years
of age

Adverse Reactions

>10%:

Central nervous system: Drowsiness, dizziness, lightheadedness, fatigue,
tiredness

Dermatologic: Rash

Gastrointestinal: Diarrhea (mild), nausea, vomiting

Neuromuscular & skeletal: Muscle weakness

1% to 10%:

Cardiovascular: Pleural effusion with pericarditis

Central nervous system: Chills, fever, headache, insomnia, nervousness,
mental depression

Gastrointestinal: Diarrhea (severe), constipation, anorexia, stomach cramps

Ocular: Blurred vision

Respiratory: Respiratory depression

<1%:

Central nervous system: Seizures, confusion

Hepatic: Hepatitis

Overdosage/Toxicology Symptoms of overdose include CNS depression,
hypotension, nausea, vomiting; for decontamination, lavage/activated charcoal
with cathartic; do not use ipecac; hypotension can be treated with isotonic I.V.
fluids with the patient placed in the Trendelenburg position; dopamine or norepinephrine can be given if hypotension is refractory to above therapy

Drug Interactions Increased toxicity: Estrogens (hepatotoxicity), CNS depressants (sedation), MAO inhibitors, phenothiazines, clindamycin (increased neuromuscular blockade), verapamil (hyperkalemia and cardiac depression), warfarin,
clofibrate and tolbutamide

Stability Reconstitute vial by adding 60 mL of sterile water for injection USP (**not
bacteriostatic water for injection**); protect from light; use within 6 hours; avoid
glass bottles for I.V. infusion

Mechanism of Action Acts directly on skeletal muscle by interfering with release
of calcium ion from the sarcoplasmic reticulum; prevents or reduces the increase
in myoplasmic calcium ion concentration that activates the acute catabolic
processes associated with malignant hyperthermia

Pharmacodynamics/Kinetics

Absorption: Slow and incomplete from GI tract

Metabolism: Slowly in liver

Half-life: 8.7 hours

Elimination: 25% excreted in urine as metabolites and unchanged drug, 45% to
50% excreted in feces via bile

(Continued)

301

Dantrolene Sodium *(Continued)*

Usual Dosage

Spasticity: Oral:

Children: Initial: 0.5 mg/kg/dose twice daily, increase frequency to 3-4 times/day at 4- to 7-day intervals, then increase dose by 0.5 mg/kg to a maximum of 3 mg/kg/dose 2-4 times/day up to 400 mg/day

Adults: 25 mg/day to start, increase frequency to 2-4 times/day, then increase dose by 25 mg every 4-7 days to a maximum of 100 mg 2-4 times/day or 400 mg/day

Malignant hyperthermia: Children and Adults:

Oral: 4-8 mg/kg/day in 4 divided doses

Preoperative prophylaxis: Begin 1-2 days prior to surgery with last dose 3-4 hours prior to surgery

I.V.: 1 mg/kg; may repeat dose up to cumulative dose of 10 mg/kg (mean effective dose is 2.5 mg/kg), then switch to oral dosage

Preoperative: 2.5 mg/kg ~1¼ hours prior to anesthesia and infused over 1 hour with additional doses as needed and individualized

Monitoring Parameters Motor performance should be monitored for therapeutic outcomes; nausea, vomiting, and liver function tests should be monitored for potential hepatotoxicity; intravenous administration requires cardiac monitor and blood pressure monitor

Test Interactions ↑ serum AST (SGOT), ALT (SGPT), alkaline phosphatase, LDH, BUN, and total serum bilirubin

Patient Information Avoid unnecessary exposure to sunlight (or use sunscreen, protective clothing); avoid alcohol and other CNS depressants; patients should use caution while driving or performing other tasks requiring alertness

Nursing Implications 36 vials needed for adequate hyperthermia therapy; exercise caution at meals on the day of administration because difficulty swallowing and choking has been reported; avoid extravasation as is a tissue irritant

Dosage Forms

Capsule: 25 mg, 50 mg, 100 mg

Powder for injection: 20 mg

Extemporaneous Preparations A 5 mg/mL suspension may be made by adding five (5) 100 mg capsules to a citric acid solution (150 mg citric acid powder in 10 mL water) and then adding syrup to a total volume of 100 mL; stable 2 days in refrigerator

Dapa® [OTC] *see* Acetaminophen *on page 17*

Dapiprazole Hydrochloride *(da' pi pray zole)*

Brand Names Rēv-Eyes™

Use Reverse dilation due to drugs (adrenergic or parasympathomimetic) after eye exams

Pregnancy Risk Factor B

Contraindications Contraindicated in the presence of conditions where miosis is unacceptable, such as acute iritis and in patients with a history of hypersensitivity to any component of the formulation

Warnings/Precautions For ophthalmic use only

Adverse Reactions

>10%: Ophthalmic: Conjunctival injection, headache, burning sensation in the eyes, lid edema, ptosis, lid erythema, chemosis, itching, punctate keratitis, corneal edema, photophobia

1% to 10%: Ophthalmic: Dry eyes, blurring of vision, tearing of eye

Stability After reconstitution, drops are stable at room temperature for 21 days. Store at room temperature (15°C to 30°C/59°F to 86°F)

Mechanism of Action Dapiprazole is a selective alpha-adrenergic blocking agent, exerting effects primarily on alpha₁-adrenoceptors. It induces miosis via relaxation of the smooth dilator (radial) muscle of the iris, which causes pupillary constriction. It is devoid of cholinergic effects. Dapiprazole also partially reverses the cycloplegia induced with parasympatholytic agents such as tropicamide. Although the drug has no significant effect on the ciliary muscle *per se*, it may increase accommodative amplitude, therefore relieving the symptoms of paralysis of accommodation.

Usual Dosage Adults: Administer 2 drops followed 5 minutes later by an additional 2 drops applied to the conjunctiva of each eye; should not be used more frequently than once a week in the same patient

Administration Shake container for several minutes to ensure mixing. Instill 2 drops into the conjunctiva of each eye followed 5 minutes later by an additional 2 drops. Administer after the ophthalmic examination to reverse the diagnostic mydriasis.

Patient Information May still be sensitive to sunlight and sensitivity may return in 2 or more hours: exercise caution when driving at night or performing other activities in poor illumination. To avoid contamination, do not touch tip of container to any surface.

Nursing Implications Finger pressure should be applied to lacrimal sac for 1-2 minutes after instillation to decrease risk of absorption and systemic reactions

Dosage Forms Powder, lyophilized: 25 mg [0.5% solution when mixed with supplied diluent]

Dapsone (dap' sone)
Brand Names Avlosulfon®
Synonyms Diaminodiphenylsulfone
Use Treatment of leprosy and dermatitis herpetiformis (infections caused by *Mycobacterium leprae*), alternative agent for *Pneumocystis carinii* pneumonia prophylaxis (given alone) and treatment (given with trimethoprim)
Pregnancy Risk Factor C
Contraindications Hypersensitivity to dapsone or any component
Warnings/Precautions Use with caution in patients with severe anemia, G-6-PD deficiency; hypersensitivity to other sulfonamides
Adverse Reactions
1% to 10%:
    Hematologic: Dose-related hemolysis, methemoglobinemia with cyanosis
    Miscellaneous: Reactional states
<1%:
    Central nervous system: Peripheral neuropathy, insomnia, headache
    Dermatologic: Exfoliative dermatitis
    Gastrointestinal: Nausea, vomiting
    Hematologic: Hemolytic anemia, methemoglobinemia, leukopenia, agranulocytosis
    Hepatic: Hepatitis, cholestatic jaundice
    Ocular: Blurred vision
    Otic: Tinnitus
Overdosage/Toxicology Symptoms of overdose include nausea, vomiting, hyperexcitability, methemoglobin-induced depression, seizures, cyanosis, hemolysis; following decontamination, methylene blue 1-2 mg/kg I.V. is treatment of choice
Drug Interactions
    Decreased effect/levels: Para-aminobenzoic acid and rifampin
    Increased toxicity: Folic acid antagonists
Stability Protect from light
Mechanism of Action Dapsone is a sulfone antimicrobial. The mechanism of action of the sulfones is similar to that of the sulfonamides. Sulfonamides are competitive antagonists of para-aminobenzoic acid (PABA) and prevent normal bacterial utilization of PABA for the synthesis of folic acid.
Pharmacodynamics/Kinetics
    Absorption: Oral: Well absorbed
    Distribution: V_d: 1.5 L/kg; throughout total body water and present in all tissues, especially liver and kidney
    Metabolism: In the liver
    Half-life, elimination: 30 hours (range: 10-50 hours)
    Elimination: In urine
Usual Dosage Oral:
    Leprosy:
        Children: 1-2 mg/kg/24 hours, up to a maximum of 100 mg/day
        Adults: 50-100 mg/day for 3-10 years
        Dermatitis herpetiformis: Adults: Start at 50 mg/day, increase to 300 mg/day, or higher to achieve full control, reduce dosage to minimum level as soon as possible
        Prophylaxis of *Pneumocystis carinii* pneumonia: Children >1 month: 1 mg/kg/day; maximum: 100 mg
        Treatment of *Pneumocystis carinii* pneumonia: Adults: 100 mg/day in combination with trimethoprim (20 mg/kg/day) for 21 days

    Dosing in renal impairment: Adjustment is necessary, but no specific guidelines are available
Monitoring Parameters Monitor patient for signs of jaundice and hemolysis
Patient Information Frequent blood tests are required during early therapy; discontinue if rash develops and contact physician if persistent sore throat, fever, malaise, or fatigue occurs; may cause photosensitivity
Dosage Forms Tablet: 25 mg, 100 mg

Daraprim® *see* Pyrimethamine *on page 962*

Darvon® *see* Propoxyphene *on page 946*

Darvon-N® *see* Propoxyphene *on page 946*

Datril® [OTC] *see* Acetaminophen *on page 17*

Daunomycin *see* Daunorubicin Hydrochloride *on this page*

Daunorubicin Hydrochloride (daw noe roo' bi sin)

Related Information

Antiemetics for Chemotherapy Induced Nausea and Vomiting *on page 1202*
Cancer Chemotherapy Regimens *on page 1218-1241*
Extravasation Management of Chemotherapeutic Agents *on page 1207-1208*

Brand Names Cerubidine®

Synonyms Daunomycin; DNR; Rubidomycin Hydrochloride

Use Treatment of ANLL and myeloblastic leukemia; questionable results in neuroblastoma

Pregnancy Risk Factor D

Contraindications Hypersensitivity to daunorubicin or any component; congestive heart failure or arrhythmias; pre-existing bone marrow suppression

Warnings/Precautions The U.S. Food and Drug Administration (FDA) currently recommends that procedures for proper handling and disposal of antineoplastic agents be considered. I.V. use only, severe local tissue necrosis will result if extravasation occurs; reduce dose in patients with impaired hepatic, renal, or biliary function; severe myelosuppression is possible when used in therapeutic doses. Total cumulative dose should take into account previous or concomitant treatment with cardiotoxic agents or irradiation of chest.

Irreversible myocardial toxicity may occur as total dosage approaches:
550 mg/m^2 in adults
400 mg/m^2 in patients receiving chest radiation
300 mg/m^2 in children >2 years of age or
10 mg/kg in children <2 years; this may occur during therapy or several months after therapy

Adverse Reactions

>10%:
Alopecia (reversible)
Discoloration of urine (red)
Gastrointestinal: Mild nausea or vomiting occurs in 50% of patients within the first 24 hours; stomatitis may occur 3-7 days after administration, but is not as severe as that caused by doxorubicin

1% to 10%:
Cardiac toxicity: Congestive heart failure; maximum lifetime dose: Refer to Warnings/Precautions
Vesicant chemotherapy
Extravasation: Daunorubicin is a vesicant; infiltration can cause severe inflammation, tissue necrosis, and ulceration; if the drug is infiltrated, consult institutional policy, apply ice to the area, and elevate the limb
Endocrine & metabolic: Hyperuricemia
Gastrointestinal: GI ulceration, diarrhea
Myelosuppressive: Dose-limiting toxicity, occurs in all patients; leukopenia is more significant than thrombocytopenia
WBC: Severe
Platelets: Severe
Onset (days): 7
Nadir (days): 14
Recovery (days): 21-28

<1%:
Dermatologic: Skin rash, pigmentation of nail beds, urticaria
Hepatic: Elevation in serum bilirubin, AST, and alkaline phosphatase
Miscellaneous: Fertility impairment, pericarditis/myocarditis, chills

Overdosage/Toxicology Symptoms of overdose include myelosuppression, nausea, vomiting, stomatitis; there are no known antidotes; treatment is primarily symptomatic and supportive

Stability Reconstituted solution is stable for 24 hours at room temperature and 48 hours when refrigerated; unstable in solutions with a pH >8; reconstituted solution should be protected from sunlight; must be dispensed in an amber bag; **incompatible** with heparin, sodium bicarbonate, 5-FU, and dexamethasone

Mechanism of Action Inhibition of DNA and RNA synthesis, by intercalating between DNA base pairs and by steric obstruction; is not cell cycle-specific for the S phase of cell division; daunomycin is preferred over doxorubicin for the treatment of ANLL because of its dose-limiting toxicity (myelosuppression) is not of concern in the therapy of this disease; has less mucositis associated with its use

Pharmacodynamics/Kinetics

Distribution: V_d: 40 L/kg; crosses the placenta; distributed to many body tissues, particularly the liver, kidneys, lung, spleen, and heart; does not distribute into the CNS

Metabolism: Primarily in the liver to daunorubicinol (active), which circulates

Half-life:

Distribution: 2 minutes

Elimination: 14-20 hours

Terminal: 18.5 hours

Daunorubicinol plasma half-life: 24-48 hours

Elimination: 40% of dose excreted in the bile; ~25% is excreted in the urine as metabolite and unchanged drug; can turn the urine red during first 24-48 hours after treatment

Usual Dosage I.V. (refer to individual protocols):

Children:

Combination therapy: Remission induction for ALL: 25-45 mg/m² on day 1 every week for 4 cycles

<2 years or <0.5 m²: 1 mg/kg per protocol with frequency dependent on regimen employed

Adults: 30-60 mg/m²/day for 3-5 days, repeat dose in 3-4 weeks; total cumulative dose should not exceed 400-600 mg/m²

Normal dose for induction remission for ANLL: 45 mg/m²/day for 3 days

Dosing adjustment in renal impairment: Cl_{cr} <10 mL/minute: Administer 75% of normal dose

Dosing adjustment in hepatic impairment:

Serum bilirubin 1.2-3 mg/dL or AST 60-180 IU: Reduce dose to 75%

Serum bilirubin 3.1-5 mg/dL or AST >180 IU: Reduce dose to 50%

Serum bilirubin >5 mg/dL: Omit use

Administration Administer IVP diluting the reconstituted dose in 10-15 mL normal saline and administering over 2-3 minutes into the tubing of a rapidly infusing I.V. solution of D_5W or NS; daunorubicin has also been diluted in 100 mL of D_5W or NS and infused over 30-45 minutes

Monitoring Parameters CBC with differential and platelet count, liver function test, EKG, ventricular ejection fraction, renal function test

Test Interactions ↑ potassium (S)

Patient Information Discoloration of urine (red) may occur transiently; immediately report any change in sensation (eg, stinging) at injection site during infusion (may be an early sign of infiltration)

Nursing Implications Daunorubicin is a vesicant and should never be administered I.M. or S.C.

Extravasation management:

Topical cooling may be achieved using ice packs or cooling pad with circulating ice water. Cooling of site for 24 hours as tolerated by the patient. Elevate and rest extremity 24-48 hours, then resume normal activity as tolerated. Application of cold inhibits vesicant's cytotoxicity.

Application of heat can be harmful and is contraindicated

If pain, erythema, and/or swelling persist beyond 48 hours, refer patient immediately to plastic surgeon for consultation and possible debridement

Dosage Forms Powder for injection, lyophilized: 20 mg

Daypro™ see Oxaprozin on page 823

DC 240® Softgels® [OTC] see Docusate on page 362

DCF see Pentostatin on page 861

DDAVP® see Desmopressin Acetate on page 311

ddC see Zalcitabine on page 1172

DDI see Didanosine on page 331

1-Deamino-8-D-Arginine Vasopressin see Desmopressin Acetate on page 311

Debrisan® [OTC] see Dextranomer on page 319

Debrox® [OTC] see Carbamide Peroxide on page 179

Decaderm® see Dexamethasone on page 314

Decadron® see Dexamethasone on page 314

Decadron®-LA see Dexamethasone on page 314

Decadron® Turbinaire® see Dexamethasone on page 314

Deca-Durabolin® see Nandrolone on page 774

Decaject-L.A.® see Dexamethasone on page 314

Decaspray® *see* Dexamethasone *on page 314*

Declomycin® *see* Demeclocycline Hydrochloride *on page 308*

Decofed® Syrup [OTC] *see* Pseudoephedrine *on page 955*

Deferoxamine Mesylate (de fer ox′ a meen)

Brand Names Desferal® Mesylate

Use Acute iron intoxication; chronic iron overload secondary to multiple transfusions; diagnostic test for iron overload; iron overload secondary to congenital anemias; hemochromatosis; removal of corneal rust rings following surgical removal of foreign bodies

Investigational use: Treatment of aluminum accumulation in renal failure

Pregnancy Risk Factor C

Contraindications Patients with anuria, primary hemochromatosis

Warnings/Precautions Use with caution in patients with severe renal disease, pyelonephritis; may increase susceptibility to *Yersinia enterocolitica*

Adverse Reactions

1% to 10%: Local: Pain and induration at injection site

<1%:

Cardiovascular: Flushing, hypotension, tachycardia, shock, swelling

Central nervous system: Fever

Dermatologic: Erythema, urticaria, pruritus, rash, cutaneous wheal formation

Gastrointestinal: Abdominal discomfort, diarrhea

Neuromuscular & skeletal: Leg cramps

Ocular: Blurred vision, cataracts

Otic: Hearing loss

Miscellaneous: Anaphylaxis

Overdosage/Toxicology Symptoms of overdose include hypotension, blurring of vision, diarrhea, leg cramps, tachycardia; treatment is symptomatic and supportive

Stability Protect from light; reconstituted solutions (sterile water) may be stored at room temperature for 7 days

Mechanism of Action Complexes with trivalent ions (ferric ions) to form ferrioxamine, which are removed by the kidneys

Pharmacodynamics/Kinetics

Absorption: Oral: <15%

Metabolism: In the liver to ferrioxamine

Half-life:

Parent drug: 6.1 hours

Ferrioxamine: 5.8 hours

Elimination: Renal excretion of the metabolite and unchanged drug

Usual Dosage

Children:

Acute iron intoxication (I.M. is preferred route for patients not in shock). Treat until urine is no longer pink salmon colored:

I.M.: 50 mg/kg/dose every 6 hours to a maximum of 6 g/day

I.V.: 15 mg/kg/hour; maximum: 6 g/day

Chronic iron overload:

I.M., I.V.: 50 mg/kg/dose to a maximum of 6 g/24 hours or 2 g/dose; do not exceed 15 mg/kg/hour I.V.

S.C.: 20-40 mg/kg/day over 8-12 hours (via a portable, controlled infusion device)

Aluminum-induced bone disease: 20-40 mg/kg every hemodialysis treatment, frequency dependent on clinical status of the patient

Adults:

Acute iron intoxication: (I.M. is preferred route for patients not in shock). Treat until urine is no longer pink salmon colored:

I.M., I.V.: 1 g stat, then 0.5 g every 4 hours for two doses, then 0.5 g every 4-12 hours up to 6 g/day; do not exceed 15 mg/kg/hour I.V.

Chronic iron overload:

I.M.: 0.5-1 g every day

I.V.: 2 g after each unit of blood infusion at 15 mg/kg/hour

S.C.: 1-2 g every day over 8-24 hours

Dosing adjustment in renal impairment: Cl_{cr} <10 mL/minute: Administer 50% of dose

Has been used investigationally as a single 40 mg/kg I.V. dose over 2 hours, to promote mobilization of aluminum from tissue stores as an aid in the diagnosis of aluminum-associated osteodystrophy

Administration I.M. is preferred route; maximum I.V. rate is 15 mg/kg/hour. Urticaria, hypotension, and shock have occurred following rapid I.V. administration; give I.M., slow S.C. or I.V. infusion. Add 2 mL sterile water to 500 mg vial; for

I.M. or S.C. administration, no further dilution is required; for I.V. infusion, dilute in dextrose, normal saline, or lactated Ringer's; 10 mg/mL (maximum: 25 mg/mL); maximum rate of infusion: 15 mg/kg/hour.

Monitoring Parameters Serum iron, total iron binding capacity; ophthalmologic exam and audiometry with chronic therapy

Patient Information May turn urine pink; blood and urine tests are necessary to follow therapy

Nursing Implications Iron chelate colors urine salmon pink

Dosage Forms Powder for injection: 500 mg

Deficol® [OTC] see Bisacodyl on page 134

Degest® 2 [OTC] see Naphazoline Hydrochloride on page 775

Dehist® see Brompheniramine Maleate on page 143

Dekasol-L.A.® see Dexamethasone on page 314

Deladiol® see Estradiol on page 407

Delatest® see Testosterone on page 1063

Delatestryl® see Testosterone on page 1063

Delaxin® see Methocarbamol on page 710

Delcort® see Hydrocortisone on page 546

Delestrogen® see Estradiol on page 407

Delsym® [OTC] see Dextromethorphan on page 321

Delta-Cortef® see Prednisolone on page 919

Deltacortisone see Prednisone on page 921

Deltadehydrocortisone see Prednisone on page 921

Deltahydrocortisone see Prednisolone on page 919

Deltasone® see Prednisone on page 921

Demadex® see Torsemide on page 1106

Demecarium Bromide (dem e kare' ee um)

Related Information
Glaucoma Drug Therapy Comparison on page 1270

Brand Names Humorsol®

Use Management of chronic simple glaucoma, chronic and acute angle-closure glaucoma; strabismus

Pregnancy Risk Factor C

Pregnancy/Breast Feeding Implications Although there are no reports of use in pregnancy, demecarium is an ophthalmic medication and transplacental passage in significant amounts would not be expected

Contraindications Hypersensitivity to demecarium or any component, acute inflammatory disease of anterior chamber; pregnancy

Adverse Reactions
1% to 10%: Ophthalmic: Stinging, burning, myopia, visual blurring
<1%:
Cardiovascular: Bradycardia, hypotension, flushing
Gastrointestinal: Nausea, vomiting, diarrhea
Neuromuscular & skeletal: Muscle weakness
Ocular: Retinal detachment, miosis, twitching eyelids, watering eyes
Respiratory: Difficulty in breathing
Miscellaneous: Diaphoresis

Overdosage/Toxicology Antidote: Atropine sulfate: Adults: 0.4-0.6 mg (1/150-1/100 grain) or more parenterally

Stability Do not freeze; protect from heat

Mechanism of Action Cholinesterase inhibitor (anticholinesterase) which causes acetylcholine to accumulate at cholinergic receptor sites and produces effects equivalent to excessive stimulation of cholinergic receptors. Demecarium mainly acts by inhibiting true (erythrocyte) cholinesterase and causes a reduction in intraocular pressure due to facilitation of outflow of aqueous humor; the reduction is likely to be particularly marked in eyes in which the pressure is elevated.

Usual Dosage Children/Adults: Ophthalmic:
Glaucoma: Instill 1 drop into eyes twice weekly to a maximum dosage of 1 or 2 drops twice daily for up to 4 months
Strabismus:
Diagnosis: Instill 1 drop daily for 2 weeks, then 1 drop every 2 days for 2-3 weeks. If eyes become straighter, an accommodative factor is demonstrated.
Therapy: Instill not more than 1 drop at a time in both eyes every day for 2-3 weeks. Then reduce dosage to 1 drop every other day for 3-4 weeks and re-
(Continued)

Demecarium Bromide *(Continued)*

evaluate. Continue at 1 drop every 2 days to 1 drop twice a week and evaluate the patient's condition every 4-12 weeks. If improvement continues, reduce dose to 1 drop once a week and eventually off of medication. Discontinue therapy after 4 months if control of the condition still requires 1 drop every 2 days.

Patient Information For the eye; do not touch dropper to eye; transient burning or stinging may occur; do not use more often than directed

Nursing Implications Finger pressure should be applied to lacrimal sac for 1-2 minutes after instillation to decrease risk of absorption and systemic reactions; patient must be under supervision and tonometric examinations performed every 3-4 hours following initiation of therapy

Dosage Forms Solution, ophthalmic: 0.125% (5 mL); 0.25% (5 mL)

Demeclocycline Hydrochloride (dem e kloe sye' kleen)

Brand Names Declomycin®

Synonyms Demethylchlortetracycline

Use Treatment of susceptible bacterial infections (acne, gonorrhea, pertussis and urinary tract infections) caused by both gram-negative and gram-positive organisms; used when penicillin is contraindicated (other agents are preferred); treatment of chronic syndrome of inappropriate secretion of antidiuretic hormone (SIADH)

Pregnancy Risk Factor D

Contraindications Hypersensitivity to demeclocycline, tetracyclines, or any component

Warnings/Precautions Do not administer to children <9 years of age; photosensitivity reactions occur frequently with this drug, avoid prolonged exposure to sunlight, do not use tanning equipment

Adverse Reactions

1% to 10%:

Dermatologic: Photosensitivity

Gastrointestinal: Nausea, diarrhea

<1%:

Cardiovascular: Pericarditis

Central nervous system: Increased intracranial pressure, bulging fontanels in infants

Dermatologic: Dermatologic effects, pruritus, exfoliative dermatitis

Endocrine & metabolic: Diabetes insipidus syndrome

Gastrointestinal: Vomiting, esophagitis, anorexia, abdominal cramps

Neuromuscular & skeletal: Paresthesia

Renal: Acute renal failure, azotemia

Miscellaneous: Superinfections, anaphylaxis, pigmentation of nails

Overdosage/Toxicology Symptoms of overdose include diabetes insipidus, nausea, anorexia, diarrhea; following GI decontamination, treatment is supportive

Drug Interactions

Decreased effect with antacids (aluminum, calcium, zinc, or magnesium), bismuth salts, sodium bicarbonate, barbiturates, carbamazepine, hydantoins

Decreased effect of oral contraceptives

Increased effect of warfarin

Mechanism of Action Inhibits protein synthesis by binding with the 30S and possibly the 50S ribosomal subunit(s) of susceptible bacteria; may also cause alterations in the cytoplasmic membrane

Pharmacodynamics/Kinetics

Onset of action for diuresis in SIADH: Several days

Absorption: ~50% to 80% from GI tract; food and dairy products reduce absorption

Protein binding: 41% to 50%

Metabolism: Small amounts metabolized in the liver to inactive metabolites; enterohepatically recycled

Half-life: Reduced renal function: 10-17 hours

Time to peak serum concentration: Oral: Within 3-6 hours

Elimination: As unchanged drug (42% to 50%) in urine

Usual Dosage Oral:

Children ≥8 years: 8-12 mg/kg/day divided every 6-12 hours

Adults: 150 mg 4 times/day or 300 mg twice daily

Uncomplicated gonorrhea (penicillin sensitive): 600 mg stat, 300 mg every 12 hours for 4 days (3 g total)

SIADH: 900-1200 mg/day or 13-15 mg/kg/day divided every 6-8 hours initially, then decrease to 0.6-0.9 g/day

Dosing adjustment/comments in renal/hepatic impairment: Should be avoided in patients with renal/hepatic dysfunction

Monitoring Parameters CBC, renal and hepatic function

Test Interactions May interfere with tests for urinary glucose (false-negative urine glucose using Clinistix®, Tes-Tape®)

Patient Information Avoid prolonged exposure to sunlight or sunlamps; avoid taking antacids before tetracyclines

Nursing Implications Administer 1 hour before or 2 hours after food or milk with plenty of fluid

Dosage Forms
Capsule: 150 mg
Tablet: 150 mg, 300 mg

Demerol® *see* Meperidine Hydrochloride *on page 684*

4-demethoxydaunorubicin *see* Idarubicin *on page 563*

Demethylchlortetracycline *see* Demeclocycline Hydrochloride *on previous page*

Demser® *see* Metyrosine *on page 735*

Demulen® *see* Ethinyl Estradiol and Ethynodiol Diacetate *on page 421*

Deodorized Opium Tincture *see* Opium Tincture *on page 819*

Deoxycoformycin *see* Pentostatin *on page 861*

2'-deoxycoformycin *see* Pentostatin *on page 861*

Depakene® *see* Valproic Acid and Derivatives *on page 1143*

Depakote® *see* Valproic Acid and Derivatives *on page 1143*

Depen® *see* Penicillamine *on page 847*

depGynogen® *see* Estradiol *on page 407*

depMedalone® *see* Methylprednisolone *on page 724*

Depo®-Estradiol *see* Estradiol *on page 407*

Depogen® *see* Estradiol *on page 407*

Depoject® *see* Methylprednisolone *on page 724*

Depo-Medrol® *see* Methylprednisolone *on page 724*

Deponit® *see* Nitroglycerin *on page 799*

Depopred® *see* Methylprednisolone *on page 724*

Depo-Provera® *see* Medroxyprogesterone Acetate *on page 677*

Depotest® *see* Testosterone *on page 1063*

Depo®-Testosterone *see* Testosterone *on page 1063*

Deprenyl *see* Selegiline Hydrochloride *on page 1001*

Dermacomb® *see* Nystatin and Triamcinolone *on page 812*

Dermacort® *see* Hydrocortisone *on page 546*

Dermarest Dricort® *see* Hydrocortisone *on page 546*

Derma-Smoothe/FS® *see* Fluocinolone Acetonide *on page 469*

Dermatop® *see* Prednicarbate *on page 919*

Dermatophytin® *see* Trichophyton Skin Test *on page 1119*

DermiCort® *see* Hydrocortisone *on page 546*

Dermolate® [OTC] *see* Hydrocortisone *on page 546*

Dermoplast® [OTC] *see* Benzocaine *on page 121*

Dermoxyl® [OTC] *see* Benzoyl Peroxide *on page 122*

Dermtex® HC with Aloe *see* Hydrocortisone *on page 546*

DES *see* Diethylstilbestrol *on page 334*

Desferal® Mesylate *see* Deferoxamine Mesylate *on page 306*

Desiccated Thyroid *see* Thyroid *on page 1088*

Desipramine Hydrochloride (dess ip' ra meen)

Related Information
Antidepressant Agents Comparison *on page 1250-1252*

Brand Names Norpramin®; Pertofrane®

Synonyms Desmethylimipramine HCl

(Continued)

Desipramine Hydrochloride *(Continued)*

Use Treatment of various forms of depression, often in conjunction with psychotherapy; analgesic adjunct in chronic pain, peripheral neuropathies

Pregnancy Risk Factor C

Contraindications Hypersensitivity to desipramine (cross-sensitivity with other tricyclic antidepressants may occur); patients receiving MAO inhibitors within past 14 days; narrow-angle glaucoma

Warnings/Precautions Use with caution in patients with cardiovascular disease, conduction disturbances, urinary retention, seizure disorders, hyperthyroidism or those receiving thyroid replacement; some formulations contain tartrazine which may cause allergic reaction; do not discontinue abruptly in patients receiving long-term high-dose therapy

Adverse Reactions

>10%:

Central nervous system: Dizziness, drowsiness, headache

Gastrointestinal: Dry mouth, constipation, increased appetite, nausea, weakness, unpleasant taste, weight gain

1% to 10%:

Cardiovascular: Arrhythmias, hypotension

Central nervous system: Confusion, delirium, hallucinations, nervousness, restlessness, parkinsonian syndrome, insomnia

Gastrointestinal: Diarrhea, heartburn

Genitourinary: Difficult urination, sexual function impairment

Neuromuscular & skeletal: Fine muscle tremors

Ocular: Blurred vision, eye pain

Miscellaneous: Excessive sweating

<1%:

Central nervous system: Anxiety, seizures

Dermatologic: Alopecia

Endocrine & metabolic: Breast enlargement, galactorrhea, SIADH

Genitourinary: Testicular swelling

Hematologic: Agranulocytosis, leukopenia, eosinophilia

Hepatic: Cholestatic jaundice, increased liver enzymes

Ocular: Photosensitivity, increased intraocular pressure

Otic: Tinnitus

Miscellaneous: Trouble with gums, decreased lower esophageal sphincter tone may cause GE reflux, allergic reactions

Overdosage/Toxicology Symptoms of overdose include agitation, confusion, hallucinations, hyperthermia, urinary retention, CNS depression, cyanosis, dry mucous membranes, cardiac arrhythmias, seizures

Following GI decontamination, treatment is supportive. Ventricular arrhythmias and EKG changes (eg, QRS widening) often respond with concurrent systemic alkalinization (sodium bicarbonate 0.5-2 mEq/kg I.V.). Arrhythmias unresponsive to phenytoin 15-20 mg/kg (adults) may respond to lidocaine 1 mg/kg I.V. followed by a titrated infusion. Physostigmine (1-2 mg I.V. slowly for adults or 0.5 mg I.V. slowly for children) may be indicated in reversing cardiac arrhythmias that are life-threatening. Seizures usually respond to diazepam I.V. boluses (5-10 mg for adults up to 30 mg or 0.25-0.4 mg/kg/dose for children up to 10 mg/dose). If seizures are unresponsive or recur, phenytoin or phenobarbital may be required.

Drug Interactions

Decreased effects: Guanethidine, clonidine; decreased effect with barbiturates, carbamazepine, phenytoin

Increased effects: Sympathomimetics, benzodiazepines

Increased toxicity: Anticholinergics; increased toxicity with MAO inhibitors (hyperpyrexia, tachycardia, hypertension, seizures, and death may occur), alcohol, CNS depressants, cimetidine

Mechanism of Action Traditionally believed to increase the synaptic concentration of norepinephrine in the central nervous system by inhibition of its reuptake by the presynaptic neuronal membrane. However, additional receptor effects have been found including desensitization of adenyl cyclase, down regulation of beta-adrenergic receptors, and down regulation of serotonin receptors.

Pharmacodynamics/Kinetics

Onset of action: 1-3 weeks (maximum antidepressant effects: after >2 weeks)

Absorption: Well absorbed (90%) from GI tract

Metabolism: In the liver

Half-life: Adults: 12-57 hours

Elimination: 70% excreted in urine

Usual Dosage Oral:

Children 6-12 years: 10-30 mg/day or 1-5 mg/kg/day in divided doses; do not exceed 5 mg/kg/day

Adolescents: Initial: 25-50 mg/day; gradually increase to 100 mg/day in single or divided doses; maximum: 150 mg/day

Adults: Initial: 75 mg/day in divided doses; increase gradually to 150-200 mg/day in divided or single dose; maximum: 300 mg/day

Elderly: Initial dose: 10-25 mg/day; increase by 10-25 mg every 3 days for inpatients and every week for outpatients if tolerated; usual maintenance dose: 75-100 mg/day, but doses up to 300 mg/day may be necessary

Hemodialysis/peritoneal dialysis effects: Supplemental dose is not necessary

Monitoring Parameters Monitor blood pressure and pulse rate prior to and during initial therapy evaluate mental status; monitor weight

Reference Range

Plasma levels do not always correlate with clinical effectiveness

Timing of serum samples: Draw trough just before next dose

Therapeutic: 100-300 ng/mL

In elderly patients the response rate is greatest with steady-state plasma concentrations >115 ng/mL

Possible toxicity: >300 ng/mL

Toxic: >1000 ng/mL

Test Interactions ↑ glucose

Patient Information Avoid alcohol ingestion; do not discontinue medication abruptly; may cause urine to turn blue-green; may cause drowsiness; avoid unnecessary exposure to sunlight; sugarless hard candy or gum can help with dry mouth; full effect may not occur for 3-4 weeks

Nursing Implications May increase appetite

Dosage Forms

Capsule (Pertofrane®): 25 mg, 50 mg

Tablet (Norpramin®): 10 mg, 25 mg, 50 mg, 75 mg, 100 mg, 150 mg

Desitin® [OTC] see Zinc Oxide, Cod Liver Oil, and Talc *on page 1176*

Desmethylimipramine HCl see Desipramine Hydrochloride *on page 309*

Desmopressin Acetate (des moe press' in)

Brand Names DDAVP®; Stimate™

Synonyms 1-Deamino-8-D-Arginine Vasopressin

Use Treatment of diabetes insipidus and controlling bleeding in mild hemophilia, von Willebrand's disease, and thrombocytopenia (eg, uremia)

Pregnancy Risk Factor B

Contraindications Hypersensitivity to desmopressin or any component; avoid using in patients with type IIB or platelet-type von Willebrand's disease; or patients with <5% factor VIII activity level

Warnings/Precautions Avoid overhydration especially when drug is used for its hemostatic effect

Adverse Reactions

1% to 10%:

Cardiovascular: Facial flushing

Central nervous system: Headache, dizziness

Gastrointestinal: Nausea, abdominal cramps

Genitourinary: Vulval pain

Local: Pain at the injection site, nasal congestion

<1%:

Cardiovascular: Increase in blood pressure

Endocrine & metabolic: Hyponatremia

Genitourinary: Water intoxication

Overdosage/Toxicology Symptoms of overdose include drowsiness, headache, confusion, anuria, water intoxication

Drug Interactions

Decreased effect: Demeclocycline, lithium → ↓ ADH effects

Increased effect: Chlorpropamide, fludrocortisone → ↑ ADH response

Stability Keep in refrigerator, avoid freezing; discard discolored solutions; nasal solution stable for 3 weeks at room temperature; injection stable for 2 weeks at room temperature

Mechanism of Action Enhances reabsorption of water in the kidneys by increasing cellular permeability of the collecting ducts; possibly causes smooth muscle constriction with resultant vasoconstriction; raises plasma levels of von Willebrand's factor and factor VIII

Pharmacodynamics/Kinetics

Intranasal administration:

Onset of ADH effects: Within 1 hour

Peak effect: Within 1-5 hours

Duration: 5-21 hours

(Continued)

311

Desmopressin Acetate *(Continued)*

I.V. infusion:
Onset of increased factor VIII activity: Within 15-30 minutes
Peak effect: 90 minutes to 3 hours
Absorption: Nasal: Slow; 10% to 20%
Metabolism: Unknown
Half-life: Elimination (terminal): 75 minutes

Usual Dosage Dilute I.V. dose in 50 mL 0.9% sodium chloride and infuse over 15-30 minutes

Children:
Diabetes insipidus: 3 months to 12 years: Intranasal: Initial: 5 mcg/day divided 1-2 times/day; range: 5-30 mcg/day divided 1-2 times/day
Von Willebrand's disease, thrombocytopathies, hemophilia: >3 months:
Intranasal: 2-4 mcg/kg/dose
I.V.: 0.3 mcg/kg by slow infusion over 15-30 minutes; usually tachyphylaxis occurs after 2-3 doses in 24 hours, recovery of response may take 48-72 hours
Nocturnal enuresis: ≥6 years: Intranasal: Initial: 20 mcg at bedtime; range: 10-40 mcg
Adults:
Diabetes insipidus: I.V., S.C.: 2-4 mcg/day in 2 divided doses or $^1/_{10}$ of the maintenance intranasal dose; intranasal: 5-40 mcg/day 1-3 times/day
Von Willebrand's disease, thrombocytopathies, hemophilia:
Intranasal: 2-4 mcg/kg/dose
I.V.: 0.3 mcg/kg by slow infusion over 15-30 minutes; usually tachyphylaxis occurs after 2-3 doses in 24 hours; recovery of responsiveness may take 48-72 hours

Administration For I.V. administration, dilute in 10-50 mL 0.9% sodium chloride and infuse over 15-30 minutes

Monitoring Parameters Blood pressure and pulse should be monitored during I.V. infusion
Diabetes insipidus: Fluid intake, urine volume, specific gravity, plasma and urine osmolality, serum electrolytes
Hemophilia: Factor VIII antigen levels, APTT, bleeding time (for von Willebrand's disease and thrombocytopathies)

Patient Information Avoid overhydration; notify physician if headache, shortness of breath, heartburn, nausea, abdominal cramps, or vulval pain occur

Dosage Forms
Injection (DDAVP®): 4 mcg/mL (1 mL, 10 mL)
Solution, nasal : 0.1 mg/mL = 10 mcg/dose (2.5 mL, 50 doses/5 mL), 1.5 mg/mL = 150 mcg/dose (25 doses/2.5 mL)

Desonide (dess' oh nide)

Related Information
Corticosteroids Comparisons *on page 1266-1268*

Brand Names DesOwen®; Tridesilon®

Use Adjunctive therapy for inflammation in acute and chronic corticosteroid responsive dermatosis (low potency corticosteroid)

Pregnancy Risk Factor C

Contraindications Known hypersensitivity to desonide, fungal infections, tuberculosis of skin, herpes simplex

Warnings/Precautions Use with caution in patients with impaired circulation, skin infections

Adverse Reactions
<1%: Topical: Burning, itching, irritation, dryness, folliculitis, hypertrichosis, acneiform eruptions, hypopigmentation, perioral dermatitis, allergic contact dermatitis, skin maceration, secondary infection, skin atrophy, striae, miliaria

Overdosage/Toxicology Symptoms of overdose include moon face, central obesity, hypertension, diabetes, hyperlipidemia, peptic ulcer, increased susceptibility to infection, electrolyte and fluid imbalance, psychosis, hallucinations. When consumed in excessive quantities, systemic hypercorticism and adrenal suppression may occur; in those cases discontinuation and withdrawal of the corticosteroid should be done judiciously

Mechanism of Action Stimulates the synthesis of enzymes needed to decrease inflammation, suppress mitotic activity, and cause vasoconstriction

Pharmacodynamics/Kinetics
Onset of effect: Commonly noted within 7 days of continued therapy
Absorption: Topical absorption extensive from the scalp, face, axilla and scrotum; adequate through epidermis on appendages; absorption can be increased with occlusion or the addition of penetrants (eg, urea, DMSO)

Metabolism: By the liver

Elimination: Primarily in urine

Usual Dosage Children and Adults: Topical: Apply 2-4 times/day sparingly

Patient Information A thin film of cream or ointment is effective, do not overuse; rub in lightly; do not use tight-fitting diapers or plastic pants on children being treated in the diaper area; use only as prescribed and for no longer than the period prescribed; avoid contact with eyes; notify physician if condition being treated persists or worsens

Nursing Implications For external use only; do not use on open wounds; apply sparingly to occlusive dressings; should not be used in the presence of open or weeping lesions

Dosage Forms

Cream, topical: 0.05% (15 g, 60 g)

Lotion: 0.05% (60 mL, 120 mL)

Ointment, topical: 0.05% (15 g, 60 g)

DesOwen® *see* Desonide *on previous page*

Desoximetasone (des ox i met' a sone)

Related Information

Corticosteroids Comparisons *on page 1266-1268*

Brand Names Topicort®; Topicort®-LP

Use Relieves inflammation and pruritic symptoms of corticosteroid-responsive dermatosis [medium to high potency topical corticosteroid]

Pregnancy Risk Factor C

Contraindications Known hypersensitivity to desoximetasone, topical fungal infections, tuberculosis of skin herpes simplex

Warnings/Precautions Use with caution in patients with impaired circulation; skin infections

Adverse Reactions

<1%: Topical: Burning, itching, irritation, dryness, folliculitis, hypertrichosis, acneiform eruptions, hypopigmentation, perioral dermatitis, allergic contact dermatitis, skin maceration, secondary infection, skin atrophy, striae, miliaria

Overdosage/Toxicology Symptoms of overdose include moon face, central obesity, hypertension, diabetes, hyperlipidemia, peptic ulcer, increased susceptibility to infection, electrolyte and fluid imbalance, psychosis, hallucinations. When consumed in excessive quantities, systemic hypercorticism and adrenal suppression may occur; in those cases discontinuation and withdrawal of the corticosteroid should be done judiciously.

Mechanism of Action Stimulates the synthesis of enzymes needed to decrease inflammation, suppress mitotic activity, and cause vasoconstriction

Pharmacodynamics/Kinetics Topical:

Absorption: Extensive from the scalp, face, axilla, and scrotum and adequate through epidermis on appendages; absorption can be increased with occlusion or the addition of penetrants

Distribution: Only small amounts reach the systemic circulation or dermal layers

Usual Dosage Topical:

Children: Apply sparingly in a very thin film to affected area 1-2 times/day

Adults: Apply sparingly in a thin film twice daily

Patient Information A thin film of cream or ointment is effective, do not overuse; rub in lightly; do not use tight-fitting diapers or plastic pants on children being treated in the diaper area; use only as prescribed and for no longer than the period prescribed; avoid contact with eyes; notify physician if condition being treated persists or worsens

Nursing Implications For external use only; apply sparingly to occlusive dressings; should not be used in the presence of open or weeping lesions

Dosage Forms Topical:

Cream:

Topicort®: 0.25% (15 g, 60 g, 120 g)

Topicort®-LP: 0.05% (15 g, 60 g)

Gel, topical: 0.05% (15 g, 60 g)

Ointment (Topicort®): 0.25% (15 g, 60 g)

Desoxyephedrine Hydrochloride *see* Methamphetamine Hydrochloride *on page 704*

Desoxyn® *see* Methamphetamine Hydrochloride *on page 704*

Desoxyphenobarbital *see* Primidone *on page 924*

Desquam-E® *see* Benzoyl Peroxide *on page 122*

Desquam-X® *see* Benzoyl Peroxide *on page 122*

Desyrel® *see* Trazodone *on page 1110*

Devrom® [OTC] *see* Bismuth *on page 134*

Dexacidin® *see* Neomycin, Polymyxin B, and Dexamethasone *on page 780*

Dex-A-Diet® [OTC] *see* Phenylpropanolamine Hydrochloride *on page 876*

Dexair® *see* Dexamethasone *on this page*

Dexamethasone (dex a meth' a sone)

Related Information
Cancer Chemotherapy Regimens *on page 1218-1241*
Corticosteroids Comparisons *on page 1266-1268*
Initial Doses in Selected Antiemetic Regimens *on page 1205*

Brand Names Aeroseb-Dex®; AK-Dex®; Alba-Dex®; Baldex®; Dalalone L.A.®; Decaderm®; Decadron®; Decadron®-LA; Decadron® Turbinaire®; Decaject-L.A.®; Decaspray®; Dekasol-L.A.®; Dexair®; Dexasone L.A.®; Dexone®; Dexone L.A.®; Dezone®; Hexadrol®; I-Methasone®; Maxidex®; Ocu-Dex®; Solurex L.A.®

Use Systemically and locally for chronic inflammation, allergic, hematologic, neoplastic, and autoimmune diseases; may be used in management of cerebral edema, septic shock, as a diagnostic agent, antiemetic

Pregnancy Risk Factor C

Pregnancy/Breast Feeding Implications Dexamethasone has been used in patients with premature labor [26-34 weeks gestation] to stimulate fetal lung maturation

Contraindications Active untreated infections; viral, fungal, or tuberculous diseases of the eye

Warnings/Precautions Fatalities have occurred due to adrenal insufficiency in asthmatic patients during and after transfer from systemic corticosteroids to aerosol steroids; aerosol steroids do **not** provide the systemic steroid needed to treat patients having trauma, surgery, or infections; use with caution in patients with hypothyroidism, cirrhosis, hypertension, congestive heart failure, ulcerative colitis, thromboembolic disorders. Because of the risk of adverse effects, systemic corticosteroids should be used cautiously in the elderly in the smallest possible dose and for the shortest possible time.

Adverse Reactions
Systemic:
>10%:
   Central nervous system: Insomnia, nervousness
   Gastrointestinal: Increased appetite, indigestion
1% to 10%:
   Endocrine & metabolic: Diabetes mellitus, hirsutism, joint pain, epistaxis
   Ocular: Cataracts
<1%:
   Central nervous system: Seizures, mood swings, headache, delirium, hallucinations, euphoria
   Dermatologic: Skin atrophy, bruising, hyperpigmentation, acne
   Endocrine & metabolic: Amenorrhea, sodium and water retention, Cushing's syndrome, hyperglycemia, bone growth suppression
   Gastrointestinal: Abdominal distention, ulcerative esophagitis, pancreatitis
   Neuromuscular & skeletal: Muscle wasting
   Miscellaneous: Hypersensitivity reactions

Topical:
<1%: Local: Burning, itching, irritation, dryness, folliculitis, hypertrichosis, acneiform eruptions, hypopigmentation, perioral dermatitis, allergic contact dermatitis, skin maceration, secondary infection, skin atrophy, striae, miliaria

Overdosage/Toxicology Symptoms of overdose include moon face, central obesity, hypertension, psychosis, hallucinations, diabetes, hyperlipidemia, peptic ulcer, increased susceptibility to infection, electrolyte and fluid imbalance, psychosis, hallucinations. When consumed in excessive quantities, systemic hypercorticism and adrenal suppression may occur; in those cases discontinuation and withdrawal of the corticosteroid should be done judiciously.

Drug Interactions Decreased effect: Barbiturates, phenytoin, rifampin → ↓ dexamethasone effects; dexamethasone decreases effect of salicylates, vaccines, toxoids

Stability
Dexamethasone 4 mg/mL injection solution is clear and colorless and dexamethasone 24 mg/mL injection solution is clear and colorless to light yellow. Injection solution should be protected from light and freezing.
Stability of injection of parenteral admixture at room temperature (25°C): 24 hours

Stability of injection of parenteral admixture at refrigeration temperature (4°C): 2 days; protect from light and freezing

Standard diluent: 4 mg/50 mL D_5W; 10 mg/50 mL D_5W

Minimum volume: 50 mL D_5W

Mechanism of Action Decreases inflammation by suppression of migration of polymorphonuclear leukocytes and reversal of increased capillary permeability; suppresses normal immune response

Pharmacodynamics/Kinetics
Duration of metabolic effect: Can last for 72 hours; acetate is a long-acting repository preparation with a prompt onset of action

Metabolism: In the liver

Half-life:
Normal renal function: 1.8-3.5 hours
Biological half-life: 36-54 hours

Time to peak serum concentration:
Oral: Within 1-2 hours
I.M.: Within 8 hours

Elimination: In the urine and bile

Usual Dosage
Children:
Antiemetic (prior to chemotherapy): I.V. (should be given as sodium phosphate): 10 mg/m²/dose (maximum: 20 mg) for first dose then 5 mg/m²/dose every 6 hours as needed

Anti-inflammatory immunosuppressant: Oral, I.M., I.V. (injections should be given as sodium phosphate): 0.08-0.3 mg/kg/day or 2.5-10 mg/m²/day in divided doses every 6-12 hours

Extubation or airway edema: Oral, I.M., I.V. (injections should be given as sodium phosphate): 0.5-2 mg/kg/day in divided doses every 6 hours beginning 24 hours prior to extubation and continuing for 4-6 doses afterwards

Cerebral edema: I.V. (should be given as sodium phosphate): Loading dose: 1-2 mg/kg/dose as a single dose; maintenance: 1-1.5 mg/kg/day (maximum: 16 mg/day) in divided doses every 4-6 hours for 5 days then taper for 5 days, then discontinue

Bacterial meningitis in infants and children >2 months: I.V. (should be given as sodium phosphate): 0.6 mg/kg/day in 4 divided doses every 6 hours for the first 4 days of antibiotic treatment; start dexamethasone at the time of the first dose of antibiotic

Adults:
Antiemetic (prior to chemotherapy): I.V. (should be given as sodium phosphate): 10 mg/m²/dose for first dose then 5 mg/m²/dose every 6 hours as needed

Anti-inflammatory:
Oral, I.M., I.V. (injections should be given as sodium phosphate): 0.5-9 mg/day in divided doses every 6-12 hours
I.M. (as acetate): 8-16 mg; may repeat in 1-3 weeks
Intralesional (as acetate): 0.8-1.6 mg
Intra-articular/soft tissue (as acetate): 4-16 mg; may repeat in 1-3 weeks
Intra-articular, intralesional or soft tissue (as sodium phosphate): 0.4-6 mg/day

Cerebral edema: I.V. 10 mg stat, 4 mg I.M./I.V. (should be given as sodium phosphate) every 6 hours until response is maximized, then switch to oral regimen, then taper off if appropriate; dosage may be reduced after 24 days and gradually discontinued over 5-7 days

Diagnosis for Cushing's syndrome: Oral: 1 mg at 11 PM, draw blood at 8 AM the following day for plasma cortisol determination

Physiological replacement: Oral, I.M., I.V. (should be given as sodium phosphate): 0.03-0.15 mg/kg/day or 0.6-0.75 mg/m²/day in divided doses every 6-12 hours

Shock therapy:
Addisonian crisis/shock (ie, adrenal insufficiency/responsive to steroid therapy): I.V. (given as sodium phosphate): 4-10 mg as a single dose, which may be repeated if necessary

Unresponsive shock (ie, unresponsive to steroid therapy): I.V. (given as sodium phosphate): 1-6 mg/kg as a single I.V. dose or up to 40 mg initially followed by repeat doses every 2-6 hours while shock persists

Ophthalmic:
Ointment: Apply thin coating into conjunctival sac 3-4 times/day; gradually taper dose to discontinue

Suspension: Instill 2 drops into conjunctival sac every hour during the day and every other hour during the night; gradually reduce dose to every 3-4 hours, then to 3-4 times/day

Topical: Apply 1-4 times/day

Monitoring Parameters Hemoglobin, occult blood loss, serum potassium, and glucose

(Continued)

Dexamethasone *(Continued)*

Reference Range Dexamethasone suppression test, overnight: 8 AM cortisol <6 µg/100 mL (dexamethasone 1 mg); plasma cortisol determination should be made on the day after giving dose

Patient Information

Notify physician of any signs of infection or injuries during therapy; inform physician or dentist before surgery if you are taking a corticosteroid; do not overuse; use only as prescribed and for no longer than the period prescribed; may cause GI upset; take with food

Topical: Thin film of cream or ointment is effective, do not overuse; do not use tight-fitting diapers or plastic pants on children being treated in the diaper area; use only as prescribed, and for no longer than the period prescribed; rub in lightly; avoid contact with eyes; notify physician if condition being treated persists or worsens

Nursing Implications Give oral formulation with meals to decrease GI upset; topical formation is for external use, do not use on open wounds; apply sparingly to occlusive dressings; should not be used in the presence of open or weeping lesions; **acetate injection is not for I.V. use**

Dosage Forms

Aerosol:

Oral, as sodium phosphate: 84 mcg dexamethasone per activation (12.6 g)

Nasal, as sodium phosphate: 84 mcg dexamethasone/spray (12.6 g)

Cream, as sodium phosphate: 0.1% (15 g, 30 g)

Elixir: 0.5 mg/5 mL (5 mL, 20 mL, 100 mL, 120 mL, 237 mL, 240 mL, 500 mL)

Injection, as acetate suspension: 8 mg/mL (1 mL, 5 mL); 16 mg/mL (1 mL, 5 mL)

Injection, as sodium phosphate: 4 mg/mL (1 mL, 5 mL, 10 mL, 25 mL, 30 mL); 10 mg/mL (1 mL, 10 mL); 20 mg/mL (5 mL); 24 mg/mL (5 mL, 10 mL)

Ointment, ophthalmic, as sodium phosphate: 0.05% (3.5 g)

Solution, oral:

Concentrate: 0.5 mg/0.5 mL (30 mL) (30% alcohol)

Oral: 0.5 mg/5 mL (5 mL, 20 mL, 500 mL)

Suspension, ophthalmic, as sodium phosphate: 0.1% with methylcellulose 0.5% (5 mL, 15 mL)

Tablet: 0.25 mg, 0.5 mg, 0.75 mg, 1 mg, 1.5 mg, 2 mg, 4 mg, 6 mg

Tablet, therapeutic pack: 6 x 1.5 mg; 8 x 0.75 mg

Topical: 0.01% (58 g); 0.04% (25 g)

Dexamethasone and Tobramycin *see* Tobramycin and Dexamethasone *on page 1100*

Dexasone L.A.® *see* Dexamethasone *on page 314*

Dexasporin® *see* Neomycin, Polymyxin B, and Dexamethasone *on page 780*

Dexatrim® [OTC] *see* Phenylpropanolamine Hydrochloride *on page 876*

Dexchlor® *see* Dexchlorpheniramine Maleate *on this page*

Dexchlorpheniramine Maleate *(dex klor fen eer′ a meen)*

Brand Names Dexchlor®; Poladex®; Polaramine®; Polargen®

Use Perennial and seasonal allergic rhinitis and other allergic symptoms including urticaria

Pregnancy Risk Factor B

Contraindications Narrow-angle glaucoma, hypersensitivity to dexchlorpheniramine or any component

Warnings/Precautions Bladder neck obstruction, symptomatic prostatic hypertrophy, asthmatic attack, and stenosing peptic ulcer

Adverse Reactions

>10%:

Central nervous system: Slight to moderate drowsiness

Miscellaneous: Thickening of bronchial secretions

1% to 10%:

Central nervous system: Headache, fatigue, nervousness, dizziness

Gastrointestinal: Appetite increase, weight increase, nausea, diarrhea, abdominal pain, dry mouth

Neuromuscular & skeletal: Arthralgia

Respiratory: Pharyngitis

<1%:

Cardiovascular: Edema, palpitations

Central nervous system: Depression, epistaxis

Dermatologic: Angioedema, photosensitivity, rash

Hepatic: Hepatitis

Neuromuscular & skeletal: Myalgia, paresthesia
Respiratory: Bronchospasm

Overdosage/Toxicology Symptoms of overdose include dry mouth, flushed skin, dilated pupils, CNS depression; there is no specific treatment for an antihistamine overdose, however, most of its clinical toxicity is due to anticholinergic effects. For anticholinergic overdose with severe life-threatening symptoms, physostigmine 1-2 mg (0.5 or 0.02 mg/kg for children) I.V., slowly may be given to reverse these effects.

Drug Interactions Increased effect/toxicity: CNS depressants, MAO inhibitors, TCAs, phenothiazines, guanabenz

Mechanism of Action Competes with histamine for H_1-receptor sites on effector cells in the gastrointestinal tract, blood vessels, and respiratory tract

Pharmacodynamics/Kinetics
Peak effect: Oral: Within 3 hours
Duration: 3-6 hours
Absorption: Well absorbed from GI tract
Distribution: Small amounts appear in breast milk
Metabolism: In the liver
Elimination: In urine within 24 hours as inactive metabolites

Usual Dosage Oral:
Children:
2-5 years: 0.5 mg every 4-6 hours (do not use timed release)
6-11 years: 1 mg every 4-6 hours or 4 mg timed release at bedtime
Adults: 2 mg every 4-6 hours or 4-6 mg timed release at bedtime or every 8-10 hours

Test Interactions May interfere with a methacholine bronchial challenge

Patient Information May cause drowsiness; swallow whole, do not crush or chew sustained release product; avoid alcohol, may impair coordination and judgment

Nursing Implications Raise bed rails, institute safety measures, assist with ambulation

Dosage Forms
Syrup (orange flavor): 2 mg/5 mL with alcohol 6% (480 mL)
Tablet: 2 mg
Tablet, sustained action: 4 mg, 6 mg

Dexedrine® see Dextroamphetamine Sulfate on page 319

Dexone ® see Dexamethasone on page 314

Dexone L.A.® see Dexamethasone on page 314

Dexpanthenol (dex pan' the nole)
Brand Names Ilopan®; Ilopan-Choline®; Panthoderm® [OTC]
Synonyms Pantothenyl Alcohol
Use Prophylactic use to minimize paralytic ileus, treatment of postoperative distention
Pregnancy Risk Factor C
Contraindications Hemophilia; mechanical obstruction of ileus
Warnings/Precautions If hypersensitivity occurs, discontinue the drug; if ileus is secondary to mechanical obstruction, therapy must be directed at the obstruction
Adverse Reactions
<1%:
Cardiovascular: Slight drop in blood pressure
Central nervous system: Tingling
Dermatologic: Dermatitis, urticaria
Gastrointestinal: Vomiting, diarrhea, hyperperistalsis
Hematologic: Prolonged bleeding time
Local: Irritation
Respiratory: Dyspnea

Overdosage/Toxicology May cause diarrhea or intestinal upset

Drug Interactions Increased/prolonged effect of succinylcholine (do not administer within 1 hour)

Mechanism of Action A pantothenic acid B vitamin analog that is converted to coenzyme A internally; coenzyme A is essential to normal fatty acid synthesis, amino acid synthesis and acetylation of choline in the production of the neurotransmitter, acetylcholine

Pharmacodynamics/Kinetics
Absorption: Well absorbed
Elimination: As pantothenic acid principally in urine with small amounts in bile

Usual Dosage
Children and Adults: Relief of itching and aid in skin healing: Topical: Apply to affected area 1-2 times/day
(Continued)

Dexpanthenol *(Continued)*

Adults:
Relief of gas retention: Oral: 2-3 tablets 3 times/day
Prevention of postoperative ileus: I.M.: 250-500 mg stat, repeat in 2 hours, followed by doses every 6 hours until danger passes
Paralyzed ileus: I.M.: 500 mg stat, repeat in 2 hours, followed by doses every 6 hours, if needed

Administration Not for direct I.V. administration; must be diluted

Dosage Forms
Cream: 2% (30 g, 60 g)
Injection (Ilopan®): 250 mg/mL (2 mL, 10 mL, 30 mL)
Tablet (Ilopan-Choline®): 50 mg with choline bitartrate 25 mg

Dextran *(dex′ tran)*

Brand Names Gentran®; LMD®; Macrodex®; Rheomacrodex®

Synonyms Dextran 40; Dextran 70; Dextran, High Molecular Weight; Dextran, Low Molecular Weight

Use Blood volume expander used in treatment of shock or impending shock when blood or blood products are not available

Pregnancy Risk Factor C

Contraindications Hypersensitivity to dextrans or components (see Dextran 1)

Warnings/Precautions Use caution in patients with CHF, renal insufficiency, thrombocytopenia, or active hemorrhage; **observe patients closely during the first minute of infusion and have other means of maintaining circulation and epinephrine and diphenhydramine available should dextran therapy result in an anaphylactoid reaction;** patients should be well hydrated at the start of therapy; discontinue dextran if urine specific gravity is low and/or if oliguria or anuria occurs or if there is a precipitous rise in central venous pressure and signs of circulatory overload

Adverse Reactions
<1%:
Cardiovascular: Mild hypotension, tightness of chest
Central nervous system: Fever
Dermatologic: Urticaria
Gastrointestinal: Nausea, vomiting
Neuromuscular & skeletal: Arthralgia
Respiratory: Nasal congestion, wheezing
Miscellaneous: Anaphylaxis

Overdosage/Toxicology Symptoms include fluid overload, pulmonary edema, increased bleeding time, decreased platelet function; treatment is supportive, blood products containing clotting factors may be necessary

Stability Store at room temperature; discard partially used containers

Mechanism of Action Produces plasma volume expansion by virtue of its highly colloidal starch structure, similar to albumin

Pharmacodynamics/Kinetics
Onset of action: I.V.: Within minutes to 1 hour (depending upon the molecular weight polysaccharide administered), infusion volume expansion occurs
Elimination: ~75% excreted in urine within 24 hours

Usual Dosage I.V.: (requires an infusion pump):
Children: Total dose should not be >20 mL/kg during first 24 hours
Adults: 500-1000 mL at rate of 20-40 mL/minute; if therapy continues beyond 24 hours, total daily dosage should not exceed 10 mL/kg and therapy should not continue beyond 5 days

Dosing in renal and/or hepatic impairment: Use with extreme caution

Administration I.V. infusion only (use an infusion pump)

Monitoring Parameters Observe patient for signs of circulatory overload and/or monitor central venous pressure; observe patients closely during the first minute of infusion and have other means of maintaining circulation should dextran therapy result in an anaphylactoid reaction

Nursing Implications Patients should be well hydrated at the start of therapy; discontinue dextran if urine specific gravity is low, and/or if oliguria or anuria occurs, or if there is a precipitous rise in central venous pressure or sign of circulatory overloading

Dosage Forms Injection:
High molecular weight:
6% dextran 75 in dextrose 5% (500 mL)
Gentran®: 6% dextran 75 in sodium chloride 0.9% (500 mL)
Gentran®, Macrodex®: 6% dextran 70 in sodium chloride 0.9% (500 mL)
Macrodex®: 6% dextran 70 in dextrose 5% (500 mL)

Low molecular weight: Gentran®, LMD®, Rheomacrodex®:
10% dextran 40 in dextrose 5% (500 mL)
10% dextran 40 in sodium chloride 0.9% (500 mL)

Dextran 1 (dex' tran)
Brand Names Promit®
Use Prophylaxis of serious anaphylactic reactions to I.V. infusion of dextran
Pregnancy Risk Factor C
Contraindications Known hypersensitivity to dextrans or any component
Warnings/Precautions If immune adverse reactions occur, do not administer large volumes of dextran solutions for clinical use
Adverse Reactions
<1%:
Cardiovascular: Mild hypotension, tightness of chest
Central nervous system: Fever
Dermatologic: Urticaria
Gastrointestinal: Nausea, vomiting
Local: Cutaneous reactions
Neuromuscular & skeletal: Arthralgia
Respiratory: Nasal congestion, wheezing
Stability Protect from freezing
Mechanism of Action Binds to dextran-reactive immunoglobulin without bridge formation and no formation of large immune complexes
Usual Dosage I.V. (time between dextran 1 and dextran solution should not exceed 15 minutes):
Children: 0.3 mL/kg 1-2 minutes before I.V. infusion of dextran
Adults: 20 mL 1-2 minutes before I.V. infusion of dextran
Nursing Implications Do not dilute or admix with dextrans
Dosage Forms Injection: 150 mg/mL (20 mL)

Dextran 40 see Dextran on previous page

Dextran 70 see Dextran on previous page

Dextran, High Molecular Weight see Dextran on previous page

Dextran, Low Molecular Weight see Dextran on previous page

Dextranomer (dex tran' oh mer)
Brand Names Debrisan® [OTC]
Use Clean exudative wounds; no controlled studies have found dextranomer to be more effective than conventional therapy
Pregnancy Risk Factor C
Contraindications Deep fistulas, sinus tracts, hypersensitivity to any component
Warnings/Precautions Do not use in deep fistulas or any area where complete removal is not assured; do not use on dry wounds (ineffective); avoid contact with eyes
Adverse Reactions 1% to 10%: Local: Maceration may occur, transitory pain, bleeding, blistering, erythema
Mechanism of Action Dextranomer is a network of dextran-sucrose beads possessing a great many exposed hydroxy groups; when this network is applied to an exudative wound surface, the exudate is drawn by capillary forces generated by the swelling of the beads, with vacuum forces producing an upward flow of exudate into the network
Usual Dosage Debride and clean wound prior to application; apply to affected area every 12 hours or more frequent as needed; removal should be done by irrigation
Patient Information For external use only; avoid contact with eyes; contact physician if condition worsens or persists beyond 14-21 days
Nursing Implications Sprinkle beads into ulcer (or apply paste) to ¼" thickness; change dressings 1-4 times/day depending on drainage; change dressing before it is completely dry to facilitate removal
Dosage Forms
Beads: 4 g, 25 g, 60 g, 120 g
Paste: 10 g foil packets

Dextroamphetamine Sulfate (dex troe am fet' a meen)
Brand Names Dexedrine®; Ferndex; Oxydess® II; Spancap® No. 1
Use Narcolepsy, exogenous obesity, abnormal behavioral syndrome in children (minimal brain dysfunction), attention deficit hyperactive disorder (ADHD)
Restrictions C-II
(Continued)

Dextroamphetamine Sulfate *(Continued)*

Pregnancy Risk Factor C

Contraindications Hypersensitivity to dextroamphetamine or any component; advanced arteriosclerosis, hypertension, hyperthyroidism, glaucoma, MAO inhibitors

Warnings/Precautions Use with caution in patients with psychopathic personalities, cardiovascular disease, HTN, angina, and glaucoma; has high potential for abuse; use in weight reduction programs only when alternative therapy has been ineffective; prolonged administration may lead to drug dependence

Adverse Reactions

>10%:
   Cardiovascular: Irregular heartbeat
   Central nervous system: False feeling of well being, nervousness, restlessness, insomnia

1% to 10%:
   Cardiovascular: Hypertension
   Central nervous system: Mood or mental changes, dizziness, lightheadedness, headache
   Endocrine & metabolic: Changes in libido
   Gastrointestinal: Diarrhea, nausea, vomiting, stomach cramps, constipation, anorexia, weight loss, dry mouth
   Ocular: Blurred vision
   Miscellaneous: Increased sweating

<1%:
   Cardiovascular: Chest pain
   Central nervous system: CNS stimulation (severe), Tourette's syndrome, hyperthermia, seizures, paranoia
   Dermatologic: Skin rash, hives
   Miscellaneous: Tolerance and withdrawal with prolonged use

Overdosage/Toxicology Symptoms of overdose include restlessness, tremor, confusion, hallucinations, panic, dysrhythmias, nausea, vomiting

There is no specific antidote for dextroamphetamine intoxication and the bulk of the treatment is supportive

Hyperactivity and agitation usually respond to reduced sensory input; however, with extreme agitation, haloperidol (2-5 mg I.M. for adults) may be required

Hyperthermia is best treated with external cooling measures, or when severe or unresponsive, muscle paralysis with pancuronium may be needed

Hypertension is usually transient and generally does not require treatment unless severe. For diastolic blood pressures >110 mm Hg, a nitroprusside infusion should be initiated.

Seizures usually respond to diazepam I.V. and/or phenytoin maintenance regimens

Drug Interactions

Decreased effect: Methyldopa decreased antihypertensive efficacy; ethosuximide; decreased effect with acidifiers, psychotropics

Increased toxicity: May precipitate hypertensive crisis in patients receiving MAO inhibitors and arrhythmias in patients receiving general anesthetics

Increased effect/toxicity of TCAs, phenytoin, phenobarbital, propoxyphene, norepinephrine and meperidine

Stability Protect from light

Mechanism of Action Blocks reuptake of dopamine and norepinephrine from the synapse, thus increases the amount of circulating dopamine and norepinephrine in cerebral cortex to reticular activating system; inhibits the action of monoamine oxidase and causes catecholamines to be released

Pharmacodynamics/Kinetics

Onset of action: 1-1.5 hours

Metabolism: In the liver

Half-life: Adults: 34 hours (pH dependent)

Time to peak serum concentration: Oral: Within 3 hours

Elimination: In urine as unchanged drug and inactive metabolites after oral dose

Usual Dosage Oral:

Children:
   Narcolepsy: 6-12 years: Initial: 5 mg/day, may increase at 5 mg increments in weekly intervals until side effects appear; maximum dose: 60 mg/day
   Attention deficit disorder:
      3-5 years: Initial: 2.5 mg/day given every morning; increase by 2.5 mg/day in weekly intervals until optimal response is obtained, usual range: 0.1-0.5 mg/kg/dose every morning with maximum of 40 mg/day
      ≥6 years: 5 mg once or twice daily; increase in increments of 5 mg/day at weekly intervals until optimal response is reached, usual range: 0.1-0.5 mg/kg/dose every morning (5-20 mg/day) with maximum of 40 mg/day

Children >12 years and Adults:

Narcolepsy: Initial: 10 mg/day, may increase at 10 mg increments in weekly intervals until side effects appear; maximum: 60 mg/day

Exogenous obesity: 5-30 mg/day in divided doses of 5-10 mg 30-60 minutes before meals

Administration Administer as single dose in morning or as divided doses with breakfast and lunch

Monitoring Parameters Growth in children and CNS activity in all

Patient Information Take during day to avoid insomnia; do not discontinue abruptly, may cause physical and psychological dependence with prolonged use

Nursing Implications Last daily dose should be given 6 hours before retiring; do not crush sustained release drug product

Dosage Forms

Capsule, sustained release: 5 mg, 10 mg, 15 mg

Elixir: 5 mg/5 mL (480 mL)

Tablet: 5 mg, 10 mg (5 mg tablets contain tartrazine)

Dextromethorphan (dex troe meth or′ fan)

Brand Names Benylin® DM [OTC]; Children's Hold® [OTC]; Delsym® [OTC]; Hold® DM [OTC]; Pertussin® CS [OTC]; Pertussin® ES [OTC]; Robitussin® Cough Calmers [OTC]; Robitussin® Pediatric [OTC]; Scot-Tussin DM® Cough Chasers [OTC]; St. Joseph® Cough Suppressant [OTC]; Sucrets® Cough Calmers [OTC]; Suppress® [OTC]; Trocal® [OTC]; Vicks Formula 44® [OTC]; Vicks Formula 44® Pediatric Formula [OTC]

Use Symptomatic relief of coughs caused by minor viral upper respiratory tract infections or inhaled irritants; most effective for a chronic nonproductive cough

Pregnancy Risk Factor C

Contraindications Hypersensitivity to dextromethorphan or any component

Warnings/Precautions Use in children <2 years of age has not been proven safe and effective

Adverse Reactions

<1%:

Central nervous system: Drowsiness, dizziness, coma, respiratory depression

Gastrointestinal: Nausea, GI upset, constipation, abdominal discomfort

Overdosage/Toxicology Symptoms of overdose include nausea, vomiting, drowsiness, blurred vision, nystagmus, urinary retention, stupor, hallucinations, ataxia, respiratory depression, convulsions; treatment is supportive

Mechanism of Action Chemical relative of morphine lacking narcotic properties except in overdose; controls cough by depressing the medullary cough center

Pharmacodynamics/Kinetics

Onset of antitussive action: Within 15-30 minutes

Duration: Up to 6 hours

Metabolism: In the liver

Elimination: Principally in urine

Usual Dosage Oral:

Children:

<2 years: Use only as directed by a physician

2-6 years (syrup): 2.5-7.5 mg every 4-8 hours; extended release is 15 mg twice daily (maximum: 30 mg/24 hours)

6-12 years: 5-10 mg every 4 hours or 15 mg every 6-8 hours; extended release is 30 mg twice daily (maximum: 60 mg/24 hours)

Children >12 years and Adults: 10-30 mg every 4-8 hours or 30 mg every 6-8 hours; extended release is 60 mg twice daily (maximum: 120 mg/24 hours)

Patient Information Shake well; do not exceed recommended dosage; take with a large glass of water; if cough lasts more than 1 week or is accompanied by a rash, fever, or headache, notify physician

Nursing Implications Raise side rails, institute safety measures

Dosage Forms

Liquid:

Pertussin® CS: 3.5 mg/5 mL (120 mL)

Robitussin® Pediatric, St. Joseph® Cough Suppressant: 7.5 mg/5 mL (60 mL, 120 mL, 240 mL)

Pertussin® ES, Vicks Formula 44®: 15 mg/5 mL (120 mL, 240 mL)

Liquid, sustained release, as polistirex (Delsym®): 30 mg/5 mL (89 mL)

Lozenges:

Scot-Tussin DM® Cough Chasers: 2.5 mg

Children's Hold®, Hold® DM, Robitussin® Cough Calmers, Sucrets® Cough Calmers: 5 mg

Suppress®, Trocal®: 7.5 mg

Syrup:

Benylin® DM: 10 mg/5 mL (120 mL, 3780 mL)

(Continued)

Dextromethorphan *(Continued)*

Vicks Formula 44® Pediatric Formula: 15 mg/15 mL (120 mL)

Dextromethorphan and Guaifenesin *see* Guaifenesin and Dextromethorphan *on page 517*

Dextropropoxyphene *see* Propoxyphene *on page 946*

Dextrothyroxine Sodium *(dex troe thye rox' een)*
Brand Names Choloxin®
Use Reduction of elevated serum cholesterol
Pregnancy Risk Factor C
Contraindications Organic heart disease, congestive heart failure, advanced renal or hepatic disease
Warnings/Precautions Use with caution in patients with a history of angina pectoris, severe hypertension, or myocardial infarction; do not use for treatment of obesity; discontinue 2 weeks prior to elective surgery
Adverse Reactions
<1%:
Cardiovascular: Myocardial infarction, angina, arrhythmias
Central nervous system: Insomnia, headache
Dermatologic: Hair loss, skin rash
Gastrointestinal: Weight loss
Neuromuscular & skeletal: Tremor, paresthesia
Ocular: Visual disturbances
Otic: Tinnitus
Miscellaneous: Sweating
Overdosage/Toxicology Symptoms of overdose include palpitations, diarrhea, abdominal cramps, sweating, heat intolerance, congestive heart failure, tachycardia, hypertension, cardiac arrhythmias, angina, restlessness, tremor, seizures; propranolol can be used to treat adrenergic adverse effects, adults rarely have severe toxicity following a single overdose
Drug Interactions
Decreased effect of beta-blockers, digitalis, hypoglycemics; decreased effect with cholestyramine
Increased effect of anticoagulants
Mechanism of Action Unclear mechanism, thought to increase the liver breakdown of cholesterol
Pharmacodynamics/Kinetics
Absorption: Poorly absorbed from GI tract (25%)
Distribution: Small amounts cross the placenta; appears in breast milk
Metabolism: In the liver
Half-life: 18 hours
Elimination: In urine and bile in approximately equal amounts as unchanged drug and metabolites
Usual Dosage Oral:
Children: 0.05 mg/kg/day, increase at 1-month intervals by 0.05 mg/kg/day to a maximum of 0.4 mg/kg/day or 4 mg/day
Adults: 1-2 mg/day, increase at 1-2 mg at intervals of 4 weeks, up to a maximum of 8 mg/day
Patient Information If chest pain, palpitations, sweating, diarrhea develop during therapy, discontinue drug
Dosage Forms Tablet: 1 mg, 2 mg, 4 mg, 6 mg

Dey-Dose® Isoproterenol *see* Isoproterenol *on page 597*

Dey-Dose® Metaproterenol *see* Metaproterenol Sulfate *on page 697*

Dey-Drop® Ophthalmic Solution *see* Silver Nitrate *on page 1004*

Dey-Lute® Isoetharine *see* Isoetharine *on page 593*

Dezocine *(dez' oh seen)*
Related Information
Narcotic Agonist Comparison Charts *on page 1274-1275*
Brand Names Dalgan®
Use Relief of moderate to severe postoperative, acute renal and ureteral colic, and cancer pain
Pregnancy Risk Factor C
Contraindications Patients experiencing immediate type hypersensitivity reactions (anaphylaxis) to dezocine or structurally related compounds should not

receive this drug. Use of other central nervous system depressants concurrently to dezocine is contraindicated.

Warnings/Precautions Use with caution in patients with head injuries or increased intracranial pressure, respiratory depression, asthma, emphysema, COPD, renal or hepatic disease, labor and delivery, biliary surgery, or in patients with a history of drug abuse; abuse potential is apparent; may be better tolerated than other opioid agonist-antagonist; does not affect cardiac performance; contains bisulfites, avoid use in those sensitive to bisulfites

Adverse Reactions

1% to 10%:
Central nervous system: Sedation, dizziness, vertigo
Gastrointestinal: Nausea, vomiting
Local: Injection site reactions

<1%:
Cardiovascular: Hypotension, palpitations, bradycardia, peripheral vasodilation
Central nervous system: Increased intracranial pressure, CNS depression, drowsiness
Endocrine & metabolic: Antidiuretic hormone release
Gastrointestinal: Constipation
Ocular: Miosis
Respiratory: Respiratory depression
Miscellaneous: Biliary or urinary tract spasm, histamine release, physical and psychological dependence with prolonged use

Overdosage/Toxicology Symptoms of overdose include CNS and respiratory depression, gastrointestinal cramping, constipation; naloxone 2 mg I.V. (0.01 mg/kg for children) with repeat administration as necessary up to a total of 10 mg

Drug Interactions Increased effect with CNS depressants

Stability Store at room temperature; protect from light

Mechanism of Action Binds to opiate receptors in the CNS, causing inhibition of ascending pain pathways, altering the perception of and response to pain; produces generalized CNS depression; it is a mixed agonist-antagonist that appears to bind selectively to CNS μ and Δ opiate receptors

Pharmacodynamics/Kinetics

Onset of analgesia: Within 15-30 minutes
Peak effect: 1 hour
Duration of analgesia: 4-6 hours
Half-life: 2.6-2.8 hours
Metabolism: Glucuronidated in liver
Elimination: Excretion of inactive metabolites and unchanged drug in the urine

Usual Dosage Adults (not recommended for patients <18 years):
I.M.: Initial: 5-20 mg; may be repeated every 3-6 hours as needed; maximum: 120 mg/day and 20 mg/dose
I.V.: Initial: 2.5-10 mg; may be repeated every 2-4 hours as needed

Dosing adjustment in renal impairment: Should be used cautiously at reduced doses

Monitoring Parameters Monitor blood pressure and heart rate during adjustment of dose

Patient Information Avoid driving or operating machinery until the effect of drug wears off; may cause physical and psychological dependence with prolonged use

Nursing Implications Watch closely for respiratory depression; induced respiratory depression is greater than that seen with morphine during the first hour after administration

Dosage Forms Injection, single dose vial: 5 mg/mL (2 mL); 10 mg/mL (2 mL); 15 mg/mL (2 mL)

Dezone® see Dexamethasone on page 314

DFMO see Eflornithine Hydrochloride on page 383

DFP see Isoflurophate on page 594

DHAD see Mitoxantrone Hydrochloride on page 749

DHC Plus® see Dihydrocodeine Compound on page 342

D.H.E. 45® see Dihydroergotamine Mesylate on page 343

DHPG Sodium see Ganciclovir on page 496

DHT™ see Dihydrotachysterol on page 344

Diaβeta® see Glyburide on page 505

Diabetic Tussin DM® [OTC] see Guaifenesin and Dextromethorphan on page 517

Diabinese® see Chlorpropamide on page 232

ALPHABETICAL LISTING OF DRUGS

Dialose® [OTC] *see* Docusate *on page 362*

Dialume® [OTC] *see* Aluminum Hydroxide *on page 48*

Diamine T.D.® [OTC] *see* Brompheniramine Maleate *on page 143*

Diaminodiphenylsulfone *see* Dapsone *on page 303*

Diamox® *see* Acetazolamide *on page 20*

Diamox Sequels® *see* Acetazolamide *on page 20*

Diapid® *see* Lypressin *on page 656*

Diasorb® [OTC] *see* Attapulgite *on page 102*

Diazepam (dye az' e pam)
Related Information
  Benzodiazepines Comparison *on page 1256*
Brand Names Valium®; Valrelease®; Zetran® Injection
Use Management of general anxiety disorders, panic disorders, and provide preoperative sedation, light anesthesia, and amnesia; treatment of status epilepticus, alcohol withdrawal symptoms; used as a skeletal muscle relaxant
Restrictions C-IV
Pregnancy Risk Factor D
Contraindications Hypersensitivity to diazepam or any component; there may be a cross-sensitivity with other benzodiazepines; do not use in a comatose patient, in those with pre-existing CNS depression, respiratory depression, narrow-angle glaucoma, or severe uncontrolled pain; do not use in pregnant women
Warnings/Precautions Use with caution in patients receiving other CNS depressants, patients with low albumin, hepatic dysfunction, and in the elderly and young infants. Due to its long-acting metabolite, diazepam is not considered a drug of choice in the elderly; long-acting benzodiazepines have been associated with falls in the elderly.
Adverse Reactions
  >10%:
    Cardiovascular: Cardiac arrest, hypotension, bradycardia, cardiovascular collapse, tachycardia, chest pain
    Central nervous system: Drowsiness, ataxia, amnesia, slurred speech, paradoxical excitement or rage, fatigue, lightheadedness, insomnia, memory impairment, headache, anxiety, depression, dysarthria
    Dermatologic: Rash
    Endocrine & metabolic: Decreased libido
    Gastrointestinal: Dry mouth, changes in salivation, constipation, nausea, vomiting, diarrhea, increased or decreased appetite
    Local: Phlebitis, pain with injection
    Neuromuscular & skeletal: Impaired coordination
    Ocular: Blurred vision, diplopia
    Respiratory: Decrease in respiratory rate, apnea, laryngospasm
    Miscellaneous: Sweating
  1% to 10%:
    Cardiovascular: Syncope, hypotension
    Central nervous system: Confusion, nervousness, dizziness, akathisia
    Dermatologic: Dermatitis
    Gastrointestinal: Weight gain or loss
    Neuromuscular & skeletal: Rigidity, tremor, muscle cramps
    Otic: Tinnitus
    Respiratory: Nasal congestion, hyperventilation
    Miscellaneous: Hiccups
  <1%:
    Endocrine & metabolic: Menstrual irregularities
    Hematologic: Blood dyscrasias
    Miscellaneous: Physical and psychological dependence with prolonged use, reflex slowing
Overdosage/Toxicology Symptoms of overdose include somnolence, confusion, coma, hypoactive reflexes, dyspnea, hypotension, slurred speech, impaired coordination; treatment for benzodiazepine overdose is supportive. Rarely is mechanical ventilation required. Flumazenil has been shown to selectively block the binding of benzodiazepines to CNS receptors, resulting in a reversal of benzodiazepine-induced CNS depression, but not respiratory depression.
Drug Interactions
  Decreased effect: Enzyme inducers may increase the metabolism of diazepam
  Increased toxicity: CNS depressants (alcohol, barbiturates, opioids) may enhance sedation and respiratory depression; cimetidine may decrease the metabolism of diazepam; cisapride can significantly increase diazepam levels;

valproic acid may displace diazepam from binding sites which may result in an increase in sedative effects; selective serotonin reuptake inhibitors (eg, fluoxetine, sertraline, paroxetine) have greatly increased diazepam levels by altering its clearance

Stability Protect parenteral dosage form from light; potency is retained for up to 3 months when kept at room temperature; most stable at pH 4-8, hydrolysis occurs at pH <3; do not mix I.V. product with other medications

Mechanism of Action Depresses all levels of the CNS, including the limbic and reticular formation, probably through the increased action of gamma-aminobutyric acid (GABA), which is a major inhibitory neurotransmitter in the brain

Pharmacodynamics/Kinetics

I.V. for status epilepticus:
  Onset of action: Almost immediate
  Duration: Short, 20-30 minutes
Absorption: Oral: 85% to 100%, more reliable than I.M.
Protein binding: 98%
Metabolism: In the liver
Half-life:
  Parent drug: Adults: 20-50 hours, increased half-life in neonates, elderly, and those with severe hepatic disorders
  Active major metabolite (desmethyldiazepam): 50-100 hours, can be prolonged in neonates

Usual Dosage Oral absorption is more reliable than I.M.

Children:
  Conscious sedation for procedures: Oral: 0.2-0.3 mg/kg (maximum: 10 mg) 45-60 minutes prior to procedure
  Sedation or muscle relaxation or anxiety:
    Oral: 0.12-0.8 mg/kg/day in divided doses every 6-8 hours
    I.M., I.V.: 0.04-0.3 mg/kg/dose every 2-4 hours to a maximum of 0.6 mg/kg within an 8-hour period if needed
  Status epilepticus:
    Infants 30 days to 5 years: I.V.: 0.05-0.3 mg/kg/dose given over 2-3 minutes, every 15-30 minutes to a maximum total dose of 5 mg; repeat in 2-4 hours as needed or 0.2-0.5 mg/dose every 2-5 minutes to a maximum total dose of 5 mg
    >5 years: I.V.: 0.05-0.3 mg/kg/dose given over 2-3 minutes every 15-30 minutes to a maximum total dose of 10 mg; repeat in 2-4 hours as needed or 1 mg/dose given over 2-3 minutes, every 2-5 minutes to a maximum total dose of 10 mg
    Rectal: 0.5 mg/kg, then 0.25 mg/kg in 10 minutes if needed

Adolescents: Conscious sedation for procedures:
  Oral: 10 mg
  I.V.: 5 mg, may repeat with ½ dose if needed

Adults:
  Anxiety/sedation/skeletal muscle relaxation:
    Oral: 2-10 mg 2-4 times/day
    I.M., I.V.: 2-10 mg, may repeat in 3-4 hours if needed
  Status epilepticus: I.V.: 5-10 mg every 10-20 minutes, up to 30 mg in an 8-hour period; may repeat in 2-4 hours if necessary

Elderly: Oral: Initial:
  Anxiety: 1-2 mg 1-2 times/day; increase gradually as needed, rarely need to use >10 mg/day
  Skeletal muscle relaxant: 2-5 mg 2-4 times/day

Hemodialysis effects: Not dialyzable (0% to 5%); supplemental dose is not necessary

Dosing adjustment in hepatic impairment: Reduce dose by 50% in cirrhosis and avoid in severe/acute liver disease

Administration In children, do not exceed 1-2 mg/minute IVP; adults 5 mg/minute

Monitoring Parameters Respiratory rate, heart rate, blood pressure with I.V. use

Reference Range Therapeutic: Diazepam: 0.2-1.5 µg/mL (SI: 0.7-5.3 µmol/L); N-desmethyldiazepam (nordiazepam): 0.1-0.5 µg/mL (SI: 0.35-1.8 µmol/L)

Test Interactions False-negative urinary glucose determinations when using Clinistix® or Diastix®

Patient Information Avoid alcohol and other CNS depressants; avoid activities needing good psychomotor coordination until CNS effects are known; drug may cause physical or psychological dependence; avoid abrupt discontinuation after prolonged use
(Continued)

Diazepam *(Continued)*

Nursing Implications Provide safety measures (ie, side rails, night light, and call button); supervise ambulation

Dosage Forms
Capsule, sustained release (Valrelease®): 15 mg
Injection: 5 mg/mL (1 mL, 2 mL, 5 mL, 10 mL)
Solution, oral (wintergreen-spice flavor): 5 mg/5 mL (5 mL, 10 mL, 500 mL)
Solution, oral concentrate: 5 mg/mL (30 mL)
Tablet: 2 mg, 5 mg, 10 mg

Diazoxide *(dye az ox' ide)*

Brand Names Hyperstat® I.V.; Proglycem®

Use
Oral: Hypoglycemia related to islet cell adenoma, carcinoma, hyperplasia, or adenomatosis, nesidioblastosis, leucine sensitivity, or extrapancreatic malignancy
I.V.: Emergency lowering of blood pressure

Pregnancy Risk Factor C

Contraindications Hypersensitivity to diazoxide, thiazides, or other sulfonamide derivatives; aortic coarctation, arteriovenous shunts, dissecting aortic aneurysm

Warnings/Precautions Diabetes mellitus, renal or liver disease, coronary artery disease, or cerebral vascular insufficiency; patients may require a diuretic with repeated I.V. doses

Adverse Reactions
1% to 10%:
Cardiovascular: Hypotension
Central nervous system: Dizziness
Gastrointestinal: Nausea, vomiting
Neuromuscular & skeletal: Weakness
<1%:
Cardiovascular: Tachycardia, flushing
Central nervous system: Seizures, headache, extrapyramidal symptoms and development of abnormal facies with chronic oral use
Dermatologic: Rash, hirsutism
Endocrine & metabolic: Hyperglycemia, ketoacidosis, sodium and water retention, hyperuricemia
Gastrointestinal: Anorexia, constipation
Hematologic: Leukopenia, thrombocytopenia
Local: Pain, burning, cellulitis/phlebitis upon extravasation
Miscellaneous: Inhibition of labor

Overdosage/Toxicology Symptoms of overdose include hyperglycemia, ketoacidosis, hypotension. Treatment: Insulin, fluid, and electrolyte restoration; I.V. pressors may be needed to support blood pressure

Drug Interactions
Decreased effect: Diazoxide may increase phenytoin metabolism or free fraction
Increased toxicity:
Diuretics and hypotensive agents may potentiate diazoxide adverse effects
Diazoxide may decrease warfarin protein binding

Stability Protect from light, heat, and freezing; avoid using darkened solutions

Mechanism of Action Inhibits insulin release from the pancreas; produces direct smooth muscle relaxation of the peripheral arterioles which results in decrease in blood pressure and reflex increase in heart rate and cardiac output

Pharmacodynamics/Kinetics
Hyperglycemic effect: Oral:
Onset of action: Within 1 hour
Duration (normal renal function): 8 hours
Hypotensive effect: I.V.:
Peak: Within 5 minutes
Duration: Usually 3-12 hours
Protein binding: 90%
Half-life:
Children: 9-24 hours
Adults: 20-36 hours
End stage renal disease: >30 hours
Elimination: 50% excreted unchanged in urine

Usual Dosage
Hypertension: Children and Adults: I.V.: 1-3 mg/kg up to a maximum of 150 mg in a single injection; repeat dose in 5-15 minutes until blood pressure adequately reduced; repeat administration at intervals of 4-24 hours; monitor the blood pressure closely; do not use longer than 10 days
Hyperinsulinemic hypoglycemia: Oral: **Note:** Use lower dose listed as initial dose

Newborns and Infants: 8-15 mg/kg/day in divided doses every 8-12 hours
Children and Adults: 3-8 mg/kg/day in divided doses every 8-12 hours

Dosing adjustment in renal impairment: None
Elimination is not enhanced via hemo- or peritoneal dialysis; supplemental dose is not necessary

Administration I.V. diazoxide is given undiluted by rapid I.V. injection over a period of 30 seconds or less but may also be given by continuous infusion

Monitoring Parameters Blood pressure, blood glucose, serum uric acid; intravenous administration requires cardiac monitor and blood pressure monitor

Test Interactions False-negative insulin response to glucagon

Patient Information Check blood glucose carefully, monitor urine glucose/ketones; shake suspension well before using

Nursing Implications Extravasation can be treated with warm compresses; monitor blood glucose daily in patients receiving I.V. therapy

Dosage Forms
Capsule (Proglycem®): 50 mg
Injection (Hyperstat®): 15 mg/mL (1 mL, 20 mL)
Suspension, oral (chocolate-mint flavor) (Proglycem®): 50 mg/mL (30 mL)

Dibent® *see* Dicyclomine Hydrochloride *on page 330*

Dibenzyline® *see* Phenoxybenzamine Hydrochloride *on page 871*

Dibucaine (dye' byoo kane)

Brand Names Nupercainal® [OTC]

Use Fast, temporary relief of pain and itching due to hemorrhoids, minor burns, or other minor skin conditions [amide derivative local anesthetic]

Pregnancy Risk Factor C

Contraindications Known hypersensitivity to amide-type anesthetics, ophthalmic use

Adverse Reactions
1% to 10%:
Local: Burning, contact dermatitis
Dermatologic: Angioedema
<1%: Local: Edema, urticaria, urethritis, cutaneous lesions, tenderness, irritation, inflammation

Overdosage/Toxicology Symptoms of overdose are due to high plasma levels and include convulsions or hypotension; treatment is supportive; maintain an airway and support ventilation; methemoglobinemia may be treated with methylene blue

Mechanism of Action Blocks both the initiation and conduction of nerve impulses by decreasing the neuronal membrane's permeability to sodium ions, which results in inhibition of depolarization with resultant blockade of conduction

Pharmacodynamics/Kinetics
Onset of action: Within 15 minutes
Duration: 2-4 hours
Absorption: Poorly through intact skin, but well absorbed through mucous membranes and excoriated skin

Usual Dosage Children and Adults:
Rectal: Hemorrhoids: Insert ointment into rectum using a rectal applicator; administer each morning, evening, and after each bowel movement
Topical: Apply gently to the affected areas; no more than 30 g for adults or 7.5 g for children should be used in any 24-hour period

Patient Information If condition worsens or if symptoms persist for >7 days, stop using the ointment and consult a physician; wash hands after use to avoid getting ointment in eyes

Nursing Implications Do not use near the eyes or over denuded surfaces or blistered areas

Dosage Forms
Cream, topical: 0.5% (45 g)
Ointment, topical: 1% (30 g, 60 g, 454 g)

DIC *see* Dacarbazine *on page 297*

Dicalcium Phosphate *see* Calcium Phosphate, Tribasic *on page 171*

Dicarbosil® [OTC] *see* Calcium Carbonate *on page 161*

Dichysterol *see* Dihydrotachysterol *on page 344*

Diclofenac (dye kloe´ fen ak)

Related Information
Nonsteroidal Anti-Inflammatories Comparison *on page 1280*

Brand Names Cataflam®; Voltaren®

Use Acute treatment of mild to moderate pain; acute and chronic treatment of rheumatoid arthritis, ankylosing spondylitis, and osteoarthritis; used for juvenile rheumatoid arthritis, gout, dysmenorrhea; ophthalmic solution for postoperative inflammation after cataract extraction

Pregnancy Risk Factor B

Contraindications Known hypersensitivity to diclofenac, any component, aspirin or other nonsteroidal anti-inflammatory drugs (NSAIDs); porphyria

Warnings/Precautions Use with caution in patients with congestive heart failure, hypertension, decreased renal or hepatic function, history of GI disease, or those receiving anticoagulants

Adverse Reactions

>10%:
  Dermatologic: Skin rash
  Gastrointestinal: Abdominal cramps, heartburn, indigestion, nausea

1% to 10%:
  Cardiovascular: Angina pectoris, arrhythmias
  Central nervous system: Dizziness, nervousness
  Dermatologic: Skin rash, itching
  Gastrointestinal: GI ulceration, vomiting
  Genitourinary: Vaginal bleeding
  Otic: Tinnitus

<1%:
  Cardiovascular: Chest pain, congestive heart failure, hypertension, tachycardia
  Central nervous system: Epistaxis, convulsions, forgetfulness, mental depression, drowsiness, nervousness, insomnia, weakness
  Dermatologic: Hives, exfoliative dermatitis, erythema multiforme, Stevens-Johnson syndrome, angioedema
  Gastrointestinal: Stomatitis
  Genitourinary: Cystitis
  Hematologic: Agranulocytosis, anemia, pancytopenia, leukopenia, thrombocytopenia
  Hepatic: Hepatitis
  Neuromuscular & skeletal: Peripheral neuropathy, trembling
  Ocular: Blurred vision, change in vision
  Otic: Decreased hearing
  Renal: Interstitial nephritis, nephrotic syndrome, renal impairment
  Respiratory: Wheezing, laryngeal edema, shortness of breath
  Miscellaneous: Anaphylaxis, increased sweating

Overdosage/Toxicology Symptoms of overdose include acute renal failure, vomiting, drowsiness, leukocytosis; management of a nonsteroidal anti-inflammatory drug (NSAID) intoxication is primarily supportive and symptomatic. Fluid therapy is commonly effective in managing the hypotension that may occur following an acute NSAID overdose, except when this is due to an acute blood loss.

Drug Interactions
Decreased effect with aspirin; decreased effect of thiazides, furosemide
Increased toxicity of digoxin, methotrexate, cyclosporine, lithium, insulin, sulfonylureas, potassium-sparing diuretics, aspirin

Mechanism of Action Inhibits prostaglandin synthesis by decreasing the activity of the enzyme, cyclo-oxygenase, which results in decreased formation of prostaglandin precursors

Pharmacodynamics/Kinetics
Onset of action: Cataflam® has a more rapid onset of action than does the sodium salt (Voltaren®), because it is absorbed in the stomach instead of the duodenum
Protein binding: 99%
Metabolism: In the liver to inactive metabolites
Half-life: 2 hours
Time to peak serum concentration:
  Cataflam®: Within 1 hour
  Voltaren®: Within 2 hours
Elimination: Primarily in urine

Usual Dosage Adults:
Oral:
  Analgesia (Cataflam®): Starting dose: 50 mg 3 times/day
  Rheumatoid arthritis: 150-200 mg/day in 2-4 divided doses
  Osteoarthritis: 100-150 mg/day in 2-3 divided doses
  Ankylosing spondylitis: 100-125 mg/day in 4-5 divided doses

Ophthalmic: Instill 1 drop into affected eye 4 times/day beginning 24 hours after cataract surgery and continuing for 2 weeks

Monitoring Parameters Monitor CBC, liver enzymes; monitor urine output and BUN/serum creatinine in patients receiving diuretics; occult blood loss

Patient Information Do not crush tablets; take with food, milk, or water; report any signs of blood in stool

Nursing Implications Do not crush tablets

Additional Information
Diclofenac potassium = Cataflam®
Diclofenac sodium = Voltaren®

Dosage Forms
Solution, ophthalmic, as sodium: 0.1% (2.5 mL, 5 mL)
Tablet, enteric coated, as sodium: 25 mg, 50 mg, 75 mg
Tablet, as potassium: 50 mg

Dicloxacillin Sodium (dye klox a sill' in)

Brand Names Dycill®; Dynapen®; Pathocil®

Use Treatment of systemic infections such as pneumonia, skin and soft tissue infections, and osteomyelitis caused by penicillinase-producing staphylococci

Pregnancy Risk Factor B

Contraindications Known hypersensitivity to dicloxacillin, penicillin, or any components

Warnings/Precautions Monitor PT if patient concurrently on warfarin; elimination of drug is slow in neonates; use with caution in patients allergic to cephalosporins; bad taste of suspension may make compliance difficult

Adverse Reactions
1% to 10%: Gastrointestinal: Diarrhea
<1%:
Central nervous system: Fever
Dermatologic: Rash
Gastrointestinal: Nausea, vomiting
Hematologic: Eosinophilia, neutropenia, leukopenia, thrombocytopenia
Hepatic: Elevation in liver enzymes
Miscellaneous: Sickness-like reaction

Overdosage/Toxicology Symptoms of penicillin overdose include neuromuscular hypersensitivity (agitation, hallucinations, asterixis, encephalopathy, confusion, and seizures) and electrolyte imbalance with potassium or sodium salts, especially in renal failure; hemodialysis may be helpful to aid in the removal of the drug from the blood, otherwise most treatment is supportive or symptom directed

Drug Interactions
Decreased effect: Efficacy of oral contraceptives may be reduced
Increased effect: Disulfiram, probenecid → ↑ penicillin levels; increased effect of anticoagulants

Stability Refrigerate suspension after reconstitution; discard after 14 days if refrigerated or 7 days if kept at room temperature; unit dose antibiotic oral syringes are stable for 48 hours

Mechanism of Action Interferes with bacterial cell wall synthesis during active multiplication, causing cell wall death and resultant bactericidal activity against susceptible bacteria

Pharmacodynamics/Kinetics
Absorption: 35% to 76% from GI tract; food decreases rate and extent of absorption
Distribution: Crosses the placenta; distributes into breast milk
Protein binding: 96%
Half-life: 0.6-0.8 hours, slightly prolonged in patients with renal impairment
Time to peak serum concentration: Within 0.5-2 hours
Elimination: Prolonged in neonates; partially eliminated by the liver and excreted in bile, 56% to 70% is eliminated in urine as unchanged drug

Usual Dosage Oral:
Children <40 kg: 12.5-50 mg/kg/day divided every 6 hours; doses of 50-100 mg/kg/day in divided doses every 6 hours have been used for therapy of osteomyelitis
Children >40 kg and Adults: 125-500 mg every 6 hours

Dosage adjustment in renal impairment: Not necessary
Not dialyzable (0% to 5%); supplemental dosage not necessary
Peritoneal dialysis effects: Supplemental dosage not necessary
Continuous arterio-venous or veno-venous hemofiltration (CAVH/CAVHD): Supplemental dosage not necessary
(Continued)

Dicloxacillin Sodium *(Continued)*

Administration Administer 1 hour before or 2 hours after meals; administer around-the-clock rather than 4 times/day to promote less variation in peak and trough serum levels

Monitoring Parameters Monitor prothrombin time if patient concurrently on warfarin

Test Interactions Positive Coombs' test [direct]

Patient Information Take until all medication used; take 1 hour before or 2 hours after meals, do not skip doses

Additional Information

Sodium content of 250 mg capsule: 13 mg (0.6 mEq)

Sodium content of suspension 65 mg/5 mL: 27 mg (1.2 mEq)

Dosage Forms

Capsule: 125 mg, 250 mg, 500 mg

Powder for oral suspension: 62.5 mg/5 mL (80 mL, 100 mL, 200 mL)

Dicyclomine Hydrochloride *(dye sye' kloe meen)*

Brand Names Antispas®; Bemote®; Bentyl® Hydrochloride; Byclomine®; Dibent®; Di-Spaz®; Neoquess® Injection; Or-Tyl®; Spasmoject®

Synonyms Dicycloverine Hydrochloride

Use Treatment of functional disturbances of GI motility such as irritable bowel syndrome

Unlabeled use: Urinary incontinence

Pregnancy Risk Factor B

Contraindications Hypersensitivity to any anticholinergic drug; narrow-angle glaucoma, myasthenia gravis; should not be used in infants <6 months of age

Warnings/Precautions Use with caution in patients with hepatic or renal disease, ulcerative colitis, hyperthyroidism, cardiovascular disease, hypertension, tachycardia, GI obstruction, obstruction of the urinary tract. The elderly are at increased risk for anticholinergic effects, confusion and hallucinations.

Adverse Reactions

>10%:

Gastrointestinal: Constipation

Local: Injection site reactions

Miscellaneous: Decreased sweating, dry mouth, nose, throat, or skin

1% to 10%: Decreased flow of breast milk, difficulty in swallowing, blurred vision, increased sensitivity to light

<1%:

Cardiovascular: Orthostatic hypotension, tachycardia, palpitations

Central nervous system: Confusion, drowsiness, headache, lightheadedness, loss of memory, weakness, tiredness, seizures, coma, nervousness, excitement, insomnia

Dermatologic: Skin rash

Gastrointestinal: Bloated feeling, nausea, vomiting

Genitourinary: Difficult urination, urinary retention

Neuromuscular & skeletal: Muscular hypotonia

Ocular: Increased intraocular pain

Respiratory: Asphyxia, respiratory distress

Overdosage/Toxicology Symptoms of overdose include CNS stimulation followed by depression, confusion, delusions, nonreactive pupils, tachycardia, hypertension; anticholinergic toxicity is caused by strong binding of the drug to cholinergic receptors. For anticholinergic overdose with severe life-threatening symptoms, physostigmine 1-2 mg (0.5 or 0.02 mg/kg for children) S.C. or I.V., slowly may be given to reverse these effects.

Drug Interactions

Decreased effect: Phenothiazines, anti-Parkinson's drugs, haloperidol, sustained release dosage forms; decreased effect with antacids

Increased toxicity: Anticholinergics, amantadine, narcotic analgesics, type I antiarrhythmics, antihistamines, phenothiazines, TCAs

Mechanism of Action Blocks the action of acetylcholine at parasympathetic sites in smooth muscle, secretory glands and the CNS

Pharmacodynamics/Kinetics

Onset of effect: 1-2 hours

Duration: Up to 4 hours

Absorption: Oral: Well absorbed

Metabolism: Extensive

Half-life:

Initial phase: 1.8 hours

Terminal phase: 9-10 hours

Elimination: In urine with only a small amount excreted as unchanged drug

Usual Dosage

Oral:

Infants >6 months: 5 mg/dose 3-4 times/day

Children: 10 mg/dose 3-4 times/day

Adults: Begin with 80 mg/day in 4 equally divided doses, then increase up to 160 mg/day

I.M. **(should not be used I.V.):** Adults: 80 mg/day in 4 divided doses (20 mg/dose)

Administration Do not administer I.V.

Monitoring Parameters Pulse, anticholinergic effect, urinary output, GI symptoms

Patient Information May cause drowsiness; avoid alcohol; may impair coordination and judgment; may cause blurred vision or dizziness; take 30-60 minutes before a meal; may cause dry mouth, difficult urination, or constipation

Nursing Implications Raise bed rails, institute safety measures

Dosage Forms

Capsule: 10 mg, 20 mg

Injection: 10 mg/mL (2 mL, 10 mL)

Syrup: 10 mg/5 mL (118 mL, 473 mL, 946 mL)

Tablet: 20 mg

Dicycloverine Hydrochloride *see* Dicyclomine Hydrochloride *on previous page*

Didanosine (dye dan' oh seen)

Brand Names Videx®

Synonyms DDI

Use Treatment of advanced HIV infection in patients who are intolerant of zidovudine therapy or who have demonstrated significant clinical or immunologic deterioration during zidovudine therapy

Pregnancy Risk Factor B

Contraindications Hypersensitivity to any component

Warnings/Precautions Didanosine is indicated for treatment of HIV infection only in patients intolerant of zidovudine or who have failed zidovudine. Patients receiving didanosine may still develop opportunistic infections. Peripheral neuropathy occurs in ~35% of patients receiving the drug; pancreatitis (sometimes fatal) occurs in ~9%; risk factors for developing pancreatitis include a previous history of the condition, concurrent cytomegalovirus or *Mycobacterium avium-intracellulare* infection, and concomitant use of pentamidine or co-trimoxazole; discontinue didanosine if clinical signs of pancreatitis occur. Didanosine may cause retinal depigmentation in children receiving doses >300 mg/m²/day. Patients should undergo retinal examination every 6-12 months. Use with caution in patients with decreased renal or hepatic function, phenylketonuria, sodium-restricted diets, or with edema, congestive heart failure or hyperuricemia; in high concentrations, didanosine is mutagenic.

Adverse Reactions

>10%:

Central nervous system: Anxiety, headache, irritability, insomnia, restlessness

Gastrointestinal: Abdominal pain, nausea, diarrhea

Neuromuscular & skeletal: Peripheral neuropathy

1% to 10%:

Central nervous system: Depression

Dermatologic: Rash, pruritus

Gastrointestinal: Pancreatitis

<1%:

Central nervous system: Seizures

Hematologic: Anemia, granulocytopenia, leukopenia, thrombocytopenia

Hepatic: Hepatitis

Ocular: Retinal depigmentation

Renal: Renal impairment

Miscellaneous: Hypersensitivity

Overdosage/Toxicology Chronic overdose may cause pancreatitis, peripheral neuropathy, diarrhea, hyperuricemia, and hepatic impairment; there is no known antidote for didanosine overdose; treatment is asymptomatic

Drug Interactions Drugs whose absorption depends on the level of acidity in the stomach such as ketoconazole, itraconazole, and dapsone should be administered at least 2 hours prior to didanosine

Decreased effect: Didanosine may decrease absorption of quinolones or tetracyclines, didanosine should be held during PCP treatment with pentamidine

(Continued)

Didanosine *(Continued)*

    Increased toxicity: Concomitant administration of other drugs which have the potential to cause peripheral neuropathy or pancreatitis may increase the risk of these toxicities

Stability Tablets should be stored in tightly closed bottles at 15°C to 30°C; undergoes rapid degradation when exposed to an acidic environment; tablets dispersed in water are stable for 1 hour at room temperature; reconstituted buffered solution is stable for 4 hours at room temperature; reconstituted pediatric solution is stable for 30 days if refrigerated; unbuffered powder for oral solution must be reconstituted and mixed with an equal volume of antacid at time of preparation

Mechanism of Action Didanosine, a purine nucleoside analogue and the deamination product of dideoxyadenosine (ddA), inhibits HIV replication *in vitro* in both T cells and monocytes. Didanosine is converted within the cell to the mono-, di-, and triphosphates of ddA. These ddA triphosphates act as substrate and inhibitor of HIV reverse transcriptase substrate and inhibitor of HIV reverse transcriptase thereby blocking viral DNA synthesis and suppressing HIV replication.

Pharmacodynamics/Kinetics

    Absorption: Subject to degradation by the acidic pH of the stomach; buffered to resist the acidic pH; as much as 50% reduction in the peak plasma concentration is observed in the presence of food

    Distribution: V_d: 54 L; children: 35.6 L/m^2

    Protein binding: <5%

    Metabolism: Has not been evaluated in man; studies conducted in dogs, shows didanosine extensively metabolized with allantoin, hypoxanthine, xanthine, and uric acid being the major metabolites found in the urine

    Bioavailability: 21% (range: 2% to 89%)

    Half-life:

        Children and Adolescents: 0.8 hour

        Adults:

            Normal renal function: 1.5 hours; however, its active metabolite ddATP has an intracellular half-life >12 hours *in vitro*; this permits the drug to be dosed at 12-hour intervals; total body clearance averages 800 mL/minute

            Impaired renal function: Half-life is increased, with values ranging from 2.5-5 hours

    Elimination: ~55% of drug is eliminated unchanged in urine

Usual Dosage Oral (administer on an empty stomach):

    Children: 180 mg/m^2/day divided every 12 hours **or** dosing is based on body surface area (m^2): See table.

Didanosine — Pediatric Dosing

Body Surface Area (m²)	Dosing (Tablets) (mg bid)
≤0.4	25
0.5-0.7	50
0.8-1	75
1.1-1.4	100

    Adults: Dosing is based on patient weight: See table.

Didanosine — Adult Dosing

Patient Weight (kg)	Dosing (Tablets) (mg bid)
35-49	125
50-74	200
≥75	300

Note: Children >1 year and Adults should receive 2 tablets per dose and children <1 year should receive 1 tablet per dose for adequate buffering and absorption; tablets should be chewed

Dosing adjustment in renal impairment: Patients with severe renal dysfunction should receive appropriate dose based on patient's weight on a once-a-day dosing schedule instead of twice daily dosing

    Cl_{cr} 10-<60 mL/minute: Adjustment should be considered

    Cl_{cr} <10 mL/minute: Administer every 24 hours

    Removed by hemodialysis (40% to 60%)

Dosing adjustment in hepatic impairment: Should be considered

Patient Information Thoroughly chew tablets or manually crush or disperse 2 tablets in 1 oz of water prior to taking; for powder, open packet and pour contents into 4 oz of liquid; do not mix with fruit juice or other acid-containing liquid; stir until dissolved, drink immediately; do not take with meals

Nursing Implications Administer liquified powder immediately after dissolving; avoid creating dust if powder spilled, use wet mop or damp sponge

Dosage Forms
Powder for oral solution:
Buffered (single dose packet): 100 mg, 167 mg, 250 mg, 375 mg
Pediatric: 2 g, 4 g
Tablet, buffered, chewable (mint flavor): 25 mg, 50 mg, 100 mg, 150 mg

Dideoxycytidine see Zalcitabine on page 1172

Didronel® see Etidronate Disodium on page 432

Dienestrol (dye en ess' trole)
Brand Names DV® Cream; Ortho® Dienestrol
Use Symptomatic management of atrophic vaginitis or kraurosis vulvae in post-menopausal women
Pregnancy Risk Factor X
Contraindications Pregnancy; should not be used during lactation or undiagnosed vaginal bleeding
Warnings/Precautions Use with caution in patients with a history of thromboembolism, stroke, myocardial infarction (especially age >40 who smoke), liver tumor, hypertension, cardiac, renal or hepatic insufficiency
Adverse Reactions
1% to 10%:
Cardiovascular: Peripheral edema
Endocrine & metabolic: Breast tenderness, breast enlargement
Gastrointestinal: Anorexia, abdominal cramping
<1%:
Cardiovascular: Hypertension, thromboembolism, myocardial infarction
Central nervous system: Stroke, migraine, dizziness, anxiety, depression, headache
Dermatologic: Chloasma, melasma, rash
Endocrine & metabolic: Decreased glucose tolerance, alterations in frequency and flow of menses, breast tenderness or enlargement, increased triglycerides and LDL
Gastrointestinal: Nausea, GI distress
Hepatic: Cholestatic jaundice
Miscellaneous: Increased susceptibility to Candida infection
Mechanism of Action Increases the synthesis of DNA, RNA, and various proteins in target tissues; reduces the release of gonadotropin-releasing hormone from the hypothalamus; reduces FSH and LH release from the pituitary
Pharmacodynamics/Kinetics
Time to peak serum concentration: Topical: Within 3-4 hours
Metabolism: In the liver
Usual Dosage Adults: Vaginal: Insert 1 applicatorful once or twice daily for 1-2 weeks and then 1/2 of that dose for 1-2 weeks; maintenance dose: 1 applicatorful 1-3 times/week for 3-6 months
Patient Information Insert applicator high into vagina. Patients should inform their physician if signs or symptoms of any of the following occur: Thromboembolic or thrombotic disorders including sudden severe headache or vomiting, disturbance of vision or speech, loss of vision, numbness or weakness in an extremity, sharp or crushing chest pain, calf pain, shortness of breath, severe abdominal pain or mass, mental depression, or unusual bleeding. Patients should discontinue taking the medication if they suspect they are pregnant or become pregnant.
Dosage Forms Cream, vaginal: 0.01% (30 g with applicator; 78 g with applicator)

Diethylpropion Hydrochloride (dye eth il proe' pee on)
Brand Names Tenuate®; Tenuate® Dospan®; Tepanil®
Synonyms Amfepramone
Use Short-term adjunct in exogenous obesity
Restrictions C-IV
Pregnancy Risk Factor B
Contraindications Known hypersensitivity to diethylpropion
Warnings/Precautions Prolonged administration may lead to dependence; use with caution in patients with mental illness or diabetes mellitus, cardiovascular
(Continued)
333

Diethylpropion Hydrochloride *(Continued)*

disease, nephritis, angina pectoris, hypertension, glaucoma, and patients with a history of drug abuse

Adverse Reactions

>10%:
Cardiovascular: Hypertension
Central nervous system: Euphoria, nervousness, insomnia

1% to 10%:
Central nervous system: Confusion, mental depression
Endocrine & metabolic: Changes in libido
Gastrointestinal: Nausea, vomiting, restlessness, constipation
Hematologic: Blood dyscrasias
Neuromuscular & skeletal: Tremor
Ocular: Blurred vision

<1%:
Cardiovascular: Tachycardia, arrhythmias
Central nervous system: Depression, headache
Dermatologic: Alopecia
Gastrointestinal: Diarrhea, abdominal cramps
Neuromuscular & skeletal: Myalgia, tremor
Renal: Dysuria, polyuria
Respiratory: Dyspnea
Miscellaneous: Increased sweating

Overdosage/Toxicology There is no specific antidote for amphetamine intoxication and the bulk of the treatment is supportive. Hyperactivity and agitation usually respond to reduced sensory input; however, with extreme agitation, haloperidol (2-5 mg I.M. for adults) may be required. Hyperthermia is best treated with external cooling measures, or when severe or unresponsive, muscle paralysis with pancuronium may be needed. Hypertension is usually transient and generally does not require treatment unless severe. For diastolic blood pressures >110 mm Hg, a nitroprusside infusion should be initiated. Seizures usually respond to diazepam I.V. and/or phenytoin maintenance regimens.

Drug Interactions

Decreased effect of guanethidine; decreased effect with phenothiazines
Increased effect/toxicity with MAO inhibitors (hypertensive crisis), CNS depressants, general anesthetics (arrhythmias), sympathomimetics

Mechanism of Action Diethylpropion is used as an anorexiant agent possessing pharmacological and chemical properties similar to those of amphetamines. The mechanism of action of diethylpropion in reducing appetite appears to be secondary to CNS effects, specifically stimulation of the hypothalamus to release catecholamines into the central nervous system; anorexiant effects are mediated via norepinephrine and dopamine metabolism. An increase in physical activity and metabolic effects (inhibition of lipogenesis and enhancement of lipolysis) may also contribute to weight loss.

Usual Dosage Adults: Oral:
Tablet: 25 mg 3 times/day before meals or food
Tablet, controlled release: 75 mg at midmorning

Monitoring Parameters Monitor CNS

Patient Information Avoid alcoholic beverages; take during day to avoid insomnia; do not discontinue abruptly, may cause physical and psychological dependence with prolonged use

Nursing Implications Do not crush 75 mg controlled release tablets; dose should not be given in evening or at bedtime

Dosage Forms

Tablet: 25 mg
Tablet, controlled release: 75 mg

Diethylstilbestrol *(dye eth il stil bess' trole)*

Brand Names Stilphostrol®

Synonyms DES; Stilbestrol

Use Palliative treatment of inoperable metastatic prostatic carcinoma and postmenopausal inoperable, progressing breast cancer

Pregnancy Risk Factor X

Contraindications Undiagnosed vaginal bleeding, during pregnancy

Warnings/Precautions Use with caution in patients with a history of thromboembolism, stroke, myocardial infarction (especially >40 of age who smoke), liver tumor, hypertension, cardiac, renal or hepatic insufficiency; estrogens have been reported to increase the risk of endometrial carcinoma; do not use estrogens during pregnancy

Adverse Reactions
>10%:
Cardiovascular: Peripheral edema
Endocrine & metabolic: Enlargement of breasts (female and male), breast tenderness
Gastrointestinal: Nausea, anorexia, bloating
1% to 10%:
Central nervous system: Headache
Endocrine & metabolic: Increased libido (female), decreased libido (male)
Gastrointestinal: Vomiting, diarrhea
<1%:
Cardiovascular: Hypertension, thromboembolism, myocardial infarction, edema
Central nervous system: Stroke, depression, dizziness, anxiety
Dermatologic: Chloasma, melasma, rash
Endocrine & metabolic: Breast tumors, amenorrhea, alterations in frequency and flow of menses
Gastrointestinal: Nausea, GI distress
Hepatic: Increased triglycerides and LDL, cholestatic jaundice
Miscellaneous: Intolerance to contact lenses, decreased glucose tolerance, increased susceptibility to *Candida* infection

Overdosage/Toxicology Nausea

Stability Intravenous solution should be stored at room temperature and away from direct light; solution is stable for 3 days as long as cloudiness or precipitation has not occurred

Mechanism of Action Competes with estrogenic and androgenic compounds for binding onto tumor cells and thereby inhibits their effects on tumor growth

Pharmacodynamics/Kinetics
Metabolism: In the liver
Elimination: In urine and feces

Usual Dosage Adults:
Male:
Prostate carcinoma (inoperable, progressing): Oral: 1-3 mg/day
Diphosphate: Inoperable progressing prostate cancer:
Oral: 50 mg 3 times/day; increase up to 200 mg or more 3 times/day; maximum daily dose: 1 g
I.V.: Give 0.5 g, dissolved in 250 mL of saline or D_5W, administer slowly the first 10-15 minutes then adjust rate so that the entire amount is given in 1 hour; repeat for ≥5 days depending on patient response, then repeat 0.25-0.5 g 1-2 times for one week or change to oral therapy
Female: Postmenopausal inoperable, progressing breast carcinoma: Oral: 15 mg/day

Test Interactions
Increased prothrombin and factors VII, VIII, IX, X
Decreased antithrombin III
Increased platelet aggregability
Increased thyroid binding globulin
Increased total thyroid hormone (T_4)
Decreased serum folate concentration
Increased serum triglycerides/phospholipids

Patient Information Patients should inform their physicians if signs or symptoms of thromboembolic or thrombotic disorders including sudden severe headache or vomiting, disturbance of vision or speech, loss of vision, numbness or weakness in an extremity, sharp or crushing chest pain, calf pain, shortness of breath, severe abdominal pain or mass, mental depression or unusual bleeding.

Dosage Forms
Injection, as diphosphate sodium (Stilphostrol®): 0.25 g (5 mL)
Tablet: 1 mg, 5 mg
Tablet, as diphosphate (Stilphostrol®): 50 mg

Diflorasone Diacetate (dye flor' a sone)
Related Information
Corticosteroids Comparisons *on page 1266-1268*
Brand Names Florone®; Florone E®; Maxiflor®; Psorcon™
Use Relieves inflammation and pruritic symptoms of corticosteroid-responsive dermatosis [high to very high potency topical corticosteroid]
Pregnancy Risk Factor C
Contraindications Known hypersensitivity to diflorasone
Warnings/Precautions Use with caution in patients with impaired circulation; skin infections
(Continued)

Diflorasone Diacetate *(Continued)*

Adverse Reactions
<1%:
Local: Burning, itching, folliculitis, dryness, maceration
Neuromuscular & skeletal: Muscle atrophy, arthralgia
Miscellaneous: Secondary infection

Overdosage/Toxicology Symptoms of overdose include moon face, central obesity, hypertension, diabetes, hyperlipidemia, peptic ulcer, increased susceptibility to infection, electrolyte and fluid imbalance, psychosis, hallucinations. When consumed in excessive quantities, systemic hypercorticism and adrenal suppression may occur; in those cases discontinuation and withdrawal of the corticosteroid should be done judiciously.

Mechanism of Action Decreases inflammation by suppression of migration of polymorphonuclear leukocytes and reversal of increased capillary permeability

Pharmacodynamics/Kinetics
Absorption: Topical: Negligible, around 1% reaches dermal layers or systemic circulation; occlusive dressings increase absorption percutaneously
Metabolism: Primarily in the liver

Usual Dosage Topical: Apply ointment sparingly 1-3 times/day; apply cream sparingly 2-4 times/day

Patient Information A thin film of cream or ointment is effective; do not overuse; do not use tight-fitting diapers or plastic pants on children being treated in the diaper area; use only as prescribed, and for no longer than the period prescribed; apply sparingly in light film; rub in lightly; avoid contact with eyes; notify physician if condition being treated persists or worsens

Nursing Implications For external use only; do not use on open wounds; apply sparingly to occlusive dressings; should not be used in the presence of open or weeping lesions

Dosage Forms
Cream: 0.05% (15 g, 30 g, 60 g)
Ointment, topical: 0.05% (15 g, 30 g, 60 g)

Diflucan® *see* Fluconazole *on page 461*

Diflunisal *(dye floo' ni sal)*

Brand Names Dolobid®

Use Management of inflammatory disorders usually including rheumatoid arthritis and osteoarthritis; can be used as an analgesic for treatment of mild to moderate pain

Pregnancy Risk Factor C (D if used in the 3rd trimester)

Contraindications Hypersensitivity to diflunisal or any component, may be a cross-sensitivity with other nonsteroidal anti-inflammatory agents including aspirin; should not be used in patients with active GI bleeding

Warnings/Precautions Peptic ulceration and GI bleeding have been reported; platelet function and bleeding time are inhibited; ophthalmologic effects; impaired renal function, use lower dosage; peripheral edema; possibility of Reye's syndrome; elevation in liver tests

Adverse Reactions
>10%:
Cardiovascular: Fluid retention
Central nervous system: Headache
1% to 10%:
Cardiovascular: Angina pectoris, arrhythmias
Central nervous system: Dizziness
Dermatologic: Skin rash, itching
Gastrointestinal: GI ulceration
Genitourinary: Vaginal bleeding
Otic: Tinnitus
<1%:
Cardiovascular: Chest pain, vasculitis, tachycardia
Central nervous system: Convulsions, hallucinations, mental depression, drowsiness, nervousness, insomnia, weakness
Dermatologic: Toxic epidermal necrolysis, hives, exfoliative dermatitis, itching, erythema multiforme, Stevens-Johnson syndrome, angioedema
Gastrointestinal: Stomatitis, esophagitis or gastritis, gastrointestinal ulceration
Genitourinary: Cystitis
Hematologic: Hemolytic anemia, agranulocytosis, thrombocytopenia
Hepatic: Hepatitis
Neuromuscular & skeletal: Peripheral neuropathy, trembling
Ocular: Blurred vision, change in vision
Otic: Decreased hearing

Renal: Interstitial nephritis, nephrotic syndrome, renal impairment
Respiratory: Wheezing, shortness of breath
Miscellaneous: Anaphylaxis, increased sweating

Overdosage/Toxicology Symptoms of overdose include drowsiness, nausea, vomiting, hyperventilation, tachycardia, tinnitus, stupor, coma, renal failure, leukocytosis; management of a nonsteroidal anti-inflammatory drug (NSAID) intoxication is primarily supportive and symptomatic. Fluid therapy is commonly effective in managing the hypotension that may occur following an acute NSAID overdose, except when this is due to an acute blood loss.

Drug Interactions
Decreased effect with antacids
Increased effect/toxicity of digoxin, methotrexate, anticoagulants, phenytoin, sulfonylureas, sulfonamides, lithium, indomethacin, hydrochlorothiazide, acetaminophen (levels)

Mechanism of Action Inhibits prostaglandin synthesis by decreasing the activity of the enzyme, cyclo-oxygenase, which results in decreased formation of prostaglandin precursors

Pharmacodynamics/Kinetics
Onset of analgesia: Within 1 hour
Duration of action: 8-12 hours
Absorption: Well absorbed from GI tract
Distribution: Appears in breast milk
Metabolism: Extensively in the liver
Half-life: 8-12 hours, prolonged with renal impairment
Time to peak serum concentration: Oral: Within 2-3 hours
Elimination: In urine within 72-96 hours, ~3% as unchanged drug and 90% as glucuronide conjugates

Usual Dosage Adults: Oral:
Pain: Initial: 500-1000 mg followed by 250-500 mg every 8-12 hours; maximum daily dose: 1.5 g
Inflammatory condition: 500-1000 mg/day in 2 divided doses; maximum daily dose: 1.5 g

Dosing adjustment in renal impairment: Cl_{cr} <50 mL/minute: Administer 50% of normal dose

Test Interactions ↑ chloride (S), glucose, ketone (U), uric acid (S), sodium (S); ↓ uric acid (S), catecholamines (U), glucose, potassium (S), prothrombin time (S), uric acid (S), ↑ bleeding time

Patient Information May cause GI upset, take with water, milk, or meals; do not take aspirin with diflunisal, swallow tablets whole, do not crush or chew

Dosage Forms Tablet: 250 mg, 500 mg

Digibind® *see* Digoxin Immune Fab *on page 342*

Digitoxin (di ji tox' in)
Brand Names Crystodigin®
Use Treatment of congestive heart failure, atrial fibrillation, atrial flutter, paroxysmal atrial tachycardia, and cardiogenic shock
Pregnancy Risk Factor C
Contraindications Hypersensitivity to digitoxin or any component (rare); digitalis toxicity, beriberi heart disease, A-V block, idiopathic hypertrophic subaortic stenosis, constrictive pericarditis, ventricular fibrillation, or tachycardia
Warnings/Precautions Use with caution in patients with hypoxia, hypothyroidism, acute myocarditis,; do not use to treat obesity; patients with incomplete A-V block (Stokes-Adams attack) may progress to complete block with digitalis drug administration; use with caution in patients with acute myocardial infarction, severe pulmonary disease, advanced heart failure, idiopathic hypertrophic subaortic stenosis, Wolff-Parkinson-White syndrome, sick-sinus syndrome (bradyarrhythmias), amyloid heart disease, and constrictive cardiomyopathies; adjust dose with renal or hepatic impairment and aged patients; elderly may develop exaggerated serum/tissue concentrations due to decreased lean body mass, total body water, and age-related reduction in renal/hepatic function; exercise will reduce serum concentrations of digoxin due to increased skeletal muscle uptake

Adverse Reactions
1% to 10%: Gastrointestinal: Anorexia, nausea, vomiting
<1%:
Cardiovascular: Sinus bradycardia, A-V block, S-A block, atrial or nodal ectopic beats, ventricular arrhythmias, bigeminy, trigeminy, atrial tachycardia with A-V block
Central nervous system: Drowsiness, headache, fatigue, lethargy, neuralgia, vertigo, disorientation
Endocrine & metabolic: Hyperkalemia with acute toxicity
(Continued)

Digitoxin *(Continued)*

Gastrointestinal: Feeding intolerance, abdominal pain, diarrhea

Ocular: Blurred vision, halos, yellow or green vision, diplopia, photophobia, flashing lights

Overdosage/Toxicology Antidote: Life-threatening digitoxin toxicity is treated with Digibind®; discontinue digitalis preparation; administer potassium 40-80 mEq in divided doses in D_5W at 20 mEq/hour I.V.; do not give potassium with complete heart block secondary to digitalis product or in cases of renal failure; digitalis-induced arrhythmias not responsive to potassium may be treated with phenytoin (0.5 mg/kg I.V. at 50 mg/minute), lidocaine (1 mg/kg over 5 minutes); cholestyramine, colestipol, activated charcoal may decrease absorption; other agents to consider, based on EKG and clinical assessment are atropine, quinidine, procainamide, and propranolol. **Note:** Other antiarrhythmics appear more dangerous to use in toxicity.

Drug Interactions

Decreased effect/levels of digitoxin/digoxin: Antacids (magnesium, aluminum), cholestyramine, colestipol, kaolin/pectin, aminosalicylic acid, metoclopramide, sulfasalazine

Decreased effect/levels of digitoxin only (eg, increased metabolism): Aminoglutethimide, barbiturates, hydantoins, rifampin, phenylbutazone, thyroid replacement

Increased effect/toxicity/levels of digitoxin/digoxin: Amiodarone, nifedipine, quinidine, quinine, verapamil, nondepolarizing muscle relaxants, succinylcholine, potassium-losing diuretics

Mechanism of Action Digitalis binds to and inhibits magnesium and adenosine triphosphate dependent sodium and potassium ATPase thereby increasing the influx of calcium ions, from extracellular to intracellular cytoplasm due to the inhibition of sodium and potassium ion movement across the myocardial membranes; this increase in calcium ions results in a potentiation of the activity of the contractile heart muscle fibers and an increase in the force of myocardial contraction (positive inotropic effect); digitalis may also increase intracellular entry of calcium via slow calcium channel influx; stimulates release and blocks re-uptake of norepinephrine; decreases conduction through the S-A and A-V nodes

Pharmacodynamics/Kinetics

Absorption: 90% to 100%

Distribution: V_d: 7 L/kg

Protein binding: 90% to 97%

Metabolism: Hepatic, 50% to 70%

Time to peak: 8-12 hours

Half-life: 7-8 days

Elimination: 30% to 50% excreted unchanged in urine/feces

Usual Dosage Oral:

Children: Doses are very individualized; **when recommended,** digitalizing dose is as follows:

<1 year: 0.045 mg/kg

1-2 years: 0.04 mg/kg

>2 years: 0.03 mg/kg which is equivalent to 0.75 mg/mm^2

Maintenance: Approximately $^1/_{10}$ of the digitalizing dose

Adults: Oral:

Rapid loading dose: Initial: 0.6 mg followed by 0.4 mg and then 0.2 mg at intervals of 4-6 hours

Slow loading dose: 0.2 mg twice daily for a period of 4 days followed by a maintenance dose

Maintenance: 0.05-0.3 mg/day

Most common dose: 0.15 mg/day

Dosing adjustment in renal impairment:

Cl_{cr} <10 mL/minute: Administer 50% to 75% of normal dose

Not dialyzable (0% to 5%)

Dosing adjustment in hepatic impairment:

Dosage reduction is necessary in severe liver disease

Reference Range Therapeutic: 20-35 ng/mL; Toxic: >45 ng/mL

Patient Information Do not discontinue medication without physician's advice; instruct patients to notify physician if they suffer loss of appetite, visual changes, nausea, vomiting, weakness, drowsiness, headache, confusion, or depression

Nursing Implications Observe patients for noncardiac signs of toxicity: anorexia, vision changes (blurred), confusion, and depression

Dosage Forms Tablet: 0.05 mg, 0.1 mg, 0.15 mg, 0.2 mg

Digoxin (di jox' in)

Related Information

Antiarrhythmic Drugs *on page 1246-1248*

Brand Names Lanoxicaps®; Lanoxin®

Use Treatment of congestive heart failure and to slow the ventricular rate in tachyarrhythmias such as atrial fibrillation, atrial flutter, and supraventricular tachycardia (paroxysmal atrial tachycardia); cardiogenic shock

Pregnancy Risk Factor C

Contraindications Hypersensitivity to digoxin or any component; A-V block, idiopathic hypertrophic subaortic stenosis, or constrictive pericarditis

Warnings/Precautions Use with caution in patients with hypoxia, myxedema, hypothyroidism, acute myocarditis; do not use to treat obesity; patients with incomplete A-V block (Stokes-Adams attack) may progress to complete block with digitalis drug administration; use with caution in patients with acute myocardial infarction, severe pulmonary disease, advanced heart failure, idiopathic hypertrophic subaortic stenosis, Wolff-Parkinson-White syndrome, sick-sinus syndrome (bradyarrhythmias), amyloid heart disease, and constrictive cardiomyopathies; adjust dose with renal impairment; elderly and neonates may develop exaggerated serum/tissue concentrations due to age-related alterations in clearance and pharmacodynamic differences; exercise will reduce serum concentrations of digoxin due to increased skeletal muscle uptake

Adverse Reactions

1% to 10%: Gastrointestinal: Anorexia, nausea, vomiting

<1%:

Cardiovascular: Sinus bradycardia, A-V block, S-A block, atrial or nodal ectopic beats, ventricular arrhythmias, bigeminy, trigeminy, atrial tachycardia with A-V block

Central nervous system: Drowsiness, headache, fatigue, lethargy, neuralgia, vertigo, disorientation

Endocrine & metabolic: Hyperkalemia with acute toxicity

Gastrointestinal: Feeding intolerance, abdominal pain, diarrhea

Ocular: Blurred vision, halos, yellow or green vision, diplopia, photophobia, flashing lights

Overdosage/Toxicology Manifested by a wide variety of signs and symptoms difficult to distinguish from effects associated with cardiac disease; nausea and vomiting are common early signs of toxicity and may precede or follow evidence of cardiotoxicity; anorexia, diarrhea, abdominal discomfort, headache, weakness, drowsiness, visual disturbances, mental depression, confusion, restlessness, disorientation, seizures, hallucinations; cardiac abnormalities include ventricular tachycardia, unifocal or multifocal PVCs (bigeminal, trigeminal); paroxysmal nodal rhythms, A-V dissociation; excessive slowing of the pulse, A-V block of varying degree; P-R prolongation, S-T depression; occasional arterial fibrillation; ventricular fibrillation is common cause of death (alterations in cardiac rate and rhythm can result in any type of known arrhythmia)

Antidote: Life-threatening digoxin toxicity is treated with Digibind®; administer potassium except in cases of complete heart block or renal failure; digitalis-induced arrhythmias not responsive to potassium may be treated with phenytoin lidocaine; cholestyramine, and colestipol may decrease absorption; other agents to consider, based on EKG and clinical assessment are atropine, quinidine, procainamide, and propranolol. **Note:** Other antiarrhythmics appear more dangerous to use in toxicity.

Drug Interactions

Decreased effect/levels of digitoxin/digoxin: Antacids (magnesium, aluminum), cholestyramine, colestipol, kaolin/pectin, aminosalicylic acid, metoclopramide, sulfasalazine

Decreased effect/levels of digitoxin only (eg, increased metabolism): Aminoglutethimide, barbiturates, hydantoins, rifampin, phenylbutazone, thyroid replacement

Increased effect/toxicity/levels of digitoxin/digoxin: Amiodarone, nifedipine, quinidine, quinine, verapamil, nondepolarizing muscle relaxants, succinylcholine, potassium-losing diuretics

Stability Protect elixir and injection from light; solution **compatibility**: D_5W, $D_{10}W$, NS, sterile water for injection (when diluted fourfold or greater)

Mechanism of Action

Congestive heart failure: Inhibition of the sodium/potassium ATPase pump which acts to increase the intracellular sodium-calcium exchange to increase intracellular calcium leading to increased contractility

Supraventricular arrhythmias: Direct suppression of the A-V node conduction to increase effective refractory period and decrease conduction velocity - positive inotropic effect, enhanced vagal tone, and decreased ventricular rate to fast atrial arrhythmias. Atrial fibrillation may decrease sensitivity and increase tolerance to higher serum digoxin concentrations.

(Continued)

339

Digoxin *(Continued)*

Pharmacodynamics/Kinetics

Onset of action:
  Oral: 1-2 hours
  I.V.: 5-30 minutes
Peak effect:
  Oral: 2-8 hours
  I.V.: 1-4 hours
Duration: Adults: 3-4 days both forms
Absorption: By passive nonsaturable diffusion in the upper small intestine; food may delay, but does not affect extent of digoxin absorption
Distribution:
  Normal renal function: 6-7 L/kg
  V_d: Extensive to peripheral tissues, with a distinct distribution phase which lasts 6-8 hours; concentrates in heart, liver, kidney, skeletal muscle and intestines. Heart/serum concentration is 70:1. Pharmacologic effects are delayed and do not correlate well with serum concentrations during distribution phase.
  Hyperthyroidism: Increased V_d
  Hyperkalemia, hyponatremia: Decreased digoxin distribution to heart and muscle
  Hypokalemia: Increased digoxin distribution to heart and muscles
  Concomitant quinidine therapy: Decreased V_d
  Chronic renal failure: 4-6 L/kg
  Decreased sodium/potassium ATPase activity - decreased tissue binding
  Neonates, full term: 7.5-10 L/kg
  Children: 16 L/kg
  Adults: 7 L/kg, decreased with renal disease
Protein binding: 30% (in uremic patients, digoxin is displaced from plasma protein binding sites)
Metabolism: By sequential sugar hydrolysis in the stomach or by reduction of lactone ring by intestinal bacteria (in ~10% of population, gut bacteria may metabolize up to 40% of digoxin dose); metabolites may contribute to therapeutic and toxic effects of digoxin; metabolism is reduced in patients with CHF
Bioavailability: Oral (dependent upon formulation):
  Elixir: 75% to 85%
  Tablets: 70% to 80%
Half-life: Dependent upon age, renal and cardiac function:
  Neonates:
    Premature: 61-170 hours
    Full-term: 35-45 hours
  Infants: 18-25 hours
  Children: 35 hours
  Adults: 38-48 hours
  Adults, anephric: 4-6 days
Half-life:
  Parent drug: 38 hours

Dosage Recommendations for Digoxin

Age	Total Digitalizing Dose† (mcg/kg)*		Daily Maintenance Dose‡ (mcg/kg*)	
	P.O.	I.V. or I.M.	P.O.	I.V. or I.M.
Preterm infant*	20-30	15-25	5-7.5	4-6
Full-term infant*	25-35	20-30	6-10	5-8
1 mo - 2 y*	35-60	30-50	10-15	7.5-12
2-5 y*	30-40	25-35	7.5-10	6-9
5-10 y*	20-35	15-30	5-10	4-8
>10 y*	10-15	8-12	2.5-5	2-3
Adults	0.75-1.5 mg	0.5-1 mg	0.125-0.5 mg	0.1-0.4 mg

†Give one-half of the total digitalizing dose (TDD) in the initial dose, then give one-quarter of the TDD in each of two subsequent doses at 8- to 12-hour intervals. Obtain EKG 6 hours after each dose to assess potential toxicity.

*Based on lean body weight and normal renal function for age. Decrease dose in patients with ↓ renal function; digitalizing dose often not recommended in infants and children.

‡Divided every 12 hours in infants and children <10 years of age. Given once daily to children >10 years of age and adults.

Metabolites:
Digoxigenin: 4 hours
Monodigitoxoside: 3-12 hours
Time to peak serum concentration: Oral: Within 1 hour
Elimination: 50% to 70% excreted unchanged in urine
Usual Dosage When changing from oral (tablets or liquid) or I.M. to I.V. therapy, dosage should be reduced by 20% to 25%. See table.

Dosing adjustment/interval in renal impairment
Cl_{cr} 10-50 mL/minute: Administer 25% to 75% of dose or every 36 hours
Cl_{cr} <10 mL/minute: Administer 10% to 25% of dose or every 48 hours
Reduce loading dose by 50% in ESRD
Not dialyzable (0% to 5%)

Monitoring Parameters
When to draw serum digoxin concentrations: Digoxin serum concentrations are monitored because digoxin possesses a narrow therapeutic serum range; the therapeutic endpoint is difficult to quantify and digoxin toxicity may be life threatening. Digoxin serum levels should be drawn **at least 4 hours after an intravenous dose** and **at least 6 hours after an oral dose (optimally 12-24 hours after a dose).**
Initiation of therapy:
If a loading dose is given: Digoxin serum concentration may be drawn within 12-24 hours after the initial loading dose administration. Levels drawn this early may confirm the relationship of digoxin plasma levels and response but are of little value in determining maintenance doses.
If a loading dose is not given: Digoxin serum concentration should be obtained after 3-5 days of therapy
Maintenance therapy:
Trough concentrations should be followed just prior to the next dose or at a minimum of 4 hours after an I.V. dose and at least 6 hours after an oral dose
Digoxin serum concentrations should be obtained within 5-7 days (approximate time to steady-state) after any dosage changes. Continue to obtain digoxin serum concentrations 7-14 days after any change in maintenance dose.
Note: In patients with end stage renal disease, it may take 15-20 days to reach steady-state.
Additionally, patients who are receiving potassium-depleting medications such as diuretics, should be monitored for potassium, magnesium, and calcium levels
Digoxin serum concentrations should be obtained whenever any of the following conditions occur:
Questionable patient compliance or to evaluate clinical deterioration following an initial good response
Changing renal function
Suspected digoxin toxicity
Initiation or discontinuation of therapy with drugs (amiodarone, quinidine, verapamil) which potentially interact with digoxin; if quinidine therapy is started; digoxin levels should be drawn within the first 24 hours after starting quinidine therapy, then 7-14 days later or empirically skip one day's digoxin dose and decrease the daily dose by 50%
Any disease changes (hypothyroidism)
Heart rate and rhythm should be monitored along with periodic EKGs to assess both desired effects and signs of toxicity
Follow closely (especially in patients receiving diuretics or amphotericin) for decreased serum potassium and magnesium or increased calcium, all of which predispose to digoxin toxicity
Assess renal function
Be aware of drug interactions

Reference Range
Digoxin therapeutic serum concentrations:
Congestive heart failure: 0.8-2 ng/mL
Arrhythmias: 1.5-2.5 ng/mL

Adults: <0.5 ng/mL; probably indicates underdigitalization unless there are special circumstances
Toxic: >2.5 ng/mL; tachyarrhythmias commonly require levels >2 ng/mL
Digoxin-like immunoreactive substance (DLIS) may crossreact with digoxin immunoassay. DLIS has been found in patients with renal and liver disease, congestive heart failure, neonates, and pregnant women (third trimester).

Patient Information Do not discontinue medication without checking with physician; notify physician if loss of appetite or visual changes occur
Nursing Implications Observe patients for noncardiac signs of toxicity, ie, anorexia, vision changes (blurred), confusion, and depression

Dosage Forms
Capsule: 50 mcg, 100 mcg, 200 mcg
(Continued)

Digoxin *(Continued)*

Elixir, pediatric (lime flavor): 50 mcg/mL with alcohol 10% (60 mL)
Injection: 250 mcg/mL (1 mL, 2 mL)
Injection, pediatric: 100 mcg/mL (1 mL)
Tablet: 125 mcg, 250 mcg, 500 mcg

Digoxin Immune Fab (di jox' in)

Brand Names Digibind®

Synonyms Antidigoxin Fab Fragments

Use Digoxin immune Fab are specific antibodies for the treatment of digitalis intoxication in carefully selected patients; use in life-threatening ventricular arrhythmias secondary to digoxin, acute digoxin ingestion (ie, >10 mg in adults or >4 mg in children), hyperkalemia (serum potassium >5 mEq/L) in the setting of digoxin toxicity

Pregnancy Risk Factor C

Contraindications Hypersensitivity to sheep products

Warnings/Precautions Use with caution in renal or cardiac failure; allergic reactions possible (sheep product)-skin testing not routinely recommended; epinephrine should be immediately available, Fab fragments may be eliminated more slowly in patients with renal failure, heart failure may be exacerbated as digoxin level is reduced; total serum digoxin concentration may rise precipitously following administration of Digibind®, but this will be almost entirely bound to the Fab fragment and not able to react with receptors in the body; Digibind® will interfere with digitalis immunoassay measurements - this will result in clinically misleading serum digoxin concentrations until the Fab fragment is eliminated from the body (several days to >1 week after Digibind® administration). Hypokalemia has been reported to occur following reversal of digitalis intoxication as has exacerbation of underlying heart failure; Serum digoxin levels drawn prior to therapy may be difficult to evaluate if 6-8 hours have not elapsed after the last dose of digoxin (time to equilibration between serum and tissue); redigitalization should not be initiated until Fab fragments have been eliminated from the body, which may occur over several days or greater than a week in patients with impaired renal function.

Adverse Reactions

<1%:

Cardiovascular: Worsening of low cardiac output or congestive heart failure, rapid ventricular response in patients with atrial fibrillation as digoxin is withdrawn

Endocrine & metabolic: Hypokalemia

Dermatologic: Urticarial rash

Miscellaneous: Allergic reactions, facial swelling and redness

Overdosage/Toxicology Symptoms of overdose include delayed serum sickness; treatment of serum sickness includes acetaminophen, histamine$_1$ and possibly histamine$_2$ blockers and corticosteroids

Stability Should be refrigerated (2°C to 8°C); reconstituted solutions should be used within 4 hours if refrigerated

Mechanism of Action Binds with molecules of digoxin or digitoxin and then is excreted by the kidneys and removed from the body

Pharmacodynamics/Kinetics

Onset of action: I.V.: Improvement in signs and symptoms occur within 2-30 minutes

Half-life: 15-20 hours; prolonged in patients with renal impairment

Elimination: Renally with levels declining to undetectable amounts within 5-7 days

Usual Dosage Each vial of Digibind® will bind approximately 0.6 mg of digoxin or digitoxin

I.V.: To determine the dose of digoxin immune Fab, first determine the total body load of digoxin (TNI using either an approximation of the amount ingested or a postdistribution serum digoxin concentration). If neither ingestion amount or serum level is known: Adult dosage is 20 vials (800 mg) I.V. infusion.

Administration Continuous I.V. infusion over 15-30 minutes is preferred; digoxin immune Fab is reconstituted by adding 4 mL sterile water, resulting in 10 mg/mL for I.V. infusion, the reconstituted solution may be further diluted with NS to a convenient volume (eg, 1 mg/mL)

Monitoring Parameters Serum potassium, serum digoxin concentration prior to first dose of digoxin immune Fab; **digoxin levels will greatly increase with Digibind® use and are not an accurate determination of body stores**

Dosage Forms Powder for injection, lyophilized: 40 mg

Dihydrocodeine Compound (dye hye droe koe' deen)

Brand Names DHC Plus®; Synalgos®-DC

Use Management of mild to moderate pain that requires relaxation

Restrictions C-III

Pregnancy Risk Factor B (D if used for prolonged periods or in high doses at term)

Contraindications Hypersensitivity to dihydrocodeine or any component

Warnings/Precautions Use with caution in patients with hypersensitivity reactions to other phenanthrene derivative opioid agonists (morphine, hydrocodone, hydromorphone, levorphanol, oxycodone, oxymorphone); respiratory diseases including asthma, emphysema, COPD, or severe liver or renal insufficiency; some preparations contain sulfites which may cause allergic reactions; may be habit-forming; dextromethorphan has equivalent antitussive activity but has much lower toxicity in accidental overdose

Adverse Reactions
>10%:
    Central nervous system: Lightheadedness, dizziness, drowsiness, sedation
    Dermatologic: Pruritus, skin reactions
    Gastrointestinal: Nausea, vomiting, constipation
1% to 10%:
    Cardiovascular: Hypotension, palpitations, bradycardia, peripheral vasodilation
    Central nervous system: Increased intracranial pressure
    Endocrine & metabolic: Antidiuretic hormone release
    Ocular: Miosis
    Respiratory: Respiratory depression
    Miscellaneous: Biliary or urinary tract spasm, histamine release, physical and psychological dependence with prolonged use

Overdosage/Toxicology Naloxone 2 mg I.V. (0.01 mg/kg for children) with repeat administration as necessary up to a total of 10 mg; see Aspirin toxicology

Drug Interactions Increased toxicity: MAO inhibitors → ↑ adverse symptoms

Mechanism of Action Binds to opiate receptors in the CNS, causing inhibition of ascending pain pathways, altering the perception of and response to pain; causes cough suppression by direct central action in the medulla; produces generalized CNS depression

Usual Dosage Adults: Oral: 1-2 capsules every 4-6 hours as needed for pain

Patient Information Avoid alcohol, may cause drowsiness, impaired judgment or coordination; may cause physical and psychological dependence with prolonged use

Nursing Implications Observe patient for excessive sedation, respiratory depression; implement safety measures, assist with ambulation

Dosage Forms Capsule:
    DHC Plus®: Dihydrocodeine bitartrate 16 mg, acetaminophen 356.4 mg, and caffeine 30 mg
    Synalgos®-DC: Dihydrocodeine bitartrate 16 mg, aspirin 356.4 mg, and caffeine 30 mg

Dihydroergotamine Mesylate (dye hye droe er got' a meen)

Brand Names D.H.E. 45®

Use Aborts or prevents vascular headaches; also as an adjunct for DVT prophylaxis for hip surgery, for orthostatic hypotension, xerostomia secondary to antidepressant use, and pelvic congestion with pain

Pregnancy Risk Factor X

Contraindications High-dose aspirin therapy, hypersensitivity to dihydroergotamine or any component

Warnings/Precautions Use with caution in hypertension, angina, peripheral vascular disease, impaired renal or hepatic function; avoid pregnancy

Adverse Reactions
>10%:
    Cardiovascular: Localized edema, peripheral vascular effects (numbness and tingling of fingers and toes)
    Central nervous system: Drowsiness, dizziness
    Gastrointestinal: Dry mouth, diarrhea, nausea, vomiting
1% to 10%:
    Cardiovascular: Precordial distress and pain, transient tachycardia or bradycardia
    Neuromuscular & skeletal: Muscle pain in the extremities, weakness in the legs

Overdosage/Toxicology Symptoms of overdose include peripheral ischemia, paresthesia, headache, nausea, vomiting; activated charcoal is effective at binding certain chemicals; this is especially true for ergot alkaloids

Drug Interactions
    Increased effect of heparin
(Continued)

343

Dihydroergotamine Mesylate *(Continued)*

Increased toxicity with erythromycin, clarithromycin, nitroglycerin, propranolol, troleandomycin

Stability Store in refrigerator

Mechanism of Action Ergot alkaloid alpha-adrenergic blocker directly stimulates vascular smooth muscle to vasoconstrict peripheral and cerebral vessels; also has effects on serotonin receptors

Pharmacodynamics/Kinetics

Onset of action: Within 15-30 minutes

Duration: 3-4 hours

Distribution: V_d: 14.5 L/kg

Protein binding: 90%

Metabolism: Extensively in the liver

Half-life: 1.3-3.9 hours

Time to peak serum concentration: I.M.: Within 15-30 minutes

Elimination: Predominately into bile and feces and 10% excreted in urine, mostly as metabolites

Usual Dosage Adults:

I.M.: 1 mg at first sign of headache; repeat hourly to a maximum dose of 3 mg total

I.V.: Up to 2 mg maximum dose for faster effects; maximum dose: 6 mg/week

Dosing adjustment in hepatic impairment: Dosage reductions are probably necessary but specific guidelines are not available

Reference Range Minimum concentration for vasoconstriction is reportedly 0.06 ng/mL

Patient Information Rare feelings of numbness or tingling of fingers, toes, or face may occur; avoid using this medication if you are pregnant, have heart disease, hypertension, liver disease, infection, itching

Dosage Forms Injection: 1 mg/mL (1 mL)

Dihydroergotoxine *see* Ergoloid Mesylates *on page 397*

Dihydromorphinone *see* Hydromorphone Hydrochloride *on page 550*

Dihydrotachysterol (dye hye droe tak iss' ter ole)

Brand Names DHT™; Hytakerol®

Synonyms Dichysterol

Use Treatment of hypocalcemia associated with hypoparathyroidism; prophylaxis of hypocalcemic tetany following thyroid surgery

Pregnancy Risk Factor A (D if used in doses above the recommended daily allowance)

Contraindications Hypercalcemia, known hypersensitivity to dihydrotachysterol

Warnings/Precautions Calcium-phosphate product (serum calcium and phosphorus) must not exceed 70; avoid hypercalcemia; use with caution in coronary artery disease, decreased renal function (especially with secondary hyperparathyroidism), renal stones, and elderly

Adverse Reactions

>10%:

Endocrine & metabolic: Hypercalcemia, hypercalciuria

Renal: Elevated serum creatinine

<1%:

Central nervous system: Convulsions

Endocrine & metabolic: Polydipsia

Gastrointestinal: Nausea, vomiting, anorexia, weight loss

Hematologic: Anemia

Neuromuscular & skeletal: Weakness, metastatic calcification

Renal: Renal damage, polyuria

Overdosage/Toxicology Symptoms of overdose include hypercalcemia, anorexia, nausea, weakness, constipation, diarrhea, vague aches, mental confusion, tinnitus, ataxia, depression, hallucinations, syncope, coma; polyuria, polydipsia, nocturia, hypercalciuria, irreversible renal insufficiency or proteinuria, azotemia; will spread tissue calcifications, hypertension. Following withdrawal of the drug, treatment consists of bed rest, liberal intake of fluids, reduced calcium intake, and cathartic administration. Severe hypercalcemia requires I.V. hydration and forced diuresis. Urine output should be monitored and maintained at >3 mL/kg/hour. I.V. saline can quickly and significantly increase excretion of calcium into the urine. Calcitonin, cholestyramine, prednisone, sodium EDTA and mithramycin have all been used successfully to treat the more resistant cases of vitamin D-induced hypercalcemia.

Drug Interactions
Decreased effect/levels of vitamin D: Cholestyramine, colestipol, mineral oil; phenytoin and phenobarbital may inhibit activation → ↓ effectiveness
Increased toxicity: Thiazide diuretics increase calcium

Stability Protect from light

Mechanism of Action Synthetic analogue of vitamin D with a faster onset of action; stimulates calcium and phosphate absorption from the small intestine, promotes secretion of calcium from bone to blood; promotes renal tubule resorption of phosphate

Pharmacodynamics/Kinetics
Peak hypercalcemic effect: Within 2-4 weeks
Duration: Can be as long as 9 weeks
Absorption: Well absorbed from the GI tract
Elimination: In bile and feces; stored in liver, fat, skin, muscle, and bone

Usual Dosage Oral:
Hypoparathyroidism:
Neonates: 0.05-0.1 mg/day
Infants and young Children: Initial: 1-5 mg/day for 4 days, then 0.1-0.5 mg/day
Older Children and Adults: Initial: 0.8-2.4 mg/day for several days followed by maintenance doses of 0.2-1 mg/day
Nutritional rickets: 0.5 mg as a single dose or 13-50 mcg/day until healing occurs
Renal osteodystrophy: Maintenance: 0.25-0.6 mg/24 hours adjusted as necessary to achieve normal serum calcium levels and promote bone healing

Monitoring Parameters Monitor renal function, serum calcium, and phosphate concentrations; if hypercalcemia is encountered, discontinue agent until serum calcium returns to normal

Reference Range Calcium (serum): 9-10 mg/dL (4.5-5 mEq/L)

Patient Information Do not take more than the recommended amount. While taking this medication, your physician may want you to follow a special diet or take a calcium supplement; follow this diet closely. Avoid taking magnesium supplements or magnesium-containing antacids. Early symptoms of hypercalcemia include weakness, fatigue, headache, metallic taste, stomach upset, muscle or bone pain, and irritability.

Nursing Implications Monitor symptoms of hypercalcemia (weakness, fatigue, somnolence, headache, anorexia, dry mouth, metallic taste, nausea, vomiting, cramps, diarrhea, muscle pain, bone pain, and irritability)

Dosage Forms
Capsule: 0.125 mg
Solution:
Concentrate: 0.2 mg/mL (30 mL)
Oral: 0.2 mg/5 mL (500 mL)
Oral, in oil: 0.25 mg/mL (15 mL)
Tablet: 0.125 mg, 0.2 mg, 0.4 mg

1,25 Dihydroxycholecalciferol see Calcitriol on page 159

Diiodohydroxyquin see Iodoquinol on page 588

Diisopropyl Fluorophosphate see Isoflurophate on page 594

Dilacor™ XR see Diltiazem on this page

Dilantin® see Phenytoin on page 877

Dilatrate®-SR see Isosorbide Dinitrate on page 599

Dilaudid® see Hydromorphone Hydrochloride on page 550

Dilaudid-HP® see Hydromorphone Hydrochloride on page 550

Dilocaine® see Lidocaine Hydrochloride on page 633

Diltiazem (dil tye' a zem)
Related Information
Antiarrhythmic Drugs on page 1246-1248
Calcium Channel Blockers Cardiovascular Adverse Reactions on page 1262
Calcium Channel Blockers Central Nervous System Adverse Reactions on page 1264
Calcium Channel Blockers Comparative Actions on page 1260
Calcium Channel Blockers Comparative Pharmacokinetics on page 1261
Calcium Channel Blockers FDA-Approved Indications on page 1263
Calcium Channel Blockers Gastrointestinal and Miscellaneous Adverse Reactions on page 1265
Brand Names Cardizem® CD; Cardizem® Injectable; Cardizem® SR; Cardizem® Tablet; Dilacor™ XR
(Continued)

Diltiazem *(Continued)*

Use
Capsule: Hypertension (alone or in combination); chronic stable angina or angina from coronary artery spasm

Injection: Atrial fibrillation or atrial flutter; paroxysmal supraventricular tachycardias (PSVT)

Pregnancy Risk Factor C

Pregnancy/Breast Feeding Implications
Teratogenic and embryotoxic effects have been demonstrated in small animals

Contraindications
Severe hypotension or second and third degree heart block; hypersensitivity to other calcium channel blockers, adenosine; atrial and ventricular arrhythmias, acute myocardial infarction, and pulmonary congestion

Warnings/Precautions
Use with caution and titrate dosages for patients with impaired renal or hepatic function; use caution when treating patients with congestive heart failure, sick-sinus syndrome, severe left ventricular dysfunction, hypertrophic cardiomyopathy (especially obstructive), concomitant therapy with beta-blockers or digoxin, edema, or increased intracranial pressure with cranial tumors; do not abruptly withdraw (may cause chest pain); elderly may experience hypotension and constipation more readily.

Adverse Reactions
>10%: Headache

1% to 10%:
Cardiovascular: Bradycardia, A-V block (first degree), edema, EKG abnormality

Central nervous system: Dizziness, asthenia

Gastrointestinal: Nausea, vomiting

<1%:
Cardiovascular: A-V block (second degree), angina

Central nervous system: Abnormal dreams, amnesia, depression, gait abnormality, insomnia, nervousness

Dermatologic: Urticaria, photosensitivity, alopecia, purpura

Gastrointestinal: Anorexia, constipation, diarrhea, dysgeusia, dyspepsia

Hematologic: Hemolytic anemia, leukopenia thrombocytopenia

Neuromuscular & skeletal: Paresthesia, tremor

Ocular: Amblyopia, retinopathy

Respiratory: Pharyngitis, cough increase

Miscellaneous: Flu syndrome

Overdosage/Toxicology
The primary cardiac symptoms of calcium blocker overdose includes hypotension and bradycardia. The hypotension is caused by peripheral vasodilation, myocardial depression, and bradycardia. Bradycardia results from sinus bradycardia, second- or third-degree atrioventricular block, or sinus arrest with junctional rhythm. Intraventricular conduction is usually not affected so QRS duration is normal (verapamil does prolong the P-R interval and bepridil prolongs the Q-T and may cause ventricular arrhythmias, including torsade de pointes).

The noncardiac symptoms include confusion, stupor, nausea, vomiting, metabolic acidosis and hyperglycemia. Following initial gastric decontamination, if possible, repeated calcium administration may promptly reverse the depressed cardiac contractility (but not sinus node depression or peripheral vasodilation); glucagon, epinephrine, and amrinone may treat refractory hypotension; glucagon and epinephrine also increase the heart rate (outside the U.S., 4-aminopyridine may be available as an antidote); dialysis and hemoperfusion are not effective in enhancing elimination although repeat-dose activated charcoal may serve as an adjunct with sustained-release preparations.

Drug Interactions
Increased toxicity/effect/levels:

H_2 blockers $\rightarrow$ ↑ bioavailability diltiazem

Beta-blockers $\rightarrow$ ↑ cardiac depressant effects on A-V conduction

Carbamazepine $\rightarrow$ ↑ carbamazepine levels

Cyclosporine $\rightarrow$ ↑ cyclosporine levels

Fentanyl $\rightarrow$ ↑ hypotension

Digitalis $\rightarrow$ ↑ digitalis levels

Quinidine $\rightarrow$ ↑ quinidine levels (hypotension, bradycardia)

Theophylline $\rightarrow$ ↑ pharmacologic actions of theophylline

Mechanism of Action
Inhibits calcium ion from entering the "slow channels" or select voltage-sensitive areas of vascular smooth muscle and myocardium during depolarization, producing a relaxation of coronary vascular smooth muscle and coronary vasodilation; increases myocardial oxygen delivery in patients with vasospastic angina

Pharmacodynamics/Kinetics
Onset of action: Oral: 30-60 minutes (including sustained release)

Absorption: 80% to 90%

Time to peak serum concentration:

Short-acting tablets: Within 2-3 hours

Sustained release: 6-11 hours

Distribution: V_d: 1.7 L/kg; appears in breast milk

Protein binding: 77% to 85%

Metabolism: Extensive first-pass metabolism; metabolized in the liver; following single I.V. injection, plasma concentrations of N-monodesmethyldiltiazem and desacetyldiltiazem are typically undetectable; however, these metabolites accumulate to detectable concentrations following 24-hour constant rate infusion. N-monodesmethyldiltiazem appears to have 20% of the potency of diltiazem; desacetyldiltiazem is about 50% as potent as the parent compound.

Bioavailability: ~40% to 60% due to significant first-pass effect

Half-life: 4-6 hours, may increase with renal impairment; 5-7 hours with sustained release

Elimination: In urine and bile mostly as metabolites

Usual Dosage Adults:

Oral: 30-120 mg 3-4 times/day; dosage should be increased gradually, at 1- to 2-day intervals until optimum response is obtained; usual maintenance dose is usually 240-360 mg/day

Sustained-release capsules: Cardizem® CD: Total daily dose of short-acting administered once daily **or** initially 180 or 240 mg once daily; maximum antihypertensive effect is usually achieved after 14 days of chronic therapy. Adjust dosage accordingly up to a maximum of 360 mg/day of Cardizem® CD.

I.V. (requires an infusion pump): See table.

Diltiazem — I.V. Dosage and Administration

Initial Bolus Dose	0.25 mg/kg actual body weight over 2 min (average adult dose: 20 mg)
Repeat Bolus Dose may be administered after 15 min if the response is inadequate	0.35 mg/kg actual body weight over 2 min (average adult dose: 25 mg)
Continuous Infusion Infusions of >24 h or infusion rates >15 mg/h are not recommended due to potential accumulation of metabolites and increased toxicity	Initial infusion rate of 10 mg/h Rate may be increased in 5 mg/h increments up to 15 mg/h as needed Some patients may respond to an initial rate of 5 mg/h

If Cardizem® injectable is administered by continuous infusion for >24 hours, the possibility of decreased diltiazem clearance, prolonged elimination half-life, and increased diltiazem and/or diltiazem metabolite plasma concentrations should be considered

Conversion from I.V. diltiazem to oral diltiazem: Start oral approximately 3 hours after bolus dose

Oral dose (mg/day) is approximately equal to [rate (mg/hour) x 3 + 3] x 10

3 mg/hour = 120 mg/day

5 mg/hour = 180 mg/day

7 mg/hour = 240 mg/day

11 mg/hour = 360 mg/day (maximum recommended dose)

Dosing comments in renal/hepatic impairment: Use with caution as extensively metabolized by the liver and excreted in the kidneys and bile

Not removed by hemo- or peritoneal dialysis; supplemental dose is not necessary

Patient Information Sustained release products should be taken with food and not crushed; limit caffeine intake; avoid alcohol; notify physician if angina pain is not reduced when taking this drug, irregular heartbeat, shortness of breath, swelling, dizziness, constipation, nausea, or hypotension occurs; do not stop therapy without advice of physician

Nursing Implications Do not crush sustained release capsules

Dosage Forms

Capsule, sustained release:

Cardizem® CD: 120 mg, 180 mg, 240 mg, 300 mg

Cardizem® SR: 60 mg, 90 mg, 120 mg

Dilacor™ XR: 180 mg, 240 mg

Injection (Cardizem®): 5 mg/mL (5 mL, 10 mL)

Tablet (Cardizem®): 30 mg, 60 mg, 90 mg, 120 mg

Dimenhydrinate (dye men hye' dri nate)

Brand Names Calm-X® [OTC]; Dimetabs®; Dinate®; Dramamine® [OTC]; Dramilin®; Hydrate®; Marmine® [OTC]; Tega-Cert® [OTC]; TripTone® Caplets® [OTC]; Wehamine®

Use Treatment and prevention of nausea, vertigo, and vomiting associated with motion sickness

Pregnancy Risk Factor B

Contraindications Hypersensitivity to dimenhydrinate or any component

Warnings/Precautions Use with caution with prostatic hypertrophy, peptic ulcer, narrow-angle glaucoma, bronchial asthma, and cardiac arrhythmias

Adverse Reactions

>10%:

Central nervous system: Slight to moderate drowsiness

Miscellaneous: Thickening of bronchial secretions

1% to 10%:

Central nervous system: Headache, fatigue, nervousness, dizziness

Gastrointestinal: Appetite increase, weight increase, nausea, diarrhea, abdominal pain, dry mouth

Neuromuscular & skeletal: Arthralgia

Respiratory: Pharyngitis

<1%:

Cardiovascular: Edema, palpitations, hypotension

Central nervous system: Depression, drowsiness, paradoxical CNS stimulation

Dermatologic: Angioedema, photosensitivity, rash

Gastrointestinal: Anorexia

Genitourinary: Urinary frequency

Hepatic: Hepatitis

Local: Pain at the injection site

Neuromuscular & skeletal: Myalgia, paresthesia

Ocular: Blurred vision

Otic: Tinnitus

Respiratory: Bronchospasm

Miscellaneous: Epistaxis

Overdosage/Toxicology Toxicity may resemble atropine overdosage; CNS depression or stimulation; there is no specific treatment for an antihistamine overdose, however, most of its clinical toxicity is due to anticholinergic effects. For anticholinergic overdose with severe life-threatening symptoms, physostigmine 1-2 mg (0.5 or 0.02 mg/kg for children) I.V., slowly may be given to reverse these effects.

Drug Interactions

Increased effect/toxicity with CNS depressants, anticholinergics, TCAs, MAO inhibitors

Increased toxicity of antibiotics, especially aminoglycosides (ototoxicity)

Stability When mixed in the same syringe, drugs reported to be **incompatible** include aminophylline, barbiturates, butorphanol, chlorpromazine, glycopyrrolate, heparin, hydrocortisone, hydroxyzine, midazolam, phenytoin, prednisolone, prochlorperazine, promethazine, tetracycline, trifluoperazine

Mechanism of Action Competes with histamine for H_1-receptor sites on effector cells in the gastrointestinal tract, blood vessels, and respiratory tract; blocks chemoreceptor trigger zone, diminishes vestibular stimulation, and depresses labyrinthine function through its central anticholinergic activity

Pharmacodynamics/Kinetics

Onset of action: Oral: Within 15-30 minutes

Absorption: Well absorbed from GI tract

Distribution: Small amounts appear in breast milk

Metabolism: Extensively in the liver

Usual Dosage

Children:

Oral:

2-5 years: 12.5-25 mg every 6-8 hours, maximum: 75 mg/day

6-12 years: 25-50 mg every 6-8 hours, maximum: 150 mg/day

I.M.: 1.25 mg/kg or 37.5 mg/m^2 4 times/day, not to exceed 300 mg/day

Adults: Oral, I.M., I.V.: 50-100 mg every 4-6 hours, not to exceed 400 mg/day

Administration I.V. injection must be diluted to 10 mL with NS and given at 25 mg/minute

Patient Information May cause drowsiness, may impair judgment and coordination; avoid alcohol; drink plenty of fluids for dry mouth and to prevent constipation

Nursing Implications Raise bed rails, institute safety measures, assist with ambulation

Dosage Forms

Capsule: 50 mg

Injection: 50 mg/mL (1 mL, 5 mL, 10 mL)

Liquid: 12.5 mg/4 mL (90 mL, 473 mL); 16.62 mg/5 mL (480 mL)
Tablet: 50 mg
Tablet, chewable: 50 mg

Dimercaprol (dye mer kap' role)

Brand Names BAL in Oil®

Synonyms BAL; British Anti-Lewisite; Dithioglycerol

Use Antidote to gold, arsenic, and mercury poisoning; adjunct to edetate calcium disodium in lead poisoning

Pregnancy Risk Factor C

Contraindications Hepatic insufficiency (unless due to arsenic poisoning); do not use on iron, cadmium, or selenium poisoning

Warnings/Precautions Potentially a nephrotoxic drug, use with caution in patients with oliguria or glucose 6-phosphate dehydrogenase deficiency; keep urine alkaline to protect kidneys; give all injections deep I.M. at different sites

Adverse Reactions
>10%:
Cardiovascular: Hypertension, tachycardia
Central nervous system: Convulsions
1% to 10%: Gastrointestinal: Nausea, vomiting
<1%:
Central nervous system: Nervousness, fever, headache
Gastrointestinal: Salivation
Hematologic: Transient neutropenia
Local: Pain at the injection site
Ocular: Blepharospasm
Renal: Nephrotoxicity
Miscellaneous: Burning sensation of the lips, mouth, throat, eyes, and penis

Drug Interactions Toxic complexes with iron, cadmium, selenium, or uranium

Mechanism of Action Sulfhydryl group combines with ions of various heavy metals to form relatively stable, nontoxic, soluble chelates which are excreted in urine

Pharmacodynamics/Kinetics
Distribution: Distributes to all tissues including the brain
Metabolism: Rapidly to inactive products
Time to peak serum concentration: 0.5-1 hour
Elimination: In urine

Usual Dosage Children and Adults: Deep I.M.:
Mild arsenic and gold poisoning: 2.5 mg/kg/dose every 6 hours for 2 days, then every 12 hours on the third day, and once daily thereafter for 10 days
Severe arsenic and gold poisoning: 3 mg/kg/dose every 4 hours for 2 days then every 6 hours on the third day, then every 12 hours thereafter for 10 days
Mercury poisoning: Initial: 5 mg/kg followed by 2.5 mg/kg/dose 1-2 times/day for 10 days
Lead poisoning (use with edetate calcium disodium):
Mild: 3 mg/kg/dose every 4 hours for 5-7 days
Severe and acute encephalopathy: 4 mg/kg/dose initially alone then every 4 hours in combination of edetate calcium disodium

Dosing adjustment in hepatic impairment: Necessary in acute hepatic insufficiency

Administration Administer deep I.M. only

Test Interactions Iodine ^{131}I thyroidal uptake values may be decreased

Patient Information Frequent blood and urine tests may be required

Nursing Implications Urine should be kept alkaline because chelate dissociates in acid media

Dosage Forms Injection: 100 mg/mL (3 mL)

Dimetabs® see Dimenhydrinate on page 347

Dimetane® [OTC] see Brompheniramine Maleate on page 143

Dimethoxyphenyl Penicillin Sodium see Methicillin Sodium on page 707

β,β-Dimethylcysteine see Penicillamine on page 847

Dimethyl Triazeno Imidazol Carboxamide see Dacarbazine on page 297

Dinate® see Dimenhydrinate on page 347

Dinoprostone (dye noe prost' one)

Brand Names Prepidil® Gel; Prostin E₂®

Synonyms PGE₂; Prostaglandin E₂

Use

Gel: Promote cervical ripening prior to labor induction; usage for gel include any patient undergoing induction of labor with an unripe cervix, most commonly for pre-eclampsia, eclampsia, postdates, diabetes, intrauterine growth retardation, and chronic hypertension

Suppositories: Terminate pregnancy from 12th through 28th week of gestation; evacuate uterus in cases of missed abortion or intrauterine fetal death; manage benign hydatidiform mole

Pregnancy Risk Factor X

Contraindications

Gel: Hypersensitivity to prostaglandins or any constituents of the cervical gel, history of asthma, contracted pelvis, malpresentation of the fetus

Gel: The following are "relative" contraindications and should only be considered by the physician under these circumstances: Patients in whom vaginal delivery is not indicated (ie, herpes genitalia with a lesion at the time of delivery), prior uterine surgery, breech presentation, multiple gestation, polyhydramnios, premature rupture of membranes

Suppository: Known hypersensitivity to dinoprostone, acute pelvic inflammatory disease, uterine fibroids, cervical stenosis

Warnings/Precautions Dinoprostone should be used only by medically trained personnel in a hospital; caution in patients with cervicitis, infected endocervical lesions, acute vaginitis, compromised (scarred) uterus or history of asthma, hypertension or hypotension, epilepsy, diabetes mellitus, anemia, jaundice, or cardiovascular, renal, or hepatic disease. Oxytocin should not be used simultaneously with Prepidil™ (>6 hours of the last dose of Prepidil™).

Adverse Reactions

>10%:

Central nervous system: Headache

Gastrointestinal: Vomiting, diarrhea, nausea

1% to 10%:

Cardiovascular: Bradycardia

Central nervous system: Fever

Neuromuscular & skeletal: Back pain

<1%:

Cardiovascular: Hypotension, cardiac arrhythmias, syncope, flushing, pain and tightness of the chest

Central nervous system: Vasomotor and vasovagal reactions, dizziness, chills, shivering

Endocrine & metabolic: Hot flashes

Respiratory: Wheezing, dyspnea, coughing, bronchospasm

Overdosage/Toxicology Vomiting, bronchospasm, hypotension, chest pain, abdominal cramps, uterine contractions; treatment is symptomatic

Drug Interactions Increased effect of oxytocics

Stability Suppositories must be kept frozen, store in freezer not above -20°F (-4°C); bring to room temperature just prior to use; cervical gel should be stored under refrigeration 2°C to 8°C (36°F to 46°F)

Mechanism of Action A synthetic prostaglandin E₂ abortifacient that stimulates uterine contractions similar to those seen during natural labor

Pharmacodynamics/Kinetics

Onset of effect (uterine contractions): Within 10 minutes

Duration: Up to 2-3 hours

Absorption: Vaginal: Slow following administration

Metabolism: In many tissues including the kidney, lungs, and spleen

Elimination: Primarily in urine with small amounts excreted in feces

Usual Dosage

Abortifacient: Insert 1 suppository high in vagina, repeat at 3- to 5-hour intervals until abortion occurs up to 240 mg (maximum dose); continued administration for longer than 2 days is not advisable

Cervical ripening:

Gel:

Intracervical: 0.25-1 mg

Intravaginal: 2.5 mg

Suppositories: Intracervical: 2-3 mg

Administration Intracervically: For cervical ripening, patient should be supine in the dorsal position

Nursing Implications Bring suppository to room temperature just prior to use; patient should remain supine for 10 minutes following insertion; commercially available suppositories should not be used for extemporaneous preparation of any other dosage form of drug

Dosage Forms
Gel, endocervical: 0.5 mg in 3 g syringes [each package contains a 10-mm and 20-mm shielded catheter]
Suppository, vaginal: 20 mg

Diocto-K® [OTC] *see* Docusate *on page 362*

Diocto® [OTC] *see* Docusate *on page 362*

Dioctyl Calcium Sulfosuccinate *see* Docusate *on page 362*

Dioctyl Sodium Sulfosuccinate *see* Docusate *on page 362*

Dioeze® [OTC] *see* Docusate *on page 362*

Dioval® *see* Estradiol *on page 407*

Dipalmitoylphosphatidylcholine *see* Colfosceril Palmitate *on page 272*

Dipentum® *see* Olsalazine Sodium *on page 815*

Diphenhydramine Hydrochloride (dye fen hye' dra meen)
Related Information
Initial Doses in Selected Antiemetic Regimens *on page 1205*
Brand Names AllerMax® [OTC]; Banophen® [OTC]; Beldin® [OTC]; Belix® [OTC]; Benadryl® [OTC]; Benylin® Cough Syrup [OTC]; Compoz® [OTC]; Diphen® Cough [OTC]; Genahist®; Nidryl® [OTC]; Nordryl®; Nytol® [OTC]; Sleep-eze 3® [OTC]; Sominex® [OTC]; Tusstat®; Twilite® [OTC]; Valdrene®
Use Symptomatic relief of allergic symptoms caused by histamine release which include nasal allergies and allergic dermatosis; can be used for mild nighttime sedation; prevention of motion sickness and as an antitussive; has antinauseant and topical anesthetic properties; treatment of phenothiazine-induced dystonic reactions
Pregnancy Risk Factor C
Contraindications Hypersensitivity to diphenhydramine or any component; should not be used in acute attacks of asthma
Warnings/Precautions Use with caution in patients with angle-closure glaucoma, peptic ulcer, urinary tract obstruction, hyperthyroidism; some preparations contain sodium bisulfite; syrup contains alcohol; diphenhydramine has high sedative and anticholinergic properties, so it may not be considered the antihistamine of choice for prolonged use in the elderly
Adverse Reactions
>10%:
Central nervous system: Slight to moderate drowsiness
Respiratory: Thickening of bronchial secretions
1% to 10%:
Central nervous system: Headache, fatigue nervousness
Gastrointestinal: Nausea, vomiting, diarrhea, abdominal pain, dry mouth, appetite increase, weight gain
Neuromuscular & skeletal: Arthralgia
Respiratory: Pharyngitis
Miscellaneous: Dry mucous membranes
<1%:
Cardiovascular: Hypotension, palpitations, edema
Central nervous system: Sedation, dizziness, paradoxical excitement, fatigue, insomnia, depression
Dermatologic: Photosensitivity, rash, angioedema
Genitourinary: Urinary retention
Hepatic: Hepatitis
Neuromuscular & skeletal: Myalgia, paresthesia, tremor
Ocular: Blurred vision
Respiratory: Bronchospasm
Miscellaneous: Epistaxis
Overdosage/Toxicology Symptoms of overdose include CNS stimulation or depression; overdose may result in death in infants and children. There is no specific treatment for an antihistamine overdose, however, most of its clinical toxicity is due to anticholinergic effects. Anticholinesterase inhibitors (eg, physostigmine, neostigmine, pyridostigmine, or edrophonium) may be useful by reducing acetylcholinesterase. For anticholinergic overdose with severe life-threatening symptoms, physostigmine 1-2 mg (0.5 or 0.02 mg/kg for children) I.V., slowly may be given to reverse these effects.
Drug Interactions Increased toxicity: CNS depressants worsens CNS and respiratory depression, monoamine oxidase inhibitors → ↑ anticholinergic effects; syrup should not be given to patients taking drugs that can cause disulfiram reactions (ie, metronidazole, chlorpropamide) due to high alcohol content
(Continued)

Diphenhydramine Hydrochloride *(Continued)*

Stability Protect from light; the following drugs are **incompatible** with diphenhydramine when mixed in the same syringe: Amobarbital, amphotericin B, cephalothin, diatrizoate, foscarnet, heparin, hydrocortisone, hydroxyzine, pentobarbital, phenobarbital, phenytoin, prochlorperazine, promazine, promethazine, tetracycline, thiopental

Mechanism of Action Competes with histamine for H_1-receptor sites on effector cells in the gastrointestinal tract, blood vessels, and respiratory tract

Pharmacodynamics/Kinetics

Maximum sedative effect: 1-3 hours

Duration of action: 4-7 hours

Absorption: Oral: 40% to 60% reaches systemic circulation due to first-pass metabolism

Metabolism: Extensive in the liver and, to smaller degrees, in the lung and kidney

Half-life: 2-8 hours; elderly: 13.5 hours

Protein binding: 78%

Time to peak serum concentration: 2-4 hours

Usual Dosage

Children:

Oral: (>10 kg): 12.5-25 mg 3-4 times/day; maximum daily dose: 300 mg

I.M., I.V.: 5 mg/kg/day or 150 mg/m²/day in divided doses every 6-8 hours, not to exceed 300 mg/day

Adults:

Oral: 25-50 mg every 6-8 hours

Nighttime sleep aid: 50 mg at bedtime

I.M., I.V.: 10-50 mg in a single dose every 2-4 hours, not to exceed 400 mg/day

Topical: For external application, not longer than 7 days

Reference Range

Antihistamine effects at levels >25 ng/mL

Drowsiness at levels 30-40 ng/mL

Mental impairment at levels >60 ng/mL

Therapeutic: Not established

Toxic: >0.1 µg/mL

Test Interactions May suppress the wheal and flare reactions to skin test antigens

Patient Information May cause drowsiness; swallow whole, do not crush or chew sustained release product; avoid alcohol, may impair coordination and judgment

Nursing Implications Raise bed rails, institute safety measures, assist with ambulation

Dosage Forms

Capsule: 25 mg, 50 mg

Cream: 1%, 2%

Elixir: 12.5 mg/5 mL (5 mL, 10 mL, 20 mL, 120 mL, 480 mL, 3780 mL)

Injection: 10 mg/mL (10 mL, 30 mL); 50 mg/mL (1 mL, 10 mL)

Lotion: 1% (75 mL)

Solution, topical spray: 1% (60 mL)

Syrup: 12.5 mg/5 mL (5 mL, 120 mL, 240 mL, 480 mL, 3780 mL)

Tablet: 25 mg, 50 mg

Diphenoxylate and Atropine *(dye fen ox' i late)*

Brand Names Lofene®; Logen®; Lomanate®; Lomodix®; Lomotil®; Lonox®; Low-Quel®

Synonyms Atropine and Diphenoxylate

Use Treatment of diarrhea

Restrictions C-V

Pregnancy Risk Factor C

Contraindications Hypersensitivity to diphenoxylate, atropine or any component; severe liver disease, jaundice, dehydrated patient, and narrow-angle glaucoma; it should not be used for children <2 years of age

Warnings/Precautions High doses may cause physical and psychological dependence with prolonged use; use with caution in patients with ulcerative colitis, dehydration, and hepatic dysfunction; reduction of intestinal motility may be deleterious in diarrhea resulting from *Shigella*, *Salmonella*, toxigenic strains of *E. coli*, and from pseudomembranous enterocolitis associated with broad spectrum antibiotics; children may develop signs of atropinism (dryness of skin and mucous membranes, thirst, hyperthermia, tachycardia, urinary retention, flushing) even at the recommended dosages; if there is no response with 48 hours, the drug is unlikely to be effective and should be discontinued; if chronic diarrhea is not improved symptomatically within 10 days at maximum dosage of 20 mg/day, control is unlikely with further use.

Adverse Reactions

1% to 10%:

Central nervous system: Nervousness, restlessness, dizziness, drowsiness, headache, mental depression

Gastrointestinal: Paralytic ileus, dry mouth

Genitourinary: Urinary retention and difficult urination

Ocular: Blurred vision

Respiratory: Respiratory depression

<1%:

Cardiovascular: Tachycardia

Central nervous system: Sedation, euphoria, weakness, hyperthermia

Dermatologic: Pruritus, urticaria

Gastrointestinal: Nausea, vomiting, abdominal discomfort, pancreatitis, stomach cramps

Neuromuscular & skeletal: Muscle cramps

Miscellaneous: Increased sweating

Overdosage/Toxicology Symptoms of overdose include drowsiness, hypotension, blurred vision, flushing, dry mouth, miosis

Administration of activated charcoal will reduce bioavailability of diphenoxylate; naloxone 2 mg I.V. (0.01 mg/kg for children) with repeat administration as necessary up to a total of 10 mg; for anticholinergic overdose with severe life-threatening symptoms, physostigmine 1-2 mg (0.5 or 0.02 mg/kg for children) S.C. or I.V., slowly may be given to reverse these effects

Drug Interactions Increased toxicity: MAO inhibitors (hypertensive crisis), CNS depressants, antimuscarinics (paralytic ileus); may prolong half-life of drugs metabolized in liver

Stability Protect from light

Mechanism of Action Diphenoxylate inhibits excessive GI motility and GI propulsion; commercial preparations contain a subtherapeutic amount of atropine to discourage abuse

Pharmacodynamics/Kinetics

Onset of action: Within 45-60 minutes

Peak effect: Within 2 hours

Duration: 3-4 hours

Absorption: Oral: Well absorbed

Metabolism: Extensively in the liver to diphenoxylic acid (active)

Half-life: Diphenoxylate: 2.5 hours

Time to peak serum concentration: 2 hours

Elimination: Primarily in feces (via bile); ~14% excreted in urine; <1% excreted unchanged in urine

Usual Dosage Oral:

Children (use with caution in young children due to variable responses): Liquid: 0.3-0.4 mg of diphenoxylate/kg/day in 2-4 divided doses **or**

<2 years: Not recommended

2-5 years: 2 mg of diphenoxylate 3 times/day

5-8 years: 2 mg of diphenoxylate 4 times/day

8-12 years: 2 mg of diphenoxylate 5 times/day

Adults: 15-20 mg/day of diphenoxylate in 3-4 divided doses; maintenance: 5-15 mg/day in 2-3 divided doses

Monitoring Parameters Watch for signs of atropinism (dryness of skin and mucous membranes, tachycardia, thirst, flushing); monitor number and consistency of stools; observe for signs of toxicity, fluid and electrolyte loss, hypotension, and respiratory depression

Patient Information Drowsiness, dizziness, dry mouth; use caution while driving or performing hazardous tasks; avoid alcohol or other CNS depressants; do not exceed prescribed dose; report persistent diarrhea, fever, or palpitations to physician

Nursing Implications Raise bed rails, institute safety measures

Dosage Forms

Solution, oral: Diphenoxylate hydrochloride 2.5 mg and atropine sulfate 0.025 mg per 5 mL (4 mL, 10 mL, 60 mL)

Tablet: Diphenoxylate hydrochloride 2.5 mg and atropine sulfate 0.025 mg

Diphen® Cough [OTC] see Diphenhydramine Hydrochloride on page 351

Diphenylan Sodium® see Phenytoin on page 877

Diphenylhydantoin see Phenytoin on page 877

Diphtheria and Tetanus Toxoid (dif theer' ee a)

Related Information

Immunization Guidelines on page 1389-1405

(Continued)

Diphtheria and Tetanus Toxoid *(Continued)*

Skin Testing for Delayed Hypersensitivity *on page 1325-1327*
Vaccines *on page 1386-1388*

Synonyms DT; Td; Tetanus and Diphtheria Toxoid

Use Active immunity against diphtheria and tetanus when pertussis vaccine is contraindicated

DT: Infants and children through 6 years of age

Td: Children and adults ≥7 years of age

Pregnancy Risk Factor C

Pregnancy/Breast Feeding Implications Td and T vaccines are not known to cause special problems for pregnant women or their unborn babies. While physicians do not usually recommend giving any drugs or vaccines to pregnant women, a pregnant women who needs Td vaccine should get it; wait until 2nd trimester if possible.

Contraindications Patients receiving immunosuppressive agents, prior anaphylactic, allergic, or systemic reactions; hypersensitivity to diphtheria and tetanus toxoid or any component; acute respiratory infection or other active infection

Warnings/Precautions History of a neurologic reaction or immediate hypersensitivity reaction following a previous dose. History of severe local reaction (Arthus-type) following previous dose (such individuals should not be given further routine or emergency doses of tetanus and diphtheria toxoids for 10 years). Do not confuse pediatric DT with adult diphtheria and tetanus toxoid (Td), absorbed (Td) is used in patients >7 years of age; primary immunization should be postponed until the second year of life due to possibility of CNS damage or convulsion; have epinephrine 1:1000 available.

Adverse Reactions Severe adverse reactions must be reported to the FDA

>10%: Central nervous system: Fretfulness, drowsiness

1% to 10%:

Gastrointestinal: Anorexia, vomiting

Miscellaneous: Persistent crying

<1%:

Cardiovascular: Tachycardia, hypotension

Central nervous system: Convulsions (rarely)

Dermatologic: Tenderness, swelling, redness, urticaria, pruritus

Miscellaneous: Pain, Arthus-type hypersensitivity reactions, transient fever

Drug Interactions Decreased effect with immunosuppressive agents, immunoglobulins if given within 1 month

Stability Refrigerate

Usual Dosage I.M.:

Infants and Children (DT):

6 weeks to 1 year: Three 0.5 mL doses at least 4 weeks apart; give a reinforcing dose 6-12 months after the third injection

1-6 years: Two 0.5 mL doses at least 4 weeks apart; reinforcing dose 6-12 months after second injection; if final dose is given after seventh birthday, use adult preparation

4-6 years (booster immunization): 0.5 mL; not necessary if all 4 doses were given after fourth birthday - routinely give booster doses at 10-year intervals with the adult preparation

Children >7 years and Adults: Should receive Td; 2 primary doses of 0.5 mL each, given at an interval of 4-6 weeks; third (reinforcing) dose of 0.5 mL 6-12 months later; boosters every 10 years

Administration Give only I.M.; do not inject the same site more than once

Patient Information DT, Td and T vaccines cause few problems (mild fever or soreness, swelling, and redness/knot at the injection site); these problems usually last 1-2 days, but this does not happen nearly as often as with DTP vaccine

Nursing Implications Shake well before giving

Additional Information Pediatric dosage form should only be used in patients ≤6 years of age. Federal law requires that the date of administration, the vaccine manufacturer, lot number of vaccine, and the administering person's name, title, and address be entered into the patient's permanent medical record.

Dosage Forms Injection:

Pediatric use:

Diphtheria 6.6 Lf units and tetanus 5 Lf units per 0.5 mL (5 mL)

Diphtheria 10 Lf units and tetanus 5 Lf units per 0.5 mL (0.5 mL, 5 mL)

Diphtheria 12.5 Lf units and tetanus 5 Lf units per 0.5 mL (5 mL)

Diphtheria 15 Lf units and tetanus 10 Lf units per 0.5 mL (5 mL)

Adult use:

Diphtheria 1.5 Lf units and tetanus 5 Lf units per 0.5 mL (0.5 mL, 5 mL)

Diphtheria 2 Lf units and tetanus 5 Lf units per 0.5 mL (5 mL)

Diphtheria 2 Lf units and tetanus 10 Lf units per 0.5 mL (5 mL)

Diphtheria and Tetanus Toxoids and Acellular Pertussis Vaccine (dif theer' ee a)

Related Information
Immunization Guidelines *on page 1389-1405*
Vaccines *on page 1386-1388*

Brand Names Acel-Imune®; Tripedia®

Synonyms DTaP

Use Fourth or fifth immunization of children 15 months to 7 years of age (prior to seventh birthday) who have been previously immunized with 3 or 4 doses of whole-cell pertussis DTP vaccine

Pregnancy Risk Factor B

Contraindications Patients >7 years of age, patients with cancer, immunodeficiencies, an acute respiratory infection, or any other active infection; children with a history of neurologic disorders should not receive the pertussis or any component; history of any of the following effects from previous administration of pertussis vaccine precludes further use: >103°F fever (39.4°C), convulsions, focal neurologic signs, screaming episodes, shock, collapse, sleepiness or encephalopathy; known hypersensitivity to diphtheria and tetanus toxoids or pertussis vaccine; do not use for treatment of actual tetanus, diphtheria, or whooping cough infections

Warnings/Precautions DTaP should not be used in children <15 months of age and should not be used in children who have received fewer than 3 doses of DTP

Adverse Reactions All serious adverse reactions must be reported to the FDA
<1%:
Central nervous system: Convulsions, screaming episodes, malaise, sleepiness, focal neurological signs, shock, collapse, fever, chills
Dermatologic: Erythema, swelling, induration, rash, urticaria, local tenderness
Neuromuscular & skeletal: Arthralgias

Drug Interactions Decreased effect with immunosuppressive agents, corticosteroids within 1 month

Stability Refrigerate at 2°C to 8°C (35°F to 46°F); do not freeze

Usual Dosage I.M.: After at least 3 doses of whole-cell DTP, give 0.5 mL at ~18 months (at least 6 months after third DTWP dose), then another dose at 4-5 years of age

Administration Give only I.M. in anterolateral aspect of thigh or deltoid muscle of upper arm

Patient Information A nodule may be palpable at the injection site for a few weeks

Nursing Implications Ensure that at least 3 doses of whole-cell DTwP vaccine have been previously given. Acetaminophen 10-15 mg/kg before and every 4 hours to 12-24 hours may reduce or prevent fever; shake well before administering; the child's medical record should document that the small risk of postvaccination seizure and the benefits of the pertussis vaccination were discussed with the patient.

Additional Information This preparation contains less endotoxin relative to DTP and, although immunogenic, it apparently is less reactogenic than DTP. Federal law requires that the date of administration, the vaccine manufacturer, lot number of vaccine, and the administering person's name, title, and address be entered into the patient's permanent medical record.

Dosage Forms Injection:
Acel-Imune®: Diphtheria 7.5 Lf units, tetanus 5 Lf units, and acellular pertussis vaccine 40 mcg per 0.5 mL (7.5 mL)
Tripedia®: Diphtheria 6.7 Lf units, tetanus 5 Lf units, and acellular pertussis vaccine 46.8 mcg per 0.5 mL (7.5 mL)

Diphtheria CRM$_{197}$ Protein Conjugate *see* Haemophilus b Conjugate Vaccine *on page 521*

Diphtheria, Tetanus Toxoids, Whole-Cell Pertussis Vaccine, and Haemophilus b Conjugate Vaccine (dif theer' ee a, tet' a nus tok' soyds, hole sel per tus' iss vak seen', & hee mof' i lus b kon' ju gate vak seen')

Brand Names Tetramune®

Use Active immunization of infants and children through 5 years of age (between 2 months and the sixth birthday) against diphtheria, tetanus, and pertussis and Haemophilus b disease when indications for immunization with DTP vaccine and HIB vaccine coincide

Pregnancy Risk Factor B

Contraindications Children with any febrile illness or active infection, known hypersensitivity to Haemophilus b polysaccharide vaccine (thimerosal), children *(Continued)*

Diphtheria, Tetanus Toxoids, Whole-Cell Pertussis Vaccine, and Haemophilus b Conjugate Vaccine (Continued)

who are immunosuppressed or receiving immunosuppressive therapy; patients >7 years of age, patients with cancer; children with a history of neurologic and seizure disorders should not receive the pertussis any component; history of any of the following effects from previous administration of pertussis vaccine precludes further use: fever >103°F (39.4°C), convulsions, focal neurologic signs, screaming episodes, shock, collapse, sleepiness or encephalopathy; known hypersensitivity to diphtheria and tetanus toxoids or pertussis vaccine; do not use DTP for treatment of actual tetanus, diphtheria, or whooping cough infections

Warnings/Precautions If adverse reactions occurred with previous doses, immunization should be completed with diphtheria and tetanus toxoid absorbed (pediatric); any febrile illness or active infection is reason for delaying use of Haemophilus b conjugate vaccine

Adverse Reactions All serious adverse reactions must be reported to the FDA

>10%:
Central nervous system: Fever, chills, irritability, restlessness, drowsiness
Local: Erythema, swelling induration, pain and warmth at injection site

1% to 10%:
Dermatologic: Rash
Gastrointestinal: Vomiting, diarrhea, loss of appetite

<1%:
Central nervous system: Convulsions, screaming episodes, malaise sleepiness, focal neurological signs, shock, collapse, chills, arthralgias
Local: Urticaria, local tenderness
Miscellaneous: Increased risk of Haemophilus b infections in the week after vaccination, rarely allergic or anaphylactic reactions

Drug Interactions Decreased effect: Immunosuppressive agents; may interfere with antigen detection tests

Stability Keep in refrigerator, may be frozen (not diluent) without affecting potency

Usual Dosage The primary immunization for children 2 months to 5 years of age, ideally beginning at the age of 2-3 months or at 6-week checkup. Administer 0.5 mL I.M. on 3 occasions at ~2-month intervals, followed by a fourth 0.5 mL dose at ~15 months of age.

Administration Give only I.M.

Patient Information A nodule may be palpable at the injection site for a few weeks

Nursing Implications
Acetaminophen 10-15 mg/kg before and every 4 hours to 12-24 hours may reduce or prevent fever
Shake well before administering
The child's medical record should document that the small risk of past vaccination seizure and the benefits of the pertussis vaccination were discussed with the patient

Additional Information Inactivated bacterial vaccine; Federal law requires that the date of administration, the vaccine manufacturer, lot number of vaccine and the administering person's name, title and address be entered into the patient's permanent medical record

Dosage Forms Injection: 5 mL

Diphtheria Toxoid Conjugate see Haemophilus b Conjugate Vaccine on page 521

Dipivalyl Epinephrine see Dipivefrin on this page

Dipivefrin (dye pi′ ve frin)

Related Information
Glaucoma Drug Therapy Comparison on page 1270

Brand Names Propine®

Synonyms Dipivalyl Epinephrine; DPE

Use Reduces elevated intraocular pressure in chronic open-angle glaucoma; also used to treat ocular hypertension, low tension, and secondary glaucomas

Pregnancy Risk Factor B

Contraindications Hypersensitivity to dipivefrin, ingredients in the formulation, or epinephrine; contraindicated in patients with angle-closure glaucoma

Warnings/Precautions Use with caution in patients with vascular hypertension or cardiac patients and in aphakic patients; contains sodium metabisulfite

Adverse Reactions
1% to 10%:
Central nervous system: Headache
Local: Burning, stinging
Ocular: Ocular congestion, photophobia, mydriasis, blurred vision, ocular pain, bulbar conjunctival follicles, blepharoconjunctivitis, cystoid macular edema
<1%: Cardiovascular: Arrhythmias, hypertension

Drug Interactions Increased or synergistic effect when used with other agents to lower intraocular pressure

Stability Avoid exposure to light and air; discolored or darkened solutions indicate loss of potency

Mechanism of Action Dipivefrin is a prodrug of epinephrine which is the active agent that stimulates alpha- and/or beta-adrenergic receptors increasing aqueous humor outflow

Pharmacodynamics/Kinetics
Ocular pressure effect:
Onset of action: Within 30 minutes
Duration: ≥12 hours
Mydriasis:
Onset of action: May occur within 30 minutes
Duration: Several hours
Absorption: Rapid into the aqueous humor
Metabolism: Converted to epinephrine

Usual Dosage Adults: Ophthalmic: Instill 1 drop every 12 hours into the eyes

Patient Information Discolored solutions should be discarded; may cause transient burning or stinging

Nursing Implications Finger pressure should be applied to lacrimal sac for 1-2 minutes after instillation to decrease risk of absorption and systemic reactions

Dosage Forms Solution, ophthalmic: 0.1% (5 mL, 10 mL, 15 mL)

Diprivan® see Propofol on page 943

Diprolene® see Betamethasone on page 129

Diprolene® AF see Betamethasone on page 129

Dipropylacetic Acid see Valproic Acid and Derivatives on page 1143

Diprosone® see Betamethasone on page 129

Dipyridamole (dye peer id' a mole)
Brand Names Persantine®

Use Maintains patency after surgical grafting procedures including coronary artery bypass; used with warfarin to decrease thrombosis in patients after artificial heart valve replacement; used with aspirin to prevent coronary artery thrombosis; in combination with aspirin or warfarin to prevent other thromboembolic disorders. Dipyridamole may also be given 2 days prior to open heart surgery to prevent platelet activation by extracorporeal bypass pump and as a diagnostic agent in CAD.

Pregnancy Risk Factor C

Contraindications Hypersensitivity to dipyridamole or any component

Warnings/Precautions Safety and effectiveness in children <12 years of age have not been established; may further decrease blood pressure in patients with hypotension due to peripheral vasodilation; use with caution in patients taking other drugs which affect platelet function or coagulation and in patients with hemostatic defects. Since evidence suggests that clinically used doses are ineffective for prevention of platelet aggregation, consideration for low-dose aspirin (81-325 mg/day) alone may be necessary; this will decrease cost as well as inconvenience.

Adverse Reactions
>10%:
Cardiovascular: Exacerbation of angina pectoris
Central nervous system: Dizziness
1% to 10%:
Cardiovascular: Hypotension, hypertension, tachycardia
Central nervous system: Headache
Dermatologic: Rash
Gastrointestinal: Abdominal distress
Respiratory: Dyspnea
<1%:
Cardiovascular: Vasodilation, flushing, syncope, edema
Central nervous system: Migraine
Neuromuscular & skeletal: Weakness, hypertonia
Respiratory: Rhinitis, hyperventilation
(Continued)

Dipyridamole *(Continued)*

Miscellaneous: Allergic reaction, pleural pain

Overdosage/Toxicology Symptoms of overdose include hypotension, peripheral vasodilation; dialysis is not effective; treatment includes fluids and vasopressors although hypotension is often transient

Drug Interactions
Increased toxicity: Heparin → ↑ anticoagulation
Decreased hypotensive effect (I.V.): Theophylline

Stability Do not freeze, protect I.V. preparation from light

Mechanism of Action Inhibits the activity of adenosine deaminase and phosphodiesterase, which causes an accumulation of adenosine, adenine nucleotides, and cyclic AMP; these mediators then inhibit platelet aggregation and may cause vasodilation; may also stimulate release of prostacyclin or PGD_2; causes coronary vasodilation

Pharmacodynamics/Kinetics
Absorption: Readily absorbed from GI tract but variable
Distribution: V_d: 2-3 L/kg in adults
Protein binding: 91% to 99%
Metabolism: Concentrated and metabolized in the liver
Half-life, terminal: 10-12 hours
Time to peak serum concentration: 2-2.5 hours
Elimination: In feces via bile as glucuronide conjugates and unchanged drug

Usual Dosage
Oral:
Children: 3-6 mg/kg/day in 3 divided doses
Doses of 4-10 mg/kg/day have been used investigationally to treat proteinuria in pediatric renal disease
Adults: 75-400 mg/day in 3-4 divided doses
I.V. 0.14 mg/kg/minute for 4 minutes; maximum dose: 60 mg

Patient Information Notify physician or pharmacist if taking other medications that affect bleeding, such as NSAIDs or warfarin

Dosage Forms
Injection: 10 mg/2 mL
Tablet: 25 mg, 50 mg, 75 mg

Disalcid® *see* Salsalate *on page 993*

Disalicylic Acid *see* Salsalate *on page 993*

Discase® *see* Chymopapain *on page 243*

Disodium Cromoglycate *see* Cromolyn Sodium *on page 280*

***d*-Isoephedrine Hydrochloride** *see* Pseudoephedrine *on page 955*

Disonate® [OTC] *see* Docusate *on page 362*

Disopyramide Phosphate *(dye soe peer' a mide)*

Related Information
Antiarrhythmic Drugs *on page 1246-1248*

Brand Names Norpace®

Use Suppression and prevention of unifocal and multifocal premature, ventricular premature complexes, coupled ventricular tachycardia; effective in the conversion of atrial fibrillation, atrial flutter, and paroxysmal atrial tachycardia to normal sinus rhythm and prevention of the reoccurrence of these arrhythmias after conversion by other methods

Pregnancy Risk Factor C

Contraindications Pre-existing second or third degree A-V block, cardiogenic shock, or known hypersensitivity to the drug

Warnings/Precautions Pre-existing urinary retention, family history, or existing angle-closure glaucoma, myasthenia gravis, hypotension during initiation of therapy, congestive heart failure unless caused by an arrhythmia, widening of QRS complex during therapy or Q-T interval (>25% to 50% of baseline QRS complex or Q-T interval), sick-sinus syndrome or WPW, renal or hepatic impairment require decrease in dosage; disopyramide ineffective in hypokalemia and potentially toxic with hyperkalemia. Due to changes in total clearance (decreased) in elderly, monitor closely; the anticholinergic action may be intolerable and require discontinuation.

Adverse Reactions
>10%: Genitourinary: Urinary retention/hesitancy
1% to 10%:
Cardiovascular: Chest pains, congestive heart failure, hypotension
Endocrine & metabolic: Hypokalemia
Gastrointestinal: Stomach pain, bloating, dry mouth

Neuromuscular & skeletal: Muscle weakness

Ocular: Blurred vision

<1%:

Cardiovascular: Syncope and conduction disturbances including A-V block, widening QRS complex and lengthening of Q-T interval

Central nervous system: Fatigue, malaise, nervousness, acute psychosis, depression, dizziness, headache, pain

Dermatologic: Generalized rashes

Endocrine & metabolic: Hypoglycemia, may initiate contractions of pregnant uterus, hyperkalemia may enhance toxicities, increased cholesterol and triglycerides

Gastrointestinal: Constipation, nausea, vomiting, diarrhea, gas, anorexia, weight gain

Hepatic: Hepatic cholestasis, elevated liver enzymes

Neuromuscular & skeletal: Weakness

Respiratory: Dyspnea

Miscellaneous: Dry nose, eyes, and throat

Overdosage/Toxicology Has a low toxic therapeutic ratio and may easily produce fatal intoxication (acute toxic dose: 1 g in adults); symptoms of overdose include sinus bradycardia, sinus node arrest or asystole, P-R, QRS or Q-T interval prolongation, torsade de pointes (polymorphous ventricular tachycardia) and depressed myocardial contractility, which along with alpha-adrenergic or ganglionic blockade, may result in hypotension and pulmonary edema; other effects are anticholinergic (dry mouth, dilated pupils, and delirium) as well as seizures, coma and respiratory arrest.

Treatment is primarily symptomatic and effects usually respond to conventional therapies (fluids, positioning, vasopressors, anticonvulsants, antiarrhythmics). **Note:** Do not use other type Ia or Ic antiarrhythmic agents to treat ventricular tachycardia; sodium bicarbonate may treat wide QRS intervals or hypotension; markedly impaired conduction or high degree A-V block, unresponsive to bicarbonate, indicates consideration of a pacemaker.

Drug Interactions

Decreased effect with hepatic microsomal enzyme-inducing agents (ie, phenytoin, phenobarbital, rifampin)

Increased effect/levels/toxicity with erythromycin; increased levels of digoxin

Mechanism of Action Class IA antiarrhythmic: Decreases myocardial excitability and conduction velocity; reduces disparity in refractory between normal and infarcted myocardium; possesses anticholinergic, peripheral vasoconstrictive, and negative inotropic effects

Pharmacodynamics/Kinetics

Onset of action: 0.5-3.5 hours

Duration of effect: 1.5-8.5 hours

Absorption: 60% to 83%

Protein binding: Concentration dependent, ranges from 20% to 60%

Metabolism: In the liver to inactive metabolites

Half-life: Adults: 4-10 hours, increased half-life with hepatic or renal disease

Elimination: 40% to 60% excreted unchanged in urine and 10% to 15% in feces

Usual Dosage Oral:

Children:

<1 year: 10-30 mg/kg/24 hours in 4 divided doses

1-4 years: 10-20 mg/kg/24 hours in 4 divided doses

4-12 years: 10-15 mg/kg/24 hours in 4 divided doses

12-18 years: 6-15 mg/kg/24 hours in 4 divided doses

Adults:

<50 kg: 100 mg every 6 hours or 200 mg every 12 hours (controlled release)

>50 kg: 150 mg every 6 hours or 300 mg every 12 hours (controlled release); if no response, may increase to 200 mg every 6 hours; maximum dose required for patients with severe refractory ventricular tachycardia is 400 mg every 6 hours

Dosing adjustment in renal impairment: 100 mg (nonsustained release) given at the following intervals: See table.

Creatinine Clearance (mL/min)	Dosage Interval
30-40	q8h
15-30	q12h
<15	q24h

(Continued)

Disopyramide Phosphate *(Continued)*

or alter the dose as follows:
Cl_{cr} 30-<40 mL/minute: Reduce dose 50%
Cl_{cr} 15-30 mL/minute: Reduce dose 75%
Not dialyzable (0% to 5%) by hemo- or peritoneal methods; supplemental dose not necessary

Dosing interval in hepatic impairment: 100 mg every 6 hours or 200 mg every 12 hours (controlled release)
Administration Administer around-the-clock rather than 4 times/day (ie, 12-6-12-6, not 9-1-5-9) to promote less variation in peak and trough serum levels
Monitoring Parameters EKG, blood pressure, disopyramide drug level, urinary retention, CNS anticholinergic effects (confusion, agitation, hallucinations, etc)
Reference Range
Therapeutic concentration:
Atrial arrhythmias: 2.8-3.2 µg/mL
Ventricular arrhythmias 3.3-7.5 µg/mL
Toxic concentration: >7 µg/mL
Patient Information Notify physician if urinary retention or worsening CHF; do not break or chew sustained release capsules
Nursing Implications Do not crush controlled release capsules
Dosage Forms
Capsule: 100 mg, 150 mg
Capsule, sustained action: 100 mg, 150 mg

Disotate® *see* Edetate Disodium *on page 381*

Di-Spaz® *see* Dicyclomine Hydrochloride *on page 330*

Dispos-a-Med® Isoproterenol *see* Isoproterenol *on page 597*

Disulfiram *(dye sul' fi ram)*
Brand Names Antabuse®
Use Management of chronic alcoholism
Pregnancy Risk Factor C
Contraindications Severe myocardial disease and coronary occlusion, hypersensitivity to disulfiram or any component, patient receiving alcohol, paraldehyde, alcohol-containing preparations like cough syrup or tonics
Warnings/Precautions Use with caution in patients with diabetes, hypothyroidism, seizure disorders, hepatic cirrhosis, or insufficiency; should never be administered to a patient when he/she is in a state of alcohol intoxication, or without his/her knowledge
Adverse Reactions
>10%: Central nervous system: Drowsiness
1% to 10%:
Central nervous system: Headache, tiredness, mood changes, neurotoxicity
Dermatologic: Skin rash
Gastrointestinal: Metallic or garlic-like aftertaste
Genitourinary: Impotence
<1%:
Hepatic: Hepatitis, encephalopathy
Disulfiram reaction with alcohol: Flushing, sweating, cardiovascular collapse, myocardial infarction, vertigo, seizures, headache, nausea, vomiting, dyspnea, chest pain, death
Overdosage/Toxicology Management of disulfiram reaction: Institute support measures to restore blood pressure (pressors and fluids); monitor for hypokalemia
Drug Interactions
Increased effect: Diazepam, chlordiazepoxide
Increased toxicity:
Alcohol and disulfiram: Antabuse® reaction
Tricyclic antidepressants, metronidazole, isoniazid: Encephalopathy
Phenytoin → ↑ serum levels and toxicity
Warfarin → ↑ prothrombin time
Mechanism of Action Disulfiram is a thiuram derivative which interferes with aldehyde dehydrogenase. When taken concomitantly with alcohol, there is an increase in serum acetaldehyde levels. High acetaldehyde causes uncomfortable symptoms including flushing, nausea, thirst, palpitations, chest pain, vertigo, and hypotension. This reaction is the basis for disulfiram use in postwithdrawal long-term care of alcoholism.
Pharmacodynamics/Kinetics
Absorption: Rapid from GI tract
Full effect: 12 hours

Metabolism: To diethylthiocarbamate

Duration: May persist for 1-2 weeks after last dose

Usual Dosage Adults: Oral: Do not administer until the patient has abstained from alcohol for at least 12 hours

Initial: 500 mg/day as a single dose for 1-2 weeks; maximum daily dose is 500 mg

Average maintenance dose: 250 mg/day; range: 125-500 mg; duration of therapy is to continue until the patient is fully recovered socially and a basis for permanent self control has been established; maintenance therapy may be required for months or even years

Patient Information Do not drink any alcohol, including products containing alcohol (cough and cold syrups), or use alcohol-containing skin products for at least 3 days and preferably 14 days after stopping this medication or while taking this medication; not for treatment of alcohol intoxication; may cause drowsiness; tablets can be crushed or mixed with water

Nursing Implications Administration of any medications containing alcohol including topicals is contraindicated

Dosage Forms Tablet: 250 mg, 500 mg

Dithioglycerol see Dimercaprol on page 349

Ditropan® see Oxybutynin Chloride on page 825

Diucardin® see Hydroflumethiazide on page 549

Diuretics, Loop Comparison see page 1269

Diurigen® see Chlorothiazide on page 227

Diuril® see Chlorothiazide on page 227

Divalproex Sodium see Valproic Acid and Derivatives on page 1143

Dizmiss® [OTC] see Meclizine Hydrochloride on page 674

dl-Alpha Tocopherol see Vitamin E on page 1164

dl-Norephedrine Hydrochloride see Phenylpropanolamine Hydrochloride on page 876

D-Mannitol see Mannitol on page 664

DNase see Dornase Alfa on page 365

DNR see Daunorubicin Hydrochloride on page 304

Dobutamine Hydrochloride (doe byoo' ta meen)

Related Information

Adrenergic Agonists, Cardiovascular Comparison on page 1242

Extravasation Treatment of Other Drugs on page 1209

Brand Names Dobutrex®

Use Short-term management of patients with cardiac decompensation

Pregnancy Risk Factor C

Contraindications Hypersensitivity to sulfites (commercial preparation contains sodium bisulfite); patients with idiopathic hypertrophic subaortic stenosis, atrial fibrillation or atrial flutter

Warnings/Precautions Hypovolemia should be corrected prior to use; infiltration causes local inflammatory changes, extravasation may cause dermal necrosis; use with extreme caution following myocardial infarction; potent drug, must be diluted prior to use

Adverse Reactions

>10%: Cardiovascular: Ectopic heartbeats, increased heart rate, chest pain, angina, palpitations, elevation in blood pressure; in higher doses ventricular tachycardia or arrhythmias may be seen; patients with atrial fibrillation or flutter are at risk of developing a rapid ventricular response

1% to 10%:

Cardiovascular: Premature ventricular beats, chest pain, angina, palpitations, shortness of breath

Central nervous system: Tingling sensation, headache

Gastrointestinal: Nausea, vomiting

Neuromuscular & skeletal: Mild leg cramps, paresthesia

Respiratory: Dyspnea

Overdosage/Toxicology Symptoms of overdose include fatigue, nervousness, tachycardia, hypertension, arrhythmias; reduce rate of administration or discontinue infusion until condition stabilizes

Drug Interactions

Decreased effect: Beta-adrenergic blockers (increased peripheral resistance)

Increased toxicity: General anesthetics (ie, halothane or cyclopropane) and usual doses of dobutamine have resulted in ventricular arrhythmias in animals

(Continued)

Dobutamine Hydrochloride *(Continued)*

Stability Remix solution every 24 hours; store reconstituted solution under refrigeration for 48 hours or 6 hours at room temperature; pink discoloration of solution indicates slight oxidation but **no** significant loss of potency.

Stability of parenteral admixture at room temperature (25°C): 48 hours; at refrigeration (4°C): 7 days

Standard adult diluent: 250 mg/500 mL D_5W; 500 mg/500 mL D_5W

Incompatible with heparin, sodium bicarbonate, cefazolin, penicillin; incompatible in alkaline solutions (sodium bicarbonate)

Compatible with dopamine, epinephrine, isoproterenol, lidocaine

Mechanism of Action Stimulates beta$_1$-adrenergic receptors, causing increased contractility and heart rate, with little effect on beta$_2$- or alpha-receptors

Pharmacodynamics/Kinetics

Onset of action: I.V.: 1-10 minutes

Peak effect: Within 10-20 minutes

Metabolism: In tissues and the liver to inactive metabolites

Half-life: 2 minutes

Elimination: Metabolites are excreted in urine

Usual Dosage I.V. infusion:

Neonates and Children: 2.5-15 mcg/kg/minute, titrate to desired response

Adults: 2.5-15 mcg/kg/minute; maximum: 40 mcg/kg/minute, titrate to desired response

Infusion Rates of Various Dilutions of Dobutamine

Desired Delivery Rate (mcg/kg/min)	Infusion Rate (mL/kg/min)	
	500 mcg/mL*	1000 mcg/mL†
2.5	0.005	0.0025
5.0	0.01	0.005
7.5	0.015	0.0075
10.0	0.02	0.01
12.5	0.025	0.0125
15.0	0.03	0.015

* 500 mg per liter or 250 mg per 500 mL of diluent.

†1000 mg per liter or 250 mg per 250 mL of diluent.

Administration Use infusion device to control rate of flow; administer into large vein

To prepare for infusion:

$$\frac{6 \times weight\ (kg) \times desired\ dose\ (mcg/kg/min)}{I.V.\ infusion\ rate\ (mL/h)} = \frac{mg\ of\ drug\ to\ be\ added\ to}{100\ mL\ of\ I.V.\ fluid}$$

Do not give through same I.V. line as heparin, hydrocortisone sodium succinate, cefazolin, or penicillin

Monitoring Parameters Blood pressure, EKG, heart rate, CVP, RAP, MAP, urine output; if pulmonary artery catheter is in place, monitor CI, PCWP, and SVR; also monitor serum glucose

Patient Information May affect serum assay of chloramphenicol

Nursing Implications Management of extravasation: Phentolamine: Mix 5 mg with 9 mL of NS; inject a small amount of this dilution into extravasation area; blanching should reverse immediately. Monitor site; if blanching should recur, additional injections of phentolamine may be needed.

Dosage Forms Injection: 250 mg (20 mL)

Dobutrex® *see* Dobutamine Hydrochloride *on previous page*

Docusate *(dok' yoo sate)*

Related Information

Laxatives, Classification and Properties *on page 1272*

Brand Names Colace® [OTC]; DC 240® Softgels® [OTC]; Dialose® [OTC]; Diocto® [OTC]; Diocto-K® [OTC]; Dioeze® [OTC]; Disonate® [OTC]; DOK® [OTC]; DOS® Softgel® [OTC]; Doxinate® [OTC]; D-S-S® [OTC]; Kasof® [OTC]; Modane® Soft [OTC]; Pro-Cal-Sof® [OTC]; Pro-Sof® [OTC]; Regulax SS® [OTC]; Regutol® [OTC]; Sulfalax® [OTC]; Surfak® [OTC]

Synonyms Dioctyl Calcium Sulfosuccinate; Dioctyl Sodium Sulfosuccinate; DOSS; DSS

Use Stool softener in patients who should avoid straining during defecation and constipation associated with hard, dry stools; prophylaxis for straining (valsalva) following myocardial infarction. A safe agent to be used in elderly; some evidence that doses <200 mg are ineffective; stool softeners are unnecessary if stool is well hydrated or "mushy" and soft; shown to be ineffective used long-term.

Pregnancy Risk Factor C

Contraindications Concomitant use of mineral oil; intestinal obstruction, acute abdominal pain, nausea, vomiting; hypersensitivity to docusate or any component

Warnings/Precautions Prolonged, frequent or excessive use may result in dependence or electrolyte imbalance

Adverse Reactions
1% to 10%:
Gastrointestinal: Intestinal obstruction, diarrhea, abdominal cramping
Miscellaneous: Throat irritation

Overdosage/Toxicology Symptoms of overdose include abdominal cramps, diarrhea, fluid loss, hypokalemia; treatment is symptomatic

Drug Interactions
Decreased effect of Coumadin®, aspirin
Increased toxicity with mineral oil, phenolphthalein

Mechanism of Action Reduces surface tension of the oil-water interface of the stool resulting in enhanced incorporation of water and fat allowing for stool softening

Pharmacodynamics/Kinetics Onset of action: 12-72 hours

Usual Dosage Docusate salts are interchangeable; the amount of sodium, calcium, or potassium per dosage unit is clinically insignificant

Infants and Children <3 years: Oral: 10-40 mg/day in 1-4 divided doses
Children: Oral:
3-6 years: 20-60 mg/day in 1-4 divided doses
6-12 years: 40-150 mg/day in 1-4 divided doses
Adolescents and Adults: Oral: 50-500 mg/day in 1-4 divided doses
Older Children and Adults: Rectal: Add 50-100 mg of docusate liquid to enema fluid (saline or water); give as retention or flushing enema

Test Interactions ↓ potassium (S), ↓ chloride (S)

Patient Information Adults: Docusate should be taken with a full glass of water; do not use if abdominal pain, nausea, or vomiting are present; laxative use should be used for a short period of time (<1 week); prolonged use may result in abuse, dependence, as well as fluid and electrolyte loss; notify physician if bleeding occurs or if constipation is not relieved

Nursing Implications Docusate liquid should be given with milk, fruit juice, or infant formula to mask the bitter taste

Dosage Forms
Capsule, as calcium:
DC 240® Softgels®, Pro-Cal-Sof®, Sulfalax®: 240 mg
Surfak®: 50 mg, 240 mg
Capsule, as potassium:
Dialose®, Diocto-K®: 100 mg
Kasof®: 240 mg
Capsule, as sodium:
Colace®: 50 mg, 100 mg
Dioeze®: 250 mg
Disonate®: 100 mg, 240 mg
DOK®: 100 mg, 250 mg
DOS® Softgel®: 100 mg, 250 mg
Doxinate®: 250 mg
D-S-S®: 100 mg
Modane® Soft: 100 mg
Pro-Sof®: 100 mg, 250 mg
Regulax SS®: 100 mg, 250 mg
Liquid, as sodium (Diocto®, Colace®, Disonate®, DOK®): 150 mg/15 mL (30 mL, 60 mL, 480 mL)
Solution, oral, as sodium (Doxinate®): 50 mg/mL with alcohol 5% (60 mL, 3780 mL)
Syrup, as sodium:
50 mg/15 mL (15 mL, 30 mL)
Colace®, Diocto®, Disonate®, DOK®, Pro-Sof®: 60 mg/15 mL (240 mL, 480 mL, 3780 mL)
Tablet, as sodium (Regutol®): 100 mg

DOK® [OTC] *see Docusate on previous page*

Doktors® Nasal Solution [OTC] *see* Phenylephrine Hydrochloride *on page 874*

Dolacet® *see* Hydrocodone and Acetaminophen *on page 543*

Dolene® *see* Propoxyphene *on page 946*

Dolobid® *see* Diflunisal *on page 336*

Dolophine® *see* Methadone Hydrochloride *on page 703*

Dome Paste Bandage *see* Zinc Gelatin *on page 1175*

Donnamor® *see* Hyoscyamine, Atropine, Scopolamine, and Phenobarbital *on page 557*

Donnapine® *see* Hyoscyamine, Atropine, Scopolamine, and Phenobarbital *on page 557*

Donna-Sed® *see* Hyoscyamine, Atropine, Scopolamine, and Phenobarbital *on page 557*

Donnatal® *see* Hyoscyamine, Atropine, Scopolamine, and Phenobarbital *on page 557*

Donphen® *see* Hyoscyamine, Atropine, Scopolamine, and Phenobarbital *on page 557*

Dopamine Hydrochloride (doe' pa meen)

Related Information

Adrenergic Agonists, Cardiovascular Comparison *on page 1242*
Extravasation Treatment of Other Drugs *on page 1209*

Brand Names Dopastat®; Intropin®

Use Adjunct in the treatment of shock which persists after adequate fluid volume replacement

Pregnancy Risk Factor C

Contraindications Hypersensitivity to sulfites (commercial preparation contains sodium bisulfite); pheochromocytoma or ventricular fibrillation

Warnings/Precautions Safety in children has not been established; hypovolemia should be corrected by appropriate plasma volume expanders before administration; extravasation may cause tissue necrosis; potent drug, must be diluted prior to use; patient's hemodynamic status should be monitored; use with caution in patients with cardiovascular disease or cardiac arrhythmias or patients with occlusive vascular disease

Adverse Reactions

>10%:
  Cardiovascular: Ectopic heartbeats, tachycardia, vasoconstriction, hypotension, cardiac conduction abnormalities, widened QRS complex, ventricular arrhythmias
  Central nervous system: Headache
  Gastrointestinal: Nausea, vomiting
  Respiratory: Dyspnea
1% to 10%: Cardiovascular: Bradycardia, hypertension, gangrene of the extremities
<1%:
  Cardiovascular: Vasoconstriction
  Central nervous system: Anxiety
  Genitourinary: Decreased urine output, azotemia
  Neuromuscular & skeletal: Piloerection

Overdosage/Toxicology Symptoms of overdose include severe hypertension, cardiac arrhythmias, acute renal failure. **Important:** Antidote for peripheral ischemia: To prevent sloughing and necrosis in ischemic areas, the area should be infiltrated as soon as possible with 10-15 mL of saline solution containing from 5-10 mg of Regitine® (brand of phentolamine), an adrenergic blocking agent. A syringe with a fine hypodermic needle should be used, and the solution liberally infiltrated throughout the ischemic area. Sympathetic blockade with phentolamine causes immediate and conspicuous local hyperemic changes if the area is infiltrated within 12 hours. Therefore, phentolamine should be given as soon as possible after the extravasation is noted.

Drug Interactions Increased effect: Dopamine's effects are prolonged and intensified by MAO inhibitors, alpha- and beta-adrenergic blockers, general anesthetics, phenytoin

Stability Protect from light; solutions that are darker than slightly yellow should not be used; **incompatible** with alkaline solutions or iron salts; **compatible** when coadministered with dobutamine, epinephrine, isoproterenol, and lidocaine

Mechanism of Action Stimulates both adrenergic and dopaminergic receptors, lower doses are mainly dopaminergic stimulating and produce renal and mesenteric vasodilation, higher doses also are both dopaminergic and beta$_1$-adrenergic stimulating and produce cardiac stimulation and renal vasodilation; large doses stimulate alpha-adrenergic receptors

Pharmacodynamics/Kinetics

Children: With medication changes, may not achieve steady-state for ~1 hour rather than 20 minutes

Adults:

Onset of action: 5 minutes

Duration: <10 minutes

Metabolism: In the plasma, kidneys, and liver 75% to inactive metabolites by monoamine oxidase and 25% to norepinephrine (active)

Half-life: 2 minutes

Elimination: Metabolites are excreted in urine; neonatal clearance varies and appears to be age related; clearance is more prolonged with combined hepatic and renal dysfunction

Dopamine has exhibited nonlinear kinetics in children

Usual Dosage I.V. infusion:

Neonates: 1-20 mcg/kg/minute continuous infusion, titrate to desired response

Children: 1-20 mcg/kg/minute, maximum: 50 mcg/kg/minute continuous infusion, titrate to desired response

Adults: 1-5 mcg/kg/minute up to 50 mcg/kg/minute, titrate to desired response; infusion may be increased by 1-4 mcg/kg/minute at 10- to 30-minute intervals until optimal response is obtained

If dosages >20-30 mcg/kg/minute are needed, a more direct-acting pressor may be more beneficial (ie, epinephrine, norepinephrine)

The hemodynamic effects of dopamine are dose-dependent:

Low-dose: 1-5 mcg/kg/minute, increased renal blood flow and urine output

Intermediate-dose: 5-15 mcg/kg/minute, increased renal blood flow, heart rate, cardiac contractility, and cardiac output

High-dose: >15 mcg/kg/minute, alpha-adrenergic effects begin to predominate, vasoconstriction, increased blood pressure

Administration

To prepare for infusion:

$$\frac{6 \times weight\ (kg) \times desired\ dose\ (mcg/kg/min)}{I.V.\ infusion\ rate\ (mL/h)} = \frac{mg\ of\ drug\ to\ be\ added\ to}{100\ mL\ of\ I.V.\ fluid}$$

Administer into large vein to prevent the possibility of extravasation; monitor continuously for free flow; use infusion device to control rate of flow; administration into an umbilical arterial catheter is not recommended; central line administration

Monitoring Parameters Blood pressure, EKG, heart rate, CVP, RAP, MAP, urine output; if pulmonary artery catheter is in place, monitor CI, PCWP, SVR, and PVR

Nursing Implications Extravasation: Due to short half-life, withdrawal of drug is often only necessary treatment Use phentolamine as antidote; mix 5 mg with 9 mL of NS; inject a small amount of this dilution into extravasated area; blanching should reverse immediately. Monitor site; if blanching should recur, additional injections of phentolamine may be needed.

Dosage Forms

Infusion, in D₅W: 0.8 mg/mL (250 mL, 500 mL); 1.6 mg/mL (250 mL, 500 mL); 3.2 mg/mL (250 mL, 500 mL)

Injection: 40 mg/mL (5 mL, 10 mL, 20 mL); 80 mg/mL (5 mL, 20 mL); 160 mg/mL (5 mL)

Dopar® see Levodopa on page 624

Dopastat® see Dopamine Hydrochloride on previous page

Dopram® see Doxapram Hydrochloride on page 367

Doral® see Quazepam on page 963

Dorcol® [OTC] see Acetaminophen on page 17

Dornase Alfa (door' nace al' fa)

Brand Names Pulmozyme®

Synonyms DNase; Recombinant Human Deoxyribonuclease

Use Management of cystic fibrosis patients to reduce the frequency of respiratory infections that require parenteral antibiotics, and to improve pulmonary function

Pregnancy Risk Factor B

(Continued)

Dornase Alfa *(Continued)*

Contraindications Contraindicated in patients with known hypersensitivity to dornase alfa, Chinese hamster ovary cell products (eg, epoetin alfa), or any component

Warnings/Precautions No clinical trials have been conducted to demonstrate safety and effectiveness of dornase in children <5 years of age, in patients with pulmonary function <40% of normal, or in patients for longer treatment periods >12 months; no data exists regarding safety during lactation

Adverse Reactions
>10%: Voice alteration, pharyngitis
1% to 10%:
Cardiovascular: Chest pain
Dermatologic: Rash
Ocular: Conjunctivitis
Respiratory: Laryngitis, cough, dyspnea, hemoptysis, rhinitis, hoarse throat, wheezing

Stability Most be stored in the refrigerator at 2°C to 8°C (36°F to 46°F) and protected from strong light; should not be exposed to room temperature for a total of 24 hours

Mechanism of Action The hallmark of cystic fibrosis lung disease is the presence of abundant, purulent airway secretions composed primarily of highly polymerized DNA. The principal source of this DNA is the nuclei of degenerating neutrophils, which is present in large concentrations in infected lung secretions. The presence of this DNA produces a viscous mucous that may contribute to the decreased mucocilliary transport and persistent infections that are commonly seen in this population. Dornase alfa is a deoxyribonuclease (DNA) enzyme produced by recombinant gene technology. Dornase selectively cleaves DNA, thus reducing mucous viscosity and as a result, airflow in the lung is improved and the risk of bacterial infection may be decreased.

Pharmacodynamics/Kinetics Following nebulization, enzyme levels are measurable in the sputum within 15 minutes and decline rapidly thereafter

Usual Dosage Children >5 years and Adults: Inhalation: 2.5 mg once daily through selected nebulizers in conjunction with a Pulmo-Aide® or a Pari-Proneb® compressor

Nursing Implications Should not be diluted or mixed with any other drugs in the nebulizer, this may inactivate the drug

Dosage Forms Solution, inhalation: 1 mg/mL (2.5 mL)

Doryx® *see Doxycycline on page 373*

DOS® Softgel® [OTC] *see Docusate on page 362*

DOSS *see Docusate on page 362*

Dovonex® *see Calcipotriene on page 157*

Doxacurium Chloride *(dox a kyoo' rium)*

Related Information
Neuromuscular Blocking Agents Comparison Charts *on page 1276-1278*

Brand Names Nuromax® Injection

Use Adjunct to general anesthesia; provides skeletal muscle relaxation during surgery. Doxacurium is a long-acting nondepolarizing neuromuscular blocker with virtually no cardiovascular side effects. The characteristics of this agent make it especially useful in procedures requiring careful maintenance of hemodynamic stability for prolonged periods.

Pregnancy Risk Factor C

Contraindications Hypersensitivity to doxacurium or any component

Warnings/Precautions Use with caution in the elderly, effects and duration are more variable; product contains benzoyl alcohol; use with caution in newborns; use with caution in patients with neuromuscular diseases such as myasthenia gravis; resistance may develop in burn patients; ensure proper electrolyte balance prior to use; use with caution in patients with renal or hepatic impairment

Adverse Reactions
<1%:
Cardiovascular: Hypotension
Central nervous system: Fever
Dermatologic: Urticaria
Neuromuscular & skeletal: Skeletal muscle weakness
Ocular: Double vision
Respiratory: Respiratory insufficiency and apnea, wheezing
Miscellaneous: **Produces little, if any, histamine release**

Overdosage/Toxicology Overdosage is manifested by prolonged neuromuscular blockage; treatment is supportive; reverse blockade with neostigmine, pyridostigmine, or edrophonium

Drug Interactions
Decreased effect: Phenytoin, carbamazepine ($\downarrow$ neuromuscular blockade)
Increased effect: Magnesium, lithium
Prolonged neuromuscular blockade:
  Corticosteroids
  Inhaled anesthetics
  Local anesthetics
  Calcium channel blockers
  Antiarrhythmics (eg, quinidine or procainamide)
  Antibiotics (eg, aminoglycosides, tetracyclines, vancomycin, clindamycin)
  Immunosuppressants (eg, cyclosporine)

Mechanism of Action Doxacurium is a long-acting nondepolarizing skeletal muscle relaxant. The drug is a bis-quaternary benzylisoquinolinium diester, with a chemical structure similar to that of atracurium. Similar to other nondepolarizing neuromuscular blocking agents, doxacurium produces muscle relaxation by competing with acetylcholine for cholinergic receptor sites on the postjunctional membrane; significant presynaptic depressant activity is also observed.

Pharmacodynamics/Kinetics
Onset of effect: 5-11 minutes
Duration: 30 minutes (range: 12-54 minutes)
Protein binding: 30%
Elimination: Primarily as unchanged drug via the kidneys and biliary tract
Recovery time is longer in elderly patients

Usual Dosage I.V. (in obese patients, use ideal body weight to calculate dose):
Children >2 years: Initial: 0.03-0.05 mg/kg followed by maintenance doses of 0.005-0.01 mg/kg after 30-45 minutes

Adults: Surgery: 0.05 mg/kg with thiopental/narcotic or 0.025 mg/kg with succinylcholine; maintenance doses of 0.005-0.01 mg/kg after 60-100 minutes

Dosing adjustment in renal or hepatic impairment: Reduce initial dose and titrate carefully as duration may be prolonged

Monitoring Parameters Blockade is monitored with a peripheral nerve stimulator, should also evaluate EKG, blood pressure, and heart rate

Dosage Forms Injection: 1 mg/mL (5 mL)

Doxapram Hydrochloride (dox' a pram)

Brand Names Dopram®

Use Respiratory and CNS stimulant; stimulates respiration in patients with drug-induced CNS depression or postanesthesia respiratory depression; in hospitalized patients with COPD associated with acute hypercapnia

Pregnancy Risk Factor B

Contraindications Hypersensitivity to doxapram or any component; epilepsy, cerebral edema, head injury, severe pulmonary disease, pheochromocytoma, cardiovascular disease, hypertension, hyperthyroidism

Warnings/Precautions Safety of doxapram in children <12 years of age has not been established; may cause severe CNS toxicity, seizures; should be used with caution in newborns as the U.S. product contains benzyl alcohol (0.9%); recommended doses of doxapram for neonates will deliver 5.4-27 mg/kg/day of benzyl alcohol; large amounts of benzyl alcohol (>100 mg/kg/day) have been associated with fatal toxicity (gasping syndrome); the use of doxapram in newborns should be reserved for neonates who are unresponsive to the treatment of apnea with therapeutic serum concentrations of theophylline or caffeine. Doxapram is neither a nonspecific CNS depressant antagonist nor an opiate antagonist.

Adverse Reactions
1% to 10%:
  Cardiovascular: Ectopic beats, hypotension, vasoconstriction, tachycardia, anginal pain, palpitations
  Central nervous system: Headache
  Gastrointestinal: Nausea, vomiting
  Respiratory: Dyspnea
<1%:
  Cardiovascular: Hypertension (dose related), arrhythmias, flushing, feeling of warmth
  Central nervous system: CNS stimulation, restlessness, lightheadedness, jitters, hallucinations, irritability, seizures, headache, hyperpyrexia
  Gastrointestinal: Abdominal distension, retching
  Hematologic: Hemolysis
  Local: Phlebitis
(Continued)

Doxapram Hydrochloride *(Continued)*

Neuromuscular & skeletal: Tremor, hyperreflexia
Ocular: Mydriasis, lacrimation
Respiratory: Coughing, laryngospasm
Miscellaneous: Sweating

Overdosage/Toxicology Symptoms of overdose include excessive increases in blood pressure, tachycardia, arrhythmias, muscle spasticity, dyspnea. Supportive care is the preferred treatment; seizures are unlikely and can be treated with benzodiazepines; **doxapram is not dialyzable.**

Drug Interactions Increased toxicity (elevated blood pressure): Sympathomimetics, MAO inhibitors

Halothane, cyclopropane, and enflurane may sensitize the myocardium to catecholamine and epinephrine which is released at the initiation of doxapram, hence, separate discontinuation of anesthetics and start of doxapram by at least 10 minutes

Stability Incompatible with aminophylline, thiopental, or sodium bicarbonate (alkali drugs)

Mechanism of Action Stimulates respiration through action on respiratory center in medulla or indirectly on peripheral carotid chemoreceptors

Pharmacodynamics/Kinetics

Onset of action (respiratory stimulation): I.V.: Within 20-40 seconds
Peak effect: Within 1-2 minutes
Duration: 5-12 minutes
Metabolism: In the liver
Half-life:
  Neonates, premature: ~7-10 hours
  Adults: 3.4 hours (mean half-life)
Elimination: In urine as metabolites within 24-48 hours

Usual Dosage Not for use in newborns since doxapram contains a significant amount of benzyl alcohol (0.9%)

Neonatal apnea (apnea of prematurity): I.V.:
  Initial: 1-1.5 mg/kg/hour
  Maintenance: 0.5-2.5 mg/kg/hour, titrated to the lowest rate at which apnea is controlled

Adults: Respiratory depression following anesthesia: I.V.:
  Initial: 0.5-1 mg/kg; may repeat at 5-minute intervals; maximum total dose: 2 mg/kg
  I.V. infusion: Initial: 5 mg/minute until adequate response or adverse effects seen; decrease to 1-3 mg/minute; usual total dose: 0.5-4 mg/kg; maximum: 300 mg

Not dialyzable

Administration Dilute to 1 mg/mL in D_5W or NS for continuous infusion

Monitoring Parameters Heart rate, blood pressure, reflexes, CNS status, apnea episodes

Nursing Implications Avoid extravasation, rapid infusion may cause hemolysis; not for use in newborns since doxapram injection contains significant amount of benzyl alcohol (0.9%)

Dosage Forms Injection: 20 mg/mL (20 mL)

Doxazosin (dox ay' zoe sin)

Brand Names Cardura®

Use Treatment of hypertension, severe congestive heart failure (in conjunction with diuretics and cardiac glycosides)

Unlabeled use: Symptoms of benign prostatic hypertrophy

Pregnancy Risk Factor B

Contraindications Hypersensitivity to doxazosin or any component

Warnings/Precautions Use with caution in patients with renal impairment. Can cause marked hypotension and syncope with sudden loss of consciousness with the first dose. Anticipate a similar effect if therapy is interrupted for a few days, if dosage is increased rapidly, or if another antihypertensive drug is introduced.

Adverse Reactions

>10%: Central nervous system: Dizziness
1% to 10%:
  Cardiovascular: Palpitations, arrhythmia
  Central nervous system: Vertigo, nervousness, somnolence, anxiety
  Endocrine & metabolic: Decreased libido
  Gastrointestinal: Nausea, vomiting, dry mouth, diarrhea, constipation
  Neuromuscular & skeletal: Shoulder, neck, back pain

Ocular: Abnormal vision
Respiratory: Rhinitis
<1%:
Cardiovascular: Hypotension, tachycardia
Central nervous system: Depression
Gastrointestinal: Abdominal discomfort, flatulence
Genitourinary: Incontinence
Ocular: Conjunctivitis
Otic: Tinnitus
Renal: Polyuria
Respiratory: Dyspnea, sinusitis
Miscellaneous: Epistaxis

Overdosage/Toxicology Symptoms of overdose include severe hypotension, drowsiness, tachycardia. Hypotension usually responds to I.V. fluids, Trendelenburg positioning, or parenteral vasoconstrictor; treatment is primarily supportive and symptomatic.

Drug Interactions
Decreased effect with NSAIDs
Increased effect with diuretics and antihypertensive medications (especially beta-blockers)

Mechanism of Action Competitively inhibits postsynaptic alpha-adrenergic receptors which results in vasodilation of veins and arterioles and a decrease in total peripheral resistance and blood pressure; approximately 50% as potent on a weight by weight basis as prazosin

Usual Dosage Oral:
Adults: 1 mg once daily, may be increased to 2 mg once daily thereafter up to 16 mg if needed
Elderly: Initial: 0.5 mg once daily

Monitoring Parameters Blood pressure, standing and sitting/supine

Test Interactions Increased urinary VMA 17%, norepinephrine metabolite 42%

Patient Information Rise from sitting/lying position carefully; may cause dizziness; report to physician if painful persistent erection occurs; take the first dose at bedtime

Nursing Implications Syncope may occur usually within 90 minutes of the initial dose

Dosage Forms Tablet: 1 mg, 2 mg, 4 mg, 8 mg

Doxepin Hydrochloride (dox' e pin)

Related Information
Antidepressant Agents Comparison on page 1250-1252

Brand Names Adapin®; Sinequan®

Use Treatment of various forms of depression, usually in conjunction with psychotherapy; treatment of anxiety disorders; analgesic for certain chronic and neuropathic pain

Pregnancy Risk Factor C

Contraindications Hypersensitivity to doxepin or any component (cross-sensitivity with other tricyclic antidepressants may occur); narrow-angle glaucoma

Warnings/Precautions Use with caution in patients with cardiovascular disease, conduction disturbances, seizure disorders, urinary retention, hyperthyroidism, or those receiving thyroid replacement; avoid use during lactation; use with caution in pregnancy; do not discontinue abruptly in patients receiving chronic high-dose therapy

Adverse Reactions
>10%:
Central nervous system: Sedation, drowsiness, dizziness, headache
Gastrointestinal: Dry mouth, constipation, increased appetite, nausea, weakness, unpleasant taste, weight gain
1% to 10%:
Cardiovascular: Hypotension, arrhythmias
Central nervous system: Confusion, delirium, hallucinations, nervousness, restlessness, parkinsonian syndrome, insomnia
Gastrointestinal: Difficult urination, diarrhea, heartburn
Genitourinary: Sexual function impairment
Neuromuscular & skeletal: Fine muscle tremors
Ocular: Blurred vision, eye pain
Miscellaneous: Excessive sweating
<1%:
Central nervous system: Anxiety, seizures
Dermatologic: Alopecia, dermal photosensitivity
Endocrine & metabolic: Breast enlargement, galactorrhea
Genitourinary: Urinary retention, testicular swelling, SIADH
Hematologic: Agranulocytosis, leukopenia, eosinophilia
(Continued)

Doxepin Hydrochloride *(Continued)*

 Hepatic: Hepatitis, cholestatic jaundice and increased liver enzymes

 Ocular: Increased intraocular pressure, photosensitivity

 Otic: Tinnitus

 Miscellaneous: Trouble with gums, decreased lower esophageal sphincter tone may cause GE reflux, allergic reactions

Overdosage/Toxicology Symptoms of overdose include confusion, hallucinations, seizures, urinary retention, hypothermia, hypotension, tachycardia, cyanosis

Following initiation of essential overdose management, toxic symptoms should be treated. Ventricular arrhythmias often respond to systemic alkalinization with or without phenytoin 15-20 mg/kg (adults) (sodium bicarbonate 0.5-2 mEq/kg I.V.). Arrhythmias unresponsive to this therapy may respond to lidocaine 1 mg/kg I.V. followed by a titrated infusion. Physostigmine (1-2 mg I.V. slowly for adults or 0.5 mg I.V. slowly for children) may be indicated in reversing cardiac arrhythmias that are life-threatening. Seizures usually respond to diazepam I.V. boluses (5-10 mg for adults up to 30 mg or 0.25-0.4 mg/kg/dose for children up to 10 mg/dose). If seizures are unresponsive or recur, phenytoin or phenobarbital may be required.

Drug Interactions

 Decreased effect of bretylium, guanethidine, clonidine, levodopa; decreased effect with ascorbic acid, cholestyramine

 Increased effect/toxicity of carbamazepine, amphetamines, thyroid preparations, sympathomimetics

 Increased toxicity with fluoxetine (seizures), thyroid preparations, MAO inhibitors, albuterol, CNS depressants (ie, benzodiazepines, opiate analgesics, phenothiazines, alcohol), anticholinergics, cimetidine

Stability Protect from light

Mechanism of Action Increases the synaptic concentration of serotonin and/or norepinephrine in the central nervous system by inhibition of their reuptake by the presynaptic neuronal membrane

Pharmacodynamics/Kinetics

 Peak effect (antidepressant): Usually more than 2 weeks; anxiolytic effects may occur sooner

 Distribution: Crosses the placenta; appears in breast milk

 Protein binding: 80% to 85%

 Metabolism: Hepatic; metabolites include desmethyldoxepin (active)

 Half-life: Adults: 6-8 hours

 Elimination: Renal

Usual Dosage Oral (entire daily dose may be given at bedtime):

 Adolescents: Initial: 25-50 mg/day in single or divided doses; gradually increase to 100 mg/day

 Adults: Initial: 30-150 mg/day at bedtime or in 2-3 divided doses; may gradually increase up to 300 mg/day; single dose should not exceed 150 mg; select patients may respond to 25-50 mg/day

 Dosing adjustment in hepatic impairment: Use a lower dose and adjust gradually

Monitoring Parameters Monitor blood pressure and pulse rate prior to and during initial therapy; monitor mental status, weight

Reference Range Therapeutic: 30-150 ng/mL; Toxic: >500 ng/mL; utility of serum level monitoring is controversial

Test Interactions ↑ glucose

Patient Information Avoid unnecessary exposure to sunlight; avoid alcohol ingestion; do not discontinue medication abruptly; may cause urine to turn blue-green; may cause drowsiness; can use sugarless gum or hard candy for dry mouth; full effect may not occur for 4-6 weeks

Nursing Implications May increase appetite; may cause drowsiness, raise bed rails, institute safety precautions

Dosage Forms

 Capsule: 10 mg, 25 mg, 50 mg, 75 mg, 100 mg, 150 mg

 Concentrate, oral: 10 mg/mL (120 mL)

Doxinate® [OTC] *see* Docusate *on page 362*

Doxorubicin Hydrochloride *(dox oh roo′ bi sin)*

Related Information

 Antiemetics for Chemotherapy Induced Nausea and Vomiting *on page 1202*

 Cancer Chemotherapy Regimens *on page 1218-1241*

 Extravasation Management of Chemotherapeutic Agents *on page 1207-1208*

Brand Names Adriamycin PFS™; Adriamycin RDF™; Rubex®

Synonyms ADR; Hydroxydaunomycin Hydrochloride

Use Treatment of leukemias, lymphomas, multiple myeloma, osseous and nonosseous sarcomas, mesotheliomas, germ cell tumors of the ovary or testis, and carcinomas of the head and neck, thyroid, lung, breast, stomach, pancreas, liver, ovary, bladder, prostate, and uterus, neuroblastoma, osteosarcoma

Pregnancy Risk Factor D

Contraindications Hypersensitivity to doxorubicin or any component, severe congestive heart failure, cardiomyopathy, pre-existing myelosuppression, patients with impaired cardiac function, patients who received previous treatment with complete cumulative doses of doxorubicin and/or daunorubicin

Warnings/Precautions The U.S. Food and Drug Administration (FDA) currently recommends that procedures for proper handling and disposal of antineoplastic agents be considered. Total dose should not exceed 550 mg/m^2 or 400 mg/m^2 in patients with previous or concomitant treatment (with daunorubicin, cyclophosphamide, or irradiation of the cardiac region); irreversible myocardial toxicity may occur as total dosage approaches 550 mg/m^2. I.V. use only, severe local tissue necrosis will result if extravasation occurs; reduce dose in patients with impaired hepatic function; severe myelosuppression is also possible.

Adverse Reactions

>10%:

Extravasation: Doxorubicin is one of the most notorious vesicants. Infiltration can cause severe inflammation, tissue necrosis, and ulceration. If the drug is infiltrated, consult institutional policy, apply ice to the area, and elevate the limb. Can have ongoing tissue destruction secondary to propagation of free radicals; may require debridement.

Vesicant chemotherapy

Gastrointestinal: Acute nausea and vomiting may be seen in 21% to 55% of patients; mucositis, ulceration, and necrosis of the colon, anorexia, and diarrhea

Emetic potential:

≤20 mg: Moderately low (10% to 30%)

>20 mg or <75 mg: Moderate (30% to 60%)

≥75 mg: Moderately high (60% to 90%)

Myelosuppressive: 60% to 80% of patients will have leukopenia; dose-limiting toxicity

WBC: Moderate

Platelets: Moderate

Onset (days): 7

Nadir (days): 10-14

Recovery (days): 21-28

Miscellaneous: Alopecia, discoloration of urine (red), stomatitis, esophagitis

1% to 10%:

Cardiac toxicity: Dose-limiting and related to cumulative dose; usually a maximum total lifetime dose of 450-550 mg/m^2 is administered; although, it has been demonstrated that if given by continuous infusion in breast cancer patients, higher doses may be tolerated. Patients may present with acute toxicity (arrhythmias, heart block, pericarditis-myocarditis) which may be fatal. More commonly, chronic toxicity is seen, in which patients present with signs of congestive heart failure. Several methods of monitoring cardiac toxicity have been utilized, including myocardial biopsy (expensive and hazardous procedure).

Dermatologic: Hyperpigmentation of nail beds, facial flushing, erythematous streaking along the vein if administered too rapidly

Miscellaneous: Hyperuricemia

<1%:

Hypersensitivity: Allergic reaction, anaphylaxis, fever, chills, urticaria

Radiation recall: Noticed in patients who have had prior irradiation; reactions include redness, warmth, erythema, and dermatitis in the radiation port. Can progress to severe desquamation and ulceration. Occurs 5-7 days after doxorubicin administration; local therapy with topical corticosteroids and cooling have given the best relief.

Miscellaneous: Conjunctivitis

Overdosage/Toxicology Symptoms of overdose include myelosuppression, nausea, vomiting, myocardial toxicity

Drug Interactions

Decreased effect: Doxorubicin may decrease digoxin plasma levels and renal excretion

Increased effect: Allopurinol may enhance the antitumor activity of doxorubicin (animal data only)

Increased toxicity:

Cyclophosphamide enhances the cardiac toxicity of doxorubicin by producing additional myocardial cell damage

(Continued)

371

Doxorubicin Hydrochloride *(Continued)*

Mercaptopurine increases toxicities

Streptozocin greatly enhances leukopenia and thrombocytopenia

Verapamil alters the cellular distribution of doxorubicin; may result in increased cell toxicity by inhibition of the P-glycoprotein pump

Stability Protect from light, must be dispensed in an amber bag; store powder vials at room temperature, refrigerate liquid vials; reconstituted powder vials stable for 24 hours at room temperature and 48 hours if refrigerated; unstable in solutions with a pH <3 or >7

Incompatible with hydrocortisone, fluorouracil, sodium bicarbonate, aminophylline, heparin, cephalothin, dexamethasone, furosemide, dexamethasone, diazepam

Y-site compatible with vincristine, cyclophosphamide, dacarbazine, bleomycin, vinblastine

Mechanism of Action Doxorubicin works through inhibition of topoisomerase-II at the point of DNA cleavage. A second mechanism of action is the production of free radicals (the hydroxy radical OH) by doxorubicin, which in turn can destroy DNA and cancerous cells. Doxorubicin is also a very powerful iron chelator, equal to deferoxamine. The iron-doxorubicin complex can bind DNA and cell membranes rapidly and produce free radicals that immediately cleave the DNA and cell membranes. Inhibits DNA and RNA synthesis by intercalating between DNA base pairs and by steric obstruction; active throughout entire cell cycle.

Pharmacodynamics/Kinetics

Absorption: Oral: Poor, <50%

Distribution: V_d: 25 L/kg; rapidly distributed into the liver, spleen, kidney, lung and heart, also distributes into breast milk

Protein binding: 70% bound to plasma proteins

Metabolism: In both the liver and in plasma to both active and inactive metabolites

Half-life, triphasic:

Primary: 30 minutes

Secondary: 3-3.5 hours for metabolites

Terminal: 17-30 hours for doxorubicin and its metabolites

Elimination, triphasic: 80% eventually excreted in bile and feces

Usual Dosage Refer to individual protocols

I.V. (patient's ideal weight should be used to calculate body surface area):

Children: 35-75 mg/m² as a single dose, repeat every 21 days; or 20 mg/m² once weekly

Adults: 60-75 mg/m² as a single dose, repeat every 21 days or other dosage regimens like 20-30 mg/m²/day for 2-3 days, repeat in 4 weeks or 20 mg/m² once weekly

The lower dose regimen should be given to patients with decreased bone marrow reserve, prior therapy or marrow infiltration with malignant cells

Currently the maximum cumulative dose is 550 mg/m²; a baseline MUGA should be performed prior to initiating treatment. If the LVEF is <30% to 40%, therapy should not be instituted; LVEF should be monitored during therapy. Doxorubicin has also been administered intraperitoneal (phase I in refractory ovarian cancer patients) and intra-arterially.

Dosing adjustment in renal impairment: Adjustments not required in mild to moderate renal failure

Cl_{cr} <10 mL/minute: Reduce dose to 75% of normal dose in severe renal failure

Hemodialysis effects: Supplemental dose is not necessary

Dosing adjustment in hepatic impairment:

Bilirubin 1.5-3 mg/dL or AST 60-180 IU: Administer 50% of dose

Bilirubin 3.1-5 mg/dL or AST >180 IU: Administer 25% of dose

Bilirubin >5 mg/dL: Avoid use

Administration May be further diluted in either NS of D_5W for I.V. administration

Monitoring Parameters CBC with differential and platelet count, echocardiogram, liver function tests

Patient Information Discolors urine red/orange; immediately report any change in sensation (eg, stinging) at injection site during infusion (may be an early sign of infiltration)

Nursing Implications Local erythematous streaking along the vein and/or facial flushing may indicate too rapid a rate of administration

Extravasation management:

Topical cooling may be achieved using ice packs or cooling pad with circulating ice water. Cooling of site for 24 hours as tolerated by the patient. Elevate and rest extremity 24-48 hours, then resume normal activity as tolerated. Application of cold inhibits vesicant's cytotoxicity.

Application of heat can be harmful and is contraindicated

If pain, erythema, and/or swelling persist beyond 48 hours, refer patient immediately to plastic surgeon for consultation and possible debridement

Dosage Forms
Injection:
Aqueous, with NS: 2 mg/mL (5 mL, 10 mL, 25 mL)
Preservative free: 2 mg/mL (5 mL, 10 mL, 25 mL, 100 mL)
Powder for injection, lyophilized: 10 mg, 20 mg, 50 mg, 100 mg
Powder for injection, lyophilized, rapid dissolution formula: 10 mg, 20 mg, 50 mg, 150 mg

Doxy® *see Doxycycline on this page*

Doxychel® *see Doxycycline on this page*

Doxycycline (dox i sye' kleen)
Related Information
Antimicrobial Drugs of Choice *on page 1298-1302*
Prevention of Malaria *on page 1405*
Brand Names Doryx®; Doxy®; Doxychel®; Vibramycin®; Vibra-Tabs®
Synonyms Doxycycline Hyclate; Doxycycline Monohydrate
Use Principally in the treatment of infections caused by susceptible *Rickettsia*, *Chlamydia*, and *Mycoplasma* along with uncommon susceptible gram-negative and gram-positive organisms; alternative to mefloquine for malaria prophylaxis

Unapproved use: Treatment for syphilis in penicillin-allergic patients; sclerosing agent for pleural effusions
Pregnancy Risk Factor D
Contraindications Hypersensitivity to doxycycline, tetracycline or any component; children <8 years of age; severe hepatic dysfunction
Warnings/Precautions Use of tetracyclines during tooth development may cause permanent discoloration of the teeth and enamel hypoplasia; prolonged use may result in superinfection; photosensitivity reaction may occur with this drug; avoid prolonged exposure to sunlight or tanning equipment
Adverse Reactions
>10%: Miscellaneous: Discoloration of teeth in children
1% to 10%: Gastrointestinal: Esophagitis
<1%:
Central nervous system: Increased intracranial pressure, bulging fontanels in infants
Dermatologic: Rash, photosensitivity
Gastrointestinal: Nausea, diarrhea
Hematologic: Neutropenia, eosinophilia
Hepatic: Hepatotoxicity
Local: Phlebitis
Overdosage/Toxicology Symptoms of overdose include nausea, anorexia, diarrhea; following GI decontamination, supportive care only; fluid support may be required for hypotension
Drug Interactions
Decreased effect with antacids containing aluminum, calcium, or magnesium
Iron and bismuth subsalicylate may decrease doxycycline bioavailability
Barbiturates, phenytoin, and carbamazepine decrease doxycycline's half-life
Increased effect of warfarin
Mechanism of Action Inhibits protein synthesis by binding with the 30S and possibly the 50S ribosomal subunit(s) of susceptible bacteria; may also cause alterations in the cytoplasmic membrane
Pharmacodynamics/Kinetics
Absorption: Almost completely from the GI tract; absorption can be reduced by food or milk by 20%
Distribution: Appears in breast milk
Protein binding: 90%
Metabolism: Not metabolized in the liver, instead is partially inactivated in the GI tract by chelate formation
Half-life: 12-15 hours (usually increases to 22-24 hours with multiple dosing)
End stage renal disease: 18-25 hours
Time to peak serum concentration: Within 1.5-4 hours
Elimination: In urine (23%) and feces (30%)
Usual Dosage Oral, I.V.:
Children ≥8 years (<45 kg): 2-5 mg/kg/day in 1-2 divided doses, not to exceed 200 mg/day
Children >8 years (>45 kg) and Adults: 100-200 mg/day in 1-2 divided doses
Sclerosing agent for pleural effusion injection: 500 mg as a single dose in 30-50 mL of NS or SWI
(Continued)

Doxycycline *(Continued)*

Dosing adjustment in renal impairment: No change is necessary

Not dialyzable; 0% to 5% by hemo- and peritoneal methods or by continuous arterio-venous or veno-venous hemofiltration (CAVH/CAVHD); no supplemental dosage necessary

Administration Infuse I.V. doxycycline over 1 hour

Test Interactions False-negative urine glucose using Clinistix®, Tes-Tape®

Patient Information Avoid unnecessary exposure to sunlight; do not take with antacids, iron products, or dairy products; finish all medication; do not skip doses

Nursing Implications Avoid extravasation; do not give orally with antacids, iron products, or dairy products, but may give with meals to decrease GI upset

Dosage Forms

Capsule, as hyclate:
Doxychel®, Vibramycin®: 50 mg
Doxy®, Doxychel®, Vibramycin®: 100 mg

Capsule, coated pellets, as hyclate (Doryx®): 100 mg

Powder for injection, as hyclate (Doxy®, Doxychel®, Vibramycin® IV): 100 mg, 200 mg

Powder for oral suspension, as monohydrate (raspberry flavor) (Vibramycin®): 25 mg/5 mL (60 mL)

Syrup, as calcium (raspberry-apple flavor) (Vibramycin®): 50 mg/5 mL (30 mL, 473 mL)

Tablet, as hyclate
Doxychel®: 50 mg
Doxychel®, Vibra-Tabs®: 100 mg

Doxycycline Hyclate *see* Doxycycline *on previous page*

Doxycycline Monohydrate *see* Doxycycline *on previous page*

DPA *see* Valproic Acid and Derivatives *on page 1143*

DPE *see* Dipivefrin *on page 356*

D-Penicillamine *see* Penicillamine *on page 847*

DPH *see* Phenytoin *on page 877*

DPPC *see* Colfosceril Palmitate *on page 272*

Dramamine® [OTC] *see* Dimenhydrinate *on page 347*

Dramilin® *see* Dimenhydrinate *on page 347*

Drisdol® *see* Ergocalciferol *on page 396*

Dristan® Long Lasting Nasal Solution [OTC] *see* Oxymetazoline Hydrochloride *on page 829*

Drithocreme® *see* Anthralin *on page 80*

Drithocreme® HP 1% *see* Anthralin *on page 80*

Dritho-Scalp® *see* Anthralin *on page 80*

Drixoral® Non-Drowsy [OTC] *see* Pseudoephedrine *on page 955*

Dronabinol *(droe nab' i nol)*

Related Information

Initial Doses in Selected Antiemetic Regimens *on page 1205*

Brand Names Marinol®

Synonyms Tetrahydrocannabinol, THC

Use When conventional antiemetics fail to relieve the nausea and vomiting associated with cancer chemotherapy, AIDS-related anorexia

Restrictions C-II

Pregnancy Risk Factor B

Contraindications Use only for cancer chemotherapy-induced nausea; should not be used in patients with a history of schizophrenia or in patients with known hypersensitivity to dronabinol or any component

Warnings/Precautions Use with caution in patients with heart disease, hepatic disease, or seizure disorders; reduce dosage in patients with severe hepatic impairment

Adverse Reactions

>10%: Central nervous system: Drowsiness, dizziness, detachment, anxiety, difficulty concentrating, mood change

1% to 10%:
Cardiovascular: Orthostatic hypotension, tachycardia
Central nervous system: Coordination impairment, depression, weakness, headache, vertigo, hallucinations, memory lapse, ataxia
Gastrointestinal: Dry mouth

Neuromuscular & skeletal: Paresthesia

<1%:
Cardiovascular: Syncope
Central nervous system: Nightmares, speech difficulties
Gastrointestinal: Diarrhea
Neuromuscular & skeletal: Muscular pains
Otic: Tinnitus
Miscellaneous: Sweating

Overdosage/Toxicology Tachycardia, hyper- and hypotension

Drug Interactions Increased toxicity (drowsiness) with alcohol, barbiturates, benzodiazepines

Stability Store in a cool place

Mechanism of Action Not well defined, probably inhibits the vomiting center in the medulla oblongata

Pharmacodynamics/Kinetics
Absorption: Oral: Erratic
Protein binding: 97% to 99%
Metabolism: Extensive first-pass metabolism; metabolized in the liver to several metabolites, some of which are active
Half-life: 19-24 hours
Time to peak serum concentration: Within 2-3 hours
Elimination: In feces and urine

Usual Dosage Oral:
Children: NCI protocol recommends 5 mg/m^2 starting 6-8 hours before chemotherapy and every 4-6 hours after to be continued for 12 hours after chemotherapy is discontinued

Adults: 5 mg/m^2 1-3 hours before chemotherapy, then give 5 mg/m^2/dose every 2-4 hours after chemotherapy for a total of 4-6 doses/day; dose may be increased up to a maximum of 15 mg/m^2/dose if needed (dosage may be increased by 2.5 mg/m^2 increments)

Appetite stimulant (AIDS-related): Initial: 2.5 mg twice daily (before lunch and dinner); titrate up to a maximum of 20 mg/day

Monitoring Parameters CNS effects, heart rate, blood pressure

Reference Range Antinauseant effects: 5-10 ng/mL

Test Interactions ↓ FSH, ↓ LH, ↓ growth hormone, ↓ testosterone

Patient Information Avoid activities such as driving which require motor coordination, avoid alcohol and other CNS depressants; may impair coordination and judgment

Nursing Implications Raise bed rails, institute safety measures, assist with ambulation

Dosage Forms Capsule: 2.5 mg, 5 mg, 10 mg

Droperidol (droe per' i dole)

Brand Names Inapsine®

Use Tranquilizer and antiemetic in surgical and diagnostic procedures; antiemetic for cancer chemotherapy; preoperative medication; has good antiemetic effect as well as sedative and antianxiety effects

Pregnancy Risk Factor C

Contraindications Hypersensitivity to droperidol or any component

Warnings/Precautions Safety in children <6 months of age has not been established; use with caution in patients with seizures, bone marrow depression, or severe liver disease

Significant hypotension may occur, especially when the drug is administered parenterally; injection contains benzyl alcohol; injection also contains sulfites which may cause allergic reaction

Tardive dyskinesia: Prevalence rate may be 40% in elderly; development of the syndrome and the irreversible nature are proportional to duration and total cumulative dose over time. May be reversible if diagnosed early in therapy.

Extrapyramidal reactions are more common in elderly with up to 50% developing these reactions after 60 years of age. Drug-induced **Parkinson's syndrome** occurs often. **Akathisia** is the most common extrapyramidal reaction in elderly.

Increased confusion, memory loss, psychotic behavior, and agitation frequently occur as a consequence of anticholinergic effects

Orthostatic hypotension is due to alpha-receptor blockade, the elderly are at greater risk for orthostatic hypotension

Antipsychotic associated sedation in nonpsychotic patients is extremely unpleasant due to feelings of depersonalization, derealization, and dysphoria

Life-threatening arrhythmias have occurred at therapeutic doses of antipsychotics

(Continued)

375

Droperidol *(Continued)*

Adverse Reactions

>10%:
Cardiovascular: Mild to moderate hypotension, tachycardia
Central nervous system: Postoperative drowsiness

1% to 10%:
Cardiovascular: Hypertension
Central nervous system: Extrapyramidal reactions
Respiratory: Respiratory depression

<1%:
Central nervous system: Dizziness, chills, shivering, postoperative hallucinations
Respiratory: Laryngospasm, bronchospasm

Overdosage/Toxicology Symptoms of overdose include hypotension, tachycardia, hallucinations, extrapyramidal symptoms.

Following initiation of essential overdose management, toxic symptom treatment and supportive treatment should be initiated. Hypotension usually responds to I.V. fluids or Trendelenburg positioning. If unresponsive to these measures, the use of a parenteral inotrope may be required (eg, norepinephrine 0.1-0.2 mcg/kg/minute titrated to response). Seizures commonly respond to diazepam (I.V. 5-10 mg bolus in adults every 15 minutes if needed up to a total of 30 mg; I.V. 0.25-0.4 mg/kg/dose up to a total of 10 mg in children) or to phenytoin or phenobarbital. Critical cardiac arrhythmias often respond to I.V. phenytoin (15 mg/kg up to 1 g), while other antiarrhythmics can be used. Neuroleptics often cause extrapyramidal symptoms (eg, dystonic reactions) requiring management with diphenhydramine 1-2 mg/kg (adults) up to a maximum of 50 mg I.M. or I.V. slow push followed by a maintenance dose for 48-72 hours. When these reactions are unresponsive to diphenhydramine, benztropine mesylate I.V. 1-2 mg (adults) may be effective. These agents are generally effective within 2-5 minutes.

Drug Interactions Increased toxicity: CNS depressants, fentanyl and other analgesics increased blood pressure; conduction anesthesia decreased blood pressure; epinephrine decreased blood pressure; atropine, lithium

Stability

Droperidol ampuls/vials should be stored at room temperature and protected from light
Stability of parenteral admixture at room temperature (25°C): 7 days
Standard diluent: 2.5 mg/50 mL D_5W
Incompatible with barbiturates

Mechanism of Action Alters the action of dopamine in the CNS, at subcortical levels, to produce sedation; reduces emesis by blocking dopamine stimulation of the chemotrigger zone

Pharmacodynamics/Kinetics

Following parenteral administration:
Peak effect: Within 30 minutes
Duration: 2-4 hours, may extend to 12 hours
Metabolism: In the liver
Half-life: Adults: 2.3 hours
Elimination: In urine (75%) and feces (22%)

Usual Dosage Titrate carefully to desired effect

Children 2-12 years:
Premedication: I.M.: 0.1-0.15 mg/kg; smaller doses may be sufficient for control of nausea or vomiting
Adjunct to general anesthesia: I.V. induction: 0.088-0.165 mg/kg
Nausea and vomiting: I.M., I.V.: 0.05-0.06 mg/kg/dose every 4-6 hours as needed

Adults:
Premedication: I.M.: 2.5-10 mg 30 minutes to 1 hour preoperatively
Adjunct to general anesthesia: I.V. induction: 0.22-0.275 mg/kg; maintenance: 1.25-2.5 mg/dose
Alone in diagnostic procedures: I.M.: Initial: 2.5-10 mg 30 minutes to 1 hour before; then 1.25-2.5 mg if needed
Nausea and vomiting: I.M., I.V.: 2.5-5 mg/dose every 3-4 hours as needed

Administration Administer I.M. or I.V.; I.V. should be administered slow IVP (over 2-5 minutes) or IVPB

Monitoring Parameters Blood pressure, heart rate, respiratory rate; observe for dystonias, extrapyramidal side effects, and temperature changes

Dosage Forms Injection: 2.5 mg/mL (1 mL, 2 mL, 5 mL, 10 mL)

Drotic® *see* Neomycin, Polymyxin B, and Hydrocortisone *on page 781*

Dryox® [OTC] *see* Benzoyl Peroxide *on page 122*

DSCG *see* Cromolyn Sodium *on page 280*

DSS *see* Docusate *on page 362*

D-S-S® [OTC] *see* Docusate *on page 362*

DT *see* Diphtheria and Tetanus Toxoid *on page 353*

DTaP *see* Diphtheria and Tetanus Toxoids and Acellular Pertussis Vaccine *on page 354*

DTIC *see* Dacarbazine *on page 297*

DTIC-Dome® *see* Dacarbazine *on page 297*

DTO *see* Opium Tincture *on page 819*

d-**Tubocurarine Chloride** *see* Tubocurarine Chloride *on page 1136*

Dulcolax® [OTC] *see* Bisacodyl *on page 134*

DuoCet™ *see* Hydrocodone and Acetaminophen *on page 543*

Duo-Trach® *see* Lidocaine Hydrochloride *on page 633*

Duotrate® *see* Pentaerythritol Tetranitrate *on page 855*

Duphalac® *see* Lactulose *on page 617*

Durabolin® *see* Nandrolone *on page 774*

Duradyne DHC® *see* Hydrocodone and Acetaminophen *on page 543*

Dura-Estrin® *see* Estradiol *on page 407*

Duragen® *see* Estradiol *on page 407*

Duragesic™ *see* Fentanyl *on page 446*

Duralone® *see* Methylprednisolone *on page 724*

Duralutin® *see* Hydroxyprogesterone Caproate *on page 553*

Duramorph® *see* Morphine Sulfate *on page 756*

Duranest® *see* Etidocaine Hydrochloride *on page 431*

Duraphyl™ *see* Theophylline/Aminophylline *on page 1072*

Duratest® *see* Testosterone *on page 1063*

Durathate® *see* Testosterone *on page 1063*

Duration® Nasal Solution [OTC] *see* Oxymetazoline Hydrochloride *on page 829*

Duricef® *see* Cefadroxil Monohydrate *on page 192*

Durrax® *see* Hydroxyzine *on page 556*

Duvoid® *see* Bethanechol Chloride *on page 132*

DV® Cream *see* Dienestrol *on page 333*

Dyazide® *see* Triamterene and Hydrochlorothiazide *on page 1116*

Dycill® *see* Dicloxacillin Sodium *on page 329*

Dyclone® *see* Dyclonine Hydrochloride *on this page*

Dyclonine Hydrochloride (dye′ kloe neen)
Brand Names Dyclone®

Use Local anesthetic prior to laryngoscopy, bronchoscopy, or endotracheal intubation; use topically for temporary relief of pain associated with oral mucosa or anogenital lesions

Pregnancy Risk Factor C

Contraindications Contraindicated in patients allergic to chlorobutanol (preservative used in dyclonine) or dyclonine

Warnings/Precautions Use with caution in patients with sepsis or traumatized mucosa in the area of application to avoid rapid systemic absorption; may impair swallowing and enhance the danger of aspiration; use with caution in patients with shock or heart block; resuscitative equipment, oxygen, and resuscitative drugs should be immediately available when dyclonine topical solution is administered to mucous membranes; **not for injection or ophthalmic use**

Adverse Reactions <1%:
Cardiovascular: Hypotension, bradycardia, respiratory arrest, cardiac arrest
Central nervous system: Excitation, drowsiness, nervousness, dizziness, seizures
Local: Slight irritation and stinging may occur when applied
Ocular: Blurred vision
Sensitivity reactions: Allergic reactions

Overdosage/Toxicology Symptoms of overdose are primarily CNS (seizures, excitation) and cardiovascular (hypotension, myocardial depression); treatment
(Continued)

Dyclonine Hydrochloride *(Continued)*

is supportive with fluids and pressors (particularly those that stimulate the myocardium); diazepam 0.1 mg/kg can be used to control seizures

Stability Store in tight, light-resistant containers

Mechanism of Action Blocks impulses at peripheral nerve endings in skin and mucous membranes by altering cell membrane permeability to ionic transfer

Pharmacodynamics/Kinetics

Onset of local anesthesia: 2-10 minutes

Duration: 30-60 minutes

Usual Dosage Use the lowest dose needed to provide effective anesthesia

Children and Adults: Topical solution:

Mouth sores: 5-10 mL of 0.5% or 1% to oral mucosa (swab or swish and then spit) 3-4 times/day as needed; maximum single dose: 200 mg (40 mL of 0.5% solution or 20 mL of 1% solution)

Bronchoscopy: Use 2 mL of the 1% solution or 4 mL of the 0.5% solution sprayed onto the larynx and trachea every 5 minutes until the reflex has been abolished

Patient Information Food should not be ingested for 60 minutes following application in the mouth or throat area; numbness of the tongue and buccal mucosa may result in increased risk of biting trauma; may impair swallowing; not for use in small infants or children

Dosage Forms Solution, topical: 0.5% (30 mL); 1% (30 mL)

Dyflos *see* Isoflurophate *on page 594*

Dymelor® *see* Acetohexamide *on page 23*

DynaCirc® *see* Isradipine *on page 604*

Dyna-Hex® [OTC] *see* Chlorhexidine Gluconate *on page 223*

Dynapen® *see* Dicloxacillin Sodium *on page 329*

Dyrenium® *see* Triamterene *on page 1115*

Easprin® *see* Aspirin *on page 92*

Echothiophate Iodide *(ek oh thye' oh fate)*

Related Information

Glaucoma Drug Therapy Comparison *on page 1270*

Brand Names Phospholine Iodide®

Synonyms Ecostigmine Iodide

Use Reverses toxic CNS effects caused by anticholinergic drugs; used as miotic in treatment of glaucoma; accommodative esotropia

Pregnancy Risk Factor C

Contraindications Hypersensitivity to echothiophate or any component; most cases of angle-closure glaucoma; active uveal inflammation or any inflammatory disease of the iris or ciliary body, glaucoma associated with iridocyclitis

Warnings/Precautions Tolerance may develop after prolonged use; a rest period restores response to the drug

Adverse Reactions

1% to 10%: Ocular: Stinging, burning, myopia, visual blurring

<1%:

Cardiovascular: Bradycardia, hypotension, flushing

Gastrointestinal: Nausea, vomiting, diarrhea

Ocular: Retinal detachment, diaphoresis, muscle weakness, browache, miosis, twitching eyelids, watering eyes

Respiratory: Difficulty in breathing

Overdosage/Toxicology Symptoms of overdose include excessive salivation, urinary incontinence, dyspnea, diarrhea, profuse sweating; if systemic effects occur, give parenteral atropine; for severe muscle weakness, pralidoxime may be used in addition to atropine

Drug Interactions Increased toxicity: Carbamate or organophosphate insecticides and pesticides; succinylcholine; systemic acetylcholinesterases → ↑ neuromuscular effects

Stability Store undiluted vials at room temperature (15°C to 30°C/59°F to 86°F); reconstituted solutions remain stable for 30 days at room temperature or 6 months when refrigerated

Mechanism of Action Produces miosis and changes in accommodation by inhibiting cholinesterase, thereby preventing the breakdown of acetylcholine; acetylcholine is, therefore, allowed to continuously stimulate the iris and ciliary muscles of the eye

Pharmacodynamics/Kinetics

Onset of action:

Miosis: 10-30 minutes

Intraocular pressure decrease: 4-8 hours
Peak intraocular pressure decrease: 24 hours
Duration: Up to 1-4 weeks

Usual Dosage Adults:

Ophthalmic: Glaucoma: Instill 1 drop twice daily into eyes with 1 dose just prior to bedtime; some patients have been treated with 1 dose daily or every other day

Accommodative esotropia:

Diagnosis: Instill 1 drop of 0.125% once daily into both eyes at bedtime for 2-3 weeks

Treatment: Use lowest concentration and frequency which gives satisfactory response, with a maximum dose of 0.125% once daily, although more intensive therapy may be used for short periods of time

Patient Information Be sure of solution expiration date; local irritation and headache may occur; notify physician if abdominal cramps, diarrhea, or salivation occur; use caution if driving at night or performing hazardous tasks

Nursing Implications Keep refrigerated; do not touch dropper to eye

Dosage Forms Powder for reconstitution, ophthalmic: 1.5 mg [0.03%] (5 mL); 3 mg [0.06%] (5 mL); 6.25 mg [0.125%] (5 mL); 12.5 mg [0.25%] (5 mL)

E-Complex-600® [OTC] *see* Vitamin E *on page 1164*

Econazole Nitrate (e kone' a zole)

Brand Names Spectazole™

Use Topical treatment of tinea pedis (athlete's foot), tinea cruris (jock itch), tinea corporis (ringworm), tinea versicolor, and cutaneous candidiasis

Pregnancy Risk Factor C

Pregnancy/Breast Feeding Implications Do not use during the first trimester of pregnancy, unless essential to a patient's welfare; use during the second and third trimesters only if clearly needed

Contraindications Known hypersensitivity to econazole or any component

Warnings/Precautions Discontinue drug if sensitivity or chemical irritation occurs; not for ophthalmic or intravaginal use

Adverse Reactions 1% to 10%: Local: Pruritus, erythema, burning, stinging

Mechanism of Action Alters fungal cell wall membrane permeability; may interfere with RNA and protein synthesis, and lipid metabolism

Pharmacodynamics/Kinetics

Absorption: Topical: <10%
Metabolism: In the liver to >20 metabolites
Elimination: <1% of applied dose recovered in urine or feces

Usual Dosage Children and Adults: Topical:

Tinea pedis, tinea cruris, tinea corporis, tinea versicolor: Apply sufficient amount to cover affected areas once daily

Cutaneous candidiasis: Apply sufficient quantity twice daily (morning and evening)

Duration of treatment: Candidal infections and tinea cruris, versicolor, and corporis should be treated for 2 weeks and tinea pedis for 1 month; occasionally, longer treatment periods may be required

Patient Information For external use only; avoid eye contact; if condition worsens or persists, or irritation occurs, notify physician

Dosage Forms Cream: 1% in water miscible base (15 g, 30 g, 85 g)

Econopred® *see* Prednisolone *on page 919*

Econopred® Plus *see* Prednisolone *on page 919*

Ecostigmine Iodide *see* Echothiophate Iodide *on previous page*

Ecotrin® [OTC] *see* Aspirin *on page 92*

Ectasule® *see* Ephedrine Sulfate *on page 388*

Edathamil Disodium *see* Edetate Disodium *on page 381*

Edecrin® *see* Ethacrynic Acid *on page 415*

Edetate Calcium Disodium (ed' e tate)

Brand Names Calcium Disodium Versenate®

Synonyms Calcium EDTA

Use Treatment of acute and chronic lead poisoning; used as an aid in the diagnosis of lead poisoning

Pregnancy Risk Factor C

Contraindications Severe renal disease, anuria

Warnings/Precautions Potentially nephrotoxic; renal tubular acidosis and fatal nephrosis may occur, especially with high doses; EKG changes may occur
(Continued)

379

Edetate Calcium Disodium *(Continued)*

during therapy; do not exceed recommended daily dose; avoid rapid I.V. infusion in the management of lead encephalopathy, may increase intracranial pressure to lethal levels. If anuria, increasing proteinuria, or hematuria occurs during therapy, discontinue calcium EDTA.

Adverse Reactions
1% to 10%: Renal: Renal tubular necrosis
<1%:
    Cardiovascular: Hypotension, arrhythmias
    Central nervous system: Numbness, tingling, fever, headache, chills
    Dermatologic: Skin lesions
    Endocrine & metabolic: Hypercalcemia
    Gastrointestinal: GI upset
    Hematologic: Transient marrow suppression
    Local: Pain at injection site following I.M. injection, thrombophlebitis following I.V. infusion (when concentration >0.5%)
    Ocular: Lacrimation
    Renal: Proteinuria, microscopic hematuria
    Respiratory: Sneezing, nasal congestion

Drug Interactions Decreased effect: Do not use simultaneously with zinc insulin preparations; do not mix in the same syringe with dimercaprol

Stability Dilute with 0.9% sodium chloride or D_5W; physically **incompatible** with $D_{10}W$, LR, Ringer's

Mechanism of Action Calcium is displaced by divalent and trivalent heavy metals, forming a nonionizing soluble complex that is excreted in urine

Pharmacodynamics/Kinetics
Absorption: I.M., S.C.: Well absorbed
Distribution: Into extracellular fluid; minimal CSF penetration
Half-life, plasma:
    I.M.: 1.5 hours
    I.V.: 20 minutes
Elimination: Rapidly excreted in urine as metal chelates or unchanged drug, decreased GFR decreases elimination; when administered I.V., urinary excretion of chelated lead begins in 1 hour and peak excretion of chelated lead occurs within 24-48 hours

Usual Dosage
Children: I.M. (preferred route of administration as rapid I.V. infusion may be lethal), I.V., S.C.:
    Asymptomatic lead poisoning: (Blood lead concentration >55 mcg/dL or blood lead concentrations of 25-55 mcg/dL with blood erythrocyte protoporphyrin concentrations ≥35 mcg/dL and positive mobilization test) or **symptomatic lead poisoning without encephalopathy** with lead level <100 mcg/dL: 1 g/m²/day I.M./I.V. in divided doses every 8-12 hours for 3-5 days (usually 5 days) with dimercaprol; maximum: 1 g/24 hours or 50 mg/kg/day
    Symptomatic lead poisoning with encephalopathy with lead level >100 mcg/dL (treatment with calcium EDTA and dimercaprol is preferred): 250 mg/m² I.M. or intermittent I.V. infusion 4 hours after dimercaprol, then at 4-hour intervals thereafter for 5 days (1.5 g/m²/day); dose (1.5 g/m²/day) can also be given as a single I.V. continuous infusion over 12-24 hours/day for 5 days; maximum: 1 g/24 hours or 75 mg/kg/day
    Note: Course of therapy may be repeated in 2-3 weeks until blood lead level is normal

Adults: Treatment: I.M., I.V.: 2-4 g/day or 1.5 g/m²/day in divided doses every 12-24 hours for 5 days; may repeat course one time after at least 2 days (usually after 2 weeks) not more than 2 courses of therapy are recommended

Dosing adjustment/comments in renal impairment: Calcium disodium EDTA is almost exclusively eliminated in urine and should not be administered during periods of anuria

Administration For intermittent I.V. infusion, administer the dose I.V. over at least 1 hour in asymptomatic patients, 2 hours in symptomatic patients; for I.V. continuous infusion, dilute to 2-4 mg/mL in D_5W or NS and infuse over at least 8 hours, usually over 12-24 hours; for I.M. injection, 1 mL of 1% procaine hydrochloride may be added to each mL of EDTA calcium to minimize pain at injection site

Monitoring Parameters BUN, creatinine, urinalysis, I & O, and EKG during therapy; intravenous administration requires a cardiac monitor

Test Interactions If calcium EDTA is given as a continuous I.V. infusion, stop the infusion for at least 1 hour before blood is drawn for lead concentration to avoid a falsely elevated value

Dosage Forms Injection: 200 mg/mL (5 mL)

Edetate Disodium (ed′ e tate)

Brand Names Chealamide®; Disotate®; Endrate®

Synonyms Edathamil Disodium; EDTA; Sodium Edetate

Use Emergency treatment of hypercalcemia; control digitalis-induced cardiac dysrhythmias (ventricular arrhythmias)

Pregnancy Risk Factor C

Contraindications Severe renal failure or anuria

Warnings/Precautions Use of this drug is recommended only when the severity of the clinical condition justifies the aggressive measures associated with this type of therapy; use with caution in patients with renal dysfunction, intracranial lesions, seizure disorders, coronary or peripheral vascular disease

Adverse Reactions

Rapid I.V. administration or excessive doses may cause a sudden drop in serum calcium concentration which may lead to hypocalcemic tetany, seizures, arrhythmias, and death from respiratory arrest. Do **not** exceed recommended dosage and rate of administration.

1% to 10%: Gastrointestinal: Nausea, vomiting, abdominal cramps, diarrhea

<1%:
Cardiovascular: Arrhythmias, transient hypotension, acute tubular necrosis
Central nervous system: Seizures, fever, headache, tetany, chills
Dermatologic: Eruptions, dermatologic lesions
Endocrine & metabolic: Hypomagnesemia, hypokalemia
Hematologic: Anemia
Local: Thrombophlebitis, pain at the site of injection
Neuromuscular & skeletal: Paresthesia may occur, back pain, muscle cramps
Renal: Nephrotoxicity
Respiratory: Death from respiratory arrest

Overdosage/Toxicology Symptoms of overdose include hypotension, dysrhythmias, tetany, seizures; treatment includes immediate I.V. calcium salts for hypocalcemia related adverse reactions; replace calcium cautiously in patients on digitalis

Drug Interactions Increased effect of insulin (edetate disodium may decrease blood glucose concentrations and reduce insulin requirements in diabetic patients treated with insulin)

Mechanism of Action Chelates with divalent or trivalent metals to form a soluble complex that is then eliminated in urine

Pharmacodynamics/Kinetics

Metabolism: Not metabolized

Half-life: 20-60 minutes

Elimination: Following chelation, 95% excreted in urine as chelates within 24-48 hours

Usual Dosage Hypercalcemia: I.V.:

Children: 40-70 mg/kg/day slow infusion over 3-4 hours or more to a maximum of 3 g/24 hours; administer for 5 days and allow 5 days between courses of therapy

Adults: 50 mg/kg/day over 3 or more hours to a maximum of 3 g/24 hours; a suggested regimen of 5 days followed by 2 days without drug and repeated courses up to 15 total doses

Administration Must be diluted before use in 500 mL D_5W or NS to <30 mg/mL

Monitoring Parameters Cardiac function (EKG monitoring); blood pressure during infusion; renal function should be assessed before and during therapy; monitor calcium, magnesium, and potassium levels; cardiac monitor required

Nursing Implications Avoid extravasation; patient should remain supine for a short period after infusion; infuse over 3-4 hours

Additional Information Sodium content of 1 g: 5.4 mEq

Dosage Forms Injection: 150 mg/mL (20 mL)

Edrophonium Chloride (ed roe foe′ nee um)

Brand Names Enlon®; Reversol®; Tensilon®

Use Diagnosis of myasthenia gravis; differentiation of cholinergic crises from myasthenia crises; reversal of nondepolarizing neuromuscular blockers; treatment of paroxysmal atrial tachycardia

Pregnancy Risk Factor C

Contraindications Hypersensitivity to edrophonium or any component, GI or GU obstruction, hypersensitivity to sulfite agents

Warnings/Precautions Use with caution in patients with bronchial asthma and those receiving a cardiac glycoside; atropine sulfate should always be readily available as an antagonist. Overdosage can cause cholinergic crisis which may be fatal. I.V. atropine should be readily available for treatment of cholinergic reactions.

(Continued)

Edrophonium Chloride *(Continued)*

Adverse Reactions
>10%:
  Gastrointestinal: Nausea, vomiting, diarrhea, excessive salivation, stomach
    cramps
  Miscellaneous: Increased sweating
1% to 10%:
  Genitourinary: Urinary frequency
  Ocular: Small pupils, lacrimation
  Respiratory: Increased bronchial secretions
<1%:
  Cardiovascular: Bradycardia, A-V block
  Central nervous system: Seizures, headache, drowsiness, dysphoria
  Neuromuscular & skeletal: Weakness, muscle cramps, muscle spasms
  Local: Thrombophlebitis
  Ocular: Diplopia, miosis
  Respiratory: Laryngospasm, bronchospasm, respiratory paralysis
  Miscellaneous: Hypersensitivity, hyper-reactive cholinergic responses

Overdosage/Toxicology Symptoms of overdose include muscle weakness,
nausea, vomiting, miosis, bronchospasm, respiratory paralysis. Maintain
adequate airway; antidote is atropine for muscarinic symptoms; pralidoxime (2-
PAM) may also be needed to reverse severe muscle weakness or paralysis;
skeletal muscle effects of edrophonium not alleviated by atropine.

Drug Interactions
Decreased effect: Atropine, nondepolarizing muscle relaxants, procainamide,
  quinidine
Increased effect: Succinylcholine, digoxin, I.V. acetazolamide, neostigmine,
  physostigmine

Mechanism of Action Inhibits destruction of acetylcholine by acetylcholinesterase. This facilitates transmission of impulses across myoneural junction and
results in increased cholinergic responses such as miosis, increased tonus of
intestinal and skeletal muscles, bronchial and ureteral constriction, bradycardia,
and increased salivary and sweat gland secretions.

Pharmacodynamics/Kinetics
I.M.:
  Onset of effect: Within 2-10 minutes
  Duration: 5-30 minutes
I.V.:
  Onset of effect: Within 30-60 seconds
  Duration: 10 minutes
Distribution: V_d: 1.1 L/kg
Half-life: 1.8 hours

Usual Dosage Usually administered I.V., however, if not possible, I.M. or S.C.
may be used:
Infants:
  I.M.: 0.5-1 mg
  I.V.: Initial: 0.1 mg, followed by 0.4 mg if no response; total dose = 0.5 mg

Children:
  Diagnosis: Initial: 0.04 mg/kg over 1 minute followed by 0.16 mg/kg if no
    response, to a maximum total dose of 5 mg for children <34 kg, or 10 mg for
    children >34 kg
  I.M.:
    <34 kg: 1 mg
    >34 kg: 5 mg
  Titration of oral anticholinesterase therapy: 0.04 mg/kg once given 1 hour after
    oral intake of the drug being used in treatment; if strength improves, an
    increase in neostigmine or pyridostigmine dose is indicated

Adults:
  Diagnosis:
    I.V.: 2 mg test dose administered over 15-30 seconds; 8 mg given 45
      seconds later if no response is seen; test dose may be repeated after 30
      minutes
    I.M.: Initial: 10 mg; if no cholinergic reaction occurs, give 2 mg 30 minutes
      later to rule out false-negative reaction
  Titration of oral anticholinesterase therapy: 1-2 mg given 1 hour after oral dose
    of anticholinesterase; if strength improves, an increase in neostigmine or
    pyridostigmine dose is indicated
  Reversal of nondepolarizing neuromuscular blocking agents (neostigmine with
    atropine usually preferred): I.V.: 10 mg over 30-45 seconds; may repeat
    every 5-10 minutes up to 40 mg
  Termination of paroxysmal atrial tachycardia: I.V. rapid injection: 5-10 mg

Differentiation of cholinergic from myasthenic crisis: I.V.: 1 mg; may repeat after 1 minute. **Note:** Intubation and controlled ventilation may be required if patient has cholinergic crisis

Dosing adjustment in renal impairment: Dose may need to be reduced in patients with chronic renal failure

Test Interactions ↑ aminotransferase [ALT (SGPT)/AST (SGOT)] (S), amylase (S)

Dosage Forms Injection: 10 mg/mL (1 mL, 10 mL, 15 mL)

EDTA *see* Edetate Disodium *on page 381*

E.E.S.® *see* Erythromycin *on page 401*

Efedron® *see* Ephedrine Sulfate *on page 388*

Effer-K™ *see* Potassium Bicarbonate and Potassium Citrate, Effervescent *on page 905*

Effer-Syllium® **[OTC]** *see* Psyllium *on page 956*

Effexor® *see* Venlafaxine *on page 1152*

Efidac/24® **[OTC]** *see* Pseudoephedrine *on page 955*

Eflornithine Hydrochloride (ee flor´ ni theen)
Brand Names Ornidyl®
Synonyms DFMO
Use Treatment of meningoencephalitic stage of *Trypanosoma brucei gambiense* infection (sleeping sickness)
Pregnancy Risk Factor C
Contraindications Hypersensitivity to eflornithine or any component
Warnings/Precautions Must be diluted before use; frequent monitoring for myelosuppression should be done; use with caution in patients with a history of seizures and in patients with renal impairment; serial audiograms should be obtained; due to the potential for relapse, patients should be followed up for at least 24 months
Adverse Reactions
>10%: Hematologic: Anemia, leukopenia, thrombocytopenia
1% to 10%:
Central nervous system: Seizures, dizziness
Dermatologic: Alopecia
Gastrointestinal: Vomiting, diarrhea
Hematologic: Eosinophilia
Otic: Hearing impairment
<1%:
Cardiovascular: Facial edema
Central nervous system: Headache, asthenia
Gastrointestinal: Abdominal pain, anorexia
Overdosage/Toxicology No known antidote; treatment is supportive
Stability Must be diluted before use and used within 24 hours of preparation
Mechanism of Action Eflornithine exerts antitumor and antiprotozoal effects through specific, irreversible ("suicide") inhibition of the enzyme ornithine decarboxylase (ODC). ODC is the rate-limiting enzyme in the biosynthesis of putrescine, spermine, and spermidine, the major polyamines in nucleated cells. Polyamines are necessary for the synthesis of DNA, RNA, and proteins and are, therefore, necessary for cell growth and differentiation. Although many microorganisms and higher plants are able to produce polyamines from alternate biochemical pathways, all mammalian cells depend on ornithine decarboxylase to produce polyamines. Eflornithine inhibits ODC and rapidly depletes animal cells of putrescine and spermidine; the concentration of spermine remains the same or may even increase. Rapidly dividing cells appear to most susceptible to the effects of eflornithine.
Usual Dosage Adults: I.V. infusion: 100 mg/kg/dose given every 6 hours (over at least 45 minutes) for 14 days

Dosing adjustment in renal impairment: Dose should be adjusted although no specific guidelines are available
Monitoring Parameters CBC with platelet counts
Patient Information Report any persistent or unusual fever, sore throat, fatigue, bleeding, or bruising; frequent blood tests are needed during therapy
Dosage Forms Injection: 200 mg/mL (100 mL)

Efodine® **[OTC]** *see* Povidone-Iodine *on page 913*

Efudex® *see* Fluorouracil *on page 473*

EHDP *see* Etidronate Disodium *on page 432*

E-IPV *see* Polio Vaccines *on page 898*

Elavil® *see* Amitriptyline Hydrochloride *on page 60*

Eldecort® *see* Hydrocortisone *on page 546*

Eldepryl® *see* Selegiline Hydrochloride *on page 1001*

Eldercaps® **[OTC]** *see* Vitamin, Multiple *on page 1166*

Eldopaque Forte® *see* Hydroquinone *on page 551*

Eldopaque® **[OTC]** *see* Hydroquinone *on page 551*

Eldoquin Forte® *see* Hydroquinone *on page 551*

Eldoquin® **[OTC]** *see* Hydroquinone *on page 551*

Electrolyte Lavage Solution *see* Polyethylene Glycol-Electrolyte Solution *on page 900*

Elimite™ *see* Permethrin *on page 864*

Elixophyllin® *see* Theophylline/Aminophylline *on page 1072*

Elixophyllin® **SR** *see* Theophylline/Aminophylline *on page 1072*

Elocon® *see* Mometasone Furoate *on page 754*

Elspar® *see* Asparaginase *on page 89*

Eltroxin™ *see* Levothyroxine Sodium *on page 629*

Emcyt® *see* Estramustine Phosphate Sodium *on page 409*

Eminase® *see* Anistreplase *on page 79*

EMLA® *see* Lidocaine and Prilocaine *on page 632*

Empirin® **[OTC]** *see* Aspirin *on page 92*

Empirin® **With Codeine** *see* Aspirin and Codeine *on page 94*

Emulsoil® **[OTC]** *see* Castor Oil *on page 190*

E-Mycin® *see* Erythromycin *on page 401*

Enalapril (e nal' a pril)

Related Information

Angiotensin-Converting Enzyme Inhibitors, Comparative Pharmacokinetics *on page 1244*

Angiotensin-Converting Enzyme Inhibitors, Comparisons of Indications and Adult Dosages *on page 1243*

Brand Names Vasotec®

Synonyms Enalaprilat

Use Management of mild to severe hypertension and congestive heart failure

    Unlabeled use: Hypertensive crisis, diabetic nephropathy, rheumatoid arthritis, diagnosis of anatomic renal artery stenosis, hypertension secondary to scleroderma renal crisis, diagnosis of aldosteronism, idiopathic edema, Bartter's syndrome, postmyocardial infarction for prevention of ventricular failure

Pregnancy Risk Factor D

Contraindications Hypersensitivity to enalapril, enalaprilat, other ACE inhibitors, or any component

Warnings/Precautions Use with caution and modify dosage in patients with renal impairment (especially renal artery stenosis), severe congestive heart failure, or with coadministered diuretic therapy, valvular stenosis, hyperkalemia (>5.7 mEq/L); experience in children is limited. Severe hypotension may occur in patients who are sodium and/or volume depleted; initiate lower doses and monitor closely when starting therapy in these patients.

Adverse Reactions

    1% to 10%:

        Cardiovascular: Chest pain, palpitations, tachycardia, syncope

        Central nervous system: Insomnia, headache dizziness, fatigue, malaise, asthenia

        Dermatologic: Rash

        Gastrointestinal: Dysgeusia, abdominal pain, vomiting, nausea, diarrhea, anorexia, constipation

        Neuromuscular & skeletal: Paresthesia

        Respiratory: Bronchitis, cough, dyspnea

    <1%:

        Cardiovascular: Angina pectoris, flushing

        Dermatologic: Alopecia, erythema multiforme, pruritus, Stevens-Johnson syndrome, urticaria, angioedema

        Endocrine & metabolic: Hypoglycemia, hyperkalemia

Genitourinary: Impotence

Hematologic: Agranulocytosis, neutropenia, anemia

Neuromuscular & skeletal: Myalgia

Ocular: Blurred vision

Otic: Tinnitus

Renal: Oliguria

Respiratory: Asthma, bronchospasm

Miscellaneous: Sweating

Overdosage/Toxicology Mild hypotension has been the only toxic effect seen with acute overdose. Bradycardia may also occur; hyperkalemia occurs even with therapeutic doses, especially in patients with renal insufficiency and those taking NSAIDs. Following initiation of essential overdose management, toxic symptom treatment and supportive treatment should be initiated. Hypotension usually responds to I.V. fluids or Trendelenburg positioning.

Drug Interactions See table.

Drug-Drug Interactions With ACEIs

Precipitant Drug	Drug (Category) and Effect	Description
Antacids	ACEIs: decreased	Decreased bioavailability of ACEIs. May be more likely with captopril. Separate administration times by 1-2 hours.
NSAIDs (indomethacin)	ACEIs: decreased	Reduced hypotensive effects of ACEIs. More prominent in low renin or volume dependent hypertensive patients.
Phenothiazines	ACEIs: increased	Pharmacologic effects of ACEIs may be increased.
ACEIs	Allopurinol: increased	Higher risk of hypersensitivity reaction possible when given concurrently. Three case reports of Stevens-Johnson syndrome with captopril.
ACEIs	Digoxin: increased	Increased plasma digoxin levels.
ACEIs	Lithium: increased	Increased serum lithium levels and symptoms of toxicity may occur.
ACEIs	Potassium preps/potassium-sparing diuretics increased	Coadministration may result in elevated potassium levels.

Stability Solutions for I.V. infusion mixed in NS or D_5W are stable for 24 hours at room temperature

Mechanism of Action Competitive inhibitor of angiotensin-converting enzyme (ACE); prevents conversion of angiotensin I to angiotensin II, a potent vasoconstrictor; results in lower levels of angiotensin II which causes an increase in plasma renin activity and a reduction in aldosterone secretion

Pharmacodynamics/Kinetics

Oral:

Onset of action: ~1 hour

Duration: 12-24 hours

Absorption: Oral: 55% to 75%

Protein binding: 50% to 60%

Metabolism: Enalapril is a prodrug and undergoes biotransformation to enalaprilat in the liver

Half-life:

Enalapril: Adults:

Healthy: 2 hours

With congestive heart failure: 3.4-5.8 hours

Enalaprilat:

Infants 6 weeks to 8 months: 6-10 hours

Adults: 35-38 hours

Time to peak serum concentration: Oral:

Enalapril: Within 0.5-1.5 hours

Enalaprilat (active): Within 3-4.5 hours

Elimination: Principally in urine (60% to 80%) with some fecal excretion

Usual Dosage Use lower listed initial dose in patients with hyponatremia, hypovolemia, severe congestive heart failure, decreased renal function, or in those receiving diuretics
(Continued)

Enalapril *(Continued)*

Children:

Investigational initial oral doses of **enalapril** of 0.1 mg/kg/day increasing over 2 weeks to 0.12-0.43 mg/kg/day have been used to treat severe congestive heart failure in infants (n=8)

Investigational I.V. doses of **enalaprilat** of 5-10 mcg/kg/dose administered every 8-24 hours (as determined by blood pressure readings) have been used for the treatment of neonatal hypertension (n=10); monitor patients carefully; select patients may require higher doses

Adults:

Oral: **Enalapril:** 2.5-5 mg/day then increase as required, usual therapeutic dose for hypertension: 10-40 mg/day in 1-2 divided doses; usual therapeutic dose for heart failure: 5-20 mg/day

I.V.: **Enalaprilat:** 1.25 mg/dose, given over 5 minutes every 6 hours; doses as high as 5 mg/dose every 6 hours have been tolerated for up to 36 hours

Dosing adjustment in renal impairment:

Oral: Enalapril:

Cl_{cr} 10-50 mL/minute: Administer 75% to 100% of usual dose

Cl_{cr} <10 mL/minute: Administer 50% of usual dose

I.V.: Enalaprilat: Cl_{cr} <30 mL/minute: Start at 0.625 mg every 6 hours and increase dose based on response

Monitoring Parameters Blood pressure, renal function, WBC, serum potassium; blood pressure monitor required during intravenous administration

Test Interactions Positive Coombs' [direct]; may cause false-positive results in urine acetone determinations using sodium nitroprusside reagent

Patient Information Notify physician if vomiting, diarrhea, excessive perspiration, or dehydration should occur; also if swelling of face, lips, tongue, or difficulty in breathing occurs or if persistent cough develops

Nursing Implications May cause depression in some patients; discontinue if angioedema of the face, extremities, lips, tongue, or glottis occurs; watch for hypotensive effects within 1-3 hours of first dose or new higher dose

Dosage Forms

Injection, as enalaprilat: 1.25 mg/mL (1 mL, 2 mL)

Tablet, as maleate: 2.5 mg, 5 mg, 10 mg, 20 mg

Enalaprilat *see* Enalapril *on page 384*

Endep® *see* Amitriptyline Hydrochloride *on page 60*

End Lice® [OTC] *see* Pyrethrins *on page 959*

Endolor® *see* Butalbital Compound *on page 153*

Endrate® *see* Edetate Disodium *on page 381*

Enduron® *see* Methyclothiazide *on page 718*

Ener-B® [OTC] *see* Cyanocobalamin *on page 282*

Engerix-B® *see* Hepatitis B Vaccine *on page 533*

Enhanced-potency Inactivated Poliovirus Vaccine *see* Polio Vaccines *on page 898*

Enlon® *see* Edrophonium Chloride *on page 381*

Enovid® *see* Mestranol and Norethynodrel *on page 696*

Enovil® *see* Amitriptyline Hydrochloride *on page 60*

Enoxacin *(en ox' a sin)*

Brand Names Penetrex™

Use Treatment of complicated and uncomplicated urinary tract infections caused by susceptible gram-negative and gram-positive bacteria

Pregnancy Risk Factor C

Contraindications Hypersensitivity to enoxacin, any component, or other quinolones

Warnings/Precautions Use with caution in patients with a history of convulsions or epilepsy, renal dysfunction, psychosis, elevated intracranial pressure, prepubertal children, and pregnancy; nalidixic acid and ciprofloxacin (related compounds) have been associated with erosions of the cartilage in weight-bearing joints and other signs of arthropathy in immature animals and children; similar precautions are advised for enoxacin although no data is available.

Adverse Reactions

1% to 10%: Gastrointestinal: Nausea, vomiting

<1%:

Central nervous system: Restlessness, dizziness, confusion, seizures, headache

Dermatologic: Rash
Gastrointestinal: Diarrhea, GI bleeding
Hematologic: Anemia
Hepatic: Increased liver enzymes
Neuromuscular & skeletal: Tremor, arthralgia
Renal: Increased serum creatinine and BUN, acute renal failure

Overdosage/Toxicology Symptoms of overdose include acute renal failure, seizures; GI decontamination and supportive care; diazepam for seizures; not removed by peritoneal or hemodialysis

Drug Interactions
Decreased effect with antacids (magnesium, aluminum), iron and zinc salts, sucralfate, bismuth salts
Increased toxicity/levels of warfarin, cyclosporine, digoxin, caffeine; increased levels with cimetidine

Mechanism of Action Exerts a broad spectrum antimicrobial effect. The primary target of the fluoroquinolones is DNA gyrase (topoisomerase II) an essential bacterial enzyme that maintains the superhelical structure of DNA. DNA gyrase is required for DNA replication and transcription, DNA repair, recombination, and transposition.

Pharmacodynamics/Kinetics
Absorption: 98%
Distribution: Penetrates well into tissues and body secretions
Bioavailability: Has essentially the same bioavailability as intravenous administration; administration with food does not affect the bioavailability of enoxacin
Half-life: 3-6 hours (average)
Elimination: Primarily in urine, however, significant drug concentrations are achieved in feces

Usual Dosage Adults: Oral: 400 mg twice daily
Dosing adjustment in renal impairment:
Cl_{cr} <50 mL/minute: Administer 50% of dose

Dosage Forms Tablet: 200 mg, 400 mg

Enoxaparin Sodium (e nox ah pair' in)

Brand Names Lovenox®

Use Prevention of deep vein thrombosis following orthopedic surgery

Pregnancy Risk Factor B

Contraindications Patients with active major bleeding, thrombocytopenia associated with a positive *in vitro* test for antiplatelet antibody or enoxaparin-induced platelet aggregation, hypersensitivity to enoxaparin, known hypersensitivity to heparin or pork products

Warnings/Precautions Do not administer intramuscularly; use with extreme caution in patients with a history of heparin-induced thrombocytopenia; bacterial endocarditis, hemorrhagic stroke, recent CNS or ophthalmological surgery, bleeding diathesis, uncontrolled arterial hypertension, or a history of recent gastrointestinal ulceration and hemorrhage. Elderly and patients with renal insufficiency may show delayed elimination of enoxaparin; avoid use in lactation.

Adverse Reactions
1% to 10%:
Central nervous system: Fever, confusion
Dermatologic: Erythema, ecchymosis
Gastrointestinal: Nausea
Hematologic: Hemorrhage, thrombocytopenia, hematoma, hypochromic anemia
Local: Local irritation, pain

At the recommended doses, single injections of enoxaparin do not significantly influence platelet aggregation or affect global clotting time (ie, prothrombin time or activated partial thromboplastin time)

Overdosage/Toxicology Symptoms of overdose include hemorrhage; protamine zinc has been used to reverse effects

Drug Interactions Increased toxicity with oral anticoagulants, platelet inhibitors

Pharmacodynamics/Kinetics
Onset of effect: Maximum anti-factor Xa and antithrombin (anti-factor IIa) activities occur 3-5 hours after S.C. administration
Duration: Following a 40 mg dose, significant anti-factor Xa activity persists in plasma for ~12 hours
Protein binding: Low molecular weight heparins do not bind to heparin binding proteins
Half-life, plasma: Low molecular weight heparin is 2-4 times longer than standard heparin independent of the dose

Usual Dosage S.C.:
Children: Safety and effectiveness have not been established
(Continued)

Enoxaparin Sodium *(Continued)*

Adults: 30 mg twice daily; first dose within 12 hours after surgery and every 12 hours for 3 days (including day of surgery); after 3 days, switch to adjusted dose heparin

A single daily dose of 40 mg has been found to be equally effective in patients undergoing orthopedic or gynecologic surgical procedures

Dosing adjustment in renal impairment: Adjustment may be necessary in elderly and patients with severe renal impairment

Monitoring Parameters Platelets, occult blood, and anti-Xa activity, if available; the monitoring of PT and/or PTT is not necessary

Dosage Forms Injection, preservative free: 30 mg/0.3 mL

Entacef® *see* Cephalexin Monohydrate *on page 210*

Entolase®-HP *see* Pancrelipase *on page 837*

Enulose® *see* Lactulose *on page 617*

Ephedrine Sulfate *(e fed′ rin)*

Brand Names Ectasule®; Efedron®; Ephedsol®; Vicks Vatronol®

Use Treatment of bronchial asthma, nasal congestion, acute bronchospasm, idiopathic orthostatic hypotension

Pregnancy Risk Factor C

Contraindications Hypersensitivity to ephedrine or any component, cardiac arrhythmias, angle-closure glaucoma, patients on other sympathomimetic agents

Warnings/Precautions Blood volume depletion should be corrected before ephedrine therapy is instituted; use caution in patients with unstable vasomotor symptoms, diabetes, hyperthyroidism, prostatic hypertrophy, or a history of seizures; also use caution in the elderly and those patients with cardiovascular disorders such as coronary artery disease, arrhythmias, and hypertension. Ephedrine may cause hypertension resulting in intracranial hemorrhage. Long-term use may cause anxiety and symptoms of paranoid schizophrenia. Avoid as a bronchodilator; generally not used as a bronchodilator since new beta$_2$ agents are less toxic. Use with caution in the elderly, since it crosses the blood-brain barrier and may cause confusion.

Adverse Reactions

>10%: Central nervous system: CNS stimulating effects, nervousness, anxiety, apprehension, fear, tension, agitation, excitation, restlessness, irritability, insomnia, hyperactivity

1% to 10%:

Cardiovascular: Hypertension, tachycardia, palpitations, elevation or depression of blood pressure

Central nervous system: Dizziness, headache, weakness

Gastrointestinal: Dry mouth, nausea, anorexia, GI upset, vomiting

Genitourinary: Painful urination

Neuromuscular & skeletal: Trembling, tremor (more common in the elderly)

Miscellaneous: Increased sweating, unusual paleness

<1%:

Cardiovascular: Chest pain, arrhythmias

Central nervous system: Anxiety, apprehension, fear, tension, agitation, excitation, restlessness, irritability

Neuromuscular & skeletal: Tremor

Respiratory: Difficulty in breathing

Overdosage/Toxicology Symptoms of overdose include dysrhythmias, CNS excitation, respiratory depression, vomiting, convulsions

There is no specific antidote for ephedrine intoxication and the bulk of the treatment is supportive. Hyperactivity and agitation usually respond to reduced sensory input; however, with extreme agitation, haloperidol (2-5 mg I.M. for adults) may be required. Hyperthermia is best treated with external cooling measures; or when severe or unresponsive, muscle paralysis with pancuronium may be needed. Hypertension is usually transient and generally does not require treatment unless severe. For diastolic blood pressures >110 mm Hg, a nitroprusside infusion should be initiated. Seizures usually respond to diazepam I.V. and/or phenytoin maintenance regimens.

Drug Interactions

Decreased effect: Alpha- and beta-adrenergic blocking agents ↓ ephedrine vasopressor effects

Increased toxicity: Additive cardiostimulation with other sympathomimetic agents; theophylline → cardiostimulation; MAO inhibitors or atropine → ↑ blood pressure; cardiac glycosides or general anesthetics → ↑ cardiac stimulation

Stability Protect all dosage forms from light

Mechanism of Action Releases tissue stores of epinephrine and thereby produces an alpha- and beta-adrenergic stimulation; longer-acting and less potent than epinephrine

Pharmacodynamics/Kinetics
Oral:
Onset of bronchodilation: Within 0.25-1 hour
Duration of action: 3-6 hours
Distribution: Crosses the placenta; appears in breast milk
Metabolism: Little hepatic metabolism
Half-life: 2.5-3.6 hours
Elimination: 60% to 77% of dose excreted as unchanged drug in urine within 24 hours

Usual Dosage
Children:
Oral, S.C.: 3 mg/kg/day or 25-100 mg/m^2/day in 4-6 divided doses every 4-6 hours
I.M., slow I.V. push: 0.2-0.3 mg/kg/dose every 4-6 hours
Adults:
Oral: 25-50 mg every 3-4 hours as needed
I.M., S.C.: 25-50 mg, parenteral adult dose should not exceed 150 mg in 24 hours
I.V.: 5-25 mg/dose slow I.V. push repeated after 5-10 minutes as needed, then every 3-4 hours not to exceed 150 mg/24 hours

Monitoring Parameters Blood pressure, pulse, urinary output, mental status; cardiac monitor and blood pressure monitor required

Test Interactions Can cause a false-positive amphetamine EMIT assay

Patient Information May cause wakefulness or nervousness; take last dose 4-6 hours before bedtime

Nursing Implications Do not administer unless solution is clear

Dosage Forms
Capsule: 25 mg, 50 mg
Injection: 25 mg/mL (1 mL); 50 mg/mL (1 mL, 10 mL)
Syrup: 11 mg/5 mL (473 mL); 20 mg/5 mL (473 mL)

Ephedsol® see Ephedrine Sulfate *on previous page*

Epifrin® see Epinephrine *on this page*

Epinal® see Epinephrine *on this page*

Epinephrine (ep i nef' rin)

Related Information
Adrenergic Agonists, Cardiovascular Comparison *on page 1242*
Extravasation Treatment of Other Drugs *on page 1209*
Glaucoma Drug Therapy Comparison *on page 1270*

Brand Names Adrenalin®; AsthmaHaler®; AsthmaNefrin® [OTC]; Bronitin®; Bronkaid® Mist [OTC]; Epifrin®; Epinal®; EpiPen®; EpiPen® Jr; Epitrate®; Eppy/N®; Glaucon®; Medihaler-Epi®; microNefrin®; Primatene® Mist [OTC]; Sus-Phrine®; Vaponefrin®

Synonyms Adrenaline; Epinephrine Bitartrate; Epinephrine Hydrochloride; Levoepinephrine; Racemic Epinephrine

Use Treatment of bronchospasms, anaphylactic reactions, cardiac arrest, management of open-angle (chronic simple) glaucoma

Pregnancy Risk Factor C

Contraindications Hypersensitivity to epinephrine or any component; cardiac arrhythmias, angle-closure glaucoma

Warnings/Precautions Use with caution in elderly patients, patients with diabetes mellitus, cardiovascular diseases (angina, tachycardia, myocardial infarction), thyroid disease, or cerebral arteriosclerosis, Parkinson's; some products contain sulfites as preservatives. Rapid I.V. infusion may cause death from cerebrovascular hemorrhage or cardiac arrhythmias. Oral inhalation of epinephrine is **not** the preferred route of administration.

Adverse Reactions
>10%:
Cardiovascular: Tachycardia (parenteral), pounding heartbeat
Central nervous system: Nervousness, restlessness
1% to 10%:
Cardiovascular: Flushing, hypertension
Central nervous system: Headache, dizziness, lightheadedness, insomnia
Gastrointestinal: Nausea, vomiting
Neuromuscular & skeletal: Weakness, trembling
Miscellaneous: Increased sweating, unusual paleness
(Continued)

389

Epinephrine *(Continued)*

<1%:

Cardiovascular: Pallor, tachycardia, hypertension, chest pain, increased myocardial oxygen consumption, cardiac arrhythmias, sudden death

Central nervous system: Anxiety

Gastrointestinal: Dry mouth or throat

Genitourinary: Decreased renal and splanchnic blood flow, acute urinary retention in patients with bladder outflow obstruction

Ocular: Precipitation of or exacerbation of narrow-angle glaucoma

Respiratory: Wheezing

Overdosage/Toxicology Hypertension which may result in subarachnoid hemorrhage and hemiplegia; symptoms of overdose include arrhythmias, unusually large pupils, pulmonary edema, renal failure, metabolic acidosis

There is no specific antidote for epinephrine intoxication and the bulk of the treatment is supportive. Hyperactivity and agitation usually respond to reduced sensory input; however, with extreme agitation, haloperidol (2-5 mg I.M. for adults) may be required. Hyperthermia is best treated with external cooling measures; or when severe or unresponsive, muscle paralysis with pancuronium may be needed. Hypertension is usually transient and generally does not require treatment unless severe. For diastolic blood pressures >110 mm Hg, a nitroprusside infusion should be initiated. Seizures usually respond to diazepam I.V. and/or phenytoin maintenance regimens.

Drug Interactions Increased toxicity: Increased cardiac irritability if administered concurrently with halogenated inhalational anesthetics, beta-blocking agents, alpha-blocking agents

Stability

Epinephrine is sensitive to light and air; protection from light is recommended

Oxidation turns drug pink, then a brown color; **solutions should not be used if they are discolored or contain a precipitate**

Stability of injection of parenteral admixture at room temperature (25°C) or refrigeration (4°C): 24 hours

Standard diluent: 1 mg/250 mL NS

Compatible with dopamine, dobutamine, diltiazem

Incompatible with aminophylline, sodium bicarbonate or other alkaline solutions

Mechanism of Action Stimulates alpha-, beta$_1$-, and beta$_2$-adrenergic receptors resulting in relaxation of smooth muscle of the bronchial tree, cardiac stimulation, and dilation of skeletal muscle vasculature; small doses can cause vasodilation via beta$_2$-vascular receptors; large doses may produce constriction of skeletal and vascular smooth muscle; decreases production of aqueous humor and increases aqueous outflow; dilates the pupil by contracting the dilator muscle

Pharmacodynamics/Kinetics

Onset of bronchodilation:

Subcutaneous: Within 5-10 minutes

Inhalation: Within 1 minute

Conjunctival instillation:

Onset of effect: Intraocular pressures fall within 1 hour

Peak effect: Within 4-8 hours

Duration of ocular effect: 12-24 hours

Absorption: Orally ingested doses are rapidly metabolized in the GI tract and liver; pharmacologically active concentrations are not achieved

Distribution: Crosses the placenta; appears in breast milk

Metabolism: Following administration, drug is taken up into the adrenergic neuron and metabolized by monoamine oxidase and catechol-o-methyltransferase; circulating drug is metabolized in the liver

Elimination: Inactive metabolites (metanephrine and the sulfate and hydroxy derivatives of mandelic acid) and a small amount of unchanged drug is excreted in urine

Usual Dosage

Bronchodilator:

Children: S.C.: 10 mcg/kg (0.01 mL/kg of 1:1000) (single doses not to exceed 0.5 mg); injection suspension (1:200): 0.005 mL/kg/dose (0.025 mg/kg/dose) to a maximum of 0.15 mL (0.75 mg for single dose) every 8-12 hours

Adults:

I.M., S.C. (1:1000): 0.1-0.5 mg every 10-15 minutes to 4 hours

Suspension (1:200) S.C.: 0.1-0.3 mL (0.5-1.5 mg)

I.V.: 0.1-0.25 mg (single dose maximum: 1 mg)

Cardiac arrest:

Neonates: I.V. or intratracheal: 0.01-0.03 mg/kg (0.1-0.3 mL/kg of 1:10,000 solution) every 3-5 minutes as needed; dilute intratracheal doses in 1-2 mL of normal saline

Infants and Children: Asystole or pulseless arrest:
  I.V., intraosseous: First dose: 0.01 mg/kg (0.1 mL/kg of a 1:10,000 solution); subsequent doses: 0.1 mg/kg (0.1 mL/kg of a 1:1000 solution); doses as high as 0.2 mg/kg may be effective; repeat every 3-5 minutes
  Intratracheal: 0.1 mg/kg (0.1 mL/kg of a 1:1000 solution); doses as high as 0.2 mg/kg may be effective

Adults: Asystole:
  I.V.: 1 mg every 3-5 minutes; if this approach fails, alternative regimens include: Intermediate: 2-5 mg every 3-5 minutes; Escalating: 1 mg, 3 mg, 5 mg at 3-minute intervals; High: 0.1 mg/kg every 3-5 minutes
  Intratracheal: Although optimal dose is unknown, doses of 2-2.5 times the I.V. dose may be needed

Bradycardia: Children:
  I.V.: 0.01 mg/kg (0.1 mL/kg of 1:10,000 solution) every 3-5 minutes as needed (maximum: 1 mg/10 mL)
  Intratracheal: 0.1 mg/kg (0.1 mL/kg of 1:1000 solution every 3-5 minutes); doses as high as 0.2 mg/kg may be effective

Refractory hypotension (refractory to dopamine/dobutamine): I.V. infusion administration requires the use of an infusion pump:
  Children: Infusion rate 0.1-4 mcg/kg/minute
  Adults: I.V. infusion: 1 mg in 250 mL NS/D$_5$W at 0.1-1 mcg/kg/minute; titrate to desired effect

Hypersensitivity reaction:
  Children: S.C.: 0.01 mg/kg every 15 minutes for 2 doses then every 4 hours as needed (single doses not to exceed 0.5 mg)
  Adults: I.M., S.C.: 0.2-0.5 mg every 20 minutes to 4 hours (single dose maximum: 1 mg)

Nebulization:
  Children <2 years: 0.25 mL of 1:1000 diluted in 3 mL NS with treatments ordered individually
  Children >2 years and Adolescents: 0.5 mL of 1:1000 concentration diluted in 3 mL NS
  Children >2 years and Adults (racemic epinephrine):
    <10 kg: 2 mL of 1:8 dilution over 15 minutes every 1-4 hours
    10-15 kg: 2 mL of 1:6 dilution over 15 minutes every 1-4 hours
    15-20 kg: 2 mL of 1:4 dilution over 15 minutes every 1-4 hours
    >20 kg: 2 mL of 1:3 dilution over 15 minutes every 1-4 hours
  Adults: Instill 8-15 drops into nebulizer reservoirs; administer 1-3 inhalations 4-6 times/day

Ophthalmic: Instill 1-2 drops in eye(s) once or twice daily

Intranasal: Children ≥6 years and Adults: Apply locally as drops or spray or with sterile swab
Administration Central line administration only; intravenous infusions require an infusion pump
  Endotracheal: Doses (2-2.5 times the I.V. dose) should be diluted to 10 mL with NS or distilled water prior to administration
  Epinephrine can be administered S.C., I.M., I.V., or intracardiac injection
  I.M. administration into the buttocks should be avoided

Desired pediatric intravenous infusion solution preparation: "RULE OF 6"
  Simplified equation: 0.6 x weight (kg) = amount (mg) of drug to be added to 100 mL of I.V. fluid
    When infused at 1 mL/hour, then it will deliver the drug at a rate of 0.1 mcg/kg/minute
  Complex equation: 0.6 x desired dose (mcg/kg/minute) x body weight (kg) divided by desired rate (mL/hour) is the mg added to make 100 mL of solution
  Preparation of adult I.V. infusion: Dilute 1 mg in 250 mL of D$_5$W or NS (4 mcg/mL); administer at an initial rate of 1 mcg/minute and increase to desired effects; at 20 mcg/minute pure alpha effects occur
    1 mcg/minute: 15 mL/hour
    2 mcg/minute: 30 mL/hour
    3 mcg/minute: 45 mL/hour, etc
Monitoring Parameters Pulmonary function, heart rate, blood pressure, site of infusion for blanching, extravasation; cardiac monitor and blood pressure monitor required
Reference Range Therapeutic: 31-95 pg/mL (SI: 170-520 pmol/L)
Test Interactions ↑ bilirubin (S), catecholamines (U), glucose, uric acid (S)
(Continued)

Epinephrine *(Continued)*

Nursing Implications Patients should be cautioned to avoid the use of over-the-counter epinephrine inhalation products; beta$_2$-adrenergic agents for inhalation are preferred

Management of extravasation: Use phentolamine as antidote; mix 5 mg with 9 mL of NS; inject a small amount of this dilution into extravasated area; blanching should reverse immediately. Monitor site; if blanching should recur, additional injections of phentolamine may be needed.

Additional Information
Epinephrine: Primatene® Mist, Bronkaid® Mist, Sus-Phrine®
Epinephrine bitartrate: AsthmaHaler®, Bronitin®, Epitrate®, Medihaler-Epi®; Primatene® Mist
Epinephrine hydrochloride: Adrenalin®, Epifrin®, EpiPen®, EpiPen® Jr
Racemic epinephrine: AsthmaHaler®, Breatheasy®, microNefrin®, Vaponefrin®
Epinephryl borate: Epinal®

Dosage Forms
Aerosol, oral:
Bitartrate (AsthmaHaler®, Bronitin®, Medihaler-Epi®, Primatene® Suspension): 0.3 mg/spray [epinephrine base 0.16 mg/spray] (10 mL, 15 mL, 22.5 mL)
Bronkaid®: 0.5% (10 mL, 15 mL, 22.5 mL)
Primatene®: 0.2 mg/spray (15 mL, 22.5 mL)
Auto-injector:
EpiPen®: Delivers 0.3 mg I.M. of epinephrine 1:1000 (2 mL)
EpiPen® Jr.: Delivers 0.15 mg I.M. of epinephrine 1:2000 (2 mL)
Solution:
Inhalation:
Adrenalin®: 1% [10 mg/mL, 1:100] (7.5 mL)
AsthmaNefrin®, microNefrin®, Nephron®, S-2®: Racepinephrine 2% [epinephrine base 1.125%] (7.5 mL, 15 mL, 30 mL)
Vaponefrin®: Racepinephrine 2% [epinephrine base 1%] (15 mL, 30 mL)
Injection:
Adrenalin®: 0.01 mg/mL [1:100,000] (5 mL); 0.1 mg/mL [1:10,000] (3 mL, 10 mL); 1 mg/mL [1:1000] (1 mL, 2 mL, 30 mL)
Suspension (Sus-Phrine®): 5 mg/mL [1:200] (0.3 mL, 5 mL)
Nasal (Adrenalin®): 0.1% [1 mg/mL, 1:1000] (30 mL)
Ophthalmic, as borate (Epinal®, Eppy/N®): 0.5% (7.5 mL); 1% (7.5 mL); 2% (7.5 mL)
Ophthalmic, as hydrochloride (Epifrin®, Glaucon®): 0.1% (1 mL, 30 mL); 0.25% (15 mL); 0.5% (15 mL); 1% (1 mL, 10 mL, 15 mL); 2% (10 mL, 15 mL)
Topical (Adrenalin®): 0.1% [1 mg/mL, 1:1000] (30 mL, 10 mL)

Epinephrine Bitartrate *see* Epinephrine *on page 389*

Epinephrine Hydrochloride *see* Epinephrine *on page 389*

EpiPen® *see* Epinephrine *on page 389*

EpiPen® Jr *see* Epinephrine *on page 389*

Epipodophyllotoxin *see* Etoposide *on page 434*

Epitol® *see* Carbamazepine *on page 177*

Epitrate® *see* Epinephrine *on page 389*

EPO *see* Epoetin Alfa *on this page*

Epoetin Alfa *(e poe' e tin al' fa)*

Brand Names Epogen®; ProCrit®
Synonyms EPO; Erythropoietin; rHuEPO-α
Use
Anemia associated with end stage renal disease (FDA-approved indication)
Anemia related to AIDS and therapy with AZT-treated in HIV-infected patients (FDA-approved indication)
Endogenous serum erythropoietin (EPO) level which are inappropriately low for hemoglobin level (eg, anemia of neoplasia); (FDA-approved indication)
Patients undergoing autologous blood donation prior to surgery - EPO may accelerate recovery of hemoglobin level and, in some cases, permit more units of blood to be donated
HuEPO is not beneficial in the acute treatment of anemia (onset of reticulocyte response does not appear until 7-10 days and hemoglobin rise appears over 2-6 weeks after starting therapy). Therefore, emergency/stat orders for the drug are not appropriate.
Pregnancy Risk Factor C

Pregnancy/Breast Feeding Implications Epoetin alpha has been shown to have adverse effects in rats when given in doses 5X the human dose. There are no adequate and well-controlled studies in pregnant women. Epoetin alpha should be used only if potential benefit justifies the potential risk to the fetus.

Contraindications Known hypersensitivity to albumin (human) or mammalian cell-derived products; uncontrolled hypertension

Warnings/Precautions Use with caution in patients with porphyria, hypertension, or a history of seizures; prior to and during therapy, iron stores must be evaluated

Pretherapy parameters:

Serum ferritin >100 ng/dL

Transferrin saturation (serum iron/iron binding capacity x 100) >20%

Iron supplementation (usual oral dosing of 325 mg of ferrous sulfate 2-3 times/day) should be given during therapy to provide for increased requirements during expansion of the red cell mass secondary to marrow stimulation by EPO

For patients with endogenous serum EPO levels which are inappropriately low for hemoglobin level, documentation of the serum EPO level will help indicate which patients may benefit from EPO therapy

If the patient fails to respond or to maintain a response to doses within the recommended dosing range, the following etiologies should be considered:

iron deficiency: all patients will require supplemental iron therapy

underlying infectious, inflammatory, or malignant processes

occult blood loss

underlying hematologic diseases (ie, thalassemia, refractory anemia, myelodysplastic disorders)

hemolysis

aluminum intoxication

osteitis fibrosa cystica

Adverse Reactions

1% to 10%:

Cardiovascular: Hypertension, chest pain, edema

Central nervous system: Fatigue, headache, asthenia, dizziness, seizures

Dermatologic: Rash

Gastrointestinal: Nausea, vomiting, diarrhea

Hematologic: Clotted access

Neuromuscular & skeletal: Arthralgias

<1%:

Cardiovascular: Myocardial infarction, CVA/TIA

Sensitivity reactions: Hypersensitivity reactions

Overdosage/Toxicology Symptoms of overdose include polycythemia; management includes adequate airway and other supportive measures; if polycythemia is of concern, phlebotomy may be indicated to decrease the hematocrit

Stability

Vials should be stored at 2°C to 8°C (36°F to 46°F); **do not freeze or shake**; vials are stable 2 weeks at room temperature

Single-dose 1 mL vial contains no preservative: Use one dose per vial; do not re-enter vial; discard unused portions

Multidose 2 mL vial contains preservative; store at 2°C to 8°C after initial entry and between doses; discard 21 days after initial entry

For minimal dilution: Mix with bacteriostatic 0.9% sodium chloride, containing 20 mL of 0.9% sodium chloride and benzyl alcohol as the bacteriostatic agent; dilutions of 1:10 and 1:20 (1 part epoetin:19 parts sodium chloride) are stable for 18 hours at room temperature; results showed no loss of epoetin alfa after a 1:20 dilution; 250 mcg/mL albumin remaining after a 1:10 dilution of formulated epoetin alfa should be sufficient to prevent it from binding to commonly encountered containers

Mechanism of Action Induces erythropoiesis by stimulating the division and differentiation of committed erythroid progenitor cells; induces the release of reticulocytes from the bone marrow into the blood stream, where they mature to erythrocytes. There is a dose response relationship with this effect. This results in an increase in reticulocyte counts followed by a rise in hematocrit and hemoglobin levels.

Pharmacodynamics/Kinetics

Onset of action: Several days

Peak effect: 2-3 weeks

Distribution: V_d: 9 L; rapid in the plasma compartment; majority of drug is taken up by the liver, kidneys, and bone marrow

Metabolism: Some metabolic degradation does occur

Bioavailability: S.C.: ~21% to 31%; intraperitoneal epoetin in a few patients demonstrated a bioavailability of only 3%

(Continued)

393

Epoetin Alfa (Continued)

Half-life: Circulating: 4-13 hours in patients with chronic renal failure; 20% shorter in patients with normal renal function

Time to peak serum concentrations: S.C.: 2-8 hours

Elimination: Small amounts recovered in the urine; majority hepatically eliminated; 10% excreted unchanged in the urine of normal volunteers

Usual Dosage

Individuals with anemia due to iron deficiency, sickle cell disease, autoimmune hemolytic anemia, and bleeding, generally have appropriate endogenous EPO levels to drive erythropoiesis and would not ordinarily be candidates for EPO therapy.

In patients on dialysis, epoetin alfa usually has been administered as an IVP 3 times/week. While the administration is independent of the dialysis procedure, it may be administered into the venous line at the end of the dialysis procedure to obviate the need for additional venous access; in patients with CRF not on dialysis, epoetin alfa may be given either as an IVP or S.C. injection.

Neonates: Anemia of prematurity: S.C.: 25-100 units/kg/dose 3 times/week

Children/Adults: Dosing recommendations:

Dosing schedules need to be individualized and careful monitoring of patients receiving the drug is mandatory

rHuEPO-α may be ineffective if other factors such as iron or B_{12}/folate deficiency limit marrow response

IVP, S.C.:

Chronic renal failure patients:

Initial dose: 50-100 units/kg 3 times/week

Dose should be reduced when the hematocrit reaches the target range of 30% to 36% or a hematocrit increase >4% points over any 2-week period

Dose should be held if the hematocrit exceeds 36% and until the hematocrit decreases to the target range (30% to 36%).

Dose should be increased not more frequently than once a month, unless clinically indicated. After any dose adjustment, the hematocrit should be determined twice weekly for at least 2-6 weeks. If a hematocrit increase of 5-6 points is not achieved after a 8-week period and iron stores are adequate, the dose may be incrementally increased. Further increases may be made at 4-6 week intervals until the desired response is obtained.

Maintenance dose: Should be individualized to maintain the hematocrit within the 30% to 33% target range. The median maintenance dose in phase III studies in chronic renal failure patients on dialysis was 75 units/kg three times weekly (range 12.5-525 units/kg 3 times/week).

Epoetin doses of 75-150 units/kg/week have been shown to maintain hematocrits of 36% to 38% for up to 6 months in patients with chronic renal failure not requiring dialysis

Zidovudine-treated HIV patients: Prior to beginning epoetin alpha, serum erythropoietin levels should be determined. Available evidence suggest that patients receiving zidovudine with endogenous serum erythropoietin levels >500 milliunits/mL are unlikely to respond to therapy with epoetin alpha.

Initial dose: For patients with serum erythropoietin levels <500 milliunits/mL who are receiving a dose of zidovudine ≤4,200 mg/week: 100 units/kg three times weekly for 8 weeks.

Dose should be held: if the hematocrit is >40% until the hematocrit drops to 36%. The dose should be reduced by 25% when the treatment is resumed and then titrated to maintain the desired hematocrit.

Dose should be reduced: if the initial dose of epoetin alpha includes a rapid rise in hematocrit (>4% points in any 2-week period).

Increase dose: by 50-100 units/kg if the response is not satisfactory in terms of reducing transfusion requirements or increasing hematocrit after 8 weeks of therapy. Response should be evaluated every 4-8 weeks thereafter and the dose adjusted and the dose adjusted accordingly by 50-100 units/kg increments three times weekly. If patients have not responded satisfactorily to a dose of 300 units/kg three times weekly, it is unlikely that they will respond to higher doses.

Maintenance dose: Dose should be titrated to maintain target hematocrit range: 36% to 40%

Cancer patients on chemotherapy: Although no specific serum erythropoietin level can be stipulated above which patients would be unlikely to respond to epoetin alpha therapy, treatment of patients with grossly elevated serum erythropoietin levels (>200 milliunits/mL) is not recommended

Initial dose: 150 units/kg 3 times/week

Increase dose: Response should be evaluated every 8 weeks thereafter and the dose adjusted and the dose adjusted accordingly by 50-100 units/kg increments three times weekly up to 300 units/kg three times weekly if the response is not satisfactory. If patients have not responded satisfactorily to a dose of 300 units/kg three times weekly, it is unlikely that they will respond to higher doses.

Dose should be held: if the hematocrit is >40% until the hematocrit drops to 36%. The dose should be reduced by 25% when the treatment is resumed and then titrated to maintain the desired hematocrit.

Dose should be reduced: if the initial dose of epoetin alpha includes a rapid rise in hematocrit (>4% points in any 2-week period), the dose should be reduced

Maintenance dose: Dose should be titrated to maintain target hematocrit range: 36% to 40%

Monitoring Parameters

Careful monitoring of blood pressure is indicated; problems with hypertension have been noted in renal failure patients treated with rHuEPO-α. Other patients are less likely to develop this complication.

Follow serum ferritin and serum transferrin saturation monthly. During epoetin alpha therapy, absolute or functional iron deficiency may develop. Transferrin saturation should be at least 20% and ferritin should be at least 100 ng/mL. All patients will eventually require supplementation to increase or maintain transferrin saturation to levels which will adequately support erythropoiesis.

Hematocrit should be determined twice weekly until stabilization within the target range (30% to 36%), and twice weekly at least 2 to 6 weeks after a dose increase; the hematocrit should then be monitored at regular intervals

CBC with differential and platelet count should be monitored regularly

In patients with chronic renal failure, serum chemistry values (BUN, uric acid, creatinine, phosphorus, and potassium) should be monitored regularly

Reference Range Guidelines should be based on the following chart or published literature

Guidelines for estimating appropriateness of endogenous EPO levels for varying levels of anemia via the EIA assay method: See figure. The reference range for erythropoietin in serum, for subjects with normal hemoglobin and hematocrit, is 4.1-22.2 mIU/mL by the EIA method. Erythropoietin levels are typically inversely related to hemoglobin (and hematocrit) levels in anemias not attributed to impaired erythropoietin production.

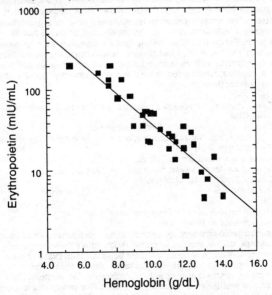

Zidovudine-treated HIV patients: Available evidence indicates patients with endogenous serum erythropoietin levels >500 mIU/mL are unlikely to respond

Cancer chemotherapy patients: Treatment of patients with endogenous serum erythropoietin levels >200 mIU/mL is not recommended

Patient Information

If necessary, the patient should be instructed as to the proper dosage and self-administration of epoetin alpha

(Continued)

Epoetin Alfa (Continued)

Frequent blood tests are needed to determine the correct dose; notify physician if any severe headache develops

Additional Information

Reimbursement Hotline (Epogen®): 1-800-272-9376
Professional Services [Amgen]: 1-800-77-AMGEN
Reimbursement Hotline (Procrit®):
   1-800-553-3851
   1-800-447-3437 Financial Assistance Program
   1-800-441-1366 Cost Sharing Program
Professional services [Ortho Biotech]: 1-800-325-7504

Dosage Forms

1 mL single-dose vials: Preservative-free solution
   2000 units/mL
   3000 units/mL
   4000 units/mL
   10,000 units/mL
2 mL multidose vials: Preserved solution: 10,000 units/mL

Epogen® see Epoetin Alfa on page 392

Eppy/N® see Epinephrine on page 389

Epsom Salts see Magnesium Sulfate on page 661

EPT see Teniposide on page 1057

Equalactin® Chewable Tablet [OTC] see Calcium Polycarbophil on page 172

Equanil® see Meprobamate on page 689

Ercaf® see Ergotamine on page 399

Ergamisol® see Levamisole Hydrochloride on page 622

Ergocalciferol (er goe kal sif' e role)

Brand Names Calciferol™; Drisdol®
Synonyms Activated Ergosterol; Viosterol; Vitamin D_2
Use Treatment of refractory rickets, hypophosphatemia, hypoparathyroidism
Pregnancy Risk Factor A (C if dose exceeds RDA recommendation)
Contraindications Hypercalcemia, hypersensitivity to ergocalciferol or any component; malabsorption syndrome; evidence of vitamin D toxicity
Warnings/Precautions Administer with extreme caution in patients with impaired renal function, heart disease, renal stones, or arteriosclerosis; must give concomitant calcium supplementation; maintain adequate fluid intake; avoid hypercalcemia; renal function impairment with secondary hyperparathyroidism

Adverse Reactions

1% to 10%:
   Cardiovascular: Hypotension, cardiac arrhythmias, hypertension, irregular heartbeat
   Central nervous system: Irritability, headache
   Gastrointestinal: Nausea, vomiting, anorexia, pancreatitis, metallic taste
   Dermatologic: Pruritus
   Endocrine & metabolic: Polydipsia
   Neuromuscular & skeletal: Bone pain, muscle pain
   Ocular: Conjunctivitis, photophobia
   Renal: Polyuria
<1%:
   Central nervous system: Overt psychosis
   Gastrointestinal: Weight loss

Overdosage/Toxicology Symptoms of chronic overdose include hypercalcemia, weakness, fatigue, lethargy, anorexia. Following withdrawal of the drug and oral decontamination, treatment consists of bedrest, liberal intake of fluids, reduced calcium intake, and cathartic administration. Severe hypercalcemia requires I.V. hydration and forced diuresis with I.V. furosemide. Urine output should be monitored and maintained at >3 mL/kg/hour. I.V. saline can quickly and significantly increase excretion of calcium into urine. Calcitonin, mithramycin, and biphosphonates have all been used successfully to treat the more resistant cases of vitamin D-induced hypercalcemia.

Drug Interactions

Decreased effect: Cholestyramine, colestipol, mineral oil → ↓ oral absorption
Increased effect: Thiazide diuretics → ↑ vitamin D effects
Increased toxicity: Cardiac glycosides → ↑ toxicity
Stability Protect from light

Mechanism of Action Stimulates calcium and phosphate absorption from the small intestine, promotes secretion of calcium from bone to blood; promotes renal tubule phosphate resorption

Pharmacodynamics/Kinetics

Peak effect: In ~1 month following daily doses

Absorption: Readily absorbed from GI tract; absorption requires intestinal presence of bile

Metabolism: Inactive until hydroxylated in the liver and the kidney to calcifediol and then to calcitriol (most active form)

Usual Dosage Oral dosing is preferred

Dietary supplementation (each mcg = 40 USP units):

Premature infants: 10-20 mcg/day (400-800 units), up to 750 mcg/day (30,000 units)

Infants and healthy Children: 10 mcg/day (400 units)

Adults: 10 mcg/day (400 units)

Renal failure:

Children: 100-1000 mcg/day (4000-40,000 units)

Adults: 500 mcg/day (20,000 units)

Hypoparathyroidism:

Children: 1.25-5 mg/day (50,000-200,000 units) and calcium supplements

Adults: 625 mcg to 5 mg/day (25,000-200,000 units) and calcium supplements

Vitamin D-dependent rickets:

Children: 75-125 mcg/day (3000-5000 units); maximum: 1500 mcg/day

Adults: 250 mcg to 1.5 mg/day (10,000-60,000 units)

Nutritional rickets and osteomalacia:

Children and Adults (with normal absorption): 25-125 mcg/day (1000-5000 units)

Children with malabsorption: 250-625 mcg/day (10,000-25,000 units)

Adults with malabsorption: 250-7500 mcg (10,000-300,000 units)

Vitamin D-resistant rickets:

Children: Initial: 1000-2000 mcg/day (400,000-800,000 units) with phosphate supplements; daily dosage is increased at 3- to 4-month intervals in 250-500 mcg (10,000-20,000 units) increments

Adults: 250-1500 mcg/day (10,000-60,000 units) with phosphate supplements

Administration Parenteral injection for I.M. use only

Monitoring Parameters Measure serum calcium, BUN, and phosphorus every 1-2 weeks

Reference Range Serum calcium times phosphorus should not exceed 70 mg/dL to avoid ectopic calcification; ergocalciferol levels: 10-60 ng/mL; serum calcium: 9-10 mg/dL, phosphorus: 2.5-5 mg/dL

Patient Information Early symptoms of hypercalcemia include weakness, fatigue, somnolence, headache, anorexia, dry mouth, metallic taste, nausea, vomiting, cramps, diarrhea, muscle pain, bone pain, and irritability. Your physician may place you on a special diet or have you take a calcium supplement. Follow this diet closely; do not take magnesium supplements or magnesium-containing antacids.

Nursing Implications Monitor serum calcium, phosphorus, and BUN every 2 weeks

Additional Information 1.25 mg ergocalciferol provides 50,000 units of vitamin D activity

Dosage Forms

Capsule (Drisdol®): 50,000 units [1.25 mg]

Injection (Calciferol™): 500,000 units/mL [12.5 mg/mL] (1 mL)

Liquid (Calciferol™, Drisdol®): 8000 units/mL [200 mcg/mL] (60 mL)

Tablet (Calciferol™): 50,000 units [1.25 mg]

Ergoloid Mesylates (er′ goe loyd mess′ i lates)

Brand Names Germinal®; Hydergine®; Hydergine® LC; Hydro-Ergoloid®; Niloric®

Synonyms Dihydroergotoxine; Hydrogenated Ergot Alkaloids

Use Treatment of cerebrovascular insufficiency in primary progressive dementia, Alzheimer's dementia, and senile onset

Pregnancy Risk Factor C

Contraindications Acute or chronic psychosis, hypersensitivity to ergot or any component

Warnings/Precautions Exclude possibility that signs and symptoms of illness are from a potentially and treatable condition

Adverse Reactions

1% to 10%:

Gastrointestinal: Transient nausea

Miscellaneous: Sublingual irritation

(Continued)

Ergoloid Mesylates *(Continued)*

<1%:
Cardiovascular: Bradycardia, orthostatic hypotension
Central nervous system: Fainting, flushing, headache
Dermatologic: Skin rash
Gastrointestinal: Anorexia, nausea, vomiting, stomach cramps
Ocular: Blurred vision
Respiratory: Stuffy nose

Overdosage/Toxicology Symptoms of overdose include sinus bradycardia, blurred vision, headache, stomach cramps; chronic overdose usually manifests as signs and symptoms of extremity or organ ischemia; nitroprusside has been shown to reverse the vasoconstriction associated with ergot toxicity

Drug Interactions Increased toxicity with dopamine

Mechanism of Action Ergot alkaloid alpha-adrenergic agonist directly stimulates vascular smooth muscle to vasoconstrict peripheral and cerebral vessels; may also have antagonist effects on serotonin

Pharmacodynamics/Kinetics
Absorption: Rapid yet incomplete
Metabolism: Significant first-pass metabolism
Half-life: 3.5 hours
Time to peak serum concentration: Within 1 hour

Usual Dosage Adults: Oral: 1 mg 3 times/day up to 4.5-12 mg/day; up to 6 months of therapy may be necessary

Monitoring Parameters Blood pressure, heart rate

Patient Information Do not chew or crush sublingual tablets, allow to dissolve under tongue

Dosage Forms
Capsule, liquid (Hydergine® LC): 1 mg
Liquid (Hydergine®): 1 mg/mL (100 mL)
Tablet:
Oral:
0.5 mg
Gerimal®, Hydergine®: 1 mg
Sublingual:
Gerimal®, Hydergine®: 0.5 mg
Gerimal®, Hydergine®, Niloric®: 1 mg

Ergometrine Maleate *see* Ergonovine Maleate *on this page*

Ergonovine Maleate (er goe noe' veen)

Brand Names Ergotrate® Maleate

Synonyms Ergometrine Maleate

Use Prevention and treatment of postpartum and postabortion hemorrhage caused by uterine atony or subinvolution

Pregnancy Risk Factor X

Contraindications Induction of labor, threatened spontaneous abortion, hypersensitivity to ergonovine or any component

Warnings/Precautions Use with caution in patients with sepsis or with hepatic or renal impairment

Adverse Reactions
1% to 10%: Gastrointestinal: Nausea, vomiting
<1%:
Cardiovascular: Palpitations, bradycardia, transient chest pain, hypertension, cerebrovascular accidents
Central nervous system: Seizures, dizziness, headache
Local: Thrombophlebitis
Otic: Tinnitus
Respiratory: Dyspnea
Miscellaneous: Diaphoresis

Overdosage/Toxicology Symptoms of overdose include gangrene, seizures, chest pain, numbness in extremities, weak pulse, confusion, excitement, delirium, hallucinations; treatment is supportive. Diazepam 0.1 mg/kg for seizures and excitement; haloperidol as needed for delirium or hallucinations; heparin for hypercoagulability; nitroprusside for arterial venospasm; nitroglycerin for coronary vasospasm

Stability Refrigerate injection, protect from light; store intact ampuls in refrigerator, stable for 60-90 days; do not use if discoloration occurs

Mechanism of Action Ergot alkaloid alpha-adrenergic agonist directly stimulates vascular smooth muscle to vasoconstrict peripheral and cerebral vessels; may also have antagonist effects on serotonin

Pharmacodynamics/Kinetics
Onset of effect:
Oral: Within 5-15 minutes
I.M.: Within 2-5 minutes
Duration: Uterine effects persist for 3 hours, except when given I.V., then effects persist for ~45 minutes

Usual Dosage Adults:
Oral: 1-2 tablets (0.2-0.4 mg) every 6-12 hours for up to 48 hours
I.M., I.V. (I.V. should be reserved for emergency use only): 0.2 mg, repeat dose in 2-4 hours as needed

Administration I.V. doses should be administered over a period of not <1 minute; dilute in NS to 5 mL for I.V. administration

Patient Information May cause nausea, vomiting, dizziness, increased blood pressure, headache, ringing in the ears, chest pain, or shortness of breath

Nursing Implications I.V. use should be limited to patients with severe uterine bleeding or other life-threatening emergency situations

Dosage Forms Injection: 0.2 mg/mL (1 mL)

Ergostat® *see* Ergotamine *on this page*

Ergotamine (er got' a meen)

Brand Names Bellergal-S®; Cafatine®; Cafatine-PB®; Cafergot®; Cafetrate®; Ercaf®; Ergostat®; Medihaler Ergotamine™; Wigraine®

Use Abort or prevent vascular headaches, such as migraine or cluster

Pregnancy Risk Factor X

Contraindications Hypersensitivity to ergotamine, caffeine, or any component; peripheral vascular disease, hepatic or renal disease, hypertension, peptic ulcer disease, sepsis; avoid during pregnancy

Warnings/Precautions Avoid prolonged administration or excessive dosage because of the danger of ergotism and gangrene; patients who take ergotamine for extended periods of time may become dependent on it. May be harmful due to reduction in cerebral blood flow; may precipitate angina, myocardial infarction, or aggravate intermittent claudication; therefore, not considered a drug of choice in the elderly.

Adverse Reactions
>10%:
Cardiovascular: Tachycardia, bradycardia, arterial spasm, claudication and vasoconstriction; rebound headache may occur with sudden withdrawal of the drug in patients on prolonged therapy; localized edema, peripheral vascular effects (numbness and tingling of fingers and toes)
Central nervous system: Drowsiness, dizziness
Gastrointestinal: Nausea, vomiting, diarrhea, dry mouth
1% to 10%:
Cardiovascular: Transient tachycardia or bradycardia, precordial distress and pain
Neuromuscular & skeletal: Weakness in the legs, abdominal or muscle pain, muscle pains in the extremities, paresthesia

Overdosage/Toxicology Symptoms include vasospastic effects, nausea, vomiting, lassitude, impaired mental function, hypotension, hypertension, unconsciousness, seizures, shock, and death. Treatment includes general supportive therapy, gastric lavage, or induction of emesis, activated charcoal, saline cathartic; keep extremities warm. Activated charcoal is effective at binding certain chemicals, and this is especially true for ergot alkaloids; treatment is symptomatic with heparin, vasodilators (nitroprusside); vasodilators should be used with caution to avoid exaggerating any pre-existing hypotension.

Drug Interactions Increased toxicity:
Propranolol: One case of severe vasoconstriction with pain and cyanosis has been reported
Erythromycin, troleandomycin and other macrolide antibiotics: Monitor for signs of ergot toxicity

Mechanism of Action Ergot alkaloid alpha-adrenergic blocker directly stimulates vascular smooth muscle to vasoconstrict peripheral and cerebral vessels; also has antagonist effects on serotonin

Pharmacodynamics/Kinetics
Absorption: Oral, rectal: Erratic; enhanced by caffeine coadministration
Metabolism: Extensively in the liver
Bioavailability: Poor overall (<5%)
Time to peak serum concentration: Within 0.5-3 hours following co-administration with caffeine
Elimination: In bile as metabolites (90%)

Usual Dosage Adults:
(Continued)

Ergotamine *(Continued)*

Oral:

Cafergot®: 2 tablets at onset of attack; then 1 tablet every 30 minutes as needed; maximum: 6 tablets per attack; do not exceed 10 tablets/week

Ergostat®: 1 tablet under tongue at first sign, then 1 tablet every 30 minutes, 3 tablets/24 hours, 5 tablets/week

Rectal (Cafergot® suppositories, Wigraine® suppositories, Cafergot P-B suppositories): 1 at first sign of an attack; follow with second dose after 1 hour, if needed; maximum dose: 2 per attack; do not exceed 5/week

Inhalation: Initial: 1 inhalation, followed by repeat inhalations 5 minutes apart to a maximum of 6 inhalations/24 hours or 15 inhalations/1 week

Patient Information Any symptoms such as nausea, vomiting, numbness or tingling, and chest, muscle, or abdominal pain should be reported to the physician. Initiate therapy at first sign of attack. Do **not** exceed recommended dosage.

Nursing Implications Do not crush sublingual drug product

Additional Information

Ergotamine tartrate: Ergostat®

Ergotamine tartrate and caffeine: Cafergot®

Dosage Forms

Aerosol, oral (Medihaler Ergotamine™): Ergotamine tartrate 360 mcg/metered spray [62.5 doses] (2.5 mL)

Suppository, rectal (Cafatine®, Cafergot®, Cafetrate®, Wigraine®): Ergotamine tartrate 2 mg and caffeine 100 mg (12s)

Tablet (Ercaf®, Wigraine®): Ergotamine tartrate 1 mg and caffeine 100 mg

Tablet:

Extended release:

Bellergal-S®: Ergotamine tartrate 0.6 mg with belladonna alkaloids 0.2 mg, and phenobarbital 40 mg

Cafatine-PB®: Ergotamine tartrate 1 mg with belladonna alkaloids 0.125 mg, caffeine 100 mg, and pentobarbital 30 mg

Sublingual (Ergostat®): Ergotamine tartrate 2 mg

Ergotrate® Maleate *see* Ergonovine Maleate *on page 398*

Eridium® *see* Phenazopyridine Hydrochloride *on page 866*

ERO Ear® [OTC] *see* Carbamide Peroxide *on page 179*

Erwiniar® *see* Asparaginase *on page 89*

Eryc® *see* Erythromycin *on next page*

EryPed® *see* Erythromycin *on next page*

Ery-Tab® *see* Erythromycin *on next page*

Erythrityl Tetranitrate *(e ri' thri till te tra nye' trate)*

Brand Names Cardilate®

Use Prophylaxis and long-term treatment of frequent or recurrent anginal pain and reduced exercise tolerance associated with angina pectoris

Unlabeled use: Reduce cardiac workload in CHF or following an MI; adjunct in treatment of Raynaud's disease

Pregnancy Risk Factor C

Contraindications Severe anemia, closed-angle glaucoma, postural hypotension, cerebral hemorrhage, head trauma, hypersensitivity to erythrityl tetranitrate or any component

Warnings/Precautions Use with caution in patients with hypertrophic cardiomyopathy, in patients with glaucoma, or volume depletion; tolerance may develop

Adverse Reactions

>10%: Central nervous system: Headache

1% to 10%: Cardiovascular: Tachycardia, hypotension, flushing

<1%:

Central nervous system: Restlessness, weakness, dizziness

Gastrointestinal: Nausea, vomiting, diarrhea

Hematologic: Methemoglobinemia

Overdosage/Toxicology Symptoms of overdose include hypotension, tachycardia, flushing, diaphoresis, dizziness, syncope, nausea, confusion, increased intracranial pressure, methemoglobinemia, cyanosis, metabolic acidosis, seizures. Following decontamination, keep patients recumbent, treat hypotension with fluids and pressors, treat methemoglobinemia with methylene-blue 1-2 mg/kg; epinephrine is ineffective in reversing hypotension.

Mechanism of Action Erythrityl tetranitrate, like other organic nitrates, induces vasodilation by dephosphorylation of the myosin light chain in smooth muscles. This is accomplished by activation of guanylate cyclase, which eventually stimulates a cyclic GMP-dependent protein kinase that alters the phosphorylation of the myosin. Venodilation causes peripheral blood pooling, which decreases venous return to the heart, central venous pressure, and pulmonary capillary wedge pressure. A reduction in pulmonary vascular resistance occurs secondary to pulmonary arteriolar dilation and afterload may be decreased by a lowering of systemic arterial pressure.

Usual Dosage Adults: Oral: 5 mg under the tongue or in the buccal pouch 3 times/day or 10 mg before meals or food, chewed 3 times/day, increasing in 2-3 days if needed; dosages of up to 100 mg/day are tolerated; some patients may need bedtime doses if they experience nocturnal symptoms

Monitoring Parameters Monitor blood pressure reduction for maximal effect and orthostatic hypotension

Test Interactions ↓ cholesterol (S)

Patient Information Do not change brands without consulting physician or pharmacist; notify physician if persistent headache, dizziness, or flushing occurs; seek medical help if chest pain is unresolved after 15 minutes; do not chew or swallow sublingual tablet; keep tablets in original container and keep container tightly closed; take sublingual and chewable tablets while sitting down

Nursing Implications Do not crush sublingual drug product

Dosage Forms Tablet, oral or sublingual: 10 mg

Erythrocin® see Erythromycin *on this page*

Erythromycin (er ith roe mye' sin)

Related Information

Prevention of Bacterial Endocarditis *on page 1285-1288*

Brand Names E.E.S.®; E-Mycin®; Eryc®; EryPed®; Ery-Tab®; Erythrocin®; Ilosone®; PCE®; Wyamycin® S

Synonyms Erythromycin Base; Erythromycin Estolate; Erythromycin Ethylsuccinate; Erythromycin Gluceptate; Erythromycin Lactobionate; Erythromycin Stearate

Use Treatment of susceptible bacterial infections including *M. pneumoniae*, *Legionella pneumophila*, diphtheria, pertussis, chancroid, *Chlamydia*, and *Campylobacter* gastroenteritis; used in conjunction with neomycin for decontaminating the bowel

Unlabeled use: Gastroparesis

Pregnancy Risk Factor B

Contraindications Hepatic impairment, known hypersensitivity to erythromycin or its components

Warnings/Precautions Hepatic impairment with or without jaundice has occurred, it may be accompanied by malaise, nausea, vomiting, abdominal colic, and fever; discontinue use if these occur; avoid using erythromycin lactobionate in neonates since formulations may contain benzyl alcohol which is associated with toxicity in neonates

Adverse Reactions

>10%: Gastrointestinal: Abdominal pain, cramping, nausea, vomiting

1% to 10%:

Gastrointestinal: Oral candidiasis

Hepatic: Cholestatic jaundice

Local: Phlebitis at the injection site

Miscellaneous: Hypersensitivity reactions

<1%:

Cardiovascular: Ventricular arrhythmias

Central nervous system: Fever

Dermatologic: Skin rash

Gastrointestinal: Hypertrophic pyloric stenosis, diarrhea

Hematologic: Eosinophilia

Local: Thrombophlebitis

Miscellaneous: Allergic reactions

Overdosage/Toxicology Symptoms of overdose include nausea, vomiting, diarrhea, prostration, reversible pancreatitis, hearing loss with or without tinnitus or vertigo; general and supportive care only

Drug Interactions Cytochrome P-450 IIIA enzyme inhibitor

Increased toxicity:

Erythromycin decreases clearance of carbamazepine, cyclosporine, and triazolam

Erythromycin may decrease theophylline clearance and increase theophylline's half-life by up to 60% (patients on high-dose theophylline and erythromycin or who have received erythromycin for >5 days may be at higher risk)

Terfenadine increases Q-T interval

(Continued)

Erythromycin *(Continued)*

Stability

Erythromycin lactobionate should be reconstituted with sterile water for injection without preservatives to avoid gel formation; the reconstituted solution is stable for 2 weeks when refrigerated or 24 hours at room temperature

Erythromycin I.V. infusion solution is stable at pH 6-8. Stability of lactobionate is pH dependent; I.V. form has the longest stability in 0.9% sodium chloride (NS) and should be prepared in this base solution whenever possible. Do not use D_5W as a diluent unless sodium bicarbonate is added to solution. If I.V. must be prepared in D_5W, 0.5 mL of the 8.4% sodium bicarbonate solution should be added per each 100 mL of D_5W.

Stability of parenteral admixture at room temperature (25°C) and at refrigeration temperature (4°C): 24 hours

Standard diluent: 500 mg/250 mL D_5W/NS; 750 mg/250 mL D_5W/NS; 1 g/250 mL D_5W/NS

Refrigerate oral suspension

Mechanism of Action
Inhibits RNA-dependent protein synthesis at the chain elongation step; binds to the 50S ribosomal subunit resulting in blockage of transpeptidation

Pharmacodynamics/Kinetics

Absorption: Variable but better with salt forms than with base form; 18% to 45% absorbed orally, ethylsuccinate may be better absorbed with food

Distribution: Crosses the placenta; appears in breast milk

Relative diffusion of antimicrobial agents from blood into cerebrospinal fluid (CSF): Minimal even with inflammation

Ratio of CSF to blood level (%):

Normal meninges: 1-12

Inflamed meninges: 7-25

Protein binding: 75% to 90%

Metabolism: In the liver by demethylation

Half-life: 1.5-2 hours (peak)

End stage renal disease: 5-6 hours

Time to peak serum concentration: 4 hours for the base, 30 minutes to 2.5 hours for the ethylsuccinate; delayed in the presence of food; due to differences in absorption, **200 mg erythromycin ethylsuccinate produces the same serum levels as 125 mg of erythromycin base**

Elimination: 2% to 15% excreted as unchanged drug in urine and major excretion in feces (via bile)

Usual Dosage
Erythromycin has been used as a prokinetic agent to improve gastric emptying time and intestinal motility. In adults, 200 mg was infused I.V. initially followed by 250 mg orally 3 times/day 30 minutes before meals. In children, erythromycin 3 mg/kg I.V. has been infused over 60 minutes initially followed by 20 mg/kg/day orally in 3-4 divided doses before meals or before meals and at bedtime

Neonates:

Oral:

Postnatal age ≤7 days: Oral: 10 mg/kg/dose every 12 hours

Postnatal age >7 days: Oral:

<1200 g: 10 mg/kg/dose every 12 hours

≥1200 g: 10 mg/kg/dose every 8 hours

Ophthalmic: Prophylaxis of neonatal gonococcal or chlamydial conjunctivitis: 0.5-1 cm ribbon of ointment should be instilled into each conjunctival sac

Infants and Children:

Oral: Do not exceed 2 g/day

Base and ethylsuccinate: 30-50 mg/kg/day divided every 6-8 hours

Endocarditis prophylaxis in penicillin-allergic patients: Oral: Base: 20 mg/kg/dose 2 hours before procedure and 10 mg/kg/dose 6 hours later

Preop bowel preparation: 20 mg/kg erythromycin base at 1, 2, and 11 PM on the day before surgery combined with mechanical cleansing of the large intestine and oral neomycin

I.V.: Lactobionate: 20-40 mg/kg/day divided every 6 hours, not to exceed 4 g/day

Adults:

Oral:

Base: 250-500 mg every 6-12 hours

Ethylsuccinate: 400-800 mg every 6-12 hours

Endocarditis prophylaxis in penicillin-allergic patients: Oral: 1 g 2 hours before procedure and 500 mg 6 hours later

Preop bowel preparation: Oral: 1 g erythromycin base at 1, 2, and 11 PM on the day before surgery combined with mechanical cleansing of the large intestine and oral neomycin

I.V.: Lactobionate: 15-20 mg/kg/day divided every 6 hours or 500 mg to 1 g every 6 hours, or given as a continuous infusion over 24 hours (maximum: 4 g/24 hours)

Children and Adults: Ophthalmic: Instill ½" (1.25 cm) 2-8 times/day depending on the severity of the infection

Slightly dialyzable (5% to 20%); no supplemental dosage necessary in hemo or peritoneal dialysis or in continuous arterio-venous or veno-venous hemofiltration (CAVH/CAVHD)

Administration Administer around-the-clock rather than 4 times/day to promote less variation in peak and trough serum levels

Test Interactions False-positive urinary catecholamines

Patient Information Refrigerate after reconstitution, take until gone, do not skip doses; chewable tablets should not be swallowed whole; report to physician if persistent diarrhea occurs; discard any unused portion after 10 days; drug absorption unaffected by food

Nursing Implications Some formulations may contain benzyl alcohol as a preservative; use with extreme care in neonates; do not crush enteric coated drug product; GI upset, including diarrhea, is common; can give with food to decrease GI upset

Dosage Forms

Capsule, as estolate: 250 mg

Gel: 2% (30 g, 60 g)

Granules, for oral suspension, ethylsuccinate: 400 mg/5 mL (60 mL, 100 mL, 200 mL)

Injection, lactobionate: 500 mg, 1 g

Ointment: 2% (25 g)

Ointment, ophthalmic: 5 mg/g (1 g, 3.5 g)

Solution: 1.5% (60 mL); 2% (60 mL)

Suspension:

Estolate: 125 mg/5 mL (480 mL); 250 mg/5 mL (480 mL)

Ethylsuccinate: 200 mg/5 mL (480 mL); 400 mg/5 mL (480 mL)

Suspension, drops, as ethylsuccinate: 100 mg/2.5 mL (50 mL)

Tablet:

Chewable, as ethylsuccinate: 200 mg

Delayed release, as base: 250 mg, 333 mg, 500 mg

Estolate: 500 mg

Ethylsuccinate: 400 mg

Film coated: 250 mg, 500 mg

Film coated, stearate: 250 mg, 500 mg

Polymer coated particles, as base: 333 mg, 500 mg

Erythromycin and Sulfisoxazole (er ith roe mye′ sin & sul fi sox′ a zole)

Brand Names Eryzole®; Pediazole®

Synonyms Sulfisoxazole and Erythromycin

Use Treatment of susceptible bacterial infections of the upper and lower respiratory tract, otitis media in children caused by susceptible strains of *Haemophilus influenzae*, and other infections in patients allergic to penicillin

Pregnancy Risk Factor C

Contraindications Hepatic dysfunction, known hypersensitivity to erythromycin or sulfonamides; infants <2 months of age (sulfas compete with bilirubin for binding sites); patients with porphyria

Warnings/Precautions Use with caution in patients with impaired renal or hepatic function, G-6-PD deficiency (hemolysis may occur)

Adverse Reactions

>10%: Gastrointestinal: Abdominal pain, cramping, nausea, vomiting

1% to 10%:

Gastrointestinal: Oral candidiasis

Hepatic: Cholestatic jaundice

Local: Phlebitis at the injection site

Miscellaneous: Hypersensitivity reactions

<1%:

Cardiovascular: Ventricular arrhythmias

Central nervous system: Fever, headache

Dermatologic: Skin rash, Stevens-Johnson syndrome, toxic epidermal necrolysis

Gastrointestinal: Hypertrophic pyloric stenosis, diarrhea

Hematologic: Eosinophilia, agranulocytosis, aplastic anemia

Hepatic: Hepatic necrosis

Local: Thrombophlebitis

(Continued)

Erythromycin and Sulfisoxazole *(Continued)*

Renal: Toxic nephrosis, crystalluria

Overdosage/Toxicology Symptoms of overdose include nausea, vomiting, diarrhea, prostration, reversible pancreatitis, hearing loss with or without tinnitus or vertigo; general and supportive care only; keep patient well hydrated

Drug Interactions Increased effect/toxicity/levels of alfentanil, anticoagulants, astemizole, terfenadine, loratadine, bromocriptine, carbamazepine, cyclosporine, digoxin, disopyramide, theophylline, triazolam, and warfarin

Stability Reconstituted suspension is stable for 14 days when refrigerated

Mechanism of Action Erythromycin inhibits bacterial protein synthesis; sulfisoxazole competitively inhibits bacterial synthesis of folic acid from para-aminobenzoic acid

Pharmacodynamics/Kinetics

Erythromycin ethylsuccinate:
Absorption: Well absorbed from GI tract
Distribution: Crosses the placenta; appears in breast milk
Protein binding: 75% to 90%
Metabolism: In the liver
Half-life: 1-1.5 hours
Elimination: Unchanged drug is excreted and concentrated in bile

Sulfisoxazole acetyl: Hydrolyzed in the GI tract to sulfisoxazole which has the following characteristics:
Absorption: Readily absorbed
Distribution: Crosses the placenta; appears in breast milk
Protein binding: 85%
Half-life: 6 hours, prolonged in renal impairment
Elimination: 50% excreted in urine as unchanged drug

Usual Dosage Oral (dosage recommendation is based on the product's erythromycin content):

Children ≥2 months: 50 mg/kg/day erythromycin and 150 mg/kg/day sulfisoxazole in divided doses every 6 hours; not to exceed 2 g erythromycin/day or 6 g sulfisoxazole/day for 10 days
Adults: 400 mg erythromycin and 1200 mg sulfisoxazole every 6 hours

Dosing adjustment in renal impairment (sulfisoxazole must be adjusted in renal impairment):
Cl_{cr} 10-50 mL/minute: Administer every 8-12 hours
Cl_{cr} <10 mL/minute: Administer every 12-24 hours

Monitoring Parameters CBC and periodic liver function test

Test Interactions False-positive urinary protein

Patient Information Maintain adequate fluid intake; avoid prolonged exposure to sunlight; discontinue if rash appears; take until gone, do not skip doses

Nursing Implications Shake well before use; refrigerate

Dosage Forms Suspension, oral: Erythromycin ethylsuccinate 200 mg and sulfisoxazole acetyl 600 mg per 5 mL (100 mL, 150 mL, 200 mL, 250 mL)

Erythromycin Base *see* Erythromycin *on page 401*

Erythromycin Estolate *see* Erythromycin *on page 401*

Erythromycin Ethylsuccinate *see* Erythromycin *on page 401*

Erythromycin Gluceptate *see* Erythromycin *on page 401*

Erythromycin Lactobionate *see* Erythromycin *on page 401*

Erythromycin Stearate *see* Erythromycin *on page 401*

Erythropoietin *see* Epoetin Alfa *on page 392*

Eryzole® *see* Erythromycin and Sulfisoxazole *on previous page*

Eserine Salicylate *see* Physostigmine *on page 881*

Esgic® *see* Butalbital Compound *on page 153*

Esidrix® *see* Hydrochlorothiazide *on page 542*

Eskalith® *see* Lithium *on page 643*

Esmolol Hydrochloride *(ess' moe lol)*

Related Information
Antiarrhythmic Drugs *on page 1246-1248*
Beta-Blockers Comparison *on page 1257-1259*

Brand Names Brevibloc®

Use Treatment of supraventricular tachycardia, atrial fibrillation/flutter (primarily to control ventricular rate), and hypertension (especially perioperatively)

Pregnancy Risk Factor C

Contraindications Sinus bradycardia or heart block; uncompensated congestive heart failure; cardiogenic shock; hypersensitivity to esmolol, any component, or other beta-blockers

Warnings/Precautions Must be diluted for continuous I.V. infusion; use with extreme caution in patients with hyper-reactive airway disease; use lowest dose possible and discontinue infusion if bronchospasm occurs; use with caution in diabetes mellitus, hypoglycemia, renal failure; avoid extravasation; caution should be exercised when discontinuing esmolol infusions to avoid withdrawal effects; esmolol shares the toxic potentials of beta-adrenergic blocking agents and the usual precautions of these agents should be observed

Adverse Reactions

>10%:
Cardiovascular: Asymptomatic and symptomatic hypotension
Miscellaneous: Diaphoresis

1% to 10%:
Cardiovascular: Peripheral ischemia
Central nervous system: Dizziness, somnolence, confusion, headache, agitation, fatigue
Gastrointestinal: Nausea, vomiting
Local: Infusion site reactions

<1%:
Cardiovascular: Pallor, flushing, bradycardia, chest pain, syncope, heart block, edema
Central nervous system: Asthenia, depression, abnormal thinking, anxiety, fever, lightheadedness, seizures
Dermatologic: Erythema, skin discoloration
Gastrointestinal: Anorexia, dyspepsia, constipation, dry mouth, abdominal discomfort
Genitourinary: Urinary retention
Local: Thrombophlebitis
Neuromuscular & skeletal: Paresthesia, rigors
Ocular: Abnormal vision
Respiratory: Bronchospasm, wheezing, dyspnea, nasal congestion, pulmonary edema
Miscellaneous: Speech disorder, midcapsular pain

Overdosage/Toxicology Symptoms of overdose include hypotension, bradycardia, heart block; sympathomimetics (eg, epinephrine or dopamine), glucagon, or a pacemaker can be used to treat the toxic bradycardia, asystole, and/or hypotension; initially, fluids may be the best treatment for hypotension

Drug Interactions

Decreased effect of beta-blockers with aluminum salts, barbiturates, calcium salts, cholestyramine, colestipol, NSAIDs, penicillins (ampicillin), rifampin, salicylates and sulfinpyrazone due to decreased bioavailability and plasma levels

Beta-blockers may decrease the effect of sulfonylureas

Increased effect/toxicity of beta-blockers with calcium blockers (diltiazem, felodipine, nicardipine), contraceptives, flecainide, haloperidol (propranolol, hypotensive effects), H_2 antagonists (metoprolol, propranolol only by cimetidine, possibly ranitidine), hydralazine (metoprolol, propranolol), loop diuretics (propranolol, not atenolol), MAO inhibitors (metoprolol, nadolol, bradycardia), phenothiazines (propranolol), propafenone (metoprolol, propranolol), quinidine (in extensive metabolizers), ciprofloxacin, thyroid hormones (metoprolol, propranolol, when hypothyroid patient is converted to euthyroid state)

Beta-blockers may increase the effect/toxicity of flecainide, haloperidol (hypotensive effects), hydralazine, phenothiazines, acetaminophen, anticoagulants (propranolol, warfarin), benzodiazepines (not atenolol), clonidine (hypertensive crisis after or during withdrawal of either agent), epinephrine (initial hypertensive episode followed by bradycardia), nifedipine and verapamil lidocaine, ergots (peripheral ischemia), prazosin (postural hypotension)

Beta-blockers may affect the action or levels of ethanol, disopyramide, nondepolarizing muscle relaxants and theophylline although the effects are difficult to predict

Stability Clear, colorless to light yellow solution which should be stored at room temperature and protected from temperatures >40°C
Stability of parenteral admixture at room temperature (25°C) and at refrigeration temperature (4°C): 24 hours
Standard diluent: 5 g/500 mL NS

Mechanism of Action Class II antiarrhythmic: Competitively blocks response to beta$_1$- and beta$_2$-adrenergic stimulation

Pharmacodynamics/Kinetics
Onset of beta blockade: I.V.: Within 2-10 minutes (onset of effect is quickest when loading doses are administered)
(Continued)

Esmolol Hydrochloride *(Continued)*

Duration of activity: Short, 10-30 minutes; prolonged following higher cumulative doses, extended duration of use

Protein binding: 55%

Metabolism: In blood by esterases

Half-life: Adults: 9 minutes

Elimination: ~69% of dose excreted in urine as metabolites and 2% as unchanged drug

Usual Dosage I.V. administration requires an infusion pump (must be adjusted to individual response and tolerance):

Children: An extremely limited amount of information regarding esmolol use in pediatric patients is currently available

Some centers have utilized doses of 100-500 mcg/kg given over 1 minute for control of supraventricular tachycardias

Loading doses of 500 mcg/kg/minute over 1 minute with maximal doses of 50-250 mcg/kg/minute (mean 173) have been used in addition to nitroprusside to treat postoperative hypertension after coarctation of aorta repair

Adults: Loading dose: 500 mcg/kg over 1 minute; follow with a 50 mcg/kg/minute infusion for 4 minutes; if response is inadequate, rebolus with another 500 mcg/kg loading dose over 1 minute, and increase the maintenance infusion to 100 mcg/kg/minute. Repeat this process until a therapeutic effect has been achieved or to a maximum recommended maintenance dose of 200 mcg/kg/minute. Usual dosage range: 50-200 mcg/kg/minute with average dose of 100 mcg/kg/minute.

Esmolol: Hemodynamic effects of beta blockade return to baseline within 20-30 minutes after discontinuing esmolol infusions

Guidelines for withdrawal of therapy:

Transfer to alternative antiarrhythmic drug (propranolol, digoxin, verapamil)

Infusion should be reduced by 50% 30 minutes following the first dose of the alternative agent

Following the second dose of the alternative drug, patient's response should be monitored and if control is adequate for the first hours, esmolol may be discontinued

Not removed by hemo- or peritoneal dialysis; supplemental dose is not necessary

Administration The 250 mg/mL ampul is **not** for direct I.V. injection, but rather must first be diluted to a final concentration of 10 mg/mL (ie, 2.5 g in 250 mL or 5 g in 500 mL); decrease or discontinue infusion if hypotension, congenital heart failure occur

Monitoring Parameters Blood pressure, heart rate, MAP, EKG, respiratory rate, I.V. site; cardiac monitor and blood pressure monitor required

Test Interactions Increases cholesterol (S), glucose

Dosage Forms Injection: 10 mg/mL (10 mL); 250 mg/mL (10 mL)

Esoterica® Facial [OTC] *see* Hydroquinone *on page 551*

Esoterica® Regular [OTC] *see* Hydroquinone *on page 551*

Esoterica® Sensitive Skin Formula [OTC] *see* Hydroquinone *on page 551*

Esoterica® Sunscreen [OTC] *see* Hydroquinone *on page 551*

Estazolam *(ess ta' zoe lam)*

Related Information

Benzodiazepines Comparison *on page 1256*

Brand Names ProSom™

Use Short-term management of insomnia; there has been little experience with this drug in the elderly, but because of its lack of active metabolites, it is a reasonable choice when a benzodiazepine hypnotic is indicated

Restrictions C-IV

Pregnancy Risk Factor X

Contraindications Hypersensitivity to estazolam, cross-sensitivity with other benzodiazepines may occur, pre-existing CNS depression, sleep apnea, pregnancy, narrow-angle glaucoma

Warnings/Precautions Abrupt discontinuance may precipitate withdrawal or rebound insomnia; use with caution in patients receiving other CNS depressants, patients with low albumin, hepatic dysfunction, and in the elderly; do not use in pregnant women; may cause drug dependency; safety and efficacy have not been established in children <15 years of age, not recommended in nursing mothers

Adverse Reactions
>10%:
Cardiovascular: Tachycardia, chest pain
Central nervous system: Drowsiness, fatigue, impaired coordination, lightheadedness, memory impairment, insomnia, anxiety, depression, headache
Dermatologic: Rash
Endocrine & metabolic: Decreased libido
Gastrointestinal: Dry mouth, constipation, decreased salivation, nausea, vomiting, diarrhea, increased or decreased appetite
Neuromuscular & skeletal: Dysarthria
Ocular: Blurred vision
Miscellaneous: Sweating
1% to 10%:
Cardiovascular: Syncope, hypotension
Central nervous system: Confusion, nervousness, dizziness, akathisia
Dermatologic: Dermatitis
Gastrointestinal: Weight gain or loss, increased salivation
Neuromuscular & skeletal: Rigidity, tremor, muscle cramps
Otic: Tinnitus
Respiratory: Nasal congestion, hyperventilation
<1%:
Central nervous system: Reflex slowing
Endocrine & metabolic: Menstrual irregularities
Hematologic: Blood dyscrasias
Miscellaneous: Drug dependence

Overdosage/Toxicology Symptoms of overdose include respiratory depression, hypoactive reflexes, unsteady gait, hypotension. Treatment for benzodiazepine overdose is supportive; rarely is mechanical ventilation required; flumazenil has been shown to selectively block the binding of benzodiazepines to CNS receptors, resulting in a reversal of benzodiazepine-induced CNS depression.

Drug Interactions
Decreased effect: Enzyme inducers may increase the metabolism of estazolam
Increased toxicity: CNS depressants may increase CNS adverse effects; cimetidine may decrease metabolism of estazolam

Mechanism of Action Benzodiazepines may exert their pharmacologic effect through potentiation of the inhibitory activity of GABA. Benzodiazepines do not alter the synthesis, release, reuptake, or enzymatic degradation of GABA.

Usual Dosage Adults: Oral: 1 mg at bedtime, some patients may require 2 mg; start at doses of 0.5 mg in debilitated or small elderly patients

Dosing adjustment in hepatic impairment: May be necessary

Monitoring Parameters Respiratory and cardiovascular status

Patient Information May cause daytime drowsiness, avoid alcohol and drugs with CNS depressant effects; avoid activities needing good psychomotor coordination until CNS effects are known; drug may cause physical or psychological dependence; avoid abrupt discontinuation after prolonged use

Nursing Implications Provide safety measures (ie, side rails, night light, and call button); remove smoking materials from area; supervise ambulation; avoid abrupt discontinuance in patients with prolonged therapy or seizure disorders

Dosage Forms Tablet: 1 mg, 2 mg

Estinyl® *see* Ethinyl Estradiol *on page 419*

Estivin® II [OTC] *see* Naphazoline Hydrochloride *on page 775*

Estrace® *see* Estradiol *on this page*

Estra-D® *see* Estradiol *on this page*

Estraderm® *see* Estradiol *on this page*

Estradiol (ess tra dye' ole)

Brand Names Deladiol®; Delestrogen®; depGynogen®; Depo®-Estradiol; Depogen®; Dioval®; Dura-Estrin®; Duragen®; Estrace®; Estra-D®; Estraderm®; Estra-L®; Estro-Cyp®; Estroject-L.A.®; Gynogen L.A.®; Valergen®

Synonyms Estradiol Cypionate; Estradiol Transdermal; Estradiol Valerate

Use Treatment of atrophic vaginitis, atrophic dystrophy of vulva, menopausal symptoms, female hypogonadism, ovariectomy, primary ovarian failure, inoperable breast cancer, inoperable prostatic cancer, mild to severe vasomotor symptoms associated with menopause

Pregnancy Risk Factor X

Contraindications Known or suspected pregnancy, undiagnosed genital bleeding, carcinoma of the breast (except in patients treated for metastatic (Continued)

Estradiol *(Continued)*

disease), estrogen-dependent tumors, history of thrombophlebitis, thrombosis, or thromboembolic disorders associated with estrogen use

Warnings/Precautions Use with caution in patients with renal or hepatic insufficiency; estrogens may cause premature closure of epiphyses in young individuals; in patients with a history of thromboembolism, stroke, myocardial infarction (especially age >40 who smoke), liver tumor, hypertension.

Estrogens have been reported to increase the risk of endometrial carcinoma; do not use estrogens during pregnancy. Before prescribing estrogen therapy to postmenopausal women, the risks and benefits must be weighed for each patient. Women should be informed of these risks and benefits, as well as possible side effects and the return of menstrual bleeding (when cycled with a progestin), and be involved in the decision to prescribe. Oral therapy may be more convenient for vaginal atrophy and stress incontinence.

Adverse Reactions

>10%:

Cardiovascular: Peripheral edema

Endocrine & metabolic: Enlargement of breasts (female and male), breast tenderness, bloating

Gastrointestinal: Nausea, anorexia

1% to 10%:

Central nervous system: Headache

Endocrine & metabolic: Increased libido (female), decreased libido (male)

Gastrointestinal: Vomiting, diarrhea

<1%:

Cardiovascular: Increase in blood pressure, edema, thromboembolic disorders, myocardial infarction

Central nervous system: Depression, dizziness, anxiety, stroke

Dermatologic: Chloasma, melasma, rash

Endocrine & metabolic: Hypercalcemia, folate deficiency, change in menstrual flow, breast tumors, amenorrhea, decreased glucose tolerance, increased triglycerides and LDL

Gastrointestinal: Nausea, GI distress

Hepatic: Cholestatic jaundice

Local: Pain at injection site

Miscellaneous: Intolerance to contact lenses, increased susceptibility to *Candida* infection

Overdosage/Toxicology Symptoms of overdose include fluid retention, nausea, vomiting; toxicity is unlikely following single exposures of excessive doses; any treatment following emesis and charcoal administration should be supportive and symptomatic

Drug Interactions

Decreased effect: Rifampin decreases estrogen serum concentrations

Increased toxicity: Hydrocortisone increases corticosteroid toxic potential; increases potential for thromboembolic events with anticoagulants

Mechanism of Action Increases the synthesis of DNA, RNA, and various proteins in target tissues; reduces the release of gonadotropin-releasing hormone from the hypothalamus; reduces FSH and LH release from the pituitary

Pharmacodynamics/Kinetics

Absorption: Readily absorbed through skin and GI tract; reabsorbed from bile in GI tract and enterohepatically recycled

Distribution: Crosses the placenta; appears in breast milk

Metabolism: Principally degraded in the liver

Protein binding: 80%

Half-life: 50-60 minutes

Elimination: In urine as conjugates; small amounts excreted in feces via bile, reabsorbed from the GI tract and enterohepatically recycled

Usual Dosage Adults (all dosage needs to be adjusted based upon the patient's response):

Male:

Prostate cancer: Valerate: I.M.: ≥30 mg or more every 1-2 weeks

Prostate cancer (androgen-dependent, inoperable, progressing): Oral: 10 mg 3 times/day for at least 3 months

Female:

Breast cancer (inoperable, progressing): Oral: 10 mg 3 times/day for at least 3 months

Osteoporosis prevention: Oral: 0.5 mg/day in a cyclic regimen (3 weeks on and 1 week off of drug)

Hypogonadism, moderate to severe vasomotor symptoms:

Oral: 1-2 mg/day in a cyclic regimen for 3 weeks on drug, then 1 week off drug

Moderate to severe vasomotor symptoms:
I.M.: Cypionate: 1-5 mg every 3-4 months
I.M.: Valerate: 10-20 mg every 4 weeks
Postpartum breast engorgement: I.M.: Valerate: 10-25 mg at end of first stage of labor
Transdermal: Apply 0.05 mg patch initially (titrate dosage to response) applied twice weekly in a cyclic regimen, for 3 weeks on drug and 1 week off drug in patients with an intact uterus and continuously in patients without a uterus
Atrophic vaginitis, kraurosis vulvae: Vaginal: Insert 2-4 g/day for 2 weeks then gradually reduce to 1/2 the initial dose for 2 weeks followed by a maintenance dose of 1 g 1-3 times/week

Administration Injection for intramuscular use only

Reference Range
Children: <10 pg/mL (SI: <37 pmol/L)
Male: 10-50 pg/mL (SI: 37-184 pmol/L)
Female:
Premenopausal: 30-400 pg/mL (SI: 110-1468 pmol/L)
Postmenopausal: 0-30 pg/mL (SI: 0-110 pmol/L)

Test Interactions
Decreased antithrombin III
Decreased serum folate concentration
Increased prothrombin and factors VII, VIII, IX, X
Increased platelet aggregability
Increased thyroid binding globulin
Increased total thyroid hormone (T_4)
Increased serum triglycerides/phospholipids

Patient Information Patients should inform their physicians if signs or symptoms of any of the following occur: Thromboembolic or thrombotic disorders including sudden severe headache or vomiting, disturbance of vision or speech, loss of vision, numbness or weakness in an extremity, sharp or crushing chest pain, calf pain, shortness of breath, severe abdominal pain or mass, mental depression, or unusual bleeding.

Patients should discontinue taking the medication if they suspect they are pregnant or become pregnant. Notify physician if area under dermal patch becomes irritated or a rash develops. Patient package insert is available with product; insert vaginal product high into the vagina.

Nursing Implications Aerosol topical corticosteroids applied under the patch may reduce allergic reactions; do not apply transdermal system to breasts, but place on trunk of body (preferably abdomen); rotate application sites

Additional Information
Estradiol: Estraderm®, Estrace®
Estradiol cypionate: Depo®-Estradiol, depGynogen®, Depogen®, Dura-Estrin®, Estra-D®, Estro-Cyp®, Estroject-L.A.®
Estradiol valerate: Delestrogen®, Dioval®, Duragen®, Estra-L®Gynogen®, Valergen®

Dosage Forms
Cream, vaginal (Estrace®): 0.1 mg/g (42.5 g)
Injection, as cypionate (in oil): 5 mg/mL (5 mL, 10 mL)
Injection, as valerate (in oil): 10 mg/mL (5 mL, 10 mL); 20 mg/mL (1 mL, 5 mL, 10 mL); 40 mg/mL (5 mL, 10 mL)
Tablet, micronized (Estrace®): 0.5 mg, 1 mg, 2 mg
Transdermal system (Estraderm®):
0.05 mg/24 hours [10 cm²], total estradiol 4 mg
0.1 mg/24 hours [20 cm²], total estradiol 8 mg

Estradiol Cypionate see Estradiol on page 407

Estradiol Transdermal see Estradiol on page 407

Estradiol Valerate see Estradiol on page 407

Estradurin® see Polyestradiol Phosphate on page 899

Estra-L® see Estradiol on page 407

Estramustine Phosphate Sodium (ess tra muss' teen)
Brand Names Emcyt®
Use Palliative treatment of prostatic carcinoma (progressive or metastatic)
Pregnancy Risk Factor C
Contraindications Active thrombophlebitis or thromboembolic disorders, hypersensitivity to estramustine or any component, estradiol or nitrogen mustard
Warnings/Precautions The U.S. Food and Drug Administration (FDA) currently recommends that procedures for proper handling and disposal of antineoplastic agents be considered. Glucose tolerance may be decreased; elevated blood
(Continued)

Estramustine Phosphate Sodium *(Continued)*

pressure may occur; exacerbation of peripheral edema or congestive heart disease may occur; use with caution in patients with impaired liver function, renal insufficiency, or metabolic bone diseases.

Adverse Reactions

>10%:

Cardiovascular: Edema

Gastrointestinal: Diarrhea, nausea, mild increases in AST (SGOT) or LDH

Endocrine & metabolic: Decreased libido, breast tenderness, breast enlargement

Respiratory: Dyspnea

1% to 10%:

Cardiovascular: Myocardial infarction

Central nervous system: Insomnia, lethargy

Gastrointestinal: Anorexia, flatulence

Hematologic: Leukopenia

Local: Thrombophlebitis

Neuromuscular & skeletal: Leg cramps

Respiratory: Pulmonary embolism

<1%:

Cardiovascular: Cardiac arrest

Central nervous system: Night sweats, depression

Dermatologic: Pigment changes

Endocrine & metabolic: Hypercalcemia, hot flashes

Otic: Tinnitus

Overdosage/Toxicology Symptoms of overdose include nausea, vomiting, myelosuppression; there are no known antidotes, treatment is primarily symptomatic and supportive

Drug Interactions Decreased effect: Milk products and calcium-rich foods/drugs may impair the oral absorption of estramustine phosphate sodium

Stability Refrigerate at 2°C to 8°C (36°F to 46°F); capsules may be stored outside of refrigerator for up to 24-48 hours without affecting potency

Mechanism of Action Mechanism is not completely clear, thought to act as an alkylating agent and as estrogen

Pharmacodynamics/Kinetics

Absorption: Oral: Well absorbed (75%)

Metabolism: Dephosphorylated in the intestines and eventually oxidized and hydrolyzed to estramustine, estrone, estradiol, and nitrogen mustard

Half-life: 20 hours

Time to peak serum concentration: Within 2-3 hours

Elimination: In feces via bile

Usual Dosage Adults: Oral: 14 mg/kg/day (range: 10-16 mg/kg/day) in 3-4 divided doses for 30-90 days; some patients have been maintained for >3 years on therapy

Patient Information Take on an empty stomach, particularly avoid taking with milk

Dosage Forms Capsule: 140 mg

Estratab® *see Estrogens, Esterified on page 412*

Estro-Cyp® *see Estradiol on page 407*

Estrogenic Substance Aqueous *see Estrone on page 413*

Estrogenic Substances, Conjugated *see Estrogens, Conjugated on this page*

Estrogens, Conjugated *(ess' troe jenz)*

Brand Names Premarin®

Synonyms C.E.S.; Estrogenic Substances, Conjugated

Use Atrophic vaginitis; hypogonadism; primary ovarian failure; vasomotor symptoms of menopause; prostatic carcinoma; osteoporosis prophylactic

Pregnancy Risk Factor X

Contraindications Undiagnosed vaginal bleeding; hypersensitivity to estrogens or any component; thrombophlebitis, liver disease, known or suspected pregnancy, carcinoma of the breast, estrogen dependent tumor

Warnings/Precautions Use with caution in patients with asthma, epilepsy, migraine, diabetes, cardiac or renal dysfunction; estrogens may cause premature closure of the epiphyses in young individuals; safety and efficacy in children have not been established; estrogens have been reported to increase the risk of endometrial carcinoma; do not use estrogens during pregnancy

Adverse Reactions

>10%:

Cardiovascular: Peripheral edema

Endocrine & metabolic: Breast tenderness, hypercalcemia, enlargement of breasts

Gastrointestinal: Nausea, anorexia, bloating

1% to 10%:

Central nervous system: Headache

Endocrine & metabolic: Increased libido

Gastrointestinal: Vomiting, diarrhea

Local: Pain at injection site

<1%:

Cardiovascular: Increase in blood pressure, edema, thromboembolic disorder, myocardial infarction, stroke, hypertension

Central nervous system: Depression, dizziness, anxiety

Dermatologic: Chloasma, melasma, rash

Endocrine & metabolic: Breast tumors, amenorrhea, alterations in frequency and flow of menses, decreased glucose tolerance, increased triglycerides and LDL

Gastrointestinal: Vomiting, GI distress

Hepatic: Cholestatic jaundice

Miscellaneous: Intolerance to contact lenses, increased susceptibility to *Candida* infection

Overdosage/Toxicology Symptoms of overdose include fluid retention, jaundice, thrombophlebitis; toxicity is unlikely following single exposures of excessive doses, any treatment following emesis and charcoal administration should be supportive and symptomatic

Drug Interactions

Decreased effect: Rifampin decreases estrogen serum concentrations

Increased toxicity:

Hydrocortisone increases corticosteroid toxic potential

Anticoagulants: Increases potential for thromboembolic events with anticoagulants

Carbamazepine, tricyclic antidepressants, and corticosteroids; ↑ thromboembolic potential with oral anticoagulants

Stability

Refrigerate injection; at room temperature, the injection is stable for 24 months

Reconstituted solution is stable for 60 days at refrigeration

Compatible with normal saline, dextrose, and inert sugar solution

Incompatible with proteins, ascorbic acid, or solutions with acidic pH

Mechanism of Action Increases the synthesis of DNA, RNA, and various proteins in target tissues; reduces the release of gonadotropin-releasing hormone from the hypothalamus; reduces FSH and LH release from the pituitary

Pharmacodynamics/Kinetics

Absorption: Readily absorbed from GI tract

Metabolism: To inactive compounds in the liver

Elimination: In bile and urine

Usual Dosage Adults:

Male: Prostate cancer: Oral: 1.25-2.5 mg 3 times/day

Female:

Hypogonadism: Oral: 2.5-7.5 mg/day for 20 days, off 10 days and repeat until menses occur

Abnormal uterine bleeding:

Oral: 2.5-5 mg/day for 7-10 days; then decrease to 1.25 mg/day for 2 weeks

I.M., I.V.: 25 mg every 6-12 hours until bleeding stops

Moderate to severe vasomotor symptoms: Oral: 0.625-1.25 mg/day

Postpartum breast engorgement: Oral: 3.75 mg every 4 hours for 5 doses, then 1.25 mg every 4 hours for 5 days

Atrophic vaginitis, kraurosis vulvae: Vaginal: 2-4 g instilled/day 3 weeks on and 1 week off

Osteoporosis: Oral: 0.625 mg/day chronically

Uremic bleeding: I.V.: 0.6 mg/kg/dose daily for 5 days

Administration May also be administered intramuscularly; when administered I.V., drug should be administered slowly to avoid the occurrence of a flushing reaction

Reference Range

Children: <10 µg/24 hour (SI: <35 µmol/day) (values at Mayo Medical Laboratories)

Adults:

Male: 15-40 µg/24 hours (SI: 52-139 µmol/day)

Female:

Menstruating: 15-80 µg/24 hour (SI: 52-277 µmol/day)

(Continued)

411

Estrogens, Conjugated *(Continued)*

Postmenopausal: <20 µg/24 hour (SI: <69 µmol/day)

Test Interactions
Decreased antithrombin III
Decreased serum folate concentration
Increased prothrombin and factors VII, VIII, IX, X
Increased platelet aggregability
Increased thyroid binding globulin
Increased total thyroid hormone (T_4)
Increased serum triglycerides/phospholipids

Patient Information Insert vaginal product high into vagina
Patient package insert available with product
Women should inform their physicians if signs or symptoms of any of the following occur: Thromboembolic or thrombotic disorders including sudden severe headache or vomiting, disturbance of vision or speech, loss of vision, numbness or weakness in an extremity, sharp or crushing chest pain, calf pain, shortness of breath, severe abdominal pain or mass, mental depression or unusual bleeding
Women should discontinue taking the medication if they suspect they are pregnant or become pregnant

Nursing Implications Give at bedtime to minimize occurrence of adverse effects

Additional Information Contains 50% to 65% sodium estrone sulfate and 20% to 35% sodium equilin sulfate

Dosage Forms
Cream, vaginal: 0.625 mg/g (42.5 g)
Injection: 25 mg (5 mL)
Tablet: 0.3 mg, 0.625 mg, 0.9 mg, 1.25 mg, 2.5 mg

Estrogens, Esterified (ess' troe jen)

Brand Names Estratab®; Menest®

Use Atrophic vaginitis; hypogonadism; primary ovarian failure; vasomotor symptoms of menopause; prostatic carcinoma; osteoporosis prophylactic

Pregnancy Risk Factor X

Contraindications Known or suspected cancer of the breast, except in appropriately selected patients being treated for metastatic disease; known or suspected estrogen-dependent neoplasia; known or suspected pregnancy; undiagnosed abnormal genital bleeding; active thrombophlebitis or thromboembolic disorders; past history of thrombophlebitis, thrombosis, or thromboembolic disorders associated with previous estrogen use except when used in the treatment of breast or prostatic malignancy

Warnings/Precautions Use with caution in patients with asthma, epilepsy, migraine, diabetes, cardiac or renal dysfunction; estrogens may cause premature closure of the epiphyses in young individuals; safety and efficacy in children have not been established; estrogens have been reported to increase the risk of endometrial carcinoma, do not use estrogens during pregnancy

Adverse Reactions
>10%:
Cardiovascular: Peripheral edema
Endocrine & metabolic: Enlargement of breasts, breast tenderness, bloating
Gastrointestinal: Nausea, anorexia
1% to 10%:
Central nervous system: Headache
Endocrine & metabolic: Increased libido
Gastrointestinal: Vomiting, diarrhea
<1%:
Cardiovascular: Hypertension, thromboembolism, myocardial infarction, edema
Central nervous system: Stroke, depression, dizziness, anxiety
Dermatologic: Chloasma, melasma, rash
Endocrine & metabolic: Breast tumors, amenorrhea, alterations in frequency and flow of menses, decreased glucose tolerance, increased triglycerides and LDL
Gastrointestinal: GI distress
Hepatic: Cholestatic jaundice
Miscellaneous: Intolerance to contact lenses, increased susceptibility to *Candida* infection

Overdosage/Toxicology Symptoms of overdose include fluid retention, jaundice, thrombophlebitis; toxicity is unlikely following single exposures of excessive doses, any treatment following emesis and charcoal administration should be supportive and symptomatic

Drug Interactions
Decreased effect: Rifampin decreases estrogen serum concentrations
Increased toxicity:
Hydrocortisone increases corticosteroid toxic potential
Anticoagulants: Increases potential for thromboembolic events with anticoagulants
Carbamazepine, tricyclic antidepressants, and corticosteroids; ↑ thromboembolic potential with oral anticoagulants

Mechanism of Action Primary effects on the interphase DNA-protein complex (chromatin) by binding to a receptor (usually located in the cytoplasm of a target cell) and initiating translocation of the hormone-receptor complex to the nucleus

Pharmacodynamics/Kinetics
Absorption: Readily absorbed from GI tract
Metabolism: Rapidly in the liver to less active metabolites
Elimination: In urine as unchanged compound and metabolites

Usual Dosage Adults: Oral:
Male: Prostate cancer (inoperable, progressing): 1.25-2.5 mg 3 times/day
Female:
Hypogonadism: 2.5-7.5 mg/day for 20 days, off 10 days and repeat until menses occur
Moderate to severe vasomotor symptoms: 0.3-1.25 mg/day
Breast cancer (inoperable, progressing): 10 mg 3 times/day for at least 3 months

Test Interactions Endocrine function test may be altered
Decreased antithrombin III
Decreased serum folate concentration
Increased prothrombin and factors VII, VIII, IX, X
Increased platelet aggregability
Increased thyroid binding globulin
Increased total thyroid hormone (T_4)
Increased serum triglycerides/phospholipids

Patient Information Patients should inform their physicians if signs or symptoms of thromboembolic or thrombotic disorders occur including sudden severe headache or vomiting, disturbance of vision or speech, loss of vision, numbness or weakness in an extremity, sharp or crushing chest pain, calf pain, shortness of breath, severe abdominal pain or mass, mental depression or unusual bleeding; patients should discontinue taking the medication if they suspect they are pregnant or become pregnant.

Additional Information Esterified estrogens are a combination of the sodium salts of the sulfate esters of estrogenic substances; the principal component is estrone, with preparations containing 75% to 85% sodium estrone sulfate and 6% to 15% sodium equilin sulfate such that the total is not <90%

Dosage Forms Tablet: 0.3 mg, 0.625 mg, 1.25 mg, 2.5 mg

Estroject-L.A.® see Estradiol on page 407

Estrone (es' trone)
Brand Names Estronol®; Kestrone®; Theelin®
Synonyms Estrogenic Substance Aqueous
Use Hypogonadism; primary ovarian failure; vasomotor symptoms of menopause; prostatic carcinoma; inoperable breast cancer, kraurosis vulvae, abnormal uterine bleeding due to hormone imbalance
Pregnancy Risk Factor X
Contraindications Thrombophlebitis, undiagnosed vaginal bleeding, hypersensitivity to estrogens or any component, pregnancy
Warnings/Precautions Use with caution in patients with asthma, epilepsy, migraine, diabetes, cardiac or renal dysfunction; estrogens may cause premature closure of the epiphyses in young individuals; safety and efficacy in children have not been established; estrogens have been reported to increase the risk of endometrial carcinoma, do not use estrogens during pregnancy

Adverse Reactions
>10%:
Cardiovascular: Peripheral edema
Endocrine & metabolic: Enlargement of breasts, breast tenderness, bloating
Gastrointestinal: Nausea, anorexia
1% to 10%:
Central nervous system: Headache
Endocrine & metabolic: Increased libido
Gastrointestinal: Vomiting, diarrhea
<1%:
Cardiovascular: Hypertension, thromboembolism, myocardial infarction, edema
(Continued)

Estrone *(Continued)*

Central nervous system: Stroke, depression, dizziness, anxiety

Dermatologic: Chloasma, melasma, rash

Endocrine & metabolic: Breast tumors, amenorrhea, alterations in frequency and flow of menses, decreased glucose tolerance, increased triglycerides and LDL

Gastrointestinal: GI distress

Hepatic: cholestatic jaundice

Miscellaneous: Intolerance to contact lenses, increased susceptibility to *Candida* infection

Overdosage/Toxicology Symptoms of overdose include fluid retention, jaundice, thrombophlebitis; toxicity is unlikely following single exposures of excessive doses, any treatment should be supportive and symptomatic

Drug Interactions

Decreased effect: Rifampin decreases estrogen serum concentrations

Increased toxicity:

Hydrocortisone increases corticosteroid toxic potential

Anticoagulants: Increases potential for thromboembolic events with anticoagulants

Carbamazepine, tricyclic antidepressants, and corticosteroids; ↑ thromboembolic potential with oral anticoagulants

Mechanism of Action Estrone is a natural ovarian estrogenic hormone that is available as an aqueous mixture of water insoluble estrone and water soluble estrone potassium sulfate; all estrogens, including estrone, act in a similar manner; there is no evidence that there are biological differences among various estrogen preparations other than their ability to bind to cellular receptors inside the target cells

Usual Dosage Adults: I.M.:

Male: Prostatic carcinoma: 2-4 mg 2-3 times/week

Female:

Senile vaginitis and kraurosis vulvae: 0.1-0.5 mg 2-3 times/week

Breast cancer (inoperable, progressing): 5 mg 3 or more times/week

Primary ovarian failure, hypogonadism: 0.1-1 mg/week, up to 2 mg/week in single or divided doses

Abnormal uterine bleeding: 2.5 mg/day for several days

Administration Intramuscular injection only

Test Interactions

Decreased antithrombin III

Decreased serum folate concentration

Increased prothrombin and factors VII, VIII, IX, X

Increased platelet aggregability

Increased thyroid binding globulin

Increased total thyroid hormone (T_4)

Increased serum triglycerides/phospholipids

Patient Information Patients should inform their physicians if signs or symptoms of any of the following occur: Thromboembolic or thrombotic disorders including sudden severe headache or vomiting, disturbance of vision or speech, loss of vision, numbness or weakness in an extremity, sharp or crushing chest pain, calf pain, shortness of breath, severe abdominal pain or mass, mental depression or unusual bleeding; patients should discontinue taking the medication if they suspect they are pregnant or become pregnant

Dosage Forms Injection: 2 mg/mL (10 mL, 30 mL); 5 mg/mL (10 mL)

Estronol® *see* Estrone *on previous page*

Estropipate *(ess' troe pih pate)*

Brand Names Ogen®; Ortho-Est®

Synonyms Piperazine Estrone Sulfate

Use Atrophic vaginitis; hypogonadism; primary ovarian failure; vasomotor symptoms of menopause; osteoporosis prophylactic

Pregnancy Risk Factor X

Contraindications Thrombophlebitis, undiagnosed vaginal bleeding, hypersensitivity to estrogens or any component

Warnings/Precautions Use with caution in patients with asthma, epilepsy, migraine, diabetes, cardiac or renal dysfunction; estrogens may cause premature closure of the epiphyses in young individuals; safety and efficacy in children have not been established; estrogens have been reported to increase the risk of endometrial carcinoma, do not use estrogens during pregnancy

Adverse Reactions

>10%:

Cardiovascular: Peripheral edema

Endocrine & metabolic: Enlargement of breasts, breast tenderness, bloating
Gastrointestinal: Nausea, anorexia

1% to 10%:
Central nervous system: Headache
Endocrine & metabolic: Increased libido
Gastrointestinal: Vomiting, diarrhea

<1%:
Cardiovascular: Hypertension, thromboembolism, myocardial infarction, edema
Central nervous system: Stroke, depression, dizziness, anxiety
Dermatologic: Chloasma, melasma, rash
Endocrine & metabolic: Breast tumors, amenorrhea, alterations in frequency and flow of menses, decreased glucose tolerance, increased triglycerides and LDL
Gastrointestinal: GI distress
Hepatic: Cholestatic jaundice
Miscellaneous: Intolerance to contact lenses, increased susceptibility to *Candida* infection

Overdosage/Toxicology Symptoms of overdose include fluid retention, jaundice, thrombophlebitis; toxicity is unlikely following single exposures of excessive doses, any treatment following emesis and charcoal administration should be supportive and symptomatic

Drug Interactions
Decreased effect: Rifampin decreases estrogen serum concentrations
Increased toxicity:
Hydrocortisone increases corticosteroid toxic potential
Anticoagulants: Increases potential for thromboembolic events with anticoagulants
Carbamazepine, tricyclic antidepressants, and corticosteroids; increased thromboembolic potential with oral anticoagulants

Mechanism of Action Crystalline estrone that has been solubilized as the sulfate and stabilized with piperazine. Primary effects on the interphase DNA-protein complex (chromatin) by binding to a receptor (usually located in the cytoplasm of a target cell) and initiating translocation of the hormone receptor complex to the nucleus.

Usual Dosage Adults: Female:
Moderate to severe vasomotor symptoms: Oral: 0.625-5 mg/day
Hypogonadism or primary ovarian failure: Oral: 1.25-7.5 mg/day for 3 weeks followed by an 8- to 10-day rest period
Osteoporosis prevention: Oral: 0.625 mg/day for 25 days of a 31-day cycle
Atrophic vaginitis or kraurosis vulvae: Vaginal: Instill 2-4 g/day 3 weeks on and 1 week off

Test Interactions
Decreased antithrombin III
Decreased serum folate concentration
Increased prothrombin and factors VII, VIII, IX, X
Increased platelet aggregability
Increased thyroid binding globulin
Increased total thyroid hormone (T_4)
Increased serum triglycerides/phospholipids

Patient Information Patients should inform their physicians if signs or symptoms of any of the following occur: Thromboembolic or thrombotic disorders including sudden severe headache or vomiting, disturbance of vision or speech, loss of vision, numbness or weakness in an extremity, sharp or crushing chest pain, calf pain, shortness of breath, severe abdominal pain or mass, mental depression or unusual bleeding; patients should discontinue taking the medication if they suspect they are pregnant or become pregnant. Patient package insert is available; insert product high into the vagina.

Dosage Forms
Cream, vaginal: 0.15% [estropipate 1.5 mg/g] (42.5 g tube)
Tablet: 0.625 mg [estropipate 0.75 mg]; 1.25 mg [estropipate 1.5 mg]; 2.5 mg [estropipate 3 mg]; 5 mg [estropipate 6 mg]

Estrovis® *see* Quinestrol *on page 966*

Ethacrynic Acid (eth a krin' ik)
Related Information
Diuretics, Loop Comparison *on page 1269*
Brand Names Edecrin®
Use Management of edema associated with congestive heart failure; hepatic cirrhosis or renal disease; short-term management of ascites due to malignancy, idiopathic edema, and lymphedema
(Continued)

415

Ethacrynic Acid (Continued)

Pregnancy Risk Factor B

Contraindications Hypersensitivity to ethacrynic acid or any component; anuria, hypotension, dehydration with low serum sodium concentrations; metabolic alkalosis with hypokalemia, or history of severe, watery diarrhea from ethacrynic acid

Warnings/Precautions Use with caution in patients with advanced hepatic cirrhosis, diabetes mellitus, hypotension, dehydration, history of watery diarrhea from ethacrynic acid, hearing impairment; ototoxicity occurs more frequently than with other loop diuretics; safety and efficacy in infants have not been established

Adverse Reactions
>10%: Diarrhea
1% to 10%:
  Central nervous system: Headache
  Endocrine & metabolic: Hyponatremia, hypochloremic alkalosis, hypokalemia
  Gastrointestinal: Loss of appetite
  Neuromuscular & skeletal: Orthostatic hypotension
  Ocular: Blurred vision
  Otic: Ototoxicity
<1%:
  Central nervous system: Nervousness
  Dermatologic: Skin rash
  Endocrine & metabolic: Hyperuricemia, gout
  Gastrointestinal: Gastrointestinal bleeding, pancreatitis, stomach cramps
  Hepatic: Hepatic dysfunction, abnormal LFTs
  Hematologic: Leukopenia, agranulocytosis, thrombocytopenia
  Local: Local irritation
  Renal: Renal injury, hematuria

Overdosage/Toxicology Symptoms of overdose include electrolyte depletion, volume depletion, dehydration, circulatory collapse; following GI decontamination, treatment is supportive; hypotension responds to fluids and Trendelenburg position

Drug Interactions
Increased toxicity:
  Hypotensive agents → additive ↓ blood pressure
  Drugs affected by or causing potassium depletion → additive ↓ potassium
  Increased nephrotoxic potential with aminoglycosides
  Digoxin increases cardiotoxic potential → arrhythmias
  Increased warfarin anticoagulant effects; increased lithium levels
Decreased effect:
  Probenecid decreases diuretic effects
  Decreased effectiveness of antidiabetic agents

Mechanism of Action Inhibits reabsorption of sodium and chloride in the ascending loop of Henle and distal renal tubule, interfering with the chloride-binding cotransport system, thus causing increased excretion of water, sodium, chloride, magnesium, and calcium

Pharmacodynamics/Kinetics
Onset of diuretic effect:
  Oral: Within 30 minutes
  I.V.: 5 minutes
Peak effect:
  Oral: 2 hours
  I.V.: 30 minutes
Duration of action:
  Oral: 12 hours
  I.V.: 2 hours
Absorption: Oral: Rapid
Metabolism: In the liver to active cysteine conjugate (35% to 40%)
Protein binding: >90%
Half-life: Normal renal function: 2-4 hours
Elimination: 30% to 60% excreted unchanged in bile and urine

Usual Dosage I.V. formulation should be diluted in D_5W or NS (1 mg/mL) and infused over several minutes

Children:
  Oral: 1 mg/kg/dose once daily; increase at intervals of 2-3 days as needed, to a maximum of 3 mg/kg/day
  I.V.: 1 mg/kg/dose, (maximum: 50 mg/dose); repeat doses not routinely recommended; however, if indicated, repeat doses every 8-12 hours
Adults:
  Oral: 50-100 mg/day in 1-2 divided doses; may increase in increments of 25-50 mg at intervals of several days to a maximum of 400 mg/24 hours
  I.V.: 0.5-1 mg/kg/dose (maximum: 100 mg/dose); repeat doses not routinely recommended; however, if indicated, repeat doses every 8-12 hours

Dosing adjustment/comments in renal impairment: Cl_{cr} <10 mL/minute: Avoid use

Not removed by hemo- or peritoneal dialysis; supplemental dose is not necessary

Administration Injection should **not** be given S.C. or I.M. due to local pain and irritation; single I.V. doses should not exceed 100 mg; if a second dose is needed, use a new injection site to avoid possible thrombophlebitis

Monitoring Parameters Blood pressure, renal function, serum electrolytes, and fluid status closely, including weight and I & O daily; hearing

Patient Information May be taken with food or milk; get up slowly from a lying or sitting position to minimize dizziness, lightheadedness, or fainting; also use extra care when exercising, standing for long periods of time, and during hot weather. Take in morning, take last dose of multiple doses before 6 PM unless instructed otherwise.

Dosage Forms
Powder for injection, as ethacrynate sodium: 50 mg (50 mL)
Tablet: 25 mg, 50 mg

Ethambutol Hydrochloride (e tham' byoo tole)

Related Information
Antimicrobial Drugs of Choice on page 1298-1302
Recommendations of the Advisory Council on the Elimination of Tuberculosis on page 1303-1304

Brand Names Myambutol®

Use Treatment of tuberculosis and other mycobacterial diseases in conjunction with other antituberculosis agents; only indicated when patients are from areas where drug-resistant M. tuberculosis is endemic, in HIV-infected elderly patients, and when drug-resistant M. tuberculosis is suspected

Pregnancy Risk Factor B

Contraindications Hypersensitivity to ethambutol or any component; optic neuritis

Warnings/Precautions Use only in children whose visual acuity can accurately be determined and monitored (not recommended for use in children <13 years of age); dosage modification required in patients with renal insufficiency

Adverse Reactions
1% to 10%:
Central nervous system: Headache, confusion, disorientation
Endocrine & metabolic: Acute gout or hyperuricemia
Gastrointestinal: Abdominal pain, anorexia, nausea, vomiting
<1%:
Central nervous system: Malaise, peripheral neuritis, mental confusion, fever
Dermatologic: Rash, pruritus
Hepatic: Abnormal liver function tests
Ocular: Optic neuritis
Miscellaneous: Anaphylaxis

Overdosage/Toxicology Symptoms of overdose include decrease in visual acuity, anorexia, joint pain, numbness of the extremities; following GI decontamination, treatment is supportive

Drug Interactions Decreased absorption with aluminum salts

Mechanism of Action Suppresses mycobacteria multiplication by interfering with RNA synthesis

Pharmacodynamics/Kinetics
Absorption: Oral: ~80%
Distribution: Well distributed throughout the body with high concentrations in kidneys, lungs, saliva, and red blood cells
Relative diffusion of antimicrobial agents from blood into CSF: Adequate with or without inflammation (exceeds usual MICs)
Ratio of CSF to blood level (%):
Normal meninges: 0
Inflamed meninges: 25
Protein binding: 20% to 30%
Metabolism: 20% metabolized by the liver to inactive metabolite
Half-life: 2.5-3.6 hours
End stage renal disease: 7-15 hours
Time to peak serum concentration: 2-4 hours
Elimination: ~50% excreted in the urine and 20% excreted in the feces as unchanged drug

Usual Dosage Oral:
Ethambutol is generally not recommended in children whose visual acuity cannot be monitored (<6 years of age). However, ethambutol should be considered for all children with organisms resistant to other drugs, when susceptibility to ethambutol has been demonstrated, or susceptibility is likely.

(Continued)

417

Ethambutol Hydrochloride *(Continued)*

Note: A four-drug regimen (isoniazid, rifampin, pyrazinamide, and either strepto-mycin or ethambutol) is preferred for the initial, empiric treatment of TB. When the drug susceptibility results are available, the regimen should be altered as appropriate.

Patients with tuberculosis and without HIV infection:
OPTION 1: Isoniazid resistance rate <4%: Administer daily isoniazid, rifampin, and pyrazinamide for 8 weeks followed by isoniazid and rifampin daily or directly observed therapy (DOT) 2-3 times/week for 16 weeks. If isoniazid resistance rate is not documented, ethambutol or streptomycin should also be administered until susceptibility to isoniazid or rifampin is demonstrated. Continue treatment for at least 6 months or 3 months beyond culture conversion.

OPTION 2: Administer daily isoniazid, rifampin, pyrazinamide, and either strepto-mycin or ethambutol for 2 weeks followed by DOT 2 times/week administration of the same drugs for 6 weeks, and subsequently, with isoniazid and rifampin DOT 2 times/week administration for 16 weeks

OPTION 3: Administer isoniazid, rifampin, pyrazinamide, and either etham-butol or streptomycin by DOT 3 times/week for 6 months

Patients with TB and with HIV infection: Administer any of the above OPTIONS 1, 2 or 3; however, treatment should be continued for a total of 9 months and at least 6 months beyond culture conversion

Note: Some experts recommend that the duration of therapy should be extended to 9 months for patients with disseminated disease, miliary disease, disease involving the bones or joints, or tuberculosis lymphadenitis

Children (>6 years) and Adults:
Daily therapy: 15-25 mg/kg/day (maximum: 2.5 g/day)
Directly observed therapy (DOT): Twice weekly: 50 mg/kg (maximum: 2.5 g)
DOT: 3 times/week: 25-30 mg/kg (maximum: 2.5 g)

Dosing interval in renal impairment:
Cl_{cr} 10-50 mL/minute: Administer every 24-36 hours
Cl_{cr} <10 mL/minute: Administer every 48 hours
Slightly dialyzable (5% to 20%); Administer dose postdialysis
Peritoneal dialysis: Dose for Cl_{cr} <10 mL/minute
Continuous arterio-venous or veno-venous hemofiltration: Administer every 24-36 hours

Monitoring Parameters Periodic visual testing in patients receiving more than 15 mg/kg/day; periodic renal, hepatic, and hematopoietic tests

Test Interactions ↑ uric acid (S)

Patient Information Report any visual changes or rash to physician; may cause stomach upset, take with food; do not take within 2 hours of aluminum-containing antacids

Dosage Forms Tablet: 100 mg, 400 mg

Ethamolin® *see* Ethanolamine Oleate *on this page*

Ethanoic Acid *see* Acetic Acid *on page 22*

Ethanolamine Oleate *(eth' a nol a meen)*

Brand Names Ethamolin®

Use Mild sclerosing agent used for bleeding esophageal varices

Pregnancy Risk Factor C

Contraindications Hypersensitivity to agent or oleic acid

Warnings/Precautions Fatal anaphylactic shock has been reported following administration; use with caution in children class C patients

Adverse Reactions
1% to 10%:
Central nervous system: Pyrexia
Gastrointestinal: Esophageal ulcer, esophageal stricture
Respiratory: Pleural effusion, pneumonia
Miscellaneous: Retrosternal pain
<1%:
Local: Injection necrosis
Renal: Acute renal failure
Miscellaneous: Aspiration, anaphylaxis

Overdosage/Toxicology Anaphylaxis after administration of larger than normal volumes, severe intramural necrosis; treatment is supportive with epinephrine, corticosteroids, fluids, and pressors

Mechanism of Action Derived from oleic acid and similar in physical properties to sodium morrhuate; however, the exact mechanism of the hemostatic effect used in endoscopic injection sclerotherapy is not known. Intravenously injected ethanolamine oleate produces a sterile inflammatory response resulting in fibrosis and occlusion of the vein; a dose-related extravascular inflammatory reaction occurs when the drug diffuses through the venous wall. Autopsy results indicate that variceal obliteration occurs secondary to mural necrosis and fibrosis. Thrombosis appears to be a transient reaction.

Usual Dosage Adults: 1.5-5 mL per varix, up to 20 mL total or 0.4 mL/kg; patients with severe hepatic dysfunction should receive less than recommended maximum dose

Nursing Implications Have epinephrine and resuscitative equipment nearby

Dosage Forms Injection: 5% [50 mg/mL] (2 mL)

Ethchlorvynol (eth klor vi' nole)

Brand Names Placidyl®

Use Short-term management of insomnia

Restrictions C-IV

Pregnancy Risk Factor C

Contraindications Porphyria, hypersensitivity to ethchlorvynol or any component

Warnings/Precautions Administer with caution to depressed or suicidal patients or to patients with a history of drug abuse; intoxication symptoms may appear with prolonged daily doses of as little as 1 g; withdrawal symptoms may be seen upon abrupt discontinuation; use with caution in the elderly and in patients with hepatic or renal dysfunction; use with caution in patients who have a history of paradoxical restlessness to barbiturates or alcohol; some products may contain tartrazine

Adverse Reactions
>10%:
　Central nervous system: Dizziness, weakness
　Gastrointestinal: Indigestion, nausea, stomach pain, unpleasant aftertaste
　Ocular: Blurred vision
1% to 10%:
　Central nervous system: Nervousness, excitement, clumsiness, confusion, drowsiness (daytime)
　Dermatologic: Skin rash
<1%:
　Cardiovascular: Bradycardia
　Central nervous system: Hyperthermia, weakness (severe), slurred speech
　Hepatic: Cholestatic jaundice
　Neuromuscular & skeletal: Trembling
　Respiratory: Shortness of breath

Overdosage/Toxicology Symptoms of overdose include prolonged deep coma, respiratory depression, hypothermia, bradycardia, hypotension, nystagmus; treatment is supportive in nature; hemoperfusion may be helpful in enhancing elimination

Drug Interactions
　Decreased effect of oral anticoagulants
　Increased toxicity (CNS depression) with alcohol, CNS depressants, MAO inhibitors, TCAs (delirium)

Stability Capsules should not be crushed and should not be refrigerated

Mechanism of Action Causes nonspecific depression of the reticular activating system

Pharmacodynamics/Kinetics
　Onset of action: 15-60 minutes
　Duration: 5 hours
　Absorption: Rapid from GI tract
　Metabolism: In the liver
　Half-life: 10-20 hours
　Time to peak serum concentration: 2 hours

Usual Dosage Adults: Oral: 500-1000 mg at bedtime
　Dosing adjustment in renal impairment: Cl_{cr} <50 mL/minute: Avoid use

Monitoring Parameters Cardiac and respiratory function and abuse potential

Reference Range Therapeutic: 2-9 µg/mL; Toxic: >20 µg/mL

Patient Information May cause drowsiness, can impair judgment and coordination; avoid alcohol and other CNS depressants; ataxia can be reduced if taken with food, do not crush or refrigerate capsules

Nursing Implications Raise bed rails, institute safety measures, assist with ambulation

Dosage Forms Capsule: 200 mg, 500 mg, 750 mg

Ethinyl Estradiol (eth' in il ess tra dye' ole)

Brand Names Estinyl®

Use Hypogonadism; primary ovarian failure; vasomotor symptoms of menopause; prostatic carcinoma; breast cancer

Pregnancy Risk Factor X

Contraindications Thrombophlebitis, undiagnosed vaginal bleeding, hypersensitivity to ethinyl estradiol or any component, known or suspected pregnancy, carcinoma of the breast, estrogen-dependent tumor

Warnings/Precautions Use with caution in patients with asthma, seizure disorders, migraine, cardiac, renal or hepatic impairment, cerebrovascular disorders or history of breast cancer, past or present thromboembolic disease, smokers >35 years of age

Adverse Reactions

>10%:

Cardiovascular: Peripheral edema

Endocrine & metabolic: Enlargement of breasts, breast tenderness, bloating

Gastrointestinal: Nausea, anorexia

1% to 10%:

Central nervous system: Headache

Endocrine & metabolic: Increased libido

Gastrointestinal: Vomiting, diarrhea

<1%:

Cardiovascular: Hypertension, thromboembolism, myocardial infarction, edema

Central nervous system: Stroke, depression, dizziness, anxiety

Dermatologic: Chloasma, melasma, rash

Endocrine & metabolic: Breast tumors, amenorrhea, alterations in frequency and flow of menses, decreased glucose tolerance, increased triglycerides and LDL

Gastrointestinal: GI distress

Hepatic: Cholestatic jaundice

Miscellaneous: Intolerance to contact lenses, increased susceptibility to *Candida* infection

Overdosage/Toxicology Symptoms of overdose include fluid retention, jaundice, thrombophlebitis, nausea; toxicity is unlikely following single exposures of excessive doses, any treatment following emesis and charcoal administration should be supportive and symptomatic

Drug Interactions

Decreased effect: Rifampin decreases estrogen serum concentrations

Increased toxicity:

Hydrocortisone increases corticosteroid toxic potential

Anticoagulants: Increases potential for thromboembolic events with anticoagulants

Carbamazepine, tricyclic antidepressants, and corticosteroids; increased thromboembolic potential with oral anticoagulants

Mechanism of Action Increases the synthesis of DNA, RNA, and various proteins in target tissues; reduces the release of gonadotropin-releasing hormone from the hypothalamus; reduces FSH and LH release from the pituitary

Pharmacodynamics/Kinetics

Absorption: Absorbed well from GI tract

Protein binding: 50% to 80%

Metabolism: Inactivated by liver

Elimination: By the kidneys

Usual Dosage Adults: Oral:

Male: Prostatic cancer (inoperable, progressing): 0.15-2 mg/day for palliation

Female:

Hypogonadism: 0.05 mg 1-3 times/day for 2 weeks of a theoretical menstrual cycle followed by progesterone for 3-6 months

Vasomotor symptoms: 0.02-0.05 mg for 21 days, off 7 days and repeat

Breast cancer (inoperable, progressing): 1 mg 3 times/day for palliation

Test Interactions

Decreased antithrombin III

Decreased serum folate concentration

Increased prothrombin and factors VII, VIII, IX, X

Increased platelet aggregability

Increased thyroid binding globulin

Increased total thyroid hormone (T_4)

Increased serum triglycerides/phospholipids

Patient Information Photosensitivity may occur

Women should inform their physicians if signs or symptoms of any of the following occur: Thromboembolic or thrombotic disorders including sudden severe headache or vomiting, disturbance of vision or speech, loss of vision, numbness or weakness in an extremity, sharp or crushing chest pain, calf pain, shortness of breath, severe abdominal pain or mass, mental depression or unusual bleeding

Women should discontinue taking the medication if they suspect they are pregnant or become pregnant

Nursing Implications Give at bedtime to minimize occurrence of adverse effects

Dosage Forms Tablet: 0.02 mg, 0.05 mg, 0.5 mg

Ethinyl Estradiol and Ethynodiol Diacetate (eth' in il ess tra dye' ole & e thye noe dye' ole)

Brand Names Demulen®

Synonyms Ethynodiol Diacetate and Ethinyl Estradiol

Use Prevention of pregnancy; treatment of hypermenorrhea, endometriosis, female hypogonadism

Pregnancy Risk Factor X

Contraindications Known or suspected pregnancy, undiagnosed genital bleeding, carcinoma of the breast, estrogen-dependent tumor

Warnings/Precautions In patients with a history of thromboembolism, stroke, myocardial infarction (especially >40 years of age who smoke), liver tumor, hypertension, cardiac, renal or hepatic insufficiency; use of any progestin during the first 4 months of pregnancy is not recommended; risk of cardiovascular side effects increases in those women who smoke cigarettes and in women >35 years of age

Adverse Reactions

>10%:

    Cardiovascular: Peripheral edema

    Endocrine & metabolic: Enlargement of breasts, breast tenderness, bloating

    Gastrointestinal: Nausea, anorexia

1% to 10%:

    Central nervous system: Headache

    Endocrine & metabolic: Increased libido

    Gastrointestinal: Vomiting, diarrhea

<1%:

    Cardiovascular: Hypertension, thromboembolism, stroke, myocardial infarction, edema

    Central nervous system: Depression, dizziness, anxiety

    Dermatologic: Chloasma, melasma, rash

    Endocrine & metabolic: Decreased glucose tolerance, breast tumors, amenorrhea, alterations in frequency and flow of menses, increased triglycerides and LDL

    Gastrointestinal: GI distress

    Hepatic: Cholestatic jaundice

    Miscellaneous: Intolerance to contact lenses, increased susceptibility to *Candida* infection

See tables.

Overdosage/Toxicology Toxicity is unlikely following single exposures of excessive doses; any treatment following emesis and charcoal administration should be supportive and symptomatic

Drug Interactions

Decreased effect of oral contraceptives with barbiturates, hydantoins - phenytoin, rifampin, antibiotics - penicillins, tetracyclines, griseofulvin

Increased toxicity of acetaminophen, anticoagulants, benzodiazepines, caffeine, corticosteroids, metoprolol, theophylline, tricyclic antidepressants

Pharmacological Effects of Progestins Used in Oral Contraceptives

	Progestin	Estrogen	Antiestrogen	Androgen
Norgestrel/levonorgestrel	+++	0	++	+++
Ethynodiol diacetate	++	+*	+*	+
Norethindrone acetate	+	+	+++	+
Norethindrone	+	+*	+*	+
Norethynodrel	+	+++	0	0

*Has estrogenic effect at low doses; may have antiestrogenic effect at higher doses.

+++ = pronounced effect

++ = moderate effect

+ = slight effect

0 = moderate effect

(Continued)

Ethinyl Estradiol and Ethynodiol Diacetate *(Continued)*
Achieving Proper Hormonal Balance in an Oral Contraceptive

Estrogen		Progestin	
Excess	**Deficiency**	**Excess**	**Deficiency**
Nausea, bloating	Early or midcycle	Increased appetite	Late breakthrough
Cervical mucorrhea,	breakthrough	Weight gain	bleeding
polyposis	bleeding	Tiredness, fatigue	Amenorrhea
Melasma	Increased spotting	Hypomenorrhea	Hypermenorrhea
Migraine headache	Hypomenorrhea	Acne, oily scalp*	
Breast fullness or		Hair loss, hirsutism*	
tenderness		Depression	
Edema		Monilial vaginitis	
Hypertension		Breast regression	

*Result of androgenic activity of progestins.

Mechanism of Action Combination oral contraceptives inhibit ovulation via a negative feedback mechanism on the hypothalamus, which alters the normal pattern of gonadotropin secretion of a follicle-stimulating hormone (FSH) and luteinizing hormone by the anterior pituitary. The follicular phase FSH and midcycle surge of gonadotropins are inhibited. In addition, oral contraceptives produce alterations in the genital tract, including changes in the cervical mucus, rendering it unfavorable for sperm penetration even if ovulation occurs. Changes in the endometrium may also occur, producing an unfavorable environment for nidation. Oral contraceptive drugs may alter the tubal transport of the ova through the fallopian tubes. Progestational agents may also alter sperm fertility.

Pharmacodynamics/Kinetics
Ethinyl estradiol:
Absorption: Absorbed well from GI tract
Protein binding: 50% to 80%
Metabolism: Inactivated by liver
Elimination: By the kidneys
Ethynodiol diacetate:
Converted to norethindrone
Metabolism: By conjugation in the liver
Half-life, terminal: 5-14 hours

Usual Dosage Adults: Female: Oral:
For 21-tablet cycle packs, with 21 active tablets (28-day packs have 21 active tablets and 7 inert tablets): Take 1 tablet daily starting on the fifth day of menstrual cycle, with day 1 being the first day of menstruation; begin taking a new cycle pack on the eighth day after taking the last tablet from the previous pack

With 28-tablet packages, dosage is 1 tablet daily without interruption; extra tablets are placebos or contain iron. If next menstrual period does not begin on schedule, rule out pregnancy before starting new dosing cycle. If menstrual period begins, start new dosing cycle 7 days after last tablet was taken. If all doses have been taken on schedule and one menstrual period is missed, continue dosing cycle. If two consecutive menstrual periods are missed, pregnancy test is required before new dosing cycle is started.
One dose missed: Take as soon as remembered or take 2 tablets next day
Two doses missed: Take 2 tablets as soon as remembered or 2 tablets next 2 days
Three doses missed: Begin new compact of tablets starting on day 1 of next cycle

Test Interactions
Decreased antithrombin III
Decreased serum folate concentration
Increased prothrombin and factors VII, VIII, IX, X
Increased platelet aggregability
Increased thyroid binding globulin
Increased total thyroid hormone (T_4)
Increased serum triglycerides/phospholipids

Patient Information Photosensitivity may occur
Inform your physician if signs or symptoms of any of the following occur: Thromboembolic or thrombotic disorders including sudden severe headache or vomiting, disturbance of vision or speech, loss of vision, numbness or weakness in an extremity, sharp or crushing chest pain, calf pain, shortness of breath, severe abdominal pain or mass, mental depression or unusual bleeding.
If any doses are missed, alternative contraceptive methods should be used for the next 2 days or until 2 days into the new cycle

Discontinue taking the medication if you suspect you are pregnant or become pregnant

Additional Information Monophasic oral contraceptive

Dosage Forms Tablet:

1/35: Ethinyl estradiol 0.035 mg and ethynodiol diacetate 1 mg (21s, 28s)

1/50: Ethinyl estradiol 0.05 mg and ethynodiol diacetate 1 mg (21s, 28s)

Ethinyl Estradiol and Levonorgestrel (lee' voe nor jess trel)

Brand Names Levlen®; Levora®; Nordette®; Tri-Levlen®; Triphasil®

Synonyms Levonorgestrel and Ethinyl Estradiol

Use Prevention of pregnancy; treatment of hypermenorrhea, endometriosis, female hypogonadism

Pregnancy Risk Factor X

Contraindications Thrombophlebitis, undiagnosed vaginal bleeding, hypersensitivity to ethinyl estradiol or any component, known or suspected pregnancy, carcinoma of the breast, estrogen-dependent tumor

Warnings/Precautions Use of any progestin during the first 4 months of pregnancy is not recommended; use with caution in patients with asthma, seizure disorders, migraine, cardiac, renal or hepatic impairment, cerebrovascular disorders or history of breast cancer, past and present thromboembolic disease, smokers >35 years of age

Adverse Reactions

>10%:

Cardiovascular: Peripheral edema

Endocrine & metabolic: Enlargement of breasts, breast tenderness, bloating

Gastrointestinal: Nausea, anorexia

1% to 10%:

Central nervous system: Headache

Endocrine & metabolic: Increased libido

Gastrointestinal: Vomiting, diarrhea

<1%:

Cardiovascular: Hypertension, thromboembolism, stroke, myocardial infarction, edema

Central nervous system: Depression, dizziness, anxiety

Dermatologic: Chloasma, melasma, rash

Endocrine & metabolic: Decreased glucose tolerance, breast tumors, amenorrhea, alterations in frequency and flow of menses, increased triglycerides and LDL

Gastrointestinal: GI distress

Hepatic: Cholestatic jaundice

Miscellaneous: Intolerance to contact lenses, increased susceptibility to *Candida* infection

See tables.

Overdosage/Toxicology Toxicity is unlikely following single exposures of excessive doses; any treatment following emesis and charcoal administration should be supportive and symptomatic

Drug Interactions

Decreased effect of oral contraceptives with barbiturates, hydantoins - phenytoin, rifampin, antibiotics - penicillins, tetracyclines, griseofulvin

Increased toxicity of acetaminophen, anticoagulants, benzodiazepines, caffeine, corticosteroids, metoprolol, theophylline, tricyclic antidepressants

Pharmacological Effects of Progestins Used in Oral Contraceptives

	Progestin	Estrogen	Antiestrogen	Androgen
Norgestrel/levonorgestrel	+++	0	++	+++
Ethynodiol diacetate	++	+*	+*	+
Norethindrone acetate	+	+	+++	+
Norethindrone	+	+*	+*	+
Norethynodrel	+	+++	0	0

*Has estrogenic effect at low doses; may have antiestrogenic effect at higher doses.

+++ = pronounced effect

++ = moderate effect

+ = slight effect

0 = moderate effect

(Continued)

423

Ethinyl Estradiol and Levonorgestrel *(Continued)*
Achieving Proper Hormonal Balance in an Oral Contraceptive

Estrogen		Progestin	
Excess	**Deficiency**	**Excess**	**Deficiency**
Nausea, bloating	Early or midcycle	Increased appetite	Late breakthrough
Cervical mucorrhea,	breakthrough	Weight gain	bleeding
polyposis	bleeding	Tiredness, fatigue	Amenorrhea
Melasma	Increased spotting	Hypomenorrhea	Hypermenorrhea
Migraine headache	Hypomenorrhea	Acne, oily scalp*	
Breast fullness or		Hair loss, hirsutism*	
tenderness		Depression	
Edema		Monilial vaginitis	
Hypertension		Breast regression	

*Result of androgenic activity of progestins.

Mechanism of Action Combination oral contraceptives inhibit ovulation via a negative feedback mechanism on the hypothalamus, which alters the normal pattern of gonadotropin secretion of a follicle-stimulating hormone (FSH) and luteinizing hormone by the anterior pituitary. The follicular phase FSH and midcycle surge of gonadotropins are inhibited. In addition, oral contraceptives produce alterations in the genital tract, including changes in the cervical mucus, rendering it unfavorable for sperm penetration even if ovulation occurs. Changes in the endometrium may also occur, producing an unfavorable environment for nidation. Oral contraceptive drugs may alter the tubal transport of the ova through the fallopian tubes. Progestational agents may also alter sperm fertility.

Pharmacodynamics/Kinetics
    Ethinyl estradiol:
        Absorption: Absorbed well from GI tract
        Protein binding: 50% to 80%
        Metabolism: Inactivated by liver
        Elimination: By the kidneys
    Levonorgestrel:
        Bioavailability: Completely
        Metabolism: Does not undergo first-pass effect; chiefly metabolized by reduction and conjugation
        Time to peak: 0.5-2 hours
        Half-life, terminal: 11-45 hours

Usual Dosage Adults: Female: Oral:
    Contraception: 1 tablet daily, beginning on day 5 of menstrual cycle (first day of menstrual flow is day 1). With 20-tablet and 21-tablet packages, new dosing cycle begins 7 days after last tablet taken. With 28-tablet packages, dosage is 1 tablet daily without interruption; extra tablets are placebos or contain iron. If next menstrual period does not begin on schedule, rule out pregnancy before starting new dosing cycle. If menstrual period begins, start new dosing cycle 7 days after last tablet was taken. If all doses have been taken on schedule and one menstrual period is missed, continue dosing cycle. If two consecutive menstrual periods are missed, pregnancy test is required before new dosing cycle is started.
    One dose missed: Take as soon as remembered or take 2 tablets next day
    Two doses missed: Take 2 tablets as soon as remembered or 2 tablets next 2 days
    Three doses missed: Begin new compact of tablets starting on day 1 of next cycle
    Triphasic oral contraceptive (Tri-Levlen®, Triphasil®): 1 tablet/day in the sequence specified by the manufacturer

Test Interactions
    Decreased antithrombin III
    Decreased serum folate concentration
    Increased prothrombin and factors VII, VIII, IX, X
    Increased platelet aggregability
    Increased thyroid binding globulin
    Increased total thyroid hormone (T_4)
    Increased serum triglycerides/phospholipids

Patient Information
    Inform your physician if signs or symptoms of any of the following occur: Thromboembolic or thrombotic disorders including sudden severe headache or vomiting, disturbance of vision or speech, loss of vision, numbness or weakness in an extremity, sharp or crushing chest pain, calf pain, shortness of breath, severe abdominal pain or mass, mental depression or unusual bleeding
    If any doses are missed, alternative contraceptive methods should be used for the next 2 days or until 2 days into the new cycle

Discontinue taking the medication if you suspect you are pregnant or become pregnant

Additional Information
Monophasic oral contraceptives: Levlen®, Levora®, Nordette®
Triphasic oral contraceptives: Tri-Levlen® and Triphasil®

Dosage Forms Tablet:
Levlen®, Levora®, Nordette®: Ethinyl estradiol 0.03 mg and levonorgestrel 0.15 mg (21s, 28s)
Tri-Levlen®, Triphasil®: Phase 1 (6 brown tablets): Ethinyl estradiol 0.03 mg and levonorgestrel 0.05 mg; Phase 2 (5 white tablets): Ethinyl estradiol 0.04 mg and levonorgestrel 0.075 mg; Phase 3 (10 yellow tablets): Ethinyl estradiol 0.03 mg and levonorgestrel 0.125 mg (21s, 28s)

Ethinyl Estradiol and Norethindrone (nor eth in' drone)

Brand Names Brevicon®; Genora®; Jenest™; Loestrin®; Modicon™; N.E.E.™; Nelova™; Norethin™; Norinyl®; Norlestrin®; Ortho-Novum™; Ovcon®; Tri-Norinyl®

Synonyms Norethindrone Acetate and Ethinyl Estradiol

Use Prevention of pregnancy; treatment of hypermenorrhea, endometriosis, female hypogonadism

Pregnancy Risk Factor X

Contraindications Thrombophlebitis, cerebral vascular disease, coronary artery disease, known or suspected breast carcinoma, undiagnosed abnormal genital bleeding

Warnings/Precautions Use of any progestin during the first 4 months of pregnancy is not recommended; in patients with a history of thromboembolism, stroke, myocardial infarction (especially >40 years of age who smoke), liver tumor, hypertension, cardiac, renal or hepatic insufficiency; risk of cardiovascular side effects increases in those women who smoke cigarettes and in women >35 years of age

Adverse Reactions
>10%:
Cardiovascular: Peripheral edema
Endocrine & metabolic: Enlargement of breasts, breast tenderness, bloating
Gastrointestinal: Nausea, anorexia
1% to 10%:
Central nervous system: Headache
Endocrine & metabolic: Increased libido
Gastrointestinal: Vomiting, diarrhea
<1%:
Cardiovascular: Hypertension, thromboembolism, stroke, myocardial infarction, edema
Central nervous system: Depression, dizziness, anxiety
Dermatologic: Chloasma, melasma, rash
Endocrine & metabolic: Decreased glucose tolerance, breast tumors, amenorrhea, alterations in frequency and flow of menses, increased triglycerides and LDL
Gastrointestinal: GI distress
Hepatic: Cholestatic jaundice
Miscellaneous: Intolerance to contact lenses, increased susceptibility to *Candida* infection
See tables.

Achieving Proper Hormonal Balance in an Oral Contraceptive

Estrogen		Progestin	
Excess	**Deficiency**	**Excess**	**Deficiency**
Nausea, bloating	Early or midcycle breakthrough bleeding	Increased appetite	Late breakthrough bleeding
Cervical mucorrhea, polyposis		Weight gain	Amenorrhea
Melasma	Increased spotting	Tiredness, fatigue	Hypermenorrhea
Migraine headache	Hypomenorrhea	Hypomenorrhea	
Breast fullness or tenderness		Acne, oily scalp*	
Edema		Hair loss, hirsutism*	
Hypertension		Depression	
		Monilial vaginitis	
		Breast regression	

*Result of androgenic activity of progestins.

Ethinyl Estradiol and Norethindrone *(Continued)*

Pharmacological Effects of Progestins Used in Oral Contraceptives

	Progestin	Estrogen	Antiestrogen	Androgen
Norgestrel/levonorgestrel	+++	0	++	+++
Ethynodiol diacetate	++	+*	+*	+
Norethindrone acetate	+	+	+++	+
Norethindrone	+	+*	+*	· +
Norethynodrel	+	+++	0	0

*Has estrogenic effect at low doses; may have antiestrogenic effect at higher doses.

+++ = pronounced effect

++ = moderate effect

+ = slight effect

0 = moderate effect

Overdosage/Toxicology Toxicity is unlikely following single exposures of excessive doses; any treatment following emesis and charcoal administration should be supportive and symptomatic

Drug Interactions

Decreased effect of oral contraceptives with barbiturates, hydantoins - phenytoin, rifampin, antibiotics - penicillins, tetracyclines, griseofulvin

Increased toxicity of acetaminophen, anticoagulants, benzodiazepines, caffeine, corticosteroids, metoprolol, theophylline, tricyclic antidepressants

Mechanism of Action Combination oral contraceptives inhibit ovulation via a negative feedback mechanism on the hypothalamus, which alters the normal pattern of gonadotropin secretion of a follicle-stimulating hormone (FSH) and luteinizing hormone by the anterior pituitary. The follicular phase FSH and midcycle surge of gonadotropins are inhibited. In addition, oral contraceptives produce alterations in the genital tract, including changes in the cervical mucus, rendering it unfavorable for sperm penetration even if ovulation occurs. Changes in the endometrium may also occur, producing an unfavorable environment for nidation. Oral contraceptive drugs may alter the tubal transport of the ova through the fallopian tubes. Progestational agents may also alter sperm fertility.

Pharmacodynamics/Kinetics

Ethinyl estradiol:

Absorption: Absorbed well from GI tract

Protein binding: 50% to 80%

Metabolism: Inactivated by liver

Elimination: By the kidneys

Norethindrone:

Time to peak: Oral: 0.5-4 hours

Bioavailability: Overall 65% with first-pass metabolism

Half-life, terminal: 5-14 hours

Usual Dosage Adults: Female: Oral:

For 21-tablet cycle packs, with 21 active tablets (28-day packs have 21 active tablets and 7 inert tablets): Take 1 tablet daily starting on the fifth day of menstrual cycle, with day 1 being the first day of menstruation; begin taking a new cycle pack on the eighth day after taking the last tablet from the previous pack

With 28-tablet packages, dosage is 1 tablet daily without interruption; extra tablets are placebos or contain iron. If next menstrual period does not begin on schedule, rule out pregnancy before starting new dosing cycle. If menstrual period begins, start new dosing cycle 7 days after last tablet was taken. If all doses have been taken on schedule and one menstrual period is missed, continue dosing cycle. If two consecutive menstrual periods are missed, pregnancy test is required before new dosing cycle is started.

One dose missed: Take as soon as remembered or take 2 tablets next day

Two doses missed: Take 2 tablets as soon as remembered or 2 tablets next 2 days

Three doses missed: Begin new compact of tablets starting on day 1 of next cycle

Biphasic oral contraceptive (Jenest™-28, Ortho-Novum™ 10/11, Nelova™ 10/11): 1 color tablet/day for 10 days, then next color tablet for 11 days

Triphasic oral contraceptive (Ortho-Novum™ 7/7/7, Tri-Norinyl®, Triphasil®): 1 tablet/day in the sequence specified by the manufacturer

Test Interactions

Decreased antithrombin III

Decreased serum folate concentration

Increased prothrombin and factors VII, VIII, IX, X

Increased platelet aggregability
Increased thyroid binding globulin
Increased total thyroid hormone (T_4)
Increased serum triglycerides/phospholipids

Patient Information

Inform your physician if signs or symptoms of any of the following occur: Thromboembolic or thrombotic disorders including sudden severe headache or vomiting, disturbance of vision or speech, loss of vision, numbness or weakness in an extremity, sharp or crushing chest pain, calf pain, shortness of breath, severe abdominal pain or mass, mental depression or unusual bleeding

If any doses are missed, alternative contraceptive methods should be used for the next 2 days or until 2 days into the new cycle

Discontinue taking the medication if you suspect you are pregnant or become pregnant

Nursing Implications Give at bedtime to minimize occurrence of adverse effects

Additional Information

Monophasic oral contraceptives: Ovcon®, Genora®, Loestrin®, N.E.E.®, Nelova®, Norethin®, Norinyl®, Ortho-Novum®

Biphasic oral contraceptives: Jenest®, Nelova™ 10/11, Ortho-Novum™ 10/11

Triphasic oral contraceptives: Tri-Norinyl®, Ortho-Novum™ 7/7/7

Dosage Forms Tablet:

Brevicon®, Genora® 0.5/35, Modicon™, Nelova® 0.5/35E: Ethinyl estradiol 0.035 mg and norethindrone 0.5 mg (21s, 28s)

Genora® 1/35, N.E.E.®1/35, Nelova® 1/35E, Norethin® 1/35E, Norinyl® 1 + 35, Ortho-Novum® 1/35: Ethinyl estradiol 0.035 mg and norethindrone 1 mg (21s, 28s)

Jenest™-28: Phase 1 (7 white tablets): Ethinyl estradiol 0.035 mg and norethindrone 0.5 mg; Phase 2 (14 peach tablets): Ethinyl estradiol 0.035 mg and norethindrone 1 mg (21s, 28s)

Loestrin® 1.5/30: Ethinyl estradiol 0.03 mg and norethindrone acetate 1.5 mg (21s, 28s)

Loestrin® Fe 1.5/30: Ethinyl estradiol 0.03 mg and norethindrone acetate 1.5 mg with ferrous fumarate 75 mg in 7 inert tablets (28s)

Loestrin® 1/20: Ethinyl estradiol 0.02 mg and norethindrone acetate 1 mg (21s)

Loestrin® Fe 1/20: Ethinyl estradiol 0.02 mg and norethindrone acetate 1 mg with ferrous fumarate 75 mg in 7 inert tablets (28s)

Nelova™ 10/11: Phase 1 (10 light yellow tablets): Ethinyl estradiol 0.035 mg and norethindrone 0.5 mg; Phase 2 (11 dark yellow tablets): Ethinyl estradiol 0.035 mg and norethindrone 1 mg (21s, 28s)

Ortho-Novum™ 10/11: Phase 1 (10 white tablets): Ethinyl estradiol 0.035 mg and norethindrone 0.5 mg; Phase 2 (11 peach tablets): Ethinyl estradiol 0.035 mg and norethindrone 1 mg (21s, 28s)

Ortho-Novum™ 7/7/7: Phase 1 (7 white tablets): Ethinyl estradiol 0.035 mg and norethindrone 0.5 mg; Phase 2 (7 light peach tablets): Ethinyl estradiol 0.035 mg and norethindrone 0.75 mg; Phase 3 (7 peach tablets): Ethinyl estradiol 0.035 mg and norethindrone 1 mg (21s, 28s)

Ovcon®-35: Ethinyl estradiol 0.035 mg and norethindrone acetate 0.4 mg (21s)

Ovcon®-50: Ethinyl estradiol 0.05 mg and norethindrone acetate 1 mg (21s, 28s)

Tri-Norinyl®: Phase 1 (7 blue tablets): Ethinyl estradiol 0.035 mg and norethindrone 0.5 mg; Phase 2 (9 yellow-green tablets): Ethinyl estradiol 0.035 mg and norethindrone 1 mg; Phase 3 (5 blue tablets): Ethinyl estradiol 0.035 mg and norethindrone 0.5 mg (21s, 28s)

Ethinyl Estradiol and Norgestrel (nor jess' trel)

Brand Names Lo/Ovral®; Ovral®

Synonyms Morning After Pill; Norgestrel and Ethinyl Estradiol

Use Prevention of pregnancy; treatment of hypermenorrhea, endometriosis, female hypogonadism; postcoital contraception

Pregnancy Risk Factor X

Contraindications Thromboembolic disorders, cerebrovascular or coronary artery disease; known or suspected breast cancer; undiagnosed abnormal vaginal bleeding; women smokers >35 years of age; all women >40 years of age

Warnings/Precautions Use of any progestin during the first 4 months of pregnancy is not recommended; in patients with a history of thromboembolism, stroke, myocardial infarction (especially >40 years of age who smoke), liver tumor, hypertension, cardiac, renal or hepatic insufficiency; risk of cardiovascular side effects increases in those women who smoke cigarettes and in women >35 years of age

Adverse Reactions

>10%:

Cardiovascular: Peripheral edema

Endocrine & metabolic: Enlargement of breasts, breast tenderness, bloating

(Continued)

Ethinyl Estradiol and Norgestrel *(Continued)*

Gastrointestinal: Nausea, anorexia

1% to 10%:

Central nervous system: Headache

Endocrine & metabolic: Increased libido

Gastrointestinal: Vomiting, diarrhea

<1%:

Cardiovascular: Hypertension, thromboembolism, stroke, myocardial infarction, edema

Central nervous system: Depression, dizziness, anxiety

Dermatologic: Chloasma, melasma, rash

Endocrine & metabolic: Decreased glucose tolerance, breast tumors, amenorrhea, alterations in frequency and flow of menses, increased triglycerides and LDL

Gastrointestinal: GI distress

Hepatic: Cholestatic jaundice

Miscellaneous: Intolerance to contact lenses, increased susceptibility to *Candida* infection

See tables.

Achieving Proper Hormonal Balance in an Oral Contraceptive

Estrogen		Progestin	
Excess	Deficiency	Excess	Deficiency
Nausea, bloating	Early or midcycle	Increased appetite	Late breakthrough
Cervical mucorrhea,	breakthrough	Weight gain	bleeding
polyposis	bleeding	Tiredness, fatigue	Amenorrhea
Melasma	Increased spotting	Hypomenorrhea	Hypermenorrhea
Migraine headache	Hypomenorrhea	Acne, oily scalp*	
Breast fullness or		Hair loss, hirsutism*	
tenderness		Depression	
Edema		Monilial vaginitis	
Hypertension		Breast regression	

*Result of androgenic activity of progestins.

Pharmacological Effects of Progestins Used in Oral Contraceptives

	Progestin	Estrogen	Antiestrogen	Androgen
Norgestrel/levonorgestrel	+++	0	++	+++
Ethynodiol diacetate	++	+*	+*	+
Norethindrone acetate	+	+	+++	+
Norethindrone	+	+*	+*	+
Norethynodrel	+	+++	0	0

*Has estrogenic effect at low doses; may have antiestrogenic effect at higher doses.

+++ = pronounced effect

++ = moderate effect

+ = slight effect

0 = moderate effect

Overdosage/Toxicology Toxicity is unlikely following single exposures of excessive doses; any treatment following emesis and charcoal administration should be supportive and symptomatic

Drug Interactions

Decreased effect of oral contraceptives with barbiturates, hydantoins - phenytoin, rifampin, antibiotics - penicillins, tetracyclines, griseofulvin

Increased toxicity of acetaminophen, anticoagulants, benzodiazepines, caffeine, corticosteroids, metoprolol, theophylline, tricyclic antidepressants

Mechanism of Action Combination oral contraceptives inhibit ovulation via a negative feedback mechanism on the hypothalamus, which alters the normal pattern of gonadotropin secretion of a follicle-stimulating hormone (FSH) and luteinizing hormone by the anterior pituitary. The follicular phase FSH and midcycle surge of gonadotropins are inhibited. In addition, oral contraceptives produce alterations in the genital tract, including changes in the cervical mucus, rendering it unfavorable for sperm penetration even if ovulation occurs. Changes in the endometrium may also occur, producing an unfavorable environment for nidation. Oral contraceptive drugs may alter the tubal transport of the ova through the fallopian tubes. Progestational agents may also alter sperm fertility.

Pharmacodynamics/Kinetics

Ethinyl estradiol:
Absorption: Absorbed well from GI tract
Protein binding: 50% to 80%
Metabolism: Inactivated by liver
Elimination: By the kidneys

Norgestrel:
Metabolism: Reduction and conjugation
Time to peak: 0.5-2 hours
Bioavailability: Complete with no first-pass effect
Half-life, terminal: 11-45 hours

Usual Dosage Adults: Female: Oral: Contraception: 1 tablet daily, beginning on day 5 of menstrual cycle (first day of menstrual flow is day 1). With 20-tablet and 21-tablet packages, new dosing cycle begins 7 days after last tablet taken; with 28-tablet packages, dosage is 1 tablet daily without interruption; extra tablets are placebos or contain iron. If next menstrual period does not begin on schedule, rule out pregnancy before starting new dosing cycle; if menstrual period begins, start new dosing cycle 7 days after last tablet was taken; if all doses have been taken on schedule and one menstrual period is missed, continue dosing cycle; if two consecutive menstrual periods are missed, pregnancy test is required before new dosing cycle is started.

One dose missed: Take as soon as remembered or take 2 tablets next day
Two doses missed: Take 2 tablets as soon as remembered or 2 tablets next 2 days
Three doses missed: Begin new compact of tablets starting on day 1 of next cycle

"Morning After" pill: Postcoital contraception (Ovral®): 2 tablets at initial visit and 2 tablets 12 hours later

Test Interactions

Decreased antithrombin III
Decreased serum folate concentration
Increased prothrombin and factors VII, VIII, IX, X
Increased platelet aggregability
Increased thyroid binding globulin
Increased total thyroid hormone (T_4)
Increased serum triglycerides/phospholipids

Patient Information

Inform your physician if signs or symptoms of any of the following occur: Thromboembolic or thrombotic disorders including sudden severe headache or vomiting, disturbance of vision or speech, loss of vision, numbness or weakness in an extremity, sharp or crushing chest pain, calf pain, shortness of breath, severe abdominal pain or mass, mental depression or unusual bleeding
If any doses are missed, alternative contraceptive methods should be used for the next 2 days or until 2 days into the new cycle
Discontinue taking the medication if you suspect you are pregnant or become pregnant

Nursing Implications Give at bedtime to minimize occurrence of adverse effects

Additional Information Monophasic oral contraceptives

Dosage Forms Tablet:
Lo/Ovral®: Ethinyl estradiol 0.03 mg and norgestrel 0.3 mg (21s and 28s)
Ovral®: Ethinyl estradiol 0.05 mg and norgestrel 0.5 mg (21s and 28s)

Ethionamide (e thye on am' ide)

Related Information

Antimicrobial Drugs of Choice *on page 1298-1302*

Brand Names Trecator®-SC

Use Treatment of tuberculosis and other mycobacterial diseases, in conjunction with other antituberculosis agents, when first-line agents have failed or resistance has been demonstrated

Pregnancy Risk Factor C

Contraindications Contraindicated in patients with severe hepatic impairment or in patients who are sensitive to the drug

Warnings/Precautions Use with caution in patients receiving cycloserine or isoniazid, in diabetics

Adverse Reactions

>10%: Gastrointestinal: Anorexia, nausea, vomiting
1% to 10%:
Cardiovascular: Postural hypotension
Central nervous system: Peripheral neuritis, psychiatric disturbances
Gastrointestinal: Metallic taste

(Continued)

Ethionamide *(Continued)*

    Hepatic: Hepatitis, jaundice
    <1%:
        Central nervous system: Drowsiness, dizziness, seizures, headache
        Dermatologic: Rash
        Endocrine & metabolic: Hypothyroidism or goiter, hypoglycemia, gynecomastia
        Gastrointestinal: Stomatitis, abdominal pain, diarrhea
        Hematologic: Thrombocytopenia
        Ocular: Optic neuritis

Overdosage/Toxicology Symptoms of overdose include peripheral neuropathy, anorexia, joint pain; following GI decontamination, treatment is supportive; pyridoxine may be given to prevent peripheral neuropathy

Mechanism of Action Inhibits peptide synthesis

Pharmacodynamics/Kinetics
    Distribution: Crosses the placenta
    Protein binding: 10%
    Bioavailability: 80%
    Half-life: 2-3 hours
    Time to peak serum concentration: Oral: Within 3 hours
    Elimination: As metabolites (active and inactive) and parent drug in urine

Usual Dosage Oral:
    Children: 15-20 mg/kg/day in 2 divided doses, not to exceed 1 g/day
    Adults: 500-1000 mg/day in 1-3 divided doses

    Dosing adjustment in renal impairment:
        Cl_{cr} <50 mL/minute: Administer 50% of dose

Monitoring Parameters Initial and periodic serum ALT and AST

Test Interactions ↓ thyroxine (S)

Patient Information Take with meals; notify physician of persistent or severe stomach upset, loss of appetite, or metallic taste; frequent blood tests are needed for monitoring; increase dietary intake of pyridoxine

Nursing Implications Neurotoxic effects may be relieved by the administration of pyridoxine

Dosage Forms Tablet, sugar coated: 250 mg

Ethmozine® *see* Moricizine Hydrochloride *on page 755*

Ethosuximide *(eth oh sux' i mide)*

Brand Names Zarontin®

Use Management of absence (petit mal) seizures, myoclonic seizures, and akinetic epilepsy; considered to be drug of choice for simple absence seizures

Pregnancy Risk Factor C

Contraindications Known hypersensitivity to ethosuximide

Warnings/Precautions Use with caution in patients with hepatic or renal disease; abrupt withdrawal of the drug may precipitate absence status; ethosuximide may increase tonic-clonic seizures in patients with mixed seizure disorders; ethosuximide must be used in combination with other anticonvulsants in patients with both absence and tonic-clonic seizures

Adverse Reactions
    >10%:
        Central nervous system: Ataxia, drowsiness, sedation, dizziness, lethargy, euphoria, hallucinations, insomnia, agitation, behavioral changes, headache
        Dermatologic: Stevens-Johnson syndrome
        Gastrointestinal: Weight loss
        Gastrointestinal: Nausea, vomiting, anorexia, abdominal pain
        Miscellaneous: Hiccups, SLE
    1% to 10%: Central nervous system: Aggressiveness, mental depression, nightmares, weakness, tiredness
    <1%:
        Central nervous system: Paranoid psychosis
        Dermatologic: Rashes, urticaria, exfoliative dermatitis
        Hematologic: Leukopenia, aplastic anemia, thrombocytopenia, agranulocytosis, pancytopenia

Overdosage/Toxicology Acute overdosage can cause CNS depression, ataxia, stupor, coma, hypotension; chronic overdose can cause skin rash, confusion, ataxia, proteinuria, hepatic dysfunction, hematuria; treatment is supportive; hemoperfusion and hemodialysis may be useful

Drug Interactions
    Decreased effect: Phenytoin, carbamazepine, primidone, phenobarbital may increase the hepatic metabolism of ethosuximide

Increased toxicity: Isoniazid may inhibit hepatic metabolism with a resultant increase in ethosuximide serum concentrations

Mechanism of Action Increases the seizure threshold and suppresses paroxysmal spike-and-wave pattern in absence seizures; depresses nerve transmission in the motor cortex

Pharmacodynamics/Kinetics

Time to peak serum concentration:
Capsule: Within 2-4 hours
Syrup: <2-4 hours
Distribution: Adults: V_d: 0.62-0.72 L/kg
Metabolism: ~80% metabolized in the liver to three inactive metabolites
Half-life:
Children: 30 hours
Adults: 50-60 hours
Elimination: Slowly excreted in urine as metabolites (50%) and as unchanged drug (10% to 20%); small amounts excreted in feces

Usual Dosage Oral:
Children 3-6 years: Initial: 250 mg/day (or 15 mg/kg/day) in 2 divided doses; increase every 4-7 days; usual maintenance dose: 15-40 mg/kg/day in 2 divided doses
Children >6 years and Adults: Initial: 250 mg twice daily; increase by 250 mg as needed every 4-7 days up to 1.5 g/day in 2 divided doses; usual maintenance dose: 20-40 mg/kg/day in 2 divided doses

Monitoring Parameters Seizure frequency, trough serum concentrations; CBC, platelets, liver enzymes, urinalysis

Reference Range Therapeutic: 40-100 µg/mL (SI: 280-710 µmol/L); Toxic: >150 µg/mL (SI: >1062 µmol/L)

Test Interactions ↑ alkaline phosphatase (S); positive Coombs' [direct]; ↓ calcium (S)

Patient Information Take with food; do not discontinue abruptly; may cause drowsiness and impair judgment

Nursing Implications Observe patient for excess sedation

Dosage Forms

Capsule: 250 mg
Syrup (raspberry flavor): 250 mg/5 mL (473 mL)

Ethoxynaphthamido Penicillin Sodium *see* Nafcillin Sodium *on page 768*

Ethyl Aminobenzoate *see* Benzocaine *on page 121*

Ethynodiol Diacetate and Ethinyl Estradiol *see* Ethinyl Estradiol and Ethynodiol Diacetate *on page 421*

Etidocaine Hydrochloride (e ti' doe kane)

Brand Names Duranest®

Use Infiltration anesthesia; peripheral nerve blocks; central neural blocks

Pregnancy Risk Factor B

Contraindications Heart block, severe hemorrhage, severe hypotension, known hypersensitivity to etidocaine or other amide local anesthetics

Warnings/Precautions Use with caution in patients with cardiac disease and hyperthyroidism; fetal bradycardia may occur up to 20% of the time; use with caution in areas of inflammation or sepsis, in debilitated or elderly patients, and those with severe cardiovascular disease or hepatic dysfunction; some products may contain sulfites

Adverse Reactions

<1%:
Cardiovascular: Myocardial depression, hypotension, bradycardia, cardiovascular collapse
Central nervous system: Anxiety, restlessness, disorientation, confusion, seizures, drowsiness, unconsciousness, chills, shivering
Dermatologic: Urticaria
Gastrointestinal: Nausea, vomiting
Local: Transient stinging or burning at injection site
Neuromuscular & skeletal: Tremor
Ocular: Blurred vision
Otic: Tinnitus
Respiratory: Respiratory arrest
Miscellaneous: Anaphylactoid reactions

Overdosage/Toxicology Symptoms of overdose include seizures, hypoventilation, apnea, hypotension, cardiac depression, arrhythmias, cardiac arrest; treatment is supportive; seizures may be treated with diazepam; hypotension, circulatory collapse respond best to fluids and Trendelenburg position
(Continued)

Etidocaine Hydrochloride *(Continued)*

Mechanism of Action Blocks nervous conduction through the stabilization of neuronal membranes. By preventing the transient increase in membrane permeability to sodium, the ionic fluxes necessary for initiation and transmission of electrical impulses are inhibited and local anesthesia is induced.

Pharmacodynamics/Kinetics

Onset of anesthesia: Within 2-5 minutes

Duration: ~4-10 hours

Absorption: Rapid

Distribution: Wide V_d allows wide distribution into neuronal tissues

Protein binding: High

Metabolism: Extensively in the liver

Elimination: Small amounts excreted in urine

Usual Dosage Varies with procedure; use 1% for peripheral nerve block, central nerve block, lumbar peridural caudal; use 1.5% for maxillary infiltration or inferior alveolar nerve block; use 1% or 1.5% for intra-abdominal or pelvic surgery, lower limb surgery, or caesarean section

Reference Range Toxic concentration: >0.1 µg/mL

Nursing Implications Before injecting withdraw syringe plunger to ensure injection is not into vein or artery; have resuscitative equipment nearby

Dosage Forms

Injection: 1% [10 mg/mL] (30 mL)

Injection, with epinephrine 1:200,000: 1% [10 mg/mL] (30 mL); 1.5% [15 mg/mL] (20 mL)

Etidronate Disodium *(e ti droe' nate)*

Brand Names Didronel®

Synonyms EHDP; Sodium Etidronate

Use Symptomatic treatment of Paget's disease and heterotopic ossification due to spinal cord injury or after total hip replacement, hypercalcemia associated with malignancy

Pregnancy Risk Factor B (oral)/C (parenteral)

Contraindications Patients with serum creatinine >5 mg/dL; hypersensitivity to biphosphonates

Warnings/Precautions Use with caution in patients with restricted calcium and vitamin D intake; dosage modification required in renal impairment; I.V. form may be nephrotoxic and should be used with caution, if at all, in patients with impaired renal function (serum creatinine: 2.5-4.9 mg/dL)

Adverse Reactions

1% to 10%:

Central nervous system: Fever, convulsions

Endocrine & metabolic: Hypophosphatemia, hypomagnesemia, fluid overload

Neuromuscular & skeletal: Bone pain

Respiratory: Dyspnea

<1%:

Dermatologic: Angioedema, skin rash

Gastrointestinal: Occult blood in stools, altered taste

Hypersensitivity: Hypersensitivity reactions

Renal: Nephrotoxicity

Miscellaneous: Pain, increased risk of fractures

Overdosage/Toxicology Symptoms of overdose include diarrhea, nausea, vomiting, paresthesias, tetany, coma; antidote is calcium

Stability Store ampuls at room temperature and avoid excess heat (>40°C/104°F); intravenous solution diluted in ≥250 mL normal saline is stable for 48 hours at room temperature or refrigerated

Mechanism of Action Decreases bone resorption by inhibiting osteocystic osteolysis; decreases mineral release and matrix or collagen breakdown in bone

Pharmacodynamics/Kinetics

Onset of therapeutic effect: Within 1-3 months of therapy

Duration: Can persist for 12 months without continuous therapy

Absorption: Dependent upon dose administered

Metabolism: Not metabolized

Elimination: As unchanged drug primarily in urine with unabsorbed drug being eliminated in feces

Usual Dosage Adults:

Paget's disease: Oral: 5 mg/kg/day given every day for no more than 6 months; may give 10 mg/kg/day for up to 3 months; daily dose may be divided if adverse GI effects occur

Heterotopic ossification with spinal cord injury: 20 mg/kg/day for 2 weeks, then 10 mg/kg/day for 10 weeks (this dosage has been used in children, however, treatment >1 year has been associated with a rachitic syndrome)

Hypercalcemia associated with malignancy:
  I.V. (Dilute dose in at least 250 mL NS): 7.5 mg/kg/day for 3 days; there should
    be at least 7 days between courses of treatment
  Oral: Start 20 mg/kg/day on the last day of infusion and continue for 30-90 days

Dosing adjustment in renal impairment:
  S_{cr} 2.5-5 mg/dL: Use with caution
  S_{cr} >5 mg/dL: Do not use
Administration Administer intravenous dose over at least 2 hours; I.V. doses
  should be diluted in at least 250 mL 0.9% sodium chloride
Monitoring Parameters Serum calcium and phosphorous; serum creatinine and
  BUN
Reference Range Calcium (total): Adults: 9.0-11.0 mg/dL
Patient Information Maintain adequate intake of calcium and vitamin D; take
  medicine on an empty stomach 2 hours before meals
Nursing Implications Ensure adequate hydration
Dosage Forms
  Injection: 50 mg/mL (6 mL)
  Tablet: 200 mg, 400 mg

Etodolac (ee toe doe' lak)
Related Information
  Nonsteroidal Anti-Inflammatories Comparison *on page 1280*
Brand Names Lodine®
Synonyms Etodolic Acid
Use Acute and long-term use in the management of signs and symptoms of
  osteoarthritis and management of pain
  Unapproved use: Rheumatoid arthritis
Pregnancy Risk Factor C
Contraindications Hypersensitivity to etodolac, aspirin, or other NSAIDs
Warnings/Precautions Use with caution in patients with congestive heart failure,
  hypertension, decreased renal or hepatic function, history of GI disease, or those
  receiving anticoagulants
Adverse Reactions
  >10%:
    Central nervous system: Dizziness
    Dermatologic: Skin rash
    Gastrointestinal: Abdominal cramps, heartburn, indigestion, nausea
  1% to 10%:
    Cardiovascular: Fluid retention
    Central nervous system: Headache, nervousness
    Dermatologic: Itching
    Gastrointestinal: Vomiting
    Otic: Ringing in ears
  <1%:
    Cardiovascular: Congestive heart failure, hypertension, arrhythmia, tachy-
      cardia
    Central nervous system: Confusion, hallucinations, aseptic meningitis, mental
      depression, drowsiness, insomnia
    Dermatologic: Hives, erythema multiforme, toxic epidermal necrolysis,
      Stevens-Johnson syndrome, angioedema
    Endocrine & metabolic: Polydipsia, hot flushes
    Gastrointestinal: Gastritis, GI ulceration
    Genitourinary: Cystitis
    Hematologic: Agranulocytosis, anemia, hemolytic anemia, bone marrow
      depression, leukopenia, thrombocytopenia
    Hepatic: Hepatitis
    Neuromuscular & skeletal: Peripheral neuropathy
    Ocular: Toxic amblyopia, blurred vision, conjunctivitis, dry eyes
    Otic: Decreased hearing
    Renal: Polyuria, acute renal failure
    Respiratory: Allergic rhinitis, shortness of breath
    Miscellaneous: Epistaxis
Overdosage/Toxicology Symptoms of overdose include acute renal failure,
  vomiting, drowsiness, leukocytes. Management of a nonsteroidal anti-inflammatory drug (NSAID) intoxication is primarily supportive and symptomatic. Fluid
  therapy is commonly effective in managing the hypotension that may occur
  following an acute NSAID overdose, except when this is due to an acute blood
  loss.
Drug Interactions
  Decreased effect with aspirin
  (Continued)

Etodolac *(Continued)*

Increased effect/toxicity with aspirin (GI irritation), probenecid; increased effect/toxicity of lithium, methotrexate, digoxin, cyclosporin (nephrotoxicity), warfarin (bleeding)

Stability Protect from moisture

Mechanism of Action Inhibits prostaglandin synthesis by decreasing the activity of the enzyme, cyclo-oxygenase, which results in decreased formation of prostaglandin precursors

Pharmacodynamics/Kinetics

Absorption: Oral: Well absorbed

Distribution: V_d: 0.4 L/kg

Protein binding: High

Half-life: 7 hours

Time to peak serum concentration: 1 hour

Usual Dosage Single dose of 76-100 mg is comparable to the analgesic effect of aspirin 650 mg; in patients ≥65 years, no substantial differences in the pharmacokinetics or side-effects profile were seen compared with the general population

Adults: Oral:

Acute pain: 200-400 mg every 6-8 hours, as needed, not to exceed total daily doses of 1200 mg; for patients weighing <60 kg, total daily dose should not exceed 20 mg/kg/day

Osteoarthritis: Initial: 800-1200 mg/day given in divided doses: 400 mg 2 or 3 times/day; 300 mg 2, 3 or 4 times/day; 200 mg 3 or 4 times/day; total daily dose should not exceed 1200 mg; for patients weighing <60 kg, total daily dose should not exceed 20 mg/kg/day

Monitoring Parameters Monitor CBC, liver enzymes; in patients receiving diuretics, monitor urine output and BUN/serum creatinine

Test Interactions False-positive for urinary bilirubin and ketone ↑ bleeding time

Patient Information Do not crush tablets; take with food, milk, or water; report any signs of blood in stool

Dosage Forms Capsule: 200 mg, 300 mg

Etodolic Acid *see* Etodolac *on previous page*

Etomidate *(e tom' i date)*

Brand Names Amidate®

Use Induction of general anesthesia

Pregnancy Risk Factor C

Contraindications Known hypersensitivity to etomidate

Warnings/Precautions Consider exogenous corticosteroid replacement in patients undergoing severe stress

Adverse Reactions

>10%:

Gastrointestinal: Nausea, vomiting

Local: Pain at injection site

Neuromuscular & skeletal: Transient skeletal movements, uncontrolled eye movements

1% to 10%: Hiccups

<1%:

Cardiovascular: Hypertension, hypotension, tachycardia, bradycardia, arrhythmias

Respiratory: Hyperventilation, hypoventilation, apnea, laryngospasm

Overdosage/Toxicology Symptoms of overdose include respiratory arrest, coma; supportive treatment

Stability Store in refrigerator

Mechanism of Action Ultrashort-acting nonbarbiturate hypnotic used for the induction of anesthesia; chemically, it is a carboxylated imidazole and has been shown to produce a rapid induction of anesthesia with minimal cardiovascular and respiratory effects

Usual Dosage Children >10 years and Adults: I.V.: 0.2-0.6 mg/kg over a period of 30-60 seconds for induction of anesthesia

Dosage Forms Injection: 2 mg/mL (10 mL, 20 mL)

Etoposide *(e toe poe' side)*

Related Information

Cancer Chemotherapy Regimens *on page 1218-1241*

Extravasation Management of Chemotherapeutic Agents *on page 1207-1208*

Brand Names VePesid®

Synonyms Epipodophyllotoxin; VP-16; VP-16-213

Use Treatment of lymphomas, ANLL, lung, testicular, bladder, and prostate carcinoma, hepatoma, rhabdomyosarcoma, uterine carcinoma, neuroblastoma, mycosis fungoides, Kaposi's sarcoma, histiocytosis, gestational trophoblastic disease, Ewing's sarcoma, Wilm's tumor, and brain tumors

Pregnancy Risk Factor D

Contraindications Hypersensitivity to etoposide or any component; **I.T. administration is contraindicated**

Warnings/Precautions The U.S. Food and Drug Administration (FDA) currently recommends that procedures for proper handling and disposal of antineoplastic agents be considered. Severe myelosuppression with resulting infection or bleeding may occur. Administer I.V. infusions over a period of at least 30-60 minutes; **must be diluted - do not give IVP**; dosage should be adjusted in patients with hepatic or renal impairment.

Adverse Reactions

>10%:

Gastrointestinal: Occasional diarrhea and infrequent nausea and vomiting at standard doses; severe mucositis occurs with high (BMT) doses

Emetic potential: Moderately low (10% to 30%)

Miscellaneous: Alopecia (reversible), anorexia

Myelosuppressive: Principal dose-limiting toxicity of VP-16. White blood cell count nadir is 5-15 days after administration and is more frequent than thrombocytopenia. Recovery is usually within 24-28 days and cumulative toxicity has not been noted with VP-16 as a single agent. No difference in toxicity is seen when VP-16 is administered over a 24-hour period or over 2 hours on 5 consecutive days.

WBC: Mild to severe

Platelets: Mild

Onset (days): 10

Nadir (days): 14-16

Recovery (days): 21-28

1% to 10%:

Central nervous system: Unusual tiredness

Gastrointestinal: Stomatitis, diarrhea, abdominal pain, hepatitic dysfunction

Hypotension: Related to drug infusion time; may be related to vehicle used in the I.V. preparation (polysorbate 80 plus polyethylene glycol). Best to administer the drug over 1 hour.

<1%:

Cardiovascular: Tachycardia

Central nervous system: Neurotoxicity, somnolence, fatigue, fever, headache, peripheral neuropathy

Irritant chemotherapy, thrombophlebitis has been reported

Hepatic: Toxic hepatitis (with high-dose therapy)

Hypersensitivity: Reports of flushing or bronchospasm, which did not reoccur in one report if patients were pretreated with corticosteroids and antihistamines

Overdosage/Toxicology Symptoms of overdose include bone marrow depression, leukopenia, thrombocytopenia, nausea, vomiting; treatment is supportive

Drug Interactions Increased toxicity:

Warfarin → increases prothrombin time with concurrent use

Methotrexate: Alteration of MTX transport has been found as a slow efflux of MTX and its polyglutamated form out of the cell, leading to intercellular accumulation of MTX

Calcium antagonists: Increases the rate of VP-16-induced DNA damage and cytotoxicity *in vitro*

Carmustine: Reports of frequent hepatic dysfunction with hyperbilirubinemia, ascites, and thrombocytopenia

Cyclosporine: Additive cytotoxic effects on tumor cells

Stability Store injection at room temperature and capsules under refrigeration; capsules are stable 3 months at room temperature; do not freeze.

VP-16 should be further diluted in D_5W, LR, or NS for administration; stability is dependent upon the concentration of the solution

At room temperature in D_5W or NS in polyvinyl chloride, the concentration is stable as follows:

0.2 mg/mL: 96 hours

0.4 mg/mL: 48 hours

0.6 mg/mL: 8 hours

1 mg/mL: 2 hours

2 mg/mL: 1 hour

20 mg/mL (undiluted): 24 hours

Y-site compatible with carboplatin, cytarabine, mesna, daunorubicin

Mechanism of Action Inhibits mitotic activity; inhibits cells from entering prophase; inhibits DNA synthesis. Initially thought to be mitotic inhibitors similar to podophyllotoxin, but actually have no effect on microtubule assembly. (Continued)

Etoposide (Continued)

However, later shown to induce DNA strand breakage and inhibition of topoisomerase II (an enzyme which breaks and repairs DNA); etoposide acts in late S or early G2 phases.

Pharmacodynamics/Kinetics

Absorption: Oral: 32% to 57%

Distribution: Poor penetration across blood-brain barrier, with concentrations in the CSF being <10% that of plasma

Average V_d: 3-36 L/m^2

Protein binding: 94% to 97%

Metabolism: In the liver (with a biphasic decay)

Half-life: Terminal: 4-15 hours

Children: 6-8 hours with normal renal and hepatic function

Time to peak serum concentration: Oral: 1-1.5 hours

Elimination: Both unchanged drug and metabolites are excreted in the urine and a small amount (2% to 16%) excreted in feces; up to 55% of an I.V. dose is excreted unchanged in urine in children

Usual Dosage Refer to individual protocols

Oral dose is twice the I.V. dose

Testicular cancer: I.V.: 50-100 mg/m^2/day on days 1-5 or 100 mg/m^2/day on days 1, 3, and 5 every 3-4 weeks for 3-4 courses

Small cell lung cancer:

I.V.: 35 mg/m^2/day for 4 days or 50 mg/m^2/day for 5 days every 3-4 weeks

Oral: Twice the I.V. dose rounded to the nearest 50 mg given once daily if total dose ≤400 mg or in divided doses if >400 mg

Higher doses may be used in bone marrow transplantation (doses up to 2400 mg/m^2)

Dosage adjustment in renal impairment:

Cl_{cr} 10-50 mL/minute: Reduce dose by 25%

Cl_{cr} <10 mL minute: Reduce dose by 50%

Hemodialysis effects: Supplemental dose is not necessary

Dosage adjustment in hepatic impairment:

Bilirubin 1.5-3 mg/dL or AST 60-180 units: Reduce dose by 50%

Bilirubin >3 mg/dL or AST >180 units: Reduce by 75%

Administration If necessary, the injection may be used for oral administration; mix with orange juice, apple juice, or lemonade to a concentration of 0.4 mg/mL or less, and use within a 3-hour period

Monitoring Parameters CBC with differential and platelet count, vital signs (blood pressure), bilirubin, and renal function tests

Patient Information Any signs of infection, easy bruising or bleeding, shortness of breath, or painful or burning urination should be brought to physician's attention. Nausea, vomiting, or hair loss sometimes occur. The drug may cause permanent sterility and may cause birth defects. The drug may be excreted in breast milk, therefore, an alternative form of feeding your baby should be used.

Nursing Implications Extravasation treatment: Inject 3-5 mL of hyaluronidase (10 units/mL) S.C. clockwise into the infiltrated area using a 25-gauge needle; change the needle with each injection; apply heat immediately for 1 hour, repeat 4 times/day for 3-5 days (application of cold and injection of hydrocortisone is contraindicated)

Dosage Forms

Capsule: 50 mg

Injection: 20 mg/mL (5 mL)

Etretinate (e tret' i nate)

Brand Names Tegison®

Use Treatment of severe recalcitrant psoriasis in patients intolerant of or unresponsive to standard therapies

Pregnancy Risk Factor X

Contraindications Pregnancy, known hypersensitivity to etretinate; because of the high likelihood of long lasting teratogenic effects, do not prescribe etretinate for women who are or who are likely to become pregnant while or after using the drug

Warnings/Precautions Not to be used in severe obesity or women of childbearing potential unless woman is capable of complying with effective contraceptive measures; therapy is normally begun on the second or third day of next normal menstrual period; effective contraception must be used for at least 1 month before beginning therapy, during therapy, and for 1 month after discontinuation of therapy; pregnancy test must be performed prior to starting therapy

Adverse Reactions
>10%:
Central nervous system: Fatigue, headache, fever, epistaxis
Dermatologic: Chapped lips, alopecia
Endocrine & metabolic: Hypercholesterolemia, hypertriglyceridemia
Gastrointestinal: Nausea, appetite change, dry mouth, sore tongue
Neuromuscular & skeletal: Hyperostosis, Bone and joint pain
Ocular: Eye irritation
1% to 10%:
Cardiovascular: Edema
Central nervous system: Dizziness, lethargy
Hepatic: Hepatitis
Neuromuscular & skeletal: Myalgia
Ocular: Blurred vision
Otic: Otitis externa
Respiratory: Dyspnea
<1%:
Cardiovascular: Syncope
Central nervous system: Amnesia, confusion, pseudotumor cerebri, depression
Dermatologic: Urticaria
Gastrointestinal: Mouth ulcers, diarrhea, constipation, flatulence, weight loss,
gingival bleeding
Endocrine & metabolic: Gout
Local: Phlebitis
Neuromuscular & skeletal: Hyperkinesia, hypertonia
Ocular: Photophobia
Otic: Ear infection
Renal: Polyuria, dysuria, kidney stones
Miscellaneous: Runny nose
Drug Interactions
Increased effect: Milk increases absorption of etretinate
Increased toxicity: Additive toxicity with vitamin A
Mechanism of Action Unknown; related to retinoic acid and retinol (vitamin A)
Pharmacodynamics/Kinetics
Absorption: Oral: Absorbed from small intestine; absorption enhanced when
coadministered with whole milk or a high lipid meal (highly lipophilic)
Protein binding: 99%
Metabolism: Undergoes significant first-pass metabolism to form acitretin (active)
Half-life: 4-8 days (with multiple doses)
Elimination: By metabolism and by excretion in feces of unchanged drug and
metabolites
Usual Dosage Adults: Oral: Individualized; Initial: 0.75-1 mg/kg/day in divided
doses, increase by 0.25 mg/kg/day at weekly intervals up to 1.5 mg/kg/day;
maintenance dose established after 8-10 weeks of therapy 0.5-0.75 mg/kg/day
Patient Information Do not become pregnant while taking this drug, use effective contraceptive measures; if severe persistent nausea, abdominal pain, or
vomiting recur stop taking the drug; if persistent or severe headache or visual
disturbance occur, stop taking the drug; take with food, do not take vitamin A
supplements while taking this drug, may have decreased tolerance to contact
lenses before and after therapy
Dosage Forms Capsule: 10 mg, 25 mg

Extravasation Management of Chemotherapeutic Agents *see page 1207*

Extravasation Treatment of Other Drugs *see page 1209*

Eye-Sed® [OTC] *see Zinc Supplements on page 1176*

Eye-Zine® [OTC] *see Tetrahydrozoline Hydrochloride on page 1071*

Ezide® *see Hydrochlorothiazide on page 542*

F₃T *see Trifluridine on page 1122*

Factor IX Complex (Human) (fak′ ter nin kom′ pleks)

Brand Names AlphaNine®; Konȳne® 80; Mononine®; Profilnine® Heat-Treated; Proplex® SX-T; Proplex® T

Use Controls bleeding in patients with factor IX deficiency (Hemophilia B or Christmas disease); prevention/control of bleeding in hemophilia A patients with inhibitors to factor VIII

Pregnancy Risk Factor C

Contraindications Liver disease with signs of intravascular coagulation or fibrinolysis, not for use in factor VII deficiencies, patients undergoing elective surgery

Warnings/Precautions Use with caution in patients with liver dysfunction; risk of viral transmission is not totally eradicated, prepared from pooled human plasma

Adverse Reactions

1% to 10%: Following rapid administration: Transient fever

Central nervous system: Tingling, fever, headache, chills

<1%:

Cardiovascular: Flushing, DIC, thrombosis following high dosages in hemophilia B patients

Central nervous system: Somnolence

Dermatologic: Urticaria

Gastrointestinal: Nausea, vomiting

Respiratory: Tightness in chest and neck

Overdosage/Toxicology Disseminated intravascular coagulation (DIC)

Drug Interactions Increased toxicity: Do not coadminister with aminocaproic acid → ↑ risk for thrombosis

Stability When stored at refrigerator temperature, 2°C to 8°C (36°F to 46°F), coagulation factor IX is stable for the period indicated by the expiration date on its label. Avoid freezing which may damage container for the diluent.

Stability of parenteral admixture at room temperature (25°C): 24 hours; do **not** refrigerate after reconstitution

Standard diluent: Dose in units/bag

Minimum volume: Use complete vial(s) for entire dose

Comments: Infusion rate should be 2 mL/minute

Mechanism of Action Replaces deficient clotting factor including factor X; hemophilia B, or Christmas disease, is an X-linked recessively inherited disorder of blood coagulation characterized by insufficient or abnormal synthesis of the clotting protein factor IX. Factor IX is a vitamin K-dependent coagulation factor which is synthesized in the liver. Factor IX is activated by factor XIa in the intrinsic coagulation pathway. Activated factor IX (IXa), in combination with factor VII:C activates factor X to Xa, resulting ultimately in the conversion of prothrombin to thrombin and the formation of a fibrin clot. The infusion of exogenous factor IX to replace the deficiency present in hemophilia B temporarily restores hemostasis.

Pharmacodynamics/Kinetics

Half-life:

VII component: Cleared rapidly from the serum in two phases; initial: 4-6 hours; terminal: 22.5 hours

IX component: 24 hours

Usual Dosage Children and Adults: Dosage is expressed in units of factor IX activity and must be individualized. I.V. only:

Factor VII deficiency: Highly individualized

0.5 unit/kg x body weight (kg) x desired increase (%)

For example, for a 70 kg adult to increase level by 25%:

0.5 unit/kg x 70 kg x 25 = 875 units

Factor IX deficiency: Highly individualized

1 unit/kg x body weight (in kg) x desired increase (%)

For example, to increase the level by 25% in a 70 kg adult:

1 unit x 70 kg x 25 = 1,750 units

Formula for units required to raise blood level %:

Total blood volume (mL blood/kg) = 70 mL/kg (adults), 80 mL/kg (children)

Plasma volume = total blood volume (mL) x [1 - Hct (in decimals)]

For example, for a 70 kg adult with a Hct = 40%: Plasma volume = [70 kg x 70 mL/kg] x [1 - 0.4] = 2940 mL

To calculate number of units needed to increase level to desired range (highly individualized and dependent on patient's condition):

Number of units = desired level increase [desired level - actual level] x plasma volume (in mL)

For example, for a 100% level in the above patient who has an actual level of 20%: Number of units needed = [1 (for a 100% level) - 0.2] x 2940 mL = 2,352 units

As a general rule, the level of factor IX required for treatment of different conditions is shown in the table.

	Minor Spontaneous Hemorrhage, Prophylaxis	Major Trauma or Surgery
Desired levels of factor IX for hemostasis	15%-25%	25%-50%
Initial loading dose to achieve desired level	<20-30 units/kg	<75 units/kg
Frequency of dosing	Once; repeated in 24 h if necessary	q18-30h, depending on half-life and measured factor IX levels
Duration of treatment	Once; repeated if necessary	Up to 10 days, depending upon nature of insult

Factor VIII inhibitor patients: 75 units/kg/dose; may be given every 6-12 hours

Anticoagulant overdosage: I.V.: 15 units/kg

Administration Solution should be infused at room temperature

I.V. administration only: Should be infused **slowly:** Start infusion at a rate of 2-3 mL/minute. If headache, flushing, changes in pulse rate or blood pressure appear, the infusion rate should be decreased. Initially, stop the infusion until the symptoms disappear, then resume the infusion at a slower rate. **Infuse at a rate not exceeding 3 mL/minute.**

Monitoring Parameters Levels of factors II, IX, and X; PT and PTT

Reference Range Average normal factor VII and factor IX levels are 50% to 150%; patients with severe hemophilia will have levels <1%, often undetectable. Moderate forms of the disease have levels of 1% to 10% while some mild cases may have 11% to 49% of normal factor IX.

Maintain factor IX plasma level at least 20% until hemostasis achieved after acute joint or muscle bleeding

In preparation for and following surgery:

Level to prevent spontaneous hemorrhage: 5%

Minimum level for hemostasis following trauma and surgery: 30% to 50%

Severe hemorrhage: >60%

Major surgery: >60% prior to procedure, 30% to 50% for several days after surgery, and >20% for 7-10 days thereafter

Dosage Forms Injection:

AlphaNine®: 500 units, 1000 units, 1500 units

Konÿne® 80: 10 mL, 20 mL

Mononine®: 250 units, 500 units, 1000 units

Profilnine® Heat-Treated: Single dose vial

Proplex® SX-T: Vial

Proplex® T: Vial

Factor VIII see Antihemophilic Factor (Human) on page 80

Factrel® see Gonadorelin on page 510

Famciclovir (fam sye' kloe veer)

Brand Names Famvir™

Use Management of acute herpes zoster (shingles)

Pregnancy Risk Factor B

Pregnancy/Breast Feeding Implications Use only if the benefit to the patient clearly exceeds the potential risk to the fetus; due to potential for excretion of famciclovir in breast milk and for its associated tumorigenicity, discontinue nursing or discontinue the drug during lactation

Contraindications Hypersensitivity to famciclovir

(Continued)

Famciclovir *(Continued)*

Warnings/Precautions Has not been studied in immunocompromised patients or patients with ophthalmic or disseminated zoster; dosage adjustment is required in patients with renal insufficiency (Cl_{cr} <60 mL/minute) and in patients with noncompensated hepatic disease; safety and efficacy have not been established in children <18 years of age; animal studies indicated increases in incidence of carcinomas, mutagenic changes, and decreases in fertility with extremely large doses

Adverse Reactions

>10%:

Central nervous system: Headache

Gastrointestinal: Nausea

1% to 10%:

Central nervous system: Fatigue, fever, dizziness, somnolence

Gastrointestinal: Diarrhea, vomiting, constipation, anorexia, abdominal pain

Neuromuscular & skeletal: Rigors, paresthesia

Overdosage/Toxicology Supportive and symptomatic care is recommended; hemodialysis may enhance elimination

Drug Interactions Increased effect/toxicity:

Cimetidine: Penciclovir AUC may increase due to impaired metabolism

Digoxin: C_{max} of digoxin increases by ~19%

Probenecid: Penciclovir serum levels significantly increase

Theophylline: Penciclovir AUC/C_{max} may increase and renal clearance decrease, although not clinically significant

Mechanism of Action After undergoing rapid biotransformation to the active compound, penciclovir, famciclovir is phosphorylated by viral thymidine kinase in HSV-1, HSV-2, and VZV-infected cells to a monophosphate form; this is then converted to penciclovir triphosphate and competes with deoxyguanosine triphosphate to inhibit HSV-2 polymerase (ie, herpes viral DNA synthesis/replication is selectively inhibited)

Pharmacodynamics/Kinetics

Absorption: Food decreases the maximum peak concentration and delays the time to peak; AUC remains the same

Distribution: V_{dss}: 0.98-1.08 L/kg

Protein binding: 20%

Metabolism: Rapidly deacetylated and oxidized to penciclovir (not by cytochrome P-450)

Bioavailability: 77%; T_{max}: 0.9 hours

Half-life: Penciclovir: 2-3 hours (10, 20, and 7 hours in HSV-1, HSV-2, and VZV-infected cells); linearly decreased with reductions in renal failure

Elimination: >90% of penciclovir is eliminated unchanged in urine; C_{max} and T_{max} are decreased and prolonged, respectively in patients with noncompensated hepatic impairment

Usual Dosage Adults: Oral: 500 mg every 8 hours for 7 days

Dosing interval in renal impairment:

Cl_{cr} ≥60 mL/minute: Administer 500 mg every 8 hours

Cl_{cr} 40-59 mL/minute: Administer 500 mg every 12 hours

Cl_{cr} 20-39 mL/minute: Administer 500 mg every 24 hours

Cl_{cr} <20 mL/minute: Unknown

Administration Initiate therapy as soon as herpes zoster is diagnosed

Patient Information May take medication with food or on an empty stomach

Additional Information Most effective if therapy is initiated within 72 hours of initial lesion

Dosage Forms Tablet: 500 mg

Famotidine *(fa moe' ti deen)*

Brand Names Pepcid® [OTC]

Use Therapy and treatment of duodenal ulcer, gastric ulcer, control gastric pH in critically ill patients, symptomatic relief in gastritis, gastroesophageal reflux, active benign ulcer, and pathological hypersecretory conditions

Pregnancy Risk Factor B

Contraindications Hypersensitivity to famotidine or other H_2 antagonists

Warnings/Precautions Modify dose in patients with renal impairment; use with caution in patients with CHF who are receiving calcium channel blockers

Adverse Reactions

1% to 10%:

Central nervous system: Dizziness, headache

Gastrointestinal: Constipation, diarrhea

<1%:

Cardiovascular: Bradycardia, tachycardia, palpitations, hypertension

Central nervous system: Fever, dizziness, weakness, fatigue, seizures, insomnia, drowsiness
Dermatologic: Acne, pruritus, urticaria, dry skin
Gastrointestinal: Abdominal discomfort, flatulence, belching, anorexia
Hematologic: Agranulocytosis, neutropenia, thrombocytopenia
Hepatic: Increases in AST, ALT
Neuromuscular & skeletal: Paresthesia
Renal: Increases in BUN, creatinine, proteinuria
Respiratory: Bronchospasm
Miscellaneous: Allergic reaction

Overdosage/Toxicology Symptoms of overdose include hypotension, tachycardia, vomiting, drowsiness; treatment is primarily symptomatic and supportive

Drug Interactions Decreased effect of ketoconazole, itraconazole

Stability Reconstituted I.V. solution is stable for 48 hours at room temperature; I.V. infusion in NS or D$_5$W solution is stable for 48 hours at room temperature; reconstituted oral solution is stable for 30 days at room temperature

Mechanism of Action Competitive inhibition of histamine at H$_2$ receptors of the gastric parietal cells, which inhibits gastric acid secretion

Pharmacodynamics/Kinetics
Onset of GI effect: Oral: Within 1 hour
Duration: 10-12 hours
Protein binding: 15% to 20%
Bioavailability: Oral: 40% to 50%
Half-life: 2.5-3.5 hours; increases with renal impairment, oliguric patients: 20 hours
Time to peak serum concentration: Oral: Within 1-3 hours
Elimination: In urine as unchanged drug

Usual Dosage
Children: Oral, I.V.: Doses of 1-2 mg/kg/day have been used; maximum dose: 40 mg
Adults:
Oral:
Duodenal ulcer, gastric ulcer: 40 mg/day at bedtime for 4-8 weeks
Hypersecretory conditions: Initial: 20 mg every 6 hours, may increase up to 160 mg every 6 hours
GERD: 20 mg twice daily for 6 weeks
I.V.: 20 mg every 12 hours

Dosing adjustment in renal impairment:
Cl$_{cr}$ 30-50 mL/minute: Administer every 24 hours or 50% of dose
Cl$_{cr}$ <30 mL/minute: Administer every 36-48 hours or 25% of dose

Administration Administer over 15-30 minutes; may be given undiluted I.V. push

Dosage Forms
Injection: 10 mg/mL (2 mL, 4 mL)
Powder for oral suspension (cherry-banana-mint flavor): 40 mg/5 mL (50 mL)
Tablet, film coated: 20 mg, 40 mg

Famvir™ see Famciclovir on page 439

Fansidar® see Sulfadoxine and Pyrimethamine on page 1041

Fastin® see Phentermine Hydrochloride on page 872

Fat Emulsion (fat e mul' shun)
Brand Names Intralipid®; Liposyn®; Nutrilipid®; Soyacal®
Synonyms Intravenous Fat Emulsion
Use Source of calories and essential fatty acids for patients requiring parenteral nutrition of extended duration
Pregnancy Risk Factor B/C
Contraindications Pathologic hyperlipidemia, lipoid nephrosis, known hypersensitivity to fat emulsion and severe egg or legume (soybean) allergies, pancreatitis with hyperlipemia
Warnings/Precautions Use caution in patients with severe liver damage, pulmonary disease, anemia, or blood coagulation disorder; use with caution in jaundiced, premature, and low birth weight children
Adverse Reactions
>10%: Local: Thrombophlebitis
1% to 10%: Endocrine & metabolic: Hyperlipemia
<1%:
Cardiovascular: Cyanosis, flushing, chest pain
Gastrointestinal: Nausea, vomiting, diarrhea
Hepatic: Hepatomegaly
Respiratory: Dyspnea
(Continued)

Fat Emulsion *(Continued)*

Miscellaneous: Sepsis

Overdosage/Toxicology Too rapid administration results in fluid or fat over-loading to cause dilution of serum electrolytes, overhydration, pulmonary edema, impaired pulmonary diffusion capacity, metabolic acidosis; treatment is supportive

Stability May be stored at room temperature; do not store partly used bottles for later use; do not use if emulsion appears to be oiling out

Mechanism of Action Essential for normal structure and function of cell membranes

Pharmacodynamics/Kinetics

Metabolism: Undergoes lipolysis to free fatty acids, which are utilized by reticulo-endothelial cells

Half-life: 0.5-1 hour

Usual Dosage Fat emulsion should not exceed 60% of the total daily calories

Infants, premature: Initial dose: 0.25-0.5 g/kg/day, increase by 0.25-0.5 g/kg/day to a maximum of 3-4 g/kg/day; maximum rate of infusion: 0.15 g/kg/hour (0.75 mL/kg/hour of 20% solution)

Infants and Children: Initial dose: 0.5-1 g/kg/day, increase by 0.5 g/kg/day to a maximum of 3-4 g/kg/day; maximum rate of infusion: 0.25 g/kg/hour (1.25 mL/kg/hour of 20% solution)

Adolescents and Adults: Initial dose: 1 g/kg/day, increase by 0.5-1 g/kg/day to a maximum of 2.5 g/kg/day of 10% and 3 g/kg/day of 20%; maximum rate of infusion: 0.25 g/kg/hour (1.25 mL/kg/hour of 20% solution); do not exceed 50 mL/hour (20%) or 100 mL/hour (10%)

Note: At the onset of therapy, the patient should be observed for any immediate allergic reactions such as dyspnea, cyanosis, and fever. Slower initial rates of infusion may be used for the first 10-15 minutes of the infusion (eg, 0.1 mL/minute of 10% or 0.05 mL/minute of 20% solution).

Prevention of fatty acid deficiency (8% to 10% of total caloric intake): 0.5-1 g/kg/24 hours

Children: 5-10 mL/kg/day at 0.1 mL/minute then up to 100 mL/hour

Adults: 500 mL twice weekly at rate of 1 mL/minute for 30 minutes, then increase to 500 mL over 4-6 hours

Can be used in both children and adults on a daily basis as a caloric source in TPN

Administration May be simultaneously infused with amino acid dextrose mixtures by means of Y-connector located near infusion site. The 10% isotonic solution which has 1.1 cal/mL (10%) and may be administered peripherally; the 20% (2 cal/mL) is not recommended for use in low birth weight infants.

Monitoring Parameters Serum triglycerides; before initiation of therapy and at least weekly during therapy

Dosage Forms Injection: 10% [100 mg/mL] (100 mL, 250 mL, 500 mL); 20% [200 mg/mL] (100 mL, 250 mL, 500 mL)

5-FC *see* Flucytosine *on page 462*

[18]FDG *see* Fludeoxyglucose F 18 *on page 465*

Feiba VH Immuno® *see* Anti-Inhibitor Coagulant Complex *on page 83*

Feldene® *see* Piroxicam *on page 893*

Felodipine *(fe loe' di peen)*

Related Information

Calcium Channel Blockers Cardiovascular Adverse Reactions *on page 1262*

Calcium Channel Blockers Central Nervous System Adverse Reactions *on page 1264*

Calcium Channel Blockers Comparative Actions *on page 1260*

Calcium Channel Blockers Comparative Pharmacokinetics *on page 1261*

Calcium Channel Blockers FDA-Approved Indications *on page 1263*

Calcium Channel Blockers Gastrointestinal and Miscellaneous Adverse Reactions *on page 1265*

Brand Names Plendil®

Use Treatment of hypertension, congestive heart failure

Pregnancy Risk Factor C

Contraindications Hypersensitivity to felodipine or any component or other calcium channel blocker; severe hypotension or second and third degree heart block

Warnings/Precautions Use with caution and titrate dosages for patients with impaired renal or hepatic function; use caution when treating patients with congestive heart failure, sick-sinus syndrome, severe left ventricular dysfunction, hypertrophic cardiomyopathy (especially obstructive), concomitant therapy with beta-blockers or digoxin, edema, or increased intracranial pressure with cranial tumors; do not abruptly withdraw (may cause chest pain); elderly may experience hypotension and constipation more readily.

Adverse Reactions
>10%: Cardiovascular: Peripheral edema
1% to 10%:
    Cardiovascular: Chest pain, tachycardia
    Central nervous system: Dizziness, lightheadedness
    Dermatologic: Skin rash
    Gastrointestinal: Constipation, diarrhea
<1%:
    Cardiovascular: Hypotension, arrhythmia, bradycardia, palpitations
    Central nervous system: Mental depression, dizziness, headache
    Dermatologic: Rash
    Gastrointestinal: Gingival hyperplasia, dry mouth, nausea
    Hepatic: Marked elevations in liver function tests
    Ocular: Blurred vision
    Respiratory: Shortness of breath

Overdosage/Toxicology The primary cardiac symptoms of calcium blocker overdose includes hypotension and bradycardia. The hypotension is caused by peripheral vasodilation, myocardial depression, and bradycardia. Bradycardia results from sinus bradycardia, second- or third-degree atrioventricular block, or sinus arrest with junctional rhythm. Intraventricular conduction is usually not affected so QRS duration is normal (verapamil does prolong the P-R interval and bepridil prolongs the Q-T and may cause ventricular arrhythmias, including torsade de pointes).

The noncardiac symptoms include confusion, stupor, nausea, vomiting, metabolic acidosis and hyperglycemia. Following initial gastric decontamination, if possible, repeated calcium administration may promptly reverse the depressed cardiac contractility (but not sinus node depression or peripheral vasodilation); glucagon, epinephrine, and amrinone may treat refractory hypotension; glucagon and epinephrine also increase the heart rate (outside the U.S., 4-aminopyridine may be available as an antidote); dialysis and hemoperfusion are not effective in enhancing elimination although repeat-dose activated charcoal may serve as an adjunct with sustained-release preparations.

Drug Interactions Increased toxicity/effect/levels:
Calcium channel blockers (CCB) and H_2 blockers → ↑ bioavailability CCB
CCB and beta-blockers → ↑ cardiac depressant effects on A-V conduction
CCB and carbamazepine → ↑ carbamazepine levels
CCB and cyclosporine → ↑ cyclosporine levels
CCB and fentanyl → ↑ hypotension
CCB and digitalis → ↑ digitalis levels
CCB and quinidine → ↑ quinidine levels (hypotension, bradycardia)
CCB and theophylline → ↑ pharmacologic actions of theophylline

Mechanism of Action Inhibits calcium ions from entering the "slow channels" or select voltage-sensitive areas of vascular smooth muscle and myocardium during depolarization, producing a relaxation of coronary vascular smooth muscle and coronary vasodilation; increases myocardial oxygen delivery in patients with vasospastic angina

Pharmacodynamics/Kinetics
    Onset of effect: 2-5 hours
    Duration: 16-24 hours
    Absorption: 100%; absolute: 20% due to first-pass effect
    Protein binding: >99%
    Metabolism: >99% in liver
    Half-life: 11-16 hours
    Elimination: In urine as metabolites

Usual Dosage Adults: Oral: 5-10 mg once daily; increase by 5 mg at 2-week intervals, as needed, to a maximum of 20 mg/day (elderly: begin with 5 mg/day)

    Dosing adjustment/comments in hepatic impairment: Do not use doses >10 mg/day

Patient Information Do not crush or chew tablets; do not discontinue abruptly; report any dizziness, shortness of breath, palpitations or edema occurs

Dosage Forms Tablet, extended release: 5 mg, 10 mg

Femcare® [OTC] see Clotrimazole on page 265

Femcet® see Butalbital Compound on page 153

Femiron® [OTC] see Ferrous Fumarate on page 450

Femstat® see Butoconazole Nitrate on page 155

Fenesin™ *see* Guaifenesin *on page 515*

Fenfluramine Hydrochloride (fen flure' a meen)
Brand Names Pondimin®
Use Short-term adjunct in exogenous obesity
Restrictions C-IV
Pregnancy Risk Factor C
Contraindications Known hypersensitivity to fenfluramine
Warnings/Precautions Cardiovascular disease, nephritis, angina pectoris, hypertension, glaucoma, patients with a history of drug abuse, known hypersensitivity to amphetamine
Adverse Reactions
>10%:
  Cardiovascular: Hypertension
  Central nervous system: Euphoria, nervousness, insomnia
1% to 10%:
  Central nervous system: Confusion, mental depression, restlessness
  Endocrine & metabolic: Changes in libido
  Gastrointestinal: Nausea, vomiting, constipation
  Hematologic: Blood dyscrasias
  Neuromuscular & skeletal: Tremor
  Ocular: Blurred vision
<1%:
  Cardiovascular: Tachycardia, arrhythmias
  Central nervous system: Restlessness, depression, headache
  Dermatologic: Alopecia
  Gastrointestinal: Diarrhea, abdominal cramps
  Neuromuscular & skeletal: Myalgia
  Renal: Dysuria, polyuria
  Respiratory: Dyspnea
  Miscellaneous: Increased sweating
Overdosage/Toxicology Symptoms of overdose include agitation, drowsiness, confusion, flushing, tremor, fever, sweating, abdominal pain, dilated nonreactive pupils

There is no specific antidote for amphetamine intoxication; the bulk of the treatment is supportive. Hyperactivity and agitation usually respond to reduced sensory input; however, with extreme agitation haloperidol (2-5 mg I.M. for adults) may be required. Hyperthermia is best treated with external cooling measures; when severe or unresponsive, muscle paralysis with pancuronium may be needed. Hypertension is usually transient and generally does not require treatment unless severe. For diastolic blood pressures >110 mm Hg, a nitroprusside infusion should be initiated. Seizures usually respond to diazepam IVP and/or phenytoin maintenance regimens.
Mechanism of Action Fenfluramine hydrochloride is a phenethylamine structurally related to amphetamine; central nervous system depression is more common than stimulation, which makes fenfluramine pharmacologically different from amphetamine. Fenfluramine's exact mechanism of action is not well understood; the drug's appetite suppressing action may be due to the stimulation of the hypothalamus; the anorectic effect may also be due to delayed gastric emptying.
Usual Dosage Adults: Oral: 20 mg 3 times/day before meals or food, up to 40 mg 3 times/day; maximum daily dose: 120 mg
Patient Information Take during day to avoid insomnia; do not discontinue abruptly, may cause physical and psychological dependence with prolonged use
Nursing Implications Monitor CNS, dose should not be given in evening or at bedtime
Dosage Forms Tablet: 20 mg

Fenofibrate (fen o fye' brate)
Brand Names Lipidil®
Synonyms Procetofene; Proctofene
Use Adjunct to dietary therapy for the treatment of adults with very high elevations of serum triglyceride levels (types IV and V hyperlipidemia) who are at risk of pancreatitis and who do not respond adequately to a determined dietary effort; its efficacy can be enhanced by combination with other hypolipidemic agents that have a different mechanism of action; safety and efficacy may be greater than that of clofibrate
Pregnancy Risk Factor C
Pregnancy/Breast Feeding Implications Although teratogenicity and mutagenicity tests in animals have been negative, significant risk has been

identified with clofibrate; use should be avoided, if possible, in pregnant women since the neonatal glucuronide conjugation pathways are immature

Warnings/Precautions The hypoprothrombinemic effect of anticoagulants is significantly increased with concomitant fenofibrate administration; use with caution in patients with severe renal dysfunction

Adverse Reactions
>10%: Gastrointestinal: Nausea, gastric discomfort
1% to 10%:
    Dermatologic: Skin reactions
    Gastrointestinal: Constipation, diarrhea
<1%:
    Central nervous system: Dizziness, headache, fatigue, insomnia
    Hepatic: Transient increases in LFTs
    Neuromuscular & skeletal: Arthralgia, myalgia

Overdosage/Toxicology Symptoms of overdose include nausea, vomiting, diarrhea, GI distress; following GI decontamination, treatment is supportive

Drug Interactions
Increased hypolipidemic effect: Cholestyramine, colestipol
Increased hypoprothrombinemic effect: Warfarin

Mechanism of Action Fenofibric acid is believed to increase VLDL catabolism by enhancing the synthesis of lipoprotein lipase; as a result of a decrease in VLDL levels, total plasma triglycerides are reduced by 30% to 60% (VLDL contains ~60% triglycerides and 10% to 15% cholesterol); apolipoprotein B, which stabilizes the structure of VLDL and LDL, decreases in a parallel fashion and plasma cholesterol levels decrease by fenofibrate's effect on LDL levels and cholesterol synthesis; modest increase in HDL occurs in some hypertriglyceridemic patients since it is involved in the storage and transport of cholesterol ester and apolipoproteins

Pharmacodynamics/Kinetics
Peak effect: 4-6 hours
Absorption: 60% to 90% when given with meals
Distribution: V_d: 0.9 L/kg; distributes well to most tissues except brain or eye; concentrates in liver, kidneys, and gut
Protein binding: >99%
Metabolism: Metabolized to its active form, fenofibric acid, by tissue and plasma esterases; then undergoes inactivation by glucuronidation in the liver or kidneys
Half-life: Fenofibrate: 21 hours (30 hours in elderly, 44-54 hours in hepatic impairment)
Elimination: 60% to 93% excreted in metabolized form; 5% to 25% excreted fecally; hemodialysis has no effect on removal of fenofibric acid from the plasma

Usual Dosage Oral:
Children >10 years: 5 mg/kg/day
Adults: 100 mg 3 times/day with meals or 200 mg in the morning and 100 mg in the evening

Dosing adjustment/comments in renal impairment: Decrease dose or increase dosing interval for patients with renal failure
Administration 6-8 weeks of therapy is required to determine efficacy
Monitoring Parameters Total serum cholesterol and triglyceride concentration and CLDL, LDL, and HDL levels should be measured periodically; if only marginal changes are noted in 6-8 weeks, the drug should be discontinued; serum transaminases should be measured every 3 months; if ALT values increase >100 units/L, therapy should be discontinued

Test Interactions
Alkaline phosphatase: May decrease by 20% with fenofibrate therapy
Bilirubin: May decrease
Creatinine: Transient increases may occur
Gamma glucuronyl transferase: Levels may decrease with long-term therapy
Serum transaminases: Transiently increased
Uric acid: Decreases of 20% to 30% may occur within 14 days of starting therapy
Aminotransaminases: Transient increases have been reported

Fenoprofen Calcium (fen oh proe' fen)
Related Information
Nonsteroidal Anti-Inflammatories Comparison *on page 1280*
Brand Names Nalfon®
Use Symptomatic treatment of acute and chronic rheumatoid arthritis and osteoarthritis; relief of mild to moderate pain
Pregnancy Risk Factor B (D if used in the 3rd trimester or near delivery)
Contraindications Known hypersensitivity to fenoprofen or other NSAIDs
(Continued)

Fenoprofen Calcium *(Continued)*

Warnings/Precautions Use with caution in patients with congestive heart failure, hypertension, decreased renal or hepatic function, history of GI disease, or those receiving anticoagulants

Adverse Reactions

>10%:

Central nervous system: Dizziness

Dermatologic: Skin rash

Gastrointestinal: Abdominal cramps, heartburn, indigestion, nausea

1% to 10%:

Cardiovascular: Fluid retention

Central nervous system: Headache, nervousness

Dermatologic: Itching

Gastrointestinal: Vomiting

Otic: Ringing in ears

<1%:

Cardiovascular: Congestive heart failure, hypertension, arrhythmias, tachycardia, hot flushes

Central nervous system: Confusion, hallucinations, aseptic meningitis, mental depression, drowsiness, insomnia

Dermatologic: Hives, erythema multiforme, toxic epidermal necrolysis, Stevens-Johnson syndrome, angioedema

Endocrine & metabolic: Polydipsia

Gastrointestinal: Gastritis, GI ulceration

Genitourinary: Cystitis

Hematologic: Agranulocytosis, anemia, hemolytic anemia, bone marrow depression, leukopenia, thrombocytopenia

Hepatic: Hepatitis

Neuromuscular & skeletal: Peripheral neuropathy

Ocular: Toxic amblyopia, blurred vision, conjunctivitis, dry eyes

Otic: Decreased hearing

Renal: Polyuria, acute renal failure

Respiratory: Allergic rhinitis, shortness of breath

Miscellaneous: Epistaxis

Overdosage/Toxicology Symptoms of overdose include acute renal failure, vomiting, drowsiness, leukocytosis. Management of a nonsteroidal anti-inflammatory drug (NSAID) intoxication is primarily supportive and symptomatic. Fluid therapy is commonly effective in managing the hypotension that may occur following an acute NSAID overdose, except when this is due to an acute blood loss.

Drug Interactions

Decreased effect with phenobarbital

Increased effect/toxicity of phenytoin, sulfonamides, sulfonylureas

Increased toxicity with salicylates, oral anticoagulants

Mechanism of Action Inhibits prostaglandin synthesis by decreasing the activity of the enzyme, cyclo-oxygenase, which results in decreased formation of prostaglandin precursors

Pharmacodynamics/Kinetics

Absorption: Rapid (to 80%) from upper GI tract

Distribution: Does not cross the placenta

Protein binding: 99%

Metabolism: Extensively in the liver

Half-life: 2.5-3 hours

Time to peak serum concentration: Within 2 hours

Elimination: In urine 2% to 5% as unchanged drug; small amounts appear in feces

Usual Dosage Adults: Oral:

Rheumatoid arthritis: 300-600 mg 3-4 times/day up to 3.2 g/day

Mild to moderate pain: 200 mg every 4-6 hours as needed

Monitoring Parameters Monitor CBC, liver enzymes; monitor urine output and BUN/serum creatinine in patients receiving diuretics

Reference Range Therapeutic: 20-65 µg/mL (SI: 82-268 µmol/L)

Test Interactions ↑ chloride (S), ↑ sodium (S)

Patient Information Do not crush tablets; take with food, milk, or water; report any signs of blood in stool

Dosage Forms

Capsule: 200 mg, 300 mg

Tablet: 600 mg

Fentanyl (fen' ta nil)

Related Information

Narcotic Agonist Comparison Charts *on page 1274-1275*

Brand Names Duragesic™; Fentanyl Oralet®; Sublimaze®

Use Sedation, relief of pain, preoperative medication, adjunct to general or regional anesthesia, management of chronic pain (transdermal product)

Restrictions C-II

Pregnancy Risk Factor B (D if used for prolonged periods or in high doses at term)

Contraindications Hypersensitivity to fentanyl or any component; increased intracranial pressure; severe respiratory depression; severe liver or renal insufficiency;

Transmucosal is contraindicated in unmonitored settings where a risk of unrecognized hypoventilation exists or in treating acute or chronic pain

Warnings/Precautions Fentanyl shares the toxic potentials of opiate agonists, and precautions of opiate agonist therapy should be observed; use with caution in patients with bradycardia; rapid I.V. infusion may result in skeletal muscle and chest wall rigidity → impaired ventilation → respiratory distress → apnea, bronchoconstriction, laryngospasm; inject slowly over 3-5 minutes; nondepolarizing skeletal muscle relaxant may be required.

Transmucosal fentanyl: Fentanyl Oralet® is not indicated for use in unmonitored settings where there is a risk of unrecognized hypoventilation or in treating acute or chronic pain. Patients should be monitored by direct visual observation and by some means of measuring respiratory function such as pulse oximetry until they are recovered. Facilities for the administration of fluids, opioid antagonists, oxygen and resuscitation equipment (including facilities for endotracheal intubation) should be readily available.

Topical patches: Serum fentanyl concentrations may increase approximately one-third for patients with a body temperature of 40°C secondary to a temperature-dependent increase in fentanyl release from the system and increased skin permeability. Patients who experience adverse reactions should be monitored for at least 12 hours after removal of the patch.

The elderly may be particularly susceptible to the CNS depressant and constipating effects of narcotics

Adverse Reactions

>10%:

Cardiovascular: Hypotension, bradycardia

Central nervous system: CNS depression, drowsiness, sedation

Gastrointestinal: Nausea, vomiting, constipation

Respiratory: Respiratory depression

1% to 10%:

Cardiovascular: Cardiac arrhythmias, orthostatic hypotension

Central nervous system: Confusion, CNS depression

Gastrointestinal: Biliary spasm

Ocular: Miosis

<1%:

Central nervous system: Convulsions, dysesthesia, paradoxical CNS excitation or delirium; cold, clammy skin; dizziness

Dermatologic: Erythema, pruritus, skin rash, hives, itching

Endocrine & metabolic: ADH release

Respiratory: Bronchospasm, circulatory depression, laryngospasm

Miscellaneous: Physical and psychological dependence with prolonged use, biliary or urinary tract spasm

Overdosage/Toxicology Symptoms of overdose include CNS depression, respiratory depression, miosis. Treatment of an overdose includes support of the patient's airway, establishment of an I.V. line, and administration of naloxone 2 mg I.V. (0.01 mg/kg for children) with repeat administration as necessary up to a total of 10 mg

Drug Interactions Increased toxicity: CNS depressants, phenothiazines, tricyclic antidepressants may potentiate fentanyl's adverse effects

Stability Protect from light; **incompatible** when mixed in the same syringe with pentobarbital

Transmucosal: Store at controlled room temperature of 15°C to 30°C (59°F to 86°F)

Mechanism of Action Binds with stereospecific receptors at many sites within the CNS, increases pain threshold, alters pain reception, inhibits ascending pain pathways

Pharmacodynamics/Kinetics Respiratory depressant effect may last longer than analgesic effect

(Continued)

Fentanyl (Continued)

I.M.:
Onset of analgesia: 7-15 minutes
Duration: 1-2 hours

I.V.:
Onset of analgesia: Almost immediate
Duration: 0.5-1 hour

Transmucosal:
Onset of effect: 5-15 minutes with a maximum reduction in activity/apprehension
Peak analgesia: Within 20-30 minutes
Duration: Related to blood level of the drug

Absorption: Transmucosal: Rapid, ~25% from the buccal mucosa; 75% swallowed with saliva and slowly absorbed from gastrointestinal tract

Distribution: Highly lipophilic, redistributes into muscle and fat

Metabolism: In the liver

Bioavailability: Transmucosal: ~50% (range: 36% to 71%)

Half-life: 2-4 hours
Transmucosal: 6.6 hours (range: 5-15 hours)

Elimination: In urine primarily as metabolites and 10% as unchanged drug

Usual Dosage Doses should be titrated to appropriate effects; wide range of doses, dependent upon desired degree of analgesia/anesthesia

Children 1-12 years:
Sedation for minor procedures/analgesia:
I.M., I.V.: 1-2 mcg/kg/dose; may repeat at 30- to 60-minute intervals. **Note:** Children 18-36 months of age may require 2-3 mcg/kg/dose
Transmucosal (dosage strength is based on patient weight): 5 mcg/kg if child is not fearful; fearful children and some younger children may require doses of 5-15 mcg/kg (which also carries an increased risk of hypoventilation); drug effect begins within 10 minutes, with sedation beginning shortly thereafter
Continuous sedation/analgesia: Initial I.V. bolus: 1-2 mcg/kg then 1 mcg/kg/hour; titrate upward; usual: 1-3 mcg/kg/hour
Pain control: Transdermal: Not recommended

Children >12 years and Adults:
Sedation for minor procedures/analgesia:
I.M., I.V.: 0.5-1 mcg/kg/dose; higher doses are used for major procedures
Transmucosal: 5 mcg/kg, suck on lozenge vigorously approximately 20-40 minutes before the start of procedure, drug effect begins within 10 minutes, with sedation beginning shortly thereafter; see table.
Preoperative sedation, adjunct to regional anesthesia, postoperative pain: I.M., I.V.: 50-100 mcg/dose
Adjunct to general anesthesia: I.M., I.V.: 2-50 mcg/kg
General anesthesia without additional anesthetic agents: I.V. 50-100 mcg/kg with O_2 and skeletal muscle relaxant
Pain control: Transdermal: Initial: 25 mcg/hour system; if currently receiving opiates, convert to fentanyl equivalent and administer equianalgesic dosage titrated to minimize the adverse effects and provide analgesia. To convert patients from oral or parenteral opioids to Duragesic™, the previous 24-hour analgesic requirement should be calculated. This analgesic requirement should be converted to the equianalgesic oral morphine dose. See tables.

The dosage should not be titrated more frequently than every 3 days after the initial dose or every 6 days thereafter. The majority of patients are controlled

Equianalgesic Doses of Opioid Agonists

Drug	Equianalgesic Dose (mg)	
	I.M.	P.O.
Codeine	130	200
Hydromorphone	1.5	7.5
Levorphanol	2	4
Meperidine	75	—
Methadone	10	20
Morphine	10	60
Oxycodone	15	30
Oxymorphone	1	10 (PR)

From N Engl J Med, 1985, 313:84-95.

Dosage Recommendations for Transmucosal Fentanyl (Oralet®)

Patient Age/Weight	5-10 mcg/kg/dose	10-15 mcg/kg/dose
Children < 2 years of age OR < 15 kg	NOT RECOMMENDED	NOT RECOMMENDED
< 15 kg	NOT AVAILABLE	200 mcg
20 kg	200 mcg	200-300 mcg
25 kg	200 mcg	300 mcg
30 kg	300 mcg	300-400 mcg
35 kg	300 mcg	400 mcg
> 40 kg	400 mcg	400 mcg
Adults	400 mcg	400 mcg

Corresponding Doses of Oral/Intramuscular Morphine and Duragesic™

Oral 24-Hour Morphine (mg/d)	I.M. 24-Hour Morphine (mg/d)	Duragesic™ Dose (mcg/h)
45-134	8-22	25
135-224	28-37	50
225-314	38-52	75
315-404	53-67	100
405-494	68-82	125
495-584	83-97	150
585-674	98-112	175
675-764	113-127	200
765-854	128-142	225
855-944	143-157	250
945-1034	158-172	275
1035-1124	173-187	300

Product information, Duragesic™ — Janssen Pharmaceutica, January, 1991.

on every 72-hour administration, however, a small number of patients require every 48-hour administration.

Elderly >65 years: Transmucosal: Dose should be reduced to 2.5-5 mcg/kg; elderly have been found to be twice as sensitive as younger patients to the effects of fentanyl

Dosing adjustment in renal impairment:
Cl_{cr} 10-50 mL/minute: Administer at 75% of normal dose
Cl_{cr} <10 mL/minute: Administer at 50% of normal dose

Administration Transmucosal product should begin 20-40 minutes prior to the anticipated start of surgery, diagnostic, or therapeutic procedure; foil overwrap should be removed just prior to administration; once removed, patient should place the unit in mouth and suck (not chew) it; unit should be removed after it is consumed or if patient has achieved an adequate sedation and anxiolytic level, and/or shows signs of respiratory depression

Monitoring Parameters Respiratory and cardiovascular status, blood pressure, heart rate

Nursing Implications

May cause rebound respiratory depression postoperatively

Patients with increased temperature may have increased fentanyl absorption transdermally, observe for adverse effects, dosage adjustment may be needed

Pharmacologic and adverse effects can be seen after discontinuation of transdermal system, observe patients for at least 12 hours after transdermal product removed; keep transdermal product (both used and unused) out of the reach of children

Do **not** use soap, alcohol, or other solvents to remove transdermal gel if it accidentally touches skin as they may increase transdermal absorption, use copious amounts of water For patients who have received transmucosal product within 6-12 hours, it is recommended that if other narcotics are required, they should be used at starting doses 1/4 to 1/3 those usually recommended.

Dosage Forms

Injection, as citrate: 0.05 mg/mL (2 mL, 5 mL, 10 mL, 20 mL, 50 mL)

Lozenge, oral transmucosal (raspberry flavored): 200 mcg, 300 mcg, 400 mcg

(Continued)

449

Fentanyl *(Continued)*

Transdermal system: 25 mcg/hour [10 cm²]; 50 mcg/hour [20 cm²]; 75 mcg/hour [30 cm²]; 100 mcg/hour [40 cm²] (all available in 5s)

Fentanyl Oralet® *see* Fentanyl *on page 446*

Feosol® [OTC] *see* Ferrous Sulfate *on page 452*

Feostat® [OTC] *see* Ferrous Fumarate *on this page*

Feratab® [OTC] *see* Ferrous Sulfate *on page 452*

Fergon® [OTC] *see* Ferrous Gluconate *on next page*

Fer-In-Sol® [OTC] *see* Ferrous Sulfate *on page 452*

Fer-Iron® [OTC] *see* Ferrous Sulfate *on page 452*

Ferndex *see* Dextroamphetamine Sulfate *on page 319*

Fero-Gradumet® [OTC] *see* Ferrous Sulfate *on page 452*

Ferospace® [OTC] *see* Ferrous Sulfate *on page 452*

Ferralet® [OTC] *see* Ferrous Gluconate *on next page*

Ferralyn® Lanacaps® [OTC] *see* Ferrous Sulfate *on page 452*

Ferra-TD® [OTC] *see* Ferrous Sulfate *on page 452*

Ferro-Sequels® [OTC] *see* Ferrous Fumarate *on this page*

Ferrous Fumarate *(fyoo' ma rate)*

Brand Names Femiron® [OTC]; Feostat® [OTC]; Ferro-Sequels® [OTC]; Fumasorb® [OTC]; Fumerin® [OTC]; Hemocyte® [OTC]; Ircon® [OTC]; Nephro-Fer™ [OTC]; Span-FF® [OTC]

Use Prevention and treatment of iron deficiency anemias

Pregnancy Risk Factor A

Contraindications Hemochromatosis, hemolytic anemia, known hypersensitivity to iron salts

Warnings/Precautions Avoid in patients with peptic ulcer, enteritis, or ulcerative colitis. Administration of iron for >6 months should be avoided except in patients with continuous bleeding or menorrhagia. Anemia in the elderly is often caused by "anemia of chronic disease" or associated with inflammation rather than blood loss. Iron stores are usually normal or increased, with a serum ferritin >50 ng/mL and a decreased total iron binding capacity. Hence, the "anemia of chronic disease" is not secondary to iron deficiency but the inability of the reticuloendothelial system to reclaim available iron stores.

Adverse Reactions
>10%: Gastrointestinal: Stomach cramping, constipation, nausea, vomiting, dark stools

1% to 10%:
Gastrointestinal: Heartburn, diarrhea
Miscellaneous: Discolored urine, staining of teeth

<1%: Ocular: Contact irritation

Overdosage/Toxicology Symptoms of overdose include acute GI irritation, erosion of GI mucosa, hepatic and renal impairment, coma, hematemesis, lethargy, acidosis, serum Fe level >300 mcg/mL requires treatment of overdose due to severe toxicity. Following treatment for fluid losses, metabolic acidosis, and shock, a severe iron overdose (when the serum iron concentration exceeds the total iron-binding capacity) may be treated with deferoxamine. Deferoxamine may be administered I.V. (80 mg/kg over 24 hours) or I.M. (40-90 mg/kg every 8 hours). Usual toxic dose of elemental iron: ≥35 mg/kg.

Drug Interactions
Decreased effect: Absorption of oral preparation of iron and tetracyclines are decreased when both of these drugs are given together; concurrent administration of antacids may decrease iron absorption; iron may decrease absorption of penicillamine when given at the same time; response to iron therapy may be delayed in patients receiving chloramphenicol
Milk may decrease absorption of iron
Increased effect: Current administration ≥200 mg vitamin C per 30 mg elemental iron increases absorption of oral iron

Mechanism of Action Replaces iron found in hemoglobin, myoglobin, and enzymes; allows the transportation of oxygen via hemoglobin

Pharmacodynamics/Kinetics
Onset of hematologic response (essentially the same to either oral or parenteral iron salts): Red blood cell form and color changes within 3-10 days
Peak reticulocytosis: Within 5-10 days; hemoglobin values increase within 2-4 weeks

Absorption: Iron is absorbed in the duodenum and upper jejunum; in persons with normal iron stores 10% of an oral dose is absorbed, this is increased to 20% to 30% in persons with inadequate iron stores; food and achlorhydria will decrease absorption

Elimination: Iron is largely bound to serum transferrin and excreted in the urine, sweat, sloughing of intestinal mucosa, and by menses

Usual Dosage Oral (dose expressed in terms of elemental iron):

Children:

Severe iron deficiency anemia: 4-6 mg Fe/kg/day in 3 divided doses

Mild to moderate iron deficiency anemia: 3 mg Fe/kg/day in 1-2 divided doses

Prophylaxis: 1-2 mg Fe/kg/day

Adults:

Iron deficiency: 60-100 mg twice daily up to 60 mg 2 times/day

Prophylaxis: 60-100 mg/day

To avoid GI upset, start with a single daily dose and increase by 1 tablet/day each week or as tolerated until desired daily dose is achieved

Elderly: 200 mg 3-4 times/day

Reference Range

Serum iron:

Male: 75-175 µg/dL (SI: 13.4-31.3 µmol/L)

Female: 65-165 µg/dL (SI: 11.6-29.5 µmol/L)

Total iron binding capacity: 230-430 µg/dL

Transferrin: 204-360 mg/dL

Percent transferrin saturation: 20% to 50%

Iron levels >300 µg/dL can be considered toxic, should be treated as an overdose

Patient Information May color stool black, take between meals for maximum absorption; may take with food if GI upset occurs, do not take with milk or antacids; keep out of reach of children

Additional Information Elemental iron content of ferrous fumarate: 33%

Dosage Forms Amount of elemental iron is listed in brackets

Capsule, controlled release (Span-FF®): 325 mg [106 mg]

Drops (Feostat®): 45 mg/0.6 mL [15 mg/0.6 mL] (60 mL)

Suspension, oral (Feostat®): 100 mg/5 mL [33 mg/5 mL] (240 mL)

Tablet:

325 mg [106 mg]

Chewable (chocolate flavor) (Feostat®): 100 mg [33 mg]

Femiron®: 63 mg [20 mg]

Fumerin®: 195 mg [64 mg]

Fumasorb®, Ircon®: 200 mg [66 mg]

Hemocyte®: 324 mg [106 mg]

Nephro-Fer™: 350 mg [115 mg]

Timed release (Ferro-Sequels®): Ferrous fumarate 150 mg [50 mg] and docusate sodium 100 mg

Ferrous Gluconate (gloo' koe nate)

Brand Names Fergon® [OTC]; Ferralet® [OTC]; Simron® [OTC]

Use Prevention and treatment of iron deficiency anemias

Pregnancy Risk Factor A

Contraindications Hemochromatosis, hemolytic anemia; known hypersensitivity to iron salts

Warnings/Precautions Administration of iron for >6 months should be avoided except in patients with continued bleeding, menorrhagia, or repeated pregnancies; avoid in patients with peptic ulcer, enteritis, or ulcerative colitis. Anemia in the elderly is often caused by "anemia of chronic disease" or associated with inflammation rather than blood loss. Iron stores are usually normal or increased, with a serum ferritin >50 ng/mL and a decreased total iron binding capacity. Hence, the "anemia of chronic disease" is not secondary to iron deficiency but the inability of the reticuloendothelial system to reclaim available iron stores.

Adverse Reactions

>10%: Gastrointestinal: Stomach cramping, constipation, nausea, vomiting, dark stools

1% to 10%:

Gastrointestinal: Heartburn, diarrhea

Miscellaneous: Discolored urine, staining of teeth

<1%: Ocular: Contact irritation

Overdosage/Toxicology Symptoms of overdose include acute GI irritation; erosion of GI mucosa, hepatic and renal impairment, coma, hematemesis, lethargy, acidosis. Following treatment for fluid losses, metabolic acidosis, and shock, a severe iron overdose (when the serum iron concentration exceeds the total iron-binding capacity) may be treated with deferoxamine. Deferoxamine
(Continued)

Ferrous Gluconate *(Continued)*

may be administered I.V. (80 mg/kg over 24 hours) or I.M. (40-90 mg/kg every 8 hours). Usual toxic dose of elemental iron: ≥35 mg/kg.

Drug Interactions Absorption of oral preparation of iron and tetracyclines is decreased when both of these drugs are given together; concurrent administration of antacids may decrease iron absorption; iron may decrease absorption of penicillamine when given at the same time. Response to iron therapy may be delayed in patients receiving chloramphenicol. Concurrent administration ≥200 mg vitamin C/30 mg elemental iron increases absorption of oral iron; milk may decrease absorption of iron.

Mechanism of Action Replaces iron found in hemoglobin, myoglobin, and enzymes; allows the transportation of oxygen via hemoglobin

Pharmacodynamics/Kinetics Onset of hematologic response (essentially the same to either oral or parenteral iron salts): Red blood cells form and color changes within 3-10 days, peak reticulocytosis occurs in 5-10 days, and hemoglobin values increase within 2-4 weeks

Usual Dosage Oral **(dose expressed in terms of elemental iron):**
Children:
Severe iron deficiency anemia: 4-6 mg Fe/kg/day in 3 divided doses
Mild to moderate iron deficiency anemia: 3 mg Fe/kg/day in 1-2 divided doses
Prophylaxis: 1-2 mg Fe/kg/day
Adults:
Iron deficiency: 60 mg twice daily up to 60 mg 4 times/day
Prophylaxis: 60 mg/day

Reference Range Therapeutic: Male: 75-175 μg/dL (SI: 13.4-31.3 μmol/L); Female: 65-165 μg/dL (SI: 11.6-29.5 μmol/L); serum iron level >300 μg/dL usually requires treatment of overdose due to severe toxicity

Test Interactions False-positive for blood in stool by the guaiac test

Patient Information May color stool black, take between meals for maximum absorption; may take with food if GI upset occurs, do not take with milk or antacids; keep out of reach of children

Additional Information Elemental iron content of gluconate: 12%

Dosage Forms Amount of elemental iron is listed in brackets
Capsule, soft gelatin (Simron®): 86 mg [10 mg]
Elixir (Fergon®): 300 mg/5 mL [34 mg/5 mL] with alcohol 7% (480 mL)
Tablet: 300 mg [34 mg]; 325 mg [38 mg]
Fergon®, Ferralet®: 320 mg [37 mg]
Sustained release (Ferralet® Slow Release): 320 mg [37 mg]

Ferrous Sulfate (fer′ us)

Brand Names Feosol® [OTC]; Feratab® [OTC]; Fer-In-Sol® [OTC]; Fer-Iron® [OTC]; Fero-Gradumet® [OTC]; Ferospace® [OTC]; Ferralyn® Lanacaps® [OTC]; Ferra-TD® [OTC]; Mol-Iron® [OTC]; Slow FE® [OTC]

Synonyms $FeSO_4$

Use Prevention and treatment of iron deficiency anemias

Pregnancy Risk Factor A

Contraindications Hemochromatosis, hemolytic anemia; known hypersensitivity to iron salts

Warnings/Precautions Administration of iron for >6 months should be avoided except in patients with continued bleeding, menorrhagia, or repeated pregnancies; avoid in patients with peptic ulcer, enteritis, or ulcerative colitis. Anemia in the elderly is often caused by "anemia of chronic disease" or associated with inflammation rather than blood loss. Iron stores are usually normal or increased, with a serum ferritin >50 ng/mL and a decreased total iron binding capacity. Hence, the "anemia of chronic disease" is not secondary to iron deficiency but the inability of the reticuloendothelial system to reclaim available iron stores.

Adverse Reactions
>10%: Gastrointestinal: GI irritation, epigastric pain, nausea, dark stool, vomiting, stomach cramping, constipation
1% to 10%:
Gastrointestinal: Heartburn, diarrhea
Miscellaneous: Liquid preparations may temporarily stain the teeth, discolored urine
<1%: Ocular: Contact irritation

Overdosage/Toxicology Symptoms of overdose include acute GI irritation; erosion of GI mucosa, hepatic and renal impairment, coma, hematemesis, lethargy, acidosis. Following treatment for fluid losses, metabolic acidosis, and shock, a severe iron overdose (when the serum iron concentration exceeds the total iron-binding capacity) may be treated with deferoxamine. Deferoxamine may be administered I.V. (80 mg/kg over 24 hours) or I.M. (40-90 mg/kg every 8 hours). Usual toxic dose of elemental iron: ≥35 mg/kg.

Drug Interactions

Decreased effect: Absorption of oral preparation of iron and tetracyclines are decreased when both of these drugs are given together; concurrent administration of antacids may decrease iron absorption; iron may decrease absorption of penicillamine when given at the same time; response to iron therapy may be delayed in patients receiving chloramphenicol; milk may decrease absorption of iron

Increased effect: Concurrent administration ≥200 mg vitamin C per 30 mg elemental Fe increases absorption of oral iron

Mechanism of Action Replaces iron, found in hemoglobin, myoglobin, and other enzymes; allows the transportation of oxygen via hemoglobin

Pharmacodynamics/Kinetics

Onset of hematologic response (essentially the same to either oral or parenteral iron salts): Red blood cell form and color changes within 3-10 days

Peak reticulocytosis: Occurs in 5-10 days, and hemoglobin values increase within 2-4 weeks

Absorption: Iron is absorbed in the duodenum and upper jejunum; in persons with normal serum iron stores, 10% of an oral dose is absorbed; this is increased to 20% to 30% in persons with inadequate iron stores. Food and achlorhydria will decrease absorption

Elimination: Iron is largely bound to serum transferrin and excreted in the urine, sweat, sloughing of the intestinal mucosa, and by menstrual bleeding

Usual Dosage Oral:

Children (dose expressed in terms of elemental iron):

Severe iron deficiency anemia: 4-6 mg Fe/kg/day in 3 divided doses

Mild to moderate iron deficiency anemia: 3 mg Fe/kg/day in 1-2 divided doses

Prophylaxis: 1-2 mg Fe/kg/day up to a maximum of 15 mg/day

Adults (dose expressed in terms of ferrous sulfate):

Iron deficiency: 300 mg twice daily up to 300 mg 4 times/day or 250 mg (extended release) 1-2 times/day

Prophylaxis: 300 mg/day

Administration Administer ferrous sulfate 2 hours prior to, or 4 hours after antacids

Reference Range

Serum iron:

Male: 75-175 µg/dL (SI: 13.4-31.3 µmol/L)

Female: 65-165 µg/dL (SI: 11.6-29.5 µmol/L)

Total iron binding capacity: 230-430 µg/dL

Transferrin: 204-360 mg/dL

Percent transferrin saturation: 20% to 50%

Test Interactions False-positive for blood in stool by the guaiac test

Patient Information May color stool black, take between meals for maximum absorption; may take with food if GI upset occurs, do not take with milk or antacids; keep out of reach of children

Additional Information Elemental iron content of iron salts in ferrous sulfate is 20% (ie, 300 mg ferrous sulfate is equivalent to 60 mg ferrous iron)

Dosage Forms Amount of elemental iron is listed in brackets

Capsule:

Exsiccated (Fer-In-Sol®): 190 mg [60 mg]

Exsiccated, timed release (Feosol®): 159 mg [50 mg]

Exsiccated, timed release (Ferralyn® Lanacaps®, Ferra-TD®): 250 mg [50 mg]

Ferospace®: 250 mg [50 mg]

Drops, oral:

Fer-In-Sol®: 75 mg/0.6 mL [15 mg/0.6 mL] (50 mL)

Fer-Iron®: 125 mg/mL [25 mg/mL] (50 mL)

Elixir (Feosol®): 220 mg/5 mL [44 mg/5 mL] with alcohol 5% (473 mL, 4000 mL)

Syrup (Fer-In-Sol®): 90 mg/5 mL [18 mg/5 mL] with alcohol 5% (480 mL)

Tablet: 324 mg [65 mg]

Exsiccated (Feosol®) 200 mg [65 mg]

Exsiccated, timed release (Slow FE®): 160 mg [50 mg]

Feratab®: 300 mg [60 mg]

Mol-Iron®: 195 mg [39 mg]

Timed release (Fero-Gradumet®): 525 mg [105 mg]

FeSO₄ see Ferrous Sulfate on previous page

Festal®ll [OTC] see Pancrelipase on page 837

Feverall™ [OTC] see Acetaminophen on page 17

Fiberall® Chewable Tablet [OTC] see Calcium Polycarbophil on page 172

Fiberall® Powder [OTC] see Psyllium on page 956

Fiberall® Wafer [OTC] *see* Psyllium *on page 956*

FiberCon® Tablet [OTC] *see* Calcium Polycarbophil *on page 172*

Fiber-Lax® Tablet [OTC] *see* Calcium Polycarbophil *on page 172*

Filgrastim (fil gra' stim)

Related Information
Cancer Chemotherapy Regimens *on page 1218-1241*
Sargramostim *on page 994*

Brand Names Neupogen®

Synonyms G-CSF; Granulocyte Colony Stimulating Factor

Use
Patients with nonmyeloid malignancies receiving myelosuppressive anticancer drugs associated with a significant incidence of neutropenia (FDA-approved indication)

Bone marrow transplant - to reduce the duration of neutropenia and neutropenia-related clinical sequelae in patients with nonmyeloid malignancies undergoing myeloablative chemotherapy followed by marrow transplantation (FDA-approved indication)

Severe chronic neutropenia - chronic administration to reduce the incidence and duration of sequelae of neutropenia in symptomatic patients with congenital neutropenia, cyclic neutropenia or idiopathic neutropenia (FDA-approved indication)

Unlabeled use: AIDS, aplastic anemia, hairy cell leukemia, myelodysplasia

Pregnancy Risk Factor C

Contraindications Patients with known hypersensitivity to *E. coli*-derived proteins or G-CSF

Warnings/Precautions Complete blood count and platelet count should be obtained prior to chemotherapy. Do not use G-CSF in the period 24 hours before to 24 hours after administration of cytotoxic chemotherapy because of the potential sensitivity of rapidly dividing myeloid cells to cytotoxic chemotherapy. Precaution should be exercised in the usage of G-CSF in any malignancy with myeloid characteristics. G-CSF can potentially act as a growth factor for any tumor type, particularly myeloid malignancies. Tumors of nonhematopoietic origin may have surface receptors for G-CSF.

Adverse Reactions Effects are generally mild and dose related
>10%:
Gastrointestinal: Nausea, vomiting, diarrhea, mucositis
Medullary bone pain (24% incidence): This occurs most commonly in lower back pain, posterior iliac crest, and sternum and is controlled with non-narcotic analgesics
Miscellaneous: Alopecia, neutropenic fever, fever
Splenomegaly: This occurs more commonly in patients with cyclic neutropenia/congenital agranulocytosis who received S.C. injections for a prolonged (>14 days) period of time; ~33% of these patients experience subclinical splenomegaly (detected by MRI or CT scan); ~3% of these patients experience clinical splenomegaly
1% to 10%:
Cardiovascular: Chest pain, fluid retention
Central nervous system: Headache, weakness
Dermatologic: Skin rash
Gastrointestinal: Anorexia, stomatitis, constipation
Local: Pain at injection site
Hematologic: Leukocytosis
Respiratory: Dyspnea, cough, sore throat
<1%:
Cardiovascular: Transient supraventricular arrhythmia, pericarditis
Local: Thrombophlebitis
Hypersensitivity: Anaphylactic reaction

Overdosage/Toxicology No clinical adverse effects seen with high dose producing ANC >10,000/mm^3; leukocytosis which was not associated with any clinical adverse effects; after discontinuing the drug there is a 50% decrease in circulating levels of neutrophils within 1-2 days, return to pretreatment levels within 1-7 days

Stability
Filgrastim is a clear, colorless solution and should be stored under refrigeration at 2°C to 8°C (36°F to 46°F) and protected from direct sunlight; filgrastim should be protected from freezing and temperatures >30°C to avoid aggregation

The solution should not be shaken since bubbles and/or foam may form. If foaming occurs, the solution should be left undisturbed for a few minutes until bubbles dissipate

Filgrastim is stable for 24 hours at 9°C to 30°C, however, the manufacturer recommends discarding after 6 hours because of microbiological concerns; the product is packaged as single-use vial without a preservative

Undiluted filgrastim is stable for 24 hours at 15°C to 30°C and 7 days at 2°C to 8°C in tuberculin syringes. However, refrigeration and use within 24 hours are recommended because of concern for bacterial contamination.

Filgrastim may be diluted in dextrose 5% in water to a concentration ≥15 mcg/mL for I.V. infusion administration

Minimum concentration is 15 mcg/mL

Concentrations <15 mcg/mL require addition of albumin (1 mL of 5%) to the bag to prevent absorption to plastics/PVC

This diluted solution is stable for 7 days under refrigeration or at room temperature

Standard diluent: ≥375 mcg/25 mL D_5W; **filgrastim is incompatible with 0.9% sodium chloride (normal saline)**

Mechanism of Action Stimulates the production, maturation, and activation of neutrophils, G-CSF activates neutrophils to increase both their migration and cytotoxicity. Natural proteins which stimulate hematopoietic stem cells to proliferate, prolong cell survival, stimulate cell differentiation, and stimulate functional activity of mature cells. CSFs are produced by a wide variety of cell types. Specific mechanisms of action are not yet fully understood, but possibly work by a second-messenger pathway with resultant protein production. See table.

Proliferation/Differentiation	G-CSF (Filgrastim)	GM-CSF (Sargramostim)
Neutrophils	Yes	Yes
Eosinophils	No	Yes
Macrophages	No	Yes
Neutrophil migration	Enhanced	Inhibited

Pharmacodynamics/Kinetics

Onset of action: Rapid elevation in neutrophil counts within the first 24 hours, reaching a plateau in 3-5 days

Duration: ANC decreases by 50% within 2 days after discontinuing G-CSF; white counts return to the normal range in 4-7 days

Absorption: S.C.: 100% absorbed; peak plasma levels can be maintained for up to 12 hours

Distribution: V_d: 150 mL/kg; no evidence of drug accumulation over a 11- to 20-day period

Metabolism: Systemically metabolized

Bioavailability: Oral: Not bioavailable

Half-life: 1.8-3.5 hours

Time to peak serum concentration: S.C.: Within 2-6 hours

Usual Dosage Children and Adults: administered S.C. or I.V. as a single daily infusion over 20-30 minutes

Myelosuppressive chemotherapy 5 mcg/kg/day S.C. or I.V.

Doses may be increased in increments of 5 mcg/kg for each chemotherapy cycle, according to the duration and severity of the absolute neutrophil count (ANC) nadir. In phase III trials, efficacy was observed at doses of 4-6 mcg/kg/day. Discontinue therapy if the ANC count is >10,000/mm³ after the ANC nadir has occurred following the expected chemotherapy-induced neutrophil nadir. Some cancer centers are stopping therapy at an ANC of 2500. Duration of therapy needed to attenuate chemotherapy-induced neutropenia may be dependent on the myelosuppressive potential of the chemotherapy regimen employed. Duration of therapy in clinical studies has ranged from 2 weeks to 3 years.

Bone marrow transplant patients

Bone marrow transplant patients: 10 mcg/kg/day as an I.V. infusion of 4 or 24 hours or as continuous 24-hour S.C. infusion. Administer first dose at least

Filgrastim Dose Based on Neutrophil Response

Absolute Neutrophil Count	Filgrastim Dose Adjustment
When ANC > 1000/mm³ for 3 consecutive days	Reduce to 5 mcg/kg/day
If ANC remains > 1000/mm³ for 3 more consecutive days	Discontinue filgrastim
If ANC decreases to < 1000/mm³	Resume at 5 mcg/kg/day

(Continued)

Filgrastim *(Continued)*

24 hours after cytotoxic chemotherapy and at least 24 hours after bone marrow infusion.

Severe chronic neutropenia:
Congenital neutropenia: 6 mcg/kg twice daily S.C.
Idiopathic/cyclic neutropenia: 5 mcg/kg/day S.C.

Chronic daily administration is required to maintain clinical benefit. Adjust dose based on the patients' clinical course as well as ANC. In phase III studies, the target ANC was 1,500-10,000/mm^3. Reduce the dose of the ANC is persistently >10,000/mm^3.

Premature discontinuation of G-CSF therapy prior to the time of recovery from the expected neutrophil is generally not recommended. A transient increase in neutrophil counts is typically seen 1-2 days after initiation of therapy.

Administration May be administered undiluted by S.C. or IVP administration; may also be administered by I.V. infusion over 15-60 minutes in D$_5$W; **incompatible with sodium chloride solutions**

Monitoring Parameters CBC and platelet count should be obtained twice weekly. Leukocytosis (white blood cell counts ≥100,000/mm^3) has been observed in ~2% of patients receiving G-CSF at doses >5 mcg/kg/day. Monitor platelets and hematocrit regularly. Monitor patients with pre-existing cardiac conditions closely as cardiac events (myocardial infarctions, arrhythmias) have been reported in premarketing clinical studies.

Reference Range No clinical benefit seen with ANC >10,000/mm^3

Patient Information Possible bone pain

Nursing Implications Do not mix with sodium chloride solutions

Additional Information
Reimbursement Hotline: 1-800-272-9376
Professional Services [AMGEN]: 1-800-77-AMGEN

Dosage Forms Injection, preservative free: 300 mcg/mL (1 mL, 1.6 mL)

Filibon® [OTC] *see* Vitamin, Multiple *on page 1166*

Finasteride *(fi nas' teer ide)*

Brand Names Proscar®

Use Early data indicate that finasteride is useful in the treatment of symptomatic benign prostatic hyperplasia (BPH)

Unlabeled use: Adjuvant monotherapy after radical prostatectomy in the treatment of prostatic cancer

Pregnancy Risk Factor X

Contraindications History of hypersensitivity to drug, pregnancy, lactation, children

Warnings/Precautions A minimum of 6 months of treatment may be necessary to determine whether an individual will respond to finasteride. Use with caution in those patients with liver function abnormalities. Carefully monitor patients with a large residual urinary volume or severely diminished urinary flow for obstructive uropathy. These patients may not be candidates for finasteride therapy.

Adverse Reactions
1% to 10%:
Endocrine & metabolic: Decreased libido
Genitourinary: <4% incidence of impotence, decreased volume of ejaculate

Mechanism of Action Finasteride is a 4-azo analog of testosterone and is a competitive inhibitor of both tissue and hepatic 5-alpha reductase. This results in inhibition of the conversion of testosterone to dihydrotestosterone and markedly suppresses serum dihydrotestosterone levels; depending on dose and duration, serum testosterone concentrations may or may not increase. Testosterone-dependent processes such as fertility, muscle strength, potency, and libido are not affected by finasteride.

Pharmacodynamics/Kinetics
Onset of clinical effect: Within 12 weeks to 6 months of ongoing therapy
Duration of action:
After a single oral dose as small as 0.5 mg: 65% depression of plasma dihydrotestosterone levels persists 5-7 days
After 6 months of treatment with 5 mg/day: Circulating dihydrotestosterone levels are reduced to castrate levels without significant effects on circulating testosterone; levels return to normal within 14 days of discontinuation of treatment
Absorption: Oral: Extent may be reduced if administered with food
Bioavailability: Mean: 63%
Time to peak serum concentration: Oral: 2-6 hours

Metabolism: Unchanged finasteride is major circulating component; two active metabolites have been identified

Half-life, serum: Parent drug: ~5-17 hours (mean: 1.9 fasting, 4.2 with breakfast)

Half-life:
Elderly: 8 hours
Adults: 6 hours (3-16)

Protein binding: 90%

Elimination: As metabolites in urine and feces; elimination rate is decreased in the elderly, but no dosage adjustment is needed

Usual Dosage Adults: Male: Benign prostatic hyperplasia: Oral: 5 mg/day as a single dose; clinical responses occur within 12 weeks to 6 months of initiation of therapy; long-term administration is recommended for maximal response

Dosing adjustment in renal impairment: No dosage adjustment is necessary

Monitoring Parameters Objective and subjective signs of relief of benign prostatic hyperplasia, including improvement in urinary flow, reduction in symptoms of urgency, and relief of difficulty in micturition

Nursing Implications Administration with food may delay the rate and reduce the extent of oral absorption

Dosage Forms Tablet, film coated: 5 mg

Fiorgen PF® see Butalbital Compound on page 153

Fioricet® see Butalbital Compound on page 153

Fiorinal® see Butalbital Compound on page 153

Fisalamine see Mesalamine on page 691

FK506 see Tacrolimus on page 1053

Flagyl® see Metronidazole on page 733

Flarex® see Fluorometholone on page 473

Flatulex® [OTC] see Simethicone on page 1006

Flavorcee® [OTC] see Ascorbic Acid on page 88

Flavoxate (fla vox′ ate)

Brand Names Urispas®

Use Antispasmodic used to provide symptomatic relief of dysuria, nocturia, suprapubic pain, urgency, and incontinence

Pregnancy Risk Factor B

Contraindications Pyloric or duodenal obstruction, GI hemorrhage, GI obstruction, obstructive uropathies of the lower urinary tract

Warnings/Precautions May cause drowsiness, vertigo, and ocular disturbances; give cautiously in patients with suspected glaucoma

Adverse Reactions
>10%:
Central nervous system: Drowsiness
Miscellaneous: Dry mouth/throat
1% to 10%:
Cardiovascular: Tachycardia, palpitations,
Central nervous system: Nervousness, fatigue, vertigo, headache, drowsiness, hyperpyrexia
Gastrointestinal: Constipation, nausea, vomiting
<1%:
Central nervous system: Confusion (especially in the elderly)
Dermatologic: Skin rash
Hematologic: Leukopenia
Ophthalmic: Increased intraocular pressure

Overdosage/Toxicology Symptoms of overdose include clumsiness, dizziness, drowsiness, flushing, hallucinations, irritability; supportive care only

Mechanism of Action Synthetic antispasmotic with similar actions to that of propantheline; it exerts a direct relaxant effect on smooth muscles via phosphodiesterase inhibition, providing relief to a variety of smooth muscle spasms; it is especially useful for the treatment of bladder spasticity, whereby it produces an increase in urinary capacity

Pharmacodynamics/Kinetics
Onset of action: 55-60 minutes
Metabolism: To methyl; flavone carboxylic acid active
Elimination: 10% to 30% of dose excreted in urine within 6 hours

Usual Dosage Children >12 years and Adults: Oral: 100-200 mg 3-4 times/day; reduce the dose when symptoms improve

Monitoring Parameters Monitor I & O closely

(Continued)

Flavoxate *(Continued)*

Patient Information May cause drowsiness, dizziness, or visual disturbances; use with caution if performing tasks requiring coordination or mental alertness; avoid other substances that may cause similar effects (eg, alcohol); may cause dry mouth

Dosage Forms Tablet, film coated: 100 mg

Flecainide Acetate *(fle kay' nide)*

Related Information

Antiarrhythmic Drugs *on page 1246-1248*

Brand Names Tambocor™

Use Prevention and suppression of documented life-threatening ventricular arrhythmias (ie, sustained ventricular tachycardia); controlling symptomatic, disabling supraventricular tachycardias in patients without structural heart disease in whom other agents fail

Pregnancy Risk Factor C

Contraindications Pre-existing second or third degree A-V block; right bundle branch block associated with left hemiblock (bifascicular block) or trifascicular block; cardiogenic shock, myocardial depression; known hypersensitivity to the drug

Warnings/Precautions

Pre-existing sinus node dysfunction, sick-sinus syndrome, history of congestive heart failure or myocardial dysfunction; increases in P-R interval $\geq$300 MS, QRS $\geq$180 MS, Q-T$_c$ interval increases, and/or new bundle branch block; patients with pacemakers, renal impairment, and/or hepatic impairment.

The manufacturer and FDA recommend that this drug be reserved for life-threatening ventricular arrhythmias unresponsive to conventional therapy. Its use for symptomatic nonsustained ventricular tachycardia, frequent premature ventricular complexes (PVCs), uniform and multiform PVCs and/or coupled PVCs is no longer recommended. Flecainide can worsen or cause arrhythmias with an associated risk of death. Proarrhythmic effects range from an increased number of PVCs to more severe ventricular tachycardias (eg, tachycardias that are more sustained or more resistant to conversion to sinus rhythm).

Adverse Reactions

>10%:

Central nervous system: Dizziness

Ocular: Visual disturbances

Respiratory: Dyspnea

1% to 10%:

Cardiovascular: Palpitations, chest pain, edema, tachycardia

Central nervous system: Headache, fatigue, asthenia, fever

Dermatologic: Rash

Gastrointestinal: Nausea, constipation, abdominal pain

Neuromuscular & skeletal: Tremor

<1%:

Cardiovascular: Bradycardia, heart block, increased P-R, QRS duration, worsening ventricular arrhythmias, congestive heart failure

Central nervous system: Nervousness, hypoesthesia

Dermatologic: Alopecia

Hematologic: Blood dyscrasias

Hepatic: Possible hepatic dysfunction

Neuromuscular & skeletal: Paresthesia

Overdosage/Toxicology Has a narrow therapeutic index and severe toxicity may occur slightly above the therapeutic range, especially if combined with other antiarrhythmic drugs. (Acute single ingestion of twice the daily therapeutic dose is life-threatening.) Symptoms of overdose include increases in P-R, QRS, Q-T intervals and amplitude of the T wave, A-V block, bradycardia, hypotension, ventricular arrhythmias (monomorphic or polymorphic ventricular tachycardia), and asystole; other symptoms include dizziness, blurred vision, headache, and GI upset.

Treatment is supportive, using conventional treatment (fluids, positioning, anticonvulsants and antiarrhythmics). **Note:** Type Ia antiarrhythmic agents should not be used to treat cardiotoxicity caused by type 1c drugs; sodium bicarbonate may reverse QRS prolongation, bradycardia and hypotension; ventricular pacing may be needed; hemodialysis only of possible benefit for tocainide or flecainide overdose in patients with renal failure.

Drug Interactions

Increased toxicity:

Digoxin, amiodarone (increased plasma concentrations)

Beta-adrenergic blockers, disopyramide, verapamil (possible additive negative inotropic effects)

Alkalinizing agents (high dose antacids, cimetidine, carbonic anhydrase inhibitors or sodium bicarbonate) may decrease flecainide clearance

Decreased toxicity: Smoking and acid urine (increases flecainide clearance)

Mechanism of Action Class IC antiarrhythmic; slows conduction in cardiac tissue by altering transport of ions across cell membranes; causes slight prolongation of refractory periods; decreases the rate of rise of the action potential without affecting its duration; increases electrical stimulation threshold of ventricle, HIS-Purkinje system; possesses local anesthetic and moderate negative inotropic effects

Pharmacodynamics/Kinetics

Absorption: Oral: Rapid

Distribution: Adults: V_d: 5-13.4 L/kg

Protein binding: 40% to 50% (alpha$_1$ glycoprotein)

Bioavailability: 85% to 90%

Metabolism: In the liver

Half-life:

Infants: 11-12 hours

Children: 8 hours

Adults: 7-22 hours, increased with congestive heart failure or renal dysfunction

End stage renal disease: 19-26 hours

Time to peak serum concentration: Within 1.5-3 hours

Elimination: 80% to 90% excreted in urine as unchanged drug and metabolites (10% to 50%)

Usual Dosage Oral:

Children:

Initial: 3 mg/kg/day or 50-100 mg/m^2/day in 3 divided doses

Usual: 3-6 mg/kg/day or 100-150 mg/m^2/day in 3 divided doses; up to 11 mg/kg/day or 200 mg/m^2/day for uncontrolled patients with subtherapeutic levels

Adults:

Life-threatening ventricular arrhythmias:

Initial: 100 mg every 12 hours

Increase by 50-100 mg/day (given in 2 doses/day) every 4 days; maximum: 400 mg/day

For patients receiving 400 mg/day who are not controlled and have trough concentrations <0.6 mcg/mL, dosage may be increased to 600 mg/day

Prevention of paroxysmal supraventricular arrhythmias in patients with disabling symptoms but no structural heart disease:

Initial: 50 mg every 12 hours

Increase by 50 mg twice daily at 4-day intervals; maximum: 300 mg/day

Dosing adjustment in severe renal impairment: Cl_{cr} <10 mL minute: Decrease usual dose by 25% to 50%

Not dialyzable (0% to 5%) via hemo- or peritoneal dialysis; no supplemental dose necessary

Dosing adjustment/comments in hepatic impairment: Monitoring of plasma levels is recommended because of significantly increased half-life

When transferring from another antiarrhythmic agent, allow for 2-4 half-lives of the agent to pass before initiating flecainide therapy

Administration Administer around-the-clock to promote less variation in peak and trough serum levels

Monitoring Parameters EKG, blood pressure, pulse, periodic serum concentrations, especially in patients with renal or hepatic impairment

Reference Range Therapeutic: 0.2-1 µg/mL; pediatric patients may respond at the lower end of the recommended therapeutic range

Patient Information Notify physician if chest pain, faintness, or palpitations occurs; take only as prescribed

Dosage Forms Tablet: 50 mg, 100 mg, 150 mg

Fleet® Phospho®-Soda [OTC] *see* Sodium Phosphates *on page 1015*

Fleet® Laxative [OTC] *see* Bisacodyl *on page 134*

Fleet® Flavored Castor Oil [OTC] *see* Castor Oil *on page 190*

Fleet® Babylax® [OTC] *see* Glycerin *on page 506*

Fleet® Mineral Oil Enema [OTC] *see* Mineral Oil *on page 743*

Fleet® Enema [OTC] *see* Sodium Phosphates *on page 1015*

Flexaphen® *see* Chlorzoxazone *on page 236*

Flexeril® *see* Cyclobenzaprine Hydrochloride *on page 285*

Flonase™ *see* Fluticasone Propionate *on page 484*

Florinef® Acetate *see* Fludrocortisone Acetate *on page 465*

Florone® *see* Diflorasone Diacetate *on page 335*

Florone E® *see* Diflorasone Diacetate *on page 335*

Floropryl® *see* Isoflurophate *on page 594*

Florvite® *see* Vitamin, Multiple *on page 1166*

Floxin® *see* Ofloxacin *on page 814*

Floxuridine (flox yoor' i deen)
Related Information
Cancer Chemotherapy Regimens *on page 1218-1241*
Brand Names FUDR®
Synonyms Fluorodeoxyuridine
Use Treatment of gastrointestinal adenocarcinoma metastatic to the liver
Pregnancy Risk Factor D
Contraindications Poor nutritional status, depressed (leukocyte count <5000/mm^3 or platelet count <100,000/mm^3) bone marrow function, potentially serious infections
Warnings/Precautions
The U.S. Food and Drug Administration (FDA) currently recommends that procedures for proper handling and disposal of antineoplastic agents be considered

Impaired kidney or liver function; the drug should be discontinued if intractable vomiting or diarrhea, precipitous fall in leukocyte or platelet counts or myocardial ischemia occurs

Use with caution in patients who have had high-dose pelvic radiation or previous use of alkylating agents. Patient should be hospitalized during initial course of therapy.

Adverse Reactions
>10%: Gastrointestinal: GI hemorrhage, stomatitis, esophagopharyngitis, diarrhea, gastritis

1% to 10%:
Dermatologic: **Alopecia**, dermatitis, rash
Gastrointestinal: **Anorexia**, glossitis

<1%:
Cardiovascular: **Myocardial ischemia**, angina
Central nervous system: Lethargy, weakness, acute cerebellar syndrome, confusion, euphoria, fever
Hematologic: Severe hematologic toxicity, leukopenia, thrombocytopenia, pancytopenia, agranulocytosis
Myelosuppressive:
WBC: Mild
Platelets: Mild
Onset (days): 7-10
Nadir (days): 9-14
Recovery (days): 21
Sensitivity reactions: Anaphylaxis, photophobia

Overdosage/Toxicology Symptoms of overdose include diarrhea, alopecia, myelosuppression, hyperpigmentation, nausea, vomiting, GI ulceration, bleeding
Stability Reconstituted solutions are stable for up to 14 days (refrigerated); FUDR® is stable in D$_5$W or NS
Mechanism of Action Mechanism of action and pharmacokinetics are very similar to 5-FU; FUDR® is the deoxyribonucleotide of 5-FU. Inhibits DNA and RNA synthesis via formation of carbonium ions; cross-links strands of DNA, causing an imbalance of growth and cell death
Pharmacodynamics/Kinetics
Metabolism: Following infusion of small doses, most of the drug appears to be metabolized in the liver (as 5-FU) to the active metabolite FUDR-MP; following rapid administration of single doses, the drug appears to be rapidly catabolized to fluorouracil; metabolic degradation is less when floxuridine is given by continuous infusion than by single injections

Elimination: As metabolites in the urine and as respiratory carbon dioxide
Usual Dosage Adults (refer to individual protocols):
Intra-arterial: Primarily by an implantable pump: 0.1-0.6 mg/kg/day continuous intra-arterial administration for 14 days then heparinized saline is given for 14 days; toxicity requires dose reduction

I.V.: 0.5-1 mg/kg/day for 6-15 days
Administration Infused for intra-arterial use, use infusion pump, either external or implanted
Patient Information Any signs of infection, easy bruising or bleeding, shortness of breath, or painful or burning urination should be brought to physician's attention. Nausea, vomiting, or hair loss sometimes occur. The drug may cause

permanent sterility and may cause birth defects. The drug may be excreted in breast milk, therefore, an alternative form of feeding your baby should be used.

Dosage Forms
Injection, preservative free: 100 mg/mL (5 mL)
Powder for injection: 500 mg (5 mL, 10 mL)

Flubenisolone *see* Betamethasone *on page 129*

Fluconazole (floo koe' na zole)
Related Information
Antifungal Agents *on page 1253-1254*
Brand Names Diflucan®
Use Oral fluconazole should be used in persons able to tolerate oral medications; parenteral fluconazole should be reserved for patients who are both unable to take oral medications and are unable to tolerate amphotericin B (eg, due to hypersensitivity or renal insufficiency)

Indications for use in adult patients:
Oral or vaginal candidiasis unresponsive to nystatin or clotrimazole
Nonlife-threatening *Candida* infections (eg, cystitis, esophagitis)
Treatment of hepatosplenic candidiasis
Treatment of other *Candida* infections in persons unable to tolerate amphotericin B
Treatment of cryptococcal infections
Secondary prophylaxis for cryptococcal meningitis in persons with AIDS
Antifungal prophylaxis in allogeneic bone marrow transplant recipients

Pregnancy Risk Factor C
Contraindications Known hypersensitivity to fluconazole or other azoles
Warnings/Precautions Should be used with caution in patients with renal and hepatic dysfunction or previous hepatotoxicity from other azole derivatives. Patients who develop abnormal liver function tests during fluconazole therapy should be monitored closely and discontinued if symptoms consistent with liver disease develop.

Adverse Reactions
1% to 10%:
Central nervous system: Headache
Dermatologic: Skin rash
Gastrointestinal: Nausea, vomiting, abdominal pain, diarrhea
<1%:
Cardiovascular: Pallor
Central nervous system: Dizziness
Endocrine & metabolic: Hypokalemia
Miscellaneous: Elevated AST, ALT, or alkaline phosphatase

Overdosage/Toxicology Symptoms of overdose include decreased lacrimation, salivation, respiration and motility, urinary incontinence, cyanosis; treatment includes supportive measures, a 3-hour hemodialysis will remove 50%

Drug Interactions Cytochrome P-450 IIIA4 enzyme inhibitor and cytochrome P-450 IIC enzyme inhibitor
Decreased effect: Rifampin ↓ concentrations of fluconazole
Increased toxicity:
May increase cyclosporine levels when high doses used
May increase phenytoin serum concentration
Fluconazole may also inhibit warfarin metabolism

Stability Parenteral admixture at room temperature (25°C): Manufacturer expiration dating; do not refrigerate
Standard diluent: 200 mg/100 mL NS (premixed); 400 mg/200 mL NS (premixed)
Incompatible with ampicillin, calcium gluconate, ceftazidime, cefotaxime, cefuroxime, ceftriaxone, clindamycin, furosemide, imipenem, ticarcillin, and piperacillin

Mechanism of Action Interferes with cytochrome P-450 activity, decreasing ergosterol synthesis (principal sterol in fungal cell membrane) and inhibiting cell membrane formation

Pharmacodynamics/Kinetics
Distribution: Relative diffusion of antimicrobial agents from blood into CSF: Adequate with or without inflammation (exceeds usual MICs)
Ratio of CSF to blood level (%):
Normal meninges: 70-80
Inflamed meninges: >70-80
Protein binding, plasma: 11% to 12%
Bioavailability: Oral: >90%
Half-life: 25-30 hours with normal renal function
Time to peak serum concentration: Oral: Within 2-4 hours
(Continued)

Fluconazole *(Continued)*

Elimination: 80% of a dose excreted unchanged in the urine

Usual Dosage The daily dose of fluconazole is the same for oral and I.V. administration

Efficacy of fluconazole has not been established in children; a small number of patients from 3-13 years of age have been treated with fluconazole using doses of 3-6 mg/kg/day once daily. Doses as high as 12 mg/kg/day once daily have been used to treat candidiasis in immunocompromised children; 10-12 mg/kg/day has been used prophylactically against fungal infections in pediatric bone marrow transplant patients.

Adults: Oral, I.V.: See table for once daily dosing.

Indication	Day 1	Daily Therapy	Minimum Duration of Therapy
Oropharyngeal candidiasis	200 mg	100 mg	14 d
Esophageal candidiasis	200 mg	100 mg	21 d
Systemic candidiasis	400 mg	200 mg	28 d
Cryptococcal meningitis			10-12 wk after CSF culture becomes negative
acute	400 mg	200 mg	
relapse	200 mg	200 mg	

Dosing adjustment/interval in renal impairment:

Cl_{cr} 21-50 mL/minute: Administer 50% of recommended dose or administer every 48 hours

Cl_{cr} <20 mL/minute: Administer 25% of recommended dose or administer every 72 hours

50% removed by hemodialysis

Administration Parenteral fluconazole must be administered by I.V. infusion over approximately 1-2 hours; do not exceed 200 mg/hour when giving I.V. infusion; maximum rate of infusion: 200 mg/hour

Monitoring Parameters Periodic liver function tests (AST, ALT, alkaline phosphatase) and renal function tests, potassium

Patient Information May take with food; complete full course of therapy; contact physician or pharmacist if side effects develop

Nursing Implications Do not use if cloudy or precipitated

Dosage Forms

Injection: 2 mg/mL (100 mL, 200 mL)

Tablet: 50 mg, 100 mg, 200 mg

Flucytosine *(floo sye' toe seen)*

Related Information

Antifungal Agents *on page 1253-1254*

Brand Names Ancobon®

Synonyms 5-FC; 5-Flurocytosine

Use Adjunctive treatment of susceptible fungal infections (usually *Candida* or *Cryptococcus*); in combination with amphotericin B, fluconazole, or itraconazole; synergy with amphotericin B for fungal infections (*Aspergillus*)

Pregnancy Risk Factor C

Contraindications Hypersensitivity to flucytosine or any component

Warnings/Precautions Use with extreme caution in patients with renal impairment or bone marrow depression; dosage modification required in patients with impaired renal function

Adverse Reactions

1% to 10%:

Dermatologic: Skin rash

Gastrointestinal: Abdominal pain, diarrhea, loss of appetite, nausea, vomiting

Hematologic: Anemia, leukopenia, thrombocytopenia

Hepatic: Hepatitis, jaundice

<1%:

Cardiovascular: Cardiac arrest

Central nervous system: Confusion, hallucinations, dizziness, drowsiness, headache, parkinsonism, psychosis, ataxia

Dermatologic: Photosensitivity

Endocrine & metabolic: Temporary growth failure, hypoglycemia, hypokalemia

Hematologic: Bone marrow depression

Hepatic: Elevated liver enzymes

Neuromuscular & skeletal: Paresthesia

Otic: Hearing loss

Respiratory: Respiratory arrest

Overdosage/Toxicology Symptoms of overdose include nausea, vomiting, diarrhea, bone marrow depression; treatment is supportive

Drug Interactions Increased effect/toxicity (enterocolitis) with concurrent amphotericin administration

Stability Protect from light

Mechanism of Action Penetrates fungal cells and is converted to fluorouracil which competes with uracil interfering with fungal RNA and protein synthesis

Pharmacodynamics/Kinetics

Absorption: Oral: 75% to 90%

Distribution: Into CSF and bronchial secretions

Metabolism: Minimal

Protein binding: 2% to 4%

Half-life: 3-8 hours

Anuria: May be as long as 200 hours

End stage renal disease: 75-200 hours

Time to peak serum concentration: Within 2-6 hours

Elimination: 75% to 90% excreted unchanged in the urine by glomerular filtration

Usual Dosage Children and Adults: Oral: 50-150 mg/kg/day in divided doses every 6 hours

Dosing interval in renal impairment:

Cl_{cr} 10-<50 mL/minute: Administer every 12 hours

Cl_{cr} <10 mL/minute: Administer every 24 hours

Dialyzable (50% to 100%); administer dose post hemodialysis; administer 0.5-1 g every 24 hours during peritoneal dialysis (adults) and during continuous arterio-venous or veno-venous hemofiltration

Administration Administer around-the-clock rather than 4 times/day to promote less variation in peak and trough serum levels

Monitoring Parameters Serum creatinine, BUN, alkaline phosphatase, AST, ALT, CBC; serum flucytosine concentrations

Reference Range

Therapeutic: 25-100 µg/mL (SI: 195-775 µmol/L); levels should not exceed 100-120 µg/mL to avoid toxic bone marrow depressive effects

Trough: Draw just prior to dose administration

Peak: Draw 2 hours after an oral dose administration

Test Interactions Flucytosine causes markedly false elevations in serum creatinine values when the Ektachem® analyzer is used

Patient Information Take capsules a few at a time with food over a 15-minute period to avoid nausea

Dosage Forms Capsule: 250 mg, 500 mg

Fludara® *see* Fludarabine Phosphate *on this page*

Fludarabine Phosphate (floo dare' a been)

Related Information

Cancer Chemotherapy Regimens *on page 1218-1241*

Brand Names Fludara®

Use Treatment of chronic lymphocytic leukemia (B-cell) in patients who have not responded to other alkylating agent regimen; low-grade non-Hodgkin's lymphoma

Pregnancy Risk Factor D

Contraindications Hypersensitivity of fludarabine; patients with severe infections

Warnings/Precautions The U.S. Food and Drug Administration (FDA) currently recommends that procedures for proper handling and disposal of antineoplastic agents be considered. Use with caution with renal insufficiency, patients with a fever documented infection or pre-existing hematological disorders (particularly granulocytopenia) or in patients with pre-existing central nervous system disorder (epilepsy), spasticity, or peripheral neuropathy.

Adverse Reactions

>10%:

Cardiovascular: Edema

Central nervous system: Fever, chills, weakness, fatigue

Dermatologic: Rash

Gastrointestinal: Mild nausea, vomiting, diarrhea, stomatitis, GI bleeding

Genitourinary: Urinary infection

Myelosuppression: Dose-limiting toxicity; myelosuppression may not be related to cumulative dose

Granulocyte nadir: 13 days (3-25)

Platelet nadir: 16 days (2-32)

WBC nadir: 8 days

Recovery: 5-7 weeks

(Continued)

Fludarabine Phosphate (Continued)

Neuromuscular & skeletal: Paresthesia, myalgia

Respiratory: Manifested as dyspnea and a nonproductive cough; lung biopsy has shown pneumonitis in some patients, pneumonia

Miscellaneous: Infection, pain

1% to 10%:

Cardiovascular: Congestive heart failure

Central nervous system: Malaise, headache

Dermatologic: Alopecia

Endocrine & metabolic: Hyperglycemia

Gastrointestinal: Anorexia

Otic: Hearing loss

<1%:

Central nervous system: Reported with higher dose levels; most patients shown to have CNS demyelination; somnolence also noted; severe neurotoxicity

Dermatologic: Skin rash

Endocrine & metabolic: Metabolic acidosis

Hematologic: Hematuria

Hepatic: Reversible hepatotoxicity

Renal: Renal failure

Respiratory: Interstitial pneumonitis

Miscellaneous: Increased serum creatinine, metallic taste, tumor lysis syndrome

Overdosage/Toxicology There are clear dose-dependent toxic neurologic effects associated with fludarabine. Doses of 96 mg/m^2/day for 5-7 days are associated with a syndrome characterized by delayed blindness, coma, and death. Symptoms appeared from 21-60 days following the last dose. The central nervous system toxicity has distinctive features of delayed onset and progressive encephalopathy resulting in fatal outcomes. It is reported at an incidence rate of 36% at high doses (≥96 mg/m^2/day for 5-7 days) and <0.2% for low doses (≤125 mg/m^2/course).

Drug Interactions Increased toxicity: Cytarabine when administered with or prior to a fludarabine dose competes for deoxycytidine kinase decreasing the metabolism of F-ara-A to the active F-ara-ATP (inhibits the antineoplastic effect of fludarabine); however, administering fludarabine prior to cytarabine may stimulate activation of cytarabine

Stability Fludarabine should be stored under refrigeration (2°C to 8°C or 36°F to 46°F). Reconstitute with 2 mL of sterile water for injection to a final concentration of 25 mg/mL; after dissolution (within 15 seconds), fludarabine should be further diluted in 100-150 mL of either dextrose 5% in water or 0.9% sodium chloride for administration by intravenous piggyback over 30 minutes; fludarabine should be used within 8 hours of reconstitution as it contains no preservatives; however, is chemically stable 48 hours at room temperature and refrigeration.

Mechanism of Action Fludarabine is analogous to that of Ara-C and Ara-A. Following systemic administration, FAMP is rapidly dephosphorylated to 2-fluoro-Ara-A. 2-Fluoro-Ara-A enters the cell by a carrier-mediated transport process, then is phosphorylated intracellularly by deoxycytidine kinase to form the active metabolite 2-fluoro-Ara-ATP. 2-Fluoro-Ara-ATP inhibits DNA synthesis by inhibition of DNA polymerase and ribonucleotide reductase.

Pharmacodynamics/Kinetics

Absorption: Oral preparation is under study

Bioavailability: Shown to be 100% in animal models

Distribution: V_d: 38-96 L/m^2; widely distributed with extensive tissue binding

Metabolism: I.V.: Fludarabine phosphate is rapidly dephosphorylated to 2-fluoro-vidarabine, which subsequently enters tumor cells and is phosphorylated to the active triphosphate derivative; rapidly dephosphorylated in the serum

Half-life, elimination: 2-fluoro-vidarabine: 9 hours

Elimination: 24% of dose recovered in urine as 2-fluoro-vidarabine

Usual Dosage I.V.:

Children:

Acute leukemia: 10 mg/m^2 bolus over 15 minutes followed by continuous infusion of 30.5 mg/m^2/day over 5 days

or

10.5 mg/m^2 bolus over 15 minutes followed by 30.5 mg/m^2/day over 48 hours followed by cytarabine has been used in clinical trials

Solid tumors: 9 mg/m^2 bolus followed by 27 mg/m^2/day continuous infusion over 5 days

Adults:

Chronic lymphocytic leukemia: 25 mg/m^2/day over a 30-minute period for 5 days; 5-day courses are repeated every 28 days

Non-Hodgkin's lymphoma: Loading dose: 20 mg/m² followed by 30 mg/m²/day for 48 hours

Dosing in renal impairment: Cl_{cr} <50 mL/minute: Monitor closely for toxicity

Administration Administer I.V. over 15-30 minutes or continuous infusion

Monitoring Parameters CBC with differential, platelet count, AST, ALT, creatinine, serum albumin, uric acid

Reference Range Peak plasma levels: 0.3-0.9 µg/mL following a short infusion of 25 mg/m²

Dosage Forms Powder for injection, lyophilized: 50 mg (6 mL)

Fludeoxyglucose F 18 (floo dee oxy' glu kose)

Brand Names [18]FDG

Use Identification of regions of abnormal glucose metabolism associated with foci of epileptic seizures, stroke, myocardial infarction, malignant tumors, and (brain, liver, thyroid) through the use of positron emission tomography; also used in cerebral imaging

Mechanism of Action Portion of the fludeoxyglucose molecule is labeled with F-18, a positron-emitting radionucleide which provides the signal for tumor identification in Positron Emission Tomography (PET) scanners

Pharmacodynamics/Kinetics Half-life: 110 minutes

Administration For I.V. use only

Additional Information Activity >37 x 10³ MBq (1 ci)/mmol

Fludrocortisone Acetate (floo droe kor' ti sone)

Brand Names Florinef® Acetate

Synonyms Fluohydrisone Acetate; Fluohydrocortisone Acetate; 9α-Fluorohydrocortisone Acetate

Use Partial replacement therapy for primary and secondary adrenocortical insufficiency in Addison's disease; treatment of salt-losing adrenogenital syndrome

Pregnancy Risk Factor C

Contraindications Known hypersensitivity to fludrocortisone; systemic fungal infections

Warnings/Precautions Taper dose gradually when therapy is discontinued; patients with Addison's disease are more sensitive to the action of the hormone and may exhibit side effects in an exaggerated degree

Adverse Reactions
1% to 10%:
Cardiovascular: Hypertension, edema, congestive heart failure
Central nervous system: Convulsions, headache, sweating, dizziness
Dermatologic: Acne, rash
Endocrine & metabolic: Hypokalemic alkalosis, suppression of growth, hyperglycemia, HPA suppression
Gastrointestinal: Peptic ulcer
Hematologic: Bruising
Neuromuscular & skeletal: Muscle weakness
Ocular: Cataracts

Overdosage/Toxicology Symptoms of overdose include hypokalemia, edema, hypertension; when consumed in excessive quantities, systemic hypercorticism and adrenal suppression may occur; in those cases, discontinuation and withdrawal of the corticosteroid should be done judiciously

Drug Interactions Decreased effect:
Anticholinesterases effects are antagonized
Decreased corticosteroid effects by rifampin, barbiturates, and hydantoins
Decreased salicylate levels

Mechanism of Action Promotes increased reabsorption of sodium and loss of potassium from renal distal tubules

Pharmacodynamics/Kinetics
Absorption: Rapid and complete from GI tract, partially absorbed through skin
Protein binding: 42%
Metabolism: In the liver
Half-life:
Plasma: 30-35 minutes
Biological: 18-36 hours
Time to peak serum concentration: Within 1.7 hours

Usual Dosage Oral:
Infants and Children: 0.05-0.1 mg/day
Adults: 0.1-0.2 mg/day with ranges of 0.1 mg 3 times/week to 0.2 mg/day

Administration Administration in conjunction with a glucocorticoid is preferable
(Continued)

465

Fludrocortisone Acetate (Continued)

Monitoring Parameters Monitor blood pressure and signs of edema when patient is on chronic therapy; very potent mineralocorticoid with high glucocorticoid activity; monitor serum electrolytes, serum renin activity, and blood pressure; monitor evidence of infection; closely monitor patients with Addison's disease and stop treatment if a significant increase in weight or blood pressure, edema or cardiac enlargement occurs

Patient Information Notify physician if dizziness, severe or continuing headaches, swelling of feet or lower legs or unusual weight gain occur

Dosage Forms Tablet: 0.1 mg

Flu-Imune® see Influenza Virus Vaccine on page 577

Flumadine® see Rimantadine Hydrochloride on page 984

Flumazenil (floo' may ze nil)

Brand Names Romazicon™

Use Benzodiazepine antagonist - reverses sedative effects of benzodiazepines used in general anesthesia; for management of benzodiazepine overdose; flumazenil does **not** antagonize the CNS effects of other GABA agonists (such as ethanol, barbiturates, or general anesthetics), **does not** reverse narcotics

Pregnancy Risk Factor C

Contraindications Known hypersensitivity to flumazenil or benzodiazepines; patients given benzodiazepines for control of potentially life-threatening conditions (eg, control of intracranial pressure or status epilepticus); patients who are showing signs of serious cyclic-antidepressant overdosage

Warnings/Precautions

Risk of seizures = high-risk patients:
Patients on benzodiazepines for long-term sedation
Tricyclic antidepressant overdose patients
Concurrent major sedative-hypnotic drug withdrawal
Recent therapy with repeated doses of parenteral benzodiazepines
Myoclonic jerking or seizure activity prior to flumazenil administration

Hypoventilation: Does not reverse respiratory depression/hypoventilation or cardiac depression

Resedation: Occurs more frequently in patients where a large single dose or cumulative dose of a benzodiazepine is administered along with a neuromuscular blocking agent and multiple anesthetic agents

Flumazenil should be used with caution in the intensive care unit because of increased risk of unrecognized benzodiazepine dependence in such settings.

Adverse Reactions

>10%:
Central nervous system: Dizziness
Gastrointestinal: Vomiting, nausea

1% to 10%:
Central nervous system: Headache, asthenia, malaise, anxiety, nervousness, dry mouth, insomnia, abnormal crying, euphoria, depression, vision, increased sweating disorders
Endocrine & metabolic: Hot flushes
Local: Pain at injection site
Neuromuscular & skeletal: Tremor
Respiratory: Dyspnea, hyperventilation

<1%:
Cardiovascular: Bradycardia, tachycardia, chest pain, hypertension, ventricular extrasystoles, altered blood pressure (increases and decreases)
Central nervous system: Anxiety and sensation of coldness, generalized convulsions, withdrawal syndrome, shivering, somnolence
Otic: Abnormal hearing
Miscellaneous: Thick tongue, hiccups

Drug Interactions Increased toxicity:
Use with caution in overdosage involving mixed drug overdose
Toxic effects may emerge (especially with cyclic antidepressants) with the reversal of the benzodiazepine effect by flumazenil

Stability For I.V. use only; **compatible** with D_5W, lactated Ringer's, or normal saline; once drawn up in the syringe or mixed with solution use within 24 hours; discard any unused solution after 24 hours

Mechanism of Action Antagonizes the effect of benzodiazepines on the GABA/benzodiazepine receptor complex. Flumazenil is benzodiazepine specific and does not antagonize other nonbenzodiazepine GABA agonists (including ethanol, barbiturates, general anesthetics); flumazenil does not reverse the effects of opiates

Pharmacodynamics/Kinetics

Onset of action: 1-3 minutes; 80% response within 3 minutes

Peak effect: 6-10 minutes

Duration: Resedation occurs usually within 1 hour; duration is related to dose given and benzodiazepine plasma concentrations; reversal effects of flumazenil may wear off before effects of benzodiazepine

Distribution: 0.63-1.06 L/kg

Initial V_d: 0.5 L/kg

V_{dss} 0.77-1.6 L/kg

Protein binding: 40% to 50%

Half-life, adults:

Alpha: 7-15 minutes

Terminal: 41-79 minutes

Elimination: Clearance dependent upon hepatic blood flow; hepatically eliminated, 0.2% unchanged in urine

Usual Dosage See table.

Flumazenil

Pediatric Dosage	
Pediatric dosage for **reversal of conscious sedation**: Intravenously through a freely running intravenous infusion into a large vein to minimize pain at the injection site	
Children Weighing <20 kg	
Initial dose	0.01 mg/kg over 15 seconds (maximum dose of 0.2 mg)
Repeat doses	0.005 mg/kg (maximum dose of 0.2 mg) repeated at 1-minute intervals
Maximum total cumulative dose	1 mg
Children Weighing 20-40 kg	
Initial dose	0.2 mg over 15 seconds
Repeat doses	0.005 mg/kg (maximum dose of 0.2 mg) repeated at 1-minute intervals
Maximum total cumulative dose	1 mg
Children weighing >40 kg: Use adult dosage recommendations.	
Adult Dosage	
Adult dosage for **reversal of conscious sedation**: Intravenously through a freely running intravenous infusion into a large vein to minimize pain at the injection site	
Initial dose	0.2 mg intravenously over 15 seconds
Repeat doses	If desired level of consciousness is not obtained, 0.2 mg may be repeated at 1-minute intervals
Maximum total cumulative dose	1 mg
Most patients respond to doses of 0.6-1 mg.	
Adult dosage for **suspected benzodiazepine overdose**: Intravenously through a freely running intravenous infusion into a large vein to minimize pain at the injection site	
Initial dose	0.2 mg intravenously over 30 seconds
Repeat doses	0.5 mg over 30 seconds repeated at 1-minute intervals
Maximum total cumulative dose	5 mg

Resedation: Repeated doses may be given at 20-minute intervals as needed; repeat treatment doses of 1 mg (at a rate of 0.5 mg/minute) should be given at any time and no more than 3 mg should be given in any hour. After intoxication with high doses of benzodiazepines, the duration of a single dose of flumazenil is not expected to exceed 1 hour; if desired, the period of wakefulness may be prolonged with repeated low intravenous doses of flumazenil, or by an infusion of 0.1-0.4 mg/hour. Most patients with benzodiazepine overdose will respond to a cumulative dose of 1-3 mg and doses >3 mg do not reliably produce additional effects. Rarely, patients with a partial response at 3 mg may require additional titration up to a total dose of 5 mg. **If a patient has not responded 5 minutes after receiving a cumulative dose of 5 mg, the major cause of sedation is not likely to be due to benzodiazepines.**

Dosing in renal impairment: Not significantly affected by renal failure (Cl_{cr} <10 mL/minute) or hemodialysis beginning 1 hour after drug administration

(Continued)

467

Flumazenil (Continued)

Dosing in hepatic impairment: Initial dose of flumazenil used for initial reversal of benzodiazepine effects is not changed; however, subsequent doses in liver disease patients should be reduced in size or frequency

Monitoring Parameters Monitor patients for return of sedation or respiratory depression

Patient Information Flumazenil does not consistently reverse amnesia; do not engage in activities requiring alertness for 18-24 hours after discharge; resedation may occur in patients on long-acting benzodiazepines (such as diazepam)

Dosage Forms Injection: 0.1 mg/mL (5 mL, 10 mL)

Flunisolide (floo niss' oh lide)

Related Information

Corticosteroids Comparisons *on page 1266-1268*

Brand Names AeroBid®; AeroBid-M®; Nasalide®

Use Steroid-dependent asthma; nasal solution is used for seasonal or perennial rhinitis

Pregnancy Risk Factor C

Contraindications Known hypersensitivity to flunisolide, acute status asthmaticus; viral, tuberculosis, fungal or bacterial respiratory infections, or infections of nasal mucosa

Warnings/Precautions Use with caution in patients with hypothyroidism, cirrhosis, hypertension, congestive heart failure, ulcerative colitis, thromboembolic disorders; do not stop medication abruptly if on prolonged therapy; fatalities have occurred due to adrenal insufficiency in asthmatic patients during and after transfer from systemic corticosteroids to aerosol steroids; several months may be required for recovery of this syndrome; during this period, aerosol steroids do **not** provide the systemic steroid needed to treat patients having trauma, surgery or infections. When consumed in excessive quantities, systemic hypercorticism and adrenal suppression may occur; withdrawal and discontinuation of the corticosteroid should be done carefully.

Adverse Reactions

>10%:

Cardiovascular: Pounding heartbeat

Central nervous system: Dizziness, headache, nervousness

Dermatologic: Itching, skin rash

Endocrine & metabolic: Adrenal suppression, menstrual problems

Gastrointestinal: GI irritation, anorexia

Local: Nasal burning, nasal congestion, nasal dryness, sore throat, bitter taste, *Candida* infections of the nose or pharynx, atrophic rhinitis

Respiratory: Sneezing, coughing, upper respiratory tract infection, bronchitis

Miscellaneous: Increased susceptibility to infections

1% to 10%:

Central nervous system: Insomnia, psychic changes

Dermatologic: Acne, hives

Gastrointestinal: Increase in appetite

Ocular: Cataracts

Miscellaneous: Epistaxis, diaphoresis, dry mouth/throat, loss of smell/taste

<1%:

Gastrointestinal: Abdominal fullness

Respiratory: Bronchospasm, shortness of breath

Overdosage/Toxicology When consumed in excessive quantities, systemic hypercorticism and adrenal suppression may occur; in those cases; discontinuation and withdrawal of the corticosteroid should be done judiciously

Drug Interactions Expected interactions similar to other corticosteroids

Mechanism of Action Decreases inflammation by suppression of migration of polymorphonuclear leukocytes and reversal of increased capillary permeability; does not depress hypothalamus

Pharmacodynamics/Kinetics

Absorption: Nasal inhalation: ~50%

Metabolism: Rapidly in the liver to active metabolites

Half-life: 1.8 hours

Elimination: Equally in urine and feces

Usual Dosage

Children >6 years:

Oral inhalation: 2 inhalations twice daily (morning and evening) up to 4 inhalations/day

Nasal: 1 spray each nostril twice daily (morning and evening), not to exceed 4 sprays/day each nostril

Adults:

Oral inhalation: 2 inhalations twice daily (morning and evening) up to 8 inhalations/day maximum

Nasal: 2 sprays each nostril twice daily (morning and evening); maximum dose: 8 sprays/day in each nostril

Patient Information Inhaler should be shaken well immediately prior to use; while activating inhaler, deep breathe for 3-5 seconds, hold breath for ~10 seconds and allow ≥1 minute between inhalations

Nursing Implications Shake well before giving; do not use Nasalide® orally; throw out product after it has been opened for 3 months

Additional Information Does not contain fluorocarbons; contains polyethylene glycol vehicle

Dosage Forms Inhalant:

Nasal (Nasalide®): 25 mcg/actuation [200 sprays] (25 mL)

Oral:

AeroBid®: 250 mcg/actuation [100 metered doses] (7 g)

AeroBid-M® (menthol flavor): 250 mcg/actuation [100 metered doses] (7 g)

Fluocinolone Acetonide (floo oh sin' oh lone)

Related Information

Corticosteroids Comparisons *on page 1266-1268*

Brand Names Derma-Smoothe/FS®; Fluonid®; Flurosyn®; FS Shampoo®; Synalar®; Synalar-HP®; Synemol®

Use Relief of susceptible inflammatory dermatosis [low, medium, high potency topical corticosteroid]

Pregnancy Risk Factor C

Contraindications Fungal infection, hypersensitivity to fluocinolone or any component, TB of skin, herpes (including varicella)

Warnings/Precautions Adverse systemic effects may occur when used on large areas of the body, denuded areas, for prolonged periods of time, with an occlusive dressing, and/or in infants or small children. Infants and small children may be more susceptible to adrenal axis suppression from topical corticosteroid therapy.

Adverse Reactions

<1%:

Dermatologic: Acne, hypopigmentation, allergic dermatitis, maceration of the skin, skin atrophy, folliculitis, hypertrichosis

Endocrine & metabolic: HPA suppression, Cushing's syndrome, growth retardation

Local: Burning, itching, irritation, dryness

Miscellaneous: Secondary infection

Overdosage/Toxicology When consumed in excessive quantities, systemic hypercorticism and adrenal suppression may occur; in those cases, discontinuation and withdrawal of the corticosteroid should be done judiciously

Mechanism of Action A synthetic corticosteroid which differs structurally from triamcinolone acetonide in the presence of an additional fluorine atom in the 6-alpha position on the steroid nucleus. The mechanism of action for all topical corticosteroids is not well defined, however, is believed to be a combination of three important properties: anti-inflammatory activity, immunosuppressive properties, and antiproliferative actions.

Pharmacodynamics/Kinetics

Absorption: Dependent on strength of preparation, amount applied, and nature of skin at application site; ranges from ~1% in thick stratum corneum areas (palms, soles, elbows, etc) to 36% in areas of thinnest stratum corneum (face, eyelids, etc); increased absorption in areas of skin damage, inflammation, or occlusion

Distribution: Throughout the local skin; absorbed drug is distributed rapidly into muscle, liver, skin, intestines, and kidneys

Metabolism: Primarily in the skin; small amount absorbed into systemic circulation is metabolized primarily in the liver to inactive compounds

Elimination: By the kidneys primarily as glucuronides and sulfate, but also as unconjugated products; small amounts of metabolites are excreted in feces

Usual Dosage Children and Adults: Topical: Apply a thin layer to affected area 2-4 times/day

Patient Information A thin film of cream or ointment is effective; do not overuse; do not use tight-fitting diapers or plastic pants on children being treated in the diaper area; use only as prescribed, and for no longer than the period prescribed; apply sparingly in light film; rub in lightly; avoid contact with eyes; notify physician if condition being treated persists or worsens

Dosage Forms

Cream:

Flurosyn®, Synalar®: 0.01% (15 g, 30 g, 60 g, 425 g)

(Continued)

Fluocinolone Acetonide *(Continued)*

Flurosyn®, Synalar®, Synemol®: 0.025% (15 g, 30 g, 60 g, 425 g)
Synalar-HP®: 0.2% (12 g)
Ointment, topical (Flurosyn®, Synalar®): 0.025% (15 g, 30 g, 60 g, 425 g)
Oil (Derma-Smoothe/FS®): 0.01% (120 mL)
Shampoo (FS Shampoo®): 0.01% (180 mL)
Solution, topical (Fluonid®, Synalar®): 0.01% (20 mL, 60 mL)

Fluocinonide (floo oh sin' oh nide)
Related Information
Corticosteroids Comparisons *on page 1266-1268*
Brand Names Fluonex®; Lidex®; Lidex-E®
Use Anti-inflammatory, antipruritic, relief of inflammatory and pruritic manifestations [high potency topical corticosteroid]
Pregnancy Risk Factor C
Contraindications Viral, fungal, or tubercular skin lesions, herpes simplex, known hypersensitivity to fluocinonide
Warnings/Precautions Adverse systemic effects may occur when used on large areas of the body, denuded areas, for prolonged periods of time, with an occlusive dressing, and/or in infants or small children
Adverse Reactions <1%:
Central nervous system: Intracranial hypertension
Dermatologic: Acne, hypopigmentation, allergic dermatitis, maceration of the skin, skin atrophy
Endocrine & metabolic: HPA suppression, Cushing's syndrome, growth retardation
Local: Burning, itching, irritation, dryness, folliculitis, hypertrichosis
Miscellaneous: Secondary infection
Mechanism of Action Not well defined for all topical corticosteroids; however, is felt to be a combination of three important properties: anti-inflammatory activity, immunosuppressive properties, and antiproliferative actions.
Pharmacodynamics/Kinetics
Absorption: Dependent on amount applied and nature of skin at application site; ranges from ~1% in areas of thick stratum corneum (palms, soles, elbows, etc) to 36% in areas of thin stratum corneum (face, eyelids, etc); absorption is increased in areas of skin damage, inflammation, or occlusion
Distribution: Distributed throughout local skin; any absorbed drug is removed rapidly from the blood and distributed into muscle, liver, skin, intestines, and kidneys
Metabolism: Primarily in the skin; small amount absorbed into systemic circulation is metabolized primarily in the liver to inactive compounds
Elimination: By the kidneys primarily as glucuronides and sulfates, but also as unconjugated products; small amounts of metabolites are excreted in feces
Usual Dosage Children and Adults: Topical: Apply thin layer to affected area 2-4 times/day depending on the severity of the condition
Patient Information Do not use tight-fitting diapers or plastic pants on children being treated in the diaper area; use only as prescribed, and for no longer than the period prescribed; apply sparingly in a light film; rub in lightly; notify physician if condition being treated persists or worsens; avoid contact with eyes
Dosage Forms
Cream:
Anhydrous, emollient (Fluonex®, Lidex®): 0.05% (15 g, 30 g, 60 g, 120 g)
Aqueous, emollient (Lidex-E®): 0.05% (15 g, 30 g, 60 g, 120 g)
Gel, topical (Lidex®): 0.05% (15 g, 30 g, 60 g, 120 g)
Ointment, topical (Lidex®): 0.05% (15 g, 30 g, 60 g, 120 g)
Solution, topical (Lidex®): 0.05% (20 mL, 60 mL)

Fluogen® *see* Influenza Virus Vaccine *on page 577*

Fluohydrisone Acetate *see* Fludrocortisone Acetate *on page 465*

Fluohydrocortisone Acetate *see* Fludrocortisone Acetate *on page 465*

Fluonex® *see* Fluocinonide *on this page*

Fluonid® *see* Fluocinolone Acetonide *on previous page*

Fluoracaine® *see* Proparacaine and Fluorescein *on page 942*

Fluorescein Sodium (flure' e seen)
Brand Names AK-Fluor; Fluorescite®; Fluorets®; Fluor-I-Strip®; Fluor-I-Strip-AT®; Fluress®; Ful-Glo®; Funduscein®; Ophthifluor®

Synonyms Soluble Fluorescein

Use Demonstrates defects of corneal epithelium; diagnostic aid in ophthalmic angiography

Pregnancy Risk Factor C (topical); X (parenteral)

Contraindications Hypersensitivity to fluorescein or any other component of the product; do not use with soft contact lenses, as this will cause them to discolor

Warnings/Precautions Use with caution in patients with history of hypersensitivity, allergies, or asthma; avoid extravasation; should not be used in patients with soft contact lenses, will cause them to discolor

Adverse Reactions

1% to 10%: Topical: Temporary stinging, burning sensation

<1%:

Cardiovascular: Syncope, hypotension, cardiac arrest, basilar artery ischemia, severe shock

Central nervous system: Headache

Gastrointestinal: Nausea, GI distress, vomiting

Local: Thrombophlebitis

Mechanism of Action Yellow, water soluble, dibasic acid xanthine dye which penetrates any break in epithelial barrier to permit rapid penetration

Usual Dosage

Ophthalmic:

Solution: Instill 1-2 drops of 2% solution and allow a few seconds for staining; wash out excess with sterile water or irrigating solution

Strips: Moisten strip with sterile water. Place moistened strip at the fornix into the lower cul-de-sac close to the punctum. For best results, patient should close lid tightly over strip until desired amount of staining is obtained. Patient should blink several times after application.

Removal of foreign bodies, sutures or tonometry (Fluress®): Instill 1 or 2 drops (single installations) into each eye before operating

Deep ophthalmic anesthesia (Fluress®): Instill 2 drops into each eye very 90 seconds up to 3 doses

Injection: Prior to use, perform intradermal skin test; have epinephrine 1:1000, an antihistamine, and oxygen available

Children: 3.5 mg/lb (7.5 mg/kg) injected rapidly into antecubital vein

Adults: 500-750 mg injected rapidly into antecubital vein

Patient Information Do not replace soft contact lenses for at least 1 hour, flush eye before replacing; skin discoloration may last 6-12 hours, urine 24-36 hours if given systemically

Nursing Implications Avoid extravasation, results in severe local tissue damage; have epinephrine 1:1000, an antihistamine, and oxygen available

Dosage Forms

Injection (AK-Fluor, Fluorescite®, Funduscein®, Ophthifluor®): 10% [100 mg/mL] (5 mL); 25% [250 mg/mL] (2 mL, 3 mL)

Ophthalmic:

Solution: 2% [20 mg/mL] (1 mL, 2 mL, 15 mL)

Fluress®: 0.25% [2.5 mg/mL] with benoxinate 0.4% (5 mL)

Strip:

Ful-Glo®: 0.6 mg

Fluorets®, Fluor-I-Strip-AT®: 1 mg

Fluor-I-Strip®: 9 mg

Fluorescite® see Fluorescein Sodium on previous page

Fluorets® see Fluorescein Sodium on previous page

Fluoride (flur´ ide)

Brand Names ACT® [OTC]; Fluorigard® [OTC]; Fluorinse®; Fluoritab®; Flura®; Flura-Drops®; Flura-Loz®; Gel Kam®; Gel-Tin® [OTC]; Karidium®; Karigel®; Karigel®-N; Listermint® with Fluoride [OTC]; Luride®; Luride® Lozi-Tab®; Luride®-SF Lozi-Tab®; Minute-Gel®; Pediaflor®; Pharmaflur®; Phos-Flur®; Point-Two®; PreviDent®; Stop® [OTC]; Thera-Flur®; Thera-Flur-N®

Synonyms Acidulated Phosphate Fluoride; Sodium Fluoride; Stannous Fluoride

Use Prevention of dental caries

Pregnancy Risk Factor C

Contraindications Hypersensitivity to fluoride or any component, or when fluoride content of drinking water exceeds 0.7 ppm

Warnings/Precautions Prolonged ingestion with excessive doses may result in dental fluorosis and osseous changes; do **not** exceed recommended dosage; some products contain tartrazine

Adverse Reactions

<1%:

Dermatologic: Rash

(Continued)

Fluoride *(Continued)*

Gastrointestinal: GI upset, nausea, vomiting

Miscellaneous: Products containing stannous fluoride may stain the teeth

Overdosage/Toxicology Symptoms of overdose include hypersalivation, salty or soapy taste, epigastric pain, nausea, vomiting, diarrhea, rash muscle weakness, tremor, seizures, cardiac failure, respiratory arrest, shock, death

Fatal dose not known. Children: 500 mg; Adults: 7-140 mg/kg

Treatment of overdose: Gastric lavage with $CaCl_2$ or $Ca(OH)_2$ solution; give large quantity of milk at frequent intervals; $Al(OH)_3$ may also bind the fluoride ion

Drug Interactions Decreased effect/absorption with magnesium-, aluminum-, and calcium-containing products

Stability Store in tight plastic containers (not glass)

Mechanism of Action Promotes remineralization of decalcified enamel; inhibits the cariogenic microbial process in dental plaque; increases tooth resistance to acid dissolution

Pharmacodynamics/Kinetics

Absorption: Absorbed in GI tract, lungs, and skin; calcium, iron, or magnesium may delay absorption

Distribution: 50% of fluoride is deposited in teeth and bone after ingestion; topical application works superficially on enamel and plaque; crosses placenta; appears in breast milk

Elimination: In urine and feces

Usual Dosage Oral:

Recommended daily fluoride supplement (2.2 mg of sodium fluoride is equivalent to 1 mg of fluoride ion): See table.

Fluoride Ion

Fluoride Content of Drinking Water	Daily Dose, Oral (mg)
<0.3 ppm	
Birth - 2 y	0.25
2-3 y	0.5
3-12 y	1
0.3-0.7 ppm	
Birth - 2 y	0
2-3 y	0.25
3-12 y	0.5

Dental rinse or gel:

Children 6-12 years: 5-10 mL rinse or apply to teeth and spit daily after brushing

Adults: 10 mL rinse or apply to teeth and spit daily after brushing

Patient Information Take with food (but not milk) to eliminate GI upset; with dental rinse or dental gel do **not** swallow, do **not** eat or drink for 30 minutes after use

Nursing Implications Avoid giving with milk or dairy products

Dosage Forms Fluoride ion content listed in brackets

Drops, oral, as sodium:

Fluoritab®, Flura-Drops®: 0.55 mg/drop [0.25 mg/drop] (22.8 mL, 24 mL)

Karidium®, Luride®: 0.275 mg/drop [0.125 mg/drop] (30 mL, 60 mL)

Pediaflor®: 1.1 mg/mL [0.5 mg/mL] (50 mL)

Gel, topical:

Acidulated phosphate fluoride (Minute-Gel): 1.23% (480 mL)

Sodium fluoride (Karigel®, Karigel®-N, PreviDent®): 1.1% [0.5%] (24 g, 30 g, 60 g, 120 g, 130 g, 250 g)

Stannous fluoride (Gel Kam®, Gel-Tin®, Stop®): 0.4% [0.1%] (60 g, 65 g, 105 g, 120 g)

Lozenge, as sodium (Flura-Loz®) (raspberry flavor): 2.2 mg [1 mg]

Rinse, topical, as sodium:

ACT®, Fluorigard®: 0.05% [0.02%] (90 mL, 180 mL, 300 mL, 360 mL, 480 mL)

Fluorinse®, Point-Two®: 0.2% [0.09%] (240 mL, 480 mL, 3780 mL)

Listermint® with Fluoride: 0.02% [0.01%] (180 mL, 300 mL, 360 mL, 480 mL, 540 mL, 720 mL, 960 mL, 1740 mL)

Solution, oral, as sodium (Phos-Flur®): 0.44 mg/mL [0.2 mg/mL] (250 mL, 500 mL, 3780 mL)

Tablet, as sodium:

Chewable:

Fluoritab®, Luride Lozi-Tab®, Pharmaflur®: 1.1 mg [0.5 mg]

Fluoritab®, Karidium®, Luride® Lozi-Tab® Luride®-SF Lozi-Tab®, Pharmaflur®: 2.2 mg [1 mg]
  Oral: Flura®, Karidium®: 2.2 mg [1 mg]

Fluorigard® [OTC] *see Fluoride on page 471*

Fluorinse® *see Fluoride on page 471*

Fluor-I-Strip® *see Fluorescein Sodium on page 470*

Fluor-I-Strip-AT® *see Fluorescein Sodium on page 470*

Fluoritab® *see Fluoride on page 471*

Fluorodeoxyuridine *see Floxuridine on page 460*

9α-Fluorohydrocortisone Acetate *see Fludrocortisone Acetate on page 465*

Fluorometholone (flure oh meth' oh lone)
Related Information
  Corticosteroids Comparisons *on page 1266-1268*
Brand Names Flarex®; Fluor-Op®; FML®; FML® Forte
Use Inflammatory conditions of the eye, including keratitis, iritis, cyclitis, and conjunctivitis
Pregnancy Risk Factor C
Contraindications Herpes simplex, keratitis, fungal diseases of ocular structures, most viral diseases, hypersensitivity to any component
Warnings/Precautions Not recommended in children <2 years of age, prolonged use may result in glaucoma, elevated intraocular pressure, or other ocular damage; some products contain sulfites
Adverse Reactions
  1% to 10%: Ophthalmic: Blurred vision
  <1%: Ophthalmic: Stinging, burning, increased intraocular pressure, open-angle glaucoma, defect in visual acuity and field of vision, cataracts
Overdosage/Toxicology When consumed in excessive quantities, systemic hypercorticism and adrenal suppression may occur; in those cases, discontinuation and withdrawal of the corticosteroid should be done judiciously
Mechanism of Action Decreases inflammation by suppression of migration of polymorphonuclear leukocytes and reversal of increased capillary permeability
Pharmacodynamics/Kinetics Absorption: Into aqueous humor with slight systemic absorption
Usual Dosage Children >2 years and Adults: Ophthalmic:
  Ointment: May be applied every 4 hours in severe cases; 1-3 times/day in mild to moderate cases
  Solution: Instill 1-2 drops into conjunctival sac every hour during day, every 2 hours at night until favorable response is obtained, then use 1 drop every 4 hours; for mild to moderate inflammation, instill 1-2 drops into conjunctival sac 2-4 times/day
Patient Information Do not discontinue use without consulting a physician; photosensitivity may occur; notify physician if improvement does not occur after 7-8 days
Nursing Implications Use a separate individual container for each patient
Dosage Forms Ophthalmic:
  Ointment (FML®): 0.1% (3.5 g)
  Suspension:
    Flarex®, Fluor-Op®, FML®: 0.1% (2.5 mL, 5 mL, 10 mL)
    FML® Forte: 0.25% (2 mL, 5 mL, 10 mL, 15 mL)

Fluor-Op® *see Fluorometholone on this page*

Fluoroplex® *see Fluorouracil on this page*

Fluorouracil (flure oh yoor' a sill)
Related Information
  Cancer Chemotherapy Regimens *on page 1218-1241*
Brand Names Adrucil®; Efudex®; Fluoroplex®
Synonyms 5-Fluorouracil; 5-FU
Use Treatment of carcinoma of stomach, colon, rectum, breast, and pancreas; also used topically for management of multiple actinic keratoses and superficial basal cell carcinomas
Pregnancy Risk Factor D (injection); X (topical)
Contraindications Hypersensitivity to fluorouracil or any component; patients with poor nutritional status, bone marrow depression
(Continued)

Fluorouracil (Continued)

Warnings/Precautions The U.S. Food and Drug Administration (FDA) currently recommends that procedures for proper handling and disposal of antineoplastic agents be considered. Use with caution in patients who have had high-dose pelvic radiation or previous use of alkylating agents. Patient should be hospitalized during initial course of therapy. Use with caution in patients with impaired kidney or liver function. The drug should be discontinued if intractable vomiting or diarrhea, precipitous fall in leukocyte or platelet counts or myocardial ischemia occurs.

Adverse Reactions Toxicity depends on route and duration of infusion

Irritant chemotherapy

>10%:

Dermatologic: Dermatitis, alopecia

Gastrointestinal (route and schedule dependent): Heartburn, stomatitis, nausea, vomiting, stomatitis, esophagitis, anorexia, and diarrhea; bolus dosing produces milder GI problems, while continuous infusion tends to produce severe mucositis and diarrhea; emesis is moderate, occurring in 30% to 60% of patients, and responds well to phenothiazines and dexamethasone

Emetic potential:

<1000 mg: Moderately low (10% to 30%)

≥1000 mg: Moderate (30% to 60%)

1% to 10%:

Dermatologic: Dry skin

Gastrointestinal: GI ulceration

Myelosuppressive: Granulocytopenia occurs around 9-14 days after 5-FU and thrombocytopenia around 7-17 days. The marrow recovers after 22 days. Myelosuppression tends to be more pronounced in patients receiving bolus dosing of 5-FU.

WBC: Mild to moderate

Platelets: Mild

Onset (days): 7-10

Nadir (days): 14

Recovery (days): 21

<1%:

Cardiovascular: Chest pain, shortness of breath, EKG changes similar to ischemic changes, and possibly cardiac enzyme abnormalities. Usually occurs within the first 2 days of therapy, and may resolve with nitroglycerin and calcium channel blockers. May be due to coronary vessel vasospasm induced by 5-FU.

Central nervous system: Headache, cerebellar ataxia, tingling of hands; somnolence, ataxia are seen primarily in intracarotid arterial infusions for head and neck tumors; this is believed to be caused by fluorocitrate, a neurotoxic metabolite of the parent compound

Dermatologic: Alopecia, hyperpigmentation of nailbeds, face, hands, and veins used in infusion; photosensitization with UV light; palmar-plantar syndrome; hand-foot syndrome, pruritic maculopapular rash

Hematologic: Coagulopathy

Hepatic: Hepatotoxicity

Ocular: Conjunctivitis, tear duct stenosis, excessive lacrimation, visual disturbances

Overdosage/Toxicology Symptoms of overdose include myelosuppression, nausea, vomiting, diarrhea, alopecia; no specific antidote exists; monitor hematologically for at least 4 weeks; supportive therapy

Drug Interactions Methotrexate: This interaction is schedule dependent; **5-FU should be given following MTX, not prior to**

If MTX is given first: The cells exposed to MTX before 5-FU have a depleted reduced folate pool which inhibits the binding of the 5dUMP to TS. However, it does not interfere with FUTP incorporation into RNA. Polyglutamines, which accumulate in the presence of MTX may be substituted for the folates and allow binding of FdUMP to TS. MTX given prior to 5-FU may actually activate 5-FU due to MTX inhibition of purine synthesis.

If 5-FU is given first: 5-FU inhibits the TS binding and thus the reduced folate pool is not depleted, thereby negating the effect of MTX

Increased effect: Leucovorin: Increases the folate pool and in certain tumors, may promote TS inhibition and increase 5-FU activity. Must be given before or with the 5-FU to prime the cells; it is not used as a rescue agent in this case.

Increased toxicity:

Allopurinol: Inhibits thymidine phosphorylase (an enzyme that activates 5-FU). The antitumor effect of 5-FU appears to be unaltered, but the toxicity is decreased.

Cimetidine: Results in increased plasma levels of 5-FU due to drug metabolism inhibition and reduction of liver blood flow induced by cimetidine

Stability Protect from light; slight discoloration of injection occurring during storage does not adversely affect potency or safety; but discard dark yellow solution; if precipitate forms, redissolve drug by heating to 140°F (60°C), shake well; allow to cool to body temperature before administration

Incompatible with cytarabine, diazepam, doxorubicin, methotrexate; **concentrations >25 mg/mL of fluorouracil and >2 mg/mL of leucovorin are incompatible (precipitation occurs)**

Compatible with vincristine, methotrexate, potassium chloride, magnesium sulfate

Mechanism of Action A pyrimidine antimetabolite that interferes with DNA synthesis by blocking the methylation of deoxyuricytic acid; 5-FU rapidly enters the cell and is activated to the nucleotide level; there it inhibits thymidylate synthetase (TS), or is incorporated into RNA (most evident during the GI phase of the cell cycle). The reduced folate cofactor is required for tight binding to occur between the 5-FdUMP and TS.

Pharmacodynamics/Kinetics

Absorption: Oral: Erratic and rarely used

Distribution: V_d: ~22% of total body water; penetrates the extracellular fluid, CSF, and third space fluids (such as pleural effusions and ascitic fluid)

Metabolism: 5-FU must be metabolized to be active. 90% metabolized; accomplished by a dehydrogenase enzyme primarily found in the liver; dose may need to be omitted in patients with liver failure (bilirubin >5 mg/dL)

Bioavailability: <75%, erratic and undependable

Half-life (biphasic): Initial: 6-20 minutes; doses of 400-600 mg/m^2 produce drug concentrations above the threshold for cytotoxicity for normal tissue and remain there for 6 hours; 2 metabolites, FdUMP and FUTP, have prolonged half-lives depending on the type of tissue; the clinical effect of these metabolites has not been determined

Elimination: 5% of dose excreted as unchanged drug in the urine in 6 hours, and a large amount excreted as CO_2 from the lung

Usual Dosage

Children and Adults (refer to individual protocols):

I.V.: Initial: 12 mg/kg/day (maximum: 800 mg/day) for 4-5 days; maintenance: 6 mg/kg every other day for 4 doses

Single weekly bolus dose of 15 mg/kg can be administered depending on the patient's reaction to the previous course of treatment; maintenance dose of 5-15 mg/kg/week as a single dose not to exceed 1 g/week

I.V. infusion: 15 mg/kg/day (maximum daily dose: 1 g) has been given by I.V. infusion over 4 hours for 5 days repeated every 4-6 weeks

Alternatively:

I.V. infusion: 1000 mg/m^2 over 24 hours for 4-5 days, **or**

I.V. infusion: 3000 mg/m^2 over 24 hours once each week

Oral: 20 mg/kg/day for 5 days every 5 weeks for colorectal cancer

Administer dose posthemodialysis

Dosing adjustment/comments in hepatic impairment:

Bilirubin >5 mg/dL: Omit use

5-FU may also be administered intra-arterially or intrahepatically (refer to specific protocols).

Topical:

Actinic or solar keratosis: Apply twice daily for 2-6 weeks

Superficial basal cell carcinomas: Apply 5% twice daily for at least 3-6 weeks and up to 10-12 weeks

Administration Direct I.V. push injection (50 mg/mL solution needs no further dilution) or by I.V. infusion; toxicity may be reduced by giving the drug as a constant infusion. Bolus doses may be administered by slow IVP or IVPB; continuous infusions may be administered in D_5W or NS. Solution should be protected from direct sunlight; 5-FU may also be administered intra-arterially or intrahepatically (refer to specific protocols).

Monitoring Parameters CBC with differential and platelet count, renal function tests, liver function tests

Test Interactions Fecal discoloration

Patient Information Avoid unnecessary exposure to sunlight; any signs of infection, easy bruising or bleeding, shortness of breath, or painful or burning urination should be brought to physician's attention. Nausea, vomiting, or hair loss sometimes occur. The drug may cause permanent sterility and may cause birth (Continued)

Fluorouracil *(Continued)*

defects. The drug may be excreted in breast milk, therefore, an alternative form of feeding your baby should be used.

Nursing Implications Cool to body temperature before using; after vial has been entered, any unused portion should be discarded within 1 hour; wash hands immediately after topical application of the 5% cream; I.V. formulation may be given orally mixed in water, grape juice, or carbonated beverage

Dosage Forms
Cream, topical:
Efudex®: 5% (25 g)
Fluoroplex®: 1% (30 g)
Injection (Adrucil®): 50 mg/mL (10 mL, 20 mL, 50 mL, 100 mL)
Solution, topical:
Efudex®: 2% (10 mL); 5% (10 mL)
Fluoroplex®: 1% (30 mL)

5-Fluorouracil *see* Fluorouracil *on page 473*

Fluostigmin *see* Isoflurophate *on page 594*

Fluoxetine Hydrochloride *(floo ox′ e teen)*

Related Information
Antidepressant Agents Comparison *on page 1250-1252*
Brand Names Prozac®
Use Treatment of major depression
Pregnancy Risk Factor B
Contraindications Hypersensitivity to fluoxetine; patients receiving MAO inhibitors currently or in past 2 weeks
Warnings/Precautions Use with caution in patients with hepatic impairment, history of seizures; MAO inhibitors should be discontinued at least 14 days before initiating fluoxetine therapy; add or initiate other antidepressants with caution for up to 5 weeks after stopping fluoxetine
Adverse Reactions Predominant adverse effects are CNS and GI
>10%:
Central nervous system: Headache, nervousness, insomnia, drowsiness
Gastrointestinal: Nausea, diarrhea, dry mouth
1% to 10%:
Central nervous system: Anxiety, dizziness, fatigue, sedation
Dermatologic: Rash, pruritus
Endocrine & metabolic: SIADH, hypoglycemia, hyponatremia (elderly or volume-depleted patients)
Gastrointestinal: Anorexia, dyspepsia, constipation
Neuromuscular & skeletal: Tremor
Miscellaneous: Excessive sweating
<1%: Central nervous system: Extrapyramidal reactions (rare)
Miscellaneous: Anaphylactoid reactions, allergies, visual disturbances, suicidal ideation
Overdosage/Toxicology Symptoms of overdose include ataxia, sedation, and coma; respiratory depression may occur, especially with coingestion of alcohol or other drugs; seizures very rarely occur
Drug Interactions
Increased effect with tricyclics (2 times ↑ plasma level)
Increased/decreased effect of lithium (both ↑ and ↓ level has been reported)
Increased toxicity of diazepam, trazodone via ↓ clearance; increased toxicity with MAO inhibitors (hyperpyrexia, tremors, seizures, delirium, coma)
Displace protein bound drugs
Mechanism of Action Inhibits CNS neuron serotonin uptake; minimal or no effect on reuptake of norepinephrine or dopamine; does not significantly bind to alpha-adrenergic, histamine or cholinergic receptors; may therefore be useful in patients at risk from sedation, hypotension, and anticholinergic effects of tricyclic antidepressants
Pharmacodynamics/Kinetics
Peak antidepressant effect: After >4 weeks
Absorption: Oral: Well absorbed
Metabolism: To norfluoxetine (active)
Half-life: Adults: 2-3 days; due to long half-life, resolution of adverse reactions after discontinuation may be slow
Time to peak serum concentration: Within 4-8 hours
Elimination: In urine as fluoxetine (2.5% to 5%) and norfluoxetine (10%)
Usual Dosage Oral:
Children <18 years: Dose and safety not established; preliminary experience in children 6-14 years using initial doses of 20 mg/day have been reported

Adults: 20 mg/day in the morning; may increase after several weeks by 20 mg/day increments; maximum: 80 mg/day; doses >20 mg should be divided into morning and noon doses

Usual dosage range:
20-80 mg/day for depression and OCD
20-60 mg/day for obesity
60-80 mg/day for bulimia nervosa
Note: Lower doses of 5 mg/day have been used for initial treatment

Elderly: Some patients may require an initial dose of 10 mg/day with dosage increases of 10 and 20 mg every several weeks as tolerated; should not be taken at night unless patient experiences sedation

Dosing adjustment in renal impairment:
Single dose studies: the pharmacokinetics of fluoxetine and norfluoxetine were similar among subjects with all levels of impaired renal function, including anephric patients on chronic hemodialysis
Chronic administration: Additional accumulation of fluoxetine or norfluoxetine may occur in patients with severely impaired renal function
Not removed by hemodialysis

Dosing adjustment in hepatic impairment: Elimination half-life of fluoxetine is prolonged in patients with hepatic impairment; a lower or less frequent dose of fluoxetine should be used in these patients
Cirrhosis patients: Administer a lower dose or less frequent dosing interval
Compensated cirrhosis without ascites: Administer 50% of normal dose

Reference Range Therapeutic levels have not been well established
Therapeutic: Fluoxetine: 100-800 ng/mL (SI: 289-2314 nmol/L); Norfluoxetine: 100-600 ng/mL (SI: 289-1735 nmol/L)
Toxic: Fluoxetine plus norfluoxetine: >2000 ng/mL

Test Interactions ↑ albumin in urine

Patient Information Avoid alcoholic beverages, take in morning to avoid insomnia; fluoxetine's potential stimulating and anorexic effects may be bothersome to some patients. Use sugarless hard candy for dry mouth; avoid alcoholic beverages, may cause drowsiness, improvement may take several weeks; rise slowly to prevent dizziness.

Nursing Implications Offer patient sugarless hard candy for dry mouth

Dosage Forms
Capsule: 10 mg, 20 mg
Liquid (mint flavor): 20 mg/5 mL (120 mL)

Extemporaneous Preparations A 20 mg capsule may be mixed with 4 oz of water, apple juice, or Gatorade® to provide a solution that is stable for 14 days under refrigeration

Fluoxymesterone (floo ox i mes' te rone)

Related Information
Cancer Chemotherapy Regimens *on page 1218-1241*

Brand Names Halotestin®

Use Replacement of endogenous testicular hormone; in female used as palliative treatment of breast cancer, postpartum breast engorgement

Restrictions C-III

Pregnancy Risk Factor X

Contraindications Serious cardiac disease, liver or kidney disease, hypersensitivity to fluoxymesterone or any component

Warnings/Precautions May accelerate bone maturation without producing compensatory gain in linear growth in children; in prepubertal children perform radiographic examination of the hand and wrist every 6 months to determine the rate of bone maturation and to assess the effect of treatment on the epiphyseal centers

Adverse Reactions
>10%:
Males: Priapism
Females: Menstrual problems (amenorrhea), virilism, breast soreness
Dermatologic: Edema, acne
1% to 10%:
Males: Prostatic carcinoma, hirsutism (increase in pubic hair growth), impotence, testicular atrophy
Dermatologic: Edema
Gastrointestinal: GI irritation, nausea, vomiting, prostatic hypertrophy
Hepatic: Hepatic dysfunction
<1%:
Males: Gynecomastia
Females: Amenorrhea
(Continued)

Fluoxymesterone *(Continued)*

    Endocrine & metabolic: Hypercalcemia
    Hematologic: Leukopenia, polycythemia
    Hepatic: Hepatic necrosis, cholestatic hepatitis
    Miscellaneous: Hypersensitivity reactions

Overdosage/Toxicology Abnormal liver function tests, water retention

Drug Interactions
  Decreased blood glucose concentrations and insulin requirements in patients with diabetes
  Increased effect of oral anticoagulants

Stability Protect from light

Mechanism of Action Synthetic androgenic anabolic hormone responsible for the normal growth and development of male sex organs and maintenance of secondary sex characteristics; stimulates RNA polymerase activity resulting in an increase in protein production; increases bone development

Pharmacodynamics/Kinetics
  Absorption: Oral: Rapid
  Protein binding: 98%
  Metabolism: In the liver
  Half-life: 10-100 minutes
  Elimination: Enterohepatic circulation and urinary excretion (90%)

  Halogenated derivative of testosterone with up to 5 times the activity of methyltestosterone

Usual Dosage Adults: Oral:
  Male:
    Hypogonadism: 5-20 mg/day
    Delayed puberty: 2.5-20 mg/day for 4-6 months
  Female:
    Inoperable breast carcinoma: 10-40 mg/day in divided doses for 1-3 months
    Breast engorgement: 2.5 mg after delivery, 5-10 mg/day in divided doses for 4-5 days

Monitoring Parameters In prepubertal children, perform radiographic examination of the head and wrist every 6 months

Test Interactions Decreased levels of thyroxine-binding globulin; decreased total T_4 serum levels; increased resin uptake of T_3 and T_4

Patient Information Men should report overly frequent or persistent penile erections; women should report menstrual irregularities; all patients should report persistent GI distress, diarrhea, or jaundice

Dosage Forms Tablet: 2 mg, 5 mg, 10 mg

Fluphenazine *(floo fen' a zeen)*

Related Information
  Antipsychotic Agents Comparison *on page 1255*

Brand Names Permitil®; Prolixin®; Prolixin Decanoate®; Prolixin Enanthate®

Synonyms Fluphenazine Decanoate; Fluphenazine Enanthate; Fluphenazine Hydrochloride

Use Management of manifestations of psychotic disorders

Pregnancy Risk Factor C

Contraindications Hypersensitivity to fluphenazine or any component, cross-sensitivity with other phenothiazines may exist; avoid use in patients with narrow-angle glaucoma

Warnings/Precautions Safety in children <6 months of age has not been established; use with caution in patients with cardiovascular disease or seizures; benefits of therapy must be weighed against risks of therapy; adverse effects may be of longer duration with Depot® form; watch for hypotension when administering I.M. or I.V.; use with caution in patients with severe liver or renal disease

Adverse Reactions
  >10%:
    Cardiovascular: Orthostatic hypotension, hypotension, tachycardia, arrhythmias
    Central nervous system: Parkinsonian symptoms, akathisia, dystonias, tardive dyskinesia (persistent), dizziness
    Gastrointestinal: Constipation
    Ocular: Pigmentary retinopathy
    Respiratory: Nasal congestion
    Miscellaneous: Decreased sweating
  1% to 10%:
    Central nervous system: Dizziness
    Dermatologic: Increased sensitivity to sun, skin rash

Endocrine & metabolic: Changes in menstrual cycle pain in breasts, amenorrhea, galactorrhea, gynecomastia, changes in libido

Gastrointestinal: Weight gain, nausea, vomiting, stomach pain

Genitourinary: Difficulty in urination, ejaculatory disturbances

Neuromuscular & skeletal: Trembling of fingers

<1%:

Anticholinergic: Dry mouth, urinary retention, constipation, blurred vision

Central nervous system: Sedation, drowsiness, restlessness, anxiety, extrapyramidal reactions, pseudoparkinsonian signs and symptoms, seizures, altered central temperature regulation

Dermatologic: Photosensitivity, hyperpigmentation, pruritus, rash, discoloration of skin (blue-gray)

Endocrine & metabolic: Galactorrhea

Gastrointestinal: GI upset

Genitourinary: Priapism

Hematologic: Agranulocytosis (more often in women between 4th and 10th weeks of therapy), leukopenia (usually in patients with large doses for prolonged periods)

Hepatic: Cholestatic jaundice, hepatotoxicity

Ocular: Retinal pigmentation, cornea and lens changes

Overdosage/Toxicology Symptoms of overdose include deep sleep, hypo- or hypertension, dystonia, seizures, extrapyramidal symptoms, respiratory failure

Following initiation of essential overdose management, toxic symptom treatment and supportive treatment should be initiated. Hypotension usually responds to I.V. fluids or Trendelenburg positioning. If unresponsive to these measures, the use of a parenteral inotrope may be required. Seizures commonly respond to diazepam (I.V. 5-10 mg bolus in adults every 15 minutes if needed up to a total of 30 mg; I.V. 0.25-0.4 mg/kg/dose up to a total of 10 mg in children) or to phenytoin or phenobarbital. Cardiac arrhythmias often respond to I.V. lidocaine while other antiarrhythmics can be used. Neuroleptics often cause extrapyramidal symptoms (eg, dystonic reactions) requiring management; benztropine mesylate I.V. 1-2 mg (adults) may be effective. These agents are generally effective within 2-5 minutes.

Drug Interactions

Decreased effect: Barbiturate levels and decreased fluphenazine effectiveness when given together

Increased toxicity: With ethanol, effects of both drugs may be increased; EPSEs and other CNS effects may be increased when coadministered with lithium; may potentiate the effects of narcotics including respiratory depression

Mechanism of Action Blocks postsynaptic mesolimbic dopaminergic D_1 and D_2 receptors in the brain; exhibits a strong alpha-adrenergic blocking and anticholinergic effect, depresses the release of hypothalamic and hypophyseal hormones; believed to depress the reticular activating system thus affecting basal metabolism, body temperature, wakefulness, vasomotor tone, and emesis

Pharmacodynamics/Kinetics

Following I.M. or S.C. administration (derivative dependent):

Decanoate (lasts the longest and requires more time for onset):

Onset of action: 24-72 hours

Peak neuroleptic effect: Within 48-96 hours

Hydrochloride salt (acts quickly and persists briefly):

Onset of activity: Within 1 hour

Duration: 6-8 hours

Distribution: Crosses the placenta; appears in breast milk

Metabolism: In the liver

Half-life: Derivative dependent:

Enanthate: 84-96 hours

Hydrochloride: 33 hours

Decanoate: 163-232 hours

Usual Dosage Adults:

Oral: 0.5-10 mg/day in divided doses at 6- to 8-hour intervals; some patients may require up to 40 mg/day

I.M.: 2.5-10 mg/day in divided doses at 6- to 8-hour intervals (parenteral dose is $^1/_3$ to $^1/_2$ the oral dose for the hydrochloride salts)

I.M., S.C. (decanoate): 12.5 mg every 3 weeks

Conversion from hydrochloride to decanoate I.M. 0.5 mL (12.5 mg) decanoate every 3 weeks is approximately equivalent to 10 mg hydrochloride/day

I.M., S.C. (enanthate): 12.5-25 mg every 3 weeks

Not dialyzable (0% to 5%)

Reference Range Therapeutic: 5-20 ng/mL; correlation of serum concentrations and efficacy is controversial; most often dosed to best response

Test Interactions ↑ cholesterol (S), ↑ glucose; ↓ uric acid (S)

(Continued)

Fluphenazine *(Continued)*

Patient Information Avoid alcoholic beverages, may cause drowsiness, do not discontinue without consulting physician

Nursing Implications Avoid contact of oral solution or injection with skin (contact dermatitis); watch for hypotension when administering I.M. or I.V.; oral liquid to be diluted in the following **only**: water, saline, 7-UP®, homogenized milk, carbonated orange beverages, pineapple, apricot, prune, orange, V8® juice, tomato, and grapefruit juices

Dosage Forms

Concentrate, as hydrochloride:
 Permitil®: 5 mg/mL with alcohol 1% (118 mL)
 Prolixin®: 5 mg/mL with alcohol 14% (120 mL)
Elixir, as hydrochloride (Prolixin®): 2.5 mg/5 mL with alcohol 14% (60 mL, 473 mL)
Injection, as decanoate (Prolixin Decanoate®): 25 mg/mL (1 mL, 5 mL)
Injection, as enanthate (Prolixin Enanthate®): 25 mg/mL (5 mL)
Injection, as hydrochloride (Prolixin®): 2.5 mg/mL (10 mL)
Tablet, as hydrochloride
 Permitil®: 2.5 mg, 5 mg, 10 mg
 Prolixin®: 1 mg, 2.5 mg, 5 mg, 10 mg

Fluphenazine Decanoate *see* Fluphenazine *on page 478*

Fluphenazine Enanthate *see* Fluphenazine *on page 478*

Fluphenazine Hydrochloride *see* Fluphenazine *on page 478*

Flura® *see* Fluoride *on page 471*

Flura-Drops® *see* Fluoride *on page 471*

Flura-Loz® *see* Fluoride *on page 471*

Flurandrenolide *(flure an dren' oh lide)*

Related Information

Corticosteroids Comparisons *on page 1266-1268*

Brand Names Cordran®; Cordran® SP

Synonyms Flurandrenolone

Use Inflammation of corticosteroid-responsive dermatoses [medium potency topical corticosteroid]

Pregnancy Risk Factor C

Contraindications Viral, fungal, or tubercular skin lesions, known hypersensitivity to flurandrenolide

Warnings/Precautions Adverse systemic effects may occur when used on large areas of the body, denuded areas, for prolonged periods of time, with an occlusive dressing, and/or in infants or small children

Adverse Reactions

<1%:
 Topical: Burning, itching, irritation, dryness, folliculitis, hypertrichosis, acneiform eruptions, hypopigmentation, perioral dermatitis, allergic contact dermatitis, skin atrophy, striae, miliaria; intracranial hypertension, acne, maceration of the skin
 Systemic: HPA suppression, Cushing's syndrome, growth retardation, burning, secondary infection

Overdosage/Toxicology When consumed in excessive quantities, systemic hypercorticism and adrenal suppression may occur; in those cases, discontinuation and withdrawal of the corticosteroid should be done judiciously

Mechanism of Action Decreases inflammation by suppression of migration of polymorphonuclear leukocytes and reversal of increased capillary permeability

Pharmacodynamics/Kinetics

Absorption: Adequate with intact skin
Metabolism: In the liver
Elimination: By the kidney with small amounts appearing in bile
Repeated applications lead to depot effects on skin, potentially resulting in enhanced percutaneous absorption

Usual Dosage Topical:

Children:
 Ointment, cream: Apply sparingly 1-2 times/day
 Tape: Apply once daily
Adults: Cream, lotion, ointment: Apply sparingly 2-3 times/day

Patient Information A thin film of cream or ointment is effective; do not overuse do not use tight-fitting diapers or plastic pants on children being treated in the diaper area; use only as prescribed, and for no longer than the period prescribed apply sparingly in light film; rub in lightly; avoid contact with eyes; notify physician if condition being treated persists or worsens

Dosage Forms
Cream, emulsified base (Cordran® SP): 0.025% (30 g, 60 g); 0.05% (15 g, 30 g, 60 g)
Lotion (Cordran®): 0.05% (15 mL, 60 mL)
Ointment, topical (Cordran®): 0.025% (30 g, 60 g); 0.05% (15 g, 30 g, 60 g)
Tape, topical (Cordran®): 4 mcg/cm^2 (7.5 cm x 60 cm, 7.5 cm x 200 cm rolls)

Flurandrenolone *see Flurandrenolide on previous page*

Flurazepam Hydrochloride (flure az′ e pam)
Related Information
Benzodiazepines Comparison *on page 1256*
Brand Names Dalmane®
Use Short-term treatment of insomnia
Restrictions C-IV
Pregnancy Risk Factor X
Contraindications Hypersensitivity to flurazepam or any component (there may be cross-sensitivity with other benzodiazepines); pregnancy, pre-existing CNS depression, respiratory depression, narrow-angle glaucoma
Warnings/Precautions Use with caution in patients receiving other CNS depressants, patients with low albumin, hepatic dysfunction, and in the elderly; do not use in pregnant women; may cause drug dependency; safety and efficacy have not been established in children <15 years of age
Adverse Reactions
>10%:
Cardiovascular: Tachycardia, chest pain
Central nervous system: Drowsiness, fatigue, impaired coordination, lightheadedness, memory impairment, insomnia, anxiety, depression, headache
Dermatologic: Rash
Endocrine & metabolic: Decreased libido
Gastrointestinal: Dry mouth, constipation, decreased salivation, nausea, vomiting, diarrhea, increased or decreased appetite
Neuromuscular & skeletal: Dysarthria
Ocular: Blurred vision
Miscellaneous: Sweating
1% to 10%:
Cardiovascular: Syncope, hypotension
Central nervous system: Confusion, nervousness, dizziness, akathisia
Dermatologic: Dermatitis
Gastrointestinal: Weight gain or loss, increased salivation
Neuromuscular & skeletal: Rigidity, tremor, muscle cramps
Otic: Tinnitus
Respiratory: Hyperventilation, nasal congestion
<1%:
Central nervous system: Reflex slowing
Endocrine & metabolic: Menstrual irregularities
Hematologic: Blood dyscrasias
Miscellaneous: Drug dependence
Overdosage/Toxicology Symptoms of overdose include respiratory depression, hypoactive reflexes, unsteady gait, hypotension. Treatment for benzodiazepine overdose is supportive. Rarely is mechanical ventilation required. Flumazenil has been shown to selectively block the binding of benzodiazepines to CNS receptors, resulting in a reversal of benzodiazepine-induced CNS depression.
Drug Interactions
Decreased effect with enzyme inducers
Increased toxicity with other CNS depressants and cimetidine
Stability Store in light-resistant containers
Mechanism of Action Depresses all levels of the CNS, including the limbic and reticular formation, probably through the increased action of gamma-aminobutyric acid (GABA), which is a major inhibitory neurotransmitter in the brain
Pharmacodynamics/Kinetics
Onset of hypnotic effect: 15-20 minutes
Peak: 3-6 hours
Duration of action: 7-8 hours
Metabolism: In the liver to N-desalkylflurazepam (active)
Half-life: Adults: 40-114 hours
Usual Dosage Oral:
Children:
<15 years: Dose not established
>15 years: 15 mg at bedtime
(Continued)

Flurazepam Hydrochloride *(Continued)*

Adults: 15-30 mg at bedtime

Monitoring Parameters Respiratory and cardiovascular status

Reference Range Therapeutic: 0-4 ng/mL (SI: 0-9 nmol/L); Metabolite N-desalkylflurazepam: 20-110 ng/mL (SI: 43-240 nmol/L); Toxic: >0.12 μg/mL

Patient Information Avoid alcohol and other CNS depressants; avoid activities needing good psychomotor coordination until CNS effects are known; drug may cause physical or psychological dependence; avoid abrupt discontinuation after prolonged use

Nursing Implications Provide safety measures (ie, side rails, night light, and call button); remove smoking materials from area; supervise ambulation; avoid abrupt discontinuance in patients with prolonged therapy or seizure disorders

Dosage Forms Capsule: 15 mg, 30 mg

Flurbiprofen Sodium *(flure bi′ proe fen)*

Related Information

Nonsteroidal Anti-Inflammatories Comparison *on page 1280*

Brand Names Ansaid®; Ocufen®

Use Inhibition of intraoperative miosis; acute or long-term treatment of signs and symptoms of rheumatoid arthritis and osteoarthritis; prevention and management of postoperative ocular inflammation and postoperative cystoid macular edema remains to be determined

Pregnancy Risk Factor C

Contraindications Dendritic keratitis, hypersensitivity to flurbiprofen or any component

Warnings/Precautions Should be used with caution in patients with a history of herpes simplex, keratitis, and patients who might be affected by inhibition of platelet aggregation; slowing of corneal wound healing patients in whom asthma, rhinitis, or urticaria is precipitated by aspirin or other NSAIDs.

Adverse Reactions

Ophthalmic:
>10%: Ocular: Slowing of corneal wound healing, mild ocular stinging, itching, burning, ocular irritation
1% to 10%: Ocular: Eye redness

Oral:
>10%:
Central nervous system: Dizziness
Dermatologic: Skin rash
Gastrointestinal: Abdominal cramps, heartburn, indigestion, nausea
1% to 10%:
Cardiovascular: Fluid retention
Central nervous system: Headache, nervousness
Dermatologic: Itching
Gastrointestinal: Vomiting
Otic: Ringing in ears
<1%:
Cardiovascular: Congestive heart failure, hypertension, arrhythmias, tachycardia
Central nervous system: Epistaxis, confusion, hallucinations, aseptic meningitis, mental depression, drowsiness, insomnia
Dermatologic: Hives, erythema multiforme, toxic epidermal necrolysis, Stevens-Johnson syndrome, angioedema
Endocrine & metabolic: Polydipsia, hot flushes
Gastrointestinal: Gastritis, GI ulceration
Genitourinary: Cystitis
Hematologic: Agranulocytosis, anemia, hemolytic anemia, bone marrow depression, leukopenia, thrombocytopenia
Hepatic: Hepatitis
Neuromuscular & skeletal: Peripheral neuropathy
Ocular: Toxic amblyopia, blurred vision, conjunctivitis, dry eyes
Otic: Decreased hearing
Renal: Polyuria, acute renal failure
Respiratory: Shortness of breath, allergic rhinitis

Overdosage/Toxicology Symptoms include apnea, metabolic acidosis, coma, and nystagmus; leukocytosis, renal failure

Management of a nonsteroidal anti-inflammatory drug (NSAID) intoxication is primarily supportive and symptomatic. Fluid therapy is commonly effective in managing the hypotension that may occur following an acute NSAIDs overdose, except when this is due to an acute blood loss. Seizures tend to be very short-lived and often do not require drug treatment; although, recurrent seizures should be treated with I.V. diazepam. Since many of the NSAID undergo enterohepatic cycling, multiple doses of charcoal may be needed to reduce the potential for delayed toxicities.

Drug Interactions Decreased effect: When used concurrently with flurbiprofen, reports acetylcholine chloride and carbachol being ineffective

Mechanism of Action Inhibits prostaglandin synthesis by decreasing the activity of the enzyme, cyclo-oxygenase, which results in decreased formation of prostaglandin precursors

Pharmacodynamics/Kinetics Onset of effect: Within 1-2 hours

Usual Dosage
Oral: Rheumatoid arthritis and osteoarthritis: 200-300 mg/day in 2, 3, or 4 divided doses
Ophthalmic: Instill 1 drop every 30 minutes, 2 hours prior to surgery (total of 4 drops to each affected eye)

Patient Information Take the oral formulation with food to decrease any abdominal complaints. Eye drops may cause mild burning or stinging, notify physician if this becomes severe or persistent; do not touch dropper to eye, visual acuity may be decreased after administration.

Nursing Implications Care should be taken to avoid contamination of the solution container tip

Dosage Forms
Solution, ophthalmic (Ocufen®): 0.03% (2.5 mL, 5 mL, 10 mL)
Tablet (Ansaid®): 50 mg, 100 mg

Fluress® see Fluorescein Sodium on page 470

5-Flurocytosine see Flucytosine on page 462

Flurosyn® see Fluocinolone Acetonide on page 469

Flutamide (floo' ta mide)
Related Information
Cancer Chemotherapy Regimens on page 1218-1241
Brand Names Eulexin®
Use In combination therapy with LHRH agonist analogues in treatment of metastatic prostatic carcinoma. A study has shown that the addition of flutamide to leuprolide therapy in patients with advanced prostatic cancer increased median actuarial survival time to 34.9 months versus 27.9 months with leuprolide alone. To achieve benefit to combination therapy, both drugs need to be started simultaneously.
Pregnancy Risk Factor D
Contraindications Known hypersensitivity to flutamide
Warnings/Precautions The U.S. Food and Drug Administration (FDA) currently recommends that procedures for proper handling and disposal of antineoplastic agents be considered. Animal data (based on using doses higher than recommended for humans) produced testicular interstitial cell adenoma. Do not discontinue therapy without physician's advice.
Adverse Reactions
>10%:
Gastrointestinal: Nausea, vomiting, diarrhea
Genitourinary: Impotence
Endocrine & metabolic: Loss of libido, hot flashes
1% to 10%:
Endocrine & metabolic: Gynecomastia
Gastrointestinal: Anorexia
Miscellaneous: Numbness in extremities
<1%:
Cardiovascular: Hypertension, edema
Central nervous system: Drowsiness, nervousness, confusion
Hepatic: Hepatitis
Overdosage/Toxicology Symptoms of overdose include hypoactivity, ataxia, anorexia, vomiting, slow respiration, lacrimation; management is supportive, dialysis not of benefit; induce vomiting
Stability Store at room temperature
Mechanism of Action Nonsteroidal antiandrogen that inhibits androgen uptake or inhibits binding of androgen in target tissues
Pharmacodynamics/Kinetics
Absorption: Rapid and complete
Metabolism: Extensively to more than 10 metabolites
Half-life: 5-6 hours
Elimination: All metabolites excreted primarily in urine
Usual Dosage Adults: Oral: 2 capsules every 8 hours for a total daily dose of 750 mg
(Continued)

Flutamide *(Continued)*

Administration Contents of capsule may be opened and mixed with applesauce, pudding, or other soft foods; mixing with a beverage is not recommended

Monitoring Parameters LFTs, tumor reduction, testosterone/estrogen, and phosphatase serum levels

Patient Information Flutamide and the drug used for medical castration should be administered concomitantly; do not interrupt or stop taking medication; frequent blood tests may be needed to monitor therapy

Dosage Forms Capsule: 125 mg

Flutex® *see* Triamcinolone *on page 1112*

Fluticasone Propionate (floo tik' a sone)

Brand Names Cutivate™; Flonase™

Use

Intranasal: Management of seasonal and perennial allergic rhinitis in patients ≥12 years of age

Topical: Relief of inflammation and pruritus associated with corticosteroid-responsive dermatoses [medium potency topical corticosteroid]

Pregnancy Risk Factor C

Contraindications Hypersensitivity to any component, bacterial infections, ophthalmic use

Warnings/Precautions Adverse systemic effects may occur when used on large areas of the body, denuded areas, for prolonged periods of time, with an occlusive dressing, and/or in infants or small children

Adverse Reactions

<1%:

Dermatologic: Acne, hypopigmentation, allergic dermatitis, maceration of the skin, skin atrophy, folliculitis, hypertrichosis

Endocrine & metabolic: HPA suppression, Cushing's syndrome, growth retardation

Local: Burning, itching, irritation, dryness

Miscellaneous: Secondary infection

Overdosage/Toxicology When consumed in excessive quantities, systemic hypercorticism and adrenal suppression may occur; in those cases, discontinuation and withdrawal of the corticosteroid should be done judiciously

Mechanism of Action Fluticasone belongs to a new group of corticosteroids which utilizes a fluorocarbothioate ester linkage at the 17 carbon position; extremely potent vasoconstrictive and anti-inflammatory activity; has a weak hypothalamic -pituitary- adrenocortical axis (HPA) inhibitory potency when applied topically, which gives the drug a high therapeutic index. The mechanism of action for all topical corticosteroids is not well defined, however, is believed to be a combination of three important properties: anti-inflammatory activity, immunosuppressive properties, and antiproliferative actions

Usual Dosage

Adolescents:

Topical: Apply sparingly in a thin film twice daily

Intranasal: Initially 1 spray (50 mcg/spray) per nostril once daily. Patients not adequately responding or patients with more severe symptoms may use 2 sprays (200 mcg) per nostril. Depending on response, dosage may be reduced to 100 mcg daily. Total daily dosage should not exceed 4 sprays (200 mcg)/day.

Adults:

Topical: Apply sparingly in a thin film twice daily

Intranasal: Initially 2 sprays (50 mcg/spray) per nostril once daily. After the first few days, dosage may be reduced to 1 spray per nostril once daily for maintenance therapy. Maximum total daily dose should not exceed 4 sprays (200 mcg)/day.

Patient Information A thin film of cream or ointment is effective; do not overuse; do not use tight-fitting diapers or plastic pants on children being treated in the diaper area; use only as prescribed, and for no longer than the period prescribed; apply sparingly in light film; rub in lightly; avoid contact with eyes; notify physician if condition being treated persists or worsens

Dosage Forms

Spray, intranasal: 50 mcg/actuation (9 g = 60 actuations, 16 g = 120 actuations)

Topical:

Cream: 0.05% (15 g, 30 g, 60 g)

Ointment, topical: 0.005% (15 g, 60 g)

Fluvastatin (flu' va stat in)

Related Information
Lipid-Lowering Agents *on page 1273*

Brand Names Lescol®

Use Adjunct to dietary therapy to decrease elevated serum total and LDL cholesterol concentrations in primary hypercholesterolemia

Pregnancy Risk Factor X

Pregnancy/Breast Feeding Implications Skeletal malformations have occurred in animals following agents with similar structure; avoid use in women of childbearing age; discontinue if pregnancy occurs; avoid use in nursing mothers; avoid use in nursing mothers

Contraindications Myopathy or marked elevations of CPK

Warnings/Precautions Avoid combination of clofibrate and fluvastatin due to possible myopathy; consider temporarily withholding therapy in patients with risk of developing renal failure; avoid prolonged exposure to the sun or other ultraviolet light

Adverse Reactions
1% to 1%:
Central nervous system: Headache, dizziness, insomnia
Dermatologic: Rash
Gastrointestinal: Dyspepsia, diarrhea, nausea, vomiting, constipation, flatulence
Neuromuscular & skeletal: Back pain, abdominal and other muscle pain, arthropathy
Miscellaneous: Cold symptoms

Overdosage/Toxicology No symptomatology has been reported in cases of significant overdosage, however, supportive measure should be instituted, as required; dialyzability is not known

Drug Interactions Anticoagulant effect of warfarin may be increased

Mechanism of Action Acts by competitively inhibiting 3-hydroxyl-3-methylglutaryl-coenzyme A (HMG-CoA) reductase, the enzyme that catalyzes the reduction of HMG-CoA to mevalonate; this is an early rate-limiting step in cholesterol biosynthesis. HDL is increased while total, LDL and VLDL cholesterols, apolipoprotein B, and plasma triglycerides are decreased.

Pharmacodynamics/Kinetics
Protein binding: >98%
Metabolism: Undergoes extensive first pass hepatic extraction; metabolized to inactive and active metabolites although the active forms do not circulate systemically
Bioavailability: Absolute (24%); T_{max}: ≤1 hour
Half-life: 1.2 hours
Elimination: Urine (5%), feces (90%)

Usual Dosage Adults: Oral:
Initial dose: 20 mg at bedtime
Usual dose: 20-40 mg at bedtime
Note: Splitting the 40 mg dose into a twice/daily regimen may provide a modest improvement in LDL response; maximum response occurs within 4-6 weeks; decrease dose and monitor effects carefully in patients with hepatic insufficiency

Administration Place patient on a standard cholesterol-lowering diet before and during treatment; fluvastatin may be taken without regard to meals; adjust dosage as needed in response to periodic lipid determinations during the first 4 weeks after a dosage change; lipid-lowering effects are additive when fluvastatin is combined with a bile-acid binding resin or niacin, however, it must be administered at least 2 hours following these drugs.

Test Interactions Increased serum transaminases, CPK, alkaline phosphatase, and bilirubin and thyroid function tests

Patient Information Avoid prolonged exposure to the sun and other ultraviolet light; report unexplained muscle pain or weakness, especially if accompanied by fever or malaise

Dosage Forms Capsule: 20 mg, 40 mg

Fluvoxamine (floo vox' ah meen)

Brand Names Luvox®

Use Treatment of obsessive-compulsive disorder (OCD); effective in the treatment of major depression; may be useful for the treatment of panic disorder

Pregnancy Risk Factor C

Contraindications Concomitant terfenadine or astemizole; during or within 14 days of MAO inhibitors; hypersensitivity to fluvoxamine or any congeners (eg, fluoxetine)
(Continued)

Fluvoxamine *(Continued)*

Warnings/Precautions Use with caution in patients with liver dysfunction, suicidal tendencies, history of seizures, mania, or drug abuse, ECT, cardiovascular disease, and the elderly

Adverse Reactions
>10%: Gastrointestinal: Nausea
1% to 10%:
  Cardiovascular: Palpitations
  Central nervous system: Somnolence, asthenia, headache, insomnia, dizziness, nervousness, mania, hypomania, vertigo, abnormal thinking, agitation, anxiety, malaise, amnesia
  Endocrine & metabolic: Decreased libido
  Gastrointestinal: Dry mouth, abdominal pain, vomiting, dyspepsia, constipation, diarrhea, dysgeusia, anorexia
  Neuromuscular & skeletal: Tremors
  Miscellaneous: Sweating
<1%:
  Central nervous system: Seizures
  Dermatologic: Toxic epidermal necrolysis
  Hematologic: Thrombocytopenia, increases in serum creatinine
  Hepatic: Hepatic dysfunction
  Miscellaneous: Extrapyramidal reactions

Overdosage/Toxicology
Symptoms of overdose include drowsiness, nausea, vomiting, abdominal pain, tremors, sinus bradycardia, and seizures
Specific antidote does not exist; treatment is supportive. Although vomiting has not been extensive in overdose to date, patients should be monitored for fluid and electrolyte loss, and appropriate replacement therapy instituted when necessary.

Drug Interactions Because fluvoxamine inhibits cytochrome P-450 isozymes IA2, IIC9, IIIA4, and possibly IID6, it is associated with numerous significant drug interactions

Increased toxicity: Terfenadine and astemizole are both metabolized by the cytochrome P-450 IIIA4 isozyme, increased levels of these drugs have been associated with prolongation of the Q-T interval and potentially fatal, torsade de pointes ventricular arrhythmias. Since fluvoxamine inhibits the enzyme responsible for their clearance, the concomitant use of these agents is contraindicated.
Potentiates triazolam and alprazolam (dose should be reduced by at least 50%), hypertensive crisis with MAO inhibitors, theophylline (doses should be reduced by 1/3 and plasma levels monitored), warfarin (reduce its dose and monitor PT/INR), carbamazepine (monitor levels), tricyclic antidepressants (monitor effects and reduce doses accordingly), methadone, beta-blockers (reduce dose of propranolol or metoprolol), diltiazem. Caution with other benzodiazepines, phenytoin, lithium, clozapine, alcohol, other CNS drugs, quinidine, ketoconazole.

Mechanism of Action Inhibits CNS neuron serotonin uptake; minimal or no effect on reuptake of norepinephrine or dopamine; does not significantly bind to alpha-adrenergic, histamine or cholinergic receptors

Usual Dosage
Adults: Initial: 50 mg at bedtime; adjust in 50 mg increments at 4- to 7-day intervals; usual dose range: 100-300 mg/day; divide total daily dose into 2 doses; give larger portion at bedtime
Elderly or hepatic impairment: Reduce dose, titrate slowly

Monitoring Parameters Signs and symptoms of depression, anxiety, weight gain or loss, nutritional intake, sleep

Patient Information Avoid alcoholic beverages; its favorable side effect profile makes it a useful alternative to the traditional agents; use sugarless hard candy for dry mouth; avoid alcoholic beverages, may cause drowsiness; improvement may take several weeks; rise slowly to prevent dizziness. As with all psychoactive drugs, fluvoxamine may impair judgment, thinking, or motor skills, so use caution when operating hazardous machinery, including automobiles, especially early on into therapy. Inform your physician of any concurrent medications you may be taking.

Dosage Forms Tablet: 50 mg, 100 mg

Fluzone® *see* Influenza Virus Vaccine *on page 577*

FML® *see* Fluorometholone *on page 473*

FML® Forte *see* Fluorometholone *on page 473*

Foille Medicated First Aid® [OTC] *see* Benzocaine *on page 121*

Foille® [OTC] *see* Benzocaine *on page 121*

Folacin *see* Folic Acid *on this page*

Folate *see* Folic Acid *on this page*

Folex® *see* Methotrexate *on page 711*

Folic Acid (foe′ lik)

Brand Names Folvite®

Synonyms Folacin; Folate; Pteroylglutamic Acid

Use Treatment of megaloblastic and macrocytic anemias due to folate deficiency; dietary supplement to prevent neural tube defects

Pregnancy Risk Factor A (C if dose exceeds RDA recommendation)

Contraindications Pernicious, aplastic, or normocytic anemias

Warnings/Precautions Doses <0.1 mg/day may obscure pernicious anemia with continuing irreversible nerve damage progression. Resistance to treatment may occur with depressed hematopoiesis, alcoholism, deficiencies of other vitamins. Injection contains benzyl alcohol (1.5%) as preservative (use care in administration to neonates).

Adverse Reactions

  <1%:

    Cardiovascular: Slight flushing

    Central nervous system: General malaise

    Dermatologic: Pruritus, rash

    Respiratory: Bronchospasm

    Miscellaneous: Allergic reaction

Drug Interactions

  Decreased effect: In folate-deficient patients, folic acid therapy may increase **phenytoin** metabolism. **Phenytoin, primidone, para-aminosalicylic acid, and sulfasalazine** may decrease serum folate concentrations and cause deficiency. **Oral contraceptives** may also impair folate metabolism producing depletion, but the effect is unlikely to cause anemia or megaloblastic changes. Concurrent administration of **chloramphenicol** and folic acid may result in antagonism of the hematopoietic response to folic acid.

Stability Incompatible with oxidizing and reducing agents and heavy metal ions

Mechanism of Action Folic acid is necessary for formation of a number of coenzymes in many metabolic systems, particularly for purine and pyrimidine synthesis; required for nucleoprotein synthesis and maintenance in erythropoiesis; stimulates WBC and platelet production in folate deficiency anemia

Pharmacodynamics/Kinetics

  Peak effect: Oral: Within 0.5-1 hour

  Absorption: In the proximal part of the small intestine

Usual Dosage Oral, I.M., I.V., S.C.:

  Infants: 0.1 mg/day

  Children: Initial: 1 mg/day

    Deficiency: 0.5-1 mg/day

    Maintenance dose:

      <4 years: Up to 0.3 mg/day

      >4 years: 0.4 mg/day

  Adults: Initial: 1 mg/day

    Deficiency: 1-3 mg/day

    Maintenance dose: 0.5 mg/day

    Women of childbearing age, pregnant, and lactating women: 0.8 mg/day

Administration Oral, but may also be administered by deep I.M., S.C., or I.V. injection; a diluted solution for oral or for parenteral administration may be prepared by diluting 1 mL of folic acid injection (5 mg/mL), with 49 mL sterile water for injection; resulting solution is 0.1 mg folic acid per 1 mL

Reference Range Therapeutic: 0.005-0.015 μg/mL

Test Interactions Falsely low serum concentrations may occur with the *Lactobacillus casei* assay method in patients on anti-infectives (eg, tetracycline)

Patient Information Take folic acid replacement only under recommendation of physician

Dosage Forms

  Injection, as sodium folate: 5 mg/mL (10 mL); 10 mg/mL (10 mL)

    Folvite®: 5 mg/mL (10 mL)

  Tablet: 0.1 mg, 0.4 mg, 0.8 mg, 1 mg

    Folvite®: 1 mg

Folinic Acid *see* Leucovorin Calcium *on page 619*

Follutein® *see* Chorionic Gonadotropin *on page 242*

Folvite® *see* Folic Acid *on previous page*

Footwork® [OTC] *see* Tolnaftate *on page 1106*

Formula Q® [OTC] *see* Quinine Sulfate *on page 970*

5-Formyl Tetrahydrofolate *see* Leucovorin Calcium *on page 619*

Fortaz® *see* Ceftazidime *on page 204*

Foscarnet (fos kar' net)

Related Information

Antimicrobial Drugs of Choice *on page 1298-1302*

Brand Names Foscavir®

Synonyms PFA; Phosphonoformate; Phosphonoformic Acid

Use Approved indications in adult patients:

Herpesvirus infections suspected to be caused by acyclovir (HSV, VZV) or ganciclovir (CMV) resistant strains (this occurs almost exclusively in persons with advanced AIDS who have received prolonged treatment for a herpesvirus infection)

CMV retinitis in persons with AIDS

Other CMV infections in persons unable to tolerate ganciclovir

Pregnancy Risk Factor C

Contraindications Hypersensitivity to foscarnet, Cl_{cr} <0.4 mL/minute/kg during therapy

Warnings/Precautions Renal impairment occurs to some degree in the majority of patients treated with foscarnet; renal impairment may occur at any time and is usually reversible within 1 week following dose adjustment or discontinuation of therapy, however, several patients have died with renal failure within 4 weeks of stopping foscarnet; therefore, renal function should be closely monitored. Foscarnet is deposited in teeth and bone of young, growing animals; it has adversely affected tooth enamel development in rats; safety and effectiveness in children have not been studied. Imbalance of serum electrolytes or minerals occurs in 6% to 18% of patients (hypocalcemia, low ionized calcium, hypo- or hyperphosphatemia, hypomagnesemia or hypokalemia). Patients with a low ionized calcium may experience perioral tingling, numbness, paresthesias, tetany, and seizures. Seizures have been experienced by up to 10% of AIDS patients. Risk factors for seizures include a low baseline absolute neutrophil count (ANC), impaired baseline renal function and low total serum calcium. Some patients who have experienced seizures have died, while others have been able to continue or resume foscarnet treatment after their mineral or electrolyte abnormality has been corrected, their underlying disease state treated, or their dose decreased. Foscarnet has been shown to be mutagenic *in vitro* and in mice at very high doses. Information on the use of foscarnet is lacking in the elderly; dose adjustments and proper monitoring must be performed because of the decreased renal function common in older patients.

Adverse Reactions

>10%:

Central nervous system: Fever, headache, seizures

Gastrointestinal: Nausea, diarrhea, vomiting

Hematologic: Anemia

Renal: Abnormal renal function, decreased creatinine clearance

1% to 10%:

Central nervous system: Fatigue, rigors, asthenia, malaise, dizziness, hypoesthesia, neuropathy, depression, confusion, anxiety

Dermatologic: Rash

Endocrine & metabolic: Electrolyte imbalance

Gastrointestinal: Anorexia

Hematologic: Granulocytopenia, leukopenia

Local: Injection site pain

Neuromuscular & skeletal: Paresthesia, involuntary muscle contractions

Ocular: Vision abnormalities

Renal: Decreased creatinine clearance

Respiratory: Coughing, dyspnea

Miscellaneous: Sepsis, increased sweating

<1%:

Cardiovascular: Cardiac failure, bradycardia, arrhythmias, cerebral edema, leg edema, peripheral edema, syncope, coma

Central nervous system: Hypothermia, abnormal crying, malignant hyperpyrexia, vertigo

Endocrine & metabolic: Gynecomastia, decreased gonadotropins

Hepatic: Cholecystitis, cholelithiasis, hepatitis, hepatosplenomegaly, ascites

Neuromuscular & skeletal: Abnormal gait, dyskinesia

Ocular: Nystagmus

Miscellaneous: Substernal chest pain, hypertonia, vocal cord paralysis, speech disorders

Overdosage/Toxicology Symptoms of overdose include seizures, renal dysfunction, perioral or limb paresthesias, hypocalcemia; treatment is supportive; I.V. calcium salts for hypocalcemia

Drug Interactions Increased toxicity: Pentamidine increases hypocalcemia

Stability

Foscarnet injection is a clear, colorless solution; it should be stored at room temperature and protected from temperatures >40°C and from freezing

Foscarnet should be diluted in D_5W or NS and transferred to PVC containers; stable for 24 hours at room temperature or refrigeration

For peripheral line administration, foscarnet **must** be diluted to 12 mg/mL with D_5W or NS

For central line administration, foscarnet may be administered undiluted

Incompatible with dextrose 30%, I.V. solutions containing calcium, magnesium, vancomycin, TPN

Mechanism of Action Pyrophosphate analogue which acts as a noncompetitive inhibitor of many viral RNA and DNA polymerases as well as HIV reverse transcriptase. Inhibitory effects occur at concentrations which do not affect host cellular DNA polymerases; however, some human cell growth suppression has been observed with high *in vitro* concentrations. Similar to ganciclovir, foscarnet is a virostatic agent. Foscarnet does not require activation by thymidine kinase.

Pharmacodynamics/Kinetics

Absorption: Oral: Poorly absorbed; I.V. therapy is needed for the treatment of viral infections in AIDS patients

Distribution: Up to 28% of cumulative I.V. dose may be deposited in bone

Metabolism: Biotransformation does not occur

Half-life: ~3 hours

Elimination: Up to 28% excreted unchanged in urine

Usual Dosage

Adolescents and Adults: I.V.:

Induction treatment: 60 mg/kg/dose every 8 hours for 14-21 days

Maintenance therapy: 90-120 mg/kg/day as a single infusion

See table.

Dose Adjustment for Renal Impairment

The induction dose of foscarnet should be adjusted according to creatinine clearance as follows:

Creatinine Clearance (mL/min/kg)	Foscarnet Induction Dose (mg/kg q8h)
1.6	60
1.5	57
1.4	53
1.3	49
1.2	46
1.1	42
1	39
0.9	35
0.8	32
0.7	28
0.6	25
0.5	21
0.4	18

The maintenance dose of foscarnet should be adjusted according to creatinine clearance as follows:

Creatinine Clearance (mL/min/kg)	Foscarnet Maintenance Dose (mg/kg/day)
1.4	90-120
1.2-1.4	78-104
1-1.2	75-100
0.8-1	71-94
0.6-0.8	63-84
0.4-0.6	57-75

(Continued)

Foscarnet *(Continued)*

Administration

Foscarnet is administered by intravenous infusion, using an infusion pump, at a rate not exceeding 1 mg/kg/minute

Adult induction doses of 60 mg/kg are administered over 1 hour

Adult maintenance doses of 90-120 mg/kg are infused over 2 hours

Undiluted (24 mg/mL) solution can be administered without further dilution when using a central venous catheter for infusion

For peripheral vein administration, the solution **must** be diluted to a final concentration **not to exceed** 12 mg/mL

The recommended dosage, frequency, and rate of infusion should not be exceeded

Patient Information Close monitoring is important and any symptom of electrolyte abnormalities should be reported immediately; maintain adequate fluid intake and hydration; regular ophthalmic examinations are necessary. Foscarnet is not a cure; disease progression may occur during or following treatment. Report any numbness in the extremities, parethesias, or perioral tingling.

Dosage Forms Injection: 24 mg/mL (250 mL, 500 mL)

Foscavir® *see Foscarnet on page 488*

Fosinopril *(foe sin' oh pril)*

Related Information

Angiotensin-Converting Enzyme Inhibitors, Comparative Pharmacokinetics *on page 1244*

Angiotensin-Converting Enzyme Inhibitors, Comparisons of Indications and Adult Dosages *on page 1243*

Brand Names Monopril®

Use Treatment of hypertension, either alone or in combination with other antihypertensive agents; congestive heart failure

Pregnancy Risk Factor D

Contraindications Renal impairment, collagen vascular disease, hypersensitivity to fosinopril, any component, or other angiotensin-converting enzyme inhibitors

Warnings/Precautions Use with caution and modify dosage in patients with renal impairment (decrease dosage) (especially renal artery stenosis), severe congestive heart failure or with coadministered diuretic therapy; experience in children is limited. Severe hypotension may occur in patients who are sodium and/or volume depleted; initiate lower doses and monitor closely when starting therapy in these patients.

Adverse Reactions

1% to 10%:

Cardiovascular: Orthostatic hypotension

Central nervous system: Headache, dizziness, fatigue

Endocrine & metabolic: Sexual dysfunction

Gastrointestinal: Diarrhea, nausea, vomiting

Drug-Drug Interactions With ACEIs

Precipitant Drug	Drug (Category) and Effect	Description
Antacids	ACEIs: decreased	Decreased bioavailability of ACEIs. May be more likely with captopril. Separate administration times by 1-2 hours.
NSAIDs (indomethacin)	ACEIs: decreased	Reduced hypotensive effects of ACEIs. More prominent in low renin or volume dependent hypertensive patients.
Phenothiazines	ACEIs: increased	Pharmacologic effects of ACEIs may be increased.
ACEIs	Allopurinol: increased	Higher risk of hypersensitivity reaction possible when given concurrently. Three case reports of Stevens-Johnson syndrome with captopril.
ACEIs	Digoxin: increased	Increased plasma digoxin levels.
ACEIs	Lithium: increased	Increased serum lithium levels and symptoms of toxicity may occur.
ACEIs	Potassium preps/potassium-sparing diuretics increased	Coadministration may result in elevated potassium levels.

Respiratory: Cough

<1%:

Cardiovascular: Syncope

Central nervous system: Vertigo, insomnia

Dermatologic: Angioedema, rash

Endocrine & metabolic: Hypoglycemia, hyperkalemia

Genitourinary: Impotence

Hematologic: Neutropenia, agranulocytosis, anemia

Neuromuscular & skeletal: Muscle cramps

Renal: Deterioration in renal function

Miscellaneous: Loss of taste perception

Overdosage/Toxicology Mild hypotension has been the only toxic effect seen with acute overdose. Bradycardia may also occur; hyperkalemia occurs even with therapeutic doses, especially in patients with renal insufficiency and those taking NSAIDs. Following initiation of essential overdose management, toxic symptom treatment and supportive treatment should be initiated. Hypotension usually responds to I.V. fluids or Trendelenburg positioning.

Drug Interactions

Increased toxicity:

Probenecid ↑ blood levels of captopril

Captopril and diuretics have additive hypotensive effects; see table.

Mechanism of Action Competitive inhibitor of angiotensin-converting enzyme (ACE); prevents conversion of angiotensin I to angiotensin II, a potent vasoconstrictor; results in lower levels of angiotensin II which causes an increase in plasma renin activity and a reduction in aldosterone secretion; a CNS mechanism may also be involved in hypotensive effect as angiotensin II increases adrenergic outflow from CNS; vasoactive kallikreins may be decreased in conversion to active hormones by ACE inhibitors, thus reducing blood pressure

Pharmacodynamics/Kinetics

Absorption: 36%

Metabolism: Fosinopril is a prodrug and is hydrolyzed to its active metabolite fosinoprilat by intestinal wall and hepatic esterases

Half-life, serum (fosinoprilat): 12 hours

Time to peak serum concentration: ~3 hours

Elimination: In the urine and bile as fosinoprilat and it conjugates in roughly equal proportions (45% to 50%)

Usual Dosage Adults: Oral: Initial: 10 mg/day and increase to a maximum dose of 80 mg/day; most patients are maintained on 20-40 mg/day

Moderately dialyzable (20% to 50%)

Monitoring Parameters Serum potassium, calcium, creatinine, BUN, WBC

Test Interactions Positive Coombs' [direct]; may cause false-positive results in urine acetone determinations using sodium nitroprusside reagent

Patient Information Notify physician if vomiting, diarrhea, excessive perspiration, or dehydration should occur; also if swelling of face, lips, tongue, or difficulty in breathing occurs or if persistent cough develops; may be taken with meals; do not stop therapy or add a potassium salt replacement without physician's advice

Nursing Implications May cause depression in some patients; discontinue if angioedema of the face, extremities, lips, tongue, or glottis occurs; watch for hypotensive effects within 1-3 hours of first dose or new higher dose

Dosage Forms Tablet: 10 mg, 20 mg

Fostex® [OTC] see Benzoyl Peroxide on page 122

Fragmin® see Dalteparin on page 299

Frusemide see Furosemide on next page

FS Shampoo® see Fluocinolone Acetonide on page 469

5-FU see Fluorouracil on page 473

FUDR® see Floxuridine on page 460

Ful-Glo® see Fluorescein Sodium on page 470

Fulvicin® P/G see Griseofulvin on page 514

Fulvicin-U/F® see Griseofulvin on page 514

Fumasorb® [OTC] see Ferrous Fumarate on page 450

Fumerin® [OTC] see Ferrous Fumarate on page 450

Funduscein® see Fluorescein Sodium on page 470

Fungatin® [OTC] see Tolnaftate on page 1106

Fungizone® see Amphotericin B on page 71

Furacin® see Nitrofurazone on page 798

Furadantin® see Nitrofurantoin on page 797

Furalan® *see* Nitrofurantoin *on page 797*

Furan® *see* Nitrofurantoin *on page 797*

Furanite® *see* Nitrofurantoin *on page 797*

Furazolidone (fur a zoe' li done)
Brand Names Furoxone®

Use Treatment of bacterial or protozoal diarrhea and enteritis caused by susceptible organisms *Giardia lamblia* and *Vibrio cholerae*

Pregnancy Risk Factor C

Contraindications Known hypersensitivity to furazolidone; concurrent use of alcohol; patients <1 month of age because of the possibility of producing hemolytic anemia

Warnings/Precautions Use caution in patients with G-6-PD deficiency when administering large doses for prolonged periods; furazolidone inhibits monoamine oxidase

Adverse Reactions
>10%: Miscellaneous: Dark yellow to brown discoloration of urine
1% to 10%:
  Central nervous system: Headache
  Gastrointestinal: Abdominal pain, diarrhea, nausea, vomiting
<1%:
  Cardiovascular: Orthostatic hypotension
  Central nervous system: Fever, dizziness, drowsiness, malaise
  Dermatologic: Skin rash
  Endocrine & metabolic: Hypoglycemia, disulfiram-like reaction after alcohol ingestion, leukopenia
  Hematologic: Agranulocytosis, hemolysis in patients with G-6-PD deficiency
  Neuromuscular & skeletal: Joint pain

Overdosage/Toxicology Symptoms of overdose include nausea, vomiting, serotonin crisis; treatment is supportive care only; serotonin crisis may require dantrolene/bromocriptine

Drug Interactions
Increased effect with sympathomimetic amines, tricyclic antidepressants, tyramine-containing foods, MAO inhibitors, meperidine, anorexiants, dextromethorphan, fluoxetine, paroxetine, sertraline, trazodone
Increased effect/toxicity of levodopa
Disulfiram-like reaction with alcohol

Mechanism of Action Inhibits several vital enzymatic reactions causing antibacterial and antiprotozoal action

Pharmacodynamics/Kinetics
Absorption: Oral: Poor
Elimination: Oral: $1/3$ of dose is excreted in urine as active drug and metabolites

Usual Dosage Oral:
Children >1 month: 5-8 mg/kg/day in 4 divided doses for 7 days, not to exceed 400 mg/day or 8.8 mg/kg/day
Adults: 100 mg 4 times/day for 7 days

Test Interactions False-positive results for urine glucose with Clinitest®

Patient Information May discolor urine to a brown tint; avoid drinking alcohol during or for 4 days after therapy or eating tyramine-containing foods; consult with physician or pharmacist for a list of these foods. Do not take any prescription or nonprescription drugs without consulting the physician or pharmacist; if result not achieved at the end of treatment contact physician.

Dosage Forms
Liquid: 50 mg/15 mL (60 mL, 473 mL)
Tablet: 100 mg

Furazosin *see* Prazosin Hydrochloride *on page 918*

Furosemide (fur oh' se mide)
Related Information
Diuretics, Loop Comparison *on page 1269*

Brand Names Lasix®

Synonyms Frusemide

Use Management of edema associated with congestive heart failure and hepatic or renal disease; used alone or in combination with antihypertensives in treatment of hypertension

Pregnancy Risk Factor C

Contraindications Hypersensitivity to furosemide, any component, or other sulfonamides

Warnings/Precautions Loop diuretics are potent diuretics; close medical supervision and dose evaluation is required to prevent fluid and electrolyte imbalance; use caution with other nephrotoxic or ototoxic drugs

Adverse Reactions

>10%:

Cardiovascular: Orthostatic hypotension

Central nervous system: Dizziness

1% to 10%:

Central nervous system: Headache

Dermatologic: Photosensitivity

Endocrine & metabolic: Electrolyte imbalance (hypokalemia, hyponatremia, hypochloremia, hypercalciuria, hyperuricemia), alkalosis, dehydration

Gastrointestinal: Diarrhea, loss of appetite, stomach cramps or pain

Ocular: Blurred vision

<1%:

Dermatologic: Skin rash

Gastrointestinal: Pancreatitis, nausea

Genitourinary: Prerenal azotemia

Hepatic: Hepatic dysfunction

Hematologic: Agranulocytosis, leukopenia, anemia, thrombocytopenia

Local: Redness at injection site

Neuromuscular & skeletal: Gout

Ocular: Xanthopsia

Otic: Ototoxicity

Renal: Nephrocalcinosis, interstitial nephritis

Overdosage/Toxicology Symptoms of overdose include electrolyte depletion, volume depletion, hypotension, dehydration, circulatory collapse; following GI decontamination, treatment is supportive; hypotension responds to fluids and Trendelenburg position

Drug Interactions

Decreased effect:

Furosemide interferes with hypoglycemic effect of antidiabetic agents

Indomethacin may reduce natriuretic and hypotensive effects of furosemide

Increased effect: Effects of antihypertensive agents may be enhanced

Increased toxicity:

Lithium → renal clearance decreased

Concomitant use of furosemide with aminoglycoside antibiotics or other ototoxic drugs should be avoided

Stability

Furosemide injection should be stored at controlled room temperature and protected from light

Exposure to light may cause discoloration; do not use furosemide solutions if they have a yellow color

Refrigeration may result in precipitation or crystallization, however, resolubilization at room temperature or warming may be performed without affecting the drugs stability

Furosemide solutions are unstable in acidic media but very stable in basic media

I.V. infusion solution mixed in NS or D_5W solution is stable for 24 hours at room temperature

Mechanism of Action Inhibits reabsorption of sodium and chloride in the ascending loop of Henle and distal renal tubule, interfering with the chloride-binding cotransport system, thus causing increased excretion of water, sodium, chloride, magnesium, and calcium

Pharmacodynamics/Kinetics

Onset of diuresis:

Oral: Within 30-60 minutes

I.M.: 30 minutes

I.V.: Within 5 minutes

Peak effect: Oral: Within 1-2 hours

Duration:

Oral: 6-8 hours

I.V.: 2 hours

Absorption: Oral: 60% to 67%

Protein binding: >98%

Half-life:

Normal renal function: 0.5-1.1 hours

End stage renal disease: 9 hours

Elimination: 50% of an oral or 80% of an I.V. dose is excreted in the urine within 24 hours; the remainder is eliminated by other nonrenal pathways, including liver metabolism and excretion of unchanged drug in the feces

(Continued)

493

Furosemide *(Continued)*

Usual Dosage

Neonates, premature:

Oral: Bioavailability is poor by this route; doses of 1-4 mg/kg/dose 1-2 times/day have been used

I.M., I.V.: 1-2 mg/kg/dose given every 12-24 hours

Infants and Children:

Oral: 1-2 mg/kg/dose increased in increments of 1 mg/kg/dose with each succeeding dose until a satisfactory effect is achieved to a maximum of 6 mg/kg/dose no more frequently than 6 hours

I.M., I.V.: 1 mg/kg/dose, increasing by each succeeding dose at 1 mg/kg/dose at intervals of 6-12 hours until a satisfactory response up to 6 mg/kg/dose

Adults:

Oral: 20-80 mg/dose initially increased in increments of 20-40 mg/dose at intervals of 6-8 hours; usual maintenance dose interval is twice daily or every day

I.M., I.V.: 20-40 mg/dose, may be repeated in 1-2 hours as needed and increased by 20 mg/dose with each succeeding dose up to 1000 mg/day; usual dosing interval: 6-12 hours

Continuous I.V. infusion: Initial I.V. bolus dose of 0.1 mg/kg followed by continuous I.V. infusion doses of 0.1 mg/kg/hour doubled every 2 hours to a maximum of 0.4 mg/kg/hour if urine output is <1 mL/kg/hour have been found to be effective and result in a lower daily requirement of furosemide than with intermittent dosing. Other studies have used 20-160 mg/hour continuous I.V. infusion.

Elderly: Oral, I.M., I.V.: Initial: 20 mg/day; increase slowly to desired response

Dosing adjustment/comments in renal impairment: Acute renal failure: Doses up to 100 mg/day may be necessary to initiate desired response; avoid use in oliguric states

Not removed by hemo- or peritoneal dialysis; supplemental dose is not necessary

Dosing adjustment/comments in hepatic disease: Diminished natriuretic effect with increased sensitivity to hypokalemia and volume depletion in cirrhosis; monitor effects, particularly with high doses

Administration I.V. injections should be given slowly over 1-2 minutes; maximum rate of administration for IVPB or infusion: 4 mg/minute; replace parenteral therapy with oral therapy as soon as possible

Monitoring Parameters Monitor weight and I & O daily; blood pressure, serum electrolytes, renal function; in high doses, monitor hearing

Patient Information May be taken with food or milk; rise slowly from a lying or sitting position to minimize dizziness, lightheadedness, or fainting; also use extra care when exercising, standing for long periods of time, and during hot weather; take last dose of day early in the evening to prevent nocturia

Additional Information Sodium content of 1 mL (injection): 0.162 mEq

Dosage Forms

Injection: 10 mg/mL (2 mL, 4 mL, 5 mL, 6 mL, 8 mL, 10 mL, 12 mL)

Solution, oral: 10 mg/mL (60 mL, 120 mL); 40 mg/5 mL (5 mL, 10 mL, 500 mL)

Tablet: 20 mg, 40 mg, 80 mg

Furoxone® see Furazolidone *on page 492*

G-1® see Butalbital Compound *on page 153*

Gabapentin *(ga' ba pen tin)*

Brand Names Neurontin®

Use Adjunct for treatment of drug-refractory partial and secondarily generalized seizures in adults with epilepsy; not effective for absence seizures

Pregnancy Risk Factor C

Contraindications Hypersensitivity to the drug or its ingredients

Warnings/Precautions Avoid abrupt withdrawal, may precipitate seizures; may be associated with a slight incidence (0.6%) of status epilepticus and sudden deaths (0.0038 deaths/patient year); use cautiously in patients with severe renal dysfunction; rat studies demonstrated an association with pancreatic adenocarcinoma in male rats; clinical implication unknown

Adverse Reactions

>10%: Central nervous system: Somnolence, dizziness, ataxia, fatigue

1% to 10%:

Cardiovascular: Peripheral edema

Central nervous system: Nervousness, amnesia, depression, anxiety, abnormal coordination

Dermatologic: Pruritus

Gastrointestinal: Dyspepsia, dry mouth/throat, nausea, constipation, appetite stimulation (weight gain)

Genitourinary: Impotence

Hematologic: Leukopenia

Neuromuscular & skeletal: Back pain, myalgia, dysarthria, tremor

Ocular: Diplopia, blurred vision, nystagmus

Respiratory: Rhinitis, bronchospasm

Miscellaneous: Hiccups

Overdosage/Toxicology

Decontamination: Lavage/activated charcoal with cathartic

Enhancement of elimination: Multiple dosing of activated charcoal may be useful; hemodialysis will be useful

Drug Interactions

Gabapentin does not modify plasma concentrations of standard anticonvulsant medications (ie, valproic acid, carbamazepine, phenytoin, or phenobarbital)

Decreased effect: Antacids reduce the bioavailability of gabapentin by 20%

Increased toxicity: Cimetidine may decrease clearance of gabapentin; gabapentin may increase levels of norethindrone by 13%

Mechanism of Action Exact mechanism of action is not known, but does have properties in common with other anticonvulsants; although structurally related to GABA, it does not interact with GABA receptors

Pharmacodynamics/Kinetics

Absorption: Oral: 50% to 60%

Distribution: V_d: 0.6-0.8 L/kg

Protein binding: 0%

Half-life: 5-6 hours

Elimination: Renal, 56% to 80%

Usual Dosage If gabapentin is discontinued or if another anticonvulsant is added to therapy, it should be done slowly over a minimum of 1 week

Children >12 years and Adults: Oral:

Initial: 300 mg on day 1 (at bedtime to minimize sedation), then 300 mg twice daily on day 2, and then 300 mg 3 times/day on day 3

Total daily dosage range: 900-1800 mg/day administered in 3 divided doses at 8-hour intervals

Dosing adjustment in renal impairment:

Cl_{cr} >60 mL/minute: Administer 1200 mg/day

Cl_{cr} 30-60 mL/minute: Administer 600 mg/day

Cl_{cr} 15-30 mL/minute: Administer 300 mg/day

Cl_{cr} <15 mL/minute: Administer 150 mg/day

Hemodialysis: 200-300 mg after each 4-hour dialysis following a loading dose of 300-400 mg

Administration Administer first dose on first day at bedtime to avoid somnolence and dizziness

Monitoring Parameters Monitor serum levels of concomitant anticonvulsant therapy; routine monitoring of gabapentin levels is not mandatory

Reference Range Minimum effective serum concentration may be 2 mcg/mL; **routine monitoring of drug levels is not required**

Patient Information Take only as prescribed; may cause dizziness, somnolence, and other symptoms and signs of CNS depression; do not operate machinery or drive a car until you have experience with the drug; may be administered without regard to meals

Nursing Implications Dosage must be adjusted for renal function and elderly often have reduced renal function

Dosage Forms Capsule: 100 mg, 300 mg, 400 mg

Gallium Nitrate (gal' ee um)

Brand Names Ganite™

Use Treatment of clearly symptomatic cancer-related hypercalcemia that has not responded to adequate hydration

Pregnancy Risk Factor C

Contraindications Should not be used in patients with a serum creatinine >2.5 mg/dL, hypersensitivity to any component

Warnings/Precautions Safety and efficacy in children have not been established. Concurrent use of gallium nitrate with other potentially nephrotoxic drugs may increase the risk for developing severe renal insufficiency in patients with cancer-related hypercalcemia; use with caution in patients with impaired renal function or dehydration

Adverse Reactions

>10%:

Endocrine & metabolic: Hypophosphatemia

(Continued)

Gallium Nitrate *(Continued)*

  Gastrointestinal: Nausea, vomiting, diarrhea, metallic taste
  Renal: Renal toxicity
  1% to 10%: Endocrine & metabolic: Hypocalcemia
  <1%:
  Hematologic: Anemia
  Ocular: Optic neuritis
  Otic: Hearing impairment

Overdosage/Toxicology Symptoms of overdose include nausea, vomiting, renal failure, hypocalcemia, tetany; supportive measures ensure adequate hydration, calcium salts

Drug Interactions Increased toxicity: Nephrotoxic drugs (eg, aminoglycosides, amphotericin B)

Stability Store at room temperature (15°C to 30°C/59°F to 86°F); when diluted in NS or D_5W, stable for 48 hours at room temperature or 7 days at refrigeration (2°C to 8°C/36°F to 46°F)

Mechanism of Action Primarily via inhibition of bone resorption with associated reduction in urinary calcium excretion. Gallium has increased the calcium content of newly mineralized bone following short-term treatment *in vitro*, and this effect combined with its ability to inhibit bone resorption has suggested the use of gallium for other disorders associated with increased bone loss.

Pharmacodynamics/Kinetics
  Metabolism: Not metabolized by liver or kidneys
  Half-life, elimination: Terminal: 25-111 hours
  Elimination: Up to 70% of dose excreted by the kidneys

Usual Dosage Adults:
  I.V. infusion (over 24 hours): 200 mg/m² for 5 consecutive days in 1 L of NS or D_5W
  Mild hypercalcemia/few symptoms: 100 mg/m²/day for 5 days in 1 L of NS or D_5W

  Dosing adjustment/comments in renal impairment:
  Cl_{cr} <30 mL/minute: Avoid use

Monitoring Parameters Serum creatinine, BUN, and calcium

Reference Range Steady-state gallium serum levels: Generally obtained within 2 days following initiation of continuous I.V. infusions of gallium nitrate

Nursing Implications Patients should have adequate I.V. hydration, serum creatinine levels should be monitored during gallium nitrate therapy

Dosage Forms Injection: 25 mg/mL (20 mL)

Gamastan® *see* Immune Globulin, Intramuscular *on page 570*

Gamimune® N *see* Immune Globulin, Intravenous *on page 571*

Gamma Benzene Hexachloride *see* Lindane *on page 636*

Gammagard® *see* Immune Globulin, Intravenous *on page 571*

Gamma Globulin *see* Immune Globulin, Intramuscular *on page 570*

Gammar® *see* Immune Globulin, Intramuscular *on page 570*

Gamulin® Rh *see* Rho(D) Immune Globulin *on page 978*

Ganciclovir *(gan sye' kloe vir)*
  Related Information
  Antimicrobial Drugs of Choice *on page 1298-1302*
  Brand Names Cytovene®
  Synonyms DHPG Sodium; GCV Sodium; Nordeoxyguanosine
  Use Treatment of CMV retinitis in immunocompromised individuals, including patients with acquired immunodeficiency syndrome; treatment of CMV pneumonia in marrow transplant recipients AIDS patients and organ transplant recipients with CMV colitis, pneumonitis, and multiorgan involvement; bone marrow transplant patients when given in combination with IVIG or CMV hyperimmune globulin

  Oral: Alternative to the I.V. formulation for maintenance treatment of CMV retinitis in immunocompromised patients, including patients with AIDS, in whom retinitis is stable following appropriate induction therapy and for whom the risk of more rapid progression is balanced by the benefit associated with avoiding daily I.V. infusions

  Pregnancy Risk Factor C
  Contraindications Absolute neutrophil count <500/mm³; platelet count <25,000/mm³; known hypersensitivity to ganciclovir or acyclovir

Warnings/Precautions Dosage adjustment or interruption of ganciclovir therapy may be necessary in patients with neutropenia and/or thrombocytopenia and patients with impaired renal function. Use with extreme caution in children since long-term safety has not been determined and due to ganciclovir's potential for long-term carcinogenic and adverse reproductive effects; ganciclovir may adversely affect spermatogenesis and fertility; due to its mutagenic potential, contraceptive precautions for female and male patients need to be followed during and for at least 90 days after therapy with the drug; take care to administer only into veins with good blood flow.

Adverse Reactions

>10%:
Central nervous system: Headache
Hematologic: Granulocytopenia, thrombocytopenia

1% to 10%:
Central nervous system: Confusion, fever
Dermatologic: Rash
Hematologic: Anemia
Hepatic: Abnormal liver function values
Miscellaneous: Sepsis

<1%:
Cardiovascular: Arrhythmia, hypertension, hypotension, coma, edema
Central nervous system: Ataxia, dizziness, nervousness, psychosis, malaise
Dermatologic: Alopecia, pruritus, urticaria
Gastrointestinal: Nausea, vomiting, diarrhea, abdominal pain
Hematologic: Eosinophilia, hemorrhage
Local: Inflammation or pain at injection site
Neuromuscular & skeletal: Paresthesia, tremor
Ocular: Retinal detachment
Respiratory: Dyspnea

Overdosage/Toxicology Symptoms of overdose include neutropenia, vomiting, hypersalivation, bloody diarrhea, cytopenia, testicular atrophy; treatment is supportive; hemodialysis removes 50% of drug; hydration may be of some benefit

Drug Interactions

Decreased effect: Didanosine: A decrease in steady-state ganciclovir AUC may occur

Increased toxicity:
Zidovudine, immunosuppressive agents → ↑ hematologic toxicity
Imipenem/cilastatin → ↑ seizure potential
Zidovudine: Oral ganciclovir increased the AUC of zidovudine. Since both drugs have the potential to cause neutropenia and anemia, some patients may not tolerate concomitant therapy with these drugs at full dosage.
Probenecid: The renal clearance of ganciclovir is decreased in the presence of probenecid

Stability

Preparation should take place in a vertical laminar flow hood with the same precautions as antineoplastic agents

Intact vials should be stored at room temperature and protected from temperatures >40°C

Reconstitute powder with sterile water **not** bacteriostatic water because parabens may cause precipitation

Reconstituted solution is stable for 12 hours at room temperature, however, conflicting data indicates that reconstituted solution is stable for 60 days under refrigeration (4°C)

Drug product should be reconstituted immediately before use and any unused portion should be discarded

Stability of parenteral admixture at room temperature (25°C) and at refrigeration temperature (4°C): 5 days

An in-line filter of 0.22-5 micron is recommended during the infusion of all ganciclovir solutions

Mechanism of Action Ganciclovir is phosphorylated to a substrate which competitively inhibits the binding of deoxyguanosine triphosphate to DNA polymerase resulting in inhibition of viral DNA synthesis

Pharmacodynamics/Kinetics

Absorption: Oral: Absolute bioavailability under fasting conditions: 5% and following food: 6% to 9%; following fatty meal: 28% to 31%

Protein binding: 1% to 2%

Half-life: 1.7-5.8 hours; increases with impaired renal function
End stage renal disease: 3.6 hours

Elimination: Majority (94% to 99%) excreted as unchanged drug in the urine

(Continued)

Ganciclovir *(Continued)*

Usual Dosage

Slow I.V. infusion (dosing is based on total body weight):

Children >3 months and Adults:

Induction therapy: 5 mg/kg/dose every 12 hours for 14-21 days followed by maintenance therapy

Maintenance therapy: 5 mg/kg/day as a single daily dose for 7 days/week or 6 mg/kg/day for 5 days/week

Oral: 1000 mg 3 times/day with food **or** 500 mg 6 times/day with food

Dosing adjustment in renal impairment:

I.V.:

Cl_{cr} 50-79 mL/minute: Administer 2.5 mg/kg/dose every 12 hours

Cl_{cr} 25-49 mL/minute: Administer 2.5 mg/kg/dose every 24 hours

Cl_{cr} <25 mL/minute: Administer 1.25 mg/kg/dose every 24 hours

Oral:

Cl_{cr} 50-69 mL/minute: Administer 1500 mg/day or 500 mg 3 times/day

Cl_{cr} 25-49 mL/minute: Administer 1000 mg/day or 500 mg twice daily

Cl_{cr} 10-24 mL/minute: Administer 500 mg/day

Cl_{cr} <10 mL/minute: Administer 500 mg 3 times/week following hemodialysis

Dialyzable (50%) following hemodialysis; administer dose postdialysis; during peritoneal dialysis, dose as for Cl_{cr} <10 mL/minute; during continuous arteriovenous or veno-venous hemofiltration (CAVH/CAVHD), administer 2.5 mg/kg/dose every 24 hours

Administration The same precautions utilized with antineoplastic agents should be followed with ganciclovir administration. Ganciclovir should not be administered by I.M., S.C., or rapid IVP administration; administer by slow I.V. infusion over at least 1 hour at a final concentration for administration not to exceed 10 mg/mL. **An IN-LINE filter of 0.22-5 micron is recommended during the infusion of all ganciclovir solutions.** Oral ganciclovir should be administered with food

Monitoring Parameters CBC with differential and platelet count, serum creatinine, ophthalmologic exams

Patient Information Ganciclovir is not a cure for CMV retinitis; regular ophthalmologic examinations should be done; close monitoring of blood counts should be done while on therapy and dosage adjustments may need to be made; take with food to increase absorption

Nursing Implications Must be prepared in vertical flow hood; use chemotherapy precautions during administration; discard appropriately

Additional Information Sodium content of 500 mg vial: 46 mg

Dosage Forms

Capsule: 250 mg

Powder for injection, lyophilized: 500 mg (10 mL)

Ganite™ *see* Gallium Nitrate *on page 495*

Gantanol® *see* Sulfamethoxazole *on page 1042*

Gantrisin® *see* Sulfisoxazole *on page 1045*

Garamycin® *see* Gentamicin Sulfate *on page 500*

Gas Relief® [OTC] *see* Simethicone *on page 1006*

Gastrocrom® Oral *see* Cromolyn Sodium *on page 280*

Gastrosed™ *see* Hyoscyamine Sulfate *on page 559*

Gas-X® [OTC] *see* Simethicone *on page 1006*

G-CSF *see* Filgrastim *on page 454*

GCV Sodium *see* Ganciclovir *on page 496*

Gee Gee® [OTC] *see* Guaifenesin *on page 515*

Gel Kam® *see* Fluoride *on page 471*

Gel-Tin® [OTC] *see* Fluoride *on page 471*

Gelucast® *see* Zinc Gelatin *on page 1175*

Gemfibrozil *(jem fi' broe zil)*

Related Information

Lipid-Lowering Agents *on page 1273*

Brand Names Lopid®

Synonyms CI-719

Use Treatment of hypertriglyceridemia in types IV and V hyperlipidemia for patients who are at greater risk for pancreatitis and who have not responded to dietary intervention; reduction of coronary heart disease in type IIB patients who have low HDL cholesterol, ↑ LDL cholesterol, and ↑ triglycerides

Pregnancy Risk Factor B

Contraindications Renal or hepatic dysfunction, gallbladder disease, hypersensitivity to gemfibrozil or any component

Warnings/Precautions Abnormal elevation of AST, ALT, LDH, bilirubin, and alkaline phosphatase has occurred; if no appreciable triglyceride or cholesterol lowering effect occurs after 3 months, the drug should be discontinued; not useful for type I hyperlipidemia; myositis may be more common in patients with poor renal function

Adverse Reactions
>10%:
    Gastrointestinal: Dyspepsia, abdominal pain
    Hepatic: Cholelithiasis
1% to 10%:
    Central nervous system: Fatigue, vertigo, headache
    Dermatologic: Eczema, rash
    Gastrointestinal: Diarrhea, nausea, vomiting, constipation, acute appendicitis
<1%:
    Cardiovascular: Atrial fibrillation
    Central nervous system: Hypesthesia, dizziness, drowsiness, somnolence, mental depression
    Gastrointestinal: Flatulence
    Neuromuscular & skeletal: Paresthesia
    Ocular: Blurred vision

Overdosage/Toxicology Symptoms of overdose include abdominal pain, diarrhea, nausea, vomiting; following GI decontamination, treatment is supportive

Drug Interactions
Increased toxicity:
    May potentiate the effects of warfarin
    Manufacturer warns against the use of gemfibrozil with concomitant lovastatin therapy

Mechanism of Action The exact mechanism of action of gemfibrozil is unknown, however, several theories exist regarding the VLDL effect; it can inhibit lipolysis and decrease subsequent hepatic fatty acid uptake as well as inhibit hepatic secretion of VLDL; together these actions decrease serum VLDL levels; increases HDL cholesterol; the mechanism behind HDL elevation is currently unknown

Pharmacodynamics/Kinetics
Absorption: Well absorbed
Protein binding: 99%
Metabolism: In the liver by oxidation to two inactive metabolites
Half-life: 1.4 hours
Time to peak serum concentration: Within 1-2 hours
Elimination: A portion of the drug undergoes enterohepatic recycling; excreted in urine, primarily as unchanged drug (70%)

Usual Dosage Adults: Oral: 1200 mg/day in 2 divided doses, 30 minutes before breakfast and dinner
Not removed by hemodialysis; supplemental dose is not necessary

Monitoring Parameters Serum cholesterol, LFTs

Patient Information May cause dizziness or blurred vision, abdominal or epigastric pain, diarrhea, nausea, or vomiting; notify physician if these become pronounced

Dosage Forms
Capsule: 300 mg
Tablet, film coated: 600 mg

Genabid® see Papaverine Hydrochloride on page 839

Genac® [OTC] see Triprolidine and Pseudoephedrine on page 1131

Genahist® see Diphenhydramine Hydrochloride on page 351

Genapap® [OTC] see Acetaminophen on page 17

Genaspor® [OTC] see Tolnaftate on page 1106

Genatuss DM® [OTC] see Guaifenesin and Dextromethorphan on page 517

Genatuss® [OTC] see Guaifenesin on page 515

Gen-K® see Potassium Chloride on page 906

Genoptic® see Gentamicin Sulfate on next page

Genora® see Ethinyl Estradiol and Norethindrone on page 425

Genora® 1/50 see Mestranol and Norethindrone on page 695

Genpril® [OTC] *see* Ibuprofen *on page 561*

Gentacidin® *see* Gentamicin Sulfate *on this page*

Gentafair® *see* Gentamicin Sulfate *on this page*

Gentak® *see* Gentamicin Sulfate *on this page*

Gentamicin Sulfate (jen ta mye' sin)

Related Information
Antimicrobial Drugs of Choice *on page 1298-1302*
Prevention of Bacterial Endocarditis *on page 1285-1288*

Brand Names Garamycin®; Genoptic®; Gentacidin®; Gentafair®; Gentak®; Gentrasul®; I-Gent®; Jenamicin®; Ocumycin®

Use Treatment of susceptible bacterial infections, normally gram-negative organisms including *Pseudomonas*, *Proteus*, *Serratia*, and gram-positive *Staphylococcus*; treatment of bone infections, respiratory tract infections, skin and soft tissue infections, as well as abdominal and urinary tract infections, endocarditis, and septicemia; used topically to treat superficial infections of the skin or ophthalmic infections caused by susceptible bacteria

Pregnancy Risk Factor C

Contraindications Hypersensitivity to gentamicin or other aminoglycosides

Warnings/Precautions
Not intended for long-term therapy due to toxic hazards associated with extended administration; pre-existing renal insufficiency, vestibular or cochlear impairment, myasthenia gravis, hypocalcemia, conditions which depress neuromuscular transmission

Parenteral aminoglycosides are associated with significant nephrotoxicity or ototoxicity; the ototoxicity may be directly proportional to the amount of drug given and the duration of treatment; tinnitus or vertigo are indications of vestibular injury and impending hearing loss; renal damage is usually reversible

Adverse Reactions
>10%:
Central nervous system: Neurotoxicity (vertigo, ataxia, gait instability)
Otic: Ototoxicity (auditory), ototoxicity (vestibular)
Renal: Nephrotoxicity, decreased creatinine clearance
1% to 10%: Dermatologic: Skin itching, redness, rash, swelling
<1%:
Central nervous system: Drowsiness, weakness, headache, pseudomotor cerebri
Dermatologic: Photosensitivity, erythema, burning, stinging
Gastrointestinal: Anorexia, nausea, vomiting, weight loss, increased salivation, enterocolitis
Hematologic: Granulocytopenia, agranulocytosis, thrombocytopenia
Hepatic: Elevated LFTs
Neuromuscular & skeletal: Tremors, muscle cramps
Respiratory: Difficulty in breathing

Overdosage/Toxicology Symptoms of overdose include ototoxicity, nephrotoxicity, and neuromuscular toxicity; serum level monitoring is recommended. The treatment of choice, following a single acute overdose, appears to be the maintenance of good urine output of at least 3 mL/kg/hour. Dialysis is of questionable value in the enhancement of aminoglycoside elimination. If required, hemodialysis is preferred over peritoneal dialysis in patients with normal renal function. Careful hydration may be all that is required to promote diuresis and therefore the enhancement of the drug's elimination. Chelation with penicillins is experimental.

Drug Interactions
Increased toxicity:
Penicillins, cephalosporins, amphotericin B, loop diuretics → ↑ nephrotoxic potential
Neuromuscular blocking agents → ↑ neuromuscular blockade

Stability
Gentamicin is a colorless to slightly yellow solution which should be stored between 2°C to 30°C, but refrigeration is not recommended
I.V. infusion solutions mixed in NS or D_5W solution are stable for 24 hours at room temperature and refrigeration
Premixed bag: Manufacturer expiration date
Out of overwrap stability: 30 days

Mechanism of Action Interferes with bacterial protein synthesis by binding to 30S and 50S ribosomal subunits resulting in a defective bacterial cell membrane

Pharmacodynamics/Kinetics
Absorption: Oral: Not absorbed
Distribution: Crosses the placenta
V_d: Increased by edema, ascites, fluid overload; decreased in patients with dehydration. See table.

Aminoglycoside Penetration Into Various Tissues

Site	Extent of Distribution
Eye	Poor
CNS	Poor (<25%)
Pleural	Excellent
Bronchial secretions	Poor
Sputum	Fair (10%-50%)
Pulmonary tissue	Excellent
Ascitic fluid	Variable (43%-132%)
Peritoneal fluid	Poor
Bile	Variable (25%-90%)
Bile with obstruction	Poor
Synovial fluid	Excellent
Bone	Poor
Prostate	Poor
Urine	Excellent
Renal tissue	Excellent

    Neonates: 0.4-0.6 L/kg
    Children: 0.3-0.35 L/kg
    Adults: 0.2-0.3 L/kg
Relative diffusion of antimicrobial agents from blood into cerebrospinal fluid (CSF): Minimal even with inflammation
Ratio of CSF to blood level (%):
    Normal meninges: Nil
    Inflamed meninges: 10-30
Protein binding: <30%
Half-life:
    Infants:
        <1 week: 3-11.5 hours
        1 week to 6 months: 3-3.5 hours
    Adults: 1.5-3 hours; end stage renal disease: 36-70 hours
Time to peak serum concentration:
    I.M.: Within 30-90 minutes
    I.V.: 30 minutes after a 30-minute infusion
Elimination: Clearance is directly related to renal function, eliminated almost completely by glomerular filtration of unchanged drug with excretion into the urine

Usual Dosage Individualization is critical because of the low therapeutic index

Use of ideal body weight (IBW) for determining the mg/kg/dose appears to be more accurate than dosing on the basis of total body weight (TBW).

In morbid obesity, dosage requirement may best be estimated using a dosing weight of IBW + 0.4 (TBW - IBW)

Initial and periodic peak and trough plasma drug levels should be determined, particularly in critically ill patients with serious infections or in disease states known to significantly alter aminoglycoside pharmacokinetics (eg, cystic fibrosis, burns, or major surgery)

Once daily dosing: Higher peak serum drug concentration to MIC ratios, demonstrated aminoglycoside postantibiotic effect, decreased renal cortex drug uptake, and improved cost-time efficiency are supportive reasons for the use of once daily dosing regimens for aminoglycosides. Current research indicates these regimens to be as effective for nonlife-threatening infections, with no higher incidence of nephrotoxicity, than those requiring multiple daily doses. Doses are determined by calculating the entire day's dose via usual multiple dose calculation techniques and administering this quantity as a single dose. Doses are then adjusted to maintain mean serum concentrations above the MIC(s) of the causative organism(s). (Example: 4.5-6 mg/kg as a single dose, adjusted to achieve an average serum level of 3-4 mcg/mL). Further research is needed for universal recommendation in all patient populations and gram-negative disease.

Neonates: I.M., I.V.:
    0-4 weeks:
        <1200 g: 2.5 mg/kg/dose every 18-24 hours
        1200-2000 g, 0-4 weeks: 2.5 mg/kg/dose every 12-18 hours
        >2000 g: 2.5 mg/kg/dose every 12 hours
(Continued)

Gentamicin Sulfate *(Continued)*

Postnatal age >7 days:
  1200-2000 g: 2.5 mg/kg/dose every 8-12 hours
  >2000 g: 2.5 mg/kg/dose every 8 hours
Newborns: Intrathecal: 1 mg every day
Infants and Children <5 years: I.M., I.V.: 2.5 mg/kg/dose every 8 hours•
  Cystic fibrosis: 2.5 mg/kg/dose every 6 hours
Children >5 years: I.M., I.V.: 1.5-2.5 mg/kg/dose every 8 hours•
  •Some patients may require larger or more frequent doses (eg, every 6 hours) if serum levels document the need (ie, cystic fibrosis or febrile granulocytopenic patients)
Intrathecal: >3 months: 1-2 mg/day

Adults: I.M., I.V.:
  Severe life-threatening infections: 2-2.5 mg/kg/dose
  Urinary tract infections: 1.5 mg/kg/dose
  Synergy (for gram-positive infections): 1 mg/kg/dose

Children and Adults:
  Intrathecal: 4-8 mg/day
  Ophthalmic:
    Ointment: Instill ½" (1.25 cm) 2-3 times/day to every 3-4 hours
    Solution: Instill 1-2 drops every 2-4 hours, up to 2 drops every hour for severe infections
  Topical: Apply 3-4 times/day to affected area

Dosing interval in renal impairment:
  Cl_{cr} ≥60 mL/minute: Administer every 8 hours
  Cl_{cr} 40-60 mL/minute: Administer every 12 hours
  Cl_{cr} 20-40 mL/minute: Administer every 24 hours
  Cl_{cr} 10-20 mL/minute: Administer every 48 hours
  Cl_{cr} <10 mL/minute: Administer every 72 hours
Dialyzable; removal by hemodialysis: 30% removal of aminoglycosides occurs during 4 hours of HD; administer dose after dialysis and follow levels
Removal by Continuous ambulatory peritoneal dialysis (CAPD):
  Administration via CAPD fluid:
  Gram-negative infection: 4-8 mg/L (4-8 mcg/mL) of CAPD fluid
  Gram-positive infection (ie, synergy): 3-4 mg/L (3-4 mcg/mL) of CAPD fluid
  Administration via I.V., I.M. route during CAPD: Dose as for Cl_{cr} <10 mL/minute and follow levels
  Removal via continuous arterio-venous or veno-venous hemofiltration (CAVH/CAVHD): Dose as for Cl_{cr} 10-15 mL/minute and follow levels

Dosing adjustment/comments in hepatic disease: Monitor plasma concentrations
Monitoring Parameters Urinalysis, urine output, BUN, serum creatinine; hearing should be tested before, during, and after treatment; particularly in those at risk for ototoxicity or who will be receiving prolonged therapy (>2 weeks)
Reference Range
Timing of serum samples: Draw peak 30 minutes after 30-minute infusion has been completed or 1 hour after I.M. injection; draw trough immediately before next dose
Sample size: 0.5-2 mL blood (red top tube) or 0.1-1 mL serum (separated)
Therapeutic levels:
  Peak:
    Serious infections: 6-8 µg/mL (12-17 µmol/L)
    Life-threatening infections: 8-10 µg/mL (17-21 µmol/L)
    Urinary tract infections: 4-6 µg/mL
    Synergy against gram-positive organisms: 3-5 µg/mL
  Trough:
    Serious infections: 0.5-1 µg/mL
    Life-threatening infections: 1-2 µg/mL
Monitor serum creatinine and urine output; obtain drug levels after the third dose unless renal dysfunction/toxicity suspected.
Test Interactions ↑ protein; ↓ magnesium; ↑ BUN, AST, GPT, alk phos, serum creatinine; ↓ potassium, sodium, calcium
Patient Information Report any dizziness or sensations of ringing or fullness in ears; do not touch ophthalmics to eye; use no other eye drops within 5-10 minutes of instilling ophthalmic
Nursing Implications Slower absorption and lower peak concentrations probably due to poor circulation in the atrophic muscle, may occur following I.M. injection in paralyzed patients (suggest I.V. route); aminoglycoside levels measured in blood taken from Silastic® central catheters can sometimes give falsely high readings (draw via separate lumen or peripheral site if possible,

otherwise flush very well). Monitor serum creatinine and urine output; obtain drug levels after the third dose unless otherwise directed (eg, suspected toxicity or renal dysfunction). Peak levels are drawn 30 minutes after the end of a 30-minute infusion or 60 minutes following I.M. injection; trough levels are drawn within 30 minutes before the next dose; give other antibiotic drugs at least 1 hour before or after gentamicin. Hearing should be tested before, during, and after treatment in patients at risk for ototoxicity.

Dosage Forms
Cream, topical: 0.1% (15 g)
Injection: 40 mg/mL (1 mL, 2 mL, 10 mL, 20 mL)
    Pediatric: 10 mg/mL (2 mL)
    Intrathecal: 2 mg/mL (2 mL)
Ointment:
    Ophthalmic: 0.3% (3.5 g)
    Topical: 0.1% (15 g)
Solution, ophthalmic: 0.3% (1 mL, 5 mL, 15 mL)

Gentian Violet (jen' shun)
Synonyms Crystal Violet; Methylrosaniline Chloride
Use Treatment of cutaneous or mucocutaneous infections caused by *Candida albicans* and other superficial skin infections - antibacterial and antifungal dye
Pregnancy Risk Factor C
Contraindications Known hypersensitivity to gentian violet; ulcerated areas; patients with porphyria
Warnings/Precautions Infants should be turned face down after application to minimize amount of drug swallowed; may result in tattooing of the skin when applied to granulation tissue; solution is for external use only; avoid contact with eyes
Adverse Reactions
1% to 10%:
    Local: Esophagitis, burning, irritation, vesicle formation, ulceration of mucous membranes
    Systemic: Sensitivity reactions, laryngitis, tracheitis, laryngeal obstruction
Overdosage/Toxicology Laryngeal obstruction
Mechanism of Action Topical antiseptic/germicide effective against some vegetative gram-positive bacteria, particularly *Staphylococcus* sp, and some yeast; it is much less effective against gram-negative bacteria and is ineffective against acid-fast bacteria
Usual Dosage Children and Adults: Topical: Apply 0.5% to 2% locally with cotton to lesion 2-3 times/day for 3 days, do not swallow and avoid contact with eyes
Patient Information Drug stains skin and clothing purple; do not apply to an ulcerative lesion; may result in "tattooing" of the skin.
Nursing Implications Should be applied to lesions only
Dosage Forms Solution, topical: 1% (30 mL); 2% (30 mL)

Glipizide (glip' i zide)
Related Information
Hypoglycemic Agents Comparison on page 1271
Brand Names Glucotrol®
Synonyms Glydiazinamide
(Continued)

503

Glipizide *(Continued)*

Use Management of noninsulin-dependent diabetes mellitus (type II)

Pregnancy Risk Factor C

Contraindications Hypersensitivity to glipizide or any component, other sulfonamides, type I diabetes mellitus

Warnings/Precautions Use with caution in patients with severe hepatic disease; a useful agent since few drug to drug interactions and not dependent upon renal elimination of active drug

Adverse Reactions
>10%:
   Central nervous system: Headache
   Gastrointestinal: Anorexia, nausea, vomiting, diarrhea, epigastric fullness, constipation, heartburn
1% to 10%: Dermatologic: Rash, hives, photosensitivity
<1%:
   Cardiovascular: Edema
   Endocrine & metabolic: Hypoglycemia, hyponatremia, hypoglycemia
   Genitourinary: Diuretic effect
   Hematologic: Blood dyscrasias, aplastic anemia, hemolytic anemia, bone marrow depression, thrombocytopenia, agranulocytosis
   Hepatic: Cholestatic jaundice

Overdosage/Toxicology Symptoms of overdose include low blood sugar, tingling of lips and tongue, nausea, yawning, confusion, agitation, tachycardia, sweating, convulsions, stupor, and coma; intoxications with sulfonylureas can cause hypoglycemia and are best managed with glucose administration (oral for milder hypoglycemia or by injection in more severe forms)

Drug Interactions
Decreased effects: Beta-blockers, cholestyramine, hydantoins, rifampin, thiazide diuretics, urinary alkalines, charcoal
Increased effects: H_2 antagonists, anticoagulants, androgens, fluconazole, salicylates, gemfibrozil, sulfonamides, tricyclic antidepressants, probenecid, MAO inhibitors, methyldopa, digitalis glycosides, urinary acidifiers
Increased toxicity: Cimetidine $\rightarrow$ ↑ hypoglycemic effects

Mechanism of Action Stimulates insulin release from the pancreatic beta cells; reduces glucose output from the liver; insulin sensitivity is increased at peripheral target sites

Pharmacodynamics/Kinetics
Duration of action: 12-24 hours
Peak blood glucose reductions: Within 1.5-2 hours
Protein binding: 92% to 99%
Absorption: Delayed when given with food
Metabolism: In the liver with metabolites (91% to 97%)
Half-life: 2-4 hours
Elimination: Metabolites (91% to 97%) excreted in urine (60% to 80%) and feces (11%)

Usual Dosage Oral (allow several days between dose titrations):
Adults: 2.5-40 mg/day; doses >15-20 mg/day should be divided and given twice daily
Elderly: Initial: 2.5-5 mg/day; increase by 2.5-5 mg/day at 1- to 2-week intervals

   Dosing adjustment/comments in renal impairment: Cl_{cr} <10 mL/minute: Some investigators recommend not using

   Dosing adjustment in hepatic impairment: Initial dosage should be 2.5 mg/day

Administration Administer 30 minutes before a meal to achieve greatest reduction in postprandial hyperglycemia

Monitoring Parameters Urine for glucose and ketones; monitor for signs and symptoms of hypoglycemia (fatigue, excessive hunger, profuse sweating, numbness of extremities), fasting blood glucose, hemoglobin A_{1c}, fructosamine

Reference Range Glucose:
Adults: 60-110 mg/dL
Elderly: 100-180 mg/dL

Patient Information Patients must be counseled by someone experienced in diabetes education, signs and symptoms of hyper- and hypoglycemia, exercise and diet, blood glucose monitoring, and other related topics; eat regularly, do not skip meals; carry quick source of sugar; medical alert bracelet

Nursing Implications Patients who are NPO may need to have their dose held to avoid hypoglycemia

Dosage Forms Tablet: 5 mg, 10 mg

Glucagon (gloo' ka gon)

Use Management of hypoglycemia; diagnostic aid in the radiologic examination of GI tract when a hypnotic state is needed; used with some success as a cardiac stimulant in management of severe cases of beta-adrenergic blocking agent overdosage

Pregnancy Risk Factor B

Contraindications Hypersensitivity to glucagon or any component

Warnings/Precautions Use with caution in patients with a history of insulinoma and/or pheochromocytoma

Adverse Reactions 1% to 10%:
Cardiovascular: Hypotension
Dermatologic: Urticaria
Gastrointestinal: Nausea, vomiting
Respiratory: Respiratory distress

Overdosage/Toxicology Symptoms of overdose include hypokalemia, nausea, vomiting

Drug Interactions Increased toxicity: Oral anticoagulant - hypoprothrombinemic effects may be increased possibly with bleeding

Stability After reconstitution, use immediately; may be kept at 5°C for up to 48 hours if necessary

Mechanism of Action Stimulates adenylate cyclase to produce increased cyclic AMP, which promotes hepatic glycogenolysis and gluconeogenesis, causing a raise in blood glucose levels

Pharmacodynamics/Kinetics
Peak effect on blood glucose levels: Parenteral: Within 5-20 minutes
Duration of action: 60-90 minutes
Metabolism: In the liver with some inactivation occurring in the kidneys and plasma
Half-life, plasma: 3-10 minutes

Usual Dosage
Hypoglycemia or insulin shock therapy: I.M., I.V., S.C.:
Neonates: 0.3 mg/kg/dose; maximum: 1 mg/dose
Children: 0.025-0.1 mg/kg/dose, not to exceed 1 mg/dose, repeated in 20 minutes as needed
Adults: 0.5-1 mg, may repeat in 20 minutes as needed
If patient fails to respond to glucagon, I.V. dextrose must be given
Diagnostic aid: Adults: I.M., I.V.: 0.25-2 mg 10 minutes prior to procedure

Administration Reconstitute powder for injection by adding 1 or 10 mL of sterile diluent to a vial containing 1 or 10 units of the drug, respectively, to provide solutions containing 1 mg of glucagon/mL; if dose to be administered is <2 mg of the drug → use only the diluent provided by the manufacturer; if >2 mg → use sterile water for injection; use immediately after reconstitution

Monitoring Parameters Blood pressure, blood glucose

Patient Information Instruct a close associate on how to prepare and administer as a treatment for insulin shock

Additional Information 1 unit = 1 mg

Dosage Forms Powder for injection, lyophilized: 1 mg [1 unit]; 10 mg [10 units]

Glucocerebrosidase see Alglucerase on page 40

Glucophage® see Metformin Hydrochloride on page 700

Glucotrol® see Glipizide on page 503

Glukor® see Chorionic Gonadotropin on page 242

Glyate® [OTC] see Guaifenesin on page 515

Glybenclamide see Glyburide on this page

Glybenzcyclamide see Glyburide on this page

Glyburide (glye' byoor ide)

Related Information
Hypoglycemic Agents Comparison on page 1271

Brand Names Diaβeta®; Glynase™ PresTab™; Micronase®

Synonyms Glibenclamide; Glybenclamide; Glybenzcyclamide

Use Management of noninsulin-dependent diabetes mellitus (type II)

Pregnancy Risk Factor D

Contraindications Hypersensitivity to glyburide or any component, or other sulfonamides; type I diabetes mellitus

Warnings/Precautions Use with caution in patients with hepatic impairment. Elderly: Rapid and prolonged hypoglycemia (>12 hours) despite hypertonic glucose injections have been reported; age and hepatic and renal impairment are
(Continued)

505

Glyburide *(Continued)*

independent risk factors for hypoglycemia; dosage titration should be made at weekly intervals. Use with caution in patients with renal and hepatic impairment.

Adverse Reactions

>10%:

Central nervous system: Headache, anorexia, dizziness

Gastrointestinal: Nausea, epigastric fullness, heartburn, constipation, diarrhea, anorexia

1% to 10%:

Dermatologic: Pruritus, rash, hives, photosensitivity reaction

<1%:

Endocrine & metabolic: Hypoglycemia

Genitourinary: Nocturia, diuretic effect

Hematologic: Leukopenia, thrombocytopenia, hemolytic anemia, aplastic anemia, bone marrow depression, agranulocytosis

Hepatic: Cholestatic jaundice

Neuromuscular & skeletal: Joint pain, paresthesia

Overdosage/Toxicology Symptoms of overdose include low blood sugar, tingling of lips and tongue, nausea, yawning, confusion, agitation, tachycardia, sweating, convulsions, stupor, and coma; intoxications with sulfonylureas can cause hypoglycemia and are best managed with glucose administration (oral for milder hypoglycemia or by injection in more severe forms)

Drug Interactions

Decreased effect: Thiazides and beta-blockers → ↓ effectiveness of glyburide

Increased toxicity:

Since this agent is highly protein bound, the toxic potential is increased when given concomitantly with other highly protein bound drugs (ie, phenylbutazole, oral anticoagulants, hydantoins, salicylates, NSAIDs, sulfonamides) - increased hypoglycemic effect

Alcohol → disulfiram reactions

Phenylbutazone can increase hypoglycemic effects

Mechanism of Action Stimulates insulin release from the pancreatic beta cells; reduces glucose output from the liver; insulin sensitivity is increased at peripheral target sites

Pharmacodynamics/Kinetics

Onset of action: Oral: Insulin levels in the serum begin to increase within 15-60 minutes after a single dose

Duration: Up to 24 hours

Metabolism: To one moderately active and several inactive metabolites

Plasma protein binding: High (>99%)

Half-life: 5-16 hours; may be prolonged with renal insufficiency or hepatic insufficiency

Time to peak serum concentration: Adults: Within 2-4 hours

Usual Dosage Oral:

Adults: 1.25-5 mg to start then increase at weekly intervals to 1.25-20 mg maintenance dose/day divided in 1-2 doses

Elderly: Initial: 1.25-2.5 mg/day, increase by 1.25-2.5 mg/day every 1-3 weeks

Prestab™: Initial: 0.75-3 mg/day, increase by 1.5 mg/day in weekly intervals, maximum: 12 mg/day

Dosing adjustment/comments in renal impairment:

Cl_{cr} 10-50 mL/minute: Use conservative initial and maintenance doses

Cl_{cr} <10 mL/minute: Avoid use

Dosing adjustment in hepatic impairment: Use conservative initial and maintenance doses and avoid use in severe disease

Monitoring Parameters Signs and symptoms of hypoglycemia, fasting blood glucose, hemoglobin A_{1c}, fructosamine

Reference Range Glucose:

Adults: 80-110 mg/dL

Elderly: 100-180 mg/dL

Patient Information Patients must be counseled by someone experienced in diabetes education, signs and symptoms of hyper- and hypoglycemia, exercise and diet, blood glucose monitoring, and other related topics; eat regularly, do not skip meals; carry quick source of sugar; medical alert bracelet

Nursing Implications Patients who are anorexic or NPO, may need to have their dose held to avoid hypoglycemia

Dosage Forms

Tablet (Diaβeta®, Micronase®): 1.25 mg, 2.5 mg, 5 mg

Tablet, micronized (Glynase™ PresTab™): 1.5 mg, 3 mg

Glycate® [OTC] *see* Calcium Carbonate *on page 161*

Glycerin (glis' er in)

Related Information
Laxatives, Classification and Properties *on page 1272*

Brand Names Fleet® Babylax® [OTC]; Ophthalgan®; Osmoglyn®; Sani-Supp® [OTC]

Synonyms Glycerol

Use Constipation; reduction of intraocular pressure; reduction of corneal edema; glycerin has been administered orally to reduce intracranial pressure

Pregnancy Risk Factor C

Contraindications Known hypersensitivity to glycerin or any ingredients, anuria, pulmonary edema, severe dehydration

Warnings/Precautions Safety and efficacy of ophthalmic solution in children have not been established. The primary use of glycerin in the elderly is as a laxative, although it is not recommended as a first-line treatment. Oral: Use cautiously in hypovolemia, confused mental state, congestive heart failure, elderly, senile, diabetic, and severely dehydrated patients.

Adverse Reactions
>10%:
  Central nervous system: Headache
  Gastrointestinal: Vomiting
1% to 10%:
  Central nervous system: Dizziness, confusion
  Endocrine & metabolic: Polydipsia
  Gastrointestinal: Diarrhea, nausea, tenesmus, dry mouth, thirst
<1%:
  Cardiovascular: Arrhythmias
  Endocrine & metabolic: Hyperglycemia
  Local: Pain, rectal irritation, burning, cramping pain

Stability
Refrigerate suppositories; protect from heat; freezing should be avoided
Ophthalmic: Keep bottle tightly closed; store at room temperature; discard 6 months after dropper is first placed in the solution

Mechanism of Action Osmotic dehydrating agent which increases osmotic pressure; draws fluid into colon and thus stimulates evacuation

Pharmacodynamics/Kinetics
Absorption:
  Oral: Well absorbed
  Rectal: Poorly absorbed
Decrease in intraocular pressure: Oral:
  Onset of action: Within 10-30 minutes
  Peak effect: Within 60-90 minutes
  Duration: 4-8 hours
Reduction of intracranial pressure: Oral:
  Onset of action: Within 10-60 minutes
  Peak effect: Within 60-90 minutes
  Duration: ~2-3 hours
Constipation: Suppository: Onset of action: 15-30 minutes
Metabolism: Primarily in the liver with 20% metabolized in the kidney
Half-life: 30-45 minutes
Elimination: Only a small percentage of drug is excreted unchanged in the urine

Usual Dosage
Constipation: Rectal:
  Neonates: 0.5 mL/kg/dose
  Children <6 years: 1 infant suppository 1-2 times/day as needed or 2-5 mL as an enema
  Children >6 years and Adults: 1 adult suppository 1-2 times/day as needed or 5-15 mL as an enema
Children and Adults:
  Reduction of intraocular pressure: Oral: 1-1.8 g/kg 1-1½ hours preoperatively; additional doses may be administered at 5-hour intervals
  Reduction of intracranial pressure: Oral: 1.5 g/kg/day divided every 4 hours; 1 g/kg/dose every 6 hours has also been used
  Reduction of corneal edema: Ophthalmic solution: Instill 1-2 drops in eye(s) prior to examination OR for lubricant effect, instill 1-2 drops in eye(s) every 3-4 hours

Patient Information Do not use if experiencing abdominal pain, nausea, or vomiting

Nursing Implications Apply topical anesthetic before instilling ophthalmic drops. Use caution during insertion of suppository to avoid intestinal perforation, especially in neonates; suppository needs to melt to provide laxative effect; primary use of glycerin in the elderly is as a laxative, although it is not recommended as a first line treatment.

(Continued)

Glycerin (Continued)

Dosage Forms
Solution:
Ophthalmic, sterile (Ophthalgan®): Glycerin with chlorobutanol 0.55% (7.5 mL)
Oral (lime flavor)(Osmoglyn®): 50% (220 mL)
Rectal (Fleet Babylax®): 4 mL/applicator (6s)
Suppository, rectal (Sani-Supp®): Glycerin with sodium stearate (infant and adult sizes)

Glycerol see Glycerin on page 506

Glycerol Guaiacolate see Guaifenesin on page 515

Glyceryl Trinitrate see Nitroglycerin on page 799

Glycopyrrolate (glye koe pye' roe late)
Brand Names Robinul®; Robinul® Forte
Synonyms Glycopyrronium Bromide
Use Adjunct in treatment of peptic ulcer disease; inhibit salivation and excessive secretions of the respiratory tract preoperatively; reversal of neuromuscular blockade; control of upper airway secretions
Pregnancy Risk Factor B
Contraindications Narrow-angle glaucoma, acute hemorrhage, tachycardia, hypersensitivity to glycopyrrolate or any component; ulcerative colitis, obstructive uropathy, paralytic ileus, obstructive disease of GI tract
Warnings/Precautions Not recommended in children <12 years of age for the management of peptic ulcer; infants, patients with Down syndrome, and children with spastic paralysis or brain damage may be hypersensitive to antimuscarine effects. Use caution in elderly, patients with autonomic neuropathy, hepatic or renal disease, ulcerative colitis may predispose megacolon, hyperthyroidism, CAD, CHF, arrhythmias, tachycardia, BPH, hiatal hernia, with reflux.
Adverse Reactions
>10%:
Gastrointestinal: Constipation
Local: Irritation at injection site
Miscellaneous: Decreased sweating, dry mouth, nose, throat, or skin
1% to 10%: Decreased flow of breast milk, difficulty in swallowing, increased sensitivity to light
<1%:
Cardiovascular: Orthostatic hypotension, ventricular fibrillation, tachycardia, palpitations
Central nervous system: Confusion, drowsiness, headache, loss of memory, weakness, tiredness, ataxia
Dermatologic: Skin rash
Gastrointestinal: Bloated feeling, nausea, vomiting
Genitourinary: Difficult urination
Ocular: Increased intraocular pain, blurred vision
Overdosage/Toxicology Symptoms of overdose include blurred vision, urinary retention, tachycardia, absent bowel sounds. Anticholinergic toxicity is caused by strong binding of the drug to cholinergic receptors. For anticholinergic overdose with severe life-threatening symptoms, physostigmine 1-2 mg (0.5 or 0.02 mg/kg for children) S.C. or I.V., slowly may be given to reverse these effects.
Drug Interactions
Decreased effect of levodopa
Increased toxicity with amantadine, cyclopropane
Stability Unstable at pH >6; **incompatible** with secobarbital (immediate precipitation), sodium bicarbonate (gas evolves), thiopental (immediate precipitation)
Mechanism of Action Blocks the action of acetylcholine at parasympathetic sites in smooth muscle, secretory glands, and the CNS
Pharmacodynamics/Kinetics
Oral:
Onset of action: Within 50 minutes
Peak effect: Within 1 hour
I.M.: Onset of action: 20-40 minutes
I.V.: Onset of action: 10-15 minutes
Absorption: Oral: Poor and erratic
Bioavailability: ~10%
Usual Dosage
Children: Control of secretions:
Oral: 40-100 mcg/kg/dose 3-4 times/day
I.M., I.V.: 4-10 mcg/kg/dose every 3-4 hours; maximum: 0.2 mg/dose or 0.8 mg/24 hours

Children:
   Intraoperative: I.V.: 4 mcg/kg not to exceed 0.1 mg; repeat at 2- to 3-minute
      intervals as needed
   Preoperative: I.M.:
      <2 years: 4.4-8.8 mcg/kg 30-60 minutes before procedure
      >2 years: 4.4 mcg/kg 30-60 minutes before procedure

Children and Adults: Reverse neuromuscular blockade: I.V.: 0.2 mg for each 1
   mg of neostigmine or 5 mg of pyridostigmine administered

Adults:
   Intraoperative: I.V.: 0.1 mg repeated as needed at 2- to 3-minute intervals
   Peptic ulcer:
      Oral: 1-2 mg 2-3 times/day
      I.M., I.V.: 0.1-0.2 mg 3-4 times/day
   Preoperative: I.M.: 4.4 mcg/kg 30-60 minutes before procedure
Administration For I.V. administration, glycopyrrolate may also be administered
   via the tubing of a running I.V. infusion of a compatible solution
Patient Information Maintain good oral hygiene habits, because lack of saliva
   may increase chance of cavities. Observe caution while driving or performing
   other tasks requiring alertness, as may cause drowsiness, dizziness, or blurred
   vision. Notify physician if skin rash, flushing or eye pain occurs; or if difficulty in
   urinating, constipation, or sensitivity to light becomes severe or persists.
Dosage Forms
   Injection (Robinul®): 0.2 mg/mL (1 mL, 2 mL, 5 mL, 20 mL)
   Tablet:
      Robinul®: 1 mg
      Robinul® Forte: 2 mg

Glycopyrronium Bromide see Glycopyrrolate on previous page

Glycotuss-DM® [OTC] see Guaifenesin and Dextromethorphan on
page 517

Glycotuss® [OTC] see Guaifenesin on page 515

Glydiazinamide see Glipizide on page 503

Glynase™ PresTab™ see Glyburide on page 505

Gly-Oxide® [OTC] see Carbamide Peroxide on page 179

Glytuss® [OTC] see Guaifenesin on page 515

GM-CSF see Sargramostim on page 994

GnRH see Gonadorelin on next page

Gold Sodium Thiomalate (gold sow' dee um thio mal' ate)
Brand Names Myochrysine®
Use Treatment of progressive rheumatoid arthritis
Pregnancy Risk Factor C
Contraindications Hypersensitivity to gold compounds or any component;
   systemic lupus erythematosus; history of blood dyscrasias; congestive heart
   failure, exfoliative dermatitis, colitis
Warnings/Precautions
   Frequent monitoring of patients for signs and symptoms of toxicity will prevent
   serious adverse reactions; nonsteroidal anti-inflammatory drugs (NSAIDs) and
   corticosteroids may be discontinued after initiating gold therapy; must not be
   injected I.V.
   Explain the possibility of adverse reactions before initiating therapy; signs of gold
   toxicity include decrease in hemoglobin, leukopenia, granulocytes and platelets; proteinuria, hematuria, pigmentation, pruritus, stomatitis or persistent diarrhea, rash, metallic taste; advise patient to report any symptoms of toxicity; use
   with caution in patients with liver or renal disease
Adverse Reactions
   >10%:
      Dermatologic: Itching, skin rash
      Gastrointestinal: Stomatitis, gingivitis, glossitis
      Ocular: Conjunctivitis
   1% to 10%:
      Dermatologic: Hives, alopecia
      Hematologic: Eosinophilia, leukopenia, thrombocytopenia, hematuria
      Renal: Proteinuria
   <1%:
      Dermatologic: Angioedema
      Gastrointestinal: Ulcerative enterocolitis, GI hemorrhage, metallic taste
      Hematologic: Agranulocytosis, anemia, aplastic anemia
(Continued)

Gold Sodium Thiomalate *(Continued)*

    Hepatic: Hepatotoxicity
    Neuromuscular & skeletal: Peripheral neuropathy
    Respiratory: Interstitial pneumonitis
    Miscellaneous: Difficulty in swallowing

Overdosage/Toxicology Symptoms of overdose include hematuria, proteinuria, fever, nausea, vomiting, diarrhea; for mild gold poisoning, dimercaprol 2.5 mg/kg 4 times/day for 2 days or for more severe forms of gold intoxication, dimercaprol 3-5 mg/kg every 4 hours for 2 days should be initiated; then after 2 days, the initial dose should be repeated twice daily on the third day, and once daily thereafter for 10 days. Other chelating agents have been used with some success.

Drug Interactions Decreased effect with penicillamine, acetylcysteine

Stability Should not be used if solution is darker than pale yellow

Mechanism of Action Unknown, may decrease prostaglandin synthesis or may alter cellular mechanisms by inhibiting sulfhydryl systems

Pharmacodynamics/Kinetics
    Half-life: 5 days; may lengthen with multiple doses
    Time to peak serum concentration: Within 4-6 hours
    Elimination: Majority (60% to 90%) excreted in urine with smaller amounts (10% to 40%) excreted in feces (via bile)

Usual Dosage I.M.:
    Children: Initial: Test dose of 10 mg is recommended, followed by 1 mg/kg/week for 20 weeks; maintenance: 1 mg/kg/dose at 2- to 4-week intervals thereafter for as long as therapy is clinically beneficial and toxicity does not develop. Administration for 2-4 months is usually required before clinical improvement is observed.
    Adults: 10 mg first week; 25 mg second week; then 25-50 mg/week until 1 g cumulative dose has been given; if improvement occurs without adverse reactions, give 25-50 mg every 2-3 weeks for 2-20 weeks, then every 3-4 weeks indefinitely

    Dosing adjustment in renal impairment:
    Cl_{cr} 50-80 mL/minute: Administer 50% of normal dose
    Cl_{cr} <50 mL/minute: Avoid use

Administration Deep I.M. injection into the upper outer quadrant of the gluteal region addition of 0.1 mL of 1% lidocaine to each injection may reduce the discomfort associated with I.M. administration

Monitoring Parameters Signs and symptoms of gold toxicity, CBC with differential and platelet count, urinalysis

Reference Range Gold: Normal: 0-0.1 μg/mL (SI: 0-0.0064 μmol/L); Therapeutic: 1-3 μg/mL (SI: 0.06-0.18 μmol/L); Urine: <0.1 μg/24 hour

Patient Information Minimize exposure to sunlight; benefits from drug therapy may take as long as 3 months to appear; notify physician of pruritus, rash, sore mouth; metallic taste may occur

Nursing Implications Explain the possibility of adverse reactions before initiating therapy

Additional Information Approximately 50% gold

Dosage Forms Injection: 25 mg/mL (1 mL); 50 mg/mL (1 mL, 10 mL)

GoLYTELY® *see* Polyethylene Glycol-Electrolyte Solution *on* page 900

Gonadorelin *(goe nad oh rell′ in)*

Brand Names Factrel®; Lutrepulse®

Synonyms GnRH; Gonadorelin Acetate; Gonadorelin HCl; Gonadotropin Releasing Hormone; LH-RH; LRH; Luteinizing Hormone Releasing Hormone

Use Evaluation of the functional capacity and response of gonadotrophic hormones; evaluate abnormal gonadotropin regulation as in precocious puberty and delayed puberty. Lutrepulse®: Induction of ovulation in females with hypothalamic amenorrhea.

Pregnancy Risk Factor B

Contraindications Known hypersensitivity to gonadorelin, women with any condition that could be exacerbated by pregnancy; patients who have ovarian cysts or causes of anovulation other than those of hypothalamic origin; any condition that may worsened by reproductive hormones

Warnings/Precautions Hypersensitivity and anaphylactic reactions have occurred following multiple-dose administration; multiple pregnancy is a possibility; use with caution in women in whom pregnancy could worsen preexisting conditions (eg, pituitary prolactinemia). Multiple pregnancy is a possibility with Lutrepulse®.

Adverse Reactions
1% to 10%: Local: Pain at injection site
<1%:
Cardiovascular: Flushing
Central nervous system: Light headedness, headache
Dermatologic: Skin rash
Gastrointestinal: Nausea, abdominal discomfort

Overdosage/Toxicology Symptoms of overdose include abdominal discomfort, nausea, headache, flushing; symptomatic treatment

Drug Interactions
Decreased levels/effect: Oral contraceptives, digoxin, phenothiazines, dopamine antagonists
Increased levels/effect: Androgens, estrogens, progestins, glucocorticoids, spironolactone, levodopa

Stability
Factrel®: Prepare immediately prior to use; after reconstitution, store at room temperature and use within 1 day; discard unused portion
Lutrepulse®: Store at room temperature; reconstitute with diluent immediately prior to use and transfer to plastic reservoir. The solution will supply 90 minute pulsatile doses for 7 consecutive days (Lutrepulse® pump).

Mechanism of Action Stimulates the release of luteinizing hormone (LH) from the anterior pituitary gland

Pharmacodynamics/Kinetics
Peak effect: Maximal LH release occurs within 20 minutes
Duration of action: 3-5 hours
Half-life: 4 minutes

Usual Dosage
Diagnostic test: Children >12 years and Adults (female): I.V., S.C. hydrochloride salt: 100 mcg administered in women during early phase of menstrual cycle (day 1-7)
Primary hypothalamic amenorrhea: Female adults: Acetate: I.V.: 5 mcg every 90 minutes via Lutrepulse® pump kit at treatment intervals of 21 days (pump will pulsate every 90 minutes for 7 days)

Administration
Factrel®: Dilute in 3 mL of normal saline; give I.V. push over 30 seconds
Lutrepulse®: A presterilized reservoir bag with the infusion catheter set supplied with the kit should be filled with the reconstituted solution and administered I.V. using the Lutrepulse® pump. Set the pump to deliver 25-50 mL of solution, based upon the dose, over a pulse period of 1 minute and at a pulse frequency of 90 minutes.

Monitoring Parameters LH, FSH

Dosage Forms
Injection, as acetate (Lutrepulse®): 0.8 mg, 3.2 mg
Injection, as hydrochloride (Factrel®): 100 mcg, 500 mcg

Gonadorelin Acetate *see* Gonadorelin *on previous page*

Gonadorelin HCl *see* Gonadorelin *on previous page*

Gonadotropin Releasing Hormone *see* Gonadorelin *on previous page*

Gonic® *see* Chorionic Gonadotropin *on page 242*

Goserelin Acetate (goe' se rel in)
Related Information
Cancer Chemotherapy Regimens *on page 1218-1241*

Brand Names Zoladex®

Use Palliative treatment of advanced prostate cancer; a synthetic analog of luteinizing hormone-releasing hormone also known as gonadotropin-releasing hormone (GnRH); GnRH has also been used to induce ovulation or to treat endometriosis.

Pregnancy Risk Factor X

Contraindications In women who are or may become pregnant, patients who are hypersensitive to the drug

Warnings/Precautions Initially, goserelin transiently increases serum levels of testosterone. Transient worsening of signs and symptoms, usually manifested by an increase in cancer-related pain which was managed symptomatically, may develop during the first few weeks of treatment. Isolated cases of ureteral obstruction and spinal cord compression have been reported; patient's symptoms may initially worsen temporarily during first few weeks of therapy, cancer-related pain can usually be controlled by analgesics.

Adverse Reactions
General: Worsening of signs and symptoms may occur during the first few weeks of therapy and are usually manifested by an increase in bone pain, increased
(Continued)

Goserelin Acetate *(Continued)*

difficulty in urinating, hot flashes, injection site irritation, and weakness; this will subside, but patients should be aware

>10%:

Endocrine & metabolic: Gynecomastia, postmenopausal symptoms, sexual dysfunction, loss of libido, hot flashes

Genitourinary: Impotence, decreased erection

1% to 10%:

Cardiovascular: Edema

Central nervous system: Headache, spinal cord compression (possible result of tumor flare), lethargy, dizziness, sweating, insomnia

Dermatologic: Rash

Gastrointestinal: Nausea and vomiting, anorexia, diarrhea, weight gain

Genitourinary: Vaginal spotting and breakthrough bleeding, breast tenderness/enlargement

Local: Pain on injection

Neuromuscular & skeletal: Bone loss, increased bone pain

Overdosage/Toxicology Symptomatic management

Stability Zoladex® should be stored at room temperature not to exceed 25°C or 77°F; must be dispensed in an amber bag

Mechanism of Action LHRH synthetic analog of luteinizing hormone-releasing hormone also known as gonadotropin-releasing hormone (GnRH) incorporated into a biodegradable depot material which allows for continuous slow release over 28 days; mechanism of action is similar to leuprolide

Pharmacodynamics/Kinetics

Absorption:

Oral: Inactive when administered orally

S.C.: Rapid and can be detected in the serum in 10 minutes

Distribution: V_d: 13.7 L

Time to peak serum concentration: S.C.: 12-15 days

Half-life: Following a bolus S.C. dose: 5 hours

Elimination: By the kidney; elimination time: 4.2 hours (prolonged in impaired renal function - 12 hours)

Usual Dosage

Adults: S.C.: 3.6 mg injected into upper abdomen every 28 days; do not try to aspirate with the goserelin syringe, if the needle is in a large vessel, blood will immediately appear in syringe chamber

Prostate carcinoma: Intended for long-term administration

Endometriosis: Recommended duration is 6 months; retreatment is not recommended since safety data is not available

Administration

Do not remove the sterile syringe until immediately before use.

After cleaning with an alcohol swab, a local anesthetic may be used on an area of skin on the upper abdominal wall.

Stretch the patient's skin with one hand, and grip the needle with fingers around the barrel of the syringe. Insert the hypodermic needle into the SC fat. Do not aspirate. If the hypodermic needle penetrates a large vessel, blood will be seen instantly in the syringe chamber.

Change the direction of the needle so it parallels the abdominal wall. Push the needle in until the barrel hub touches the patient's skin. Withdraw the needle 1 cm to create a space to discharge the drug; fully depress the plunger to discharge.

Withdraw needle and bandage the site. Confirm discharge by ensuring tip of the plunger is visible within the tip of the needle.

Test Interactions Serum alkaline phosphatase, serum acid phosphatase, serum testosterone, serum LH and FSH, serum estradiol

Patient Information Females must use reliable contraception during therapy; symptoms may worsen temporarily during first weeks of therapy

Dosage Forms Injection: 3.6 mg single dose disposable syringe with 16-gauge hypodermic needle

Granisetron (gra ni' se tron)

Brand Names Kytril®

Use Prophylaxis and treatment of chemotherapy-related emesis; may be prescribed for patients who are refractory to or have severe adverse reactions to standard antiemetic therapy. Granisetron may be prescribed for young patients (ie, <45 years of age who are more likely to develop extrapyramidal reactions to high-dose metoclopramide) who are to receive highly emetogenic chemotherapeutic agents as listed:

Agents with high emetogenic potential (>90%) (dose/m^2):
  Carmustine ≥200 mg
  Cisplatin ≥75 mg
  Cyclophosphamide ≥1000 mg
  Cytarabine ≥1000 mg
  Dacarbazine ≥500 mg
  Ifosfamide ≥1000 mg
  Lomustine ≥60 mg
  Mechlorethamine
  Pentostatin
  Streptozocin

or two agents classified as having high or moderately high emetogenic potential as listed:

Agents with moderately high emetogenic potential (60% to 90%) (dose/m^2):
  Carmustine <200 mg
  Cisplatin <75 mg
  Cyclophosphamide 1000 mg
  Cytarabine 250-1000 mg
  Dacarbazine <500 mg
  Doxorubicin ≥75 mg
  Ifosfamide
  Lomustine <60 mg
  Methotrexate ≥250 mg
  Mitomycin
  Mitoxantrone
  Procarbazine

Granisetron should not be prescribed for chemotherapeutic agents with a low emetogenic potential (eg, bleomycin, busulfan, cyclophosphamide <1000 mg, etoposide, 5-fluorouracil, vinblastine, vincristine)

Contraindications Previous hypersensitivity to granisetron

Warnings/Precautions Use with caution in patients with liver disease or in pregnant patients

Adverse Reactions
>10%: Central nervous system: Headache
1% to 10%:
  Central nervous system: Asthenia, dizziness, insomnia, anxiety
  Gastrointestinal: Constipation, abdominal pain, diarrhea
  Hematologic: Transient blood pressure changes
<1%:
  Cardiovascular: Arrhythmias
  Central nervous system: Somnolence, agitation, weakness
  Endocrine & metabolic: Hot flashes
  Hepatic: Liver enzyme elevations

Stability IV: Stable when mixed in NS or D$_5$W for 24 hours at room temperature; protect from light; do not freeze vials

Mechanism of Action Selective 5-HT$_3$ receptor antagonist, blocking serotonin, both peripherally on vagal nerve terminals and centrally in the chemoreceptor trigger zone

Pharmacodynamics/Kinetics
Onset of action: Commonly controls emesis within 1-3 minutes of administration
Duration: Effects generally last no more than 24 hours maximum
Distribution: V$_d$: 2-3 L/kg; widely distributed throughout the body
Half-life:
  Cancer patients: 10-12 hours
  Healthy volunteers: 3-4 hours
Elimination: Primarily nonrenal, 8% to 15% of a dose is excreted unchanged in urine

Usual Dosage
  I.V.: Children and Adults: 10 mcg/kg for 1-3 doses. Doses should be administered as a single IVPB over 5 minutes to 1 hour, given just prior to chemotherapy (15-60 minutes before); as intervention therapy for breakthrough nausea and vomiting, during the first 24 hours following chemotherapy, 2 or 3 repeat infusions (same dose) have been administered, separated by at least 10 minutes
  Oral: Adults: 1 mg twice daily; the first 1 mg dose should be given up to 1 hour before chemotherapy, and the second tablet, 12 hours after the first
  Note: Granisetron should only be given on the day(s) of chemotherapy

Dosing interval in renal impairment: Creatinine clearance values have no relationship to granisetron clearance
(Continued)

Granisetron *(Continued)*

Dosing interval in hepatic impairment: Kinetic studies in patients with hepatic impairment showed that total clearance was approximately halved, however, standard doses were very well tolerated

Nursing Implications Doses should be given at least 15 minutes prior to initiation of chemotherapy

Dosage Forms
Injection: 1 mg/mL
Tablet: 1 mg (2s), (20s)

Granulocyte Colony Stimulating Factor *see* Filgrastim *on page 454*

Granulocyte-Macrophage Colony Stimulating Factor *see* Sargramostim *on page 994*

Grifulvin® V *see* Griseofulvin *on this page*

Grisactin® *see* Griseofulvin *on this page*

Grisactin® Ultra *see* Griseofulvin *on this page*

Griseofulvin *(gri see oh ful' vin)*

Brand Names Fulvicin® P/G; Fulvicin-U/F®; Grifulvin® V; Grisactin®; Grisactin® Ultra; Gris-PEG®

Synonyms Griseofulvin Microsize; Griseofulvin Ultramicrosize

Use Treatment of susceptible tinea infections of the skin, hair, and nails

Pregnancy Risk Factor C

Contraindications Hypersensitivity to griseofulvin or any component; severe liver disease, porphyria (interferes with porphyrin metabolism)

Warnings/Precautions Safe use in children <2 years of age has not been established; during long-term therapy, periodic assessment of hepatic, renal, and hematopoietic functions should be performed; may cause fetal harm when administered to pregnant women; avoid exposure to intense sunlight to prevent photosensitivity reactions; hypersensitivity cross reaction between penicillins and griseofulvin is possible

Adverse Reactions
>10%: Dermatologic: Skin rash, urticaria
1% to 10%:
 Central nervous system: Headache, fatigue, dizziness, insomnia, mental confusion
 Dermatologic: Photosensitivity
 Gastrointestinal: Nausea, vomiting, epigastric distress, diarrhea
 Miscellaneous: Oral thrush
<1%:
 Endocrine & metabolic: Menstrual toxicity
 Gastrointestinal: GI bleeding
 Hematologic: Leukopenia
 Hepatic: Hepatic toxicity
 Renal: Proteinuria, nephrosis
 Miscellaneous: Angioneurotic edema

Overdosage/Toxicology Symptoms of overdose include lethargy, vertigo, blurred vision, nausea, vomiting, diarrhea; following GI decontamination, treatment is supportive

Drug Interactions
Decreased effect:
 Barbiturates → ↓ levels
 Decreased warfarin activity
 Decreased oral contraceptive effectiveness
Increased toxicity: With alcohol → tachycardia and flushing

Mechanism of Action Inhibits fungal cell mitosis at metaphase; binds to human keratin making it resistant to fungal invasion

Pharmacodynamics/Kinetics
Absorption: Ultramicrosize griseofulvin absorption is almost complete; absorption of microsize griseofulvin is variable (25% to 70% of an oral dose); absorption is enhanced by ingestion of a fatty meal
Distribution: Crosses the placenta
Metabolism: Extensive in the liver
Half-life: 9-22 hours
Elimination: <1% excreted unchanged in urine; also excreted in feces and perspiration

Usual Dosage Oral:
Children:
 Microsize: 10-15 mg/kg/day in single or divided doses
 Ultramicrosize: >2 months: 5.5-7.3 mg/kg/day in single or divided doses

Adults:
Microsize: 500-1000 mg/day in single or divided doses
Ultramicrosize: 330-375 mg/day in single or divided doses; doses up to 750 mg/day have been used for infections more difficult to eradicate such as tinea unguium and tinea pedis

Duration of therapy depends on the site of infection:
Tinea corporis: 2-4 weeks
Tinea capitis: 4-6 weeks or longer
Tinea pedis: 4-8 weeks
Tinea unguium: 4-6 months

Monitoring Parameters Periodic renal, hepatic, and hematopoietic function tests

Test Interactions False-positive urinary VMA levels

Patient Information Avoid exposure to sunlight, take with fatty meal; if patient gets headache, it usually goes away with continued therapy; may cause dizziness, drowsiness, and impair judgment; do not take if pregnant; if you become pregnant, discontinue immediately

Additional Information
Microsize: Fulvicin-U/F®, Grifulvin® V, Grisactin®
Ultramicrosize: Fulvicin® P/G, Grisactin® Ultra, Gris-PEG®; GI absorption of ultramicrosize is ~1.5 times that of microsize

Dosage Forms
Microsize:
Capsule (Grisactin®): 125 mg, 250 mg
Suspension, oral (Grifulvin® V): 125 mg/5 mL with alcohol 0.2% (120 mL)
Tablet:
Fulvicin-U/F®, Grifulvin® V: 250 mg
Fulvicin-U/F®, Grifulvin® V, Grisactin-500®: 500 mg
Ultramicrosize:
Tablet:
Fulvicin® P/G: 165 mg, 330 mg
Fulvicin® P/G, Grisactin® Ultra, Gris-PEG®: 125 mg, 250 mg
Grisactin® Ultra: 330 mg

Griseofulvin Microsize *see* Griseofulvin *on previous page*

Griseofulvin Ultramicrosize *see* Griseofulvin *on previous page*

Gris-PEG® *see* Griseofulvin *on previous page*

Growth Hormone *see* Human Growth Hormone *on page 538*

Guaifenesin (gwye fen' e sin)

Brand Names Amonidrin® [OTC]; Anti-Tuss® Expectorant [OTC]; Breonesin® [OTC]; Fenesin™; Gee Gee® [OTC]; Genatuss® [OTC]; GG-Cen® [OTC]; Glyate® [OTC]; Glycotuss® [OTC]; Glytuss® [OTC]; Guiatuss® [OTC]; Halotussin® [OTC]; Humibid® L.A.; Humibid® Sprinkle; Hytuss-2X® [OTC]; Hytuss® [OTC]; Malotuss® [OTC]; Mytussin® [OTC]; Naldecon® Senior EX [OTC]; Robitussin® [OTC]; Scot-Tussin® [OTC]; Sinumist®-SR Capsulets®; Uni-Tussin® [OTC]

Synonyms GG; Glycerol Guaiacolate

Use Temporary control of cough due to minor throat and bronchial irritation

Pregnancy Risk Factor C

Contraindications Hypersensitivity to guaifenesin or any component

Warnings/Precautions Not for persistent cough such as occurs with smoking, asthma, or emphysema or cough accompanied by excessive secretions

Adverse Reactions
1% to 10%:
Central nervous system: Drowsiness, headache
Dermatologic: Rash
Gastrointestinal: Nausea, vomiting, stomach pain

Overdosage/Toxicology Symptoms of overdose include vomiting, lethargy, coma, respiratory depression; treatment is supportive

Stability Protect from light

Mechanism of Action Thought to act as an expectorant by irritating the gastric mucosa and stimulating respiratory tract secretions, thereby increasing respiratory fluid volumes and decreasing phlegm viscosity

Pharmacodynamics/Kinetics
Absorption: Well absorbed from GI tract
Metabolism: Hepatic, 60%
Elimination: Renal excretion of changed and unchanged drug

Usual Dosage Oral:
(Continued)

515

Guaifenesin *(Continued)*

Children:

<2 years: 12 mg/kg/day in 6 divided doses

2-5 years: 50-100 mg every 4 hours, not to exceed 600 mg/day

6-11 years: 100-200 mg every 4 hours, not to exceed 1.2 g/day

Children >12 years and Adults: 200-400 mg every 4 hours to a maximum of 2.4 g/day

Test Interactions Possible color interference with determination of 5-HIAA and VMA

Patient Information Take with a large quantity of fluid to ensure proper action; if cough persists for more than 1 week or is accompanied by fever, rash, or persistent headache, physician should be consulted

Additional Information Syrup contains 3.5% alcohol

Dosage Forms

Capsule (Breonesin®, GG-Cen®, Hytuss-2X®): 200 mg

Capsule, sustained release (Humibid® Sprinkle): 300 mg

Liquid (Naldecon® Senior EX): 200 mg/5 mL (118 mL, 480 mL)

Syrup (Anti-Tuss® Expectorant, Genatuss®, Glyate®, Guiatuss®, Halotussin®, Malotuss®, Mytussin®, Robitussin®, Scot-Tussin®, Uni-Tussin®): 100 mg/5 mL (5 mL, 10 mL, 15 mL, 30 mL, 118 mL, 120 mL, 240 mL, 473 mL, 946 mL)

Tablet:

Amonidrin®, Gee Gee®, Glytuss®: 200 mg

Glycotuss®, Hytuss®: 100 mg

Sustained release:

Fenesin™, Humibid® L.A., Sinumist®-SR Capsulets®: 600 mg

Guaifenesin and Codeine *(gwye fen' e sin & koe' deen)*

Brand Names Cheracol®; Guaituss AC®; Guiatussin® with Codeine; Halotussin® AC; Mytussin® AC; Robafen® AC; Robitussin® A-C

Synonyms Codeine and Guaifenesin

Use Temporary control of cough due to minor throat and bronchial irritation

Restrictions C-V

Pregnancy Risk Factor C

Contraindications Hypersensitivity to guaifenesin, codeine or any component

Warnings/Precautions Should not be used for chronic productive coughs

Adverse Reactions

Codeine:

>10%:

Central nervous system: Drowsiness

Gastrointestinal: Constipation

1% to 10%:

Cardiovascular: Hypotension, palpitations, tachycardia or bradycardia, peripheral vasodilation

Central nervous system: CNS depression, drowsiness, sedation, confusion, headache, increased intracranial pressure, dizziness, lightheadedness, false feeling of well being, restlessness, paradoxical CNS stimulation, weakness, malaise

Dermatologic: Skin rash, hives

Endocrine & metabolic: Antidiuretic hormone release

Gastrointestinal: Nausea, vomiting, anorexia, dry mouth

Genitourinary: Decreased urination

Ocular: Miosis, blurred vision

Respiratory: Respiratory depression, shortness of breath, troubled breathing

Miscellaneous: Histamine release, physical and psychological dependence with prolonged use, biliary or urinary tract spasm

<1%:

Central nervous system: Convulsions, hallucinations, mental depression, nightmares, insomnia

Gastrointestinal: Biliary spasm, stomach cramps, paralytic ileus

Neuromuscular & skeletal: Trembling, muscle rigidity

Guaifenesin:

1% to 10%:

Central nervous system: Drowsiness, headache

Dermatologic: Rash

Gastrointestinal: Nausea, vomiting, stomach pain

Drug Interactions Increased toxicity: CNS depressant medications produce additive sedative properties

Mechanism of Action Refer to individual monographs for Guaifenesin and Codeine

Pharmacodynamics/Kinetics Refer to individual monographs for Guaifenesin and Codeine

Usual Dosage Oral:

Children:

2-6 years: 1-1.5 mg/kg codeine/day divided into 4 doses administered every 4-6 hours (maximum: 30 mg/24 hours)

6-12 years: 5 mL every 4 hours, not to exceed 30 mL/24 hours

Children >12 years and Adults: 5-10 mL every 4-8 hours not to exceed 60 mL/24 hours

Patient Information Take with a large quantity of fluid to ensure proper action; if cough persists for more than 1 week or is accompanied by fever, rash, or persistent headache, physician should be consulted; avoid CNS depressants and alcohol; do not use for chronic or persistent coughs

Dosage Forms Syrup: Guaifenesin 100 mg and codeine phosphate 10 mg per 5 mL (60 mL, 120 mL, 480 mL)

Guaifenesin and Dextromethorphan (gwye fen' e sin & dex troe meth or' fan)

Brand Names Benylin® Expectorant [OTC]; Cheracol D® [OTC]; Contac® Cough Formula Liquid [OTC]; Diabetic Tussin DM® [OTC]; Extra Action Cough Syrup [OTC]; Genatuss DM® [OTC]; Glycotuss-DM® [OTC]; GuiaCough [OTC]; Guiatuss DM® [OTC]; Halotussin® DM [OTC]; Humibid® DM [OTC]; Iophen DM® [OTC]; Kolephrin® GG/DM [OTC]; Mytussin® DM [OTC]; Naldecon® Senior DX [OTC]; Rhinosyn-DMX® [OTC]; Robafen DM® [OTC]; Robitussin®-DM [OTC]; Safe Tussin 30 Liquid® [OTC]; Syracol-CF® [OTC]; Tolu-Sed® DM [OTC]; Tuss-DM® [OTC]; Uni-tussin® DM [OTC]

Synonyms Dextromethorphan and Guaifenesin

Use Temporary control of cough due to minor throat and bronchial irritation

Pregnancy Risk Factor C

Contraindications Hypersensitivity to guaifenesin, dextromethorphan or any component

Warnings/Precautions Should not be used for persistent or chronic cough such as that occurring with smoking, asthma, chronic bronchitis, or emphysema or for cough associated with excessive phlegm

Adverse Reactions

1% to 10%:

Central nervous system: Drowsiness, headache

Dermatologic: Rash

Gastrointestinal: Nausea, vomiting

Pharmacodynamics/Kinetics Refer to Dexamethasone and Guaifenesin monographs

Usual Dosage Oral:

Children: Dextromethorphan: 1-2 mg/kg/24 hours divided 3-4 times/day

Children >12 years and Adults: 5 mL every 4 hours or 10 mL every 6-8 hours not to exceed 40 mL/24 hours

Patient Information Take with a large quantity of fluid to ensure proper action; if cough persists for more than one week, is recumbent, or is accompanied by fever, rash or persistent headache, physician should be consulted

Dosage Forms

Syrup:

Cheracol D®, Diabetic Tussin DM®, Guiatuss DM®, Genatuss DM®, Halotussin-DM®, Robafen DM®, Mytussin® DM, Robitussin®-DM, Tolu-Sed® DM, Uni-tussin DM®: Guaifenesin 100 mg and dextromethorphan hydrobromide 10 mg per 5 mL (5 mL, 10 mL, 118 mL, 120 mL, 240 mL, 360 mL, 473 mL, 480 mL, 3780 mL)

Rhinosyn-DMX®, SafeTussin®: Guaifenesin 100 mg and dextromethorphan hydrobromide 15 mg per 5 mL (120 mL, 480 mL)

Kolephrin® GG/DM: Guaifenesin 150 mg and dextromethorphan hydrobromide 10 mg per 5 mL (120 mL)

Naldecon® Senior DX: Guaifenesin 200 mg and dextromethorphan hydrobromide 10 mg per 5 mL (120 mL)

Tablet:

Extended release (Humibid® DM): Guaifenesin 600 mg and dextromethorphan hydrobromide 30 mg

Humibid DM Sprinkle Capsules®: Guaifenesin 300 mg and dextromethorphan hydrobromide 15 mg

Tuss-DM®: Guaifenesin 200 mg and dextromethorphan hydrobromide 10 mg

Glycotuss-dM®: Guaifenesin 100 mg and dextromethorphan hydrobromide 10 mg

Guaituss AC® see Guaifenesin and Codeine *on previous page*

Guanabenz Acetate (gwahn' a benz)

Brand Names Wytensin®

Use Management of hypertension

Pregnancy Risk Factor C

Contraindications Hypersensitivity to guanabenz or any component

Warnings/Precautions Use with caution in patients with severe coronary insufficiency, recent myocardial infarction, severe renal or hepatic impairment

Adverse Reactions

>10%:

Central nervous system: Drowsiness or sedation, dizziness

Gastrointestinal: Dry mouth

Neuromuscular & skeletal: Weakness

1% to 10%:

Cardiovascular: Chest pain, edema

Central nervous system: Headache

Endocrine & metabolic: Decreased sexual ability

Gastrointestinal: Nausea

<1%:

Cardiovascular: Arrhythmias, palpitations

Central nervous system: Anxiety, ataxia, depression, sleep disturbances

Dermatologic: Rash, pruritus

Endocrine & metabolic: Disturbances of sexual function, gynecomastia

Gastrointestinal: Diarrhea, vomiting, constipation

Genitourinary: Urinary frequency

Neuromuscular & skeletal: Muscle aches

Ocular: Blurring of vision

Respiratory: Nasal congestion, dyspnea

Miscellaneous: Taste disorders

Overdosage/Toxicology Symptoms of overdose include CNS depression, hypothermia, apnea, lethargy, diarrhea, hypotension, bradycardia; treatment is primarily supportive and symptomatic. Hypotension usually responds to I.V. fluids, Trendelenburg positioning, or vasoconstrictors. CNS depression and/or apnea may respond to naloxone I.V. 0.4-2 mg, with repeats as needed.

Drug Interactions

Decreased hypotensive effect of guanabenz with tricyclic antidepressants

Increased effect: Other hypotensive agents

Stability Protect from light

Mechanism of Action Stimulates alpha$_2$-adrenoreceptors in the brain stem, thus activating an inhibitory neuron, resulting in reduced sympathetic outflow, producing a decrease in vasomotor tone and heart rate

Pharmacodynamics/Kinetics

Onset of antihypertensive effect: Within 1 hour

Absorption: ~75%

Metabolism: Extensive

Half-life: 7-10 hours

Elimination: <1% of dose excreted as unchanged drug in urine

Usual Dosage Adults: Oral: Initial: 4 mg twice daily, increase in increments of 4-8 mg/day every 1-2 weeks to a maximum of 32 mg twice daily

Dosing adjustment in hepatic impairment: Probably necessary

Monitoring Parameters Blood pressure, standing and sitting/supine

Patient Information May cause drowsiness; rise from sitting/lying position carefully, may cause dizziness; do not discontinue without notifying physician

Dosage Forms Tablet: 4 mg, 8 mg

Guanadrel Sulfate (gwahn' a drel)

Brand Names Hylorel®

Use Considered a second line agent in the treatment of hypertension, usually with a diuretic

Pregnancy Risk Factor B

Contraindications Known hypersensitivity to guanadrel, pheochromocytoma, patients taking MAO inhibitors

Warnings/Precautions Orthostatic hypotension can occur frequently; use with caution in patients with CHF, in patients with regional vascular disease, and in patients with asthma or active peptic ulcer

Adverse Reactions

>10%:

Cardiovascular: Palpitations, chest pain, peripheral edema

Central nervous system: Fatigue, headache, faintness, drowsiness, confusion

Gastrointestinal: Increased bowel movements, gas pain, constipation, anorexia, weight gain/loss

Genitourinary: Nocturia, urinary frequency, ejaculation disturbances

Neuromuscular & skeletal: Paresthesia, aching limbs, leg cramps, backache, joint pain

Ocular: Visual disturbances

Respiratory: Shortness of breath, coughing

1% to 10%:

Cardiovascular: Orthostatic hypotension

Central nervous system: Psychological problems, depression, sleep disorders

Gastrointestinal: Increased bowel movements, glossitis, nausea, vomiting, dry mouth

Genitourinary: Impotence

Renal: Hematuria

<1%: Cardiovascular: Syncope, angina

Overdosage/Toxicology Symptoms of overdose include hypotension, blurred vision, dizziness, syncope; treatment is primarily supportive and symptomatic; hypotension usually responds to I.V. fluids, Trendelenburg positioning or vasoconstrictors

Drug Interactions

Decreased effect with tricyclic antidepressants, indirect-acting amines (ephedrine, phenylpropanolamine), phenothiazines

Increased toxicity of direct-acting amines (epinephrine, norepinephrine)

Increased effect of beta-blockers, vasodilators

Mechanism of Action Acts as a false neurotransmitter that blocks the adrenergic actions of norepinephrine; it displaces norepinephrine from its presynaptic storage granules and thus exposes it to degradation; it thereby produces a reduction in total peripheral resistance and, therefore, blood pressure

Pharmacodynamics/Kinetics

Peak effect: Within 4-6 hours

Duration: 4-14 hours

Absorption: Oral: Rapid

Distribution: Crosses the placenta; hydrophilic, therefore, does not cross the blood-brain barrier

Protein binding: 20%

Half-life, biphasic:

Initial: 1-4 hours

Terminal: 5-45 hours

Time to peak serum concentration: Within 1.5-2 hour

Elimination: In urine, 40% as unchanged drug

Usual Dosage

Adults: Oral: Initial: 10 mg/day (5 mg twice daily); adjust dosage until blood pressure is controlled, usual dosage: 20-75 mg/day, given twice daily

Elderly: Initial: 5 mg once daily

Dosing interval in renal impairment:

Cl_{cr} 10-50 mL/minute: Administer every 12-24 hours

Cl_{cr} <10 mL/minute: Administer every 24-48 hours

Monitoring Parameters Blood pressure, standing and sitting/supine

Patient Information May cause orthostatic hypotension, rise slowly from sitting or lying; take no new prescription or OTC medication without contacting your physician or pharmacist

Nursing Implications Tablet may be crushed; assist patient with rising and ambulation; monitor for orthostasis

Dosage Forms Tablet: 10 mg, 25 mg

Guanethidine Sulfate (gwahn eth' i deen)

Brand Names Ismelin®

Use Treatment of moderate to severe hypertension

Pregnancy Risk Factor C

Contraindications Pheochromocytoma, patients taking MAO inhibitors, hypersensitivity to guanethidine or any component

Warnings/Precautions Orthostatic hypotension can occur frequently; use with caution in patients with CHF, in patients with regional vascular disease, and in patients with asthma or active peptic ulcer; withdraw therapy 2 weeks prior to surgery to decrease chance of vascular collapse and cardiac arrest during anesthesia

Adverse Reactions

>10%:

Cardiovascular: Palpitations, chest pain, peripheral edema

Central nervous system: Fatigue, headache, faintness, drowsiness, confusion

Endocrine & metabolic: Ejaculation disturbances

Gastrointestinal: Increased bowel movements, gas pain, constipation, anorexia, weight gain/loss

(Continued)

519

Guanethidine Sulfate *(Continued)*

    Genitourinary: Nocturia, urinary frequency, impotence

    Neuromuscular & skeletal: Paresthesia, aching limbs, leg cramps, backache, joint pain

    Ocular: Visual disturbances

    Respiratory: Shortness of breath, coughing

  1% to 10%:

    Cardiovascular: Orthostatic hypotension

    Central nervous system: Psychological problems, depression, sleep disorders

    Gastrointestinal: Increased bowel movements, glossitis, nausea, vomiting, dry mouth

    Renal: Hematuria

  <1%: Cardiovascular: Syncope, angina

Overdosage/Toxicology Symptoms of overdose include hypotension, blurred vision, dizziness, syncope; hypotension usually responds to I.V. fluids, Trendelenburg positioning or vasoconstrictors; treatment is primarily supportive and symptomatic

Drug Interactions

  Decreased effect with tricyclic antidepressants, indirect-acting amines (ephedrine, phenylpropanolamine)

  Increased toxicity of direct-acting amines (epinephrine, norepinephrine)

Mechanism of Action Acts as a false neurotransmitter that blocks the adrenergic actions of norepinephrine; it displaces norepinephrine from its presynaptic storage granules and thus exposes it to degradation; it thereby produces a reduction in total peripheral resistance and, therefore, blood pressure

Pharmacodynamics/Kinetics

  Onset of effect: Within 0.5-2 hours

  Peak antihypertensive effect: Within 6-8 hours

  Duration: 24-48 hours

  Absorption: Irregular (3% to 55%)

  Metabolism: Hepatic; metabolites inactive

  Half-life: 5-10 days

  Elimination: 25% to 60% of dose excreted unchanged in urine; small amounts also appear in feces

Usual Dosage Oral:

  Children: Initial: 0.2 mg/kg/day, increase by 0.2 mg/kg/day at 7- to 10-day intervals to a maximum of 3 mg/kg/day

  Adults:

    Ambulatory patients: Initial: 10 mg/day, increase at 5- to 7-day intervals to a maximum of 25-50 mg/day

    Hospitalized patients: Initial: 25-50 mg/day, increase by 25-50 mg/day or every other day to desired therapeutic response

  Elderly: Initial: 5 mg once daily

  Dosing interval in renal impairment: Cl_{cr} <10 mL/minute: Administer every 24-36 hours

Monitoring Parameters Blood pressure, standing and sitting/supine; monitor for orthostasis

Patient Information May cause drowsiness; rise from sitting/lying carefully, may cause dizziness; do not take any OTC or prescription cough or cold medication without consulting physician

Nursing Implications Tablet may be crushed

Dosage Forms Tablet: 10 mg, 25 mg

Guanfacine Hydrochloride *(gwahn' fa seen)*

Brand Names Tenex®

Use Management of hypertension

Pregnancy Risk Factor B

Contraindications Hypersensitivity to guanfacine or any component

Warnings/Precautions Use with caution in patients with severe coronary insufficiency, recent myocardial infarction, severe renal or hepatic impairment

Adverse Reactions

  >10%:

    Central nervous system: Somnolence, dizziness

    Gastrointestinal: Dry mouth, constipation

  1% to 10%:

    Central nervous system: Fatigue, headache, insomnia

    Endocrine & metabolic: Decreased sexual ability

    Gastrointestinal: Nausea, vomiting

    Ocular: Conjunctivitis

<1%:
Cardiovascular: Bradycardia, palpitations
Central nervous system: Amnesia, confusion, depression, malaise
Dermatologic: Dermatitis, pruritus, purpura
Gastrointestinal: Abdominal pain, diarrhea, dyspepsia, dysphagia, taste perversion
Genitourinary: Testicular disorder, urinary incontinence
Neuromuscular & skeletal: Leg cramps, hypokinesia, paresthesia
Otic: Tinnitus
Respiratory: Rhinitis, dyspnea
Miscellaneous: Substernal pain, sweating

Overdosage/Toxicology Symptoms of overdose include CNS depression, hypothermia, apnea, lethargy, diarrhea, hypotension, bradycardia; treatment is primarily supportive and symptomatic. Hypotension usually responds to I.V. fluids, Trendelenburg positioning or vasoconstrictors. Naloxone may be utilized in treating CNS depression and/or apnea.

Drug Interactions
Increased effect: Other hypotensive agents
Decreased hypotensive effect of guanfacine with tricyclic antidepressants

Mechanism of Action Stimulates alpha$_2$-adrenoreceptors in the brain stem, thus activating an inhibitory neuron, resulting in reduced sympathetic outflow, producing a decrease in vasomotor tone and heart rate

Pharmacodynamics/Kinetics
Peak effect: Within 8-11 hours
Duration: 24 hours following a single dose
Protein binding: 20% to 30%
Metabolism: In the liver to glucuronide and sulfate metabolites
Bioavailability: 80% to 100%
Half-life: 17 hours
Time to peak serum concentration: Within 1-4 hours
Elimination: Renal excretion of changed and unchanged drug (30%)

Usual Dosage Adults: Oral: 1 mg usually at bedtime, may increase if needed at 3- to 4-week intervals to a maximum of 3 mg/day; 1 mg/day is most common dose

Monitoring Parameters Blood pressure, standing and sitting/supine

Patient Information May cause drowsiness, dizziness; do not discontinue this medication without consulting your physician; take at bedtime; do not abruptly quit taking this medication

Nursing Implications Administer dose at bedtime; observe for orthostasis

Dosage Forms Tablet: 1 mg

GuiaCough® [OTC] *see* Guaifenesin and Dextromethorphan *on page 517*

Guiatuss DM® [OTC] *see* Guaifenesin and Dextromethorphan *on page 517*

Guiatussin® with Codeine *see* Guaifenesin and Codeine *on page 516*

Guiatuss® [OTC] *see* Guaifenesin *on page 515*

G-well® *see* Lindane *on page 636*

Gynecort® [OTC] *see* Hydrocortisone *on page 546*

Gyne-Lotrimin® [OTC] *see* Clotrimazole *on page 265*

Gyne-Sulf® *see* Sulfabenzamide, Sulfacetamide, and Sulfathiazole *on page 1039*

Gynogen L.A.® *see* Estradiol *on page 407*

Habitrol™ *see* Nicotine *on page 792*

Haemophilus b Conjugate Vaccine (hem off' fil us)
Related Information
Immunization Guidelines *on page 1389-1405*
Vaccines *on page 1386-1388*
Brand Names HibTITER®; PedvaxHIB™; ProHIBiT®
Synonyms Diphtheria CRM$_{197}$ Protein Conjugate; Diphtheria Toxoid Conjugate; Haemophilus b Oligosaccharide Conjugate Vaccine; Haemophilus b Polysaccharide Vaccine; HbCV; Hib Polysaccharide Conjugate; PRP-D
Use Routine immunization of children 2 months to 5 years of age against invasive disease caused by *H. influenzae*

Unimmunized children ≥5 years of age with a chronic illness known to be associated with increased risk of *Haemophilus influenzae* type b disease, specifically,
(Continued)

521

Haemophilus b Conjugate Vaccine *(Continued)*

persons with anatomic or functional asplenia or sickle cell anemia or those who have undergone splenectomy, should receive Hib vaccine.

Haemophilus b conjugate vaccines are not indicated for prevention of bronchitis or other infections due to *H. influenzae* in adults; adults with specific dysfunction or certain complement deficiencies who are at especially high risk of *H. influenzae* type b infection (HIV-infected adults); patients with Hodgkin's disease (vaccinated at least 2 weeks before the initiation of chemotherapy or 3 months after the end of chemotherapy)

Pregnancy Risk Factor C

Contraindications Children with any febrile illness or active infection, known hypersensitivity to Haemophilus b polysaccharide vaccine (thimerosal), children who are immunosuppressed or receiving immunosuppressive therapy

Warnings/Precautions Have epinephrine 1:1000 available; children in whom DTP or DT vaccination is deferred: The carrier proteins used in HbOC (but not PRP-OMP) are chemically and immunologically related to toxoids contained in DTP vaccine. Earlier or simultaneous vaccination with diphtheria or tetanus toxoids may be required to elicit an optimal anti-PRP antibody response to HbOC. In contrast, the immunogenicity of PRP-OMP is not affected by vaccination with DTP. In infants in whom DTP or DT vaccination is deferred, PRP-OMP may be advantageous for *Haemophilus influenzae* type b vaccination.

Children with immunologic impairment: Children with chronic illness associated with increased risk of *Haemophilus influenzae* type b disease may have impaired anti-PRP antibody responses to conjugate vaccination. Examples include those with HIV infection, immunoglobulin deficiency, anatomic or functional asplenia, and sickle cell disease, as well as recipients of bone marrow transplants and recipients of chemotherapy for malignancy. Some children with immunologic impairment may benefit from more doses of conjugate vaccine than normally indicated.

Adverse Reactions When administered during the same visit that DTP vaccine is given, the rates of systemic reactions do not differ from those observed only when DTP vaccine is administered

25%: Local: Increased risk of Haemophilus b infections in the week after vaccination, swelling, local erythema, warmth

>10%: Acute febrile reactions

1% to 10%:

Central nervous system: Fever (up to 102.2°F), irritability, lethargy

Gastrointestinal: Anorexia, diarrhea

Local: Irritation at injection site

<1%:

Central nervous system: Convulsions, fever >102.2°F

Gastrointestinal: Vomiting

Miscellaneous: Allergic or anaphylactic reactions (difficulty in breathing, hives, itching, swelling of eyes, face, unusual tiredness or weakness)

Drug Interactions Decreased effect with immunosuppressive agents, immunoglobulins within 1 month may decrease antibody production; may interfere with antigen detection tests

Vaccination Schedule for Haemophilus b Conjugate Vaccines

Age at 1st Dose (mo)	HibTITER®		PedvaxHIB®		ProHIBiT®	
	Primary Series	Booster	Primary Series	Booster	Primary Series	Booster
2-6*	3 doses, 2 months apart	15 mo†	2 doses, 2 months apart	12 mo†		
7-11	2 doses, 2 months apart	15 mo†	2 doses, 2 months apart	15 mo†		
12-14	1 dose	15 mo†	1 dose	15 mo†		
15-60	1 dose	—	1 dose	—	1 dose	—

*It is not currently recommended that the various Haemophilus b conjugate vaccines be interchanged (ie, the same brand should be used throughout the entire vaccination series). If the health care provider does not know which vaccine was previously used, it is prudent that an infant, 2-6 months of age, be given a primary series of three doses.

†At least 2 months after previous dose.

Stability Keep in refrigerator, may be frozen (not diluent) without affecting potency; reconstituted Hib-Imune® remains stable for only 8 hours, whereas HibVAX® remain stable for 30 days when refrigerated

Mechanism of Action Stimulates production of anticapsular antibodies and provides active immunity to *Haemophilus influenzae*; Hib conjugate vaccines use covalent binding of capsular polysaccharide of *Haemophilus influenzae* type b to diphtheria CRM 197 (HibTITER®) to produce an antigen which is postulated to convert a T-independent antigen into a T-dependent antigen to result in enhanced antibody response and on immunologic memory

Pharmacodynamics/Kinetics

The seroconversion following one dose of Hib vaccine for children 18 months or 24 months of age or older is 75% to 90% respectively

Onset of serum antibody responses: 1-2 weeks after vaccination

Duration: Immunity appears to last 1.5 years

Usual Dosage Children: I.M.: 0.5 mL as a single dose should be administered according to one of the following "brand-specific" schedules; do not inject I.V.

Test Interactions May interfere with interpretation of antigen detection tests

Patient Information May use acetaminophen for post-dose fever

Nursing Implications Defer immunization if infection or febrile illness present. Do not give I.V.

Additional Information Federal law requires that the date of administration, the vaccine manufacturer, lot number of vaccine, and the administering person's name, title, and address be entered into the patient's permanent medical record

Haemophilus Influenzae type b Conjugate Vaccines

Manufacturer	Abbreviation	Trade Name	Carrier Protein
Connaught Laboratories	PRP-D•	ProHiBit®	Diphtheria toxoid
Lederle Laboratories	HbOC	HibTITER®	CRM_{197} (a nontoxic mutant diphtheria toxin)
Merck and Company	PRP-OMP	PedvaxHIB	OMP (an outer membrane protein complex of *Neisseria meningitidis*)
Pasteur Merieux Vaccines (Distributed by Connaught Laboratories, Inc, and SmithKline Beecham)	PRP-T••	ActHIB OmniHIB	Tetanus toxoid

•PRP-D is recommended by the American Academy of Pediatrics for only infants ≥12 months of age. HbOC, PRP-OMP, and PRP-T are recommended for infants beginning at approximately 2 months of age.

••PRP-T may be reconstituted with DTP, manufactured by Connaught Laboratories. Other licensed formulations of DTP have not been approved by the FDA for reconstitution and may not be used for this purpose.

Dosage Forms Injection:

HibTITER®: Capsular oligosaccharide 10 mcg and diphtheria CRM_{197} protein ~25 mcg per 0.5 mL (0.5 mL, 2.5 mL, 5 mL)

PedvaxHIB™: Purified capsular polysaccharide 15 mcg and *Neisseria meningitidis* OMPC 250 mcg per dose (0.5 mL)

ProHIBiT®: Purified capsular polysaccharide 25 mcg and conjugated diphtheria toxoid protein 18 mcg per dose (0.5 mL, 2.5 mL, 5 mL)

Haemophilus b Oligosaccharide Conjugate Vaccine *see* Haemophilus b Conjugate Vaccine *on page 521*

Haemophilus b Polysaccharide Vaccine *see* Haemophilus b Conjugate Vaccine *on page 521*

Halcinonide (hal sin' oh nide)
Related Information
Corticosteroids Comparisons *on page 1266-1268*
Brand Names Halog®; Halog®-E
(Continued)

Halcinonide *(Continued)*

Use Inflammation of corticosteroid-responsive dermatoses [high potency topical corticosteroid]

Pregnancy Risk Factor C

Contraindications Viral, fungal, or tubercular skin lesions, known hypersensitivity to halcinonide or any component

Warnings/Precautions Adverse systemic effects may occur when used on large areas of the body, denuded areas, for prolonged periods of time, with an occlusive dressing, and/or in infants or small children

Adverse Reactions <1%: Topical: Burning, itching, irritation, dryness, folliculitis, hypertrichosis, acneiform eruptions, hypopigmentation, perioral dermatitis, allergic contact dermatitis, skin maceration, secondary infection, skin atrophy, striae, miliaria

Overdosage/Toxicology When consumed in excessive quantities, systemic hypercorticism and adrenal suppression may occur; in those cases, discontinuation and withdrawal of the corticosteroid should be done judiciously

Mechanism of Action Decreases inflammation by suppression of migration of polymorphonuclear leukocytes and reversal of increased capillary permeability

Pharmacodynamics/Kinetics

Absorption: Percutaneous absorption varies by location of topical application and the use of occlusive dressings

Metabolism: Primarily in the liver

Elimination: By the kidneys

Usual Dosage Children and Adults: Topical: Apply sparingly 1-3 times/day, occlusive dressing may be used for severe or resistant dermatoses; a thin film of cream or ointment is effective; do not overuse

Patient Information A thin film of cream or ointment is effective; do not overuse; do not use tight-fitting diapers or plastic pants on children being treated in the diaper area; use only as prescribed, and for no longer than the period prescribed; apply sparingly in light film; rub in lightly; avoid contact with eyes; notify physician if condition being treated persists or worsens

Dosage Forms

Cream (Halog®): 0.025% (15 g, 60 g); 0.1% (15 g, 30 g, 60 g, 240 g)

Cream, emollient base (Halog®-E) : 0.1% (15 g, 30 g, 60 g)

Ointment, topical (Halog®): 0.1% (15 g, 30 g, 60 g, 240 g)

Solution (Halog®): 0.1% (20 mL, 60 mL)

Halcion® *see Triazolam on page 1117*

Haldol® *see Haloperidol on next page*

Haldol® Decanoate *see Haloperidol on next page*

Halenol® [OTC] *see Acetaminophen on page 17*

Halfan® *see Halofantrine on next page*

Halobetasol Propionate *(hal oh bay' ta sol)*

Brand Names Ultravate™

Use Relief of inflammatory and pruritic manifestations of corticosteroid-response dermatoses [very high potency topical corticosteroid]

Pregnancy Risk Factor C

Contraindications Hypersensitivity to halobetasol or any component; viral, fungal, or tubercular skin lesions

Warnings/Precautions Not for ophthalmic use; may cause adrenal suppression or insufficiency; application to abraded or inflamed areas or too large of areas of the body may increase the risk of systemic absorption and the risk of adrenal suppression, as may prolonged use or the use of >50 g/week. Topical halobetasol should not be used for the treatment of rosacea or perioral dermatitis.

Adverse Reactions <1%: Topical: Burning, itching, irritation, dryness, folliculitis, hypertrichosis, acneiform eruptions, hypopigmentation, perioral dermatitis, allergic contact dermatitis, skin maceration, secondary infection, skin atrophy, striae, miliaria

Overdosage/Toxicology When consumed in excessive quantities, systemic hypercorticism and adrenal suppression may occur; in those cases, discontinuation and withdrawal of the corticosteroid should be done judiciously

Mechanism of Action Corticosteroids inhibit the initial manifestations of the inflammatory process (ie, capillary dilation and edema, fibrin deposition, and migration and diapedesis of leukocytes into the inflamed site) as well as later sequelae (angiogenesis, fibroblast proliferation)

Pharmacodynamics/Kinetics
  Absorption: Percutaneous absorption varies by location of topical application and
    the use of occlusive dressings; ~3% of a topically applied dose of ointment
    enters the circulation within 96 hours
  Metabolism: Primarily in the liver
  Elimination: By the kidneys

Usual Dosage Children and Adults: Topical: Apply sparingly to skin twice daily,
rub in gently and completely; treatment should not exceed 2 consecutive weeks
and total dosage should not exceed 50 g/week

Patient Information A thin film of cream or ointment is effective; do not overuse;
do not use tight-fitting diapers or plastic pants on children being treated in the
diaper area; use only as prescribed, and for no longer than the period prescribed;
apply sparingly in light film; rub in lightly; avoid contact with eyes; notify physician
if condition being treated persists or worsens

Dosage Forms
  Cream: 0.05% (15 g, 45 g)
  Ointment, topical: 0.05% (15 g, 45 g)

Halofantrine (ha loe fan' trin)
Brand Names Halfan®
Use Treatment of mild to moderate acute malaria caused by susceptible strains of
Plasmodium falciparum and *Plasmodium vivax*
Pregnancy Risk Factor X
Contraindications Pregnancy
Warnings/Precautions Monitor closely for decreased hematocrit and hemo-
globin, patients with chronic liver disease
Adverse Reactions
  >10%: Dermatologic: Pruritus
  1% to 10%:
    Cardiovascular: Edema
    Central nervous system: Malaise, headache
    Gastrointestinal: Nausea, vomiting
    Hematologic: Leukocytosis
    Hepatic: Elevated LFTs
    Local: Tenderness
    Neuromuscular & skeletal: Myalgia
    Respiratory: Cough
    Miscellaneous: Lymphadenopathy
  <1%:
    Cardiovascular: Tachycardia, hypotension
    Dermatologic: Urticaria
    Endocrine & metabolic: Hypoglycemia
    Local: Sterile abscesses
    Respiratory: Asthma
    Miscellaneous: Anaphylactic shock
Mechanism of Action Similar to mefloquine; destruction of asexual blood forms,
possible inhibition of proton pump
Pharmacodynamics/Kinetics
  Mean time to parasite clearance: 40-84 hours
  Absorption: Erratic and variable; serum levels are proportional to dose up to 1000
    mg; doses greater than this should be divided; may be increased 60% with high
    fat meals
  Distribution: V_d: 570 L/kg; widely distributed in most tissues
  Metabolism: To active metabolite in liver
  Half-life: 23 hours; metabolite: 82 hours; may be increased in active disease
  Elimination: Essentially unchanged in urine
Usual Dosage Oral:
  Children <40 kg: 8 mg/kg every 6 hours for 3 doses
  Adults: 500 mg every 6 hours for 3 doses
Monitoring Parameters CBC, LFTs, parasite counts
Test Interactions Increased serum transaminases, bilirubin
Patient Information Take with food, avoid high fat meals; notify physician of
persistent nausea, vomiting, abdominal pain, light stools, dark urine
Nursing Implications Monitor closely for jaundice, other signs of hepatotoxicity
Dosage Forms
  Suspension: 100 mg/5 mL
  Tablet: 250 mg

Halog® *see* Halcinonide *on page 523*
Halog®-E *see* Halcinonide *on page 523*

Haloperidol (ha loe per' i dole)

Related Information
Antipsychotic Agents Comparison *on page 1255*

Brand Names Haldol®; Haldol® Decanoate

Use Treatment of psychoses, Tourette's disorder, and severe behavioral problems in children; may be used for the emergency sedation of severely agitated or delirious patients

Pregnancy Risk Factor C

Contraindications Hypersensitivity to haloperidol or any component; narrow-angle glaucoma, bone marrow depression, CNS depression, severe liver or cardiac disease, subcortical brain damage; circulatory collapse; severe hypotension or hypertension

Warnings/Precautions Safety and efficacy have not been established in children <3 years of age; watch for hypotension when administering I.M. or I.V.; use with caution in patients with cardiovascular disease or seizures; benefits of therapy must be weighed against risks of therapy; decanoate form should never be given I.V.; some tablets contain tartrazine which may cause allergic reactions; use caution with CNS depression and severe liver or cardiac disease

Adverse Reactions Sedation and anticholinergic effects are more pronounced than extrapyramidal effects; EKG changes, retinal pigmentation are more common than with chlorpromazine

>10%:
  Central nervous system: Sedation, drowsiness, restlessness, anxiety, extrapyramidal reactions, dystonic reactions, pseudoparkinsonian signs and symptoms, tardive dyskinesia, neuroleptic malignant syndrome, seizures, altered central temperature regulation, akathisia
  Endocrine & metabolic: Swelling of breasts
  Gastrointestinal: Weight gain, constipation

1% to 10%:
  Cardiovascular: Hypotension (especially orthostatic), tachycardia, arrhythmias, abnormal T waves with prolonged ventricular repolarization
  Central nervous system: Hallucinations, persistent tardive dyskinesia, drowsiness
  Gastrointestinal: Nausea, vomiting
  Genitourinary: Difficult urination

<1%:
  Central nervous system: Tardive dystonia, neuroleptic malignant syndrome (NMS)
  Dermatologic: Hyperpigmentation, pruritus, rash, contact dermatitis, alopecia, photosensitivity (rare)
  Endocrine & metabolic: Amenorrhea, galactorrhea, gynecomastia
  Gastrointestinal: Adynamic ileus, GI upset, dry mouth (problem for denture user)
  Genitourinary: Urinary retention, overflow incontinence, priapism, sexual dysfunction
  Hematologic: Agranulocytosis, leukopenia (usually inpatients with large doses for prolonged periods)
  Hepatic: Cholestatic jaundice, obstructive jaundice
  Ocular: Blurred vision, retinal pigmentation, decreased visual acuity (may be irreversible)
  Respiratory: Laryngospasm, respiratory depression
  Miscellaneous: Heat stroke, altered temperature regulation

Overdosage/Toxicology Symptoms of overdose include deep sleep, dystonia, agitation, dysrhythmias, extrapyramidal symptoms

Following initiation of essential overdose management, toxic symptom treatment and supportive treatment should be initiated. Critical cardiac arrhythmias often respond to I.V. lidocaine, while other antiarrhythmics can be used. Neuroleptics often cause extrapyramidal symptoms (eg, dystonic reactions) requiring management with benztropine mesylate I.V. 1-2 mg (adult) may be effective. These agents are generally effective within 2-5 minutes.

Drug Interactions Cytochrome P-450 IID6 enzyme inhibitor
  Decreased effect: Carbamazepine and phenobarbital may increase metabolism and decreased effectiveness of haloperidol
  Increased toxicity: CNS depressants may increase adverse effects; epinephrine may cause hypotension; haloperidol and anticholinergic agents → ↑ intraocular pressure; concurrent use with lithium has occasionally caused acute encephalopathy-like syndrome

Stability
  Protect oral dosage forms from light
  Haloperidol lactate injection should be stored at controlled room temperature and protected from light, freezing and temperatures >40°C; exposure to light may

cause discoloration and the development of a grayish-red precipitate over several weeks

Haloperidol lactate may be administered IVPB or I.V. infusion in D_5W solutions; NS solutions should not be used due to reports of decreased stability and incompatibility

Standardized dose: 0.5-100 mg/50-100 mL D_5W

Stability of standardized solutions is 38 days at room temperature (24°C)

Mechanism of Action Blocks postsynaptic mesolimbic dopaminergic D_1 and D_2 receptors in the brain; exhibits a strong alpha-adrenergic blocking and anticholinergic effect, depresses the release of hypothalamic and hypophyseal hormones; believed to depress the reticular activating system thus affecting basal metabolism, body temperature, wakefulness, vasomotor tone, and emesis

Pharmacodynamics/Kinetics

Onset of sedation: I.V.: Within 1 hour

Duration of action: ~3 weeks for decanoate form

Distribution: Crosses the placenta; appears in breast milk

Protein binding: 90%

Metabolism: In the liver to inactive compounds

Bioavailability: Oral: 60%

Half-life: 20 hours

Time to peak serum concentration: 20 minutes

Elimination: 33% to 40% excreted in urine within 5 days; an additional 15% excreted in feces

Usual Dosage

Children: 3-12 years (15-40 kg): Oral:

Initial: 0.05 mg/kg/day or 0.25-0.5 mg/day given in 2-3 divided doses; increase by 0.25-0.5 mg every 5-7 days; maximum: 0.15 mg/kg/day

Usual maintenance:

Agitation or hyperkinesia: 0.01-0.03 mg/kg/day once daily

Nonpsychotic disorders: 0.05-0.075 mg/kg/day in 2-3 divided doses

Psychotic disorders: 0.05-0.15 mg/kg/day in 2-3 divided doses

Children 6-12 years: I.M. (as lactate): 1-3 mg/dose every 4-8 hours to a maximum of 0.15 mg/kg/day; change over to oral therapy as soon as able

Adults:

Oral: 0.5-5 mg 2-3 times/day; usual maximum: 30 mg/day; some patients may require up to 100 mg/day

I.M. (as lactate): 2-5 mg every 4-8 hours as needed

I.M. (as decanoate): Initial: 10-15 times the daily oral dose administered at 3- to 4-week intervals

Sedation in the Intensive Care Unit:

I.M./IVP/IVPB: May repeat bolus doses after 30 minutes until calm achieved then administer 50% of the maximum dose every 6 hours

Mild agitation: 0.5-2 mg

Moderate agitation: 2-5 mg

Severe agitation: 10-20 mg

Continuous intravenous infusion (100 mg/100 mL D_5W): Rates of 1-40 mg/hour have been used

Elderly (nonpsychotic patients, dementia behavior):

Initial: Oral: 0.25-0.5 mg 1-2 times/day; increase dose at 4- to 7-day intervals by 0.25-0.5 mg/day; increase dosing intervals (twice daily, 3 times/day, etc) as necessary to control response or side effects

Maximum daily dose: 50 mg; gradual increases (titration) may prevent side effects or decrease their severity

Hemodialysis/peritoneal dialysis effects: Supplemental dose is not necessary

Administration The decanoate injectable formulation should be administered I.M. only, **do not give decanoate I.V.** Dilute the oral concentrate with water or juice before administration

Monitoring Parameters Monitor orthostatic blood pressures 3-5 days after initiation of therapy or a dose increase; observe for tremor and abnormal movement or posturing (extrapyramidal symptoms)

Reference Range

Therapeutic: 5-15 ng/mL (SI: 10-30 nmol/L) (psychotic disorders - less for Tourette's and mania)

Toxic: >42 ng/mL (SI: >84 nmol/L)

Test Interactions ↓ cholesterol (S)

Patient Information May cause drowsiness, restlessness, avoid alcohol and other CNS depressants, rise slowly from recumbent position; use of supportive stockings may help prevent orthostatic hypotension; do not alter dosage or discontinue without consulting physician; oral concentrate must be diluted in 2-4 oz of liquid (water, fruit juice, carbonated drinks, milk, or pudding)

Nursing Implications Avoid skin contact with oral suspension or solution; may cause contact dermatitis

(Continued)

Haloperidol *(Continued)*
Dosage Forms
Concentrate, oral, as lactate: 2 mg/mL (5 mL, 10 mL, 15 mL, 120 mL, 240 mL)
Injection, as decanoate: 50 mg/mL (1 mL, 5 mL); 100 mg/mL (1 mL, 5 mL)
Injection, as lactate: 5 mg/mL (1 mL, 2 mL, 2.5 mL, 10 mL)
Tablet: 0.5 mg, 1 mg, 2 mg, 5 mg, 10 mg, 20 mg

Haloprogin *(ha loe proe' jin)*
Brand Names Halotex®
Use Topical treatment of tinea pedis (athlete's foot), tinea cruris (jock itch), tinea corporis (ring worm), tinea manuum caused by *Trichophyton rubrum*, *Trichophyton tonsurans*, *Trichophyton mentagrophytes*, *Microsporum canis*, or *Epidermophyton floccosum*. Topical treatment of *Malassezia furfur*.
Pregnancy Risk Factor B
Contraindications Hypersensitivity to haloprogin or any component
Warnings/Precautions Safety and efficacy have not been established in children
Adverse Reactions <1%: Topical: Pruritus, folliculitis, irritation, burning sensation, vesicle formation, erythema
Mechanism of Action Interferes with fungal DNA replication to inhibit yeast cell respiration and disrupt its cell membrane
Pharmacodynamics/Kinetics
Absorption: Poorly through the skin (~11%)
Metabolism: To trichlorophenol
Elimination: In urine, 75% as unchanged drug
Usual Dosage Topical: Children and Adults: Apply liberally twice daily for 2-3 weeks; intertriginous areas may require up to 4 weeks of treatment
Patient Information Avoid contact with eyes; for external use only; improvement should occur within 4 weeks; discontinue use if sensitization or irritation occur
Dosage Forms
Cream: 1% (15 g, 30 g)
Solution, topical: 1% with alcohol 75% (10 mL, 30 mL)

Halotestin® *see* Fluoxymesterone *on page 477*

Halotex® *see* Haloprogin *on this page*

Halotussin® AC *see* Guaifenesin and Codeine *on page 516*

Halotussin® [OTC] *see* Guaifenesin *on page 515*

Halotussin® DM [OTC] *see* Guaifenesin and Dextromethorphan *on page 517*

Haltran® [OTC] *see* Ibuprofen *on page 561*

Havrix® *see* Hepatitis A Vaccine *on page 531*

HbCV *see* Haemophilus b Conjugate Vaccine *on page 521*

H-BIG® *see* Hepatitis B Immune Globulin *on page 532*

25-HCC *see* Calcifediol *on page 156*

hCG *see* Chorionic Gonadotropin *on page 242*

HCTZ *see* Hydrochlorothiazide *on page 542*

HDCV *see* Rabies Virus Vaccine *on page 972*

Healon® *see* Sodium Hyaluronate *on page 1014*

Heavy Mineral Oil *see* Mineral Oil *on page 743*

Hemabate™ *see* Carboprost Tromethamine *on page 184*

Hemocyte® [OTC] *see* Ferrous Fumarate *on page 450*

Hemofil® M *see* Antihemophilic Factor (Human) *on page 80*

Hemril-HC™ *see* Hydrocortisone *on page 546*

Heparin *(hep' a rin)*
Brand Names Calciparine®; HepFlush®; Hep-Lock®; Liquaemin®
Synonyms Heparin Lock Flush; Heparin Sodium, Heparin Calcium
Use Prophylaxis and treatment of thromboembolic disorders
Pregnancy Risk Factor C
Contraindications Hypersensitivity to heparin or any component; severe thrombocytopenia, subacute bacterial endocarditis, suspected intracranial hemorrhage, uncontrollable bleeding (unless secondary to disseminated intravascular coagulation)

Warnings/Precautions

Use with caution as hemorrhaging may occur; risk factors for hemorrhage include I.M. injections, peptic ulcer disease, increased capillary permeability, menstruation; severe renal, hepatic or biliary disease; use with caution in patients with shock, severe hypotension

Some preparations contain benzyl alcohol as a preservative. In neonates, large amounts of benzyl alcohol (>100 mg/kg/day) have been associated with fatal toxicity (gasping syndrome). The use of preservative-free heparin is, therefore, recommended in neonates. Some preparations contain sulfite which may cause allergic reactions.

Heparin does not possess fibrinolytic activity and, therefore, cannot lyse established thrombi; discontinue heparin if hemorrhage occurs; severe hemorrhage or overdosage may require protamine

Use caution with white clot syndrome (new thrombus associated with thrombocytopenia) and heparin resistance

Adverse Reactions

>10%:

Gastrointestinal: Constipation, vomiting of blood

Hematologic: Hemorrhage, blood in urine, bleeding from gums

Miscellaneous: Unexplained bruising

1% to 10%:

Cardiovascular: Chest pain

Genitourinary: Frequent or persistent erection

Neuromuscular & skeletal: Peripheral neuropathy

Miscellaneous: Allergic reactions

<1%:

Central nervous system: Fever, headache, chills

Dermatologic: Urticaria

Gastrointestinal: Nausea, vomiting

Hematologic: Thrombocytopenia (heparin-associated thrombocytopenia occurs in <1% of patients; immune thrombocytopenia occurs with progressive fall in platelet counts and, in some cases, thromboembolic complications; daily platelet counts for 5-7 days at initiation of therapy may help detect the onset of this complication)

Hepatic: Elevation of liver enzymes

Local: Irritation, ulceration, cutaneous necrosis have been rarely reported with deep S.C. injections

Neuromuscular & skeletal: Osteoporosis (chronic therapy effect)

Overdosage/Toxicology
The primary symptom of overdose is bleeding. Antidote is protamine; dose 1 mg per 1 mg (100 units) of heparin. Discontinue all heparin if evidence of progressive immune thrombocytopenia occurs.

Drug Interactions

Decreased effect with digoxin, TCN, nicotine, antihistamine, I.V. NTG

Increased toxicity with NSAIDs, ASA, dipyridamole, dextran, hydroxychloroquine

Stability

Heparin solutions are colorless to slightly yellow; minor color variations do not affect therapeutic efficacy

Heparin should be stored at controlled room temperature and protected from freezing and temperatures >40°C

Stability at room temperature and refrigeration:

Prepared bag: 24 hours

Premixed bag: After seal is broken 4 days

Out of overwrap stability: 30 days

Standard diluent: 25,000 units/500 mL D_5W (premixed)

Minimum volume: 250 mL D_5W

Mechanism of Action
Potentiates the action of antithrombin III and thereby inactivates thrombin (as well as activated coagulation factors IX, X, XI, XII, and plasmin) and prevents the conversion of fibrinogen to fibrin; heparin also stimulates release of lipoprotein lipase (lipoprotein lipase hydrolyzes triglycerides to glycerol and free fatty acids)

Pharmacodynamics/Kinetics

Onset of anticoagulation:

I.V.: Immediate with use

S.C.: Within 20-30 minutes

Absorption: Oral, rectal, sublingual, I.M.: Erratic

Distribution: Does not cross placenta; does not appear in breast milk

Metabolism: Hepatic; believed to be partially metabolized in the reticuloendothelial system

Half-life:

Mean: 1.5 hours

Range: 1-2 hours; affected by obesity, renal function, hepatic function, malignancy, presence of pulmonary embolism, and infections

Elimination: Renal excretion, small amount excreted unchanged in urine

(Continued)

Heparin *(Continued)*

Usual Dosage

Line flushing: When using daily flushes of heparin to maintain patency of single and double lumen central catheters, 10 units/mL is commonly used for younger infants (eg, <10 kg) while 100 units/mL is used for older infants, children, and adults. Capped PVC catheters and peripheral heparin locks require flushing more frequently (eg, every 6-8 hours). Volume of heparin flush is usually similar to volume of catheter (or slightly greater). Additional flushes should be given when stagnant blood is observed in catheter, after catheter is used for drug or blood administration, and after blood withdrawal from catheter.

Addition of heparin (0.5-1 unit/mL) to peripheral and central TPN has been shown to increase duration of line patency. The final concentration of heparin used for TPN solutions may need to be decreased to 0.5 units/mL in small infants receiving larger amounts of volume in order to avoid approaching therapeutic amounts. Arterial lines are heparinized with a final concentration of 1 unit/mL.

Children:
Intermittent I.V.: Initial: 50-100 units/kg, then 50-100 units/kg every 4 hours
I.V. infusion: Initial: 50 units/kg, then 15-25 units/kg/hour; increase dose by 2-4 units/kg/hour every 6-8 hours as required

Adults:
Prophylaxis (low-dose heparin): S.C.: 5000 units every 8-12 hours
Intermittent I.V.: Initial: 10,000 units, then 50-70 units/kg (5000-10,000 units) every 4-6 hours
I.V. infusion: 50 units/kg to start, then 15-25 units/kg/hour as continuous infusion; increase dose by 5 units/kg/hour every 4 hours as required according to PTT results, usual range: 10-30 units/hour
Weight-based protocol: 80 units/kg I.V. push followed by continuous infusion of 18 units/kg/hour. See table.

Standard Heparin Solution
(25,000 units/500 mL D$_5$ W)

To Administer a Dose of	Set Infusion Rate at
400 units/h	8 mL/h
500 units/h	10 mL/h
600 units/h	12 mL/h
700 units/h	14 mL/h
800 units/h	16 mL/h
900 units/h	18 mL/h
1000 units/h	20 mL/h
1100 units/h	22 mL/h
1200 units/h	24 mL/h
1300 units/h	26 mL/h
1400 units/h	28 mL/h
1500 units/h	30 mL/h
1600 units/h	32 mL/h
1700 units/h	34 mL/h
1800 units/h	36 mL/h
1900 units/h	38 mL/h
2000 units/h	40 mL/h

Administration Do not administer I.M. due to pain, irritation, and hematoma formation; central venous catheters must be flushed with heparin solution when newly inserted, daily (at the time of tubing change), after blood withdrawal or transfusion, and after an intermittent infusion through an injectable cap. A volume of at least 10 mL of blood should be removed and discarded from a heparinized line before blood samples are sent for coagulation testing.

Monitoring Parameters Platelet counts, PTT, hemoglobin, hematocrit, signs of bleeding

For intermittent I.V. injections, PTT is measured 3.5-4 hours after I.V. injection

Note: Continuous I.V. infusion is preferred vs I.V. intermittent injections. For full-dose heparin (ie, nonlow-dose), the dose should be titrated according to PTT results. For anticoagulation, an APTT 1.5-2.5 times normal is usually desired. APTT is usually measured prior to heparin therapy, 6-8 hours after initiation of a continuous infusion (following a loading dose), and 6-8 hours after changes in the infusion rate; increase or decrease infusion by 2-4 units/kg/hour dependent on PTT. See table.

Heparin Infusion Dose Adjustment

APTT	Adjustment
>3 x control	↓ Infusion rate 50%
2-3 x control	↓ Infusion rate 25%
1.5-2 x control	No change
<1.5 x control	↑ Rate of infusion 25% Max 2,500 units/h

Reference Range Heparin: 0.3-0.5 unit/mL; APTT: 1.5-2.5 times **the patient's baseline**

Test Interactions ↑ thyroxine (S) (competitive protein binding methods); ↑ PT, ↑ PTT, ↑ bleeding time

Dosage Forms
Heparin sodium:
Lock flush injection:
Beef lung source: 10 units/mL (1 mL, 2 mL, 2.5 mL, 3 mL, 5 mL, 10 mL, 30 mL); 100 units/mL (1 mL, 2 mL, 2.5 mL, 3 mL, 5 mL, 10 mL, 30 mL)
Porcine intestinal mucosa source: 10 units/mL (1 mL, 2 mL, 10 mL, 30 mL); 100 units/mL (1 mL, 2 mL, 10 mL, 30 mL)
Porcine intestinal mucosa source, preservative free: 10 units/mL (1 mL); 100 units/mL (1 mL)
Multiple-dose vial injection:
Beef lung source, with preservative: 1000 units/mL (5 mL, 10 mL, 30 mL); 5000 units/mL (10 mL); 10,000 units/mL (4 mL, 5 mL, 10 mL); 20,000 units/mL (2 mL, 5 mL, 10 mL); 40,000 units/mL (5 mL)
Porcine intestinal mucosa source, with preservative: 1000 units/mL (10 mL, 30 mL); 5000 units/mL (10 mL); 10,000 units/mL (4 mL); 20,000 units/mL (2 mL, 5 mL)
Single-dose vial injection:
Beef lung source: 1000 units/mL (1 mL); 5000 units/mL (1 mL); 10,000 units/mL (1 mL); 20,000 units/mL (1 mL); 40,000 units/mL (1 mL)
Porcine intestinal mucosa: 1000 units/mL (1 mL); 5000 units/mL (1 mL); 10,000 units/mL (1 mL); 20,000 units/mL (1 mL); 40,000 units/mL (1 mL)
Unit dose injection:
Porcine intestinal mucosa source, with preservative: 1000 units/dose (1 mL, 2 mL); 2500 units/dose (1 mL); 5000 units/dose (0.5 mL, 1 mL); 7500 units/dose (1 mL); 10,000 units/dose (1 mL); 15,000 units/dose (1 mL); 20,000 units/dose (1 mL)

Heparin sodium infusion, porcine intestinal mucosa source:
D_5W: 40 units/mL (500 mL); 50 units/mL (250 mL, 500 mL); 100 units/mL (100 mL, 250 mL)
NaCl 0.45%: 2 units/mL (500 mL, 1000 mL); 50 units/mL (250 mL); 100 units/mL (250 mL)
NaCl 0.9%: 2 units/mL (500 mL, 1000 mL); 5 units/mL (1000 mL); 50 units/mL (250 mL, 500 mL, 1000 mL)

Heparin calcium:
Unit dose injection, porcine intestinal mucosa, preservative free (Calciparine®): 5000 units/dose (0.2 mL); 12,500 units/dose (0.5 mL); 20,000 units/dose (0.8 mL)

Heparin Lock Flush *see* Heparin *on page 528*

Heparin Sodium, Heparin Calcium *see* Heparin *on page 528*

Hepatitis A Vaccine (hep a ti' tis a vak seen')
Related Information
Immunization Guidelines *on page 1389-1405*
Brand Names Havrix®
Use For populations desiring protection against hepatitis A or for populations at high risk of exposure to hepatitis A virus (travelers to developing countries, household and sexual contacts of persons infected with hepatitis A), child day care employees, illicit drug users, male homosexuals, institutional workers (eg, institutions for the mentally and physically handicapped persons, prisons, etc), and healthcare workers who may be exposed to hepatitis A virus (eg, laboratory employees)
Pregnancy Risk Factor C
Contraindications Hypersensitivity to any component of hepatitis A vaccine
(Continued)

Hepatitis A Vaccine *(Continued)*

Adverse Reactions
Central nervous system: Headache, fatigue, fever (rare)
Hepatic: Transient liver function test abnormalities
Local: Cutaneous reactions at the injection site (pain, soreness, tenderness, swelling, warmth, and redness)

Drug Interactions No interference of immunogenicity was reported when mixed with hepatitis B vaccine

Mechanism of Action As an inactivated virus vaccine, hepatitis A vaccine offers active immunization against hepatitis A virus infection at an effective immune response rate in up to 99% of subjects

Pharmacodynamics/Kinetics
Onset of action (protection): 3 weeks after a single dose
Duration: Neutralizing antibodies have persisted for >3 years; unconfirmed evidence indicates that antibody levels may persist for 5-10 years

Usual Dosage I.M.:
Children: 0.5 mL (360 units) on days 1 and 30, with a booster dose 6-12 months later (completion of the first 2 doses [ie, the primary series] should be accomplished at least 2 weeks before anticipated exposure to hepatitis A)
Adults: 1 mL (1440 units), with a booster dose at 6-12 months

Administration Inject I.M. into the deltoid muscle, if possible

Monitoring Parameters Liver function tests

Reference Range Seroconversion for Havrix®: Antibody >20 milli-international units/mL

Additional Information Some investigators suggest simultaneous or sequential administration of inactivated hepatitis A vaccine and immune globulin for postexposure protection, especially for travelers requiring rapid immunization, although a slight decrease in vaccine immunogenicity may be observed with this technique

Dosage Forms Injection: 0.5 mL (260 units/0.5 mL); 1 mL (1440 units/mL)

Hepatitis B Immune Globulin (hep a ti′ tis b i myun′ glob′ yoo lin)

Related Information
Immunization Guidelines *on page 1389-1405*
Vaccines *on page 1386-1388*

Brand Names H-BIG®; Hep-B-Gammagee®; HyperHep®

Use Provide prophylactic passive immunity to hepatitis B infection to those individuals exposed; newborns of mothers known to be hepatitis B surface antigen positive; hepatitis B immune globulin is not indicated for treatment of active hepatitis B infections and is ineffective in the treatment of chronic active hepatitis B infection

Pregnancy Risk Factor C

Contraindications Hypersensitivity to hepatitis B immune globulin or any component; allergies to gamma globulin or anti-immunoglobulin antibodies; allergies to thimerosal; IgA deficiency; I.M. injections in patients with thrombocytopenia or coagulation disorders

Adverse Reactions
1% to 10%:
Central nervous system: Dizziness, malaise,
Dermatologic: Urticaria, angioedema, rash, erythema
Local: Pain and tenderness at injection site
Neuromuscular & skeletal: Joint pains
<1%: Miscellaneous: Anaphylaxis

Drug Interactions Increased toxicity: Live virus vaccines

Stability Refrigerate at 2°C to 8°C (36°F to 46°F); do not freeze

Mechanism of Action Hepatitis B immune globulin (HBIG) is a nonpyrogenic sterile solution containing 10% to 18% protein of which at least 80% is monomeric immunoglobulin G (IgG). HBIG differs from immune globulin in the amount of anti-HB$_s$. Immune globulin is prepared from plasma that is not preselected for anti-HB$_s$ content. HBIG is prepared from plasma preselected for high titer anti-HB$_s$. In the U.S., HBIG has an anti-HB$_s$ high titer >1:100,000 by IRA. There is no evidence that the causative agent of AIDS (HTLV-III/LAV) is transmitted by HBIG.

Pharmacodynamics/Kinetics
Absorption: Slow
Time to peak serum concentration: 1-6 days

Usual Dosage I.M.:
Newborns: Hepatitis B: 0.5 mL as soon after birth as possible (within 12 hours)
Adults: Postexposure prophylaxis: 0.06 mL/kg; usual dose: 3-5 mL; maximum dose: 5 mL as soon as possible after exposure (within 96 hours); repeat at 28-30 days after exposure

Administration I.M. injection only in gluteal or deltoid region; to prevent injury from injection, care should be taken when giving to patients with thrombocytopenia or bleeding disorders; **do not administer I.V.**

Dosage Forms Injection:
H-BIG®: 4 mL, 5 mL
Hep-B-Gammagee®: 5 mL
HyperHep®: 0.5 mL, 1 mL, 5 mL

Hepatitis B Inactivated Virus Vaccine (plasma derived) *see* Hepatitis B Vaccine *on this page*

Hepatitis B Inactivated Virus Vaccine (recombinant DNA) *see* Hepatitis B Vaccine *on this page*

Hepatitis B Vaccine (hep a ti′ tis b vak seen′)

Related Information
Immunization Guidelines *on page 1389-1405*
Vaccines *on page 1386-1388*

Brand Names Engerix-B®; Recombivax HB®

Synonyms Hepatitis B Inactivated Virus Vaccine (plasma derived); Hepatitis B Inactivated Virus Vaccine (recombinant DNA)

Use Immunization against infection caused by all known subtypes of hepatitis B virus in individuals considered at high risk of potential exposure to hepatitis B virus or HB₅Ag-positive materials; see chart.

Pre-exposure Prophylaxis for Hepatitis B
Health care workers*
Special patient groups
Hemodialysis patients†
Recipients of certain blood products‡
Lifestyle factors
Homosexual and bisexual men
Intravenous drug abusers
Heterosexually active persons with multiple sexual partners or recently acquired sexually transmitted diseases
Environmental factors
Household and sexual contacts of HBV carriers
Prison inmates
Clients and staff of institutions for the mentally retarded
Residents, immigrants and refugees from areas with endemic HBV infection
International travelers at increased risk of acquiring HBV infection

*The risk of hepatitis B virus (HBV) infection for health care workers varies both between hospitals and within hospitals. Hepatitis B vaccination is recommended for all health care workers with blood exposure.

†Hemodialysis patients often respond poorly to hepatitis B vaccination; higher vaccine doses or increased number of doses are required. A special formulation of one vaccine is now available for such persons (Recombivax HB®, 40 mcg/mL) .The anti-Hbs (antibody to hepatitis B surface antigen) response of such persons should be tested after they are vaccinated, and those who have not responded should be revaccinated with 1-3 additional doses

Patients with chronic renal disease should be vaccinated as early as possible, ideally before they require hemodialysis. In addition, their anti- HBs levels should be monitored at 6-12 month intervals to assess the need for revaccination.

‡Patients with hemophilia should be immunized subcutaneously, not intramuscularly.

Pregnancy Risk Factor C

Contraindications Hypersensitivity to yeast, hypersensitivity to hepatitis B vaccine or any component

Adverse Reactions
>10%:
Central nervous system: Fever, malaise, fatigue, headache
Local: Mild local tenderness, local inflammatory reaction
1% to 10%:
Gastrointestinal: Nausea, diarrhea
Respiratory: Pharyngitis
<1%:
Cardiovascular: Tachycardia, hypotension, sensation of warmth, flushing,
Central nervous system: Lightheadedness, chills, somnolence, insomnia, irritability, agitation
Dermatologic: Pruritus, rash, erythema, urticaria
(Continued)

Hepatitis B Vaccine *(Continued)*

Gastrointestinal: Vomiting, GI disturbances, constipation, abdominal cramps, dyspepsia, anorexia

Neuromuscular & skeletal: Arthralgia, myalgia, stiffness in back/neck/arm or shoulder

Otic: Earache

Renal: Dysuria

Respiratory: Rhinitis, cough, nosebleed

Miscellaneous: Sweating

Drug Interactions Decreased effect: Immunosuppressive agents

Stability Refrigerate, do not freeze

Mechanism of Action Recombinant hepatitis B vaccine is a noninfectious subunit viral vaccine. The vaccine is derived from hepatitis B surface antigen (HB_sAg) produced through recombinant DNA techniques from yeast cells. The portion of the hepatitis B gene which codes for HB_sAg is cloned into yeast which is then cultured to produce hepatitis B vaccine.

Pharmacodynamics/Kinetics Duration of action: Following all 3 doses of hepatitis B vaccine, immunity will last approximately 5-7 years

Usual Dosage See tables.

Immunization Regimen of Three I.M. Hepatitis B Vaccine Doses

Age	Initial		1 mo		6 mo	
	Recombivax HB® (mL)	Engerix-B® (mL)	Recombivax HB® (mL)	Engerix-B® (mL)	Recombivax HB® (mL)	Engerix-B® (mL)
Birth* - 10 y	0.25	0.5	0.25	0.5	0.25	0.5
11-19 y	0.5	1	0.5	1	0.5	1
≥20 y	1	1	1	1	1	1
Dialysis or immuno-compromised patients		2†		2†		2†

*Infants born of HB_sAg negative mothers.

†Two 1 mL doses given at different sites.

Recommended Dosage for Infants Born to HB_sAg Positive Mothers

Treatment	Birth	Within 7 d	1 mo	6 mo
Engerix-B® (pediatric dose 10 mcg/0.5 mL)	*	0.5 mL*	0.5 mL	0.5 mL
Recombivax HB® (pediatric dose 5 mcg/0.5 mL)	*	0.5 mL*	0.5 mL	0.5 mL
Hepatitis B immune globulin	0.5 mL	—	—	—

*The first dose may be given at birth at the same time as HBIG, but give in the opposite anterolateral thigh. This may better ensure vaccine absorption.

Administration I.M. injection only; in adults, the deltoid muscle is the preferred site; the anterolateral thigh is the recommended site in infants and young children

Patient Information Must complete full course of injections for adequate immunization

Nursing Implications Rare chance of anaphylactoid reaction; have epinephrine available

Additional Information Inactivated virus vaccine; federal law requires that the date of administration, the vaccine manufacturer, lot number of vaccine, and the administering person's name, title and address be entered into the patient's permanent medical record

Dosage Forms Injection:

Recombinant DNA (Engerix-B®): Hepatitis B surface antigen 20 mcg/mL (1 mL)

Pediatric, recombinant DNA (Engerix-B®): Hepatitis B surface antigen 10 mcg/0.5 mL (0.5 mL)

Recombinant DNA (Recombivax HB®): Hepatitis B surface antigen 10 mcg/mL (1 mL, 3 mL)

Dialysis formulation, recombinant DNA (Recombivax HB®): Hepatitis B surface antigen 40 mcg/mL (1 mL)

Hep-B-Gammagee® *see* Hepatitis B Immune Globulin *on page 532*

HepFlush® *see* Heparin *on page 528*

Hep-Lock® *see* Heparin *on page 528*

Heptalac® *see* Lactulose *on page 617*

Herplex® *see* Idoxuridine *on page 564*

HES *see* Hetastarch *on this page*

Hespan® *see* Hetastarch *on this page*

Hetastarch (het′ a starch)
Brand Names Hespan®
Synonyms HES; Hydroxyethyl Starch
Use Blood volume expander used in treatment of shock or impending shock when blood or blood products are not available; does not have oxygen-carrying capacity and is not a substitute for blood or plasma
Pregnancy Risk Factor C
Contraindications Severe bleeding disorders, renal failure with oliguria or anuria, or severe congestive heart failure
Warnings/Precautions Anaphylactoid reactions have occurred; use with caution in patients with thrombocytopenia (may interfere with platelet function); large volume may cause drops in hemoglobin concentrations; use with caution in patients at risk from overexpansion of blood volume, including the very young or aged patients, those with congestive heart failure or pulmonary edema; large volumes may interfere with platelet function and prolong PT and PTT times
Adverse Reactions
   <1%:
   Cardiovascular: Peripheral edema, heart failure, circulatory overload
   Central nervous system: Fever, chills, headaches
   Dermatologic: Itching, pruritus
   Gastrointestinal: Vomiting
   Hematologic: Bleeding, prolongation of PT, PTT, clotting time, and bleeding time
   Neuromuscular & skeletal: Muscle pains
   Miscellaneous: Hypersensitivity
Overdosage/Toxicology Symptoms of overdose include heart failure, nausea, vomiting, circulatory overload, bleeding; treatment is supportive
Stability Do not use if crystalline precipitate forms or is turbid deep brown
Mechanism of Action Produces plasma volume expansion by virtue of its highly colloidal starch structure, similar to albumin
Pharmacodynamics/Kinetics
   Onset of volume expansion: I.V.: Within 30 minutes
   Duration: 24-36 hours
   Metabolism: Molecules >50,000 daltons require enzymatic degradation by the reticuloendothelial system or amylases in the blood prior to urinary and fecal excretion
   Elimination: Smaller molecular weight molecules are readily excreted in urine
Usual Dosage I.V. infusion (requires an infusion pump):
   Children: Safety and efficacy have not been established
   Adults: 500-1000 mL (up to 1500 mL/day) or 20 mL/kg/day (up to 1500 mL/day); larger volumes (15,000 mL/24 hours) have been used safely in small numbers of patients

   Dosing adjustment in renal impairment: Cl$_{cr}$ <10 mL/minute: Initial dose is the same but subsequent doses should be reduced by 20% to 50% of normal
Administration I.V. only; may administer up to 1.2 g/kg/hour (20 mL/kg/hour)
Nursing Implications Anaphylactoid reactions can occur, have epinephrine and resuscitative equipment available
Dosage Forms Infusion, in sodium chloride 0.9%: 6% (500 mL)

Hexachlorocyclohexane *see* Lindane *on page 636*

Hexachlorophene (hex a klor′ oh feen)
Brand Names pHisoHex®; pHiso® Scrub; Septisol®
Use Surgical scrub and as a bacteriostatic skin cleanser; control an outbreak of gram-positive infection when other procedures have been unsuccessful
Pregnancy Risk Factor C
Contraindications Known hypersensitivity to halogenated phenol derivatives or hexachlorophene; use in premature infants; use on burned or denuded skin; occlusive dressing; application to mucous membranes
Warnings/Precautions Discontinue use if signs of cerebral irritability occur; exposure of preterm infants or patients with extensive burns has been associated
(Continued)

Hexachlorophene *(Continued)*

with apnea, convulsions, agitation and coma; do not use for bathing infants, premature infants are particularly susceptible to hexachlorophene topical absorption

Adverse Reactions
<1%:
Central nervous system: CNS injury, seizures, irritability
Dermatologic: Photosensitivity, dermatitis, redness, dry skin

Overdosage/Toxicology Symptoms of overdose include anorexia, vomiting, abdominal cramps, diarrhea, dehydration, seizures, hypotension, shock; treatment is supportive

Stability Store in nonmetallic container (**incompatible** with many metals); prolonged direct exposure to strong light may cause brownish surface discoloration, but this does not affect its action

Mechanism of Action Bacteriostatic polychlorinated biphenyl which inhibits membrane-bound enzymes and disrupts the cell membrane

Pharmacodynamics/Kinetics
Absorption: Percutaneously through inflamed, excoriated, and intact skin
Distribution: Crosses the placenta
Half-life: Infants: 6.1-44.2 hours

Usual Dosage Children and Adults: Topical: Apply 5 mL cleanser and water to area to be cleansed; lather and rinse thoroughly under running water

Patient Information Do not leave on skin for prolonged contact; for external use only; discontinue product if condition persists or worsens and call physician; if suds enter eye, rinse out thoroughly with water

Dosage Forms
Foam: 0.23% (180 mL, 600 mL)
Liquid: 3% (8 mL, 150 mL, 473 mL, 946 mL)

Hexadrol® *see* Dexamethasone *on page 314*

Hexalen® *see* Altretamine *on page 47*

Hexamethylenetetramine *see* Methenamine *on page 706*

Hexamethylmelamine *see* Altretamine *on page 47*

Hexavitamin *see* Vitamin, Multiple *on page 1166*

Hibiclens® [OTC] *see* Chlorhexidine Gluconate *on page 223*

Hibistat® [OTC] *see* Chlorhexidine Gluconate *on page 223*

Hib Polysaccharide Conjugate *see* Haemophilus b Conjugate Vaccine *on page 521*

HibTITER® *see* Haemophilus b Conjugate Vaccine *on page 521*

Hi-Cor 1.0® *see* Hydrocortisone *on page 546*

Hi-Cor-2.5® *see* Hydrocortisone *on page 546*

Hiprex® *see* Methenamine *on page 706*

Hismanal® *see* Astemizole *on page 95*

Histaject® *see* Brompheniramine Maleate *on page 143*

Histerone® *see* Testosterone *on page 1063*

Histrelin *(his trel' in)*

Brand Names Supprelin™

Use Treatment of central idiopathic precocious puberty; treatment of estrogen associated gynecological disorders such as acute intermittent porphyria, endometriosis, leiomyomata uteri, and premenstrual syndrome

Pregnancy Risk Factor X

Contraindications Hypersensitivity to histrelin, pregnancy, breast-feeding

Warnings/Precautions The site of injection should be varied daily; the dose should be administered at the same time each day. In precocious puberty changing the dosage schedule or noncompliance may result in inadequate control of the pubertal process.

Adverse Reactions
>10%:
Cardiovascular: Vasodilation
Central nervous system: Headache
Gastrointestinal: Abdominal pain
Genitourinary: Vaginal bleeding, vaginal dryness
Local: Skin reaction at injection site
1% to 10%:
Central nervous system: Mood swings, headache

Dermatologic: Skin rashes, hives
Endocrine & metabolic: Breast tenderness, hot flashes
Gastrointestinal: Nausea, vomiting
Genitourinary: Increased urinary calcium excretion
Neuromuscular & skeletal: Joint stiffness, pain

Stability Refrigerate at 2°C to 8°C (36°F to 46°F) and protect from light; allow vial to reach room temperature before injecting contents

Mechanism of Action Histrelin is a synthetic long-acting gonadotropin-releasing hormone analog; with daily administration, it desensitizes the pituitary to endogenous gonadotropin-releasing hormone (ie, suppresses gonadotropin release by causing down regulation of the pituitary); this results in a decrease in gonadal sex steroid production which stops the secondary sexual development

Pharmacodynamics/Kinetics

Precocious puberty: Onset of hormonal responses: Within 3 months of initiation of therapy

Acute intermittent porphyria associated with menses: Amelioration of symptoms: After 1-2 months of therapy

Treatment of endometriosis or leiomyomata uteri: Onset of responses: After 3-6 months of treatment

Usual Dosage

Central idiopathic precocious puberty: S.C.: Usual dose is 10 mcg/kg/day given as a single daily dose at the same time each day

Acute intermittent porphyria in women: S.C.: 5 mcg/day

Endometriosis: S.C.: 100 mcg/day

Leiomyomata uteri: S.C.: 20-50 mcg/day or 4 mcg/kg/day

Administration Injection site should be varied daily; dose should be administered at the same time each day

Monitoring Parameters Precocious puberty: Prior to initiating therapy: Height and weight, hand and wrist x-rays, total sex steroid levels, beta-hCG level, adrenal steroid level, gonadotropin-releasing hormone stimulation test, pelvic/adrenal/testicular ultrasound/head CT; during therapy monitor 3 months after initiation and then every 6-12 months; serial levels of sex steroids and gonadotropin-releasing hormone testing; physical exam; secondary sexual development; histrelin may be discontinued when the patient reaches the appropriate age for puberty

Dosage Forms Injection: 7-day kits of single use: 120 mcg/0.6 mL; 300 mcg/0.6 mL; 600 mcg/0.6 mL

Hivid® *see* Zalcitabine *on page 1172*

HMS Liquifilm® *see* Medrysone *on page 678*

HN₂ *see* Mechlorethamine Hydrochloride *on page 672*

Hold® DM [OTC] *see* Dextromethorphan *on page 321*

Homatropine and Hydrocodone *see* Hydrocodone and Homatropine *on page 545*

Homatropine Hydrobromide (hoe ma' troe peen)

Related Information
Cycloplegic Mydriatics Comparison *on page 1269*

Brand Names AK-Homatropine®; Isopto® Homatropine

Use Producing cycloplegia and mydriasis for refraction; treatment of acute inflammatory conditions of the uveal tract

Pregnancy Risk Factor C

Contraindications Narrow-angle glaucoma, acute hemorrhage or hypersensitivity to the drug or any component in the formulation

Warnings/Precautions Use with caution in patients with hypertension, cardiac disease, or increased intraocular pressure; safety and efficacy not established in infants and young children, therefore, use with extreme caution due to susceptibility of systemic effects; use with caution in obstructive uropathy, paralytic ileus, ulcerative colitis, unstable cardiovascular status in acute hemorrhage

Adverse Reactions
>10%: Ocular: Blurred vision, photophobia
1% to 10%:
Local: Stinging, local irritation
Ocular: Increased intraocular pressure
Respiratory: Congestion
<1%:
Cardiovascular: Vascular congestion, edema
Central nervous system: Drowsiness
Dermatologic: Exudate, eczematoid dermatitis
Ocular: Follicular conjunctivitis
(Continued)

Homatropine Hydrobromide *(Continued)*

Overdosage/Toxicology Symptoms of overdose include blurred vision, urinary retention, tachycardia; anticholinergic toxicity is caused by strong binding of the drug to cholinergic receptors. For anticholinergic overdose with severe life-threatening symptoms, physostigmine 1-2 mg (0.5 or 0.02 mg/kg for children) S.C. or I.V., slowly may be given to reverse these effects.

Stability Protect from light

Mechanism of Action Blocks response of iris sphincter muscle and the accommodative muscle of the ciliary body to cholinergic stimulation resulting in dilation and loss of accommodation

Pharmacodynamics/Kinetics
Onset of accommodation and pupil effect: Ophthalmic:
Maximum mydriatic effect: Within 10-30 minutes
Maximum cycloplegic effect: Within 30-90 minutes
Duration:
Mydriasis: 6 hours to 4 days
Cycloplegia: 10-48 hours

Usual Dosage
Children:
Mydriasis and cycloplegia for refraction: Instill 1 drop of 2% solution immediately before the procedure; repeat at 10-minute intervals as needed
Uveitis: Instill 1 drop of 2% solution 2-3 times/day

Adults:
Mydriasis and cycloplegia for refraction: Instill 1-2 drops of 2% solution or 1 drop of 5% solution before the procedure; repeat at 5- to 10-minute intervals as needed
Uveitis: Instill 1-2 drops of 2% or 5% 2-3 times/day up to every 3-4 hours as needed

Patient Information May cause blurred vision; if irritation persists or increases, discontinue use

Nursing Implications Finger pressure should be applied to lacrimal sac for 1-2 minutes after instillation to decrease risk of absorption and systemic reactions

Dosage Forms Solution, ophthalmic: 2% (1 mL, 5 mL); 5% (1 mL, 2 mL, 5 mL)
AK-Homatropine®: 5% (15 mL)
Isopto® Homatropine 2% (5 mL, 15 mL); 5% (5 mL, 15 mL)

Horse Anti-human Thymocyte Gamma Globulin *see* Lymphocyte Immune Globulin *on page 655*

H.P. Acthar® Gel *see* Corticotropin *on page 274*

Human Diploid Cell Cultures Rabies Vaccine *see* Rabies Virus Vaccine *on page 972*

Human Diploid Cell Cultures Rabies Vaccine (Intradermal use) *see* Rabies Virus Vaccine *on page 972*

Human Growth Hormone

Brand Names Humatrope®; Nutropin®; Protropin®

Synonyms Growth Hormone; Somatrem; Somatropin

Use
Long-term treatment of growth failure from lack of adequate endogenous growth hormone secretion
Nutropin®: Treatment of children who have growth failure associated with chronic renal insufficiency up until the time of renal transplantation

Pregnancy Risk Factor C

Contraindications Closed epiphyses, known hypersensitivity to drug, benzyl alcohol (somatrem), or M-cresol or glycerin (somatropin); progression of any underlying intracranial lesion or actively growing intracranial tumor

Warnings/Precautions Use with caution in patients with diabetes; when administering to newborns, reconstitute with sterile water for injection

Adverse Reactions S.C. administration can cause local lipoatrophy or lipodystrophy and may enhance the development of neutralizing antibodies
1% to 10%: Hypothyroidism
<1%:
Dermatologic: Skin rash, itching
Local: Pain at injection site
Miscellaneous: Hypoglycemia, small risk for developing leukemia, pain in hip/knee

Overdosage/Toxicology Symptoms include hypoglycemia, hyperglycemia, acromegaly

Drug Interactions Decreased effect: Glucocorticoid therapy may inhibit growth-promoting effects.

Stability

Sumatrem (Protropin®): Store vials at 2°C to 8°C/36°F to 46°F; reconstitute each 5 mg vial with 1-5 mL of bacteriostatic water for injection; use reconstituted vials within 7 days; avoid freezing

Somatropin (Humatrope®/Nutropin®): Store vials at 2°C to 8°C/36°C to 46°F; avoid freezing; reconstitute each 5 mg vial with 1-5 mL of bacteriostatic water for injection; use reconstituted vials within 14 days; avoid freezing

Mechanism of Action Somatrem and somatropin are purified polypeptide hormones of recombinant DNA origin; somatrem contains the identical sequence of amino acids found in human growth hormone while somatropin's amino acid sequence is identical plus an additional amino acid, methionine; human growth hormone stimulates growth of linear bone, skeletal muscle, and organs; stimulates erythropoietin which increases red blood cell mass; exerts both insulin-like and diabetogenic effects

Pharmacodynamics/Kinetics Somatrem and somatropin have equivalent pharmacokinetic properties

Duration of action: Maintains supraphysiologic levels for 18-20 hours

Absorption: I.M.: Well absorbed

Metabolism: ~90% in the liver

Half-life: 15-50 minutes

Elimination: 0.1% excreted in urine unchanged

Usual Dosage Children (individualize dose):

Somatrem (Protropin®): I.M., S.C.: Up to 0.1 mg (0.26 units)/kg/dose 3 times/week

Somatropin (Humatrope®): I.M., S.C.: Up to 0.06 mg (0.16 units)/kg/dose 3 times/week

Somatropin (Nutropin®): S.C.:

Growth hormone inadequacy: Weekly dosage of 0.3 mg/kg (0.78 IU/kg) administered daily

Chronic renal insufficiency: Weekly dosage of 0.35 mg/kg (0.91 IU/kg) administered daily

Therapy should be discontinued when patient has reached satisfactory adult height, when epiphyses have fused, or when the patient ceases to respond

Growth of 5 cm/year or more is expected, if growth rate does not exceed 2.5 cm in a 6-month period, double the dose for the next 6 months, if there is still no satisfactory response, discontinue therapy

Administration Do not shake; administer S.C. or I.M.; refer to product labeling; when administering to newborns, reconstitute with sterile water for injection

Monitoring Parameters Growth curve, periodic thyroid function tests, bone age (annually), periodical urine testing for glucose, somatomedin C levels

Nursing Implications Watch for glucose intolerance

Dosage Forms Injection:

Somatropin: 5 mg ~13 units (5 mL), 10 mg ~26 units (10 mL)

Somatrem: 5 mg ~13 units (10 mL), 10 mg ~26 units (10 mL)

Humate-P® see Antihemophilic Factor (Human) on page 80

Humatin® see Paromomycin Sulfate on page 841

Humatrope® see Human Growth Hormone on previous page

Humibid® L.A. see Guaifenesin on page 515

Humibid® DM [OTC] see Guaifenesin and Dextromethorphan on page 517

Humibid® Sprinkle see Guaifenesin on page 515

HuMIST® [OTC] see Sodium Chloride on page 1012

Humorsol® see Demecarium Bromide on page 307

Humulin® 50/50 [OTC] see Insulin Preparations on page 578

Humulin® 70/30 [OTC] see Insulin Preparations on page 578

Humulin® L [OTC] see Insulin Preparations on page 578

Humulin® N [OTC] see Insulin Preparations on page 578

Humulin® R [OTC] see Insulin Preparations on page 578

Humulin® U Utralente [OTC] see Insulin Preparations on page 578

Hurricaine® see Benzocaine on page 121

Hyaluronic Acid see Sodium Hyaluronate on page 1014

Hyaluronidase (hye al yoor on' i dase)

Related Information
Extravasation Treatment of Other Drugs *on page 1209*

Brand Names Wydase®

Use Increases the dispersion and absorption of other drugs; increases rate of absorption of parenteral fluids given by hypodermoclysis; enhances diffusion of locally irritating or toxic drugs in the management of I.V. extravasation

Pregnancy Risk Factor C

Contraindications Hypersensitivity to hyaluronidase or any component; do not inject in or around infected, inflamed, or cancerous areas

Warnings/Precautions Drug infiltrates in which hyaluronidase is contraindicated: Dopamine, alpha-adrenergic agonists; an intradermal skin test for sensitivity should be performed before actual administration using 0.02 mL of a 150 units/mL of hyaluronidase solution

Adverse Reactions
<1%:
Cardiovascular: Tachycardia, hypotension
Central nervous system: Dizziness, chills
Dermatologic: Urticaria, erythema
Gastrointestinal: Nausea, vomiting

Overdosage/Toxicology Local edema, urticaria, erythema, chills, nausea, vomiting, hypotension

Drug Interactions Decreased effect: Salicylates, cortisone, ACTH, estrogens, antihistamines

Stability Reconstituted hyaluronidase solution remains stable for only 24 hours when stored in the refrigerator; do not use discolored solutions

Mechanism of Action Modifies the permeability of connective tissue through hydrolysis of hyaluronic acid, one of the chief ingredients of tissue cement which offers resistance to diffusion of liquids through tissues

Pharmacodynamics/Kinetics
Onset of action: Immediate by the subcutaneous or intradermal routes for the treatment of extravasation
Duration: 24-48 hours

Usual Dosage
Infants and Children:
Management of I.V. extravasation: Reconstitute the 150 unit vial of lyophilized powder with 1 mL normal saline; take 0.1 mL of this solution and dilute with 0.9 mL normal saline to yield 15 units/mL; using a 25- or 26-gauge needle, five 0.2 mL injections are made subcutaneously or intradermally into the extravasation site at the leading edge, changing the needle after each injection
Hypodermoclysis:
S.C.: 1 mL (150 units) is added to 1000 mL of infusion fluid and 0.5 mL (75 units) in injected into each clysis site at the initiation of the infusion
I.V.: 15 units is added to each 100 mL of I.V. fluid to be administered
Children <3 years: Limit volume of single clysis to 200 mL
Premature Infants and Neonates: Do not exceed 25 mL/kg/day and not >2 mL/minute
Adults: Absorption and dispersion of drugs: 150 units are added to the vehicle containing the drug

Administration Administer hyaluronidase within the first few minutes to 1 hour after the extravasation of a necrotizing agent is recognized; do not administer I.V.

Nursing Implications Appropriate drugs for the management of an acute hypersensitivity (epinephrine, corticosteroids, and antihistamines) should be readily available

Additional Information The USP hyaluronidase unit is equivalent to the turbidity-reducing (TR) unit and the International Unit; each unit is defined as being the activity contained in 100 mcg of the International Standard Preparation

Dosage Forms
Injection, stabilized solution: 150 units/mL (1 mL, 10 mL)
Powder for injection, lyophilized: 150 units, 1500 units

Hyate®:C *see* Antihemophilic Factor (Porcine) *on page 82*

Hybalamin® *see* Hydroxocobalamin *on page 552*

Hybolin™ Decanoate *see* Nandrolone *on page 774*

Hybolin™ Improved *see* Nandrolone *on page 774*

Hycodan® *see* Hydrocodone and Homatropine *on page 545*

Hycort® *see* Hydrocortisone *on page 546*

Hydeltrasol® *see* Prednisolone *on page 919*

Hydeltra-T.B.A.® *see* Prednisolone *on page 919*

Hydergine® *see Ergoloid Mesylates on page 397*

Hydergine® LC *see Ergoloid Mesylates on page 397*

Hydralazine Hydrochloride (hye dral' a zeen)

Brand Names Apresoline®

Use Management of moderate to severe hypertension, congestive heart failure, hypertension secondary to pre-eclampsia/eclampsia; also used to treat primary pulmonary hypertension

Pregnancy Risk Factor C

Contraindications Hypersensitivity to hydralazine or any component, dissecting aortic aneurysm, mitral valve rheumatic heart disease

Warnings/Precautions Discontinue hydralazine in patients who develop SLE-like syndrome or positive ANA. Use with caution in patients with severe renal disease or cerebral vascular accidents or with known or suspected coronary artery disease; monitor blood pressure closely with I.V. use; some formulations may contain tartrazines or sulfites. Slow acetylators, patients with decreased renal function, and patients receiving >200 mg/day (chronically) are at higher risk for SLE. Titrate dosage to patient's response. Usually administered with diuretic and a beta-blocker to counteract side effects of sodium and water retention and reflex tachycardia.

Adverse Reactions

>10%:
  Cardiovascular: Palpitations, flushing, tachycardia, angina pectoris
  Central nervous system: Headache
  Gastrointestinal: Nausea, vomiting, diarrhea, anorexia
1% to 10%:
  Cardiovascular: Hypotension, redness or flushing of face
  Gastrointestinal: Constipation
  Ocular: Lacrimation
  Respiratory: Dyspnea, nasal congestion
<1%:
  Central nervous system: Malaise, peripheral neuritis, fever, dizziness
  Dermatologic: Rash, edema
  Neuromuscular & skeletal: Arthralgias, weakness
  Miscellaneous: Positive ANA, positive LE cells
  Note: Because of blunted beta-receptor response, the elderly are less likely to experience reflex tachycardia; this puts them at greater risk for orthostatic hypotension

Overdosage/Toxicology Symptoms of overdose include hypotension, tachycardia, shock; hypotension usually responds to I.V. fluid, Trendelenburg positioning or vasoconstrictors; treatment is primarily supportive and symptomatic

Drug Interactions Increased toxicity: MAO inhibitors → significant decrease in blood pressure; indomethacin → ↓ hypotensive effects

Stability

Intact ampuls/vials of hydralazine should not be stored under refrigeration because of possible precipitation or crystallization
Hydralazine should be diluted in NS for IVPB administration due to decreased stability in D_5W
Stability of IVPB solution in NS: 4 days at room temperature

Mechanism of Action Direct vasodilation of arterioles (with little effect on veins) with decreased systemic resistance

Pharmacodynamics/Kinetics

Onset of action:
  Oral: 20-30 minutes
  I.V.: 5-20 minutes
Duration:
  Oral: 2-4 hours
  I.V.: 2-6 hours
Distribution: Crosses placenta; appears in breast milk
Metabolism: Large first-pass effect orally, acetylated in liver
Protein binding: 85% to 90%
Bioavailability: 30% to 50%; enhanced by concurrent administration with food
Half-life:
  Normal renal function: 2-8 hours
  End stage renal disease: 7-16 hours
Elimination: 14% excreted unchanged in urine

Usual Dosage

Children:
  Oral: Initial: 0.75-1 mg/kg/day in 2-4 divided doses, not to exceed 25 mg/dose; increase over 3-4 weeks to maximum of 7.5 mg/kg/day in 2-4 divided doses; maximum daily dose: 200 mg/day

(Continued)

Hydralazine Hydrochloride *(Continued)*

I.M., I.V.: 0.1-0.2 mg/kg/dose (not to exceed 20 mg) every 4-6 hours as needed, up to 1.7-3.5 mg/kg/day in 4-6 divided doses

Adults:

Oral: Hypertension:
Initial dose: 10 mg 4 times/day
Increase by 10-25 mg/dose every 2-5 days
Maximum dose: 300 mg/day

Oral: Congestive heart failure:
Initial dose: 10-25 mg TID
Target dose: 75 mg TID
Maximum dose: 100 mg TID

I.M., I.V.:
Hypertensive Initial: 10-20 mg/dose every 4-6 hours as needed, may increase to 40 mg/dose; change to oral therapy as soon as possible
Pre-eclampsia/eclampsia: 5 mg/dose then 5-10 mg every 20-30 minutes as needed

Elderly: Oral: Initial: 10 mg 2-3 times/day; increase by 10-25 mg/day every 2-5 days

Dosing interval in renal impairment:
Cl_{cr} 10-50 mL/minute: Administer every 8 hours
Cl_{cr} <10 mL/minute: Administer every 8-16 hours in fast acetylators and every 12-24 hours in slow acetylators
Hemodialysis effects: Supplemental dose is not necessary
Peritoneal dialysis effects: Supplemental dose is not necessary

Monitoring Parameters Blood pressure (monitor closely with I.V. use), standing and sitting/supine, heart rate, ANA titer

Patient Information Report flu-like symptoms, rise slowly from sitting/lying position; take with meals

Nursing Implications Aid with ambulation, rising may cause orthostasis

Dosage Forms
Injection: 20 mg/mL (1 mL)
Tablet: 10 mg, 25 mg, 50 mg, 100 mg

Hydrate® *see* Dimenhydrinate *on page 347*

Hydrated Chloral *see* Chloral Hydrate *on page 217*

Hydrea® *see* Hydroxyurea *on page 554*

Hydrex® *see* Benzthiazide *on page 123*

Hydrisalic™ *see* Salicylic Acid *on page 991*

Hydrobexan® *see* Hydroxocobalamin *on page 552*

Hydrocet® *see* Hydrocodone and Acetaminophen *on next page*

Hydrochlorothiazide *(hye droe klor oh thye' a zide)*

Brand Names Esidrix®; Ezide®; HydroDIURIL®; Hydro-Par®; Oretic®

Synonyms HCTZ

Use Management of mild to moderate hypertension; treatment of edema in congestive heart failure and nephrotic syndrome

Pregnancy Risk Factor D

Contraindications Anuria, renal decompensation, hypersensitivity to hydrochlorothiazide or any component, cross-sensitivity with other thiazides and sulfonamide derivatives

Warnings/Precautions Use with caution in renal disease, hepatic disease, gout, lupus erythematosus, diabetes mellitus; some products may contain tartrazine. Hydrochlorothiazide is not effective in patients with a Cl_{cr} <30 mL/minute, therefore, it may not be a useful agent in many elderly patients.

Adverse Reactions
1% to 10%: Endocrine & metabolic: Hypokalemia
<1%:
Cardiovascular: Hypotension
Dermatologic: Photosensitivity
Endocrine & metabolic: Fluid and electrolyte imbalances (hypocalcemia, hypomagnesemia, hyponatremia), hyperglycemia
Hematologic: Rarely blood dyscrasias
Renal: Prerenal azotemia

Overdosage/Toxicology Symptoms of overdose include hypermotility, diuresis, lethargy, confusion, muscle weakness; following GI decontamination, therapy is supportive with I.V. fluids, electrolytes, and I.V. pressors if needed

Drug Interactions
Decreased effect: Decreased antidiabetic drug efficacy
Increased toxicity:
Hypotensive agents → ↑ hypotensive potential
Increased digoxin related arrhythmias
Increased lithium levels
Tetracyclines → ↑ uremia
Mechanism of Action Inhibits sodium reabsorption in the distal tubules causing increased excretion of sodium and water as well as potassium and hydrogen ions
Pharmacodynamics/Kinetics
Onset of diuretic action: Oral: Within 2 hours
Peak effect: 4 hours
Duration: 6-12 hours
Absorption: Oral: ~60% to 80%
Elimination: Excreted unchanged in urine
Usual Dosage Oral (effect of drug may be decreased when used every day):
Children (In pediatric patients, chlorothiazide may be preferred over hydrochlorothiazide as there are more dosage formulations (eg, suspension) available):
<6 months: 2-3 mg/kg/day in 2 divided doses
>6 months: 2 mg/kg/day in 2 divided doses
Adults: 25-100 mg/day in 1-2 doses
Maximum: 200 mg/day
Elderly: 12.5-25 mg once daily
Minimal increase in response and more electrolyte disturbances are seen with doses >50 mg/day

Dosing adjustment/comments in renal impairment: Cl_{cr} <50 mL/minute: Not effective
Monitoring Parameters Assess weight, I & O reports daily to determine fluid loss; blood pressure, serum electrolytes, BUN, creatinine
Test Interactions ↑ creatine phosphokinase [CPK] (S), ammonia (B), amylase (S), calcium (S), chloride (S), cholesterol (S), glucose, ↑ acid (S), ↓ chloride (S), magnesium, potassium, sodium (S); Tyramine and phentolamine tests, histamine tests for pheochromocytoma
Patient Information May be taken with food or milk; take early in day to avoid nocturia; take the last dose of multiple doses no later than 6 PM unless instructed otherwise. A few people who take this medication become more sensitive to sunlight and may experience skin rash, redness, itching, or severe sunburn, especially if sun block SPF ≥15 is not used on exposed skin areas. May increase blood glucose levels in diabetics.
Nursing Implications Take blood pressure with patient lying down and standing
Dosage Forms
Solution, oral (mint flavor): 50 mg/5 mL (50 mL)
Tablet: 25 mg, 50 mg, 100 mg

Hydrocil® [OTC] *see* Psyllium *on page 956*

Hydro-Cobex® *see* Hydroxocobalamin *on page 552*

Hydrocodone and Acetaminophen (hye droe koe' done)
Related Information
Narcotic Agonist Comparison Charts *on page 1274-1275*
Brand Names Anexsia®; Anodynos-DHC®; Bancap HC®; Co-Gesic®; Dolacet®; DuoCet™; Duradyne DHC®; Hydrocet®; Hydrogesic®; Hy-Phen®; Lorcet®; Lorcet®-HD; Lorcet® Plus; Lortab®; Margesic® H; Norcet®; Stagesic®; T-Gesic®; Vicodin®; Vicodin® ES; Zydone®
Synonyms Acetaminophen and Hydrocodone
Use Relief of moderate to severe pain; antitussive (hydrocodone)
Restrictions C-III
Pregnancy Risk Factor C
Contraindications CNS depression, hypersensitivity to hydrocodone, acetaminophen or any component; severe respiratory depression
Warnings/Precautions Use with caution in patients with hypersensitivity reactions to other phenanthrene derivative opioid agonists (morphine, hydrocodone, hydromorphone, levorphanol, oxycodone, oxymorphone); tablets contain metabisulfite which may cause allergic reactions
Adverse Reactions
>10%:
Cardiovascular: Hypotension
Central nervous system: Lightheadedness, dizziness, sedation, drowsiness, weakness, tiredness
1% to 10%:
Cardiovascular: Bradycardia
(Continued)

Hydrocodone and Acetaminophen *(Continued)*

    Central nervous system: Confusion
    Gastrointestinal: Nausea, vomiting
    Genitourinary: Decreased urination
    Respiratory: Shortness of breath, troubled breathing
<1%:
    Cardiovascular: Hypertension
    Central nervous system: Hallucinations
    Gastrointestinal: Dry mouth, anorexia
    Ocular: Double vision, miosis
    Miscellaneous: Biliary or urinary tract spasm, histamine release, physical and psychological dependence with prolonged use

Overdosage/Toxicology Symptoms of overdose include hepatic necrosis, blood dyscrasias, respiratory depression. Acetylcysteine 140 mg/kg orally (loading) followed by 70 mg/kg every 4 hours for 17 doses. Therapy should be initiated based upon laboratory analysis suggesting high probability of hepatotoxic potential. Naloxone (2 mg I.V.) can also be used to reverse the toxic effects of the opiate. Activated charcoal is effective at binding certain chemicals, and this is especially true for acetaminophen.

Drug Interactions
    Decreased effect with phenothiazines
    Increased effect with dextroamphetamine
    Increased toxicity with CNS depressants, TCAs

Mechanism of Action See individual agents

Pharmacodynamics/Kinetics
    Onset of narcotic analgesia: Within 10-20 minutes
    Duration: 3-6 hours
    Distribution: Crosses the placenta
    Metabolism: In the liver
    Half-life: 3.8 hours
    Elimination: In urine

Usual Dosage Oral (doses should be titrated to appropriate analgesic effect):
    Children:
        Antitussive (hydrocodone): 0.6 mg/kg/day in 3-4 divided doses
            A single dose should not exceed 10 mg in children >12 years, 5 mg in children 2-12 years, and 1.25 mg in children <2 years of age
        Analgesic (acetaminophen): Refer to Acetaminophen monograph

    Adults: Analgesic: 1-2 tablets or capsules every 4-6 hours or 5-10 mL solution every 4-6 hours as needed for pain

Monitoring Parameters Pain relief, respiratory and mental status, blood pressure

Patient Information May cause drowsiness; do not exceed recommended dose; do not take for more than 10 days without physician's advice

Nursing Implications Observe patient for excessive sedation, respiratory depression

Dosage Forms
    Capsule:
        Bancap HC®, Dolacet®, Hydrocet®, Hydrogesic®, Lorcet®-HD, Margesic® H, Norcet®, Stagesic®, T-Gesic®, Zydone®: Hydrocodone bitartrate 5 mg and acetaminophen 500 mg
    Solution, oral (tropical fruit punch flavor) (Lortab®): Hydrocodone bitartrate 2.5 mg and acetaminophen 120 mg per 5 mL with alcohol 7% (480 mL)
    Tablet:
        Lortab® 2.5/500: Hydrocodone bitartrate 2.5 mg and acetaminophen 500 mg
        Anexsia® 5/500, Anodynos-DHC®, Co-Gesic®, DuoCet™, Duradyne DHC®, Hy-Phen®, Lorcet®, Lortab®® 5/500, Vicodin®: Hydrocodone bitartrate 5 mg and acetaminophen 500 mg
        Lortab® 7.5/500: Hydrocodone bitartrate 7.5 mg and acetaminophen 500 mg
        Anexsia® 7.5/650, Lorcet® Plus: Hydrocodone bitartrate 7.5 mg and acetaminophen 650 mg
        Vicodin® ES: Hydrocodone bitartrate 7.5 mg and acetaminophen 750 mg
        Lortab® 10/650: Hydrocodone bitartrate 10 mg and acetaminophen 650 mg

Hydrocodone and Aspirin *(hye droe koe' done)*

Related Information
    Narcotic Agonist Comparison Charts *on page 1274-1275*

Brand Names Azdone®; Damason-P®; Lortab® ASA

Use Relief of moderate to moderately severe pain

Restrictions C-III

Pregnancy Risk Factor D

Warnings/Precautions Use with caution in patients with impaired renal function, erosive gastritis, or peptic ulcer disease; children and teenagers should not use for chickenpox or flu symptoms before a physician is consulted about Reye's syndrome

Adverse Reactions

>10%:

Cardiovascular: Hypotension

Central nervous system: Lightheadedness, dizziness, sedation, drowsiness, weakness, tiredness

Gastrointestinal: Nausea, heartburn, stomach pains, dyspepsia, epigastric discomfort

1% to 10%:

Cardiovascular: Bradycardia

Central nervous system: Confusion

Dermatologic: Skin rash

Gastrointestinal: Vomiting, gastrointestinal ulceration

Genitourinary: Decreased urination

Hematologic: Hemolytic anemia

Respiratory: Shortness of breath, troubled breathing

Miscellaneous: Anaphylactic shock

<1%:

Cardiovascular: Hypertension

Central nervous system: Hallucinations, insomnia, nervousness, jitters

Gastrointestinal: Dry mouth, anorexia

Hematologic: Occult bleeding, prolongation of bleeding time, leukopenia, thrombocytopenia, iron deficiency anemia

Hepatic: Hepatotoxicity

Ocular: Double vision, miosis

Renal: Impaired renal function

Respiratory: Bronchospasm

Miscellaneous: Biliary or urinary tract spasm, histamine release, physical and psychological dependence with prolonged use

Overdosage/Toxicology

Antidote is naloxone for codeine. Naloxone 2 mg I.V. (0.01 mg/kg for children) with repeat administration as necessary up to a total of 10 mg

The "Done" nomogram is very helpful for estimating the severity of aspirin poisoning and directing treatment using serum salicylate levels. Treatment can also be based upon symptomatology; see Aspirin.

Drug Interactions Increased toxicity with CNS depressants, warfarin (bleeding)

Mechanism of Action Refer to individual agents

Usual Dosage Adults: Oral: 1-2 tablets every 4-6 hours as needed for pain

Administration Administer with food or a full glass of water to minimize GI distress

Monitoring Parameters Observe patient for excessive sedation, respiratory depression

Test Interactions Urine glucose, urinary 5-HIAA, serum uric acid

Patient Information May cause drowsiness; avoid alcohol; watch for bleeding gums or any signs of GI bleeding; take with food or milk to minimize GI distress, notify physician if ringing in ears or persistent GI pain occurs

Dosage Forms Tablet: Hydrocodone bitartrate 5 mg and aspirin 500 mg

Hydrocodone and Homatropine (hoe ma' toe peen)

Related Information

Narcotic Agonist Comparison Charts *on page 1274-1275*

Brand Names Hycodan®; Hydromet®; Hydropane®; Hydrotropine®; Tussigon®

Synonyms Homatropine and Hydrocodone

Use Symptomatic relief of cough

Restrictions C-III

Pregnancy Risk Factor C

Contraindications Increased intracranial pressure, narrow-angle glaucoma, depressed ventilation, hypersensitivity to hydrocodone, homatropine, or any component

Warnings/Precautions Use with caution in patients with hypersensitivity to other phenanthrene derivatives; use with caution in patients with respiratory diseases, or severe liver or renal failure; use with caution in children with spastic paralysis, in the elderly, and in patients with prostatic hypertrophy

Adverse Reactions

>10%:

Cardiovascular: Hypotension

Central nervous system: Lightheadedness, dizziness, sedation, drowsiness, weakness, tiredness

(Continued)

Hydrocodone and Homatropine *(Continued)*

1% to 10%:
  Cardiovascular: Bradycardia, tachycardia
  Central nervous system: Confusion
  Gastrointestinal: Nausea, vomiting
  Genitourinary: Decreased urination
  Respiratory: Shortness of breath, troubled breathing

<1%:
  Central nervous system: Hallucinations
  Cardiovascular: Hypertension
  Dermatologic: Dry hot skin
  Gastrointestinal: Dry mouth, anorexia, impaired GI motility
  Ocular: Double vision, miosis, mydriasis, blurred vision
  Miscellaneous: Biliary or urinary tract spasm, histamine release, physical and
    psychological dependence with prolonged use

Overdosage/Toxicology Symptoms of overdose include CNS and respiratory
depression; gastrointestinal cramping; dilated, unreactive pupils; blurred vision;
hot, dry flushed skin; dryness of mucous membranes; difficulty in swallowing, foul
breath, diminished or absent bowel sounds, urinary retention, tachycardia, hyperthermia, hypertension, increased respiratory rate

CNS depression is an extension of pharmacologic effect; treatment is supportive;
naloxone 0.4 mg I.V. (0.01 mg/kg for children) with repeat administrations as
necessary; anticholinergic toxicity is caused by strong binding of the drug to
cholinergic receptors. For anticholinergic overdose with severe life-threatening
symptoms, physostigmine 1-2 mg (0.5 or 0.02 mg/kg for children) S.C. or I.V.,
slowly may be given to reverse these effects.

Usual Dosage Oral (based on hydrocodone component):
  Children: 0.6 mg/kg/day in 3-4 divided doses; do not administer more frequently
    than every 4 hours
    A single dose should not exceed 1.25 mg in children <2 years of age, 5 mg in
      children 2-12 years, and 10 mg in children >12 years
  Adults: 5-10 mg every 4-6 hours, a single dose should not exceed 15 mg; do not
    administer more frequently than every 4 hours

Test Interactions ↑ ALT, AST (S)

Patient Information Avoid alcohol; may cause drowsiness and impair judgment
or coordination; may cause physical and psychological dependence with
prolonged use; lack of saliva may enhance cavities; maintain good oral hygiene;
use caution while driving; may cause blurred vision; notify physician if difficulty in
urinating or constipation becomes severe

Nursing Implications Dispense in light-resistant container; observe patient for
excessive sedation, respiratory depression, implement safety measures, assist
with ambulation

Dosage Forms
  Syrup (Hycodan®, Hydromet®, Hydropane®, Hydrotropine®): Hydrocodone
    bitartrate 5 mg and homatropine methylbromide 1.5 mg per 5 mL (120 mL, 480
    mL, 4000 mL)
  Tablet (Hycodan®, Tussigon®): Hydrocodone bitartrate 5 mg and homatropine
    methylbromide 1.5 mg

Hydrocort® *see Hydrocortisone on this page*

Hydrocortisone *(hye droe kor' ti sone)*

Related Information
  Corticosteroids Comparisons *on page 1266-1268*

Brand Names Acticort™; Aeroseb-HC®; A-HydroCort®; Ala-Cort®; Ala-Scalp™;
Anucort-HC®; Anumed HC™; Anusol-HC® [OTC]; Caldecort® Anti-Itch Spray
[OTC]; Caldecort® [OTC]; Cetacort®; Clocort® Maximum Strength; CortaGel®
[OTC]; Cortaid® Maximum Strength [OTC]; Cortaid® with Aloe [OTC]; Cort-
Dome®; Cortef®; Cortef® Feminine Itch [OTC]; Cortenema®; Corticaine®
[OTC]; Cortizone®-5 [OTC]; Cortizone®-10 [OTC]; Delcort®; Dermacort®;
Dermarest Dricort®; DermiCort®; Dermolate® [OTC]; Dermtex® HC with Aloe;
Eldecort®; Gynecort® [OTC]; Hemril-HC™; Hi-Cor 1.0®; Hi-Cor-2.5®; Hycort®;
Hydrocort®; Hydrocortone® Acetate; Hydrocortone® Phosphate; HydroSKIN®;
Hydro-Tex® [OTC]; Hytone®; LactiCare-HC®; Lanacort® [OTC]; Locoid®;
Maximum Strength Bactimne™ [OTC]; Nutracort®; Orabase® HCA; Penecort®;
Proctocort™; ProctoCream-HC™; Scalpicin®; Solu-Cortef®; S-T Cort®;
Synacort®; Tegrin®-HC; Texacort™; U-Cort™ Cortifoam®; Westcort®

Synonyms Compound F; Cortisol; Hydrocortisone Acetate; Hydrocortisone Cypionate; Hydrocortisone Sodium Phosphate; Hydrocortisone Sodium Succinate;
Hydrocortisone Valerate

Use Management of adrenocortical insufficiency; relief of inflammation of corticosteroid-responsive dermatoses (low and medium potency topical corticosteroid); adjunctive treatment of ulcerative colitis

Pregnancy Risk Factor C

Contraindications Serious infections, except septic shock or tuberculous meningitis; known hypersensitivity to hydrocortisone; viral, fungal, or tubercular skin lesions

Warnings/Precautions

Use with caution in patients with hyperthyroidism, cirrhosis, nonspecific ulcerative colitis, hypertension, osteoporosis, thromboembolic tendencies, CHF, convulsive disorders, myasthenia gravis, thrombophlebitis, peptic ulcer, diabetes

Acute adrenal insufficiency may occur with abrupt withdrawal after long-term therapy or with stress; young pediatric patients may be more susceptible to adrenal axis suppression from topical therapy

Because of the risk of adverse effects, systemic corticosteroids should be used cautiously in the elderly, in the smallest possible dose, and for the shortest possible time

Adverse Reactions

>10%:

Central nervous system: Insomnia, nervousness

Gastrointestinal: Increased appetite, indigestion

1% to 10%:

Central nervous system: Epistaxis

Dermatologic: Hirsutism

Endocrine & metabolic: Diabetes mellitus

Neuromuscular & skeletal: Joint pain

Ocular: Cataracts

<1%:

Cardiovascular: Hypertension, edema

Central nervous system: Euphoria, headache, delirium, hallucinations, seizures, mood swings

Dermatologic: Acne, dermatitis, skin atrophy, bruising, hyperpigmentation

Endocrine & metabolic: Hypokalemia, hyperglycemia, Cushing's syndrome, sodium and water retention, bone growth suppression, amenorrhea

Gastrointestinal: Peptic ulcer, abdominal distention, ulcerative esophagitis, pancreatitis

Hematologic: Immunosuppression

Neuromuscular & skeletal: Muscle wasting

Miscellaneous: Hypersensitivity reactions

Overdosage/Toxicology Symptoms of overdose include cushingoid appearance (systemic), muscle weakness (systemic), osteoporosis (systemic) all with long-term use only. When consumed in excessive quantities for prolonged periods, systemic hypercorticism and adrenal suppression may occur. In those cases, discontinuation and withdrawal of the corticosteroid should be done judiciously.

Drug Interactions

Decreased effect:

Insulin decreased hypoglycemic effect

Phenytoin, phenobarbital, ephedrine, and rifampin ↑ metabolism of hydrocortisone and ↓ steroid blood level

Increased toxicity:

Oral anticoagulants change prothrombin time; potassium depleting diuretics increase risk of hypokalemia

Cardiac glucosides increase risk of arrhythmias or digitalis toxicity secondary to hypokalemia

Stability

Hydrocortisone sodium phosphate and hydrocortisone sodium succinate are clear, light yellow solutions which are heat labile

After initial reconstitution, hydrocortisone sodium succinate solutions are stable for 3 days at room temperature and refrigeration if protected from light

Stability of parenteral admixture (Solu-Cortef®) at room temperature (25°C) and at refrigeration temperature (4°C) is concentration dependent

Minimum volume: Concentration should not exceed 1 mg/mL

Stability of concentration ≤1 mg/mL: 24 hours; concentration >1 mg/mL to <25 mg/mL: Unpredictable, 4-6 hours; concentration ≥25 mg/mL: 3 days

Standard diluent (Solu-Cortef®): 50 mg/50 mL D_5W; 100 mg/100 mL D_5W

Comments: Should be administered in a 0.1-1 mg/mL concentration due to stability problems

Mechanism of Action Decreases inflammation by suppression of migration of polymorphonuclear leukocytes and reversal of increased capillary permeability

Pharmacodynamics/Kinetics

Absorption: Rapid by all routes, except rectally

(Continued)

547

Hydrocortisone *(Continued)*

Metabolism: In the liver

Half-life, biologic: 8-12 hours

Elimination: Renally, mainly as 17-hydroxysteroids and 17-ketosteroids

Hydrocortisone acetate salt has a slow onset but long duration of action when compared with more soluble preparations

Hydrocortisone sodium phosphate salt is a water soluble salt with a rapid onset but short duration of action

Hydrocortisone sodium succinate salt is a water soluble salt with is rapidly active

Usual Dosage

Acute adrenal insufficiency: I.M., I.V.:

Infants and young Children: Succinate: 1-2 mg/kg/dose bolus, then 25-150 mg/day in divided doses

Older Children: Succinate: 1-2 mg/kg bolus then 150-250 mg/day in divided doses

Physiologic replacement: Children:

Oral: 0.5-0.75 mg/kg/day or 20-25 mg/m^2/day every 8 hours

I.M.: Succinate: 0.25-0.35 mg/kg/day or 12-15 mg/m^2/day once daily

Adrenal corticoid insufficiency: Adults: Oral: 20-30 mg/day

Anti-inflammatory or immunosuppressive:

Infants and Children:

Oral: 2.5-10 mg/kg/day or 75-300 mg/m^2/day every 6-8 hours

I.M., I.V.: Succinate: 1-5 mg/kg/day or 30-150 mg/m^2/day divided every 12-24 hours

Adults:

Oral: 20-240 mg/day in 2-4 divided doses;

I.M., I.V.: Succinate: 100-500 mg every 2-10 hours

I.M., I.V.,S.C.: Sodium phosphate: Initially 15-240 mg/day (approximately $^1/_3$ to $^1/_2$ of the oral dose) in divided doses every 12 hours. In acute diseases, doses >240 mg may be required.

Congenital adrenal hyperplasia: Oral: Initial: 30-36 mg/m^2/day with $^1/_3$ of dose every morning and $^2/_3$ every evening or $^1/_4$ every morning and mid-day and $^1/_2$ every evening; maintenance: 20-25 mg/m^2/day in divided doses

Status asthmaticus: Children and Adults: I.V.: Succinate: 1-2 mg/kg/dose every 6 hours for 24 hours, then maintenance of 0.5-1 mg/kg every 6 hours

Shock: I.M., I.V.: Succinate:

Children: Initial: 50 mg/kg, then 50-75 mg/kg/day every 6 hours

Adults: 500 mg to 2 g every 2-6 hours

Rheumatic diseases:

Adults: Intralesional, intra-articular, soft tissue injection: Acetate:

Large joints: 25 mg (up to 37.5 mg)

Small joints: 10-25 mg

Tendon sheaths: 5-12.5 mg

Soft tissue infiltration: 25-50 mg (up to 75 mg)

Bursae: 25-37.5 mg

Ganglia: 12.5-25 mg

Dermatosis: Children >2 years and Adults: Topical: Apply to affected area 2-4 times/day

Anorectal: Adults: Rectal: 10-100 mg 1-2 times/day for 2-3 weeks

Administration

Hydrocortisone sodium succinate may be administered by I.M. or I.V. routes

I.V. bolus: Dilute to 50 mg/mL and give over 30 seconds to several minutes (depending on the dose)

I.V. intermittent infusion: Dilute to 1 mg/mL and give over 20-30 minutes

Monitoring Parameters Blood pressure, weight, serum glucose, and electrolytes

Reference Range Therapeutic: AM: 5-25 µg/dL (SI: 138-690 nmol/L), PM: 2-9 µg/dL (SI: 55-248 nmol/L) depending on test, assay

Patient Information Notify surgeon or dentist before surgical repair; oral formulation may cause GI upset, take with food; notify physician if any sign of infection occurs; avoid abrupt withdrawal when on long-term therapy. Before applying, gently wash area to reduce risk of infection; apply a thin film to cleansed area and rub in gently and thoroughly until medication vanishes; avoid exposure to sunlight, severe sunburn may occur.

Additional Information

Sodium content of 1 g (sodium succinate injection): 47.5 mg (2.07 mEq)

Hydrocortisone base topical cream, lotion, and ointments in concentrations of 0.25%, 0.5%, and 1% may be OTC or prescription depending on the product labeling

Dosage Forms

Hydrocortisone acetate:

Cream, topical: 0.5% (15 g, 22.5 g, 30 g); 1% (15 g, 30 g, 120 g)

Ointment, topical: 0.5% (15 g, 30 g); 1% (15 g, 21 g, 30 g)

Injection, suspension: 25 mg/mL (5 mL, 10 mL); 50 mg/mL (5 mL, 10 mL)
Suppositories, rectal: 10 mg, 25 mg
Hydrocortisone base:
Aerosol, topical: 0.5% (45 g, 58 g); 1% (45 mL)
Cream, rectal: 1% (30 g); 2.5% (30 g)
Cream, topical: 0.5% (15 g, 30 g, 60 g, 120 g, 454 g); 1% (15 g, 20 g, 30 g, 60 g, 90 g, 120 g, 240 g, 454 g); 2.5% (15 g, 20 g, 30 g, 60 g, 120 g, 240 g, 454 g)
Gel, topical: 0.5% (15 g, 30 g); 1% (15 g, 30 g)
Lotion, topical: 0.25% (120 mL); 0.5% (30 mL, 60 mL, 120 mL); 1% (60 mL, 118 mL, 120 mL); 2% (30 mL) ; 2.5% (60 mL, 120 mL)
Ointment, rectal: 1% (30 g)
Ointment, topical: 0.5% (30 g) ; 1% (15 g, 20 g, 28 g, 30 g, 60 g, 120 g, 240 g, 454 g); 2.5% (20 g, 30 g)
Suspension, rectal: 100 mg/60 mL (7s)
Tablet, oral: 5 mg, 10 mg, 20 mg
Hydrocortisone cypionate:
Suspension, oral: 10 mg/5 mL (120 mL)
Hydrocortisone sodium phosphate:
Injection, IM/IV/SC: 50 mg/mL (2 mL, 10 mL)
Hydrocortisone sodium succinate:
Injection, IM/IV: 100 mg, 250 mg, 500 mg, 1000 mg
Hydrocortisone valerate:
Cream, topical: 0.2% (15 g, 45 g, 60 g)
Ointment, topical: 0.2% (15 g, 45 g, 60 g, 120 g)

Hydrocortisone Acetate *see* Hydrocortisone *on page 546*

Hydrocortisone Cypionate *see* Hydrocortisone *on page 546*

Hydrocortisone Sodium Phosphate *see* Hydrocortisone *on page 546*

Hydrocortisone Sodium Succinate *see* Hydrocortisone *on page 546*

Hydrocortisone Valerate *see* Hydrocortisone *on page 546*

Hydrocortone® Acetate *see* Hydrocortisone *on page 546*

Hydrocortone® Phosphate *see* Hydrocortisone *on page 546*

Hydro-Crysti-12® *see* Hydroxocobalamin *on page 552*

HydroDIURIL® *see* Hydrochlorothiazide *on page 542*

Hydro-Ergoloid® *see* Ergoloid Mesylates *on page 397*

Hydroflumethiazide (hye droe floo meth eye' a zide)
Brand Names Diucardin®; Saluron®
Use Management of mild to moderate hypertension; treatment of edema in congestive heart failure and nephrotic syndrome
Pregnancy Risk Factor D
Contraindications Anuria, renal decompensation, hypersensitivity to hydrochlorothiazide or any component, cross-sensitivity with other thiazides and sulfonamide derivatives
Warnings/Precautions Use with caution in renal disease, hepatic disease, gout, lupus erythematosus, diabetes mellitus; some products may contain tartrazine
Adverse Reactions
1% to 10%: Endocrine & metabolic: Hypokalemia
<1%:
Cardiovascular: Hypotension
Central nervous system: Drowsiness
Dermatologic: Photosensitivity, rash
Endocrine & metabolic: Fluid and electrolyte imbalances (hypocalcemia, hypomagnesemia, hyponatremia), hyperglycemia
Gastrointestinal: Anorexia
Genitourinary: Uremia
Hematologic: Aplastic anemia, hemolytic anemia, leukopenia, agranulocytosis, thrombocytopenia, rarely blood dyscrasias
Hepatic: Hepatitis
Neuromuscular & skeletal: Paresthesia
Renal: Polyuria, prerenal azotemia
Overdosage/Toxicology Symptoms of overdose include hypermotility, diuresis, lethargy; following GI decontamination, therapy is supportive with I.V. fluids, electrolytes, and I.V. pressors if needed
Drug Interactions
Decreased effect of oral hypoglycemics; decreased absorption with cholestyramine and colestipol
Increased effect with furosemide and other loop diuretics
(Continued)

Hydroflumethiazide *(Continued)*

Increased toxicity/levels of lithium

Mechanism of Action The diuretic mechanism of action is primarily inhibition of sodium, chloride, and water reabsorption in the renal distal tubules, thereby producing diuresis with a resultant reduction in plasma volume

Pharmacodynamics/Kinetics

Onset of diuretic effect: Within ~2 hours

Peak effect: Within ~4 hours

Duration of action: 12-24 hours

Usual Dosage Oral:

Children: 1 mg/kg/24 hours

Adults: 50-200 mg/day

Monitoring Parameters Assess weight, I & O reports daily to determine fluid loss; blood pressure, serum electrolytes, BUN, creatinine

Test Interactions ↑ ammonia (B), ↑ amylase (S), ↑ calcium (S), ↑ chloride (S), ↑ glucose, ↑ uric acid (S); ↓ chloride (S), ↓ magnesium, ↓ potassium (S), ↓ sodium (S)

Patient Information May be taken with food or milk; take early in day to avoid nocturia; take the last dose of multiple doses no later than 6 PM unless instructed otherwise. A few people who take this medication become more sensitive to sunlight and may experience skin rash, redness, itching or severe sunburn, especially if sun block SPF ≥15 is not used on exposed skin areas.

Nursing Implications Take blood pressure with patient lying down and standing

Dosage Forms Tablet: 50 mg

Hydrogenated Ergot Alkaloids *see* Ergoloid Mesylates *on page 397*

Hydrogesic® *see* Hydrocodone and Acetaminophen *on page 543*

Hydromet® *see* Hydrocodone and Homatropine *on page 545*

Hydromorphone Hydrochloride *(hye droe mor' fone)*

Related Information

Narcotic Agonist Comparison Charts *on page 1274-1275*

Brand Names Dilaudid®; Dilaudid-HP®

Synonyms Dihydromorphinone

Use Management of moderate to severe pain; antitussive at lower doses

Restrictions C-II

Pregnancy Risk Factor B (D if used for prolonged periods or in high doses at term)

Contraindications Hypersensitivity to hydromorphone or any component or other phenanthrene derivative

Warnings/Precautions Tablet and cough syrup contain tartrazine which may cause allergic reactions; hydromorphone shares toxic potential of opiate agonists, and precaution of opiate agonist therapy should be observed; extreme caution should be taken to avoid confusing the highly concentrated injection with the less concentrated injectable product, injection contains benzyl alcohol; use with caution in patients with hypersensitivity to other phenanthrene opiates, in patients with respiratory disease, or severe liver or renal failure

Adverse Reactions

Endocrine & metabolic: Antidiuretic hormone release

Ocular: Miosis

Sensitivity reactions: Histamine release

Miscellaneous: Physical and psychological dependence, biliary or urinary tract spasm

>10%:

Cardiovascular: Palpitations, hypotension, peripheral vasodilation

Central nervous system: Dizziness, lightheadedness, drowsiness

Gastrointestinal: Anorexia

1% to 10%:

Cardiovascular: Tachycardia, bradycardia, flushing of face

Central nervous system: CNS depression, increased intracranial pressure, weakness, tiredness, headache, nervousness, restlessness

Gastrointestinal: Nausea, vomiting, constipation, stomach cramps, dry mouth

Genitourinary: Decreased urination, ureteral spasm

Neuromuscular & skeletal: Trembling

Respiratory: Respiratory depression, troubled breathing, shortness of breath

<1%:

Central nervous system: Hallucinations, mental depression, paralytic ileus

Dermatologic: Pruritus, skin rash, hives

Overdosage/Toxicology Symptoms of overdose include CNS depression, respiratory depression, miosis, apnea, pulmonary edema, convulsions. Maintain airway, establish I.V. line; naloxone 2 mg I.V. (0.01 mg/kg for children) with repeat administration as necessary up to a total of 10 mg.

Drug Interactions Increased toxicity: CNS depressants, phenothiazines, tricyclic antidepressants may potentiate the adverse effects of hydromorphone

Stability Protect tablets from light; do not store intact ampuls in refrigerator; a slightly yellowish discoloration has not been associated with a loss of potency; I.V. is **incompatible** when mixed with minocycline, prochlorperazine, sodium bicarbonate, tetracycline, thiopental

Mechanism of Action Binds to opiate receptors in the CNS, causing inhibition of ascending pain pathways, altering the perception of and response to pain; causes cough supression by direct central action in the medulla; produces generalized CNS depression

Pharmacodynamics/Kinetics
Onset of analgesic effect: Within 15-30 minutes
Peak effect: Within 0.5-1.5 hours
Duration: 4-5 hours
Metabolism: Primarily in the liver
Bioavailability: 62%
Half-life: 1-3 hours
Elimination: In urine, principally as glucuronide conjugates

Usual Dosage
Doses should be titrated to appropriate analgesic effects; when changing routes of administration, note that oral doses are less than half as effective as parenteral doses (may be only one-fifth as effective)

Pain: Older Children and Adults:
Oral, I.M., I.V., S.C.: 1-4 mg/dose every 4-6 hours as needed; usual adult dose: 2 mg/dose
Rectal: 3 mg every 6-8 hours

Antitussive: Oral:
Children 6-12 years: 0.5 mg every 3-4 hours as needed
Children >12 years and Adults: 1 mg every 3-4 hours as needed

Dosing adjustment in hepatic impairment: Should be considered

Monitoring Parameters Pain relief, respiratory and mental status, blood pressure

Test Interactions ↑ aminotransferase [ALT (SGPT)/AST (SGOT)] (S)

Patient Information May cause drowsiness; avoid alcohol; take with food or milk to minimize GI distress

Nursing Implications Observe patient for oversedation, respiratory depression, implement safety measures

Additional Information Equianalgesic doses: Morphine 10 mg I.M. = hydromorphone 1.5 mg I.M.

Dosage Forms
Injection: 1 mg/mL (1 mL); 2 mg/mL (1 mL, 20 mL); 3 mg/mL (1 mL); 4 mg/mL (1 mL); 10 mg/mL (1 mL, 2 mL, 5 mL)
Suppository, rectal: 3 mg
Tablet: 2 mg, 4 mg

Hydromox® see Quinethazone on page 967

Hydropane® see Hydrocodone and Homatropine on page 545

Hydro-Par® see Hydrochlorothiazide on page 542

Hydroquinone (hye′ droe kwin one)

Brand Names Eldopaque® [OTC]; Eldopaque Forte®; Eldoquin® [OTC]; Eldoquin Forte®; Esoterica® Facial [OTC]; Esoterica® Regular [OTC]; Esoterica® Sensitive Skin Formula [OTC]; Esoterica® Sunscreen [OTC]; Melanex®; Porcelana® [OTC]; Solaquin® [OTC]; Solaquin Forte®

Use Gradual bleaching of hyperpigmented skin conditions

Pregnancy Risk Factor C

Contraindications Sunburn, depilatory usage, known hypersensitivity to hydroquinone

Warnings/Precautions Limit application to area no larger than face and neck or hands and arms

Adverse Reactions 1% to 10%: Dermatologic: Dermatitis, dryness, erythema, stinging, irritation, inflammatory reaction, sensitization

Mechanism of Action Produces reversible depigmentation of the skin by suppression of melanocyte metabolic processes, in particular the inhibition of the
(Continued)

551

Hydroquinone *(Continued)*

enzymatic oxidation of tyrosine to DOPA (3,4-dihydroxyphenylalanine); sun exposure reverses this effect and will cause repigmentation.

Pharmacodynamics/Kinetics Onset and duration of depigmentation produced by hydroquinone varies among individuals

Usual Dosage Children >12 years and Adults: Topical: Apply thin layer and rub in twice daily

Patient Information Use sunscreens or clothing; do not use on irritated or denuded skin; stop using if rash or irritation develops; for external use only, avoid eye contact

Dosage Forms

Cream, topical:

Esoterica® Sensitive Skin Formula: 1.5% (85 g)

Eldopaque®, Eldoquin®, Esoterica® Facial, Esoterica® Regular, Porcelana®, Esoterica® Sunscreen, Porcelana®, Solaquin®: 2% (14.2 g, 28.4 g, 60 g, 85 g, 120 g)

Eldopaque Forte®, Eldoquin Forte®, Solaquin Forte®: 4% (14.2 g, 28.4 g)

Gel, topical, with sunscreen (Solaquin Forte®): 4% (14.2 g, 28.4 g)

Lotion (Eldoquin®): 2% (15 mL)

Solution, topical (Melanex®): 3% (30 mL)

HydroSKIN® *see* Hydrocortisone *on page 546*

Hydro-Tex® [OTC] *see* Hydrocortisone *on page 546*

Hydrotropine® *see* Hydrocodone and Homatropine *on page 545*

Hydroxacen® *see* Hydroxyzine *on page 556*

Hydroxocobalamin *(hye drox oh koe bal′ a min)*

Brand Names Alphamin®; Codroxomin®; Hybalamin®; Hydrobexan®; Hydro-Cobex®; Hydro-Crysti-12®; LA-12®

Synonyms Vitamin B_{12}

Use Treatment of pernicious anemia, vitamin B_{12} deficiency, increased B_{12} requirements due to pregnancy, thyrotoxicosis, hemorrhage, malignancy, liver or kidney disease

Pregnancy Risk Factor C

Contraindications Hypersensitivity to cyanocobalamin or any component, cobalt; patients with hereditary optic nerve atrophy

Warnings/Precautions Some products contain benzoyl alcohol; avoid use in premature infants; an intradermal test dose should be performed for hypersensitivity; use only if oral supplementation not possible or when treating pernicious anemia

Adverse Reactions

1% to 10%:

Dermatologic: Itching

Gastrointestinal: Diarrhea

<1%:

Cardiovascular: Peripheral vascular thrombosis

Dermatologic: Urticaria

Miscellaneous: Anaphylaxis

Mechanism of Action Coenzyme for various metabolic functions, including fat and carbohydrate metabolism and protein synthesis, used in cell replication and hematopoiesis

Usual Dosage Vitamin B_{12} deficiency: I.M.:

Children: 1-5 mg given in single doses of 100 mcg over 2 or more weeks, followed by 30-50 mcg/month

Adults: 30 mcg/day for 5-10 days, followed by 100-200 mcg/month

Administration Administer I.M. only; may require coadministration of folic acid

Patient Information Therapy is required throughout life; do not take folic acid instead of B_{12} to prevent anemia

Dosage Forms Injection: 1000 mcg/mL (10 mL, 30 mL)

Hydroxycarbamide *see* Hydroxyurea *on page 554*

Hydroxychloroquine Sulfate *(hye drox ee klor′ oh kwin)*

Related Information

Prevention of Malaria *on page 1405*

Brand Names Plaquenil®

Use Suppresses and treats acute attacks of malaria; treatment of systemic lupus erythematosus and rheumatoid arthritis

Pregnancy Risk Factor C

Contraindications Retinal or visual field changes attributable to 4-aminoquinolines; hypersensitivity to hydroxychloroquine, 4-aminoquinoline derivatives, or any component

Warnings/Precautions Use with caution in patients with hepatic disease, G-6-PD deficiency, psoriasis, and porphyria; long-term use in children is not recommended; perform baseline and periodic (6 months) ophthalmologic examinations; test periodically for muscle weakness

Adverse Reactions

>10%:

Central nervous system: Headache

Dermatologic: Itching

Gastrointestinal: Diarrhea, loss of appetite, nausea, stomach cramps, vomiting

Ocular: Ciliary muscle dysfunction

1% to 10%:

Central nervous system: Dizziness, lightheadedness, nervousness, restlessness

Dermatologic: Bleaching of hair, skin rash blue-black discoloration of skin

Ocular: Ocular toxicity, keratopathy, retinopathy

<1%:

Central nervous system: Emotional changes, seizures

Hematologic: Agranulocytosis, aplastic anemia, neutropenia, thrombocytopenia

Neuromuscular & skeletal: Neuromyopathy

Otic: Ototoxicity

Overdosage/Toxicology Symptoms of overdose include headache, drowsiness, visual changes, cardiovascular collapse, and seizures followed by respiratory and cardiac arrest; treatment is symptomatic; urinary alkalinization will enhance renal elimination

Mechanism of Action Interferes with digestive vacuole function within sensitive malarial parasites by increasing the pH and interfering with lysosomal degradation of hemoglobin; inhibits locomotion of neutrophils and chemotaxis of eosinophils; impairs complement-dependent antigen-antibody reactions

Pharmacodynamics/Kinetics

Absorption: Oral: Complete

Protein binding: 55%

Metabolism: In the liver

Elimination: Metabolites and unchanged drug slowly excreted in urine, may be enhanced by urinary acidification

Usual Dosage Oral:

Children:

Chemoprophylaxis of malaria: 5 mg/kg (base) once weekly; should not exceed the recommended adult dose; begin 2 weeks before exposure; continue for 4-6 weeks after leaving endemic area

Acute attack: 10 mg/kg (base) initial dose; followed by 5 mg/kg at 6, 24, and 48 hours

JRA or SLE: 3-5 mg/kg/day divided 1-2 times/day to a maximum of 400 mg/day; not to exceed 7 mg/kg/day

Adults:

Chemoprophylaxis of malaria: 2 tablets weekly on same day each week; begin 2 weeks before exposure; continue for 4-6 weeks after leaving endemic area

Acute attack: 4 tablets first dose day 1; 2 tablets in 6 hours day 1; 2 tablets in 1 dose day 2; and 2 tablets in 1 dose on day 3

Rheumatoid arthritis: 2-3 tablets/day to start taken with food or milk; increase dose until optimum response level is reached; usually after 4-12 weeks dose should be reduced by ½ and a maintenance dose of 1-2 tablets/day given

Lupus erythematosus: 2 tablets every day or twice daily for several weeks depending on response; 1-2 tablets/day for prolonged maintenance therapy

Monitoring Parameters Ophthalmologic exam, CBC

Patient Information Take with food or milk; complete full course of therapy; wear sunglasses in bright sunlight; notify physician if blurring or other vision changes, ringing in the ears, or hearing loss occurs

Nursing Implications Periodic blood counts and eye examinations are recommended when patient is on chronic therapy; give with food or milk

Dosage Forms Tablet: 200 mg [base 155 mg]

25-Hydroxycholecalciferol see Calcifediol on page 156

Hydroxydaunomycin Hydrochloride see Doxorubicin Hydrochloride on page 370

Hydroxyethyl Starch see Hetastarch on page 535

Hydroxyprogesterone Caproate (hye drox ee proe jess' te rone)

Brand Names Duralutin®; Gesterol® L.A.; Hy-Gestrone®; Hylutin®; Hyprogest®

Use Treatment of amenorrhea, abnormal uterine bleeding, endometriosis, uterine carcinoma

Pregnancy Risk Factor D

Contraindications Thrombophlebitis, thromboembolic disorders, cerebral hemorrhage, liver impairment, carcinoma of the breast, hypersensitivity to hydroxyprogesterone or any component, undiagnosed vaginal bleeding

Warnings/Precautions Use with caution in patients with asthma, seizure disorders, migraine, cardiac or renal impairment, history of mental depression; use of any progestin during the first 4 months of pregnancy is not recommended; observe patients closely for signs and symptoms of thrombotic disorders

Adverse Reactions
>10%:
　Cardiovascular: Edema
　Central nervous system: Weakness
　Endocrine & metabolic: Breakthrough bleeding, spotting, changes in menstrual flow, amenorrhea
　Gastrointestinal: Anorexia
　Local: Pain at injection site
1% to 10%:
　Cardiovascular: Edema
　Central nervous system: Mental depression, insomnia, fever
　Dermatologic: Melasma or chloasma, allergic rash with or without pruritus
　Gastrointestinal: Weight gain or loss
　Genitourinary: Changes in cervical erosion and secretions, increased breast tenderness
　Hepatic: Cholestatic jaundice

Overdosage/Toxicology Toxicity is unlikely following single exposures of excessive doses; supportive treatment is adequate in most cases

Drug Interactions Decreased effect: Rifampin → ↑ clearance of hydroxyprogesterone

Stability Store at <40°C (15°C to 30°C); avoid freezing

Mechanism of Action Natural steroid hormone that induces secretory changes in the endometrium, promotes mammary gland development, relaxes uterine smooth muscle, blocks follicular maturation and ovulation and maintains pregnancy

Pharmacodynamics/Kinetics
　Metabolism: Hepatic
　Peak serum concentration: I.M.: 3-7 days; concentrations are measurable for 3-4 weeks after injection
　Elimination: Renal

Usual Dosage Adults: Female: I.M.:
　Amenorrhea: 375 mg; if no bleeding, begin cyclic treatment with estradiol valerate
　Production of secretory endometrium and desquamation: (Medical D and C): 125-250 mg administered on day 10 of cycle; repeat every 7 days until supression is no longer desired.
　Uterine carcinoma: 1 g one or more times/day (1-7 g/week) for up to 12 weeks

Administration Administer deep I.M. only

Test Interactions Thyroid function tests and liver function tests and endocrine function tests

Patient Information Take this medicine only as directed; do not exceed recommended dosage nor take it for a longer period of time; if you suspect you may have become pregnant, stop taking this medicine; take with food; patient package insert is available upon request; notify physician of pain in calves along with swelling and warmth, severe headache, visual disturbance

Nursing Implications Patients should receive a copy of the patient labeling for the drug

Dosage Forms Injection (in oil): 125 mg/mL (10 mL); 250 mg/mL (5 mL)

Hydroxyurea (hye drox ee yoor ee' a)

Related Information
　Cancer Chemotherapy Regimens on page 1218-1241

Brand Names Hydrea®

Synonyms Hydroxycarbamide

Use CML in chronic phase; radiosensitizing agent in the treatment of primary brain tumors; head and neck tumors; uterine cervix and nonsmall cell lung cancer; psoriasis; sickle cell anemia and other hemoglobinopathies; hematologic conditions such as essential thrombocythemia, polycythemia vera, hypereosinophilia, and hyperleukocytosis due to acute leukemia. Has shown activity against renal cell cancer, malignant melanoma, ovarian cancer, head and neck cancer, and prostate cancer. Reduce the frequency of the painful crises caused by sickle cell anemia.

Pregnancy Risk Factor D

Contraindications Severe anemia, severe bone marrow depression; WBC <2500/mm³ or platelet count <100,000/mm³; hypersensitivity to hydroxyurea

Warnings/Precautions The U.S. Food and Drug Administration (FDA) currently recommends that procedures for proper handling and disposal of antineoplastic agents be considered. Use with caution in patients with renal impairment, in patients who have received prior irradiation therapy, and in the elderly.

Adverse Reactions
>10%:
  Central nervous system: Drowsiness
  Gastrointestinal: Mild to moderate nausea and vomiting may occur, as well as diarrhea, constipation, mucositis, ulceration of the GI tract, anorexia, and stomatitis
  Myelosuppression: Dose-limiting toxicity, causes a rapid drop in leukocyte count (seen in 4-5 days in nonhematologic malignancy and more rapidly in leukemia). Thrombocytopenia and anemia occur less often; reversal of WBC count occurs rapidly, but the platelet count may take 7-10 days to recover.
    WBC: Moderate
    Platelets: Moderate
    Onset (days): 7
    Nadir (days): 10
    Recovery (days): 21
1% to 10%:
  Dermatologic: Dermatologic changes (hyperpigmentation, erythema of the hands and face, maculopapular rash, or dry skin), alopecia
  Hepatic: Abnormal LFTs and hepatitis
  Renal: Increased creatinine and BUN
  Miscellaneous: Carcinogenic potential
<1%:
  Central nervous system: Neurotoxicity, renal tubular function impairment, dizziness, disorientation, hallucination, seizures, headache
  Dermatologic: Facial erythema
  Genitourinary: Hyperuricemia, dysuria
  Hepatic: Elevation of hepatic enzymes

Overdosage/Toxicology Symptoms of overdose include myelosuppression, facial swelling, hallucinations, disorientation; treatment is supportive

Drug Interactions Increased toxicity: Fluorouracil: The potential for neurotoxicity may be increased with concomitant administration

Stability Store capsules at room temperature; capsules may be opened and emptied into water (will not dissolve completely)

Mechanism of Action Interferes with synthesis of DNA, during the S phase of cell division, without interfering with RNA synthesis; inhibits ribonucleoside diphosphate reductase, preventing conversion of ribonucleotides to deoxyribonucleotides; cell-cycle specific for the S phase and may hold other cells in the G_1 phase of the cell cycle.

Pharmacodynamics/Kinetics
Absorption: Readily absorbed from GI tract (≥80%)
Distribution: Readily crosses the blood-brain barrier; well distributed into intestine, brain, lung, and kidney tissues; appears in breast milk
Metabolism: In the liver
Half-life: 3-4 hours
Time to peak serum concentration: Within 2 hours
Elimination: Renal excretion of urea (metabolite) and respiratory excretion of CO_2 (metabolic end product); 50% of the drug is excreted unchanged in urine

Usual Dosage Oral (refer to individual protocols):
Children: No dosage regimens have been established. Dosages of 1500-3000 mg/m² as a single dose in combination with other agents every 4-6 weeks have been used in the treatment of pediatric astrocytoma, medulloblastoma, and primitive neuroectodermal tumors

Adults: Dose should always be titrated to patient response and WBC counts. Usual oral doses range from 10-30 mg/kg/day or 500-3000 mg/day; if WBC count falls to <2500 cells/mm³, or the platelet count to <100,000/mm³, therapy should be stopped for at least 3 days and resumed when values rise toward normal
  Solid tumors: Intermittent therapy: 80 mg/kg as a single dose every third day; continuous therapy: 20-30 mg/kg/day given as a single dose/day
  Concomitant therapy with irradiation: 80 mg/kg as a single dose every third day starting at least 7 days before initiation of irradiation
  Resistant chronic myelocytic leukemia: 20-30 mg/kg/day divided daily
(Continued)

Hydroxyurea *(Continued)*

Sickle cell anemia (moderate/severe disease):

Initial: 15 mg/kg/day, increased by 5 mg/kg every 12 weeks unless toxicity is observed or the maximum tolerated dose of 35 mg/kg/day is achieved. Monitor for toxicity every 2 weeks. If toxicity occurs, stop treatment until the bone marrow recovers. Restart at 2.5 mg/kg/day less than the dose at which toxicity occurs. If no toxicity occurs over the next 12 weeks, then the subsequent dose should be increased by 2.5 mg/kg/day.

Dosing adjustment in renal impairment:

Cl_{cr} 10-50 mL/minute: Administer 50% of normal dose

Cl_{cr} <10 mL/minute: Administer 20% of normal dose

Monitoring Parameters CBC with differential, platelets, renal function and liver function tests, serum uric acid

Patient Information Contents of capsule may be emptied into a glass of water if taken immediately; inform the physician if you develop fever, sore throat, bruising, or bleeding; may cause drowsiness, constipation, and loss of hair

Dosage Forms Capsule: 500 mg

25-Hydroxyvitamin D₃ *see* Calcifediol *on page 156*

Hydroxyzine *(hye drox' i zeen)*

Brand Names Anxanil®; Atarax®; Atozine®; Durrax®; E-Vista®; Hydroxacen®; Hy-Pam®; Hyzine-50®; Neucalm®; Quiess®; Vamate®; Vistacon-50®; Vistaject-25®; Vistaject-50®; Vistaquel®; Vistaril®; Vistazine®

Synonyms Hydroxyzine Hydrochloride; Hydroxyzine Pamoate

Use Treatment of anxiety, as a preoperative sedative, an antipruritic, an antiemetic, and in alcohol withdrawal symptoms

Pregnancy Risk Factor C

Contraindications Hypersensitivity to hydroxyzine or any component

Warnings/Precautions S.C., intra-arterial and I.V. administration **not** recommended since thrombosis and digital gangrene can occur; extravasation can result in sterile abscess and marked tissue induration; should be used with caution in patients with narrow-angle glaucoma, prostatic hypertrophy, and bladder neck obstruction; should also be used with caution in patients with asthma or COPD

Anticholinergic effects are not well tolerated in the elderly. Hydroxyzine may be useful as a short-term antipruritic, but it is not recommended for use as a sedative or anxiolytic in the elderly.

Adverse Reactions

>10%:

Central nervous system: Slight to moderate drowsiness

Miscellaneous: Thickening of bronchial secretions

1% to 10%:

Central nervous system: Headache, fatigue, nervousness, dizziness

Gastrointestinal: Appetite increase, weight increase, nausea, diarrhea, abdominal pain, dry mouth

Neuromuscular & skeletal: Arthralgia

Respiratory: Pharyngitis

<1%:

Cardiovascular: Palpitations, hypotension, edema

Central nervous system: Depression, sedation, paradoxical excitement, insomnia

Dermatologic: Angioedema, photosensitivity, rash

Genitourinary: Urinary retention

Hepatic: Hepatitis

Neuromuscular & skeletal: Myalgia, tremor, paresthesia

Ocular: Blurred vision

Respiratory: Bronchospasm

Miscellaneous: Epistaxis

Overdosage/Toxicology Symptoms of overdose include seizures, sedation, hypotension. There is no specific treatment for an antihistamine overdose, however, most of its clinical toxicity is due to anticholinergic effects. Anticholinesterase inhibitors may be useful by reducing acetylcholinesterase. For anticholinergic overdose with severe life-threatening symptoms, physostigmine 1-2 mg (0.5 or 0.02 mg/kg for children) I.V., slowly may be given to reverse these effects.

Drug Interactions

Decreased effect: Epinephrine decreased vasopressor effect

Increased toxicity: CNS depressants, anticholinergics

Stability Protect from light; store at 15°C to 30°C and protected from freezing; I.V. is **incompatible** when mixed with aminophylline, amobarbital, chloramphenicol, dimenhydrinate, heparin, penicillin G, pentobarbital, phenobarbital, phenytoin, ranitidine, sulfisoxazole, vitamin B complex with C

Mechanism of Action Competes with histamine for H_1-receptor sites on effector cells in the gastrointestinal tract, blood vessels, and respiratory tract

Pharmacodynamics/Kinetics

Onset of effect: Within 15-30 minutes

Duration: 4-6 hours

Absorption: Oral: Rapid

Metabolism: Exact fate is unknown

Half-life: 3-7 hours

Time to peak serum concentration: Within 2 hours

Usual Dosage

Children:

Oral: 0.6 mg/kg/dose every 6 hours

I.M.: 0.5-1 mg/kg/dose every 4-6 hours as needed

Adults:

Antiemetic: I.M.: 25-100 mg/dose every 4-6 hours as needed

Anxiety: Oral: 25-100 mg 4 times/day; maximum dose: 600 mg/day

Preoperative sedation:

Oral: 50-100 mg

I.M.: 25-100 mg

Management of pruritus: Oral: 25 mg 3-4 times/day

Dosing interval in hepatic impairment: Change dosing interval to every 24 hours in patients with primary biliary cirrhosis

Administration For I.M. administration in children, injections should be made into the midlateral muscles of the thigh; S.C., intra-arterial, and I.V. administration **not** recommended since thrombosis and digital gangrene can occur

Monitoring Parameters Relief of symptoms, mental status, blood pressure

Patient Information Will cause drowsiness, avoid alcohol and other CNS depressants, avoid driving and other hazardous tasks until the CNS effects are known

Nursing Implications Extravasation can result in sterile abscess and marked tissue induration; provide safety measures (ie, side rails, night light, and call button); remove smoking materials from area; supervise ambulation

Additional Information

Hydroxyzine hydrochloride: Anxanil®, Atarax®, E-Vista®, Hydroxacen®, Quiess®, Vistaril® injection, Vistazine®

Hydroxyzine pamoate: Hy-Pam®, Vistaril® capsule and suspension

Dosage Forms

Hydroxyzine hydrochloride:

Injection:

Vistaject-25®, Vistaril®: 25 mg/mL (1 mL, 2 mL, 10 mL)

E-Vista®, Hydroxacen®, Hyzine-50®, Neucalm®, Quiess®, Vistacon-50®, Vistaject-50®, Vistaquel®, Vistaril®, Vistazine®: 50 mg/mL (1 mL, 2 mL, 10 mL)

Syrup (Atarax®): 10 mg/5 mL (120 mL, 480 mL, 4000 mL)

Tablet:

Anxanil®: 25 mg

Atarax®: 10 mg, 25 mg, 50 mg, 100 mg

Atozine®: 10 mg, 25 mg, 50 mg

Durrax®: 10 mg, 25 mg

Hydroxyzine pamoate:

Capsule:

Hy-Pam®: 25 mg, 50 mg

Vamate®: 25 mg, 50 mg, 100 mg

Vistaril®: 25 mg, 50 mg, 100 mg

Suspension, oral (Vistaril®:) 25 mg/5 mL (120 mL, 480 mL)

Hydroxyzine Hydrochloride see Hydroxyzine on previous page

Hydroxyzine Pamoate see Hydroxyzine on previous page

Hy-Gestrone® see Hydroxyprogesterone Caproate on page 553

Hygroton® see Chlorthalidone on page 235

Hylorel® see Guanadrel Sulfate on page 518

Hylutin® see Hydroxyprogesterone Caproate on page 553

Hyoscine see Scopolamine on page 997

Hyoscyamine, Atropine, Scopolamine, and Phenobarbital (hye oh sye' a meen, a' troe peen, skoe pol' a meen & fee noe bar' bi tal)

(Continued)

Hyoscyamine, Atropine, Scopolamine, and Phenobarbital *(Continued)*

Brand Names Barbidonna®; Barophen®; Donnamor®; Donnapine®; Donna-Sed®; Donnatal®; Donphen®; Hyosophen®; Kinesed®; Malatal®; Relaxadon®; Spaslin®; Spasmolin®; Spasmophen®; Spasquid®; Susano®

Use Adjunct in treatment of peptic ulcer disease, irritable bowel, spastic colitis, spastic bladder, and renal colic

Pregnancy Risk Factor C

Contraindications Hypersensitivity to hyoscyamine, atropine, scopolamine, phenobarbital, or any component; narrow-angle glaucoma, tachycardia, GI and GU obstruction, myasthenia gravis

Warnings/Precautions Use with caution in patients with hepatic or renal disease, hyperthyroidism, cardiovascular disease, hypertension, prostatic hypertrophy, autonomic neuropathy in the elderly; abrupt withdrawal may precipitate status epilepticus. Because of the anticholinergic effects of this product, it is not recommended for use in the elderly.

Adverse Reactions

>10%:

Gastrointestinal: Constipation

Local: Irritation at injection site

Miscellaneous: Decreased sweating, dry mouth, nose, throat, or skin

1% to 10%: Decreased flow of breast milk, difficulty in swallowing, increased sensitivity to light

<1%:

Cardiovascular: Orthostatic hypotension, ventricular fibrillation, tachycardia, palpitations

Central nervous system: Confusion, drowsiness, headache, loss of memory, tiredness, ataxia

Dermatologic: Skin rash

Ocular: Increased intraocular pain, blurred vision

Gastrointestinal: Bloated feeling, nausea, vomiting

Genitourinary: Difficult urination

Overdosage/Toxicology Symptoms of overdose include unsteady gait, slurred speech, confusion, hypotension, respiratory collapse, dilated unreactive pupils, hot or flushed skin, diminished bowel sounds, urinary retention. Anticholinergic toxicity is caused by strong binding of the drug to cholinergic receptors. Anticholinesterase inhibitors reduce acetylcholinesterase, the enzyme that breaks down acetylcholine and thereby allows acetylcholine to accumulate and compete for receptor binding with the offending anticholinergic. For anticholinergic overdose with severe life-threatening symptoms, physostigmine 1-2 mg (0.5 or 0.02 mg/kg for children) S.C. or I.V., slowly may be given to reverse these effects.

Drug Interactions Increased toxicity: CNS depressants, coumarin anticoagulants, amantadine, antihistamine, phenothiazides, antidiarrheal suspensions, corticosteroids, digitalis, griseofulvin, tetracyclines, anticonvulsants, MAO inhibitors, tricyclic antidepressants

Mechanism of Action Refer to individual agents

Pharmacodynamics/Kinetics Absorption: Well absorbed from GI tract

Usual Dosage Oral:

Children 2-12 years: Kinesed® dose: ½ to 1 tablet 3-4 times/day

Children: Donnatal® elixir: 0.1 mL/kg/dose every 4 hours; maximum dose: 5 mL **or** see table for alternative.

Weight (kg)	Dose (mL)	
	q4h	q6h
4.5	0.5	0.75
10	1	1.5
14	1.5	2
23	2.5	3.8
34	3.8	5
≥45	5	7.5

Adults: 1-2 capsules or tablets 3-4 times/day; or 1 Donnatal® Extentab® in sustained release form every 12 hours; or 5-10 mL elixir 3-4 times/day or every 8 hours

Patient Information Maintain good oral hygiene habits, because lack of saliva may increase chance of cavities. Observe caution while driving or performing other tasks requiring alertness, as may cause drowsiness, dizziness, or blurred vision. Notify physician if skin rash, flushing or eye pain occurs; or if difficulty in urinating, constipation, or sensitivity to light becomes severe or persists. Do not attempt tasks requiring mental alertness or physical coordination until you know the effects of the drug. Swallow extended release tablet whole, do not crush or chew.

Dosage Forms

Capsule (Donnatal®, Spasmolin®): Hyoscyamine sulfate 0.1037 mg, atropine sulfate 0.0194 mg, scopolamine hydrobromide 0.0065 mg, and phenobarbital 16.2 mg

Elixir (Barophen®, Donnamor®, Donna-Sed®, Donnatal®, Hyosophen®, Spasmophen®, Spasquid®, Susano®): Hyoscyamine sulfate 0.1037 mg, atropine sulfate 0.0194 mg, scopolamine hydrobromide 0.0065 mg, and phenobarbital 16.2 mg per 5 mL (120 mL, 480 mL, 4000 mL)

Tablet:

Barbidonna®: Hyoscyamine hydrobromide 0.1286 mg, atropine sulfate 0.025 mg, scopolamine hydrobromide 0.0074 mg, and phenobarbital 16 mg

Barbidonna® No. 2: Hyoscyamine hydrobromide 0.1286 mg, atropine sulfate 0.025 mg, scopolamine hydrobromide 0.0074 mg, and phenobarbital 32 mg

Chewable (Kinesed®): Hyoscyamine hydrobromide 0.12 mg, atropine sulfate 0.12 mg, scopolamine hydrobromide 0.007 mg, and phenobarbital 16 mg

Donnapine®, Donnatal®, Hyosophen®, Malatal®, Relaxadon®, Spaslin®, Susano®: Hyoscyamine sulfate 0.1037 mg, atropine sulfate 0.0194 mg, scopolamine hydrobromide 0.0065 mg, and phenobarbital 16.2 mg

Donnatal® No. 2: Hyoscyamine sulfate 0.1037 mg, atropine sulfate 0.0194 mg, scopolamine hydrobromide 0.0065 mg, and phenobarbital 32.4 mg

Donphen®: Hyoscyamine sulfate 0.1 mg, atropine sulfate 0.02 mg, scopolamine hydrobromide 0.006 mg, and phenobarbital 15 mg

Long-acting (Donnatal®): Hyoscyamine sulfate 0.3111 mg, atropine sulfate 0.0582 mg, scopolamine hydrobromide 0.0195 mg, and phenobarbital 48.6 mg

Spasmophen®: Hyoscyamine sulfate 0.1037 mg, atropine sulfate 0.0194 mg, scopolamine hydrobromide 0.0065 mg, and phenobarbital 15 mg

Hyoscyamine Sulfate (hye oh sye' a meen)

Brand Names Anaspaz®; Cystospaz®; Cystospaz-M®; Gastrosed™; Levsin®; Levsinex®; Neoquess® Tablet

Synonyms l-Hyoscyamine Sulfate

Use Treatment of GI tract disorders caused by spasm, adjunctive therapy for peptic ulcers

Pregnancy Risk Factor C

Contraindications Narrow-angle glaucoma, obstructive uropathy, obstructive GI tract disease, myasthenia gravis, known hypersensitivity to belladonna alkaloids

Warnings/Precautions Use with caution in children with spastic paralysis; use with caution in elderly patients. Low doses cause a paradoxical decrease in heart rates. Some commercial products contain sodium metabisulfite, which can cause allergic-type reactions. May accumulate with multiple inhalational administration, particularly in the elderly. Heat prostration may occur in hot weather. Use with caution in patients with autonomic neuropathy, prostatic hypertrophy, hyperthyroidism, congestive heart failure, cardiac arrhythmias, chronic lung disease, biliary tract disease.

Adverse Reactions

>10%:

Local: Irritation at injection site

Miscellaneous: Decreased sweating, dry mouth, nose, throat, or skin

1% to 10%:

Dermatologic: Photosensitivity

Gastrointestinal: Constipation

Ocular: Blurred vision, mydriasis

Miscellaneous: Difficulty in swallowing

<1%:

Cardiovascular: Palpitations, orthostatic hypotension

Central nervous system: Headache, lightheadedness, memory loss, fatigue, delirium, restlessness, ataxia

Dermatologic: Skin rash

Genitourinary: Difficult urination

Neuromuscular & skeletal: Tremor

Ocular: Increased intraocular pressure

Overdosage/Toxicology Symptoms of overdose include dilated, unreactive pupils; blurred vision; hot, dry flushed skin; dryness of mucous membranes; difficulty in swallowing, foul breath, diminished or absent bowel sounds, urinary retention, tachycardia, hyperthermia, hypertension, increased respiratory rate. Anticholinergic toxicity is caused by strong binding of the drug to cholinergic receptors. Anticholinesterase inhibitors reduce acetylcholinesterase, the enzyme (Continued)

Hyoscyamine Sulfate *(Continued)*

that breaks down acetylcholine and thereby allows acetylcholine to accumulate and compete for receptor binding with the offending anticholinergic. For anticholinergic overdose with severe life-threatening symptoms, physostigmine 1-2 mg (0.5 or 0.02 mg/kg for children) S.C. or I.V., slowly may be given to reverse these effects.

Drug Interactions

Decreased effect with antacids

Increased toxicity with amantadine, antimuscarinics, haloperidol, phenothiazines, TCAs, MAO inhibitors

Mechanism of Action Blocks the action of acetylcholine at parasympathetic sites in smooth muscle, secretory glands and the CNS; increases cardiac output, dries secretions, antagonizes histamine and serotonin

Pharmacodynamics/Kinetics

Onset of effect: 2-3 minutes

Duration: 4-6 hours

Absorption: Oral: Absorbed well

Distribution: Crosses the placenta; small amounts appear in breast milk

Protein binding: 50%

Metabolism: In the liver

Half-life: 13% to 38%

Elimination: In urine

Usual Dosage

Children: Oral, S.L.: Dose as per table repeated every 4 hours as needed

Hyoscyamine

Weight (kg)	Dose (mcg)	Maximum 24-Hour Dose (mcg)
Children <2 y		
2.3	12.5	75
3.4	16.7	100
5	20.8	125
7	25	150
10	31.3-33.3	200
15	45.8	275
Children 2-10 y		
10	31.3-33.3	
20	62.5	Do not exceed
40	93.8	0.75 mg
50	125	

Adults:

Oral or S.L.: 0.125-0.25 mg 3-4 times/day before meals or food and at bedtime

Oral: 0.375-0.75 mg (timed release) every 12 hours

I.M., I.V., S.C.: 0.25-0.5 mg every 6 hours

Patient Information Maintain good oral hygiene habits, because lack of saliva may increase chance of cavities. Observe caution while driving or performing other tasks requiring alertness, as may cause drowsiness, dizziness, or blurred vision. Notify physician if skin rash, flushing or eye pain occurs; or if difficulty in urinating, constipation or sensitivity to light becomes severe or persists.

Nursing Implications Observe for tachycardia if patient has cardiac problems.

Dosage Forms

Capsule, timed release (Cystospaz-M®, Levsinex®): 0.375 mg

Elixir (Levsin®): 0.125 mg/5 mL with alcohol 20% (480 mL)

Injection (Levsin®): 0.5 mg/mL (1 mL, 10 mL)

Solution, oral (Gastrosed™, Levsin®): 0.125 mg/mL (15 mL)

Tablet:

Anaspaz®, Gastrosed™, Levsin®, Neoquess®: 0.125 mg

Cystospaz®: 0.15 mg

Hyosophen® *see* Hyoscyamine, Atropine, Scopolamine, and Phenobarbital *on page 557*

Hy-Pam® *see* Hydroxyzine *on page 556*

Hyperab® *see* Rabies Immune Globulin, Human *on page 971*

HyperHep® *see* Hepatitis B Immune Globulin *on page 532*

Hyperstat® I.V. *see* Diazoxide *on page 326*

Hyper-Tet® *see* Tetanus Immune Globulin, Human *on page 1065*

Hy-Phen® *see* Hydrocodone and Acetaminophen *on page 543*

Hypoglycemic Agents Comparison *see page 1271*

HypRho®-D *see* Rho(D) Immune Globulin *on page 978*

HypRho®-D Mini-Dose *see* Rho(D) Immune Globulin *on page 978*

Hyprogest® *see* Hydroxyprogesterone Caproate *on page 553*

Hytakerol® *see* Dihydrotachysterol *on page 344*

Hytone® *see* Hydrocortisone *on page 546*

Hytrin® *see* Terazosin *on page 1059*

Hytuss-2X® [OTC] *see* Guaifenesin *on page 515*

Hytuss® [OTC] *see* Guaifenesin *on page 515*

Hyzine-50® *see* Hydroxyzine *on page 556*

Iberet-Folic-500® *see* Vitamin, Multiple *on page 1166*

Ibidomide Hydrochloride *see* Labetalol Hydrochloride *on page 614*

Ibuprin® [OTC] *see* Ibuprofen *on this page*

Ibuprofen (eye byoo proe' fen)
Related Information
Ibuprofen Toxicity Nomogram *on page 1385*
Nonsteroidal Anti-Inflammatories Comparison *on page 1280*
Brand Names Aches-N-Pain® [OTC]; Advil® [OTC]; Excedrin® IB [OTC]; Genpril® [OTC]; Haltran® [OTC]; Ibuprin® [OTC]; Ibuprohm® [OTC]; Ibu-Tab®; Medipren® [OTC]; Menadol® [OTC]; Midol® 200 [OTC]; Motrin®; Motrin® IB [OTC]; Nuprin® [OTC]; Pamprin IB® [OTC]; PediaProfen™; Rufen®; Saleto-200® [OTC]; Saleto-400®; Trendar® [OTC]; Uni-Pro® [OTC]
Synonyms *p*-Isobutylhydratropic Acid
Use Inflammatory diseases and rheumatoid disorders including juvenile rheumatoid arthritis, mild to moderate pain, fever, dysmenorrhea, gout, ankylosing spondylitis, acute migraine headache
Pregnancy Risk Factor B (D if used in the 3rd trimester)
Contraindications Hypersensitivity to ibuprofen, any component, aspirin, or other nonsteroidal anti-inflammatory drugs (NSAIDs)
Warnings/Precautions Do not exceed 3200 mg/day; use with caution in patients with congestive heart failure, hypertension, decreased renal or hepatic function, history of GI disease (bleeding or ulcers), or those receiving anticoagulants; safety and efficacy in children <6 months of age have not yet been established; elderly are a high-risk population for adverse effects from nonsteroidal anti-inflammatory agents. As much as 60% of elderly can develop peptic ulceration and/or hemorrhage asymptomatically.

Use lowest effective dose for shortest period possible. Use of NSAIDs can compromise existing renal function especially when Cl$_{cr}$ is <30 mL/minute. CNS adverse effects such as confusion, agitation, and hallucination are generally seen in overdose or high dose situations; but elderly may demonstrate these adverse effects at lower doses than younger adults.
Adverse Reactions
>10%:
  Central nervous system: Dizziness, fatigue
  Dermatologic: Rash, urticaria
  Gastrointestinal: Abdominal cramps, heartburn, indigestion, nausea
1% to 10%:
  Central nervous system: Headache, nervousness
  Dermatologic: Itching
  Gastrointestinal: Dyspepsia, heartburn, vomiting, abdominal pain, peptic ulcer, GI bleed, GI perforation
  Otic: Tinnitus
  Miscellaneous: Fluid retention
<1%:
  Cardiovascular: Edema, congestive heart failure, arrhythmias, tachycardia, hypertension
  Central nervous system: Confusion, hallucinations, mental depression, drowsiness, insomnia
  Dermatologic: Hives, erythema multiforme, toxic epidermal necrolysis, Stevens-Johnson syndrome
  Endocrine & metabolic: Polydipsia, hot flushes
  Gastrointestinal: Gastritis, GI ulceration
  Genitourinary: Acute renal failure, cystitis, polyuria
(Continued)

Ibuprofen *(Continued)*

Hematologic: Neutropenia, anemia, agranulocytosis, inhibition of platelet aggregation, hemolytic anemia, bone marrow depression, leukopenia, thrombocytopenia

Hepatic: Hepatitis

Neuromuscular & skeletal: Peripheral neuropathy

Ocular: Vision changes, blurred vision, conjunctivitis, dry eyes, toxic amblyopia

Otic: Decreased hearing

Respiratory: Allergic rhinitis, shortness of breath

Miscellaneous: Epistaxis, aseptic meningitis

Overdosage/Toxicology Symptoms include apnea, metabolic acidosis, coma, and nystagmus; leukocytosis, renal failure

Management of a nonsteroidal anti-inflammatory drug (NSAID) intoxication is primarily supportive and symptomatic. Fluid therapy is commonly effective in managing the hypotension that may occur following an acute NSAID overdose, except when this is due to an acute blood loss. Seizures tend to be very short-lived and often do not require drug treatment; although, recurrent seizures should be treated with I.V. diazepam. Since many of the NSAIDs undergo enterohepatic cycling, multiple doses of charcoal may be needed to reduce the potential for delayed toxicities.

Drug Interactions

Decreased effect: Aspirin may decrease ibuprofen serum concentrations

Increased toxicity: May increase digoxin, methotrexate, and lithium serum concentrations; other nonsteroidal anti-inflammatories may increase adverse gastrointestinal effects

Mechanism of Action Inhibits prostaglandin synthesis by decreasing the activity of the enzyme, cyclo-oxygenase, which results in decreased formation of prostaglandin precursors

Pharmacodynamics/Kinetics

Onset of analgesia: 30-60 minutes

Duration: 4-6 hours

Onset of anti-inflammatory effect: Up to 7 days

Peak action: 1-2 weeks

Absorption: Oral: Rapid (85%)

Time to peak serum concentration: Within 1-2 hours

Protein binding: 90% to 99%

Metabolism: In the liver by oxidation

Half-life: 2-4 hours

End stage renal disease: Unchanged

Elimination: In urine (1% as free drug); some biliary excretion occurs

Usual Dosage Oral:

Children:

Antipyretic: 6 months to 12 years: Temperature <102.5°F (39°C): 5 mg/kg/dose; temperature >102.5°F: 10 mg/kg/dose given every 6-8 hours; maximum daily dose: 40 mg/kg/day

Juvenile rheumatoid arthritis: 30-70 mg/kg/24 hours divided every 6-8 hours

<20 kg: Maximum: 400 mg/day

20-30 kg: Maximum: 600 mg/day

30-40 kg: Maximum: 800 mg/day

>40 kg: Adult dosage

Start at lower end of dosing range and titrate upward; maximum: 2.4 g/day

Analgesic: 4-10 mg/kg/dose every 6-8 hours

Adults:

Inflammatory disease: 400-800 mg/dose 3-4 times/day; maximum dose: 3.2 g/day

Analgesia/pain/fever/dysmenorrhea: 200-400 mg/dose every 4-6 hours; maximum daily dose: 1.2 g (unless directed by physician)

Dosing adjustment/comments in severe hepatic impairment: Avoid use

Administration Administer with food

Monitoring Parameters CBC; occult blood loss and periodic liver function tests; monitor response (pain, range of motion, grip strength, mobility, ADL function), inflammation; observe for weight gain, edema; monitor renal function (urine output, serum BUN and creatinine); observe for bleeding, bruising; evaluate gastrointestinal effects (abdominal pain, bleeding, dyspepsia); mental confusion, disorientation; with long-term therapy, periodic ophthalmic exams

Reference Range Plasma concentrations >200 µg/mL may be associated with severe toxicity

Test Interactions ↑ chloride (S), ↑ sodium (S), ↑ bleeding time

Patient Information Serious gastrointestinal bleeding can occur as well as ulceration and perforation. Pain may or may not be present. Avoid aspirin and aspirin-containing products while taking this medication. If gastric upset occurs, take with food, milk, or antacid. If gastric adverse effects persist, contact physician. May cause drowsiness, dizziness, blurred vision, and confusion. Use caution when performing tasks that require alertness (eg, driving). Do not take for more than 3 days for fever or 10 days for pain without physician's advice.

Nursing Implications Do not crush tablet
Additional Information Sucrose content of 5 mL (suspension): 2.5 g
Dosage Forms
Suspension, oral: 100 mg/5 mL (120 mL, 480 mL)
Tablet: 200 mg [OTC], 300 mg, 400 mg, 600 mg, 800 mg

Ibuprofen Toxicity Nomogram *see page 1385*

Ibuprohm® [OTC] *see Ibuprofen on page 561*

Ibu-Tab® *see Ibuprofen on page 561*

Idamycin® *see Idarubicin on this page*

Idarubicin (eye da rue' bi sin)
Related Information
Cancer Chemotherapy Regimens *on page 1218-1241*
Brand Names Idamycin®
Synonyms 4-demethoxydaunorubicin; IDR
Use In combination treatment of acute myeloid leukemia (AML), this includes classifications M1 through M7 of the French-American-British (FAB) classification system and acute lymphocytic leukemia (ALL) in children
Pregnancy Risk Factor D
Contraindications Hypersensitivity to idarubicin, daunorubicin, or any component
Warnings/Precautions The U.S. Food and Drug Administration (FDA) currently recommends that procedures for proper handling and disposal of antineoplastic agents be considered. Give I.V. slowly into a freely flowing I.V. infusion; do not give I.M. or S.C., severe necrosis can result if extravasation occurs; can cause myocardial toxicity and is more common in patients who have previously received anthracyclines or have pre-existing cardiac disease; reduce dose in patients with impaired hepatic function; irreversible myocardial toxicity may occur as total dosage approaches 137.5 mg/m^2; severe myelosuppression is also possible.
Adverse Reactions
>10%:
Central nervous system: Headache
Miscellaneous: Infection, hemorrhage, mucositis, reddish urine, fever
Local: Tissue necrosis upon extravasation, erythematous streaking
Vesicant chemotherapy
Dermatologic: Alopecia, rash, urticaria
Gastrointestinal: Nausea, vomiting, diarrhea, stomatitis
Hematologic:
Leukopenia (nadir: 8-29 days)
Thrombocytopenia (nadir: 10-15 days)
Anemia
1% to 10%:
Central nervous system: Seizures, peripheral neuropathy
Miscellaneous: Pulmonary allergy
<1%:
Cardiovascular: Arrhythmias, EKG changes, cardiomyopathy, congestive heart failure, myocardial toxicity, acute life-threatening arrhythmias
Endocrine & metabolic: Hyperuricemia
Hepatic: Elevations in liver enzymes or bilirubin
Overdosage/Toxicology Symptoms of overdose include severe myelosuppression and increased GI toxicity; treatment is supportive
Stability Reconstituted solutions are physically and chemically stable for at least 7 days under refrigeration at 2°C to 8°C (36°F to 46°F) and 72 hours at controlled room temperature at 15°C to 30°C (59°F to 86°F); prolonged contact with any solution of an alkaline pH will result in degradation of idarubicin

Incompatible with fluorouracil, etoposide, dexamethasone, heparin, hydrocortisone, methotrexate, vincristine
Mechanism of Action Similar to daunorubicin, idarubicin exhibits inhibitory effects on DNA and RNA polymerase *in vitro*. Idarubicin has an affinity for DNA similar to daunorubicin and somewhat higher efficacy in stabilizing the DNA double helix against heat denaturation. Idarubicin has been as active or more active than daunorubicin in inhibiting 3H-TdR uptake by DNA or RNA of mouse embryo fibroblasts.
(Continued)

Idarubicin (Continued)

Pharmacodynamics/Kinetics
Absorption: Oral: Rapid but erratic (20% to 30%) from GI tract
Distribution: Large volume due to extensive tissue binding and distributes into CSF
Protein binding: 94% to 97%
Metabolism: In the liver to idarubicinol, which is pharmacologically active
Half-life, elimination:
Oral: 14-35 hours
I.V.: 12-27 hours
Time to peak serum concentration: Within 2-4 hours and varies considerably
Elimination: ~15% of an I.V. dose has been recovered in urine as idarubicin and idarubicinol; urinary recovery of idarubicin and idarubicinol is lower following oral doses; similar amounts are excreted via bile

Usual Dosage I.V.:
Children:
Leukemia: 10 mg/m² once daily for 3 days and repeat every 3 weeks
Solid tumors: 5 mg/m² once daily for 3 days and repeat every 3 weeks
Adults: 12 mg/m²/day for 3 days in combination with Ara-C or 25 mg/m² bolus

Dosing adjustment in renal impairment: Dose reduction is recommended

Dosing adjustment/comments in hepatic impairment:
Bilirubin 1.5-5.0 mg/dL or AST 60-180 units: Reduce dose 50%
Bilirubin >5 mg/dL or AST >180 units: Do not administer

Administration Administer by intermittent infusion over 10-30 minutes into a free flowing I.V. solution of NS or D₅W; administer at a final concentration of 1 mg/mL

Monitoring Parameters CBC with differential, platelet count, ECHO, EKG, serum electrolytes, creatinine, uric acid, ALT, AST, bilirubin, signs of extravasation

Patient Information May cause hair loss; notify physician if pain, burning, or stinging around injection site occur

Nursing Implications
Local erythematous streaking along the vein may indicate too rapid a rate of administration
Unless specific data available, do not mix with other drugs
Extravasation management:
Topical cooling may be achieved using ice packs or cooling pad with circulating ice water. Cooling of site for 24 hours as tolerated by the patient. Elevate and rest extremity 24-48 hours, then resume normal activity as tolerated. Application of cold inhibits vesicant's cytotoxicity.
Application of heat can be harmful and is contraindicated
If pain, erythema, and/or swelling persist beyond 48 hours, refer patient immediately to plastic surgeon for consultation and possible debridement

Dosage Forms Powder for injection, lyophilized: 5 mg, 10 mg

Idoxuridine (eye dox yoor' i deen)
Brand Names Herplex®
Synonyms IDU; IUDR
Use Treatment of herpes simplex keratitis
Pregnancy Risk Factor C
Contraindications Hypersensitivity to idoxuridine or any component; concurrent use in patients receiving corticosteroids with superficial dendritic keratitis
Warnings/Precautions Use with caution in patients with corneal ulceration or patients receiving corticosteroid applications; if no response in epithelial infections within 14 days, consider a second form of therapy

Adverse Reactions
1% to 10%:
Dermatologic: Pruritus, follicular conjunctivitis
Local: Irritation, pain, inflammation, mild edema of the eyelids and cornea
Ocular: Visual haze, corneal clouding, photophobia, small punctate defects on the corneal epithelium
<1%: Ocular: Small punctate defects on the corneal epithelium

Overdosage/Toxicology Due to frequent dosing, small defects on the epithelium may result. Mutagenic and cytotoxic and should be considered as being potentially carcinogenic; no treatment is indicated for accidental ingestion

Drug Interactions Increased toxicity: Do not coadminister with boric acid containing solutions

Stability Store in tight, light-resistant containers at 2°C to 8°C until dispensed; do not mix with other medications; solution must be refrigerated

Mechanism of Action Incorporated into viral DNA in place of thymidine resulting in mutations and inhibition of viral replication

Pharmacodynamics/Kinetics

Absorption: Ophthalmic: Poorly absorbed following instillation; tissue uptake is a function of cellular metabolism, which is inhibited by high concentrations of the drug (absorption decreases as the concentration of drug increases)

Distribution: Crosses the placenta

Metabolism: To iodouracil, uracil, and iodide

Elimination: Unchanged drug and metabolites excreted in the urine

Usual Dosage Adults: Ophthalmic: Solution: Instill 1 drop in eye(s) every hour during day and every 2 hours at night, continue until definite improvement is noted, then reduce daytime dose to 1 drop every 2 hours and every 4 hours at night; continue for 5-7 days after healing appears complete

Patient Information May cause sensitivity to bright light; minimize by wearing sunglasses; notify physician if improvement is not seen in 7-8 days, if condition worsens, or if pain, decreased vision, itching, or swelling of the eye occur; do not exceed recommended dose

Nursing Implications Idoxuridine solution should not be mixed with other medications

Dosage Forms Solution, ophthalmic: 0.1% (15 mL)

IDR see Idarubicin on page 563

IDU see Idoxuridine on previous page

Ifex® see Ifosfamide on this page

IFLrA see Interferon Alfa-2a on page 581

IFN see Interferon Alfa-2a on page 581

IFN-alpha 2 see Interferon Alfa-2b on page 583

Ifosfamide (eye foss' fa mide)

Related Information

Antiemetics for Chemotherapy Induced Nausea and Vomiting on page 1202

Cancer Chemotherapy Regimens on page 1218-1241

Brand Names Ifex®

Use In combination with certain other antineoplastics in treatment of lung cancer, Hodgkin's and non-Hodgkin's lymphoma, breast cancer, acute and chronic lymphocytic leukemia, ovarian cancer, testicular cancer, and sarcomas, pancreatic and gastric carcinoma

Pregnancy Risk Factor D

Contraindications Patients who have demonstrated a previous hypersensitivity to ifosfamide; patients with severely depressed bone marrow function

Warnings/Precautions The U.S. Food and Drug Administration (FDA) currently recommends that procedures for proper handling and disposal of antineoplastic agents be considered. Used in combination with mesna as a prophylactic agent to protect against hemorrhagic cystitis. Use with caution in patients with impaired renal function or those with compromised bone marrow reserve. May require therapy cessation if confusion or coma occurs; carcinogenic in rats.

Adverse Reactions

>10%:

Dermatologic: Alopecia occurs in 50% to 83% of patients 2-4 weeks after initiation of therapy; may be as high as 100% in combination therapy

Gastrointestinal: Nausea and vomiting in 58% of patients is dose and schedule related (more common with higher doses and after bolus regimens); nausea and vomiting can persist up to 3 days after therapy; also anorexia, diarrhea, constipation, transient increase in LFTs and stomatitis noted.

Emetic potential: Moderate (58%)

Genitourinary: Hemorrhagic cystitis has been frequently associated with the use of ifosfamide. A urinalysis prior to each dose should be obtained. **Ifosfamide should never be administered without a uroprotective agent (MESNA).** Hematuria has been reported in 6% to 92% of patients. Renal toxicity occurs in 6% of patients and is manifested as an increase in BUN or serum creatinine and is most likely related to tubular damage. Metabolic acidosis may occur in up to 31% of patients.

1% to 10%:

Central nervous system: Somnolence, confusion, hallucinations in 12% and coma (rare) have occurred and are usually reversible; usually occur with higher doses; depressive psychoses, polyneuropathy

Dermatologic: Phlebitis, dermatitis, nail ridging, skin hyperpigmentation, impaired wound healing

Endocrine & metabolic: SIADH

Hepatic: Elevated liver enzymes

(Continued)

Ifosfamide *(Continued)*

Myelosuppression: Less of a problem than with cyclophosphamide if used alone. Leukopenia is mild to moderate, thrombocytopenia and anemia are rare. However, myelosuppression can be severe when used with other chemotherapeutic agents. Be cautious with patients with compromised bone marrow reserve.

WBC: Moderate

Platelets: Mild

Onset (days): 7

Nadir (days): 10-14

Respiratory: Nasal stuffiness, pulmonary fibrosis

Miscellaneous: Immunosuppression, sterility, possible secondary malignancy, allergic reactions

<1%:

Cardiovascular: Cardiotoxicity

Respiratory: Pulmonary toxicity

Overdosage/Toxicology Symptoms of overdose include myelosuppression, nausea, vomiting, diarrhea, alopecia; direct extension of the drug's pharmacologic effect; treatment is supportive

Drug Interactions Decreased effect: Because ifosfamide undergoes hepatic activation by microsomal enzymes, induction of these enzymes is potentially possible by pretreatment with various enzyme-inducers such as phenobarbital, phenytoin, and chloral hydrate

Stability Reconstituted solution is stable for 7 days at room temperature and 21 days when refrigerated; for I.V. infusion in NS or D_5W, solution is stable for 7 days at room temperature and 6 weeks when refrigerated. **Compatible** with mesna.

Mechanism of Action Causes cross-linking of strands of DNA by binding with nucleic acids and other intracellular structures; inhibits protein synthesis and DNA synthesis; an analogue of cyclophosphamide, and like cyclophosphamide, it undergoes activation by microsomal enzymes in the liver. Ifosfamide is metabolized to active compounds, ifosfamide mustard, and acrolein

Pharmacodynamics/Kinetics Pharmacokinetics are dose-dependent

Absorption: Oral: Peak plasma levels occur within 1 hour

Bioavailability: Estimated at 100%

Distribution: V_d: Has been calculated to be 5.7-49 L; does penetrate CNS, but not in therapeutic levels

Protein binding: Not appreciably protein bound

Metabolism: In the liver to active species; requires biotransformation in the liver before it can act as an alkylating agent; the metabolite acrolein is the toxic agent implicated in the development of hemorrhagic cystitis

Half-life: Beta phase: 11-15 hours with high-dose (3800-5000 mg/m^2) or 4-7 hours with lower doses (1800 mg/m^2)

Elimination: 15% to 50% excreted unchanged in urine

Usual Dosage I.V. (refer to individual protocols):

Children: 1800 mg/m^2/day for 3-5 days every 21-28 days or 5 g/m^2 as a single 24-hour infusion or 3 g/m^2/day for 2 days

Adults:

Doses may be given as 50 mg/kg/day or 1200-2000 mg/m^2/day for 5 days

Alternatives include 2400 mg/m^2/day for 3 days or 5000 mg/m^2 as a single dose

Doses of 700-900 mg/m^2/day for 5 days may be given IVP; courses may be repeated every 3-4 weeks

To prevent bladder toxicity, ifosfamide should be given with extensive hydration consisting of at least 2 L of oral or I.V. fluid per day. A protector, such as mesna, should also be used to prevent hemorrhagic cystitis. The dose-limiting toxicity is hemorrhagic cystitis and ifosfamide should be used in conjunction with a uroprotective agent.

Dosing adjustment in renal impairment:

S_{cr} 2.1-3.0 mg/dL: Reduce dose by 25% to 50%

S_{cr} >3.0 mg/dL: Withhold drug

Dosing adjustment in hepatic impairment: Although no specific guidelines are available, it is possible that higher doses are indicated in hepatic disease

Administration Administer as a slow I.V. intermittent infusion over at least 30 minutes at a final concentration for administration not to exceed 40 mg/mL (usual concentration for administration is between 0.6-20 mg/mL) or administer as a 24-hour infusion

Monitoring Parameters CBC with differential and platelet count, urine output, urinalysis, liver function, and renal function tests

Patient Information Drink plenty of fluids after dose; notify physician if persistent sore throat, fever, sores on mucous membranes, fatigue, or unusual bleeding or bruising occur

Nursing Implications Mesna to be used concomitantly for prophylaxis against hemorrhagic cystitis

Dosage Forms Powder for injection: 1 g, 3 g

IG *see* Immune Globulin, Intramuscular *on page 570*

I-Gent® *see* Gentamicin Sulfate *on page 500*

IGIM *see* Immune Globulin, Intramuscular *on page 570*

IL-2 *see* Aldesleukin *on page 35*

Ilopan® *see* Dexpanthenol *on page 317*

Ilopan-Choline® *see* Dexpanthenol *on page 317*

Ilosone® *see* Erythromycin *on page 401*

Ilozyme® *see* Pancrelipase *on page 837*

Imdur™ *see* Isosorbide Mononitrate *on page 601*

I-Methasone® *see* Dexamethasone *on page 314*

Imidazole Carboxamide *see* Dacarbazine *on page 297*

Imipemide *see* Imipenem/Cilastatin *on this page*

Imipenem/Cilastatin (i mi pen' em/sye la stat' in)

Related Information
Antimicrobial Drugs of Choice *on page 1298-1302*

Brand Names Primaxin®

Synonyms Imipemide

Use Treatment of documented multidrug resistant gram-negative infection due to organisms proven or suspected to be susceptible to imipenem/cilastatin; treatment of multiple organism infection in which other agents have an insufficient spectrum of activity or are contraindicated due to toxic potential; Antibacterial activity includes resistant gram-negative bacilli (*Pseudomonas aeruginosa* and *Enterococcus* sp), gram-positive bacteria (methicillin-sensitive *Staphylococcus aureus* and *Enterococcus* sp) and anaerobes

Pregnancy Risk Factor C

Contraindications Hypersensitivity to imipenem/cilastatin or any component

Warnings/Precautions Dosage adjustment required in patients with impaired renal function; safety and efficacy in children <12 years of age have not yet been established; prolonged use may result in superinfection; use with caution in patients with a history of seizures or hypersensitivity to beta-lactams; elderly patients often require lower doses

Adverse Reactions
1% to 10%:
  Gastrointestinal: Nausea, diarrhea, vomiting
  Local: Phlebitis
<1%:
  Cardiovascular: Hypotension, palpitations
  Central nervous system: Seizures
  Dermatologic: Rash
  Gastrointestinal: Pseudomembranous colitis
  Hematologic: Neutropenia, eosinophilia
  Local: Pain at injection site
  Miscellaneous: Emergence of resistant strains of *P. aeruginosa*

Overdosage/Toxicology Symptoms of overdose include neuromuscular hypersensitivity, seizures; hemodialysis may be helpful to aid in the removal of the drug from the blood; otherwise most treatment is supportive or symptom directed

Drug Interactions Increased toxicity: Beta-lactam antibiotics, probenecid → ↑ toxic potential

Stability
Imipenem/cilastatin powder for injection should be stored at <30°C
Reconstituted solutions are stable 10 hours at room temperature and 48 hours at refrigeration (4°C) with NS
If reconstituted with 5% or 10% dextrose injection, 5% dextrose and sodium bicarbonate, 5% dextrose and 0.9% sodium chloride, is stable for 4 hours at room temperature and 24 hours when refrigerated
Imipenem/cilastatin is most stable at a pH of 6.5-7.5; imipenem is inactivated at acidic or alkaline pH
Standard diluent: 500 mg/100 mL NS; 1 g/250 mL NS
Comments: All IVPB should be prepared fresh; do not use dextrose as a diluent due to limited stability

(Continued)

Imipenem/Cilastatin *(Continued)*

Mechanism of Action

A carbapenem with broad-spectrum antibacterial activity including resistant gram-negative bacilli (*Pseudomonas aeruginosa* and *Enterococcus* sp), gram-positive bacteria (methicillin-sensitive *Staphylococcus aureus* and *Enterococcus* sp) and anaerobes

Inhibits cell wall synthesis by binding to penicillin-binding proteins on the bacterial outer membrane; cilastatin prevents renal metabolism of imipenem by competitive inhibition of dehydropeptidase along the brush border of the proximal renal tubules

Pharmacodynamics/Kinetics

Imipenem:

Distribution: Appears in breast milk; crosses the placenta

Metabolism: In the kidney by dehydropeptidase

Half-life: 1 hour, extended with renal insufficiency

Elimination: When given with cilastatin, urinary excretion of unchanged imipenem increases to 70%

Cilastatin:

Metabolism: Partially in the kidneys

Half-life: 1 hour, extended with renal insufficiency

Elimination: 70% to 80% of dose excreted in urine as unchanged cilastatin

Usual Dosage I.M. and I.V. (dosing based on imipenem component):

Neonates: I.V.:

0-4 weeks, <1200 g: 20 mg/kg/dose every 18-24 hours

Postnatal age:

≤7 days, ≥1200 g: 20 mg/kg/dose every 12 hours

>7 days, 1200-2000 g: 20 mg/kg/dose every 12 hours

>7 days, >2000 g: 20 mg/kg/dose every 8 hours

Children: I.V.: 60-100 mg/kg/24 hours divided every 6 hours (maximum: 4 g/day)

Adults: I.V.: 500 mg every 6-8 hours (1 g every 6-8 hours for severe *Pseudomonas* infection); infuse each 250-500 mg dose over 20-30 minutes; infuse each 1 g dose over 40-60 minutes

Mild to moderate infection **only**: I.M.: 500-750 mg every 12 hours (**Note:** 750 mg is recommended for intra-abdominal and more severe respiratory, dermatologic, or gynecologic infections; total daily I.M. dosages >1500 mg are not recommended; deep I.M. injection should be carefully made into a large muscle mass only)

Dosing adjustment in renal impairment: See table.

CreatinineClearance mL/min/1.73 m^2	Frequency	% Decrease in Daily Maximum Dose
30-70	q6-8h	50
20-30	q8-12h	63
5-20	q12h	75

Imipenem (**not cilastatin**) is moderately dialyzable (20% to 50%) by hemodialysis; administer dose postdialysis; during peritoneal dialysis, dose as for Cl_{cr} <10 mL/minute

Continuous arterio-venous or veno-venous hemofiltration (CAVH/CAVHD): Removes 20 mg of imipenem/L of filtrate per day

Administration

Not for direct infusion; vial contents must be transferred to 100 mL of infusion solution; final concentration should not exceed 5 mg/mL; infuse over 30-60 minutes; watch for convulsions. If nausea and/or vomiting occur during administration, decrease the rate of I.V. infusion; do not mix with or physically add to other antibiotics; however, may administer concomitantly

Monitoring Parameters Periodic renal, hepatic, and hematologic function tests

Test Interactions Interferes with urinary glucose determination using Clinitest®

Additional Information Sodium content of 1 g: 3.2 mEq

Dosage Forms Powder for injection:

I.M.:

Imipenem 500 mg and cilastatin 500 mg

Imipenem 750 mg and cilastatin 750 mg

I.V.:

Imipenem 250 mg and cilastatin 250 mg

Imipenem 500 mg and cilastatin 500 mg

Imipramine *(im ip' ra meen)*

Related Information

Antidepressant Agents Comparison *on page 1250-1252*

Brand Names Janimine®; Tofranil®; Tofranil-PM®

Synonyms Imipramine Hydrochloride; Imipramine Pamoate

Use Treatment of various forms of depression, often in conjunction with psycho-therapy; enuresis in children; analgesic for certain chronic and neuropathic pain

Pregnancy Risk Factor D

Contraindications Hypersensitivity to imipramine (cross-sensitivity with other tricyclics may occur); patients receiving MAO inhibitors or fluoxetine within past 14 days; narrow-angle glaucoma

Warnings/Precautions Use with caution in patients with cardiovascular disease, conduction disturbances, seizure disorders, urinary retention, hyperthyroidism or those receiving thyroid replacement; do not discontinue abruptly in patients receiving long-term, high-dose therapy; some oral preparations contain tartrazine and injection contains sulfites, both of which can cause allergic reactions

Orthostatic hypotension is a concern with this agent, especially in patients taking other medications that may affect blood pressure; may precipitate arrhythmias in predisposed patients; may aggravate seizures; a less anticholinergic antidepressant may be a better choice

Adverse Reactions Less sedation and anticholinergic effects than amitriptyline

>10%:
    Anticholinergic: Dry mouth, constipation, urinary retention
    Central nervous system: Dizziness, drowsiness, headache
    Gastrointestinal: Increased appetite, nausea, weakness, unpleasant taste, weight gain

1% to 10%:
    Cardiovascular: Postural hypotension, arrhythmias, tachycardia, sudden death
    Central nervous system: Confusion, delirium, hallucinations, nervousness, restlessness, parkinsonian syndrome, insomnia
    Gastrointestinal: Diarrhea, heartburn
    Genitourinary: Difficult urination, sexual dysfunction
    Neuromuscular & skeletal: Fine muscle tremors
    Ocular: Blurred vision, eye pain
    Miscellaneous: Excessive sweating

<1%:
    Central nervous system: Anxiety, seizures
    Dermatologic: Alopecia, photosensitivity
    Endocrine & metabolic: Breast enlargement, galactorrhea, SIADH
    Genitourinary: Testicular swelling
    Hematologic: Leukopenia, eosinophilia, rarely agranulocytosis
    Hepatic: Increased liver enzymes, cholestatic jaundice
    Ocular: Increased intraocular pressure
    Otic: Tinnitus
    Miscellaneous: Allergic reactions, trouble with gums, decreased lower esophageal sphincter tone may cause GE reflux, has been associated with falls

Overdosage/Toxicology Symptoms of overdose include confusion, hallucinations, constipation, cyanosis, tachycardia, urinary retention, ventricular tachycardia, seizures

Following initiation of essential overdose management, toxic symptoms should be treated. Ventricular arrhythmias often respond to concurrent systemic alkalinization (sodium bicarbonate 0.5-2 mEq/kg I.V.). Arrhythmias unresponsive to this therapy may respond to lidocaine 1 mg/kg I.V. followed by a titrated infusion. Physostigmine (1-2 mg I.V. slowly for adults or 0.5 mg I.V. slowly for children) may be indicated in reversing cardiac arrhythmias that are life-threatening. Seizures usually respond to diazepam I.V. boluses (5-10 mg for adults up to 30 mg or 0.25-0.4 mg/kg/dose for children up to 10 mg/dose). If seizures are unresponsive or recur, phenytoin or phenobarbital may be required.

Drug Interactions
    Decreased effect: Clonidine, blocks uptake of guanethidine and prevents its hypotensive effects
    Increased toxicity: MAO inhibitors: Hyperpyrexia, hypertension, tachycardia, confusion, seizures, and death have been reported; may increase the prothrombin time in patients stabilized on warfarin; may potentiate the action of other CNS depressants; potentiates the pressor and cardiac effects of sympathomimetic agents such as isoproterenol, epinephrine, etc; additive anticholinergic effects seen with other anticholinergic agents; cimetidine reduces the hepatic metabolism of imipramine

Stability Solutions stable at a pH of 4-5; turns yellowish or reddish on exposure to light. Slight discoloration does not affect potency; marked discoloration is associated with loss of potency. Capsules stable for 3 years following date of manufacture.

Mechanism of Action Traditionally believed to increase the synaptic concentration of serotonin and/or norepinephrine in the central nervous system by inhibition of their reuptake by the presynaptic neuronal membrane. However, (Continued)

Imipramine *(Continued)*

additional receptor effects have been found including desensitization of adenyl cyclase, down regulation of beta-adrenergic receptors, and down regulation of serotonin receptors.

Pharmacodynamics/Kinetics

Peak antidepressant effect: Usually after ≥2 weeks

Absorption: Oral: Well absorbed

Distribution: Crosses the placenta

Metabolism: In the liver by microsomal enzymes to desipramine (active) and other metabolites; significant first-pass metabolism

Half-life: 6-18 hours

Elimination: Almost all compounds following metabolism are excreted in urine

Usual Dosage Maximum antidepressant effect may not be seen for 2 or more weeks after initiation of therapy.

Children: Oral:

Depression: 1.5 mg/kg/day with dosage increments of 1 mg/kg every 3-4 days to a maximum dose of 5 mg/kg/day in 1-4 divided doses; monitor carefully especially with doses ≥3.5 mg/kg/day

Enuresis: ≥6 years: Initial: 10-25 mg at bedtime, if inadequate response still seen after 1 week of therapy, increase by 25 mg/day; dose should not exceed 2.5 mg/kg/day or 50 mg at bedtime if 6-12 years of age or 75 mg at bedtime if ≥12 years of age

Adjunct in the treatment of cancer pain: Initial: 0.2-0.4 mg/kg at bedtime; dose may be increased by 50% every 2-3 days up to 1-3 mg/kg/dose at bedtime

Adolescents: Oral: Initial: 25-50 mg/day; increase gradually; maximum: 100 mg/day in single or divided doses

Adults:

Oral: Initial: 25 mg 3-4 times/day, increase dose gradually, total dose may be given at bedtime; maximum: 300 mg/day

I.M.: Initial: Up to 100 mg/day in divided doses; change to oral as soon as possible

Elderly: Initial: 10-25 mg at bedtime; increase by 10-25 mg every 3 days for inpatients and weekly for outpatients if tolerated; average daily dose to achieve a therapeutic concentration: 100 mg/day; range: 50-150 mg/day

Monitoring Parameters Monitor blood pressure and pulse rate prior to and during initial therapy; EKG, CBC; evaluate mental status

Reference Range Therapeutic: Imipramine and desipramine: 150-250 ng/mL (SI: 530-890 nmol/L); desipramine: 150-300 ng/mL (SI: 560-1125 nmol/L); Toxic: >500 ng/mL (SI: 446-893 nmol/L); utility of serum level monitoring controversial

Test Interactions ↑ glucose

Patient Information May require 2-4 weeks to achieve desired effect; avoid alcohol ingestion; do not discontinue medication abruptly; may cause urine to turn blue-green; may cause drowsiness, avoid alcohol and other CNS depressants; dry mouth may be helped by sips of water, sugarless gum, or hard candy; rise slowly to avoid dizziness

Nursing Implications Raise bed rails, institute safety measures

Additional Information

Imipramine hydrochloride: Tofranil®, Janimine®

Imipramine pamoate: Tofranil-PM®

Dosage Forms

Capsule, as pamoate (Tofranil-PM®): 75 mg, 100 mg, 125 mg, 150 mg

Injection, as hydrochloride (Tofranil®): 12.5 mg/mL (2 mL)

Tablet, as hydrochloride (Janimine®, Tofranil®): 10 mg, 25 mg, 50 mg

Imipramine Hydrochloride *see Imipramine on page 568*

Imipramine Pamoate *see Imipramine on page 568*

Imitrex® *see Sumatriptan Succinate on page 1049*

Immune Globulin, Intramuscular (i myun' glob' yoo lin, in' tra mus' kyou lar)

Related Information

Immunization Guidelines *on page 1389-1405*

Vaccines *on page 1386-1388*

Brand Names Gamastan®; Gammar®

Synonyms Gamma Globulin; IG; IGIM; Immune Serum Globulin; ISG

Use Household and sexual contacts of persons with hepatitis A, measles, varicella, and possibly rubella; travelers to high-risk areas outside tourist routes; staff, attendees, and patients of diapered attendees in day-care center outbreaks

For travelers, IG is not an alternative to careful selection of foods and water; immune globulin can interfere with the antibody response to parenterally administered live virus vaccines. Frequent travelers should be tested for hepatitis A antibody, immune hemolytic anemia, and neutropenia (with ITP, I.V. route is usually used).

Pregnancy Risk Factor C

Contraindications Thrombocytopenia, hypersensitivity to immune globulin, thimerosal, IgA deficiency

Warnings/Precautions Skin testing should not be performed as local irritation can occur and be misinterpreted as a positive reaction; do not administer I.V.; IG should **not** be used to control outbreaks of measles; epidemiologic and laboratory data indicate current IMIG products do not have a discernible risk of transmitting HIV

Adverse Reactions
>10%: Local: Pain, tenderness, muscle stiffness at I.M. site
1% to 10%:
  Cardiovascular: Flushing
  Central nervous system: Chills
  Gastrointestinal: Nausea
<1%:
  Central nervous system: Lethargy, fever
  Dermatologic: Urticaria, angioedema, erythema
  Gastrointestinal: Emesis
  Neuromuscular & skeletal: Myalgia
  Miscellaneous: Hypersensitivity reactions

Drug Interactions Increased toxicity: Live virus, vaccines (measles, mumps, rubella); do not administer within 3 months after administration of these vaccines

Stability Keep in refrigerator; do not freeze

Mechanism of Action Provides passive immunity by increasing the antibody titer and antigen-antibody reaction potential

Pharmacodynamics/Kinetics
Duration of immune effect: Usually 3-4 weeks
Half-life: 23 days
Time to peak serum concentration: I.M.: Within 24-48 hours

Usual Dosage I.M.:
Hepatitis A:
  Pre-exposure prophylaxis upon travel into endemic areas:
    0.02 mL/kg for anticipated risk 1-3 months
    0.06 mL/kg for anticipated risk >3 months
    Repeat approximate dose every 4-6 months if exposure continues
  Postexposure prophylaxis: 0.02 mL/kg given within 2 weeks of exposure
Measles:
  Prophylaxis: 0.25 mL/kg/dose (maximum dose: 15 mL) given within 6 days of exposure followed by live attenuated measles vaccine in 3 months or at 15 months of age (whichever is later)
  For patients with leukemia, lymphoma, immunodeficiency disorders, generalized malignancy, or receiving immunosuppressive therapy: 0.5 mL/kg (maximum dose: 15 mL)
Poliomyelitis: Prophylaxis: 0.3 mL/kg/dose as a single dose
Rubella: Prophylaxis: 0.55 mL/kg/dose within 72 hours of exposure
Varicella:: Prophylaxis: 0.6-1.2 mL/kg (varicella zoster immune globulin preferred) within 72 hours of exposure
IgG deficiency: 1.3 mL/kg, then 0.66 mL/kg in 3-4 weeks
Hepatitis B: Prophylaxis: 0.06 mL/kg/dose (HBIG preferred)

Administration Intramuscular injection only

Test Interactions Skin tests should **not** be done

Nursing Implications Do not mix with other medications; skin testing should not be performed as local irritation can occur and be misinterpreted as a positive reaction

Dosage Forms Injection: I.M.: 165±15 mg (of protein)/mL (2 mL, 10 mL)

Immune Globulin, Intravenous (i myun' glob' yoo lin, in' tra vee' nus)

Related Information
Immunization Guidelines *on page 1389-1405*
Vaccines *on page 1386-1388*
Brand Names Gamimune® N; Gammagard®; Iveegam®; Polygam®; Sandoglobulin®; Venoglobulin®-I
(Continued)

Immune Globulin, Intravenous *(Continued)*

Synonyms IVIG

Use Treatment of immunodeficiency sufficiency (hypogammaglobulinemia, agammaglobulinemia, IgG subclass deficiencies, severe combined immunodeficiency syndromes (SCIDS), Wiskott-Aldrich syndrome), idiopathic thrombocytopenic purpura; used in conjunction with appropriate anti-infective therapy *to prevent or modify acute bacterial or viral infections* in patients with iatrogenically-induced or disease-associated immunodepression; *chronic lymphocytic leukemia (CLL) - chronic prophylaxis autoimmune neutropenia, bone marrow transplantation patients, autoimmune hemolytic anemia or neutropenia, refractory dermatomyositis/polymyositis, autoimmune diseases* (myasthenia gravis, SLE, bullous pemphigoid, severe rheumatoid arthritis), *Kawasaki disease, Guillain-Barré syndrome.* Therapy should be guided by clinical observation and serial determination of serum IgG levels.

Pregnancy Risk Factor C

Contraindications Hypersensitivity to immune globulin or any component, IgA deficiency (except with the use of Gammagard®, Polygam®)

Warnings/Precautions Anaphylactic hypersensitivity reactions can occur, especially in IgA-deficient patients; studies indicate that the currently available products have no discernible risk of transmitting HIV or hepatitis B

Adverse Reactions

1% to 10%:
  Cardiovascular: Flushing of the face, tachycardia
  Central nervous system: Chills
  Gastrointestinal: Nausea
  Respiratory: Dyspnea

<1%:
  Cardiovascular: Hypotension, tightness in the chest
  Central nervous system: Dizziness, fever, headache
  Miscellaneous: Diaphoresis, hypersensitivity reactions

Drug Interactions Increased toxicity: Live virus, vaccines (measles, mumps, rubella); do not administer within 3 months after administration of these vaccines

Stability Stability and dilution is dependent upon the manufacturer and brand; do not mix with other drugs

Mechanism of Action Replacement therapy for primary and secondary immunodeficiencies; interference with F_c receptors on the cells of the reticuloendothelial system for autoimmune cytopenias and ITP; possible role of contained antiviral-type antibodies

Pharmacodynamics/Kinetics I.V. provides immediate antibody levels
  Half-life: 21-24 days

Usual Dosage Children and Adults: I.V.:
  Dosages should be based on ideal body weight and not actual body weight in morbidly obese patients
  Primary immunodeficiency disorders: 200-400 mg/kg every 4 weeks or as per monitored serum IgG concentrations
  Chronic lymphocytic leukemia (CLL): 400 mg/kg/dose every 3 weeks
  Idiopathic thrombocytopenic purpura (ITP): Maintenance dose:
    400 mg/kg/day for 5 consecutive days
    800 mg/kg/day for 2 consecutive days
  Chronic ITP: 400-1000 mg/kg/dose every 7 or 14 days
  Kawasaki disease:
    400 mg/kg/day for 4 days within 10 days of onset of fever
    800 mg/kg/day for 1-2 days within 10 days of onset of fever
    2 g/kg for one dose only
  Acquired immunodeficiency syndrome (patients must be symptomatic):
    200-250 mg/kg/dose every 2 weeks
    400-500 mg/kg/dose every month or every 4 weeks
  Autoimmune hemolytic anemia and neutropenia: 1000 mg/kg/dose for 2-3 days
  Autoimmune diseases: 400 mg/kg/day for 4 days
  Post allogeneic bone marrow transplant: 500 mg/kg/week for 4 months post-transplant
  Adjuvant to severe cytomegalovirus infections: 500 mg/kg/dose every other day for 7 doses
  Severe systemic viral and bacterial infections:
    Neonates: 500 mg/kg/day for 2-6 days then once weekly
    Children: 500-1000 mg/kg/week
  Prevention of gastroenteritis: Infants and Children: Oral: 50 mg/kg/day divided every 6 hours
  Guillain-Barré syndrome:
    400 mg/kg/day for 4 days
    1000 mg/kg/day for 2 days
    2000 mg/kg/day for one day

INTRAVENOUS IMMUNE GLOBULIN PRODUCT COMPARISON

	Gamimune® N	Gammagard®	Gammar® -IV	Iveegam®	Polygam®	Sandoglobulin®	Venoglobulin® -I
FDA indication	Primary immunodeficiency, ITP	Primary immunodeficiency, ITP, CLL prophylaxis	Primary immunodeficiency	Primary immunodeficiency, Kawasaki syndrome	Primary immunodeficiency, ITP, CLL	Primary immunodeficiency, ITP	Primary immunodeficiency, ITP
Contraindication	IgA deficiency	None (caution with IgA deficiency)	IgA deficiency	IgA deficiency	None (caution with IgA deficiency)	IgA deficiency	IgA deficiency
IgA content	270 mcg/mL	0.92-1.6 mcg/mL	<20 mcg/mL	10 mcg/mL	0.74±0.33 mcg/mL	720 mcg/mL	20-24 mcg/mL
Adverse reactions (%)	5.2	6	15	1	6	2.5-6.6	6
Plasma source	>2000 paid donors	4000-5000 paid donors	>8000 paid donors	>6000 paid donors	50,000 voluntary donors	8000-15,000 voluntary donors	6000-9000 paid donors
Half-life	21 d	24 d	21-24 d	26-29 d	21-25 d	21-23 d	29 d
IgG subclass (%)							
IgG$_1$ (60-70)	60	67 (66.8)[1]	69	64.1[2]	67	60.5 (55.3)[1]	62.3[2]
IgG$_2$ (19-31)	29.4	25 (25.4)	23	30.3	25	30.2 (35.7)	32.8
IgG$_3$ (5-8.4)	6.5	5 (7.4)	6	4	5	6.6 (6.3)	2.9
IgG$_4$ (0.7-4)	4.1	3 (0.3)	2	1.5	3	2.6 (2.6)	2
Monomers (%)	>95	>95	>98	93.8	>95	>92	>98
Gammaglobulin (%)	>98	>90	>98	100	>90	>96	>98
Storage	Refrigerate	Room temp	Room temp	Refrigerate	Room temp	Room temp	Room temp
Recommendations for initial infusion rate	0.01-0.02 mL/kg/min	0.5 mL/kg/h	0.01-0.02 mL/kg/min	1 mL/min	0.5 mL/kg/h	0.01-0.03 mL/kg/min	0.01-0.02 mL/kg/min
Maximum infusion rate	0.08 mL/kg/min	4 mL/kg/h	0.06 mL/kg/min	2 mL/min	4 mL/kg/h	2.5 mL/min	0.04 mL/kg/min
Maximum concentration for infusion (%)	10	5	5	5	10	12	10

[1] Skvaril F and Gardi A, 'Differences Among Available Immunoglobulin Preparations for Intravenous Use,' *Pediatr Infect Dis J,* 1988, 7:543-48.
[2] Roomer J, Morgenthaler JJ, Scherz R, et al, 'Characterization of Various Immunoglobulin Preparations for Intravenous Application,' *Vox Sang,* 1982, 42:62-73.
[3] ASHP Commission on Therapeutics, ASHP Therapeutic Guidelines for Intravenous Immune Globulin, *Clin Pharm,* 1992, 11:117-36.
[4] Manufacturer's Product Information/Personal Communication.

Immune Globulin, Intravenous *(Continued)*

Refractory dermatomyositis: 2 g/kg/dose every month x 3-4 doses
Refractory polymyositis: 1 g/kg/day x 2 days every month x 4 doses
Chronic inflammatory demyelinating polyneuropathy:
400 mg/kg/day for 5 doses once each month
800 mg/kg/day for 3 doses once each month
1000 mg/kg/day for 2 days once each month

Dosing adjustment/comments in renal impairment: Cl_{cr} <10 mL/minute: Avoid use

Administration I.V. use only; for initial treatment, a lower concentration and/or a slower rate of infusion should be used

Dosage Forms

Injection: Gamimune® N: 5% [50 mg/mL] with maltose 10% (10 mL, 50 mL, 100 mL)

Powder for injection, lyophilized:
Gammagard®, Polygam®: 0.5 g, 2.5 g, 5 g, 10 g
Gammar®-IV: 2.5 g
Iveegam®: 0.5 g, 1 g, 2.5 g, 5 g
Polygam®: 5 g, 10 g
Sandoglobulin®: 1 g, 3 g, 6 g
Venoglobulin®-I: 2.5 g, 5 g

Parenteral: See table for administration information

Immune Serum Globulin *see* Immune Globulin, Intramuscular *on page 570*

Immunization Guidelines *see page 1389*

Imodium® *see* Loperamide Hydrochloride *on page 647*

Imodium® A-D [OTC] *see* Loperamide Hydrochloride *on page 647*

Imogam® *see* Rabies Immune Globulin, Human *on page 971*

Imovax® Rabies I.D. Vaccine *see* Rabies Virus Vaccine *on page 972*

Imovax® Rabies Vaccine *see* Rabies Virus Vaccine *on page 972*

Imuran® *see* Azathioprine *on page 106*

I-Naphline® *see* Naphazoline Hydrochloride *on page 775*

Inapsine® *see* Droperidol *on page 375*

Indanyl Sodium *see* Carbenicillin *on page 180*

Indapamide *(in dap' a mide)*

Brand Names Lozol®

Use Management of mild to moderate hypertension; treatment of edema in congestive heart failure and nephrotic syndrome

Pregnancy Risk Factor D

Contraindications Anuria, hypersensitivity to hydrochlorothiazide or any component, cross-sensitivity with other thiazides and sulfonamide derivatives

Warnings/Precautions Use with caution in patients with renal or hepatic disease, gout, lupus erythematosus, or diabetes mellitus

Adverse Reactions

1% to 10%: Endocrine & metabolic: Hypokalemia

<1%:
Cardiovascular: Irregular heartbeats, weak pulse, hypotension
Central nervous system: Mood changes
Dermatologic: Photosensitivity
Endocrine & metabolic: Fluid and electrolyte imbalances (hypocalcemia, hypomagnesemia, hyponatremia), hyperglycemia
Gastrointestinal: Dry mouth
Hematologic: Rarely blood dyscrasias
Neuromuscular & skeletal: Numbness or tingling in hands, feet or lips, muscle cramps or pain, unusual weakness
Renal: Prerenal azotemia
Respiratory: Shortness of breath
Miscellaneous: Increased thirst

Overdosage/Toxicology Symptoms of overdose include lethargy, diuresis, hypermotility, confusion, muscle weakness; following GI decontamination, therapy is supportive with I.V. fluids, electrolytes, and I.V. pressors if needed

Drug Interactions

Decreased effect of oral hypoglycemics; decreased absorption with cholestyramine and colestipol

Increased effect with furosemide and other loop diuretics

Increased toxicity/levels of lithium; when given with digoxin, diuretic-induced hypokalemia increases the risk of digoxin toxicity

Mechanism of Action Diuretic effect is localized at the proximal segment of the distal tubule of the nephron; it does not appear to have significant effect on glomerular filtration rate nor renal blood flow; like other diuretics, it enhances sodium, chloride, and water excretion by interfering with the transport of sodium ions across the renal tubular epithelium

Pharmacodynamics/Kinetics
Absorption: Completely from GI tract
Plasma protein binding: 71% to 79%
Metabolism: Extensively in the liver
Half-life: 14-18 hours
Time to peak serum concentration: 2-2.5 hours
Elimination: ~60% of dose excreted in urine within 48 hours, ~16% to 23% excreted via bile in feces

Usual Dosage Adults: Oral: 2.5-5 mg/day. **Note:** There is little therapeutic benefit to increasing the dose >5 mg/day; there is, however, an increased risk of electrolyte disturbances.

Monitoring Parameters Blood pressure (both standing and sitting/supine), serum electrolytes, renal function, assess weight, I & O reports daily to determine fluid loss

Patient Information May be taken with food or milk; take early in day to avoid nocturia; take the last dose of multiple doses no later than 6 PM unless instructed otherwise. A few people who take this medication become more sensitive to sunlight and may experience skin rash, redness, itching, or severe sunburn, especially if sun block SPF ≥15 is not used on exposed skin areas.

Nursing Implications Take blood pressure with patient lying down and standing; may increase serum glucose in diabetic patients

Dosage Forms Tablet: 1.25 mg, 2.5 mg

Inderal® see Propranolol Hydrochloride on page 947

Inderal® LA see Propranolol Hydrochloride on page 947

Indochron E-R® see Indomethacin on this page

Indocin® see Indomethacin on this page

Indocin® I.V. see Indomethacin on this page

Indocin® SR see Indomethacin on this page

Indometacin see Indomethacin on this page

Indomethacin (in doe meth' a sin)
Related Information
Nonsteroidal Anti-Inflammatories Comparison on page 1280
Brand Names Indochron E-R®; Indocin®; Indocin® I.V.; Indocin® SR
Synonyms Indometacin
Use Management of inflammatory diseases and rheumatoid disorders; moderate pain; acute gouty arthritis; I.V. form used as alternative to surgery for closure of patent ductus arteriosus in neonates
Pregnancy Risk Factor B (D if used longer than 48 hours or after 34-week gestation)
Contraindications Hypersensitivity to indomethacin, any component, aspirin, or other nonsteroidal anti-inflammatory drugs (NSAIDs); active GI bleeding, ulcer disease; premature neonates with necrotizing enterocolitis, impaired renal function, active bleeding, thrombocytopenia
Warnings/Precautions Use with caution in patients with cardiac dysfunction, hypertension, renal or hepatic impairment, epilepsy, history of GI bleeding, patients receiving anticoagulants, and for treatment of JRA in children (fatal hepatitis has been reported); may have adverse effects on fetus; may affect platelet and renal function in neonates; elderly are a high-risk population for adverse effects from nonsteroidal anti-inflammatory agents. As much as 60% of elderly can develop peptic ulceration and/or hemorrhage asymptomatically.

Use lowest effective dose for shortest period possible. Use of NSAIDs can compromise existing renal function especially when Cl_{cr} is <30 mL/minute.

CNS adverse effects such as confusion, agitation, and hallucination are generally seen in overdose or high-dose situations; but elderly may demonstrate these adverse effects at lower doses than younger adults.

Adverse Reactions
>10%:
Central nervous system: Dizziness
Dermatologic: Rash
(Continued)

575

Indomethacin *(Continued)*

Gastrointestinal: Nausea, epigastric pain, abdominal pain, anorexia, GI bleeding, ulcers, perforation, abdominal cramps, heartburn, indigestion

1% to 10%:

Central nervous system: Headache, nervousness, fluid retention

Dermatologic: Itching

Gastrointestinal: Vomiting

Otic: Tinnitus

<1%:

Cardiovascular: Hypertension, congestive heart failure, arrhythmias, tachycardia

Central nervous system: Somnolence, fatigue, depression, confusion, drowsiness, hallucinations

Dermatologic: Hives, erythema multiforme, toxic epidermal necrolysis, Stevens-Johnson syndrome, angioedema

Endocrine & metabolic: Hyperkalemia, dilutional hyponatremia (I.V.), oliguria, hypoglycemia (I.V.), hot flushes, polydipsia

Gastrointestinal: Gastritis, GI ulceration

Genitourinary: Renal failure, cystitis

Hematologic: Hemolytic anemia, bone marrow depression, agranulocytosis, thrombocytopenia, inhibition of platelet aggregation, anemia, leukopenia

Hepatic: Hepatitis

Neuromuscular & skeletal: Peripheral neuropathy

Ocular: Corneal opacities, blurred vision, conjunctivitis, dry eyes, toxic amblyopia

Otic: Decreased hearing

Renal: Polyuria

Respiratory: Shortness of breath, allergic rhinitis

Miscellaneous: Epistaxis, aseptic meningitis, hypersensitivity reactions

Overdosage/Toxicology Symptoms of overdose include drowsiness, lethargy, nausea, vomiting, seizures, paresthesia, headache, dizziness, GI bleeding, cerebral edema, tinnitus, leukocytosis, renal failure

Management of a nonsteroidal anti-inflammatory drug (NSAID) intoxication is primarily supportive and symptomatic. Fluid therapy is commonly effective in managing the hypotension that may occur following an acute NSAID overdose, except when this is due to an acute blood loss. Seizures tend to be very short-lived and often do not require drug treatment. Although, recurrent seizures should be treated with I.V. diazepam.

Drug Interactions

Decreased effect: May decrease antihypertensive effects of beta-blockers, hydralazine and captopril; aspirin may decrease antihypertensive and diuretic effects of furosemide and thiazides

Increased toxicity: May increase serum potassium with potassium-sparing diuretics; probenecid may increase indomethacin serum concentrations; other NSAIDs may increase GI adverse effects; may increase nephrotoxicity of cyclosporin

Indomethacin may increase serum concentrations of digoxin, methotrexate, lithium, and aminoglycosides (reported with I.V. use in neonates)

Stability I.V.: Protect from light; not stable in alkaline solution; reconstitute just prior to administration; discard any unused portion; do not use preservative-containing diluents for reconstitution; suppositories do not require refrigeration

Mechanism of Action Inhibits prostaglandin synthesis by decreasing the activity of the enzyme, cyclo-oxygenase, which results in decreased formation of prostaglandin precursors

Pharmacodynamics/Kinetics

Onset of action: Within 30 minutes

Duration: 4-6 hours

Absorption: Prompt and extensive

Distribution: V_d: 0.34-1.57 L/kg; crosses the placenta; appears in breast milk

Protein binding: 90%

Metabolism: In the liver with significant enterohepatic cycling

Half-life: 4.5 hours, longer in neonates

Time to peak serum concentration: Oral: Within 3-4 hours

Elimination: Significant enterohepatic recycling; excreted in urine principally as glucuronide conjugates

Usual Dosage

Patent ductus arteriosus:

Neonates: I.V.: Initial: 0.2 mg/kg; followed with: 2 doses of 0.1 mg/kg at 12- to 24-hour intervals if age <48 hours at time of first dose; 0.2 mg/kg 2 times if 2-7 days old at time of first dose; or 0.25 mg/kg 2 times if over 7 days at time of first dose; discontinue if significant adverse effects occur. Dose should be withheld if patient has anuria or oliguria.

Analgesia:
  Children: Oral: Initial: 1-2 mg/kg/day in 2-4 divided doses; maximum: 4 mg/kg/day; not to exceed 150-200 mg/day
  Adults: Oral, rectal: 25-50 mg/dose 2-3 times/day; maximum dose: 200 mg/day; extended release capsule should be given on a 1-2 times/day schedule

Administration I.V.: Administer over 20-30 minutes at a concentration of 0.5-1 mg/mL in preservative-free sterile water for injection or normal saline. Reconstitute I.V. formulation just prior to administration; discard any unused portion; avoid I.V. bolus administration or infusion via an umbilical catheter into vessels near the superior mesenteric artery as these may cause vasoconstriction and can compromise blood flow to the intestines. Do not give intra-arterially.

Monitoring Parameters Monitor response (pain, range of motion, grip strength, mobility, ADL function), inflammation; observe for weight gain, edema; monitor renal function (serum creatinine, BUN); observe for bleeding, bruising; evaluate gastrointestinal effects (abdominal pain, bleeding, dyspepsia); mental confusion, disorientation, CBC, liver function tests

Test Interactions Positive Coombs' [direct]; ↑ sodium, ↑ chloride, ↑ bleeding time

Patient Information Take with food, milk, or with antacids; extended release capsules must be swallowed whole/intact, can cause dizziness or drowsiness

Nursing Implications Administer orally with food, milk, or antacids to decrease GI adverse effects; extended release capsules must be swallowed intact

Dosage Forms
  Capsule: 25 mg, 50 mg
  Capsule, sustained release: 75 mg
  Powder for injection, as sodium trihydrate: 1 mg
  Suppository, rectal: 50 mg
  Suspension, oral: 25 mg/5 mL (237 mL, 500 mL)

InFed™ *see* Iron Dextran Complex *on page 591*

Inflamase® *see* Prednisolone *on page 919*

Inflamase® Mild *see* Prednisolone *on page 919*

Influenza Virus Vaccine (in floo en' za)
Related Information
  Immunization Guidelines *on page 1389-1405*
  Vaccines *on page 1386-1388*

Brand Names Flu-Imune®; Fluogen®; Fluzone®

Synonyms Influenza Virus Vaccine (inactivated whole-virus); Influenza Virus Vaccine (split-virus) Influenza Virus Vaccine (purified surface antigen)

Use Provide active immunity to influenza virus strains contained in the vaccine; for high risk persons, previous year vaccines should not be to prevent present year influenza

Those at risk for influenza injection:
  Persons ≥65 years of age
  Institutionalized patients
  Persons of any age with chronic disorders of pulmonary and/or cardiovascular system
  Persons who have required medical follow-up following hospitalization for other chronic diseases such as diabetes, renal disease, immunodepressive disorders, etc
  Travelers, especially those at risk (above)

Pregnancy Risk Factor C

Contraindications Persons with allergy history to eggs or egg products, chicken, chicken feathers or chicken dander, hypersensitivity to thimerosal, influenza virus vaccine or any component, presence of acute respiratory disease or other active infections or illnesses, delay immunization in a patient with an active neurological disorder

Warnings/Precautions Waiting until the second or third trimester to vaccinate the pregnant woman with a high-risk condition may be reasonable. Antigenic response may not be as great as expected in patients requiring immunosuppressive drug; hypersensitivity reactions may occur; because of potential for febrile reactions, risks and benefits must carefully be considered in patients with history of febrile convulsions; influenza vaccines from previous seasons must not be used; patients with sulfite sensitivity may be affected by this product.

Adverse Reactions
  1% to 10%:
    Central nervous system: Fever, malaise
    Local: Tenderness, redness, or induration at the site of injection
(Continued)

Influenza Virus Vaccine *(Continued)*

<1%:
Central nervous system: Guillain-Barré syndrome, fever
Dermatologic: Hives, angioedema
Neuromuscular & skeletal: Myalgia
Respiratory: Asthma
Miscellaneous: Anaphylactoid reactions (most likely to residual egg protein), allergic reactions

Drug Interactions
Decreased effect with immunosuppressive agents; do not administer within 7 days after administration of diphtheria and tetanus toxoids and pertussis vaccine adsorbed (DTP)
Increased effect/toxicity of theophylline and warfarin

Stability Refrigerate

Usual Dosage Adults: I.M.: 0.5 mL each year of appropriate vaccine for the year, one dose is all that is necessary; administer in late fall to allow maximum titers to develop by peak epidemic periods usually occurring in early December

Administration Inspect for particulate matter and discoloration prior to administration; for I.M. administration only

Additional Information Pharmacies will stock the formulations(s) standardized according to the USPHS requirements for the season. Influenza vaccines from previous seasons must not be used. Federal law requires that the date of administration, the vaccine manufacturer, lot number of vaccine, and the administering person's name, title and address be entered into the patient's permanent medical record.

Dosage Forms Injection:
Purified surface antigen (Flu-Imune®): 5 mL
Split-virus (Fluogen®, Fluzone®): 0.5 mL, 5 mL
Whole-virus (Fluzone®): 5 mL

Influenza Virus Vaccine (inactivated whole-virus) *see* Influenza Virus Vaccine *on previous page*

Influenza Virus Vaccine (split-virus) Influenza Virus Vaccine (purified surface antigen) *see* Influenza Virus Vaccine *on previous page*

INH™ *see* Isoniazid *on page 595*

Initial Doses in Selected Antiemetic Regimens *see page 1205*

Inocor® *see* Amrinone Lactate *on page 76*

Insta-Char® [OTC] *see* Charcoal *on page 214*

Insulin Preparations *(in' su lin)*

Brand Names Humulin® 50/50 [OTC]; Humulin® 70/30 [OTC]; Humulin® L [OTC]; Humulin® N [OTC]; Humulin® R [OTC]; Humulin® U Utralente [OTC]; Lente® Iletin® I [OTC]; Lente® Iletin® II [OTC]; Lente® Insulin [OTC]; Lente® L [OTC]; Novolin® 70/30 [OTC]; Novolin® 70/30 PenFil® [OTC]; Novolin® L [OTC]; Novolin® N [OTC]; Novolin® N PenFil® [OTC]; Novolin® R [OTC]; Novolin® R PenFil® [OTC]; NPH Iletin® I [OTC]; NPH Insulin [OTC]; NPH-N [OTC]; Pork NPH Iletin® II [OTC]; Pork Regular Iletin® II [OTC]; Regular Concentrated Iletin® II; Regular Iletin® I [OTC]; Regular Insulin [OTC]; Regular Purified Pork Insulin [OTC]; Ultralente® U [OTC]; Velosulin® Human [OTC]

Use Treatment of insulin-dependent diabetes mellitus, also noninsulin-dependent diabetes mellitus unresponsive to treatment with diet and/or oral hypoglycemics; to assure proper utilization of glucose and reduce glucosuria in nondiabetic patients receiving parenteral nutrition whose glucosuria cannot be adequately controlled with infusion rate adjustments or those who require assistance in achieving optimal caloric intakes; hyperkalemia (use with glucose to shift potassium into cells to lower serum potassium levels)

Pregnancy Risk Factor B

Warnings/Precautions Any change of insulin should be made cautiously; changing manufacturers, type and/or method of manufacture, may result in the need for a change of dosage; human insulin differs from animal-source insulin; hypoglycemia may result from increased work or exercise without eating; use with caution in patients with a previous hypersensitivity reaction; S.C. doses used in insulin-resistant patients must be reduced if given I.V., only regular insulin should be given I.V.

Adverse Reactions
1% to 10%:
Cardiovascular: Perspiration, palpitation, tachycardia
Central nervous system: Fatigue, tingling of fingers, mental confusion, loss of consciousness, headache

Dermatologic: Urticaria, anaphylaxis
Endocrine & metabolic: Hypoglycemia, hypothermia
Gastrointestinal: Hunger, pallor, nausea, numbness of mouth
Local: Itching, redness, swelling, stinging, or warmth at injection site, atrophy or hypertrophy of S.C. fat tissue
Neuromuscular & skeletal: Muscle weakness, tremor
Ocular: Transient presbyopia or blurred vision, blurred vision

Overdosage/Toxicology Symptoms of overdose include tachycardia, anxiety, hunger, tremors, pallor, headache, motor dysfunction, speech disturbances, sweating, palpitations, coma, death; antidote is glucose and glucagon if necessary

Drug Interactions See table.

Drug Interactions With Insulin Injection

Decrease Hypoglycemic Effect of Insulin	Increase Hypoglycemic Effect of Insulin
Contraceptives, oral	Alcohol
Corticosteroids	Alpha blockers
Dextrothyroxine	Anabolic steroids
Diltiazem	Beta-blockers*
Dobutamine	Clofibrate
Epinephrine	Fenfluramine
Smoking	Guanethidine
Thiazide diuretics	MAO inhibitors
Thyroid hormone	Pentamidine
Niacin	Phenylbutazone
	Salicylates
	Sulfinpyrazone
	Tetracyclines

*Nonselective beta-blockers may delay recovery from hypoglycemic episodes and mask signs/symptoms of hypoglycemia. Cardioselective agents may be alternatives.

Stability Bottle in use is stable at room temperature up to 1 month; cold (freezing) causes more damage to insulin than room temperatures up to 100°F; avoid direct sunlight; cold injections should be avoided

Mechanism of Action Replacement therapy for persons unable to produce the hormone naturally or in insufficient amounts to maintain glycemic control

Pharmacodynamics/Kinetics
Onset and duration of hypoglycemic effects depend upon preparation administered. See table.

Pharmacokinetics/Pharmacodynamics: Onset and Duration of Hypoglycemic Effects Depend Upon Preparation Administered

	Onset (h)	Peak (h)	Duration (h)
Insulin, regular (Novolin® R)	1/2-1 (1/2)	5-10 (21/2-5)	6-8 (8)
Prompt insulin zinc suspension (Semilente®)	1-11/2	5-10	12-16
Insulin zinc suspension (NPH) (Novolin® N)	1-11/2 (11/2)	4-12 (4-12)	24 (24)
Isophane insulin suspension (Lente®)	1-21/2	7-15	24
Isophane insulin suspension and regular insulin injection (Novolin® 70/30)	1/2 (1/2)	4-8 (2-12)	24 (24)
Prompt zinc insulin suspension (PZI)	4-8	14-24	36
Extended insulin zinc suspension (Ultralente®)	4-8	10-30	>36

Onset and duration: Biosynthetic NPH human insulin shows a more rapid onset and shorter duration of action than corresponding porcine insulins; human insulin and purified porcine regular insulin are similarly efficacious following S.C. administration. The duration of action of highly purified porcine insulins is shorter than that of conventional insulin equivalents. Duration depends on type of preparation and route of administration as well as patient related variables. In general, the larger the dose of insulin, the longer the duration of activity.
(Continued)

Insulin Preparations *(Continued)*

Absorption: Biosynthetic regular human insulin is absorbed from the S.C. injection site more rapidly than insulins of animal origin (60-90 minutes peak vs 120-150 minutes peak respectively) and lowers the initial blood glucose much faster. Human Ultralente® insulin is absorbed about twice as quickly as its bovine equivalent, and bioavailability is also improved. Human Lente® insulin preparations are also absorbed more quickly than their animal equivalents.

Bioavailability: Medium-acting S.C. Lente®-type human insulins did not differ from the corresponding porcine insulins

Usual Dosage Dose requires continuous medical supervision; may administer I.V. (regular), I.M., S.C.

Diabetes mellitus:
Children and Adults: 0.5-1 unit/kg/day in divided doses
Adolescents (growth spurts): 0.8-1.2 units/kg/day in divided doses
Adjust dose to maintain premeal and bedtime blood glucose of 80-140 mg/dL (children <5 years: 100-200 mg/dL)

Hyperkalemia: Give calcium gluconate and $NaHCO_3$ first then 50% dextrose at 0.5-1 mL/kg and insulin 1 unit for every 4-5 g dextrose given

Diabetic ketoacidosis: Children and Adults: I.V. loading dose: 0.1 unit/kg, then maintenance continuous infusion: 0.1 unit/kg/hour (range: 0.05-0.2 units/kg/hour depending upon the rate of decrease of serum glucose - too rapid decrease of serum glucose may lead to cerebral edema).
Optimum rate of decrease (serum glucose): 80-100 mg/dL/hour
Note: Newly diagnosed patients with IDDM presenting in DKA and patients with blood sugars <800 mg/dL may be relatively "sensitive" to insulin and should receive loading and initial maintenance doses approximately ¹/₂ of those indicated above.

Dosing adjustment in renal impairment (regular):
Cl_{cr} 10-50 mL/minute: Administer at 75% of normal dose
Cl_{cr} <10 mL/minute: Administer at 25% to 50% of normal dose and monitor glucose closely

Hemodialysis effects: Because of a large molecular weight (6000 daltons), insulin is not significantly removed by either peritoneal or hemodialysis
Supplemental dose is not necessary
Peritoneal dialysis effects: Supplemental dose is not necessary
Continuous arterio-venous or veno-venous hemofiltration effects: Supplemental dose is not necessary

Administration

Regular insulin may be administered by S.C., I.M., or I.V. routes
S.C. administration is usually made into the thighs, arms, buttocks, or abdomen, with sites rotated
When mixing regular insulin with other preparations of insulin, regular insulin should be drawn into syringe first
I.V. administration (requires use of an infusion pump): **Only regular insulin** may be administered I.V.
I.V. infusions: To minimize adsorption problems to I.V. solution bag:
If new tubing is **not** needed: Wait a minimum of 30 minutes between the preparation of the solution and the initiation of the infusion
If new tubing is needed: After receiving the insulin drip solution, the administration set should be attached to the I.V. container and the line should be flushed with the insulin solution. The nurse should then wait 30 minutes, then flush the line again with the insulin solution prior to initiating the infusion
If insulin is required prior to the availability of the insulin drip, regular insulin should be administered by I.V. push injection
Because of adsorption, the actual amount of insulin being administered could be substantially less than the apparent amount. Therefore, adjustment of the insulin drip rate should be based on effect and not solely on the apparent insulin dose. Furthermore, the apparent dose should not be used as the basis for determining the subsequent insulin dose upon discontinuing the insulin drip. Dose requires continuous medical supervision.
To be ordered as units/hour
Example: Standard diluent of regular insulin only: 100 units/100 mL NS (can be given as a more diluted solution, ie, 100 units/250 mL NS)
Insulin rate of infusion (100 units regular/100 mL NS)
1 unit/hour: 1 mL/hour
2 units/hour: 2 mL/hour
3 units/hour: 3 mL/hour
4 units/hour: 4 mL/hour

5 units/hour: 5 mL/hour, etc

Monitoring Parameters Urine sugar and acetone, serum glucose, electrolytes

Reference Range

Therapeutic, serum insulin (fasting): 5-20 µIU/mL (SI: 35-145 pmol/L)

Glucose, fasting:

Newborns: 60-110 mg/dL

Adults: 60-110 mg/dL

Elderly: 100-180 mg/dL

Patient Information Do not change insulins without physician's approval; titrate vials to mix, do not shake; store in a cool place; when mixing insulins, draw up regular insulin into syringe first and use as soon as possible after mixing. Patients must be counseled by someone experienced in diabetes education, signs and symptoms of hyper- and hypoglycemia, exercise and diet, blood glucose monitoring, and other related topics.

Nursing Implications Patients using human insulin may be less likely to recognize hypoglycemia than if they use pork insulin, patients on pork insulin that have low blood sugar exhibit hunger and sweating; regular insulin is the only form for I.V. use. Patients who are unable to accurately draw up their dose will need assistance such as prefilled syringes.

Additional Information The term "purified" refers to insulin preparations containing no more than 10 ppm proinsulin (purified and human insulins are less immunogenic)

Dosage Forms All insulins are 100 units/mL (10 mL) except where indicated:

Insulin injection (Regular Insulin)

Beef and pork: Regular Iletin® I [Lilly]

Human:

rDNA: Humulin® R [Lilly], Novolin® R [Novo Nordisk], Novolin® R PenFil® (1.5 mL) [Novo Nordisk]

Semisynthetic: Velosulin® Human [Novo Nordisk]

Pork: Regular Insulin [Novo Nordisk]

Purified pork: Pork Regular Iletin® II [Lilly], Regular Purified Pork Insulin [Novo Nordisk]

Insulin zinc suspension (Lente®)

Beef: Lente® Insulin [Novo Nordisk]

Beef and pork: Lente® Iletin® I [Lilly]

Human, rDNA: Humulin® L [Lilly], Novolin® L [Novo Nordisk]

Purified pork: Lente® Iletin® II [Lilly], Lente® L [Novo Nordisk]

Insulin zinc suspension, extended (Ultralente®)

Beef: Ultralente® U [Novo Nordisk]

Human, rDNA: Humulin® U Utralente [Lilly]

Isophane Insulin Suspension (NPH)

Beef: NPH Insulin [Novo Nordisk]

Beef and pork: NPH Iletin® I [Lilly]

Human, rDNA: Humulin® N [Lilly], Novolin® N [Novo Nordisk], Novolin® N PenFil® (1.5 mL) [Novo Nordisk]

Purified pork: Pork NPH Iletin® II [Lilly], NPH-N [Novo Nordisk]

Isophane insulin suspension and insulin injection

Isophane insulin suspension (50%) and insulin injection (50%) human (rDNA): Humulin® 50/50 [Lilly]

Isophane insulin suspension (70%) and insulin injection (30%) human (rDNA): Humulin® 70/30 [Lilly], Novolin® 70/30 [Novo Nordisk], Novolin® 70/30 PenFil® (1.5 mL) [Novo Nordisk]

Regular (concentrated) Iletin® II U-500 injection: Purified pork: 500 units/mL (20 mL)

Intal® Inhalation Capsule *see* Cromolyn Sodium *on page 280*

Intal® Nebulizer Solution *see* Cromolyn Sodium *on page 280*

Intal® Oral Inhaler *see* Cromolyn Sodium *on page 280*

α-2-interferon *see* Interferon Alfa-2b *on page 583*

Interferon Alfa-2a (in ter feer' on)

Related Information

Antimicrobial Drugs of Choice *on page 1298-1302*

Brand Names Roferon-A®

Synonyms IFLrA; IFN; rIFN-A

Use FDA approved: Patients >18 years of age: Hairy cell leukemia, AIDS related Kaposi's sarcoma; multiple unlabeled uses; indications and dosage regimens are specific for a particular brand of interferon

Pregnancy Risk Factor C

Contraindications Hypersensitivity to alfa-2a interferon or any component of the product

(Continued)

Interferon Alfa-2a *(Continued)*

Warnings/Precautions The U.S. Food and Drug Administration (FDA) currently recommends that procedures for proper handling and disposal of antineoplastic agents be considered. Use with caution in patients with seizure disorders, brain metastases, compromised CNS, multiple sclerosis, and patients with pre-existing cardiac disease, severe renal or hepatic impairment, or myelosuppression; safety and efficacy in children <18 years of age have not been established. Higher doses in the elderly or in malignancies other than hairy cell leukemia may result in severe obtundation.

Adverse Reactions

>10%:

Central nervous system: Dizziness, tiredness, fatigue, malaise, fever (usually within 4-6 hours), chills

Dermatologic: Skin rash

Gastrointestinal: Dry mouth, sweating, nausea, vomiting, diarrhea, dizziness, abdominal cramps, weight loss, metallic taste

Hematologic: Mildly myelosuppressive and well tolerated if used without adjunct antineoplastic agents; thrombocytosis has been reported, leukopenia (mainly neutropenia), anemia, thrombocytopenia, decreased hemoglobin, hematocrit, platelets

Myelosuppressive:

WBC: Mild

Platelets: Mild

Onset (days): 7-10

Nadir (days): 14

Recovery (days): 21

Neuromuscular & skeletal: Rigors, arthralgia

Miscellaneous: Flu-like syndrome

1% to 10%:

Central nervous system: Headache, delirium, somnolence neurotoxicity

Dermatologic: alopecia, dry skin

Gastrointestinal: Anorexia, stomatitis

Hepatic: Hepatotoxicity

Neuromuscular & skeletal: Peripheral neuropathy, leg cramps

Ocular: Blurred vision

Miscellaneous: Diaphoresis

<1%:

Cardiovascular: Tachycardia, arrhythmias, chest pain, hypotension, SVT, edema

Central nervous system: Confusion, sensory neuropathy, fever, headache, psychiatric effects, EEG abnormalities, depression, chills

Dermatologic: Partial alopecia, rash

Gastrointestinal: Weight loss, change in taste

Hematologic: Decreased hemoglobin, hematocrit, platelets

Hepatic: Increased hepatic transaminase

Neuromuscular & skeletal: Myalgia, arthralgia, rigors

Ocular: Blurred vision, visual disturbances

Renal: Proteinuria, increased uric acid level, increased Cr, increased BUN

Respiratory: Coughing, chest pain, dyspnea, nasal congestion

Miscellaneous: Hypothyroidism, neutralizing antibodies, local sensitivity to injection; usually patient can build up a tolerance to side effects

Overdosage/Toxicology Symptoms of overdose include CNS depression, obtundation, flu-like symptoms, myelosuppression; treatment is supportive

Drug Interactions

Increased effect:

Cimetidine: May augment the antitumor effects of interferon in melanoma

Theophylline: Clearance has been reported to be decreased in hepatitis patients receiving interferon

Increased toxicity: Vinblastine: Enhances interferon toxicity in several patients; increased incidence of paresthesia has also been noted

Stability Refrigerate (2°C to 8°C/36°F to 46°F); do not freeze; do not shake; after reconstitution, the solution is stable for 24 hours at room temperature and for 1 month when refrigerated

Pharmacodynamics/Kinetics

Absorption: Filtered and absorbed at the renal tubule

Distribution: The V_d of interferon is 31 L; but has been noted to be much greater (370-720 L) in leukemia patients receiving continuous infusion IFN; IFN does not penetrate the CSF

Metabolism: Majority of dose thought to be metabolized in the kidney

Bioavailability:

I.M.: 83%

S.C.: 90%

Half-life: Elimination:
I.M., I.V.: 2 hours after administration
S.C.: 3 hours
Time to peak serum concentration: I.M., S.C.: ~6-8 hours

Usual Dosage Refer to individual protocols

Infants and Children: Hemangiomas of infancy, pulmonary hemangiomatosis: S.C.: 1-3 million units/m^2/day once daily

Adults >18 years: I.M., S.C.:

Hairy cell leukemia:

Induction: 3 million units/day for 16-24 weeks.

Maintenance: 3 million units 3 times/week (may be treated for up to 20 consecutive weeks)

AIDS-related Kaposi's sarcoma:

Induction: 36 million units/day for 10-12 weeks

Maintenance: 36 million units 3 times/week (may begin with dose escalation from 3-9-18 million units each day over 3 consecutive days followed by 36 million units/day for the remainder of the 10-12 weeks of induction)

If severe adverse reactions occur, modify dosage (50% reduction) or temporarily discontinue therapy until adverse reactions abate

Administration S.C. administration is suggested for those who are at risk for bleeding or are thrombocytopenic; rotate S.C. injection site; patient should be well hydrated

Monitoring Parameters Baseline chest x-ray, EKG, CBC with differential, liver function tests, electrolytes, platelets, weight; patients with pre-existing cardiac abnormalities, or in advanced stages of cancer should have EKGs taken before and during treatment

Patient Information Do not change brands as changes in dosage may result; possible mental status changes may occur while on therapy; report to physician any persistent or severe sore throat, fever, fatigue, unusual bleeding, or bruising; do not operate heavy machinery while on therapy since changes in mental status may occur

Nursing Implications Do not freeze or shake solution; a flu-like syndrome (fever, chills) occurs in the majority of patients 2-6 hours after a dose; pretreatment with nonsteroidal anti-inflammatory drug (NSAID) or acetaminophen can decrease fever and its severity and alleviate headache

Dosage Forms

Injection: 3 million units/mL (1 mL); 6 million units/mL (3 mL); 36 million units/mL (1 mL)

Powder for injection: 6 million units/mL when reconstituted

Interferon Alfa-2b (in ter feer' on)

Related Information

Antimicrobial Drugs of Choice on page 1298-1302
Cancer Chemotherapy Regimens on page 1218-1241

Brand Names Intron® A

Synonyms IFN-alpha 2; α-2-interferon; rIFN-α2

Use FDA approved: Patients >18 years of age: Hairy cell leukemia, condylomata acuminata, AIDS-related Kaposi's sarcoma, chronic hepatitis non-A, non-B(C), chronic hepatitis B; indications and dosage regimens are specific for a particular brand of interferon

Pregnancy Risk Factor C

Contraindications Known hypersensitivity to interferon alfa-2b or any component

Warnings/Precautions The U.S. Food and Drug Administration (FDA) currently recommends that procedures for proper handling and disposal of antineoplastic agents be considered. Use with caution in patients with seizure disorders, brain metastases, compromised CNS, multiple sclerosis, and patients with pre-existing cardiac disease, severe renal or hepatic impairment, or myelosuppression; safety and efficacy in children <18 years of age have not been established. Higher doses in the elderly or in malignancies other than hairy cell leukemia may result in severe obtundation.

Adverse Reactions

>10%:

Central nervous system: Dizziness, tiredness, fatigue, malaise, fever (usually within 4-6 hours). chills

Dermatologic: Skin rash

Gastrointestinal: Dry mouth, sweating, nausea, vomiting, diarrhea, dizziness, abdominal cramps, weight loss, metallic taste, anorexia

Hematologic: Mildly myelosuppressive and well tolerated if used without adjunct antineoplastic agents; thrombocytosis has been reported, leukopenia (mainly neutropenia), anemia, thrombocytopenia, decreased hemoglobin, hematocrit, platelets

(Continued)

Interferon Alfa-2b *(Continued)*

Myelosuppressive:
  WBC: Mild
  Platelets: Mild
  Onset (days): 7-10
  Nadir (days): 14
  Recovery (days): 21
Neuromuscular & skeletal: Rigors, arthralgia
Miscellaneous: Flu-like syndrome
1% to 10%:
  Central nervous system: Neurotoxicity
  Dermatologic: Dry skin, alopecia
  Gastrointestinal: Stomatitis
  Hepatic: Hepatotoxicity
  Neuromuscular & skeletal: Peripheral neuropathy, leg cramps
  Ocular: Blurred vision
  Miscellaneous: Diaphoresis
<1%:
  Cardiovascular: Cardiotoxicity, tachycardia, arrhythmias, hypotension, SVT, arrhythmias, chest pain, edema
  Central nervous system: EEG abnormalities, confusion, sensory neuropathy, fever, headache, psychiatric effects, delirium, somnolence, chills
  Dermatologic: Partial alopecia, rash
  Gastrointestinal: Weight loss, change in taste
  Hematologic: Decreased hemoglobin, hematocrit, platelets
  Hepatic: Increased hepatic transaminase, increased ALT and AST
  Neuromuscular & skeletal: Myalgia, arthralgia, rigors
  Ocular: Visual disturbances, blurred vision
  Renal: Proteinuria, increased uric acid level, increased Cr, increased BUN
  Respiratory: Coughing, dyspnea, nasal congestion
  Miscellaneous: Local sensitivity to injection, hypothyroidism, neutralizing antibodies; usually patient can build up a tolerance to side effects

Overdosage/Toxicology Symptoms of overdose include CNS depression, obtundation, flu-like symptoms, myelosuppression; treatment is supportive

Drug Interactions
Increased effect: Cimetidine: May augment the antitumor effects of interferon in melanoma
Increased toxicity:
  Theophylline: Clearance has been reported to be decreased in hepatitis patients receiving interferon
  Vinblastine: Enhances interferon toxicity in several patients; increased incidence of paresthesia has also been noted

Stability Refrigerate (2°C to 8°C/36°F to 46°F); reconstituted solution is stable for 1 month when refrigerated

Mechanism of Action Alpha interferons are a family of proteins, produced by nucleated cells, that have antiviral, antiproliferative, and immune-regulating activity. There are 16 known subtypes of alpha interferons. Interferons interact with cells through high affinity cell surface receptors. Following activation, multiple effects can be detected including induction of gene transcription. Inhibit cellular growth, alters the state of cellular differentiation, interferes with oncogene expression, alters cell surface antigen expression, increases phagocytic activity of macrophages, and augments cytotoxicity of lymphocytes for target cells

Pharmacodynamics/Kinetics
Absorption: Filtered and absorbed at the renal tubule
Distribution: The V_d of interferon is 31 L; but has been noted to be much greater (370-720 L) in leukemia patients receiving continuous infusion IFN; IFN does not penetrate the CSF
Metabolism: Majority of dose thought to be metabolized in the kidney
Bioavailability:
  I.M.: 83%
  S.C.: 90%
Half-life: Elimination:
  I.M., I.V.: 2 hours
  S.C.: 3 hours
Time to peak serum concentration: I.M., S.C.: ~6-8 hours

Usual Dosage Adults (refer to individual protocols):
Hairy cell leukemia: I.M., S.C.: 2 million IU/m² 3 times/week for 2-≥6 months therapy
AIDS-related Kaposi's sarcoma: I.M., S.C. (use 50 million IU vial): 30 million units/m² 3 times/week
Condylomata acuminata: Intralesionally (use 10 million IU vial): 1 million units/lesion 3 times/week for 4-8 weeks; not to exceed 5 million units per treatment (maximum: 5 lesions at one time)

Chronic hepatitis C (non-A, non-B): I.M., S.C.: 3 million IU 3 times/week for approximately a 6-month course

Chronic hepatitis B: I.M., S.C.: 5 million IU/day or 10 million IU 3 times/week for 16 weeks

If severe adverse reactions occur, reduce dosage 50% or temporarily discontinue therapy until adverse reactions abate

See table.

Decreased Granulocyte or Platelet Counts

Granulocyte Count	Platelet Count	Interferon 2b dose
<750/mm^3	<50,000/mm^3	Decrease by 50%
<500/mm^3	<30,000/mm^3	Interrupt

When platelet/granulocyte count returns to normal, reinstitute therapy

Monitoring Parameters Baseline chest x-ray, EKG, CBC with differential, liver function tests, electrolytes, platelets, weight; patients with pre-existing cardiac abnormalities, or in advanced stages of cancer should have EKGs taken before and during treatment

Patient Information Do not change brands of interferon as changes in dosage may result; do not operate heavy machinery while on therapy since changes in mental status may occur; report to physician any persistent or severe sore throat, fever, fatigue, unusual bleeding, or bruising

Nursing Implications Use acetaminophen to prevent or partially alleviate headache and fever; do not use 3, 5, and 25 million unit strengths intralesionally, solutions are hypertonic; 50 million unit strength is not for use in condylomata

Dosage Forms Powder for injection, lyophilized: 3 million IU, 5 million IU, 10 million IU, 18 million IU, 25 million IU, 50 million IU

Interferon Alfa-N3 (in ter feer' on al fa n3)

Brand Names Alferon® N

Use FDA approved (Patients ≥18 years of age): Condylomata acuminata, intralesional treatment of refractory or recurring genital or venereal warts; useful in patients who do not respond or are not candidates for usual treatments; indications and dosage regimens are specific for a particular brand of interferon

Pregnancy Risk Factor C

Contraindications Patients with known hypersensitivity to alpha interferon, mouse immunoglobulin, or any component of the product

Warnings/Precautions The U.S. Food and Drug Administration (FDA) currently recommends that procedures for proper handling and disposal of antineoplastic agents be considered. Use with caution in patients with seizure disorders, brain metastases, compromised CNS function, cardiac disease, severe renal or hepatic impairment, multiple sclerosis; safety and efficacy in children <18 years have not been established.

Adverse Reactions

>10%:

Central nervous system: Fatigue, malaise, fever (usually within 4-6 hours), rigors, chills, tiredness

Dermatologic: Skin rash

Gastrointestinal: Dry mouth, sweating, nausea, vomiting, diarrhea, dizziness, abdominal cramps, weight loss, metallic tastes, anorexia

Hematologic: Mildly myelosuppressive and well tolerated if used without adjunct antineoplastic agents; thrombocytosis has been reported, leukopenia (mainly neutropenia), anemia, thrombocytopenia, decreased hemoglobin, hematocrit, platelets

Myelosuppressive:

WBC: Mild

Platelets: Mild

Onset (days): 7-10

Nadir (days): 14

Recovery (days): 21

Neuromuscular & skeletal: Arthralgia

Miscellaneous: Flu-like syndrome

1% to 10%:

Central nervous system: Headache, delirium, somnolence, neurotoxicity

Dermatologic: Alopecia, dry skin

Gastrointestinal: Stomatitis, hepatotoxicity

Neuromuscular & skeletal: Peripheral neuropathy

Miscellaneous: Diaphoresis, leg cramps, blurred vision

(Continued)

585

Interferon Alfa-N3 *(Continued)*

<1%:

Cardiovascular: Tachycardia, arrhythmias, chest pain, hypotension, SVT, edema

Central nervous system: EEG abnormalities, confusion, sensory neuropathy, fever, headache, confusion, psychiatric effects, depression, chills

Dermatologic: Rash, partial alopecia, local sensitivity to injection

Gastrointestinal: Weight loss, change in taste

Hematologic: Decreased hemoglobin, hematocrit, platelets

Hepatic: Increased hepatic transaminase, increased ALT and AST

Neuromuscular & skeletal: Arthralgia, rigors, myalgia

Ocular: Visual disturbances, blurred vision

Renal: Proteinuria, increased uric acid level, increased Cr, increased BUN, proteinuria

Respiratory: Coughing, chest pain, dyspnea, cough, nasal congestion

Miscellaneous: Hypothyroidism, neutralizing antibodies, usually patient can build up a tolerance to side effects

Overdosage/Toxicology Symptoms of overdose include CNS depression, obtundation, flu-like symptoms, myelosuppression; treatment is supportive

Drug Interactions

Increased effect: Cimetidine: May augment the antitumor effects of interferon in melanoma

Increased toxicity:

Vinblastine: Enhances interferon toxicity in several patients; increased incidence of paresthesia has also been noted

Theophylline: Clearance has been reported to be decreased in hepatitis patients receiving interferon

Stability Store solution at 2°C to 8°C (36°F to 46°F); do not freeze or shake solution

Mechanism of Action Interferons interact with cells through high affinity cell surface receptors. Following activation, multiple effects can be detected including induction of gene transcription. Inhibits cellular growth, alters the state of cellular differentiation, interferes with oncogene expression, alters cell surface antigen expression, increases phagocytic activity of macrophages, and augments cytotoxicity of lymphocytes for target cells

Usual Dosage Adults: Inject 250,000 units (0.05 mL) in each wart twice weekly for a maximum of 8 weeks; therapy should not be repeated for at least 3 months after the initial 8-week course of therapy

Administration Inject into base of wart with a small 30-gauge needle

Patient Information Warts are highly contagious until they completely disappear, abstain from sexual activity or use barrier protection; inform nurse or physician if allergy exists to eggs, neomycin, mouse immunoglobulin, or to human interferon alpha; acetaminophen can be used to treat flu-like symptoms

Dosage Forms Injection: 5 million IU (1 mL)

Interferon Beta-1b *(in ter feer' on bay ta 1b)*

Brand Names Betaseron®

Synonyms rIFN-b

Use Reduces the frequency of clinical exacerbations in ambulatory patients with relapsing-remitting multiple sclerosis (MS)

Pregnancy Risk Factor C

Contraindications Hypersensitivity to *E. coli* derived products, natural or recombinant interferon beta, albumin human or any other component of the formulation

Warnings/Precautions The safety and efficacy of interferon beta-1b in chronic progressive MS have not been evaluated; use with caution in women who are breast feeding; flu-like symptoms complex (ie, myalgia, fever, chills, malaise, sweating) is reported in 53% of patients who receive interferon beta-1b

Adverse Reactions Due to the pivotal position of interferon in the immune system, toxicities can affect nearly every organ system. Injection site reactions, injection site necrosis, flu-like symptoms, menstrual disorders, depression (with suicidal ideations), somnolence, palpitations, peripheral vascular disorders, hypertension, blood dyscrasias, dyspnea, laryngitis, cystitis, gastrointestinal complaints

Overdosage/Toxicology Symptoms of overdose include CNS depression, obtundation, flu-like symptoms, myelosuppression; treatment is supportive

Stability Store solution at 2°C to 8°C (36°F to 46°F); do not freeze or shake solution; use product within 3 hours of reconstitution

Mechanism of Action Interferon beta-1b differs from naturally occurring human protein by a single amino acid substitution and the lack of carbohydrate side chains; alters the expression and response to surface antigens and can enhance immune cell activities. Properties of interferon beta-1b that modify biologic responses are mediated by cell surface receptor interactions; mechanism in the treatment of MS is unknown.

Usual Dosage S.C.:
Children <18 years: Not recommended
Adults >18 years: 0.25 mg (8 million IU) every other day

Administration Withdraw 1 mL of reconstituted solution from the vial into a sterile syringe fitted with a 27-gauge needle and inject the solution subcutaneously; sites for self-injection include arms, abdomen, hips, and thighs

Monitoring Parameters Hemoglobin, liver function, and blood chemistries

Patient Information Instruct patients on self-injection technique and procedures. If possible, perform first injection under the supervision of an appropriately qualified healthcare professional. Injection site reactions may occur during therapy. They are usually transient and do not require discontinuation of therapy, but careful assessment of the nature and severity of all reported reactions. Flu-like symptoms are not uncommon following initiation of therapy. Acetaminophen may reduce these symptoms. Do not change the dosage or schedule of administration without medical consultation. Report depression or suicide ideation to physicians. Avoid prolonged exposure to sunlight or sunlamps.

Nursing Implications Patient should be informed of possible side effects, especially depression, suicidal ideations, and the risk of abortion; flu-like symptoms such as chills, fever, malaise, sweating, and myalgia are common

Additional Information May be available only in small supplies; for information on availability and distribution, call the patient information line at 800-580-3837

Dosage Forms Powder for injection, lyophilized: 0.3 mg [9.6 million IU units]

Interleukin-2 *see* Aldesleukin *on page 35*

Intralipid® *see* Fat Emulsion *on page 441*

Intravenous Fat Emulsion *see* Fat Emulsion *on page 441*

Intron® A *see* Interferon Alfa-2b *on page 583*

Intropin® *see* Dopamine Hydrochloride *on page 364*

Inversine® *see* Mecamylamine Hydrochloride *on page 672*

Iodex® Regular *see* Povidone-Iodine *on page 913*

Iodinated Glycerol (eye′ oh di nay ted gli′ ser ole)

Brand Names Iophen®; Organidin®; Par Glycerol®; R-Gen®

Use Mucolytic expectorant in adjunctive treatment of bronchitis, bronchial asthma, pulmonary emphysema, cystic fibrosis, or chronic sinusitis

Pregnancy Risk Factor X

Contraindications Hypersensitivity to inorganic iodides, iodinated glycerol, or any component; pregnancy; newborns

Warnings/Precautions Use with caution in patients with thyroid disease or renal impairment

Adverse Reactions
1% to 10%: Gastrointestinal: Diarrhea, nausea, vomiting
<1%:
Central nervous system: Headache
Dermatologic: Acne, dermatitis
Endocrine & metabolic: Acute parotitis
Gastrointestinal: GI irritation
Respiratory: Pulmonary edema
Miscellaneous: Thyroid gland enlargement, swelling of the eyelids, hypersensitivity

Overdosage/Toxicology Symptoms include metallic taste, swollen eyelids, sneezing, nausea, vomiting, diarrhea

Drug Interactions Increased toxicity: Disulfiram, metronidazole, procarbazine, MAO inhibitors, CNS depressants, lithium

Mechanism of Action Increases respiratory tract secretions by decreasing surface tension and thereby decreases the viscosity of mucus, which aids in removal of the mucus

Pharmacodynamics/Kinetics
Absorption: From GI tract
Distribution: Accumulates in the thyroid gland
Elimination: In urine

Usual Dosage Oral:
Children: Up to 30 mg 4 times/day
Adults: 60 mg 4 times/day

Test Interactions Thyroid function tests may be altered

Patient Information Take with a full glass of water; not for use in coughs lasting longer than 1 week or associated with a fever
(Continued)

Iodinated Glycerol *(Continued)*

Nursing Implications Give with plenty of fluids; elixir contains 21.75% alcohol; watch for sedation; avoid elixir in children due to high alcohol content

Dosage Forms Organically bound iodine in brackets
Elixir: 60 mg/5 mL [30 mg/5 mL] (120 mL, 480 mL)
Solution: 50 mg/mL [25 mg/mL] (30 mL)
Tablet: 30 mg [15 mg]

Iodochlorhydroxyquin (eye oh doe klor' hye drox ee kwin)

Brand Names Vioform® [OTC]

Synonyms Clioquinol

Use Topically in the treatment of tinea pedis, tinea cruris, and skin infections caused by dermatophytic fungi (ring worm)

Pregnancy Risk Factor C

Contraindications Not effective in the treatment of scalp or nail fungal infections; children <2 years of age, hypersensitivity to any component

Warnings/Precautions May irritate sensitized skin; topical application poses a potential risk of toxicity to infants and children; known to cause serious and irreversible optic atrophy and peripheral neuropathy with muscular weakness, sensory loss, spastic paraparesis, and blindness; use with caution in patients with iodine intolerance

Adverse Reactions
1% to 10%:
Dermatologic: Skin irritation, rash
Neuromuscular & skeletal: Peripheral neuropathy
Ocular: Optic atrophy

Mechanism of Action Chelates bacterial surface and trace metals needed for bacterial growth

Pharmacodynamics/Kinetics
Absorption: With an occlusive dressing, up to 40% of dose can be absorbed systemically during a 12-hour period; absorption is enhanced when applied under diapers
Half-life: 11-14 hours
Elimination: Conjugated and excreted in urine

Usual Dosage Children and Adults: Topical: Apply 2-3 times/day; do not use for longer than 7 days

Test Interactions Thyroid function tests (decreased ^{131}I uptake); false-positive ferric chloride test for phenylketonuria

Patient Information Cleanse affected area before application; can stain skin and fabrics; for external use only; avoid contact with eyes and mucous membranes

Nursing Implications Watch affected area for increased irritation

Dosage Forms
Cream: 3% (30 g)
Ointment, topical: 3% (30 g)

Iodoquinol (eye oh doe kwin' ole)

Brand Names Sebaquin® [OTC]; Yodoxin®

Synonyms Diiodohydroxyquin

Use Treatment of acute and chronic intestinal amebiasis; asymptomatic cyst passers; *Blastocystis hominis* infections; ineffective for amebic hepatitis or hepatic abscess

Pregnancy Risk Factor C

Contraindications Known hypersensitivity to iodine or iodoquinol; hepatic damage; pre-existing optic neuropathy

Warnings/Precautions Optic neuritis, optic atrophy, and peripheral neuropathy have occurred following prolonged use; avoid long-term therapy

Adverse Reactions
>10%: Gastrointestinal: Diarrhea, nausea, vomiting, stomach pain
1% to 10%:
Central nervous system: Fever, chills, agitation, retrograde amnesia, headache
Dermatologic: Skin rash, hives
Endocrine & metabolic: Thyroid gland enlargement
Neuromuscular & skeletal: Peripheral neuropathy, weakness
Ocular: Optic neuritis, optic atrophy, visual impairment
Miscellaneous: Itching of rectal area

Overdosage/Toxicology
Chronic overdose can result in vomiting, diarrhea, abdominal pain, metallic taste, paresthesias, paraplegia, and loss of vision; can lead to destruction of the long fibers of the spinal cord and optic nerve

Acute overdose: Delirium, stupor, coma, amnesia
Following GI decontamination, treatment is symptomatic
Mechanism of Action Contact amebicide that works in the lumen of the intestine by an unknown mechanism
Pharmacodynamics/Kinetics
Absorption: Oral: Poor and irregular
Metabolism: In the liver
Elimination: High percentage of the dose excreted in feces
Usual Dosage Oral:
Children: 30-40 mg/kg/day (maximum: 650 mg/dose) in 3 divided doses for 20 days; not to exceed 1.95 g/day
Adults: 650 mg 3 times/day after meals for 20 days; not to exceed 2 g/day
Monitoring Parameters Ophthalmologic exam
Test Interactions May increase protein-bound serum iodine concentrations reflecting a decrease in ^{131}I uptake; false-positive ferric chloride test for phenylketonuria
Patient Information May take with food or milk to reduce stomach upset; complete full course of therapy
Nursing Implications Tablets may be crushed and mixed with applesauce or chocolate syrup
Dosage Forms
Powder: 25 g
Shampoo: 3% (120 mL)
Tablet: 210 mg, 650 mg

Ionamin® see Phentermine Hydrochloride on page 872

Ionil® [OTC] see Salicylic Acid on page 991

Iophen® see Iodinated Glycerol on page 587

Iophen DM® [OTC] see Guaifenesin and Dextromethorphan on page 517

Iopidine® see Apraclonidine Hydrochloride on page 84

Iosat® see Potassium Iodide on page 909

I-Paracaine® see Proparacaine Hydrochloride on page 943

I-Parescein® see Proparacaine and Fluorescein on page 942

Ipecac Syrup (ip′ e kak)

Use Treatment of acute oral drug overdosage and in certain poisonings
Pregnancy Risk Factor C
Contraindications Do not use in unconscious patients, patients with no gag reflex; ingestion of strong bases or acids, volatile oils; seizures
Warnings/Precautions Do not confuse ipecac syrup with ipecac fluid extract, which is 14 times more potent; use with caution in patients with cardiovascular disease and bulimics; may not be effective in antiemetic overdose
Adverse Reactions
1% to 10%:
Cardiovascular: Cardiotoxicity
Central nervous system: Lethargy
Gastrointestinal: Protracted vomiting, diarrhea
Neuromuscular & skeletal: Myopathy
Overdosage/Toxicology Contains cardiotoxin; symptoms of overdose include tachycardia, CHF, atrial fibrillation, depressed myocardial contractility, myocarditis, diarrhea, persistent vomiting, hypotension; treatment is activated charcoal, gastric lavage
Drug Interactions
Decreased effect: Activated charcoal, milk, carbonated beverages
Increased toxicity: Phenothiazines (chlorpromazine has been associated with serious dystonic reactions)
Mechanism of Action Irritates the gastric mucosa and stimulates the medullary chemoreceptor trigger zone to induce vomiting
Pharmacodynamics/Kinetics
Onset of action: Within 15-30 minutes
Duration: 20-25 minutes; can last longer, 60 minutes in some cases
Absorption: Significant amounts, mainly when it does not produce emesis
Elimination: Emetine (alkaloid component) may be detected in urine 60 days after excess dose or chronic use
Usual Dosage Oral:
Children:
6-12 months: 5-10 mL followed by 10-20 mL/kg of water; repeat dose one time if vomiting does not occur within 20 minutes
(Continued)

Ipecac Syrup *(Continued)*

1-12 years: 15 mL followed by 10-20 mL/kg of water; repeat dose one time if vomiting does not occur within 20 minutes

If emesis does not occur within 30 minutes after second dose, ipecac must be removed from stomach by gastric lavage

Adults: 15-30 mL followed by 200-300 mL of water; repeat dose one time if vomiting does not occur within 20 minutes

Patient Information Call Poison Center before administering. Patients should be kept active and moving following administration of ipecac; follow dose with 8 oz of water following initial episode; if vomiting, no food or liquids should be ingested for 1 hour

Nursing Implications Do **not** administer to unconscious patients; patients should be kept active and moving following administration of ipecac; if vomiting does not occur after second dose, gastric lavage may be considered to remove ingested substance

Dosage Forms Syrup: 70 mg/mL (15 mL, 30 mL, 473 mL, 4000 mL)

I-Pentolate® *see* Cyclopentolate Hydrochloride *on page 286*

I-Phrine® Ophthalmic Solution *see* Phenylephrine Hydrochloride *on page 874*

IPOL™ *see* Polio Vaccines *on page 898*

Ipratropium Bromide (i pra troe' pee um)

Brand Names Atrovent®

Use Anticholinergic bronchodilator in bronchospasm associated with COPD, bronchitis, and emphysema

Pregnancy Risk Factor B

Contraindications Hypersensitivity to atropine or its derivatives

Warnings/Precautions Not indicated for the initial treatment of acute episodes of bronchospasm; use with caution in patients with narrow-angle glaucoma, prostatic hypertrophy, or bladder neck obstruction; ipratropium has not been specifically studied in the elderly, but it is poorly absorbed from the airways and appears to be safe in this population.

Adverse Reactions Note: Ipratropium is poorly absorbed from the lung, so systemic effects are rare

>10%:
Central nervous system: Nervousness, dizziness, fatigue, headache
Gastrointestinal: Nausea, dry mouth, stomach upset
Respiratory: Cough

1% to 10%:
Cardiovascular: Palpitations, hypotension
Central nervous system: Insomnia
Genitourinary: Urinary retention
Neuromuscular & skeletal: Trembling
Ocular: Blurred vision
Respiratory: Nasal congestion

<1%:
Dermatologic: Skin rash, hives
Gastrointestinal: Stomatitis

Overdosage/Toxicology Symptoms of overdose include dry mouth, drying of respiratory secretions, cough, nausea, GI distress, blurred vision or impaired visual accommodation, headache, nervousness. Acute overdosage with ipratropium by inhalation is unlikely since it is so poorly absorbed. However, if poisoning occurs, it can be treated like any other anticholinergic toxicity. An anticholinergic overdose with severe life-threatening symptoms may be treated with physostigmine 1-2 mg (0.5 or 0.02 mg/kg for children) S.C. or I.V., slowly.

Drug Interactions
Increased effect with albuterol
Increased toxicity with anticholinergics or drugs with anticholinergic properties, dronabinol

Mechanism of Action Blocks the action of acetylcholine at parasympathetic sites in bronchial smooth muscle causing bronchodilation

Pharmacodynamics/Kinetics
Onset of bronchodilation: 1-3 minutes after administration
Peak effect: Within 1.5-2 hours
Duration: Up to 4-6 hours
Absorption: Not readily absorbed into the systemic circulation from the surface of the lung or from the GI tract
Distribution: Inhalation: 15% of dose reaches the lower airways

Usual Dosage
Children:
<2 years: Nebulization: 250 mcg 3 times/day
3-14 years: Metered dose inhaler: 1-2 inhalations 3 times/day, up to 6 inhalations/24 hours
Children >12 years and Adults: Nebulization: 500 mcg (1 unit-dose vial) administered 3-4 times/day by oral nebulization, with doses 6-8 hours apart
Children >14 years and Adults: Metered dose inhaler: 2 inhalations 4 times/day every 4-6 hours up to 12 inhalations in 24 hours

Patient Information
Inhaler directions: Effects are enhanced by breath-holding 10 seconds after inhalation; temporary blurred vision may occur if sprayed into eyes; shake canister well before each use of the inhaler; follow instructions for use accompanying the product; close eyes when administering ipratropium; wait at least one full minute between inhalations
Nebulizer directions: Twist open the top of one unit dose vial and squeeze the contents into the nebulizer reservoir. Connect the nebulizer reservoir to the mouthpiece or face mask. Connect the nebulizer to the compressor. Sit in a comfortable, upright position; place the mouthpiece in your mouth or put on the face mask and turn on the compressor. If a face mask is used, care should be taken to avoid leakage around the mask as temporary blurring of vision, precipitation or worsening of narrow-angle glaucoma, or eye pain may occur if the solution comes into direct contact with the eyes. Breathe as calmly, deeply, and evenly as possible until no more mist is formed in the nebulizer chamber (about 5-15 minutes). At this point, the treatment is finished. Clean the nebulizer.

Dosage Forms
Nebulization: 0.02% solution (500 mcg/2.5 mL vial in a foil pouch)
Solution, inhalation: 18 mcg/actuation (14 g)

Iproveratril Hydrochloride see Verapamil Hydrochloride on page 1153
Ircon® [OTC] see Ferrous Fumarate on page 450

Iron Dextran Complex (i' run de' tran kom' pleks)
Brand Names InFed™
Use Treatment of microcytic hypochromic anemia resulting from iron deficiency in whom oral administration is infeasible or ineffective
Pregnancy Risk Factor C
Contraindications Hypersensitivity to iron dextran, all anemias that are not involved with iron deficiency, hemochromatosis, hemolytic anemia
Warnings/Precautions Use with caution in patients with history of asthma, hepatic impairment, rheumatoid arthritis; not recommended in children <4 months of age; deaths associated with parenteral administration following anaphylactic-type reactions have been reported; use only in patients where the iron deficient state is not amenable to oral iron therapy. A test dose of 0.5 mL I.V. or I.M. should be given to observe for adverse reactions. Anemia in the elderly is often caused by "anemia of chronic disease" or associated with inflammation rather than blood loss. Iron stores are usually normal or increased, with a serum ferritin >50 ng/mL and a decreased total iron binding capacity. I.V. administration of iron dextran is often preferred over I.M. in the elderly secondary to a decreased muscle mass and the need for daily injections.
Adverse Reactions
Cardiovascular: Cardiovascular collapse, hypotension
Dermatologic: Urticaria
Hematologic: Leukocytosis

>10%:
Central nervous system: Dizziness, fever, headache, sweating
Gastrointestinal: Nausea, vomiting, metallic taste
Local: Pain, staining of skin at the site of I.M. injection, phlebitis, flushing
1% to 10%: Discolored urine, diarrhea
<1%:
Cardiovascular: Flushing
Local: Phlebitis
Neuromuscular & skeletal: Arthralgia
Respiratory: Respiratory difficulty
Miscellaneous: Chills, lymphadenopathy

Note: Sweating, urticaria, arthralgia, fever, chills, dizziness, headache, and nausea may be delayed 24-48 hours after I.V. administration or 3-4 days after I.M. administration
(Continued)
591

Iron Dextran Complex *(Continued)*

Anaphylactoid reactions: Respiratory difficulties and cardiovascular collapse have been reported and occur most frequently within the first several minutes of administration

Overdosage/Toxicology Symptoms of overdose include erosion of GI mucosa, pulmonary edema, hyperthermia, convulsions, tachycardia, hepatic and renal impairment, coma, hematemesis, lethargy, tachycardia, acidosis, serum Fe level >300 mcg/mL requires treatment of overdose due to severe toxicity. Although rare, if a severe iron overdose (when the serum iron concentration exceeds the total iron-binding capacity) occurs, it may be treated with deferoxamine. Deferoxamine may be administered I.V. (80 mg/kg over 24 hours) or I.M. (40-90 mg/kg every 8 hours).

Drug Interactions Decreased effect with chloramphenicol

Stability Store at room temperature

Stability of parenteral admixture at room temperature (25°C): 3 months

Standard diluent: Dose/250-1000 mL NS

Minimum volume: 250 mL NS

Mechanism of Action The released iron, from the plasma, eventually replenishes the depleted iron stores in the bone marrow where it is incorporated into hemoglobin

Pharmacodynamics/Kinetics

Absorption:

I.M.: 50% to 90% is promptly absorbed, the balance is slowly absorbed over month

I.V.: Uptake of iron by the reticuloendothelial system appears to be constant at about 10-20 mg/hour

Elimination: By the reticuloendothelial system and excreted in the urine and feces (via bile)

Usual Dosage I.M. (Z-track method should be used for I.M. injection), I.V.:

A 0.5 mL test dose (0.25 mL in infants) should be given prior to starting iron dextran therapy; total dose should be divided into a daily schedule for I.M., total dose may be given as a single continuous infusion

Iron deficiency anemia: Dose (mL) = 0.0476 x wt (kg) x (normal hemoglobin - observed hemoglobin) + (1 mL/5 kg) to maximum of 14 mL for iron stores

Iron replacement therapy for blood loss: Replacement iron (mg) = blood loss (mL) x hematocrit

Maximum daily dose (can give total dose at one time I.V.):

Infants <5 kg: 25 mg iron (0.5 mL)

Children:

5-10 kg: 50 mg iron (1 mL)

10-50 kg: 100 mg iron (2 mL)

Adults >50 kg: 100 mg iron (2 mL)

Administration Use Z-track technique for I.M. administration (deep into the upper outer quadrant of buttock); may be administered I.V. bolus at rate ≤50 mg/minute or diluted in 250-1000 mL NS and infused over 1-6 hours; infuse initial 25 mL slowly, observe for allergic reactions; have epinephrine nearby

Monitoring Parameters Hemoglobin, hematocrit, reticulocyte count, serum ferritin

Reference Range

Hemoglobin 14.8 mg % (for weight >15 kg), hemoglobin 12.0 mg % (for weight <15 kg)

Serum iron: 40-160 µg/dL

Total iron binding capacity: 230-430 µg/dL

Transferrin: 204-360 mg/dL

Percent transferrin saturation: 20% to 50%

Test Interactions May cause falsely elevated values of serum bilirubin and falsely decreased values of serum calcium

Dosage Forms Injection: 50 mg/mL (2 mL, 10 mL)

Isobamate *see* Carisoprodol *on page 185*

Iso-Bid® *see* Isosorbide Dinitrate *on page 599*

Isocaine® HCl *see* Mepivacaine Hydrochloride *on page 688*

Isocarboxazid (eye soe kar box' a zid)

Brand Names Marplan®

Use Symptomatic treatment of atypical, nonendogenous or neurotic depression

Pregnancy Risk Factor C

Contraindications Uncontrolled hypertension, known hypersensitivity to isocarboxazid, pheochromocytoma, congestive heart failure, severe renal or hepatic impairment

Warnings/Precautions Avoid tyramine-containing foods: red wine, cheese (except cottage, ricotta, and cream), smoked or pickled fish, beef or chicken liver, dried sausage, fava or broad bean pods, yeast vitamin supplements; avoid use with patients <16 or >60 years of age

Adverse Reactions
>10%:
  Cardiovascular: Orthostatic hypotension
  Central nervous system: Drowsiness, weakness
  Endocrine & metabolic: Decreased sexual ability
  Neuromuscular & skeletal: Trembling
  Ocular: Blurred vision
1% to 10%:
  Cardiovascular: Tachycardia, peripheral edema
  Central nervous system: Nervousness, chills
  Gastrointestinal: Diarrhea, anorexia, dry mouth, constipation
<1%:
  Central nervous system: Parkinsonian syndrome
  Hematologic: Leukopenia
  Hepatic: Hepatitis

Overdosage/Toxicology Symptoms of overdose include tachycardia, palpitations, muscle twitching, seizures. Competent supportive care is the most important treatment for an overdose with a monoamine oxidase (MAO) inhibitor. Both hypertension or hypotension can occur with intoxication. Hypotension may respond to I.V. fluids or vasopressors, and hypertension usually responds to an alpha-adrenergic blocker. While treating the hypertension, care is warranted to avoid sudden drops in blood pressure, since this may worsen the MAO inhibitor toxicity. Muscle irritability and seizures often respond to diazepam, while hyperthermia is best treated with antipyretics and cooling blankets. Cardiac arrhythmias are best treated with phenytoin or procainamide.

Drug Interactions
Decreased effect of antihypertensives
Increased toxicity with disulfiram (possible seizures), fluoxetine (and other serotonin active agents), TCAs (cardiovascular instability), meperidine (cardiovascular instability), phenothiazines (hyperpyretic crisis), levodopa, sympathomimetics (hyperpyretic crisis), barbiturates, rauwolfia alkaloids (eg, reserpine), dextroamphetamine (psychoses), foods containing tyramine

Mechanism of Action Thought to act by increasing endogenous concentrations of epinephrine, norepinephrine, dopamine, and serotonin through inhibition of the enzyme (monoamine oxidase) responsible for the breakdown of these neurotransmitters

Usual Dosage Adults: Oral: 10 mg 3 times/day; reduce to 10-20 mg/day in divided doses when condition improves

Test Interactions ↓ glucose

Patient Information Avoid tyramine-containing foods and drinks

Nursing Implications Watch for postural hypotension; monitor blood pressure carefully, especially at therapy onset or if other CNS drugs or cardiovascular drugs are added; check for dietary and drug restriction

Dosage Forms Tablet: 10 mg

Isodine® [OTC] *see* Povidone-Iodine *on page 913*

Isoetharine (eye soe eth' a reen)

Brand Names Arm-a-Med® Isoetharine; Beta-2®; Bronkometer®; Bronkosol®; Dey-Lute® Isoetharine

Synonyms Isoetharine Hydrochloride; Isoetharine Mesylate

Use Bronchodilator in bronchial asthma and for reversible bronchospasm occurring with bronchitis and emphysema

Pregnancy Risk Factor C

Contraindications Known hypersensitivity to isoetharine
(Continued)

Isoetharine *(Continued)*

Warnings/Precautions Excessive or prolonged use may result in decreased effectiveness

Adverse Reactions

1% to 10%:

Cardiovascular: Tachycardia, hypertension, pounding heartbeat

Central nervous system: Dizziness, lightheadedness, headache, nervousness, insomnia, weakness

Gastrointestinal: Dry mouth, nausea, vomiting

Neuromuscular & skeletal: Trembling

<1%: Respiratory: Paradoxical bronchospasm

Overdosage/Toxicology Symptoms of overdose include nausea, vomiting, hypertension, tremors; beta-adrenergic stimulation can cause ↑ heart rate, ↓ blood pressure, and CNS excitation; heart rate can be treated with beta-blockers, ↓ blood pressure can be treated with pure alpha-adrenergic agents, diazepam 0.07 mg/kg can be used for excitation, seizures

Drug Interactions

Decreased effect with beta-blockers

Increased toxicity with other sympathomimetics (eg, epinephrine)

Stability Do not use if solution is discolored or a precipitation is present; **compatible** with sterile water, 0.45% sodium chloride, and 0.9% sodium chloride; protect from light

Mechanism of Action Relaxes bronchial smooth muscle by action on beta$_2$-receptors with very little effect on heart rate

Pharmacodynamics/Kinetics

Peak effect: Inhaler: Within 5-15 minutes

Duration: 1-4 hours

Metabolism: In many tissues including the liver and lungs

Elimination: Renal, primarily (90%) as metabolites

Usual Dosage Treatments are usually not repeated more often than every 4 hours, except in severe cases

Nebulizer: Children: 0.01 mL/kg; minimum dose 0.1 mL; maximum dose: 0.5 mL diluted in 2-3 mL normal saline

Inhalation: Oral: Adults: 1-2 inhalations every 4 hours as needed

Administration Administer around-the-clock to promote less variation in peak and trough serum levels

Monitoring Parameters Heart rate, blood pressure, respiratory rate

Test Interactions ↓ potassium (S)

Patient Information Do not exceed recommended dosage - excessive use may lead to adverse effects or loss of effectiveness. Shake canister well before use. Administer pressurized inhalation during the second half of inspiration, as the airways are open wider and the aerosol distribution is more extensive. If more than one inhalation per dose is necessary, wait at least 1 full minute between inhalations - second inhalation is best delivered after 10 minutes. May cause nervousness, restlessness, insomnia; if these effects continue after dosage reduction, notify physician. Also notify physician if palpitations, tachycardia, chest pain, muscle tremors, dizziness, headache, flushing, or if breathing difficulty persists.

Additional Information

Isoetharine hydrochloride: Arm-a-Med® isoetharine, Beta-2®, Bronkosol®, Dey-Lute® isoetharine

Isoetharine mesylate: Bronkometer®

Dosage Forms

Aerosol, oral, as mesylate: 340 mcg/metered spray

Solution, inhalation, as hydrochloride: 0.062% (4 mL); 0.08% (3.5 mL); 0.1% (2.5 mL, 5 mL); 0.125% (4 mL); 0.167% (3 mL); 0.17% (3 mL); 0.2% (2.5 mL); 0.25% (2 mL, 3.5 mL); 0.5% (0.5 mL); 1% (0.5 mL, 0.25 mL, 10 mL, 14 mL, 30 mL)

Isoetharine Hydrochloride *see* Isoetharine *on previous page*

Isoetharine Mesylate *see* Isoetharine *on previous page*

Isoflurophate *(eye soe flure' oh fate)*

Related Information

Glaucoma Drug Therapy Comparison *on page 1270*

Brand Names Floropryl®

Synonyms DFP; Diisopropyl Fluorophosphate; Dyflos; Fluostigmin

Use Treat primary open-angle glaucoma and conditions that obstruct aqueous outflow and to treat accommodative convergent strabismus

Pregnancy Risk Factor X

Contraindications Active uveal inflammation, angle-closure (narrow-angle) glaucoma, known hypersensitivity to isoflurophate, pregnancy

Warnings/Precautions May retard corneal healing; because of the tendency to produce more severe adverse effects, use the lowest dose possible; keep frequency of use to a minimum to avoid cyst formation; some products may contain sulfites

Adverse Reactions
1% to 10%: Ocular: Stinging, burning, myopia, visual blurring
<1%:
  Cardiovascular: Bradycardia, hypotension, flushing
  Gastrointestinal: Nausea, vomiting, diarrhea
  Neuromuscular & skeletal: Muscle weakness
  Ocular: Retinal detachment, browache, miosis, twitching eyelids, watering eyes
  Respiratory: Difficulty in breathing
  Miscellaneous: Diaphoresis

Overdosage/Toxicology Symptoms of overdose include excessive salivation, urinary incontinence, dyspnea, diarrhea, profuse sweating; if systemic effects occur, give parenteral atropine; for severe muscle weakness; pralidoxime may be used in addition to atropine

Drug Interactions Increased toxicity: Succinylcholine, systemic anticholinesterases, carbamate or organic phosphate insecticides, → ↓ cholinesterase levels

Stability Protect from moisture, freezing, excessive heat

Mechanism of Action Cholinesterase inhibitor that causes contraction of the iris and ciliary muscles producing miosis, reduced intraocular pressure, and increased aqueous humor outflow

Pharmacodynamics/Kinetics
Peak IOP reduction: 24 hours
  Duration: 1 week
Onset of miosis: Within 5-10 minutes
  Duration: Up to 4 weeks

Usual Dosage Adults: Ophthalmic:
Glaucoma: Instill 0.25" strip in eye every 8-72 hours
Strabismus: Instill 0.25" strip to each eye every night for 2 weeks then reduce to 0.25" every other night to once weekly for 2 months

Patient Information Notify physician if abdominal cramps, diarrhea, or salivation occur

Nursing Implications Keep tube tightly closed to prevent absorption of moisture and loss of potency

Dosage Forms Ointment, ophthalmic: 0.025% in polyethylene mineral oil gel (3.5 g)

Isollyl Improved® *see* Butalbital Compound *on page 153*

Isonate® *see* Isosorbide Dinitrate *on page 599*

Isoniazid (eye soe nye' a zid)
Related Information
Recommendations of the Advisory Council on the Elimination of Tuberculosis *on page 1303-1304*

Brand Names INH™; Laniazid®; Nydrazid®

Synonyms Isonicotinic Acid Hydrazide

Use Treatment of susceptible tuberculosis infections and prophylactically to those individuals exposed to tuberculosis

Pregnancy Risk Factor C

Contraindications Acute liver disease; hypersensitivity to isoniazid or any component; previous history of hepatic damage during isoniazid therapy

Warnings/Precautions Use with caution in patients with renal impairment and chronic liver disease. Severe and sometimes fatal hepatitis may occur or develop even after many months of treatment; patients must report any prodromal symptoms of hepatitis, such as fatigue, weakness, malaise, anorexia, nausea, or vomiting. Children with low milk and low meat intake should receive concomitant pyridoxine therapy. Periodic ophthalmic examinations are recommended even when usual symptoms do not occur; pyridoxine is recommended in individuals likely to develop peripheral neuropathies; dose is 10-50 mg/day.

Adverse Reactions
>10%:
  Central nervous system: Peripheral neuritis
  Gastrointestinal: Loss of appetite, nausea, vomiting, stomach pain
  Hepatic: Hepatitis
  Neuromuscular & skeletal: Weakness
1% to 10%:
  Central nervous system: Dizziness, slurred speech, lethargy
(Continued)

Isoniazid *(Continued)*

    Neuromuscular & skeletal: Hyperreflexia
<1%:
    Central nervous system: Fever, seizures, mental depression, psychosis
    Dermatologic: Skin rash
    Hematologic: Blood dyscrasias
    Neuromuscular & skeletal: Arthralgia
    Ocular: Blurred vision, loss of vision

Overdosage/Toxicology Symptoms of overdose include nausea, vomiting, slurred speech, dizziness, blurred vision, hallucinations, stupor, coma, intractable seizures, onset of metabolic acidosis is 30 minutes to 3 hours. Because of the severe morbidity and high mortality rates with isoniazid overdose, patients who are asymptomatic after an overdose, should be monitored for 4-6 hours. Pyridoxine has been shown to be effective in the treatment of intoxication, especially when seizures occur. Pyridoxine I.V. is administered on a milligram to milligram dose. If the amount of isoniazid ingested is unknown, 5 g of pyridoxine should be given over 3-5 minutes and may be followed by an additional 5 g in 30 minutes. Treatment is supportive; may require airway protection, ventilation; diazepam for seizures, sodium bicarbonate for acidosis; forced diuresis and hemodialysis can result in more rapid removal.

Drug Interactions
Decreased effect/levels of isoniazid with aluminum salts
Increased toxicity/levels of oral anticoagulants, carbamazepines, cycloserine, hydantoins, hepatically metabolized benzodiazepines; reaction with disulfiram

Stability Protect oral dosage forms from light

Mechanism of Action Unknown, but may include the inhibition of myocolic acid synthesis resulting in disruption of the bacterial cell wall

Pharmacodynamics/Kinetics
    Absorption: Oral, I.M.: Rapid and complete; rate can be slowed when orally administered with food
    Distribution: Crosses the placenta; appears in breast milk; distributes into all body tissues and fluids including the CSF
    Protein binding: 10% to 15%
    Metabolism: By the liver with decay rate determined genetically by acetylation phenotype
    Half-life:
        Fast acetylators: 30-100 minutes
        Slow acetylators: 2-5 hours; half-life may be prolonged in patients with impaired hepatic function or severe renal impairment
    Time to peak serum concentration: Within 1-2 hours
    Elimination: In urine (75% to 95%), feces, and saliva

Usual Dosage Oral, I.M. (recommendations often change due to resistant strains and newly developed information; consult *MMWR* for current CDC recommendations):

    Children: 10-20 mg/kg/day in 1-2 divided doses (maximum: 300 mg total dose)
        Prophylaxis: 10 mg/kg/day given daily (up to 300 mg total dose) for 6 months

    Adults: 5 mg/kg/day given daily (usual dose is 300 mg)
        Disseminated disease: 10 mg/kg/day in 1-2 divided doses
        Treatment should be continued for 9 months with rifampin or for 6 months with rifampin and pyrazinamide
        Prophylaxis: 300 mg/day given daily for 6 months

    American Thoracic Society and CDC currently recommend twice weekly therapy as part of a short-course regimen which follows 1-2 months of daily treatment for uncomplicated pulmonary tuberculosis in compliant patients
        Children: 20-40 mg/kg/dose (up to 900 mg) twice weekly
        Adults: 15 mg/kg/dose (up to 900 mg) twice weekly

    Dosing adjustment in hepatic impairment: Dose should be reduced in severe hepatic disease
    Dialyzable (50% to 100%)

Monitoring Parameters Monitor transaminase levels at baseline 1, 3, 6, and 9 months

Reference Range Therapeutic: 1-7 µg/mL (SI: 7-51 µmol/L); Toxic: 20-710 µg/mL (SI: 146-5176 µmol/L)

Test Interactions False-positive urinary glucose with Clinitest®

Patient Information Report any prodromal symptoms of hepatitis (fatigue, weakness, nausea, vomiting, dark urine, or yellowing of eyes) or any burning, tingling, or numbness in the extremities

Dosage Forms
    Injection: 100 mg/mL (10 mL)

Syrup (orange flavor): 50 mg/5 mL (473 mL)
Tablet: 50 mg, 100 mg, 300 mg

Isonicotinic Acid Hydrazide *see* Isoniazid *on page 595*

Isonipecaine Hydrochloride *see* Meperidine Hydrochloride *on page 684*

Isoprenaline Hydrochloride *see* Isoproterenol *on this page*

Isopro® *see* Isoproterenol *on this page*

Isoproterenol (eye soe proe ter' e nole)

Related Information
Adrenergic Agonists, Cardiovascular Comparison *on page 1242*

Brand Names Arm-a-Med® Isoproterenol; Dey-Dose® Isoproterenol; Dispos-a-Med® Isoproterenol; Isopro®; Isuprel®; Medihaler-Iso®; Norisodrine®; Vapo-Iso®

Synonyms Isoprenaline Hydrochloride; Isoproterenol Hydrochloride; Isoproterenol Sulfate

Use Treatment of reversible airway obstruction as in asthma or COPD; used parenterally in ventricular arrhythmias due to A-V nodal block; hemodynamically compromised bradyarrhythmias or atropine-resistant bradyarrhythmias; temporary use in third degree A-V block until pacemaker insertion; low cardiac output; vasoconstrictive shock states

Pregnancy Risk Factor C

Contraindications Angina, pre-existing cardiac arrhythmias (ventricular); tachycardia or A-V block caused by cardiac glycoside intoxication; allergy to sulfites or isoproterenol or other sympathomimetic amines

Warnings/Precautions Elderly patients, diabetics, renal or cardiovascular disease, hyperthyroidism; excessive or prolonged use may result in decreased effectiveness

Adverse Reactions
>10%:
Central nervous system: Insomnia, restlessness
Miscellaneous: Discoloration of saliva (pinkish-red), dry mouth or throat
1% to 10%:
Cardiovascular: Sweating, flushing of the face or skin, ventricular arrhythmias, tachycardias, profound hypotension, hypertension
Central nervous system: Nervousness, anxiety, dizziness, headache, weakness, lightheadedness
Gastrointestinal: Vomiting, nausea
Neuromuscular & skeletal: Trembling, tremor
<1%:
Cardiovascular: Arrhythmias, chest pain
Respiratory: Paradoxical bronchospasm

Overdosage/Toxicology Symptoms of overdose include tremors, nausea, vomiting, hypotension; beta-adrenergic stimulation can cause ↑ heart rate, ↓ blood pressure, and CNS excitation, heart rate can be treated with beta-blockers, ↓ blood pressure can be treated with pure alpha-adrenergic agents, diazepam 0.07 mg/kg can be used for excitation, seizures

Drug Interactions Increased toxicity: Sympathomimetic agents → headaches and ↑ blood pressure; general anesthetics → arrhythmias

Stability
Isoproterenol solution should be stored at room temperature; it should not be used if a color or precipitate is present
Exposure to air, light, or increased temperature may cause a pink to brownish pink color to develop
Stability of parenteral admixture at room temperature (25°C) or at refrigeration (4°C): 24 hours
Standard diluent: 2 mg/500 mL D_5W; 4 mg/500 mL D_5W
Minimum volume: 1 mg/100 mL D_5W
Incompatible with alkaline solutions, aminophylline and furosemide

Mechanism of Action Stimulates $beta_1$- and $beta_2$-receptors resulting in relaxation of bronchial, GI, and uterine smooth muscle, increased heart rate and contractility, vasodilation of peripheral vasculature

Pharmacodynamics/Kinetics
Onset of bronchodilation: Oral inhalation: Immediately
Time to peak serum concentration: Oral: Within 1-2 hours
Duration:
Oral inhalation: 1 hour
S.C.: Up to 2 hours
Metabolism: By conjugation in many tissues including the liver and lungs
Half-life: 2.5-5 minutes
(Continued)

Isoproterenol *(Continued)*

Elimination: In urine principally as sulfate conjugates

Usual Dosage

Children:

Bronchodilation: Inhalation: Metered dose inhaler: 1-2 metered doses up to 5 times/day

Bronchodilation (using 1:200 inhalation solution) 0.01 mL/kg/dose every 4 hours as needed (maximum: 0.05 mL/dose) diluted with NS to 2 mL

Sublingual: 5-10 mg every 3-4 hours, not to exceed 30 mg/day

Cardiac arrhythmias: I.V.: Start 0.1 mcg/kg/minute (usual effective dose 0.2-2 mcg/kg/minute)

Adults:

Bronchodilation: Inhalation: Metered dose inhaler: 1-2 metered doses 4-6 times/day

Bronchodilation: 1-2 inhalations of a 0.25% solution, no more than 2 inhalations at any one time (1-5 minutes between inhalations); no more than 6 inhalations in any hour during a 24-hour period; maintenance therapy: 1-2 inhalations 4-6 times/day. Alternatively: 0.5% solution via hand bulb nebulizer is 5-15 deep inhalations repeated once in 5-10 minutes if necessary; treatments may be repeated up to 5 times/day.

Sublingual: 10-20 mg every 3-4 hours; not to exceed 60 mg/day

Cardiac arrhythmias: I.V.: 5 mcg/minute initially, titrate to patient response (2-20 mcg/minute)

Shock: I.V.: 0.5-5 mcg/minute; adjust according to response

Administration Administer around-the-clock to promote less variation in peak and trough serum levels; I.V. infusion administration requires the use of an infusion pump

To prepare for infusion:

$$\frac{6 \times weight\ (kg) \times desired\ dose\ (mcg/kg/min)}{I.V.\ infusion\ rate\ (mL/h)} = \begin{array}{l} mg\ of\ drug\ to\ be\ added\ to \\ 100\ mL\ of\ I.V.\ fluid \end{array}$$

Monitoring Parameters EKG, heart rate, respiratory rate, arterial blood gas, arterial blood pressure, CVP

Patient Information Do not exceed recommended dosage; excessive use may lead to adverse effects or loss of effectiveness. Shake canister well before use. Administer pressurized inhalation during the second half of inspiration, as the airways are open wider and the aerosol distribution is more extensive. If more than one inhalation per dose is necessary, wait at least 1 full minute between inhalations - second inhalation is best delivered after 10 minutes. May cause nervousness, restlessness, insomnia; if these effects continue after dosage reduction, notify physician. Notify physician if palpitations, tachycardia, chest pain, muscle tremors, dizziness, headache, flushing or if breathing difficulty persists. Do not chew or swallow sublingual tablet.

Nursing Implications Elderly may find it useful to utilize a spacer device when using a metered dose inhaler

Additional Information

Isoproterenol hydrochloride: Aerolone®, Dey-Dose® isoproterenol, Dispos-a-Med® isoproterenol, Isopro®, Isuprel®, Norisodrine®, Vapo-Iso®

Isoproterenol sulfate: Medihaler-Iso®

Dosage Forms

Inhalation:

Aerosol: 0.2% (1:500) (15 mL, 22.5 mL); 0.25% (1:400) (15 mL)

Solution for nebulization: 0.031% (4 mL); 0.062% (4 mL); 0.25% (0.5 mL, 30 mL); 0.5% (0.5 mL, 10 mL, 60 mL); 1% (10 mL)

Injection: 0.2 mg/mL (1:5000) (1 mL, 5 mL, 10 mL)

Tablet, sublingual: 10 mg, 15 mg

Isoproterenol Hydrochloride *see* Isoproterenol *on previous page*

Isoproterenol Sulfate *see* Isoproterenol *on previous page*

Isoptin® *see* Verapamil Hydrochloride *on page 1153*

Isopto® Atropine *see* Atropine Sulfate *on page 100*

Isopto® Carbachol *see* Carbachol *on page 176*

Isopto® Carpine *see* Pilocarpine *on page 883*

Isopto® Eserine *see* Physostigmine *on page 881*

Isopto® Frin Ophthalmic Solution *see* Phenylephrine Hydrochloride *on page 874*

Isopto® Homatropine *see* Homatropine Hydrobromide *on page 537*

Isopto® Hyoscine *see* Scopolamine *on page 997*

Isordil® see Isosorbide Dinitrate on this page

Isosorbide (eye soe sor' bide)

Brand Names Ismotic®

Use Short-term emergency treatment of acute angle-closure glaucoma and short-term reduction of intraocular pressure prior to and following intraocular surgery; may be used to interrupt an acute glaucoma attack; preferred agent when need to avoid nausea and vomiting

Pregnancy Risk Factor B

Contraindications Severe renal disease, anuria, severe dehydration, acute pulmonary edema, severe cardiac decompensation, known hypersensitivity to isosorbide

Warnings/Precautions Use with caution in patients with impending pulmonary edema and in the elderly due to the elderly's predisposition to dehydration and the fact that they frequently have concomitant diseases which may be aggravated by the use of isosorbide; hypernatremia and dehydration may begin to occur after 72 hours of continuous administration. Maintain fluid/electrolyte balance with multiple doses; monitor urinary output; if urinary output declines, need to review clinical status.

Adverse Reactions

1% to 10%:
  Central nervous system: Headache, confusion, disorientation
  Gastrointestinal: Vomiting

<1%:
  Cardiovascular: Syncope
  Central nervous system: Lethargy, vertigo, dizziness, lightheadedness, irritability
  Dermatologic: Rash
  Endocrine & metabolic: Hypernatremia, hyperosmolarity, thirst
  Gastrointestinal: Nausea, abdominal/gastric discomfort (infrequently), anorexia
  Miscellaneous: Hiccups

Overdosage/Toxicology Symptoms of overdose include dehydration, hypotension, hyponatremia; general supportive care, fluid administration, electrolyte balance, discontinue agent

Mechanism of Action Elevates osmolarity of glomerular filtrate to hinder the tubular resorption of water and increase excretion of sodium and chloride to result in diuresis; creates an osmotic gradient between plasma and ocular fluids

Pharmacodynamics/Kinetics
  Onset of action: Within 10-30 minutes
  Peak action: 1-1.5 hours
  Duration: 5-6 hours
  Distribution: In total body water
  Metabolism: Not metabolized
  Half-life: 5-9.5 hours
  Elimination: By glomerular filtration; see Mechanism of Action

Usual Dosage Adults: Oral: Initial: 1.5 g/kg with a usual range of 1-3 g/kg 2-4 times/day as needed

Monitoring Parameters Monitor for signs of dehydration, blood pressure, renal output, intraocular pressure reduction

Nursing Implications Palatability may be improved if poured over ice and sipped

Additional Information Each 220 mL contains isosorbide 100 g, sodium 4.6 mEq, and potassium 0.9 mEq

Dosage Forms Solution: 45% [450 mg/mL] (100 g per 220 mL)

Isosorbide Dinitrate (eye soe sor' bide)

Related Information
  Nitrates Comparison on page 1279

Brand Names Dilatrate®-SR; Iso-Bid®; Isonate®; Isordil®; Isotrate®; Sorbitrate®

Synonyms ISD; ISDN

Use Prevention and treatment of angina pectoris; for congestive heart failure; to relieve pain, dysphagia, and spasm in esophageal spasm with GE reflux

Pregnancy Risk Factor C

Contraindications Severe anemia, closed-angle glaucoma, postural hypotension, cerebral hemorrhage, head trauma, hypersensitivity to isosorbide dinitrate or any component

Warnings/Precautions Use with caution in patients with increased intracranial pressure, hypotension, hypovolemia, glaucoma; sustained release products may be absorbed erratically in patients with GI hypermotility or malabsorption
(Continued)

Isosorbide Dinitrate *(Continued)*

syndrome; do not crush or chew sublingual dosage form; abrupt withdrawal may result in angina; tolerance may develop (adjust dose or change agent)

Adverse Reactions

>10%:

Cardiovascular: Flushing, postural hypotension

Central nervous system: Headache, lightheadedness, dizziness

Neuromuscular & skeletal: Weakness

1% to 10%: Dermatologic: Drug rash, exfoliative dermatitis

<1%:

Gastrointestinal: Nausea, vomiting

Hematologic: Methemoglobinemia (overdose)

Overdosage/Toxicology Symptoms of overdose include hypotension, throbbing headache, palpitations, visual disturbances, tachycardia, methemoglobinemia, flushing, diaphoresis, metabolic acidosis, coma. High levels or methemoglobinemia can cause signs and symptoms of hypoxemia; treatment consists of placing patient in recumbent position and administering fluids; alpha-adrenergic vasopressors may be required; treat methemoglobinemia with oxygen and methylene blue at a dose of 1-2 mg/kg I.V. slowly

Mechanism of Action Stimulation of intracellular cyclic-GMP results in vascular smooth muscle relaxation of both arterial and venous vasculature. Increased venous pooling decreases left ventricular pressure (preload) and arterial dilatation decreases arterial resistance (afterload). Therefore, this reduces cardiac oxygen demand by decreasing left ventricular pressure and systemic vascular resistance by dilating arteries. Additionally, coronary artery dilation improves collateral flow to ischemic regions; esophageal smooth muscle is relaxed via the same mechanism.

Pharmacodynamics/Kinetics See table.

Dosage Form	Onset of Action	Duration
Sublingual tablet	2-10 min	1-2 h
Chewable tablet	3 min	0.5-2 h
Oral tablet	45-60 min	4-6 h
Sustained release tablet	30 min	6-12 h

Metabolism: Extensive in the liver to conjugated metabolites, including isosorbide 5-mononitrate (active) and 2-mononitrate (active)

Half-life:

Parent drug: 1-4 hours

Metabolite (5-mononitrate): 4 hours

Elimination: In urine and feces

Usual Dosage Adults (elderly should be given lowest recommended daily doses initially and titrate upward):

Oral: Angina: 5-40 mg 4 times/day or 40 mg every 8-12 hours in sustained released dosage form

Oral: Congestive heart failure:

Initial dose: 10 mg 3 times/day

Target dose: 40 mg 3 times/day

Maximum dose: 80 mg 3 times/day

Sublingual: 2.5-10 mg every 4-6 hours

Chew: 5-10 mg every 2-3 hours

Tolerance to nitrate effects develops with chronic exposure

Dose escalation does not overcome this effect. Tolerance can only be overcome by short periods of nitrate absence from the body. Short periods (10-12 hours) or nitrate withdrawal help minimize tolerance.

During hemodialysis, administer dose postdialysis or administer supplemental 10-20 mg dose; during peritoneal dialysis, supplemental dose is not necessary

Administration Do not administer around-the-clock; the first dose of nitrates should be administered in a physician's office to observe for maximal cardiovascular dynamic effects and adverse effects (orthostatic blood pressure drop, headache)

Monitoring Parameters Monitor for orthostasis

Test Interactions ↓ cholesterol (S)

Patient Information Do not chew or crush sublingual or sustained release dosage form; do not change brands without consulting your pharmacist or physician; keep tablets or capsules in original container and keep container tightly closed; if no relief from sublingual tablets after 15 minutes, report to nearest emergency room or seek emergency help

Nursing Implications 8- to 12-hour nitrate-free interval is needed each day to prevent tolerance

Dosage Forms

Capsule, sustained release: 40 mg

Tablet:

Chewable: 5 mg, 10 mg

Oral: 5 mg, 10 mg, 20 mg, 30 mg, 40 mg

Sublingual: 2.5 mg, 5 mg, 10 mg

Sustained release: 40 mg

Isosorbide Mononitrate (eye' soe sor bide mon oh ni' trate)

Related Information

Nitrates Comparison *on page 1279*

Brand Names Imdur™; Ismo™; Monoket®

Synonyms ISMN

Use Long-acting metabolite of the vasodilator isosorbide dinitrate used for the prophylactic treatment of angina pectoris

Contraindications Contraindicated due to potential increases in intracranial pressure in patients with head trauma or cerebral hemorrhage; hypersensitivity or idiosyncrasy to nitrates

Warnings/Precautions Postural hypotension, transient episodes of weakness, dizziness, or syncope may occur even with small doses; alcohol accentuates these effects; tolerance and cross-tolerance to nitrate antianginal and hemodynamic effects may occur during prolonged isosorbide mononitrate therapy; (minimized by using the smallest effective dose, by alternating coronary vasodilators or offering drug-free intervals of as little as 12 hours). Excessive doses may result in severe headache, blurred vision, or dry mouth; increased anginal symptoms may be a result of dosage increases.

Adverse Reactions

>10%: Central nervous system: Headache

1% to 10%: Gastrointestinal: Dizziness, nausea, vomiting

<1%:

Cardiovascular: Angina pectoris, arrhythmias, atrial fibrillation, hypotension, palpitations, postural hypotension, premature ventricular contractions, supraventricular tachycardia, syncope, edema

Central nervous system: Asthenia, malaise, agitation, anxiety, confusion, hypoesthesia, insomnia, nervousness, nightmares

Dermatologic: Pruritus, rash

Gastrointestinal: Abdominal pain, diarrhea, dyspepsia, tenesmus, increased appetite

Genitourinary: Impotence, urinary frequency

Hematologic: Methemoglobinemia (rarely)

Neuromuscular & skeletal: Neck stiffness, rigors, arthralgia, dyscoordination

Ocular: Blurred vision, diplopia

Renal: Dysuria

Respiratory: Bronchitis, pneumonia, upper respiratory tract infection

Miscellaneous: Tooth disorder, cold sweat

Overdosage/Toxicology Symptoms of overdose include hypotension, throbbing headache, palpitations, visual disturbances, tachycardia, methemoglobinemia, flushing, diaphoresis, metabolic acidosis, coma. High levels or methemoglobinemia can cause signs and symptoms of hypoxemia; treatment consists of placing patient in recumbent position and administering fluids; alpha-adrenergic vasopressors may be required; treat methemoglobinemia with oxygen and methylene blue at a dose of 1-2 mg/kg I.V. slowly.

Stability Tablets should be stored in a tight container at room temperature of 15°C to 30°C (59°F to 86°F)

Mechanism of Action Prevailing mechanism of action for nitroglycerin (and other nitrates) is systemic venodilation, decreasing preload as measured by pulmonary capillary wedge pressure and left ventricular end diastolic volume and pressure; the average reduction in LVEDV is 25% at rest, with a corresponding increase in ejection fractions of 50% to 60%. This effect improves congestive symptoms in heart failure and improves the myocardial perfusion gradient in patients with coronary artery disease.

Pharmacodynamics/Kinetics

Absorption: Oral: Nearly complete and low intersubject variability in its pharmacokinetic parameters and plasma concentrations

Metabolism: Metabolite of isosorbide dinitrate

Half-life: Mononitrate: ~4 hours (8 times that of dinitrate)

Usual Dosage Adults: Oral:

Regular tablet: 20 mg twice daily separated by 7 hours; maintenance doses as high as 120 mg have been used

(Continued)

Isosorbide Mononitrate *(Continued)*

Extended release tablet (Imdur™): Initial: 30-60 mg once daily; after several days the dosage may be increased to 120 mg/day (given as two 60 mg tablets); daily dose should be taken in the morning upon arising; maximum: 240 mg/day
Asymmetrical dosing regimen of 7 AM and 3 PM or 9 AM and 5 PM to allow for a nitrate-free dosing interval to minimize nitrate tolerance

Dosing adjustment in renal impairment: Not necessary for elderly or patients with altered renal or hepatic function

Administration Do not administer around-the-clock

Monitoring Parameters Monitor for orthostasis

Patient Information Dispense drug in easy-to-open container; do not change brands without consulting pharmacist or physician; keep tablets or capsules tightly closed in original container; extended release tablets should not be chewed or crushed and should be swallowed together with a half-glassful of fluid; the antianginal efficacy of tablets can be maintained by carefully following the prescribed schedule of dosing (2 doses taken 7 hours apart); headaches are sometimes a marker of the activity of the drug

Nursing Implications Do not crush; 8- to 12-hour nitrate-free interval is needed each day to prevent tolerance

Dosage Forms
Tablet (Ismo™, Monoket®): 10 mg, 20 mg
Tablet, extended release (Imdur™): 60 mg

Isotrate® *see* Isosorbide Dinitrate *on page 599*

Isotretinoin (eye soe tret' i noyn)

Brand Names Accutane®

Synonyms 13-*cis*-Retinoic Acid

Use Treatment of severe recalcitrant cystic and/or conglobate acne unresponsive to conventional therapy

Investigational use: Treatment of children with metastatic neuroblastoma or leukemia that does not respond to conventional therapy

Pregnancy Risk Factor X

Contraindications Sensitivity to parabens, vitamin A, or other retinoids; patients who are pregnant or intend to become pregnant during treatment

Warnings/Precautions Use with caution in patients with diabetes mellitus, hypertriglyceridemia; **not to be used in women of childbearing potential** unless woman is capable of complying with effective contraceptive measures; therapy is normally begun on the second or third day of next normal menstrual period; effective contraception must be used for at least 1 month before beginning therapy, during therapy, and for 1 month after discontinuation of therapy. Because of the high likelihood of teratogenic effects (~20%), do not prescribe isotretinoin for women who are or who are likely to become pregnant while using the drug.

Adverse Reactions
>10%:
Cardiovascular: Epistaxis
Dermatologic: Burning, redness, itching of eye, cheilitis, dry mouth/nose, inflammation of lips, dry skin, pruritus, photosensitivity
Endocrine/metabolic: Increased serum concentration of triglycerides
Neuromuscular & skeletal: Bone or joint pain, muscle aches, myalgia
1% to 10%:
Central nervous system: Fatigue, headache, mental depression, tiredness
Dermatologic: Skin peeling on hands or soles of feet, skin rash
Gastrointestinal: Stomach upset
Ocular: Dry eyes, photophobia
<1%:
Central nervous system: Mood changes, pseudomotor cerebri
Dermatologic: Hair loss, pruritus
Endocrine & metabolic: Hyperuricemia
Gastrointestinal: Xerostomia, anorexia, nausea, vomiting, inflammatory bowel syndrome, bleeding of gums
Hematologic: Increase in erythrocyte sedimentation rate, decrease in hemoglobin and hematocrit
Hepatic: Hepatitis
Ocular: Conjunctivitis, corneal opacities, optic neuritis, cataracts

Overdosage/Toxicology Symptoms of overdose include headache, vomiting, flushing, abdominal pain, ataxia; all signs and symptoms have been transient

Drug Interactions
Increased effect: Increased clearance of carbamazepine

Increased toxicity: Avoid other vitamin A products; may interfere with medications used to treat hypertriglyceridemia

Stability Store at room temperature and protect from light

Mechanism of Action Reduces sebaceous gland size and reduces sebum production; regulates cell proliferation and differentiation

Pharmacodynamics/Kinetics

Absorption: Oral: Demonstrates biphasic absorption

Distribution: Crosses the placenta; appears in breast milk

Protein binding: 99% to 100%

Metabolism: In the liver; major metabolite: 4-oxo-isotretinoin (active)

Half-life, terminal:

Parent drug: 10-20 hours

Metabolite: 11-50 hours

Time to peak serum concentration: Within 3 hours

Elimination: Equally in urine and feces

Usual Dosage Oral:

Children: Maintenance therapy for neuroblastoma: 100-250 mg/m²/day in 2 divided doses has been used investigationally

Children and Adults: 0.5-2 mg/kg/day in 2 divided doses (dosages as low as 0.05 mg/kg/day have been reported to be beneficial) for 15-20 weeks or until the total cyst count decreases by 70%, whichever is sooner

Dosing adjustment in hepatic impairment: Dose reductions empirically are recommended in hepatitis disease

Monitoring Parameters CBC with differential and platelet count, baseline sed rate, serum triglycerides, liver enzymes

Patient Information Avoid pregnancy during therapy; effective contraceptive measures must be used since this drug may harm the fetus; there is information from manufacturers about this product that you should receive; discontinue therapy if visual difficulties, abdominal pain, rectal bleeding, diarrhea; exacerbation of acne may occur during first weeks of therapy; avoid use of other vitamin A products; decreased tolerance to contact lenses may occur; do not donate blood for at least 1 month following stopping of the drug; loss of night vision may occur, avoid prolonged exposure to sunlight; do not double next dose if dose is skipped

Nursing Implications Capsules can be swallowed, or chewed and swallowed. The capsule may be opened with a large needle and the contents placed on apple sauce or ice cream for patients unable to swallow the capsule.

Dosage Forms Capsule: 10 mg, 20 mg, 40 mg

Isoxazolyl Penicillin *see* Oxacillin Sodium *on page 821*

Isoxsuprine Hydrochloride (eye sox′ syoo preen)

Brand Names Vasodilan®

Use Treatment of peripheral vascular diseases, such as arteriosclerosis obliterans and Raynaud's disease

Pregnancy Risk Factor C

Contraindications Presence of arterial bleeding; do not administer immediately postpartum

Adverse Reactions

1% to 10%: Gastrointestinal: Nausea, vomiting

<1%:

Cardiovascular: Chest pain, hypotension

Dermatologic: Rash

Respiratory: Pulmonary edema

Overdosage/Toxicology Symptoms of overdose include hypotension, flushing; vasodilation mediated second to alpha-adrenergic stimulation or direct smooth muscle effects; treat with I.V. fluids, alpha-adrenergic pressors may be required

Mechanism of Action In studies on normal human subjects, isoxsuprine increases muscle blood flow, but skin blood flow is usually unaffected. Rather than increasing muscle blood flow by beta-receptor stimulation, isoxsuprine probably has a direct action on vascular smooth muscle. The generally accepted mechanism of action of isoxsuprine on the uterus is beta-adrenergic stimulation. Isoxsuprine was shown to inhibit prostaglandin synthetase at high serum concentrations, with low concentrations there was an increase in the P-G synthesis.

Pharmacodynamics/Kinetics

Absorption: Nearly complete

Metabolism: Partially conjugated in the liver

Half-life, serum: 1.25 hours mean

Time to peak serum concentration: Oral, I.M.: Within 1 hour

Elimination: Primarily in urine

(Continued)

Isoxsuprine Hydrochloride *(Continued)*

Usual Dosage Adults: 10-20 mg 3-4 times/day; start with lower dose in elderly due to potential hypotension

Patient Information May cause skin rash; discontinue use if rash occurs; arise slowly from prolonged sitting or lying position

Dosage Forms Tablet: 10 mg, 20 mg

Isradipine *(is ra' di peen)*

Related Information

Calcium Channel Blockers Cardiovascular Adverse Reactions *on page 1262*

Calcium Channel Blockers Central Nervous System Adverse Reactions *on page 1264*

Calcium Channel Blockers Comparative Actions *on page 1260*

Calcium Channel Blockers Comparative Pharmacokinetics *on page 1261*

Calcium Channel Blockers FDA-Approved Indications *on page 1263*

Calcium Channel Blockers Gastrointestinal and Miscellaneous Adverse Reactions *on page 1265*

Brand Names DynaCirc®

Use Treatment of hypertension, congestive heart failure, migraine prophylaxis

Pregnancy Risk Factor C

Contraindications Sinus bradycardia; advanced heart block; ventricular tachycardia; cardiogenic shock, hypotension, congestive heart failure; hypersensitivity to isradipine or any component, hypersensitivity to calcium channel blockers and adenosine; atrial fibrillation or flutter associated with accessory conduction pathways; not to be given within a few hours of I.V. beta-blocking agents

Warnings/Precautions Avoid use in hypotension, congestive heart failure, cardiac conduction defects, PVCs, idiopathic hypertrophic subaortic stenosis; may cause platelet inhibition; do not abruptly withdraw (chest pain); may cause hepatic dysfunction or increased angina; increased intracranial pressure with cranial tumors; elderly may have greater hypotensive effect

Adverse Reactions

>10%: Headache

1% to 10%:

Cardiovascular: Edema, palpitations, flushing, chest pain, tachycardia, hypotension

Central nervous system: Dizziness, fatigue, weakness

Dermatologic: Rash

Gastrointestinal: Nausea, abdominal discomfort, vomiting, diarrhea

Respiratory: Dyspnea

<1%:

Cardiovascular: Heart failure, atrial and ventricular fibrillation, TIAs, A-V block, myocardial infarction, abnormal EKG

Central nervous system: Disturbed sleep

Dermatologic: Pruritus, urticaria, rash

Genitourinary: Nocturia

Hematologic: Leukopenia

Neuromuscular & skeletal: Foot cramps, paresthesia

Ocular: Visual disturbance

Respiratory: Cough

Miscellaneous: Dry mouth, numbness

Overdosage/Toxicology The primary cardiac symptoms of calcium blocker overdose includes hypotension and bradycardia. The hypotension is caused by peripheral vasodilation, myocardial depression, and bradycardia. Bradycardia results from sinus bradycardia, second- or third-degree atrioventricular block, or sinus arrest with junctional rhythm. Intraventricular conduction is usually not affected so QRS duration is normal (verapamil does prolong the P-R interval and bepridil prolongs the Q-T and may cause ventricular arrhythmias, including torsade de pointes).

The noncardiac symptoms include confusion, stupor, nausea, vomiting, metabolic acidosis and hyperglycemia. Following initial gastric decontamination, if possible, repeated calcium administration may promptly reverse the depressed cardiac contractility (but not sinus node depression or peripheral vasodilation); glucagon, epinephrine, and amrinone may treat refractory hypotension; glucagon and epinephrine also increase the heart rate (outside the U.S., 4-aminopyridine may be available as an antidote); dialysis and hemoperfusion are not effective in enhancing elimination although repeat-dose activated charcoal may serve as an adjunct with sustained-release preparations.

Drug Interactions

Increased toxicity/effect/levels:

H_2 blockers → ↑ bioavailability isradipine

Cardiac depressant effects on A-V conduction

Carbamazepine → ↑ carbamazepine levels
Cyclosporine → ↑ cyclosporine levels
Fentanyl → ↑ hypotension
Digitalis → ↑ digitalis levels
Quinidine → increased quinidine levels (hypotension, bradycardia, and arrhythmias)
Theophylline → ↑ pharmacologic actions of theophylline

Mechanism of Action Inhibits calcium ion from entering the "slow channels" or select voltage-sensitive areas of vascular smooth muscle and myocardium during depolarization, producing a relaxation of coronary vascular smooth muscle and coronary vasodilation; increases myocardial oxygen delivery in patients with vasospastic angina

Pharmacodynamics/Kinetics
Absorption: Oral: 90% to 95%
Protein binding: 95%
Metabolism: In the liver
Bioavailability: Absolute due to first-pass elimination 15% to 24%
Half-life: 8 hours
Time to peak: Serum concentration: 1-1.5 hours
Elimination: Renal excretion by metabolites (cyclic lactone and monoacids)

Usual Dosage Adults: 2.5 mg twice daily; antihypertensive response seen in 2-3 hours; maximal response in 2-4 weeks; increase dose at 2- to 4-week intervals at 2.5-5 mg increments; usual dose range: 5-20 mg/day. **Note**: Most patients show no improvement with doses >10 mg/day except adverse reaction rate increases; therefore, maximal dose in elderly should be 10 mg/day.

Patient Information Do not discontinue abruptly; report any dizziness, shortness of breath, palpitations, or edema

Dosage Forms Capsule: 2.5 mg, 5 mg

Isuprel® *see* Isoproterenol *on page 597*

Itch-X® [OTC] *see* Pramoxine Hydrochloride *on page 915*

Itraconazole (i tra koe′ na zole)
Related Information
Antifungal Agents *on page 1253-1254*
Brand Names Sporanox®
Use Treatment of susceptible fungal infections in immunocompromised and immunocompetent patients including blastomycosis and histoplasmosis; also has activity against *Aspergillus, Candida, Coccidioides, Cryptococcus, Sporothrix,* and chromomycosis
Pregnancy Risk Factor C
Contraindications Known hypersensitivity to itraconazole or other azoles; terfenadine
Warnings/Precautions Rare cases of serious cardiovascular adverse event, including death, ventricular tachycardia and torsade de pointes have been observed due to increased terfenadine concentrations induced by itraconazole; patients who develop abnormal liver function tests during fluconazole therapy should be monitored and therapy discontinued if symptoms of liver disease develop
Adverse Reactions
>10%: Gastrointestinal: Nausea
1% to 10%:
Central nervous system: Headache
Dermatologic: Rash
Gastrointestinal: Abdominal pain, vomiting
<1%:
Cardiovascular: Edema, hypertension
Central nervous system: Fatigue, fever, malaise, dizziness, somnolence
Dermatologic: Pruritus
Endocrine & metabolic: Hypokalemia
Gastrointestinal: Diarrhea, anorexia
Genitourinary: Albuminuria, impotence, decreased libido
Hepatic: Abnormal hepatic function
Overdosage/Toxicology Overdoses are well tolerated; following decontamination, if possible, supportive measures only are required; dialysis is not effective
Drug Interactions
Decreased effect:
Decreased serum levels with isoniazid and phenytoin
Decreased/undetectable serum levels with rifampin - **should not be administered concomitantly with rifampin**
(Continued)

Itraconazole *(Continued)*

Absorption requires gastric acidity; therefore, antacids, H₂ antagonists (cimetidine and ranitidine), omeprazole, and sucralfate significantly reduce bioavailability resulting in treatment failures and should not be administered concomitantly; amphotericin B or fluconazole should be used instead

Increased toxicity:

May increase cyclosporine levels (by 50%) when high doses are used

May increase phenytoin serum concentration

May inhibit warfarins metabolism

May increase digoxin serum levels

May increase terfenadine levels - **concomitant administration is not recommended**

Pharmacodynamics/Kinetics

Absorption: Enhanced by food and requires gastric acidity

Distribution: Apparent volume averaged 796±185 L or 10 L/kg; highly lipophilic and tissue concentrations are higher than plasma concentrations. The highest itraconazole concentrations are achieved in adipose, omentum, endometrium, cervical and vaginal mucus, and skin/nails. Aqueous fluids, such as cerebrospinal fluid and urine, contain negligible amounts of itraconazole; steady-state concentrations are achieved in 13 days with multiple administration of itraconazole 100-400 mg/day.

Protein binding: 99.9% bound to plasma proteins; metabolite hydroxy-itraconazole is 99.5% bound to plasma proteins

Metabolism: Extensive by the liver into >30 metabolites including hydroxy-itraconazole which is the major metabolite and appears to have *in vitro* antifungal activity. The main metabolic pathway is oxidation; may undergo saturation metabolism with multiple dosing

Bioavailability: Increased from 40% fasting to 100% postprandial; absolute oral bioavailability: 55%; hypochlorhydria has been reported in HIV-infected patients; therefore, oral absorption in these patients may be decreased

Half-life: After single 200 mg dose: 21±5 hours

Elimination: ~3% to 18% excreted in feces; ~0.03% of parent drug excreted renally and 40% of dose excreted as inactive metabolites in urine

Usual Dosage Oral (absorption is best if taken with food, therefore, it is best to administer itraconazole after meals):

Children: Efficacy and safety have not been established; a small number of patients 3-16 years of age have been treated with 100 mg/day for systemic fungal infections with no serious adverse effects reported

Adults: 200 mg once daily, if obvious improvement or there is evidence of progressive fungal disease, increase the dose in 100 mg increments to a maximum of 400 mg/day; doses >200 mg/day are given in 2 divided doses

Life-threatening infections: Loading dose: 200 mg 3 times/day (600 mg/day) should be given for the first 3 days of therapy

Dosing adjustment in renal impairment: Not necessary
Not dialyzable

Dosing adjustment in hepatic impairment: May be necessary, but specific guidelines are not available

Administration Doses >200 mg/day are given in 2 divided doses; do not administer with antacids

Patient Information Take with food; report any signs and symptoms that may suggest liver dysfunction so that the appropriate laboratory testing can be done; signs and symptoms may include unusual fatigue, anorexia, nausea and/or vomiting, jaundice, dark urine, or pale stool

Dosage Forms Capsule: 100 mg

Kanamycin Sulfate (kan a mye' sin)

Related Information
Antimicrobial Drugs of Choice *on page 1298-1302*

Brand Names Kantrex®

Use
Oral: Preoperative bowel preparation in the prophylaxis of infections and adjunctive treatment of hepatic coma (oral kanamycin is not indicated in the treatment of systemic infections); treatment of susceptible bacterial infection including gram-negative aerobes, gram-positive *Bacillus* as well as some mycobacteria
Parenteral: Rarely used in antibiotic irrigations during surgery

Pregnancy Risk Factor D

Contraindications Hypersensitivity to kanamycin or any component or other aminoglycosides

Warnings/Precautions Use with caution in patients with pre-existing renal insufficiency, vestibular or cochlear impairment, myasthenia gravis, conditions which depress neuromuscular transmission
Parenteral aminoglycosides are associated with nephrotoxicity or ototoxicity; the ototoxicity may be proportional to the amount of drug given and the duration of treatment; tinnitus or vertigo are indications of vestibular injury and impending hearing loss; renal damage is usually reversible

Adverse Reactions
>10%: Renal: Nephrotoxicity
1% to 10%:
Cardiovascular: Swelling
Central nervous system: Neurotoxicity
Dermatologic: Skin itching, redness, rash
Otic: Ototoxicity (auditory), ototoxicity (vestibular)
<1%:
Central nervous system: Drowsiness, headache, pseudomotor cerebri
Dermatologic: Photosensitivity, erythema
Gastrointestinal: Anorexia, nausea, vomiting, weight loss, increased salivation, enterocolitis
Hematologic: Granulocytopenia, agranulocytosis, thrombocytopenia
Local: Burning, stinging
Neuromuscular & skeletal: Weakness, tremors, muscle cramps
Respiratory: Difficulty in breathing

Overdosage/Toxicology Symptoms of overdose include ototoxicity, nephrotoxicity, and neuromuscular toxicity. The treatment of choice following a single acute overdose appears to be the maintenance of good urine output of at least 3 mL/kg/hour. Dialysis is of questionable value in the enhancement of aminoglycoside elimination. If required, hemodialysis is preferred over peritoneal dialysis in patients with normal renal function. Careful hydration may be all that is required to promote diuresis and, therefore, the enhancement of the drug's elimination.

Drug Interactions
Increased toxicity:
Penicillins, cephalosporins, amphotericin B, diuretics → ↑ nephrotoxicity
Neuromuscular blocking agents → ↑ neuromuscular blockade

Stability Darkening of vials does not indicate loss of potency

Mechanism of Action Interferes with protein synthesis in bacterial cell by binding to ribosomal subunit

Pharmacodynamics/Kinetics
Absorption: Oral: Not absorbed following administration
Relative diffusion of antimicrobial agents from blood into cerebrospinal fluid (CSF): Good only with inflammation (exceeds usual MICs)
Ratio of CSF to blood level (%):
Normal meninges: Nil
Inflamed meninges: 43
Half-life: 2-4 hours, increases in anuria to 80 hours
End stage renal disease: 40-96 hours
Time to peak serum concentration: I.M.: 1-2 hours
Elimination: Entirely in the kidney, principally by glomerular filtration

Usual Dosage
Neonates: I.M., I.V.:
Postnatal age <7 days:
<2000 g: 7.5 mg/kg/dose every 12 hours
>2000 g: 10 mg/kg/dose every 12 hours
Postnatal age >7 days:
<2000 g: 7.5 mg/kg/dose every 8 hours
>2000 g: 10 mg/kg/dose every 8 hours
Children:
Infections: I.M., I.V.: 15-30 mg/kg/day in divided doses every 8 hours
Suppression of bowel flora: Oral: 150-250 mg/kg/day in divided doses administered every 1-6 hours
(Continued)

Kanamycin Sulfate *(Continued)*

Adults:
   Infections: I.M., I.V.: 5-7.5 mg/kg/dose in divided doses every 8-12 hours
   Preoperative intestinal antisepsis: Oral: 1 g every 4-6 hours for 36-72 hours
   Hepatic coma: Oral: 8-12 g/day in divided doses

Dosing adjustment/interval in renal impairment:
   Cl_{cr} 50-80 mL/minute: Administer 60% to 90% of dose or administer every 8-12 hours
   Cl_{cr} 10-50 mL/minute: Administer 30% to 70% of dose or administer every 12 hours
   Cl_{cr} <10 mL/minute: Administer 20% to 30% of dose or administer every 24-48 hours
Dialyzable (50% to 100%)

Administration Adults: Dilute to 100-200 mL and infuse over 30 minutes; administer around-the-clock to promote less variation in peak and trough serum levels

Monitoring Parameters Serum creatinine and BUN every 2-3 days; peak and trough concentrations; hearing

Reference Range Therapeutic: Peak: 25-35 µg/mL; Trough: 4-8 µg/mL; Toxic: Peak: >35 µg/mL; Trough: >10 µg/mL

Patient Information Report any dizziness or sensations of ringing or fullness in ears

Nursing Implications Aminoglycoside levels in blood taken from Silastic® central catheters can sometime give falsely high readings (sample from alternative lumen or via peripheral stick if possible; otherwise flush very well following administration); hearing should be tested before, during, and after treatment

Dosage Forms
Capsule: 500 mg
Injection:
   Pediatric: 75 mg (2 mL)
   Adults: 500 mg (2 mL); 1 g (3 mL)

Kestrone® *see* Estrone *on page 413*

Ketalar® *see* Ketamine Hydrochloride *on this page*

Ketamine Hydrochloride (keet' a meen)
Brand Names Ketalar®
Use Induction of anesthesia; short surgical procedures; dressing changes
Pregnancy Risk Factor D
Contraindications Elevated intracranial pressure; patients with hypertension, aneurysms, thyrotoxicosis, congestive heart failure, angina, psychotic disorders; hypersensitivity to ketamine or any component
Warnings/Precautions Should be used by or under the direct supervision of physicians experienced in administering general anesthetics and in maintenance of an airway, and in the control of respiration. Resuscitative equipment should be available for use.

Postanesthetic emergence reactions which can manifest as vivid dreams, hallucinations and/or frank delirium occur in 12% of patients; these reactions are less common in patients >65 years of age and when given I.M.; emergence reactions, confusion, or irrational behavior may occur up to 24 hours postoperatively and may be reduced by minimization of verbal, tactile, and visual patient stimulation during recovery or by pretreatment with a benzodiazepine.
Adverse Reactions
>10%:
  Cardiovascular: Hypertension, tachycardia, increased cardiac output, paradoxical direct myocardial depression
  Central nervous system: Increased intracranial pressure, vivid dreams, visual hallucinations
  Neuromuscular & skeletal: Tonic-clonic movements, tremors
  Miscellaneous: Emergence reactions, vocalization
1% to 10%:
  Cardiovascular: Bradycardia, hypotension
  Dermatologic: Pain at injection site, skin rash
  Gastrointestinal: Vomiting, anorexia, nausea
  Ocular: Nystagmus, diplopia
  Respiratory: Respiratory depression
<1%:
  Cardiovascular: Cardiac arrhythmias, myocardial depression
  Central nervous system: Increased intracranial pressure, increases in cerebral blood, fasciculations
  Endocrine & metabolic: Increased metabolic rate, increased intraocular pressure
  Neuromuscular & skeletal: Increased skeletal muscle tone
  Ocular: Increased intraocular pressure
  Respiratory: Increased airway resistance, cough reflex may be depressed, decreased bronchospasm, respiratory depression or apnea with large doses or rapid infusions, laryngospasm
  Miscellaneous: Hypersalivation
Overdosage/Toxicology Respiratory depression with excessive dosing or too rapid administration; supportive care is the treatment of choice; mechanical support of respiration is preferred
Drug Interactions
Increased effect: Nondepolarizing agents → ↑ effect
Increased toxicity:
  Barbiturates, narcotics, hydroxyzine increase prolonged recovery
  Muscle relaxants, thyroid hormones → ↑ blood pressure and heart rate
  Halothane → ↓ blood pressure
Stability Do not mix with barbiturates or diazepam → precipitation may occur
Mechanism of Action Produces dissociative anesthesia by direct action on the cortex and limbic system
Pharmacodynamics/Kinetics Duration of action (following a single dose):
Unconsciousness: 10-15 minutes
Analgesia: 30-40 minutes
Amnesia: May persist for 1-2 hours
Usual Dosage Used in combination with anticholinergic agents to ↓ hypersalivation
Children: Initial induction:
  Oral: 6-10 mg/kg for 1 dose (mixed in 0.2-0.3 mL/kg of cola or other beverage) given 30 minutes before the procedure
  I.M.: 3-7 mg/kg
  I.V.: Range: 0.5-2 mg/kg, use smaller doses (0.5-1 mg/kg) for sedation for minor procedures; usual induction dosage: 1-2 mg/kg
  Continuous I.V. infusion: Sedation: 5-20 mcg/kg/minute
(Continued)

Ketamine Hydrochloride *(Continued)*

Adults: Initial induction:
I.M.: 3-8 mg/kg
I.V.: Range: 1-4.5 mg/kg; usual induction dosage: 1-2 mg/kg
Children and Adults: Maintenance: Supplemental doses of ½ to the full induction dose; repeat as needed

Administration I.V.: Do not exceed 0.5 mg/kg/minute or give faster than 60 seconds; do not exceed final concentration of 2 mg/mL

Monitoring Parameters Cardiovascular effects, heart rate, blood pressure, respiratory rate, transcutaneous O_2 saturation

Dosage Forms Injection: 10 mg/mL (20 mL, 25 mL, 50 mL); 50 mg/mL (10 mL); 100 mg/mL (5 mL)

Ketoconazole (kee toe koe' na zole)

Related Information

Antifungal Agents *on page 1253-1254*

Brand Names Nizoral®

Use Treatment of susceptible fungal infections, including candidiasis, oral thrush, blastomycosis, histoplasmosis, paracoccidioidomycosis, chronic mucocutaneous candidiasis, as well as, certain recalcitrant cutaneous dermatophytoses; used topically for treatment of tinea corporis, tinea cruris, tinea versicolor, and cutaneous candidiasis, seborrheic dermatitis

Pregnancy Risk Factor C

Contraindications Hypersensitivity to ketoconazole or any component; CNS fungal infections (due to poor CNS penetration); coadministration with terfenadine is contraindicated

Warnings/Precautions Rare cases of serious cardiovascular adverse event, including death, ventricular tachycardia and torsade de pointes have been observed due to increased terfenadine concentrations induced by ketoconazole. Use with caution in patients with impaired hepatic function; has been associated with hepatotoxicity, including some fatalities; perform periodic liver function tests; high doses of ketoconazole may depress adrenocortical function.

Adverse Reactions

Oral:
1% to 10%:
Dermatologic: Pruritus
Gastrointestinal: Nausea, vomiting, abdominal pain
<1%:
Central nervous system: Headache, dizziness, somnolence, fever, chills, bulging fontanelles
Endocrine & metabolic: Gynecomastia
Gastrointestinal: Diarrhea
Genitourinary: Impotence
Hematologic: Thrombocytopenia, leukopenia, hemolytic anemia
Ocular: Photophobia
Cream: Severe irritation, pruritus, stinging (~5%)
Shampoo: Increases in normal hair loss, irritation (<1%), abnormal hair texture, scalp pustules, mild dryness of skin, itching, oiliness/dryness of hair

Overdosage/Toxicology Symptoms of overdose include dizziness, headache, nausea, vomiting, diarrhea. Overdoses are well tolerated; treatment includes supportive measures and gastric decontamination

Drug Interactions

Decreased effect:
Decreased serum levels with isoniazid and phenytoin
Decreased/undetectable serum levels with rifampin - **should not be administered concomitantly with rifampin**
Absorption requires gastric acidity; therefore, antacids, H_2 antagonists (cimetidine and ranitidine), omeprazole, and sucralfate significantly reduce bioavailability resulting in treatment failures and should not be administered concomitantly; amphotericin B or fluconazole should be used instead
Increased toxicity:
May increase cyclosporine levels (by 50%) when high doses are used
May increase phenytoin serum concentration
May inhibit warfarins metabolism
May increase digoxin serum levels
May increase terfenadine levels - **concomitant administration is not recommended**

Mechanism of Action Alters the permeability of the cell wall; inhibits biosynthesis of triglycerides and phospholipids by fungi; inhibits several fungal enzymes that results in a build-up of toxic concentrations of hydrogen peroxide

Pharmacodynamics/Kinetics
  Absorption: Oral: Rapid (~75%); no detectable absorption following use of the shampoo
  Distribution: Minimal distribution into the CNS
  Protein binding: 93% to 96%
  Metabolism: Partially in the liver by enzymes to inactive compounds
  Bioavailability: Decreases as pH of the gastric contents increases
  Half-life, biphasic:
    Initial: 2 hours
    Terminal: 8 hours
  Time to peak serum concentration: 1-2 hours
  Elimination: Primarily in feces (57%) with smaller amounts excreted in urine (13%)

Usual Dosage
  Oral:
    Children >2 years: 5-10 mg/kg/day divided every 12-24 hours for 2-4 weeks
    Adults: 200-400 mg/day as a single daily dose
  Shampoo: Apply twice weekly for 4 weeks with at least 3 days between each shampoo
  Topical: Rub gently into the affected area once daily to twice daily

  Dosing adjustment in hepatic impairment: Dose reductions should be considered in patients with severe liver disease
  Not dialyzable (0% to 5%)
Monitoring Parameters Liver function tests
Patient Information Cream is for topical application to the skin only; avoid contact with the eye; avoid taking antacids at the same time as ketoconazole; may take with food; may cause drowsiness, impair judgment or coordination. Notify physician of unusual fatigue, anorexia, vomiting, dark urine, or pale stools.
Nursing Implications Administer 2 hours prior to antacids to prevent decreased absorption due to the high pH of gastric contents
Dosage Forms
  Cream: 2% (15 g, 30 g, 60 g)
  Shampoo: 2% (120 mL)
  Tablet: 200 mg

Ketoprofen (kee toe proe' fen)
Related Information
  Nonsteroidal Anti-Inflammatories Comparison *on page 1280*
Brand Names Orudis®; Oruvail®
Use Acute or long-term treatment of rheumatoid arthritis and osteoarthritis; primary dysmenorrhea; mild to moderate pain
Pregnancy Risk Factor B
Contraindications Known hypersensitivity to ketoprofen or other NSAIDs/aspirin
Warnings/Precautions Use with caution in patients with congestive heart failure, hypertension, decreased renal or hepatic function, history of GI disease (bleeding or ulcers), or those receiving anticoagulants; safety and efficacy in children <6 months of age have not yet been established
Adverse Reactions
  >10%:
    Central nervous system: Dizziness
    Dermatologic: Skin rash
    Gastrointestinal: Abdominal cramps, heartburn, indigestion, nausea
  1% to 10%:
    Cardiovascular: Fluid retention
    Central nervous system: Headache, nervousness
    Dermatologic: Itching
    Gastrointestinal: Vomiting
    Otic: Ringing in ears
  <1%:
    Cardiovascular: Congestive heart failure, hypertension, arrhythmias, tachycardia
    Central nervous system: Confusion, hallucinations, mental depression, drowsiness, insomnia
    Dermatologic: Hives, erythema multiforme, toxic epidermal necrolysis, Stevens-Johnson syndrome, angioedema
    Endocrine & metabolic: Polydipsia, hot flushes
    Gastrointestinal: Gastritis, GI ulceration
    Genitourinary: Cystitis
    Hematologic: Agranulocytosis, anemia, hemolytic anemia, bone marrow depression, leukopenia, thrombocytopenia
    Hepatic: Hepatitis
(Continued)

Ketoprofen *(Continued)*

  Neuromuscular & skeletal: Peripheral neuropathy
  Ocular: Toxic amblyopia, blurred vision, conjunctivitis, dry eyes
  Otic: Decreased hearing
  Renal: Polyuria, acute renal failure
  Respiratory: Allergic rhinitis, shortness of breath
  Miscellaneous: Aseptic meningitis, epistaxis

Overdosage/Toxicology Symptoms include apnea, metabolic acidosis, coma, and nystagmus; leukocytosis, renal failure. Management of a nonsteroidal anti-inflammatory drug (NSAID) intoxication is primarily supportive and symptomatic. Fluid therapy is commonly effective in managing the hypotension that may occur following an acute NSAID overdose, except when this is due to an acute blood loss. Seizures tend to be very short-lived and often do not require drug treatment. Although, recurrent seizures should be treated with I.V. diazepam. Since many of the NSAIDs undergo enterohepatic cycling, multiple doses of charcoal may be needed to reduce the potential for delayed toxicities.

Drug Interactions
  Decreased effect of diuretics
  Increased effect/toxicity with probenecid, lithium
  Increased toxicity of methotrexate

Mechanism of Action Inhibits prostaglandin synthesis by decreasing the activity of the enzyme, cyclo-oxygenase, which results in decreased formation of prostaglandin precursors

Pharmacodynamics/Kinetics
  Absorption: Almost completely
  Metabolism: In the liver
  Half-life: 1-4 hours
  Time to peak serum concentration: 0.5-2 hours
  Elimination: Renal excretion (60% to 75%), primarily as glucuronide conjugates

Usual Dosage Oral:
  Children 3 months to 14 years: Fever: 0.5-1 mg/kg every 6-8 hours

  Children >12 years and Adults:
   Rheumatoid arthritis or osteoarthritis: 50-75 mg 3-4 times/day up to a maximum of 300 mg/day
   Mild to moderate pain: 25-50 mg every 6-8 hours up to a maximum of 300 mg/day

Test Interactions $\uparrow$ chloride (S), $\uparrow$ sodium (S), $\uparrow$ bleeding time

Patient Information Take with food; may cause dizziness or drowsiness

Nursing Implications Do not crush tablet

Dosage Forms
  Capsule: 25 mg, 50 mg, 75 mg
  Capsule, extended release: 200 mg

Ketorolac Tromethamine (kee' toe role ak)

Related Information
  Nonsteroidal Anti-Inflammatories Comparison *on page 1280*

Brand Names Acular®; Toradol®

Use Short-term (<5 days) management of pain; first parenteral NSAID for analgesia; 30 mg provides the analgesia comparable to 12 mg of morphine or 100 mg of meperidine

Pregnancy Risk Factor B (D if used in the 3rd trimester)

Contraindications In patients who have developed nasal polyps, angioedema, or bronchospastic reactions to other NSAIDs, active peptic ulcer disease, recent GI bleeding or perforation, patients with advanced renal disease or risk of renal failure, labor and delivery, nursing mothers, patients with hypersensitivity to ketorolac, aspirin, or other NSAIDs, **prophylaxis before major surgery**, suspected or confirmed cerebrovascular bleeding, hemorrhagic diathesis, concurrent ASA or other NSAIDs, epidural or intrathecal administration, concomitant probenecid

Warnings/Precautions Use extra caution and reduce dosages in the elderly because it is cleared renally somewhat slower, and the elderly are also more sensitive to the renal effects of NSAIDs; use with caution in patients with congestive heart failure, hypertension, decreased renal or hepatic function, history of GI disease (bleeding or ulcers), or those receiving anticoagulants

Adverse Reactions
  Genitourinary: Renal impairment
  Hematologic: Postoperative hematomas, wound bleeding (with I.M.)

  1% to 10%:
   Cardiovascular: Edema

Central nervous system: Drowsiness, dizziness, headache
Gastrointestinal: Pain, nausea, dyspepsia, diarrhea, gastric ulcers, indigestion
Local: Pain at injection site
Miscellaneous: Increased sweating

<1%:
Central nervous system: Mental depression
Dermatologic: Purpura
Gastrointestinal: Aphthous stomatitis, rectal bleeding, peptic ulceration
Ocular: Change in vision
Renal: Oliguria
Respiratory: Dyspnea

Overdosage/Toxicology Symptoms of overdose include diarrhea, pallor, vomiting, labored breathing, apnea, metabolic acidosis, leukocytosis, renal failure

Management of a nonsteroidal anti-inflammatory drug (NSAID) intoxication is primarily supportive and symptomatic. Fluid therapy is commonly effective in managing the hypotension that may occur following an acute NSAID overdose, except when this is due to an acute blood loss. Seizures tend to be very short-lived and often do not require drug treatment; although, recurrent seizures should be treated with I.V. diazepam. Since many of the NSAIDs undergo enterohepatic cycling, multiple doses of charcoal may be needed to reduce the potential for delayed toxicities; NSAIDs are highly bound to plasma proteins; therefore, hemodialysis and peritoneal dialysis are not useful.

Drug Interactions
Decreased effect of diuretics
Increased toxicity: Lithium, methotrexate increased drug level; increased effect/toxicity with salicylates, probenecid

Stability
Ketorolac tromethamine injection should be stored at controlled room temperature and protected from light; injection is clear and has a slight yellow color; precipitation may occur at relatively low pH values
Compatible with NS, D_5W, D_5NS, LR
Incompatible with meperidine, morphine, promethazine, and hydroxyzine

Mechanism of Action Inhibits prostaglandin synthesis by decreasing the activity of the enzyme, cyclo-oxygenase, which results in decreased formation of prostaglandin precursors

Pharmacodynamics/Kinetics
Analgesic effect:
Onset of action: I.M.: Within 10 minutes
Peak effect: Within 75-150 minutes
Duration of action: 6-8 hours
Absorption: Oral: Well absorbed
Time to peak serum concentration: I.M.: 30-60 minutes
Distribution: Crosses placenta; crosses into breast milk; poor penetration into CSF
Protein binding: 99%
Metabolism: In the liver
Half-life: 2-8 hours; increased 30% to 50% in elderly
Elimination: Renal excretion, 61% appearing in the urine as unchanged drug

Usual Dosage
Adults (pain relief usually begins within 10 minutes with parenteral forms):
Oral: 10 mg every 4-6 hours as needed for a maximum of 40 mg/day; on day of transition from I.M. to oral: maximum oral dose: 40 mg (or 120 mg combined oral and I.M.); maximum 5 days administration
I.M.: Initial: 30-60 mg, then 15-30 mg every 6 hours as needed for up to 5 days maximum; maximum dose in the first 24 hours: 150 mg with 120 mg/24 hours for up to 5 days total
I.V.: Initial: 30 mg, then 15-30 mg every 6 hours as needed for up to 5 days maximum; maximum daily dose: 120 mg for up to 5 days total
Ophthalmic: Instill 1 drop in eye(s) 4 times/day
Elderly >65 years: Renal insufficiency or weight <50 kg:
I.M.: 30 mg, then 15 mg every 6 hours
I.V.: 15 mg every 6 hours as needed for up to 5 days total; maximum daily dose: 120 mg

Monitoring Parameters Monitor response (pain, range of motion, grip strength, mobility, ADL function), inflammation; observe for weight gain, edema; monitor renal function (serum creatinine, BUN, urine output); observe for bleeding, bruising; evaluate gastrointestinal effects (abdominal pain, bleeding, dyspepsia); mental confusion, disorientation, CBC, liver function tests

Reference Range Serum concentration: Therapeutic: 0.3-5 μg/mL; Toxic: >5 μg/mL

Test Interactions ↑ chloride (S), ↑ sodium (S), ↑ bleeding time
(Continued)

Ketorolac Tromethamine *(Continued)*

Patient Information Serious gastrointestinal bleeding can occur as well as ulceration and perforation. Pain may or may not be present. Avoid aspirin and aspirin-containing products while taking this medication. If gastric adverse effects persist, contact physician. May cause drowsiness, dizziness, blurred vision, and confusion. Use caution when performing tasks which require alertness (eg, driving).

Nursing Implications Monitor for signs of pain relief, such as an increased appetite and activity

Dosage Forms
Injection: 15 mg/mL (1 mL); 30 mg/mL (1 mL, 2 mL)
Solution, ophthalmic: 0.5% (5 mL)
Tablet: 10 mg

Key-Pred® *see* Prednisolone *on page 919*

Key-Pred-SP® *see* Prednisolone *on page 919*

K-G® Elixir *see* Potassium Gluconate *on page 908*

KI *see* Potassium Iodide *on page 909*

K-Ide® *see* Potassium Bicarbonate and Potassium Citrate, Effervescent *on page 905*

Kinesed® *see* Hyoscyamine, Atropine, Scopolamine, and Phenobarbital *on page 557*

Kinevac® *see* Sincalide *on page 1007*

Klonopin™ *see* Clonazepam *on page 261*

K-Lor™ *see* Potassium Chloride *on page 906*

Klor-con® *see* Potassium Chloride *on page 906*

Klor-con®/EF *see* Potassium Bicarbonate and Potassium Citrate, Effervescent *on page 905*

Kloromin® [OTC] *see* Chlorpheniramine Maleate *on page 229*

Klorvess® *see* Potassium Chloride *on page 906*

Klotrix® *see* Potassium Chloride *on page 906*

K-Lyte® *see* Potassium Bicarbonate and Potassium Citrate, Effervescent *on page 905*

K-Lyte/CL® *see* Potassium Chloride *on page 906*

Koāte®-HP *see* Antihemophilic Factor (Human) *on page 80*

Koāte®-HS *see* Antihemophilic Factor (Human) *on page 80*

Kolephrin® GG/DM [OTC] *see* Guaifenesin and Dextromethorphan *on page 517*

Konakion® *see* Phytonadione *on page 882*

Kondremul® [OTC] *see* Mineral Oil *on page 743*

Konsyl-D® [OTC] *see* Psyllium *on page 956*

Konsyl® [OTC] *see* Psyllium *on page 956*

Konȳne® 80 *see* Factor IX Complex (Human) *on page 438*

K-Phos® Neutral *see* Potassium Phosphate and Sodium Phosphate *on page 912*

K-Phos® Original *see* Potassium Acid Phosphate *on page 904*

K-Tab® *see* Potassium Chloride *on page 906*

Ku-Zyme® HP *see* Pancrelipase *on page 837*

K-Vescent® *see* Potassium Bicarbonate and Potassium Citrate, Effervescent *on page 905*

Kwell® *see* Lindane *on page 636*

Kytril® *see* Granisetron *on page 512*

***L*-3-Hydroxytyrosine** *see* Levodopa *on page 624*

LA-12® *see* Hydroxocobalamin *on page 552*

Labetalol Hydrochloride *(la bet' a lole)*

Related Information
Beta-Blockers Comparison *on page 1257-1259*

Brand Names Normodyne®; Trandate®

Synonyms Ibidomide Hydrochloride

Use Treatment of mild to severe hypertension; I.V. for hypertensive emergencies

Pregnancy Risk Factor C

Contraindications Cardiogenic shock, uncompensated congestive heart failure, bradycardia, pulmonary edema, or heart block

Warnings/Precautions Paradoxical increase in blood pressure has been reported with treatment of pheochromocytoma or clonidine withdrawal syndrome; use with caution in patients with hyper-reactive airway disease, congestive heart failure, diabetes mellitus, hepatic dysfunction; orthostatic hypotension may occur with I.V. administration; patient should remain supine during and for up to 3 hours after I.V. administration; use with caution in impaired hepatic function (discontinue if signs of liver dysfunction occur); may mask the signs and symptoms of hypoglycemia; a lower hemodynamic response rate and higher incidence of toxicity may be observed with administration to elderly patients.

Adverse Reactions

1% to 10%:

Cardiovascular: Congestive heart failure, irregular heartbeat, reduced peripheral circulation, orthostatic hypotension

Central nervous system: Mental depression, dizziness, drowsiness

Dermatologic: Itching, numbness of skin

Endocrine & metabolic: Decreased sexual ability

Gastrointestinal: Nausea, vomiting, stomach discomfort

Neuromuscular & skeletal: Weakness

Respiratory: Breathing difficulty, stuffy nose

Miscellaneous: Changes in taste

<1%:

Cardiovascular: Bradycardia, chest pain

Dermatologic: Skin rash

Gastrointestinal: Diarrhea

Hepatic: Hepatotoxicity

Neuromuscular & skeletal: Joint pain

Ocular: Dry eyes

Overdosage/Toxicology Symptoms of intoxication include cardiac disturbances, CNS toxicity, bronchospasm, hypoglycemia and hyperkalemia. The most common cardiac symptoms include hypotension and bradycardia; atrioventricular block, intraventricular conduction disturbances, cardiogenic shock, and systole may occur with severe overdose, especially with membrane-depressant drugs (eg, propranolol); CNS effects include convulsions, coma, and respiratory arrest is commonly seen with propranolol and other membrane-depressant and lipid-soluble drugs.

Treatment includes symptomatic treatment of seizures, hypotension, hyperkalemia and hypoglycemia; bradycardia and hypotension resistant to atropine, isoproterenol or pacing may respond to glucagon; wide QRS defects caused by the membrane-depressant poisoning may respond to hypertonic sodium bicarbonate; repeat-dose charcoal, hemoperfusion, or hemodialysis may be helpful in removal of only those beta-blockers with a small V_d, long half-life or low intrinsic clearance (acebutolol, atenolol, nadolol, sotalol)

Drug Interactions

Decreased effect of beta-blockers with aluminum salts, barbiturates, calcium salts, cholestyramine, colestipol, NSAIDs, penicillins (ampicillin), rifampin, salicylates and sulfinpyrazone due to decreased bioavailability and plasma levels

Beta-blockers may decrease the effect of sulfonylureas

Increased effect/toxicity of beta-blockers with calcium blockers (diltiazem, felodipine, nicardipine), contraceptives, flecainide, haloperidol (propranolol, hypotensive effects), H_2 antagonists (metoprolol, propranolol only by cimetidine, possibly ranitidine), hydralazine (metoprolol, propranolol), loop diuretics (propranolol, not atenolol), MAO inhibitors (metoprolol, nadolol, bradycardia), phenothiazines (propranolol), propafenone (metoprolol, propranolol), quinidine (in extensive metabolizers), ciprofloxacin, thyroid hormones (metoprolol, propranolol, when hypothyroid patient is converted to euthyroid state)

Beta-blockers may increase the effect/toxicity of flecainide, haloperidol (hypotensive effects), hydralazine, phenothiazines, acetaminophen, anticoagulants (propranolol, warfarin), benzodiazepines (not atenolol), clonidine (hypertensive crisis after or during withdrawal of either agent), epinephrine (initial hypertensive episode followed by bradycardia), nifedipine and verapamil lidocaine, ergots (peripheral ischemia), prazosin (postural hypotension)

Beta-blockers may affect the action or levels of ethanol, disopyramide, nondepolarizing muscle relaxants and theophylline although the effects are difficult to predict

Stability

Labetalol should be stored at room temperature or under refrigeration and should be protected from light and freezing; the solution is clear to slightly yellow

(Continued)

Labetalol Hydrochloride *(Continued)*

Stability of parenteral admixture at room temperature (25°C) and refrigeration temperature (4°C): 3 days
Standard diluent: 500 mg/250 mL D_5W
Minimum volume: 250 mL D_5W
Incompatible with sodium bicarbonate, most stable at pH of 2-4; **incompatible** with alkaline solutions

Mechanism of Action Blocks alpha-, beta$_1$-, and beta$_2$-adrenergic receptor sites; elevated renins are reduced

Pharmacodynamics/Kinetics
Onset of action:
Oral: 20 minutes to 2 hours
I.V.: 2-5 minutes
Peak effect:
Oral: 1-4 hours
I.V.: 5-15 minutes
Duration:
Oral: 8-24 hours (dose-dependent)
I.V.: 2-4 hours
Distribution: Crosses placenta; small amounts in breast milk; moderately lipid soluble, therefore, can enter CNS
V_d: Adults: 3-16 L/kg; mean: <9.4 L/kg
Protein binding: 50%
Metabolism: Extensive first-pass effect; metabolized in liver primarily via glucuronide conjugation
Bioavailability: Oral: 25%; increased with liver disease, elderly, and concurrent cimetidine
Half-life, normal renal function: 6-8 hours
Elimination: <5% excreted in urine unchanged; possible decreased clearance in neonates/infants

Usual Dosage Due to limited documentation of its use, labetalol should be initiated cautiously in pediatric patients with careful dosage adjustment and blood pressure monitoring

Children:
Oral: Limited information regarding labetalol use in pediatric patients is currently available in literature. Some centers recommend initial oral doses of 4 mg/kg/day in 2 divided doses. Reported oral doses have started at 3 mg/kg/day and 20 mg/kg/day and have increased up to 40 mg/kg/day.
I.V., intermittent bolus doses of 0.3-1 mg/kg/dose have been reported
For treatment of pediatric hypertensive emergencies, initial continuous infusions of 0.4-1 mg/kg/hour with a maximum of 3 mg/kg/hour have been used; administration requires the use of an infusion pump

Adults:
Oral: Initial: 100 mg twice daily, may increase as needed every 2-3 days by 100 mg until desired response is obtained; usual dose: 200-400 mg twice daily; not to exceed 2.4 g/day
I.V.: 20 mg or 1-2 mg/kg whichever is lower, IVP over 2 minutes, may give 40-80 mg at 10-minute intervals, up to 300 mg total dose
I.V. infusion: Initial: 2 mg/minute; titrate to response up to 300 mg total dose; administration requires the use of an infusion pump
I.V. infusion (500 mg/250 mL D_5) rates:
1 mg/minute: 30 mL/hour
2 mg/minute: 60 mL/hour
3 mg/minute: 90 mL/hour
4 mg/minute: 120 mL/hour
5 mg/minute: 150 mL/hour
6 mg/minute: 180 mL/hour

Not removed by hemo- or peritoneal dialysis; supplemental dose is not necessary

Dosage adjustment in hepatic impairment: Dosage reduction may be necessary

Monitoring Parameters Blood pressure, standing and sitting/supine, pulse, cardiac monitor and blood pressure monitor required for I.V. administration

Test Interactions False-positive urine catecholamines, VMA if measured by fluorometric or photometric methods; use HPLC or specific catecholamine radioenzymatic technique

Patient Information Do not stop medication without aid of physician; may mask signs and symptoms of diabetes

Dosage Forms
Injection: 5 mg/mL (20 mL, 40 mL, 60 mL)

Tablet: 100 mg, 200 mg, 300 mg

LaBID® *see* Theophylline/Aminophylline *on page 1072*

LactiCare-HC® *see* Hydrocortisone *on page 546*

Lactinex® [OTC] *see* Lactobacillus acidophilus and Lactobacillus bulgaricus *on this page*

Lactobacillus acidophilus and *Lactobacillus bulgaricus*
(lak toe ba sil' us)

Brand Names Bacid® [OTC]; Lactinex® [OTC]; More-Dophilus® [OTC]

Use Treatment of uncomplicated diarrhea particularly that caused by antibiotic therapy; re-establish normal physiologic and bacterial flora of the intestinal tract

Contraindications Allergy to milk or lactose

Warnings/Precautions Discontinue if high fever present; do not use in children <3 years of age

Adverse Reactions 1% to 10%: Gastrointestinal: Intestinal flatus

Stability Store in the refrigerator

Mechanism of Action Creates an environment unfavorable to potentially pathogenic fungi or bacteria through the production of lactic acid, and favors establishment of an aciduric flora, thereby suppressing the growth of pathogenic microorganisms; helps re-establish normal intestinal flora

Pharmacodynamics/Kinetics
Absorption: Oral: Not absorbed
Distribution: Locally, primarily in the colon
Elimination: In feces

Usual Dosage Children >3 years and Adults: Oral:
Capsules: 2 capsules 2-9 times/day
Granules: 1 packet added to or taken with cereal, food, milk, fruit juice, or water, 3-4 times/day
Powder: 1 teaspoonful daily with liquid
Tablet, chewable: 4 tablets 3-4 times/day; may follow each dose with a small amount of milk, fruit juice, or water

Administration Granules may be added to or given with cereal, food, milk, fruit juice, or water

Patient Information Refrigerate; granules may be added to or taken with cereal, food, milk, fruit juice, or water

Dosage Forms
Capsule: 50s, 100s
Granules: 1 g/packet (12 packets/box)
Powder: 12 oz
Tablet, chewable: 50s

Lactoflavin *see* Riboflavin *on page 980*

Lactulose (lak' tyoo lose)
Related Information
Laxatives, Classification and Properties *on page 1272*

Brand Names Cephulac®; Cholac®; Chronulac®; Constilac®; Constulose®; Duphalac®; Enulose®; Evalose®; Heptalac®; Lactulose PSE®

Use Adjunct in the prevention and treatment of portal-systemic encephalopathy (PSE); treatment of chronic constipation

Pregnancy Risk Factor C

Contraindications Patients with galactosemia and require a low galactose diet, hypersensitivity to any component

Warnings/Precautions Use with caution in patients with diabetes mellitus; monitor periodically for electrolyte imbalance when lactulose is used >6 months or in patients predisposed to electrolyte abnormalities (eg, elderly); patients receiving lactulose and an oral anti-infective agent should be monitored for possible inadequate response to lactulose

Adverse Reactions
>10%: Gastrointestinal: Flatulence, diarrhea (excessive dose)
1% to 10%: Gastrointestinal: Abdominal discomfort, nausea, vomiting

Overdosage/Toxicology Symptoms of overdose include diarrhea, abdominal pain, hypochloremic alkalosis, dehydration, hypotension, hypokalemia; treatment includes supportive care

Drug Interactions Decreased effect: Oral neomycin, laxatives, antacids

Stability Keep solution at room temperature to reduce viscosity; discard solution if cloudy or very dark
(Continued)

617

Lactulose *(Continued)*

Mechanism of Action The bacterial degradation of lactulose resulting in an acidic pH inhibits the diffusion of NH_3 into the blood by causing the conversion of NH_3 to NH_4+; also enhances the diffusion of NH_3 from the blood into the gut where conversion to NH_4+ occurs; produces an osmotic effect in the colon with resultant distention promoting peristalsis

Pharmacodynamics/Kinetics

Absorption: Oral: Not absorbed appreciably following administration; this is desirable since the intended site of action is within the colon

Metabolism: By colonic flora to lactic acid and acetic acid, requires colonic flora for primary drug activation

Elimination: Primarily in feces and urine (~3%)

Usual Dosage Diarrhea may indicate overdosage and responds to dose reduction

Prevention of portal systemic encephalopathy (PSE): Oral:

Infants: 2.5-10 mL/day divided 3-4 times/day; adjust dosage to produce 2-3 stools/day

Older Children: Daily dose of 40-90 mL divided 3-4 times/day; if initial dose causes diarrhea, then reduce it immediately; adjust dosage to produce 2-3 stools/day

Constipation:

Children: 5 g/day (7.5 mL) after breakfast

Adults:

Acute PSE:

Oral: 20-30 g (30-45 mL) every 1-2 hours to induce rapid laxation; adjust dosage daily to produce 2-3 soft stools; doses of 30-45 mL may be given hourly to cause rapid laxation, then reduce to recommended dose; usual daily dose: 60-100 g or 20-30 g (30-45 mL), 3-4 times/day

Rectal administration: 200 g (300 mL) diluted with 700 mL of H_2O or NS; administer rectally via rectal balloon catheter and retain 30-60 minutes every 4-6 hours

Constipation: Oral: 15-30 mL/day increased to 60 mL/day if necessary

Monitoring Parameters Blood pressure, standing/supine; serum potassium, bowel movement patterns, fluid status, serum ammonia

Patient Information Lactulose can be taken "as is" or diluted with water, fruit juice or milk, or taken in a food; laxative results may not occur for 24-48 hours

Nursing Implications Dilute lactulose in water, usually 60-120 mL, prior to administering through a gastric or feeding tube

Dosage Forms Syrup: 10 g/15 mL (15 mL, 30 mL, 237 mL, 473 mL, 946 mL, 1890 mL)

Lactulose PSE® *see* Lactulose *on previous page*

Lamictal® *see* Lamotrigine *on this page*

Lamisil® *see* Terbinafine *on page 1059*

Lamotrigine *(la moe′ tri jeen)*

Brand Names Lamictal®

Synonyms BW-430C; LTG

Use Partial/secondary generalized seizures in adults; childhood epilepsy (not approved for use in children <16 years of age)

Pregnancy Risk Factor C

Contraindications History of hypersensitivity to lamotrigine or any component

Warnings/Precautions Lactation, impaired renal, hepatic, or cardiac function; avoid abrupt cessation, taper over at least 2 weeks if possible

Adverse Reactions

1% to 10%:

Central nervous system: Dizziness, sedation, ataxia

Dermatologic: Hypersensitivity rash, Stevens-Johnson syndrome, angioedema

Hematologic: Hematuria

Ocular: Nystagmus, diplopia

Overdosage/Toxicology

Decontamination: Lavage/activated charcoal with cathartic

Enhancement of elimination: Multiple dosing of activated charcoal may be useful

Drug Interactions

Decreased effect: Acetaminophen (↑ renal clearance); carbamazepine, phenobarbital, and phenytoin (↑ metabolic clearance)

Increased effect: Valproic acid increases half-life of lamotrigine (↓ metabolic clearance)

Mechanism of Action A triazine derivative which inhibits release of glutamate (an excitatory amino acid) and inhibits voltage-sensitive sodium channels, which stabilizes neuronal membranes

Pharmacodynamics/Kinetics

Distribution: V_d: 1.1 L/kg

Protein binding: 55%

Metabolism: Hepatic and renal

Half-life: 24 hours; increases to 59 hours with concomitant valproic acid therapy; decreases with concomitant phenytoin or carbamazepine therapy to 15 hours

Peak levels: Within 1-4 hours

Elimination: In urine as the glucuronide conjugate

Usual Dosage Oral:

Children: 2-15 mg/kg/day in 2 divided doses

Adults: Initial dose: 50-100 mg/day then titrate to daily maintenance dose of 100-400 mg/day in 1-2 divided daily doses

With concomitant valproic acid therapy: Start initial dose at 25 mg/day then titrate to maintenance dose of 50-200 mg/day in 1-2 divided daily doses

Monitoring Parameters Seizure, frequency and duration, serum levels of concurrent anticonvulsants, hypersensitivity reactions, especially rash

Reference Range Therapeutic range: 2-4 mcg/mL

Additional Information Low water solubility

Dosage Forms Tablet: 25 mg, 100 mg, 150 mg, 200 mg

Lamprene® *see* Clofazimine Palmitate *on page 257*

Lanacane® [OTC] *see* Benzocaine *on page 121*

Lanacort® [OTC] *see* Hydrocortisone *on page 546*

Laniazid® *see* Isoniazid *on page 595*

Lanorinal® *see* Butalbital Compound *on page 153*

Lanoxicaps® *see* Digoxin *on page 338*

Lanoxin® *see* Digoxin *on page 338*

Lariam® *see* Mefloquine Hydrochloride *on page 679*

Larodopa® *see* Levodopa *on page 624*

Larotid® *see* Amoxicillin Trihydrate *on page 68*

Lasan™ *see* Anthralin *on page 80*

Lasan HP-1™ *see* Anthralin *on page 80*

Lasix® *see* Furosemide *on page 492*

L-asparaginase *see* Asparaginase *on page 89*

Lassar's Zinc Paste *see* Zinc Oxide *on page 1175*

Laxatives, Classification and Properties *see page 1272*

LazerSporin-C® *see* Neomycin, Polymyxin B, and Hydrocortisone *on page 781*

l-Bunolol Hydrochloride *see* Levobunolol Hydrochloride *on page 623*

LCR *see* Vincristine Sulfate *on page 1159*

L-Deprenyl *see* Selegiline Hydrochloride *on page 1001*

L-Dopa *see* Levodopa *on page 624*

Ledercillin® VK *see* Penicillin V Potassium *on page 854*

Legatrin® [OTC] *see* Quinine Sulfate *on page 970*

Lente® Iletin® I [OTC] *see* Insulin Preparations *on page 578*

Lente® Iletin® II [OTC] *see* Insulin Preparations *on page 578*

Lente® Insulin [OTC] *see* Insulin Preparations *on page 578*

Lente® L [OTC] *see* Insulin Preparations *on page 578*

Lescol® *see* Fluvastatin *on page 484*

Leucovorin Calcium (loo koe vor' in)

Related Information

Cancer Chemotherapy Regimens *on page 1218-1241*

Brand Names Wellcovorin®

Synonyms Calcium Leucovorin; Citrovorum Factor; Folinic Acid; 5-Formyl Tetrahydrofolate

Use Antidote for folic acid antagonists (methotrexate [>100 mg/m^2], trimethoprim, pyrimethamine); treatment of megaloblastic anemias when folate is deficient as

(Continued)

Leucovorin Calcium *(Continued)*

in infancy, sprue, pregnancy, and nutritional deficiency when oral folate therapy is not possible; in combination with fluorouracil in the treatment of malignancy

Pregnancy Risk Factor C

Contraindications Pernicious anemia or other megaloblastic anemias where a deficiency of B_{12} is present

Warnings/Precautions Use with caution in patients with a history of hypersensitivity

Adverse Reactions

<1%:

Dermatologic: Rash, pruritus, erythema, urticaria

Hematologic: Thrombocytosis

Respiratory: Wheezing

Stability

Leucovorin injection should be stored at room temperature and protected from light

Reconstituted solution is stated to be chemically stable for 7 days

Stability of parenteral admixture at room temperature (25°C): 24 hours

Stability of parenteral admixture at refrigeration temperature (4°C): 4 days

Standard diluent: 50-100 mg/50 mL D_5W

Minimum volume: 50 mL D_5W

Concentrations >2 mg/mL of leucovorin and >25 mg/mL of fluorouracil are **incompatible** (precipitation occurs)

Mechanism of Action A reduced form of folic acid, but does not require a reduction reaction by an enzyme for activation, allows for purine and thymidine synthesis, a necessity for normal erythropoiesis; leucovorin supplies the necessary cofactor blocked by MTX, enters the cells via the same active transport system as MTX

Pharmacodynamics/Kinetics

Onset of activity:

Oral: Within 30 minutes

I.V.: Within 5 minutes

Absorption: Oral, I.M.: Rapid

Metabolism: Rapidly converted to (5MTHF) 5-methyl-tetrahydrofolate (active) in the intestinal mucosa and by the liver

Half-life:

Leucovorin: 15 minutes

5MTHF: 33-35 minutes

Elimination: Primarily in urine (80% to 90%) with small losses appearing in feces (5% to 8%)

Usual Dosage Children and Adults:

Adjunctive therapy with antimicrobial agents (pyrimethamine or trimethoprim): Oral, I.V.: 2-15 mg/day for 3 days or until blood counts are normal or 5 mg every 3 days; doses of 6 mg/day are needed for patients with platelet counts <100,000/mm^3 <graphic gr-name="leuco" title="leucovorin graph" width=250 height=180>

Folate deficient megaloblastic anemia: I.M.: 1 mg/day

Megaloblastic anemia secondary to congenital deficiency of dihydrofolate reductase: I.M.: 3-6 mg/day

Rescue dose (rescue therapy should start within 24 hours of MTX therapy): Oral, I.V.: 10 mg/m^2 to start, then 10 mg/m^2 every 6 hours orally for 72 hours until serum MTX concentration is <10^{-8}M; if serum creatinine 24 hours after methotrexate is elevated 50% or more above the pre-MTX serum creatinine **or** the serum MTX concentration is >5 x 10^{-6}M (see graph), increase dose to 100 mg/m^2/dose every 3 hours until serum methotrexate level is <1 x 10^{-8}M

The drug should be given parenterally instead or orally in patients with GI toxicity, nausea, vomiting, and when individual doses are >25 mg

Administration Leucovorin calcium should be administered I.M. or I.V.; rate of I.V. infusion should not exceed 160 mg/minute; I.V. infusion should not exceed 160 mg/minute of leucovorin

Monitoring Parameters Plasma MTX concentration as a therapeutic guide to high-dose MTX therapy with leucovorin factor rescue

Leucovorin is continued until the plasma MTX level is <1 x 10^{-7} molar

Each dose of leucovorin is increased if the plasma MTX concentration is excessively high (see table)

With 4- to 6-hour high-dose MTX infusions, plasma drug values in excess of 5 x 10^{-5} and 10^{-6} molar at 24 and 48 hours after starting the infusion, respectively, are often predictive of delayed MTX clearance; see table.

Patient Information Take exactly as directed; take at evenly spaced times day and night

Dosage Forms
Injection: 3 mg/mL (1 mL)
Powder for injection: 50 mg, 100 mg, 350 mg
Powder for oral solution: 1 mg/mL (60 mL)
Tablet: 5 mg, 15 mg, 25 mg

Leukeran® see Chlorambucil on page 218

Leukine™ see Sargramostim on page 994

Leuprolide Acetate (loo proe' lide)
Related Information
Cancer Chemotherapy Regimens on page 1218-1241
Brand Names Lupron®; Lupron Depot®; Lupron Depot-Ped™
Synonyms Leuprorelin Acetate
Use Palliative treatment of advanced prostate carcinoma (alternative when orchi-ectomy or estrogen administration are not indicated or are unacceptable to the patient); combination therapy with flutamide for treating metastatic prostatic carcinoma; endometriosis (3.75 mg depot only); central precocious puberty (may be used an agent to treat precocious puberty because of its effect in lowering levels of LH and FSH, testosterone, and estrogen).
   Unlabeled uses: Treatment of breast, ovarian, and endometrial cancer; leio-myoma uteri; infertility; prostatic hypertrophy
Pregnancy Risk Factor X
Contraindications Hypersensitivity to leuprolide; spinal cord compression (orchi-ectomy suggested); undiagnosed abnormal vaginal bleeding; women who are or may be pregnant should not receive Lupron® Depot
Warnings/Precautions Use with caution in patients hypersensitive to benzyl alcohol; after 6 months use of Depot® leuprolide, vertebral bone density decreased (average 13.5%); long-term safety of leuprolide in children has not been established; urinary tract obstruction may occur upon initiation of therapy. Closely observe patients for weakness, paresthesias, and urinary tract obstruc-tion in first few weeks of therapy. Tumor flare and bone pain may occur at initiation of therapy; transient weakness and paresthesia of lower limbs, hema-turia, and urinary tract obstruction in first week of therapy; animal studies have shown dose-related benign pituitary hyperplasia and benign pituitary adenomas after 2 years of use.
Adverse Reactions
   >10%:
      Central nervous system: Depression
      Endocrine & metabolic: Hot flashes
      Gastrointestinal: Weight gain, nausea, vomiting
      Miscellaneous: Pain
   1% to 10%:
      Cardiovascular: Cardiac arrhythmias, edema
      Central nervous system: Dizziness, lethargy, insomnia, headache
      Dermatologic: Rash
      Endocrine: Estrogenic effects (gynecomastia, breast tenderness)
      Gastrointestinal: Nausea, vomiting, diarrhea, GI bleed
      Hematologic: Decreased hemoglobin and hematocrit
      Neuromuscular & skeletal: Paresthesia, myalgia
      Ocular: Blurred vision
   <1%:
      Cardiovascular: Pulmonary embolism, myocardial infarction
      Local: Thrombophlebitis
Overdosage/Toxicology General supportive care
Stability
   Store unopened vials of injection in refrigerator, vial in use can be kept at room temperature (≤30°C/86°F) for several months with minimal loss of potency. Protect from light and store vial in carton until use. Do not freeze.
   Depot® may be stored at room temperature. Upon reconstitution, the suspension is stable for 24 hours; does not contain a preservative.
Mechanism of Action Continuous daily administration results in suppression of ovarian and testicular steroidogenesis due to decreased levels of LH and FSH with subsequent decrease in testosterone (male) and estrogen (female) levels
Pharmacodynamics/Kinetics
   Onset of action: Serum testosterone levels first increase within 3 days of therapy
   Duration: Levels decrease after 2-4 weeks with continued therapy
   Metabolism: Destroyed within the GI tract
   Bioavailability: Orally not bioavailable; S.C. and I.V. doses are comparable
   Half-life: 3-4.25 hours
   Elimination: Not well defined
Usual Dosage Requires parenteral administration
   (Continued)

Leuprolide Acetate *(Continued)*

Children: Precocious puberty:
  S.C.: 20-45 mcg/kg/day
  I.M. (Depot®) formulation: 0.3 mg/kg/dose given every 28 days
    ≤25 kg: 7.5 mg
    >25-37.5 kg: 11.25 mg
    >37.5 kg: 15 mg
Adults:
  Male: Advanced prostatic carcinoma:
    S.C.: 1 mg/day **or**
    I.M., Depot® (suspension): 7.5 mg/dose given monthly (every 28-33 days)
  Female: Endometriosis: I.M., Depot® (suspension): 3.75 mg monthly for up to 6 months

Administration When administering the Depot® form, do not use needles smaller than 22-gauge; reconstitute only with diluent provided

Monitoring Parameters Precocious puberty: GnRH testing (blood LH and FSH levels), testosterone in males and estradiol in females; closely monitor patients with prostatic carcinoma for weakness, paresthesias, and urinary tract obstruction in first few weeks of therapy

Test Interactions Interferes with pituitary gonadotropic and gonadal function tests during and up to 4-8 weeks after therapy

Patient Information Patient must be taught aseptic technique and S.C. injection technique. Rotate S.C. injection sites frequently. Disease flare (increased bone pain, urinary retention) can briefly occur with initiation of therapy. Store vials under refrigeration but do not freeze. Do not discontinue medication without physician's advice.

Nursing Implications Patient must be taught aseptic technique and S.C. injection technique. Rotate S.C. injection sites frequently. Disease flare (increased bone pain, urinary retention) can briefly occur with initiation of therapy.

Dosage Forms
  Injection: 5 mg/mL (2.8 mL)
  Powder for injection (depot):
    Depot®: 3.75 mg, 7.5 mg
    Depot-Ped™: 7.5 mg, 11.25 mg, 15 mg

Leuprorelin Acetate *see* Leuprolide Acetate *on previous page*

Leurocristine *see* Vincristine Sulfate *on page 1159*

Leustatin™ *see* Cladribine *on page 251*

Levamisole Hydrochloride *(lee vam' i sole)*

Brand Names Ergamisol®
Use Adjuvant treatment with fluorouracil in Dukes stage C colon cancer
Pregnancy Risk Factor C
Contraindications Previous hypersensitivity to the drug
Warnings/Precautions Agranulocytosis can occur asymptomatically and flu-like symptoms can occur without hematologic adverse effects; frequent hematologic monitoring is necessary
Adverse Reactions
  >10%: Gastrointestinal: Nausea, diarrhea
  1% to 10%:
    Cardiovascular: Edema
    Central nervous system: Fatigue, fever, dizziness, headache, somnolence, depression, nervousness, insomnia
    Dermatologic: Dermatitis, alopecia
    Gastrointestinal: Stomatitis, vomiting, anorexia, abdominal pain, constipation, taste perversion
    Hematologic: Leukopenia
    Neuromuscular & skeletal: Rigors, arthralgia, myalgia, paresthesia
    Miscellaneous: Infection
  <1%:
    Cardiovascular: Chest pain
    Central nervous system: Anxiety
    Dermatologic: Pruritus, urticaria
    Gastrointestinal: Flatulence, dyspepsia
    Hematologic: Thrombocytopenia, anemia, granulocytopenia
    Ocular: Abnormal tearing, blurred vision, conjunctivitis
    Miscellaneous: Epistaxis, altered sense of smell
Overdosage/Toxicology Treatment following decontamination is symptomatic and supportive

Drug Interactions
Increased toxicity/serum levels of phenytoin
Disulfiram-like reaction with alcohol
Mechanism of Action Clinically, combined therapy with levamisole and 5-fluoro-uracil has been effective in treating colon cancer patients, whereas demonstrable activity has been. Due to the broad range of pharmacologic activities of levamisole, it has been suggested that the drug may act as a biochemical modulator (of fluorouracil, for example, in colon cancer), an effect entirely independent of immune modulation. Further studies are needed to evaluate the mechanisms of action of the drug in cancer patients.

Pharmacodynamics/Kinetics
Absorption: Well absorbed
Metabolism: In the liver, >70%
Half-life, elimination: 2-6 hours
Time to peak serum concentration: 1-2 hours
Elimination: In urine and feces; elimination is virtually complete within 48 hours after an oral dose

Usual Dosage Adults: Oral: Initial: 50 mg every 8 hours for 3 days, then 50 mg every 8 hours for 3 days every 2 weeks (fluorouracil is always given concomitantly)

Dosing adjustment in hepatic impairment: May be necessary in patients with liver disease, but no specific guidelines are available
Monitoring Parameters CBC with platelet count prior to therapy and weekly prior to treatment; LFTs every 3 months
Patient Information Notify physician immediately if flu-like symptoms appear; may cause dizziness, drowsiness, impair judgment or coordination
Dosage Forms Tablet, as base: 50 mg

Levarterenol Bitartrate *see* Norepinephrine Bitartrate *on page 804*

Levlen® *see* Ethinyl Estradiol and Levonorgestrel *on page 423*

Levobunolol Hydrochloride (lee voe byoo' noe lole)
Related Information
Glaucoma Drug Therapy Comparison *on page 1270*
Brand Names AKBeta®; Betagan®
Synonyms *l*-Bunolol Hydrochloride
Use To lower intraocular pressure in chronic open-angle glaucoma or ocular hypertension
Pregnancy Risk Factor C
Contraindications Known hypersensitivity to levobunolol; bronchial asthma, severe COPD, sinus bradycardia, second or third degree A-V block, cardiac failure, cardiogenic shock
Warnings/Precautions Use with caution in patients with congestive heart failure, diabetes mellitus, hyperthyroidism; contains metabisulfite. Because systemic absorption does occur with ophthalmic administration, the elderly with other disease states or syndromes that may be affected by a beta-blocker (CHF, COPD, etc) should be monitored closely.
Adverse Reactions
>10%: Ocular: Stinging/burning of eye
1% to 10%:
Cardiovascular: Bradycardia, arrhythmia, hypotension
Central nervous system: Dizziness, headache
Dermatologic: Alopecia, erythema
Local: Stinging, burning
Ocular: Blepharoconjunctivitis, conjunctivitis
Respiratory: Bronchospasm
<1%:
Dermatologic: Skin rash
Local: Itching
Ocular: Visual disturbances, keratitis, decreased visual acuity
Overdosage/Toxicology Symptoms of intoxication include cardiac disturbances, CNS toxicity, bronchospasm, hypoglycemia and hyperkalemia. The most common cardiac symptoms include hypotension and bradycardia; atrioventricular block, intraventricular conduction disturbances, cardiogenic shock, and systole may occur with severe overdose, especially with membrane-depressant drugs (eg, propranolol); CNS effects include convulsions, coma, and respiratory arrest is commonly seen with propranolol and other membrane-depressant and lipid-soluble drugs

Treatment includes symptomatic treatment of seizures, hypotension, hyperkalemia and hypoglycemia; bradycardia and hypotension resistant to atropine, (Continued)

Levobunolol Hydrochloride (Continued)

isoproterenol or pacing may respond to glucagon; wide QRS defects caused by the membrane-depressant poisoning may respond to hypertonic sodium bicarbonate; repeat-dose charcoal, hemoperfusion, or hemodialysis may be helpful in removal of only those beta-blockers with a small V_d, long half-life or low intrinsic clearance (acebutolol, atenolol, nadolol, sotalol).

Drug Interactions

Increased toxicity:

Systemic beta-adrenergic blocking agents

Ophthalmic epinephrine (increased blood pressure/loss of IOP effect)

Quinidine (sinus bradycardia)

Verapamil (bradycardia and asystole have been reported)

Mechanism of Action A nonselective beta-adrenergic blocking agent that lowers intraocular pressure by reducing aqueous humor production and possibly increases the outflow of aqueous humor

Pharmacodynamics/Kinetics

Onset of action: Decreases in intraocular pressure (IOP) can be noted within 1 hour

Peak effect: 2-6 hours

Duration: 1-7 days

· Elimination: Not well defined

Usual Dosage Adults: Instill 1 drop in the affected eye(s) 1-2 times/day

Monitoring Parameters Intraocular pressure, heart rate, funduscopic exam, visual field testing

Patient Information May sting on instillation, do not touch dropper to eye; visual acuity may be decreased after administration; night vision may be decreased; distance vision may be altered; apply finger pressure between the bridge of the nose and corner of the eye to decrease systemic absorption; assess patient's or caregiver's ability to administer

Nursing Implications Apply finger pressure over nasolacrimal duct to decrease systemic absorption

Dosage Forms Solution: 0.25% [2.5 mg/mL] (5 mL, 10 mL); 0.5% [5 mg/mL] (2 mL, 5 mL, 10 mL, 15 mL)

Levocabastine Hydrochloride (lee' voe kab as teen hye droe klor' ide)

Brand Names Livostin®

Use Treatment of allergic conjunctivitis

Pregnancy Risk Factor B

Contraindications Hypersensitivity to any component of product; while soft contact lenses are being worn

Warnings/Precautions Safety and efficacy in children <12 years of age have not been established; not for injection; not for use in patients wearing soft contact lenses during treatment

Adverse Reactions

>10%: Local: Transient burning, stinging, discomfort

1% to 10%:

Central nervous system: Headache, somnolence, fatigue

Dermatologic: Rash

Genitourinary: Dry mouth

Ocular: Blurred vision, eye pain, somnolence, red eyes, eyelid edema

Respiratory: Dyspnea

Mechanism of Action Potent, selective histamine H_1-receptor antagonist for topical ophthalmic use

Pharmacodynamics/Kinetics Absorption: Topical: Systemically absorbed

Usual Dosage Children >12 years and Adults: Instill 1 drop in affected eye(s) 4 times/day for up to 2 weeks

Dosage Forms Solution, ophthalmic: 0.05% (2.5 mL, 5 mL, 10 mL)

Levodopa (lee voe doe' pa)

Brand Names Dopar®; Larodopa®

Synonyms L-3-Hydroxytyrosine; L-Dopa

Use Treatment of Parkinson's disease; used as a diagnostic agent for growth hormone deficiency

Pregnancy Risk Factor C

Contraindications Hypersensitivity to levodopa or any component; narrow-angle glaucoma, MAO inhibitor therapy, melanomas or any undiagnosed skin lesions

Warnings/Precautions Use with caution in patients with history of myocardial infarction, arrhythmias, asthma, wide-angle glaucoma, peptic ulcer disease;

sudden discontinuation of levodopa may cause a worsening of Parkinson's disease; some products may contain tartrazine. Elderly may be more sensitive to CNS effects of levodopa.

Adverse Reactions

>10%:

Cardiovascular: Orthostatic hypotension, arrhythmias

Central nervous system: Choreiform and involuntary movements, dizziness, anxiety, confusion, nightmares

Gastrointestinal: Anorexia, nausea, vomiting, constipation

Ophthalmic: Blepharospasm

Renal: Difficult urination

1% to 10%:

Central nervous system: Headache

Gastrointestinal: Anorexia, diarrhea, dry mouth

Neuromuscular & skeletal: Muscle twitching

Ocular: Eyelid spasms

Renal: Discoloration of urine/sweat

<1%:

Cardiovascular: Hypertension

Gastrointestinal: Duodenal ulcer, GI bleeding

Hematologic: Hemolytic anemia

Ocular: Blurred vision

Overdosage/Toxicology Symptoms of overdose include palpitations, arrhythmias, spasms, hypertension or hypotension; use fluids judiciously to maintain pressures; may precipitate a variety of arrhythmias

Drug Interactions

Decreased effect:

Hydantoins → ↓ effectiveness

Phenothiazines and hypotensive agents → ↓ effect of levodopa

Pyridoxine → ↑ peripheral conversion, → ↓ levodopa effectiveness

Increased toxicity:

Monoamine oxidase inhibitors → hypertensive reactions

Antacids → ↑ levodopa

Mechanism of Action Increases dopamine levels in the brain, then stimulates dopaminergic receptors in the basal ganglia to improve the balance between cholinergic and dopaminergic activity

Pharmacodynamics/Kinetics

Time to peak serum concentration: Oral: 1-2 hours

Metabolism: Majority of drug is peripherally decarboxylated to dopamine; small amounts of levodopa reach the brain where it is also decarboxylated to active dopamine

Half-life: 1.2-2.3 hours

Elimination: Primarily in urine (80%) as dopamine, norepinephrine, and homovanillic acid

Usual Dosage Oral:

Children (given as a single dose to evaluate growth hormone deficiency): 0.5 g/m^2 **or**

<30 lbs: 125 mg

30-70 lbs: 250 mg

>70 lbs: 500 mg

Adults (administer with food): 500-1000 mg/day in divided doses every 6-12 hours; increase by 100-750 mg/day every 3-7 days until response or total dose of 8000 mg/day is reached

Significant therapeutic response may not be obtained for 6 months

Monitoring Parameters Serum growth hormone concentration

Test Interactions False-positive reaction for urinary glucose with Clinitest®; false-negative reaction using Clinistix®; false-positive urine ketones with Acetest®, Ketostix®, Labstix®

Patient Information Avoid vitamins with B_6 (pyridoxine); can take with food to prevent GI upset; do not stop taking this drug even if you do not think it is working; dizziness, lightheadedness, fainting may occur when you get up from a sitting or lying position.

Nursing Implications Give with meals to decrease GI upset; sustained release product should not be crushed

Dosage Forms

Capsule: 100 mg, 250 mg, 500 mg

Tablet: 100 mg, 250 mg, 500 mg

Levodopa and Carbidopa (lee voe doe' pa & kar bi doe' pa

Brand Names Sinemet®

Synonyms Carbidopa and Levodopa

(Continued)

Levodopa and Carbidopa *(Continued)*

Use
Treatment of parkinsonian syndrome

50-100 mg/day of carbidopa is needed to block the peripheral conversion of levodopa to dopamine. "On-off" can be managed by giving smaller, more frequent doses of Sinemet® or adding a dopamine agonist or selegiline; when adding a new agent, doses of Sinemet® should usually be decreased.

Pregnancy Risk Factor C

Contraindications
Narrow-angle glaucoma, MAO inhibitors, hypersensitivity to levodopa, carbidopa, or any component; do not use in patients with malignant melanoma or undiagnosed skin lesions

Warnings/Precautions
Use with caution in patients with history of myocardial infarction, arrhythmias, asthma, wide angle glaucoma, peptic ulcer disease; sudden discontinuation of levodopa may cause a worsening of Parkinson's disease; some tablets may contain tartrazine. The elderly may be more sensitive to the CNS effects of levodopa. Protein in the diet should be distributed throughout the day to avoid fluctuations in levodopa absorption.

Adverse Reactions
>10%:
- Cardiovascular: Orthostatic hypotension, palpitations, cardiac arrhythmias
- Central nervous system: Confusion, nightmares, dizziness, anxiety
- Gastrointestinal: Nausea, vomiting, anorexia, constipation
- Neuromuscular & skeletal: Dystonic movements, "on-off", choreiform and involuntary movements
- Ocular: Blepharospasm
- Renal: Difficult urination

1% to 10%:
- Gastrointestinal: Anorexia, diarrhea, dry mouth
- Central nervous system: Headache, muscle twitching
- Ocular: Eyelid spasms
- Miscellaneous: Discoloration of urine/sweat

<1%:
- Cardiovascular: Hypertension
- Central nervous system: Memory loss, nervousness, anxiety, insomnia, fatigue, hallucinations, ataxia
- Gastrointestinal: Duodenal ulcer, GI bleeding
- Hematologic: Hemolytic anemia
- Ocular: Blurred vision

Overdosage/Toxicology
Symptoms of overdose include palpitations, arrhythmias, spasms, hypotension; may cause hypertension or hypotension; treatment is supportive; initiate gastric lavage, administer I.V. fluids judiciously and monitor EKG; use fluids judiciously to maintain pressures; may precipitate a variety of arrhythmias

Drug Interactions
Decreased effect:
- Hydantoins → ↓ effectiveness
- Phenothiazines and hypotensive agents → ↓ effect of levodopa

Increased toxicity:
- Monoamine oxidase inhibitors → hypertensive reactions
- Antacids → ↑ levodopa

Mechanism of Action
Parkinson's symptoms are due to a lack of striatal dopamine; levodopa circulates in the plasma to the blood-brain-barrier (BBB), where it crosses, to be converted by striatal enzymes to dopamine; carbidopa inhibits the peripheral plasma breakdown of levodopa by inhibiting its decarboxylation, and thereby increases available levodopa at the BBB

Pharmacodynamics/Kinetics
Carbidopa:
- Absorption: Oral: 40% to 70%
- Protein binding: 36%
- Half-life: 1-2 hours
- Elimination: Excreted unchanged

Levodopa:
- Absorption: May be decreased if given with a high protein meal
- Half-life: 1.2-2.3 hours
- Elimination: Primarily in urine (80%) as dopamine, norepinephrine, and homovanillic acid

Usual Dosage
Oral:
- Adults: Initial: 25/100 2-4 times/day, increase as necessary to a maximum of 200/2000 mg/day
- Elderly: Initial: 25/100 twice daily, increase as necessary

Conversion from Sinemet® to Sinemet® CR (50/200): (Sinemet® [total daily dose of levodopa] / Sinemet® CR)
300-400 mg / 1 tablet twice daily
500-600 mg / 1½ tablets twice daily or one 3 times/day
700-800 mg / 4 tablets in 3 or more divided doses
900-1000 mg / 5 tablets in 3 or more divided doses
Intervals between doses of Sinemet® CR should be 4-8 hours while awake

Monitoring Parameters Blood pressure, standing and sitting/supine; symptoms of parkinsonism, dyskinesias, mental status

Test Interactions False-positive reaction for urinary glucose with Clinitest®; false-negative reaction using Clinistix®; false-positive urine ketones with Acetest®, Ketostix®, Labstix®

Patient Information Do not stop taking this drug even if you do not think it is working; take on an empty stomach if possible; if GI distress occurs, take with meals; rise carefully from lying or sitting position as dizziness, lightheadedness, or fainting may occur; do not crush or chew sustained release product

Nursing Implications Space doses evenly over the waking hours; give with meals to decrease GI upset; sustained release product should not be crushed

Dosage Forms Tablet:
10/100: Carbidopa 10 mg and levodopa 100 mg
25/100: Carbidopa 25 mg and levodopa 100 mg
25/250: Carbidopa 25 mg and levodopa 250 mg
Sustained release: Carbidopa 50 mg and levodopa 200 mg

Levo-Dromoran® see Levorphanol Tartrate *on next page*

Levo-epinephrine *see* Epinephrine *on page 389*

Levomepromazine *see* Methotrimeprazine Hydrochloride *on page 715*

Levomethadyl Acetate Hydrochloride (lee voe meth' a dil)
Brand Names ORLAAM®
Use Management of opiate dependence
Restrictions C-II; must be dispensed in a designated clinic setting only
Warnings/Precautions Not recommended for uses outside of the treatment of opiate addiction; shall be dispensed only by treatment programs approved by FDA, DEA, and the designated state authority. Approved treatment programs shall dispense and use levomethadyl in oral form only and according to the treatment requirements stipulated in federal regulations. Failure to abide by these requirements may result in injunction precluding operation of the program, seizure of the drug supply, revocation of the program approval, and possible criminal prosecution.
Adverse Reactions
>10%:
Cardiovascular: Bradycardia, hypotension
Central nervous system: Drowsiness
Gastrointestinal: Nausea, vomiting
Respiratory: Respiratory depression
1% to 10%:
Cardiovascular: Peripheral vasodilation, orthostatic hypotension, increased intracranial pressure
Central nervous system: Dizziness/vertigo, CNS depression, confusion, sedation
Endocrine & metabolic: Antidiuretic hormone release
Gastrointestinal: Constipation
Ocular: Miosis, blurred vision
Miscellaneous: Biliary or urinary tract spasm
Drug Interactions Decreased effect/levels with phenobarbital
Usual Dosage Adults: Oral: 20-40 mg 3 times/week, with ranges of 10 mg to as high as 140 mg 3 times/week; always dilute before administration and mix with diluent prior to dispensing
Monitoring Parameters Patient adherence with regimen and avoidance of illicit substances; random drug testing is recommended
Nursing Implications Drug administration and dispensing is to take place in an authorized clinic setting only; can potentially cause Q-T prolongation on EKG (not dose related)
Dosage Forms Solution, oral: 10 mg/mL (474 mL)

Levonorgestrel (lee' voe nor jess trel)
Brand Names Norplant®
Use Prevention of pregnancy. The net cumulative 5 year pregnancy rate for levonorgestrel implant use has been reported to be from 1.5-3.9 pregnancies/100
(Continued)
627

Levonorgestrel *(Continued)*

users. Norplant® is a very efficient, yet reversible, method of contraception. The long duration of action may be particularly advantageous in women who desire an extended period of contraceptive protection without sacrificing the possibility of future fertility.

Pregnancy Risk Factor X

Contraindications Women with undiagnosed abnormal uterine bleeding, hemorrhagic diathesis, known or suspected pregnancy, active hepatic disease, active thrombophlebitis, thromboembolic disorders, or known or suspected carcinoma of the breast

Warnings/Precautions Patients presenting with lower abdominal pain should be evaluated for follicular atresia and ectopic pregnancy

Adverse Reactions

>10%: Hormonal: Prolonged menstrual flow, spotting

1% to 10%:

Central nervous system: Headache, nervousness, dizziness

Dermatologic: Dermatitis, acne

Endocrine & metabolic: Amenorrhea, irregular menstrual cycles, scanty bleeding, breast discharge

Gastrointestinal: Nausea, change in appetite, weight gain

Genitourinary: Vaginitis, leukorrhea

Neuromuscular & skeletal: Myalgia

Miscellaneous: Pain or itching at implant site

<1%: Miscellaneous: Infection at implant site

Overdosage/Toxicology Can result if >6 capsules are *in situ*; symptoms include uterine bleeding irregularities and fluid retention; treatment includes removal of all implanted capsules

Drug Interactions Decreased effect: Carbamazepine/phenytoin

Mechanism of Action First, ovulation is inhibited in about 50% to 60% of implant users from a negative feedback mechanism on the hypothalamus, leading to reduced secretion of follicle stimulating hormone (FSH) and luteinizing hormone (LH). An insufficient luteal phase has also been demonstrated with levonorgestrel administration and may result from defective gonadotropin stimulation of the ovary or from a direct effect of the drug on progesterone synthesis by the corpora lutea.

Pharmacodynamics/Kinetics

Protein binding: Following release from the implant, levonorgestrel enters the blood stream highly bound to sex hormone binding globulin (SHBG), albumin, and alpha$_1$ glycoprotein

Metabolism: In the liver

Half-life, terminal: 11-45 hours

Elimination: In urine primarily as conjugates of sulfate and glucuronide

Usual Dosage Total administration doses (implanted): 216 mg in 6 capsules which should be implanted during the first 7 days of onset of menses subdermally in the upper arm; each Norplant® silastic capsule releases 80 mcg of drug/day for 6-18 months, following which a rate of release of 25-30 mcg/day is maintained for ≤5 years; capsules should be removed by end of 5th year

Patient Information Notify physician if unusual or persistent nausea, vomiting, abdominal pain, dark urine, or pale stools; may cause changes in vision or contact lens tolerability

Dosage Forms Capsule, subdermal implantation: 36 mg (6s)

Levonorgestrel and Ethinyl Estradiol *see* Ethinyl Estradiol and Levonorgestrel *on page 423*

Levophed® *see* Norepinephrine Bitartrate *on page 804*

Levoprome® *see* Methotrimeprazine Hydrochloride *on page 715*

Levora® *see* Ethinyl Estradiol and Levonorgestrel *on page 423*

Levorphanol Tartrate *(lee vor' fa nole)*

Related Information

Narcotic Agonist Comparison Charts *on page 1274-1275*

Brand Names Levo-Dromoran®

Synonyms Levorphan Tartrate

Use Relief of moderate to severe pain; also used parenterally for preoperative sedation and an adjunct to nitrous oxide/oxygen anesthesia; 2 mg levorphanol produces analgesia comparable to that produced by 10 mg of morphine

Restrictions C-II

Pregnancy Risk Factor B (D if used for prolonged periods or in high doses at term)

Contraindications Hypersensitivity to levorphanol or any component

Warnings/Precautions Use with caution in patients with hypersensitivity reactions to other phenanthrene derivative opioid agonists (morphine, hydrocodone, hydromorphone, levorphanol, oxycodone, oxymorphone); respiratory diseases including asthma, emphysema, COPD or severe liver or renal insufficiency; some preparations contain sulfites which may cause allergic reactions; may be habit-forming; dextromethorphan has equivalent antitussive activity but has much lower toxicity in accidental overdose. Elderly may be particularly susceptible to the CNS depressant and constipating effects of narcotics.

Adverse Reactions
>10%:
  Cardiovascular: Palpitations, hypotension, bradycardia, peripheral vasodilation
  Central nervous system: CNS depression, weakness, tiredness, drowsiness, dizziness
  Dermatologic: Pruritus
  Gastrointestinal: Nausea, vomiting
1% to 10%:
  Central nervous system: Nervousness, headache, restlessness, anorexia, malaise, confusion
  Gastrointestinal: Stomach cramps, dry mouth, constipation
  Endocrine & metabolic: Antidiuretic hormone release
  Genitourinary: Decreased urination
  Local: Pain at injection site
  Ocular: Miosis
  Respiratory: Respiratory depression
  Miscellaneous: Biliary or urinary tract spasm
<1%:
  Central nervous system: Paralytic ileus, mental depression, histamine release, hallucinations, paradoxical CNS stimulation, increased intracranial pressure
  Dermatologic: Skin rash, hives
  Sensitivity reactions: Histamine release
  Miscellaneous: Physical and psychological dependence

Overdosage/Toxicology Symptoms of overdose include CNS depression, respiratory depression, miosis, apnea, pulmonary edema, convulsions; naloxone 2 mg I.V. (0.01 mg/kg for children) with repeat administration as necessary up to a total of 10 mg

Drug Interactions Increased toxicity: CNS depressants ↑ CNS depression

Stability Store at room temperature, protect from freezing; I.V. is **incompatible** when mixed with aminophylline, barbiturates, heparin, methicillin, phenytoin, sodium bicarbonate

Mechanism of Action Levorphanol tartrate is a synthetic opioid agonist that is classified as a morphinan derivative. Opioids interact with stereospecific opioid receptors in various parts of the central nervous system and other tissues. Analgesic potency parallels the affinity for these binding sites. These drugs do not alter the threshold or responsiveness to pain, but the perception of pain.

Usual Dosage Adults:
  Oral: 2 mg every 6-24 hours as needed
  S.C.: 2 mg, up to 3 mg if necessary, every 6-8 hours

  Dosing adjustment in hepatic disease: Reduction is necessary in patients with liver disease

Monitoring Parameters Pain relief, respiratory and mental status, blood pressure

Patient Information Avoid alcohol, may cause drowsiness, impaired judgment or coordination; may cause physical and psychological dependence with prolonged use

Nursing Implications Observe patient for excessive sedation, respiratory depression; implement safety measures, assist with ambulation

Dosage Forms
  Injection: 2 mg/mL (1 mL, 10 mL)
  Tablet: 2 mg

Levorphan Tartrate see Levorphanol Tartrate on previous page

Levo-T™ see Levothyroxine Sodium on this page

Levothroid® see Levothyroxine Sodium on this page

Levothyroxine Sodium (lee voe thye rox' een)
Brand Names Eltroxin™; Levo-T™; Levothroid®; Levoxyl™; Synthroid®
Synonyms L-Thyroxine Sodium; T_4
Use Replacement or supplemental therapy in hypothyroidism; some clinicians suggest levothyroxine is the drug of choice for replacement therapy
Pregnancy Risk Factor A
(Continued)

Levothyroxine Sodium *(Continued)*

Contraindications Recent myocardial infarction or thyrotoxicosis, uncorrected adrenal insufficiency, hypersensitivity to levothyroxine sodium or any component

Warnings/Precautions Ineffective for weight reduction; high doses may produce serious or even life-threatening toxic effects particularly when used with some anoretic drugs. Use with caution and reduce dosage in patients with angina pectoris or other cardiovascular disease; levothyroxine tablets contain tartrazine dye which may cause allergic reactions in susceptible individuals; use cautiously in elderly since they may be more likely to have compromised cardiovascular functions. Patients with adrenal insufficiency, myxedema, diabetes mellitus and insipidus may have symptoms exaggerated or aggravated; thyroid replacement requires periodic assessment of thyroid status. Chronic hypothyroidism predisposes patients to coronary artery disease.

Adverse Reactions

<1%:

Cardiovascular: Palpitations, cardiac arrhythmias, tachycardia, chest pain

Central nervous system: Nervousness, sweating, headache, insomnia, fever, clumsiness

Dermatologic: Hair loss

Endocrine: Changes in menstrual cycle

Gastrointestinal: Weight loss, increased appetite, diarrhea, abdominal cramps, constipation

Neuromuscular & skeletal: Muscle aches, hand tremors, tremor

Respiratory: Shortness of breath

Overdosage/Toxicology Chronic overdose may cause weight loss, nervousness, sweating, tachycardia, insomnia, heat intolerance, menstrual irregularities, palpitations, psychosis, fever; acute overdose may cause fever, hypoglycemia, CHF, unrecognized adrenal insufficiency. Chronic overdose is treated by withdrawal of the drug; massive overdose may require beta-blockers for increased sympathomimetic activity. Reduce dose or temporarily discontinue therapy; normal hypothalamic-pituitary-thyroid axis will return to normal in 6-8 weeks serum T_4 levels do not correlate well with toxicity. In massive acute ingestion reduce GI absorption, give general supportive care; treat congestive heart failure with digitalis glycosides; excessive adrenergic activity (tachycardia) requires propranolol 1-3 mg I.V. over 10 minutes or 80-160 mg orally/day; fever may be treated with acetaminophen.

Drug Interactions

Decreased effect:

Phenytoin → ↓ levothyroxine levels

Cholestyramine → ↓ absorption of levothyroxine

Increases oral hypoglycemic requirements

Increased effect: Increased effects of oral anticoagulants

Increased toxicity: Tricyclic antidepressants → ↑ toxic potential of both drugs

Stability Protect tablets from light; do not mix I.V. solution with other I.V. infusion solutions; reconstituted solutions should be used immediately and any unused portions discarded

Mechanism of Action Exact mechanism of action is unknown; however, it is believed the thyroid hormone exerts its many metabolic effects through control of DNA transcription and protein synthesis; involved in normal metabolism, growth and development; promotes gluconeogenesis, increases utilization and mobilization of glycogen stores, and stimulates protein synthesis, increases basal metabolic rate

Pharmacodynamics/Kinetics

Onset of therapeutic effect:

Oral: 3-5 days

I.V. Within 6-8 hours

Peak effect: I.V.: Within 24 hours

Absorption: Oral: Erratic

Metabolism: In the liver to tri-iodothyronine (active)

Time to peak serum concentration: 2-4 hours

Elimination: In feces and urine

Usual Dosage

Children:

Oral:

0-6 months: 8-10 mcg/kg/day or 25-50 mcg/day

6-12 months: 6-8 mcg/kg/day or 50-75 mcg/day

1-5 years: 5-6 mcg/kg/day or 75-100 mcg/day

6-12 years: 4-5 mcg/kg/day or 100-150 mcg/day

>12 years: 2-3 mcg/kg/day or ≥150 mcg/day

I.M., I.V.: 50% to 75% of the oral dose

Adults:

Oral: 12.5-50 mcg/day to start, then increase by 25-50 mcg/day at intervals of 2-4 weeks; average adult dose: 100-200 mcg/day

I.V., I.M.: 50% of the oral dose

Myxedema coma or stupor: I.V.: 200-500 mcg one time, then 100-300 mcg the next day if necessary

Administration Dilute vial with 5 mL normal saline; use immediately after reconstitution; give by direct I.V. infusion over a 2- to 3-minute period; I.V. form must be prepared immediately prior to administration; should not be admixed with other solutions

Monitoring Parameters Thyroid function test (serum thyroxine, thyrotropin concentrations), resin tri-iodothyronine uptake (RT_3U), free thyroxine index (FTI), T_4, TSH, heart rate, blood pressure, clinical signs of hypo- and hyperthyroidism; TSH is the most reliable guide for evaluating adequacy of thyroid replacement dosage. TSH may be elevated during the first few months of thyroid replacement despite patients being clinically euthyroid. In cases where T_4 remains low and TSH is within normal limits, an evaluation of "free" (unbound) T_4 is needed to evaluate further increase in dosage

Reference Range Pediatrics: Cord T_4 and values in the first few weeks are much higher, falling over the first months and years. ≥10 years: ~5.8-11 µg/dL (SI: 75-142 nmol/L). Borderline low: ≤4.5-5.7 µg/dL (SI: 58-73 nmol/L); low: ≤4.4 µg/dL (SI: 57 nmol/L); results <2.5 µg/dL (SI: <32 nmol/L) are strong evidence for hypothyroidism.

Approximate adult normal range: 4-12 µg/dL (SI: 51-154 nmol/L). Borderline high: 11.1-13 µg/dL (SI: 143-167 nmol/L); high: ≥13.1 µg/dL (SI: 169 nmol/L). Normal range is increased in women on birth control pills (5.5-12 µg/dL); normal range in pregnancy: ~5.5-16 µg/dL (SI: ~71-206 nmol/L). TSH: 0.4-10 (for those ≥80 years) mIU/L; T_4: 4-12 µg/dL (SI: 51-154 nmol/L); T_3 (RIA) (total T_3): 80-230 ng/dL (SI: 1.2-3.5 nmol/L); T_4 free (free T_4): 0.7-1.8 ng/dL (SI: 9-23 pmol/L).

Test Interactions Many drugs may have effects on thyroid function tests; para-aminosalicylic acid, aminoglutethimide, amiodarone, barbiturates, carbamazepine, chloral hydrate, clofibrate, colestipol, corticosteroids, danazol, diazepam, estrogens, ethionamide, fluorouracil, I.V. heparin, insulin, lithium, methadone, methimazole, mitotane, nitroprusside, oxyphenbutazone, phenylbutazone, PTU, perphenazine, phenytoin, propranolol, salicylates, sulfonylureas, and thiazides

Patient Information Do not change brands without physician's knowledge; report immediately to physician any chest pain, increased pulse, palpitations, heat intolerances, excessive sweating; do not discontinue without notifying your physician

Nursing Implications I.V. form must be prepared immediately prior to administration; should not be admixed with other solutions

Additional Information Levothroid® tablets contain lactose and tartrazine dye

To convert doses: Levothyroxine 0.05-0.06 mg is equivalent to 60 mg thyroid USP; 60 mg thyroglobulin; 4.5 mg thyroid strong; 1 grain (60 mg) liotrix

Dosage Forms

Injection: 0.2 mg/vial (6 mL, 10 mL); 0.5 mg/vial (6 mL, 10 mL)

Tablet: 0.025 mg, 0.05 mg, 0.075 mg, 0.088 mg, 0.1 mg, 0.112 mg, 0.125 mg, 0.137 mg, 0.15 mg, 0.175 mg, 0.2 mg, 0.3 mg

Levoxyl™ see Levothyroxine Sodium on page 629

Levsin® see Hyoscyamine Sulfate on page 559

Levsinex® see Hyoscyamine Sulfate on page 559

LH-RH see Gonadorelin on page 510

l-Hyoscyamine Sulfate see Hyoscyamine Sulfate on page 559

Libritabs® see Chlordiazepoxide on page 221

Librium® see Chlordiazepoxide on page 221

Lidex® see Fluocinonide on page 470

Lidex-E® see Fluocinonide on page 470

Lidocaine and Epinephrine (lye' doe kane & ep i nef' rin)

Brand Names Xylocaine® With Epinephrine

Use Local infiltration anesthesia; AVS for nerve block

Pregnancy Risk Factor B

Contraindications Hypersensitivity to local anesthetics of the amide type, myasthenia gravis, shock, or cardiac conduction disease

Warnings/Precautions Do not use solutions in distal portions of the body (digits, nose, ears, penis); use with caution in endocrine, heart, hepatic, or thyroid disease

(Continued)

Lidocaine and Epinephrine *(Continued)*

Adverse Reactions Refer to Lidocaine monograph

Overdosage/Toxicology Refer to Lidocaine monograph

Drug Interactions MAO inhibitors, tricyclic antidepressants, vasopressors, ergot-type anesthetics

Stability Solutions with epinephrine should be protected from light

Mechanism of Action Lidocaine blocks both the initiation and conduction of nerve impulses via decreased permeability of sodium ions; epinephrine increases the duration of action of lidocaine by causing vasoconstriction (via alpha effects) which slows the vascular absorption of lidocaine

Pharmacodynamics/Kinetics

Peak effect: Within 5 minutes

Duration: ~2 hours, dependent on dose and anesthetic procedure

Usual Dosage

Children: Use lidocaine concentrations of 0.5% to 1% (or even more diluted) to decrease possibility of toxicity; lidocaine dose should not exceed 7 mg/kg/dose; do not repeat within 2 hours

Adults: Dosage varies with the anesthetic procedure, degree of anesthesia needed, vascularity of tissue, duration of anesthesia required, and physical condition of patient

Nursing Implications Before injecting, withdraw syringe plunger to ensure injection is not into vein or artery

Additional Information Contains metabisulfites

Dosage Forms Injection with epinephrine:

1:200,000: Lidocaine hydrochloride 0.5% [5 mg/mL] (50 mL); 1% [10 mg/mL] (30 mL); 1.5% [15 mg/mL] (5 mL, 10 mL, 30 mL); 2% [20 mg/mL] (20 mL)

1:100,000: Lidocaine hydrochloride 1% [10 mg/mL] (20 mL, 50 mL); 2% [20 mg/mL] (1.8 mL, 20 mL, 50 mL)

1:50,000: Lidocaine hydrochloride 2% [20 mg/mL] (1.8 mL)

Lidocaine and Prilocaine *(lye' doe kane & pril' oh kane)*

Brand Names EMLA®

Use Topical anesthetic for use on normal intact skin to provide local analgesia for minor procedures such as I.V. cannulation or venipuncture; has also been used for painful procedures such as lumbar puncture and skin graft harvesting

Pregnancy Risk Factor B

Contraindications Known hypersensitivity to lidocaine, prilocaine, any component or local anesthetics of the amide type; patients with congenital or idiopathic methemoglobinemia, infants <1 month of age, infants <12 months of age who are receiving concurrent treatment with methemoglobin-inducing agents (ie, sulfas acetaminophen, benzocaine, chloroquine, dapsone, nitrofurantoin, nitroglycerin nitroprusside, phenobarbital, phenytoin)

Adverse Reactions

1% to 10%:

Dermatologic: Angioedema

Local: Contact dermatitis, burning, stinging

<1%:

Cardiovascular: Bradycardia, hypotension, shock

Central nervous system: Nervousness, euphoria, confusion, dizziness, drowsiness, convulsions, CNS excitation

Hematologic: Methemoglobinemia in infants

Local: Erythema, edema, blanching, itching, rash, alteration in temperature sensation, urticaria, tenderness

Neuromuscular & skeletal: Tremors

Ocular: Blurred vision

Otic: Tinnitus

Respiratory: Respiratory depression, bronchospasm

Drug Interactions

Increased toxicity:

Class I antiarrhythmic drugs (tocainide, mexiletine): Effects are additive and potentially synergistic

Drugs known to induce methemoglobinemia

Stability Store at room temperature

Mechanism of Action Local anesthetic action occurs by stabilization of neuronal membranes and inhibiting the ionic fluxes required for the initiation and conduction of impulses

Pharmacodynamics/Kinetics

Onset of action: 1 hour for sufficient dermal analgesia

Peak effect: 2-3 hours

Duration: 1-2 hours after removal of the cream

Absorption: Related to the duration of application and to the area over which it is applied
3-hour application: 3.6% lidocaine and 6.1% prilocaine were absorbed
24-hour application: 16.2% lidocaine and 33.5% prilocaine were absorbed
Distribution: Both cross the blood-brain barrier
V_d:
Lidocaine: 1.1-2.1 L/kg
Prilocaine: 0.7-4.4 L/kg
Protein binding:
Lidocaine: 70%
Prilocaine: 55%
Metabolism:
Lidocaine: Metabolized by the liver to inactive and active metabolites
Prilocaine: Metabolized in both the liver and kidneys
Half-life:
Lidocaine: 65-150 minutes, prolonged with cardiac or hepatic dysfunction
Prilocaine: 10-150 minutes, prolonged in hepatic or renal dysfunction

Usual Dosage Children and Adults:
EMLA® cream should not be used in infants under the age of 1 month or in infants, under the age of 12 months, who are receiving treatment with methemogloblin-inducing agents
Choose 2 application sites available for intravenous access
Apply a thick layer (2.5 g/site - ½ of a 5 g tube) of cream to each designated site of intact skin
Cover each site with the occlusive dressing (Tegaderm®)
Mark the time on the dressing
Allow at least 1-hour for optimum therapeutic effect. Remove the dressing and wipe off excess EMLA® cream (gloves should be worn).

EMLA® Cream Maximum Recommended Application Area* for Infants and Children Based on Application to Intact Skin

Body Weight (kg)	Maximum Application Area (cm²)†
<10 kg	100
10-20 kg	600
>20 kg	2000

*These are broad guidelines for avoiding systemic toxicity in applying EMLA® to patients with normal intact skin and with normal renal and hepatic function.
†For more individualized calculation of how much lidocaine and prilocaine may be absorbed, use the following estimates of lidocaine and prilocaine absorption for children and adults:
Estimated mean (±SD) absorption of lidocaine: 0.045 (±0.016) mg/cm² /h.
Estimated mean (±SD) absorption of prilocaine: 0.077 (±0.036) mg/cm² /h.

Debilitated patients, small children or patients with impaired elimination (ie, hepatic or renal dysfunction): Smaller areas of treatment are recommended
Patient Information Not for ophthalmic use; for external use only. EMLA® may block sensation in the treated skin.
Nursing Implications In small infants and children, an occlusive bandage should be placed over the EMLA® cream to prevent the child from placing the cream in his mouth
Dosage Forms Cream: Lidocaine 2.5% and prilocaine 2.5% [2 Tegaderm® dressings] (5 g, 30 g)

Lidocaine Hydrochloride (lye′ doe kane)
Related Information
Antiarrhythmic Drugs *on page 1246-1248*
Brand Names Anestacon®; Dalcaine®; Dilocaine®; Duo-Trach®; LidoPen®; Nervocaine®; Octocaine®; Xylocaine®
Synonyms Lignocaine Hydrochloride
Use Local anesthetic and acute treatment of ventricular arrhythmias from myocardial infarction, cardiac manipulation, digitalis intoxication; topical local anesthetic; drug of choice for ventricular ectopy, ventricular tachycardia, ventricular fibrillation; for pulseless VT or VF preferably give **after** defibrillation and epinephrine; control of premature ventricular contractions, wide-complex PSVT
Pregnancy Risk Factor C
Contraindications Known hypersensitivity to amide-type local anesthetics; patients with Adams-Stokes syndrome or with severe degree of S-A, A-V, or intraventricular heart block (without a pacemaker)
Warnings/Precautions Avoid use of preparations containing preservatives for spinal or epidural (including caudal) anesthesia. Use extreme caution in patients
(Continued)

Lidocaine Hydrochloride *(Continued)*

with hepatic disease, heart failure, marked hypoxia, severe respiratory depression, hypovolemia or shock, incomplete heart block or bradycardia, and atrial fibrillation.

Due to decreases in phase I metabolism and possibly decrease in splanchnic perfusion with age, there may be a decreased clearance or increased half-life in elderly and increased risk for CNS side effects and cardiac effects

Adverse Reactions

1% to 10%:
Cardiovascular: Hypotension
Central nervous system: Positional headache, shivering

<1%:
Cardiovascular: Heart block, arrhythmias, cardiovascular collapse
Central nervous system: Lethargy, coma, agitation, slurred speech, seizures, anxiety, euphoria, hallucinations
Dermatologic: Itching, skin rash, swelling of skin
Gastrointestinal: Nausea, vomiting
Neuromuscular & skeletal: Paresthesias
Ocular: Blurred or double vision
Respiratory: Difficulty in breathing, respiratory depression or arrest

Overdosage/Toxicology Has a narrow therapeutic index and severe toxicity may occur slightly above the therapeutic range, especially with other antiarrhythmic drugs; symptoms of overdose includes sedation, confusion, coma, seizures, respiratory arrest and cardiac toxicity (sinus arrest, A-V block, asystole, and hypotension); the QRS and Q-T intervals are usually normal, although they may be prolonged after massive overdose; other effects include dizziness, paresthesias, tremor, ataxia, and GI disturbance. Treatment is supportive, using conventional therapies (fluids, positioning, vasopressors, antiarrhythmics, anticonvulsants); sodium bicarbonate may reverse QRS prolongation, bradyarrhythmias and hypotension; enhanced elimination with dialysis, hemoperfusion or repeat charcoal is not effective.

Drug Interactions

Increased toxicity:
Concomitant cimetidine or propranolol may result in increased serum concentrations of lidocaine with resultant toxicity
Effect of succinylcholine may be enhanced

Stability

Lidocaine injection is stable at room temperature
Stability of parenteral admixture at room temperature (25°C): Expiration date on premixed bag; out of overwrap stability: 30 days
Standard diluent: 2 g/250 mL D_5W

Mechanism of Action Class IB antiarrhythmic; suppresses automaticity of conduction tissue, by increasing electrical stimulation threshold of ventricle, HIS-Purkinje system, and spontaneous depolarization of the ventricles during diastole by a direct action on the tissues; blocks both the initiation and conduction of nerve impulses by decreasing the neuronal membrane's permeability to sodium ions, which results in inhibition of depolarization with resultant blockade of conduction

Pharmacodynamics/Kinetics

Onset of action (single bolus dose): 45-90 seconds
Duration: 10-20 minutes
Distribution: V_d: Alterable by many patient factors; decreased in CHF and liver disease
Protein binding: 60% to 80%; binds to alpha$_1$ acid glycoprotein
Metabolism: 90% metabolized in liver; active metabolites monoethylglycinexylidide (MEGX) and glycinexylidide (GX) can accumulate and may cause CNS toxicity
Half-life (biphasic): Increased with CHF, liver disease, shock, severe renal disease
Initial: 7-30 minutes
Terminal:
Infants, premature: 3.2 hours
Adults: 1.5-2 hours

Usual Dosage

Topical: Apply to affected area as needed; maximum: 3 mg/kg/dose; do not repeat within 2 hours
Injectable local anesthetic: Varies with procedure, degree of anesthesia needed, vascularity of tissue, duration of anesthesia required, and physical condition of patient; maximum: 4.5 mg/kg/dose; do not repeat within 2 hours

Children: Endotracheal, I.O., I.V.: Loading dose: 1 mg/kg; may repeat in 10-15 minutes x 2 doses; after loading dose, start I.V. continuous infusion 20-50 mcg/kg/minute

Use 20 mcg/kg/minute in patients with shock, hepatic disease, mild congestive heart failure (CHF)

Moderate to severe CHF may require ½ loading dose and lower infusion rates to avoid toxicity

Adults: Antiarrhythmic:

I.V.: 1-1.5 mg/kg bolus over 2-3 minutes; may repeat doses of 0.5-0.75 mg/kg in 5-10 minutes up to a total of 3 mg/kg; continuous infusion: 1-4 mg/minute

I.V. (2 g/250 mL D_5W) infusion rates (infusion pump should be used for I.V. infusion administration):

   1 mg/minute: 7 mL/hour
   2 mg/minute: 15 mL/hour
   3 mg/minute: 21 mL/hour
   4 mg/minute: 30 mL/hour

Ventricular fibrillation (after defibrillation and epinephrine): Initial dose: 1.5 mg/kg, may repeat boluses as above; follow with continuous infusion after return of perfusion

Prevention of ventricular fibrillation: I.V.: Initial bolus: 0.5 mg/kg; repeat every 5-10 minutes to a total dose of 2 mg/kg

   Refractory ventricular fibrillation: Repeat 1.5 mg/kg bolus may be given 3-5 minutes after initial dose

   Endotracheal: 2-2.5 times the I.V. dose

Decrease dose in patients with CHF, shock, or hepatic disease

Dosing adjustment/comments in hepatic disease: Reduce dose in acute hepatitis and decompensated cirrhosis by 50%

Not dialyzable (0% to 5%) by hemo- or peritoneal dialysis; supplemental dose not necessary; supplemental dose is not necessary

Reference Range

Therapeutic: 1.5-5.0 µg/mL (SI: 6-21 µmol/L)
Potentially toxic: >6 µg/mL (SI: >26 µmol/L)
Toxic: >9 µg/mL (SI: >38 µmol/L)

Nursing Implications Local thrombophlebitis may occur in patients receiving prolonged I.V. infusions

Dosage Forms

Injection: 0.5% [5 mg/mL] (50 mL); 1% [10 mg/mL] (2 mL, 5 mL, 10 mL, 20 mL, 30 mL, 50 mL); 1.5% [15 mg/mL] (20 mL); 2% [20 mg/mL] (2 mL, 5 mL, 10 mL, 20 mL, 30 mL, 50 mL); 4% [40 mg/mL] (5 mL); 10% [100 mg/mL] (10 mL); 20% [200 mg/mL] (10 mL, 20 mL)

Injection:
I.M. use: 10% [100 mg/mL] (3 mL, 5 mL)
Direct I.V.: 1% [10 mg/mL] (5 mL, 10 mL); 20 mg/mL (5 mL)
I.V. admixture, preservative free: 4% [40 mg/mL] (25 mL, 30 mL); 10% [100 mg/mL] (10 mL); 20% [200 mg/mL] (5 mL, 10 mL)
I.V. infusion, in D_5W: 0.2% [2 mg/mL] (500 mL); 0.4% [4 mg/mL] (250 mL, 500 mL, 1000 mL); 0.8% [8 mg/mL] (250 mL, 500 mL)
Jelly, topical: 2% (30 mL)
Liquid, viscous: 2% (20 mL, 100 mL)
Ointment, topical: 2.5% [OTC], 5% (35 g)
Solution, topical: 2% [20 mg/mL] (15 mL, 240 mL); 4% [40 mg/mL] (50 mL)

LidoPen® see Lidocaine Hydrochloride on page 633

Lignocaine Hydrochloride see Lidocaine Hydrochloride on page 633

Lincocin® see Lincomycin on this page

Lincomycin (lin koe mye' sin)

Brand Names Lincocin®

Use Treatment of susceptible bacterial infections, mainly those caused by streptococci and staphylococci resistant to other agents

Pregnancy Risk Factor B

Contraindications Minor bacterial infections or viral infections, hypersensitivity to lincomycin or any component or clindamycin

Warnings/Precautions Can cause severe and possibly fatal colitis; characterized by severe persistent diarrhea, severe abdominal cramps and, possibly, the passage of blood and mucus; discontinue drug if significant diarrhea occurs; severe hepatic disease

Adverse Reactions

1% to 10%: Gastrointestinal: Nausea, vomiting, diarrhea
<1%:
Cardiovascular: Hypotension
(Continued)

Lincomycin *(Continued)*

    Central nervous system: Vertigo
    Dermatologic: Urticaria, rash, Stevens-Johnson syndrome
    Gastrointestinal: Pseudomembranous colitis, glossitis, stomatitis, pruritus ani
    Genitourinary: Vaginitis
    Hematologic: Granulocytopenia, thrombocytopenia, pancytopenia
    Hepatic: Elevation of liver enzymes
    Local: Sterile abscess at I.M. injection site, thrombophlebitis
    Otic: Tinnitus

Overdosage/Toxicology Symptoms of overdose include diarrhea, abdominal cramps; following oral decontamination, treatment is supportive

Drug Interactions
    Decreased effect with erythromycin
    Increased activity/toxicity of neuromuscular blocking agents

Mechanism of Action Lincosamide antibiotic which was isolated from a strain of *Streptomyces lincolnensis*; lincomycin, like clindamycin, inhibits bacterial protein synthesis by specifically binding on the 50S subunit and affecting the process of peptide chain initiation. Other macrolide antibiotics (erythromycin) also bind to the 50S subunit. Since only one molecule of antibiotic can bind to a single ribosome, the concomitant use of erythromycin and lincomycin is not recommended.

Pharmacodynamics/Kinetics
    Absorption: Oral: ~20% to 30%
    Distribution: V_d: 23-38 L; CSF levels are higher with inflamed meninges; CSF penetration is poor
    Protein binding: 72%
    Metabolism: Hepatic
    Half-life, elimination: 2-11.5 hours
    Time to peak serum concentration:
        Oral: 2-4 hours
        I.M.: 1 hour
    Elimination: 5% to 10% excreted unchanged in urine, with 30% to 40% (oral) and 4% to 14% (parenteral) excreted unchanged in feces

Usual Dosage
    Children >1 month:
        Oral: 30-60 mg/kg/day in divided doses every 8 hours
        I.M.: 10 mg/kg every 8-12 hours
        I.V.: 10-20 mg/kg/day in divided doses every 8-12 hours

    Adults:
        Oral: 500 mg every 6-8 hours
        I.M.: 600 mg every 12-24 hours
        I.V.: 600-1 g every 8-12 hours up to 8 g/day

    Dosing interval in renal impairment:
        Cl_{cr} 10-50 mL/minute: Administer every 6-12 hours
        Cl_{cr} <10 mL/minute: Administer every 12 hours

    Dosing adjustment in hepatic impairment: Reductions are indicated

Administration Administer oral dosage form with a full glass of water to minimize esophageal ulceration; administer around-the-clock to promote less variation in peak and trough serum levels

Patient Information Report any severe diarrhea immediately and do not take antidiarrheal medication; take each oral dose with a full glass of water; finish all medication; do not skip doses; store capsules in a light-proof container

Dosage Forms
    Capsule: 250 mg, 500 mg
    Injection: 300 mg/mL (2 mL, 10 mL)

Lindane *(lin' dane)*

Brand Names G-well®; Kwell®; Scabene®

Synonyms Benzene Hexachloride; Gamma Benzene Hexachloride; Hexachloro-cyclohexane

Use Treatment of scabies (*Sarcoptes scabiei*), *Pediculus capitis* (head lice), and *Pediculus pubis* (crab lice)

Pregnancy Risk Factor B

Pregnancy/Breast Feeding Implications There are no well controlled studies in pregnant women; treat no more than twice during a pregnancy

Contraindications Hypersensitivity to lindane or any component; premature neonates; acutely inflamed skin or raw, weeping surfaces

Warnings/Precautions Use with caution in infants and small children, and patients with a history of seizures; avoid contact with face, eyes, mucous membranes, and urethral meatus. Because of the potential for systemic absorption and CNS side effects, lindane should be used with caution; not considered a drug of first choice; consider permethrin or crotamiton agent first.

Adverse Reactions
<1%:
Cardiovascular: Cardiac arrhythmia
Central nervous system: Dizziness, restlessness, seizures, headache, ataxia
Dermatologic: Eczematous eruptions, contact dermatitis, skin and adipose tissue may act as repositories
Gastrointestinal: Nausea, vomiting
Hematologic: Aplastic anemia
Hepatic: Hepatitis
Local: Burning and stinging
Neuromuscular & skeletal: Ataxia
Renal: Hematuria
Respiratory: Pulmonary edema

Overdosage/Toxicology Symptoms of overdose include vomiting, restlessness, ataxia, seizures, arrhythmias, pulmonary edema, hematuria, hepatitis. Absorbed through skin and mucous membranes and GI tract, has occasionally caused serious CNS, hepatic and renal toxicity when used excessively for prolonged periods, or when accidental ingestion has occurred; if ingested, perform gastric lavage and general supportive measures; diazepam 0.01 mg/kg can be used to control seizures.

Drug Interactions Increased toxicity: Oil-based hair dressing → ↑ toxic potential

Mechanism of Action Directly absorbed by parasites and ova through the exoskeleton; stimulates the nervous system resulting in seizures and death of parasitic arthropods

Pharmacodynamics/Kinetics
Absorption: Systemic absorption of up to 13% may occur
Distribution: Stored in body fat and accumulates in brain; skin and adipose tissue may act as repositories
Metabolism: By the liver
Half-life: Children: 17-22 hours
Time to peak serum concentration: Topical: Children: 6 hours
Elimination: In urine and feces

Usual Dosage Children and Adults: Topical:
Scabies: Apply a thin layer of lotion or cream and massage it on skin from the neck to the toes (head to toe in infants). For adults, bathe and remove the drug after 8-12 hours; for children, wash off 6-8 hours after application (for infants, wash off 6 hours after application); repeat treatment in 7 days if lice or nits are still present
Pediculosis, capitis and pubis: 15-30 mL of shampoo is applied and lathered for 4-5 minutes; rinse hair thoroughly and comb with a fine tooth comb to remove nits; repeat treatment in 7 days if lice or nits are still present

Administration Drug should not be administered orally, for topical use only; apply to dry, cool skin

Patient Information Topical use only, do not apply to face, avoid getting in eyes; do **not** apply lotion immediately after a hot, soapy bath. Clothing and bedding should be washed in hot water or by dry cleaning to kill the scabies mite. Combs and brushes may be washed with lindane shampoo then thoroughly rinsed with water. Notify physician if condition worsens; treat sexual contact simultaneously.

Dosage Forms
Cream: 1% (60 g)
Lotion: 1% (60 mL, 473 mL, 480 mL, 3800 mL)
Shampoo: 1% (30 mL, 59 mL, 60 mL, 473 mL, 3800 mL)

Lioresal® see Baclofen on page 114

Liothyronine Sodium (lye oh thye′ roe neen)

Brand Names Cytomel®; Triostat™
Synonyms Sodium L-Triiodothyronine; T₃ Sodium
Use Replacement or supplemental therapy in hypothyroidism, management of nontoxic goiter, chronic lymphocytic thyroiditis, as an adjunct in thyrotoxicosis and as a diagnostic aid; **levothyroxine is recommended for chronic therapy**
Pregnancy Risk Factor A
Contraindications Recent myocardial infarction or thyrotoxicosis, hypersensitivity to liothyronine sodium or any component, undocumented or uncorrected adrenal insufficiency
Warnings/Precautions Ineffective for weight reduction; high doses may produce serious or even life-threatening toxic effects particularly when used with some anorectic drugs. Use with extreme caution in patients with angina pectoris or other cardiovascular disease (including hypertension) or coronary artery disease; (Continued)

Liothyronine Sodium *(Continued)*

use with caution in elderly patients since they may be more likely to have compromised cardiovascular function. Patients with adrenal insufficiency, myxedema, diabetes mellitus and insipidus may have symptoms exaggerated or aggravated; thyroid replacement requires periodic assessment or thyroid status. Chronic hypothyroidism predisposes patients to coronary artery disease.

Adverse Reactions

<1%:

Cardiovascular: Palpitations, sweating, tachycardia, cardiac arrhythmias, chest pain

Central nervous system: Nervousness, insomnia, fever, headache, insomnia, clumsiness

Dermatologic: Hair loss

Gastrointestinal: Weight loss, increased appetite, diarrhea, abdominal cramps, constipation

Endocrine & metabolic: Changes in menstrual cycle

Neuromuscular & skeletal: Muscle aches, hand tremors, tremor

Respiratory: Shortness of breath

Overdosage/Toxicology

Chronic overdose may cause hyperthyroidism, weight loss, nervousness, sweating, tachycardia, insomnia, heat intolerance, menstrual irregularities, palpitations, psychosis, fever; acute overdose may cause fever, hypoglycemia, CHF, unrecognized adrenal insufficiency.

Reduce dose or temporarily discontinue therapy; normal hypothalamic-pituitary-thyroid axis will return to normal in 6-8 weeks; serum T_4 levels do not correlate well with toxicity.

In massive acute ingestion, reduce GI absorption, give general supportive care; treat congestive heart failure with digitalis glycosides; excessive adrenergic activity (tachycardia) requires propranolol 1-3 mg I.V. over 10 minutes or 80-160 mg orally/day; fever may be treated with acetaminophen.

Drug Interactions

Decreased effect:

Cholestyramine resin → ↓ absorption

Antidiabetic drug requirements are ↑

Estrogens → ↑ thyroid requirements

Increased effect: Increased oral anticoagulant effects

Stability Vials must be stored under refrigeration at 2°C to 8°C (36°F to 46°F)

Mechanism of Action Primary active compound is T_3 (tri-iodothyronine), which may be converted from T_4 (thyroxine) and then circulates throughout the body to influence growth and maturation of various tissues; exact mechanism of action is unknown; however, it is believed the thyroid hormone exerts its many metabolic effects through control of DNA transcription and protein synthesis; involved in normal metabolism, growth, and development; promotes gluconeogenesis, increases utilization and mobilization of glycogen stores, and stimulates protein synthesis, increases basal metabolic rate

Pharmacodynamics/Kinetics

Onset of effect: Within 24-72 hours

Duration: Up to 72 hours

Absorption: Oral: Well absorbed (~85% to 90%)

Metabolism: In the liver to inactive compounds

Half-life: 16-49 hours

Elimination: In urine

Usual Dosage

Congenital hypothyroidism: Children: Oral: 5 mcg/day increase by 5 mcg every 3 days to 20 mcg/day for infants, 50 mcg/day for children 1-3 years of age, and give adult dose for children >3 years.

Hypothyroidism: Oral:

Adults: 25 mcg/day increase by 12.5-25 mcg/day every 1-2 weeks to a maximum of 100 mcg/day

Elderly: Initial: 5 mcg/day, increase by 5 mcg/day every 1-2 weeks; usual maintenance dose: 25-75 mcg/day

T_3 suppression test: Oral: 75-100 mcg/day for 7 days; use lowest dose for elderly

Myxedema coma: I.V.: 25-50 mcg

Patients with known or suspected cardiovascular disease: 10-20 mcg

Note: Normally, at least 4 hours should be allowed between doses to adequately assess therapeutic response and no more than 12 hours should elapse between doses to avoid fluctuations in hormone levels. Oral therapy should be resumed as soon as the clinical situation has been stabilized and the patient is able to take oral medication. If levothyroxine rather than liothyronine sodium is used in initiating oral therapy, the physician should bear in mind that there is a delay of several days in the onset of levothyroxine activity and that I.V. therapy should be discontinued gradually.

Administration For I.V. use only - **do not administer I.M. or S.C.**

Administer doses at least 4 hours, and no more than 12 hours, apart

Resume oral therapy as soon as the clinical situation has been stabilized and the patient is able to take oral medication

When switching to tablets, discontinue the injectable, initiate oral therapy at a low dosage and increase gradually according to response

If levothyroxine is used for oral therapy, there is a delay of several days in the onset of activity; therefore, discontinue IV therapy gradually

Monitoring Parameters T_4, TSH, heart rate, blood pressure, clinical signs of hypo- and hyperthyroidism; TSH is the most reliable guide for evaluating adequacy of thyroid replacement dosage. TSH may be elevated during the first few months of thyroid replacement despite patients being clinically euthyroid. In cases where T_4 remains low and TSH is within normal limits, an evaluation of "free" (unbound) T_4 is needed to evaluate further increase in dosage.

Reference Range Free T_3, serum: 250-390 pg/dL; TSH: 0.4 and up to 10 (≥80 years of age) mIU/L; remains normal in pregnancy

Test Interactions Many drugs may have effects on thyroid function tests; para-aminosalicylic acid, aminoglutethimide, amiodarone, barbiturates, carbamazepine, chloral hydrate, clofibrate, colestipol, corticosteroids, danazol, diazepam, estrogens, ethionamide, fluorouracil, I.V. heparin, insulin, lithium, methadone, methimazole, mitotane, nitroprusside, oxyphenbutazone, phenylbutazone, PTU, perphenazine, phenytoin, propranolol, salicylates, sulfonylureas, and thiazides

Patient Information Do not change brands without physician's knowledge; report immediately to physician any chest pain, increased pulse, palpitations, heat intolerances, excessive sweating; do not discontinue without notifying physician

Additional Information 15-37.5 mcg is equivalent to 0.05-0.06 mg levothyroxine; 60 mg thyroid USP; 45 mg Thyroid Strong®, and 60 mg thyroglobulin

Dosage Forms

Injection: 10 mcg/mL (1 mL)

Tablet: 5 mcg, 25 mcg, 50 mcg

Liotrix (lye' oh trix)

Brand Names Euthroid®; Thyrolar®

Synonyms T_3/T_4 Liotrix

Use Replacement or supplemental therapy in hypothyroidism (uniform mixture of T_4:T_3 in 4:1 ratio by weight); little advantage to this product exists and cost is not justified

Pregnancy Risk Factor A

Contraindications Hypersensitivity to liotrix or any component; recent myocardial infarction or thyrotoxicosis, uncomplicated by hypothyroidism; uncorrected adrenal insufficiency, hypersensitivity to active or extraneous constituents

Warnings/Precautions Ineffective for weight reduction; high doses may produce serious or even life-threatening toxic effects particularly when used with some anorectic drugs; use cautiously in patients with pre-existing cardiovascular disease (angina, CHD), elderly since they may be more likely to have compromised cardiovascular function

Adverse Reactions

<1%:

Cardiovascular: Palpitations, tachycardia, cardiac arrhythmias, chest pain

Central nervous system: Nervousness, sweating, headache, insomnia, fever, clumsiness

Dermatologic: Hair loss

Endocrine & metabolic: Excessive bone loss with over-treatment (excess thyroid replacement), heat intolerance, changes in menstrual cycle

Gastrointestinal: Weight loss, increased appetite, diarrhea, abdominal cramps, vomiting, constipation

Neuromuscular & skeletal: Tremor, muscle aches, hand tremors

Respiratory: Shortness of breath

Overdosage/Toxicology

Chronic overdose may cause weight loss, nervousness, sweating, tachycardia, insomnia, heat intolerance, menstrual irregularities, palpitations, psychosis, fever; acute overdose may cause fever, hypoglycemia, CHF, unrecognized adrenal insufficiency

Reduce dose or temporarily discontinue therapy; normal hypothalamic-pituitary-thyroid axis will return to normal in 6-8 weeks; serum T_4 levels do not correlate well with toxicity

In massive acute ingestion, reduce GI absorption, give general supportive care; treat congestive heart failure with digitalis glycosides; excessive adrenergic activity (tachycardia) require propranolol 1-3 mg I.V. over 10 minutes or 80-160 mg orally/day; fever may be treated with acetaminophen

(Continued)

Liotrix (Continued)

Drug Interactions
Decreased effect:
  Thyroid hormones increase hypoglycemic drug requirements
  Phenytoin → clinical lymphothyroidism
  Cholestyramine → ↓ drug absorption
Increased effect: Increased oral anticoagulant effect
Increased toxicity: Tricyclic antidepressants → ↑ potential of both drugs

Mechanism of Action The primary active compound is T_3 (tri-iodothyronine), which may be converted from T_4 (thyroxine) and then circulates throughout the body to influence growth and maturation of various tissues. Liotrix is uniform mixture of synthetic T_4 and T_3 in 4:1 ratio; exact mechanism of action is unknown; however, it is believed the thyroid hormone exerts its many metabolic effects through control of DNA transcription and protein synthesis; involved in normal metabolism, growth, and development; promotes gluconeogenesis, increases utilization and mobilization of glycogen stores and stimulates protein synthesis, increases basal metabolic rate

Pharmacodynamics/Kinetics
Absorption: 50% to 95% from GI tract
Time to peak serum concentration: 12-48 hours
Metabolism: Partially in the liver, kidneys, and intestines
Half-life: 6-7 days
Elimination: Partially in feces and bile as conjugated metabolites

Usual Dosage Oral:
Congenital hypothyroidism:
  Children (dose of T_4 or levothyroxine/day):
    0-6 months: 8-10 mcg/kg or 25-50 mcg/day
    6-12 months: 6-8 mcg/kg or 50-75 mcg/day
    1-5 years: 5-6 mcg/kg or 75-100 mcg/day
    6-12 years: 4-5 mcg/kg or 100-150 mcg/day
    >12 years: 2-3 mcg/kg or >150 mcg/day
Hypothyroidism (dose of thyroid equivalent):
  Adults: 30 mg/day, increasing by 15 mg/day at 2- to 3-week intervals to a maximum of 180 mg/day (usual maintenance dose: 60-120 mg/day)
  Elderly: Initial: 15 mg, adjust dose at 2- to 4-week intervals by increments of 15 mg

Monitoring Parameters T_4, TSH, heart rate, blood pressure, clinical signs of hypo- and hyperthyroidism; TSH is the most reliable guide for evaluating adequacy of thyroid replacement dosage. TSH may be elevated during the first few months of thyroid replacement despite patients being clinically euthyroid. In cases where T_4 remains low and TSH is within normal limits, an evaluation of "free" (unbound) T_4 is needed to evaluate further increase in dosage.

Reference Range
TSH: 0.4-10 (for those ≥80 years) mIU/L
T_4: 4-12 µg/dL (SI: 51-154 nmol/L)

Comparison of Liotrix Products

Liotrix Product	T_4 Content (mcg)	T_3 Content (mcg)	Thyroid Equivalent (mg)
Euthroid® 1/2 grain	30	7.5	30
Euthroid® 1 grain	60	15	60
Euthroid® 2 grain	120	30	120
Euthroid® 3 grain	180	45	180
Thyrolar® 1/4 grain	12.5	3.1	15
Thyrolar® 1/2 grain	25	6.25	30
Thyrolar® 1 grain	50	12.5	60
Thyrolar® 2 grain	100	25	120
Thyrolar® 3 grain	150	37.5	180

T$_3$ (RIA) (total T$_3$): 80-230 ng/dL (SI: 1.2-3.5 nmol/L)

T$_4$ free (Free T$_4$): 0.7-1.8 ng/dL (SI: 9-23 pmol/L)

Test Interactions Many drugs may have effects on thyroid function tests; para-aminosalicylic acid, aminoglutethimide, amiodarone, barbiturates, carbamazepine, chloral hydrate, clofibrate, colestipol, corticosteroids, danazol, diazepam, estrogens, ethionamide, fluorouracil, I.V. heparin, insulin, lithium, methadone, methimazole, mitotane, nitroprusside, oxyphenbutazone, phenylbutazone, PTU, perphenazine, phenytoin, propranolol, salicylates, sulfonylureas, and thiazides

Patient Information Do not change brands without physician's knowledge; report immediately to physician any chest pain, increased pulse, palpitations, heat intolerances, excessive sweating; do not discontinue without notifying your physician; replacement therapy will be for life; take as a single dose before breakfast

Additional Information Since T$_3$ is produced by monodeiodination of T$_4$ in peripheral tissues (80%) and since elderly have decreased T$_3$ (25% to 40%), little advantage to this product exists and cost is not justified; no advantage over synthetic levothyroxine sodium; 1 grain (60 mg) liotrix is equivalent to 0.05-0.06 mg levothyroxine; 60 mg thyroid USP and thyroglobulin; and 45 mg of Thyroid Strong®

Dosage Forms Tablet: 15 mg, 30 mg, 60 mg, 120 mg, 180 mg [thyroid equivalent]

Lipancreatin *see* Pancrelipase *on page 837*

Lipidil® *see* Fenofibrate *on page 444*

Lipid-Lowering Agents *see page 1273*

Liposyn® *see* Fat Emulsion *on page 441*

Liquaemin® *see* Heparin *on page 528*

Liqui-Char® [OTC] *see* Charcoal *on page 214*

Liquid Antidote *see* Charcoal *on page 214*

Liquid Paraffin *see* Mineral Oil *on page 743*

Liquid Pred® *see* Prednisone *on page 921*

Lisinopril (lyse in' oh pril)
Related Information
Angiotensin-Converting Enzyme Inhibitors, Comparative Pharmacokinetics *on page 1244*
Angiotensin-Converting Enzyme Inhibitors, Comparisons of Indications and Adult Dosages *on page 1243*

Brand Names Prinivil®; Zestril®

Use Treatment of hypertension, either alone or in combination with other antihypertensive agents; adjunctive therapy in treatment of CHF (afterload reduction)

Pregnancy Risk Factor D

Contraindications Hypersensitivity to lisinopril or any component or other ACE inhibitors

Warnings/Precautions Use with caution and modify dosage in patients with renal impairment (decrease dosage) (especially renal artery stenosis), severe congestive heart failure, or with coadministered diuretic therapy; experience in children is limited. Severe hypotension may occur in patients who are sodium and/or volume depleted, initiate lower doses and monitor closely when starting therapy in these patients.

Adverse Reactions
1% to 10%:
Cardiovascular: Hypotension
Central nervous system: Dizziness, headache, fatigue
Gastrointestinal: Diarrhea
Renal: Increased BUN and serum creatinine
Respiratory: Upper respiratory symptoms, cough
<1%:
Cardiovascular: Chest discomfort, flushing, myocardial infarction, angina pectoris, orthostatic hypotension, rhythm disturbances, tachycardia, peripheral edema, vasculitis, palpitations, syncope
Central nervous system: Fever, malaise, depression, somnolence, insomnia
Dermatologic: Urticaria, pruritus, angioedema
Endocrine & metabolic: Gout
Gastrointestinal: Pancreatitis, abdominal pain, anorexia, constipation, flatulence, dry mouth
Hematologic: Neutropenia, bone marrow depression
Hepatic: Hepatitis
Neuromuscular & skeletal: Joint pain, shoulder pain
Ocular: Blurred vision

(Continued)

Lisinopril *(Continued)*

Respiratory: Bronchitis, sinusitis, pharyngeal pain

Miscellaneous: Diaphoresis

Overdosage/Toxicology Mild hypotension has been the only toxic effect seen with acute overdose. Bradycardia may also occur; hyperkalemia occurs even with therapeutic doses, especially in patients with renal insufficiency and those taking NSAIDs. Following initiation of essential overdose management, toxic symptom treatment and supportive treatment should be initiated. Hypotension usually responds to I.V. fluids or Trendelenburg positioning.

Drug Interactions

Increased toxicity:

Probenecid ↑ blood levels of captopril

Captopril and diuretics have additive hypotensive effects; see table.

Drug-Drug Interactions With ACEIs

Precipitant Drug	Drug (Category) and Effect	Description
Antacids	ACEIs: decreased	Decreased bioavailability of ACEIs. May be more likely with captopril. Separate administration times by 1-2 hours.
NSAIDs (indomethacin)	ACEIs: decreased	Reduced hypotensive effects of ACEIs. More prominent in low renin or volume dependent hypertensive patients.
Phenothiazines	ACEIs: increased	Pharmacologic effects of ACEIs may be increased.
ACEIs	Allopurinol: increased	Higher risk of hypersensitivity reaction possible when given concurrently. Three case reports of Stevens-Johnson syndrome with captopril.
ACEIs	Digoxin: increased	Increased plasma digoxin levels.
ACEIs	Lithium: increased	Increased serum lithium levels and symptoms of toxicity may occur.
ACEIs	Potassium preps/potassium-sparing diuretics increased	Coadministration may result in elevated potassium levels.

Mechanism of Action Competitive inhibitor of angiotensin-converting enzyme (ACE); prevents conversion of angiotensin I to angiotensin II, a potent vasoconstrictor; results in lower levels of angiotensin II which causes an increase in plasma renin activity and a reduction in aldosterone secretion; a CNS mechanism may also be involved in hypotensive effect as angiotensin II increases adrenergic outflow from CNS; vasoactive kallikreins may be decreased in conversion to active hormones by ACE inhibitors, thus reducing blood pressure

Pharmacodynamics/Kinetics

Peak hypotensive effect: Oral: Within 6 hours

Absorption: Well absorbed; unaffected by food

Distribution: protein binding :25%

Half-life: 11-12 hours

Elimination: Almost entirely excreted in urine as unchanged drug

Usual Dosage

Adults: Initial: 10 mg/day; increase doses 5-10 mg/day at 1- to 2-week intervals; maximum daily dose: 40 mg

Elderly: Initial: 2.5-5 mg/day; increase doses 2.5-5 mg/day at 1- to 2-week intervals; maximum daily dose: 40 mg

Patients taking diuretics should have them discontinued 2-3 days prior to initiating lisinopril if possible; restart diuretic after blood pressure is stable if needed; in patients with hyponatremia (<130 mEq/L), start dose at 2.5 mg/day

Dosing adjustment in renal impairment:

Cl$_{cr}$ 10-50 mL/minute: Administer 50% to 75% of normal dose

Cl$_{cr}$ <10 mL/minute: Administer 25% to 50% of normal dose

Dialyzable (50%)

Monitoring Parameters Serum calcium levels, BUN, serum creatinine, renal function, WBC, and potassium

Test Interactions May cause false-positive results in urine acetone determinations using sodium nitroprusside reagent; ↑ potassium (S); ↑ serum creatinine/BUN

Patient Information Notify physician if vomiting, diarrhea, excessive perspiration, or dehydration should occur; also if swelling of face, lips, tongue or difficulty in breathing occurs or if persistent cough develops; do not stop therapy without the advise of the prescriber; do not add a salt substitute (potassium) without physician advice

Nursing Implications May cause depression in some patients; discontinue if angioedema of the face, extremities, lips, tongue, or glottis occurs; watch for hypotensive effects within 1-3 hours of first dose or new higher dose

Dosage Forms Tablet: 5 mg, 10 mg, 20 mg, 40 mg

Listermint® with Fluoride [OTC] see Fluoride on page 471

Lithane® see Lithium on this page

Lithium (lith' ee um)

Brand Names Cibalith-S®; Eskalith®; Lithane®; Lithobid®; Lithonate®; Litho-tabs®

Synonyms Lithium Carbonate; Lithium Citrate

Use Management of acute manic episodes, bipolar disorders, and depression

Pregnancy Risk Factor D

Contraindications Hypersensitivity to lithium or any component; severe cardiovascular or renal disease

Warnings/Precautions Lithium toxicity is closely related to serum levels and can occur at therapeutic doses; serum lithium determinations are required to monitor therapy. Use with caution in patients with cardiovascular or thyroid disease, severe debilitation, dehydration or sodium depletion, or in patients receiving diuretics. Some elderly patients may be extremely sensitive to the effects of lithium; see dosage and therapeutic levels.

Adverse Reactions

>10%:
 Endocrine & metabolic: Polydipsia, stress
 Gastrointestinal: Nausea, diarrhea, impaired taste
 Neuromuscular & skeletal: Trembling

1% to 10%:
 Central nervous system: Weakness, tiredness
 Dermatologic: Skin rash
 Gastrointestinal: Bloated feeling, weight gain
 Neuromuscular: Muscle twitching

<1%:
 Central nervous system: Lethargy, fatigue, dizziness, vertigo, pseudotumor cerebri
 Dermatologic: Eruptions
 Endocrine & metabolic: Hypothyroidism, goiter, acneiform
 Gastrointestinal: Anorexia, dry mouth
 Genitourinary: Diabetes insipidus, nonspecific nephron atrophy, renal tubular acidosis
 Hematologic: Leukocytosis
 Neuromuscular & skeletal: Muscle weakness, cogwheel rigidity, chronic movements of the limbs, tremor
 Ocular: Vision problems
 Miscellaneous: Discoloration of fingers and toes

Overdosage/Toxicology Symptoms of overdose include sedation, confusion, tremors, joint pain, visual changes, seizures, coma

There is no specific antidote for lithium poisoning. In the acute ingestion following initiation of essential overdose management, correction of fluid and electrolyte imbalances should be commenced. Hemodialysis and whole bowel irrigation is the treatment of choice for severe intoxications; charcoal is ineffective.

Drug Interactions
Decreased effect with xanthines (eg, theophylline, caffeine)
Increased effect/toxicity of CNS depressants, alfentanil, iodide salts increased hypothyroid effect
Increased toxicity with thiazide diuretics (dose may need to be reduced by 30%), NSAIDs, haloperidol, phenothiazines (neurotoxicity), neuromuscular blockers, carbamazepine, fluoxetine, ACE inhibitors

Mechanism of Action Alters cation transport across cell membrane in nerve and muscle cells and influences reuptake of serotonin and/or norepinephrine

Pharmacodynamics/Kinetics
Distribution: V_d: Initial: 0.3-0.4 L/kg; V_{dss}: 0.7-1 L/kg; crosses the placenta; appears in breast milk at 35% to 50% the concentrations in serum
Half-life: 18-24 hours; can increase to more than 36 hours in elderly or patients with renal impairment
Time to peak serum concentration (nonsustained release product): Within 0.5-2 hours following oral absorption

(Continued)

Lithium *(Continued)*

Elimination: 90% to 98% of dose excreted in urine as unchanged drug; other excretory routes include feces (1%) and sweat (4% to 5%)

Usual Dosage Oral: Monitor serum concentrations and clinical response (efficacy and toxicity) to determine proper dose

Children 6-12 years: 15-60 mg/kg/day in 3-4 divided doses; dose not to exceed usual adult dosage

Adults: 300-600 mg 3-4 times/day; usual maximum maintenance dose: 2.4 g/day or 450-900 mg of sustained release twice daily

Elderly: Initial dose: 300 mg twice daily; increase weekly in increments of 300 mg/day, monitoring levels; rarely need to go >900-1200 mg/day

Dosing adjustment in renal impairment:

Cl_{cr} 10-50 mL/minute: Administer 50% to 75% of normal dose

Cl_{cr} <10 mL/minute: Administer 25% to 50% of normal dose

Dialyzable (50% to 100%)

Monitoring Parameters Serum lithium every 3-4 days during initial therapy; draw lithium serum concentrations 8-12 hours postdose; renal, hepatic, thyroid, and cardiovascular function; fluid status; serum electrolytes; CBC with differential, urinalysis; monitor for signs of toxicity

Reference Range Levels should be obtained twice weekly until both patient's clinical status and levels are stable then levels may be obtained every 1-2 months

Timing of serum samples: Draw trough just before next dose

Therapeutic levels:

Acute mania: 0.6-1.2 mEq/L (SI: 0.6-1.2 mmol/L)

Protection against future episodes in most patients with bipolar disorder: 0.8-1 mEq/L (SI: 0.8-1.0 mmol/L); a higher rate of relapse is described in subjects who are maintained at <0.4 mEq/L (SI: 0.4 mmol/L)

Elderly patients can usually be maintained at lower end of therapeutic range (0.6-0.8 mEq/L)

Toxic concentration: >2 mEq/L (SI: >2 mmol/L)

Adverse effect levels:

GI complaints/tremor: 1.5-2 mEq/L

Confusion/somnolence: 2-2.5 mEq/L

Seizures/death: >2.5 mEq/L

Test Interactions ↑ calcium (S), glucose, magnesium, potassium (S); ↓ thyroxine (S)

Patient Information Avoid tasks requiring psychomotor coordination until the CNS effects are known, blood level monitoring is required to determine the proper dose; maintain a steady salt and fluid intake especially during the summer months; do not crush or chew slow or extended release dosage form, swallow whole

Nursing Implications Give with meals to decrease GI upset; avoid dehydration

Additional Information

Lithium citrate: Cibalith-S®

Lithium carbonate: Eskalith®, Lithane®, Lithobid®, Lithonate®, Lithotabs®

Dosage Forms

Capsule, as carbonate: 150 mg, 300 mg, 600 mg

Syrup, as citrate: 300 mg/5 mL (5 mL, 10 mL, 480 mL)

Tablet, as carbonate: 300 mg

Tablet:

Controlled release, as carbonate: 450 mg

Slow release, as carbonate: 300 mg

Lodoxamide Tromethamine (loe dox' a mide)

Brand Names Alomide®

Use Treatment of vernal keratoconjunctivitis, vernal conjunctivitis, and vernal keratitis

Pregnancy Risk Factor B

Contraindications Hypersensitivity to any component of product

Warnings/Precautions Safety and efficacy in children <2 years of age have not been established; not for injection; not for use in patients wearing soft contact lenses during treatment

Adverse Reactions

>10%: Local: Transient burning, stinging, discomfort

1% to 10%:
Central nervous system: Headache
Ocular: Blurred vision, corneal erosion/ulcer, eye pain, corneal abrasion, blepharitis

<1%:
Central nervous system: Dizziness, somnolence
Dermatologic: Rash
Gastrointestinal: Nausea, stomach discomfort
Ocular: Blepharitis
Respiratory: Sneezing
Miscellaneous: Dry nose

Overdosage/Toxicology Symptoms include feeling of warmth of flushing, headache, dizziness, fatigue, sweating, nausea, loose stools, and urinary frequency/urgency; consider emesis in the event of accidental ingestion

Mechanism of Action Mast cell stabilizer that inhibits the *in vivo* type I immediate hypersensitivity reaction to increase cutaneous vascular permeability associated with IgE and antigen-mediated reactions

Pharmacodynamics/Kinetics Absorption: Topical: Very small and undetectable

Usual Dosage Children >2 years and Adults: Instill 1-2 drops in eye(s) 4 times/day for up to 3 months

Dosage Forms Solution, ophthalmic: 0.1% (10 mL)

Loestrin® *see* Ethinyl Estradiol and Norethindrone *on page 425*

Lofene® *see* Diphenoxylate and Atropine *on page 352*

Logen® *see* Diphenoxylate and Atropine *on page 352*

Lomanate® *see* Diphenoxylate and Atropine *on page 352*

Lomefloxacin Hydrochloride (loe me flox' a sin)

Brand Names Maxaquin®

Use Quinolone antibiotic for skin and skin structure, lower respiratory and urinary tract infections, and sexually transmitted diseases

Pregnancy Risk Factor C

Contraindications Hypersensitivity to lomefloxacin or other members of the quinolone group such as nalidixic acid, oxolinic acid, cinoxacin, norfloxacin, and ciprofloxacin; avoid use in children <18 years of age due to association of other quinolones with transient arthropathies

Warnings/Precautions Use with caution in patients with epilepsy or other CNS diseases which could predispose them to seizures

Adverse Reactions

1% to 10%:
Central nervous system: Headache, dizziness
Dermatologic: Photosensitivity
Gastrointestinal: Nausea, dizziness

<1%:
Cardiovascular: Flushing, chest pain, hypotension, hypertension, edema, syncope, tachycardia, bradycardia, arrhythmia, extrasystoles, cyanosis, cardiac failure, angina pectoris, myocardial infarction, coma
Central nervous system: Fatigue, malaise, asthenia, chills, convulsions, vertigo
Dermatologic: Purpura, rash
Endocrine & metabolic: Gout, hypoglycemia
Gastrointestinal: Abdominal pain, vomiting, flatulence, constipation, dry mouth
Genitourinary: Micturition disorder
Hematologic: Thrombocytopenia
Neuromuscular & skeletal: Back pain, hyperkinesia, tremor, paresthesias, leg cramps, myalgia
Otic: Earache
Renal: Dysuria, hematuria, anuria
Respiratory: Dyspnea, cough

(Continued)

Lomefloxacin Hydrochloride *(Continued)*

Miscellaneous: Increased sweating, allergic reaction, face edema, flu-like symptoms, decreased heat tolerance, tongue discoloration, increased fibrinolysis, thirst, epistaxis, taste perversion

Overdosage/Toxicology Symptoms of overdose include acute renal failure, seizures; GI decontamination and supportive care; diazepam for seizures; not removed by peritoneal or hemodialysis

Drug Interactions

Decreased effect: Decreased absorption with antacids containing aluminum, magnesium, and/or calcium (by up to 98% if given at the same time)

Increased toxicity/serum levels: Quinolones cause increased levels of caffeine, warfarin, cyclosporine, and theophylline; azlocillin, cimetidine, probenecid increase quinolone levels

Mechanism of Action Inhibits DNA-gyrase in susceptible organisms thereby inhibits relaxation of supercoiled DNA and promotes breakage of DNA strands. DNA gyrase (topoisomerase II), is an essential bacterial enzyme that maintains the superhelical structure of DNA and is required for DNA replication and transcription, DNA repair, recombination, and transposition.

Pharmacodynamics/Kinetics

Absorption: Well absorbed

Distribution: V_d: 2.4-3.5 L/kg

Protein binding: 20%

Half-life, elimination: 5-7.5 hours

Elimination: Primarily unchanged in urine

Usual Dosage Oral: Adults: 400 mg once daily for 10-14 days

Patient Information Take 1 hour before or 2 hours after meals

Dosage Forms Tablet: 400 mg

Lomodix® *see* Diphenoxylate and Atropine *on page 352*

Lomotil® *see* Diphenoxylate and Atropine *on page 352*

Lomustine (loe mus' teen)

Related Information

Antiemetics for Chemotherapy Induced Nausea and Vomiting *on page 1202*

Cancer Chemotherapy Regimens *on page 1218-1241*

Brand Names CeeNU®

Synonyms CCNU

Use Treatment of brain tumors, Hodgkin's and non-Hodgkin's lymphomas, melanoma, renal carcinoma, lung cancer, colon cancer

Pregnancy Risk Factor D

Contraindications Hypersensitivity to lomustine or any component

Warnings/Precautions The U.S. Food and Drug Administration (FDA) currently recommends that procedures for proper handling and disposal for antineoplastic agents be considered. Use with caution in patients with depressed platelet, leukocyte or erythrocyte counts. Bone marrow depression, notably thrombocytopenia and leukopenia, may lead to bleeding and overwhelming infections in an already compromised patient; will last for at least 6 weeks after a dose, do not give courses more frequently than every 6 weeks because the toxicity is cumulative. Use with caution in patients with liver function abnormalities.

Adverse Reactions

>10%:

Gastrointestinal: Nausea and vomiting occur 3-6 hours after oral administration; this is due to a centrally mediated mechanism, not a direct effect on the GI lining; if vomiting occurs, it is not necessary to replace the dose unless it occurs immediately after drug administration

Emetic potential:

<60 mg: Moderately high (60% to 90%)

≥60 mg: High (>90%)

Myelosuppression: Anemia; effects occur 4-6 weeks after a dose and may persist for 1-2 weeks

WBC: Moderate

Platelets: Severe

Onset (days): 14

Nadir (weeks): 4-5

Recovery (weeks): 6

1% to 10%:

Central nervous system: Neurotoxicity

Dermatologic: Skin rash

Gastrointestinal: Stomatitis, diarrhea

Hematologic: Anemia

<1%:
  Central nervous system: Disorientation, lethargy, ataxia, dysarthria
  Dermatologic: Alopecia
  Hepatic: Hepatotoxicity
  Renal: Renal failure
  Respiratory: Pulmonary fibrosis with cumulative doses >600 mg

Overdosage/Toxicology Symptoms of overdose include nausea, vomiting, leukopenia; there are no known antidotes; treatment is primarily symptomatic and supportive

Drug Interactions
  Decreased effect with phenobarbital, resulting in decreased efficacy of both drugs
  Increased toxicity with cimetidine, reported to cause bone marrow depression or to potentiate the myelosuppressive effects of lomustine

Stability Refrigerate (<40°C/<104°F)

Mechanism of Action Inhibits DNA and RNA synthesis via carbamylation of DNA polymerase, alkylation of DNA, and alteration of RNA, proteins, and enzymes

Pharmacodynamics/Kinetics
  Absorption: Complete from GI tract; appears in plasma within 3 minutes after administration
  Distribution: Crosses blood-brain barrier to a greater degree than BNCU and CNS concentrations are equal to that of plasma
  Protein binding: 50%
  Metabolism: Rapid in the liver by hydroxylation produces at least 2 active metabolites
  Half-life: Parent drug: 16-72 hours
    Active metabolite: Terminal half-life: 1.3-2 days
  Time to peak serum concentration: Active metabolite: Within 3 hours
  Elimination: Enterohepatically recycled; excreted in the urine, feces (<5%), and in the expired air (<10%)

Usual Dosage Oral (refer to individual protocols):
  Children: 75-150 mg/m² as a single dose every 6 weeks. Subsequent doses are readjusted after initial treatment according to platelet and leukocyte counts.
  Adults: 100-130 mg/m² as a single dose every 6 weeks; readjust after initial treatment according to platelet and leukocyte counts
    Subsequent dosing adjustment based on nadir:
      Leukocytes 2,000-2,900/mm³, platelets 25,000-74,999/mm³: Administer 70% of prior dose
      Leukocytes <2,000/mm³, platelets <25,000/mm³: Administer 50% of prior dose

    Dosage adjustment in renal impairment:
      Cl_cr 10-50 mL/minute: Administer 75% of normal dose
      Cl_cr <10 mL/minute: Administer 50% of normal dose
    Hemodialysis effects: Supplemental dose is not necessary

Monitoring Parameters CBC with differential and platelet count, hepatic and renal function tests, pulmonary function tests

Test Interactions Liver function tests

Patient Information Take with fluids on an empty stomach; no food or drink for 2 hours after administration; notify physician if unusual or persistent fever, sore throat, bleeding, bruising, or fatigue occur; contraceptive measures are recommended during therapy

Dosage Forms
  Capsule: 10 mg, 40 mg, 100 mg
  Dose Pack: 10 mg (2s); 100 mg (2s); 40 mg (2s)

Loniten® *see* Minoxidil *on page 744*

Lonox® *see* Diphenoxylate and Atropine *on page 352*

Lo/Ovral® *see* Ethinyl Estradiol and Norgestrel *on page 427*

Loperamide Hydrochloride (loe per' a mide)
Brand Names Imodium®; Imodium® A-D [OTC]; Kaopectate® II [OTC]; Pepto® Diarrhea Control [OTC

Use Treatment of acute diarrhea and chronic diarrhea associated with inflammatory bowel disease; chronic functional diarrhea (idiopathic), chronic diarrhea caused by bowel resection or organic lesions; to decrease the volume of ileostomy discharge
  Unlabeled use: Treatment of traveler's diarrhea in combination with trimethoprim-sulfamethoxazole (co-trimoxazole) (3 days therapy)

Pregnancy Risk Factor B
(Continued)

647

Loperamide Hydrochloride *(Continued)*

Contraindications Patients who must avoid constipation, diarrhea resulting from some infections, or in patients with pseudomembranous colitis, hypersensitivity to specific drug or component, bloody diarrhea

Warnings/Precautions Large first-pass metabolism, use with caution in hepatic dysfunction; should not be used if diarrhea accompanied by high fever, blood in stool

Adverse Reactions

Central nervous system: Sedation, fatigue, dizziness, drowsiness

Dermatologic: Rash

Gastrointestinal: Nausea, vomiting, constipation, abdominal cramping, dry mouth, abdominal distention

Overdosage/Toxicology Symptoms of overdose include CNS and respiratory depression, gastrointestinal cramping, constipation, GI irritation, nausea, vomiting; overdosage is noted when daily doses approximate 60 mg of loperamide

Treatment of overdose: Gastric lavage followed by 100 g activated charcoal through a nasogastric tube. Monitor for signs of CNS depression; if they occur, administer naloxone 2 mg I.V. (0.01 mg/kg for children) with repeat administration as necessary up to a total of 10 mg.

Drug Interactions Increased toxicity: CNS depressants, phenothiazines, tricyclic antidepressants may potentiate the adverse effects

Mechanism of Action Acts directly on intestinal muscles to inhibit peristalsis and prolongs transit time enhancing fluid and electrolyte movement through intestinal mucosa; reduces fecal volume, increases viscosity, and diminishes fluid and electrolyte loss; demonstrates antisecretory activity; exhibits peripheral action

Pharmacodynamics/Kinetics

Onset of action: Oral: Within 0.5-1 hour

Absorption: Oral: <40%; levels in breast milk expected to be very low

Protein binding: 97%

Metabolism: Hepatic (>50%) to inactive compounds

Half-life: 7-14 hours

Elimination: Fecal and urinary (1%) excretion of metabolites and unchanged drug (30% to 40%)

Usual Dosage Oral:

Children:

Acute diarrhea: Initial doses (in first 24 hours):

2-6 years: 1 mg three times/day

6-8 years: 2 mg twice daily

8-12 years: 2 mg three times/day

Maintenance: After initial dosing, 0.1 mg/kg doses after each loose stool, but not exceeding initial dosage

Chronic diarrhea: 0.08-0.24 mg/kg/day divided 2-3 times/day, maximum: 2 mg/dose

Adults: Initial: 4 mg (2 capsules), followed by 2 mg after each loose stool, up to 16 mg/day (8 capsules)

Patient Information Do not take more than 8 capsules or 80 mL in 24 hours; may cause drowsiness; if acute diarrhea lasts longer than 48 hours, consult physician

Nursing Implications Therapy for chronic diarrhea should not exceed 10 days

Dosage Forms

Capsule: 2 mg

Liquid, oral: 1 mg/5 mL (60 mL, 90 mL, 120 mL)

Tablet: 2 mg

Lopid® *see* Gemfibrozil *on page 498*

Lopremone *see* Protirelin *on page 952*

Lopressor® *see* Metoprolol Tartrate *on page 731*

Loprox® *see* Ciclopirox Olamine *on page 244*

Lorabid™ *see* Loracarbef *on this page*

Loracarbef *(loe ra kar' bef)*

Brand Names Lorabid™

Use Infections caused by susceptible organisms involving the respiratory tract, acute otitis media, sinusitis, skin and skin structure, bone and joint, and urinary tract and gynecologic

Pregnancy Risk Factor B

Contraindications Patients with a history of hypersensitivity to loracarbef or cephalosporins

Warnings/Precautions Use with caution in patients with a previous history of hypersensitivity to other beta-lactam antibiotics (eg, penicillins, cephalosporins)

Adverse Reactions
1% to 10%:
　　Central nervous system: Headache
　　Dermatologic: Skin rashes
　　Gastrointestinal: Diarrhea, nausea, vomiting, abdominal pain, anorexia
　　Genitourinary: Vaginitis, vaginal moniliasis
<1%:
　　Cardiovascular: Vasodilation
　　Central nervous system: Somnolence, nervousness, dizziness
　　Hematologic: Transient thrombocytopenia, leukopenia, and eosinophilia
　　Miscellaneous: Transient elevations of ALT, AST, alkaline phosphatase and BUN, creatinine

Overdosage/Toxicology Symptoms of overdose include abdominal discomfort, diarrhea; supportive care only

Drug Interactions Increased serum levels with probenecid

Stability Suspension may be kept at room temperature for 14 days

Mechanism of Action Inhibits bacterial cell wall synthesis by binding to one or more of the penicillin binding proteins (PBPs); inhibits the final transpeptidation step of peptidoglycan synthesis in bacterial cell walls, thus inhibiting cell wall biosynthesis. It is thought that beta-lactam antibiotics inactivate transpeptidase via acylation of the enzyme with cleavage of the CO-N bond of the beta-lactam ring. Upon exposure to beta-lactam antibiotics, bacteria eventually lyse due to ongoing activity of cell wall autolytic enzymes (autolysins and murein hydrolases) while cell wall assembly is arrested.

Pharmacodynamics/Kinetics
Absorption: Oral: Rapid
Half-life, elimination: ~1 hour
Time to peak serum concentration: Oral: Within 1 hour
Elimination: Plasma clearance: ~200-300 mL/minute

Usual Dosage Oral:
Children:
　　Acute otitis media: 15 mg/kg twice daily for 10 days
　　Pharyngitis: 7.5-15 mg/kg twice daily for 10 days
Adults: Women:
　　Uncomplicated urinary tract infections: 200 mg once daily for 7 days
　　Skin and soft tissue: 200-400 mg every 12-24 hours
　　Uncomplicated pyelonephritis: 400 mg every 12 hours for 14 days

Dosing comments in renal impairment:
　　Cl_{cr} ≥50 mL/minute: Give usual dose
　　Cl_{cr} 10-49 mL/minute: 50% of usual dose at usual interval or usual dose given half as often
　　Cl_{cr} <10 mL/minute: Give usual dose every 3-5 days
　　Hemodialysis: Doses should be administered after dialysis sessions

Patient Information Take on an empty stomach at least 1 hour before or 2 hours after meals; finish all medication

Dosage Forms
Capsule: 200 mg
Suspension, oral: 100 mg/5 mL; 200 mg/5 mL

Loratadine (lor at' a deen)

Brand Names Claritin®

Use Relief of nasal and non-nasal symptoms of seasonal allergic rhinitis

Pregnancy Risk Factor B

Contraindications Patients hypersensitive to loratadine or any of its components

Warnings/Precautions Patients with liver impairment should start with a lower dose (10 mg every other day), since their ability to clear the drug will be reduced; use with caution in lactation, safety in children <12 years of age has not been established

Adverse Reactions
>10%:
　　Central nervous system: Headache, somnolence, fatigue
　　Gastrointestinal: Dry mouth
1% to 10%:
　　Cardiovascular: Hypotension, hypertension, palpitations, tachycardia
　　Central nervous system: Anxiety, depression
　　Endocrine & metabolic: Breast pain
　　Neuromuscular & skeletal: Hyperkinesia, arthralgias
　　Respiratory: Nasal dryness, pharyngitis, dyspnea
　　Miscellaneous: Sweating
(Continued)

Loratadine *(Continued)*

Overdosage/Toxicology Symptoms of overdose include somnolence, tachycardia, headache; no specific antidote is available, treatment is first decontamination, then symptomatic and supportive; loratadine is not eliminated by dialysis

Drug Interactions
Increased plasma concentrations of loratadine and its active metabolite with ketoconazole; erythromycin increases the AUC of loratadine and its active metabolite; no change in Q-T$_c$ interval was seen
Increased toxicity: Procarbazine, other antihistamines, alcohol

Mechanism of Action Long-acting tricyclic antihistamine with selective peripheral histamine H$_1$ receptor antagonistic properties

Pharmacodynamics/Kinetics
Onset of action: Within 1-3 hours
Peak effect: 8-12 hours
Duration: >24 hours
Absorption: Rapid
Metabolism: Extensive to an active metabolite
Half-life: 12-15 hours
Elimination: Significant excretion into breast milk

Usual Dosage Children >12 years and Adults: Oral: 10 mg/day on an empty stomach

Dosing interval in hepatic impairment: 10 mg every other day to start

Patient Information Drink plenty of water; may cause dry mouth, sedation, drowsiness, and can impair judgment and coordination

Dosage Forms Tablet: 10 mg

Lorazepam *(lor a' ze pam)*

Related Information
Benzodiazepines Comparison *on page 1256*
Initial Doses in Selected Antiemetic Regimens *on page 1205*

Brand Names Ativan®

Use Management of anxiety, status epilepticus, preoperative sedation, for desired amnesia, and as an antiemetic adjunct

Unapproved uses: Alcohol detoxification, insomnia, psychogenic catatonia, partial complex seizures

Restrictions C-IV

Pregnancy Risk Factor D

Contraindications Hypersensitivity to lorazepam or any component; there may be a cross-sensitivity with other benzodiazepines; do not use in a comatose patient, those with pre-existing CNS depression, narrow-angle glaucoma, severe uncontrolled pain, severe hypotension

Warnings/Precautions Use caution in patients with renal or hepatic impairment, organic brain syndrome, myasthenia gravis, or Parkinson's disease. Dilute injection prior to I.V. use with equal volume of compatible diluent (D$_5$W, 0.9% sodium chloride, sterile water for injection); do **not** inject intra-arterially, arteriospasm and gangrene may occur; injection contains benzyl alcohol 2%, polyethylene glycol and propylene glycol, which may be toxic to newborns in high doses, may reduce effectiveness of ECT; oral doses >0.09 mg/kg produced increased ataxia without increased sedative benefit versus lower doses

Adverse Reactions
Respiratory: Decrease in respiratory rate, apnea, laryngospasm
>10%:
Cardiovascular: Tachycardia, chest pain
Central nervous system: Drowsiness, confusion, ataxia, amnesia, slurred speech, paradoxical excitement, rage, headache, depression, anxiety, fatigue, lightheadedness, insomnia
Dermatologic: Rash
Endocrine & metabolic: Decreased libido
Gastrointestinal: Dry mouth, constipation, diarrhea, nausea, vomiting, increased or decreased appetite
Local: Phlebitis, pain with injection
Neuromuscular & skeletal: Impaired coordination, dysarthria
Ocular: Blurred vision, diplopia
Miscellaneous: Decreased salivation, sweating
1% to 10%:
Cardiovascular: Cardiac arrest, hypotension, bradycardia, cardiovascular collapse, syncope
Central nervous system: Confusion, nervousness, dizziness, akathisia
Neuromuscular & skeletal: Rigidity, tremor, muscle cramps
Dermatologic: Dermatitis

Gastrointestinal: Weight gain or loss
Otic: Tinnitus
Respiratory: Nasal congestion, hyperventilation
<1%:
Endocrine & metabolic: Menstrual irregularities
Hematologic: Blood dyscrasias
Miscellaneous: Reflex slowing, physical and psychological dependence with prolonged use, increased salivation

Overdosage/Toxicology Symptoms of overdose include confusion, coma, hypoactive reflexes, dyspnea, labored breathing. Treatment for benzodiazepine overdose is supportive. Rarely is mechanical ventilation required.

Flumazenil has been shown to selectively block the binding of benzodiazepines to CNS receptors, resulting in a reversal of benzodiazepine-induced CNS depression but not respiratory depression. Treatment requires support of blood pressure and respiration until drug effects subside.

Drug Interactions
Decreased effect with oral contraceptives (combination products), cigarette smoking; decreased effect of levodopa
Increased effect with morphine
Increased toxicity with alcohol, CNS depressants, MAO inhibitors, loxapine, TCAs

Stability
Intact vials should be refrigerated, protected from light; do not use discolored or precipitate containing solutions
May be stored at room temperature for up to 60 days
Stability of parenteral admixture at room temperature (25°C): 24 hours
Standard diluent: 1 mg/100 mL D_5W
I.V. is **incompatible** when administered in the same line with foscarnet, ondansetron, sargramostim

Mechanism of Action Depresses all levels of the CNS, including the limbic and reticular formation, probably through the increased action of gamma-aminobutyric acid (GABA), which is a major inhibitory neurotransmitter in the brain

Pharmacodynamics/Kinetics
Onset of hypnosis: I.M.: 20-30 minutes
Duration: 6-8 hours
Absorption: Oral, I.M.: Prompt following administration
Distribution: Crosses the placenta; appears in breast milk
V_d:
Neonates: 0.76 L/kg
Adults: 1.3 L/kg
Protein binding: 85%, free fraction may be significantly higher in elderly
Metabolism: In the liver to inactive compounds
Half-life:
Neonates: 40.2 hours
Older Children: 10.5 hours
Adults: 12.9 hours
Elderly: 15.9 hours
End stage renal disease: 32-70 hours
Elimination: Urinary excretion and minimal fecal clearance

Usual Dosage
Antiemetic:
Children 2-15 years: I.V.: 0.05 mg/kg (up to 2 mg/dose) prior to chemotherapy
Adults: Oral, I.V.: 0.5-2 mg every 4-6 hours as needed

Anxiety and sedation:
Infants and Children: Oral, I.V.: Usual: 0.05 mg/kg/dose (range: 0.02-0.09 mg/kg) every 4-8 hours
Adults: Oral: 1-10 mg/day in 2-3 divided doses; usual dose: 2-6 mg/day in divided doses

Insomnia: Adults: Oral: 2-4 mg at bedtime

Preoperative: Adults:
I.M.: 0.05 mg/kg administered 2 hours before surgery; maximum: 4 mg/dose
I.V.: 0.044 mg/kg 15-20 minutes before surgery; usual maximum: 2 mg/dose

Operative amnesia: Adults: I.V.: up to 0.05 mg/kg; maximum: 4 mg/dose

Status epilepticus: I.V.:
Neonates: 0.05 mg/kg over 2-5 minutes; may repeat in 10-15 minutes (see warning regarding benzyl alcohol)
Infants and Children: 0.1 mg/kg slow I.V. over 2-5 minutes, do not exceed 4 mg/single dose; may repeat second dose of 0.05 mg/kg slow I.V. in 10-15 minutes if needed
(Continued)

Lorazepam *(Continued)*

Adolescents: 0.07 mg/kg slow I.V. over 2-5 minutes; maximum: 4 mg/dose; may repeat in 10-15 minutes

Adults: 4 mg/dose given slowly over 2-5 minutes; may repeat in 10-15 minutes; usual maximum dose: 8 mg

Administration
Lorazepam may be administered by I.M. or I.V.
I.M.: Should be administered deep into the muscle mass
I.V.: Do not exceed 2 mg/minute or 0.05 mg/kg over 2-5 minutes
Dilute I.V. dose with equal volume of compatible diluent (D_5W, NS, SWI)
Injection must be made slowly with repeated aspiration to make sure the injection is not intra-arterial and that perivascular extravasation has not occurred

Monitoring Parameters Respiratory and cardiovascular status, blood pressure, heart rate, symptoms of anxiety

Reference Range Therapeutic: 50-240 ng/mL (SI: 156-746 nmol/L)

Test Interactions May increase the results of liver function tests

Patient Information Advise patient of potential for physical and psychological dependence with chronic use; advise patient of possible retrograde amnesia after I.V. or I.M. use; will cause drowsiness, impairment of judgment or coordination

Nursing Implications Keep injectable form in the refrigerator; **inadvertent intra-arterial injection may produce arteriospasm resulting in gangrene which may require amputation;** emergency resuscitative equipment should be available when administering by I.V.; prior to I.V. use, lorazepam injection must be diluted with an equal amount of compatible diluent; injection must be made slowly with repeated aspiration to make sure the injection is not intra-arterial and that perivascular extravasation has not occurred; provide safety measures (ie, side rails, night light, and call button); supervise ambulation

Dosage Forms
Injection: 2 mg/mL (1 mL, 10 mL); 4 mg/mL (1 mL, 10 mL)
Solution, oral concentrated: 2 mg/mL (30 mL)
Tablet: 0.5 mg, 1 mg, 2 mg

Lorcet® *see* Hydrocodone and Acetaminophen *on page 543*

Lorcet®-HD *see* Hydrocodone and Acetaminophen *on page 543*

Lorcet® Plus *see* Hydrocodone and Acetaminophen *on page 543*

Lorelco® *see* Probucol *on page 927*

Loroxide® [OTC] *see* Benzoyl Peroxide *on page 122*

Lortab® *see* Hydrocodone and Acetaminophen *on page 543*

Lortab® ASA *see* Hydrocodone and Aspirin *on page 544*

Losec® *see* Omeprazole *on page 816*

Lotensin® *see* Benazepril Hydrochloride *on page 118*

Lotrimin® *see* Clotrimazole *on page 265*

Lotrimin AF® [OTC] *see* Clotrimazole *on page 265*

Lovastatin *(loe′ va sta tin)*

Related Information
Lipid-Lowering Agents *on page 1273*

Brand Names Mevacor®

Synonyms Mevinolin; Monacolin K

Use Adjunct to dietary therapy to decrease elevated serum total and LDL cholesterol concentrations in primary hypercholesterolemia

Pregnancy Risk Factor X

Contraindications Active liver disease, hypersensitivity to lovastatin or any component

Warnings/Precautions May elevate aminotransferases; LFTs should be performed before and every 4- 6 weeks during the first 12-15 months of therapy and periodically thereafter; can also cause myalgia and rhabdomyolysis; use with caution in patients who consume large quantities of alcohol or who have a history of liver disease

Adverse Reactions
Endocrine & metabolic: Gynecomastia

1% to 10%: Elevated creatine phosphokinase (CPK)
Central nervous system: Headache, dizziness
Dermatologic: Rash, pruritus
Gastrointestinal: Flatulence, abdominal pain, cramps, diarrhea, pancreatitis constipation, nausea, dyspepsia, heartburn

Neuromuscular & skeletal: Myalgia
<1%:
Central nervous system: Dizziness
Gastrointestinal: Dysgeusia
Ocular: Blurred vision, myositis, lenticular opacities

Overdosage/Toxicology Very few adverse events; treatment is symptomatic

Drug Interactions
Increased toxicity: Gemfibrozil (musculoskeletal effects such as myopathy, myalgia and/or muscle weakness accompanied by markedly elevated CK concentrations, rash and/or pruritus); clofibrate, niacin (myopathy), erythromycin, cyclosporine, oral anticoagulants (elevated PT)
Increased effect/toxicity of levothyroxine

Mechanism of Action Lovastatin acts by competitively inhibiting 3-hydroxyl-3-methylglutaryl-coenzyme A (HMG-CoA) reductase, the enzyme that catalyzes the rate-limiting step in cholesterol biosynthesis

Pharmacodynamics/Kinetics
Onset of effect: 3 days of therapy required for LDL cholesterol concentration reductions
Absorption: Oral: 30%
Protein binding: 95%
Half-life: 1.1-1.7 hours
Time to peak serum concentration: Oral: 2-4 hours
Elimination: ~80% to 85% of dose excreted in feces and 10% in urine following liver hydrolysis

Usual Dosage Adults: Oral: Initial: 20 mg with evening meal, then adjust at 4-week intervals; maximum dose: 80 mg/day; before initiation of therapy, patients should be placed on a standard cholesterol-lowering diet for 3-6 months and the diet should be continued during drug therapy

Administration Administer with meals

Monitoring Parameters Plasma triglycerides, cholesterol, and liver function tests

Test Interactions ↑ liver transaminases (S), altered thyroid function tests

Patient Information Promptly report any unexplained muscle pain, tenderness or weakness, especially if accompanied by malaise or fever; do not interrupt, increase, or decrease dose without advice of physician; take with meals

Nursing Implications Urge patient to adhere to cholesterol-lowering diet

Dosage Forms Tablet: 10 mg, 20 mg, 40 mg

Lovenox® see Enoxaparin Sodium on page 387

Low-Quel® see Diphenoxylate and Atropine on page 352

Loxapine (lox' a peen)

Related Information
Antipsychotic Agents Comparison on page 1255

Brand Names Loxitane®

Synonyms Loxapine Hydrochloride; Loxapine Succinate; Oxilapine Succinate

Use Management of psychotic disorders

Pregnancy Risk Factor C

Contraindications Hypersensitivity to chlorpromazine or any component, cross-sensitivity with other phenothiazines may exist; avoid use in patients with narrow-angle glaucoma, bone marrow depression, severe liver or cardiac disease, severe CNS depression, coma

Warnings/Precautions Watch for hypotension when administering I.M.; safety in children <6 months of age has not been established; use with caution in patients with cardiovascular disease or seizures; benefits of therapy must be weighed against risks of therapy; should not be given I.V.

Adverse Reactions
>10%:
Cardiovascular: Orthostatic hypotension
Central nervous system: Drowsiness, extrapyramidal effects (parkinsonian), confusion, persistent tardive dyskinesia
Gastrointestinal: Dry mouth
Ocular: Blurred vision
1% to 10%:
Dermatologic: Skin rash
Endocrine & metabolic: Enlargement of breasts
Gastrointestinal: Constipation, nausea, vomiting
<1%:
Cardiovascular: Tachycardia, arrhythmias, abnormal T-waves with prolonged ventricular repolarization
(Continued)

653

Loxapine *(Continued)*

Central nervous system: Neuroleptic malignant syndrome (NMS), sedation, drowsiness, restlessness, anxiety, seizures

Dermatologic: Hyperpigmentation, pruritus, rash, photosensitivity

Endocrine & metabolic: Galactorrhea, amenorrhea, galactorrhea, gynecomastia

Gastrointestinal: Weight gain, adynamic ileus

Genitourinary: Urinary retention, overflow incontinence, priapism, sexual dysfunction

Hematologic: Agranulocytosis (more often in women between fourth and tenth week of therapy), leukopenia (usually in patients with large doses for prolonged periods)

Hepatic: Cholestatic jaundice

Ocular: Retinal pigmentation

Miscellaneous: Altered central temperature regulation

Overdosage/Toxicology Symptoms of overdose include deep sleep, dystonia, agitation, dysrhythmias, extrapyramidal symptoms, hypotension, seizures

Following initiation of essential overdose management, toxic symptom treatment and supportive treatment should be initiated. Hypotension usually responds to I.V. fluids or Trendelenburg positioning. If unresponsive to these measures, the use of a parenteral inotrope may be required (eg, norepinephrine 0.1-0.2 mcg/kg/minute titrated to response). Seizures commonly respond to diazepam (I.V. 5-10 mg bolus in adults every 15 minutes if needed up to a total of 30 mg; I.V. 0.25-0.4 mg/kg/dose up to a total of 10 mg in children) or to phenytoin or phenobarbital. Critical cardiac arrhythmias often respond to I.V. phenytoin (15 mg/kg up to 1 g), while other antiarrhythmics can be used. Neuroleptics often cause extrapyramidal symptoms (eg, dystonic reactions) requiring management with diphenhydramine 1-2 mg/kg (adults) up to a maximum of 50 mg I.M. or I.V. slow push followed by a maintenance dose for 48-72 hours. When these reactions are unresponsive to diphenhydramine, benztropine mesylate I.V. 1-2 mg (adults) may be effective. These agents are generally effective within 2-5 minutes.

Drug Interactions

Decreased effect of guanethidine, phenytoin

Increased toxicity with CNS depressants, metrizamide ($\uparrow$ seizure potential), guanabenz, MAO inhibitors

Mechanism of Action Unclear, thought to be similar to chlorpromazine

Pharmacodynamics/Kinetics

Onset of neuroleptic effect: Oral: Within 20-30 minutes

Peak effect: 1.5-3 hours

Duration: ~12 hours

Metabolism: Hepatic to glucuronide conjugates

Half-life, biphasic:

Initial: 5 hours

Terminal: 12-19 hours

Elimination: In urine, and to a smaller degree, feces

Usual Dosage Adults:

Oral: 10 mg twice daily, increase dose until psychotic symptoms are controlled; usual dose range: 60-100 mg/day in divided doses 2-4 times/day; dosages >250 mg/day are not recommended

I.M.: 12.5-50 mg every 4-6 hours or longer as needed and change to oral therapy as soon as possible

Administration Injectable is for I.M. use only

Test Interactions False-positives for phenylketonuria, amylase, uroporphyrins, urobilinogen, $\uparrow$ liver function tests

Patient Information May cause drowsiness; avoid alcoholic beverages; may impair judgment or coordination; may cause photosensitivity; avoid excessive sunlight; do not stop taking without consulting physician

Additional Information

Loxapine hydrochloride: Loxitane® C oral concentrate, Loxitane® IM

Loxapine succinate: Loxitane® capsule

Dosage Forms

Capsule: 5 mg, 10 mg, 25 mg, 50 mg

Concentrate, oral: 25 mg/mL (120 mL dropper bottle)

Injection: 50 mg/mL (1 mL)

Loxapine Hydrochloride *see Loxapine on previous page*

Loxapine Succinate *see Loxapine on previous page*

Loxitane® *see Loxapine on previous page*

Lozol® *see Indapamide on page 574*

L-PAM *see* Melphalan *on page 681*

LRH *see* Gonadorelin *on page 510*

L-Sarcolysin *see* Melphalan *on page 681*

LTG *see* Lamotrigine *on page 618*

***L*-Thyroxine Sodium** *see* Levothyroxine Sodium *on page 629*

Ludiomil® *see* Maprotiline Hydrochloride *on page 665*

Lugol's Solution *see* Potassium Iodide *on page 909*

Luminal® *see* Phenobarbital *on page 869*

Lupron® *see* Leuprolide Acetate *on page 621*

Lupron Depot® *see* Leuprolide Acetate *on page 621*

Lupron Depot-Ped™ *see* Leuprolide Acetate *on page 621*

Luride® *see* Fluoride *on page 471*

Luride® Lozi-Tab® *see* Fluoride *on page 471*

Luride®-SF Lozi-Tab® *see* Fluoride *on page 471*

Luteinizing Hormone Releasing Hormone *see* Gonadorelin *on page 510*

Lutrepulse® *see* Gonadorelin *on page 510*

Luvox® *see* Fluvoxamine *on page 485*

Lymphocyte Immune Globulin (lim' foe site i myun' glob' yoo lin)

Brand Names Atgam®

Synonyms Antithymocyte Globulin (Equine); Antithymocyte Immunoglobulin; ATG; Horse Anti-human Thymocyte Gamma Globulin

Use Prevention and treatment of acute renal allograft rejection; treatment of moderate to severe aplastic anemia in patients not considered suitable candidates for bone marrow transplantation; prevention of graft-versus-host disease following bone marrow transplantation

Pregnancy Risk Factor C

Contraindications Known hypersensitivity to ATG, thimerosal, or other equine gamma globulins; severe, unremitting leukopenia and/or thrombocytopenia

Warnings/Precautions Must be administered via central line due to chemical phlebitis; should only be used by physicians experienced in immunosuppressive therapy or management of renal transplant patients; adequate laboratory and supportive medical resources must be readily available in the facility for patient management; rash, dyspnea, hypotension, or anaphylaxis precludes further administration of the drug. Dose must be administered over at least 4 hours; patient may need to be pretreated with an antipyretic, antihistamine, and/or corticosteroid.

Adverse Reactions
>10%:
　Central nervous system: Fever, chills
　Dermatologic: Rash
　Hematologic: Leukopenia, thrombocytopenia
　Miscellaneous: Systemic infection
1% to 10%:
　Cardiovascular: Hypotension, hypertension, tachycardia, edema, chest pain
　Central nervous system: Headache, malaise
　Gastrointestinal: Diarrhea, nausea, stomatitis, GI bleeding
　Respiratory: Dyspnea
　Local: Pain, swelling, or redness at injection site, thrombophlebitis
　Neuromuscular & skeletal: Myalgia, back pain
　Renal: Abnormal renal function tests
　Sensitivity reactions: Anaphylaxis may be indicated by hypotension, respiratory distress, serum sickness
　Miscellaneous: Viral infection
<1%:
　Central nervous system: Seizures, weakness
　Dermatologic: Pruritus, urticaria
　Genitourinary: Acute renal failure
　Hematologic: Hemolysis, anemia
　Neuromuscular & skeletal: Arthralgia, lymphadenopathy

Stability
　Ampuls must be refrigerated
　Dose must be diluted in 0.45% or 0.9% sodium chloride
　Diluted solution is stable for 12 hours (including infusion time) at room temperature and 24 hours (including infusion time) at refrigeration

(Continued)

Lymphocyte Immune Globulin (Continued)

The use of dextrose solutions is not recommended (precipitation may occur)

Standard diluent: Dose/1000 mL NS or 0.45% sodium chloride

Minimum volume: Concentration should not exceed 1 mg/mL for a peripheral line or 4 mg/mL for a central line

Mechanism of Action May involve elimination of antigen-reactive T-lymphocytes (killer cells) in peripheral blood or alteration of T-cell function

Pharmacodynamics/Kinetics

Distribution: Poorly distributed into lymphoid tissues; binds to circulating lymphocytes, granulocytes, platelets, bone marrow cells

Half-life, plasma: 1.5-12 days

Elimination: ~1% of dose excreted in urine

Usual Dosage An intradermal skin test is recommended prior to administration of the initial dose of ATG; use 0.1 mL of a 1:1000 dilution of ATG in normal saline

Children and Adults: I.V.:

Aplastic anemia protocol: 10-20 mg/kg/day for 8-14 days, then give every other day for 7 more doses

Rejection prevention: 15 mg/kg/day for 14 days, then give every other day for 7 more doses for a total of 21 doses in 28 days; initial dose should be administered within 24 hours before or after transplantation

Rejection treatment: 10-15 mg/kg/day for 14 days, then give every other day for 7 more doses

Graft-vs-host disease treatment (following allogeneic bone marrow transplant): Doses have ranged from 15 mg/kg/dose twice daily for 5 days to 15 mg/kg/dose every other day for 6 doses have been used

Administration For I.V. use only; administer via central line; use of high flow veins will minimize the occurrence of phlebitis and thrombosis; administer by slow I.V. infusion through an inline filter with pore size of 0.2-1 micrometer over 4-8 hours at a final concentration not to exceed 4 mg ATG/mL

Monitoring Parameters Lymphocyte profile, CBC with differential and platelet count, vital signs during administration

Nursing Implications Mild itching and erythema can be treated with antihistamines; infuse dose over at least 4 hours; any severe systemic reaction to the skin test such as generalized rash, tachycardia, dyspnea, hypotension, or anaphylaxis should preclude further therapy; **epinephrine and resuscitative equipment should be nearby.** Patient may need to be pretreated with an antipyretic antihistamine, and/or corticosteroid.

Dosage Forms Injection: 50 of equine IgG/mL (5 mL)

Lyphocin® see Vancomycin Hydrochloride on page 1145

Lypressin (lye press' in)

Brand Names Diapid®

Synonyms 8-L-Lysine Vasopressin

Use Controls or prevents signs and complications of neurogenic diabetes insipidus

Pregnancy Risk Factor C

Contraindications Known hypersensitivity to lypressin

Warnings/Precautions Use with caution in patients with coronary artery disease

Adverse Reactions

1% to 10%:

Central nervous system: Dizziness, headache

Gastrointestinal: Abdominal cramping, increased bowel movements

Local: Rhinorrhea, nasal congestion, irritation or burning

Respiratory: Chest tightness, coughing, dyspnea

<1%: Miscellaneous: Water intoxication, inadvertent inhalation

Overdosage/Toxicology Symptoms of overdose include drowsiness, headache, confusion, weight gain, hypertension; systemic toxicity is unlikely to occur from the nasal spray

Drug Interactions Increased effect: Chlorpropamide, clofibrate, carbamazepine → prolongation of antidiuretic effects

Mechanism of Action Increases cyclic adenosine monophosphate (cAMP) which increases water permeability at the renal tubule resulting in decreased urine volume and increased osmolality; causes peristalsis by directly stimulating the smooth muscle in the GI tract

Pharmacodynamics/Kinetics

Onset of antidiuretic effect: Intranasal spray: Within 0.5-2 hours

Duration: 3-8 hours

Metabolism: In the liver and kidneys

Half-life: 15-20 minutes

Elimination: Urinary excretion

Usual Dosage Children and Adults: Instill 1-2 sprays into one or both nostrils whenever frequency of urination increases or significant thirst develops; usual dosage is 1-2 sprays 4 times/day; range: 1 spray/day at bedtime to 10 sprays each nostril every 3-4 hours

Patient Information To control nocturia, an additional dose may be given at bedtime; notify physician if drowsiness, fatigue, headache, shortness of breath, abdominal cramps, or severe nasal irritation occurs

Additional Information Approximately 2 USP posterior pituitary pressor units per spray

Dosage Forms Spray: 0.185 mg/mL (equivalent to 50 USP posterior pituitary units/mL) (8 mL)

Lysodren® *see* Mitotane *on page 748*

Macrobid® *see* Nitrofurantoin *on page 797*

Macrodantin® *see* Nitrofurantoin *on page 797*

Macrodex® *see* Dextran *on page 318*

Mafenide Acetate (ma′ fe nide)

Brand Names Sulfamylon®

Use Adjunct in the treatment of second and third degree burns to prevent septicemia caused by susceptible organisms such as *Pseudomonas aeruginosa*; prevention of graft loss of meshed autografts on excised burn wounds

Pregnancy Risk Factor C

Contraindications Hypersensitivity to mafenide, sulfites, or any component

Warnings/Precautions Use with caution in patients with renal impairment and in patients with G-6-PD deficiency; prolonged use may result in superinfection

Adverse Reactions
>10%: Local: Burning sensation, excoriation, pain
1% to 10%:
  Dermatologic: Skin rash
  Miscellaneous: Swelling of face, troubled breathing
<1%:
  Dermatologic: Erythema
  Endocrine & metabolic: Hyperchloremia, metabolic acidosis
  Hematologic: Bone marrow suppression, hemolytic anemia, bleeding
  Hepatic: Porphyria
  Respiratory: Hyperventilation, tachypnea
  Sensitivity reactions: Hypersensitivity

Mechanism of Action Interferes with bacterial folic acid synthesis through competitive inhibition of para-aminobenzoic acid

Pharmacodynamics/Kinetics
Absorption: Diffuses through devascularized areas and is rapidly absorbed from burned surface
Time to peak serum concentration: Topical: 2-4 hours
Metabolism: To para-carboxybenzene sulfonamide which is a carbonic anhydrase inhibitor
Elimination: In urine as metabolites

Usual Dosage Children and Adults: Topical: Apply once or twice daily with a sterile gloved hand; apply to a thickness of approximately 16 mm; the burned area should be covered with cream at all times

Monitoring Parameters Acid base balance

Patient Information Discontinue and call physician immediately if rash, blisters, or swelling appear while using cream; discontinue if condition persists or worsens while using this product; for external use only

Dosage Forms Cream, topical: 85 mg/g (37 g, 114 g, 411 g)

Magnesia Magma *see* Magnesium Hydroxide *on page 659*

Magnesium Citrate (mag nee′ ze um cit′ rate)

Related Information
Laxatives, Classification and Properties *on page 1272*

Brand Names Citroma® [OTC]; Citro-Nesia™ [OTC]; Evac-Q-Mag® [OTC]

Synonyms Citrate of Magnesia

Use Evacuation of bowel prior to certain surgical and diagnostic procedures or overdose situations

Pregnancy Risk Factor B

(Continued)

Magnesium Citrate *(Continued)*

Contraindications Renal failure, appendicitis, abdominal pain, intestinal impaction, obstruction or perforation, diabetes mellitus, complications in gastrointestinal tract, patients with colostomy, ileostomy, ulcerative colitis or diverticulitis

Warnings/Precautions Use with caution in patients with impaired renal function, especially if Cl_{cr} <30 mL/minute (accumulation of magnesium which may lead to magnesium intoxication); use with caution in digitalized patients (may alter cardiac conduction leading to heart block); use with caution in patients with lithium administration; use with caution with neuromuscular blocking agents, CNS depressants

Adverse Reactions

1% to 10%:
Cardiovascular: Hypotension
Endocrine & metabolic: Hypermagnesemia
Gastrointestinal: Abdominal cramps, diarrhea, gas formation
Respiratory: Respiratory depression

Overdosage/Toxicology

Serious, potentially life-threatening electrolyte disturbances may occur with long-term use or overdosage due to diarrhea; hypermagnesemia may occur

CNS depression, confusion, hypotension, muscle weakness, blockage of peripheral neuromuscular transmission

Serum level >4 mEq/L (4.8 mg/dL): deep tendon reflexes may be depressed

Serum level ≥10 mEq/L (12 mg/dL): deep tendon reflexes may disappear, respiratory paralysis may occur, heart block may occur

I.V. calcium (5-10 mEq) will reverse respiratory depression or heart block; in extreme cases, peritoneal dialysis or hemodialysis may be required.

Serum level >12 mEq/L may be fatal, serum level ≥10 mEq/L may cause complete heart block

Mechanism of Action Promotes bowel evacuation by causing osmotic retention of fluid which distends the colon with increased peristaltic activity

Pharmacodynamics/Kinetics

Absorption: Oral: 15% to 30%
Elimination: Renal

Usual Dosage Cathartic: Oral:

Children:
<6 years: 0.5 mL/kg up to a maximum of 200 mL repeated every 4-6 hours until stools are clear
6-12 years: 100-150 mL
Adults ≥12 years: ½ to 1 full bottle (120-300 mL)

Reference Range Serum magnesium:

Children: 1.5-1.9 mg/dL ~1.2-1.6 mEq/L
Adults: 2.2-2.8 mg/dL ~1.8-2.3 mEq/L

Test Interactions ↑ magnesium; ↓ protein, ↓ calcium (S), ↓ potassium (S)

Patient Information Take with a glass of water, fruit juice, or citrus flavored carbonated beverage to improve taste, chill before using; report severe abdominal pain to physician

Nursing Implications To increase palatability, manufacturer suggests chilling the solution prior to administration

Additional Information Magnesium content of 5 mL: 3.85-4.71 mEq

Dosage Forms Solution, oral: 300 mL

Magnesium Gluconate *(mag nee' ze um gloo' ko nate)*

Brand Names Magonate® [OTC]

Use Dietary supplement for treatment of magnesium deficiencies

Contraindications Patients with heart block, severe renal disease

Warnings/Precautions Use with caution in patients with impaired renal function; hypermagnesemia and toxicity may occur due to decreased renal clearance of absorbed magnesium

Adverse Reactions

1% to 10%: Gastrointestinal: Diarrhea (excessive dose)
<1%:
Cardiovascular: Hypotension
Endocrine & metabolic: Hypermagnesemia
Gastrointestinal: Abdominal cramps
Neuromuscular & skeletal: Muscle weakness
Respiratory: Respiratory depression

Overdosage/Toxicology Hypermagnesemia rarely occurs after acute or chronic overexposure except in patients with renal insufficiency or massive overdose; moderate toxicity causes nausea, vomiting, weakness, and cutaneous flushing; larger doses cause cardiac conduction abnormalities, hypotension, severe muscle weakness, and lethargy; very high levels cause coma, respiratory arrest, and asystole. Treatment includes replacing fluid and electrolyte losses caused by excessive catharsis; while there is no specific antidote and treatment is supportive, administration of I.V. calcium may temporarily alleviate respiratory depression; hemodialysis rapidly removes magnesium and is the only route of elimination in anuric patients (hemoperfusion and repeat-dose charcoal are not effective).

Drug Interactions Increased effect of nondepolarizing neuromuscular blockers

Mechanism of Action Magnesium is important as a cofactor in many enzymatic reactions in the body involving protein synthesis and carbohydrate metabolism, (at least 300 enzymatic reactions require magnesium). Actions on lipoprotein lipase have been found to be important in reducing serum cholesterol and on sodium/potassium ATPase in promoting polarization (ie, neuromuscular functioning).

Pharmacodynamics/Kinetics
Absorption: Oral: 15% to 30%
Elimination: Renal

Usual Dosage The recommended dietary allowance (RDA) of magnesium is 4.5 mg/kg which is a total daily allowance of 350-400 mg for adult men and 280-300 mg for adult women. During pregnancy the RDA is 300 mg and during lactation the RDA is 355 mg. Average daily intakes of dietary magnesium have declined in recent years due to processing of food. The latest estimate of the average American dietary intake was 349 mg/day.

Dietary supplement: Oral:
Children: 3-6 mg/kg/day in divided doses 3-4 times/day; maximum: 400 mg/day
Adults: 27-54 mg 2-3 times/day or 100 mg 4 times/day

Dosing in renal impairment: Patients in severe renal failure should not receive magnesium due to toxicity from accumulation. Patients with a Cl_{cr} <25 mL/minute receiving magnesium should be monitored by serum magnesium levels.

Reference Range Serum magnesium:
Children: 1.5-1.9 mg/dL ~1.2-1.6 mEq/L
Adults: 2.2-2.8 mg/dL ~1.8-2.3 mEq/L

Additional Information Magnesium content of 500 mg: 27 mg elemental magnesium

Dosage Forms Tablet: 500 mg [elemental magnesium 27 mg]

Magnesium Hydroxide (mag nee' ze um hye drok' side)

Related Information
Laxatives, Classification and Properties *on page 1272*

Brand Names Phillips'® Milk of Magnesia [OTC]

Synonyms Magnesia Magma; Milk of Magnesia; MOM

Use Short-term treatment of occasional constipation and symptoms of hyperacidity, magnesium replacement therapy

Pregnancy Risk Factor B

Contraindications Patients with colostomy or an ileostomy, intestinal obstruction, fecal impaction, renal failure, appendicitis, hypersensitivity to any component

Warnings/Precautions Use with caution in patients with severe renal impairment, (especially when doses are >50 mEq magnesium/day); hypermagnesemia and toxicity may occur due to decreased renal clearance of absorbed magnesium. Decreased renal function (Cl_{cr} <30 mL/minute) may result in toxicity; monitor for toxicity.

Adverse Reactions
>10%: Diarrhea
1% to 10%:
  Cardiovascular: Hypotension
  Endocrine & metabolic: Hypermagnesemia
  Gastrointestinal: Abdominal cramps
  Neuromuscular & skeletal: Muscle weakness
  Respiratory: Respiratory depression

Overdosage/Toxicology Magnesium antacids are also laxative and may cause diarrhea and hypokalemia; in patients with renal failure, magnesium may accumulate to toxic levels. I.V. calcium (5-10 mEq) will reverse respiratory depression or heart block; in extreme cases, peritoneal dialysis or hemodialysis may be required.

Drug Interactions Decreased effect: Decreased absorption of tetracyclines, digoxin, indomethacin, or iron salts

Mechanism of Action Promotes bowel evacuation by causing osmotic retention of fluid which distends the colon with increased peristaltic activity; reacts with hydrochloric acid in stomach to form magnesium chloride
(Continued)

Magnesium Hydroxide *(Continued)*

Pharmacodynamics/Kinetics
Onset of laxative action: 4-8 hours

Elimination: Absorbed magnesium ions (up to 30%) are usually excreted by kidneys, unabsorbed drug is excreted in feces

Usual Dosage Oral:
Laxative:
>   <2 years: 0.5 mL/kg/dose
>   2-5 years: 5-15 mL/day or in divided doses
>   6-12 years: 15-30 mL/day or in divided doses
>   ≥12 years: 30-60 mL/day or in divided doses

Antacid:
>   Children: 2.5-5 mL as needed up to 4 times/day
>   Adults: 5-15 mL or 650 mg to 1.3 g tablets up to 4 times/day as needed

Dosing in renal impairment: Patients in severe renal failure should not receive magnesium due to toxicity from accumulation. Patients with a Cl_{cr} <25 mL/minute receiving magnesium should be monitored by serum magnesium levels.

Reference Range Serum magnesium:
Children: 1.5-1.9 mg/dL (1.2-1.6 mEq/L)

Adults: 1.5-2.5 mg/dL (1.2-2.0 mEq/L)

Test Interactions ↑ magnesium; ↓ protein, calcium (S), ↓ potassium (S)

Patient Information Dilute dose in water or juice, shake well

Nursing Implications MOM concentrate is 3 times as potent as regular strength product

Additional Information Magnesium content of 30 mL: 1.05 g (87 mEq)

Dosage Forms
Liquid: 390 mg/5 mL (10 mL, 15 mL, 20 mL, 30 mL, 100 mL, 120 mL, 180 mL, 360 mL, 720 mL)

Liquid, concentrate: 10 mL equivalent to 30 mL milk of magnesia USP

Suspension, oral: 2.5 g/30 mL (10 mL, 15 mL, 30 mL)

Tablet: 300 mg, 600 mg

Magnesium Oxide *(mag nee' ze um ok' side)*

Brand Names Maox®

Use Short-term treatment of occasional constipation and symptoms of hyperacidity

Pregnancy Risk Factor B

Contraindications Patients with colostomy or an ileostomy, appendicitis, ulcerative colitis, diverticulitis, heart block, myocardial damage, serious renal impairment, hepatitis, Addison's disease, hypersensitivity to any component

Warnings/Precautions Hypermagnesemia and toxicity may occur due to decreased renal clearance (Cl_{cr} <30 mL/minute) of absorbed magnesium; monitor serum magnesium level, respiratory rate, deep tendon reflex, renal function when $MgSO_4$ is administered parenterally; use with caution in digitalized patients (may alter cardiac conduction leading heart block); use with caution in patients with lithium administration; elderly, due to disease or drug therapy, may be predisposed to diarrhea; diarrhea may result in electrolyte imbalance; monitor for toxicity

Adverse Reactions
>10%: Diarrhea

1% to 10%:
>   Cardiovascular: Hypotension, EKG changes
>   Central nervous system: Mental depression, coma
>   Gastrointestinal: Nausea, vomiting
>   Respiratory: Respiratory depression

Overdosage/Toxicology Magnesium antacids are also laxative and may cause diarrhea and hypokalemia. In patients with renal failure, magnesium may accumulate to toxic levels. I.V. calcium (5-10 mEq) will reverse respiratory depression or heart block; in extreme cases, peritoneal dialysis or hemodialysis may be required.

Drug Interactions Decreased effect: Tetracyclines, digoxin, indomethacin, iron salts, isoniazid, quinolones

Mechanism of Action Promotes bowel evacuation by causing osmotic retention of fluid which distends the colon with increased peristaltic activity

Pharmacodynamics/Kinetics
Onset of laxative action: 4-8 hours

Elimination: Absorbed magnesium ions (up to 30%) are usually excreted by kidneys, unabsorbed drug is excreted in feces

Usual Dosage Magnesium RDA: 4.5 mg/kg, which is a total daily allowance of 350 mg for adult men and 280-300 mg for adult women. During pregnancy, the RDA is 200 mg and during lactation it is 355 mg. Average daily intakes of dietary magnesium have declined in recent years due to processing of food. The latest estimate of the average American dietary intake was 349 mg/day.

Adults: Oral:
Dietary supplement: 27-54 mEq (1-2 tablets) 2-3 times
Antacid: ½ to 3 tablets (0.21-1.68 g) with water or milk 4 times/day after meals and at bedtime
Laxative: 2-4 g at bedtime with full glass of water

Dosing in renal impairment: Patients in severe renal failure should not receive magnesium due to toxicity from accumulation. Patients with a Cl$_{cr}$ <25 mL/minute should be monitored by serum magnesium levels.

Oral magnesium is not generally adequate for repletion in patients with serum magnesium concentrations <1.5 mEq/L

Reference Range Serum magnesium:
Children: 1.5-1.9 mg/dL (1.2-1.6 mEq/L)
Adults: 1.5-2.5 mg/dL (1.2-2.0 mEq/L)

Test Interactions ↑ magnesium; ↓ protein, calcium (S), ↓ potassium (S)

Patient Information Chew tablets before swallowing; take with full glass of water; notify physician if relief not obtained or if any signs of bleeding occur (black tarry stools, "coffee ground" vomit)

Additional Information 60% elemental magnesium; 49.6 mEq magnesium/g; 25 mmol magnesium/g

Dosage Forms
Capsule: 140 mg
Tablet: 400 mg, 425 mg

Magnesium Sulfate (mag nee' ze um sul' fate)

Synonyms Epsom Salts

Use Treatment and prevention of hypomagnesemia and in seizure prevention in severe pre-eclampsia or eclampsia, pediatric acute nephritis; also used as short-term treatment of constipation, postmyocardial infarction, and torsade de pointes

Pregnancy Risk Factor B

Contraindications Heart block, serious renal impairment, myocardial damage, hepatitis, Addison's disease

Warnings/Precautions Use with caution in patients with impaired renal function (accumulation of magnesium which may lead to magnesium intoxication); use with caution in digitalized patients (may alter cardiac conduction leading to heart block); monitor serum magnesium level, respiratory rate, deep tendon reflex, renal function when MgSO$_4$ is administered parenterally

Adverse Reactions
1% to 10%:
Serum magnesium levels >3 mg/dL:
Central nervous system: Depressed CNS, blocked peripheral neuromuscular transmission leading to anticonvulsant effects
Gastrointestinal: Diarrhea
Serum magnesium levels >5 mg/dL:
Cardiovascular: Flushing
Central nervous system: Somnolence
Serum magnesium levels >12.5 mg/dL:
Cardiovascular: Complete heart block
Respiratory: Respiratory paralysis

Overdosage/Toxicology Toxic symptoms usually present with serum level >4 mEq/L

Serum magnesium >4: Deep tendon reflexes may be depressed
Serum magnesium ≥10: Deep tendon reflexes may disappear, respiratory paralysis may occur, heart block may occur
Serum level >12 mEq/L may be fatal, serum level ≥10 mEq/L may cause complete heart block

I.V. calcium (5-10 mEq) 1-2 g calcium gluconate will reverse respiratory depression or heart block; in extreme cases, peritoneal dialysis or hemodialysis may be required

Drug Interactions
Decreased effect: Nifedipine decreased blood pressure and neuromuscular blockade
(Continued)

Magnesium Sulfate *(Continued)*

Increased toxicity: Aminoglycosides increased neuromuscular blockade; CNS depressants increased CNS depression; neuromuscular antagonists, beta-methasone (pulmonary edema), colistin (neuromuscular blockade), ritodrine increased cardiotoxicity

Stability Refrigeration of intact ampuls may result in precipitation or crystallization
Stability of parenteral admixture at room temperature (25°C): 60 days
I.V. is **incompatible** when mixed with fat emulsion (flocculation), calcium glucep-tate, clindamycin, dobutamine, hydrocortisone (same syringe), polymyxin B, procaine hydrochloride, nafcillin, tetracyclines, thiopental

Mechanism of Action Promotes bowel evacuation by causing osmotic retention of fluid which distends the colon with increased peristaltic activity when taken orally; parenterally, decreases acetylcholine in motor nerve terminals and acts on myocardium by slowing rate of S-A node impulse formation and prolonging conduction time

Pharmacodynamics/Kinetics

Oral: Onset of cathartic action: Within 1-2 hours
I.M.:
 Onset of action: 1 hour
 Duration: 3-4 hours
I.V.:
 Onset of action: Immediate
 Duration: 30 minutes
Elimination: Primarily in feces; absorbed magnesium is rapidly eliminated by the kidneys

Usual Dosage The recommended dietary allowance (RDA) of magnesium is 4.5 mg/kg which is a total daily allowance of 350-400 mg for adult men and 280-300 mg for adult women. During pregnancy the RDA is 300 mg and during lactation the RDA is 355 mg. Average daily intakes of dietary magnesium have declined in recent years due to processing of food. The latest estimate of the average American dietary intake was 349 mg/day. Dose represented as $MgSO_4$ unless stated otherwise.

Note: Serum magnesium is poor reflection of repletional status as the majority of magnesium is intracellular; serum levels may be transiently normal for a few hours after a dose is given, therefore, aim for consistently high normal serum levels in patients with normal renal function for most efficient repletion

Hypomagnesemia:
 Neonates: I.V.: 25-50 mg/kg/dose (0.2-0.4 mEq/kg/dose) every 8-12 hours for 2-3 doses
 Children: I.M., I.V.: 25-50 mg/kg/dose (0.2-0.4 mEq/kg/dose) every 4-6 hours for 3-4 doses, maximum single dose: 2000 mg (16 mEq), may repeat if hypomagnesemia persists (higher dosage up to 100 mg/kg/dose $MgSO_4$ I.V. has been used); maintenance: I.V.: 30-60 mg/kg/day (0.25-0.5 mEq/kg/day)

Management of seizures and hypertension:
 Children:
  Oral: 100-200 mg/kg/dose 4 times/day
  I.M., I.V.: 20-100 mg/kg/dose every 4-6 hours as needed; in severe cases doses as high as 200 mg/kg/dose have been used
 Adults:
  Oral: 3 g every 6 hours for 4 doses as needed
  I.M., I.V.: 1 g every 6 hours for 4 doses; for severe hypomagnesemia: 8-12 g $MgSO_4$/day in divided doses has been used

Eclampsia, pre-eclampsia: Adults:
 I.M.: 1-4 g every 4 hours
 I.V.: Initial: 4 g, then switch to I.M. or 1-4 g/hour by continuous infusion

Maximum dose should not exceed 30-40 g/day; maximum rate of infusion: 1-2 g/hour

Maintenance electrolyte requirements:
 Daily requirements: 0.2-0.5 mEq/kg/24 hours or 3-10 mEq/1000 kcal/24 hours
 Maximum: 8-16 mEq/24 hours

Cathartic: Oral:
 Children: 0.25 g/kg every 4-6 hours
 Adults: 10-15 g in a glass of water

Dosing adjustment/comments in renal impairment: Cl_{cr} <25 mL/minute: Do not administer or monitor serum magnesium levels carefully

Administration

Magnesium sulfate may be administered I.M. or I.V.

I.M.: A 25% or 50% concentration may be used for adults and a 20% solution is recommended for children

I.V.: Magnesium may be administered IVP, IVPB or I.V. infusion in an auxiliary medication infusion solution (eg, TPN); when giving I.V. push, must dilute first and should not be given any faster than 150 mg/minute

Maximal rate of infusion: 2 g/hour to avoid hypotension; doses of 4 g/hour have been given in emergencies (eclampsia, seizures); optimally, should add magnesium to I.V. fluids or to IVH, but bolus doses are also effective

For I.V., a concentration <20% should be used and the rate of injection should not exceed 1.5 mL of a 10% solution (or equivalent) per minute

Monitoring Parameters Monitor blood pressure when administering MgSO$_4$ I.V.; serum magnesium levels should be monitored to avoid overdose; monitor for diarrhea; monitor for arrhythmias, hypotension, respiratory and CNS depression during rapid I.V. administration

Reference Range Serum magnesium:
Children: 1.5-1.9 mg/dL (1.2-1.6 mEq/L)
Adults: 1.5-2.5 mg/dL (1.2-2.0 mEq/L)

Note: Serum magnesium is poor reflection of repletional status as the majority of magnesium is intracellular; serum levels may be transiently normal for a few hours after a dose is given, therefore, aim for consistently high normal serum levels in patients with normal renal function for most efficient repletion

Test Interactions ↑ magnesium; ↓ protein, calcium (S), ↓ potassium (S)

Additional Information 10% elemental magnesium
8.1 mEq magnesium/g
4 mmol magnesium/g
500 mg MgSO$_4$ = 4.06 mEq magnesium = 49.3 mg elemental magnesium

Dosage Forms
Granules: ~40 mEq magnesium/5 g (240 g)
Injection: 100 mg/mL (20 mL); 125 mg/mL (8 mL); 250 mg/mL (150 mL); 500 mg/mL (2 mL, 5 mL, 10 mL, 30 mL, 50 mL)
Solution, oral: 50% [500 mg/mL] (30 mL)

Magonate® [OTC] *see* Magnesium Gluconate *on page 658*

Maigret-50 *see* Phenylpropanolamine Hydrochloride *on page 876*

Malatal® *see* Hyoscyamine, Atropine, Scopolamine, and Phenobarbital *on page 557*

Malotuss® [OTC] *see* Guaifenesin *on page 515*

Mandelamine® *see* Methenamine *on page 706*

Mandol® *see* Cefamandole Nafate *on page 193*

Mandrake *see* Podophyllum Resin *on page 897*

Manganese (man' ga nees)

Brand Names Chelated Manganese® [OTC]

Synonyms Manganese Chloride; Manganese Sulfate

Use Trace element added to TPN (total parenteral nutrition) solution to prevent manganese deficiency; orally as a dietary supplement

Pregnancy Risk Factor C

Contraindications High manganese levels; patients with severe liver dysfunction or cholestasis (conjugated bilirubin >2 mg/dL) due to reduced biliary excretion

Overdosage/Toxicology Acute poisoning due to ingestion of manganese or manganese salts is rare owing to poor absorption of manganese. The main symptoms of chronic poisoning, either from injection or usually inhalation of manganese dust or fumes in air, include extrapyramidal symptoms that can lead to progressive deterioration in the central nervous system.

Stability Compatible with electrolytes usually present in amino acid/dextrose solution used for TPN solutions

Mechanism of Action Cofactor in many enzyme systems, stimulates synthesis of cholesterol and fatty acids in liver, and influences mucopolysaccharide synthesis

Pharmacodynamics/Kinetics
Distribution: Concentrated in mitochondria of pituitary gland, pancreas, liver, kidney, and bone
Elimination: Mainly in bile, urinary excretion is negligible

Usual Dosage
Infants: I.V.: 2-10 mcg/kg/day usually administered in TPN solutions
Adults:
Oral: 20-50 mg/day
RDA: 2-5 mg/day
I.V.: 150-800 mcg/day usually administered in TPN solutions

(Continued)

Manganese *(Continued)*

Administration Do not give I.M. or by direct I.V. injection since the acidic pH of the solution may cause tissue irritations and it is hypotonic

Monitoring Parameters Periodic manganese plasma level

Reference Range 4-14 µg/L

Dosage Forms

Injection, as chloride: 0.1 mg/mL (10 mL)

Injection, as sulfate: 0.1 mg/mL (10 mL, 30 mL)

Tablet: 20 mg, 50 mg

Manganese Chloride *see* Manganese *on previous page*

Manganese Sulfate *see* Manganese *on previous page*

Mannitol *(man' i tole)*

Brand Names Osmitrol®; Resectisol®

Synonyms *D*-Mannitol

Use Reduction of increased intracranial pressure associated with cerebral edema; promotion of diuresis in the prevention and/or treatment of oliguria or anuria due to acute renal failure; reduction of increased intraocular pressure; promoting urinary excretion of toxic substances; genitourinary irrigant in transurethral prostatic resection or other transurethral surgical procedures

Pregnancy Risk Factor C

Contraindications Severe renal disease (anuria), dehydration, or active intracranial bleeding, severe pulmonary edema or congestion, hypersensitivity to any component

Warnings/Precautions Should not be administered until adequacy of renal function and urine flow is established; cardiovascular status should also be evaluated; do not administer electrolyte-free mannitol solutions with blood

Adverse Reactions

>10%:

Central nervous system: Headache

Gastrointestinal: Nausea, vomiting

Genitourinary: Increased urination

1% to 10%:

Central nervous system: Dizziness

Dermatologic: Skin rash

Ocular: Blurred vision

<1%:

Cardiovascular: Circulatory overload, congestive heart failure

Central nervous system: Convulsions, headache, chills

Endocrine & metabolic: Fluid and electrolyte imbalance, water intoxication, dehydration and hypovolemia secondary to rapid diuresis

Gastrointestinal: Dry mouth

Genitourinary: Difficult urination

Local: Tissue necrosis

Respiratory: Pulmonary edema

Miscellaneous: Allergic reactions

Overdosage/Toxicology Symptoms of overdose include polyuria, hypotension, cardiovascular collapse, pulmonary edema, hyponatremia, hypokalemia, oliguria, seizures; increased electrolyte excretion and fluid overload can occur; hemodialysis will clear mannitol and reduce osmolality

Stability Should be stored at room temperature (15°C to 30°C) and protected from freezing; crystallization may occur at low temperatures; do not use solutions that contain crystals, heating in a hot water bath and vigorous shaking may be utilized for resolubilization; cool solutions to body temperature before using

Mechanism of Action Increases the osmotic pressure of glomerular filtrate, which inhibits tubular reabsorption of water and electrolytes and increases urinary output

Pharmacodynamics/Kinetics

Onset of diuresis: Injection: Within 1-3 hours

Onset of reduction in intracerebral pressure: Within 15 minutes

Duration of reduction in intracerebral pressure: 3-6 hours

Distribution: Remains confined to extracellular space (except in extreme concentrations) and does not penetrate the blood-brain barrier

Metabolism: Minimal amounts metabolized in the liver to glycogen

Half-life: 1.1-1.6 hours

Elimination: Primarily excreted unchanged in urine by glomerular filtration

Usual Dosage I.V.:

Children:

Test dose (to assess adequate renal function): 200 mg/kg over 3-5 minutes to produce a urine flow of at least 1 mL/kg for 1-3 hours

Initial: 0.5-1 g/kg

Maintenance: 0.25-0.5 g/kg given every 4-6 hours

Adults:

Test dose: 12.5 g (200 mg/kg) over 3-5 minutes to produce a urine flow of at least 30-50 mL of urine per hour over the next 2-3 hours

Initial: 0.5-1 g/kg

Maintenance: 0.25-0.5 g/kg every 4-6 hours; usual adult dose: 20-200 g/24 hours

Intracranial pressure: Cerebral edema: 1.5-2 g/kg/dose I.V. as a 15% to 20% solution over ≥30 minutes; maintain serum osmolality 310-320 mOsm/kg

Preoperative for neurosurgery: 1.5-2 g/kg administered 1-1.5 hours prior to surgery

Transurethral irrigation: Use urogenital solution as required for irrigation

Administration In-line 5-micron filter set should always be used for mannitol infusion with concentrations ≥20%; administer test dose (for oliguria) I.V. push over 3-5 minutes; for cerebral edema or elevated ICP, administer over 20-30 minutes

Monitoring Parameters Renal function, daily fluid I & O, serum electrolytes, serum and urine osmolality; for treatment of elevated intracranial pressure, maintain serum osmolality 310-320 mOsm/kg

Nursing Implications Avoid extravasation; crenation and agglutination of red blood cells may occur if administered with whole blood

Additional Information May autoclave or heat to redissolve crystals; mannitol 20% has an approximate osmolality of 1100 mOsm/L and mannitol 25% has an approximate osmolality of 1375 mOsm/L

Dosage Forms

Injection: 5% [50 mg/mL] (1000 mL); 10% [100 mg/mL] (500 mL, 1000 mL); 15% [150 mg/mL] (150 mL, 500 mL); 20% [200 mg/mL] (150 mL, 250 mL, 500 mL); 25% [250 mg/mL] (50 mL)

Solution, urogenital: 0.54% [5.4 mg/mL] (2000 mL)

Mantoux *see* Tuberculin Purified Protein Derivative *on page 1135*

Maox® *see* Magnesium Oxide *on page 660*

Maprotiline Hydrochloride (ma proe' ti leen)

Related Information

Antidepressant Agents Comparison *on page 1250-1252*

Brand Names Ludiomil®

Use Treatment of depression and anxiety associated with depression

Pregnancy Risk Factor B

Contraindications Narrow-angle glaucoma, hypersensitivity to maprotiline or any component

Warnings/Precautions Use with caution in patients with cardiac conduction disturbances, history of hyperthyroid, renal, or hepatic dysfunction; safe use of tricyclic antidepressants in children <12 years of age has not been established; to avoid cholinergic crisis do not discontinue abruptly in patients receiving high doses chronically

Adverse Reactions

>10%:

Cardiovascular: Orthostatic hypotension

Central nervous system: Drowsiness, weakness

Dermatologic: Skin rash

Gastrointestinal: Dry mouth

Genitourinary: Urinary retention

1% to 10%:

Central nervous system: Insomnia

Gastrointestinal: Constipation, nausea, vomiting, increased appetite and weight gain, weight loss

Neuromuscular & skeletal: Trembling

<1%:

Central nervous system: Confusion

Endocrine & metabolic: Breast enlargement

Genitourinary: Swelling of testicles

Hepatic: Cholestatic hepatitis

Ocular: Blurred vision, increased intraocular pressure

Otic: Tinnitus

Overdosage/Toxicology Symptoms of overdose include agitation, confusion, hallucinations, urinary retention, hypothermia, hypotension, seizures, ventricular tachycardia

Following initiation of essential overdose management, toxic symptoms should be treated. Ventricular arrhythmias often respond to systemic alkalinization

(Continued)

Maprotiline Hydrochloride *(Continued)*

(sodium bicarbonate 0.5-2 mEq/kg I.V.). Arrhythmias unresponsive to this therapy may respond to lidocaine 1 mg/kg I.V. followed by a titrated infusion. Physostigmine (1-2 mg I.V. slowly for adults or 0.5 mg I.V. slowly for children) may be indicated in reversing cardiac arrhythmias that are life-threatening. Seizures usually respond to diazepam I.V. boluses (5-10 mg for adults up to 30 mg or 0.25-0.4 mg/kg/dose for children up to 10 mg/dose). If seizures are unresponsive or recur, phenytoin or phenobarbital may be required.

Drug Interactions
Decreased effect: Barbiturates, phenytoin, carbamazepine
Increased toxicity: CNS depressants, MAO inhibitors (hyperpyretic crisis), anticholinergics, sympathomimetics, thyroid increases cardiotoxicity, phenothiazines (seizures), benzodiazepines

Mechanism of Action Traditionally believed to increase the synaptic concentration of norepinephrine in the central nervous system by inhibition of their reuptake by the presynaptic neuronal membrane. However, additional receptor effects have been found including desensitization of adenyl cyclase, down regulation of beta-adrenergic receptors, and down regulation of serotonin receptors.

Pharmacodynamics/Kinetics
Absorption: Slow
Protein binding: 88%
Metabolism: In the liver to active and inactive compounds
Half-life: 27-58 hours (mean, 43 hours)
Time to peak serum concentration: Within 12 hours
Elimination: In urine (70%) and feces (30%)

Usual Dosage Oral:
Children 6-14 years: 10 mg/day, increase to a maximum daily dose of 75 mg
Adults: 75 mg/day to start, increase by 25 mg every 2 weeks up to 150-225 mg/day; given in 3 divided doses or in a single daily dose
Elderly: Initial: 25 mg at bedtime, increase by 25 mg every 3 days for inpatients and weekly for outpatients if tolerated; usual maintenance dose: 50-75 mg/day, higher doses may be necessary in nonresponders

Monitoring Parameters Monitor blood pressure and pulse rate prior to and during initial therapy; evaluate mood and somatic complaints; monitor appetite and weight

Reference Range Therapeutic: 200-600 ng/mL (SI: 721-2163 nmol/L); not well established

Patient Information Avoid alcohol ingestion; do not discontinue medication abruptly; may cause drowsiness; full effect may not occur for 3-6 weeks; dry mouth may be helped by sips of water, sugarless gum, or hard candy; rise slowly to avoid dizziness

Nursing Implications May increase appetite and possibly a craving for sweets; often requires 2-3 weeks for therapeutic effects to be seen; severe constipation and urinary retention are possible; urge patient to report symptoms of stomatitis, sialadenitis, and xerostomia; observe seizure precautions

Dosage Forms Tablet: 25 mg, 50 mg, 75 mg

Marazide® *see* Benzthiazide *on page 123*

Marbaxin® *see* Methocarbamol *on page 710*

Marcaine® *see* Bupivacaine Hydrochloride *on page 147*

Marezine® [OTC] *see* Cyclizine *on page 284*

Margesic® H *see* Hydrocodone and Acetaminophen *on page 543*

Marinol® *see* Dronabinol *on page 374*

Marmine® [OTC] *see* Dimenhydrinate *on page 347*

Marnal® *see* Butalbital Compound *on page 153*

Marplan® *see* Isocarboxazid *on page 593*

Masoprocol *(may so pro' kol)*

Brand Names Actinex®
Use Treatment of actinic keratosis
Pregnancy Risk Factor B
Contraindications Hypersensitivity to masoprocol or any component
Warnings/Precautions Occlusive dressings should not be used; for external use only
Adverse Reactions
>10%: Dermatologic: Erythema, flaking, dryness, burning, itching
1% to 10%: Soreness, eye irritation, rash, tingling
<1%: Blistering, excoriation, skin roughness, wrinkling

Mechanism of Action Antiproliferative activity against keratinocytes

Pharmacodynamics/Kinetics Absorption: Topical: <1% to 2%

Usual Dosage Adults: Topical: Wash and dry area; gently massage into affected area every morning and evening for 28 days

Patient Information For external use only; may stain clothing or fabrics; avoid eyes and mucous membranes; do not use occlusive dressings; transient local burning sensation may occur immediately after application; contact physician if oozing or blistering occurs; wash hands immediately after use.

Dosage Forms Cream: 10% (30 g)

Matulane® *see* Procarbazine Hydrochloride *on page 931*

Maxair™ *see* Pirbuterol Acetate *on page 892*

Maxaquin® *see* Lomefloxacin Hydrochloride *on page 645*

Max-Caro® [OTC] *see* Beta-Carotene *on page 129*

Maxidex® *see* Dexamethasone *on page 314*

Maxiflor® *see* Diflorasone Diacetate *on page 335*

Maximum Strength Anbesol® [OTC] *see* Benzocaine *on page 121*

Maximum Strength Bactimne™ [OTC] *see* Hydrocortisone *on page 546*

Maximum Strength Orajel® [OTC] *see* Benzocaine *on page 121*

Maxitrol® *see* Neomycin, Polymyxin B, and Dexamethasone *on page 780*

Maxivate® *see* Betamethasone *on page 129*

Maxolon® *see* Metoclopramide *on page 728*

Maxzide® *see* Triamterene and Hydrochlorothiazide *on page 1116*

May Apple *see* Podophyllum Resin *on page 897*

Mazicon™ *see* Flumazenil *on page 466*

MCH *see* Microfibrillar Collagen Hemostat *on page 739*

Measles and Rubella Vaccines, Combined (mee' zels & rue bell' a)

Related Information

Immunization Guidelines *on page 1389-1405*

Vaccines *on page 1386-1388*

Brand Names M-R-VAX® II

Synonyms Rubella and Measles Vaccines, Combined

Use Simultaneous immunization against measles and rubella

Pregnancy Risk Factor X

Contraindications Immune deficiency condition, pregnancy

Warnings/Precautions Pregnancy, immunocompromised persons, history of anaphylactic reaction following receipt of neomycin

Adverse Reactions All serious adverse reactions must be reported to the FDA

>10%:

Central nervous system: Fever <100°F

Dermatologic: Urticaria, rash

Local: Burning at injection site, local tenderness and erythema

Neuromuscular & skeletal: Arthralgias

1% to 10%:

Central nervous system: Fever between 100°F and 103°F, malaise, headache

Miscellaneous: Allergic reaction (delayed type), sore throat, lymphadenopathy

<1%:

Central nervous system: Tiredness, convulsions, encephalitis, confusion, severe headache, fever >103°F (prolonged)

Dermatologic: Hives, itching, reddening of skin (especially around ears and eyes)

Gastrointestinal: Vomiting

Hematologic: Thrombocytopenic purpura

Neuromuscular & skeletal: Stiff neck

Ocular: Diplopia, optic neuritis

Respiratory: Difficulty of breathing

Miscellaneous: Hypersensitivity

The chance of a child having a convulsion after receiving the measles vaccine is small. The risk is up to 5 times greater if the child has ever had a convulsion before or if the child's brother, sister, or parent has ever had a convulsion.

(Continued)

Measles and Rubella Vaccines, Combined *(Continued)*

Drug Interactions Whole blood, immune globulin, immunosuppressive drugs should not be given within 1 month of other live virus vaccines except monovalent or trivalent polio vaccine; may temporarily depress tuberculin skin test sensitivity; decreased effect when immune globulin is given within 3 months and with concurrent use of corticosteroids and other immunosuppressant agents

Stability Refrigerate prior to use, use as soon as possible; discard if not used within 8 hours of reconstitution

Usual Dosage Children at 15 months and Adults: S.C.: Inject 0.5 mL into outer aspect of upper arm; no routine booster for rubella

Administration Not for I.V. administration

Patient Information Parents should monitor children closely for fever 5-11 days after vaccination

Females should not become pregnant within 3 months of vaccination

Measles vaccine:

A rash may occur from 1-2 weeks after receiving the measles vaccine; about 5 children out of every 100 will get a rash

A fever $\geq 103°F$ after receiving the first shot of measles vaccine, even though the child may not act sick. About 5-15 young children out of every 100 who receive the vaccine get such a fever. This could happen from 1-2 weeks after receiving the vaccine and usually lasts 1-2 days. The fever occurs less often after a second injection.

Rubella vaccine:

Swelling of the lymph glands in the neck or a rash that lasts 1-2 days; this could happen 1-2 weeks after getting the rubella vaccine in about 1/7 children who get the vaccine

Mild pain or stiffness in the joints that may last up to 3 days; this could happen from 1-3 weeks after getting the shot. this problem happens to about 1/100 children and 25/100 adults who are vaccinated. Women have this problem more than men and it may happen in up to 40 women out of every 100. Rarely, pain or stiffness can last for months or longer and can come and go.

Painful swelling of the joints (arthritis) happens to <1/100 children who get the rubella vaccine. About 10/100 adults can also have this problem, which usually lasts a few days to a week. Rarely, this swelling has been reported to last longer, or to come and go. Damage to the joints is very rare.

Pain or numbness, or "pins and needles" feeling in the hands and feet that lasts for a short time; this happens rarely

More serious problems: Children 6 months through 6 years of age who get the vaccines can, in rare cases, have a brief convulsion (fits, seizures, spasms, twitching, jerking, or staring spells). This usually occurs 1-2 weeks later, and usually comes from the fever caused by the measles vaccine. Very rarely, hearing loss has been reported, but it is not known whether hearing loss is caused by these vaccines. Rarely, a person can have inflammation of the brain after receiving the vaccine; this usually clears up completely.

Additional Information Federal law requires that the date of administration, the vaccine manufacturer, lot number of vaccine, and the administering person's name, title and address be entered into the patient's permanent medical record

Adults born before 1957 are generally considered to be immune to measles; all born in or after 1957 without documentation of live vaccine on or after first birthday, physician-diagnosed measles, or laboratory evidence of immunity should be vaccinated with two doses separated by or less than 1 month. For those previously vaccinated with one dose of measles vaccine, revaccination is indicated for students entering institutions of higher learning, for health care workers at time of employment, and for travelers to endemic areas. Guidelines for rubella vaccination are the same with the exception of birth year. All adults should be vaccinated against rubella. A booster dose of rubella vaccine is not necessary. Women who are pregnant when vaccinated or become pregnant within 3 months of vaccination should be consulted on the risks to the fetus; although the risks appear negligible. MMR is the vaccine of choice if recipients are likely to be susceptible to mumps as well as measles and rubella.

Dosage Forms Injection: 1000 $TCID_{50}$ each of live attenuated measles virus vaccine and live rubella virus vaccine

Measles, Mumps, and Rubella Vaccines, Combined (mee' zels, mumps & rue bell' a)

Related Information
Immunization Guidelines *on page 1389-1405*
Vaccines *on page 1386-1388*

Brand Names M-M-R® II

Synonyms MMR; Mumps, Measles and Rubella Vaccines, Combined; Rubella, Measles and Mumps Vaccines, Combined

Use
Measles, mumps, and rubella prophylaxis in children (≥15 months) and adults
For HIV-infected children, MMR should routinely be administered at 15 months of age

Pregnancy Risk Factor X

Contraindications Blood dyscrasias, cancers affecting the bone marrow or lymphatic systems, known hypersensitivity to measles, mumps and rubella vaccine, known hypersensitivity to neomycin, acute infections, and respiratory illness, pregnancy; known hypersensitivity to eggs, chicken or chicken feathers, severely immunocompromised persons

Warnings/Precautions
Females should not become pregnant within 3 months of vaccination
MMR vaccine should not be given within 3 months of immune globulin or whole blood
Have epinephrine available during and after administration
MMR vaccine should not be administered to severely immunocompromised persons
Severely immunocompromised patients and symptomatic HIV-infected patients who are exposed to measles should receive immune globulin, regardless of prior vaccination status
The immunogenicity of measles virus vaccine is decreased if vaccine is administered <6 months after immune globulin

Adverse Reactions All serious adverse reactions must be reported to the FDA
1% to 10%:
Dermatologic: Transient rash, tenderness erythema and swelling
Miscellaneous: Sore throat, allergic reactions
<1%: Central nervous system: Seizures, malaise, fever
The chance of a child having a convulsion after receiving the measles vaccine is small. The risk is up to 5 times greater if the child has ever had a convulsion before or if the child's brother, sister, or parent has ever had a convulsion.

Drug Interactions Decreased effect when immune globulin is given within 3 months and with concurrent use of corticosteroids and other immunosuppressant agents; decreased effect with concurrent infection, immunoglobulin within 1 month, other live vaccines with the exception of attenuated measles, rubella, or polio

Stability Refrigerate, protect from light prior to reconstitution; use as soon as possible; discard 8 hours after reconstitution

Usual Dosage
Infants <12 months of age: If there is risk of exposure to measles, single-antigen measles vaccine should be administered at 6-11 months of age with a second dose (of MMR) at >12 months of age
Give S.C. in outer aspect of the upper arm to children ≥15 months of age:
0.5 mL at 15 months of age and then repeated at 4-6 years• of age
In some areas, MMR vaccine may be given at 12 months
•Many experts recommend that this dose of MMR be given at entry to middle school or junior high school

Administration Not for I.V. administration

Test Interactions Temporary suppression of TB skin test reactivity with onset approximately 3 days after administration

Patient Information Females should not become pregnant within 3 months of vaccination
Measles vaccine:
A rash may occur from 1-2 weeks after receiving the measles vaccine; about 5 children out of every 100 will get a rash
A fever ≥103°F after receiving the first shot of measles vaccine, even though the child may not act sick. About 5-15 young children out of every 100 who receive the vaccine get such a fever. This could happen from 1-2 weeks after receiving the vaccine and usually lasts 1-2 days. The fever occurs less often after a second injection.
Mumps vaccine: A little swelling of the glands in the cheeks and under the jaw that lasts for a few days; this could happen from 1-2 weeks after getting the mumps vaccine; this happens rarely
Rubella vaccine: Swelling of the lymph glands in the neck or a rash that lasts 1-2 days; this could happen 1-2 weeks after getting the rubella vaccine in about 1/7 children who get the vaccine
Mild pain or stiffness in the joints that may last up to 3 days; this could happen from 1-3 weeks after getting the shot. This problem happens to about 1/100 children and 25/100 adults who are vaccinated. Women have this problem more than men and it may happen in up to 40 women out of every 100. Rarely, pain or stiffness can last for months or longer and can come and go.
Painful swelling of the joints (arthritis) happens to <1/100 children who get the rubella vaccine. About 10/100 adults can also have this problem, which
(Continued)

Measles, Mumps, and Rubella Vaccines, Combined
(Continued)

usually lasts a few days to a week. Rarely, this swelling has been reported to last longer, or to come and go. Damage to the joints is very rare.

Pain or numbness, or "pins and needles" feeling in the hands and feet that lasts for a short time; this happens rarely

More serious problems: Children 6 months through 6 years of age who get the vaccines can, in rare cases, have a brief convulsion (fits, seizures, spasms, twitching, jerking, or staring spells). This usually occurs 1-2 weeks later, and usually comes from the fever caused by the measles vaccine. Very rarely, hearing loss has been reported, but it is not known whether hearing loss is ever caused by these vaccines. Rarely, a person can have inflammation of the brain after receiving the vaccine. This usually clears up completely. These brain problems have been reported in 1/one million MMR injections.

Additional Information Live, attenuated vaccine. Federal law requires that the date of administration, the vaccine manufacturer, lot number of vaccine, and the administering person's name, title and address be entered into the patient's permanent medical record

Adults born before 1957 are generally considered to be immune to measles and mumps; all born in or after 1957 without documentation of live vaccine on or after first birthday, physician-diagnosed measles or mumps, or laboratory evidence of immunity should be vaccine with two doses separated by no less than 1 month; for those previously vaccinated with one dose of measles vaccine, revaccination is indicated for students entering institutions of higher learning, health care workers at time of employment, and for travelers to endemic areas. Guidelines for rubella vaccination are the same with the exception of birth year; all adults should be vaccinated against rubella. Booster doses of mumps and rubella are not necessary; women who are pregnant when vaccinated or become pregnant within 3 months should be counseled on the risks to the fetus; although the risks appear negligible.

Dosage Forms Injection: 1000 $TCID_{50}$ each of measles virus vaccine and rubella virus vaccine, 5000 $TCID_{50}$ mumps virus vaccine

Measles Virus Vaccine, Live
Related Information
Immunization Guidelines *on page 1389-1405*
Vaccines *on page 1386-1388*
Brand Names Attenuvax®
Synonyms More Attenuated Enders Strain; Rubeola vaccine
Use Adults born before 1957 are generally considered to be immune. All those born in or after 1957 without documentation of live vaccine on or after first birthday, physician-diagnosed measles, or laboratory evidence of immunity should be vaccinated, ideally with two doses of vaccine separated by no less than 1 month. For those previously vaccinated with one dose of measles vaccine, revaccination is recommended for students entering colleges and other institutions of higher education, for health care workers at the time of employment, and for international travelers who visit endemic areas.

MMR is the vaccine of choice if recipients are likely to be susceptible to rubella and/or mumps as well as to measles. Persons vaccinated between 1963 and 1967 with a killed measles vaccine, followed by live vaccine within 3 months, or with a vaccine of unknown type should be revaccinated with live measles virus vaccine.

Pregnancy Risk Factor X
Contraindications Pregnant females, known anaphylactoid reaction to eggs, known hypersensitivity to neomycin, acute respiratory infections, activated tuberculosis, immunosuppressed patients
Warnings/Precautions Avoid use in immunocompromised patients; defer administration in presence of acute respiratory or other active infections or inactive, untreated tuberculosis; avoid pregnancy for 3 months following vaccination; history of febrile seizures, hypersensitivity reactions may occur
Adverse Reactions All serious adverse reactions must be reported to the FDA
Central nervous system: Rarely encephalitis, fever, headache
Dermatologic: Rarely urticaria, erythema

>10%: Fever <100°F
  Local: Burning or stinging, swelling, induration
1% to 10%: Fever between 100°F and 103°F, allergic reaction (delayed type)
<1%:
  Dermatologic: Hives, itching, reddening of skin (especially around ears and eyes)

Central nervous system: Tiredness, convulsions, encephalitis, confusion, severe headache, fever >103°F (prolonged)

Gastrointestinal: Vomiting

Hematologic: Thrombocytopenic purpura

Ocular: Diplopia

Neuromuscular & skeletal: Stiff neck

Respiratory: Difficulty of breathing

Miscellaneous: Lymphadenopathy, sore throat, coryza

Drug Interactions Whole blood, immune globulin, immunosuppressive drugs should not be given within 1 month of other live virus vaccines except monovalent or trivalent polio vaccine; may temporarily depress tuberculin skin test sensitivity

Stability Refrigerate at 2°C to 8°C (36°F to 46°F); discard if left at room temperature for over 8 hours; protect from light

Usual Dosage Children >15 months and Adults: S.C.: 0.5 mL in outer aspect of the upper arm, no routine boosters

Administration Vaccine should not be given I.V.; S.C. injection preferred

Test Interactions May temporarily depress tuberculin skin test sensitivity

Patient Information Parents should monitor children closely for fever for 5-11 days after vaccination; females should not become pregnant within 3 months of vaccination

Measles vaccine:

A rash may occur from 1-2 weeks after receiving the measles vaccine; about 5 children out of every 100 will get a rash

A fever ≥103°F after receiving the first shot of measles vaccine, even though the child may not act sick. About 5-15 young children out of every 100 who receive the vaccine get such a fever. This could happen from 1-2 weeks after receiving the vaccine and usually lasts 1-2 days. The fever occurs less often after a second injection.

Additional Information Federal law requires that the date of administration, the vaccine manufacturer, lot number of vaccine, and the administering person's name, title and address be entered into the patient's permanent medical record

Dosage Forms Injection: 1000 TCID$_{50}$ per dose

Measurin® [OTC] see Aspirin on page 92

Mebaral® see Mephobarbital on page 687

Mebendazole (me ben' da zole)

Brand Names Vermox®

Use Treatment of pinworms, whipworms, roundworms, and hookworms

Pregnancy Risk Factor C

Contraindications Hypersensitivity to mebendazole or any component

Warnings/Precautions Pregnancy and children <2 years of age are relative contraindications since safety has not been established; not effective for hydatid disease

Adverse Reactions

1% to 10%: Gastrointestinal: Abdominal pain, diarrhea, nausea, vomiting

<1%:

Central nervous system: Fever, dizziness, headache

Dermatologic: Skin rash, itching, alopecia (with high doses)

Hematologic: Neutropenia (sore throat, unusual tiredness and weakness)

Overdosage/Toxicology Symptoms of overdose include abdominal pain, altered mental status; GI decontamination and supportive care

Drug Interactions Decreased effect: Anticonvulsants such as carbamazepine and phenytoin may increase metabolism of mebendazole

Mechanism of Action Selectively and irreversibly blocks glucose uptake and other nutrients in susceptible adult intestine-dwelling helminths

Pharmacodynamics/Kinetics

Absorption: Only 2% to 10%

Protein binding: High, 95%

Metabolism: Extensive in the liver

Half-life: 1-11.5 hours

Time to peak serum concentration: Within 2-4 hours

Elimination: Primarily excreted in feces with 5% to 10% eliminated in urine

Usual Dosage Children and Adults: Oral:

Pinworms: 100 mg as a single dose; may need to repeat after 2 weeks; treatment should include family members in close contact with patient

Whipworms, roundworms, hookworms: One tablet twice daily, morning and evening on 3 consecutive days; if patient is not cured within 3-4 weeks, a second course of treatment may be administered

(Continued)

Mebendazole *(Continued)*

Capillariasis: 200 mg twice daily for 20 days

Dosing adjustment in hepatic impairment: Dosage reduction may be necessary in patients with liver dysfunction

Not dialyzable (0% to 5%)

Monitoring Parameters Check for helminth ova in feces within 3-4 weeks following the initial therapy

Test Interactions ↑ LFTs

Patient Information Tablets may be chewed, swallowed whole, or crushed and mixed with food; hygienic precautions should be taken to prevent reinfection such as wearing shoes and washing hands

Dosage Forms Tablet, chewable: 100 mg

Mecamylamine Hydrochloride *(mek a mill' a meen)*

Brand Names Inversine®

Use Treatment of moderately severe to severe hypertension and in uncomplicated malignant hypertension

Pregnancy Risk Factor C

Contraindications Coronary insufficiency, pyloric stenosis, glaucoma, uremia, recent myocardial infarction, unreliable, uncooperative patients

Warnings/Precautions Use with caution in patients receiving sulfonamides or antibiotics that cause neuromuscular blockade; use with caution in patients with impaired renal function, previous CNS abnormalities, prostatic hypertrophy, bladder obstruction, or urethral strictive; do not abruptly discontinue

Adverse Reactions

>10%:

Cardiovascular: Postural hypotension

Central nervous system: Drowsiness

Endocrine & metabolic: Decreased sexual ability

Gastrointestinal: Dryness of mouth

Ocular: Blurred vision, enlarged pupils

1% to 10%:

Gastrointestinal: Loss of appetite, nausea, vomiting

Renal: Difficult urination

<1%:

Central nervous system: Convulsions, confusion, mental depression,

Gastrointestinal: Bloating, frequent stools, followed by severe constipation

Neuromuscular & skeletal: Uncontrolled movements of hands, arms, legs, or face, trembling

Respiratory: Shortness of breath

Overdosage/Toxicology Symptoms of overdose include hypotension, nausea, vomiting, urinary retention, constipation. Signs and symptoms are a direct result of ganglionic blockade; treatment is supportive; pressor amines may be used to correct hypotension; use caution as patients will be unusually sensitive to these agents.

Drug Interactions Increased effect with sulfonamides and antibiotics that cause neuromuscular blockade

Mechanism of Action Mecamylamine is a ganglionic blocker. This agent inhibits acetylcholine at the autonomic ganglia, causing a decrease in blood pressure. Mecamylamine also blocks central nicotinic cholinergic receptors, which inhibits the effects of nicotine and may suppress the desire to smoke.

Usual Dosage Adults: Oral: 2.5 mg twice daily after meals for 2 days; increased by increments of 2.5 mg at intervals ≥2 days until desired blood pressure response is achieved; average daily dose: 25 mg

Dosing adjustment/comments in renal impairment: Use with caution, if at all, although no specific guidelines are available

Patient Information Take after meals at the same time each day; notify physician immediately if frequent loose bowel movements occur; rise slowly from sitting or lying for prolonged periods; do not restrict salt intake

Nursing Implications Check frequently for orthostatic hypotension; aid with ambulation

Dosage Forms Tablet: 2.5 mg

Mechlorethamine Hydrochloride *(me klor eth' a meen)*

Related Information

Antiemetics for Chemotherapy Induced Nausea and Vomiting *on page 1202*
Cancer Chemotherapy Regimens *on page 1218-1241*
Extravasation Management of Chemotherapeutic Agents *on page 1207-1208*

Brand Names Mustargen®

Synonyms HN_2; Mustine; Nitrogen Mustard

Use Combination therapy of Hodgkin's disease and malignant lymphomas; non-Hodgkin's lymphoma; palliative treatment of bronchogenic, breast and ovarian carcinoma; may be used by intracavitary injection for treatment of metastatic tumors; pleural and other malignant effusions; topical treatment of mycosis fungoides

Pregnancy Risk Factor D

Contraindications Hypersensitivity to mechlorethamine or any component; pre-existing profound myelosuppression or infection

Warnings/Precautions The U.S. Food and Drug Administration (FDA) currently recommends that procedures for proper handling and disposal of antineoplastic agents be considered. Extravasation of the drug into subcutaneous tissues results in painful inflammation and induration; sloughing may occur. Patients with lymphomas should receive prophylactic allopurinol 2-3 days prior to therapy to prevent complications resulting from tumor lysis.

Adverse Reactions

>10%:

Gastrointestinal: Nausea and vomiting usually occur in nearly 100% of patients and onset is within 30 minutes to 2 hours after administration

Emetic potential: High (>90%)

Myelosuppressive: Leukopenia and thrombocytopenia can be severe; caution should be used with patients who are receiving radiotherapy, secondary leukemia

WBC: Severe

Platelets: Severe

Onset (days): 4-7

Nadir (days): 14

Recovery (days): 21

Reproductive: Delayed menses, oligomenorrhea, temporary or permanent amenorrhea, impaired spermatogenesis, azoospermia; spermatogenesis may return in patients in remission several years after the discontinuation of chemotherapy, chromosomal abnormalities

Miscellaneous: Precipitation of herpes zoster, ototoxicity

1% to 10%:

Central nervous system: Fever, weakness, vertigo

Dermatologic: Alopecia

Gastrointestinal: Diarrhea, anorexia, metallic taste

Local: Thrombophlebitis/extravasation: May cause local vein discomfort which may be relieved by warm soaks and pain medication. A brown discoloration of veins may occur. Mechlorethamine is a strong vesicant and can cause tissue necrosis and sloughing.

Vesicant chemotherapy

Secondary malignancies: Have been reported after several years in 1% to 6% of patients treated

Otic: Tinnitus

Miscellaneous: Hypersensitivity, anaphylaxis, hyperuricemia

<1%:

Central nervous system: Vertigo, weakness

Dermatologic: Rash

Gastrointestinal: Hepatotoxicity, peptic ulcer

Hematologic: Myelosuppression, hemolytic anemia

Neuromuscular & skeletal: Peripheral neuropathy

Overdosage/Toxicology Suppression of all formed elements of the blood, uric acid crystals, nausea, vomiting, diarrhea; sodium thiosulfate is the specific antidote for nitrogen mustard extravasations; treatment of systemic overdose is supportive

Stability Prepare solution immediately before each injection, since decomposition will occur upon standing; highly unstable in neutral or alkaline solutions; discard any unused drug after 15 minutes

Mechanism of Action Alkylating agent that inhibits DNA and RNA synthesis via formation of carbonium ions; produces interstrand and intrastrand cross-links in DNA resulting in miscoding, breakage, and failure of replication

Pharmacodynamics/Kinetics

Absorption: Incomplete absorption into blood stream following intracavitary administration secondary to rapid deactivation by body fluids

Metabolism: I.V.: Drug undergoes rapid chemical transformation; unchanged drug is undetectable in the blood within a few minutes

Half-life: <1 minute

Elimination: <0.01% of unchanged drug is recovered in urine

Usual Dosage Dosage should be based on ideal body weight and ideal BSA (refer to individual protocols)

(Continued)

Mechlorethamine Hydrochloride *(Continued)*

Children and Adults: MOPP: I.V.: 6 mg/m² on days 1 and 8 of a 28-day cycle

Adults:

I.V.: 0.4 mg/kg or 12-16 mg/m² for one dose or divided into 0.1 mg/kg/day for 4 days

Intracavitary: 10-20 mg diluted in 10 mL of SWI or 0.9% sodium chloride

Intrapericardially: 0.2-0.4 mg/kg diluted in up to 100 mL of 0.9% sodium chloride

Topical mechlorethamine has been used in the treatment of cutaneous lesions of mycosis fungoides. A skin test should be performed prior to treatment with the topical preparation to detect sensitivity and possible irritation (use fresh mechlorethamine 0.1 mg/mL and apply over a 3 x 5 cm area of normal skin).

Administration Administer I.V. push through a free flowing I.V. over 1-3 minutes at a concentration not to exceed 1 mg/mL

Monitoring Parameters CBC with differential and platelet count

Patient Information Protect skin from contact, will burn and irritate. Any signs of infection, easy bruising or bleeding, shortness of breath, or painful or burning urination should be brought to physician's attention. Nausea, vomiting, or hair loss sometimes occur. The drug may cause permanent sterility and may cause birth defects. The drug may be excreted in breast milk, therefore, an alternative form of feeding your baby should be used.

Nursing Implications Use within 1 hour of preparation; for I.V. and intracavitary administration only; avoid extravasation since mechlorethamine is a potent vesicant

Extravasation treatment: Sodium thiosulfate ⅙ molar solution is the specific antidote for nitrogen mustard extravasations and should be used as follows: Mix 4 mL of 10% sodium thiosulfate with 6 mL of sterile water for injection; inject 4 mL of this solution into the existing I.V. line; remove the needle; inject 2-3 mL of the solution S.C. clockwise into the infiltrated area using a 25-gauge needle; change the needle with each new injection; apply ice immediately for 6-12 hours

Dosage Forms Powder for injection: 10 mg

Meclan® *see* Meclocycline Sulfosalicylate *on next page*

Meclizine Hydrochloride (mek' li zeen)

Brand Names Antivert®; Antrizine®; Bonine® [OTC]; Dizmiss® [OTC]; Meni-D®; Ru-Vert-M®; Vergon® [OTC]

Synonyms Meclozine Hydrochloride

Use Prevention and treatment of symptoms of motion sickness; management of vertigo with diseases affecting the vestibular system

Pregnancy Risk Factor B

Contraindications Hypersensitivity to meclizine or any component; pregnancy

Warnings/Precautions Use with caution in patients with angle-closure glaucoma, prostatic hypertrophy, pyloric or duodenal obstruction, or bladder neck obstruction; use with caution in hot weather, and during exercise; elderly may be at risk for anticholinergic side effects such as glaucoma, prostatic hypertrophy, constipation, gastrointestinal obstructive disease; if vertigo does not respond in 1-2 weeks, it is advised to discontinue use

Adverse Reactions

>10%:

Central nervous system: Slight to moderate drowsiness

Respiratory: Thickening of bronchial secretions

1% to 10%:

Central nervous system: Headache, fatigue, nervousness, dizziness

Gastrointestinal: Appetite increase, weight increase, nausea, diarrhea, abdominal pain, dry mouth

Neuromuscular & skeletal: Arthralgia

Respiratory: Pharyngitis

<1%:

Cardiovascular: Palpitations, hypotension

Central nervous system: Depression, sedation

Dermatologic: Photosensitivity, rash, angioedema

Genitourinary: Urinary retention

Hepatic: Hepatitis

Neuromuscular & skeletal: Myalgia, tremor, paresthesia

Ocular: Blurred vision

Respiratory: Bronchospasm

Miscellaneous: Epistaxis

Overdosage/Toxicology Symptoms of overdose include CNS depression, confusion, nervousness, hallucinations, dizziness, blurred vision, nausea, vomiting, hyperthermia. There is no specific treatment for an antihistamine overdose, however, most of its clinical toxicity is due to anticholinergic effects. For anticholinergic overdose with severe life-threatening symptoms, physostigmine 1-2 mg (0.5 or 0.02 mg/kg for children) I.V., slowly may be given to reverse these effects.

Drug Interactions Increased toxicity: CNS depressants, neuroleptics, anticholinergics

Mechanism of Action Has central anticholinergic action by blocking chemoreceptor trigger zone; decreases excitability of the middle ear labyrinth and blocks conduction in the middle ear vestibular-cerebellar pathways

Pharmacodynamics/Kinetics
Onset of action: Oral: Within 1 hour
Duration: 8-24 hours
Metabolism: Reportedly in the liver
Half-life: 6 hours
Elimination: As metabolites in urine and as unchanged drug in feces

Usual Dosage Children >12 years and Adults: Oral:
Motion sickness: 12.5-25 mg 1 hour before travel, repeat dose every 12-24 hours if needed; doses up to 50 mg may be needed
Vertigo: 25-100 mg/day in divided doses

Patient Information Take after meals; do not discontinue drug abruptly; notify physician if adverse GI effects, fever, or heat intolerance occurs; may cause drowsiness; avoid alcohol; adequate fluid intake, sugar free gum or hard candy may help dry mouth; adequate fluid and exercise may help constipation

Dosage Forms
Capsule: 15 mg, 25 mg, 30 mg
Tablet: 12.5 mg, 25 mg, 50 mg
Tablet:
Chewable: 25 mg
Film coated: 25 mg

Meclocycline Sulfosalicylate (me kloe sye′ kleen)
Brand Names Meclan®
Use Topical treatment of inflammatory acne vulgaris
Pregnancy Risk Factor B
Contraindications Known hypersensitivity to tetracyclines or any component
Warnings/Precautions Use with caution in patients allergic to formaldehyde; for external use only
Adverse Reactions
>10%: Topical: Follicular staining, yellowing of the skin, burning/stinging feeling
1% to 10%: Topical: Pain, redness, skin irritation, dermatitis
Mechanism of Action Inhibits bacterial protein synthesis by binding with the 30S and possibly the 50S ribosomal subunit(s) of susceptible bacteria; may also cause alterations in the cytoplasmic membrane
Pharmacodynamics/Kinetics Absorption: Topical: Very little
Usual Dosage Children >11 years and Adults: Topical: Apply generously to affected areas twice daily
Patient Information Apply generously until skin is wet; avoid contact with eyes, nose, and mouth; stinging may occur with application, but soon stops; if skin is discolored yellow, washing will remove the color
Dosage Forms Cream, topical: 1% (20 g, 45 g)

Meclofenamate Sodium (me kloe fen am′ ate)
Related Information
Nonsteroidal Anti-Inflammatories Comparison *on page 1280*
Brand Names Meclomen®
Use Treatment of inflammatory disorders
Pregnancy Risk Factor B (D if used in the 3rd trimester)
Contraindications Active GI bleeding, ulcer disease, hypersensitivity to aspirin, meclofenamate, or other NSAIDs
Warnings/Precautions May have adverse effects on fetus
Adverse Reactions
>10%:
Central nervous system: Dizziness
Dermatologic: Skin rash
Gastrointestinal: Abdominal cramps, heartburn, indigestion, nausea
1% to 10%:
Cardiovascular: Fluid retention
(Continued)
675

Meclofenamate Sodium *(Continued)*

    Central nervous system: Headache, nervousness
    Dermatologic: Itching
    Gastrointestinal: Vomiting
    Otic: Ringing in ears
  <1%:
    Cardiovascular: Congestive heart failure, hypertension, arrhythmia, tachycardia
    Central nervous system: Epistaxis, confusion, hallucinations, aseptic meningitis, mental depression, drowsiness, insomnia
    Dermatologic: Hives, erythema multiforme, toxic epidermal necrolysis, Stevens-Johnson syndrome, angioedema
    Endocrine & metabolic: Polydipsia, hot flushes
    Gastrointestinal: Gastritis, GI ulceration
    Genitourinary: Cystitis
    Hematologic: Agranulocytosis, anemia, hemolytic anemia, bone marrow depression, leukopenia, thrombocytopenia
    Hepatic: Hepatitis
    Neuromuscular & skeletal: Peripheral neuropathy
    Ocular: Toxic amblyopia, blurred vision, conjunctivitis, dry eyes
    Otic: Decreased hearing
    Renal: Polyuria, acute renal failure
    Respiratory: Allergic rhinitis, shortness of breath

Overdosage/Toxicology Symptoms of overdose include drowsiness, lethargy, nausea, vomiting, seizures, paresthesia, headache, dizziness, GI bleeding, cerebral edema, cardiac arrest, tinnitus

Management of a nonsteroidal anti-inflammatory drug (NSAID) intoxication is primarily supportive and symptomatic. Fluid therapy is commonly effective in managing the hypotension that may occur following an acute NSAID overdose, except when this is due to an acute blood loss. Seizures tend to be very short-lived and often do not require drug treatment. Although, recurrent seizures should be treated with I.V. diazepam. Since many of the NSAID undergo enterohepatic cycling, multiple doses of charcoal may be needed to reduce the potential for delayed toxicities.

Drug Interactions
  Decreased effect with aspirin; decreased effect of diuretics, antihypertensives
  Increased effect/toxicity of warfarin, methotrexate

Mechanism of Action Inhibits prostaglandin synthesis by decreasing the activity of the enzyme, cyclo-oxygenase, which results in decreased formation of prostaglandin precursors

Pharmacodynamics/Kinetics
  Duration of action: 2-4 hours
  Distribution: Crosses the placenta
  Protein binding: 99%
  Half-life: 2-3.3 hours
  Time to peak serum concentration: Within 0.5-1.5 hours
  Elimination: Principally in urine and in feces as glucuronide conjugates

Usual Dosage Children >14 years and Adults: Oral:
  Mild to moderate pain: 50 mg every 4-6 hours, not to exceed 400 mg/day
  Rheumatoid arthritis/osteoarthritis: 200-400 mg/day in 3-4 equal doses

Test Interactions ↑ chloride (S), ↑ sodium (S)

Patient Information Take with food, milk, or with antacids

Nursing Implications Should be used for short-term only (<7 days); advise patient to report persistent GI discomfort, sore throat, fever, or malaise

Dosage Forms Capsule: 50 mg, 100 mg

Meclomen® *see* Meclofenamate Sodium *on previous page*

Meclozine Hydrochloride *see* Meclizine Hydrochloride *on page 674*

Medicinal Carbon *see* Charcoal *on page 214*

Medicinal Charcoal *see* Charcoal *on page 214*

Medigesic® *see* Butalbital Compound *on page 153*

Medihaler-Epi® *see* Epinephrine *on page 389*

Medihaler Ergotamine™ *see* Ergotamine *on page 399*

Medihaler-Iso® *see* Isoproterenol *on page 597*

Medipren® [OTC] *see* Ibuprofen *on page 561*

Medi-Quick® Ointment [OTC] *see* Bacitracin, Neomycin, and Polymyxin B *on page 113*

Medralone® *see* Methylprednisolone *on page 724*

Medrol® see Methylprednisolone *on page 724*

Medroxyprogesterone Acetate (me drox' ee proe jess' te rone)

Brand Names Amen®; Curretab®; Cycrin®; Depo-Provera®; Provera®

Synonyms Acetoxymethylprogesterone; Methylacetoxyprogesterone

Use Endometrial carcinoma or renal carcinoma as well as secondary amenorrhea or abnormal uterine bleeding due to hormonal imbalance; prevention of pregnancy

Pregnancy Risk Factor X

Contraindications Pregnancy, thrombophlebitis; hypersensitivity to medroxyprogesterone or any component; cerebral apoplexy, undiagnosed vaginal bleeding, liver dysfunction

Warnings/Precautions Use with caution in patients with depression, diabetes, epilepsy, asthma, migraines, renal or cardiac dysfunction; pretreatment exams should include PAP smear, physical exam of breasts and pelvic areas. May increase serum cholesterol, LDL, decrease HDL and triglycerides; use of any progestin during the first 4 months of pregnancy is not recommended; monitor patient closely for loss of vision, sudden onset of proptosis, diplopia, migraine, and signs and symptoms of thromboembolic disorders.

Adverse Reactions

>10%:

Cardiovascular: Edema

Central nervous system: Weakness

Endocrine & metabolic: Breakthrough bleeding, spotting, changes in menstrual flow, amenorrhea

Gastrointestinal: Anorexia

Local: Pain at injection site

1% to 10%:

Cardiovascular: Embolism, central thrombosis

Central nervous system: Mental depression, fever, insomnia

Dermatologic: Melasma or chloasma, allergic rash with or without pruritus

Endocrine & metabolic: Changes in cervical erosion and secretions, weight gain or loss, increased breast tenderness

Hepatic: Cholestatic jaundice

Local: Thrombophlebitis

Overdosage/Toxicology Toxicity is unlikely following single exposures of excessive doses; supportive treatment is adequate in most cases

Drug Interactions Decreased effect: Aminoglutethimide may decrease effects by increasing hepatic metabolism

Mechanism of Action Inhibits secretion of pituitary gonadotropins, which prevents follicular maturation and ovulation, stimulates growth of mammary tissue

Pharmacodynamics/Kinetics

Absorption: I.M.: Slow

Metabolism: Oral: In the liver

Elimination: Oral: In urine and feces

Usual Dosage

Adolescents and Adults: Oral:

Amenorrhea: 5-10 mg/day for 5-10 days or 2.5 mg/day

Abnormal uterine bleeding: 5-10 mg for 5-10 days starting on day 16 or 21 of cycle

Accompanying cyclic estrogen therapy, postmenopausal: 2.5-10 mg the last 10-13 days of estrogen dosing each month

Adults: I.M.:

Endometrial or renal carcinoma: 400-1000 mg/week

Contraception: 150 mg every 3 months or 450 mg every 6 months

Dosing adjustment in hepatic impairment: Dose needs to be lowered in patients with alcoholic cirrhosis

Monitoring Parameters Monitor patient closely for loss of vision, sudden onset of proptosis, diplopia, migraine, and signs and symptoms of thromboembolic disorders

Test Interactions Altered thyroid and liver function tests

Patient Information Take this medicine only as directed; do not take more of it and do not take it for a longer period of time; if you suspect you may have become pregnant, stop taking this medicine; notify physician if sudden loss of vision or migraine headache occurs; may cause photosensitivity, wear protective clothing or sunscreen

Nursing Implications Patients should receive a copy of the patient labeling for the drug

(Continued)

Medroxyprogesterone Acetate *(Continued)*

Dosage Forms
Injection, suspension: 100 mg/mL (5 mL); 150 mg/mL (1 mL); 400 mg/mL (1 mL, 2.5 mL, 10 mL)

Tablet: 2.5 mg, 5 mg, 10 mg

Medrysone *(me' dri sone)*

Brand Names HMS Liquifilm®

Use Treatment of allergic conjunctivitis, vernal conjunctivitis, episcleritis, ophthalmic epinephrine sensitivity reaction

Pregnancy Risk Factor C

Contraindications Fungal, viral, or untreated pus-forming bacterial ocular infections; not for use in iritis and uveitis

Warnings/Precautions Prolonged use has been associated with the development of corneal or scleral perforation and posterior subcapsular cataracts; may mask or enhance the establishment of acute purulent untreated infections of the eye; effectiveness and safety have not been established in children. Medrysone is a synthetic corticosteroid; structurally related to progesterone; if no improvement after several days of treatment, discontinue medrysone and institute other therapy; duration of therapy: 3-4 days to several weeks dependent on type and severity of disease; taper dose to avoid disease exacerbation.

Adverse Reactions
1% to 10%: Ocular: Temporary mild blurred vision
<1%: Ocular: Stinging, burning, corneal thinning, increased intraocular pressure, glaucoma, damage to the optic nerve, defects in visual activity, cataracts, secondary ocular infection

Overdosage/Toxicology Systemic toxicity is unlikely from the ophthalmic preparation

Mechanism of Action Decreases inflammation by suppression of migration of polymorphonuclear leukocytes and reversal of increased capillary permeability

Pharmacodynamics/Kinetics
Absorption: Through aqueous humor
Metabolism: Any drug absorbed is metabolized in the liver
Elimination: By the kidneys and feces

Usual Dosage Children and Adults: Ophthalmic: Instill 1 drop in conjunctival sac 2-4 times/day up to every 4 hours; may use every 1-2 hours during first 1-2 days

Monitoring Parameters Intraocular pressure and periodic examination of lens (with prolonged use)

Patient Information Shake well before using, do not touch dropper to the eye

Dosage Forms Solution, ophthalmic: 1% (5 mL, 10 mL)

Mefenamic Acid *(me fe nam' ik)*

Related Information
Nonsteroidal Anti-Inflammatories Comparison *on page 1280*

Brand Names Ponstel®

Use Short-term relief of mild to moderate pain including primary dysmenorrhea

Pregnancy Risk Factor C

Contraindications Known hypersensitivity to mefenamic acid or other NSAIDs

Warnings/Precautions May have adverse effects on fetus

Adverse Reactions
>10%:
  Central nervous system: Dizziness
  Dermatologic: Skin rash
  Gastrointestinal: Abdominal cramps, heartburn, indigestion, nausea
1% to 10%:
  Cardiovascular: Fluid retention
  Central nervous system: Headache, nervousness
  Dermatologic: Itching
  Gastrointestinal: Vomiting
  Otic: Ringing in ears
<1%:
  Cardiovascular: Congestive heart failure, hypertension, arrhythmias, tachycardia
  Central nervous system: Epistaxis, confusion, hallucinations, aseptic meningitis, mental depression, drowsiness, insomnia
  Dermatologic: Hives, erythema multiforme, toxic epidermal necrolysis, Stevens-Johnson syndrome, angioedema
  Endocrine & metabolic: Polydipsia, hot flushes
  Gastrointestinal: Gastritis, GI ulceration
  Genitourinary: Cystitis

Hematologic: Agranulocytosis, anemia, hemolytic anemia, bone marrow depression, leukopenia, thrombocytopenia

Hepatic: Hepatitis

Neuromuscular & skeletal: Peripheral neuropathy

Ocular: Toxic amblyopia, blurred vision, conjunctivitis, dry eyes

Otic: Decreased hearing

Renal: Polyuria, acute renal failure

Respiratory: Shortness of breath, allergic rhinitis

Overdosage/Toxicology Symptoms of overdose include CNS stimulation, agitation, seizures

Management of a nonsteroidal anti-inflammatory drug (NSAID) intoxication is primarily supportive and symptomatic. Fluid therapy is commonly effective in managing the hypotension that may occur following an acute NSAIDs overdose, except when this is due to an acute blood loss. Seizures tend to be very short-lived and often do not require drug treatment. Although, recurrent seizures should be treated with I.V. diazepam. Since many of the NSAID undergo entero-hepatic cycling, multiple doses of charcoal may be needed to reduce the potential for delayed toxicities.

Drug Interactions

Decreased effect of diuretics, antihypertensives; decreased effect with aspirin

Increased effect/toxicity with oral anticoagulants, methotrexate

Mechanism of Action Inhibits prostaglandin synthesis by decreasing the activity of the enzyme, cyclo-oxygenase, which results in decreased formation of prostaglandin precursors

Pharmacodynamics/Kinetics

Peak effect: Oral: Within 2-4 hours

Duration of action: Up to 6 hours

Protein binding: High

Metabolism: Conjugated in the liver

Half-life: 3.5 hours

Elimination: In urine (50%) and feces as unchanged drug and metabolites

Usual Dosage Children >14 years and Adults: Oral: 500 mg to start then 250 mg every 4 hours as needed; maximum therapy: 1 week

Dosing adjustment/comments in renal impairment: Not recommended for use

Test Interactions ↑ chloride (S), ↑ sodium (S), positive Coombs' [direct], false-positive urinary bilirubin

Patient Information Take with food, milk, or with antacids; extended release capsules must be swallowed intact

Dosage Forms Capsule: 250 mg

Mefloquine Hydrochloride (me' floe kwin)

Related Information

Prevention of Malaria on page 1405

Brand Names Lariam®

Use Treatment of acute malarial infections and prevention of malaria

Pregnancy Risk Factor C

Contraindications Hypersensitivity to any component

Warnings/Precautions Caution is warranted with lactation; discontinue if unexplained neuropsychiatric disturbances occur, caution in epilepsy patients or in patients with significant cardiac disease. If mefloquine is to be used for a prolonged period, periodic evaluations including liver function tests and ophthalmic examinations should be performed. (Retinal abnormalities have not been observed with mefloquine in humans; however, it has with long-term administration to rats). In cases of life-threatening, serious, or overwhelming malaria infections due to *Plasmodium falciparum*, patients should be treated with intravenous antimalarial drug. Mefloquine may be given orally to complete the course. Caution should be exercised with regard to driving, piloting airplanes, and operating machines since dizziness, disturbed sense of balance; neuropsychiatric reactions have been reported with mefloquine.

Adverse Reactions

1% to 10%:

Central nervous system: Difficulty concentrating, headache, insomnia, light-headedness, vertigo

Gastrointestinal: Vomiting, diarrhea, stomach pain, nausea

Ocular: Visual disturbances

Otic: Tinnitus

<1%:

Cardiovascular: Bradycardia, extrasystoles, syncope

(Continued)

Mefloquine Hydrochloride *(Continued)*

Central nervous system: Anxiety, dizziness, confusion, seizures, hallucinations, mental depression, psychosis

Overdosage/Toxicology Symptoms of overdose include vomiting, diarrhea; cardiotoxic; following GI contamination supportive care only

Drug Interactions

Decreased effect of valproic acid

Increased toxicity with beta-blockers; increased toxicity/levels of chloroquine, quinine, quinidine (hold treatment until at least 12 hours after these drugs)

Mechanism of Action Mefloquine is a quinoline-methanol compound structurally similar to quinine; mefloquine's effectiveness in the treatment and prophylaxis of malaria is due to the destruction of the asexual blood forms of the malarial pathogens that affect humans, *Plasmodium falciparum, P. vivax, P. malariae, P. ovale*

Pharmacodynamics/Kinetics

Absorption: Oral: Well absorbed

Distribution: V_d: 19 L/kg; concentrates in erythrocytes; appears in breast milk

Protein binding: 98%

Half-life: 21-22 days

Elimination: ~1.5% to 9% of dose excreted unchanged in urine

Usual Dosage Oral:

Children: Malaria prophylaxis:

15-19 kg: 1/4 tablet

20-30 kg: 1/2 tablet

31-45 kg: 3/4 tablet

>45 kg: 1 tablet

Administer weekly starting 1 week before travel, continuing weekly during travel and for 4 weeks after leaving endemic area

Adults:

Treatment of mild to moderate malaria infection: 5 tablets (1250 mg) as a single dose with at least 8 oz of water

Malaria prophylaxis: 1 tablet (250 mg) once weekly for 4 weeks, then 1 tablet every other week; start treatment 1 week prior to departure to an endemic area; to avoid development of malaria after return from an endemic area, continue prophylaxis for 4 additional weeks; for prolonged stays in an endemic area, this prophylaxis can be achieved by continuing the recommended dosage schedule once weekly for 4 weeks, then once every other week, until traveler has taken 3 doses following return to a malaria-free area

Patient Information Begin therapy before trip and continue after; do not take drug on empty stomach; take with food and at least 8 oz of water; women of childbearing age should use reliable contraception during prophylaxis treatment and for 2 months after the last dose; be aware of signs and symptoms of malaria when traveling to an endemic area. Caution should be exercised with regard to driving, piloting airplanes, and operating machines since dizziness, disturbed sense of balance, or neuropsychiatric reactions have been reported with mefloquine.

Dosage Forms Tablet: 250 mg

Mefoxin® *see* Cefoxitin Sodium *on page 201*

Mega-B® **[OTC]** *see* Vitamin, Multiple *on page 1166*

Megace® *see* Megestrol Acetate *on this page*

Megestrol Acetate *(me jess' trole)*

Brand Names Megace®

Use Palliative treatment of breast and endometrial carcinomas, appetite stimulation, and promotion of weight gain in cachexia

Pregnancy Risk Factor X

Contraindications Hypersensitivity to megestrol or any component

Warnings/Precautions The U.S. Food and Drug Administration (FDA) currently recommends that procedures for proper handling and disposal of antineoplastic agents be considered. Use during the first few months of pregnancy is not recommended. Use with caution in patients with a history of thrombophlebitis. Elderly females may have vaginal bleeding or discharge and need to be forewarned of this side effect and inconvenience.

Adverse Reactions

>10%:

Cardiovascular: Edema

Central nervous system: Weakness

Endocrine & metabolic: Breakthrough bleeding and amenorrhea, spotting, changes in menstrual flow

1% to 10%:
   Central nervous system: Insomnia, depression, fever, headache
   Dermatologic: Allergic rash with or without pruritus, melasma or chloasma, skin rash, and rarely alopecia
   Endocrine & metabolic: Changes in cervical erosion and secretions, increased breast tenderness, amenorrhea, changes in vaginal bleeding pattern, edema, fluid retention, hyperglycemia
   Gastrointestinal: Weight gain (not attributed to edema or fluid retention), nausea, vomiting, stomach cramps
   Hepatic: Cholestatic jaundice, hepatotoxicity
   Myelosuppressive:
      WBC: None
      Platelets: None
   Local: Thrombophlebitis
   Miscellaneous: Hyperpnea, carpal tunnel syndrome

Overdosage/Toxicology Toxicity is unlikely following simple exposures of excessive doses

Mechanism of Action Megestrol is an antineoplastic progestin thought to act through an antileutenizing effect mediated via the pituitary

Pharmacodynamics/Kinetics
   Onset of action: At least 2 months of continuous therapy is necessary
   Absorption: Oral: Well absorbed
   Metabolism: Completely metabolized in the liver to free steroids and glucuronide conjugates
   Time to peak serum concentration: Oral: Within 1-3 hours
   Half-life, elimination: 15-20 hours
   Elimination: In urine as steroid metabolites and inactive compound, some in feces and bile

Usual Dosage Adults: Oral (refer to individual protocols):
   Female:
      Breast carcinoma: 40 mg 4 times/day
      Endometrial: 40-320 mg/day in divided doses; use for 2 months to determine efficacy; maximum doses used have been up to 800 mg/day
      Uterine bleeding: 40 mg 2-4 times/day
   Male and Female: HIV-related cachexia: Initial dose: 800 mg/day; daily doses of 400 and 800 mg/day were found to be clinically effective

Monitoring Parameters Monitor for tumor response; observe for signs of thromboembolic phenomena; monitor for thromboembolism

Test Interactions Altered thyroid and liver function tests

Patient Information Exposure to megestrol during the first 4 months of pregnancy may pose risks to the fetus; notify physician if sudden loss of vision, double vision, migraine headache occur, or if pain in calves with warmth and tenderness develops; may cause photosensitivity, wear protective clothing or sunscreen

Dosage Forms
   Suspension, oral: 40 mg/mL with alcohol 0.06% (236.6 mL)
   Tablet: 20 mg, 40 mg

Melanex® see Hydroquinone on page 551

Mellaril® see Thioridazine on page 1084

Mellaril-S® see Thioridazine on page 1084

Melphalan (mel' fa lan)
Related Information
   Cancer Chemotherapy Regimens on page 1218-1241
Brand Names Alkeran®
Synonyms L-PAM; L-Sarcolysin; Phenylalanine Mustard
Use Palliative treatment of multiple myeloma and nonresectable epithelial ovarian carcinoma; neuroblastoma, rhabdomyosarcoma, breast cancer; I.V. formulation: Use in patients in whom oral therapy is not appropriate
Pregnancy Risk Factor D
Contraindications Hypersensitivity to melphalan or any component; severe bone marrow depression; patients whose disease was resistant to prior therapy
Warnings/Precautions The U.S. Food and Drug Administration (FDA) currently recommends that procedures for proper handling and disposal for antineoplastic agents be considered. Is potentially mutagenic, carcinogenic, and teratogenic; produces amenorrhea. Reduce dosage or discontinue therapy if leukocyte count <3000/mm³ or platelet count <100,000/mm³; use with caution in patients with bone marrow suppression, impaired renal function, or who have received prior chemotherapy or irradiation; will cause amenorrhea. Toxicity to immunosuppressives is increased in elderly. Start with lowest recommended adult doses. Signs (Continued)

Melphalan *(Continued)*

of infection, such as fever and WBC rise, may not occur. Lethargy and confusion may be more prominent signs of infection.

Adverse Reactions

>10%

Myelosuppressive: Leukopenia and thrombocytopenia are the most common effects of melphalan. Irreversible bone marrow failure has been reported.

WBC: Moderate

Platelets: Moderate

Onset (days): 7

Nadir (days): 8-10 and 27-32

Recovery (days): 42-50

Second malignancies: Reported are melphalan more frequently

1% to 10%:

Dermatologic: Vesiculation of skin, alopecia, pruritus, rash

Endocrine & metabolic: SIADH, sterility, amenorrhea

Gastrointestinal: Nausea and vomiting are mild; stomatitis and diarrhea are infrequent

Hematologic: Anemia, agranulocytosis, hemolytic anemia

Renal: Bladder irritation, hemorrhagic cystitis

Respiratory: Pulmonary fibrosis, interstitial pneumonitis

Miscellaneous: Hypersensitivity, vasculitis

Overdosage/Toxicology Symptoms of overdose include hypocalcemia, pulmonary fibrosis, nausea and vomiting, bone marrow suppression

Drug Interactions

Decreased effect: Cimetidine and other H_2 antagonists: The reduction in gastric pH has been reported to reduce the bioavailability of melphalan by 30%

Increased toxicity: Cyclosporine: Increased incidence of nephrotoxicity

Stability Tablets/injection: Protect from light, store at room temperature

Injection: Preparation:

The time between reconstitution/dilutation and administration of parenteral melphalan must be kept to a minimum (<60 minutes) because reconstituted and diluted solutions are unstable

1) Melphalan for injection must be reconstituted by rapidly injecting 10 mL of the supplied diluent directly into the vial of lyophilized powder. Immediately shake vial vigorously until a clear solution is obtained. This provides a 5 mg/mL solution of melphalan. Rapid addition of the diluent followed by immediate vigorous shaking is important for proper dissolution.

2) Immediately dilute the dose to be administered in 0.9% sodium chloride in water to a concentration ≥0.45 mg/mL

3) Administer the diluted product over a minimum of 15 minutes

4) Complete the administration within 60 minutes of reconstitution

Mechanism of Action Alkylating agent which is a derivative of mechlorethamine that inhibits DNA and RNA synthesis via formation of carbonium ions; cross-links strands of DNA

Pharmacodynamics/Kinetics

Absorption: Oral: Variable and incomplete from the GI tract; food interferes with absorption

Distribution: V_d: 0.5-0.6 L/kg throughout total body water

Bioavailability: Unpredictable, decreasing from 85% to 58%

Half-life, terminal: 1.5 hours

Time to peak serum concentration: Reportedly within 2 hours

Elimination: 10% to 15% excreted unchanged in urine; 20% to 50% excreted in stool after oral administration

Usual Dosage

Oral (refer to individual protocols; dose should always be adjusted to patient response and weekly blood counts):

Children: 4-20 mg/m²/day for 1-21 days

Adults:

Multiple myeloma: 6 mg/day for 2-3 weeks or 10 mg/day for 7-10 days or 0.15 mg/kg/day for 7 days; labs should be carefully monitored during therapy and the drug may need to be discontinued after 2-3 weeks of treatment. Maintenance doses of 1-3 mg/day may be instituted after WBC recovery.

Ovarian carcinoma: 0.2 mg/kg/day for 5 days, repeat every 4-5 weeks

Intravenous:

Pediatric rhabdomyosarcoma: 10-35 mg/m² bolus every 21-28 days

Chemoradiotherapy supported by marrow infusions for neuroblastoma: 70-140 mg/m² on day 7 and 6 before BMT or 140-220 mg/m² single dose before BMT

Multiple myeloma: 16 mg/m² administered at 2 week intervals for 4 doses; then, after adequate recovery from toxicity, administer at 4 week intervals

High-dose therapy with bone marrow or stem cell rescue: Doses of 40-260 mg/m^2 have been used; however, refer to protocol

Dosing adjustment in renal impairment:
Cl$_{cr}$ 10-50 mL/minute: Administer at 75% of normal dose
Cl$_{cr}$ <10 mL/minute: Administer at 50% of normal dose

Administration I.V. dose should be administered as a single infusion over 15-20 minutes

Monitoring Parameters CBC with differential and platelet count, serum electrolytes, serum uric acid

Test Interactions False-positive Coombs' test [direct]

Patient Information Any signs of infection, easy bruising or bleeding, shortness of breath, or painful or burning urination should be brought to physician's attention. Nausea, vomiting, or hair loss sometimes occurs; drug may cause permanent sterility and birth defects. The drug may be excreted in breast milk, therefore, an alternative form of feeding your baby should be used.

Nursing Implications Avoid skin contact with I.V. formulation

Dosage Forms
Powder for injection: 50 mg
Tablet: 2 mg

Menadol® [OTC] *see* Ibuprofen *on page 561*

Menest® *see* Estrogens, Esterified *on page 412*

Meni-D® *see* Meclizine Hydrochloride *on page 674*

Meningococcal Polysaccharide Vaccine, Groups A, C, Y, and W-135 (me ninge' oh kock al poly sack' a ride)

Related Information
Immunization Guidelines *on page 1389-1405*
Vaccines *on page 1386-1388*

Brand Names Menomune®-A/C/Y/W-135

Use
Immunization of persons 2 years of age and above in epidemic or endemic areas as might be determined in a population delineated by neighborhood, school, dormitory, or other reasonable boundary. The prevalent serogroup in such a situation should match a serogroup in the vaccine. Individuals at particular high-risk includes persons with terminal component complement deficiencies and those with anatomic or functional asplenia.
Travelers visiting areas of a country that are recognized as having hyperendemic or epidemic meningococcal disease
Vaccinations should be considered for household or institutional contacts of persons with meningococcal disease as an adjunct to appropriate antibiotic chemoprophylaxis as well as medical and laboratory personnel at risk of exposure to meningococcal disease

Pregnancy Risk Factor C

Contraindications Children <2 years of age

Warnings/Precautions Patients who undergo splenectomy secondary to trauma or nonlymphoid tumors respond well; however, those asplenic patients with lymphoid tumors who receive either chemotherapy or irradiation respond poorly; pregnancy, unless there is substantial risk of infection.

Adverse Reactions
>10%: Local: Tenderness, pain, erythema and induration
1% to 10%: Central nervous system: Headache, malaise, fever, chills

Drug Interactions Decreased effect with administration of immunoglobulin within 1 month

Stability Discard remainder of vaccine within 5 days after reconstitution; store reconstituted vaccine in refrigerator

Mechanism of Action Induces the formation of bactericidal antibodies to meningococcal antigens; the presence of these antibodies is strongly correlated with immunity to meningococcal disease caused by *Neisseria meningitidis* groups A, C, Y and W-135.

Pharmacodynamics/Kinetics
Onset: Antibody levels are achieved within 10-14 days after administration
Duration: Antibodies against group A and C polysaccharides decline markedly (to prevaccination levels) over the first 3 years following a single dose of vaccine, especially in children <4 years of age

Usual Dosage One dose I.M. (0.5 mL); the need for booster is unknown

Nursing Implications Epinephrine 1:1000 should be available to control allergic reaction

Dosage Forms Injection: 10 dose, 50 dose

Menomune®-A/C/Y/W-135 *see* Meningococcal Polysaccharide Vaccine, Groups A, C, Y, and W-135 *on previous page*

Menotropins (men oh troe' pins)

Brand Names Pergonal®

Use Sequentially with hCG to induce ovulation and pregnancy in the infertile woman with functional anovulation; used with hCG in men to stimulate spermatogenesis in those with primary hypogonadotropic hypogonadism

Pregnancy Risk Factor X

Contraindications Primary ovarian failure, overt thyroid and adrenal dysfunction, abnormal bleeding, pregnancy, men with normal urinary gonadotropin concentrations, elevated gonadotropin levels indicating primary testicular failure

Warnings/Precautions Advise patient of frequency and potential hazards of multiple pregnancy; to minimize the hazard of abnormal ovarian enlargement, use the lowest possible dose

Adverse Reactions
Male:
>10%: Gynecomastia
1% to 10%: Erythrocytosis (shortness of breath, dizziness, anorexia, fainting, epistaxis)
Female:
>10%: Ovarian enlargement, abdominal distention, pain/rash at injection site
1% to 10%: Ovarian hyperstimulation syndrome
<1%: Thromboembolism, pain, febrile reactions

Overdosage/Toxicology Symptoms of overdose include ovarian hyperstimulation

Stability Lyophilized powder may be refrigerated or stored at room temperature; after reconstitution inject immediately, discard any unused portion

Mechanism of Action Actions occur as a result of both follicle stimulating hormone (FSH) effects and luteinizing hormone (LH) effects; menotropins stimulate the development and maturation of the ovarian follicle (FSH), cause ovulation (LH), and stimulate the development of the corpus luteum (LH); in males it stimulates spermatogenesis (LH)

Pharmacodynamics/Kinetics Elimination: ~10% of dose is excreted in the urine unchanged

Usual Dosage Adults: I.M.:
Male: Following pretreatment with hCG, 1 ampul 3 times/week and hCG 2000 units twice weekly until sperm is detected in the ejaculate (4-6 months) then may be increased to 2 ampuls of menotropins (150 units FSH/150 units LH) 3 times/week
Female: 1 ampul/day (75 units of FSH and LH) for 9-12 days followed by 10,000 units hCG 1 day after the last dose; repeated at least twice at same level before increasing dosage to 2 ampuls (150 units FSH/150 units LH)

Administration I.M. administration only

Patient Information Multiple ovulations resulting in plural gestations have been reported

Dosage Forms Injection:
Follicle stimulating hormone activity 75 units and luteinizing hormone activity 75 units per 2 mL ampul
Follicle stimulating hormone activity 150 units and luteinizing hormone activity 150 units per 2 mL ampul

Meperidine Hydrochloride (me per' i deen)

Related Information
Narcotic Agonist Comparison Charts *on page 1274-1275*

Brand Names Demerol®

Synonyms Isonipecaine Hydrochloride; Pethidine Hydrochloride

Use Management of moderate to severe pain; adjunct to anesthesia and preoperative sedation

Restrictions C-II

Pregnancy Risk Factor B (D if used for prolonged periods or in high doses at term)

Contraindications Hypersensitivity to meperidine or any component; patients receiving MAO inhibitors presently or in the past 14 days

Warnings/Precautions Use with caution in patients with pulmonary, hepatic, renal disorders, or increased intracranial pressure; use with caution in patients with renal failure or seizure disorders or those receiving high-dose meperidine; normeperidine (an active metabolite and CNS stimulant) may accumulate and precipitate twitches, tremors, or seizures; some preparations contain sulfites which may cause allergic reaction; not recommended as a drug of first choice for the treatment of chronic pain in the elderly due to the accumulation of normeperidine; for acute pain, its use should be limited to 1-2 doses

Adverse Reactions
>10%:
  Cardiovascular: Hypotension
  Central nervous system: Weakness, tiredness, drowsiness, dizziness
  Gastrointestinal: Nausea, vomiting, constipation
  Miscellaneous: Histamine release
1% to 10%:
  Central nervous system: Nervousness, headache, restlessness, malaise, confusion
  Gastrointestinal: Anorexia stomach cramps, dry mouth, biliary spasm
  Genitourinary: Ureteral spasms, decreased urination
  Local: Pain at injection site
  Respiratory: Troubled breathing, shortness of breath
<1%:
  Central nervous system: Mental depression, hallucinations, paradoxical CNS stimulation, increased intracranial pressure
  Dermatologic: Skin rash, hives
  Gastrointestinal: Paralytic ileus
  Miscellaneous: Physical and psychological dependence

Overdosage/Toxicology Symptoms of overdose include CNS depression, respiratory depression, mydriasis, bradycardia, pulmonary edema, chronic tremors, CNS excitability, seizures. Treatment of an overdose includes support of the patient's airway, establishment of an I.V. line, and administration of naloxone 2 mg I.V. (0.01 mg/kg for children) with repeat administration as necessary up to a total of 10 mg.

Drug Interactions
Decreased effect: Phenytoin may decrease the analgesic effects
Increased toxicity: May aggravate the adverse effects of isoniazid; MAO inhibitors, fluoxetine, and other serotonin uptake inhibitors greatly potentiate the effects of meperidine; acute opioid overdosage symptoms can be seen, including severe toxic reactions; CNS depressants, tricyclic antidepressants, phenothiazines may potentiate the effects of meperidine

Stability Meperidine injection should be stored at room temperature and protected from light and freezing; protect oral dosage forms from light
  Incompatible with aminophylline, heparin, phenobarbital, phenytoin, and sodium bicarbonate

Mechanism of Action Binds to opiate receptors in the CNS, causing inhibition of ascending pain pathways, altering the perception of and response to pain; produces generalized CNS depression

Pharmacodynamics/Kinetics
Oral, S.C., I.M.:
  Onset of analgesic effect: Within 10-15 minutes
  Peak effect: Within 1 hour
  Duration: 2-4 hours
I.V.: Onset of effects: Within 5 minutes
Distribution: Crosses the placenta; appears in breast milk
Protein binding: 65% to 75%
Metabolism: In the liver
Bioavailability: ~50% to 60%; increased with liver disease
Half-life:
  Parent drug: Terminal phase:
    Neonates: 23 hours; range: 12-39 hours
    Adults: 2.5-4 hours
    Adults with liver disease: 7-11 hours
  Normeperidine (active metabolite): 15-30 hours; is dependent on renal function and can accumulate with high doses or in patients with decreased renal function

Usual Dosage Doses should be titrated to appropriate analgesic effect; when changing route of administration, note that oral doses are about half as effective as parenteral dose
Children: Oral, I.M., I.V., S.C.: 1-1.5 mg/kg/dose every 3-4 hours as needed; 1-2 mg/kg as a single dose preoperative medication may be used; maximum 100 mg/dose
Adults: Oral, I.M., I.V.: S.C.: 50-150 mg/dose every 3-4 hours as needed
Elderly:
  Oral: 50 mg every 4 hours
  I.M.: 25 mg every 4 hours

Dosing adjustment in renal impairment:
  Cl$_{cr}$ 10-50 mL/minute: Administer at 75% of normal dose
  Cl$_{cr}$ <10 mL/minute: Administer at 50% of normal dose
(Continued)

Meperidine Hydrochloride *(Continued)*

Dosing adjustment/comments in hepatic disease: Increased narcotic effect in cirrhosis; reduction in dose more important for oral than I.V. route

Administration
Meperidine may be administered I.M. (preferably), S.C., or I.V.
I.V. push should be given slowly, use of a 10 mg/mL concentration has been recommended

Monitoring Parameters Pain relief, respiratory and mental status, blood pressure; observe patient for excessive sedation, CNS depression, seizures, respiratory depression

Reference Range Therapeutic: 70-500 ng/mL (SI: 283-2020 nmol/L); Toxic: >1000 ng/mL (SI: >4043 nmol/L)

Test Interactions ↑ amylase (S), ↑ BSP retention, ↑ CPK (I.M. injections)

Patient Information Avoid alcohol, may cause drowsiness

Dosage Forms
Injection:
Multiple dose vials: 50 mg/mL (30 mL); 100 mg/mL (20 mL)
Single dose: 10 mg/mL (5 mL, 10 mL, 30 mL); 25 mg/dose (0.5 mL, 1 mL); 50 mg/dose (1 mL); 75 mg/dose (1 mL, 1.5 mL); 100 mg/dose (1 mL)
Syrup: 50 mg/5 mL (500 mL)
Tablet: 50 mg, 100 mg

Mephenytoin *(me fen' i toyn)*

Brand Names Mesantoin®

Synonyms Methoin; Methylphenylethylhydantoin; Phenantoin

Use Treatment of tonic-clonic and partial seizures in patients who are uncontrolled with less toxic anticonvulsants

Pregnancy Risk Factor C

Contraindications Hypersensitivity to mephenytoin, other hydantoins, or any component

Warnings/Precautions Fatal irreversible aplastic anemia has occurred; abrupt withdrawal may precipitate seizures; may increase frequency of petit mal seizures; use with caution in patients with liver disease or porphyria; usually listed in combination with other anticonvulsants

Adverse Reactions
>10%:
Central nervous system: Psychiatric changes, slurred speech, dizziness, drowsiness
Gastrointestinal: Constipation, nausea, vomiting
Neuromuscular & skeletal: Trembling
1% to 10%:
Central nervous system: Drowsiness, headache, insomnia
Dermatologic: Skin rash
Gastrointestinal: Anorexia, weight loss
Hematologic: Leukopenia
Hepatic: Hepatitis
Miscellaneous: Increase in serum creatinine
<1%:
Cardiovascular: Hypotension, bradycardia, cardiac arrhythmias, cardiovascular collapse
Central nervous system: Confusion, fever, ataxia
Dermatologic: Stevens-Johnson syndrome or SLE-like syndrome
Gastrointestinal: Gingival hyperplasia
Hematologic: Blood dyscrasias
Hepatic: Hepatitis
Local: Venous irritation and pain, thrombophlebitis
Neuromuscular & skeletal: Paresthesia, peripheral neuropathy
Ocular: Diplopia, nystagmus, blurred vision, photophobia
Miscellaneous: Lymphadenopathy, Hodgkin's disease-like syndrome, serum sickness

Overdosage/Toxicology Symptoms of overdose include Restlessness, dizziness, drowsiness, nausea, vomiting, nystagmus, ataxia, dysarthria, tremor, slurred speech, hypotension, respiratory depression, coma; treatment is supportive

Drug Interactions
Decreased effect with carbamazepine, TCAs, calcium antacids; decreased effect of oral anticoagulants, oral contraceptives, steroids, quinidine, vitamin D, vitamin K, doxycycline, furosemide, TCAs
Increased effect/toxicity with alcohol, sulfonamides, chloramphenicol, cimetidine, isoniazid, disulfiram, phenothiazines, benzodiazepines

Mechanism of Action Stabilizes neuronal membranes and decreases seizure activity by increasing efflux or decreasing influx of sodium ions across cell membranes in the motor cortex during generation of nerve impulses; prolongs effective refractory period and suppresses ventricular pacemaker automaticity, shortens action potential in the heart

Pharmacodynamics/Kinetics
Onset of action: 30 minutes
Duration: 24-48 hours
Absorption: Oral: Rapid
Metabolism: In the liver
Half-life: 144 hours
Elimination: In urine

Usual Dosage Oral:
Children: 3-15 mg/kg/day in 3 divided doses; usual maintenance dose: 100-400 mg/day in 3 divided doses
Adults: Initial dose: 50-100 mg/day given daily; increase by 50-100 mg at weekly intervals; usual maintenance dose: 200-600 mg/day in 3 divided doses; maximum: 800 mg/day

Monitoring Parameters CBC and platelet count

Reference Range Total mephenytoin (mephenytoin plus 5-ethyl-5-phenylhydantoin) of 25-40 μg/mL

Test Interactions ↑ alkaline phosphatase (S); ↓ calcium (S)

Patient Information Take with food, avoid alcoholic beverages; may cause dizziness, drowsiness, and impair coordination or judgment

Dosage Forms Tablet: 100 mg

Mephobarbital (me foe bar' bi tal)

Brand Names Mebaral®
Synonyms Methylphenobarbital
Use Sedative; treatment of grand mal and petit mal epilepsy
Restrictions C-IV
Pregnancy Risk Factor D
Contraindications Hypersensitivity to mephobarbital, other barbiturates, or any component; pre-existing CNS depression; respiratory depression; severe uncontrolled pain; history of porphyria
Warnings/Precautions Use with caution in patients with renal impairment, pulmonary insufficiency, or hepatic dysfunction; sometimes used in specific patients who have excessive sedation or hyperexcitability from phenobarbital; abrupt withdrawal may precipitate status epilepticus

Adverse Reactions
>10%: Central nervous system: Dizziness, lightheadedness, drowsiness, "hangover" effect
1% to 10%:
Central nervous system: Confusion, mental depression, unusual excitement, nervousness, faint feeling, headache, insomnia, nightmares
Gastrointestinal: Constipation, nausea, vomiting
<1%:
Cardiovascular: Hypotension
Central nervous system: Hallucinations
Dermatologic: Skin rash, exfoliative dermatitis, Stevens-Johnson syndrome, angioedema
Hematologic: Agranulocytosis, megaloblastic anemia, thrombocytopenia
Local: Thrombophlebitis
Respiratory: Respiratory depression
Miscellaneous: Dependence

Overdosage/Toxicology Symptoms of overdose include CNS depression, respiratory depression, hypothermia, tachycardia, hypotension
Repeated oral doses of activated charcoal significantly reduce the half-life of barbiturates resulting from an enhancement of nonrenal elimination. The usual dose is 30-60 g every 4-6 hours for 3-4 days unless the patient has no bowel movement causing the charcoal to remain in the GI tract. Assure adequate hydration and renal function.
Urinary alkalinization with I.V. sodium bicarbonate also helps to enhance elimination
Hemodialysis or hemoperfusion is of uncertain value. Patients in stage IV coma due to high serum barbiturate levels may require charcoal hemoperfusion.

Drug Interactions
Decreased effect: Phenothiazines, haloperidol, quinidine, cyclosporine, TCAs, corticosteroids, theophylline, ethosuximide, warfarin, oral contraceptives, chloramphenicol, griseofulvin, doxycycline, beta-blockers
Increased effect/toxicity: Propoxyphene, benzodiazepines, CNS depressants, valproic acid, methylphenidate, chloramphenicol
(Continued)

Mephobarbital (Continued)

Mechanism of Action Increases seizure threshold in the motor cortex; depresses monosynaptic and polysynaptic transmission in the CNS

Pharmacodynamics/Kinetics
Onset of action: 20-60 minutes
Duration: 6-8 hours
Absorption: Oral: ~50%
Metabolism: By the liver to phenobarbital
Half-life: 34 hours
Elimination: In urine

Usual Dosage Oral:
Epilepsy:
Children: 6-12 mg/kg/day in 2-4 divided doses
Adults: 200-600 mg/day in 2-4 divided doses

Sedation:
Children:
<5 years: 16-32 mg 3-4 times/day
>5 years: 32-64 mg 3-4 times/day
Adults: 32-100 mg 3-4 times/day

Dosing adjustment in renal or hepatic impairment: Use with caution and reduce dosages
Reference Range Phenobarbital level should be in the range of 15-40 µg/mL
Test Interactions ↑ alk phos (S), ↑ ammonia (B), ↓ bilirubin (S), ↓ calcium (S)
Patient Information May cause drowsiness, may impair coordination and judgment; do not discontinue abruptly; notify physician of dark urine, pale stools, jaundice, abdominal pain, persistent nausea, and vomiting; do not skip doses
Nursing Implications Observe patient for excessive sedation, respiratory depression; raise bed rails, institute safety precautions, assist with ambulation
Dosage Forms Tablet: 32 mg, 50 mg, 100 mg

Mephyton® see Phytonadine on page 882

Mepivacaine Hydrochloride (me piv′ a kane)

Brand Names Carbocaine®; Isocaine® HCl; Polocaine®
Use Local anesthesia by nerve block; infiltration in dental procedures; **not** for use in spinal anesthesia
Pregnancy Risk Factor C
Contraindications Hypersensitivity to mepivacaine or any component or other amide anesthetics, allergy to sodium bisulfate
Warnings/Precautions Use with caution in patients with cardiac disease, renal disease, and hyperthyroidism; convulsions due to systemic toxicity leading to cardiac arrest have been reported presumably due to intravascular injection
Adverse Reactions
<1%:
Cardiovascular: Bradycardia, myocardial depression, hypotension, cardiovascular collapse, edema
Central nervous system: Anxiety, restlessness, disorientation, confusion, seizures, drowsiness, unconsciousness, chills, shivering
Dermatologic: Urticaria
Gastrointestinal: Nausea, vomiting
Local: Transient stinging or burning at injection site
Neuromuscular & skeletal: Tremors
Ocular: Blurred vision
Otic: Tinnitus
Respiratory: Respiratory arrest
Miscellaneous: Anaphylactoid reactions
Overdosage/Toxicology Symptoms of overdose include dizziness, cyanosis, tremors, bronchial spasm. Treatment is primarily symptomatic and supportive. Termination of anesthesia by pneumatic tourniquet inflation should be attempted when the agent is administered by infiltration or regional injection. Seizures commonly respond to diazepam, while hypotension responds to I.V. fluids and Trendelenburg positioning. Bradyarrhythmias (when the heart rate is <60) can be treated with I.V., I.M., or S.C. atropine 15 mcg/kg. With the development of metabolic acidosis, I.V. sodium bicarbonate 0.5-2 mEq/kg and ventilatory assistance should be instituted.
Mechanism of Action Mepivacaine is an amino amide local anesthetic similar to lidocaine; like all local anesthetics, mepivacaine acts by preventing the generation and conduction of nerve impulses
Pharmacodynamics/Kinetics
Onset of action: Epidural: Within 7-15 minutes

Duration: 2-2.5 hours; similar onset and duration is seen following infiltration

Protein binding: 70% to 85%

Metabolism: Chiefly in the liver by N-demethylation, hydroxylation, and glucuronidation

Half-life: 1.9 hours

Elimination: Urinary excretion (95% as metabolites)

Usual Dosage Children and Adults: Injectable local anesthetic: Varies with procedure, degree of anesthesia needed, vascularity of tissue, duration of anesthesia required, and physical condition of patient

Nursing Implications Before injecting, withdraw syringe plunger to ensure injection is not into vein or artery

Dosage Forms Injection: 1% [10 mg/mL] (30 mL, 50 mL); 1.5% [15 mg/mL] (30 mL); 2% [20 mg/mL] (20 mL, 50 mL); 3% [30 mg/mL] (1.8 mL)

Meprobamate (me proe ba' mate)

Brand Names Equanil®; Meprospan®; Miltown®; Neuramate®

Use Management of anxiety disorders

Unlabeled use: Demonstrated value for muscle contraction, headache, premenstrual tension, external sphincter spasticity, muscle rigidity, opisthotonos-associated with tetanus

Restrictions C-IV

Pregnancy Risk Factor D

Contraindications Acute intermittent porphyria; hypersensitivity to meprobamate or any component; do not use in patients with pre-existing CNS depression, narrow-angle glaucoma, or severe uncontrolled pain

Warnings/Precautions Physical and psychological dependence and abuse may occur; not recommended in children <6 years of age; allergic reaction may occur in patients with history of dermatological condition (usually by fourth dose); use with caution in patients with renal or hepatic impairment, or with a history of seizures

Adverse Reactions

>10%: Central nervous system: Drowsiness, clumsiness, ataxia

1% to 10%:

Central nervous system: Dizziness

Dermatologic: Skin rashes

Gastrointestinal: Diarrhea, vomiting

Ocular: Blurred vision

Respiratory: Wheezing

<1%:

Cardiovascular: Syncope, peripheral edema

Central nervous system: Paradoxical excitement, confusion, slurred speech, headache, euphoria, chills

Dermatologic: Purpura, dermatitis, Stevens-Johnson syndrome

Gastrointestinal: Stomatitis

Hematologic: Thrombocytopenia, leukopenia

Renal: Renal failure

Respiratory: Troubled breathing, bronchospasm

Overdosage/Toxicology Symptoms of overdose include drowsiness, lethargy, ataxia, coma, hypotension, shock, death; treatment is supportive following attempts to enhance drug elimination. Hypotension should be treated with I.V. fluids and/or Trendelenburg positioning. Dialysis and hemoperfusion have not demonstrated significant reductions in blood drug concentrations.

Drug Interactions Increased toxicity: CNS depressants → ↑ CNS depression

Mechanism of Action Precise mechanism is not yet clear, but many effects have been ascribed to its central depressant actions

Pharmacodynamics/Kinetics

Onset of sedation: Oral: Within 1 hour

Distribution: Crosses the placenta; appears in breast milk

Metabolism: Promptly in the liver

Half-life: 10 hours

Elimination: In urine (8% to 20% as unchanged drug) and feces (10% as metabolites)

Usual Dosage Oral:

Children 6-12 years:

100-200 mg 2-3 times/day

Sustained release: 200 mg twice daily

Adults:

400 mg 3-4 times/day, up to 2400 mg/day

Sustained release: 400-800 mg twice daily

(Continued)

Meprobamate *(Continued)*

Dosing interval in renal impairment:
Cl$_{cr}$ 10-50 mL/minute: Administer every 9-12 hours
Cl$_{cr}$ <10 mL/minute: Administer every 12-18 hours
Moderately dialyzable (20% to 50%)

Dosing adjustment in hepatic impairment: Probably necessary in patients with liver disease

Monitoring Parameters Mental status

Reference Range Therapeutic: 6-12 µg/mL (SI: 28-55 µmol/L); Toxic: >60 µg/mL (SI: >275 µmol/L)

Patient Information May cause drowsiness; avoid alcoholic beverages

Dosage Forms
Capsule, sustained release: 200 mg, 400 mg
Tablet: 200 mg, 400 mg, 600 mg

Mepron™ *see* Atovaquone *on page 98*

Meprospan® *see* Meprobamate *on previous page*

Mercaptopurine *(mer kap toe pyoor' een)*

Related Information
Cancer Chemotherapy Regimens *on page 1218-1241*

Brand Names Purinethol®

Synonyms 6-Mercaptopurine; 6-MP

Use Treatment of leukemias (ALL or AML) maintenance therapy

Pregnancy Risk Factor D

Contraindications Hypersensitivity to mercaptopurine or any component; patients whose disease showed prior resistance to mercaptopurine or thioguanine; severe liver disease, severe bone marrow depression

Warnings/Precautions The U.S. Food and Drug Administration (FDA) currently recommends that procedures for proper handling and disposal of antineoplastic agents be considered. Mercaptopurine may cause birth defects; potentially carcinogenic; adjust dosage in patients with renal impairment or hepatic failure; use with caution in patients with prior bone marrow suppression; patients may be at risk for pancreatitis. Toxicity to immunosuppressives is increased in elderly. Start with lowest recommended adult doses. Signs of infection, such as fever and WBC rise, may not occur. Lethargy and confusion may be more prominent signs of infection.

Adverse Reactions
>10%:
Hepatic: 6-MP can cause an intrahepatic cholestasis and focal centralobular necrosis manifested as hyperbilirubinemia, increased alkaline phosphatase, and increased AST. This may be dose related, occurring more frequently at doses >2.5 mg/kg/day; jaundice is noted 1-2 months into therapy, but has ranged from 1 week to 8 years.

1% to 10%:
Dermatologic: Hyperpigmentation, rash
Gastrointestinal: Nausea, vomiting, diarrhea, stomatitis, anorexia, stomach pain, and mucositis may require parenteral nutrition and dose reduction; 6-TG is less GI toxic than 6-MP
Hematologic: Leukopenia, thrombocytopenia, anemia may occur at high doses
Myelosuppressive:
WBC: Moderate
Platelets: Moderate
Onset (days): 7-10
Nadir (days): 14
Recovery (days): 21
Renal: Renal toxicity, hyperuricemia

<1%:
Dermatologic: Dry, scaling rash
Gastrointestinal: Glossitis, tarry stools
Hematologic: Eosinophilia
Miscellaneous: Drug fever

Overdosage/Toxicology Symptoms of overdose include:
Immediate: Nausea, vomiting
Delayed: Bone marrow suppression, hepatic necrosis, gastroenteritis

Drug Interactions
Decreased effect: Warfarin: 6-MP inhibits the anticoagulation effect of warfarin by an unknown mechanism

Increased toxicity:

Allopurinol: Can cause increased levels of 6-MP by inhibition of xanthine oxidase; reduce dose of 6-MP by 75% when both drugs are used concomitantly; seen only with oral 6-MP usage, not with I.V.; may potentiate effect of bone marrow suppression (reduce 6-MP to 25% of dose)

Doxorubicin: Synergistic liver toxicity with 6-MP in >50% of patients, which resolved with discontinuation of the 6-MP

Hepatotoxic drugs: Any agent which could potentially alter the metabolic function of the liver could produce higher drug levels and greater toxicities from either 6-MP or 6-TG

Stability Store at room temperature

Mechanism of Action Purine antagonist which inhibits DNA and RNA synthesis; acts as false metabolite and is incorporated into DNA and RNA, eventually inhibiting their synthesis. 6-MP is substituted for hypoxanthine; must be metabolized to active nucleotides once inside the cell.

Pharmacodynamics/Kinetics

Absorption: Variable and incomplete (16% to 50%)

Distribution: V_d = total body water; CNS penetration is poor

Protein binding: 19%

Metabolism: Undergoes first-pass metabolism in the GI mucosa and liver; metabolized in the liver by xanthine oxidase and methylation to sulfate conjugates, 6-thiouric acid and other inactive compounds

Half-life (age-dependent):

Children: 21 minutes

Adults: 47 minutes

Time to peak serum concentration: Within 2 hours

Elimination: Prompt excretion in the urine; with high doses of I.V. 6-MP, the renal excretion of unchanged drug is 20% to 40% and can produce hematuria and crystalluria; at conventional doses renal elimination is minor

Usual Dosage Oral (refer to individual protocols):

Children:

Induction: 2.5-5 mg/kg/day given once daily or 60-75 mg/m²/day given once daily

Maintenance: 1.5-2.5 mg/kg/day given once daily

Adults:

Induction: 2.5-5 mg/kg/day (100-200 mg) or 80-100 mg/m²/day given once daily

Maintenance: 1.5-2.5 mg/kg/day

Elderly: Due to renal decline with age, start with lower recommended doses for adults

Dosing adjustment in renal or hepatic impairment: Dose should be reduced to avoid accumulation, but specific guidelines are not available

Monitoring Parameters CBC with differential and platelet count, liver function tests, uric acid, urinalysis

Patient Information Should not be taken with meals. Nausea and vomiting are rare with usual doses. Any signs of infection, easy bruising or bleeding, shortness of breath, or painful or burning urination should be brought to physician's attention. Nausea, vomiting, or hair loss sometimes occur. The drug may cause permanent sterility and may cause birth defects. The drug may be excreted in breast milk, therefore, an alternative form of feeding your baby should be used. Contraceptive measures are recommended during therapy.

Nursing Implications Adjust dosage in patients with renal insufficiency

Dosage Forms Tablet, scored: 50 mg

6-Mercaptopurine *see* Mercaptopurine *on previous page*

Mercapturic Acid *see* Acetylcysteine *on page 25*

Meruvax® II *see* Rubella Virus Vaccine, Live *on page 989*

Mesalamine (me sal' a meen)

Brand Names Asacol®; Pentasa®; Rowasa®

Synonyms 5-Aminosalicylic Acid; 5-ASA; Fisalamine; Mesalazine

Use Treatment of ulcerative colitis, proctosigmoiditis, and proctitis

Pregnancy Risk Factor B

Contraindications Known hypersensitivity to mesalamine, sulfasalazine, sulfites, or salicylates

Warnings/Precautions Pericarditis should be considered in patients with chest pain; pancreatitis should be considered in any patient with new abdominal complaints. Elderly may have difficulty administering and retaining rectal suppositories. Given renal function decline with aging, monitor serum creatinine often during therapy.

(Continued)

Mesalamine *(Continued)*

Adverse Reactions

>10%:

Central nervous system: Headache, malaise

Gastrointestinal: Abdominal pain, cramps, flatulence, gas

1% to 10%: Dermatologic: Alopecia, rash

<1%: Anal irritation, acute intolerance syndrome (bloody diarrhea, severe abdominal cramps, severe headache)

Overdosage/Toxicology Symptoms of overdose include decreased motor activity, diarrhea, vomiting, renal function impairment. Treatment is supportive; emesis, gastric lavage, and follow with activated charcoal slurry.

Drug Interactions Decreased effect: Decreased digoxin bioavailability

Stability Unstable in presence of water or light; once foil has been removed, unopened bottles have an expiration of 1 year following the date of manufacture

Mechanism of Action Mesalamine (5-aminosalicylic acid) is the active component of sulfasalazine; the specific mechanism of action of mesalamine is unknown; however, it is thought that it modulates local chemical mediators of the inflammatory response, especially leukotrienes; action appears topical rather than systemic

Pharmacodynamics/Kinetics

Absorption: Rectal: ~15%; variable and dependent upon retention time, underlying GI disease, and colonic pH

Metabolism: In the liver by acetylation to acetyl-5-aminosalicylic acid (active) and to glucuronide conjugates; intestinal metabolism may also occur

Half-life:

5-ASA: 0.5-1.5 hours

Acetyl 5-ASA: 5-10 hours

Time to peak serum concentration: Within 4-7 hours

Elimination: Most metabolites are excreted in urine with <2% appearing in feces

Usual Dosage Adults (usual course of therapy is 3-6 weeks):

Oral:

Capsule: 1 g 4 times/day

Tablet: 800 mg 3 times/day

Retention enema: 60 mL (4 g) at bedtime, retained overnight, approximately 8 hours

Rectal suppository: Insert 1 suppository in rectum twice daily

Some patients may require rectal and oral therapy concurrently

Patient Information Retain enemas for 8 hours or as long as practical; shake bottle well; do not chew or break oral tablets; for suppositories, remove foil wrapper, avoid excessive handling

Nursing Implications Provide patient with copy of mesalamine administration instructions

Dosage Forms

Capsule, controlled release: 250 mg

Suppository, rectal: 500 mg

Suspension, rectal: 4 g/60 mL

Tablet, enteric coated, delayed release: 400 mg

Mesalazine *see* Mesalamine *on previous page*

Mesantoin® *see* Mephenytoin *on page 686*

Mesna *(mes' na)*

Related Information

Cancer Chemotherapy Regimens *on page 1218-1241*

Brand Names Mesnex™

Synonyms Sodium 2-Mercaptoethane Sulfonate

Use Detoxifying agent used as a protectant against hemorrhagic cystitis induced by ifosfamide and cyclophosphamide

Pregnancy Risk Factor B

Contraindications Hypersensitivity to mesna or other thiol compounds

Warnings/Precautions Examine morning urine specimen for hematuria prior to ifosfamide or cyclophosphamide treatment; if hematuria develops, reduce the ifosfamide/cyclophosphamide dose or discontinue the drug; will not prevent or alleviate other toxicities associated with ifosfamide or cyclophosphamide and will not prevent hemorrhagic cystitis in all patients

Adverse Reactions

1% to 10%:

Cardiovascular: Hypotension

Central nervous system: Malaise, headache

Gastrointestinal: Diarrhea, nausea, vomiting, bad taste in mouth, soft stools

Neuromuscular & skeletal: Limb pain

<1%: Dermatologic: Skin rash, itching

Drug Interactions Decreased effect: Warfarin: Questionable alterations in coagulation control

Stability Diluted solutions are chemically and physically stable for 24 hours at room temperature; polypropylene syringes are stable for 9 days at refrigeration or room temperature; injection diluted for oral administration is stable 24 hours at refrigeration

Incompatible with cisplatin

Compatible with cyclophosphamide, etoposide, ifosfamide, lorazepam, potassium chloride, bleomycin, dexamethasone

Mechanism of Action Binds with and detoxifies acrolein and other urotoxic metabolites of ifosfamide and cyclophosphamide; detoxifying agent used to prevent hemorrhagic cystitis induced by ifosfamide and cyclophosphamide. In the kidney, mesna is reduced to a free thiol compound which reacts chemically with the acrolein and 4-hydroxy-ifosfamide resulting in detoxification.

Pharmacodynamics/Kinetics

Absorption: From the GI tract

Peak plasma levels: 2-3 hours after administration

Distribution: No tissue penetration; following glomerular filtration, mesna disulfide is reduced in renal tubules back to mesna

Metabolism: Rapidly oxidized intravascularly to mesna disulfide

Half-life:

Parent drug: 24 minutes

Mesna disulfide: 72 minutes

Elimination: Unchanged drug and metabolite are excreted primarily in the urine; time it takes for maximum urinary mesna excretion: 1 hour after I.V. and 2-3 hours after an oral mesna dose

Usual Dosage Children and Adults (refer to individual protocols): Oral dose is ~2 times the I.V. dose:

Ifosfamide: I.V.: 20% W/W of ifosfamide dose at time of administration and 4 and 8 hours after each dose of ifosfamide; for high dose ifosfamide: 20% W/W at time of administration and 3, 6, 9, 12 hours after dose **(total daily dose is 60% to 100% of ifosfamide)**

Cyclophosphamide: I.V.: 20% W/W of cyclophosphamide dose prior to administration and 3, 6, 9, 12 hours after cyclophosphamide dose **(total daily dose is 120% to 200% of cyclophosphamide dose)**

Oral dose: 40% W/W of the ifosfamide or cyclophosphamide agent dose in 3 doses at 4-hour intervals or 20 mg/kg/dose every 3-4 hours for 3 doses

Administration

For oral administration, injection may be diluted in 1:1, 1:2, 1:10, 1:100 concentrations in carbonated beverages (cola, ginger ale, Pepsi®, Sprite®, Dr Pepper®, etc), juices (apple or orange), or whole milk (chocolate or white), and is stable 24 hours at refrigeration; used in conjunction with ifosfamide; examine morning urine specimen for hematuria prior to ifosfamide or cyclophosphamide treatment

Administer by I.V. infusion over 15-30 minutes or per protocol; mesna can be diluted in D_5W or NS to a final concentration of 1-20 mg/mL

Monitoring Parameters Urinalysis

Test Interactions False-positive urinary ketones with Multistix® or Labstix®

Dosage Forms Injection: 100 mg/mL (2 mL, 4 mL, 10 mL)

Mesnex™ *see* Mesna *on previous page*

Mesoridazine Besylate (mez oh rid' a zeen)

Related Information

Antipsychotic Agents Comparison *on page 1255*

Brand Names Serentil®

Use Symptomatic management of psychotic disorders, including schizophrenia, behavioral problems, alcoholism as well as reducing anxiety and tension occurring in neurosis

Pregnancy Risk Factor C

Contraindications Hypersensitivity to mesoridazine or any component, cross-sensitivity with other phenothiazines may exist

Warnings/Precautions Safety in children <6 months of age has not been established; use with caution in patients with cardiovascular disease or seizures; benefits of therapy must be weighed against risks of therapy; doses >1 g/day frequently cause pigmentary retinopathy; some products contain sulfites and/or tartrazine; use with caution in patients with narrow-angle glaucoma, bone marrow depression, severe liver disease

Adverse Reactions

>10%:

Cardiovascular: Hypotension, orthostatic hypotension

(Continued)

Mesoridazine Besylate *(Continued)*

Central nervous system: Pseudoparkinsonism, akathisia, dystonias, tardive dyskinesia (persistent), dizziness
Gastrointestinal: Constipation
Ocular: Pigmentary retinopathy
Respiratory: Nasal congestion
Miscellaneous: Decreased sweating

1% to 10%:
Dermatologic: Increased sensitivity to sun, skin rash
Endocrine & metabolic: Changes in menstrual cycle, changes in libido, pain in breasts
Gastrointestinal: Weight gain, nausea, vomiting, stomach pain
Genitourinary: Difficulty in urination, ejaculatory disturbances
Neuromuscular & skeletal: Trembling of fingers

<1%:
Central nervous system: Neuroleptic malignant syndrome (NMS)
Dermatologic: Discoloration of skin (blue-gray)
Endocrine & metabolic: Galactorrhea
Genitourinary: Priapism
Hematologic: Agranulocytosis, leukopenia
Hepatic: Cholestatic jaundice, hepatotoxicity
Ocular: Cornea and lens changes, pigmentary retinopathy
Miscellaneous: Impairment of temperature regulation, lowering of seizures threshold

Overdosage/Toxicology Symptoms of overdose include deep sleep, coma, extrapyramidal symptoms, abnormal involuntary muscle movements, hypotension

Following initiation of essential overdose management, toxic symptom treatment and supportive treatment should be initiated; hypotension usually responds to I.V. fluids or Trendelenburg positioning. If unresponsive to these measures, the use of a parenteral inotrope may be required. Seizures commonly respond to diazepam (I.V. 5-10 mg bolus in adults every 15 minutes if needed up to a total of 30 mg; I.V. 0.25-0.4 mg/kg/dose up to a total of 10 mg in children) or to phenytoin or phenobarbital. Critical cardiac arrhythmias often respond to I.V. phenytoin (15 mg/kg up to 1 g), while other antiarrhythmics can be used. Extrapyramidal symptoms (eg, dystonic reactions) can be managed with benztropine mesylate I.V. 1-2 mg (adults).

Drug Interactions
Decreased effect with anticonvulsants, anticholinergics
Increased toxicity with CNS depressants, metrizamide (↑ seizures), propranolol

Mechanism of Action Blockade of postsynaptic CNS dopamine receptors

Pharmacodynamics/Kinetics
Duration of action: 4-6 hours
Absorption: Very erratic with oral tablet; oral liquids much more dependable
Protein binding: 91% to 99%
Half-life: 24-48 hours
Time to peak serum concentration: 2-4 hours
Time to steady-state serum: 4-7 days
Elimination: In urine

Usual Dosage Concentrate may be diluted just prior to administration with distilled water, acidified tap water, orange or grape juice; do not prepare and store bulk dilutions

Adults:
Oral: 25-50 mg 3 times/day; maximum: 100-400 mg/day
I.M.: 25 mg initially, repeat in 30-60 minutes as needed; optimal dosage range: 25-200 mg/day

Not dialyzable (0% to 5%)

Administration Watch for hypotension when administering I.M. or I.V., dilute oral concentration before administering; do not mix oral solutions of mesoridazine and lithium, these oral liquids are incompatible when mixed

Test Interactions ↑ cholesterol (S), ↑ glucose; ↓ uric acid (S)

Patient Information May cause drowsiness or restlessness, avoid alcohol and other CNS depressants; do not alter dosage or discontinue without consulting physician; avoid excessive sunlight, yearly ophthalmic examinations are necessary

Dosage Forms
Injection: 25 mg/mL (1 mL)
Liquid, oral: 25 mg/mL (118 mL)
Tablet: 10 mg, 25 mg, 50 mg, 100 mg

Mestinon® *see* Pyridostigmine Bromide *on page 960*

Mestranol and Norethindrone (mes' tra nole & nor eth in' drone)

Brand Names Genora® 1/50; Nelova™ 1/50M; Norethin™ 1/50M; Norinyl® 1+50; Ortho-Novum™ 1/50

Synonyms Norethindrone and Mestranol

Use Prevention of pregnancy; treatment of hypermenorrhea, endometriosis, female hypogonadism [monophasic oral contraceptive]

Pregnancy Risk Factor X

Contraindications Known or suspected breast cancer, undiagnosed abnormal vaginal bleeding, carcinoma of the breast, estrogen-dependent tumor

Warnings/Precautions Use with caution in patients with a history of thromboembolism, stroke, myocardial infarction, liver tumor, hypertension, cardiac, renal or hepatic insufficiency; use of any progestin during the first 4 months of pregnancy is not recommended; risk of cardiovascular side effects increases in those women who smoke cigarettes and in women >35 years of age

Adverse Reactions

>10%:
  Cardiovascular: Peripheral edema
  Central nervous system: Headache
  Endocrine: Enlargement of breasts, breast tenderness, bloating, increased libido
  Gastrointestinal: Nausea, anorexia

1% to 10%: Gastrointestinal: Vomiting, diarrhea

<1%:
  Cardiovascular: Hypertension, thromboembolism, edema, stroke, myocardial infarction
  Central nervous system: Depression, dizziness, anxiety
  Dermatologic: Chloasma, melasma, rash
  Endocrine: Decreased glucose tolerance, breast tumors, amenorrhea, alterations in frequency and flow of menses, increased triglycerides and LDL
  Gastrointestinal: GI distress
  Hepatic: Cholestatic jaundice,
  Miscellaneous: Intolerance to contact lenses, increased susceptibility to *Candida* infection

See tables.

Achieving Proper Hormonal Balance in an Oral Contraceptive

Estrogen		Progestin	
Excess	**Deficiency**	**Excess**	**Deficiency**
Nausea, bloating	Early or midcycle	Increased appetite	Late breakthrough
Cervical mucorrhea,	breakthrough	Weight gain	bleeding
polyposis	bleeding	Tiredness, fatigue	Amenorrhea
Melasma	Increased spotting	Hypomenorrhea	Hypermenorrhea
Migraine headache	Hypomenorrhea	Acne, oily scalp*	
Breast fullness or		Hair loss, hirsutism*	
tenderness		Depression	
Edema		Monilial vaginitis	
Hypertension		Breast regression	

*Result of androgenic activity of progestins.

Pharmacological Effects of Progestins Used in Oral Contraceptives

	Progestin	Estrogen	Antiestrogen	Androgen
Norgestrel/levonorgestrel	+++	0	++	+++
Ethynodiol diacetate	++	+*	+*	+
Norethindrone acetate	+	+	+++	+
Norethindrone	+	+*	+*	+
Norethynodrel	+	+++	0	0

*Has estrogenic effect at low doses; may have antiestrogenic effect at higher doses.

+++ = pronounced effect
++ = moderate effect
+ = slight effect
0 = moderate effect

(Continued)

Mestranol and Norethindrone *(Continued)*

Overdosage/Toxicology Toxicity is unlikely following single exposures of excessive doses; any treatment following emesis and charcoal administration should be supportive and symptomatic

Drug Interactions

Decreased effect of oral contraceptives with barbiturates, hydantoins - phenytoin, rifampin, antibiotics - penicillins, tetracyclines, griseofulvin

Increased toxicity of acetaminophen, anticoagulants, benzodiazepines, caffeine, corticosteroids, metoprolol, theophylline, tricyclic antidepressants

Mechanism of Action Inhibits ovulation via a negative feedback mechanism on the hypothalamus, which alters the normal pattern of gonadotropin secretion of a follicle-stimulating hormone (FSH) and luteinizing hormone by the anterior pituitary. Follicular phase FSH and midcycle surge of gonadotropins are inhibited. Produces alterations in the genital tract, including changes in the cervical mucus, rendering it unfavorable for sperm penetration even if ovulation occurs. Changes in the endometrium may also occur, producing an unfavorable environment for nidation. May alter the tubal transport of the ova through the fallopian tubes. Progestational agents may also alter sperm fertility.

Usual Dosage Adults: Female: Oral:

Contraception: 1 tablet daily, beginning on day 5 of menstrual cycle (first day of menstrual flow is day 1). With 20-tablet and 21-tablet packages, new dosing cycle begins 7 days after last tablet taken. With 28-tablet packages, dosage is 1 tablet daily without interruption; extra tablets are placebos or contain iron. If next menstrual period does not begin on schedule, rule out pregnancy before starting new dosing cycle. If menstrual period begins, start new dosing cycle 7 days after last tablet was taken. If all doses have been taken on schedule and one menstrual period is missed, continue dosing cycle. If two consecutive menstrual periods are missed, pregnancy test is required before new dosing cycle is started.

One dose missed: Take as soon as remembered or take 2 tablets next day

Two doses missed: Take 2 tablets as soon as remembered or 2 tablets next 2 days

Three doses missed: Begin new compact of tablets starting on day 1 of next cycle

Patient Information Take exactly as directed; use additional method of birth control during first week of administration of first cycle; photosensitivity may occur

Patients should inform their physicians if signs or symptoms of any of the following occur: Thromboembolic or thrombotic disorders including sudden severe headache or vomiting, disturbance of vision or speech, loss of vision, numbness or weakness in an extremity, sharp or crushing chest pain, calf pain, shortness of breath, severe abdominal pain or mass, mental depression, or unusual bleeding.

Patients should be advised that if they miss one daily dose, they should take the tablet as soon as remembered. If 2 daily doses are missed, 2 tablets should be taken daily for 2 days and the regular schedule resumed. If 3 or more daily doses are missed, therapy should be discontinued. Therapy with a new cycle can be resumed in 7 or 8 days. When any doses are missed, alternative contraceptive methods should be used for the next 2 days or until 2 days into the new cycle. Patients should discontinue taking the medication if they suspect they are pregnant or become pregnant.

Nursing Implications Give at bedtime to minimize occurrence of adverse effects

Additional Information 80 mcg of mestranol is approximately equivalent to 50 mcg of ethinyl estradiol

Dosage Forms Tablet: Mestranol 0.05 mg and norethindrone 1 mg (21s and 28s)

Mestranol and Norethynodrel *(nor e thye′ noe drel)*

Brand Names Enovid®

Synonyms Norethynodrel and Mestranol

Use Treatment of hypermenorrhea, endometriosis, female hypogonadism

Pregnancy Risk Factor X

Contraindications Known or suspected breast cancer, undiagnosed abnormal vaginal bleeding, carcinoma of the breast, estrogen-dependent tumors

Warnings/Precautions In patients with a history of thromboembolism, stroke, myocardial infarction, liver tumor, hypertension, cardiac, renal or hepatic insufficiency; use of any progestin during the first 4 months of pregnancy is not recommended; risk of cardiovascular side effects increases in those women who smoke cigarettes and in women >35 years of age

Adverse Reactions
>10%:
- Cardiovascular: Peripheral edema
- Endocrine & metabolic: Enlargement of breasts, breast tenderness, bloating
- Gastrointestinal: Nausea, anorexia

1% to 10%:
- Central nervous system: Headache
- Endocrine & metabolic: Increased libido
- Gastrointestinal: Vomiting, diarrhea

<1%:
- Cardiovascular: Hypertension, thromboembolism, stroke, myocardial infarction, edema
- Central nervous system: Depression, dizziness, anxiety
- Dermatologic: Chloasma, melasma, rash
- Endocrine & metabolic: Decreased glucose tolerance, breast tumors, amenorrhea, alterations in frequency and flow of menses, increased triglycerides and LDL
- Gastrointestinal: GI distress
- Hepatic: Cholestatic jaundice
- Miscellaneous: Intolerance to contact lenses, increased susceptibility to *Candida* infection

Overdosage/Toxicology Toxicity is unlikely following single exposures of excessive doses; any treatment following emesis and charcoal administration should be supportive and symptomatic

Drug Interactions
Decreased effect with barbiturates, hydantoins - phenytoin, rifampin, antibiotics - penicillins, tetracyclines, griseofulvin

Increased toxicity of acetaminophen, anticoagulants, benzodiazepines, caffeine, corticosteroids, metoprolol, theophylline, tricyclic antidepressants

Mechanism of Action Inhibits ovulation via a negative feedback mechanism on the hypothalamus, which alters the normal pattern of gonadotropin secretion of a follicle-stimulating hormone (FSH) and luteinizing hormone by the anterior pituitary. The follicular phase FSH and midcycle surge of gonadotropins are inhibited. Oral contraceptives produce alterations in the genital tract, including changes in the cervical mucus, rendering it unfavorable for sperm penetration even if ovulation occurs. Changes in the endometrium may also occur, producing an unfavorable environment for nidation. May alter the tubal transport of the ova through the fallopian tubes. Progestational agents may also alter sperm fertility.

Pharmacodynamics/Kinetics
Mestranol:
- Demethylated to ethinyl estradiol
- Protein binding: 93% bound to plasma albumin
- Half-life: 6-20 hours
- Elimination: In bile, urine as conjugates and undergoes enterohepatic recirculation

Norethynodrel:
- Converted to norethindrone
- Metabolism: Chiefly by conjugation
- Half-life, terminal: 5-14 hours

Usual Dosage Adults: Female: Oral:
Endometriosis: 5-10 mg/day for 2 weeks beginning on day 5 of menstrual cycle; increase by 5-10 mg increments at 2-week intervals up to 20 mg/day for 6-9 months

Hypermenorrhea: 20-30 mg/day until bleeding is controlled, then reduce to 10 mg/day and continue through day 24 of cycle; administer 5-10 mg/day from day 5 through day 24 of next 2-3 cycles

Patient Information Patients should inform their physicians if signs or symptoms of any of the following occur: Thromboembolic or thrombotic disorders including sudden severe headache or vomiting, disturbance of vision or speech, loss of vision, numbness or weakness in an extremity, sharp or crushing chest pain, calf pain, shortness of breath, severe abdominal pain or mass, mental depression, or unusual bleeding.

Dosage Forms Tablet:
Enovid® 5 mg: Mestranol 0.075 mg and norethynodrel 5 mg
Enovid® 10 mg: Mestranol 0.150 mg and norethynodrel 9.85 mg

Metacortandralone *see* Prednisolone *on page 919*

Metahydrin® *see* Trichlormethiazide *on page 1118*

Metamucil® [OTC] *see* Psyllium *on page 956*

Metamucil® Instant Mix [OTC] *see* Psyllium *on page 956*

Metandren® *see* Methyltestosterone *on page 726*

Metaprel® *see* Metaproterenol Sulfate *on this page*

Metaproterenol Sulfate (met a proe ter' e nol)

Brand Names Alupent®; Arm-a-Med® Metaproterenol; Dey-Dose® Metaproterenol; Metaprel®; Prometa®

Synonyms Orciprenaline Sulfate

Use Bronchodilator in reversible airway obstruction due to asthma or COPD; because of its delayed onset of action (1 hour) and prolonged effect (4 or more hours), this may not be the drug of choice for assessing response to a bronchodilator

Pregnancy Risk Factor C

Contraindications Hypersensitivity to metaproterenol or any components, pre-existing cardiac arrhythmias associated with tachycardia

Warnings/Precautions Use with caution in patients with hypertension, CHF, hyperthyroidism, CAD, diabetes, or sensitivity to sympathomimetics; excessive prolonged use may result in decreased efficacy or increased toxicity and death; use caution in patients with pre-existing cardiac arrhythmias associated with tachycardia. Metaproterenol has more beta$_1$ activity than other sympathomimetics such as albuterol and, therefore, may no longer be the beta agonist of first choice. All patients should utilize a spacer device when using a metered dose inhaler. Oral use should be avoided due to the increased incidence of adverse effects.

Adverse Reactions
>10%:
   Central nervous system: Nervousness
   Neuromuscular & skeletal: Tremor
1% to 10%:
   Cardiovascular: Tachycardia, palpitations, hypertension
   Central nervous system: Weakness, headache, dizziness
   Gastrointestinal: Nausea, vomiting, bad taste
   Neuromuscular & skeletal: Trembling, muscle cramps
   Respiratory: Coughing
   Miscellaneous: Increased sweating
<1%: Paradoxical bronchospasm

Overdosage/Toxicology Symptoms of overdose includes, angina, arrhythmias, tremor, dry mouth, insomnia; beta-adrenergic stimulation can increase and cause increased heart rate, decreased blood pressure, decreased CNS excitation. In cases of overdose, supportive therapy should be instituted, and prudent use of a cardioselective beta-adrenergic blocker (eg, atenolol or metoprolol) should be considered, keeping in mind the potential for induction of bronchoconstriction in an asthmatic individual. Dialysis has not been shown to be of value in the treatment of an overdose with this agent. Diazepam 0.07 mg/kg can be used for excitation seizures

Drug Interactions
Decreased effect: Beta-blockers
Increased toxicity: Sympathomimetics, TCAs, MAO inhibitors

Stability Store in tight, light-resistant container; do not use if brown solution or contains a precipitate

Mechanism of Action Relaxes bronchial smooth muscle by action on beta$_2$-receptors with very little effect on heart rate

Pharmacodynamics/Kinetics
Oral:
   Onset of bronchodilation: Within 15 minutes
   Peak effect: Within 1 hour
   Duration of action: ~1-5 hours
Inhalation:
   Onset of effects: Within 60 seconds
   Duration of action: Similar (~1-5 hours) regardless of route administered

Usual Dosage
Oral:
   Children:
      <2 years: 0.4 mg/kg/dose given 3-4 times/day; in infants, the dose can be given every 8-12 hours
      2-6 years: 1-2.6 mg/kg/day divided every 6 hours
      6-9 years: 10 mg/dose 3-4 times/day
   Children >9 years Adults: 20 mg 3-4 times/day
   Elderly: Initial: 10 mg 3-4 times/day, increasing as necessary up to 20 mg 3-4 times/day
Inhalation: Children >12 years and Adults: 2-3 inhalations every 3-4 hours, up to 12 inhalations in 24 hours
Nebulizer:
   Infants and Children: 0.01-0.02 mL/kg of 5% solution; minimum dose: 0.1 mL; maximum dose: 0.3 mL diluted in 2-3 mL normal saline every 4-6 hours (may be given more frequently according to need)

Adolescents and Adults: 5-20 breaths of full strength 5% metaproterenol **or** 0.2 to 0.3 mL 5% metaproterenol in 2.5-3 mL normal saline until nebulized every 4-6 hours (can be given more frequently according to need)

Administration Administer around-the-clock to promote less variation in peak and trough serum levels

Monitoring Parameters Assess lung sounds, pulse, and blood pressure before administration and during peak of medication; observe patient for wheezing after administration, if this occurs, call physician; monitor heart rate, respiratory rate, blood pressure, and arterial or capillary blood gases if applicable

Test Interactions ↑ potassium (S)

Patient Information Do not exceed recommended dosage - excessive use may lead to adverse effects or loss of effectiveness. Shake canister well before use. Administer pressurized inhalation during the second half of inspiration, as the airways are open wider and the aerosol distribution is more extensive. If more than one inhalation per dose is necessary, wait at least 1 full minute between inhalations - second inhalation is best delivered after 10 minutes for Alupent®. May cause nervousness, restlessness, insomnia - if these effects continue after dosage reduction, notify physician. Also notify physician if palpitations, tachycardia, chest pain, muscle tremors, dizziness, headache, flushing, or if breathing difficulty persists.

Nursing Implications Do not use solutions for nebulization if they are brown or contain a precipitate; before using, the inhaler must be shaken well

Dosage Forms
Aerosol, oral: 0.65 mg/dose (5 mL, 10 mL)
Solution for inhalation, preservative free: 0.4% [4 mg/mL] (2.5 mL); 0.6% [6 mg/mL] (2.5 mL); 5% [50 mg/mL] (10 mL, 30 mL)
Syrup: 10 mg/5 mL (480 mL)
Tablet: 10 mg, 20 mg

Metaraminol Bitartrate (met a ram' i nole)

Related Information
Adrenergic Agonists, Cardiovascular Comparison *on page 1242*

Brand Names Aramine®

Use Acute hypotensive crisis in the treatment of shock

Pregnancy Risk Factor D

Contraindications Hypersensitivity to metaraminol or any component, cyclopropane or halothane anesthesia, or MAO inhibitors

Warnings/Precautions Can cause cardiac arrhythmias; use with caution in patients with a previous myocardial infarction, hypertension, hyperthyroidism; prolonged use may produce cumulative effects

Adverse Reactions
1% to 10%: Cardiovascular: Tachycardia
<1%:
Cardiovascular: Hypertension, cardiac arrhythmias, flushing
Dermatologic: Blanching of skin, sloughing of tissue, abscess formation
Gastrointestinal: Nausea
Miscellaneous: Sweating

Overdosage/Toxicology Hypertension, cerebral hemorrhage, cardiac arrest, seizures

Drug Interactions
Decreased effect with TCAs
Increased toxicity with cyclopropane, halothane, MAO inhibitors (hypertensive crisis), digoxin, oxytocin, rauwolfia alkaloids, reserpine

Stability Infusion solutions are stable for 24 hours; I.V. metaraminol is **incompatible** when mixed with amphotericin B, dexamethasone, erythromycin, hydrocortisone, methicillin, penicillin G, prednisolone, thiopental

Mechanism of Action Stimulates alpha-adrenergic receptors to cause vasoconstriction, reflex bradycardia, inhibits GI smooth muscle and vascular smooth muscle supplying skeletal muscle, increases heart rate and force of heart muscle contraction

Pharmacodynamics/Kinetics
Onset of pressor effect:
I.M.: Within 10 minutes
I.V.: Within 1-2 minutes
S.C.: Within 5-20 minutes
Elimination: Has not yet been fully elucidated

Usual Dosage
Children:
I.M.: 0.01 mg/kg as a single dose
I.V.: 0.01 mg/kg as a single dose or intravenous infusion of 5 mcg/kg/minute
(Continued)

Metaraminol Bitartrate *(Continued)*

Adults:
Prevention of hypotension: I.M., S.C.: 2-10 mg
Adjunctive treatment of hypotension: I.V.: 15-100 mg in 250-500 mL NS or 5% dextrose in water
Severe shock: I.V.: 0.5-5 mg direct I.V. injection followed by intravenous infusion of 15-100 mg in 250-500 mL NS or D_5W; may also be administered endotracheally

Administration May be given I.M., I.V., S.C.; however, I.V. is the preferred route because extravasation or local injection can cause necrosis; to prevent necrosis infiltrate area with 10-15 mL of saline containing 5-10 mg of phentolamine

Monitoring Parameters Blood pressure, EKG, PCWP, CVP, pulse, and urine output

Dosage Forms Injection: 10 mg/mL (10 mL)

Metastron® *see* Strontium-89 Chloride *on page 1033*

Metaxalone (me tax' a lone)

Brand Names Skelaxin®
Use Relief of discomfort associated with acute, painful musculoskeletal conditions
Pregnancy Risk Factor C
Contraindications Impaired hepatic or renal function, known hypersensitivity to metaxalone, history of drug-induced hemolytic anemias or other anemias
Warnings/Precautions Use with caution in patients with impaired hepatic function

Adverse Reactions
>10%:
Central nervous system: Paradoxical stimulation, headache, drowsiness, dizziness
Gastrointestinal: Nausea, vomiting, stomach cramps
<1%:
Dermatologic: Allergic dermatitis
Hematologic: Leukopenia, hemolytic anemia
Hepatic: Hepatotoxicity
Miscellaneous: Anaphylaxis

Overdosage/Toxicology No major toxicities have been reported
Drug Interactions Increased effect of alcohol, CNS depressants
Mechanism of Action Does not have a direct effect on skeletal muscle; most of its therapeutic effect comes from actions on the central nervous system
Pharmacodynamics/Kinetics
Onset of action: ~1 hour
Duration: ~4-6 hours
Half-life: 2-3 hours
Elimination: In urine as metabolites

Usual Dosage Children >12 years and Adults: Oral: 800 mg 3-4 times/day
Test Interactions False-positive Benedict's test
Patient Information Avoid alcohol and other CNS depressants; may cause drowsiness, impairment of judgment, or coordination; notify physician of dark urine, pale stools, yellowing of eyes, severe nausea, vomiting, or abdominal pain
Nursing Implications Raise bed rails, institute safety measures, assist with ambulation
Dosage Forms Tablet: 400 mg

Metformin Hydrochloride (met for' min hye droe klor' ide)

Brand Names Glucophage®
Use Management of noninsulin-dependent diabetes mellitus (type II) as monotherapy when hyperglycemia cannot be managed on diet alone. May be used concomitantly with a sulfonylurea when diet and metformin or sulfonylurea alone do not result in adequate glycemic control.
Pregnancy Risk Factor B
Contraindications Hypersensitivity to metformin or any component; renal disease or renal dysfunction (serum creatinine ≥1.5 mg/dL in males or ≥1.4 mg/dL in females or abnormal clearance) which may also result from conditions such as cardiovascular collapse, acute myocardial infarction, and septicemia; acute or chronic metabolic acidosis with or without coma (including diabetic ketoacidosis); should be temporarily withheld in patients undergoing radiologic studies involving the parenteral administration of iodinated contrast materials (potential for acute alteration in renal function).

Warnings/Precautions Administration of oral antidiabetic drugs has been reported to be associated with increased cardiovascular mortality as compared to treatment with diet alone or diet plus insulin. Metformin is substantially excreted by the kidney - the risk of accumulation and lactic acidosis increases with the degree of impairment of renal function. Patients with renal function below the limit of normal for their age should not receive metformin. In elderly patients, renal function should be monitored regularly. Use of concomitant medications that may affect renal function (ie, affect tubular secretion) may affect metformin disposition. Therapy should be suspended for any surgical procedures. Avoid use in patients with impaired liver function.

Adverse Reactions

>10%: Gastrointestinal: Anorexia, nausea, vomiting, diarrhea, epigastric fullness, constipation, heartburn

1% to 10%:

Dermatologic: Rash, hives, photosensitivity

Miscellaneous: Decreased vitamin B_{12} levels

<1%: Hematologic: Blood dyscrasias, aplastic anemia, hemolytic anemia, bone marrow depression, thrombocytopenia, agranulocytosis

Overdosage/Toxicology

Hypoglycemia has not been observed with ingestions of up to 85 g of metformin, although lactic acidosis has occurred in such circumstances

Metformin is dialyzable with a clearance of up to 170 mL/minute; hemodialysis may be useful for removal of accumulated drug from patients in whom metformin overdosage is suspected

Drug Interactions

Decreased effects: Drugs which tend to produce hyperglycemia (eg, diuretics, corticosteroids, phenothiazines, thyroid products, estrogens, oral contraceptives, phenytoin, nicotinic acid, sympathomimetics, calcium channel blocking drugs, isoniazid) may lead to a loss of glycemic control

Increased effects: Furosemide increased the metformin plasma and blood C_{max} without altering metformin renal clearance in a single dose study

Increased toxicity:

Cationic drugs (eg, amiloride, digoxin, morphine, procainamide, quinidine, quinine, ranitidine, triamterene, trimethoprim, and vancomycin) which are eliminated by renal tubular secretion could have the potential for interaction with metformin by competing for common renal tubular transport systems

Cimetidine increases (by 60%) peak metformin plasma and whole blood concentrations

Mechanism of Action Decreases hepatic glucose production, decreasing intestinal absorption of glucose and improves insulin sensitivity (increases peripheral glucose uptake and utilization)

Pharmacodynamics/Kinetics

Distribution: V_d: 654±358 L

Protein binding: 92% to 99%

Protein binding, plasma: negligible

Bioavailability, absolute: 50% to 60% under fasting conditions; food decreases the extent and slightly delays the absorption; the clinical relevance is unknown

Half-life, plasma elimination: 6.2 hours

Elimination: Renal; tubular secretion is major route

Usual Dosage Oral (allow 1-2 weeks between dose titrations):

Adults:

500 mg tablets: Initial: 500 mg twice daily (given with the morning and evening meals). Dosage increases should be made in increments of one tablet every week, given in divided doses, up to a maximum of 2,500 mg/day. Doses of up to 2000 mg/day may be given twice daily. If a dose of 2,500 mg daily is required, it may be better tolerated three times daily (with meals).

850 mg tablets: Initial: 850 mg once daily (given with the morning meal). Dosage increases should be made in increments of one tablet every OTHER week, given in divided doses, up to a maximum of 2550 mg daily. The usual maintenance dose is 850 mg twice daily (with the morning and evening meals). Some patients may be given 850 mg three times daily (with meals).

Elderly patients: The initial and maintenance dosing should be conservative, due to the potential for decreased renal function. Generally, elderly patients should not be titrated to the maximum dose of metformin.

Transfer from other antidiabetic agents: No transition period is generally necessary except when transferring from chlorpropamide. When transferring from chlorpropamide, care should be exercised during the first 2 weeks because of the prolonged retention of chlorpropamide in the body, leading to overlapping drug effects and possible hypoglycemia.

Concomitant metformin and oral sulfonylurea therapy: If patients have not responded to 4 weeks of the maximum dose of metformin monotherapy, consideration to a gradually addition of an oral sulfonylurea while continuing

(Continued)

Metformin Hydrochloride *(Continued)*

metformin at the maximum dose, even if prior primary or secondary failure to a sulfonylurea has occurred.

Dosing adjustment/comments in renal impairment: The plasma and blood half-life of metformin is prolonged and the renal clearance is decreased in proportion to the decrease in creatinine clearance

Dosing adjustment in hepatic impairment: No studies have been conducted

Monitoring Parameters Urine for glucose and ketones, fasting blood glucose, hemoglobin A_{1c}, and fructosamine. Initial and periodic monitoring of hematologic parameters (eg, hemoglobin/hematocrit and red blood cell indices) and renal function should be performed, at least annually. While megaloblastic anemia has been rarely seen with metformin, if suspected, vitamin B_{12} deficiency should be excluded.

Reference Range Glucose:
Adults: 60-110 mg/dL
Elderly: 100-180 mg/dL

Patient Information Patients must be counseled by someone experienced in diabetes education, signs and symptoms of hyper- and hypoglycemia, exercise and diet, blood glucose monitoring, and other related topics; eat regularly, do not skip meals; carry quick source of sugar; medical alert bracelet. Patients should be counselled against excessive alcohol intake while receiving metformin. Metformin alone does not usually cause hypoglycemia, although it may occur in conjunction with oral sulfonylureas.

Nursing Implications Patients who are NPO may need to have their dose held to avoid hypoglycemia

Dosage Forms Tablet: 500 mg, 850 mg

Methacholine Chloride (meth a kol' leen)

Brand Names Provocholine®

Use Diagnosis of bronchial airway hyperactivity in subjects who do not have clinically apparent asthma

Pregnancy Risk Factor C

Contraindications Concomitant use of beta-blockers; hypersensitivity to the drug; because of the potential for severe bronchoconstriction, methacholine challenge should not be performed on any patient with clinically apparent asthma, wheezing, or very low baseline pulmonary function tests (forced expiratory volume in one second less than 70% of predicted value).

Warnings/Precautions Methacholine is a bronchoconstrictor for diagnostic purposes only. Perform inhalation challenge under the supervision of a physician trained in and thoroughly familiar with all aspects of the technique, all contraindications, warnings, and precautions of methacholine challenge and the management of respiratory distress. Have emergency equipment and medication immediately available to treat acute respiratory distress. Administer only by inhalation; severe bronchoconstriction and reduction in respiratory function can result. Patients with severe hyperreactivity of the airways can experience bronchoconstriction at a dosage as low as 0.025 mg/mL (0.125 cumulative units). If severe bronchoconstriction occurs, reverse immediately by administration of a rapid-acting inhaled bronchodilator (beta-agonist).

Adverse Reactions
<1%:
Cardiovascular: Hypotension, complete heart block
Central nervous system: Headache, lightheadedness, fainting
Respiratory: Throat irritation, itching, cough, dyspnea, tightness of the chest, wheezing
Miscellaneous: Substernal pain

Stability Store unreconstituted powder at 59°F to 86°F; store dilutions in refrigerator (36°F to 46°F) for up to 2 weeks

Mechanism of Action Methacholine chloride is a cholinergic (parasympathomimetic) synthetic analogue of acetylcholine. The drug stimulates muscarinic, postganglionic parasympathetic receptors, which results in smooth muscle contraction of the airways and increased tracheobronchial secretions.

Pharmacodynamics/Kinetics
Onset of action: Rapid
Peak effect: Within 1-4 minutes
Duration: 15-75 minutes or 5 minutes if the methacholine challenge is followed with a beta-agonist agent

Usual Dosage Before inhalation challenge, perform baseline pulmonary function tests; the patient must have an FEV_1 of at least 70% of the predicted value. The following is a suggested schedule for administration of methacholine challenge.

Calculate cumulative units by multiplying number of breaths by concentration given. Total cumulative units is the sum of cumulative units for each concentration given. See table.

Vial	Serial Concentration (mg/mL)	No. of Breaths	Cumulative Units per Concentration	Total Cumulative Units
E	0.025	5	0.125	0.125
D	0.25	5	1.25	1.375
C	2.5	5	12.5	13.88
B	10	5	50	63.88
A	25	5	125	188.88

Determine FEV_1 within 5 minutes of challenge, a postive challenge is a 20% reduction in FEV_1

Dosage Forms Powder for reconstitution, inhalation: 100 mg/5 mL

Methadone Hydrochloride (meth' a done)
Related Information
Narcotic Agonist Comparison Charts *on page 1274-1275*
Brand Names Dolophine®
Use Management of severe pain, used in narcotic detoxification maintenance programs
Restrictions C-II
Pregnancy Risk Factor B (D if used for prolonged periods or in high doses at term)
Contraindications Hypersensitivity to methadone or any component
Warnings/Precautions Tablets are to be used only for oral administration and **must not** be used for injection; use with caution in patients with respiratory diseases including asthma, emphysema, or COPD and in patients with severe liver disease; because methadone's effects on respiration last much longer than its analgesic effects, the dose must be titrated slowly; because of its long half-life and risk of accumulation, it is not considered a drug of first choice in the elderly, who may be particularly susceptible to its CNS depressant and constipating effects
Adverse Reactions
Central nervous system: CNS depression
Endocrine & metabolic: Antidiuretic hormone release
Ocular: Miosis
Respiratory: Respiratory depression

>10%:
  Cardiovascular: Palpitations, hypotension, bradycardia, peripheral vasodilation
  Central nervous system: Weakness, tiredness, drowsiness, dizziness
  Gastrointestinal: Nausea, vomiting, constipation
  Miscellaneous: Histamine release
1% to 10%:
  Central nervous system: Nervousness, headache, restlessness, anorexia, malaise, confusion, increased intracranial pressure
  Gastrointestinal: Stomach cramps, dry mouth
  Genitourinary: Decreased urination
  Local: Pain at injection site
  Respiratory: Troubled breathing, shortness of breath
  Miscellaneous: Biliary or urinary tract spasm
<1%:
  Central nervous system: Mental depression, hallucinations, paradoxical CNS stimulation
  Dermatologic: Pruritus, skin rash, hives
  Gastrointestinal: Paralytic ileus
  Miscellaneous: Physical and psychological dependence
Overdosage/Toxicology Symptoms of overdose include respiratory depression, CNS depression, miosis, hypothermia, circulatory collapse, convulsions; naloxone 2 mg I.V. (0.01 mg/kg for children) with repeat administration as necessary up to a total of 10 mg
Drug Interactions
Decreased effect: Phenytoin, pentazocine and rifampin may increase the metabolism of methadone and may precipitate withdrawal
Increased toxicity: CNS depressants, phenothiazines, tricyclic antidepressants, MAO inhibitors may potentiate the adverse effects of methadone
Stability Highly **incompatible** with all other I.V. agents when mixed together
(Continued)

Methadone Hydrochloride *(Continued)*

Mechanism of Action Binds to opiate receptors in the CNS, causing inhibition of ascending pain pathways, altering the perception of and response to pain; produces generalized CNS depression

Pharmacodynamics/Kinetics

Oral:
Onset of analgesia: Within 0.5-1 hour
Duration: 6-8 hours, increases to 22-48 hours with repeated doses

Parenteral:
Onset of effect: Within 10-20 minutes
Peak effect: Within 1-2 hours

Distribution: Crosses the placenta; appears in breast milk

Protein binding: 80% to 85%

Metabolism: In the liver (N-demethylation)

Half-life: 15-29 hours, may be prolonged with alkaline pH

Elimination: In urine (<10% as unchanged drug); increased renal excretion with urine pH <6

Usual Dosage Doses should be titrated to appropriate effects

Children: Analgesia:
Oral, I.M., S.C.: 0.7 mg/kg/24 hours divided every 4-6 hours as needed or 0.1-0.2 mg/kg every 4-12 hours as needed; maximum: 10 mg/dose
I.V.: 0.1 mg/kg every 4 hours initially for 2-3 doses, then every 6-12 hours as needed; maximum: 10 mg/dose

Adults:
Analgesia: Oral, I.M., I.V., S.C.: 2.5-10 mg every 3-8 hours as needed, up to 5-20 mg every 6-8 hours
Detoxification: Oral: 15-40 mg/day; should not exceed 21 days and may not be repeated earlier than 4 weeks after completion of preceding course
Maintenance of opiate dependence: Oral: 20-120 mg/day

Dosing adjustment in renal impairment: Cl_{cr} <10 mL/minute: Administer at 50% to 75% of normal dose

Dosing adjustment/comments in hepatic disease: Avoid in severe liver disease

Important note: Methadone accumulates with repeated doses and dosage may need to be adjusted downward after 3-5 days to prevent toxic effects. Some patients may benefit from every 8- to 12-hour dosing interval (pain control).

Monitoring Parameters Pain relief, respiratory and mental status, blood pressure

Reference Range Therapeutic: 100-400 ng/mL (SI: 0.32-1.29 µmol/L); Toxic: >2 µg/mL (SI: >6.46 µmol/L)

Test Interactions ↑ thyroxine (S), ↑ aminotransferase [ALT (SGPT)/AST (SGOT)] (S)

Patient Information May cause drowsiness, avoid alcohol and other CNS depressants

Nursing Implications Observe patient for excessive sedation, respiratory depression, implement safety measures, assist with ambulation

Dosage Forms

Injection: 10 mg/mL (1 mL, 10 mL, 20 mL)
Solution:
Oral: 5 mg/5 mL (5 mL, 500 mL); 10 mg/5 mL (500 mL)
Oral, concentrate: 10 mg/mL (30 mL)
Tablet: 5 mg, 10 mg
Tablet, dispersible: 40 mg

Methaminodiazepoxide Hydrochloride *see* Chlordiazepoxide *on page 221*

Methamphetamine Hydrochloride *(meth am fet' a meen)*

Brand Names Desoxyn®

Synonyms Desoxyephedrine Hydrochloride

Use Treatment of narcolepsy, exogenous obesity, abnormal behavioral syndrome in children (minimal brain dysfunction)

Restrictions C-II

Pregnancy Risk Factor C

Contraindications Known hypersensitivity to methamphetamine

Warnings/Precautions Cardiovascular disease, nephritis, angina pectoris hypertension, glaucoma, patients with a history of drug abuse, known hypersensitivity to amphetamine

Adverse Reactions
>10%:
Cardiovascular: Irregular heartbeat
Central nervous system: False feeling of well being, nervousness, restlessness, insomnia
1% to 10%:
Cardiovascular: Hypertension
Central nervous system: Mood or mental changes, dizziness, lightheadedness, headache
Endocrine & metabolic: Changes in libido
Gastrointestinal: Diarrhea, nausea, vomiting, stomach cramps, constipation, anorexia, weight loss dry mouth
Ocular: Blurred vision
Miscellaneous: Increased sweating
<1%:
Cardiovascular: Chest pain
Central nervous system: CNS stimulation (severe), Tourette's syndrome, hyperthermia, seizures, paranoia
Dermatologic: Skin rash, hives
Miscellaneous: Tolerance and withdrawal with prolonged use

Overdosage/Toxicology Symptoms of overdose include seizures, hyperactivity, coma, hypertension

There is no specific antidote for amphetamine intoxication and the bulk of the treatment is supportive. Hyperactivity and agitation usually respond to reduced sensory input, however with extreme agitation haloperidol (2-5 mg I.M. for adults) may be required. Hyperthermia is best treated with external cooling measures, or when severe or unresponsive, muscle paralysis with pancuronium may be needed. Hypertension is usually transient and generally does not require treatment unless severe. For diastolic blood pressures >110 mm Hg, a nitroprusside infusion should be initiated. Seizures usually respond to diazepam IVP and/or phenytoin maintenance regimens.

Drug Interactions Increased toxicity with MAO inhibitors (hypertensive crisis)
Usual Dosage
Attention deficit disorder: Children >6 years: 2.5-5 mg 1-2 times/day, may increase by 5 mg increments weekly until optimum response is achieved, usually 20-25 mg/day

Exogenous obesity: Children >12 years and Adults: 5 mg, 30 minutes before each meal; long-acting formulation: 10-15 mg in morning; treatment duration should not exceed a few weeks

Monitoring Parameters Heart rate, respiratory rate, blood pressure, and CNS activity
Patient Information Take during day to avoid insomnia; do not discontinue abruptly, may cause physical and psychological dependence with prolonged use; do not crush or chew extended release tablet
Nursing Implications Dose should not be given in evening or at bedtime; do not crush extended release tablet
Dosage Forms
Tablet: 5 mg
Tablet, extended release (Gradumet®): 5 mg, 10 mg, 15 mg

Methazolamide (meth a zoe′ la mide)
Related Information
Glaucoma Drug Therapy Comparison on page 1270
Brand Names Neptazane®
Use Adjunctive treatment of open-angle or secondary glaucoma; short-term therapy of narrow-angle glaucoma when delay of surgery is desired
Pregnancy Risk Factor C
Contraindications Marked kidney or liver dysfunction, severe pulmonary obstruction, hypersensitivity to methazolamide or any component
Warnings/Precautions Sulfonamide-type reactions, melena, anorexia, nausea, vomiting, constipation, hematuria, glycosuria, urinary frequency, renal colic, renal calculi, crystalluria, polyuria, hepatic insufficiency, various CNS effects, transient myopia, bone marrow depression, thrombocytopenia/purpura, hemolytic anemia, leukopenia, pancytopenia, agranulocytosis, urticaria, pruritus, rash, Stevens-Johnson syndrome, weight loss, fever, acidosis; use with caution in patients with respiratory acidosis and diabetes mellitus; impairment of mental alertness and/or physical coordination. Malaise and complaints of tiredness and myalgia are signs of excessive dosing and acidosis in the elderly.
(Continued)

Methazolamide *(Continued)*

Adverse Reactions
>10%:
  Central nervous system: Malaise, weakness
  Gastrointestinal: Metallic taste, anorexia
  Genitourinary: Increased urination
1% to 10%:
  Central nervous system: Mental depression, drowsiness, dizziness
  Renal: Crystalluria
<1%:
  Central nervous system: Fever, headache, seizures, unsteadiness, fatigue
  Dermatologic: Rash, sulfonamide rash, Stevens-Johnson syndrome
  Endocrine & metabolic: Hyperchloremic metabolic acidosis, hypokalemia, elevation of blood glucose
  Gastrointestinal: GI irritation, constipation, anorexia, dry mouth, black tarry stools
  Hematologic: Bone marrow suppression
  Neuromuscular & skeletal: Paresthesia, trembling
  Ocular: Myopia
  Otic: Tinnitus
  Renal: Dysuria
  Miscellaneous: Loss of smell, hypersensitivity

Drug Interactions
Increased toxicity:
  May induce hypokalemia which would sensitize a patient to digitalis toxicity
  May increase the potential for salicylate toxicity
  Hypokalemia may be compounded with concurrent diuretic use or steroids
  Primidone absorption may be delayed
Decreased effect: Increased lithium excretion and altered excretion of other drugs by alkalinization of the urine, such as amphetamines, quinidine, procainamide, methenamine, phenobarbital, salicylates

Mechanism of Action Noncompetitive inhibition of the enzyme carbonic anhydrase; thought that carbonic anhydrase is located at the luminal border of cells of the proximal tubule. When the enzyme is inhibited, there is an increase in urine volume and a change to an alkaline pH with a subsequent decrease in the excretion of titratable acid and ammonia.

Pharmacodynamics/Kinetics
Onset of action: Slow in comparison with acetazolamide (2-4 hours)
Peak effect: 6-8 hours
Duration: 10-18 hours
Absorption: Slowly from GI tract
Distribution: Distributes well into tissue
Protein binding: ~55%
Half-life: ~14 hours
Elimination: ~25% excreted unchanged in urine

Usual Dosage Adults: Oral: 50-100 mg 2-3 times/day

Patient Information Take with food, report any numbness or tingling in extremities to physician; may cause drowsiness, impaired judgment or coordination

Nursing Implications May cause an alteration in taste, especially when drinking carbonated beverages

Dosage Forms Tablet: 25 mg, 50 mg

Methenamine *(meth en' a meen)*

Brand Names Hiprex®; Mandelamine®; Urex®; Urised®

Synonyms Hexamethylenetetramine

Use Prophylaxis or suppression of recurrent urinary tract infections; urinary tract discomfort secondary to hypermotility; should not be used to treat infections outside of urinary tract

Pregnancy Risk Factor C

Contraindications Severe dehydration, renal insufficiency, hepatic insufficiency in patients receiving hippurate salt, hypersensitivity to methenamine or any component

Warnings/Precautions Use with caution in patients with hepatic disease, gout and the elderly; doses of 8 g/day may cause bladder irritation, some products may contain tartrazine; methenamine should not be used to treat infections outside of the lower urinary tract

Adverse Reactions
1% to 10%:
  Dermatologic: Skin rash
  Gastrointestinal: Nausea, vomiting, diarrhea, anorexia, abdominal cramping

<1%:
Central nervous system: Headache
Genitourinary: Bladder irritation
Hepatic: Elevation in AST and ALT
Renal: Hematuria, dysuria, crystalluria

Overdosage/Toxicology Well tolerated; treatment includes GI decontamination, if possible, and supportive care

Drug Interactions
Decreased effect: Sodium bicarbonate and acetazolamide will decrease effect secondary to alkalinization of urine
Increased toxicity: Sulfonamides (may precipitate)

Stability Protect from excessive heat

Mechanism of Action Methenamine is hydrolyzed to formaldehyde and ammonia in acidic urine; formaldehyde has nonspecific bactericidal action

Pharmacodynamics/Kinetics
Absorption: Readily absorbed from GI tract
Metabolism: 10% to 30% of the drug will be hydrolyzed by gastric juices unless it is protected by an enteric coating; ~10% to 25% is metabolized in the liver
Half-life: 3-6 hours
Elimination: Occurs via glomerular filtration and tubular secretion with ~70% to 90% of dose excreted unchanged in urine within 24 hours

Usual Dosage Oral:
Children: 6-12 years:
Hippurate: 25-50 mg/kg/day divided every 12 hours
Mandelate: 50-75 mg/kg/day divided every 6 hours

Children >12 years and Adults:
Hippurate: 1 g twice daily
Mandelate: 1 g 4 times/day after meals and at bedtime

Dosing adjustment/comments in renal impairment: Cl_{cr} <50 mL/minute: Avoid use

Administration Administer around-the-clock rather than 4 times/day to promote less variation in peak and trough serum levels

Monitoring Parameters Urinalysis, periodic liver function tests in patients

Test Interactions ↑ catecholamines and VMA (U); ↓ HIAA (U)

Patient Information Take with food to minimize GI upset; take with ascorbic acid to acidify urine; drink sufficient fluids to ensure adequate urine flow. Avoid excessive intake of alkalinizing foods (citrus fruits and milk products) or medication (bicarbonate, acetazolamide); notify physician is skin rash, painful urination or excessive abdominal pain occur.

Nursing Implications Urine should be acidic (pH <5.5) for maximum effect

Dosage Forms
Granules (orange flavor): 1 g (56s)
Suspension, oral, as mandelate (Mandelamine®): 250 mg/5 mL (coconut flavor), 500 mg/5 mL (cherry flavor)
Tablet, as hippurate (Hiprex®, Urex®): 1 g (Hiprex® contains tartrazine dye)
Tablet, as mandelate, enteric coated (Mandelamine®): 250 mg, 500 mg, 1 g

Methergine® see Methylergonovine Maleate on page 721

Methicillin Sodium (meth i sill' in)
Brand Names Staphcillin®
Synonyms Dimethoxyphenil Penicillin Sodium; Sodium Methicillin
Use Treatment of susceptible bacterial infections such as osteomyelitis, septicemia, endocarditis, and CNS infections due to penicillinase-producing strains of *Staphylococcus*; other antistaphylococcal penicillins are usually preferred
Pregnancy Risk Factor B
Contraindications Known hypersensitivity to methicillin or any penicillin
Warnings/Precautions Elimination rate will be slow in neonates; modify dosage in patients with renal impairment and in the elderly; use with caution in patients with cephalosporin hypersensitivity
Adverse Reactions
1% to 10%:
Dermatologic: Skin rash
Renal: Acute interstitial nephritis
<1%:
Central nervous system: Fever
Dermatologic: Rash
Hematologic: Eosinophilia, anemia, leukopenia, neutropenia, thrombocytopenia
Local: Phlebitis
(Continued)

Methicillin Sodium *(Continued)*

Renal: Hemorrhagic cystitis

Miscellaneous: Serum sickness-like reactions

Overdosage/Toxicology Symptoms of penicillin overdose include neuromuscular hypersensitivity (agitation, hallucinations, asterixis, encephalopathy, confusion, and seizures) and electrolyte imbalance with potassium or sodium salts, especially in renal failure; hemodialysis may be helpful to aid in the removal of the drug from the blood, otherwise most treatment is supportive or symptom directed

Drug Interactions

Decreased effect: Efficacy of oral contraceptives may be reduced

Increased effect: Disulfiram, probenecid → ↑ penicillin levels, increased effect of anticoagulants

Stability Reconstituted solution is stable for 24 hours at room temperature and 4 days when refrigerated; discard solutions if it has a distinctive hydrogen sulfide odor and/or color turns to a deep orange; **incompatible** with aminoglycosides and tetracyclines

Mechanism of Action Inhibits bacterial cell wall synthesis by binding to one or more of the penicillin binding proteins (PBPs); which in turn inhibits the final transpeptidation step of peptidoglycan synthesis in bacterial cell walls, thus inhibiting cell wall biosynthesis. Bacteria eventually lyse due to ongoing activity of cell wall autolytic enzymes (autolysins and murein hydrolases) while cell wall assembly is arrested.

Pharmacodynamics/Kinetics

Distribution: Crosses the placenta; distributes into milk

Protein binding: 40%

Metabolism: Only partially

Half-life (with normal renal function):

Neonates:

<2 weeks: 2-3.9 hours

>2 weeks: 0.9-3.3 hours

Children 2-16 years: 0.8 hour

Adults: 0.4-0.5 hour

Time to peak serum concentration:

I.M.: 0.5-1 hour

I.V. infusion: Within 5 minutes

Elimination: ~60% to 70% of dose eliminated unchanged in urine within 4 hours by tubular secretion and glomerular filtration

Usual Dosage I.M., I.V.:

Neonates:

0-4 weeks, <1200 g: 25 mg/kg/dose every 12 hours; meningitis: 50 mg/kg/dose every 12 hours

<7 days:

1200-2000 g: 25 mg/kg/dose every 12 hours; meningitis: 50 mg/kg/dose every 12 hours

>2000 g: 25 mg/kg/dose every 8 hours; meningitis: 50 mg/kg/dose every 8 hours

>7 days:

1200-2000 g: 25 mg/kg/dose every 8 hours; meningitis: 50 mg/kg/dose every 8 hours

>2000 g: 25 mg/kg/dose every 6 hours; meningitis: 50 mg/kg/dose every 6 hours

Children: 150-200 mg/kg/day divided every 6 hours; 200-400 mg/kg/day divided every 4-6 hours has been used for treatment of severe infections; maximum dose: 12 g/day

Adults: 4-12 g/day in divided doses every 4-6 hours

Dosing interval in renal impairment:

Cl_{cr} 10-50 mL/minute: Administer every 6-8 hours

Cl_{cr} <10 mL/minute: Administer every 8-12 hours

Not dialyzable (0% to 5%)

Administration Can be administered IVP at a rate not to exceed 200 mg/minute or intermittent infusion over 20-30 minutes; final concentration for administration should not exceed 20 mg/mL

Test Interactions Interferes with tests for urinary and serum proteins, uric acid, urinary steroids; may cause false-positive Coombs' test; may inactivate aminoglycosides *in vitro*

Dosage Forms Powder for injection: 1 g, 4 g, 6 g, 10 g

Methimazole (meth im′ a zole)

Brand Names Tapazole®

Synonyms Thiamazole

Use Palliative treatment of hyperthyroidism, return the hyperthyroid patient to a normal metabolic state prior to thyroidectomy, and to control thyrotoxic crisis that may accompany thyroidectomy. The use of antithyroid thioamides is as effective in elderly as they are in younger adults; however, the expense, potential adverse effects, and inconvenience (compliance, monitoring) make them undesirable. The use of radioiodine due to ease of administration and less concern for long-term side effects and reproduction problems (some older males) makes it a more appropriate therapy.

Pregnancy Risk Factor D

Contraindications Hypersensitivity to methimazole or any component, nursing mothers

Warnings/Precautions Use with extreme caution in patients receiving other drugs known to cause myelosuppression particularly agranulocytosis, patients >40 years of age; avoid doses >40 mg/day (↑ myelosuppression); may cause acneiform eruptions or worsen the condition of the thyroid

Adverse Reactions

>10%:
  Central nervous system: Fever
  Dermatologic: Skin rash
  Hematologic: Leukopenia

1% to 10%:
  Central nervous system: Dizziness
  Gastrointestinal: Nausea, vomiting, stomach pain, loss of taste
  Hematologic: Agranulocytosis
  Miscellaneous: SLE-like syndrome

<1%:
  Cardiovascular: Edema
  Central nervous system: Drowsiness, vertigo, headache
  Dermatologic: Rash, urticaria, pruritus, hair loss
  Endocrine & metabolic: Goiter
  Gastrointestinal: Constipation, weight gain
  Genitourinary: Nephrotic syndrome
  Hematologic: Thrombocytopenia, aplastic anemia
  Hepatic: Cholestatic jaundice
  Neuromuscular & skeletal: Arthralgia, paresthesia
  Miscellaneous: Swollen salivary glands

Overdosage/Toxicology Symptoms of overdose include nausea, vomiting, epigastric distress, headache, fever, arthralgia, pruritus, edema, pancytopenia, and signs of hypothyroidism; management of overdose is supportive

Drug Interactions Increased toxicity: Iodinated glycerol, lithium, potassium iodide; anticoagulant activity increased

Stability Protect from light

Mechanism of Action Inhibits the synthesis of thyroid hormones by blocking the oxidation of iodine in the thyroid gland, blocking iodine's ability to combine with tyrosine to form thyroxine and tri-iodothyronine (T_3), does not inactivate circulating T_4 and T_3

Pharmacodynamics/Kinetics

Bioavailability: 80% to 95%

Onset of antithyroid effect: Oral: Within 30-40 minutes

Duration: 2-4 hours

Distribution: Crosses the placenta; appears in breast milk (1:1)

Protein binding: No plasma protein binding

Half-life: 4-13 hours

Elimination: Renally with ~12% excreted in urine within 24 hours

Usual Dosage Oral: Administer in 3 equally divided doses at approximately 8-hour intervals

Children: Initial: 0.4 mg/kg/day in 3 divided doses; maintenance: 0.2 mg/kg/day in 3 divided doses up to 30 mg/24 hours maximum

Adults: Initial: 5 mg every 8 hours; maintenance dose: 5-15 mg/day up to 60 mg/day for severe hyperthyroidism

Adjust dosage as required to achieve and maintain serum T_3, T_4, and TSH levels in the normal range. An elevated T_3 may be the sole indicator of inadequate treatment. An elevated TSH indicates excessive antithyroid treatment.

Monitoring Parameters Monitor for signs of hypothyroidism, hyperthyroidism, T_4, T_3; CBC with differential, liver function (baseline and as needed), serum thyroxine, free thyroxine index

(Continued)

Methimazole *(Continued)*

Patient Information Take with meals, take at regular intervals around-the-clock; notify physician if persistent fever, sore throat, fatigue, unusual bleeding or bruising occurs

Dosage Forms Tablet: 5 mg, 10 mg

Methocarbamol *(meth oh kar' ba mole)*

Brand Names Delaxin®; Marbaxin®; Robaxin®; Robomol®

Use Treatment of muscle spasm associated with acute painful musculoskeletal conditions, supportive therapy in tetanus

Pregnancy Risk Factor C

Contraindications Renal impairment, hypersensitivity to methocarbamol or any component

Warnings/Precautions Rate of injection should not exceed 3 mL/minute; solution is hypertonic; avoid extravasation; use with caution in patients with a history of seizures

Adverse Reactions

>10%: Central nervous system: Drowsiness, dizziness, lightheadedness

1% to 10%:

Cardiovascular: Flushing of face, bradycardia

Dermatologic: Allergic dermatitis

Gastrointestinal: Nausea, vomiting

Ocular: Nystagmus

Respiratory: Nasal congestion

<1%:

Central nervous system: Convulsions, fainting

Hematologic: Leukopenia

Local: Pain at place of injection, thrombophlebitis

Ocular: Blurred vision, renal impairment

Miscellaneous: Allergic manifestations

Overdosage/Toxicology Symptoms of overdose include cardiac arrhythmias, nausea, vomiting, drowsiness, coma

Treatment is supportive following attempts to enhance drug elimination

Hypotension should be treated with I.V. fluids and/or Trendelenburg positioning

Dialysis and hemoperfusion and osmotic diuresis have all been useful in reducing serum drug concentrations

The patient should be observed for possible relapses due to incomplete gastric emptying

Drug Interactions Increased effect/toxicity with CNS depressants

Mechanism of Action Causes skeletal muscle relaxation by reducing the transmission of impulses from the spinal cord to skeletal muscle

Pharmacodynamics/Kinetics

Onset of muscle relaxation: Oral: Within 30 minutes

Metabolism: In the liver

Half-life: 1-2 hours

Time to peak serum concentration: ~2 hours

Elimination: Metabolites renally excreted

Usual Dosage

Children: Recommended **only** for use in tetanus I.V.: 15 mg/kg/dose or 500 mg/m^2/dose, may repeat every 6 hours if needed; maximum dose: 1.8 g/m^2/day for 3 days only

Adults: Muscle spasm:

Oral: 1.5 g 4 times/day for 2-3 days, then decrease to 4-4.5 g/day in 3-6 divided doses

I.M., I.V.: 1 g every 8 hours if oral not possible

Dosing adjustment/comments in renal impairment: Do not administer parenteral formulation to patients with renal dysfunction

Administration Maximum rate: 3 mL/minute

Patient Information May cause drowsiness, impair judgment or coordination; avoid alcohol or other CNS depressants; may turn urine brown, black, or green; notify physician of rash, itching, or nasal congestion

Nursing Implications Monitor closely for extravasation of I.V. injection

Dosage Forms

Injection: 100 mg/mL in polyethylene glycol 50% (10 mL)

Tablet: 500 mg, 750 mg

Methohexital Sodium (meth oh hex' i tal)

Brand Names Brevital® Sodium

Synonyms Methylphenobarbital

Use Induction and maintenance of general anesthesia for short procedures

Restrictions C-IV

Pregnancy Risk Factor C

Contraindications Porphyria, hypersensitivity to methohexital or any component

Warnings/Precautions Use with extreme caution in patients with liver impairment, asthma, cardiovascular instability

Adverse Reactions

>10%: Local: Pain on I.M. injection

1% to 10%: Gastrointestinal: Cramping, diarrhea, rectal bleeding

<1%:

Cardiovascular: Hypotension, peripheral vascular collapse

Central nervous system: Radial nerve palsy, seizures, headache

Gastrointestinal: Nausea, vomiting

Hematologic: Hemolytic anemia

Local: Thrombophlebitis

Neuromuscular & skeletal: Tremor, twitching, rigidity, involuntary muscle movement

Respiratory: Apnea, respiratory depression, laryngospasm, coughing

Miscellaneous: Hiccups

Overdosage/Toxicology Symptoms of overdose include apnea, tachycardia, hypotension; treatment is primarily supportive with mechanical ventilation if needed

Drug Interactions CNS depressants worsen CNS depression

Stability Do not dilute with solutions containing bacteriostatic agents; solutions are alkaline (pH 9.5-11) and **incompatible** with acids (eg, atropine sulfate, succinylcholine, silicone), also **incompatible** with phenol containing solutions and silicone

Mechanism of Action Ultra short-acting I.V. barbiturate anesthetic

Usual Dosage Doses must be titrated to effect

Children 3-12 years:

I.M.: Preop: 5-10 mg/kg/dose

I.V.: Induction: 1-2 mg/kg/dose

Rectal: Preop/induction: 20-35 mg/kg/dose; usual 25 mg/kg/dose; give as 10% aqueous solution

Adults: I.V.: Induction: 50-120 mg to start; 20-40 mg every 4-7 minutes

Dosing adjustment/comments in hepatic impairment: Lower dosage and monitor closely

Nursing Implications Avoid extravasation or intra-arterial administration

Dosage Forms Injection: 500 mg, 2.5 g, 5 g

Methoin see Mephenytoin on page 686

Methotrexate (meth oh trex' ate)

Related Information

Cancer Chemotherapy Regimens on page 1218-1241

Brand Names Folex®; Rheumatrex®

Synonyms Amethopterin; MTX

Use Treatment of trophoblastic neoplasms; leukemias; psoriasis; rheumatoid arthritis; breast, head, and lung carcinomas; osteosarcoma; sarcomas; carcinoma of gastric, esophagus, testes; lymphomas

Pregnancy Risk Factor D

Contraindications Hypersensitivity to methotrexate or any component; severe renal or hepatic impairment; pre-existing profound bone marrow depression in patients with psoriasis or rheumatoid arthritis, alcoholic liver disease, AIDS, pre-existing blood dyscrasias

Warnings/Precautions

The U.S. Food and Drug Administration (FDA) currently recommends that procedures for proper handling and disposal of antineoplastic agents be considered.

May cause photosensitivity type reaction; reduce dosage in patients with renal or hepatic impairment, ascites, and pleural effusion; use with caution in patients with peptic ulcer disease, ulcerative colitis, pre-existing bone marrow suppression; monitor closely for pulmonary disease; use with caution in the elderly

Because of the possibility of severe toxic reactions, fully inform patient of the risks involved; do not use in women of childbearing age unless benefit outweighs risks; may cause hepatotoxicity, fibrosis and cirrhosis, along with marked bone marrow depression; death from intestinal perforation may occur

(Continued)

Methotrexate (Continued)

Toxicity to methotrexate or any immunosuppressive is increased in elderly. Must monitor carefully. For rheumatoid arthritis and psoriasis, immunosuppressive therapy should only be used when disease is active and less toxic; traditional therapy is ineffective. Recommended doses should be reduced when initiating therapy in elderly due to possible decreased metabolism, reduced renal function, and presence of interacting diseases and drugs.

Adverse Reactions

>10%:

Mucositis: Dose-dependent; appears in 3-7 days after therapy, resolving within 2 weeks

Cardiovascular: Vasculitis

Central nervous system (with I.T. administration only):

Arachnoiditis: Acute reaction manifested as severe headache, nuchal rigidity, vomiting, and fever; may be alleviated by reducing the dose

Subacute toxicity: 10% of patients treated with 12-15 mg/m^2 of I.T. MTX may develop this in the second or third week of therapy; consists of motor paralysis of extremities, cranial nerve palsy, seizures, or coma. This has also been seen in pediatric cases receiving very high-dose MTX (when enough MTX can get across into the CSF).

Demyelinating encephalopathy: Seen months or years after receiving MTX; usually in association with cranial irradiation or other systemic chemotherapy

Dermatologic: Reddening of skin

Gastrointestinal: Ulcerative stomatitis, pharyngitis, glossitis, gingivitis, nausea, vomiting, diarrhea, anorexia, intestinal perforation

Emetic potential:

<100 mg: Moderately low (10% to 30%)

≥100 mg or <250 mg: Moderate (30% to 60%)

≥250 mg: Moderately high (60% to 90%)

Hematologic: Leukopenia, thrombocytopenia

Renal: Renal failure, azotemia, hyperuricemia, nephropathy

1% to 10%:

Central nervous system: Dizziness, malaise, encephalopathy, seizures, fever, chills

Dermatitis: Alopecia, rash, photosensitivity, depigmentation or hyperpigmentation of skin

Endocrine & metabolic: Diabetes

Hematologic: Hemorrhage

Hepatic abnormalities: Cirrhosis and portal fibrosis have been associated with chronic MTX therapy; acute elevation of liver enzymes are common after high-dose MTX, and usually resolve within 10 days

Myelosuppressive: This is the primary dose-limiting factor (along with mucositis) of MTX; occurs about 5-7 days after MTX therapy, and should resolve within 2 weeks

WBC: Mild

Platelets: Moderate

Onset (days): 7

Nadir (days): 10

Recovery (days): 21

Ocular: Blurred vision

Neuromuscular & skeletal: Arthralgia

Pneumonitis: Associated with fever, cough, and interstitial pulmonary infiltrates; treatment is to withhold MTX during the acute reaction

Renal dysfunction: Manifested by an abrupt rise in serum creatinine and BUN and a fall in urine output; more common with high-dose MTX, and may be due to precipitation of the drug. The best treatment is prevention: Aggressively hydrate with 3 L/m^2/day starting 12 hours before therapy and continue for 24-36 hours; alkalinize the urine by adding 50 mEq of bicarbonate to each liter of fluid; keep urine flow over 100 mL/hour and urine pH >7.

Renal: Vasculitis, cystitis

Miscellaneous: Anaphylaxis, decreased resistance to infection

Overdosage/Toxicology Symptoms of overdose include bone marrow depression, nausea, vomiting, alopecia, melena, renal failure; severe bone marrow toxicity can result from overdose. Antidote is leucovorin. Leucovorin should be administered as soon as toxicity is seen; administer 10 mg/m^2 orally or parenterally; follow with 10 mg/m^2 orally every 6 hours for 72 hours. After 24 hours following methotrexate administration, if the serum creatinine is ≥50% premethotrexate serum creatinine, increase leucovorin dose to 100 mg/m^2 every 3 hours until serum MTX level is <5 x 10^{-8}M. Hydration and alkalinization may be used to prevent precipitation of MTX or MTX metabolites in the renal tubules. Toxicity in low dose range is negligible, but may present mucositis and mild bone marrow suppression.

Drug Interactions

Decreased effect: Decreased phenytoin, 5-FU, nonsteroidal anti-inflammatory drugs (NSAIDs)

Increased toxicity:

Live virus vaccines → vaccinia infections

Vincristine: Inhibits MTX efflux from the cell, leading to increased and prolonged MTX levels in the cell; the dose of VCR needed to produce this effect is not achieved clinically

Organic acids: Salicylates, sulfonamides, probenecid, and high doses of penicillins compete with MTX for transport and reduce renal tubular secretion. Salicylates and sulfonamides may also displace MTX from plasma proteins, increasing MTX levels.

Ara-C: Increased formation of the Ara-C nucleotide can occur when MTX precedes Ara-C, thus promoting the action of Ara-C

Cyclosporine: CSA and MTX interfere with each others renal elimination, which may result in increased toxicity

Stability Store intact vials at room temperature; reconstituted solutions remain stable for 4 weeks at room temperature and 3 months when refrigerated; intrathecal solutions should be diluted immediately prior to use

Mechanism of Action Antimetabolite that inhibits DNA synthesis and cell reproduction in cancerous cells

Folates must be in the reduced form (FH_4) to be active; activated by dihydrofolate reductase (DHFR)

DHFR is inhibited by MTX (by binding irreversibly), causing an increase in the intracellular dihydrofolate pool (the inactive cofactor) and inhibition of both purine and thymidylate synthesis (TS)

MTX enters the cell through an energy-dependent and temperature-dependent process which is mediated by an intramembrane protein; this carrier mechanism is also used by naturally occurring reduced folates, including folinic acid (leucovorin), making this a competitive process

At high drug concentrations (>20 µM), MTX enters the cell by a second mechanism which is not shared by reduced folates; the process may be passive diffusion or a specific, saturable process, and provides a rationale for high-dose MTX; a small fraction of MTX is converted intracellularly to polyglutamates, which leads to a prolonged inhibition of DHFR

Pharmacodynamics/Kinetics

Absorption:

Oral: Rapid; well absorbed orally at low doses (<30 mg/m²), incomplete absorption after large doses

I.M.: Completely absorbed

Time to peak serum concentration:

Oral: 1-2 hours

Parenteral: 30-60 minutes

Distribution: Drug penetrates slowly into third space fluids, such as pleural effusions or ascites, and exits slowly from these compartments (slower than from plasma); crosses the placenta with small amounts appearing in breast milk; does not achieve therapeutic concentrations in the CSF and must be given intrathecally if given for CNS prophylaxis or treatment; sustained concentrations are retained in the kidney and liver

Protein binding: 50%

Metabolism: <10% metabolized; degraded by intestinal flora to DAMPA by carboxypeptidase; aldehyde oxidase in the liver converts MTX to 7-OH MTX; polyglutamates are produced intracellularly and are just as potent as MTX; their production is dose and duration dependent and are slowly eliminated by the cell once they are formed

Half-life: 8-12 hours with high doses and 3-10 hours with low doses

Elimination: Small amounts excreted in the feces; primarily excreted in the urine (44% to 100%) via glomerular filtration and active transport

Miscellaneous: Cytotoxicity is determined by both drug concentration and duration of cell exposure; extracellular drug concentrations of 1×10^{-8} M are required to inhibit thymidylate synthesis; reduced folates are able to rescue cells and reverse MTX toxicity if given within 48 hours of the MTX dose; at concentrations >10 µM MTX, reduced folates are no longer effective

Usual Dosage May be administered orally, I.M., intra-arterially, intrathecally, I.V., or S.C. (refer to individual protocols)

Leucovorin may be administered concomitantly or within 24 hours of methotrexate

Doses not requiring leucovorin rescue range from 30-40 mg/m² I.V. or I.M. repeated weekly, or oral regimens of 10 mg/m² twice weekly

Children:

I.V.:

Meningeal leukemia: Loading dose: 6 g/m² followed by I.V. continuous infusion of 1.2 g/m²/hour for 23 hours

(Continued)

Methotrexate *(Continued)*

Acute lymphocytic leukemia (high dose): Loading: 200 mg/m² followed by a
24-hour infusion of 1200 mg/m²/day

ANLL: 7.5 mg/m²/day on days 1-5

Resistant ANLL: 100 mg/m²/dose on day 1

Hodgkin's lymphoma: 200-300 mg/m²

Acute lymphoblastic leukemias:

Oral, I.M., I.V. induction: 3.3 mg/m²/day for 4-6 weeks; remission maintenance: 20-30 mg/m² twice weekly

I.T.: Repeat at 2- to 5-day intervals. 10-15 mg/m² (maximum dose: 15 mg)
by protocol; ≤3 months: 3 mg; 4-11 months: 6 mg; 1-2 years: 8 mg; 2-3
years: 10 mg; >3 years: 12 mg

Note: I.T. doses are prepared with preservative-free MTX **only**

Hydrocortisone may be added to the I.T. preparation; total volume should
range from 3-6 mL.

Osteosarcoma: I.V.: <12 years: 12 g/m² (12-18 g); >12 years: 8 g/m² (18 g
maximum dose)

Juvenile rheumatoid arthritis: Oral: 5-15 mg/m²/week as a single dose or as 3
divided doses given 12 hours apart

Adults: I.V.: Range is wide from 30-40 mg/m²/week to 100-7500 mg/m² with
leucovorin rescue

High-dose MTX is considered to be >100 mg/m² and can be as high as
1500-7500 mg/m²; these doses require leucovorin rescue

Patients receiving doses ≥1000 mg/m² should have their urine alkalinized with
bicarbonate or Bicitra® prior to and following MTX therapy

Rheumatoid arthritis: Oral: 7.5 mg once weekly or 2.5 mg every 12 hours for 3
doses/week; not to exceed 20 mg/week

Elderly: Rheumatoid arthritis/psoriasis: Oral: Initial: 5 mg once weekly; if nausea
occurs, split dose to 2.5 mg every 12 hours for the day of administration. Dose
may be increased to 7.5 mg/week based on response, not to exceed 20
mg/week.

Dosing adjustment in renal impairment:

Cl$_{cr}$ 10-50 mL/minute: Reduce dose to 50%

Cl$_{cr}$ <10 mL/minute: Avoid use

Not dialyzable (0% to 5%); supplemental dose is not necessary

Peritoneal dialysis effects: Supplemental dose is not necessary

Dosing adjustment in hepatic impairment:

Bilirubin 3.1-5 mg/dL or AST >180 units: Administer 75% of dose

Bilirubin >5 mg/dL: Do not use

Administration Methotrexate can be administered I.V. push, I.V. intermittent
infusion, or I.V. continuous infusion at a concentration <25 mg/mL; doses >100-
300 mg/m² are usually given by I.V. continuous infusion and are followed by a
course of leucovorin rescue

Rate of I.V. administration:

Doses of 5-149 mg: Slow I.V. push

Doses of 150-499 mg: I.V. drip over 20 minutes

Doses of 500-1500 mg: I.V. infusion

Monitoring Parameters CBC with differential and platelet count, creatinine
clearance, serum creatinine, BUN, and hepatic function tests, LFTs every 3-4
months, chest x-ray; for prolonged use (especially rheumatoid arthritis, psoriasis) a baseline liver biopsy, repeated at each 1-1.5 g cumulative dose interval,
should be performed

Reference Range Refer to chart in Leucovorin Calcium monograph. Therapeutic
levels: Variable; Toxic concentration: Variable; therapeutic range is dependent
upon therapeutic approach. High-dose regimens produce drug levels between
10⁻⁶M and 10⁻⁷M 24-72 hours after drug infusion. Toxic: Low-dose therapy: >9.1
ng/mL; high-dose therapy: >454 ng/mL

Patient Information Any signs of infection, easy bruising or bleeding, shortness
of breath, or painful or burning urination should be brought to physician's attention. Nausea, vomiting or hair loss sometimes occur. The drug may cause
permanent sterility and may cause birth defects. The drug may be excreted in
breast milk; therefore, an alternative form of feeding your baby should be used.
Food may decrease absorption, therefore, take on an empty stomach; avoid
alcohol; avoid prolonged exposure to sun

Additional Information

Sodium content of 100 mg injection: 20 mg (0.86 mEq)

Sodium content of 100 mg (low sodium) injection: 15 mg (0.65 mEq)

Dosage Forms

Injection, as sodium: 2.5 mg/mL (2 mL); 25 mg/mL (2 mL, 4 mL, 8 mL, 10 mL)

Injection, as sodium, preservative free: 25 mg (2 mL, 4 mL, 8 mL, 10 mL)

Powder, for injection, as sodium: 20 mg, 25 mg, 50 mg, 100 mg, 250 mg, 1 g
Tablet: 2.5 mg
Tablet, dose pack: 2.5 mg (4 cards with 2, 3, 4, 5, or 6 tablets each)

Methotrimeprazine Hydrochloride (meth oh trye mep' ra zeen)

Brand Names Levoprome®

Synonyms Levomepromazine

Use Relief of moderate to severe pain in nonambulatory patients; for analgesia and sedation when respiratory depression is to be avoided, as in obstetrics; preanesthetic for producing sedation, somnolence and relief of apprehension and anxiety

Pregnancy Risk Factor C

Contraindications Severe cardiac, renal or hepatic disease, history of convulsive disorders, concurrent use of MAO inhibitors, significant hypotension, children <12 years of age, known hypersensitivity to methotrimeprazine or phenothiazines, sulfite sensitivity

Warnings/Precautions Use with caution in patients receiving antihypertensive agents and in the elderly; if used longer than 30 days monitor for hematologic adverse effects

Adverse Reactions
>10%:
 Cardiovascular: Hypotension, orthostatic hypotension
 Central nervous system: Pseudoparkinsonism, akathisia, dystonias, tardive dyskinesia (persistent), dizziness
 Gastrointestinal: Constipation
 Ocular: Pigmentary retinopathy
 Respiratory: Nasal congestion
 Miscellaneous: Decreased sweating
1% to 10%:
 Central nervous system: Dizziness
 Dermatologic: Increased sensitivity to sun, skin rash
 Endocrine & metabolic: Changes in menstrual cycle, changes in libido, pain in breasts
 Gastrointestinal: Weight gain, nausea, vomiting, stomach pain
 Genitourinary: Difficulty in urination, ejaculatory disturbances
 Neuromuscular & skeletal: Trembling of fingers
<1%:
 Central nervous system: Neuroleptic malignant syndrome (NMS)
 Dermatologic: Discoloration of skin (blue-gray)
 Endocrine & metabolic: Galactorrhea
 Genitourinary: Priapism
 Hematologic: Agranulocytosis, leukopenia
 Hepatic: Cholestatic jaundice, hepatotoxicity
 Ocular: Cornea and lens changes, pigmentary retinopathy
 Miscellaneous: Impairment of temperature regulation, lowering of seizures threshold

Mechanism of Action Methotrimeprazine is a phenothiazine with sites of action thought to be in the thalamus, hypothalamus, reticular and limbic systems, producing suppression of sensory impulses. This results with sedation, an elevated pain threshold, and induction of amnesia. The analgesic effect of methotrimeprazine is comparable to meperidine and morphine without the respiratory suppression. This agent also has antihistamine, anticholinergic, and antiepinephrine effects.

Pharmacodynamics/Kinetics
Peak effect: Within 20-40 minutes
Duration: 4 hours
Distribution: V_d: 29.8 L/kg
Metabolism: Hepatic to sulfoxide metabolites
Half-life, elimination: 20 hours
Time to peak serum concentration: Within 0.5-1.5 hours
Elimination: 50% excreted unchanged in urine

Usual Dosage Adults: I.M.:
Sedation analgesia: 10-20 mg every 4-6 hours as needed
Preoperative medication: 2-20 mg, 45 minutes to 3 hours before surgery
Postoperative analgesia: 2.5-7.5 mg every 4-6 hours is suggested as necessary since residual effects of anesthetic may be present
Pre- and postoperative hypotension: I.M.: 5-10 mg

Dosing adjustment/comments in renal or hepatic impairment: Administer cautiously although no specific guidelines are available

Test Interactions ↑ cholesterol (S), ↑ glucose; ↓ uric acid (S)
(Continued)

Methotrimeprazine Hydrochloride *(Continued)*

Patient Information May cause drowsiness, rise slowly after sitting or lying after administration

Nursing Implications Observe for orthostasis for up to 6 hours postdose; raise bed rails, institute safety measures, assist with ambulation

Dosage Forms Injection: 20 mg/mL (10 mL)

Methoxamine Hydrochloride (meth ox′ a meen)

Brand Names Vasoxyl®

Use Treatment of hypotension occurring during general anesthesia; to terminate episodes of supraventricular tachycardia; treatment of shock

Pregnancy Risk Factor C

Contraindications Hypersensitivity to methoxamine or any component

Adverse Reactions

1% to 10%:
Cardiovascular: Hypertension (severe)
Gastrointestinal: Vomiting

<1%:
Cardiovascular: Ventricular ectopic beats, fetal bradycardia
Central nervous system: Headache
Genitourinary: Urinary urgency
Miscellaneous: Sweating

Overdosage/Toxicology Hypertension, bradycardia

Mechanism of Action Direct-acting sympathomimetic amine with similar actions as phenylephrine; causes vasoconstriction primarily via alpha-adrenergic stimulation

Pharmacodynamics/Kinetics

Adrenergic effect:
Onset of action: I.M.: Within 15 minutes
Duration:
I.M.: 1.5 hours
I.V.: ~1 hour
Pressor activity:
Onset of action:
I.M.: 15-20 minutes
I.V.: Within 1-2 minutes
Duration: ~1-1.5 hours
Elimination: Not well defined

Usual Dosage Adults:
Emergencies: I.V.: 3-5 mg
Supraventricular tachycardia: I.V.: 10 mg
During spinal anesthesia: I.M.: 10-20 mg

Dosage Forms Injection: 20 mg/mL (1 mL)

Methoxsalen (meth ox′ a len)

Brand Names 8-MOP®; Oxsoralen®; Oxsoralen-Ultra®

Synonyms Methoxypsoralen; 8-Methoxypsoralen; 8-MOP

Use

Oral: Symptomatic control of severe, recalcitrant disabling psoriasis, not responsive to other therapy when to diagnosis has been supported by biopsy. Administer only in conjunction with a schedule of controlled doses of long wave ultraviolet (UV) radiation; also used with long wave ultraviolet (UV) radiation for repigmentation of idiopathic vitiligo.

Topical: Repigmenting agent in vitiligo, used in conjunction with controlled doses of UVA or sunlight

Pregnancy Risk Factor C

Contraindications Diseases associated with photosensitivity, cataract, invasive squamous cell cancer, known hypersensitivity to methoxsalen (psoralens), and children <12 years of age

Warnings/Precautions Family history of sunlight allergy or chronic infections; lotion should only be applied under direct supervision of a physician and should not be dispensed to the patient; for use only if inadequate response to other forms of therapy, serious burns may occur from UVA or sunlight even through glass if dose and or exposure schedule is not maintained; some products may contain tartrazine; use caution in patients with hepatic or cardiac disease

Adverse Reactions

>10%:
Gastrointestinal: Nausea
Local: Itching

1% to 10%:
    Cardiovascular: Severe edema, hypotension
    Central nervous system: Nervousness, vertigo, depression
    Dermatologic: Painful blistering, burning, and peeling of skin; pruritus, freckling, hypopigmentation, rash, cheilitis, erythema
    Neuromuscular: Loss of muscle coordination

Overdosage/Toxicology Symptoms of overdose include nausea, severe burns; follow accepted treatment of severe burns; keep room darkened until reaction subsides (8-24 hours or more)

Drug Interactions Increased toxicity: Concomitant therapy with other photosensitizing agents such as anthralin, coal tar, griseofulvin, phenothiazines, nalidixic acid, sulfanilamides, tetracyclines, thiazides

Mechanism of Action Bonds covalently to pyrimidine bases in DNA, inhibits the synthesis of DNA, and suppresses cell division. The augmented sunburn reaction involves excitation of the methoxsalen molecule by radiation in the long-wave ultraviolet light (UVA), resulting in transference of energy to the methoxsalen molecule producing an excited state ("triplet electronic state"). The molecule, in this "triplet state", then reacts with cutaneous DNA.

Pharmacodynamics/Kinetics
    Metabolism: In the liver with >90% of dose appearing in urine as metabolites
    Bioavailability: May be less with the capsule than with the liquid-encapsulated preparation
    Time to peak serum concentration: Oral: 2-4 hours

Usual Dosage
    Psoriasis: Adults: Oral: 10-70 mg 1½-2 hours before exposure to ultraviolet light, 2-3 times at least 48 hours apart; dosage is based upon patient's body weight and skin type

    Vitiligo: Children >12 years and Adults:
        Oral: 20 mg 2-4 hours before exposure to UVA light or sunlight; limit exposure to 15-40 minutes based on skin basic color and exposure
        Topical: Apply lotion 1-2 hours before exposure to UVA light, no more than once weekly

Patient Information To reduce nausea, oral drug can be taken with food or milk or in 2 divided doses 30 minutes apart. If burning or blistering or intractable pruritus occurs, discontinue therapy until effects subside. Do not sunbathe for at least 24 hours prior to therapy or 48 hours after PUVA therapy. Avoid direct and indirect sunlight for 8 hours after oral and 12-48 hours after topical therapy. **If sunlight cannot be avoided, protective clothing and/or sunscreens must be worn.** Following oral therapy, wraparound sunglasses with UVA-absorbing properties must be worn for 24 hours. Avoid furocoumarin-containing foods (limes, figs, parsley, celery, cloves, lemon, mustard, carrots); do not exceed prescribed dose or exposure times.

Dosage Forms
    Capsule: 10 mg
    Lotion: 1% (30 mL)

Methoxypsoralen *see* Methoxsalen *on previous page*

8-Methoxypsoralen *see* Methoxsalen *on previous page*

Methscopolamine Bromide (meth skoe pol' a meen)

Brand Names Pamine®
Use Adjunctive therapy in the treatment of peptic ulcer
Pregnancy Risk Factor C
Contraindications Anticholinergic drugs decrease both esophageal and gastric motility and relax the lower esophageal sphincter and are contraindicated in the presence of reflux esophagitis; glaucoma, obstructed uropathy, obstructed disease of the GI tract (pyloroduodenal stenosis), paralytic ileus, intestinal atony of elderly or debilitated individuals, unstable cardiovascular status in acute hemorrhage, severe ulcerative colitis, toxic megacolon, complicated ulcerative colitis, and myasthenia gravis; hypersensitivity to this agent or related drugs

Adverse Reactions
    >10%:
        Gastrointestinal: Constipation
        Miscellaneous: Decreased sweating, dry mouth, skin, nose, or throat
    1% to 10%: Difficulty in swallowing
    <1%:
        Cardiovascular: Tachycardia
        Central nervous system: Confusion, drowsiness, nervousness, insomnia, headache, loss of memory, weakness, tiredness
        Dermatologic: Rash
        Gastrointestinal: Bloated feeling, nausea, vomiting
(Continued)

Methscopolamine Bromide *(Continued)*

Genitourinary: Urinary retention
Ocular: Increased intraocular pressure, blurred vision

Mechanism of Action Methscopolamine is a peripheral anticholinergic agent that does not cross the blood-brain barrier and provides a peripheral blockade of muscarinic receptors. This agent reduces the volume and the total acid content of gastric secretions, inhibits salivation, and reduces gastrointestinal motility.

Usual Dosage Adults: Oral: 2.5 mg 30 minutes before meals or food and 2.5-5 mg at bedtime

Dosage Forms Tablet: 2.5 mg

Methsuximide *(meth sux' i mide)*

Brand Names Celontin®

Use Control of absence (petit mal) seizures; useful adjunct in refractory, partial complex (psychomotor) seizures

Pregnancy Risk Factor C

Contraindications Known hypersensitivity to methsuximide

Warnings/Precautions Use with caution in patients with hepatic or renal disease; abrupt withdrawal of the drug may precipitate absence status; ethosuximide may increase tonic-clonic seizures in patients with mixed seizure disorders; ethosuximide must be used in combination with other anticonvulsants in patients with both absence and tonic-clonic seizures

Adverse Reactions

>10%:
Central nervous system: Ataxia, dizziness, drowsiness, headache
Dermatologic: Stevens-Johnson syndrome or SLE
Gastrointestinal: Anorexia, nausea, vomiting, weight loss
Miscellaneous: Hiccups

1% to 10%: Central nervous system: Aggressiveness, mental depression, nightmares, weakness, tiredness

<1%:
Central nervous system: Paranoid psychosis
Dermatologic: Urticaria, exfoliative dermatitis
Hematologic: Agranulocytosis, leukopenia, aplastic anemia, thrombocytopenia, pancytopenia

Overdosage/Toxicology Acute overdosage can cause CNS depression, ataxia, stupor, coma, hypotension; chronic overdose can cause skin rash, confusion, ataxia, proteinuria, hepatic dysfunction, hematuria. Treatment is supportive; hemoperfusion and hemodialysis may be useful.

Stability Protect from high temperature

Mechanism of Action Increases the seizure threshold and suppresses paroxysmal spike-and-wave pattern in absence seizures; depresses nerve transmission in the motor cortex

Pharmacodynamics/Kinetics

Metabolism: Rapidly demethylated in the liver to N-desmethylmethsuximide (active metabolite)
Half-life: 2-4 hours
Time to peak serum concentration: Oral: Within 1-3 hours
Elimination: <1% excreted in urine as unchanged drug

Usual Dosage Oral:
Children: Initial: 10-15 mg/kg/day in 3-4 divided doses; increase weekly up to maximum of 30 mg/kg/day

Adults: 300 mg/day for the first week; may increase by 300 mg/day at weekly intervals up to 1.2 g/day in 2-4 divided doses/day

Monitoring Parameters CBC, hepatic function tests, urinalysis

Reference Range Therapeutic: 10-40 μg/mL (SI: 53-212 μmol/L); Toxic: >40 μg/mL (SI: >212 μmol/L)

Test Interactions ↑ alkaline phosphatase (S); positive Coombs' [direct]; ↓ calcium (S)

Patient Information Take with food; do not discontinue abruptly; may cause drowsiness and impair judgment

Nursing Implications Observe patient for excess sedation

Dosage Forms Capsule: 150 mg, 300 mg

Methyclothiazide *(meth i kloe thye' a zide)*

Brand Names Aquatensen®; Enduron®

Use Management of mild to moderate hypertension; treatment of edema in congestive heart failure and nephrotic syndrome

Pregnancy Risk Factor D

Contraindications Hypersensitivity to methyclothiazide, other thiazides or sulfonamides, or any component, anuria

Warnings/Precautions Use with caution in renal disease, hepatic disease, gout, lupus erythematosus, diabetes mellitus; some products may contain tartrazine

Adverse Reactions

1% to 10%: Endocrine & metabolic: Hypokalemia

<1%:

Cardiovascular: Hypotension

Central nervous system: Drowsiness

Dermatologic: Photosensitivity, rash

Endocrine & metabolic: Fluid and electrolyte imbalances (hypocalcemia, hypomagnesemia, hyponatremia), hyperglycemia

Gastrointestinal: Nausea, vomiting, anorexia

Genitourinary: Uremia

Hematologic: Rarely blood dyscrasias, aplastic anemia, hemolytic anemia, leukopenia, agranulocytosis, thrombocytopenia

Hepatic: Hepatitis

Neuromuscular & skeletal: Paresthesia

Renal: Polyuria, prerenal azotemia

Overdosage/Toxicology Symptoms of overdose include hypermotility, diuresis, lethargy; GI decontamination and supportive care; fluids for hypovolemia

Drug Interactions Increased toxicity/levels of lithium

Mechanism of Action Inhibits sodium reabsorption in the distal tubules causing increased excretion of sodium and water, as well as, potassium and hydrogen ions

Pharmacodynamics/Kinetics

Onset of diuresis: Oral: 2 hours

Peak effect: 6 hours

Duration: ~1 day

Distribution: Crosses the placenta; appears in breast milk

Elimination: Unchanged in urine

Usual Dosage Oral:

Children: 0.05-0.2 mg/kg/day

Adults:

Edema: 2.5-10 mg/day

Hypertension: 2.5-5 mg/day

Monitoring Parameters Blood pressure, fluids, weight loss, serum potassium

Patient Information May be taken with food or milk; take early in day to avoid nocturia; take the last dose of multiple doses no later than 6 PM unless instructed otherwise. A few people who take this medication become more sensitive to sunlight and may experience skin rash, redness, itching, or severe sunburn, especially if sun block SPF ≥15 is not used on exposed skin areas.

Nursing Implications Assess weight, I & O reports daily to determine fluid loss; take blood pressure with patient lying down and standing

Dosage Forms Tablet: 2.5 mg, 5 mg

Methylacetoxyprogesterone see Medroxyprogesterone Acetate on page 677

Methyldopa (meth ill doe' pa)

Brand Names Aldomet®

Use Management of moderate to severe hypertension

Pregnancy Risk Factor B

Contraindications Hypersensitivity to methyldopa or any component; (oral suspension contains benzoic acid and sodium bisulfite; injection contains sodium bisulfite); liver disease, pheochromocytoma

Warnings/Precautions May rarely produce hemolytic anemia and liver disorders; positive Coombs' test occurs in 10% to 20% of patients (perform periodic CBCs); sedation usually transient may occur during initial therapy or whenever the dose is increased. Use with caution in patients with previous liver disease or dysfunction, the active metabolites of methyldopa accumulate in uremia. Patients with impaired renal function may respond to smaller doses. Elderly patients may experience syncope (avoid by giving smaller doses). Tolerance may occur usually between the second and third month of therapy. Adding a diuretic or increasing the dosage of methyldopa frequently restores blood pressure control. Because of its CNS effects, methyldopa is not considered a drug of first choice in the elderly.

Adverse Reactions

>10%: Cardiovascular: Peripheral edema

(Continued)

Methyldopa *(Continued)*

1% to 10%:
Central nervous system: Drug fever, mental depression, anxiety, nightmares, drowsiness, headache
Gastrointestinal: Dry mouth

<1%:
Cardiovascular: Orthostatic hypotension, bradycardia (sinus)
Central nervous system: Fever, chills, sedation, vertigo, depression, memory lapse
Dermatologic: Rash
Endocrine & metabolic: Sodium retention, sexual dysfunction, gynecomastia
Gastrointestinal: Colitis, pancreatitis, diarrhea, nausea, vomiting
Genitourinary: Decreased libido
Hematologic: Thrombocytopenia, hemolytic anemia, positive Coombs' test, leukopenia, transient leukopenia or granulocytopenia
Hepatic: Cholestasis or hepatitis and heptocellular injury, increased liver enzymes, jaundice, cirrhosis
Neuromuscular & skeletal: Paresthesias, weakness
Respiratory: Troubled breathing
Miscellaneous: SLE-like syndrome, hyperprolactinemia, "black" tongue

Overdosage/Toxicology Symptoms of overdose include hypotension, sedation, bradycardia, dizziness, constipation or diarrhea, flatus, nausea, vomiting. Hypotension usually responds to I.V. fluids, Trendelenburg positioning, or vasoconstrictors. Treatment is primarily supportive and symptomatic; can be removed by hemodialysis.

Drug Interactions
Decreased effect: Iron supplements can interact and cause a significant **increase** in blood pressure
Increased toxicity: Lithium → ↑ lithium toxicity; tolbutamide and levodopa effects/toxicity increased

Stability Injectable dosage form is most stable at acid to neutral pH; stability of parenteral admixture at room temperature (25°C): 24 hours; stability of parenteral admixture at refrigeration temperature (4°C): 4 days; standard diluent: 250-500 mg/100 mL D_5W

Mechanism of Action Stimulation of central alpha-adrenergic receptors by a false transmitter that results in a decreased sympathetic outflow to the heart, kidneys, and peripheral vasculature

Pharmacodynamics/Kinetics
Peak hypotensive effect: Oral, parenteral: Within 3-6 hours
Duration: 12-24 hours
Distribution: Crosses the placenta; appears in breast milk
Protein binding: <15%
Metabolism: Intestinally and in the liver
Half-life: 75-80 minutes
End stage renal disease: 6-16 hours
Elimination: Most (85%) metabolites appearing in the urine within 24 hours

Usual Dosage
Children:
Oral: Initial: 10 mg/kg/day in 2-4 divided doses; increase every 2 days as needed to maximum dose of 65 mg/kg/day; do not exceed 3 g/day
I.V.: 5-10 mg/kg/dose every 6-8 hours up to a total dose of 65 mg/kg/24 hours or 3 g/24 hours

Adults:
Oral: Initial: 250 mg 2-3 times/day; increase every 2 days as needed; usual dose 1-1.5 g/day in 2-4 divided doses; maximum dose: 3 g/day
I.V.: 250-1000 mg every 6-8 hours; maximum dose: 1 g every 6 hours

Dosing interval in renal impairment:
Cl_{cr} >50 mL/minute: Administer every 8 hours
Cl_{cr} 10-50 mL/minute: Administer every 8-12 hours
Cl_{cr} <10 mL/minute: Administer every 12-24 hours
Slightly dialyzable (5% to 20%)

Monitoring Parameters Blood pressure, standing and sitting/lying down, CBC, liver enzymes, Coombs' test (direct); blood pressure monitor required during I.V. administration

Test Interactions Methyldopa interferes with the following laboratory tests: urinary uric acid, serum creatinine (alkaline picrate method), AST (colorimetric method), and urinary catecholamines (falsely high levels)

Patient Information May cause transient drowsiness; may cause urine discoloration; notify physician of unexplained prolonged general tiredness, fever, or jaundice; rise slowly from prolonged sitting or lying position

Nursing Implications Transient sedation or depression may be common for first 72 hours of therapy; usually disappears over time; infuse over 30 minutes; assist with ambulation

Dosage Forms
Injection, as methyldopate hydrochloride: 50 mg/mL (5 mL, 10 mL)
Suspension, oral: 250 mg/5 mL (5 mL, 473 mL)
Tablet: 125 mg, 250 mg, 500 mg

Methylene Blue (meth′ i leen)

Brand Names Urolene Blue®

Use Antidote for cyanide poisoning and drug-induced methemoglobinemia, indicator dye, chronic urolithiasis.

    Unlabeled use: Has been used topically (0.1% solutions) in conjunction with polychromatic light to photoinactivate viruses such as herpes simplex; has been used alone or in combination with vitamin C for the management of chronic urolithiasis

Pregnancy Risk Factor C (D if injected intra-amniotically)

Contraindications Renal insufficiency, hypersensitivity to methylene blue or any component, intraspinal injection

Warnings/Precautions Do not inject S.C. or intrathecally; use with caution in young patients and in patients with G-6-PD deficiency; continued use can cause profound anemia

Adverse Reactions
>10%: Discolors urine/feces (blue-green)
1% to 10%: Hematologic: Anemia
<1%:
    Cardiovascular: Hypertension, sweating
    Central nervous system: Dizziness, mental confusion, headache, fever
    Dermatologic: Stains skin
    Gastrointestinal: Nausea, vomiting, abdominal pain
    Genitourinary: Bladder irritation
    Respiratory: Precordial pain

Overdosage/Toxicology Symptoms of overdose include nausea, vomiting, precordial pain, hypertension, methemoglobinemia, cyanosis; overdosage has resulted in methemoglobinemia and cyanosis; treatment is symptomatic and supportive

Mechanism of Action Weak germicide in low concentrations, hastens the conversion of methemoglobin to hemoglobin; has opposite effect at high concentrations by converting ferrous ion of reduced hemoglobin to ferric ion to form methemoglobin; in cyanide toxicity, it combines with cyanide to form cyanmethemoglobin preventing the interference of cyanide with the cytochrome system

Pharmacodynamics/Kinetics
Absorption: Oral: 53% to 97%
Elimination: In bile, feces, and urine

Usual Dosage
Children: NADPH-methemoglobin reductase deficiency: Oral: 1-1.5 mg/kg/day (maximum: 300 mg/day) given with 5-8 mg/kg/day of ascorbic acid
Children and Adults: Methemoglobinemia: I.V.: 1-2 mg/kg or 25-50 mg/m^2 over several minutes; may be repeated in 1 hour if necessary
Adults: Genitourinary antiseptic: Oral: 65-130 mg 3 times/day with a full glass of water (maximum: 390 mg/day)

Administration Administer I.V. undiluted by direct I.V. injection over several minutes

Patient Information May discolor urine and feces blue-green; take oral formulation after meals with a glass of water; skin stains may be removed using a hypochlorite solution

Additional Information Skin stains may be removed using a hypochlorite solution

Dosage Forms
Injection: 10 mg/mL (1 mL, 10 mL)
Tablet: 65 mg

Methylergometrine Maleate see Methylergonovine Maleate on this page

Methylergonovine Maleate (meth ill er goe noe′ veen)

Brand Names Methergine®

Synonyms Methylergometrine Maleate

Use Prevention and treatment of postpartum and postabortion hemorrhage caused by uterine atony or subinvolution

(Continued)

Methylergonovine Maleate (Continued)

Pregnancy Risk Factor C

Contraindications Induction of labor, threatened spontaneous abortion, hypertension, toxemia, hypersensitivity to methylergonovine or any component, pregnancy

Warnings/Precautions Use caution in patients with sepsis, obliterative vascular disease, hepatic, or renal involvement, hypertension; give with extreme caution if using I.V.

Adverse Reactions

>10%:
Cardiovascular: Hypertension
Central nervous system: Headache, seizures
1% to 10%: Gastrointestinal: Nausea, vomiting
<1%:
Cardiovascular: Temporary chest pain, palpitations
Central nervous system: Hallucinations, dizziness
Gastrointestinal: Diarrhea
Local: Thrombophlebitis
Neuromuscular & skeletal: Leg cramps
Otic: Tinnitus
Renal: Hematuria, water intoxication
Respiratory: Dyspnea, nasal congestion
Miscellaneous: Diaphoresis, foul taste

Overdosage/Toxicology Symptoms of overdose include prolonged gangrene, numbness in extremities, acute nausea, vomiting, abdominal pain, respiratory depression, hypotension, seizures; treatment is symptomatic and supportive; hypotension may require pressors; seizures can be treated with benzodiazepines

Mechanism of Action Similar smooth muscle actions as seen with ergotamine; however, it affects primarily uterine smooth muscles producing sustained contractions and thereby shortens the third stage of labor

Pharmacodynamics/Kinetics

Onset of oxytocic effect:
Oral: 5-10 minutes
I.M.: 2-5 minutes
I.V.: Immediately
Duration of action:
Oral: ~3 hours
I.M.: ~3 hours
I.V.: 45 minutes
Absorption: Rapid
Distribution: Rapidly distributed primarily to plasma and extracellular fluid following I.V. administration; distribution to tissues also occurs rapidly
Metabolism: In the liver
Half-life (biphasic):
Initial: 1-5 minutes
Terminal: 30 minutes to 2 hours
Time to peak serum concentration: Within 30 minutes to 3 hours
Elimination: In urine and feces

Usual Dosage Adults:
Oral: 0.2 mg 3-4 times/day for 2-7 days
I.M.: 0.2 mg after delivery of anterior shoulder, after delivery of placenta, or during puerperium; may be repeated as required at intervals of 2-4 hours
I.V.: Same dose as I.M., but should not be routinely administered I.V. because of possibility of inducing sudden hypertension and cerebrovascular accident

Administration Administer over no less than 60 seconds

Patient Information May cause nausea, vomiting, dizziness, increased blood pressure, headache, ringing in the ears, chest pain, or shortness of breath

Nursing Implications Ampuls containing discolored solution should not be used

Dosage Forms
Injection: 0.2 mg/mL (1 mL)
Tablet: 0.2 mg

Methylmorphine see Codeine on page 269

Methylone® see Methylprednisolone on page 724

Methylphenidate Hydrochloride (meth ill fen' i date)

Brand Names Ritalin®; Ritalin-SR®

Use Treatment of attention deficit disorder and symptomatic management of narcolepsy; many unlabeled uses

Restrictions C-II

Pregnancy Risk Factor C

Contraindications Hypersensitivity to methylphenidate or any components; glaucoma, motor tics, Tourette's syndrome, patients with marked agitation, tension, and anxiety

Warnings/Precautions Use with caution in patients with hypertension, dementia (may worsen agitation or confusion) seizures; has high potential for abuse. Treatment should include "drug holidays" or periodic discontinuation in order to assess the patient's requirements and to decrease tolerance and limit suppression of linear growth and weight; it is often useful in treating elderly patients who are discouraged, withdrawn, apathetic, or disinterested in their activities. In particular, it is useful in patients who are starting a rehabilitation program but have resigned themselves to fail; these patients may not have a major depressive disorder; will not improve memory or cognitive function.

Adverse Reactions
>10%:
Cardiovascular: Tachycardia
Central nervous system: Nervousness, insomnia
Gastrointestinal: Anorexia
1% to 10%:
Central nervous system: Dizziness, drowsiness
Gastrointestinal: Stomach pain
Miscellaneous: Hypersensitivity reactions
<1%:
Cardiovascular: Hypertension, hypotension, palpitations, cardiac arrhythmias
Central nervous system: Movement disorders, precipitation of Tourette's syndrome, and toxic psychosis (rare), fever, headache, convulsions
Dermatologic: Rash
Gastrointestinal: Nausea, weight loss, vomiting
Endocrine & metabolic: Growth retardation
Hematologic: Thrombocytopenia, anemia, leukopenia
Ocular: Blurred vision

Overdosage/Toxicology Symptoms of overdose include vomiting, agitation, tremors, hyperpyrexia, muscle twitching, hallucinations, tachycardia, mydriasis, sweating, palpitations. There is no specific antidote for methylphenidate intoxication and the bulk of the treatment is supportive. Hyperactivity and agitation usually respond to reduced sensory input or benzodiazepines, however, with extreme agitation haloperidol (2-5 mg I.M. for adults) may be required. Hyperthermia is best treated with external cooling measures, or when severe or unresponsive, muscle paralysis with pancuronium may be needed. Hypertension is usually transient and generally does not require treatment unless severe. For diastolic blood pressures >110 mm Hg, a nitroprusside infusion should be initiated. Seizures usually respond to diazepam I.V. and/or phenytoin maintenance regimens.

Drug Interactions
Decreased effect: Effects of guanethidine, bretylium may be antagonized by methylphenidate
Increased toxicity: May increase serum concentrations of tricyclic antidepressants, warfarin, phenytoin, phenobarbital, and primidone; MAO inhibitors may potentiate effects of methylphenidate

Mechanism of Action Blocks the reuptake mechanism of dopaminergic neurons; appears to stimulate the cerebral cortex and subcortical structures similar to amphetamines

Pharmacodynamics/Kinetics
Immediate release tablet:
Peak cerebral stimulation effect: Within 2 hours
Duration: 3-6 hours
Sustained release tablet:
Peak effect: Within 4-7 hours
Duration: 8 hours
Absorption: Slow and incomplete from GI tract
Metabolism: In liver via hydroxylation to ritolinic acid
Half-life: 2-4 hours
Elimination: In urine as metabolites and unchanged drug with 45% to 50% excreted in feces via bile

Usual Dosage Oral: (Discontinue periodically to re-evaluate or if no improvement occurs within 1 month)

Children ≥6 years: Attention deficit disorder: Initial: 0.3 mg/kg/dose or 2.5-5 mg/dose given before breakfast and lunch; increase by 0.1 mg/kg/dose or by 5-10 mg/day at weekly intervals; usual dose: 0.5-1 mg/kg/day; maximum dose: 2 mg/kg/day or 60 mg/day

Adults:
Narcolepsy: 10 mg 2-3 times/day, up to 60 mg/day
(Continued)

Methylphenidate Hydrochloride *(Continued)*

Depression: Initial: 2.5 mg every morning before 9 AM; dosage may be increased by 2.5-5 mg every 2-3 days as tolerated to a maximum of 20 mg/day; may be divided (ie, 7 AM and 12 noon), but should not be given after noon; do not use sustained release product

Patient Information Last daily dose should be given several hours before retiring; do not abruptly discontinue; prolonged use may cause dependence

Nursing Implications Do not crush or allow patient to chew sustained release dosage form; to effectively avoid insomnia, dosing should be completed by noon

Dosage Forms
Tablet: 5 mg, 10 mg, 20 mg
Tablet, sustained release: 20 mg

Methylphenobarbital *see* Mephobarbital *on page 687*

Methylphenobarbital *see* Methohexital Sodium *on page 710*

Methylphenyl *see* Oxacillin Sodium *on page 821*

Methylphenylethylhydantoin *see* Mephenytoin *on page 686*

Methylphytyl Napthoquinone *see* Phytonadione *on page 882*

Methylprednisolone (meth ill pred niss' oh lone)
Related Information
Corticosteroids Comparisons *on page 1266-1268*
Brand Names Adlone®; A-Methapred®; depMedalone®; Depoject®; Depo-Medrol®; Depopred®; Duralone®; Medralone®; Medrol®; Methylone®; Solu-Medrol®
Synonyms 6-α-Methylprednisolone; Methylprednisolone Acetate; Methylprednisolone Sodium Succinate
Use Primarily as an anti-inflammatory or immunosuppressant agent in the treatment of a variety of diseases including those of hematologic, allergic, inflammatory, neoplastic, and autoimmune origin
Pregnancy Risk Factor C
Contraindications Serious infections, except septic shock or tuberculous meningitis; known hypersensitivity to methylprednisolone; viral, fungal, or tubercular skin lesions; administration of live virus vaccines
Warnings/Precautions
Use with caution in patients with hyperthyroidism, cirrhosis, nonspecific ulcerative colitis, hypertension, osteoporosis, thromboembolic tendencies, CHF, convulsive disorders, myasthenia gravis, thrombophlebitis, peptic ulcer, diabetes
Acute adrenal insufficiency may occur with abrupt withdrawal after long-term therapy or with stress; young pediatric patients may be more susceptible to adrenal axis suppression from topical therapy
Because of the risk of adverse effects, systemic corticosteroids should be used cautiously in the elderly, in the smallest possible dose, and for the shortest possible time.
Adverse Reactions
>10%:
Central nervous system: Insomnia, nervousness
Gastrointestinal: Increased appetite, indigestion
1% to 10%:
Central nervous system: Epistaxis
Dermatologic: Hirsutism
Endocrine & metabolic: Diabetes mellitus
Neuromuscular & skeletal: Joint pain
Ocular: Cataracts, glaucoma
<1%:
Cardiovascular: Edema, hypertension
Central nervous system: Vertigo, seizures, psychoses, pseudotumor cerebri, headache, mood swings, delirium, hallucinations, euphoria
Dermatologic: Acne, skin atrophy, bruising, hyperpigmentation
Endocrine & metabolic: Cushing's syndrome, pituitary-adrenal axis suppression, growth suppression, glucose intolerance, hypokalemia, alkalosis, amenorrhea, sodium and water retention, hyperglycemia
Gastrointestinal: Peptic ulcer, nausea, vomiting, abdominal distention, ulcerative esophagitis, pancreatitis
Neuromuscular & skeletal: Muscle weakness, osteoporosis, fractures
Miscellaneous: Hypersensitivity reactions
Overdosage/Toxicology Symptoms of overdose include cushingoid appearance (systemic), muscle weakness (systemic), osteoporosis (systemic) all with long-term use only. When consumed in excessive quantities for prolonged

periods, systemic hypercorticism and adrenal suppression may occur; in those cases, discontinuation and withdrawal of the corticosteroid should be done judiciously

Drug Interactions

Decreased effect:

Phenytoin, phenobarbital, rifampin increases clearance of methylprednisolone

Potassium depleting diuretics enhance potassium depletion

Increased toxicity:

Skin test antigens, immunizations increase response and increase potential infections

Methylprednisolone may increase circulating glucose levels → may need adjustments of insulin or oral hypoglycemics

Stability

Intact vials of methylprednisolone sodium succinate should be stored at controlled room temperature

Reconstituted solutions of methylprednisolone sodium succinate should be stored at room temperature (15°C to 30°C) and used within 48 hours

Stability of parenteral admixture at room temperature (25°C) and at refrigeration temperature (4°C): 48 hours

Mechanism of Action Decreases inflammation by suppression of migration of polymorphonuclear leukocytes and reversal of increased capillary permeability

Pharmacodynamics/Kinetics

Time to obtain peak effect and the duration of these effects is dependent upon the route of administration. See table.

Route	Peak Effect	Duration
Oral	1-2 h	30-36 h
I.M.	4-8 d	1-4 wk
Intra-articular	1 wk	1-5 wk

Distribution: V_d: 0.7 L/kg

Half-life: 3-3.5 hours

Methylprednisolone sodium succinate is highly soluble and has a rapid effect by I.M. and I.V. routes; methylprednisolone acetate has a low solubility and has a sustained I.M. effect

Usual Dosage Only sodium succinate salt may be given I.V. Methylprednisolone sodium succinate is highly soluble and has a rapid effect by I.M. and I.V. routes. Methylprednisolone acetate has a low solubility and has a sustained I.M. effect.

Children:

Anti-inflammatory or immunosuppressive: Oral, I.M., I.V. (sodium succinate): 0.12-1.7 mg/kg/day or 5-25 mg/m²/day in divided doses every 6-12 hours

Status asthmaticus: I.V. (sodium succinate): Loading dose: 2 mg/kg/dose, then 0.5-1 mg/kg/dose every 6 hours for up to 5 days

Acute spinal cord injury: I.V. (sodium succinate): 30 mg/kg over 15 minutes followed in 45 minutes by a continuous infusion of 5.4 mg/kg/hour for 23 hours

Lupus nephritis: I.V. (sodium succinate): 30 mg/kg every other day for 6 doses

Topical: Apply sparingly 2-4 times/day

Adults:

Anti-inflammatory or immunosuppressive: Oral: 2-60 mg/day in 1-4 divided doses to start, followed by gradual reduction in dosage to the lowest possible level consistent with maintaining an adequate clinical response

I.M. (sodium succinate): 10-80 mg/day once daily

I.M. (acetate): 40-120 mg every 1-2 weeks

I.V. (sodium succinate): 10-40 mg over a period of several minutes and repeated I.V. or I.M. at intervals depending on clinical response; when high dosages are needed, give 30 mg/kg over a period of 10-20 minutes and may be repeated every 4-6 hours for 48 hours

Status asthmaticus: I.V. (sodium succinate): Loading dose: 2 mg/kg/dose, then 0.5-1 mg/kg/dose every 6 hours for up to 5 days

Lupus nephritis: I.V. (sodium succinate): 1 g/day for 3 days

Slightly dialyzable (5% to 20%)

Administer dose posthemodialysis

Intra-articular/Intralesional:

Intra-articular (acetate): 4-80 mg every 1-5 weeks

Intralesional (acetate): 20-60 mg every 1-5 weeks

Topical: Apply sparingly 2-4 times/day

Administration Methylprednisolone sodium succinate may be administered I.M. or I.V.; I.V. administration may be IVP over one to several minutes or IVPB or continuous I.V. infusion

(Continued)

Methylprednisolone *(Continued)*

Monitoring Parameters Blood pressure, blood glucose, electrolytes

Test Interactions Interferes with skin tests

Patient Information Notify surgeon or dentist before surgical repair; may cause GI upset; take oral formulation with food; notify physician if any sign of infection occurs; avoid abrupt withdrawal when on long-term therapy. Before applying topically, gently wash area to reduce risk of infection; apply a thin film to cleansed area and rub in gently and thoroughly until medication vanishes; avoid exposure to sunlight, severe sunburn may occur

Nursing Implications Give oral formulation with meals to decrease GI upset; **acetate salt should not be given I.V.**

Additional Information
Sodium content of 1 g sodium succinate injection: 2.01 mEq; 53 mg of sodium succinate salt is equivalent to 40 mg of methylprednisolone base
Methylprednisolone acetate: Depo-Medrol®
Methylprednisolone sodium succinate: Solu-Medrol®

Dosage Forms
Injection, as sodium succinate: 40 mg (1 mL, 3 mL); 125 mg (2 mL, 5 mL); 500 mg (1 mL, 4 mL, 8 mL, 20 mL); 1000 mg (1 mL, 8 mL, 50 mL); 2000 mg (30.6 mL)
Injection, as acetate: 20 mg/mL (5 mL, 10 mL); 40 mg/mL (1 mL, 5 mL, 10 mL); 80 mg/mL (1 mL, 5 mL)
Ointment, topical, as acetate: 0.25% (30 g); 1% (30 g)
Tablet: 2 mg, 4 mg, 8 mg, 16 mg, 24 mg, 32 mg
Tablet, dose pack: 4 mg (21s)

6-α-Methylprednisolone *see* Methylprednisolone *on page 724*

Methylprednisolone Acetate *see* Methylprednisolone *on page 724*

Methylprednisolone Sodium Succinate *see* Methylprednisolone *on page 724*

Methylrosaniline Chloride *see* Gentian Violet *on page 503*

Methyltestosterone *(meth ill tess toss' te rone)*

Brand Names Android®; Metandren®; Oreton® Methyl; Testred®; Virilon®

Use
Male: Hypogonadism; delayed puberty; impotence and climacteric symptoms
Female: Palliative treatment of metastatic breast cancer; postpartum breast pain and/or engorgement

Restrictions C-III

Pregnancy Risk Factor X

Contraindications Hypersensitivity to methyltestosterone or any component, known or suspected carcinoma of the breast or the prostate

Warnings/Precautions Use with extreme caution in patients with liver or kidney disease or serious heart disease; may accelerate bone maturation without producing compensatory gain in linear growth

Adverse Reactions
>10%:
Males: Virilism, priapism
Females: Virilism, menstrual problems (amenorrhea), breast soreness
Dermatologic: Edema, acne
1% to 10%:
Males: Prostatic hypertrophy, prostatic carcinoma, impotence, testicular
Females: Hirsutism (increase in pubic hair growth) atrophy
Gastrointestinal: GI irritation, nausea, vomiting
Hepatic: Hepatic dysfunction
<1%:
Endocrine & metabolic: Gynecomastia, amenorrhea, hypercalcemia
Hematologic: Leukopenia, polycythemia
Hepatic: Hepatic necrosis, cholestatic hepatitis
Miscellaneous: Hypersensitivity reactions

Overdosage/Toxicology Abnormal liver function tests

Drug Interactions Decreased effect: Oral anticoagulant effect or insulin requirements may be increased

Mechanism of Action Stimulates receptors in organs and tissues to promote growth and development of male sex organs and maintains secondary sex characteristics in androgen-deficient males

Pharmacodynamics/Kinetics
Absorption: From GI tract and oral mucosa
Metabolism: Hepatic
Elimination: In urine

Usual Dosage Adults (buccal absorption produces twice the androgenic activity of oral tablets):
Male:
  Oral: 10-40 mg/day
  Buccal: 5-25 mg/day

Female:
  Breast pain/engorgement:
    Oral: 80 mg/day for 3-5 days
    Buccal: 40 mg/day for 3-5 days
  Breast cancer:
    Oral: 50-200 mg/day
    Buccal: 25-100 mg/day

Patient Information Men should report overly frequent or persistent penile erections; women should report menstrual irregularities; all patients should report persistent GI distress, diarrhea, or jaundice; buccal tablet should not be chewed or swallowed

Nursing Implications In prepubertal children, perform radiographic examination of the hand and wrist every 6 months to determine the rate of bone maturation and to assess the effect of treatment on the epiphyseal centers

Dosage Forms
Capsule: 10 mg
Tablet: 10 mg, 25 mg
Tablet, buccal: 5 mg, 10 mg

Methysergide Maleate (meth i ser' jide)

Brand Names Sansert®

Use Prophylaxis of vascular headache

Pregnancy Risk Factor X

Contraindications Peripheral vascular disease, severe arteriosclerosis, pulmonary disease, severe hypertension, phlebitis, serious infections, pregnancy

Warnings/Precautions Patients receiving long-term therapy may develop retroperitoneal fibrosis, pleuropulmonary fibrosis and fibrotic thickening of the cardiac valves. Fibrosis occurs rarely when therapy is interrupted for 3-4 weeks every 6 months. Use caution in patients with impairment of renal of hepatic function; some products may contain tartrazine.

Adverse Reactions
>10%:
  Cardiovascular: Postural hypotension, peripheral ischemia
  Central nervous system: Insomnia
  Gastrointestinal: Nausea, vomiting, abdominal pain, diarrhea
1% to 10%:
  Cardiovascular: Peripheral edema, tachycardia, bradycardia
  Dermatologic: Skin rash
  Gastrointestinal: Heartburn
<1%:
  Central nervous system: Insomnia, overstimulation, drowsiness, mild euphoria, lethargy, mental depression, vertigo, unsteadiness, confusion, hyperesthesia, rebound headache may occur if methysergide is discontinued abruptly
  Ocular: Visual disturbances
  Respiratory: Fibrosis

Overdosage/Toxicology Hyperactivity, spasms in limbs, impaired mental function, impaired circulation

Mechanism of Action Ergotamine congener, however actions appear to differ; methysergide has minimal ergotamine-like oxytocic or vasoconstrictive properties, and has significantly greater serotonin-like properties

Pharmacodynamics/Kinetics
Metabolism: Undergoes liver metabolism
Half-life, plasma elimination: ~10 hours
Elimination: Not well defined

Usual Dosage Adults: Oral: 4-8 mg/day with meals; if no improvement is noted after 3 weeks, drug is unlikely to be beneficial; must not be given continuously for longer than 6 months, and a drug-free interval of 3-4 weeks must follow each 6-month course

Patient Information Do not take increased doses per day or for longer time than prescribed; take with meals; may cause drowsiness, impair judgment and coordination; arise slowly from prolonged sitting or lying; notify physician if cold, numbness, painful extremities, chest pain, or painful urination occurs

Nursing Implications Advise patient to make position changes slowly

Dosage Forms Tablet: 2 mg

Meticorten® *see* Prednisone *on page 921*

Metimyd® *see* Sodium Sulfacetamide and Prednisolone Acetate *on page 1019*

Metipranolol Hydrochloride (met i pran' oh lol)

Related Information

Glaucoma Drug Therapy Comparison *on page 1270*

Brand Names OptiPranolol®

Use Agent for lowering intraocular pressure in patients with chronic open-angle glaucoma

Pregnancy Risk Factor C

Contraindications Bronchial asthma, sinus bradycardia, second and third degree A-V block, cardiac failure, cardiogenic shock, hypersensitivity to betaxolol or any component, pregnancy

Warnings/Precautions Use with caution in patients with cardiac failure or diabetes mellitus, asthma, bradycardia, or A-V block

Adverse Reactions

>10%: Ocular: Mild ocular stinging and discomfort, eye irritation

1% to 10%: Ocular: Blurred vision, browache

<1%:

Cardiovascular: Bradycardia, A-V block, congestive heart failure,

Central nervous system: Asthenia

Ocular: Conjunctivitis, blepharitis, tearing, erythema, itching, keratitis, photophobia, decreased corneal sensitivity

Respiratory: Bronchospasm

Overdosage/Toxicology Symptoms of overdose include bradycardia, hypotension, A-V block; sympathomimetics (eg, epinephrine or dopamine), glucagon or a pacemaker can be used to treat the toxic bradycardia, asystole, and/or hypotension; initially, fluids may be the best treatment for toxic hypotension

Mechanism of Action Beta-adrenoceptor-blocking agent; lacks intrinsic sympathomimetic activity and membrane-stabilizing effects and possesses only slight local anesthetic activity; mechanism of action of metipranolol in reducing intraocular pressure appears to be via reduced production of aqueous humor. This effect may be related to a reduction in blood flow to the iris root-ciliary body. It remains unclear if the reduction in intraocular pressure observed with beta-blockers is actually secondary to beta-adrenoceptor blockade.

Pharmacodynamics/Kinetics

Onset of action: ≤30 minutes

Maximum effects: ~2 hours

Duration of action: Intraocular pressure reduction has persisted for 24 hours following ocular instillation

Metabolism: Rapid and complete to deacetyl metipranolol, an active metabolite

Half-life, elimination: ~3 hours

Usual Dosage Ophthalmic: Adults: Instill 1 drop in the affected eye(s) twice daily

Patient Information Intended for twice daily dosing; keep eye open and do not blink for 30 seconds after instillation; wear sunglasses to avoid photophobic discomfort

Nursing Implications Monitor for systemic effect of beta blockade

Dosage Forms Solution, ophthalmic: 0.3% (5 mL, 10 mL)

Metoclopramide (met oh kloe pra' mide)

Related Information

Initial Doses in Selected Antiemetic Regimens *on page 1205*

Brand Names Clopra®; Maxolon®; Octamide®; Reglan®

Use Symptomatic treatment of diabetic gastric stasis, gastroesophageal reflux; prevention of nausea associated with chemotherapy or postsurgery and facilitates intubation of the small intestine

Pregnancy Risk Factor B

Contraindications Hypersensitivity to metoclopramide or any component; GI obstruction, perforation or hemorrhage, pheochromocytoma, history of seizure disorder

Warnings/Precautions Use with caution in patients with Parkinson's disease and in patients with a history of mental illness; dosage and/or frequency of administration should be modified in response to degree of renal impairment; extrapyramidal reactions, depression; may exacerbate seizures in seizure patients; to prevent extrapyramidal reactions, patients may be pretreated with diphenhydramine; elderly are more likely to develop dystonic reactions than younger adults; use lowest recommended doses initially

Adverse Reactions
>10%:
Central nervous system: Weakness, restlessness, drowsiness
Gastrointestinal: Diarrhea
1% to 10%:
Central nervous system: Insomnia, depression
Dermatologic: Skin rash
Endocrine & metabolic: Breast tenderness, prolactin stimulation
Gastrointestinal: Nausea, dry mouth
<1%:
Cardiovascular: Tachycardia, hypertension or hypotension
Central nervous system: Extrapyramidal reactions•, tardive dyskinesia, fatigue, anxiety, agitation
Gastrointestinal: Constipation
Hematologic: Methemoglobinemia
•Note: A recent study suggests the incidence of extrapyramidal reactions due to metoclopramide may be as high as 34% and the incidence appears more often in the elderly

Overdosage/Toxicology Symptoms of overdose include drowsiness, ataxia, extrapyramidal reactions, seizures, methemoglobinemia (in infants); disorientation, muscle hypertonia, irritability, and agitation are common. Metoclopramide often causes extrapyramidal symptoms (eg, dystonic reactions) requiring management with diphenhydramine 1-2 mg/kg (adults) up to a maximum of 50 mg I.M. or I.V. slow push followed by a maintenance dose for 48-72 hours. When these reactions are unresponsive to diphenhydramine, benztropine mesylate I.V. 1-2 mg (adults) may be effective. These agents are generally effective within 2-5 minutes.

Drug Interactions
Decreased effect: Anticholinergic agents antagonize metoclopramide's actions
Increased toxicity: Opiate analgesics → ↑ CNS depression

Stability
Injection is a clear, colorless solution and should be stored at controlled room temperature and protected from freezing; injection is photosensitive and should be protected from light during storage; dilutions do not require light protection if used within 24 hours
Stability of parenteral admixture at room temperature (25°C) and at refrigeration temperature (4°C): 24 hours
Standard diluent: 10-150 mg/50 mL D_5W or NS
Minimum volume: 50 mL D_5W or NS; send 10 mg unmixed to nursing unit
Compatible with diphenhydramine

Mechanism of Action Blocks dopamine receptors in chemoreceptor trigger zone of the CNS; enhances the response to acetylcholine of tissue in upper GI tract causing enhanced motility and accelerated gastric emptying without stimulating gastric, biliary, or pancreatic secretions

Pharmacodynamics/Kinetics
Onset of effect:
Oral: Within 0.5-1 hour
I.V.: Within 1-3 minutes
Duration of therapeutic effect: 1-2 hours, regardless of route administered
Distribution: Crosses the placenta; appears in breast milk
Protein binding: 30%
Half-life, normal renal function: 4-7 hours (may be dose-dependent)
Elimination: Primarily as unchanged drug in urine and feces

Usual Dosage
Children:
Gastroesophageal reflux: Oral: 0.1-0.2 mg/kg/dose up to 4 times/day; efficacy of continuing metoclopramide beyond 12 weeks in reflux has not been determined; total daily dose should not exceed 0.5 mg/kg/day
Gastrointestinal hypomotility (gastroparesis): Oral, I.M., I.V.: 0.1 mg/kg/dose up to 4 times/day, not to exceed 0.5 mg/kg/day
Antiemetic (chemotherapy-induced emesis): I.V.: 1-2 mg/kg 30 minutes before chemotherapy and every 2-4 hours
Facilitate intubation: I.V.:
<6 years: 0.1 mg/kg
6-14 years: 2.5-5 mg

Adults:
Gastroesophageal reflux: Oral: 10-15 mg/dose up to 4 times/day 30 minutes before meals or food and at bedtime; single doses of 20 mg are occasionally needed for provoking situations; efficacy of continuing metoclopramide beyond 12 weeks in reflux has not been determined
Gastrointestinal hypomotility (gastroparesis):
Oral: 10 mg 30 minutes before each meal and at bedtime for 2-8 weeks
(Continued)

Metoclopramide (Continued)

I.V. (for severe symptoms): 10 mg over 1-2 minutes; 10 days of I.V. therapy may be necessary for best response

Antiemetic (chemotherapy-induced emesis): I.V.: 1-2 mg/kg 30 minutes before chemotherapy and every 2-4 hours to every 4-6 hours (and usually given with diphenhydramine 25-50 mg I.V./oral)

Postoperative nausea and vomiting: I.M.: 10 mg near end of surgery; 20 mg doses may be used

Facilitate intubation: I.V.: 10 mg

Elderly:

Gastroesophageal reflux: Oral: 5 mg 4 times/day (30 minutes before meals and at bedtime); increase dose to 10 mg 4 times/day if no response at lower dose

Gastrointestinal hypomotility:

Oral: Initial: 5 mg 30 minutes before meals and at bedtime for 2-8 weeks; increase if necessary to 10 mg doses

I.V.: Initiate at 5 mg over 1-2 minutes; increase to 10 mg if necessary

Postoperative nausea and vomiting: I.M.: 5 mg near end of surgery; may repeat dose if necessary

Dosing adjustment in renal impairment:

Cl_{cr} 10-40 mL/minute: Administer at 50% of normal dose

Cl_{cr} <10 mL/minute: Administer at 25% of normal dose

Not dialyzable (0% to 5%); supplemental dose is not necessary

Administration Lower doses of metoclopramide can be given I.V. push undiluted over 1-2 minutes; parenteral doses of up to 10 mg should be given I.V. push; higher doses to be given IVPB; infuse over at least 15 minutes

Monitoring Parameters Periodic renal function test; monitor for dystonic reactions; monitor for signs of hypoglycemia in patients using insulin and those being treated for gastroparesis; monitor for agitation and irritable confusion

Test Interactions ↑ aminotransferase [ALT (SGPT)/AST (SGOT)] (S), ↑ amylase (S)

Patient Information May impair mental alertness or physical coordination; avoid alcohol, barbiturates or other CNS depressants; take 30 minutes before meals; notify physician if involuntary movements occur

Dosage Forms

Injection: 5 mg/mL (2 mL, 10 mL, 30 mL, 50 mL, 100 mL)

Solution, oral, concentrated: 10 mg/mL (10 mL, 30 mL)

Syrup, sugar free: 5 mg/5 mL (10 mL, 480 mL)

Tablet: 5 mg, 10 mg

Metolazone (me tole' a zone)

Brand Names Mykrox®; Zaroxolyn®

Use Management of mild to moderate hypertension; treatment of edema in congestive heart failure and nephrotic syndrome, impaired renal function

Pregnancy Risk Factor D

Contraindications Hypersensitivity to metolazone or any component, other thiazides, and sulfonamide derivatives; patients with hepatic coma, anuria

Warnings/Precautions Use with caution in renal disease, hepatic disease, gout, lupus erythematosus, diabetes mellitus; some products may contain tartrazine. **Mykrox® is not bioequivalent to Zaroxolyn® and should not be interchanged for one another.**

Adverse Reactions

1% to 10%: Endocrine & metabolic: Hypokalemia

<1%:

Cardiovascular: Hypotension

Central nervous system: Drowsiness

Dermatologic: Photosensitivity, rash

Endocrine & metabolic: Fluid and electrolyte imbalances (hypocalcemia, hypomagnesemia, hyponatremia), hyperglycemia

Gastrointestinal: Nausea, vomiting, anorexia

Genitourinary: Uremia

Hematologic: Rarely blood dyscrasias, aplastic anemia, hemolytic anemia, leukopenia, agranulocytosis, thrombocytopenia

Hepatic: Hepatitis

Neuromuscular & skeletal: Paresthesia

Renal: Prerenal azotemia, polyuria

Overdosage/Toxicology Symptoms of overdose include orthostatic hypotension, dizziness, drowsiness, syncope, hemoconcentration and hemodynamic changes due to plasma volume depletion; treatment is primarily symptomatic and supportive

Drug Interactions
Increased toxicity: Concurrent administration with furosemide may cause excessive volume and electrolyte depletion; increased digitalis glycosides toxicity; increased lithium toxicity

Mechanism of Action Inhibits sodium reabsorption in the distal tubules causing increased excretion of sodium and water, as well as, potassium and hydrogen ions

Pharmacodynamics/Kinetics Same for all routes:
Onset of diuresis: Within 60 minutes
Duration: 12-24 hours
Absorption: Oral: Incomplete
Distribution: Crosses the placenta; appears in breast milk
Protein binding: 95%
Bioavailability: Mykrox® reportedly has highest
Half-life: 6-20 hours, renal function dependent
Elimination: Enterohepatic recycling; 80% to 95% excreted in urine

Usual Dosage Oral:
Children: 0.2-0.4 mg/kg/day divided every 12-24 hours
Adults:
Edema: 5-20 mg/dose every 24 hours
Hypertension: 2.5-5 mg/dose every 24 hours
Hypertension (Mykrox®): 0.5 mg/day; if response is not adequate, increase dose to maximum of 1 mg/day

Not dialyzable (0% to 5%) via hemo- or peritoneal dialysis; supplemental dose is not necessary

Monitoring Parameters Serum electrolytes (potassium, sodium, chloride, bicarbonate), renal function, blood pressure (standing, sitting/supine)

Patient Information May be taken with food or milk; take early in day to avoid nocturia; take the last dose of multiple doses no later than 6 PM unless instructed otherwise. A few people who take this medication become more sensitive to sunlight and may experience skin rash, redness, itching, or severe sunburn, especially if sun block SPF ≥15 is not used on exposed skin areas.

Nursing Implications Assess weight, I & O reports daily to determine fluid loss; take blood pressure with patient lying down and standing

Dosage Forms Tablet:
Zaroxolyn®: 2.5 mg, 5 mg, 10 mg
Mykrox®: 0.5 mg

Metoprolol Tartrate (me toe′ proe lole)
Related Information
Beta-Blockers Comparison *on page 1257-1259*
Brand Names Lopressor®; Toprol XL®
Use Treatment of hypertension and angina pectoris; prevention of myocardial infarction, atrial fibrillation, flutter, symptomatic treatment of hypertrophic subaortic stenosis
Unlabeled use: Treatment of ventricular arrhythmias, atrial ectopy, migraine prophylaxis, essential tremor, aggressive behavior
Pregnancy Risk Factor B
Contraindications Hypersensitivity to beta-blocking agents, uncompensated congestive heart failure; cardiogenic shock; bradycardia (heart rate <45 bpm) or heart block; sinus node dysfunction; A-V conduction abnormalities, systolic blood pressure <100 mm Hg; diabetes mellitus. Although metoprolol primarily blocks beta$_1$-receptors, high doses can result in beta$_2$-receptor blockage; therefore, use with caution in elderly with bronchospastic lung disease.
Warnings/Precautions Use with caution in patients with inadequate myocardial function; those undergoing anesthesia, patients with CHF, myasthenia gravis, impaired hepatic or renal function, severe peripheral vascular disease, bronchospastic disease, diabetes mellitus or hyperthyroidism. Abrupt withdrawal of the drug should be avoided (may result in an exaggerated cardiac beta-adrenergic response, tachycardia, hypertension, ischemia, angina, myocardial infarction, and sudden death), drug should be discontinued over 1-2 weeks; do not use in pregnant or nursing women; may potentiate hypoglycemia in a diabetic patient and mask signs and symptoms; sweating will continue.
Adverse Reactions
>10%: Central nervous system: Mental depression, tiredness, weakness, dizziness
1% to 10%:
Cardiovascular: Bradycardia, irregular heartbeat, reduced peripheral circulation
Gastrointestinal: Heartburn
Respiratory: Wheezing
(Continued)

Metoprolol Tartrate *(Continued)*

<1%:

   Cardiovascular: Chest pain, heart failure, Raynaud's phenomena

   Central nervous system: Insomnia, nightmares, confusion, headache

   Dermatologic: Rash, itching

   Endocrine & metabolic: Decreased sexual activity

   Gastrointestinal: Constipation, nausea, vomiting, stomach discomfort

   Genitourinary: Impotence

   Miscellaneous: Cold extremities

Overdosage/Toxicology Symptoms of intoxication include cardiac disturbances, CNS toxicity, bronchospasm, hypoglycemia and hyperkalemia. The most common cardiac symptoms include hypotension and bradycardia; atrioventricular block, intraventricular conduction disturbances, cardiogenic shock, and asystole may occur with severe overdose, especially with membrane-depressant drugs (eg, propranolol); CNS effects include convulsions, coma, and respiratory arrest.

Treatment includes symptomatic treatment of seizures, hypotension, hyperkalemia and hypoglycemia; bradycardia and hypotension resistant to atropine, isoproterenol or pacing, may respond to glucagon; wide QRS defects caused by the membrane-depressant poisoning may respond to hypertonic sodium bicarbonate; repeat-dose charcoal, hemoperfusion, or hemodialysis may be helpful in removal of only those beta-blockers with a small V_d, long half-life or low intrinsic clearance (acebutolol, atenolol, nadolol, sotalol)

Drug Interactions

Decreased effect of beta-blockers with aluminum salts, barbiturates, calcium salts, cholestyramine, colestipol, NSAIDs, penicillins (ampicillin), rifampin, salicylates and sulfinpyrazone due to decreased bioavailability and plasma levels

Beta-blockers may decrease the effect of sulfonylureas

Increased effect/toxicity of beta-blockers with calcium blockers (diltiazem, felodipine, nicardipine), contraceptives, flecainide, haloperidol (propranolol, hypotensive effects), H_2 antagonists (metoprolol, propranolol only by cimetidine, possibly ranitidine), hydralazine (metoprolol, propranolol), loop diuretics (propranolol, not atenolol), MAO inhibitors (metoprolol, nadolol, bradycardia), phenothiazines (propranolol), propafenone (metoprolol, propranolol), quinidine (in extensive metabolizers), ciprofloxacin, thyroid hormones (metoprolol, propranolol, when hypothyroid patient is converted to euthyroid state)

Beta-blockers may increase the effect/toxicity of flecainide, haloperidol (hypotensive effects), hydralazine, phenothiazines, acetaminophen, anticoagulants (propranolol, warfarin), benzodiazepines (not atenolol), clonidine (hypertensive crisis after or during withdrawal of either agent), epinephrine (initial hypertensive episode followed by bradycardia), nifedipine and verapamil lidocaine, ergots (peripheral ischemia), prazosin (postural hypotension)

Beta-blockers may affect the action or levels of ethanol, disopyramide, nondepolarizing muscle relaxants and theophylline although the effects are difficult to predict

Mechanism of Action Selective inhibitor of beta$_1$-adrenergic receptors; competitively blocks beta$_1$-receptors, with little or no effect on beta$_2$-receptors at doses <100 mg; does not exhibit any membrane stabilizing or intrinsic sympathomimetic activity

Pharmacodynamics/Kinetics

Peak antihypertensive effect: Oral: Within 1.5-4 hours

Duration: 10-20 hours

Absorption: 95%

Protein binding: 8%

Metabolism: Significant first-pass metabolism; extensively metabolized in the liver

Bioavailability: Oral: 40% to 50%

Half-life: 3-4 hours

   End stage renal disease: 2.5-4.5 hours

Elimination: In urine (3% to 10% as unchanged drug)

Usual Dosage

Children: Oral: 1-5 mg/kg/24 hours divided twice daily; allow 3 days between dose adjustments

Adults:

   Oral: 100-450 mg/day in 2-3 divided doses, begin with 50 mg twice daily and increase doses at weekly intervals to desired effect

   I.V.: 5 mg every 2 minutes for 3 doses in early treatment of myocardial infarction; thereafter give 50 mg orally every 6 hours 15 minutes after last I.V. dose and continue for 48 hours; then administer a maintenance dose of 100 mg twice daily

Elderly: Oral: Initial: 25 mg/day; usual range: 25-300 mg/day

Administer dose posthemodialysis or administer 50 mg supplemental dose supplemental dose is not necessary following peritoneal dialysis

Dosing adjustment/comments in hepatic disease: Reduced dose probably necessary

Monitoring Parameters Blood pressure, apical and radial pulses, fluid I & O, daily weight, respirations, mental status, and circulation in extremities before and during therapy

Patient Information Do not discontinue medication abruptly, sudden stopping of medication may precipitate or cause angina; consult pharmacist or physician before taking with other adrenergic drugs (eg, cold medications); use with caution while driving or performing tasks requiring alertness; may mask signs of hypoglycemia in diabetics; may be taken without regard to meals

Dosage Forms
Injection: 1 mg/mL (5 mL)
Tablet: 50 mg, 100 mg
Tablet, sustained release: 50 mg, 100 mg, 200 mg

Metreton® see Prednisolone on page 919

Metrodin® see Urofollitropin on page 1140

MetroGel® see Metronidazole on this page

Metro I.V.® see Metronidazole on this page

Metronidazole (me troe ni' da zole)
Related Information
Antimicrobial Drugs of Choice on page 1298-1302
Brand Names Flagyl®; MetroGel®; Metro I.V.®; Protostat®
Use Treatment of susceptible anaerobic bacterial and protozoal infections in the following conditions: amebiasis, symptomatic and asymptomatic trichomoniasis; skin and skin structure infections; CNS infections; intra-abdominal infections; systemic anaerobic infections; topically for the treatment of acne rosacea; treatment of antibiotic-associated pseudomembranous colitis (AAPC)
Pregnancy Risk Factor B
Contraindications Hypersensitivity to metronidazole or any component, 1st trimester of pregnancy
Warnings/Precautions Use with caution in patients with liver impairment, blood dyscrasias; history of seizures, congestive heart failure, or other sodium retaining states; reduce dosage in patients with severe liver impairment, CNS disease, and severe renal failure (Cl_{cr} <10 mL/minute). Has been shown to be carcinogenic in rodents.
Adverse Reactions
>10%:
   Central nervous system: Dizziness, headache
   Gastrointestinal: Nausea, diarrhea, loss of appetite, vomiting
1% to 10%:
   Central nervous system: Seizures
   Neuromuscular & skeletal: Peripheral neuropathy
<1%:
   Central nervous system: Ataxia
   Endocrine & metabolic: Disulfiram-type reaction with alcohol
   Gastrointestinal: Pancreatitis, dry mouth, metallic taste
   Genitourinary: Vaginal candidiasis
   Hematologic: Leukopenia
   Local: Thrombophlebitis
   Miscellaneous: Hypersensitivity, change in taste sensation, furry tongue, dark urine
Overdosage/Toxicology Symptoms of overdose include nausea, vomiting, ataxia, seizures, peripheral neuropathy; treatment is symptomatic and supportive
Drug Interactions
Decreased effect: Phenytoin, phenobarbital →↓ metronidazole half-life
Increased toxicity: Alcohol, disulfiram → disulfiram-like reactions; warfarin increases PT prolongation
Stability
Metronidazole injection should be stored at 15°C to 30°C and protected from light
Product may be refrigerated but crystals may form; crystals redissolve on warming to room temperature
Prolonged exposure to light will cause a darkening of the product. However, short-term exposure to normal room light does not adversely affect metronidazole stability. Direct sunlight should be avoided.
Stability of parenteral admixture at room temperature (25°C): Out of overwrap stability: 30 days
(Continued)

Metronidazole *(Continued)*

Standard diluent: 500 mg/100 mL NS

Mechanism of Action Reduced to a product which interacts with DNA to cause a loss of helical DNA structure and strand breakage resulting in inhibition of protein synthesis and cell death in susceptible organisms

Pharmacodynamics/Kinetics

Absorption:

Oral: Well absorbed

Topical: Concentrations achieved systemically after application of 1 g topically are 10 times less than those obtained after a 250 mg oral dose

Time to peak serum concentration: Within 1-2 hours

Distribution: Excreted in breast milk

Relative diffusion of antimicrobial agents from blood into cerebrospinal fluid (CSF): Adequate with or without inflammation (exceeds usual MICs)

Ratio of CSF to blood level (%):

Normal meninges: 16-43

Inflamed meninges: 100

Protein binding: <20%

Metabolism: 30% to 60% in the liver

Half-life:

Neonates: 25-75 hours

Others: 6-8 hours, increases with hepatic impairment

End stage renal disease: 21 hours

Elimination: Final excretion via the urine (20% as unchanged drug) and feces (6% to 15%)

Usual Dosage

Neonates: Anaerobic infections: Oral, I.V.:

0-4 weeks: <1200 g: 7.5 mg/kg/dose every 48 hours

Postnatal age <7 days:

1200-2000 g: 7.5 mg/kg/dose every 24 hours

>2000 g: 7.5 mg/kg/dose every 12 hours

Postnatal age >7 days:

1200-2000 g: 7.5 mg/kg/dose every 12 hours

>2000 g: 15 mg/kg/dose every 12 hours

Infants and Children:

Amebiasis: Oral: 35-50 mg/kg/day in divided doses every 8 hours for 10 days

Trichomoniasis: Oral: 15-30 mg/kg/day in divided doses every 8 hours for 7 days

Anaerobic infections:

Oral: 15-35 mg/kg/day in divided doses every 8 hours

I.V.: 30 mg/kg/day in divided doses every 6 hours

Clostridium difficile (antibiotic-associated colitis): Oral: 20 mg/kg/day divided every 6 hours

Maximum dose: 2 g/day

Adults:

Amebiasis: Oral: 500-750 mg every 8 hours for 5-10 days

Trichomoniasis: Oral: 250 mg every 8 hours for 7 days or 2 g as a single dose

Anaerobic infections: Oral, I.V.: 500 mg every 6-8 hours, not to exceed 4 g/day

Antibiotic-associated pseudomembranous colitis: Oral: 250-500 mg 3-4 times/day for 10-14 days

Elderly: Use lower end of dosing recommendations for adults, do not give as a single dose

Topical (acne rosacea therapy): Apply and rub a thin film twice daily, morning and evening, to entire affected areas after washing. Significant therapeutic results should be noticed within 3 weeks. Clinical studies have demonstrated continuing improvement through 9 weeks of therapy.

Dosing adjustment in renal impairment: Cl_{cr} <10 mL/minute: Administer at 50% of dose or every 12 hours

Extensively removed by hemodialysis and peritoneal dialysis (50% to 100%); administer dose post hemodialysis; during peritoneal dialysis and continuous arterio-venous or veno-venous hemofiltration (CAVH/CAVHD), dose as for Cl_{cr} <10 mL/minute

Dosing adjustment/comments in hepatic disease: Unchanged in mild liver disease; reduce dosage in severe liver disease

Test Interactions May cause falsely decreased AST and ALT levels

Patient Information Urine may be discolored to a dark or reddish-brown; do not take alcohol for at least 24 hours after the last dose; avoid beverage alcohol or any topical products containing alcohol during therapy; may cause metallic taste; may be taken with food to minimize stomach upset; notify physician if numbness or tingling in extremities; avoid contact of the topical product with the eyes; cleanse areas to be treated well before application

Nursing Implications No Antabuse®-like reactions have been reported after **topical** application, although metronidazole can be detected in the blood; avoid contact between the drug and aluminum in the infusion set

Additional Information Sodium content of 500 mg (I.V.): 322 mg (14 mEq)

Dosage Forms
Gel, topical: 0.75% [7.5 mg/mL] (30 g)
Injection, ready to use: 5 mg/mL (100 mL)
Powder for injection, as hydrochloride: 500 mg
Tablet: 250 mg, 500 mg

Metyrosine (me tye' roe seen)
Brand Names Demser®
Synonyms AMPT; OGMT
Use Short-term management of pheochromocytoma before surgery, long-term management when surgery is contraindicated or when malignant
Pregnancy Risk Factor C
Contraindications Hypertension of unknown etiology, known hypersensitivity to metyrosine
Warnings/Precautions Maintain fluid volume during and after surgery; use with caution in patients with impaired renal or hepatic function
Adverse Reactions
>10%:
Central nervous system: Drowsiness, extrapyramidal symptoms
Gastrointestinal: Diarrhea
1% to 10%:
Endocrine & metabolic: Impotence, galactorrhea, swelling of breasts
Gastrointestinal: Nausea, vomiting
Respiratory: Dry mouth, stuffy nose
<1%:
Central nervous system: Depression, hallucinations, disorientation
Dermatologic: Urticaria
Hematologic: Anemia, eosinophilia
Renal: Hematuria, urinary problems
Miscellaneous: Parkinsonism, swelling of lower extremities, hyperstimulation after withdrawal
Overdosage/Toxicology Signs of overdose include sedation, fatigue, tremor; reducing dose or discontinuation of therapy usually results in resolution of symptoms
Mechanism of Action Blocks the rate-limiting step in the biosynthetic pathway of catecholamines. It is a tyrosine hydroxylase inhibitor, blocking the conversion of tyrosine to dihydroxyphenylalanine. This inhibition results in decreased levels of endogenous catecholamines. Catecholamine biosynthesis is reduced by 35% to 80% in patients treated with metyrosine 1-4 g/day.
Pharmacodynamics/Kinetics
Half-life: 7.2 hours
Elimination: Following oral absorption, excreted primarily unchanged in urine
Usual Dosage Children >12 years and Adults: Oral: Initial: 250 mg 4 times/day, increased by 250-500 mg/day up to 4 g/day; maintenance: 2-3 g/day in 4 divided doses; for preoperative preparation, give optimum effective dosage for 5-7 days

Dosing adjustment in renal impairment: Adjustment should be considered
Patient Information Take plenty of fluids each day; may cause drowsiness, impair coordination and judgment; notify physician if drooling, tremors, speech difficulty, or diarrhea occurs; avoid alcohol and central nervous system depressants
Dosage Forms Capsule: 250 mg

Mevacor® see Lovastatin on page 652

Mevinolin see Lovastatin on page 652

Mexiletine (mex' i le teen)
Related Information
Antiarrhythmic Drugs on page 1246-1248
Brand Names Mexitil®
Use Management of serious ventricular arrhythmias; suppression of PVCs
Unlabeled use: Diabetic neuropathy
Pregnancy Risk Factor C
(Continued)

Mexiletine (Continued)

Contraindications Cardiogenic shock, second or third degree heart block, hypersensitivity to mexiletine or any component

Warnings/Precautions Exercise extreme caution in patients with pre-existing sinus node dysfunction; mexiletine can worsen CHF, bradycardias, and other arrhythmias; mexiletine, like other antiarrhythmic agents, is proarrhythmic; CAST study indicates a trend toward increased mortality with antiarrhythmics in the face of cardiac disease (myocardial infarction); elevation of AST/ALT; hepatic necrosis reported; leukopenia, agranulocytopenia, and thrombocytopenia; seizures; alterations in urinary pH may change urinary excretion; electrolyte disturbances (hypokalemia, hyperkalemia, etc) after drug response

Adverse Reactions

>10%:
  Central nervous system: Lightheadedness, dizziness, nervousness
  Neuromuscular & skeletal: Trembling, unsteady gait

1% to 10%:
  Cardiovascular: Chest pain, premature ventricular contractions
  Central nervous system: Confusion, headache, numbness of fingers or toes, insomnia
  Dermatologic: Rash
  Gastrointestinal: Constipation or diarrhea
  Hepatic: Increased LFTs
  Neuromuscular & skeletal: Weakness
  Ocular: Blurred vision
  Otic: Tinnitus
  Respiratory: Shortness of breath

<1%:
  Hematologic: Leukopenia, agranulocytosis, thrombocytopenia, positive antinuclear antibody
  Ocular: Diplopia

Overdosage/Toxicology Has a narrow therapeutic index and severe toxicity may occur slightly above the therapeutic range, especially with other antiarrhythmic drugs; acute ingestion of twice the daily therapeutic dose is potentially life-threatening; symptoms of overdose includes sedation, confusion, coma, seizures, respiratory arrest and cardiac toxicity (sinus arrest, A-V block, asystole, and hypotension); the QRS and Q-T intervals are usually normal, although they may be prolonged after massive overdose; other effects include dizziness, paresthesias, tremor, ataxia, and GI disturbance; Treatment is supportive, using conventional therapies (fluids, positioning, vasopressors, antiarrhythmics, anticonvulsants); sodium bicarbonate may reverse the QRS prolongation, bradyarrhythmias and hypotension; enhanced elimination with dialysis, hemoperfusion or repeat charcoal is not effective.

Drug Interactions
  Decreased plasma levels: Phenobarbital, phenytoin, rifampin, and other hepatic enzyme inducers, cimetidine and drugs which make the urine acidic
  Increased effect: Allopurinol
  Increased toxicity/levels of caffeine and theophylline

Mechanism of Action Class IB antiarrhythmic, structurally related to lidocaine, which inhibits inward sodium current, decreases rate of rise of phase 0, increases effective refractory period/action potential duration ratio

Pharmacodynamics/Kinetics
  Absorption: Elderly have a slightly slower rate of absorption but extent of absorption is the same as young adults
  Distribution: V_d: 5-7 L/kg
  Protein binding: 50% to 70%
  Metabolism: Extensive first-pass metabolism; extensively metabolized in liver (some minor active metabolites)
  Bioavailability: Oral: 88%
  Half-life: Adults: 10-14 hours (average: 14.4 hours elderly, 12 hours in younger adults); increase in half-life with hepatic or heart failure
  Time to peak: Peak levels attained in 2-3 hours
  Elimination: 10% to 15% excreted unchanged in urine; urinary acidification increases excretion, alkalinization decreases excretion

Usual Dosage Adults: Oral: Initial: 200 mg every 8 hours (may load with 400 mg if necessary); adjust dose every 2-3 days; usual dose: 200-300 mg every 8 hours; maximum dose: 1.2 g/day (some patients respond to every 12-hour dosing); patients with hepatic impairment or CHF may require dose reduction; when switching from another antiarrhythmic, initiate a 200 mg dose 6-12 hours after stopping former agents, 3-6 hours after stopping procainamide

Administration Administer around-the-clock rather than 3 times/day to promote less variation in peak and trough serum levels

Reference Range Therapeutic range: 0.5-2 µg/mL; potentially toxic: >2 µg/mL

Test Interactions Abnormal liver function test, positive ANA, thrombocytopenia

Patient Information Take with food or antacid; notify physician of severe or persistent abdominal pain, nausea, vomiting, yellowing of eyes or skin, pale stools, dark urine, or if persistent fever, sore throat, bleeding, or bruising occurs

Dosage Forms Capsule: 150 mg, 200 mg, 250 mg

Mexitil® see Mexiletine on page 735

Mezlin® see Mezlocillin Sodium on this page

Mezlocillin Sodium (mez loe sill' in)

Related Information

Antimicrobial Drugs of Choice on page 1298-1302

Brand Names Mezlin®

Use Treatment of infections caused by susceptible gram-negative aerobic bacilli (*Klebsiella*, *Proteus*, *Escherichia coli*, *Enterobacter*, *Pseudomonas aeruginosa*, *Serratia*) involving the skin and skin structure, bone and joint, respiratory tract, urinary tract, gastrointestinal tract, as well as, septicemia

Pregnancy Risk Factor B

Contraindications Hypersensitivity to mezlocillin, any component, or penicillins

Warnings/Precautions If bleeding occurs during therapy, mezlocillin should be discontinued; dosage modification required in patients with impaired renal function; use with caution in patients with renal impairment or biliary obstruction, or history of allergy to cephalosporins

Adverse Reactions

1% to 10%: Gastrointestinal: Nausea, diarrhea

<1%:

Central nervous system: Fever, seizures, dizziness, headache

Dermatologic: Rash, exfoliative dermatitis

Endocrine & metabolic: Hypokalemia, hypernatremia

Gastrointestinal: Vomiting

Hematologic: Eosinophilia, leukopenia, neutropenia, thrombocytopenia, agranulocytosis, hemolytic anemia, prolonged bleeding time, positive Coombs' [direct]

Hepatic: Hepatotoxicity, elevated liver enzymes

Renal: Hematuria, elevated serum creatinine and BUN, interstitial nephritis

Miscellaneous: Serum sickness-like reactions

Overdosage/Toxicology Symptoms of penicillin overdose include neuromuscular hypersensitivity (agitation, hallucinations, asterixis, encephalopathy, confusion, and seizures) and electrolyte imbalance with potassium or sodium salts, especially in renal failure; hemodialysis may be helpful to aid in the removal of the drug from the blood, otherwise most treatment is supportive or symptom directed

Drug Interactions Aminoglycosides (synergy), probenecid (decreased clearance), vecuronium (increased duration of neuromuscular blockade), heparin (increased risk of bleeding)

Stability Reconstituted solution is stable for 48 hours at room temperature and 7 days when refrigerated; for I.V. infusion in NS or D_5W solution is stable for 48 hours at room temperature, 7 days when refrigerated or 28 days when frozen; after freezing, thawed solution is stable for 48 hours at room temperature or 7 days when refrigerated; if precipitation occurs under refrigeration, warm in water bath (37°C) for 20 minutes and shake well

Mechanism of Action Interferes with bacterial cell wall synthesis during active multiplication causing cell death and resultant bactericidal activity against susceptible bacteria

Pharmacodynamics/Kinetics

Absorption: I.M.: 63%

Distribution: Into bile, heart, peritoneal fluid, sputum, bone; does not cross the blood-brain barrier well unless meninges are inflamed; crosses the placenta; distributes into breast milk at low concentrations

Protein binding: 30%

Metabolism: Minimal

Half-life: Dose dependent:

Neonates:

<7 days: 3.7-4.4 hours

>7 days: 2.5 hours

Children 2-19 years: 0.9 hour

Adults: 50-70 minutes, increased in renal impairment

Time to peak serum concentration:

I.M.: 45-90 minutes after administration

I.V. infusion: Within 5 minutes

Elimination: Principally as unchanged drug in urine, also excreted via bile

(Continued)

Mezlocillin Sodium *(Continued)*

Usual Dosage I.M., I.V.:

Neonates:
Postnatal age <7 days: 75 mg/kg/dose every 12 hours
Postnatal age >7 days: 75 mg/kg/dose every 8 hours

Children: 200-300 mg/kg/day divided every 4-6 hours; maximum: 24 g/day

Adults:
Uncomplicated urinary tract infection: 1.5-2 g every 6 hours
Serious infections: 3-4 g every 4-6 hours

Dosing interval in renal impairment:
Cl_{cr} 10-30 mL/minute: Administer every 6-8 hours
Cl_{cr} <10 mL/minute: Administer every 8 hours
Moderately dialyzable (20% to 50%)

Dosing adjustment in hepatic impairment: Reduce dose by 50%

Administration Administer around-the-clock rather than 4 times/day, 3 times/day, etc, (ie, 12-6-12-6, not 9-1-5-9) to promote less variation in peak and trough serum levels; administer I.M. injections in large muscle mass, not more than 2 g/injection. I.M. injections given over 12-15 seconds will be less painful

Test Interactions False-positive direct Coombs'; false-positive urinary protein

Nursing Implications Dosage modification is required in patients with impaired renal function

Additional Information Sodium content of 1 g: 42.6 mg (1.85 mEq)

Dosage Forms Powder for injection: 1 g, 2 g, 3 g, 4 g, 20 g

Miacalcin® *see* Calcitonin *on page 158*

Micatin® [OTC] *see* Miconazole *on this page*

Miconazole *(mi kon' a zole)*

Related Information
Antifungal Agents *on page 1253-1254*

Brand Names Micatin® [OTC]; Monistat™; Monistat-Derm™; Monistat i.v.™

Synonyms Miconazole Nitrate

Use
I.V.: Treatment of severe systemic fungal infections and fungal meningitis that are refractory to standard treatment
Topical: Treatment of vulvovaginal candidiasis and a variety of skin and mucous membrane fungal infections

Pregnancy Risk Factor C

Contraindications Hypersensitivity to miconazole, fluconazole, ketoconazole, or polyoxyl 35 castor oil or any component

Warnings/Precautions Administer I.V. with caution to patients with hepatic insufficiency; the safety of miconazole in patients <1 year of age has not been established; cardiorespiratory and anaphylaxis have occurred with excessively rapid administration

Adverse Reactions
>10%:
Central nervous system: Fever, chills
Dermatologic: Skin rash, itching
Gastrointestinal: Anorexia, diarrhea, nausea, vomiting
Local: Pain at injection site
1% to 10%: Hematologic: Anemia, thrombocytopenia
<1%:
Cardiovascular: Flushing of face or skin
Central nervous system: Drowsiness,

Overdosage/Toxicology Symptoms of overdose include nausea, vomiting, drowsiness; following GI decontamination, supportive care only

Drug Interactions Warfarin (increased anticoagulant effect), oral sulfonylureas, amphotericin B (decreased antifungal effect of both agents), phenytoin (levels may be increased)

Stability Protect from heat; darkening of solution indicates deterioration; stability of parenteral admixture at room temperature (25°C): 2 days

Mechanism of Action Inhibits biosynthesis of ergosterol, damaging the fungal cell wall membrane, which increases permeability causing leaking of nutrients

Pharmacodynamics/Kinetics
Protein binding: 91% to 93%
Metabolism: In the liver

Half-life, multiphasic:
  Initial: 40 minutes
  Secondary: 126 minutes
  Terminal phase: 24 hours
Elimination: ~50% excreted in feces and <1% in urine as unchanged drug

Usual Dosage
Children:
  I.V.: 20-40 mg/kg/day divided every 8 hours
  Topical: Apply twice daily for up to 1 month
Adults:
  Topical: Apply twice daily for up to 1 month
  I.T.: 20 mg every 1-2 days
  I.V.: Initial: 200 mg, then 1.2-3.6 g/day divided every 8 hours for up to 20 weeks
  Bladder candidal infections: 200 mg diluted solution instilled in the bladder
  Vaginal: Insert contents of 1 applicator of vaginal cream (100 mg) or 100 mg
    suppository at bedtime for 7 days, or 200 mg suppository at bedtime for 3
    days

Not dialyzable (0% to 5%)

Administration Administer I.V. dose over 2 hours; administer around-the-clock to promote less variation in peak and trough serum levels

Test Interactions ↑ protein

Patient Information Avoid contact with the eyes; for vaginal product, insert high into vagina and complete full course of therapy; notify physician if itching or burning occur; refrain from intercourse to prevent reinfection

Additional Information
Miconazole: Monistat i.v.™
Miconazole nitrate: Micatin®, Monistat™, Monistat-Derm™

Dosage Forms
Cream:
  Topical, as nitrate: 2% [20 mg/g] (15 g, 30 g, 85 g)
  Vaginal, as nitrate: 2% [20 mg/g] (45 g is equivalent to 7 doses)
Injection: 1% [10 mg/mL] (20 mL)
Lotion, as nitrate: 2% [20 mg/g] (30 mL, 60 mL)
Powder, topical: 2% [20 mg/g] (45 g, 90 g)
Spray, topical: 2% [20 mg/g] (105 mL)
Suppository, vaginal, as nitrate: 100 mg (7s); 200 mg (3s)

Miconazole Nitrate see Miconazole on previous page

MICRhoGAM™ see Rho(D) Immune Globulin on page 978

Microfibrillar Collagen Hemostat (mi kro fi' bri lar kol' la jen hee' moe stat)

Brand Names Avitene®

Synonyms Collagen; MCH

Use Adjunct to hemostasis when control of bleeding by ligature is ineffective or impractical

Pregnancy Risk Factor C

Contraindications Closure of skin incisions, contaminated wounds

Warnings/Precautions Fragments of MCH may pass through filters of blood scavenging systems; avoid reintroduction of blood from operative sites treated with MCH; after several minutes remove excess material

Adverse Reactions
1% to 10%:
  Local: Adhesion formation
  Miscellaneous: Potentiation of infection, allergic reaction

Mechanism of Action Microfibrillar collagen hemostat is an absorbable topical hemostatic agent prepared from purified bovine corium collagen and shredded into fibrils. Physically, microfibrillar collagen hemostat yields a large surface area. Chemically, it is collagen with hydrochloric acid noncovalently bound to some of the available amino groups in the collagen molecules. When in contact with a bleeding surface, microfibrillar collagen hemostat attracts platelets which adhere to its fibrils and undergo the release phenomenon. This triggers aggregation of the platelets into thrombi in the interstices of the fibrous mass, initiating the formation of a physiologic platelet plug.

Pharmacodynamics/Kinetics Absorption: By animal tissue in 3 months

Usual Dosage Apply dry directly to source of bleeding

Dosage Forms
Fibrous: 1 g, 5 g
Nonwoven web: 70 mm x 70 mm x 1 mm; 70 mm x 35 mm x 1 mm

Micro-K® see Potassium Chloride on page 906

Micronase® *see* Glyburide *on page 505*

microNefrin® *see* Epinephrine *on page 389*

Micronor® *see* Norethindrone *on page 805*

Microsulfon® *see* Sulfadiazine *on page 1040*

Midamor® *see* Amiloride Hydrochloride *on page 54*

Midazolam Hydrochloride (mid' ay zoe lam)

Related Information
Benzodiazepines Comparison *on page 1256*

Brand Names Versed®

Use Preoperative sedation and provides conscious sedation prior to diagnostic or radiographic procedures

Restrictions C-IV

Pregnancy Risk Factor D

Contraindications Hypersensitivity to midazolam or any component (cross-sensitivity with other benzodiazepines may occur); uncontrolled pain; existing CNS depression; shock; narrow-angle glaucoma

Warnings/Precautions Use with caution in patients with congestive heart failure, renal impairment, pulmonary disease, hepatic dysfunction, the elderly, and those receiving concomitant narcotics; midazolam may cause respiratory depression/arrest; deaths and hypoxic encephalopathy have resulted when these were not promptly recognized and treated appropriately

Adverse Reactions
>10%: Hiccups

Local: Pain and local reactions at injection site (severity less than diazepam)

1% to 10%:

Cardiovascular: Cardiac arrest, hypotension, bradycardia

Central nervous system: Drowsiness, ataxia, amnesia, dizziness, paradoxical excitement, sedation, headache

Gastrointestinal: Nausea, vomiting

Ocular: Blurred vision, diplopia

Respiratory: Respiratory depression, apnea, laryngospasm, bronchospasm

Miscellaneous: Physical and psychological dependence with prolonged use

<1%:

Cardiovascular: Tachycardia

Central nervous system: Delirium

Dermatologic: Skin rash

Respiratory: Wheezing

Overdosage/Toxicology Symptoms of overdose include respiratory depression, hypotension, coma, stupor, confusion, apnea. Treatment for benzodiazepine overdose is supportive. Rarely is mechanical ventilation required. Flumazenil has been shown to selectively block the binding of benzodiazepines to CNS receptors, resulting in a reversal of benzodiazepine-induced CNS depression; respiratory reaction to hypoxia may not be restored.

Drug Interactions
Decreased effect: Theophylline may antagonize the sedative effects of midazolam

Increased toxicity: CNS depressants, → ↑ sedation and respiratory depression; doses of anesthetic agents should be reduced when used in conjunction with midazolam; cimetidine may increase midazolam serum concentrations

If narcotics or other CNS depressants are administered concomitantly, the midazolam dose should be reduced by 30%, if <65 years of age or by at least 50%, if >65 years of age.

Stability Stable for 24 hours at room temperature/refrigeration; admixtures do not require protection from light for short-term storage; **compatible** with NS, D$_5$W

Standardized dose for continuous infusion: 100 mg/250 mL D$_5$W or NS; maximum concentration: 0.5 mg/mL

Mechanism of Action Depresses all levels of the CNS, including the limbic and reticular formation, probably through the increased action of gamma-aminobutyric acid (GABA), which is a major inhibitory neurotransmitter in the brain

Pharmacodynamics/Kinetics
I.M.:

Onset of sedation: Within 15 minutes

Peak effect: 0.5-1 hour

Duration: 2 hours mean, up to 6 hours

I.V.: Onset of action: Within 1-5 minutes

Absorption: Oral: Rapid

Distribution: V$_d$: 0.8-2.5 L/kg; increased with congestive heart failure (CHF) and chronic renal failure

Protein binding: 95%

Metabolism: Extensively in the liver (microsomally)

Bioavailability: 45% mean

Half-life, elimination: 1-4 hours, increased with cirrhosis, CHF, obesity, elderly

Elimination: As glucuronide conjugated metabolites in urine, ~2% to 10% excreted in feces

Usual Dosage The dose of midazolam needs to be individualized based on the patient's age, underlying diseases, and concurrent medications. Personnel and equipment needed for standard respiratory resuscitation should be immediately available during midazolam administration.

Children:
 Preoperative sedation:
  I.M.: 0.07-0.08 mg/kg 30-60 minutes presurgery
  I.V.: 0.035 mg/kg/dose, repeat over several minutes as required to achieve the desired sedative effect up to a total dose of 0.1-0.2 mg/kg
 Conscious sedation during mechanical ventilation: I.V.: Loading dose: 0.05-0.2 mg/kg then follow with initial continuous infusion: 1-2 mcg/kg/minute; titrate to the desired effect; usual range: 0.4-6 mcg/kg/minute
 Conscious sedation for procedures:
  Oral, Intranasal: 0.2-0.4 mg/kg (maximum: 15 mg) 30-45 minutes before the procedure
  I.V.: 0.05 mg/kg 3 minutes before procedure

Adolescents >12 years: I.V.: 0.5 mg every 3-4 minutes until effect achieved

Adults:
 Preoperative sedation: I.M.: 0.07-0.08 mg/kg 30-60 minutes presurgery; usual dose: 5 mg
 Conscious sedation: I.V.: Initial: 0.5-2 mg slow I.V. over at least 2 minutes; slowly titrate to effect by repeating doses every 2-3 minutes if needed; usual total dose: 2.5-5 mg; use decreased doses in elderly

Healthy Adults <60 years: Some patients respond to doses as low as 1 mg; no more than 2.5 mg should be administered over a period of 2 minutes. Additional doses of midazolam may be administered after a 2-minute waiting period and evaluation of sedation after each dose increment. A total dose >5 mg is generally not needed. If narcotics or other CNS depressants are administered concomitantly, the midazolam dose should be reduced by 30%.

Monitoring Parameters Respiratory and cardiovascular status, blood pressure, blood pressure monitor required during I.V. administration

Nursing Implications Midazolam is a short-acting benzodiazepine; recovery occurs within 2 hours in most patients, however, may require up to 6 hours in some cases

Additional Information Sodium content of 1 mL: 0.14 mEq

Dosage Forms Injection: 1 mg/mL (2 mL, 5 mL, 10 mL); 5 mg/mL (1 mL, 2 mL, 5 mL, 10 mL)

Midol® 200 [OTC] *see* Ibuprofen *on page 561*

Miflex® *see* Chlorzoxazone *on page 236*

Milkinol® [OTC] *see* Mineral Oil *on page 743*

Milk of Magnesia *see* Magnesium Hydroxide *on page 659*

Milrinone Lactate (mil' ri none)

Brand Names Primacor®

Use Short-term I.V. therapy of congestive heart failure; used for calcium antagonist intoxication

Pregnancy Risk Factor C

Contraindications Hypersensitivity to drug or amrinone

Warnings/Precautions Severe obstructive aortic or pulmonic valvular disease, history of ventricular arrhythmias; atrial fibrillation, flutter; renal dysfunction

Adverse Reactions

>10%: Cardiovascular: Ventricular arrhythmias

1% to 10%:
 Cardiovascular: Supraventricular arrhythmias, hypotension, angina, chest pain
 Central nervous system: Headache

<1%:
 Cardiovascular: Ventricular fibrillation
 Endocrine & metabolic: Hypokalemia
 Hematologic: Thrombocytopenia
 Neuromuscular & skeletal: Tremor

(Continued)

Milrinone Lactate *(Continued)*

Overdosage/Toxicology Hypotension should respond to I.V. fluids and Trendelenburg position; use of vasopressors may be required

Stability Colorless to pale yellow solution; store at room temperature and protect from light; stable at 0.2 mg/mL in 0.9% sodium chloride or D_5W for 72 hours at room temperature in normal light

Incompatible with furosemide and procainamide; **compatible** with atropine, calcium chloride, digoxin, epinephrine, lidocaine, morphine, propranolol, and sodium bicarbonate

Standardized dose: 20 mg in 80 mL of 0.9% sodium chloride or D_5W (0.2 mg/mL)

Mechanism of Action Phosphodiesterase inhibitor resulting in vasodilation

Pharmacodynamics/Kinetics

Serum level: I.V.: Following a 125 mcg/kg dose, peak plasma concentrations of ~1000 ng/mL were observed at 2 minutes postinjection, decreasing to <100 ng/mL in 2 hours

Therapeutic effect: Oral: Following doses of 7.5-15 mg, peak hemodynamic effects occurred at 90 minutes

Drug concentration levels:

Therapeutic:

Serum levels of 166 ng/mL, achieved during I.V. infusions of 0.25-1 mcg/kg/minute, were associated with sustained hemodynamic benefit in severe congestive heart failure patients over a 24-hour period

Maximum beneficial effects on cardiac output and pulmonary capillary wedge pressure following I.V. infusion have been associated with plasma milrinone concentrations of 150-250 ng/mL

Toxic: Serum concentrations >250-300 ng/mL have been associated with marked reductions in mean arterial pressure and tachycardia; however, more studies are required to determine the toxic serum levels for milrinone

Distribution: Not known if distributed into breast milk

V_d at steady-state following I.V. administration as a single bolus: 0.32 L/kg; not significantly bound to tissues

In patients with severe congestive heart failure (CHF), V_d has been 0.33-0.47 L/kg

Protein binding: ~70% in plasma

Metabolism: 12% hepatic

Half-life, elimination: I.V.: 136 minutes in patients with CHF; patients with severe CHF have a more prolonged half-life, with values ranging from 1.7-2.7 hours. Patients with CHF have a reduction in the systemic clearance of milrinone, resulting in a prolonged elimination half-life. Alternatively, one study reported that 1 month of therapy with milrinone did not change the pharmacokinetic parameters for patients with CHF despite improvement in cardiac function.

Elimination: Following I.V. administration, 85% of dose excreted unchanged in urine within 24 hours; active tubular secretion is a major elimination pathway for milrinone; bolus doses of I.V. milrinone produced systemic clearance values of 25.9±5.7 L/hour (0.37 L/hour/kg); however, in patients with severe congestive heart failure, the clearance is reduced to 0.11-0.13 L/hour/kg. The reduction in clearance may be a result of reduced renal function. Creatinine clearance values were 1/2 those reported for healthy adults in patients with severe congestive heart failure (52 vs 119 mL/minute).

Usual Dosage Adults: I.V.: Loading dose: 50 mcg/kg administered over 10 minutes followed by a maintenance dose titrated according to the hemodynamic and clinical response, see table.

Maintenance Dosage	Dose Rate (mcg/kg/min)	Total Dose (mg/kg/24 h)
Minimum	0.375	0.59
Standard	0.500	0.77
Maximum	0.750	1.13

Dosing adjustment in renal impairment:

Cl_{cr} 50 mL/minute/1.73 m^2: Administer 0.43 mcg/kg/minute

Cl_{cr} 40 mL/minute/1.73 m^2: Administer 0.38 mcg/kg/minute

Cl_{cr} 30 mL/minute/1.73 m^2: Administer 0.33 mcg/kg/minute

Cl_{cr} 20 mL/minute/1.73 m^2: Administer 0.28 mcg/kg/minute

Cl_{cr} 10 mL/minute/1.73 m^2: Administer 0.23 mcg/kg/minute

Cl_{cr} 5 mL/minute/1.73 m^2: Administer 0.2 mcg/kg/minute

Monitoring Parameters Cardiac monitor and blood pressure monitor required; serum potassium

Therapeutic: Patients should be monitored for improvement in the clinical signs and symptoms of congestive heart failure

Toxic: Patients should be monitored for ventricular arrhythmias and exacerbation of anginal symptoms; during I.V. therapy with milrinone, blood pressure and heart rate should be monitored

Nursing Implications Monitor closely, titrate to blood pressure cardiac index

Dosage Forms Injection: 1 mg/mL (5 mL, 10 mL, 20 mL)

Miltown® see Meprobamate on page 689

Mineral Oil (min' er al oyl)
Related Information
Laxatives, Classification and Properties on page 1272

Brand Names Agoral® Plain [OTC]; Fleet® Mineral Oil Enema [OTC]; Kondremul® [OTC]; Milkinol® [OTC]; Neo-Cultol® [OTC]; Zymenol® [OTC]

Synonyms Heavy Mineral Oil; Liquid Paraffin; White Mineral Oil

Use Temporary relief of constipation, to relieve fecal impaction, preparation for bowel studies or surgery

Pregnancy Risk Factor C

Contraindications Patients with colostomy or an ileostomy, appendicitis, ulcerative colitis, diverticulitis

Warnings/Precautions Oral form should be avoided in children <4 years of age; do not give with food or meals because of the risk of aspiration; prolonged administration of mineral oil may decrease absorption of lipid-soluble vitamins A, D, E, and K.

Adverse Reactions
1% to 10%:
Gastrointestinal: Nausea, vomiting, diarrhea, abdominal cramps, anal itching
Respiratory: Lipid pneumonitis with aspiration

Overdosage/Toxicology Aspiration of oils may cause chemical pneumonitis with fever, leukocytosis, x-ray changes

Drug Interactions
Decreased effect of docusate
May impair absorption of fat-soluble vitamins (A,D,K), oral contraceptives, coumarin, sulfonamides

Mechanism of Action Eases passage of stool by decreasing water absorption and lubricating the intestine

Pharmacodynamics/Kinetics
Onset of action: ~6-8 hours
Metabolism: Site of action is the colon
Elimination: In feces

Usual Dosage
Children:
Oral: 5-11 years: 5-20 mL once daily or in divided doses
Rectal: 2-11 years: 30-60 mL as a single dose

Children >12 years and Adults:
Oral: 15-45 mL/day once daily or in divided doses
Rectal: Retention enema, contents of one enema (range 60-150 mL)/day as a single dose

Administration Administer on an empty stomach

Patient Information Do not take with food or meals; do not use if experiencing abdominal pain, nausea, or vomiting; avoid use of stool softeners at the same time

Dosage Forms
Emulsion, oral: 1.4 g/5 mL (480 mL); 2.5 mL/5 mL (420 mL); 2.75 mL/5 mL (480 mL); 4.75 mL/5 mL (240 mL)
Jelly, oral: 2.75 mL/5 mL (180 mL)
Liquid:
Oral: 30 mL, 180 mL, 500 mL, 1000 mL, 4000 mL
Rectal: 133 mL

Mini-Gamulin® Rh see Rho(D) Immune Globulin on page 978

Minipress® see Prazosin Hydrochloride on page 918

Minitran® see Nitroglycerin on page 799

Minocin® see Minocycline Hydrochloride on this page

Minocin® IV see Minocycline Hydrochloride on this page

Minocycline Hydrochloride (mi noe sye' kleen)
Related Information
Antimicrobial Drugs of Choice on page 1298-1302
(Continued)

Minocycline Hydrochloride *(Continued)*

Brand Names Minocin®; Minocin® IV

Use Treatment of susceptible bacterial infections of both gram-negative and gram-positive organisms; acne, meningococcal carrier state

Pregnancy Risk Factor D

Contraindications Hypersensitivity to minocycline, other tetracyclines, or any component; children <8 years of age

Warnings/Precautions Should be avoided in renal insufficiency, children ≤8 years of age, pregnant and nursing women; photosensitivity reactions can occur with minocycline

Adverse Reactions

>10%: Miscellaneous: Discoloration of teeth in children

1% to 10%:
   Dermatologic: Photosensitivity
   Gastrointestinal: Nausea, diarrhea

<1%:
   Cardiovascular: Pericarditis
   Central nervous system: Increased intracranial pressure, bulging fontanels in infants
   Dermatologic: Dermatologic effects, pruritus, exfoliative dermatitis, rash, pigmentation of nails
   Endocrine & metabolic: Diabetes insipidus syndrome
   Gastrointestinal: Vomiting, esophagitis, anorexia, abdominal cramps
   Neuromuscular & skeletal: Paresthesia
   Renal: Acute renal failure, azotemia
   Miscellaneous: Superinfections, anaphylaxis

Overdosage/Toxicology Symptoms of overdose include diabetes insipidus, nausea, anorexia, diarrhea; following GI decontamination, supportive care only; fluid support may be required

Drug Interactions

Decreased effect with antacids (aluminum, calcium, zinc, or magnesium), bismuth salts, sodium bicarbonate, barbiturates, carbamazepine, hydantoins; decreased effect of oral contraceptives

Increased effect of warfarin

Mechanism of Action Inhibits bacterial protein synthesis by binding with the 30S and possibly the 50S ribosomal subunit(s) of susceptible bacteria; cell wall synthesis is not affected

Pharmacodynamics/Kinetics

Absorption: Well absorbed

Distribution: Crosses placenta; appears in breast milk; majority of a dose deposits for extended periods in fat

Protein binding: 70% to 75%

Half-life: 15 hours

Elimination: Eventually cleared renally

Usual Dosage

Children >8 years: Oral, I.V.: Initial: 4 mg/kg followed by 2 mg/kg/dose every 12 hours

Adults:
   Infection: Oral, I.V.: 200 mg stat, 100 mg every 12 hours not to exceed 400 mg/24 hours
   Acne: Oral: 50 mg 1-3 times/day

Not dialyzable (0% to 5%)

Administration Infuse I.V. minocycline over 1 hour

Patient Information Avoid unnecessary exposure to sunlight; do not take with antacids, iron products, or dairy products; finish all medication; do not skip doses; take 1 hour before or 2 hours after meals

Dosage Forms

Capsule, pellet-filled: 50 mg, 100 mg

Injection: 100 mg

Suspension, oral: 50 mg/5 mL (60 mL)

Minodyl® *see* Minoxidil *on this page*

Minoxidil *(mi nox' i dill)*

Brand Names Loniten®; Minodyl®; Rogaine®

Use Management of severe hypertension (usually in combination with a diuretic and beta-blocker); treatment of male pattern baldness (alopecia androgenetica)

Pregnancy Risk Factor C

Contraindications Pheochromocytoma, hypersensitivity to minoxidil or any component

Warnings/Precautions Use with caution in patients with pulmonary hypertension, significant renal failure, or congestive heart failure; use with caution in patients with coronary artery disease or recent myocardial infarction; renal failure or dialysis patients may require smaller doses; usually used with a beta-blocker (to treat minoxidil-induced tachycardia) and a diuretic (for treatment of water retention/edema); may take 1-6 months for hypertrichosis to totally reverse after minoxidil therapy is discontinued.

Adverse Reactions

>10%:

Cardiovascular: EKG changes, tachycardia, congestive heart failure, edema

Dermatologic: Hypertrichosis (commonly occurs within 1-2 months of therapy)

1% to 10%: Endocrine & metabolic: Fluid and electrolyte imbalance

<1%:

Cardiovascular: Angina, pericardial effusion tamponade

Central nervous system: Dizziness

Endocrine & metabolic: Breast tenderness

Dermatologic: Rashes, headache, coarsening facial features, dermatologic reactions, Stevens-Johnson syndrome, sunburn

Gastrointestinal: Weight gain

Hematologic: Thrombocytopenia, leukopenia

Overdosage/Toxicology Symptoms of overdose include hypotension, tachycardia, headache, nausea, dizziness, weakness syncope, warm flushed skin and palpitations; lethargy and ataxia may occur in children; hypotension usually responds to I.V. fluids, Trendelenburg positioning or vasoconstrictor; treatment is primarily supportive and symptomatic

Drug Interactions Increased toxicity:

Concurrent administration with guanethidine may cause profound orthostatic hypotensive effects

Additive hypotensive effects with other hypotensive agents or diuretics

Mechanism of Action Produces vasodilation by directly relaxing arteriolar smooth muscle, with little effect on veins; effects may be mediated by cyclic AMP; stimulation of hair growth is secondary to vasodilation, increased cutaneous blood flow and stimulation of resting hair follicles

Pharmacodynamics/Kinetics

Onset of hypotensive effect: Oral: Within 30 minutes

Peak effect: Within 2-8 hours

Duration: Up to 2-5 days

Protein binding: None

Metabolism: 88% primarily via glucuronidation

Bioavailability: Oral: 90%

Half-life: Adults: 3.5-4.2 hours

Elimination: 12% excreted unchanged in urine

Usual Dosage

Children <12 years: Hypertension: Oral: Initial: 0.1-0.2 mg/kg once daily; maximum: 5 mg/day; increase gradually every 3 days; usual dosage: 0.25-1 mg/kg/day in 1-2 divided doses; maximum: 50 mg/day

Children >12 years and Adults:

Hypertension: Oral: Initial: 5 mg once daily, increase gradually every 3 days; usual dose: 10-40 mg/day in 1-2 divided doses; maximum: 100 mg/day

Alopecia: Topical: Apply twice daily; 4 months of therapy may be necessary for hair growth

Elderly: Initial: 2.5 mg once daily; increase gradually

Supplemental dose is not necessary via hemo- or peritoneal dialysis

Monitoring Parameters Blood pressure, standing and sitting/supine; fluid and electrolyte balance and body weight should be monitored

Patient Information Topical product must be used every day. Hair growth usually takes 4 months. Notify physician if any of the following occur: Heart rate ≥20 beats per minute over normal; rapid weight gain >5 lb (2 kg); unusual swelling of extremities, face, or abdomen; breathing difficulty, especially when lying down; rise slowly from prolonged lying or sitting; new or aggravated angina symptoms (chest, arm, or shoulder pain); severe indigestion; dizziness, light-headedness, or fainting; nausea or vomiting may occur. Do not make up for missed doses.

Nursing Implications May cause hirsutism or hypertrichosis; observe for fluid retention and orthostatic hypotension

Dosage Forms

Solution, topical: 2% = 20 mg/metered dose (60 mL)

Tablet: 2.5 mg, 10 mg

Mintezol® see Thiabendazole on page 1078

Minute-Gel® *see* Fluoride *on page 471*

Miochol® *see* Acetylcholine Chloride *on page 25*

Miostat® *see* Carbachol *on page 176*

Misoprostol (mye soe prost' ole)

Brand Names Cytotec®

Use Prevention of NSAID-induced gastric ulcers

Pregnancy Risk Factor X

Contraindications Hypersensitivity to misoprostol or any component

Warnings/Precautions Safety and efficacy have not been established in children <18 years of age; use with caution in patients with renal impairment and the elderly; not to be used in pregnant women or women of childbearing potential unless woman is capable of complying with effective contraceptive measures; therapy is normally begun on the second or third day of next normal menstrual period

Adverse Reactions
>10%: Gastrointestinal: Diarrhea, abdominal pain
1% to 10%:
    Central nervous system: Headache
    Gastrointestinal: Constipation, flatulence
<1%:
    Gastrointestinal: Nausea, vomiting
    Genitourinary: Uterine stimulation, vaginal bleeding

Overdosage/Toxicology Sedation, tremor, convulsions, dyspnea, abdominal pain, diarrhea, hypotension, bradycardia

Mechanism of Action Misoprostol is a synthetic prostaglandin E_1 analog that replaces the protective prostaglandins consumed with prostaglandin-inhibiting therapies eg, nonsteroidal anti-inflammatory drugs

Pharmacodynamics/Kinetics
Absorption: Oral: Rapid
Metabolism: Rapidly de-esterified to misoprostol acid
Half-life (parent and metabolite combined): 1.5 hours
Time to peak serum concentration (active metabolite): Within 15-30 minutes
Elimination: In urine (64% to 73% in 24 hours) and feces (15% in 24 hours)

Usual Dosage Adults: Oral: 200 mcg 4 times/day with food; if not tolerated, may decrease dose to 100 mcg 4 times/day with food or 200 mcg twice daily with food

Patient Information May cause diarrhea when first being used; take after meals and at bedtime; avoid taking with magnesium-containing antacids

Nursing Implications Incidence of diarrhea may be lessened by having patient take dose right after meals

Dosage Forms Tablet: 100 mcg, 200 mcg

Mithracin® *see* Plicamycin *on page 895*

Mithramycin *see* Plicamycin *on page 895*

Mitomycin (mye toe mye' sin)

Related Information
Antiemetics for Chemotherapy Induced Nausea and Vomiting *on page 1202*
Cancer Chemotherapy Regimens *on page 1218-1241*
Extravasation Management of Chemotherapeutic Agents *on page 1207-1208*

Brand Names Mutamycin®

Synonyms Mitomycin-C; MTC

Use Therapy of disseminated adenocarcinoma of stomach or pancreas in combination with other approved chemotherapeutic agents; bladder cancer, colorectal cancer

Pregnancy Risk Factor C

Contraindications Platelet counts <75,000/mm³; leukocyte counts <3,000/mm³ or serum creatinine >1.7 mg/dL; thrombocytopenia, hypersensitivity to mitomycin or any component

Warnings/Precautions The U.S. Food and Drug Administration (FDA) currently recommends that procedures for proper handling and disposal of antineoplastic agents be considered. Use with caution in patients with impaired renal or hepatic function, myelosuppression. Follow hemoglobin, hematocrit, BUN, and creatinine closely after therapy especially after second and subsequent cycles. Bone marrow depression, notably thrombocytopenia and leukopenia, may contribute to the development of a secondary infection; hemolytic uremic syndrome, a serious and often fatal syndrome, has occurred in patients receiving long-term therapy and is correlated with total dose and total duration of therapy; mitomycin is potentially carcinogenic and teratogenic.

Adverse Reactions

>10%:

Gastrointestinal: **Nausea and vomiting (mild to moderate) seen in almost 100% of patients**; usually begins 1-2 hours after treatment and persists for 3 hours to 4 days; other toxicities include stomatitis, hepatic toxicity, diarrhea, anorexia

Emetic potential: Moderately high (60% to 90%)

Extravasation: May cause severe tissue irritation if infiltrated; can progress to cellulitis, ulceration, and sloughing of tissue

Vesicant chemotherapy

Myelosuppressive: Dose-related toxicity and may be cumulative; related to both total dose (incidence higher at doses >50 mg) and schedule

WBC: Moderate

Platelets: Severe

Onset (days): 21

Nadir (days): 36

Recovery (days): 42-56

1% to 10%:

Central nervous system: Extremity tingling

Dermatologic: Discolored fingernails (violet), alopecia

Gastrointestinal: Mouth ulcers

Respiratory: Interstitial pneumonitis or pulmonary fibrosis have been noticed in 7% of patients, and it occurs independent of dosing. Manifested as dry cough and progressive dyspnea; usually is responsive to steroid therapy.

Renal: Elevation of creatinine seen in 2% of patients; hemolytic uremic syndrome observed in <10% of patients and is dose-dependent (doses >30 mg have higher risk)

<1%:

Cardiovascular: Cardiac failure (in patients treated with doses >30 mg)

Central nervous system: Malaise, fever, weakness

Dermatologic: Pruritus, alopecia, rash

Gastrointestinal: Mouth ulcers

Hematologic: Bone marrow suppression (leukopenia, thrombocytopenia), microangiopathic hemolytic anemia

Local: Thrombophlebitis

Neuromuscular & skeletal: Paresthesia

Overdosage/Toxicology Symptoms of overdose include bone marrow depression, nausea, vomiting, alopecia

Drug Interactions Increased toxicity: *Vinca* alkaloids; doxorubicin may enhance cardiac toxicity

Stability

Stability of constituted solutions at room temperature (25°C): 1 week

Stability of constituted solutions at refrigeration temperature (4°C): 2 weeks

Must be dispensed in an amber bag

Mechanism of Action Isolated from *Streptomyces caespitosus*; acts primarily as an alkylating agent and produces DNA cross-linking (primarily with guanine and cytosine pairs); cell-cycle nonspecific; inhibits DNA and RNA synthesis by alkylation and cross-linking the strands of DNA

Pharmacodynamics/Kinetics

Absorption: Fairly well from the GI tract

Distribution: V_d: 22 L/m^2; high drug concentrations found in kidney, tongue, muscle, heart, and lung tissue; probably not distributed into the CNS

Metabolism: Hepatic

Half-life: 23-78 minutes

Terminal: 50 minutes

Elimination: Primarily in metabolism, followed by urinary excretion (<10% as unchanged drug) and to a small extent biliary excretion

Usual Dosage Children and Adults: I.V. (refer to individual protocols: 10-20 mg/m^2/dose every 6-8 weeks, or 2 mg/m^2/day for 5 days, stop for 2 days then repeat; subsequent doses should be adjusted to platelet and leukocyte response. Total cumulative dose should not exceed 50 mg/m^2. See table.

Nadir After Prior Dose per mm^3		% of Prior Dose to Be Given
Leukocytes	Platelets	
4000	>100,000	100
3000-3999	75,000-99,999	100
2000-2999	25,000-74,999	70
2000	<25,000	50

(Continued)

Mitomycin *(Continued)*

Dosing adjustment in renal impairment:
Cl_{cr} <10 mL/minute: Administer 75% of normal dose
Not removed by hemodialysis

Intravesicular instillations for bladder carcinoma: 40 mg/dose (1 mg/mL in sterile aqueous solution)

Administration Administer by short I.V. infusion over 30-60 minutes or by slow I.V. push over 5-10 minutes via a running I.V.; short I.V. infusions are usually administered at a final concentration of 20-40 mcg/mL (in 50-250 mL of D_5W or NS) or I.V. slow push can be administered at a concentration not to exceed 0.5 mg/mL

Monitoring Parameters Platelet count, CBC with differential, prothrombin time, renal and pulmonary function tests

Patient Information Any signs of infection, easy bruising or bleeding, shortness of breath, or painful or burning urination should be brought to physician's attention. Nausea, vomiting, or hair loss sometimes occur. The drug may cause permanent sterility and may cause birth defects. The drug may be excreted in breast milk, therefore, an alternative form of feeding your baby should be used.

Nursing Implications
Extravasation management:
Care should be taken to avoid extravasation. If extravasation occurs, the site should be observed closely; these injuries frequently cause necrosis; a plastic surgery consult may be required.
Few agents have been effective as antidotes, but there are reports in the literature of some benefit with dimethylsulfoxide (DSMO). Delayed dermal reactions with mitomycin are possible, even in patients who are asymptomatic at time of drug administration.

Dosage Forms Powder for injection: 5 mg, 20 mg, 40 mg

Mitomycin-C *see* Mitomycin *on page 746*

Mitotane *(mye' toe tane)*

Brand Names Lysodren®
Synonyms o,p'-DDD
Use Treatment of inoperable adrenal cortical carcinoma
Pregnancy Risk Factor C
Contraindications Known hypersensitivity to mitotane
Warnings/Precautions The U.S. Food and Drug Administration (FDA) currently recommends that procedures for proper handling and disposal of antineoplastic agents be considered. Patients should be hospitalized when mitotane therapy is initiated until a stable dose regimen is established. Discontinue temporarily following trauma or shock since the prime action of mitotane is adrenal suppression; exogenous steroids may be indicated since adrenal function may not start immediately. Administer with care to patients with severe hepatic impairment; observe patients for neurotoxicity with prolonged (2 years) use.

Adverse Reactions
>10%:
Central nervous system: Visual disturbances, double vision, blurred vision, vertigo, mental depression, dizziness; all are reversible with discontinuation of the drug and can occur in 15% to 26% of patients
Dermatologic: Rash (15%) which may subside without discontinuation of therapy, hyperpigmentation
Gastrointestinal: 75% to 80% will experience nausea, vomiting, and anorexia; diarrhea can occur in 20% of patients
1% to 10%:
Cardiovascular: Orthostatic hypotension
Central nervous system: Fever
Endocrine & metabolic: Flushing of skin
Neuromuscular & skeletal: Myalgia
Renal: Hemorrhagic cystitis
<1%:
Adrenal insufficiency: May develop and may require steroid replacement
Cardiovascular: Hypertension, flushing
Central nervous system: Lethargy, somnolence, mental depression, irritability, confusion, weakness, fatigue, headache, fever, hyperpyrexia
Dermatologic: Rash
Genitourinary: Albuminuria
Myelosuppressive:
WBC: None
Platelets: None
Neuromuscular & skeletal: Tremor

Ocular: Lens opacities, toxic retinopathy
Renal: Hypouricemia, hematuria, hemorrhagic cystitis
Respiratory: Shortness of breath, wheezing
Miscellaneous: Hypercholesterolemia

Overdosage/Toxicology Symptoms of overdose include diarrhea, vomiting, numbness of limbs, weakness

Drug Interactions
Decreased effect:
Barbiturates, warfarin may be accelerated by induction of the hepatic microsomal enzyme system
Spironolactone has resulted in negation of mitotane's effect
Phenytoin → ↑ clearance of these drugs by microsomal enzyme stimulation by mitotane
Increased toxicity: CNS depressants → ↑ CNS depression

Stability Protect from light, store at room temperature

Mechanism of Action Causes adrenal cortical atrophy; drug affects mitochondria in adrenal cortical cells and decreases production of cortisol; also alters the peripheral metabolism of steroids

Pharmacodynamics/Kinetics
Absorption: Oral: ~35% to 40%
Time to peak serum concentration: Within 3-5 hours
Distribution: Stored mainly in fat tissue but is found in all body tissues
Metabolism: Primarily in the liver by hydroxylation and oxidation and other tissues
Half-life: 18-159 days
Elimination: Metabolites excreted in urine and bile

Usual Dosage Oral:
Children: 0.1-0.5 mg/kg or 1-2 g/day in divided doses increasing gradually to a maximum of 5-7 g/day
Adults: Start at 1-6 g/day in divided doses, then increase incrementally to 8-10 g/day in 3-4 divided doses; dose is changed on basis of side effect with aim of giving as high a dose as tolerated; maximum daily dose: 18 g

Dosing adjustment in hepatic impairment: Dose may need to be decreased in patients with liver disease

Patient Information Patients should be warned that mitotane may impair ability to operate hazardous equipment or drive; avoid alcohol and other CNS depressants; notify physician if rash or darkening of skin, severe nausea, vomiting, depression, flushing, or fever occurs; contraceptive measures are recommended during therapy

Dosage Forms Tablet, scored: 500 mg

Mitoxantrone Hydrochloride (mye toe zan' trone)

Related Information
Cancer Chemotherapy Regimens on page 1218-1241

Brand Names Novantrone®

Synonyms DHAD

Use FDA approved for the treatment of acute nonlymphocytic leukemia (ANLL) in adults; mitoxantrone is also found to be very active against various leukemias, lymphoma, and breast cancer, and moderately active against pediatric sarcoma

Pregnancy Risk Factor D

Contraindications Hypersensitivity to mitoxantrone or any component

Warnings/Precautions The FDA currently recommends that procedures for proper handling and disposal of antineoplastic agents be considered. Dosage should be reduced in patients with impaired hepatobiliary function; use with caution in patients with pre-existing myelosuppression. Predisposing factors for mitoxantrone-induced cardiotoxicity include prior anthracycline therapy, prior cardiovascular disease, and mediastinal irradiation. The risk of developing cardiotoxicity is <3% when the cumulative doses are <100-120 mg/m² in patients with predisposing factors and <160 mg/m² in patients with no predisposing factors.

Adverse Reactions
>10%:
Central nervous system: Headache
Dermatologic: Alopecia
Gastrointestinal: Nausea, vomiting, diarrhea, abdominal pain, mucositis, stomatitis, GI bleeding
Hepatic: Abnormal LFTs
Emetic potential: Moderate (31% to 72%)
Respiratory: Coughing, shortness of breath
Miscellaneous: Discoloration of urine (blue-green)

(Continued)

749

Mitoxantrone Hydrochloride *(Continued)*

1% to 10%:
 Cardiac toxicity: Much reduced compared to doxorubicin and has been reported primarily in patients who have received prior anthracycline therapy, congestive heart failure, hypotension
 Central nervous system: Seizures, fever
 Dermatologic: Pruritus, skin desquamation
 Hematologic: Myelosuppressive effects of chemotherapy:
  WBC: Mild
  Platelets: Mild
  Onset (days): 7-10
  Nadir (days): 14
  Recovery (days): 21
 Hepatic: Transient elevation of liver enzymes, jaundice
 Ocular: Conjunctivitis
 Renal: Renal failure
<1%:
 Local: Pain or redness at injection site
 Irritant chemotherapy

Overdosage/Toxicology Symptoms of overdose include leukopenia, tachycardia, marrow hypoplasia; no known antidote

Stability After penetration of the stopper, undiluted mitoxantrone solution is stable for 7 days at room temperature or 14 days when refrigerated; **incompatible** with heparin and hydrocortisone

Mechanism of Action Analogue of the anthracyclines, but different in mechanism of action, cardiac toxicity, and potential for tissue necrosis; mitoxantrone does intercalate DNA; binds to nucleic acids and inhibits DNA and RNA synthesis by template disordering and steric obstruction; replication is decreased by binding to DNA topoisomerase II (enzyme responsible for DNA helix supercoiling); active throughout entire cell cycle; does not appear to produce free radicals

Pharmacodynamics/Kinetics
 Absorption: Oral: Poor
 Distribution: V_d: 14 L/kg; distributes into pleural fluid, kidney, thyroid, liver, heart, and red blood cells
 Protein binding: >95%
 Albumin binding: 76%
 Metabolism: In the liver
 Half-life: Terminal: 37 hours; may be prolonged with liver impairment
 Elimination: Slowly excreted in urine (6% to 11%) and bile as unchanged drug and metabolites

Usual Dosage I.V. (may dilute in D_5W or NS) (refer to individual protocols):

ANLL leukemias:
 Children ≤2 years: 0.4 mg/kg/day once daily for 3-5 days
 Children >2 years and Adults: 8-12 mg/m^2/day once daily for 5 days or 12 mg/m^2/day once daily for 3 days
Solid tumors:
 Children: 18-20 mg/m^2 every 3-4 weeks or 5-8 mg/m^2 every week
 Adults: 12-14 mg/m^2 every 3-4 weeks or 2-4 mg/m^2/day for 5 days
 Maximum total dose: 80-120 mg/m^2 in patients with predisposing factor and <160 mg in patients with no predisposing factors

Dosing adjustment in hepatic impairment:
 Patients with severe dysfunction (bilirubin >3.4 mg/dL) have a lower total body clearance and may require a dosage adjustment to 8 mg/m^2; starting dose: 12 mg/m^2 every 21 days
 If bilirubin is 3.1-5 mg/dL or ALT >180 units: Administer a reduced dose

Dose modifications based on degree of leukopenia or thrombocytopenia; see table.

Granulocyte Count Nadir (cells/mm^3)	Platelet Count Nadir (cells/mm^3)	Total Bilirubin (mg/dL)	Dose Adjustment
>2000	>150,000	<1.5	Increase by 1 mg/m^2
1000-2000	75,000-150,000	<1.5	Maintain same dose
<1000	<75,000	1.5-3	Decrease by 1 mg/m^2

Administration Do **not** give I.V. bolus over <3 minutes; can be administered I.V. intermittent infusion over 15-30 minutes at a concentration of 0.02-0.5 mg/mL in D_5W or normal saline

Monitoring Parameters CBC, serum uric acid, liver function tests, ECHO

Patient Information May impart a blue-green color to the urine for 24 hours after administration, and patients should be advised to expect this during therapy. Bluish discoloration of the sclera may also occur. Patients should be advised of the signs and symptoms of myelosuppression; report to physician if persistent fever, malaise, sore throat, fatigue, or unusual bleeding or bruising

Nursing Implications Vesicant; avoid extravasation

Dosage Forms Injection, as base: 2 mg/mL (10 mL, 12.5 mL, 15 mL)

Mitran® see Chlordiazepoxide on page 221

Mitrolan® Chewable Tablet [OTC] see Calcium Polycarbophil on page 172

Mivacron® see Mivacurium Chloride on this page

Mivacurium Chloride (mye va kyoo' ree um)

Related Information

Neuromuscular Blocking Agents Comparison Charts on page 1276-1278

Brand Names Mivacron®

Use Short-acting nondepolarizing neuromuscular blocking agent; an adjunct to general anesthesia; facilitates endotracheal intubation; provides skeletal muscle relaxation during surgery or mechanical ventilation

Pregnancy Risk Factor C

Contraindications Hypersensitivity to mivacurium chloride or other benzylisoquinolinium agents; pre-existing tachycardia

Adverse Reactions

>10%: Cardiovascular: Flushing of face

1% to 10%: Cardiovascular: Hypotension

<1%:

Cardiovascular: Bradycardia, tachycardia

Central nervous system: Dizziness

Dermatologic: Cutaneous erythema, rash

Hematologic: Hypoxemia

Local: Injection site reaction

Neuromuscular & skeletal: Muscle spasms

Respiratory: Bronchospasm, wheezing

Miscellaneous: Endogenous histamine release

Drug Interactions

Prolonged neuromuscular blockade:

Inhaled anesthetics

Local anesthetics

Calcium channel blockers

Antiarrhythmics (eg, quinidine or procainamide)

Antibiotics (eg, aminoglycosides, tetracyclines, vancomycin, clindamycin)

Immunosuppressants (eg, cyclosporine)

Mechanism of Action Mivacurium is a short-acting, nondepolarizing, neuromuscular-blocking agent. Like other nondepolarizing drugs, mivacurium antagonizes acetylcholine by competitively binding to cholinergic sites on motor endplates in skeletal muscle. This inhibits contractile activity in skeletal muscle leading to muscle paralysis. This effect is reversible with cholinesterase inhibitors such as edrophonium, neostigmine, and physostigmine.

Pharmacodynamics/Kinetics

Onset of neuromuscular blockade effect: I.V.: Within 2-3 minutes

Peak effect: 1.5-8 minutes

Duration of action: Short due to rapid hydrolysis by plasma cholinesterases; recovery from muscular paralysis occurs within 15-30 minutes

Usual Dosage Continuous infusion requires an infusion pump; dose should be based on ideal body weight

Children 2-12 years (duration of action is shorter and dosage requirements are higher): 200 mcg/kg I.V. bolus; 5-31 mcg/kg/minute I.V. infusion

Adults: Initial: I.V.: 0.15 mg/kg bolus; for prolonged neuromuscular block, infusions of 1-15 mcg/kg/minute are used

Dosing adjustment in renal impairment: 150 mcg/kg I.V. bolus; duration of action of blockade: 1.5 times longer in ESRD, may decrease infusion rates by as much as 50%, dependent on degree of renal impairment

Dosing adjustment in hepatic impairment: 150 mcg/kg I.V. bolus; duration of blockade: 3 times longer in ESLD, may decrease rate of infusion by as much as 50% in ESLD, dependent on the degree of impairment

(Continued)

Mivacurium Chloride *(Continued)*

Administration Children require higher mivacurium infusion rates than adults; during opioid/nitrous oxide/oxygen anesthesia, the infusion rate required to maintain 89% to 99% neuromuscular block averages 14 mcg/kg/minute (range: 5-31). For adults and children, the amount of infusion solution required per hour depends upon the clinical requirements of the patient, the concentration of mivacurium in the infusion solution, and the patient's weight. The contribution of the infusion solution to the fluid requirements of the patient must be considered. The following tables provide guidelines for delivery in mL/hour (equivalent to microdrops/minute when 60 microdrops = 1 mL) of mivacurium premixed infusion (0.5 mg/mL) and of mivacurium injection (2 mg/mL).

Infusion Rates for Maintenance of Neuromuscular Block During Opioid/Nitrous Oxide/Oxygen Anesthesia Using Mivacurium Premixed Infusion (0.5 mg/mL)

Patient Weight (kg)	Drug Delivery Rate (mcg/kg/min)									
	4	5	6	7	8	10	14	16	18	20
	Infusion Delivery Rate (mL/h)									
10	5	6	7	8	10	12	17	19	22	24
15	7	9	11	13	14	18	25	29	32	36
20	10	12	15	17	19	24	34	38	43	48
25	12	15	18	21	24	30	42	48	54	60
35	17	21	26	29	34	42	59	67	76	84
50	24	30	36	42	46	60	84	96	108	120
60	29	36	43	50	58	72	101	115	130	144
70	34	42	50	59	67	84	118	134	151	168
80	39	48	58	67	77	96	134	154	173	192
90	44	54	65	76	86	108	151	173	194	216
100	48	60	72	84	96	120	168	192	216	240

Infusion Rates for Maintenance of Neuromuscular Block During Opioid/Nitrous Oxide/Oxygen Anesthesia Using Mivacurium Injection (2 mg/mL)

Patient Weight (kg)	Drug Delivery Rate (mcg/kg/min)									
	4	5	6	7	8	10	14	16	18	20
	Infusion Delivery Rate (mL/h)									
10	1.2	1.5	1.8	2.1	2.4	3	4.2	4.8	5.4	6
15	1.8	2.3	2.7	3.2	3.6	4.5	6.3	7.2	8.1	9
20	2.4	3	3.6	4.2	4.8	6	8.4	9.5	10.8	12
25	3	3.8	4.5	5.3	6	7.5	10.5	12	13.5	15
35	4.2	5.3	6.3	7.4	8.4	10.5	14.7	16.8	18.9	21
50	6	7.5	9	10.5	12	15	21	24	27	30
60	7.2	9	10.8	12.8	14.4	18	25.2	28.8	32.4	36
70	8.4	10.5	12.6	14.7	16.8	21	29.4	33.6	37.8	42
80	9.6	12	14.4	16.8	19.2	24	33.6	38.4	43.2	48
90	10.8	13.5	16.2	18.9	21.6	27	37.8	43.2	48.6	54
100	12	15	18	21	24	30	42	48	54	60

Nursing Implications Use with caution in patients in whom histamine release would be detrimental (eg, patients with severe cardiovascular disease or asthma)

Dosage Forms
Infusion, in D$_5$W: 0.5 mg/mL (50 mL)
Injection: 2 mg/mL (5 mL, 10 mL)

M-KYA® [OTC] *see* Quinine Sulfate *on page 970*

MMR *see* Measles, Mumps, and Rubella Vaccines, Combined *on page 668*

M-M-R® II *see* Measles, Mumps, and Rubella Vaccines, Combined *on page 668*

Moban® *see* Molindone Hydrochloride *on next page*

Moctanin® *see* Monooctanoin *on page 755*

Modane® Soft [OTC] *see* Docusate *on page 362*

Modane® Bulk [OTC] *see* Psyllium *on page 956*

Modicon™ *see* Ethinyl Estradiol and Norethindrone *on page 425*

Modified Dakin's Solution *see* Sodium Hypochlorite Solution *on page 1015*

Modified Shohl's Solution *see* Sodium Citrate and Citric Acid *on page 1013*

Molindone Hydrochloride (moe lin' done)

Related Information
Antipsychotic Agents Comparison *on page 1255*

Brand Names Moban®

Use Management of psychotic disorder

Pregnancy Risk Factor C

Contraindications Narrow-angle glaucoma, hypersensitivity to molindone or any component

Warnings/Precautions Use with caution in patients with cardiovascular disease or seizures, CNS depression, or hepatic impairment

Adverse Reactions
>10%:
  Cardiovascular: Orthostatic hypotension
  Central nervous system: Akathisia, extrapyramidal effects, persistent tardive dyskinesia
  Gastrointestinal: Constipation
  Ocular: Blurred vision
  Miscellaneous: Decreased sweating, dry mouth
1% to 10%:
  Central nervous system: Mental depression
  Endocrine & metabolic: Change in menstrual periods, swelling of breasts
<1%:
  Cardiovascular: Tachycardia, arrhythmias
  Central nervous system: Sedation, drowsiness, restlessness, anxiety, seizures, neuroleptic malignant syndrome (NMS)
  Dermatologic: Hyperpigmentation, pruritus, rash, photosensitivity
  Endocrine & metabolic: Galactorrhea, gynecomastia
  Gastrointestinal: Weight gain, dry mouth
  Genitourinary: Urinary retention
  Hematologic: Agranulocytosis (more often in women between fourth and tenth weeks of therapy), leukopenia (usually in patients with large doses for prolonged periods)
  Ocular: Retinal pigmentation
  Miscellaneous: Altered central temperature regulation

Overdosage/Toxicology Symptoms of overdose include deep sleep, extrapyramidal symptoms, cardiac arrhythmias, seizures, hypotension

Following initiation of essential overdose management, toxic symptom treatment and supportive treatment should be initiated. Hypotension usually responds to I.V. fluids or Trendelenburg positioning. If unresponsive to these measures, the use of a parenteral inotrope may be required (eg, norepinephrine 0.1-0.2 mcg/kg/minute titrated to response). Seizures commonly respond to diazepam (I.V. 5-10 mg bolus in adults every 15 minutes if needed up to a total of 30 mg; I.V. 0.25-0.4 mg/kg/dose up to a total of 10 mg in children) or to phenytoin or phenobarbital. Critical cardiac arrhythmias often respond to I.V. phenytoin (15 mg/kg up to 1 g), while other antiarrhythmics can be used. Neuroleptics often cause extrapyramidal symptoms (eg, dystonic reactions) requiring management with diphenhydramine 1-2 mg/kg (adults) up to a maximum of 50 mg I.M. or I.V. slow push followed by a maintenance dose for 48-72 hours. When these reactions are unresponsive to diphenhydramine, benztropine mesylate I.V. 1-2 mg (adults) may be effective. These agents are generally effective within 2-5 minutes.

Drug Interactions Increased toxicity: CNS depressants, antihypertensives, anticonvulsants

Mechanism of Action Mechanism of action mimics that of chlorpromazine; however, it produces more extrapyramidal effects and less sedation than chlorpromazine

Pharmacodynamics/Kinetics
Metabolism: In the liver
Half-life: 1.5 hours
Time to peak serum concentration: Oral: Within 1.5 hours
Elimination: Principally in urine and feces (90% within 24 hours)

Usual Dosage Oral:
(Continued)

Molindone Hydrochloride (Continued)

Children:
  3-5 years: 1-2.5 mg/day divided into 4 doses
  5-12 years: 0.5-1 mg/kg/day in 4 divided doses

Adults: 50-75 mg/day increase at 3- to 4-day intervals up to 225 mg/day

Monitoring Parameters Monitor blood pressure and pulse rate prior to and during initial therapy evaluate mental status; monitor weight

Patient Information Dry mouth may be helped by sips of water, sugarless gum or hard candy; avoid alcohol; very important to maintain established dosage regimen; photosensitivity to sunlight can occur, do not discontinue abruptly; full effect may not occur for 3-4 weeks; full dosage may be taken at bedtime to avoid daytime sedation; report to physician any involuntary movements or feelings of restlessness

Nursing Implications May increase appetite and possibly a craving for sweets; recognize signs of neuroleptic malignant syndrome and tardive dyskinesia

Dosage Forms
  Concentrate, oral: 20 mg/mL (120 mL)
  Tablet: 5 mg, 10 mg, 25 mg, 50 mg, 100 mg

Mol-Iron® [OTC] see Ferrous Sulfate on page 452

MOM see Magnesium Hydroxide on page 659

Mometasone Furoate (moe met' a sone)

Brand Names Elocon®

Use Relief of the inflammatory and pruritic manifestations of corticosteroid-responsive dermatoses (medium potency topical corticosteroid)

Pregnancy Risk Factor C

Contraindications Hypersensitivity to mometasone or any component; fungal, viral, or tubercular skin lesions, herpes simplex or zoster

Warnings/Precautions Adverse systemic effects may occur when used on large areas of the body, denuded areas, for prolonged periods of time, with an occlusive dressing, and/or in infants or small children

Adverse Reactions
  <1%:
    Dermatologic: Acne, hypopigmentation, allergic dermatitis, maceration of the skin, skin atrophy, striae, miliaria
    Endocrine & metabolic: HPA suppression, Cushing's syndrome, growth retardation
    Local: Burning, itching, irritation, dryness, folliculitis, hypertrichosis
    Miscellaneous: Secondary infection

Mechanism of Action May depress the formation, release, and activity of endogenous chemical mediators of inflammation (kinins, histamine, liposomal enzymes, prostaglandins). Leukocytes and macrophages may have to be present for the initiation of responses mediated by the above substances. Inhibits the margination and subsequent cell migration to the area of injury, and also reverses the dilatation and increased vessel permeability in the area resulting in decreased access of cells to the sites of injury.

Usual Dosage Adults: Topical: Apply sparingly to area once daily, do not use occlusive dressings

Patient Information Before applying, gently wash area to reduce risk of infection; apply a thin film to cleansed area and rub in gently and thoroughly until medication vanishes; avoid exposure to sunlight, severe sunburn may occur

Nursing Implications For external use only; do not use on open wounds; should not be used in the presence of open or weeping lesions; use sparingly

Dosage Forms
  Cream: 0.1% (15 g, 45 g)
  Lotion: 0.1% (27.5 mL, 55 mL)
  Ointment, topical: 0.1% (15 g, 45 g)

Monacolin K see Lovastatin on page 652

Monistat™ see Miconazole on page 738

Monistat-Derm™ see Miconazole on page 738

Monistat i.v.™ see Miconazole on page 738

Monocid® see Cefonicid Sodium on page 197

Monoclate-P® see Antihemophilic Factor (Human) on page 80

Monoclonal Antibody see Muromonab-CD3 on page 761

Mono-Gesic® see Salsalate on page 993

Monoket® *see* Isosorbide Mononitrate *on page 601*

Mononine® *see* Factor IX Complex (Human) *on page 438*

Monooctanoin (mon oh ock' ta noyn)
Brand Names Moctanin®
Use Solubilizes cholesterol gallstones that are retained in the biliary tract after cholecystectomy
Pregnancy Risk Factor C
Contraindications Jaundice, significant biliary tract infection
Warnings/Precautions Use with caution in patients with impaired hepatic function as metabolic acidosis may occur during perfusion
Adverse Reactions
>10%: Gastrointestinal: Abdominal pain, nausea, vomiting, diarrhea
1% to 10%: Anorexia
<1%:
Cardiovascular: Flushing of face
Gastrointestinal: Metallic taste
Neuromuscular & skeletal: Back pain
Mechanism of Action Monooctanoin (glyceryl-1-monooctanoate) is a digestion product of medium-chain triglycerides. It is an excellent solvent for cholesterol-rich gallstones. The solubility of cholesterol in monooctanoin is 11.7 g/100 mL at 37°C. The drug dissolves cholesterol gallstones 2.5 times faster than sodium cholate which is also used for dissolution of retained cholesterol bile duct stones.
Pharmacodynamics/Kinetics
Onset of action/duration: Complete stone dissolution usually occurs in 15 days or less
Following infusion into the biliary tract, the drug is hydrolyzed by pancreatic and other digestive lipases to fatty acids and glycerol which are absorbed rapidly via the portal vein; fatty acids are oxidized to carbon dioxide in the liver and are not esterified in the intestine or liver or stored in peripheral tissue
Usual Dosage Adults: Administer via T-tube into common bile duct at rate of 3-5 mL/hour at pressure of 10 mL water for 2-10 days (not longer than 26 days); avoid use in patients with severely impaired liver
Administration Solution must be diluted prior to use; do not administer I.M. or I.V.
Dosage Forms Solution: 120 mL

Monopril® *see* Fosinopril *on page 490*

8-MOP *see* Methoxsalen *on page 716*

8-MOP® *see* Methoxsalen *on page 716*

More Attenuated Enders Strain *see* Measles Virus Vaccine, Live *on page 670*

More-Dophilus® [OTC] *see* Lactobacillus acidophilus and Lactobacillus bulgaricus *on page 617*

Moricizine Hydrochloride (mor i' siz een)
Related Information
Antiarrhythmic Drugs *on page 1246-1248*
Brand Names Ethmozine®
Use For treatment of ventricular tachycardia and life-threatening ventricular arrhythmias
Unlabeled use: PVCs, complete and nonsustained ventricular tachycardia
Pregnancy Risk Factor B
Contraindications Pre-existing second or third degree A-V block and in patients with right bundle branch block when associated with left hemiblock, unless pacemaker is present; cardiogenic shock; known hypersensitivity to the drug
Warnings/Precautions Considering the known proarrhythmic properties and lack of evidence of improved survival for any antiarrhythmic drug in patients without life-threatening arrhythmias, it is prudent to reserve the use for patients with life-threatening ventricular arrhythmias; CAST II trial demonstrated a trend towards decreased survival for patients treated with moricizine; proarrhythmic effects occur as with other antiarrhythmic agents; hypokalemia, hyperkalemia, hypomagnesemia may effect response to class I agents; use with caution in patients with sick-sinus syndrome, hepatic, and renal impairment
Adverse Reactions
>10%: Central nervous system: Dizziness
(Continued)

755

Moricizine Hydrochloride *(Continued)*

1% to 10%:
Cardiovascular: Proarrhythmia, palpitations, cardiac death, EKG abnormalities, congestive heart failure
Central nervous system: Headache, fatigue, insomnia
Gastrointestinal: Nausea, diarrhea, ileus
Genitourinary: Decreased libido
Ocular: Blurred vision, periorbital edema
Respiratory: Dyspnea

<1%:
Cardiovascular: Ventricular tachycardia, cardiac chest pain, hypotension or hypertension, syncope, supraventricular arrhythmias, myocardial infarction
Central nervous system: Anxiety, drug fever, confusion, loss of memory, vertigo, anorexia
Dermatologic: Rash, dry skin
Gastrointestinal: GI upset, vomiting, dyspepsia, flatulence, bitter taste
Genitourinary: Urinary retention, urinary incontinence, impotence
Neuromuscular & skeletal: Tremor
Otic: Tinnitus
Respiratory: Apnea
Miscellaneous: Sweating

Overdosage/Toxicology Has a narrow therapeutic index and severe toxicity may occur slightly above the therapeutic range, especially if combined with other antiarrhythmic drugs. (Acute single ingestion of twice the daily therapeutic dose is life-threatening). Symptoms of overdose include increases in P-R, QRS, Q-T intervals and amplitude of the T wave, A-V block, bradycardia, hypotension, ventricular arrhythmias (monomorphic or polymorphic ventricular tachycardia), and asystole; other symptoms include dizziness, blurred vision, headache, and GI upset.

Treatment is supportive, using conventional treatment (fluids, positioning, anti-convulsants, antiarrhythmics). **Note:** Type 1a antiarrhythmic agents should not be used to treat cardiotoxicity caused by type 1c drugs; sodium bicarbonate may reverse QRS prolongation, bradycardia and hypotension; ventricular pacing may be needed.

Drug Interactions
Decreased levels of theophylline (50%)
Increased levels with cimetidine (50%)

Mechanism of Action Class I antiarrhythmic agent; reduces the fast inward current carried by sodium ions, shortens Phase I and Phase II repolarization, resulting in decreased action potential duration and effective refractory period

Pharmacodynamics/Kinetics
Protein binding, plasma: 95%
Metabolism: Undergoes significant first-pass metabolism absolute
Bioavailability: 38%
Half-life:
Normal patients: 3-4 hours
Cardiac disease patients: 6-13 hours
Elimination: Some enterohepatic recycling occurs; 56% is excreted in feces and 39% in urine

Usual Dosage Adults: Oral: 200-300 mg every 8 hours, adjust dosage at 150 mg/day at 3-day intervals. See table for dosage recommendations of transferring from other antiarrhythmic agents to Ethmozine®.

Moricizine

Transferred From	Start Ethmozine®
Encainide, propafenone, tocainide, or mexiletine	8-12 hours after last dose
Flecainide	12-24 hours after last dose
Procainamide	3-6 hours after last dose
Quinidine, disopyramide	6-12 hours after last dose

Dosing interval in renal or hepatic impairment: Start at 600 mg/day or less
Patient Information Take as directed; do not change dose except from advice of your physician; report any chest pain and irregular heartbeats
Nursing Implications Giving 30 minutes after a meal delays the rate of absorption, resulting in lower peak plasma concentrations
Dosage Forms Tablet: 200 mg, 250 mg, 300 mg

Morning After Pill *see* Ethinyl Estradiol and Norgestrel *on page 427*

Morphine Sulfate (mor' feen)

Related Information

Narcotic Agonist Comparison Charts *on page 1274-1275*

Brand Names Astramorph™ PF; Duramorph®; MS Contin®; MSIR®; OMS®; Oramorph SR®; RMS®; Roxanol™; Roxanol SR™

Synonyms MS

Use Relief of moderate to severe acute and chronic pain; pain of myocardial infarction; relieves dyspnea of acute left ventricular failure and pulmonary edema; preanesthetic medication

Restrictions C-II

Pregnancy Risk Factor B (D if used for prolonged periods or in high doses at term)

Contraindications Known hypersensitivity to morphine sulfate; increased intracranial pressure; severe respiratory depression

Warnings/Precautions Some preparations contain sulfites which may cause allergic reactions; infants <3 months of age are more susceptible to respiratory depression, use with caution and generally in reduced doses in this age group; use with caution in patients with impaired respiratory function or severe hepatic dysfunction and in patients with hypersensitivity reactions to other phenanthrene derivative opioid agonists (codeine, hydrocodone, hydromorphone, levorphanol, oxycodone, oxymorphone). Morphine shares the toxic potential of opiate agonists and usual precautions of opiate agonist therapy should be observed; may cause hypotension in patients with acute myocardial infarction.

Elderly may be particularly susceptible to the CNS depressant and constipating effects of narcotics

Adverse Reactions

Central nervous system: CNS depression, drowsiness, sedation, sweating, flushing, increased intracranial pressure

Endocrine & metabolic: Antidiuretic hormone release

Miscellaneous: Physical and psychological dependence

>10%:

Cardiovascular: Palpitations, hypotension, bradycardia

Central nervous system: Weakness, dizziness

Gastrointestinal: Nausea, vomiting, constipation, dry mouth

Local: Pain at injection site

Miscellaneous: Histamine release

1% to 10%:

Central nervous system: Restlessness, headache, false feeling of well being, confusion

Gastrointestinal: Anorexia, GI irritation, dry mouth, paralytic ileus

Genitourinary: Decreased urination

Neuromuscular & skeletal: Trembling

Ocular: Vision problems

Respiratory: Respiratory depression, shortness of breath

<1%:

Cardiovascular: Peripheral vasodilation

Central nervous system: Insomnia, mental depression, hallucinations, paradoxical CNS stimulation, increased intracranial pressure

Dermatologic: Pruritus

Neuromuscular & skeletal: Muscle rigidity

Ocular: Miosis

Miscellaneous: Biliary or urinary tract spasm

Overdosage/Toxicology Symptoms of overdose include respiratory depression, miosis, hypotension, bradycardia, apnea, pulmonary edema. Treatment of an overdose includes support of the patient's airway, establishment of an I.V. line, and administration of naloxone 2 mg I.V. (0.01 mg/kg for children) with repeat administration as necessary up to a total of 10 mg. Primary attention should be directed to ensuring adequate respiratory exchange.

Drug Interactions

Decreased effect: Phenothiazines may antagonize the analgesic effect of morphine and other opiate agonists

Increased toxicity: CNS depressants, tricyclic antidepressants may potentiate the effects of morphine and other opiate agonists; dextroamphetamine may enhance the analgesic effect of morphine and other opiate agonists

Stability Refrigerate suppositories; do not freeze; degradation depends on pH and presence of oxygen; relatively stable in pH ≤4; darkening of solutions indicate degradation; usual concentration for continuous I.V. infusion = 0.1-1 mg/mL in D_5W

Mechanism of Action Binds to opiate receptors in the CNS, causing inhibition of ascending pain pathways, altering the perception of and response to pain; produces generalized CNS depression

(Continued)

Morphine Sulfate *(Continued)*

Pharmacodynamics/Kinetics
Absorption: Oral: Variable
Metabolism: In the liver via glucuronide conjugation
Half-life:
  Neonates: 4.5-13.3 hours (mean 7.6 hours)
  Adults: 2-4 hours
Elimination: Unchanged in urine; see table.

Dosage Form/Route	Analgesia	
	Peak	Duration
Tablets	1 h	4-5 h
Oral solution	1 h	4-5 h
Extended release tablets	1 h	8-12 h
Suppository	20-60 min	3-7 h
Subcutaneous injection	50-90 min	4-5 h
I.M. injection	30-60 min	4-5 h
I.V. injection	20 min	4-5 h

Usual Dosage Doses should be titrated to appropriate effect; when changing routes of administration in chronically treated patients, please note that oral doses are approximately one-half as effective as parenteral dose

Infants and Children:
  Oral: Tablet and solution (prompt release): 0.2-0.5 mg/kg/dose every 4-6 hours as needed; tablet (controlled release): 0.3-0.6 mg/kg/dose every 12 hours
  I.M., I.V., S.C.: 0.1-0.2 mg/kg/dose every 2-4 hours as needed; usual maximum: 15 mg/dose; may initiate at 0.05 mg/kg/dose
  I.V., S.C. continuous infusion: Sickle cell or cancer pain: 0.025-2 mg/kg/hour; postoperative pain: 0.01-0.04 mg/kg/hour
  Sedation/analgesia for procedures: I.V.: 0.05-0.1 mg/kg 5 minutes before the procedure

Adolescents >12 years: Sedation/analgesia for procedures: I.V.: 3-4 mg and repeat in 5 minutes if necessary

Adults:
  Oral: Prompt release: 10-30 mg every 4 hours as needed; controlled release: 15-30 mg every 8-12 hours
  I.M., I.V., S.C.: 2.5-20 mg/dose every 2-6 hours as needed; usual: 10 mg/dose every 4 hours as needed
  I.V., S.C. continuous infusion: 0.8-10 mg/hour; may increase depending on pain relief/adverse effects; usual range: up to 80 mg/hour
  Epidural: Initial: 5 mg in lumbar region; if inadequate pain relief within 1 hour, give 1-2 mg, maximum dose: 10 mg/24 hours
  Intrathecal ($^1/_{10}$ of epidural dose): 0.2-1 mg/dose; repeat doses **not** recommended
  Rectal: 10-20 mg every 4 hours

Dosing adjustment in renal impairment:
Cl_{cr} 10-50 mL/minute: Administer at 75% of normal dose
Cl_{cr} <10 mL/minute: Administer at 50% of normal dose

Dosing adjustment/comments in hepatic disease: Unchanged in mild liver disease; substantial extrahepatic metabolism may occur; excessive sedation may occur in cirrhosis

Administration When giving morphine I.V. push, it is best to first dilute in 4-5 mL of sterile water, and then to administer slowly (eg, 15 mg over 3-5 minutes)

Monitoring Parameters Pain relief, respiratory and mental status, blood pressure

Reference Range Therapeutic: Surgical anesthesia: 65-80 ng/mL (SI: 227-280 nmol/L); Toxic: 200-5000 ng/mL (SI: 700-17,500 nmol/L)

Test Interactions ↑ aminotransferase [ALT (SGPT)/AST (SGOT)] (S)

Patient Information Avoid alcohol, may cause drowsiness, impaired judgment or coordination; may cause physical and psychological dependence with prolonged use

Nursing Implications Do not crush controlled release drug product, observe patient for excessive sedation, respiratory depression; implement safety measures, assist with ambulation; use preservative-free solutions for intrathecal or epidural use

Dosage Forms
Injection: 0.5 mg/mL (10 mL); 1 mg/mL (10 mL, 30 mL, 60 mL); 2 mg/mL (1 mL, 2 mL, 60 mL); 3 mg/mL (50 mL); 4 mg/mL (1 mL, 2 mL); 5 mg/mL (1 mL, 30 mL); 8 mg/mL (1 mL, 2 mL); 10 mg/mL (1 mL, 2 mL, 10 mL); 15 mg/mL (1 mL, 2 mL, 20 mL)
Injection:
  Preservative free: 0.5 mg/mL (2 mL, 10 mL); 1 mg/mL (2 mL, 10 mL)
  I.V. via PCA pump: 1 mg/mL (10 mL, 30 mL, 60 mL); 5 mg/mL (30 mL)
  I.V. infusion preparation: 25 mg/mL (4 mL, 10 mL, 20 mL)
Solution, oral: 10 mg/5 mL (5 mL, 10 mL, 100 mL, 120 mL, 500 mL); 20 mg/5 mL (5 mL, 100 mL, 120 mL, 500 mL); 20 mg/mL (30 mL)
Suppository, rectal: 5 mg, 10 mg, 20 mg, 30 mg
Tablet: 15 mg, 30 mg
Tablet:
  Controlled release: 15 mg, 30 mg, 60 mg, 100 mg
  Soluble: 10 mg, 15 mg, 30 mg
  Sustained release: 30 mg, 60 mg, 100 mg

Morrhuate Sodium (mor' yoo ate)
Brand Names Scleromate™
Use Treatment of small, uncomplicated varicose veins of the lower extremities
Contraindications Arterial disease, thrombophlebitis, hypersensitivity to morrhuate sodium or any component
Warnings/Precautions Sloughing and necrosis of tissue may occur following extravasation; anaphylactoid and allergic reactions have occurred; this drug should only be administered by a physician familiar with proper injection techniques; a test dose of 0.25-5 mL of a 5% injection should be given 24 hours before full-dose treatment
Adverse Reactions
>10%:
  Cardiovascular: Thrombosis, valvular incompetency
  Dermatologic: Urticaria
  Local: Burning at the site of injection, severe extravasation effects
<1%:
  Cardiovascular: Vascular collapse
  Central nervous system: Drowsiness, headache, dizziness
  Gastrointestinal: Nausea, vomiting
  Neuromuscular & skeletal: Weakness
  Respiratory: Asthma
  Miscellaneous: Anaphylaxis
Stability Refrigerate
Mechanism of Action Both varicose veins and esophageal varices are treated by the thrombotic action of morrhuate sodium. By causing inflammation of the vein's intima, a thrombus is formed. Occlusion secondary to the fibrous tissue and the thrombus results in the obliteration of the vein.
Pharmacodynamics/Kinetics
Onset of action: ~5 minutes
Absorption: Most of the dose stays at the site of injection
Distribution: After treatment of esophageal varices, ~20% of dose distributes to the lungs
Usual Dosage I.V.:
Children 1-18 years: Esophageal hemorrhage: 2, 3, or 4 mL of 5% repeated every 3-4 days until bleeding is controlled, then every 6 weeks until varices obliterated

Adults: 50-250 mg, repeated at 5- to 7-day intervals (50-100 mg for small veins, 150-250 mg for large veins)
Administration For I.V. use only
Nursing Implications Avoid extravasation; use only clear solutions, solution should become clear when warmed
Dosage Forms Injection: 50 mg/mL (5 mL)

Motrin® see Ibuprofen on page 561

Motrin® IB [OTC] see Ibuprofen on page 561

6-MP see Mercaptopurine on page 690

M-R-VAX® II see Measles and Rubella Vaccines, Combined on page 667

MS see Morphine Sulfate on page 756

MS Contin® *see* Morphine Sulfate *on page 756*

MSIR® *see* Morphine Sulfate *on page 756*

MTC *see* Mitomycin *on page 746*

MTX *see* Methotrexate *on page 711*

Mucomyst® *see* Acetylcysteine *on page 25*

Mucosil™ *see* Acetylcysteine *on page 25*

Multiple Vitamins *see* Vitamin, Multiple *on page 1166*

Multitest CMI® *see* Skin Test Antigens, Multiple *on page 1008*

Multivitamins/Fluoride *see* Vitamin, Multiple *on page 1166*

Multi Vit® Drops [OTC] *see* Vitamin, Multiple *on page 1166*

Mumps, Measles and Rubella Vaccines, Combined *see* Measles, Mumps, and Rubella Vaccines, Combined *on page 668*

Mumpsvax® *see* Mumps Virus Vaccine, Live, Attenuated *on this page*

Mumps Virus Vaccine, Live, Attenuated (mumpsz)
Related Information
  Immunization Guidelines *on page 1389-1405*
  Skin Testing for Delayed Hypersensitivity *on page 1325-1327*
Brand Names Mumpsvax®
Use Mumps prophylaxis by promoting active immunity
Pregnancy Risk Factor X
Warnings/Precautions Pregnancy, immunocompromised persons, history of anaphylactic reaction following egg ingestion or receipt of neomycin
Adverse Reactions
  >10%: Local: Burning or stinging at injection site
  1% to 10%:
    Central nervous system: Fever ≤100°F
    Dermatologic: Skin rash
    Endocrine & metabolic: Parotitis
  <1%:
    Central nervous system: Convulsions, confusion, severe or continuing headache, fever >103°F
    Genitourinary: Orchitis in postpubescent and adult males
    Hematologic: Thrombocytopenic purpura
    Miscellaneous: Anaphylactic reactions
Drug Interactions Decreased effect with concurrent infection, immunoglobulin with in 1 month, other live vaccines with the exception of attenuated measles, rubella, or polio
Stability Refrigerate, protect from light, discard within 8 hours after reconstitution
Usual Dosage 1 vial (5000 units) S.C. in outer aspect of the upper arm, no booster
Administration Reconstitute only with diluent provided; administer only S.C. on outer aspect of upper arm
Test Interactions Temporary suppression of tuberculosis skin test
Patient Information Pregnancy should be avoided for 3 months following vaccination; a little swelling of the glands in the cheeks and under the jaw may occur that lasts for a few days; this could happen from 1-2 weeks after getting the mumps vaccine; this happens rarely
Additional Information Federal law requires that the date of administration, the vaccine manufacturer, lot number of vaccine, and the administering person's name, title and address be entered into the patient's permanent medical record; all adults without documentation of live vaccine on or after the first birthday or physician-diagnosed mumps, or laboratory evidence or immunity (particularly males and young adults who work in or congregate in hospitals, colleges, and on military bases) should be vaccinated. It is reasonable to consider persons born before 1957 immune, but there is no contraindication to vaccination of older persons. Susceptible travelers should be vaccinated.
Dosage Forms Injection: Single dose

Mupirocin (myoo peer′ oh sin)
Brand Names Bactroban®
Synonyms Pseudomonic Acid A
Use Topical treatment of impetigo due to *Staphylococcus aureus*, beta-hemolytic *Streptococcus*, and *S. pyogenes*
Pregnancy Risk Factor B
Contraindications Known hypersensitivity to mupirocin or polyethylene glycol

Warnings/Precautions Potentially toxic amounts of polyethylene glycol contained in the vehicle may be absorbed percutaneously in patients with extensive burns or open wounds; prolonged use may result in over growth of nonsusceptible organisms; for external use only; not for treatment of pressure sores

Adverse Reactions
1% to 10%:
Dermatologic: Pruritus, rash, erythema, dry skin
Local: Burning, stinging, pain, tenderness, swelling

Stability Do not mix with Aquaphor®, coal tar solution, or salicylic acid

Mechanism of Action Binds to bacterial isoleucyl transfer-RNA synthetase resulting in the inhibition of protein and RNA synthesis

Pharmacodynamics/Kinetics
Absorption: Topical: Penetrates the outer layers of the skin; systemic absorption minimal through intact skin
Protein binding: 95%
Metabolism: Extensively to monic acid, principally in the liver and skin
Half-life: 17-36 minutes
Elimination: In urine

Usual Dosage Children and Adults: Topical: Apply small amount to affected area 2-5 times/day for 5-14 days

Patient Information For topical use only; do not apply into the eye; discontinue if rash, itching, or irritation occurs; improvement should be seen in 5 days

Additional Information Not for treatment of pressure sores in elderly; contains polyethylene glycol vehicle

Dosage Forms Ointment, topical: 2% (15 g)

Murine® Ear Drops [OTC] see Carbamide Peroxide on page 179

Murine® Plus [OTC] see Tetrahydrozoline Hydrochloride on page 1071

Muro 128® Ophthalmic [OTC] see Sodium Chloride on page 1012

Muromonab-CD3 (myoo roe moe' nab)
Brand Names Orthoclone® OKT3
Synonyms Monoclonal Antibody; OKT3
Use Treatment of acute allograft rejection in renal transplant patients; effective in reversing acute hepatic, cardiac, and bone marrow transplant rejection episodes resistant to conventional treatment
Pregnancy Risk Factor C
Contraindications Patients with known hypersensitivity to OKT3 or any murine product; patients in fluid overload or those with >3% weight gain within 1 week prior to start of OKT3
Warnings/Precautions May result in an increased susceptibility to infection; dosage of concomitant immunosuppressants should be reduced during OKT3 therapy; cyclosporine should be discontinued or decreased to 50% usual maintenance dose and maintenance therapy resumed about 3 days before stopping OKT3; severe pulmonary edema has occurred in patients with fluid overload
First dose effect (flu-like symptoms, anaphylactic-type reaction) may occur within 30 minutes to 6 hours, up to 24 hours after the first dose and may be minimized by using the recommended regimens. See table.

Suggested Prevention/Treatment of Muromonab-CD3 First-Dose Effects

Adverse Reaction	Effective Prevention or Palliation	Supportive Treatment
Severe pulmonary edema	Clear chest x-ray within 24 h preinjection Weight restriction to ≤3% gain over 7 days preinjection	Prompt intubation and oxygenation 24 h close observation
Fever, chills	1 mg/kg methylprednisolone sodium succinate preinjection Fever reduction <37.8°C (100°F) preinjection	Cooling blanket Acetaminophen prn
Respiratory effects	100 mg hydrocortisone sodium succinate 30 min postinjection	Additional 100 mg hydrocortisone sodium succinate prn

Cardiopulmonary resuscitation may be needed. If the patient's temperature is >37.8°C, reduce before administering OKT3.

Adverse Reactions
>10%:
Cardiovascular: Tachycardia
Central nervous system: Dizziness, faintness
Gastrointestinal: Diarrhea, nausea, vomiting
(Continued)

Muromonab-CD3 *(Continued)*

Neuromuscular & skeletal: Trembling
Respiratory: Shortness of breath
1% to 10%:
Central nervous system: Headache, stiff neck
Ocular: Photophobia
Respiratory: Pulmonary edema
<1%:
Cardiovascular: Hypertension, hypotension, chest pain
Central nervous system: Aseptic meningitis, seizures, tiredness, confusion, coma, hallucinations
Dermatologic: Pruritus, rash
Hepatic: Increased BUN and creatinine
Neuromuscular & skeletal: Joint pain, tremor
Respiratory: Dyspnea, tightness, wheezing
Sensitivity reactions: Anaphylactic-type reactions
Miscellaneous: Pyrexia, flu-like symptoms (ie, fever, chills), infection

Drug Interactions Recommend decreasing dose of prednisone to 0.5 mg/kg, azathioprine to 0.5 mg/kg (approximate 50% decrease in dose), and discontinuing cyclosporine while patient is receiving OKT3

Decreased effect: Immunosuppressive drugs

Stability Refrigerate; do not shake or freeze; stable in Becton Dickinson syringe for 16 hours at room temperature or refrigeration

Mechanism of Action Reverses graft rejection by binding to T-cells and interfering with their function

Pharmacodynamics/Kinetics

Absorption: I.V.: Immediate
Time to steady-state: Trough level: 3-14 days; pretreatment levels are restored within 7 days after treatment is terminated

Usual Dosage I.V. (refer to individual protocols):
Children <30 kg: 2.5 mg/day once daily for 7-14 days
Children >30 kg: 5 mg/day once daily for 7-14 days
  or
Children <12 years: 0.1 mg/kg/day once daily for 10-14 days
Children >12 years and Adults: 5 mg/day once daily for 10-14 days

Removal by dialysis: Molecular size of OKT3 is 150,000 daltons; not dialyzed by most standard dialyzers; however, may be dialyzed by high flux dialysis; OKT3 will be removed by plasmapheresis; administer following dialysis treatments

Administration Filter each dose through a low protein-binding 0.22 micron filter (Millex GV) before administration; give I.V. push over <1 minute at a final concentration of 1 mg/mL; **do not give I.M.**

Children and Adults:
Methylprednisolone sodium succinate 1 mg/kg I.V. given prior to first muromonab-CD3 administration and I.V. hydrocortisone sodium succinate 50-100 mg given 30 minutes after administration are strongly recommended to decrease the incidence of reactions to the first dose
Patient temperature should not exceed 37.8°C (100°F) at time of administration

Monitoring Parameters

Chest x-ray, weight gain, CBC with differential, temperature, vital signs (blood pressure, temperature, pulse, respiration); immunologic monitoring of T cells, serum levels of OKT3

Clinical Guidelines - OKT3 Serum Concentration Monitoring: Serum level monitoring should be performed in conjunction with lymphocyte subset determinations. Trough concentrations correlate best with clinical outcome.

Clinical Guidelines for Lymphocyte Subset Monitoring: Trough sample measurement is preferable
Absolute # or % of CD3+ cells should be guided by the following:
OKT3-FITC: <10-50 cells/mm³ or 3% to 5%
  Strongly recommended!
CD3 (IgG₁)-FITC: Similar to OKT3-FITC
Leu-4a: Higher # of CD3+ cells appears acceptable
Frequency of monitoring based on indication of use for OKT3:
  Rejection: Daily monitoring
  Induction (high risk - retransplant, black race, pediatric, high PRA, poor HLA match, low anti-OKT3 antibody titer): Daily monitoring
  Induction (low-dose): Daily monitoring
  Induction (first course): Delay of initial monitoring by 2-3 days with additional monitoring every 2-3 days as indicated by clinical and laboratory parameters

Several clinical studies have established absolute CD3⁺ cell counts ≤10-50/mm³ or % of total lymphocyte ≤3% to 5% indicate adequate immunosuppression

Reference Range Mean serum trough levels rise during the first 3 days, then average 0.9 µg/mL on days 3-14

Patient Information Inform patient of expected first dose effects which are markedly reduced with subsequent treatments

Nursing Implications Monitor patient closely for 24 hours after the first dose; drugs and equipment for treating pulmonary edema and anaphylaxis should be on hand

Dosage Forms Injection: 5 mg/5 mL

Muro's Opcon® *see* Naphazoline Hydrochloride *on page 775*

Mus-Lac® *see* Chlorzoxazone *on page 236*

Mustargen® *see* Mechlorethamine Hydrochloride *on page 672*

Mustine *see* Mechlorethamine Hydrochloride *on page 672*

Mutamycin® *see* Mitomycin *on page 746*

M.V.I.® *see* Vitamin, Multiple *on page 1166*

M.V.I.®-12 *see* Vitamin, Multiple *on page 1166*

M.V.I.® Concentrate *see* Vitamin, Multiple *on page 1166*

M.V.I.® Pediatric *see* Vitamin, Multiple *on page 1166*

Myambutol® *see* Ethambutol Hydrochloride *on page 417*

Mycelex® *see* Clotrimazole *on page 265*

Mycelex-7® **[OTC]** *see* Clotrimazole *on page 265*

Mycelex®-G *see* Clotrimazole *on page 265*

Mycelex OTC® **[OTC]** *see* Clotrimazole *on page 265*

Mycelex Twin Pack® *see* Clotrimazole *on page 265*

Mycifradin® Sulfate *see* Neomycin Sulfate *on page 783*

Mycinettes® **[OTC]** *see* Benzocaine *on page 121*

Mycitracin® **[OTC]** *see* Bacitracin, Neomycin, and Polymyxin B *on page 113*

Mycobutin® *see* Rifabutin *on page 981*

Mycogen® II *see* Nystatin and Triamcinolone *on page 812*

Mycolog®-II *see* Nystatin and Triamcinolone *on page 812*

Myconel® *see* Nystatin and Triamcinolone *on page 812*

Mycostatin® *see* Nystatin *on page 811*

Myco-Triacet® II *see* Nystatin and Triamcinolone *on page 812*

Mydfrin® Ophthalmic Solution *see* Phenylephrine Hydrochloride *on page 874*

Mydriacyl® *see* Tropicamide *on page 1134*

Mykrox® *see* Metolazone *on page 730*

Mylanta® Gas [OTC] *see* Simethicone *on page 1006*

Myleran® *see* Busulfan *on page 151*

Mylicon® [OTC] *see* Simethicone *on page 1006*

Myochrysine® *see* Gold Sodium Thiomalate *on page 509*

Myotonachol™ *see* Bethanechol Chloride *on page 132*

Mysoline® *see* Primidone *on page 924*

Mytrex® *see* Nystatin and Triamcinolone *on page 812*

Mytussin® AC *see* Guaifenesin and Codeine *on page 516*

Mytussin® [OTC] *see* Guaifenesin *on page 515*

Mytussin® DM [OTC] *see* Guaifenesin and Dextromethorphan *on page 517*

Nabilone (na' bi lone)

Brand Names Cesamet®

Use Treatment of nausea and vomiting associated with cancer chemotherapy

Restrictions C-II

Pregnancy Risk Factor C

Contraindications Nausea and vomiting not secondary to cancer chemotherapy

(Continued)

Nabilone *(Continued)*

Warnings/Precautions Use with caution in the elderly, those with pre-existing CNS depression, or a history of mental illness

Adverse Reactions

>10%:

Central nervous system: Dizziness, drowsiness, vertigo, euphoria, clumsiness

Gastrointestinal: Dry mouth

1% to 10%:

Cardiovascular: Orthostatic hypotension

Central nervous system: Ataxia, depression

Ocular: Blurred vision

<1%:

Central nervous system: Changes of mood, confusion, hallucinations, headache

Gastrointestinal: Loss of appetite

Respiratory: Difficulty in breathing

Overdosage/Toxicology Symptoms of overdose include nausea, vomiting, disorientation, CNS, respiratory depression, dysphoria, euphoria; treatment is supportive and symptomatic

Mechanism of Action Nabilone is a synthetic cannabinoid utilized as an antiemetic drug in the control of nausea and vomiting in patients receiving cancer chemotherapy; like delta-9-tetrahydrocannabinol (the active principal of marijuana), nabilone is a dibenzo(b,d)pyrans

Pharmacodynamics/Kinetics

Absorption: Rapid

Distribution: Rapidly and extensive to body tissues

Metabolism: Undergoes rapid metabolism to one or more active metabolites

Bioavailability: 95.8%

Half-life: 35 hours

Usual Dosage Oral:

Children >4 years:

<18 kg: 0.5 mg twice daily

18-30 kg: 1 mg twice daily

>30 kg: 1 mg 3 times/day

Adults: 1-2 mg twice daily beginning 1-3 hours before chemotherapy is administered and continuing around-the-clock until 1 dose after chemotherapy is completed; maximum daily dose: 6 mg divided in 3 doses

Patient Information May cause drowsiness, impair judgment, coordination; avoid alcohol and other CNS depressants; can cause disorientation

Nursing Implications May cause drowsiness, euphoria; institute safety precautions

Dosage Forms Capsule: 1 mg

Nabumetone *(na byoo' me tone)*

Related Information

Nonsteroidal Anti-Inflammatories Comparison *on page 1280*

Brand Names Relafen®

Use Management of osteoarthritis and rheumatoid arthritis

Unlabeled use: Sunburn, mild to moderate pain

Pregnancy Risk Factor C

Contraindications Hypersensitivity to nabumetone; should not be administered to patients with active peptic ulceration and those with severe hepatic impairment or in patients in whom nabumetone, aspirin, or other NSAIDs have induced asthma, urticaria, or other allergic-type reactions; fatal asthmatic reactions have occurred following NSAID administration

Warnings/Precautions Elderly patients may sometimes require lower doses; patients with impaired renal function may need a dose reduction; use with caution in patients with severe hepatic impairment

Adverse Reactions

>10%:

Central nervous system: Dizziness

Dermatologic: Skin rash

Gastrointestinal: Abdominal cramps, heartburn, indigestion, nausea

1% to 10%:

Cardiovascular: Fluid retention

Central nervous system: Headache, nervousness

Dermatologic: Itching

Gastrointestinal: Vomiting

Otic: Ringing in ears

<1%:

Cardiovascular: Congestive heart failure, hypertension, arrhythmia, tachycardia

Central nervous system: Epistaxis, confusion, hallucinations, aseptic meningitis, mental depression, drowsiness, insomnia

Dermatologic: Angioedema, hives, erythema multiforme, toxic epidermal necrolysis, Stevens-Johnson syndrome

Endocrine & metabolic: Polydipsia, hot flushes

Gastrointestinal: Gastritis, GI ulceration

Genitourinary: Cystitis

Hematologic: Agranulocytosis, anemia, hemolytic anemia, bone marrow depression, leukopenia, thrombocytopenia

Hepatic: Hepatitis

Neuromuscular & skeletal: Peripheral neuropathy

Ocular: Toxic amblyopia, blurred vision, conjunctivitis, dry eyes

Otic: Decreased hearing

Renal: Polyuria, acute renal failure

Respiratory: Allergic rhinitis, shortness of breath

Mechanism of Action Nabumetone is a nonacidic, nonsteroidal anti-inflammatory drug that is rapidly metabolized after absorption to a major active metabolite, 6-methoxy-2-naphthylacetic acid. As found with previous nonsteroidal anti-inflammatory drugs, nabumetone's active metabolite inhibits the cyclo-oxygenase enzyme which is indirectly responsible for the production of inflammation and pain during arthritis by way of enhancing the production of endoperoxides and prostaglandins E_2 and I_2 (prostacyclin). The active metabolite of nabumetone is felt to be the compound primarily responsible for therapeutic effect. Comparatively, the parent drug is a poor inhibitor of prostaglandin synthesis.

Pharmacodynamics/Kinetics

Distribution: Diffusion occurs readily into synovial fluid with peak concentrations in 4-12 hours

Protein binding: >99%

Metabolism: A prodrug being rapidly metabolized to an active metabolite (6-methoxy-2-naphthylacetic acid); extensive first-pass hepatic metabolism

Half-life, elimination: Major metabolite: 24 hours

Time to peak serum concentration: Metabolite: Oral: Within 3-6 hours

Elimination: 80% recovered in urine and 10% in feces, with very little excreted as unchanged compound

Usual Dosage Adults: Oral: 1000 mg/day; an additional 500-1000 mg may be needed in some patients to obtain more symptomatic relief; may be administered once or twice daily

Dosing adjustment in renal impairment: None necessary; however, adverse effects due to accumulation of inactive metabolites of nabumetone that are renally excreted have not been studied and should be considered

Patient Information Take this medication at meal times or with food or milk to minimize gastric irritation; inform your physician if you develop stomach disturbances, blurred vision, or other eye symptoms, rash, weight gain, or edema; inform your physician if you pass dark-colored or tarry stools; concomitant use of alcohol should be avoided if possible since it may add to the irritant action of nabumetone in the stomach; aspirin should be avoided

Dosage Forms Tablet: 500 mg, 750 mg

NAC *see* Acetylcysteine *on page 25*

***N*-Acetylcysteine** *see* Acetylcysteine *on page 25*

***N*-Acetyl-L-cysteine** *see* Acetylcysteine *on page 25*

N-Acetyl-P-Aminophenol *see* Acetaminophen *on page 17*

NaCl *see* Sodium Chloride *on page 1012*

Nadolol (nay doe' lole)

Related Information

Beta-Blockers Comparison *on page 1257-1259*

Brand Names Corgard®

Use Treatment of hypertension and angina pectoris; prevention of myocardial infarction; prophylaxis of migraine headaches

Pregnancy Risk Factor C

Contraindications Uncompensated congestive heart failure, cardiogenic shock, bradycardia or heart block, hypersensitivity to any component, bronchial asthma, bronchospasms, diabetes mellitus

Warnings/Precautions Increase dosing interval in patients with renal dysfunction; abrupt withdrawal of beta-blockers may result in an exaggerated cardiac

(Continued)

Nadolol *(Continued)*

beta-adrenergic responsiveness; symptomatology has included reports of tachycardia, hypertension, ischemia, angina, myocardial infarction, and sudden death; it is recommended that patients be tapered gradually off of beta-blockers over a period of 1-2 weeks rather than via abrupt discontinuation; use with caution in patients with bronchial asthma, bronchospasms, CHF, or diabetes mellitus

Adverse Reactions

>10%: Cardiovascular: Bradycardia

1% to 10%:

Cardiovascular: Reduced peripheral circulation

Central nervous system: Mental depression, dizziness

Endocrine & metabolic: Decreased sexual ability

Gastrointestinal: Constipation

Neuromuscular & skeletal: Weakness

Respiratory: Breathing difficulty, wheezing

<1%:

Cardiovascular: Congestive heart failure, chest pain, orthostatic hypotension, Raynaud's syndrome, congestive heart failure, edema, Raynaud's phenomena

Central nervous system: Drowsiness, nightmares, vivid dreams, tingling of toes and fingers, insomnia, lethargy, dizziness, fatigue, confusion, headache

Dermatologic: Itching, rash

Gastrointestinal: Vomiting, stomach discomfort, diarrhea, nausea

Genitourinary: Impotence

Hematologic: Thrombocytopenia

Ocular: Dry eyes

Respiratory: Stuffy nose

Miscellaneous: Cold extremities

Overdosage/Toxicology Symptoms of intoxication include cardiac disturbances, CNS toxicity, bronchospasm, hypoglycemia and hyperkalemia. The most common cardiac symptoms include hypotension and bradycardia; atrioventricular block, intraventricular conduction disturbances, cardiogenic shock, and asystole may occur with severe overdose; CNS effects include convulsions, coma, and respiratory arrest

Treatment includes symptomatic treatment of seizures, hypotension, hyperkalemia and hypoglycemia; bradycardia and hypotension resistant to atropine, isoproterenol or pacing may respond to glucagon; wide QRS defects caused by the membrane-depressant poisoning may respond to hypertonic sodium bicarbonate; repeat-dose charcoal, hemoperfusion, or hemodialysis may be helpful in removal of only those beta-blockers with a small V_d, long half-life or low intrinsic clearance (acebutolol, atenolol, nadolol, sotalol).

Drug Interactions

Decreased effect of beta-blockers with aluminum salts, barbiturates, calcium salts, cholestyramine, colestipol, NSAIDs, penicillins (ampicillin), rifampin, salicylates and sulfinpyrazone due to decreased bioavailability and plasma levels

Beta-blockers may decrease the effect of sulfonylureas

Increased effect/toxicity of beta-blockers with calcium blockers (diltiazem, felodipine, nicardipine), contraceptives, flecainide, haloperidol (propranolol, hypotensive effects), H_2 antagonists (metoprolol, propranolol only by cimetidine, possibly ranitidine), hydralazine (metoprolol, propranolol), loop diuretics (propranolol, not atenolol), MAO inhibitors (metoprolol, nadolol, bradycardia), phenothiazines (propranolol), propafenone (metoprolol, propranolol), quinidine (in extensive metabolizers), ciprofloxacin, thyroid hormones (metoprolol, propranolol, when hypothyroid patient is converted to euthyroid state)

Beta-blockers may increase the effect/toxicity of flecainide, haloperidol (hypotensive effects), hydralazine, phenothiazines, acetaminophen, anticoagulants (propranolol, warfarin), benzodiazepines (not atenolol), clonidine (hypertensive crisis after or during withdrawal of either agent), epinephrine (initial hypertensive episode followed by bradycardia), nifedipine and verapamil lidocaine, ergots (peripheral ischemia), prazosin (postural hypotension)

Beta-blockers may affect the action or levels of ethanol, disopyramide, nondepolarizing muscle relaxants and theophylline although the effects are difficult to predict

Mechanism of Action Competitively blocks response to beta$_1$- and beta$_2$-adrenergic stimulation; does not exhibit any membrane stabilizing or intrinsic sympathomimetic activity

Pharmacodynamics/Kinetics

Duration of effect: 24 hours

Absorption: Oral: 30% to 40%

Time to peak serum concentration: Within 2-4 hours persisting for 17-24 hours

Distribution: Concentration in human breast milk is 4.6 times higher than serum

Protein binding: 28%

Half-life: Adults: 10-24 hours; increased half-life with decreased renal function
End stage renal disease: 45 hours

Elimination: Renally unchanged

Usual Dosage Oral:

Children: No information regarding pediatric dosage is currently available in the literature

Adults: Initial: 40-80 mg/day, increase dosage gradually by 40-80 mg increments at 3- to 7-day intervals until optimum clinical response is obtained with profound slowing of heart rate; doses up to 160-240 mg/day in angina and 240-320 mg/day in hypertension may be necessary; doses as high as 640 mg/day have been used

Elderly: Initial: 20 mg/day; increase doses by 20 mg increments at 3- to 7-day intervals; usual dosage range: 20-240 mg/day

Dosing adjustment in renal impairment:

Cl_{cr} 31-40 mL/minute: Administer every 24-36 hours or administer 50% of normal dose

Cl_{cr} 10-30 mL/minute: Administer every 24-48 hours or administer 50% of normal dose

Cl_{cr} <10 mL/minute: Administer every 40-60 hours or administer 25% of normal dose

Moderately dialyzable (20% to 50%) via hemodialysis; administer dose postdialysis or administer 40 mg supplemental dose; supplemental dose is not necessary following peritoneal dialysis

Dosing adjustment/comments in hepatic disease: Reduced dose probably necessary

Patient Information Adhere to dosage regimen; watch for postural hypotension; abrupt withdrawal of the drug should be avoided; take at the same time each day; may mask symptoms of diabetes; sweating will continue

Nursing Implications Patient's therapeutic response may be evaluated by looking at blood pressure, apical and radial pulses

Dosage Forms Tablet: 20 mg, 40 mg, 80 mg, 120 mg, 160 mg

Nafarelin Acetate (naf' a re lin)

Brand Names Synarel®

Use Treatment of endometriosis, including pain and reduction of lesions; treatment of central precocious puberty (gonadotropin-dependent precocious puberty) in children of both sexes

Pregnancy Risk Factor X

Contraindications Hypersensitivity to GnRH, GnRH-agonist analogs or any components of this product; undiagnosed abnormal vaginal bleeding; pregnancy; lactation

Warnings/Precautions Use with caution in patients with risk factors for decreased bone mineral content, nafarelin therapy may pose an additional risk; hypersensitivity reactions occur in 0.2% of the patients; safety and efficacy in children have not been established

Adverse Reactions

>10%:

Central nervous system: Headache, emotional lability

Dermatologic: Acne

Endocrine & metabolic: Hot flashes, decreased libido, decreased breast size

Genitourinary: Vaginal dryness

Neuromuscular & skeletal: Myalgia

Respiratory: Nasal irritation

1% to 10%:

Cardiovascular: Edema

Central nervous system: Insomnia

Dermatologic: Urticaria, rash, pruritus

Respiratory: Shortness of breath, chest pain

Miscellaneous: Seborrhea

<1%:

Endocrine & metabolic: Increased libido

Gastrointestinal: weight loss

Stability Store at room temperature; protect from light

Mechanism of Action Potent synthetic decapeptide analogue of gonadotropin-releasing hormone (GnRH; LHRH) which is approximately 200 times more potent than GnRH in terms of pituitary release of luteinizing hormone (LH) and follicle-stimulating hormone (FSH). Effects on the pituitary gland and sex hormones are dependent upon its length of administration. After acute administration, an initial stimulation of the release of LH and FSH from the pituitary is observed; an
(Continued)

Nafarelin Acetate *(Continued)*

increase in androgens and estrogens subsequently follows. Continued administration of nafarelin, however, suppresses gonadotrope responsiveness to endogenous GnRH resulting in reduced secretion of LH and FSH and, secondarily, decreased ovarian and testicular steroid production.

Pharmacodynamics/Kinetics
Absorption: Not absorbed from GI tract
Maximum serum concentration: 10-45 minutes
Protein binding: 80% bound to plasma proteins

Usual Dosage
Endometriosis: Adults: Female: 1 spray (200 mcg) in 1 nostril each morning and the other nostril each evening starting on days 2-4 of menstrual cycle for 6 months
Central precocious puberty: Children: Males/Females: 2 sprays (400 mcg) into each nostril in the morning 2 sprays (400 mcg) into each nostril in the evening. If inadequate suppression, may increase dose to 3 sprays (600 mcg) into alternating nostrils 3 times/day.

Patient Information Begin treatment between days 2 and 4 of menstrual cycle; usually menstruation will stop (as well as ovulation), but is not a reliable contraceptive, use of a nonhormonal contraceptive is suggested; full compliance with taking the medicine is very important; do not use nasal decongestant for at least 30 minutes after using nafarelin spray; notify physician if regular menstruation persists

Nursing Implications Do not give to pregnant or breast-feeding patients; topical nasal decongestant should be used at least 30 minutes after nafarelin use

Additional Information Each spray delivers 200 mcg

Dosage Forms Solution, nasal: 2 mg/mL (10 mL)

Nafazair® *see* Naphazoline Hydrochloride *on page 775*

Nafcil™ *see* Nafcillin Sodium *on this page*

Nafcillin Sodium (naf sill' in)

Related Information
Extravasation Treatment of Other Drugs *on page 1209*

Brand Names Nafcil™; Nallpen®; Unipen®

Synonyms Ethoxynaphthamido Penicillin Sodium; Sodium Nafcillin

Use Treatment of susceptible bacterial infections such as osteomyelitis, septicemia, endocarditis, and CNS infections due to penicillinase-producing strains of *Staphylococcus*

Pregnancy Risk Factor B

Contraindications Hypersensitivity to nafcillin or any component or penicillins

Warnings/Precautions Extravasation of I.V. infusions should be avoided; modification of dosage is necessary in patients with both severe renal and hepatic impairment; elimination rate will be slow in neonates; use with caution in patients with cephalosporin hypersensitivity

Adverse Reactions
<1%:
Central nervous system: Fever, pain
Dermatologic: Skin rash
Gastrointestinal: Nausea, diarrhea
Hematologic: Neutropenia
Local: Thrombophlebitis; oxacillin (less likely to cause phlebitis) is often preferred in pediatric patients
Renal: Acute interstitial nephritis
Miscellaneous: Hypersensitivity reactions

Overdosage/Toxicology Symptoms of penicillin overdose include neuromuscular hypersensitivity (agitation, hallucinations, asterixis, encephalopathy, confusion, and seizures) and electrolyte imbalance with potassium or sodium salts, especially in renal failure; hemodialysis may be helpful to aid in the removal of the drug from the blood, otherwise most treatment is supportive or symptom directed

Drug Interactions
Decreased effect: Chloramphenicol → ↓ nafcillin levels; oral contraceptive may have a decreased effectiveness
Increased effect: Probenecid → ↑ nafcillin levels
Increased toxicity: Oral anticoagulants, heparin ↑ risk of bleeding

Stability Refrigerate oral solution after reconstitution; discard after 7 days; reconstituted parenteral solution is stable for 3 days at room temperature and 7 days when refrigerated or 12 weeks when frozen; for I.V. infusion in NS or D_5W, solution is stable for 24 hours at room temperature and 96 hours when refrigerated

Mechanism of Action Interferes with bacterial cell wall synthesis during active multiplication, causing cell wall death and resultant bactericidal activity against susceptible bacteria

Pharmacodynamics/Kinetics

Absorption: Oral: Poor and erratic

Distribution: Crosses the placenta

Protein binding: 90%

Half-life:

Neonates:

<3 weeks: 2.2-5.5 hours

4-9 weeks: 1.2-2.3 hours

Children 1 month to 14 years: 0.75-1.9 hours

Adults: 0.5-1.5 hours, with normal hepatic function

End stage renal disease: 1.2 hours

Time to peak serum concentration:

Oral: Within 2 hours

I.M.: Within 0.5-1 hour

Elimination: Primarily in bile, and 10% to 30% in urine as unchanged drug; undergoes enterohepatic recycling

Usual Dosage

Neonates: I.V.:

0-4 weeks: <1200 g: 25 mg/kg/dose every 12 hours

Postnatal age <7 days:

1200-2000 g: 25 mg/kg/dose every 12 hours

>2000 g: 25 mg/kg/dose every 8 hours

Postnatal age >7 days:

1200-2000 g: 25 mg/kg/dose every 8 hours

>2000 g: 25 mg/kg/dose every 6 hours

Children: I.M., I.V.:

Mild to moderate infections: 50-100 mg/kg/day in divided doses every 6 hours

Severe infections: 100-200 mg/kg/day in divided doses every 4-6 hours

Maximum dose: 12 g/day

Adults:

I.M.: 500 mg every 4-6 hours

I.V.: 500-2000 mg every 4-6 hours

Dosing adjustment in renal impairment: Not necessary

Not dialyzable (0% to 5%) via hemodialysis; supplemental dosage not necessary with hemo- or peritoneal dialysis or continuous arterio-venous or veno-venous hemofiltration (CAVH/CAVHD)

Administration Administer around-the-clock to promote less variation in peak and trough serum levels

Test Interactions Positive Coombs' test (direct)

Nursing Implications

Extravasation: Use cold packs

Hyaluronidase (Wydase®): Add 1 mL NS to 150 unit vial to make 150 units/mL of concentration; mix 0.1 mL of above with 0.9 mL NS in 1 mL syringe to make final concentration = 15 units/mL

Additional Information Sodium content of 1 g: 66.7 mg (2.9 mEq)

Dosage Forms

Capsule: 250 mg

Powder for injection: 500 mg, 1 g, 2 g, 4 g, 10 g

Solution: 250 mg/5 mL (100 mL)

Tablet: 500 mg

Naftifine Hydrochloride (naf′ ti feen)

Brand Names Naftin®

Use Topical treatment of tinea cruris (jock itch), tinea corporis (ring worm), and tinea pedis (athlete's foot)

Pregnancy Risk Factor B

Contraindications Hypersensitivity to any component

Warnings/Precautions For external use only

Adverse Reactions

>10%: Local: Burning, stinging

1% to 10%: Local: Dryness, erythema, itching, irritation

Mechanism of Action Synthetic, broad-spectrum antifungal agent in the allylamine class; appears to have both fungistatic and fungicidal activity. Exhibits antifungal activity by selectively inhibiting the enzyme squalene epoxidase in a dose-dependent manner which results in the primary sterol, ergosterol, within the fungal membrane not being synthesized.

Pharmacodynamics/Kinetics

Absorption: Systemic, 6% for cream, ≤4% for gel

(Continued)

Naftifine Hydrochloride *(Continued)*

Half-life: 2-3 days
Elimination: Metabolites excreted in urine and feces

Usual Dosage Adults: Topical: Apply cream once daily and gel twice daily (morning and evening) for up to 4 weeks

Patient Information External use only; avoid eyes, mouth, and other mucous membranes; do not use occlusive dressings unless directed to do so; discontinue if irritation or sensitivity develops; wash hands after application

Dosage Forms
Cream, topical: 1% (15 g, 30 g, 60 g)
Gel, topical: 1% (20 g, 40 g, 60 g)

Naftin® *see* Naftifine Hydrochloride *on previous page*

NaHCO₃ *see* Sodium Bicarbonate *on page 1010*

Nalbuphine Hydrochloride (nal′ byoo feen)

Related Information
Narcotic Agonist Comparison Charts *on page 1274-1275*

Brand Names Nubain®

Use Relief of moderate to severe pain; preoperative analgesia, postoperative and surgical anesthesia, and obstetrical analgesia during labor and delivery

Pregnancy Risk Factor B (D if used for prolonged periods or in high doses at term)

Contraindications Hypersensitivity to nalbuphine or any component, including sulfites

Warnings/Precautions Use with caution in patients with recent myocardial infarction, biliary tract surgery, or sulfite sensitivity; may produce respiratory depression; use with caution in women delivering premature infants; use with caution in patients with a history of drug dependence, head trauma or increased intracranial pressure, decreased hepatic or renal function, or pregnancy

Adverse Reactions
>10%:
Central nervous system: Drowsiness, CNS depression
Miscellaneous: Histamine release, narcotic withdrawal
1% to 10%:
Cardiovascular: Hypotension, flushing
Central nervous system: Dry mouth, dizziness, headache, weakness
Dermatologic: Urticaria, skin rash
Gastrointestinal: Nausea, vomiting, anorexia
Local: Pain at injection site
Respiratory: Pulmonary edema
<1%:
Cardiovascular: Hypertension, tachycardia
Central nervous system: Mental depression, hallucinations, confusion, paradoxical CNS stimulation, nervousness, restlessness, nightmares, insomnia
Gastrointestinal: GI irritation, ureteral spasm, biliary spasm
Genitourinary: Decreased urination, toxic megacolon
Ocular: Blurred vision
Respiratory: Shortness of breath, respiratory depression

Overdosage/Toxicology Symptoms of overdose include CNS depression, respiratory depression, miosis, hypotension, bradycardia. Treatment of an overdose includes support of the patient's airway, establishment of an I.V. line and administration of naloxone 2 mg I.V. (0.01 mg/kg for children) with repeat administration as necessary up to a total of 10 mg.

Drug Interactions Increased toxicity: Barbiturate anesthetics → ↑ CNS depression

Mechanism of Action Binds to opiate receptors in the CNS, causing inhibition of ascending pain pathways, altering the perception of and response to pain; produces generalized CNS depression

Pharmacodynamics/Kinetics
Peak effect:
I.M.: 30 minutes
I.V.: 1-3 minutes
Metabolism: In the liver
Half-life: 3.5-5 hours
Elimination: Metabolites excreted primarily in feces (via bile) and in urine (~7%)

Usual Dosage I.M., I.V., S.C.:
Children 10 months to 14 years: Premedication: 0.2 mg/kg; maximum: 20 mg/dose

Adults: 10 mg/70 kg every 3-6 hours; maximum single dose: 20 mg; maximum daily dose: 160 mg

Dosing adjustment/comments in hepatic impairment: Use with caution and reduce dose

Monitoring Parameters Relief of pain, respiratory and mental status, blood pressure

Patient Information Avoid alcohol, may cause drowsiness, impaired judgment or coordination; may cause physical and psychological dependence with prolonged use; will cause withdrawal in patients currently dependent on narcotics

Nursing Implications Observe patient for excessive sedation, respiratory depression, implement safety measures, assist with ambulation; observe for narcotic withdrawal

Dosage Forms Injection: 10 mg/mL (1 mL, 10 mL); 20 mg/mL (1 mL, 10 mL)

Naldecon® Senior EX [OTC] *see* Guaifenesin *on page 515*

Naldecon® Senior DX [OTC] *see* Guaifenesin and Dextromethorphan *on page 517*

Nalfon® *see* Fenoprofen Calcium *on page 445*

Nalidixic Acid (nal i dix' ik)

Related Information

Antimicrobial Drugs of Choice *on page 1298-1302*

Brand Names NegGram®

Synonyms Nalidixinic Acid

Use Treatment of urinary tract infections

Pregnancy Risk Factor B

Contraindications Hypersensitivity to nalidixic acid or any component; infants <3 months of age

Warnings/Precautions Use with caution in patients with impaired hepatic or renal function and prepubertal children; has been shown to cause cartilage degeneration in immature animals; may induce hemolysis in patients with G-6-PD deficiency

Adverse Reactions

>10%: Central nervous system: Dizziness, drowsiness, headache

1% to 10%: Gastrointestinal: Nausea, vomiting

<1%:

Central nervous system: Increased intracranial pressure, malaise, vertigo, confusion, toxic psychosis, convulsions, fever, chills

Dermatologic: Rash, urticaria, photosensitivity reactions

Endocrine & metabolic: Metabolic acidosis

Hematologic: Leukopenia, thrombocytopenia

Hepatic: Hepatotoxicity

Ocular: Visual disturbances

Overdosage/Toxicology Symptoms of overdose include nausea, vomiting, toxic psychosis, convulsions, increased intracranial pressure, metabolic acidosis; severe overdose, intracranial hypertension, increased pressure, and seizures have occurred; after GI decontamination, treatment is symptomatic

Drug Interactions

Decreased effect with antacids

Increased effect of warfarin

Mechanism of Action Inhibits DNA polymerization in late stages of chromosomal replication

Pharmacodynamics/Kinetics

Distribution: Crosses the placenta; appears in breast milk; achieves significant antibacterial concentrations only in the urinary tract

Protein binding: 90%

Metabolism: Partly in the liver

Half-life: 6-7 hours; increases significantly with renal impairment

Time to peak serum concentration: Oral: Within 1-2 hours

Elimination: In urine as unchanged drug and 80% as metabolites; small amounts appear in feces

Usual Dosage Oral:

Children 3 months to 12 years: 55 mg/kg/day divided every 6 hours; suppressive therapy is 33 mg/kg/day divided every 6 hours

Adults: 1 g 4 times/day for 2 weeks; then suppressive therapy of 500 mg 4 times/day

Dosing comments in renal impairment: Cl_{cr} <50 mL/minute: Avoid use

Test Interactions False-positive urine glucose with Clinitest®, false increase in urinary VMA

(Continued)

Nalidixic Acid *(Continued)*

Patient Information Avoid undue exposure to direct sunlight or use a sunscreen; take 1 hour before meals, but can take with food to decrease GI upset, finish all medication, do not skip doses; if persistent cough occurs, notify physician

Dosage Forms
Suspension, oral (raspberry flavor): 250 mg/5 mL (473 mL)
Tablet: 250 mg, 500 mg, 1 g

Nalidixinic Acid *see* Nalidixic Acid *on previous page*

Nallpen® *see* Nafcillin Sodium *on page 768*

***N*-allylnoroxymorphine Hydrochloride** *see* Naloxone Hydrochloride *on this page*

Naloxone Hydrochloride (nal ox′ one)

Related Information
Narcotic Agonist Comparison Charts *on page 1274-1275*

Brand Names Narcan®

Synonyms *N*-allylnoroxymorphine Hydrochloride

Use Reverses CNS and respiratory depression in suspected narcotic overdose; neonatal opiate depression; coma of unknown etiology
Investigational use: Shock, PCP and alcohol ingestion

Pregnancy Risk Factor B

Contraindications Hypersensitivity to naloxone or any component

Warnings/Precautions Use with caution in patients with cardiovascular disease; excessive dosages should be avoided after use of opiates in surgery, because naloxone may cause an increase in blood pressure and reversal of anesthesia; may precipitate withdrawal symptoms in patients addicted to opiates, including pain, hypertension, sweating, agitation, irritability, shrill cry, failure to feed

Adverse Reactions
1% to 10%:
Cardiovascular: Sweating, hypertension, hypotension, tachycardia, ventricular arrhythmias
Central nervous system: Insomnia, irritability, anxiety
Dermatologic: Rash
Gastrointestinal: Nausea, vomiting
Ocular: Blurred vision
Miscellaneous: Narcotic withdrawal

Overdosage/Toxicology Naloxone is the drug of choice for respiratory depression that is known or suspected to be caused by an overdose of an opiate or opioid. **Caution:** Naloxone's effects are due to its action on narcotic reversal, not due to any direct effect upon opiate receptors. Therefore, adverse events occur secondarily to reversal (withdrawal) of narcotic analgesia and sedation, which can cause severe reactions.

Drug Interactions Decreased effect of narcotic analgesics

Stability Protect from light; stable in 0.9% sodium chloride and D_5W at 4 mcg/mL for 24 hours; do not mix with alkaline solutions

Mechanism of Action Competes and displaces narcotics at narcotic receptor sites

Pharmacodynamics/Kinetics
Onset of effect:
Endotracheal, I.M., S.C.: Within 2-5 minutes
I.V.: Within 2 minutes
Duration: 20-60 minutes; since shorter than that of most opioids, repeated doses are usually needed
Distribution: Crosses the placenta
Metabolism: Primarily by glucuronidation in the liver
Half-life:
Neonates: 1.2-3 hours
Adults: 1-1.5 hours
Elimination: In urine as metabolites

Usual Dosage I.M., I.V. (preferred), intratracheal, S.C.:
Neonates: Narcotic-induced asphyxia: 0.01 mg/kg every 2-3 minutes as needed; may need to repeat every 1-2 hours
Infants and Children: Postanesthesia narcotic reversal: 0.01 mg/kg; may repeat every 2-3 minutes as needed based on response
Opiate intoxication: Birth (including premature infants) to 5 years or <20 kg: 0.1 mg/kg; repeat every 2-3 minutes if needed; may need to repeat doses every 20-60 minutes
>5 years or ≥20 kg: 2 mg/dose; if no response, repeat every 2-3 minutes; may need to repeat doses every 20-60 minutes

Children and Adults: Continuous infusion: I.V.: If continuous infusion is required, calculate dosage/hour based on effective intermittent dose used and duration of adequate response seen, titrate dose 0.04-0.16 mg/kg/hour for 2-5 days in children, up to 0.8 mg/kg/hour in adults; alternatively, continuous infusion utilizes $\frac{2}{3}$ of the initial naloxone bolus on an hourly basis; add 10 times this dose to each liter of D_5W and infuse at a rate of 100 mL/hour; $\frac{1}{2}$ of the initial bolus dose should be readministered 15 minutes after initiation of the continuous infusion to prevent a drop in naloxone levels; increase infusion rate as needed to assure adequate ventilation

Adults: Narcotic overdose: I.V.: 0.4-2 mg every 2-3 minutes as needed; may need to repeat doses every 20-60 minutes, if no response is observed after 10 mg, question the diagnosis. **Note:** Use 0.1-0.2 mg increments in patients who are opioid dependent and in postoperative patients to avoid large cardiovascular changes.

Monitoring Parameters Respiratory rate, heart rate, blood pressure

Nursing Implications The use of neonatal naloxone (0.02 mg/mL) is no longer recommended because unacceptable fluid volumes will result, especially to small neonates; the 0.4 mg/mL preparation is available and can be accurately dosed with appropriately sized syringes (1 mL)

Dosage Forms Injection: 0.02 mg/mL (2 mL); 0.4 mg/mL (1 mL, 2 mL, 10 mL); 1 mg/mL (2 mL, 10 mL)

Naltrexone Hydrochloride (nal trex' one)

Brand Names Trexan™

Use Adjunct to the maintenance of an opioid-free state in detoxified individual

Pregnancy Risk Factor C

Contraindications Acute hepatitis, liver failure, known hypersensitivity to naltrexone

Warnings/Precautions Dose-related hepatocellular injury is possible; the margin of separation between the apparent safe and hepatotoxic doses appear to be only fivefold or less

Adverse Reactions

>10%:

Central nervous system: Insomnia, nervousness, headache

Gastrointestinal: Abdominal cramping, nausea, vomiting

Neuromuscular & skeletal: Joint pain

1% to 10%:

Central nervous system: Dizziness, anorexia

Dermatologic: Skin rash

Endocrine & metabolic: Polydipsia

Respiratory: Sneezing

<1%:

Central nervous system: Insomnia, irritability, anxiety

Hematologic: Thrombocytopenia, agranulocytosis, hemolytic anemia

Ocular: Blurred vision

Miscellaneous: Narcotic withdrawal

Overdosage/Toxicology Symptoms of overdose include clonic-tonic convulsions, respiratory failure; patients receiving up to 800 mg/day for 1 week have shown no toxicity; seizures and respiratory failure have been seen in animals

Mechanism of Action Naltrexone is a cyclopropyl derivative of oxymorphone similar in structure to naloxone and nalorphine (a morphine derivative); it acts as a competitive antagonist at opioid receptor sites

Pharmacodynamics/Kinetics

Duration of action:

50 mg: 24 hours

100 mg: 48 hours

150 mg: 72 hours

Absorption: Oral: Almost completely

Distribution: V_d: 19 L/kg; distributed widely throughout the body but considerable interindividual variation exists

Protein binding: 21%

Metabolism: Undergoes extensive first-pass metabolism to 6-β-naltrexol

Half-life: 4 hours; 6-β-naltrexol: 13 hours

Time to peak serum concentration: Within 60 minutes

Elimination: Principally in urine as metabolites and unchanged drug

Usual Dosage Do not give until patient is opioid-free for 7-10 days as required by urine analysis

Adults: Oral: 25 mg; if no withdrawal signs within 1 hour give another 25 mg; maintenance regimen is flexible, variable and individualized (50 mg/day to 100-150 mg 3 times/week)

(Continued)

Naltrexone Hydrochloride *(Continued)*

Patient Information Will cause narcotic withdrawal; serious overdose can occur after attempts to overcome the blocking effect of naltrexone

Nursing Implications Monitor for narcotic withdrawal

Dosage Forms Tablet: 50 mg

Nandrolone *(nan' droe lone)*

Brand Names Androlone®; Androlone®-D; Deca-Durabolin®; Durabolin®; Hybolin™ Decanoate; Hybolin™ Improved; Neo-Durabolic

Synonyms Nandrolone Decanoate; Nandrolone Phenpropionate

Use Control of metastatic breast cancer; management of anemia of renal insufficiency

Restrictions C-III

Pregnancy Risk Factor X

Contraindications Carcinoma of breast or prostate, nephrosis, pregnancy and infants, hypersensitivity to any component

Warnings/Precautions Monitor diabetic patients carefully; anabolic steroids may cause peliosis hepatis, liver cell tumors, and blood lipid changes with increased risk of arteriosclerosis; use with caution in elderly patients, they may be at greater risk for prostatic hypertrophy; use with caution in patients with cardiac, renal, or hepatic disease or epilepsy

Adverse Reactions

Male:

Postpubertal:

>10%:

Dermatologic: Acne

Endocrine & metabolic: Bladder irritability, priapism, gynecomastia

1% to 10%:

Central nervous system: Insomnia

Endocrine & metabolic: Decreased libido, hepatic dysfunction, chills, prostatic hypertrophy (elderly)

Gastrointestinal: Nausea, diarrhea

Hematologic: Iron deficiency anemia, suppression of clotting factors

<1%: Hepatic: Hepatic necrosis, hepatocellular carcinoma

Prepubertal:

>10%:

Dermatologic: Acne

Endocrine & metabolic: Virilism

1% to 10%:

Central nervous system: Chills, insomnia, factors

Dermatologic: Hyperpigmentation

Gastrointestinal: Diarrhea, nausea

Hematologic: Iron deficiency anemia, suppression of clotting

<1%: Hepatic: necrosis, hepatocellular carcinoma

Female:

>10%: Endocrine & metabolic: Virilism

1% to 10%:

Central nervous system: Chills, insomnia

Endocrine & metabolic: Hypercalcemia

Gastrointestinal: Nausea, diarrhea

Hematologic: Iron deficiency anemia, suppression of clotting factors

Hepatic: Hepatic dysfunction

<1%: Hepatic: Hepatic necrosis, hepatocellular carcinoma

Drug Interactions Increased toxicity: Oral anticoagulants, insulin, oral hypoglycemic agents, adrenal steroids, ACTH

Mechanism of Action Promotes tissue-building processes, increases production of erythropoietin, causes protein anabolism; increases hemoglobin and red blood cell volume

Pharmacodynamics/Kinetics

Metabolism: In the liver

Elimination: In urine

Usual Dosage Deep I.M. (into gluteal muscle):

Children 2-13 years: (decanoate): 25-50 mg every 3-4 weeks

Adults:

Male:

Breast cancer (phenpropionate): 50-100 mg/week

Anemia of renal insufficiency (decanoate): 100-200 mg/week

Female: 50-100 mg/week

Breast cancer (phenproprionate): 50-100 mg/week

Anemia of renal insufficiency (decanoate): 50-100 mg/week

Administration Inject deeply I.M., preferably into the gluteal muscle

Test Interactions Altered glucose tolerance tests

Patient Information Virilization may occur in female patients; report menstrual irregularities; male patients report persistent penile erections; all patients should report persistent GI distress, diarrhea, dark urine, pale stools, yellow coloring of skin or sclera; diabetic patients should monitor glucose closely

Additional Information Both phenpropionate and decanoate are Injections in oil

Dosage Forms
Injection, as phenpropionate, in oil: 25 mg/mL (5 mL); 50 mg/mL (2 mL)
Injection, as decanoate, in oil: 50 mg/mL (1 mL, 2 mL); 100 mg/mL (1 mL, 2 mL); 200 mg/mL (1 mL)

Nandrolone Decanoate *see* Nandrolone *on previous page*

Nandrolone Phenpropionate *see* Nandrolone *on previous page*

Naphazoline Hydrochloride (naf az' oh leen)

Brand Names AK-Con®; Albalon® Liquifilm®; Allerest® Eye Drops [OTC]; Clear Eyes® [OTC]; Comfort® [OTC]; Degest® 2 [OTC]; Estivin® II [OTC]; I-Naphline®; Muro's Opcon®; Nafazair®; Naphcon Forte®; Naphcon® [OTC]; Opcon®; Privine®; VasoClear® [OTC]; Vasocon Regular®

Use Topical ocular vasoconstrictor; will temporarily relieve congestion, itching, and minor irritation, and to control hyperemia in patients with superficial corneal vascularity

Pregnancy Risk Factor C

Contraindications Hypersensitivity to naphazoline or any component, narrow-angle glaucoma, prior to peripheral iridectomy (in patients susceptible to angle block)

Warnings/Precautions Rebound congestion may occur with extended use; use with caution in the presence of hypertension, diabetes, hyperthyroidism, heart disease, coronary artery disease, cerebral arteriosclerosis, or long-standing bronchial asthma

Adverse Reactions
1% to 10%:
Cardiovascular: Systemic cardiovascular stimulation
Central nervous system: Dizziness, headache, nervousness
Gastrointestinal: Nausea
Local: Transient stinging, nasal mucosa irritation, dryness, sneezing, rebound congestion
Ocular: Mydriasis, increased intraocular pressure, blurring of vision

Overdosage/Toxicology Symptoms of overdose include CNS depression, hypothermia, bradycardia, cardiovascular collapse, apnea, coma. Following initiation of essential overdose management, toxic symptoms should be treated. The patient should be kept warm and monitored for alterations in vital functions. Seizures commonly respond to diazepam (5-10 mg I.V. bolus in adults every 15 minutes if needed up to a total of 30 mg; I.V. 0.25-0.4 mg/kg/dose up to a total of 10 mg for children) or to phenytoin or phenobarbital. Hypotension should be treated with fluids.

Drug Interactions Increased toxicity: Anesthetics (discontinue mydriatic prior to use of anesthetics that sensitize the myocardium to sympathomimetics, ie, cyclopropane, halothane), MAO inhibitors, tricyclic antidepressants → hypertensive reactions

Stability Store in tight, light-resistant containers

Mechanism of Action Stimulates alpha-adrenergic receptors in the arterioles of the conjunctiva and the nasal mucosa to produce vasoconstriction

Pharmacodynamics/Kinetics
Onset of decongestant action: Topical: Within 10 minutes
Duration: 2-6 hours
Elimination: Not well defined

Usual Dosage
Nasal:
Children:
<6 years: Intranasal: Not recommended (especially infants) due to CNS depression
6-12 years: 1 spray of 0.05% into each nostril every 6 hours if necessary; therapy should not exceed 3-5 days
Children >12 years and Adults: 0.05%, instill 1-2 drops or sprays every 6 hours if needed; therapy should not exceed 3-5 days

Ophthalmic:
Children <6 years: Not recommended for use due to CNS depression (especially in infants)
(Continued)

Naphazoline Hydrochloride *(Continued)*

Children >6 years and Adults: Instill 1-2 drops into conjunctival sac of affected eye(s) every 3-4 hours; therapy generally should not exceed 3-4 days

Patient Information Do not use discolored solutions; discontinue eye drops if visual changes or ocular pain occur; notify physician of insomnia, tremor, or irregular heartbeat; stinging, burning, or drying of the nasal mucosa may occur; do not use beyond 72 hours

Nursing Implications Rebound congestion can result with continued use

Dosage Forms Solution:
Drops, nasal: 0.05% (25 mL)
Ophthalmic: 0.012% (7.5 mL, 15 mL, 30 mL); 0.02% (15 mL); 0.03% (15 mL); 0.1% (15 mL)
Spray: 0.05% (20 mL, 473 mL)

Naphcon Forte® *see* Naphazoline Hydrochloride *on previous page*

Naphcon® [OTC] *see* Naphazoline Hydrochloride *on previous page*

Naprosyn® *see* Naproxen *on this page*

Naproxen (na prox′ en)

Related Information
Nonsteroidal Anti-Inflammatories Comparison *on page 1280*

Brand Names Aleve® (OTC); Anaprox®; Naprosyn®

Synonyms Naproxen Sodium

Use Management of inflammatory disease and rheumatoid disorders (including juvenile rheumatoid arthritis); acute gout; mild to moderate pain; dysmenorrhea; fever, migraine headache

Pregnancy Risk Factor B (D if used in the 3rd trimester or near delivery)

Contraindications Hypersensitivity to naproxen, aspirin, or other nonsteroidal anti-inflammatory drugs (NSAIDs)

Warnings/Precautions Use with caution in patients with GI disease (bleeding or ulcers), cardiovascular disease (CHF, hypertension), renal or hepatic impairment, and patients receiving anticoagulants; perform ophthalmologic evaluation for those who develop eye complaints during therapy (blurred vision, diminished vision, changes in color vision, retinal changes); NSAIDs may mask signs/symptoms of infections; photosensitivity reported; elderly are at especially high-risk for adverse effects

Adverse Reactions
>10%:
Central nervous system: Dizziness
Dermatologic: Pruritus, rash
Gastrointestinal: Abdominal discomfort, nausea, heartburn, constipation, GI bleeding, ulcers, perforation, indigestion
1% to 10%:
Central nervous system: Headache, nervousness
Dermatologic: Itching
Gastrointestinal: Vomiting
Otic: Tinnitus
Miscellaneous: Fluid retention
<1%:
Cardiovascular: Edema, congestive heart failure, arrhythmias, tachycardia, hypertension
Central nervous system: Confusion, hallucinations, mental depression, fatigue, drowsiness, insomnia
Dermatologic: Hives, erythema multiforme, toxic epidermal necrolysis, Stevens-Johnson syndrome, angioedema, allergic rhinitis
Endocrine & metabolic: Polydipsia, hot flushes
Gastrointestinal: Gastritis, GI ulceration
Genitourinary: Cystitis, renal dysfunction
Hematologic: Anemia, hemolytic anemia, bone marrow depression, leukopenia, thrombocytopenia, inhibits platelet aggregation, prolongs bleeding time, agranulocytosis
Hepatic: Hepatitis
Neuromuscular & skeletal: Peripheral neuropathy
Ocular: Toxic amblyopia, blurred vision, conjunctivitis, dry eyes
Otic: Decreased hearing
Renal: Polyuria, acute renal failure
Respiratory: Shortness of breath
Miscellaneous: Epistaxis, aseptic meningitis

Overdosage/Toxicology Symptoms of overdose include drowsiness, heartburn, vomiting, CNS depression, leukocytosis, renal failure

Management of a nonsteroidal anti-inflammatory drug (NSAID) intoxication is primarily supportive and symptomatic; fluid therapy is commonly effective in managing the hypotension that may occur following an acute NSAID overdose, except when this is due to an acute blood loss. Seizures tend to be very short-lived and often do not require drug treatment; although, recurrent seizures should be treated with I.V. diazepam; since many of the NSAIDs undergo enterohepatic cycling, multiple doses of charcoal may be needed to reduce the potential for delayed toxicities.

Drug Interactions
Decreased effect of furosemide
Increased toxicity:
Naproxen could displace other highly protein bound drugs, such as oral anticoagulants, hydantoins, salicylates, sulfonamides, and sulfonylureas
Naproxen and warfarin → slight increase in free warfarin
Naproxen and probenecid → increased plasma half-life of naproxen
Naproxen and methotrexate → significantly increased and prolonged blood methotrexate concentration, which may be severe or fatal

Mechanism of Action Inhibits prostaglandin synthesis by decreasing the activity of the enzyme, cyclo-oxygenase, which results in decreased formation of prostaglandin precursors

Pharmacodynamics/Kinetics
Analgesia:
Onset of action: 1 hour
Duration: Up to 7 hours
Anti-inflammatory:
Onset of action: Within 2 weeks
Peak: 2-4 weeks
Absorption: Oral: Almost 100%
Time to peak serum concentration: Within 1-2 hours and persisting for up to 12 hours
Protein binding: Highly protein bound (>90%); increased free fraction in elderly
Half-life:
Normal renal function: 12-15 hours
End stage renal disease: Unchanged

Usual Dosage Oral as naproxen:
Children >2 years:
Fever: 2.5-10 mg/kg/dose; maximum: 10 mg/kg/day
Juvenile arthritis: 10 mg/kg/day in 2 divided doses

Adults:
Rheumatoid arthritis, osteoarthritis, and ankylosing spondylitis: 500-1000 mg/day in 2 divided doses; may increase to 1.5 g/day of naproxen base for limited time period
Mild to moderate pain or dysmenorrhea: Initial: 500 mg, then 250 mg every 6-8 hours; maximum: 1250 mg/day naproxen base

Dosing adjustment in hepatic impairment: Reduce dose to 50%
Administration Administer with food, milk, or antacids to decrease GI adverse effects
Monitoring Parameters Occult blood loss, periodic liver function test, CBC, BUN, serum creatinine
Test Interactions ↑ chloride (S), ↑ sodium (S), ↑ bleeding time
Patient Information Serious gastrointestinal bleeding can occur as well as ulceration and perforation. Pain may or may not be present. Avoid aspirin and aspirin-containing products while taking this medication. If gastric upset occurs, take with food, milk, or antacid. If gastric adverse effects persist, contact physician. May cause drowsiness, dizziness, blurred vision, and confusion. Use caution when performing tasks which require alertness (eg, driving). Do not take for more than 3 days for fever or 10 days for pain without physician's advice.
Additional Information Naproxen: Naprosyn®; naproxen sodium: Anaprox®; 275 mg of Anaprox® equivalent to 250 mg of Naprosyn®
Dosage Forms
Suspension, oral: 125 mg/5 mL (480 mL)
Tablet, as sodium: 275 mg (250 mg base); 550 mg (500 mg base)
Tablet: 250 mg, 375 mg, 500 mg

Naproxen Sodium see Naproxen on previous page

Naqua® see Trichlormethiazide on page 1118

Narcan® see Naloxone Hydrochloride on page 772

Narcotic Agonist Comparison Charts see page 1274

Nardil® see Phenelzine Sulfate on page 867

Nasacort® see Triamcinolone on page 1112

Nasahist B® *see* Brompheniramine Maleate *on page 143*

Nasalcrom® Nasal Solution *see* Cromolyn Sodium *on page 280*

Nasalide® *see* Flunisolide *on page 468*

Natabec® [OTC] *see* Vitamin, Multiple *on page 1166*

Natabec® FA [OTC] *see* Vitamin, Multiple *on page 1166*

Natabec® Rx *see* Vitamin, Multiple *on page 1166*

Natacyn® *see* Natamycin *on this page*

Natalins® [OTC] *see* Vitamin, Multiple *on page 1166*

Natalins® Rx *see* Vitamin, Multiple *on page 1166*

Natamycin (na ta mye' sin)
Brand Names Natacyn®
Synonyms Pimaricin
Use Treatment of blepharitis, conjunctivitis, and keratitis caused by susceptible fungi (*Aspergillus, Candida*), *Cephalosporium, Curvularia, Fusarium, Penicillium, Microsporum, Epidermophyton, Blastomyces dermatitidis, Coccidioides immitis, Cryptococcus neoformans, Histoplasma capsulatum, Sporothrix schenckii*, and *Trichomonas vaginalis*
Pregnancy Risk Factor C
Contraindications Known hypersensitivity to natamycin or any component
Warnings/Precautions Failure to improve (keratitis) after 7-10 days of administration suggests infection caused by a microorganism not susceptible to natamycin; inadequate as a single agent in fungal endophthalmitis
Adverse Reactions <1%: Ocular: Blurred vision, photophobia, eye pain, eye irritation not present before therapy
Drug Interactions Increased toxicity: Topical corticosteroids (concomitant use contraindicated)
Stability Store at room temperature (8°C to 24°C/46°F to 75°F); protect from excessive heat and light; do not freeze
Mechanism of Action Increases cell membrane permeability in susceptible fungi
Pharmacodynamics/Kinetics
Absorption: Ophthalmic: <2% systemically absorbed
Distribution: Adheres to cornea and is retained in the conjunctival fornices
Usual Dosage Adults: Ophthalmic: Instill 1 drop in conjunctival sac every 1-2 hours, after 3-4 days reduce to one drop 6-8 times/day; usual course of therapy is 2-3 weeks.
Patient Information Shake well before using, do not touch dropper to eye; notify physician if condition worsens or does not improve after 3-4 days
Dosage Forms Suspension, ophthalmic: 5% (15 mL)

Natural Lung Surfactant *see* Beractant *on page 128*

Navane® *see* Thiothixene *on page 1087*

Navelbine® *see* Vinorelbine Tartrate *on page 1160*

ND-Stat® *see* Brompheniramine Maleate *on page 143*

Nebcin® *see* Tobramycin *on page 1097*

NebuPent™ *see* Pentamidine Isethionate *on page 856*

N.E.E.™ *see* Ethinyl Estradiol and Norethindrone *on page 425*

Nefazodone (nef az' oh done)
Related Information
Antidepressant Agents Comparison *on page 1250-1252*
Brand Names Serzone®
Use Treatment of depression
Pregnancy Risk Factor C
Contraindications Hypersensitivity to nefazodone or any component; concomitant use of any MAO inhibitors, astemizole, or terfenadine
Warnings/Precautions Safety and efficacy in children <18 years of age have not been established; monitor closely and use with extreme caution in patients with cardiac disease, cerebrovascular disease or seizures; very sedating and can be dehydrating; therapeutic effects may take up to 4 weeks to occur; therapy is normally maintained for several months and optimum response is reached to prevent recurrence of depression, discontinue therapy and reevaluate if priapism occurs

Adverse Reactions
<10%:
  Central nervous system: Headache, drowsiness, insomnia, agitation, dizziness, confusion
  Gastrointestinal: Dry mouth, nausea
  Neuromuscular & skeletal: Tremor
1% to 10%:
  Cardiovascular: Postural hypotension
  Central nervous system: Asthenia
  Gastrointestinal: Constipation, vomiting
  Ocular: Blurred vision, amblyopia
<1%:
  Gastrointestinal: Diarrhea
  Genitourinary: Prolonged priapism

Overdosage/Toxicology Symptoms of overdose include drowsiness, vomiting, hypotension, tachycardia, incontinence, coma, priapism

Following initiation of essential overdose management, toxic symptoms should be treated. Ventricular arrhythmias often respond to lidocaine 1.5 mg/kg bolus followed by 2 mg/minute infusion with concurrent systemic alkalinization (sodium bicarbonate 0.5-2 mEq/kg I.V.). Seizures usually respond to diazepam I.V. boluses (5-10 mg for adults up to 30 mg or 0.25-0.4 mg/kg/dose for children up to 10 mg/dose). If seizures are unresponsive or recur, phenytoin or phenobarbital may be required. Hypotension is best treated by I.V. fluids and by placing the patient in the Trendelenburg position.

Drug Interactions
Decreased effect: Clonidine, methyldopa, diuretics, oral hypoglycemics, anticoagulants
Increased toxicity: Terfenadine and astemizole (increased concentrations have been associated with serious ventricular arrhythmias and death), fluoxetine, triazolam (reduce triazolam dose by 75%), alprazolam (reduce alprazolam dose by 50%), phenytoin, CNS depressants, MAO inhibitors (allow 14 days after MAO inhibitors are stopped or 7 days after nefazodone is stopped); digoxin serum levels may increase

Mechanism of Action Inhibits reuptake of serotonin and norepinephrine by the presynaptic neuronal membrane and desensitization of adenyl cyclase, down regulation of beta-adrenergic receptors, and down regulation of serotonin receptors

Pharmacodynamics/Kinetics
Onset of effect: Therapeutic effects take at least 3 weeks to appear
Metabolism: In the liver to 3 active metabolites; triazoledione, hydroxynefazodone and m-chlorophenylpiperazine (mCPP)
Half-life: 2-4 hours (parent compound), active metabolites persist longer
Time to peak serum concentration: 30 minutes, prolonged in presence of food
Elimination: Primarily as metabolites in urine and secondarily in feces

Usual Dosage Oral: Therapeutic effects may take up to 3-4 weeks to occur; therapy is normally maintained for several months after optimum response is reached to prevent recurrence of depression

Adults: Initial: 200 mg/day in 2 divided doses; may increase by 100-200 mg/day every 7 days up to 150-300 mg twice daily (usual effective range)
Elderly: 50 mg twice daily with 50 mg/day dose increase weekly, if tolerated; usual dose: 100-400 mg/day in 2 divided doses

Dosage adjustment in hepatic impairment: Dosage adjustment may be required

Reference Range Therapeutic plasma levels have not yet been defined

Patient Information Take shortly after a meal or light snack; can be given at bedtime dose if drowsiness occurs; optimum effect may take 2-4 weeks to be achieved; avoid alcohol; may cause painful erections (contact physician if this should occur); avoid sudden changes in position

Nursing Implications Dosing after meals may decrease lightheadedness and postural hypotension, but may also decrease absorption and therefore effectiveness; use side rails on bed if administered to the elderly; observe patient's activity and compare with admission level; assist with ambulation; sitting and standing blood pressure and pulse

Dosage Forms
Tablet: 200 mg, 250 mg
Tablet, scored: 100 mg, 150 mg

NegGram® see Nalidixic Acid on page 771
Nelova™ see Ethinyl Estradiol and Norethindrone on page 425
Nelova™ 1/50M see Mestranol and Norethindrone on page 695

Nembutal® *see* Pentobarbital *on page 859*

Neo-Calglucon® [OTC] *see* Calcium Glubionate *on page 166*

Neo-Cultol® [OTC] *see* Mineral Oil *on page 743*

Neo-Durabolic *see* Nandrolone *on page 774*

Neofed® [OTC] *see* Pseudoephedrine *on page 955*

Neo-fradin® *see* Neomycin Sulfate *on page 783*

Neoloid® [OTC] *see* Castor Oil *on page 190*

Neomixin® *see* Bacitracin, Neomycin, and Polymyxin B *on page 113*

Neomycin and Polymyxin B (pol i mix' in)

Brand Names Neosporin® G.U. Irrigant; Neosporin® Cream [OTC]; Statrol®

Synonyms Polymyxin and Neomycin; Polymyxin B and Neomycin

Use Short-term as a continuous irrigant or rinse in the urinary bladder to prevent bacteriuria and gram-negative rod septicemia associated with the use of indwelling catheters; to help prevent infection in minor cuts, scrapes, and burns; treatment of superficial ocular infections involving the conjunctiva or cornea

Pregnancy Risk Factor C (D G.U. irrigant)

Contraindications Known hypersensitivity to neomycin or polymyxin B or any component; ophthalmic use for topical cream

Warnings/Precautions Use with caution in patients with impaired renal function, infants with diaper rash involving large area of abraded skin, dehydrated patients, burn patients, and patients receiving a high-dose for prolonged periods; topical neomycin is a contact sensitizer; contains methylparaben

Adverse Reactions
1% to 10%:
Dermatologic: Contact dermatitis, erythema, rash, urticaria
Genitourinary: Nephrotoxicity, bladder irritation
Local: Burning
Neuromuscular & skeletal: Neuromuscular blockade
Otic: Ototoxicity

Overdosage/Toxicology Refer to individual monographs for Neomycin and Polymyxin B

Stability Store irrigation solution in refrigerator; aseptic prepared dilutions (1 mL/1 L) should be stored in the refrigerator and discarded after 48 hours

Mechanism of Action Refer to individual monographs for Neomycin and Polymyxin

Pharmacodynamics/Kinetics Absorption: Topical: Not absorbed following application to intact skin; absorbed through denuded or abraded skin, peritoneum, wounds, or ulcers

Usual Dosage Children and Adults:
Bladder irrigation: **Not for injection**; add 1 mL irrigant to 1 liter isotonic saline solution and connect container to the inflow of lumen of 3-way catheter. Continuous irrigant or rinse in the urinary bladder for up to a maximum of 10 days with administration rate adjusted to patient's urine output; usually no more than 1 L of irrigant is used per day.
Ophthalmic:
Ointment: Instill ½" ribbon into the conjunctival sac every 3-4 hours for acute infections or 2-3 times/day for mild to moderate infections for 7-10 days
Solution: Instill 1-2 drops every 15-30 minutes for acute infections; 1-2 drops every 3-6 hours for mild-moderate infections.
Topical: Apply cream 1-4 times/day to affected area

Monitoring Parameters Urinalysis

Patient Information Notify physician if condition worsens or if rash or irritation develops

Nursing Implications Do not inject irrigant solution; connect irrigation container to the inflow lumen of a 3-way catheter to permit continuous irrigation of the urinary bladder

Dosage Forms
Cream, topical: Neomycin sulfate 3.5 mg and polymyxin B sulfate 10,000 units per g (0.94 g, 15 g)
Ointment, ophthalmic: Neomycin sulfate 3.5 mg/g and polymyxin B sulfate 10,000 units/g
Solution:
Irrigant: Neomycin sulfate 40 mg and polymyxin B sulfate 200,000 units per mL (1 mL, 20 mL)
Ophthalmic: Neomycin sulfate 3.5 mg/mL and polymyxin B sulfate 16,250 units/mL (5 mL)

Neomycin, Polymyxin B, and Dexamethasone (dex a meth′ a sone)

Brand Names AK-Trol®; Dexacidin®; Dexasporin®; Maxitrol®

Use Steroid-responsive inflammatory ocular conditions in which a corticosteroid is indicated and where bacterial infection or a risk of bacterial infection exists

Pregnancy Risk Factor C

Contraindications Hypersensitivity to dexamethasone, polymyxin B, neomycin or any component; herpes simplex, vaccinia, and varicella

Warnings/Precautions Prolonged use may result in glaucoma, defects in visual acuity, posterior subcapsular cataract formation, and secondary ocular infections

Adverse Reactions 1% to 10%: Ocular: Cutaneous sensitization, pain, development of glaucoma, cataract, increased intraocular pressure, optic nerve damage, contact dermatitis, delayed wound healing

Overdosage/Toxicology Refer to individual monographs for Neomycin Sulfate, Polymyxin B Sulfate, and Dexamethasone

Mechanism of Action Refer to individual monographs for Neomycin Sulfate, Polymyxin B Sulfate, and Dexamethasone

Pharmacodynamics/Kinetics Refer to individual monographs for Neomycin Sulfate, Polymyxin B Sulfate, and Dexamethasone

Usual Dosage Children and Adults: Ophthalmic:

Ointment: Place a small amount (~½") in the affected eye 3-4 times/day or apply at bedtime as an adjunct with drops

Solution: Instill 1-2 drops into affected eye(s) every 3-4 hours; in severe disease, drops may be used hourly and tapered to discontinuation

Monitoring Parameters Intraocular pressure with use >10 days

Patient Information For the eye; shake well before using; tilt head back, place medication in conjunctival sac, and close eyes; do not touch dropper to eye; apply finger pressure on lacrimal sac for 1 minute following instillation; notify physician if condition worsens or does not improve in 3-4 days

Dosage Forms Ophthalmic:

Ointment: Neomycin sulfate 3.5 mg, polymyxin B sulfate 10,000 units and dexamethasone 0.1% per g (3.5 g, 5 g)

Suspension: Neomycin sulfate 3.5 mg, polymyxin B sulfate 10,000 units and dexamethasone 0.1% per mL (5 mL, 10 mL)

Neomycin, Polymyxin B, and Gramicidin (gram i si′ din)

Brand Names AK-Spore® Ophthalmic Solution; Neosporin® Ophthalmic Solution; Ocutricin® Ophthalmic Solution

Use Treatment of superficial ocular infection, infection prophylaxis in minor skin abrasions

Pregnancy Risk Factor C

Contraindications Hypersensitivity to neomycin, polymyxin B, gramicidin or any component

Warnings/Precautions Symptoms of neomycin sensitization include itching, reddening, edema, failure to heal; prolonged use may result in glaucoma, defects in visual acuity, posterior subcapsular cataract formation, and secondary ocular infections

Adverse Reactions 1% to 10%:

Local: Itching, reddening, failure to heal, edema

Ocular: Low grade conjunctivitis

Mechanism of Action Interferes with bacterial protein synthesis by binding to 30S ribosomal subunits; binds to phospholipids, alters permeability, and damages the bacterial cytoplasmic membrane permitting leakage of intracellular constituents

Usual Dosage Children and Adults: Ophthalmic: Instill 1-2 drops 4-6 times/day or more frequently as required for severe infections

Patient Information Tilt head back, place medication in conjunctival sac, and close eyes; apply finger pressure on lacrimal sac for 1 minute following instillation

Dosage Forms Solution, ophthalmic: Polymyxin B sulfate 10,000 units, neomycin sulfate 1.75 mg, and gramicidin 0.025 mg per mL (2 mL, 5 mL, 10 mL)

Neomycin, Polymyxin B, and Hydrocortisone (nee oh mye′ sin, pol i mix′ in b, & hye droe kor′ ti sone)

Brand Names AK-Spore H.C.®; AntibiOtic®; Bacticort®; Cortatrigen®; Cortisporin® Ophthalmic Suspension; Cortisporin® Otic; Cortisporin® Topical Cream; Drotic®; LazerSporin-C®; Octicair®; Ocutricin® HC; Otocort®; Otomycin-HPN®; Otosporin®; PediOtic®

Use Steroid-responsive inflammatory condition for which a corticosteroid is indicated and where bacterial infection or a risk of bacterial infection exists

(Continued)

Neomycin, Polymyxin B, and Hydrocortisone
(Continued)

Pregnancy Risk Factor C

Contraindications Known hypersensitivity to hydrocortisone, polymyxin B sulfate or neomycin sulfate; otic use when drum is perforated; herpes simplex, vaccinia, and varicella

Warnings/Precautions Prolonged use can lead to skin thinning, atrophy, sensitization, and development of resistant infections; neomycin may cause cutaneous and conjunctival sensitization; children are more susceptible to topical corticosteroid-induced hypothalamic - pituitary - adrenal axis suppression and Cushing's syndrome. Otic suspension is the preferred otic preparation; otic suspension can be used for the treatment of infections of mastoidectomy and fenestration cavities caused by susceptible organisms; otic solution is used **only** for superficial infections of the external auditory canal (ie, swimmer's ear).

Adverse Reactions
>10%: Hypersensitivity
1% to 10%:
  Local: Contact dermatitis, erythema, rash, urticaria, burning, itching, swelling, pain, stinging
  Neuromuscular & skeletal: Neuromuscular blockade
  Ocular: Elevation of intraocular pressure, glaucoma, cataracts, conjunctival erythema
  Otic: Ototoxicity
  Renal: Nephrotoxicity
  Miscellaneous: Sensitization to neomycin, secondary infections, bladder irritation

Overdosage/Toxicology Refer to individual monographs for Neomycin, Polymyxin B, and Hydrocortisone

Usual Dosage
Ophthalmic: Children and Adults: Instill 1-2 drops 2-4 times/day, or more frequently as required for severe infections; in acute infections, instill 1-2 drops every 15-30 minutes gradually reducing the frequency of administration as the infection is controlled
Otic: Suspension:
  Children: Instill 3 drops into affected ear 3-4 times/day
  Adults: Instill 4 drops 3-4 times/day
Topical: Apply a thin layer 1-4 times/day

Patient Information
Ophthalmic: May cause sensitivity to bright light; may cause temporary blurring of vision or stinging following administration, but discontinue product and see physician if problems persist or increase; to use, tilt head back and place medication in conjunctival sac and close eyes; apply light pressure on lacrimal sac for 1 minute
Otic: Hold container in hand to warm; if drops are in suspension form, shake well for approximately 10 seconds, lie on your side with affected ear up; for adults hold the ear lobe up and back, for children hold the ear lobe down and back; instill drops in ear without inserting dropper into ear; maintain tilted ear for 2 minutes

Dosage Forms
Cream, topical: Neomycin sulfate 5 mg, polymyxin b sulfate 10,000 units, and hydrocortisone 10 mg per mL (7.5 g)
Solution, otic: Neomycin sulfate 5 mg, polymyxin B sulfate 10,000 units, and hydrocortisone 10 mg per mL (10 mL)
Suspension:
  Ophthalmic: Neomycin sulfate 3.5 mg, polymyxin B sulfate 10,000 units, and hydrocortisone 10 mg per mL (7.5 mL)
  Otic: Neomycin sulfate 5 mg, polymyxin B sulfate 10,000 units, and hydrocortisone 10 mg per mL (7.5 mL, 10 mL)

Neomycin, Polymyxin B, and Prednisolone (nee oh mye' sin, pol i mix' in b, & pred niss' oh lone)

Brand Names Poly-Pred®

Use Steroid-responsive inflammatory ocular condition in which bacterial infection or a risk of bacterial ocular infection exists

Pregnancy Risk Factor C

Contraindications Known hypersensitivity to neomycin, polymyxin B, or prednisolone; dendritic keratitis, viral disease of the cornea and conjunctiva, mycobacterial infection of the eye, fungal disease of the ocular structure, or after uncomplicated removal of a corneal foreign body

Warnings/Precautions Prolonged use may result in overgrowth of nonsusceptible organisms, glaucoma, damage to the optic nerve, defects in visual acuity, and cataract formation; symptoms of neomycin sensitization include itching, reddening, edema, or failure to heal

Adverse Reactions
1% to 10%:
    Dermatologic: Cutaneous sensitization, skin rash, delayed wound healing
    Ocular: Increased intraocular pressure, glaucoma, optic nerve damage, cataracts, conjunctival sensitization

Overdosage/Toxicology Refer to individual monographs for Neomycin, Polymyxin B, and Prednisolone

Mechanism of Action Refer to individual monographs for Neomycin, Polymyxin B, and Prednisolone

Pharmacodynamics/Kinetics Refer to individual monographs for Neomycin Sulfate, Polymyxin B Sulfate, and Prednisolone

Usual Dosage Children and Adults: Ophthalmic: Instill 1-2 drops every 3-4 hours; acute infections may require every 30-minute instillation initially with frequency of administration reduced as the infection is brought under control. To treat the lids: Instill 1-2 drops every 3-4 hours, close the eye and rub the excess on the lids and lid margins.

Patient Information Ophthalmic: May cause sensitivity to bright light; may cause temporary blurring of vision or stinging following administration, but discontinue product and see physician if problems persist or increase; to use, tilt head back and place medication in conjunctival sac and close eyes; apply light pressure on lacrimal sac for 1 minute

Nursing Implications Shake suspension before using

Dosage Forms Suspension: Neomycin sulfate 0.35%, polymyxin B sulfate 10,000 units, and prednisolone acetate 0.5% per mL (5 mL, 10 mL)

Neomycin Sulfate (nee oh mye′ sin)

Brand Names Mycifradin® Sulfate; Neo-fradin®; Neo-Tabs®

Use Prepares GI tract for surgery; treat minor skin infections; treat diarrhea caused by *E. coli*; adjunct in the treatment of hepatic encephalopathy, as irrigant during surgery

Pregnancy Risk Factor C

Contraindications Hypersensitivity to neomycin or any component, or other aminoglycosides; patients with intestinal obstruction

Warnings/Precautions Use with caution in patients with renal impairment, pre-existing hearing impairment, neuromuscular disorders; neomycin is more toxic than other aminoglycosides when given parenterally; **do not administer parenterally**; topical neomycin is a contact sensitizer with sensitivity occurring in 5% to 15% of patients treated with the drug; symptoms include itching, reddening, edema, and failure to heal

Adverse Reactions
1% to 10%:
    Dermatologic: Dermatitis, rash, urticaria, erythema
    Local: Burning
    Ocular: Contact conjunctivitis
<1%:
    Gastrointestinal: Nausea, vomiting, diarrhea
    Neuromuscular & skeletal: Neuromuscular blockade
    Otic: Ototoxicity
    Renal: Nephrotoxicity

Overdosage/Toxicology Symptoms of overdose (rare due to poor oral bioavailability) include ototoxicity, nephrotoxicity, and neuromuscular toxicity. The treatment of choice following a single acute overdose appears to be the maintenance of good urine output of at least 3 mL/kg/hour. Dialysis is of questionable value in the enhancement of aminoglycoside elimination. If required, hemodialysis is preferred over peritoneal dialysis in patients with normal renal function. Chelation with penicillin may be of benefit.

Drug Interactions
Decreased effect: May decrease GI absorption of digoxin and methotrexate
Increased effect: Synergistic effects with penicillins
Increased toxicity:
    Oral neomycin may potentiate the effects of oral anticoagulants
    Increased adverse effects with other neurotoxic, ototoxic, or nephrotoxic drugs

Stability Use reconstituted parenteral solutions within 7 days of mixing, when refrigerated

Mechanism of Action Interferes with bacterial protein synthesis by binding to 30S ribosomal subunits

Pharmacodynamics/Kinetics
Absorption: Oral, percutaneous: Poor (3%)
Distribution: V_d: 0.36 L/kg
(Continued)

Neomycin Sulfate (Continued)

Metabolism: Slight hepatic
Half-life: 3 hours (age and renal function dependent)
Time to peak serum concentration:
Oral: 1-4 hours
I.M.: Within 2 hours
Elimination: In urine (30% to 50% as unchanged drug); 97% of an oral dose eliminated unchanged in feces

Usual Dosage

Neonates: Oral: Necrotizing enterocolitis: 50-100 mg/kg/day divided every 6 hours

Children: Oral:
Preoperative intestinal antisepsis: 90 mg/kg/day divided every 4 hours for 2 days; or 25 mg/kg at 1 PM, 2 PM, and 11 PM on the day preceding surgery as an adjunct to mechanical cleansing of the intestine and in combination with erythromycin base
Hepatic coma: 50-100 mg/kg/day in divided doses every 6-8 hours or 2.5-7 g/m^2/day divided every 4-6 hours for 5-6 days not to exceed 12 g/day

Children and Adults: Topical: Apply ointment 1-4 times/day; topical solutions containing 0.1% to 1% neomycin have been used for irrigation

Adults: Oral:
Preoperative intestinal antisepsis: 1 g each hour for 4 doses then 1 g every 4 hours for 5 doses; or 1 g at 1 PM, 2 PM, and 11 PM on day preceding surgery as an adjunct to mechanical cleansing of the bowel and oral erythromycin; or 6 g/day divided every 4 hours for 2-3 days
Hepatic coma: 500-2000 mg every 6-8 hours or 4-12 g/day divided every 4-6 hours for 5-6 days
Chronic hepatic insufficiency: 4 g/day for an indefinite period

Dialyzable (50% to 100%)
Monitoring Parameters Renal function tests
Patient Information Notify physician if redness, burning, or itching occurs of if condition does not improve in 3-4 days
Dosage Forms
Cream: 0.5% (15 g)
Injection: 500 mg
Ointment, topical: 0.5% (15 g, 30 g, 120 g)
Solution, oral: 125 mg/5 mL (480 mL)
Tablet: 500 mg

Neopap® [OTC] see Acetaminophen on page 17

Neoquess® Injection see Dicyclomine Hydrochloride on page 330

Neoquess® Tablet see Hyoscyamine Sulfate on page 559

Neosar® see Cyclophosphamide on page 286

Neosporin® G.U. Irrigant see Neomycin and Polymyxin B on page 780

Neosporin® Ophthalmic Ointment see Bacitracin, Neomycin, and Polymyxin B on page 113

Neosporin® Ophthalmic Solution see Neomycin, Polymyxin B, and Gramicidin on page 781

Neosporin® Topical Ointment [OTC] see Bacitracin, Neomycin, and Polymyxin B on page 113

Neosporin® Cream [OTC] see Neomycin and Polymyxin B on page 780

Neostigmine (nee oh stig' meen)

Brand Names Prostigmin®
Synonyms Neostigmine Bromide; Neostigmine Methylsulfate
Use Diagnosis and treatment of myasthenia gravis and prevent and treat postoperative bladder distention and urinary retention; reversal of the effects of nondepolarizing neuromuscular blocking agents after surgery
Pregnancy Risk Factor C
Contraindications Hypersensitivity to neostigmine, bromides or any component; GI or GU obstruction
Warnings/Precautions Does **not** antagonize and may prolong the phase I block of depolarizing muscle relaxants (eg, succinylcholine); use with caution in

patients with epilepsy, asthma, bradycardia, hyperthyroidism, cardiac arrhythmias, or peptic ulcer; adequate facilities should be available for cardiopulmonary resuscitation when testing and adjusting dose for myasthenia gravis; have atropine and epinephrine ready to treat hypersensitivity reactions; overdosage may result in cholinergic crisis, this must be distinguished from myasthenic crisis; anticholinesterase insensitivity can develop for brief or prolonged periods

Adverse Reactions
Respiratory: Bronchoconstriction
>10%:
Central nervous system: Increased sweating
Gastrointestinal: Hyperperistalsis, nausea, vomiting, salivation, diarrhea, stomach cramps
1% to 10%:
Genitourinary: Urge to urinate
Ocular: Small pupils, lacrimation
Respiratory: Increased bronchial secretions
<1%:
Cardiovascular: A-V block, bradycardia, hypotension, bradyarrhythmias, asystole
Central nervous system: Dysphoria, restlessness, agitation, seizures, fasciculations, weakness, headache, drowsiness
Local: Thrombophlebitis
Neuromuscular & skeletal: Muscle spasms, tremor
Ocular: Diplopia, miosis
Respiratory: Laryngospasm, respiratory paralysis
Miscellaneous: Hypersensitivity, hyper-reactive cholinergic responses

Overdosage/Toxicology Symptoms of overdose include muscle weakness, blurred vision, excessive sweating, tearing and salivation, nausea, vomiting, diarrhea, hypertension, bradycardia, muscle weakness, paralysis. Atropine sulfate injection should be readily available as an antagonist for the effects of neostigmine

Drug Interactions
Decreased effect: Antagonizes effects of nondepolarizing muscle relaxants (eg, pancuronium, tubocurarine); atropine antagonizes the muscarinic effects of neostigmine
Increased effect: Neuromuscular blocking agents effects are increased

Mechanism of Action Inhibits destruction of acetylcholine by acetylcholinesterase which facilitates transmission of impulses across myoneural junction

Pharmacodynamics/Kinetics
Onset of effect:
I.M.: Within 20-30 minutes
I.V.: Within 1-20 minutes
Duration:
I.M.: 2.5-4 hours
I.V.: 1-2 hours
Absorption: Oral: Poor, <2%
Metabolism: In the liver
Half-life:
Normal renal function: 0.5-2.1 hours
End stage renal disease: Prolonged
Elimination: 50% excreted renally as unchanged drug

Usual Dosage
Myasthenia gravis: Diagnosis: I.M.:
Children: 0.04 mg/kg as a single dose
Adults: 0.02 mg/kg as a single dose

Myasthenia gravis: Treatment:
Children:
Oral: 2 mg/kg/day divided every 3-4 hours
I.M., I.V., S.C.: 0.01-.04 mg/kg every 2-4 hours
Adults:
Oral: 15 mg/dose every 3-4 hours up to 375 mg/day maximum
I.M., I.V., S.C.: 0.5-2.5 mg every 1-3 hours up to 10 mg/24 hours maximum

Reversal of nondepolarizing neuromuscular blockade after surgery in conjunction with atropine: I.V.:
Infants: 0.025-0.1 mg/kg/dose
Children: 0.025-0.08 mg/kg/dose
Adults: 0.5-2.5 mg; total dose not to exceed 5 mg

Bladder atony: Adults: I.M., S.C.:
Prevention: 0.25 mg every 4-6 hours for 2-3 days
Treatment: 0.5-1 mg every 3 hours for 5 doses after bladder has emptied
(Continued)

Neostigmine *(Continued)*

Dosing adjustment in renal impairment:
Cl$_{cr}$ 10-50 mL/minute: Administer 50% of normal dose
Cl$_{cr}$ <10 mL/minute: Administer 25% of normal dose

Test Interactions ↑ aminotransferase [ALT (SGPT)/AST (SGOT)] (S), ↑ amylase (S)

Patient Information Side effects are generally due to exaggerated pharmacologic effects; most common are salivation and muscle fasciculations; notify physician if nausea, vomiting, muscle weakness, severe abdominal pain, or difficulty breathing occurs

Nursing Implications In the diagnosis of myasthenia gravis, all anticholinesterase medications should be discontinued for at least 8 hours before administering neostigmine

Additional Information
Neostigmine bromide: Prostigmin® tablet
Neostigmine methylsulfate: Prostigmin® injection

Dosage Forms
Injection, as methylsulfate: 0.25 mg/mL (1 mL); 0.5 mg/mL (1 mL, 10 mL); 1 mg/mL (10 mL)
Tablet, as bromide: 15 mg

Neostigmine Bromide *see* Neostigmine *on page 784*

Neostigmine Methylsulfate *see* Neostigmine *on page 784*

Neo-Synephrine® 12 Hour Nasal Solution [OTC] *see* Oxymetazoline Hydrochloride *on page 829*

Neo-Synephrine® Ophthalmic Solution *see* Phenylephrine Hydrochloride *on page 874*

Neo-Synephrine® Nasal Solution [OTC] *see* Phenylephrine Hydrochloride *on page 874*

Neo-Tabs® *see* Neomycin Sulfate *on page 783*

NeoVadrin® [OTC] *see* Vitamin, Multiple *on page 1166*

Nephrocaps® [OTC] *see* Vitamin, Multiple *on page 1166*

Nephro-Fer™ [OTC] *see* Ferrous Fumarate *on page 450*

Nephrox Suspension [OTC] *see* Aluminum Hydroxide *on page 48*

Neptazane® *see* Methazolamide *on page 705*

Nervocaine® *see* Lidocaine Hydrochloride *on page 633*

Nesacaine® *see* Chloroprocaine Hydrochloride *on page 224*

Nesacaine®-MPF *see* Chloroprocaine Hydrochloride *on page 224*

Nestrex® *see* Pyridoxine Hydrochloride *on page 961*

1-N-Ethyl Sisomicin *see* Netilmicin Sulfate *on this page*

Netilmicin Sulfate *(ne til mye′ sin)*

Brand Names Netromycin®

Synonyms 1-N-Ethyl Sisomicin

Use Short-term treatment of serious or life-threatening infections including septicemia, peritonitis, intra-abdominal abscess, lower respiratory tract infections, urinary tract infections; skin, bone, and joint infections caused by sensitive *Pseudomonas aeruginosa*, *Escherichia coli*, *Proteus*, *Klebsiella*, *Serratia*, *Enterobacter*, *Citrobacter*, and *Staphylococcus*

Pregnancy Risk Factor D

Contraindications Known hypersensitivity to netilmicin (aminoglycosides, bisulfites)

Warnings/Precautions
Use with caution in patients with pre-existing renal insufficiency, vestibular or cochlear impairment, myasthenia gravis, hypocalcemia, conditions which depress neuromuscular transmission
Parenteral aminoglycosides are associated with nephrotoxicity or ototoxicity; the ototoxicity may be proportional to the amount of drug given and the duration of treatment; tinnitus or vertigo are indications of vestibular injury and impending hearing loss; renal damage is usually reversible

Adverse Reactions
>10%:
Central nervous system: Neurotoxicity
Otic: Ototoxicity (auditory), ototoxicity (vestibular)
Renal: Decreased creatinine clearance, nephrotoxicity

1% to 10%:
   Cardiovascular: Swelling
   Dermatologic: Skin itching, redness, rash
<1%:
   Central nervous system: Drowsiness, headache, pseudomotor cerebri
   Dermatologic: Photosensitivity, erythema
   Gastrointestinal: Anorexia, nausea, vomiting, weight loss, increased salivation, enterocolitis
   Hematologic: Granulocytopenia, agranulocytosis, thrombocytopenia
   Local: Burning, stinging
   Neuromuscular & skeletal: Weakness, tremors, muscle cramps
   Respiratory: Difficulty in breathing

Overdosage/Toxicology Serum level monitoring is recommended. Symptoms of overdose include ototoxicity, nephrotoxicity, and neuromuscular toxicity. Treatment of choice following a single acute overdose appears to be the maintenance of good urine output of at least 3 mL/kg/hour. Dialysis is of questionable value in the enhancement of aminoglycoside elimination. If required, hemodialysis is preferred over peritoneal dialysis in patients with normal renal function. Careful hydration may be all that is required to promote diuresis and, therefore, the enhancement of the drug's elimination. Chelation with penicillins is experimental.

Drug Interactions Increased toxicity:
   Penicillins, cephalosporins, amphotericin B, loop diuretics, vancomycin → ↑ nephrotoxic potential
   Neuromuscular blocking agents → ↑ neuromuscular blockade

Mechanism of Action Interferes with protein synthesis in bacterial cell by binding to ribosomal subunit

Pharmacodynamics/Kinetics
   Absorption: I.M.: Well absorbed
   Distribution: V_d: 0.16-0.34 L/kg; distributes into extracellular fluid including serum, abscesses, ascitic, pericardial, pleural, synovial, lymphatic, and peritoneal fluids; high concentrations in urine; crosses placenta
   Half-life: 2-3 hours (age and renal function dependent)
   Time to peak serum concentration: I.M.: Within 0.5-1 hour
   Elimination: By glomerular filtration

Usual Dosage Individualization is critical because of the low therapeutic index. Use of ideal body weight (IBW) for determining the mg/kg/dose appears to be more accurate than dosing on the basis of total body weight (TBW). In morbid obesity, dosage requirement may best be estimated using a dosing weight of IBW + 0.4 (TBW - IBW). Peak and trough plasma drug levels should be determined, particularly in critically ill patients with serious infections or in disease states known to significantly alter aminoglycoside pharmacokinetics (eg, cystic fibrosis, burns, or major surgery).

Once daily dosing: Higher peak serum drug concentration to MIC ratios, demonstrated aminoglycoside postantibiotic effect, decreased renal cortex drug uptake, and improved cost-time efficiency are supportive reasons for the use of once daily dosing regimens for aminoglycosides. Current research indicates these regimens to be as effective for nonlife-threatening infections, with no higher incidence of nephrotoxicity, than those requiring multiple daily doses. Doses are determined by calculating the entire day's dose via usual multiple dose calculation techniques and administering this quantity as a single dose. Doses are then adjusted to maintain mean serum concentrations above the MIC(s) of the causative organism(s). (Example: 4.5-6 mg/kg as a single dose, adjusted to achieve an average serum level of 3-4 mcg/mL). Further research is needed for universal recommendation in all patient populations and gram-negative disease.

I.M., I.V.:
   Neonates <6 weeks: 2-3.25 mg/kg/dose every 12 hours
   Children 6 weeks to 12 years: 1-2.5 mg/kg/dose every 8 hours
   Children >12 years and Adults: 1.5-2 mg/kg/dose every 8-12 hours
   Some clinicians suggest a daily dose of 4-7 mg/kg for all patients with normal renal function. This dose is at least as efficacious with similar, if not less, toxicity than conventional dosing.

Dosing adjustment in renal impairment: Initial dose:
   All patients should receive a loading dose of at least 2 mg/kg (subsequent dosing should be base on serum concentrations)
      Cl_{cr} ≥60 mL/minute: Administer every 8 hours
      Cl_{cr} 40-60 mL/minute: Administer every 12 hours
      Cl_{cr} 20-40 mL/minute: Administer every 24 hours

Reference Range
   Therapeutic: Peak: 4-10 µg/mL (SI: 8-21 µmol/L); Trough: <2 µg/mL (SI: 4 µmol/L)
(Continued)

Netilmicin Sulfate (Continued)

Toxic: Peak: >10 µg/mL (SI: >21 µmol/L); Trough: >2 µg/mL (SI: >4.2 µmol/L)

Patient Information Report any dizziness or sensations of ringing or fullness in ears

Nursing Implications When injected into the muscles of paralyzed patients, the results are different than in normal patients, slower absorption and lower peak concentrations probably due to poor circulation in the atrophic muscles, suggest I.V. route; aminoglycoside levels measured in blood taken from Silastic® central catheters can sometime give falsely high readings (draw from alternate lumen or via peripheral stick; otherwise flush well following administration). Monitor serum creatinine and urine output; obtain drug levels after the third dose unless otherwise directed (eg, toxicity suspected, renal dysfunction). Peak levels are drawn 30 minutes after the end of a 30-minute infusion or 1 hour after I.M. injection; trough levels are drawn within 30 minutes before the next dose; give other antibiotic drugs at least 1 hour before or after gentamicin. Hearing should be tested before, during, and after treatment in high-risk patients.

Dosage Forms
Injection: 100 mg/mL (1.5 mL)
Injection:
Neonatal: 10 mg/mL (2 mL)
Pediatric: 25 mg/mL (2 mL)

Netromycin® see Netilmicin Sulfate on page 786

Neucalm® see Hydroxyzine on page 556

Neupogen® see Filgrastim on page 454

Neuramate® see Meprobamate on page 689

Neuromuscular Blocking Agents Comparison Charts see page 1276

Neurontin® see Gabapentin on page 494

Neut® see Sodium Bicarbonate on page 1010

Neutra-Phos® see Potassium Phosphate and Sodium Phosphate on page 912

Neutra-Phos®-K see Potassium Phosphate on page 910

Neutrexin™ see Trimetrexate Glucuronate on page 1127

Neutrogena® [OTC] see Benzoyl Peroxide on page 122

N.G.T.® see Nystatin and Triamcinolone on page 812

Niacels™ [OTC] see Niacin on this page

Niacin (nye' a sin)

Related Information
Lipid-Lowering Agents on page 1273

Brand Names Niac® [OTC]; Niacels™ [OTC]; Nicobid® [OTC]; Nicolar® [OTC]; Nicotinex [OTC]; Slo-Niacin® [OTC]

Synonyms Nicotinic Acid; Vitamin B_3

Use Adjunctive treatment of hyperlipidemias; peripheral vascular disease and circulatory disorders; treatment of pellagra; dietary supplement

Pregnancy Risk Factor A (C if used in doses greater than RDA suggested doses)

Contraindications Liver disease, peptic ulcer, severe hypotension, arterial hemorrhaging, hypersensitivity to niacin

Warnings/Precautions Monitor liver function tests, blood glucose; may elevate uric acid levels; use with caution in patients predisposed to gout; large doses should be administered with caution to patients with gallbladder disease, jaundice, liver disease, or diabetes; some products may contain tartrazine

Adverse Reactions
1% to 10%:
Cardiovascular: Generalized flushing with sensation of warmth
Central nervous system: Headache
Gastrointestinal: Bloating, flatulence, nausea
Hepatic: Abnormalities of hepatic function tests, jaundice
Neuromuscular & skeletal: Tingling in extremities
Miscellaneous: Increased sebaceous gland activity
<1%:
Cardiovascular: Tachycardia, syncope, vasovagal attacks
Central nervous system: Dizziness
Dermatologic: Skin rash
Hepatic: Chronic liver damage
Ocular: Blurred vision

Respiratory: Wheezing

Overdosage/Toxicology Symptoms of acute overdose include flushing, GI distress, pruritus; chronic excessive use has been associated with hepatitis; antihistamines may relieve niacin-induced histamine release; otherwise treatment is symptomatic

Drug Interactions

Decreased effect of oral hypoglycemics; may inhibit uricosuric effects of sulfinpyrazone and probenecid

Decreased toxicity (flush) with aspirin

Increased toxicity with lovastatin (myopathy) and possibly with other HMG-CoA reductase inhibitors; adrenergic blocking agents → additive vasodilating effect and postural hypotension

Mechanism of Action Component of two coenzymes which is necessary for tissue respiration, lipid metabolism, and glycogenolysis; inhibits the synthesis of very low density lipoproteins

Pharmacodynamics/Kinetics

Peak serum concentrations: Oral: Within 45 minutes

Metabolism: Depending upon the dose, niacin converts to niacinamide; following this conversion, niacinamide is 30% metabolized in the liver

Half-life: 45 minutes

Elimination: In urine; with larger doses, a greater percentage is excreted unchanged in urine

Usual Dosage Give I.M., I.V., or S.C. only if oral route is unavailable and use only for vitamin deficiencies (not for hyperlipidemia)

Children: Pellagra: Oral: 50-100 mg/dose 3 times/day

Oral: Recommended daily allowances:

0-0.5 years: 5 mg/day
0.5-1 year: 6 mg/day
1-3 years: 9 mg/day
4-6 years: 12 mg/day
7-10 years: 13 mg/day

Males:

11-14 years: 17 mg/day
15-18 years: 20 mg/day
19-24 years: 19 mg/day

Females: 11-24 years: 15 mg/day

Adults: Oral:

Recommended daily allowances:

Males: 25-50 years: 19 mg/day; >51 years: 15 mg/day
Females: 25-50 years: 15 mg/day; >51 years: 13 mg/day
Hyperlipidemia: 1.5-6 g/day in 3 divided doses with or after meals
Pellagra: 50-100 mg 3-4 times/day, maximum: 500 mg/day
Niacin deficiency: 10-20 mg/day, maximum: 100 mg/day

Monitoring Parameters Blood glucose, liver function tests (with large doses or prolonged therapy), serum cholesterol

Test Interactions False elevations in some fluorometric determinations of urinary catecholamines; false-positive urine glucose (Benedict's reagent)

Patient Information May experience transient cutaneous flushing and sensation of warmth, especially of face and upper body; itching or tingling, and headache may occur, these adverse effects may be decreased by increasing the dose slowly or by taking aspirin or a NSAID 30 minutes to 1 hour prior to taking niacin; may cause GI upset, take with food; if dizziness occurs, avoid sudden changes in posture; report any persistent nausea, vomiting, abdominal pain, dark urine, or pale stools to the physician; do not crush sustained release capsule

Nursing Implications Monitor closely for signs of hepatotoxicity and myositis; avoid sudden changes in posture; give with food

Dosage Forms

Capsule, timed release: 125 mg, 250 mg, 300 mg, 400 mg, 500 mg
Elixir: 50 mg/5 mL (473 mL, 4000 mL)
Injection: 100 mg/mL (30 mL)
Tablet: 25 mg, 50 mg, 100 mg, 250 mg, 500 mg
Tablet, timed release: 150 mg, 250 mg, 500 mg, 750 mg

Niacinamide (nye a sin' a mide)

Synonyms Nicotinamide; Vitamin B₃

Use Prophylaxis and treatment of pellagra

Pregnancy Risk Factor A (C if used in doses greater than RDA suggested doses)

Contraindications Liver disease, peptic ulcer, known hypersensitivity to niacin

(Continued)

Niacinamide *(Continued)*

Warnings/Precautions Large doses should be administered with caution to patients with gallbladder disease or diabetes; monitor blood glucose; may elevate uric acid levels; use with caution in patients predisposed to gout; some products may contain tartrazine

Adverse Reactions
1% to 10%:
Gastrointestinal: Bloating, flatulence, nausea
Neuromuscular & skeletal: Tingling in extremities
Miscellaneous: Increased sebaceous gland activity
<1%:
Cardiovascular: Tachycardia
Dermatologic: Skin rash
Ocular: Blurred vision
Respiratory: Wheezing

Overdosage/Toxicology Symptoms of overdose include GI distress

Mechanism of Action Used by the body as a source of niacin; is a component of two coenzymes which is necessary for tissue respiration, lipid metabolism, and glycogenolysis; inhibits the synthesis of very low density lipoproteins

Pharmacodynamics/Kinetics
Absorption: Rapid from GI tract
Metabolism: In the liver
Half-life: 45 minutes
Time to peak serum concentration: 20-70 minutes
Elimination: In urine

Usual Dosage Oral:
Children: Pellagra: 100-300 mg/day in divided doses

Adults: 50 mg 3-10 times/day
Pellagra: 300-500 mg/day
Recommended daily allowance: 13-19 mg/day

Test Interactions False elevations of urinary catecholamines in some fluorometric determinations

Dosage Forms Tablet: 50 mg, 100 mg, 125 mg, 250 mg, 500 mg

Niac® [OTC] *see* Niacin *on page 788*

Nicardipine Hydrochloride *(nye kar' de peen)*

Related Information
Calcium Channel Blockers Cardiovascular Adverse Reactions *on page 1262*
Calcium Channel Blockers Central Nervous System Adverse Reactions *on page 1264*
Calcium Channel Blockers Comparative Actions *on page 1260*
Calcium Channel Blockers Comparative Pharmacokinetics *on page 1261*
Calcium Channel Blockers FDA-Approved Indications *on page 1263*
Calcium Channel Blockers Gastrointestinal and Miscellaneous Adverse Reactions *on page 1265*

Brand Names Cardene®; Cardene® SR

Use Chronic stable angina; management of essential hypertension, migraine prophylaxis
Unlabeled use: Congestive heart failure

Pregnancy Risk Factor C

Contraindications Contraindicated in severe hypotension or second and third degree heart block, sinus bradycardia, advanced heart block, ventricular tachycardia, cardiogenic shock, atrial fibrillation or flutter associated with accessory conduction pathways, CHF; hypersensitivity to nicardipine or any component, calcium channel blockers, and adenosine; not to be given within a few hours of I.V. beta-blocking agents

Warnings/Precautions Use with caution in titrating dosages for impaired renal or hepatic function patients; may increase frequency, severity, and duration of angina during initiation of therapy; do not abruptly withdraw (chest pain); elderly may have a greater hypotensive effect

Adverse Reactions
1% to 10%:
Cardiovascular: Flushing, palpitations, tachycardia
Central nervous system: Headache, asthenia, dizziness, nausea, somnolence
Miscellaneous: Pedal edema
<1%:
Cardiovascular: Edema, tachycardia, syncope, abnormal EKG
Central nervous system: Insomnia, malaise, abnormal dreams
Dermatologic: Rash

Gastrointestinal: Vomiting, constipation, dyspepsia, dry mouth

Genitourinary: Nocturia

Neuromuscular & skeletal: Tremor

Overdosage/Toxicology The primary cardiac symptoms of calcium blocker overdose includes hypotension and bradycardia. The hypotension is caused by peripheral vasodilation, myocardial depression, and bradycardia. Bradycardia results from sinus bradycardia, second- or third-degree atrioventricular block, or sinus arrest with junctional rhythm. Intraventricular conduction is usually not affected so QRS duration is normal (verapamil does prolong the P-R interval and bepridil prolongs the Q-T and may cause ventricular arrhythmias, including torsade de pointes).

The noncardiac symptoms include confusion, stupor, nausea, vomiting, metabolic acidosis and hyperglycemia. Following initial gastric decontamination, if possible, repeated calcium administration may promptly reverse the depressed cardiac contractility (but not sinus node depression or peripheral vasodilation); glucagon, epinephrine, and amrinone may treat refractory hypotension; glucagon and epinephrine also increase the heart rate (outside the U.S., 4-aminopyridine may be available as an antidote); dialysis and hemoperfusion are not effective in enhancing elimination although repeat-dose activated charcoal may serve as an adjunct with sustained-release preparations.

Drug Interactions

Increased toxicity/effect/levels:

H_2 blockers → ↑ bioavailability of nicardipine

Beta-blockers → ↑ cardiac depressant effects on A-V conduction

Carbamazepine → ↑ carbamazepine levels

Cyclosporine → ↑ cyclosporine levels

Fentanyl → ↑ hypotension

Digitalis → ↑ digitalis levels

Quinidine→ increased quinidine levels (hypotension, bradycardia, and arrhythmias)

Theophylline → ↑ pharmacologic actions of theophylline

Stability Compatible with D_5W, $D_5^1/_2NS$, D_5NS, and D_5W with 40 mEq potassium chloride; 0.45% and 0.9% NS; **do not** mix with 5% sodium bicarbonate and lactated Ringer's solution; store at room temperature; protect from light; stable for 24 hours at room temperature

Mechanism of Action Inhibits calcium ion from entering the "slow channels" or select voltage-sensitive areas of vascular smooth muscle and myocardium during depolarization, producing a relaxation of coronary vascular smooth muscle and coronary vasodilation; increases myocardial oxygen delivery in patients with vasospastic angina

Pharmacodynamics/Kinetics

Absorption: Oral: Well absorbed, ~100%

Protein binding: 95%

Metabolism: Extensive first-pass metabolism; only metabolized in the liver

Bioavailability: Absolute, 35%

Half-life: 2-4 hours

Time to peak: Peak serum levels occur within 20-120 minutes and an onset of hypotension occurs within 20 minutes

Elimination: As metabolites in urine

Usual Dosage Adults:

Oral: 40 mg 3 times/day (allow 3 days between dose increases)

Oral, sustained release: Initial: 30 mg twice daily, titrate up to 60 mg twice daily

I.V. (dilute to 0.1 mg/mL): Initial: 5 mg/hour increased by 2.5 mg/hour every 15 minutes to a maximum of 15 mg/hour

Patient Information Sustained release products should be taken with food (not fatty meal); do not crush; limit caffeine intake; avoid alcohol; notify physician if angina pain is not reduced when taking this drug, irregular heartbeat, shortness of breath, swelling, dizziness, constipation, nausea, or hypotension occur; do not stop therapy without advice of physician

Nursing Implications Monitor closely for orthostasis; ampuls must be diluted before use; do not crush sustained release product

Dosage Forms

Capsule: 20 mg, 30 mg

Capsule, sustained release: 30 mg, 45 mg, 60 mg

Injection: 2.5 mg/mL (10 mL)

Niclocide® *see Niclosamide on this page*

Niclosamide (ni kloe' sa mide)

Brand Names Niclocide®

Use Treatment of intestinal beef and fish tapeworm infections and dwarf tapeworm infections

Pregnancy Risk Factor B

Contraindications Known hypersensitivity to niclosamide; treatment of cysticercosis

Warnings/Precautions Affects cestodes of the intestine only; it is without effect in cysticercosis

Adverse Reactions

1% to 10%:

Central nervous system: Drowsiness, dizziness, headache

Gastrointestinal: Nausea, vomiting, loss of appetite, diarrhea

<1%:

Cardiovascular: Palpitations

Central nervous system: Fever

Dermatologic: Rash, pruritus ani, alopecia

Gastrointestinal: Constipation

Neuromuscular & skeletal: Weakness, backache

Miscellaneous: Oral irritation, rectal bleeding, bad taste in mouth, sweating, edema in the arm

Overdosage/Toxicology Symptoms of overdose include nausea, vomiting, anorexia; in the event of an overdose, do not administer ipecac; decontaminate with lavage or laxatives

Mechanism of Action Inhibits the synthesis of ATP through inhibition of oxidative phosphorylation in the mitochondria of cestodes

Pharmacodynamics/Kinetics

Absorption: Oral: Not significant

Metabolism: Not appreciably metabolized by mammalian host, but may be metabolized in GI tract by the worm

Elimination: In feces

Usual Dosage Oral:

Beef and fish tapeworm:

Children:

11-34 kg: 1 g (2 tablets) as a single dose

>34 kg: 1.5 g (3 tablets) as a single dose

Adults: 2 g (4 tablets) in a single dose

May require a second course of treatment 7 days later

Dwarf tapeworm:

Children:

11-34 g: 1 g (2 tablets) chewed thoroughly in a single dose the first day, then 500 mg/day (1 tablet) for next 6 days

>34 g: 1.5 g (3 tablets) in a single dose the first day, then 1 g/day for 6 days

Adults: 2 g (4 tablets) in a single daily dose for 7 days

Monitoring Parameters Stool cultures

Patient Information Chew tablets thoroughly; tablets can be pulverized and mixed with water to form a paste for administration to children; can be taken with food; a mild laxative can be used for constipation

Nursing Implications Administer a laxative 2-3 hours after the niclosamide dose if treating *Taenia solium* infections to prevent the development of cysticercosis

Dosage Forms Tablet, chewable (vanilla flavor): 500 mg

Nicobid® [OTC] *see* Niacin *on page 788*

Nicoderm® *see* Nicotine *on this page*

Nicolar® [OTC] *see* Niacin *on page 788*

Nicorette® *see* Nicotine *on this page*

Nicotinamide *see* Niacinamide *on page 789*

Nicotine (nik oh teen')

Brand Names Habitrol™; Nicoderm®; Nicorette®; Nicotrol®; ProStep®

Use Treatment aid to smoking cessation while participating in a behavioral modification program under medical supervision

Pregnancy Risk Factor D (transdermal)/X (chewing gum)

Contraindications Nonsmokers, patients with a history of hypersensitivity or allergy to nicotine or any components used in the transdermal system, pregnant or nursing women, patients who are smoking during the postmyocardial infarction period, patients with life-threatening arrhythmias, or severe or worsening angina pectoris, active temporomandibular joint disease (gum)

Warnings/Precautions Use with caution in oropharyngeal inflammation and in patients with history of esophagitis, peptic ulcer, coronary artery disease, vasospastic disease, angina, hypertension, hyperthyroidism, diabetes, and hepatic dysfunction; nicotine is known to be one of the most toxic of all poisons; while the gum is being used to help the patient overcome a health hazard, it also must be considered a hazardous drug vehicle

Adverse Reactions

Chewing gum:

>10%:

Cardiovascular: Tachycardia

Central nervous system: Headache (mild)

Gastrointestinal: Nausea, vomiting, indigestion, excessive salivation, belching, increased appetite

Miscellaneous: Mouth or throat soreness, jaw muscle ache, hiccups

1% to 10%:

Central nervous system: Insomnia, dizziness, nervousness

Endocrine & metabolic: Dysmenorrhea

Gastrointestinal: GI distress, eructation

Neuromuscular & skeletal: Muscle pain

Respiratory: Hoarseness

Miscellaneous: Hiccups

<1%:

Cardiovascular: Atrial fibrillation

Dermatologic: Erythema, itching, hypersensitivity reactions

Transdermal systems:

>10%:

Cardiovascular: Tachycardia

Central nervous system: Headache (mild)

Dermatologic: Pruritus, erythema

Gastrointestinal: Increased appetite

1% to 10%:

Central nervous system: Insomnia, nervousness

Endocrine & metabolic: Dysmenorrhea

Neuromuscular & skeletal: Muscle pain

<1%:

Cardiovascular: Atrial fibrillation

Dermatologic: Itching, hypersensitivity reactions

Overdosage/Toxicology Symptoms of overdose include nausea, vomiting, abdominal pain, mental confusion, diarrhea, salivation, tachycardia, respiratory and cardiovascular collapse. Treatment after decontamination is symptomatic and supportive; remove patch, rinse area with water and dry, do not use soap as this may increase absorption.

Mechanism of Action Nicotine is one of two naturally-occurring alkaloids which exhibit their primary effects via autonomic ganglia stimulation. The other alkaloid is lobeline which has many actions similar to those of nicotine but is less potent. Nicotine is a potent ganglionic and central nervous system stimulant, the actions of which are mediated via nicotine-specific receptors. Biphasic actions are observed depending upon the dose administered. The main effect of nicotine in small doses is stimulation of all autonomic ganglia; with larger doses, initial stimulation is followed by blockade of transmission. Biphasic effects are also evident in the adrenal medulla; discharge of catecholamines occurs with small doses, whereas prevention of catecholamines release is seen with higher doses as a response to splanchnic nerve stimulation. Stimulation of the central nervous system (CNS) is characterized by tremors and respiratory excitation. However, convulsions may occur with higher doses, along with respiratory failure secondary to both central paralysis and peripheral blockade to respiratory muscles.

Pharmacodynamics/Kinetics Intranasal nicotine may more closely approximate the time course of plasma nicotine levels observed after cigarette smoking than other dosage forms

Duration of action: Transdermal: 24 hours

Absorption: Transdermal: Slow

Metabolism: In the liver, primarily to cotinine, which is $\frac{1}{5}$ as active.

Half-life, elimination: 4 hours

Time to peak serum concentration: Transdermal: 8-9 hours

Elimination: Via the kidneys; renal clearance is pH-dependent

Usual Dosage

Gum: Chew 1 piece of gum when urge to smoke, up to 30 pieces/day; most patients require 10-12 pieces of gum/day

Transdermal patch (patients should be advised to completely stop smoking upon initiation of therapy): Apply new patch every 24 hours to nonhairy, clean, dry skin on the upper body or upper outer arm; each patch should be applied to a different site

(Continued)

Nicotine *(Continued)*

Initial starting dose: 21 mg/day for 4-8 weeks for most patients

First weaning dose: 14 mg/day for 2-4 weeks

Second weaning dose: 7 mg/day for 2-4 weeks

Initial starting dose for patients <100 pounds, smoke <10 cigarettes/day, have a history of cardiovascular disease: 14 mg/day for 4-8 weeks followed by 7 mg/day for 2-4 weeks

In patients who are receiving >600 mg/day of cimetidine: Decrease to the next lower patch size

Benefits of use of nicotine transdermal patches beyond 3 months have not been demonstrated

Patient Information Instructions for the proper use of the patch should be given to the patient; notify physician if persistent rash, itching, or burning may occur with the patch; do not smoke while wearing patches

Nursing Implications Patients should be instructed to chew slowly to avoid jaw ache and to maximize benefit; patches cannot be cut; use of an aerosol corticosteroid may diminish local irritation under patches

Dosage Forms

Patch, transdermal:

Habitrol™: 21 mg/day; 14 mg/day; 7 mg/day (30 systems/box)

Nicoderm®: 21 mg/day; 14 mg/day; 7 mg/day (14 systems/box)

ProStep®: 22 mg/day; 11 mg/day (7 systems/box)

Pieces, chewing gum, as polacrilex: 2 mg/square (96 pieces/box)

Nicotinex [OTC] *see* Niacin *on page 788*

Nicotinic Acid *see* Niacin *on page 788*

Nicotrol® *see* Nicotine *on page 792*

Nidryl® [OTC] *see* Diphenhydramine Hydrochloride *on page 351*

Nifedipine *(nye fed′ i peen)*

Related Information

Calcium Channel Blockers Cardiovascular Adverse Reactions *on page 1262*

Calcium Channel Blockers Central Nervous System Adverse Reactions *on page 1264*

Calcium Channel Blockers Comparative Actions *on page 1260*

Calcium Channel Blockers Comparative Pharmacokinetics *on page 1261*

Calcium Channel Blockers FDA-Approved Indications *on page 1263*

Calcium Channel Blockers Gastrointestinal and Miscellaneous Adverse Reactions *on page 1265*

Brand Names Adalat®; Adalat® CC; Procardia®; Procardia XL®

Use Angina, hypertrophic cardiomyopathy, hypertension (sustained release only), pulmonary hypertension

Pregnancy Risk Factor C

Pregnancy/Breast Feeding Implications Use in pregnancy only when clearly needed and when the benefits outweigh the potential hazard to the fetus

Contraindications Known hypersensitivity to nifedipine or any other calcium channel blocker and adenosine; sick-sinus syndrome, 2nd or 3rd degree A-V block, hypotension (<90 mm Hg systolic)

Warnings/Precautions Use with caution and titrate dosages for patients with impaired renal or hepatic function; use caution when treating patients with congestive heart failure, sick-sinus syndrome, severe left ventricular dysfunction, hypertrophic cardiomyopathy (especially obstructive), concomitant therapy with beta-blockers or digoxin, edema, or increased intracranial pressure with cranial tumors; do not abruptly withdraw (may cause chest pain); elderly may experience hypotension and constipation more readily.

Adverse Reactions

>10%:

Cardiovascular: Flushing

Central nervous system: Dizziness, lightheadedness, giddiness, headache

Gastrointestinal: Nausea, heartburn

Neuromuscular & skeletal: Weakness

Miscellaneous: Heat sensation

1% to 10%:

Cardiovascular: Peripheral edema, palpitations, hypotension

Central nervous system: Nervousness, mood changes

Neuromuscular & skeletal: Muscle cramps, tremor

Respiratory: Dyspnea, cough, nasal congestion

Miscellaneous: Sore throat

<1%:

Cardiovascular: Tachycardia, syncope, peripheral edema

Central nervous system: Giddiness, fever, chills
Dermatologic: Dermatitis, urticaria, purpura
Gastrointestinal: Diarrhea, constipation, gingival hyperplasia
Hematologic: Thrombocytopenia, leukopenia, anemia
Neuromuscular & skeletal: Joint stiffness, arthritis with increased ANA
Ocular: Blurred vision, transient blindness
Respiratory: Shortness of breath
Miscellaneous: Sweating

Overdosage/Toxicology The primary cardiac symptoms of calcium blocker overdose includes hypotension and bradycardia. The hypotension is caused by peripheral vasodilation, myocardial depression, and bradycardia. Bradycardia results from sinus bradycardia, second- or third-degree atrioventricular block, or sinus arrest with junctional rhythm. Intraventricular conduction is usually not affected so QRS duration is normal.

The noncardiac symptoms include confusion, stupor, nausea, vomiting, metabolic acidosis and hyperglycemia. Following initial gastric decontamination, if possible, repeated calcium administration may promptly reverse the depressed cardiac contractility (but not sinus node depression or peripheral vasodilation); glucagon, epinephrine, and amrinone may treat refractory hypotension; glucagon and epinephrine also increase the heart rate (outside the U.S., 4-aminopyridine may be available as an antidote); dialysis and hemoperfusion are not effective in enhancing elimination although repeat-dose activated charcoal may serve as an adjunct with sustained-release preparations.

Drug Interactions
Increased toxicity/effect/levels:
H_2 blockers → ↑ bioavailability of nifedipine
Beta-blockers → ↑ cardiac depressant effects on A-V conduction
Carbamazepine → ↑ carbamazepine levels
Cyclosporine → ↑ cyclosporine levels
Fentanyl → ↑ hypotension
Digitalis → ↑ digitalis levels
Quinidine→ increased quinidine levels (hypotension, bradycardia, and arrhythmias)
Theophylline → ↑ pharmacologic actions of theophylline

Mechanism of Action Inhibits calcium ion from entering the "slow channels" or select voltage-sensitive areas of vascular smooth muscle and myocardium during depolarization, producing a relaxation of coronary vascular smooth muscle and coronary vasodilation; increases myocardial oxygen delivery in patients with vasospastic angina

Pharmacodynamics/Kinetics
Onset of action:
Oral: Within 20 minutes
S.L.: Within 1-5 minutes
Protein binding: 92% to 98% (concentration-dependent)
Metabolism: In the liver to inactive metabolites
Bioavailability:
Capsules: 45% to 75%
Sustained release: 65% to 86%
Half-life:
Adults, normal: 2-5 hours
Adults with cirrhosis: 7 hours
Elimination: In urine

Usual Dosage Capsule may be punctured and drug solution administered sublingually to reduce blood pressure

Children: Oral, S.L.:
Hypertensive emergencies: 0.25-0.5 mg/kg/dose
Hypertrophic cardiomyopathy: 0.6-0.9 mg/kg/24 hours in 3-4 divided doses

Adults:
Initial: 10 mg 3 times/day as capsules or 30 mg once daily as sustained release
Usual dose: 10-30 mg 3 times/day as capsules or 30-60 mg once daily as sustained release
Maximum dose: 120-180 mg/day
Increase sustained release at 7- to 14-day intervals

Not removed by hemo- or peritoneal dialysis; supplemental dose is not necessary

Dosing adjustment in hepatic impairment: Reduce oral dose by 50% to 60% in patients with cirrhosis

Monitoring Parameters Heart rate, blood pressure, signs and symptoms of CHF, peripheral edema
(Continued)

Nifedipine *(Continued)*

Patient Information Sustained release products should be taken with food and not crushed or chewed; limit caffeine intake; avoid alcohol; notify physician if angina pain is not reduced when taking this drug, irregular heartbeat, shortness of breath, swelling, dizziness, constipation, nausea, or hypotension occurs; do not stop therapy without advice of physician

Nursing Implications May cause some patients to urinate frequently at night; may cause inflamed gums; capsule may be punctured and drug solution administered sublingually or orally to reduce blood pressure in recumbent patient

Dosage Forms

Capsule, liquid-filled (Adalat®, Procardia®): 10 mg, 20 mg
Tablet, extended release (Adalat® CC): 30 mg, 60 mg, 90 mg
Tablet, sustained release (Procardia XL®): 30 mg, 60 mg, 90 mg

Niferex®-PN *see* Vitamin, Multiple *on page 1166*

Niloric® *see* Ergoloid Mesylates *on page 397*

Nilstat® *see* Nystatin *on page 811*

NIM *see* Bleomycin Sulfate *on page 138*

Nimodipine (nye moe' di peen)

Related Information

Calcium Channel Blockers Cardiovascular Adverse Reactions *on page 1262*
Calcium Channel Blockers Central Nervous System Adverse Reactions *on page 1264*
Calcium Channel Blockers Comparative Actions *on page 1260*
Calcium Channel Blockers Comparative Pharmacokinetics *on page 1261*
Calcium Channel Blockers FDA-Approved Indications *on page 1263*
Calcium Channel Blockers Gastrointestinal and Miscellaneous Adverse Reactions *on page 1265*

Brand Names Nimotop®

Use Improvement of neurological deficits due to spasm following subarachnoid hemorrhage from ruptured congenital intracranial aneurysms in patients who are in good neurological condition postictus

Pregnancy Risk Factor C

Pregnancy/Breast Feeding Implications Use in pregnancy only when clearly needed and when the benefits outweigh the potential hazard to the fetus

Contraindications Hypersensitivity to nimodipine or any component

Warnings/Precautions Use with caution and titrate dosages for patients with impaired renal or hepatic function; use caution when treating patients with congestive heart failure, sick-sinus syndrome, PVCs, severe left ventricular dysfunction, hypertrophic cardiomyopathy (especially obstructive, IHSS), concomitant therapy with beta-blockers or digoxin, edema, or increased intracranial pressure with cranial tumors; do not abruptly withdraw (may cause chest pain); elderly may experience hypotension and constipation more readily

Adverse Reactions

1% to 10%: Cardiovascular: Reductions in systemic blood pressure

<1%:

Cardiovascular: Edema, EKG abnormalities, tachycardia, bradycardia
Central nervous system: Headache, depression
Dermatologic: Rash, acne
Gastrointestinal: Diarrhea, nausea
Hematologic: Hemorrhage
Hepatic: Hepatitis
Neuromuscular & skeletal: Muscle cramps
Respiratory: Dyspnea

Overdosage/Toxicology The primary cardiac symptoms of calcium blocker overdose includes hypotension and bradycardia. The hypotension is caused by peripheral vasodilation, myocardial depression, and bradycardia. Bradycardia results from sinus bradycardia, second- or third-degree atrioventricular block, or sinus arrest with junctional rhythm. Intraventricular conduction is usually not affected so QRS duration is normal.

The noncardiac symptoms include confusion, stupor, nausea, vomiting, metabolic acidosis and hyperglycemia. Following initial gastric decontamination, if possible, repeated calcium administration may promptly reverse the depressed cardiac contractility (but not sinus node depression or peripheral vasodilation); glucagon, epinephrine, and amrinone may treat refractory hypotension; glucagon and epinephrine also increase the heart rate (outside the U.S., 4-aminopyridine may be available as an antidote); dialysis and hemoperfusion are not effective in enhancing elimination although repeat-dose activated charcoal may serve as an adjunct with sustained-release preparations.

Drug Interactions

Increased toxicity/effect/levels:

H$_2$ blockers → ↑ bioavailability of nimodipine
Beta-blockers → ↑ cardiac depressant effects on A-V conduction
Carbamazepine → ↑ carbamazepine levels
Cyclosporine → ↑ cyclosporine levels
Fentanyl → ↑ hypotension
Digitalis → ↑ digitalis levels
Quinidine→ ↑ quinidine levels (hypotension, bradycardia)
Theophylline → ↑ pharmacologic actions of theophylline

Mechanism of Action Nimodipine shares the pharmacology of other calcium channel blockers; animal studies indicate that nimodipine has a greater effect on cerebral arterials than other arterials; this increased specificity may be due to the drug's increased lipophilicity and cerebral distribution as compared to nifedipine; inhibits calcium ion from entering the "slow channels" or select voltage sensitive areas of vascular smooth muscle and myocardium during depolarization

Pharmacodynamics/Kinetics

Metabolism: Extensive in the liver
Half-life: 3 hours, increases with reduced renal function
Protein binding: >95%
Bioavailability: 13%
Time to peak serum concentration: Oral: Within 1 hour
Elimination: In feces (32%) and in urine (50% within 4 days)

Usual Dosage Adults: Oral: 60 mg every 4 hours for 21 days, start therapy within 96 hours after subarachnoid hemorrhage

Not removed by hemo- or peritoneal dialysis; supplemental dose is not necessary

Dosing adjustment in hepatic impairment: Reduce dosage to 30 mg every 4 hours in patients with liver failure

Nursing Implications If the capsules cannot be swallowed, the liquid may be removed by making a hole in each end of the capsule with an 18-gauge needle and extracting the contents into a syringe; if given via NG tube, follow with a flush of 30 mL NS

Dosage Forms Capsule, liquid-filled: 30 mg

Nimotop® see Nimodipine *on previous page*

Nipent™ see Pentostatin *on page 861*

Nipride® see Nitroprusside Sodium *on page 801*

Nitrates Comparison see page 1279

Nitro-Bid® see Nitroglycerin *on page 799*

Nitrocine® see Nitroglycerin *on page 799*

Nitrodisc® see Nitroglycerin *on page 799*

Nitro-Dur® see Nitroglycerin *on page 799*

Nitrofural see Nitrofurazone *on next page*

Nitrofurantoin (nye troe fyoor an' toyn)

Related Information

Antimicrobial Drugs of Choice *on page 1298-1302*

Brand Names Furadantin®; Furalan®; Furan®; Furanite®; Macrobid®; Macrodantin®

Use Prevention and treatment of urinary tract infections caused by susceptible gram-negative and some gram-positive organisms; *Pseudomonas*, *Serratia*, and most species of *Proteus* are generally resistant to nitrofurantoin

Pregnancy Risk Factor B

Contraindications Hypersensitivity to nitrofurantoin or any component; renal impairment; infants <1 month (due to the possibility of hemolytic anemia)

Warnings/Precautions Use with caution in patients with G-6-PD deficiency, patients with anemia, vitamin B deficiency, diabetes mellitus or electrolyte abnormalities; therapeutic concentrations of nitrofurantoin are not attained in urine of patients with Cl$_{cr}$ <40 mL/minute (elderly); use with caution if prolonged therapy is anticipated due to possible pulmonary toxicity

Adverse Reactions

>10%:

Cardiovascular: Chest pains
Central nervous system: Chills, fever
Gastrointestinal: Stomach upset, diarrhea, loss of appetite, vomiting
Respiratory: Cough, difficult breathing

(Continued)

Nitrofurantoin *(Continued)*

1% to 10%:

Central nervous system: Tiredness, drowsiness, headache, dizziness, numbness

Neuromuscular & skeletal: Weakness, tingling

Miscellaneous: Sore throat

<1%:

Dermatologic: Skin rash, itching

Hematologic: Hemolytic anemia

Hepatic: Hepatitis

Neuromuscular & skeletal: Arthralgia

Overdosage/Toxicology Symptoms of overdose include vomiting; supportive care only

Drug Interactions

Decreased effect: Antacids (decreases absorption of nitrofurantoin)

Increased toxicity: Probenecid (decreases renal excretion of nitrofurantoin)

Mechanism of Action Inhibits several bacterial enzyme systems including acetyl coenzyme A interfering with metabolism and possibly cell wall synthesis

Pharmacodynamics/Kinetics

Absorption: Well absorbed from GI tract; the macrocrystalline form is absorbed more slowly due to slower dissolution, but causes less GI distress

Distribution: V_d: 0.8 L/kg; crosses the placenta; appears in breast milk

Protein binding: ~40%

Metabolism: 60% of drug metabolized by body tissues throughout the body, with exception of plasma, to inactive metabolites

Bioavailability: Increased by presence of food

Half-life: 20-60 minutes; prolonged with renal impairment

Elimination: As metabolites and unchanged drug (40%) in urine and small amounts in bile; renal excretion via glomerular filtration and tubular secretion

Usual Dosage Oral:

Children >1 month: 5-7 mg/kg/day in divided doses every 6 hours; maximum: 400 mg/day

Chronic therapy: 1-2 mg/kg/day in divided doses every 24 hours; maximum dose: 400 mg/day

Adults: 50-100 mg/dose every 6 hours (not to exceed 400 mg/24 hours)

Prophylaxis: 50-100 mg/dose at at bedtime

Dosing adjustment in renal impairment: Cl_{cr} <50 mL/minute: Avoid use

Avoid use in hemo and peritoneal dialysis and continuous arterio-venous or veno-venous hemofiltration (CAVH/CAVHD)

Administration Administer around-the-clock rather than 4 times/day to promote less variation in peak and trough serum levels

Monitoring Parameters Signs of pulmonary reaction, signs of numbness or tingling of the extremities, periodic liver function tests

Test Interactions Causes false-positive urine glucose with Clinitest®

Patient Information Take with food or milk; may discolor urine to a dark yellow or brown color; notify physician if fever, chest pain, persistent, nonproductive cough, or difficulty breathing occurs

Nursing Implications Higher peak serum levels may cause increased GI upset; give with meals to slow the rate of absorption and decrease adverse effects

Dosage Forms

Capsule: 50 mg, 100 mg

Capsule:

Extended release: 100 mg

Macrocrystal: 25 mg, 50 mg, 100 mg

Macrocrystal/monohydrate: 100 mg

Suspension, oral: 25 mg/5 mL (470 mL)

Nitrofurazone *(nye troe fyoor′ a zone)*

Brand Names Furacin®

Synonyms Nitrofural

Use Antibacterial agent in second and third degree burns and skin grafting

Pregnancy Risk Factor C

Contraindications Hypersensitivity to nitrofurazone or any component

Warnings/Precautions Use with caution in patients with renal impairment and patients with G-6-PD deficiency

Adverse Reactions Women should inform their physicians if signs or symptoms of any of the following occur thromboembolic or thrombotic disorders including sudden severe headache or vomiting, disturbance of vision or speech, loss of vision, numbness or weakness in an extremity, sharp or crushing chest pain, calf pain, shortness of breath, severe abdominal pain or mass, mental depression or unusual bleeding

Women should discontinue taking the medication if they suspect they are pregnant or become pregnant. Notify physician if area under dermal patch becomes irritated or a rash develops.

Drug Interactions Decreased effect: Sutilains decrease activity of nitrofurazone

Stability Avoid exposure to direct sunlight; excessive heat, strong fluorescent lighting, and alkaline materials

Mechanism of Action A broad antibacterial spectrum; it acts by inhibiting bacterial enzymes involved in carbohydrate metabolism; effective against a wide range of gram-negative and gram-positive organisms; bactericidal against most bacteria commonly causing surface infections including *Staphylococcus aureus*, *Streptococcus*, *Escherichia coli*, *Enterobacter cloacae*, *Clostridium perfringens*, *Aerobacter aerogenes*, and *Proteus* sp; not particularly active against most *Pseudomonas aeruginosa* strains and does not inhibit viruses or fungi. Topical preparations of nitrofurazone are readily soluble in blood, pus, and serum and are nonmacerating.

Usual Dosage Children and Adults: Topical: Apply once daily or every few days to lesion or place on gauze

Patient Information Notify physician if condition worsens or if irritation develops

Dosage Forms
Cream: 0.2% (28 g)
Ointment, Soluble dressing, topical: 0.2% (28 g, 56 g, 454 g, 480 g)
Solution, topical: 0.2% (480 mL, 4000 mL)

Nitrogard® *see* Nitroglycerin *on this page*

Nitrogen Mustard *see* Mechlorethamine Hydrochloride *on page 672*

Nitroglycerin (nye troe gli′ ser in)
Related Information
Nitrates Comparison *on page 1279*

Brand Names Deponit®; Minitran®; Nitro-Bid®; Nitrocine®; Nitrodisc®; Nitro-Dur®; Nitrogard®; Nitroglyn®; Nitrol®; Nitrolingual®; Nitrong®; Nitrostat®; Transdermal-NTG®; Transderm-Nitro®; Tridil®

Synonyms Glyceryl Trinitrate; Nitroglycerol; NTG

Use Treatment of angina pectoris; I.V. for congestive heart failure (especially when associated with acute myocardial infarction); pulmonary hypertension; hypertensive emergencies occurring perioperatively (especially during cardiovascular surgery)

Pregnancy Risk Factor C

Contraindications Hypersensitivity to nitroglycerin or any component; closed-angle glaucoma; severe anemia, early myocardial infarction, head trauma, cerebral hemorrhage, allergy to adhesive (transdermal), uncorrected hypovolemia (I.V.), inadequate cerebral circulation, increased intracranial pressure, constrictive pericarditis and pericardial tamponade; transdermal NTG is not effective for immediate relief of angina

Warnings/Precautions Do not use extended release preparations in patients with GI hypermotility or malabsorptive syndrome; use with caution in patients with hepatic impairment; available preparations of I.V. nitroglycerin differ in concentration or volume; pay attention to dilution and dosage; I.V. preparations contain alcohol and/or propylene glycol

Adverse Reactions
>10%:
  Cardiovascular: Postural hypotension
  Central nervous system: Headache, flushing, lightheadedness, dizziness
  Neuromuscular & skeletal: Weakness
1% to 10%: Dermatologic: Drug rash, exfoliative dermatitis
<1%:
  Cardiovascular: Reflex tachycardia, bradycardia, coronary vascular insufficiency, arrhythmias
  Dermatologic: Allergic contact dermatitis, exfoliative dermatitis
  Gastrointestinal: Nausea, vomiting
  Hematologic: Methemoglobinemia (overdose)
  Miscellaneous: Sweating, collapse, alcohol intoxication

Overdosage/Toxicology Symptoms of overdose include hypotension, throbbing headache, palpitations, bloody diarrhea, bradycardia, cyanosis, tissue hypoxia, metabolic acidosis, clonic convulsions, circulatory collapse, methemoglobinemia with extremely large overdoses; treatment is supportive and symptomatic; hypotension is treated with fluids and alpha-adrenergic pressors if needed

(Continued)

ALPHABETICAL LISTING OF DRUGS

Nitroglycerin *(Continued)*

Drug Interactions
Decreased effect: I.V. nitroglycerin may antagonize the anticoagulant effect of heparin, monitor closely; may need to decrease heparin dosage when nitroglycerin is discontinued

Increased toxicity: Alcohol, beta-blockers, calcium channel blockers may enhance nitroglycerin's hypotensive effect

Stability Doses should be made in glass bottles, Excell® or PAB® containers; adsorption occurs to soft plastic (ie, PVC)

Nitroglycerin diluted in D_5W or NS in glass containers is physically and chemically stable for 48 hours at room temperature and 7 days under refrigeration; in D_5W or NS in Excell®/PAB® containers is physically and chemically stable for 24 hours at room temperature and 14 days under refrigeration

Premixed bottles are stable according to the manufacturer's expiration dating

Standard diluent: 50 mg/250 mL D_5W; 50 mg/500 mL D_5W

Minimum volume: 100 mg/250 mL D_5W; concentration should not exceed 400 mcg/mL

Store sublingual tablets and ointment in tightly closed containers at 15°C to 30°C

Mechanism of Action Reduces cardiac oxygen demand by decreasing left ventricular pressure and systemic vascular resistance; dilates coronary arteries and improves collateral flow to ischemic regions

Pharmacodynamics/Kinetics
Onset and duration of action is dependent upon dosage form administered; see table.

Dosage Form	Onset of Effect	Peak Effect	Duration
Sublingual tablet	1-3 min	4-8 min	30-60 min
Translingual spray	2 min	4-10 min	30-60 min
Buccal tablet	2-5 min	4-10 min	2 h
Sustained release	20-45 min	45-120 min	4-8 h
Topical	15-60 min	30-120 min	2-12 h
Transdermal	40-60 min	60-180 min	18-24 h
I.V. drip	Immediate	Immediate	3-5 min

Protein binding: 60%

Metabolism: Extensive first-pass metabolism

Half-life: 1-4 minutes

Elimination: Excretion of inactive metabolites in urine

Usual Dosage Note: Hemodynamic and antianginal tolerance often develop within 24-48 hours of continuous nitrate administration

Children: Pulmonary hypertension: Continuous infusion: Start 0.25-0.5 mcg/kg/minute and titrate by 1 mcg/kg/minute at 20- to 60-minute intervals to desired effect; usual dose: 1-3 mcg/kg/minute; maximum: 5 mcg/kg/minute

Adults:
Buccal: Initial: 1 mg every 3-5 hours while awake (3 times/day); titrate dosage upward if angina occurs with tablet in place

Oral: 2.5-9 mg 2-4 times/day (up to 26 mg 4 times/day)

I.V.: 5 mcg/minute, increase by 5 mcg/minute every 3-5 minutes to 20 mcg/minute; if no response at 20 mcg/minute increase by 10 mcg/minute every 3-5 minutes, up to 200 mcg/minute

Ointment: 1" to 2" every 8 hours up to 4" to 5" every 4 hours

Patch, transdermal: 0.2-0.4 mg/hour initially and titrate to doses of 0.4-0.8 mg/hour; tolerance is minimized by using a patch-on period of 12-14 hours and patch-off period of 10-12 hours

Sublingual: 0.2-0.6 mg every 5 minutes for maximum of 3 doses in 15 minutes; may also use prophylactically 5-10 minutes prior to activities which may provoke an attack

Translingual: 1-2 sprays into mouth under tongue every 3-5 minutes for maximum of 3 doses in 15 minutes, may also be used 5-10 minutes prior to activities which may provoke an attack prophylactically

May need to use nitrate-free interval (10-12 hours/day) to avoid tolerance development; tolerance may possibly be reversed with acetylcysteine; gradually decrease dose in patients receiving NTG for prolonged period to avoid withdrawal reaction

Monitoring Parameters Blood pressure, heart rate

Patient Information Go to hospital if no relief after 3 sublingual doses; do not swallow or chew sublingual form; do not change brands without notifying your physician or pharmacist; take oral nitrates on an empty stomach; keep tablets and capsules in original container; keep tightly closed; use spray only when lying down; highly flammable; do not inhale spray; do not chew sustained release products; a treatment-free interval of 8-12 hours is recommended each day; take 3 times/day rather than every 8 hours

Nursing Implications I.V. must be prepared in glass bottles and use special sets intended for nitroglycerin; transdermal patches labeled as mg/hour; do not crush sublingual drug product

Dosage Forms
Capsule, sustained release: 2.5 mg, 6.5 mg, 9 mg
Injection: 0.5 mg/mL (10 mL); 0.8 mg/mL (10 mL); 5 mg/mL (1 mL, 5 mL, 10 mL, 20 mL); 10 mg/mL (5 mL, 10 mL)
Ointment, topical (Nitrol®): 2% [20 mg/g] (30 g, 60 g)
Patch, transdermal, topical: Systems designed to deliver 2.5, 5, 7.5, 10, or 15 mg NTG over 24 hours
Spray, translingual: 0.4 mg/metered spray (13.8 g)
Tablet:
Buccal, controlled release: 1 mg, 2 mg, 3 mg
Sublingual (Nitrostat®): 0.15 mg, 0.3 mg, 0.4 mg, 0.6 mg
Sustained release: 2.6 mg, 6.5 mg, 9 mg

Nitroglycerol *see* Nitroglycerin *on page 799*

Nitroglyn® *see* Nitroglycerin *on page 799*

Nitrol® *see* Nitroglycerin *on page 799*

Nitrolingual® *see* Nitroglycerin *on page 799*

Nitrong® *see* Nitroglycerin *on page 799*

Nitropress® *see* Nitroprusside Sodium *on this page*

Nitroprusside Sodium (nye troe pruss' ide)

Brand Names Nipride®; Nitropress®
Synonyms Sodium Nitroferricyanide; Sodium Nitroprusside
Use Management of hypertensive crises; congestive heart failure; used for controlled hypotension to reduce bleeding during surgery
Pregnancy Risk Factor C
Contraindications Hypersensitivity to nitroprusside or components; decreased cerebral perfusion; arteriovenous shunt or coarctation of the aorta (ie, compensatory hypertension)
Warnings/Precautions Use with caution in patients with increased intracranial pressure (head trauma, cerebral hemorrhage); severe renal impairment, hepatic failure, hypothyroidism; use only as an infusion with 5% dextrose in water; continuously monitor patient's blood pressure; excessive amounts of nitroprusside can cause cyanide toxicity (usually in patients with decreased liver function) or thiocyanate toxicity (usually in patients with decreased renal function, or in patients with normal renal function but prolonged nitroprusside use)
Adverse Reactions
1% to 10%:
Cardiovascular: Excessive hypotensive response, palpitations
Central nervous system: Disorientation, psychosis, headache, restlessness
Endocrine & metabolic: Thyroid suppression
Gastrointestinal: Nausea, vomiting
Hematologic: Thiocyanate toxicity
Neuromuscular & skeletal: Weakness, muscle spasm
Otic: Tinnitus
Respiratory: Hypoxia
Miscellaneous: Sweating, substernal distress
Overdosage/Toxicology Symptoms of overdose include hypotension, vomiting, hyperventilation, tachycardia, muscular twitching, hypothyroidism, cyanide or thiocyanate toxicity. Thiocyanate toxicity includes psychosis, hyperreflexia, confusion, weakness, tinnitus, seizures, and coma; cyanide toxicity includes acidosis (decreased HCO_3, decreased pH, increased lactate), increase in mixed venous blood oxygen tension, tachycardia, altered consciousness, coma, convulsions, and almond smell on breath.

Nitroprusside has been shown to release cyanide *in vivo* with hemoglobin. Cyanide toxicity does not usually occur because of the rapid uptake of cyanide by erythrocytes and its eventual incorporation into cyanocobalamin. However, prolonged administration of nitroprusside or its reduced elimination can lead to cyanide intoxication. In these situations, airway support with oxygen therapy is
(Continued)
801

Nitroprusside Sodium *(Continued)*

germane, followed closely with antidotal therapy of amyl nitrate perles, sodium nitrate 300 mg I.V. for adults and sodium thiosulfate 12.5 g I.V. (1.5 mL/kg for children); nitrates should not be administered to neonates and small children. Thiocyanate is dialyzable. May be mixed with sodium thiosulfate in I.V. to prevent cyanide toxicity.

Stability

Nitroprusside sodium should be reconstituted freshly by diluting 50 mg in 250-1000 mL of D_5W

Use only clear solutions; solutions of nitroprusside exhibit a color described as brownish, brown, brownish-pink, light orange, and straw. Solutions are highly sensitive to light. Exposure to light causes decomposition, resulting in a highly colored solution of orange, dark brown or blue. **A blue color indicates almost complete degradation and breakdown to cyanide.**

Solutions should be wrapped with aluminum foil or other opaque material to protect from light (do as soon as possible)

Stability of parenteral admixture at room temperature (25°C) and at refrigeration temperature (4°C): 24 hours

Mechanism of Action Causes peripheral vasodilation by direct action on venous and arteriolar smooth muscle, thus reducing peripheral resistance; will increase cardiac output by decreasing afterload; reduces aortal and left ventricular impedance

Pharmacodynamics/Kinetics

Onset of hypotensive effect: <2 minutes

Duration: Within 1-10 minutes following discontinuation of therapy, effects cease

Metabolism: Nitroprusside is converted to cyanide ions in the bloodstream; decomposes to prussic acid which in the presence of sulfur donor is converted to thiocyanate (liver and kidney rhodanase systems)

Half-life:

Parent drug: <10 minutes

Thiocyanate: 2.7-7 days

Elimination: Thiocyanate renally eliminated

Usual Dosage Administration requires the use of an infusion pump. Average dose: 5 mcg/kg/minute

Children: Pulmonary hypertension: I.V.: Initial: 1 mcg/kg/minute by continuous I.V. infusion; increase in increments of 1 mcg/kg/minute at intervals of 20-60 minutes; titrating to the desired response; usual dose: 3 mcg/kg/minute, rarely need >4 mcg/kg/minute; maximum: 5 mcg/kg/minute.

Adults: I.V. Initial: 0.3-0.5 mcg/kg/minute; increase in increments of 0.5 mcg/kg/minute, titrating to the desired hemodynamic effect or the appearance of headache or nausea; usual dose: 3 mcg/kg/minute; rarely need >4 mcg/kg/minute; maximum: 10 mcg/kg/minute. When >500 mcg/kg is administered by prolonged infusion of faster than 2 mcg/kg/minute, cyanide is generated faster than an unaided patient can handle.

Administration I.V. infusion only, not for direct injection

Monitoring Parameters Blood pressure, heart rate; monitor for cyanide and thiocyanate toxicity; monitor acid-base status as acidosis can be the earliest sign of cyanide toxicity; monitor thiocyanate levels if requiring prolonged infusion (>3 days) or dose ≥4 mcg/kg/minute or patient has renal dysfunction; monitor cyanide blood levels in patients with decreased hepatic function; cardiac monitor and blood pressure monitor required

Reference Range Monitor thiocyanate levels if requiring prolonged infusion (>4 days) or ≥4 μg/kg/minute; not to exceed 100 μg/mL (or 10 mg/dL) plasma thiocyanate

Thiocyanate:

Therapeutic: 6-29 μg/mL

Toxic: 35-100 μg/mL

Fatal: >200 μg/mL

Cyanide: Normal <0.2 μg/mL; normal (smoker): <0.4 μg/mL

Toxic: >2 μg/mL

Potentially lethal: >3 μg/mL

Nursing Implications Brownish solution is usable, discard if bluish in color

Dosage Forms Injection: 10 mg/mL (5 mL); 25 mg/mL (2 mL)

Nitrostat® *see* Nitroglycerin *on page 799*

Nix™ [OTC] *see* Permethrin *on page 864*

Nizatidine (ni za' ti deen)

Brand Names Axid®

Use Treatment and maintenance of duodenal ulcer; treatment of gastroesophageal reflux disease (GERD)

Pregnancy Risk Factor C

Contraindications Hypersensitivity to nizatidine or any component of the preparation; hypersensitivity to other H_2 antagonists since a cross-sensitivity has been observed with this class of drugs

Warnings/Precautions Use with caution in children <12 years of age; use with caution in patients with liver and renal impairment; dosage modification required in patients with renal impairment

Adverse Reactions

1% to 10%:
    Central nervous system: Dizziness, headache
    Gastrointestinal: Constipation, diarrhea

<1%:
    Cardiovascular: Bradycardia, tachycardia, palpitations, hypertension
    Central nervous system: Fever, dizziness, weakness, fatigue, seizures, insomnia, drowsiness
    Dermatologic: Acne, pruritus, urticaria, dry skin
    Gastrointestinal: Abdominal discomfort, flatulence, belching, anorexia
    Hematologic: Agranulocytosis, neutropenia, thrombocytopenia
    Hepatic: Increases in AST, ALT
    Neuromuscular & skeletal: Paresthesia
    Renal: Increases in BUN, creatinine, proteinuria
    Respiratory: Bronchospasm
    Miscellaneous: Allergic reaction

Overdosage/Toxicology Symptoms of overdose include muscular tremors, vomiting, rapid respiration. LD_{50} ~80 mg/kg; treatment is primarily symptomatic and supportive.

Mechanism of Action Nizatidine is an H_2-receptor antagonist. In healthy volunteers, nizatidine has been effective in suppressing gastric acid secretion induced by pentagastrin infusion or food. Nizatidine reduces gastric acid secretion by 29.4% to 78.4%. This compares with a 60.3% reduction by cimetidine. Nizatidine 100 mg is reported to provide equivalent acid suppression as cimetidine 300 mg.

Usual Dosage Adults: Active duodenal ulcer: Oral:
Treatment: 300 mg at bedtime or 150 mg twice daily
Maintenance: 150 mg/day

Dosing adjustment in renal impairment:
    Cl_{cr} 50-80 mL/minute: Administer 75% of normal dose
    Cl_{cr} 10-50 mL/minute: Administer 50% of normal dose or 150 mg/day for active treatment and 150 mg every other day for maintenance treatment
    Cl_{cr} <10 mL/minute: Administer 25% of normal dose or 150 mg every other day for treatment and 150 mg every 3 days for maintenance treatment

Test Interactions False-positive urine protein using Multistix®, gastric acid secretion test, skin tests allergen extracts, serum creatinine and serum transaminase concentrations, urine protein test

Patient Information May take several days before medication begins to relieve stomach pain; antacids may be taken with nizatidine unless physician has instructed you not to use them; wait 30-60 minutes between taking the antacid and nizatidine; avoid aspirin, cough and cold preparations; avoid use of black pepper, caffeine, alcohol, and harsh spices; may cause drowsiness or impair coordination and judgment

Nursing Implications Giving dose at 6 PM may better suppress nocturnal acid secretion than 10 PM

Dosage Forms Capsule: 150 mg, 300 mg

Nizoral® *see* Ketoconazole *on page 610*

NāSal™ [OTC] *see* Sodium Chloride *on page 1012*

N-Methylhydrazine *see* Procarbazine Hydrochloride *on page 931*

Noctec® *see* Chloral Hydrate *on page 217*

Nolvadex® *see* Tamoxifen Citrate *on page 1055*

Nonsteroidal Anti-Inflammatories Comparison *see page 1280*

Noradrenaline *see* Norepinephrine Bitartrate *on next page*

Noradrenaline Acid Tartrate *see* Norepinephrine Bitartrate *on next page*

Norcet® *see* Hydrocodone and Acetaminophen *on page 543*

Norcuron® *see* Vecuronium *on page 1151*

Nordeoxyguanosine *see* Ganciclovir *on page 496*

Nordette® *see* Ethinyl Estradiol and Levonorgestrel *on page 423*

Nordryl® *see* Diphenhydramine Hydrochloride *on page 351*

Norepinephrine Bitartrate (nor ep i nef' rin)
Related Information
Adrenergic Agonists, Cardiovascular Comparison *on page 1242*
Extravasation Treatment of Other Drugs *on page 1209*
Brand Names Levophed®
Synonyms Levarterenol Bitartrate; Noradrenaline; Noradrenaline Acid Tartrate
Use Treatment of shock which persists after adequate fluid volume replacement
Pregnancy Risk Factor D
Contraindications Hypersensitivity to norepinephrine or sulfites
Warnings/Precautions Blood/volume depletion should be corrected, if possible, before norepinephrine therapy; extravasation may cause severe tissue necrosis, give into a large vein. The drug should not be given to patients with peripheral or mesenteric vascular thrombosis because ischemia may be increased and the area of infarct extended; use with caution during cyclopropane and halothane anesthesia; use with caution in patients with occlusive vascular disease; some products may contain sulfites
Adverse Reactions
1% to 10%:
  Central nervous system: Dizziness, anxiety, headache, insomnia
  Endocrine & metabolic: Thyroid gland enlargement
  Neuromuscular & skeletal: Trembling
<1%:
  Cardiovascular: Cardiac arrhythmias, palpitations, bradycardia, tachycardia, hypertension, chest pain
  Dermatologic: Pallor
  Endocrine & metabolic: Uterine contractions
  Gastrointestinal: Vomiting
  Local: Sloughing at the infusion site
  Ocular: Photophobia
  Respiratory: Respiratory distress, diaphoresis
  Miscellaneous: Gangrene of extremities
Overdosage/Toxicology Symptoms of overdose include hypertension, sweating, cerebral hemorrhage, convulsions. Treatment of extravasation: Infiltrate area of extravasation with phentolamine 5-10 mg in 10-15 mL of saline solution.
Drug Interactions
Increased effect with tricyclic antidepressants, MAO inhibitors, antihistamines (diphenhydramine, tripelennamine), guanethidine, ergot alkaloids, and methyldopa
Atropine sulfate may block the reflex bradycardia caused by norepinephrine and enhances the pressor response
Stability Readily oxidized, protect from light, do not use if brown coloration; dilute with D₅W or DS/NS, but not recommended to dilute in normal saline; not stable with alkaline solutions; stability of parenteral admixture at room temperature (25°C): 24 hours
Mechanism of Action Stimulates beta₁-adrenergic receptors and alpha-adrenergic receptors causing increased contractility and heart rate as well as vasoconstriction, thereby increasing systemic blood pressure and coronary blood flow; clinically alpha effects (vasoconstriction) are greater than beta effects (inotropic and chronotropic effects)
Pharmacodynamics/Kinetics
Onset of action: I.V.: Very rapid-acting
Duration: Limited
Metabolism: By catechol-o-methyltransferase (COMT) and monoamine oxidase (MAO)
Elimination: In urine (84% to 96% as inactive metabolites)
Usual Dosage Note: Norepinephrine dosage is stated in terms of norepinephrine base and intravenous formulation is norepinephrine bitartrate

Norepinephrine bitartrate 2 mg = norepinephrine base 1 mg

Continuous I.V. infusion:
  Children:
    Initial: 0.05-0.1 mcg/kg/minute; titrate to desired effect
    Maximum dose: 1-2 mcg/kg/minute
  Adults: Initiate at 4 mcg/minute and titrate to desired response; 8-12 mcg/minute is usual range

ACLS dosing range: 0.5-30 mcg/minute
Rate of infusion: 4 mg in 500 mL D$_5$W
2 mcg/minute = 15 mL/hour
4 mcg/minute = 30 mL/hour
6 mcg/minute = 45 mL/hour
8 mcg/minute = 60 mL/hour
10 mcg/minute = 75 mL/hour
12 mcg/minute = 90 mL/hour
14 mcg/minute = 105 mL/hour
16 mcg/minute = 120 mL/hour
18 mcg/minute = 135 mL/hour
20 mcg/minute = 150 mL/hour

Administration Administer into large vein to avoid the potential for extravasation; potent drug, must be diluted prior to use. Rate (mL/hour) = dose (mcg/kg/minute) x weight (kg) x 60 minutes/hour divided by concentration (mcg/mL)

"Rule of 6" method for infusion preparation:
Simplified equation: 0.6 x weight (kg) = amount (mg) of drug to be added to 100 mL of I.V. fluid
When infused at 1 mL/hour, then it will deliver the drug at a rate of 0.1 mcg/kg/minute
Complex equation: 0.6 x desired dose (mcg/kg/minute) x body weight (kg) divided by desired rate (mL/hour) is the mg added to make 100 mL of solution

Nursing Implications Central line administration required; do not administer NaHCO$_3$ through an I.V. line containing norepinephrine; administer into large vein to avoid the potential for extravasation; potent drug, must be diluted prior to use

Extravasation: Use phentolamine as antidote; mix 5 mg with 9 mL of NS; inject a small amount of this dilution into extravasated area; blanching should reverse immediately. Monitor site; if blanching should recur, additional injections of phentolamine may be needed.
Dosage Forms Injection: 1 mg/mL (4 mL)

Norethin™ see Ethinyl Estradiol and Norethindrone on page 425

Norethin™ 1/50M see Mestranol and Norethindrone on page 695

Norethindrone (nor eth in' drone)
Brand Names Aygestin®; Micronor®; Norlutate®; Norlutin®; Nor-Q.D.®
Synonyms Norethindrone Acetate; Norethisterone
Use Treatment of amenorrhea; abnormal uterine bleeding; endometriosis, oral contraceptive; **higher rate of failure with progestin only contraceptives**
Pregnancy Risk Factor X
Contraindications Known hypersensitivity to norethindrone; thromboembolic disorders, severe hepatic disease, breast cancer, undiagnosed vaginal bleeding
Warnings/Precautions Use of any progestin during the first 4 months of pregnancy is not recommended; use with caution in patients with asthma, diabetes, seizure disorders, migraine, cardiac or renal dysfunction; progestin-induced withdrawal bleeding occurs within 3-7 days after discontinuation of drug
Adverse Reactions
>10%:
Cardiovascular: Edema
Central nervous system: Weakness
Endocrine & metabolic: Breakthrough bleeding, spotting, changes in menstrual flow, amenorrhea
Gastrointestinal: Anorexia
1% to 10%:
Cardiovascular: Embolism, central thrombosis
Central nervous system: Mental depression, fever, insomnia
Dermatologic: Melasma or chloasma, allergic rash with or without pruritus
Endocrine & metabolic: Changes in cervical erosion and secretions, weight gain or loss, increased breast tenderness
Hepatic: Cholestatic jaundice
Local: Thrombophlebitis
Overdosage/Toxicology Toxicity is unlikely following single exposures of excessive doses; supportive treatment is adequate in most cases
Drug Interactions Decreased effect: Aminoglutethimide may decrease effects by increasing hepatic metabolism
Mechanism of Action Inhibits secretion of pituitary gonadotropin (LH) which prevents follicular maturation and ovulation
(Continued)

Norethindrone *(Continued)*

Pharmacodynamics/Kinetics
Protein binding: 80%
Metabolism: In the liver
Half-life: 10 hours
Elimination: In urine and feces

Usual Dosage Adolescents and Adults: Female: Oral:
Contraception: Progesterone only: Norethindrone 0.35 mg every day of the year starting on first day of menstruation; if one dose is missed take as soon as remembered; then next tablet at regular time; if two doses are missed, take one of the missed doses, discard the other, and take daily dose at usual time; if three doses are missed, use another form of birth control until menses appear or pregnancy is ruled out

Amenorrhea and abnormal uterine bleeding:
Norethindrone: 5-20 mg/day on days 5-25 of menstrual cycle
Acetate salt: 2.5-10 mg on days 5-25 of menstrual cycle

Endometriosis:
Norethindrone: 10 mg/day for 2 weeks; increase at increments of 5 mg/day every 2 weeks until 30 mg/day; continue for 6-9 months or until breakthrough bleeding demands temporary termination
Acetate salt: 5 mg/day for 14 days; increase at increments of 2.5 mg/day every 2 weeks up to 15 mg/day; continue for 6-9 months or until breakthrough bleeding demands temporary termination

Test Interactions Thyroid function test, metyrapone test, liver function tests

Patient Information Take this medicine only as directed; do not take more of it and do not take it for a longer period of time; if you suspect you may have become pregnant, stop taking this medicine; report any loss of vision or vision changes immediately; avoid excessive exposure to sunlight

Nursing Implications Patients should receive a copy of the patient labeling for the drug

Additional Information Norethindrone acetate is ~2 times as potent as norethindrone

Dosage Forms
Tablet: 0.35 mg, 5 mg
Tablet, as acetate: 5 mg

Norethindrone Acetate *see* Norethindrone *on previous page*

Norethindrone Acetate and Ethinyl Estradiol *see* Ethinyl Estradiol and Norethindrone *on page 425*

Norethindrone and Mestranol *see* Mestranol and Norethindrone *on page 695*

Norethisterone *see* Norethindrone *on previous page*

Norethynodrel and Mestranol *see* Mestranol and Norethynodrel *on page 696*

Norflex™ *see* Orphenadrine Citrate *on page 820*

Norfloxacin (nor flox' a sin)

Related Information
Antimicrobial Drugs of Choice *on page 1298-1302*

Brand Names Chibroxin™; Noroxin®

Use Complicated and uncomplicated urinary tract infections caused by susceptible gram-negative and gram-positive bacteria; ophthalmic solution for conjunctivitis

Pregnancy Risk Factor C

Contraindications Known hypersensitivity to quinolones

Warnings/Precautions Not recommended in children <18 years of age; other quinolones have caused transient arthropathy in children; CNS stimulation may occur which may lead to tremor, restlessness, confusion, and very rarely to hallucinations or convulsive seizures. Use with caution in patients with known or suspected CNS disorders.

Adverse Reactions
1% to 10%:
Central nervous system: Headache, dizziness, fatigue
Gastrointestinal: Nausea
<1%:
Central nervous system: Somnolence, depression, insomnia, fever, asthenia
Dermatologic: Pruritus, hyperhidrosis, erythema, rash

Gastrointestinal: Abdominal pain, dyspepsia, constipation, flatulence, heartburn, dry mouth, diarrhea, vomiting, loose stools, anorexia, bitter taste, GI bleeding

Hepatic: Increased liver enzymes

Neuromuscular & skeletal: Back pain

Renal: Increased serum creatinine and BUN, acute renal failure

Overdosage/Toxicology Symptoms of overdose include acute renal failure, seizures; following GI decontamination, use supportive measures

Drug Interactions

Decreased effect: Decreased absorption with antacids containing aluminum, magnesium, and/or calcium (by up to 98% if given at the same time)

Increased toxicity/serum levels: Quinolones cause increased levels of caffeine, warfarin, cyclosporine, and theophylline; azlocillin, cimetidine, probenecid increase quinolone levels

Mechanism of Action Norfloxacin is a DNA gyrase inhibitor. DNA gyrase is an essential bacterial enzyme that maintains the superhelical structure of DNA. DNA gyrase is required for DNA replication and transcription, DNA repair, recombination, and transposition; bactericidal

Pharmacodynamics/Kinetics

Absorption: Oral: Rapid, up to 40%

Distribution: Crosses the placenta; small amounts appear in breast milk

Protein binding: 15%

Metabolism: In the liver

Half-life: 4.8 hours (can be higher with reduced glomerular filtration rates)

Time to peak serum concentration: Within 1-2 hours

Elimination: In urine and feces (30%)

Usual Dosage

Ophthalmic: Children >1 year and Adults: Instill 1-2 drops in affected eye(s) 4 times/day for up to 7 days

Oral: Adults: 400 mg twice daily for 7-21 days depending on infection; maximum: 800 mg/day

Dosing interval in renal impairment:

Cl_{cr} 10-30 mL/minute: Administer every 24 hours

Cl_{cr} <10 mL/minute: Do not use

Patient Information Tablets should be taken at least 1 hour before or at least 2 hours after a meal with a glass of water; patients receiving norfloxacin should be well hydrated; take all the medication, do not skip doses; Do not take with antacids

Nursing Implications Hold antacids, sucralfate for 3-4 hours after giving

Dosage Forms

Solution, ophthalmic: 0.3% [3 mg/mL] (5 mL)

Tablet: 400 mg

Norgestrel (nor jess' trel)

Brand Names Ovrette®

Use Prevention of pregnancy; **progestin only products have higher risk of failure in contraceptive use**

Pregnancy Risk Factor X

Contraindications Known hypersensitivity to norgestrel; thromboembolic disorders, severe hepatic disease, breast cancer, undiagnosed vaginal bleeding

Warnings/Precautions Discontinue if sudden loss of vision or if diplopia or proptosis occur; use with caution in patients with a history of mental depression; use of any progestin during the first 4 months of pregnancy is not recommended

Adverse Reactions

>10%:

Cardiovascular: Edema

Central nervous system: Weakness

Endocrine & metabolic: Breakthrough bleeding, spotting, changes in menstrual flow, amenorrhea

Gastrointestinal: Anorexia

1% to 10%:

Cardiovascular: Embolism, central thrombosis

Central nervous system: Mental depression, fever, insomnia

Dermatologic: Melasma or chloasma, allergic rash with or without pruritus

Endocrine & metabolic: Changes in cervical erosion and secretions, weight gain or loss, increased breast tenderness

Hepatic: Cholestatic jaundice

Local: Thrombophlebitis

Overdosage/Toxicology Toxicity is unlikely following single exposures of excessive doses; supportive treatment is adequate in most cases

(Continued)

Norgestrel *(Continued)*

Drug Interactions Decreased effect: Aminoglutethimide may decrease effects by increasing hepatic metabolism

Mechanism of Action Inhibits secretion of pituitary gonadotropin (LH) which prevents follicular maturation and ovulation

Usual Dosage Administer daily, starting the first day of menstruation, take one tablet at the same time each day, every day of the year. If one dose is missed, take as soon as remembered, then next tablet at regular time; if two doses are missed, take one tablet and discard the other, then take daily at usual time; if three doses are missed, use an additional form of birth control until menses or pregnancy is ruled out

Test Interactions Thyroid function tests, metyrapone test, liver function tests

Patient Information Take this medicine only as directed; do not take more of it and do not take it for a longer period of time; if you suspect you may have become pregnant, stop taking this medicine; report any loss of vision or vision changes immediately; avoid excessive exposure to sunlight

Nursing Implications Patients should receive a copy of the patient labeling

Dosage Forms Tablet: 0.075 mg

Norgestrel and Ethinyl Estradiol *see* Ethinyl Estradiol and Norgestrel *on page 427*

Norinyl® *see* Ethinyl Estradiol and Norethindrone *on page 425*

Norinyl® 1+50 *see* Mestranol and Norethindrone *on page 695*

Norisodrine® *see* Isoproterenol *on page 597*

Norlestrin® *see* Ethinyl Estradiol and Norethindrone *on page 425*

Norlutate® *see* Norethindrone *on page 805*

Norlutin® *see* Norethindrone *on page 805*

Normal Human Serum Albumin *see* Albumin, Human *on page 32*

Normal Saline *see* Sodium Chloride *on page 1012*

Normal Serum Albumin (Human) *see* Albumin, Human *on page 32*

Normodyne® *see* Labetalol Hydrochloride *on page 614*

Noroxin® *see* Norfloxacin *on page 806*

Norpace® *see* Disopyramide Phosphate *on page 358*

Norplant® *see* Levonorgestrel *on page 627*

Norpramin® *see* Desipramine Hydrochloride *on page 309*

Nor-Q.D.® *see* Norethindrone *on page 805*

Nor-tet® *see* Tetracycline *on page 1069*

Nortriptyline Hydrochloride *(nor trip′ ti leen)*

Related Information

Antidepressant Agents Comparison *on page 1250-1252*

Brand Names Aventyl® Hydrochloride; Pamelor®

Use Treatment of various forms of depression, often in conjunction with psychotherapy. Maximum antidepressant effect may not be seen for 2 or more weeks after initiation of therapy; has also demonstrated effectiveness for chronic pain.

Pregnancy Risk Factor D

Contraindications Narrow-angle glaucoma, avoid use during pregnancy and lactation, hypersensitivity to tricyclic antidepressants

Warnings/Precautions Use with caution in patients with cardiac conduction disturbances, history of hyperthyroid; should not be abruptly discontinued in patients receiving high doses for prolonged periods; use with caution with renal or hepatic impairment

Adverse Reactions

Neuromuscular & skeletal: Tremor

>10%:
Central nervous system: Dizziness, drowsiness, headache, weakness
Gastrointestinal: Dry mouth, constipation, increased appetite, nausea unpleasant taste, weight gain
1% to 10%:
Anticholinergic: Dry mouth, blurred vision, constipation, urinary retention increased intraocular pressure
Cardiovascular: Postural hypotension, arrhythmias, tachycardia, sudden death
Central nervous system: Confusion, delirium, hallucinations, nervousness restlessness, parkinsonian syndrome, excessive sweating, insomnia
Gastrointestinal: Diarrhea, heartburn

Genitourinary: Difficult urination, sexual dysfunction
Ocular: Blurred vision, eye pain
Neuromuscular & skeletal: Fine muscle tremors
<1%:
Central nervous system: Anxiety, seizures
Dermatologic: Alopecia, photosensitivity
Endocrine & metabolic: Breast enlargement, galactorrhea, SIADH
Genitourinary: Testicular swelling trouble with gums, decreased lower esophageal sphincter tone may cause GE reflux
Hematologic: Leukopenia, rarely agranulocytosis, eosinophilia
Hepatic: Increased liver enzymes, cholestatic jaundice
Ocular: Increased intraocular pressure
Otic: Tinnitus
Miscellaneous: Allergic reactions

Overdosage/Toxicology Symptoms of overdose include agitation, confusion, hallucinations, urinary retention, hypothermia, hypotension, seizures, ventricular tachycardia

Following initiation of essential overdose management, toxic symptoms should be treated. Ventricular arrhythmias and EKG changes (QRS widening) often respond to phenytoin 15-20 mg/kg (adults) with concurrent systemic alkalinization (sodium bicarbonate 0.5-2 mEq/kg I.V.). Arrhythmias unresponsive to this therapy may respond to lidocaine 1 mg/kg I.V. followed by a titrated infusion. Physostigmine (1-2 mg I.V. slowly for adults or 0.5 mg I.V. slowly for children) may be indicated in reversing cardiac arrhythmias that are life-threatening. Seizures usually respond to diazepam I.V. boluses (5-10 mg for adults up to 30 mg or 0.25-0.4 mg/kg/dose for children up to 10 mg/dose). If seizures are unresponsive or recur, phenytoin or phenobarbital may be required.

Drug Interactions
Blocks the uptake of guanethidine and thus prevents the hypotensive effect of guanethidine; may be additive with or may potentiate the action of other CNS depressants such as sedatives or hypnotics; potentiates the pressor and cardiac effects of sympathomimetic agents such as isoproterenol, epinephrine, etc
With MAO inhibitors, hyperpyrexia, hypertension, tachycardia, confusion, seizures, and death have been reported
Additive anticholinergic effect seen with other anticholinergic agents
Cimetidine reduces the metabolism of nortriptyline
May increase prothrombin time in patients stabilized on warfarin

Stability Protect from light

Mechanism of Action Traditionally believed to increase the synaptic concentration of serotonin and/or norepinephrine in the central nervous system by inhibition of their reuptake by the presynaptic neuronal membrane. However, additional receptor effects have been found including desensitization of adenyl cyclase, down regulation of beta-adrenergic receptors, and down regulation of serotonin receptors.

Pharmacodynamics/Kinetics
Onset of action: 1-3 weeks before therapeutic effects are seen
Distribution: V_d: 21 L/kg
Protein binding: 93% to 95%
Metabolism: Undergoes significant first-pass metabolism; primarily detoxified in the liver
Half-life: 28-31 hours
Time to peak serum concentration: Oral: Within 7-8.5 hours
Elimination: As metabolites and small amounts of unchanged drug in urine; small amounts of biliary elimination occur

Usual Dosage Oral:
Nocturnal enuresis:
Children:
6-7 years (20-25 kg): 10 mg/day
8-11 years (25-35 kg): 10-20 mg/day
>11 years (35-54 kg): 25-35 mg/day
Depression:
Adolescents: 30-50 mg/day in divided doses
Adults: 25 mg 3-4 times/day up to 150 mg/day
Elderly:
Initial: 10-25 mg at bedtime
Dosage can be increased by 25 mg every 3 days for inpatients and weekly for outpatients if tolerated
Usual maintenance dose: 75 mg as a single bedtime dose, however, lower or higher doses may be required to stay within the therapeutic window

Dosing adjustment in hepatic impairment: Lower doses and slower titration dependent on individualization of dosage is recommended
(Continued)

Nortriptyline Hydrochloride *(Continued)*

Monitoring Parameters Monitor blood pressure and pulse rate prior to and during initial therapy; evaluate mental status; monitor weight

Reference Range
Plasma levels do not always correlate with clinical effectiveness
Therapeutic: 50-150 ng/mL (SI: 190-570 nmol/L)
Toxic: >500 ng/mL (SI: >1900 nmol/L)

Test Interactions ↑ glucose

Patient Information Avoid alcohol ingestion; do not discontinue medication abruptly; may cause urine to turn blue-green; may cause drowsiness; full effect may not occur for 3-6 weeks; dry mouth may be helped by sips of water, sugarless gum, or hard candy

Nursing Implications May increase appetite and possibly a craving for sweets

Dosage Forms
Capsule: 10 mg, 25 mg, 50 mg, 75 mg
Solution: 10 mg/5 mL (473 mL)

Norvasc® *see* Amlodipine *on page 62*

Nōstrilla® *see* Oxymetazoline Hydrochloride *on page 829*

Nōstrilla® Long-Acting Nasal Solution [OTC] *see* Oxymetazoline Hydrochloride *on page 829*

Nostril® Nasal Solution [OTC] *see* Phenylephrine Hydrochloride *on page 874*

Novafed® *see* Pseudoephedrine *on page 955*

Novantrone® *see* Mitoxantrone Hydrochloride *on page 749*

Novocain® *see* Procaine Hydrochloride *on page 930*

Novolin® 70/30 [OTC] *see* Insulin Preparations *on page 578*

Novolin® 70/30 PenFil® [OTC] *see* Insulin Preparations *on page 578*

Novolin® L [OTC] *see* Insulin Preparations *on page 578*

Novolin® N [OTC] *see* Insulin Preparations *on page 578*

Novolin® N PenFil® [OTC] *see* Insulin Preparations *on page 578*

Novolin® R [OTC] *see* Insulin Preparations *on page 578*

Novolin® R PenFil® [OTC] *see* Insulin Preparations *on page 578*

NP-27® [OTC] *see* Tolnaftate *on page 1106*

NPH Iletin® I [OTC] *see* Insulin Preparations *on page 578*

NPH Insulin [OTC] *see* Insulin Preparations *on page 578*

NPH-N [OTC] *see* Insulin Preparations *on page 578*

NTG *see* Nitroglycerin *on page 799*

NTZ® Nasal Solution [OTC] *see* Oxymetazoline Hydrochloride *on page 829*

Nubain® *see* Nalbuphine Hydrochloride *on page 770*

NuLytely® *see* Polyethylene Glycol-Electrolyte Solution *on page 900*

Numorphan® *see* Oxymorphone Hydrochloride *on page 831*

Numzitdent® [OTC] *see* Benzocaine *on page 121*

Numzit Teething® [OTC] *see* Benzocaine *on page 121*

Nupercainal® [OTC] *see* Dibucaine *on page 327*

Nuprin® [OTC] *see* Ibuprofen *on page 561*

Nuromax® Injection *see* Doxacurium Chloride *on page 366*

Nutracort® *see* Hydrocortisone *on page 546*

Nutraplus® [OTC] *see* Urea *on page 1139*

Nutrilipid® *see* Fat Emulsion *on page 441*

Nutropin® *see* Human Growth Hormone *on page 538*

Nydrazid® *see* Isoniazid *on page 595*

Nylidrin Hydrochloride *(nye' li drin)*

Brand Names Arlidin®

Use Considered "possibly effective" for increasing blood supply to treat peripheral disease (arteriosclerosis obliterans, diabetic vascular disease, nocturnal leg cramps, Raynaud's disease, frost bite, ischemic ulcer, thrombophlebitis) and circulatory disturbances of the inner ear (cochlear ischemia, macular or ampullar ischemia, etc)

Pregnancy Risk Factor C

Contraindications Paroxysmal tachycardia, acute myocardial infarction, progressive angina pectoris, thyrotoxicosis

Warnings/Precautions Use with caution in patients with tachyarrhythmias or uncompensated CHF, may cause maternal hyperglycemia

Adverse Reactions

1% to 10%:
Central nervous system: Nervousness
Neuromuscular & skeletal: Trembling

<1%:
Cardiovascular: Palpitations, postural hypotension
Central nervous system: Dizziness
Gastrointestinal: Nausea, vomiting
Neuromuscular & skeletal: Weakness

Overdosage/Toxicology Symptoms of overdose include tremors, hypotension; hypotension can be treated by fluids and alpha-adrenergic pressors if needed

Mechanism of Action Nylidrin is a peripheral vasodilator; this results from direct relaxation of vascular smooth muscle and beta agonist action. Nylidrin does not appear to affect cutaneous blood flow; it reportedly increases heart rate and cardiac output; cutaneous blood flow is not enhanced to any appreciable extent.

Usual Dosage Adults: Oral: 3-12 mg 3-4 times/day; start with lower dose in elderly due to hypotensive effect

Monitoring Parameters Monitor for orthostasis

Patient Information May cause dizziness, rise slowly from prolonged sitting or lying; may impair judgment and coordination

Dosage Forms Tablet: 6 mg, 12 mg

Nystatin (nye stat' in)

Brand Names Mycostatin®; Nilstat®; Nystat-Rx®; Nystex®; O-V Staticin®

Use Treatment of susceptible cutaneous, mucocutaneous, and oral cavity fungal infections normally caused by the *Candida* species

Pregnancy Risk Factor B/C (oral)

Contraindications Hypersensitivity to nystatin or any component

Adverse Reactions

1% to 10%: Gastrointestinal: Nausea, vomiting, diarrhea, stomach pain
<1%: Miscellaneous: Hypersensitivity reactions
Dermatologic: Contact dermatitis, Stevens-Johnson syndrome

Overdosage/Toxicology Symptoms of overdose include nausea, vomiting, diarrhea

Stability Keep vaginal inserts in refrigerator; protect from temperature extremes, moisture, and light

Mechanism of Action Binds to sterols in fungal cell membrane, changing the cell wall permeability allowing for leakage of cellular contents

Pharmacodynamics/Kinetics

Onset of symptomatic relief from candidiasis: Within 24-72 hours
Absorption: Not absorbed through mucous membranes or intact skin; poorly absorbed from the GI tract
Elimination: In feces as unchanged drug

Usual Dosage

Oral candidiasis: Suspension (swish and swallow orally):
Neonates: 100,000 units 4 times/day or 50,000 units to each side of mouth 4 times/day
Infants: 200,000 units 4 times/day or 100,000 units to each side of mouth 4 times/day
Children and Adults: 400,000-600,000 units 4 times/day; troche: 200,000-400,000 units 4-5 times/day
Adults: 400,000-600,000 units 4 times/day; pastilles: 200,000-400,000 units 4-5 times/day

Mucocutaneous infections: Children and Adults: Topical: Apply 2-3 times/day to affected areas; very moist topical lesions are treated best with powder
Intestinal infections: Adults: Oral tablets: 500,000-1,000,000 units every 8 hours
Vaginal infections: Adults: Vaginal tablets: Insert 1 tablet/day at bedtime for 2 weeks

Patient Information The oral suspension should be swished about the mouth and retained in the mouth for as long as possible (several minutes) before swallowing. For neonates and infants, paint nystatin suspension into recesses of the mouth. Troches must be allowed to dissolve slowly and should not be chewed or swallowed whole. If topical irritation occurs, discontinue; for external use only; do not discontinue therapy even if symptoms are gone

(Continued)

Nystatin *(Continued)*

Dosage Forms
Cream: 100,000 units/g (15 g, 30 g)

Ointment, topical: 100,000 units/g (15 g, 30 g)

Powder, for preparation of oral suspension: 50 million units, 1 billion units, 2 billion units, 5 billion units

Powder, topical: 100,000 units/g (15 g)

Suspension, oral: 100,000 units/mL (5 mL, 60 mL, 480 mL)

Tablet:
 Oral: 500,000 units
 Vaginal: 100,000 units (15 and 30/box with applicator)

Troche: 200,000 units

Nystatin and Triamcinolone *(nye stat' in)*

Brand Names Dermacomb®; Mycogen® II; Mycolog®-II; Myconel®; Myco-Triacet® II; Mytrex®; N.G.T.®; Tri-Statin® II

Synonyms Triamcinolone and Nystatin

Use Treatment of cutaneous candidiasis

Pregnancy Risk Factor C

Contraindications Known hypersensitivity to nystatin or triamcinolone

Warnings/Precautions Avoid use of occlusive dressings; limit therapy to least amount necessary for effective therapy, pediatric patients may be more susceptible to HPA axis suppression due to larger BSA to weight ratio

Adverse Reactions
1% to 10%:
 Dermatologic: Dryness, folliculitis, hypertrichosis, acne, hypopigmentation, allergic dermatitis, maceration of the skin, skin atrophy
 Local: Burning, itching, irritation
 Miscellaneous: Increased incidence of secondary infection

Overdosage/Toxicology Refer to individual monographs for Nystatin and Triamcinolone

Mechanism of Action Refer to individual monographs for Nystatin and Triamcinolone

Pharmacodynamics/Kinetics Refer to individual monographs for Nystatin and Triamcinolone

Usual Dosage Children and Adults: Topical: Apply sparingly 2-4 times/day

Patient Information Before applying, gently wash area to reduce risk of infection; apply a thin film to cleansed area and rub in gently and thoroughly until medication vanishes; avoid exposure to sunlight, severe sunburn may occur

Nursing Implications External use only; do not use on open wounds; apply sparingly to occlusive dressings; should not be used in the presence of open or weeping lesions

Dosage Forms
Cream: Nystatin 100,000 units and triamcinolone acetonide 0.1% (1.5 g, 15 g, 30 g, 60 g, 120 g)

Ointment, topical: Nystatin 100,000 units and triamcinolone acetonide 0.1% (15 g, 30 g, 60 g, 120 g)

Nystat-Rx® *see* Nystatin *on previous page*

Nystex® *see* Nystatin *on previous page*

Nytol® [OTC] *see* Diphenhydramine Hydrochloride *on page 351*

Ocean Nasal Mist [OTC] *see* Sodium Chloride *on page 1012*

OCL® *see* Polyethylene Glycol-Electrolyte Solution *on page 900*

Octamide® *see* Metoclopramide *on page 728*

Octicair® *see* Neomycin, Polymyxin B, and Hydrocortisone *on page 781*

Octocaine® *see* Lidocaine Hydrochloride *on page 633*

Octreotide Acetate *(ok tree' oh tide)*

Brand Names Sandostatin®

Use Control of symptoms in patients with metastatic carcinoid and vasoactive intestinal peptide-secreting tumors (VIPomas); pancreatic tumors, gastrinoma, secretory diarrhea

 Unlabeled uses: Acromegaly, AIDS-associated secretory diarrhea, control of bleeding of esophageal varices, breast cancer, cryptosporidiosis, Cushing's syndrome, insulinomas, small bowel fistulas, postgastrectomy dumping syndrome, chemotherapy-induced diarrhea, GVHD-induced diarrhea, Zollinger-Ellison syndrome

Pregnancy Risk Factor B

Contraindications Known hypersensitivity to octreotide or any component

Warnings/Precautions Dosage adjustment may be required to maintain symptomatic control; insulin requirements may be reduced as well as sulfonylurea requirements; monitor patients for cholelithiasis, hyper- or hypoglycemia; use with caution in patients with renal impairment

Adverse Reactions

1% to 10%:

Cardiovascular: Flushing, edema

Central nervous system: Fatigue, weakness, headache, dizziness, vertigo, fatigue, anorexia, depression

Endocrine & metabolic: Hypoglycemia or hyperglycemia (1%), hypothyroidism, galactorrhea

Gastrointestinal/hepatic: Cholelithiasis has occurred, presumably by altering fat absorption and decreasing the motility of the gallbladder, nausea, vomiting, diarrhea, constipation, abdominal pain, cramping, discomfort, fat malabsorption, loose stools, flatulence

Hepatic: Jaundice, hepatitis, increase LFTs

Local: Pain at injection site

<1%:

Cardiovascular: Chest pain, flushing, edema, hypertensive reaction

Central nervous system: Dizziness, fatigue, anxiety, headache, fever, weakness, hyperesthesia

Dermatologic: Hair loss, wheal/erythema, rash

Endocrine & metabolic: Hypoglycemia, hyperglycemia, galactorrhea

Gastrointestinal: Constipation, flatulence

Hepatic: Hepatitis

Local: Injection site pain, thrombophlebitis

Neuromuscular & skeletal: Leg cramps, Bell's palsy, muscle cramping

Ocular: Burning eyes

Respiratory: Throat discomfort, rhinorrhea, shortness of breath

Overdosage/Toxicology Symptoms of overdose include hypo- or hyperglycemia, blurred vision, dizziness, drowsiness, loss of motor function; well tolerated bolus doses up to 1000 mcg have failed to produce adverse effects

Drug Interactions Decreased effect: Cyclosporine (case report of a transplant rejection due to reduction of serum cyclosporine levels)

Stability

Octreotide is a clear solution and should be stored under refrigeration; ampuls may be stored at room temperature for up to 14 days when protected from light

Stability of parenteral admixture in NS at room temperature (25°C) and at refrigeration temperature (4°C): 48 hours

Common diluent: 50-100 mcg/50 mL NS; common diluent for continuous I.V. infusion: 1200 mcg/250 mL NS

Minimum volume: 50 mL NS

Mechanism of Action Mimics natural somatostatin by inhibiting serotonin release, and the secretion of gastrin, VIP, insulin, glucagon, secretin, motilin, and pancreatic polypeptide

Pharmacodynamics/Kinetics

Duration of action: 6-12 hours

Absorption:

Oral: Absorbed but still under study

S.C.: Rapid

Bioavailability: S.C.: 100%

Distribution: V_d: 14 L; 65% bound to lipoproteins

Metabolism: Extensive by the liver

Half-life: 60-110 minutes

Elimination: 32% by the kidney

Usual Dosage Adults: S.C.: Initial: 50 mcg 1-2 times/day and titrate dose based on patient tolerance and response

Carcinoid: 100-600 mcg/day in 2-4 divided doses

VIPomas: 200-300 mcg/day in 2-4 divided doses

Diarrhea: Initial: I.V.: 50-100 mcg every 8 hours; increase by 100 mcg/dose at 48-hour intervals; maximum dose: 500 mcg every 8 hours

Esophageal variced bleeding: I.V. bolus: 25-50 mcg followed by continuous I.V. infusion of 25-50 mcg/hour

Administration

Administer S.C. or I.V.

I.V. administration may be IVP, IVPB, or continuous I.V. infusion

IVP should be administered undiluted over 3 minutes

IVPB should be administered over 15-30 minutes

(Continued)

Octreotide Acetate *(Continued)*

Continuous I.V. infusion rates have ranged from 25-50 mcg/hour for the treatment of esophageal variceal bleeding

Reference Range Vasoactive intestinal peptide: <75 ng/L; levels vary considerably between laboratories

Nursing Implications Do not use if solution contains particles or is discolored

Dosage Forms Injection: 0.05 mg (1 mL); 0.1 mg (1 mL); 0.5 mg (1 mL)

Ocu-Carpine® *see* Pilocarpine *on page 883*

OcuClear® [OTC] *see* Oxymetazoline Hydrochloride *on page 829*

Ocu-Dex® *see* Dexamethasone *on page 314*

Ocu-Drop® [OTC] *see* Tetrahydrozoline Hydrochloride *on page 1071*

Ocufen® *see* Flurbiprofen Sodium *on page 482*

Ocuflox™ *see* Ofloxacin *on this page*

Oculinum® *see* Botulinum Toxin Type A *on page 139*

Ocumycin® *see* Gentamicin Sulfate *on page 500*

Ocu-Pentolate® *see* Cyclopentolate Hydrochloride *on page 286*

Ocupress® *see* Carteolol Hydrochloride *on page 188*

Ocusert® Pilo *see* Pilocarpine *on page 883*

Ocusert Pilo-20® *see* Pilocarpine *on page 883*

Ocusert Pilo-40® *see* Pilocarpine *on page 883*

Ocutricin® HC *see* Neomycin, Polymyxin B, and Hydrocortisone *on page 781*

Ocutricin® Ophthalmic Solution *see* Neomycin, Polymyxin B, and Gramicidin *on page 781*

Ocutricin® Topical Ointment *see* Bacitracin, Neomycin, and Polymyxin B *on page 113*

Ocu-Tropine® *see* Atropine Sulfate *on page 100*

Ofloxacin *(oh floks' a sin)*

Brand Names Floxin®; Ocuflox™

Use Quinolone antibiotic for skin and skin structure, lower respiratory and urinary tract infections, and sexually transmitted diseases, bacterial conjunctivitis caused by susceptible organisms

Pregnancy Risk Factor C

Contraindications Hypersensitivity to ofloxacin or other members of the quinolone group such as nalidixic acid, oxolinic acid, cinoxacin, norfloxacin, and ciprofloxacin

Warnings/Precautions Use with caution in patients with epilepsy or other CNS diseases which could predispose seizures; use with caution in patients with renal impairment; failure to respond to an ophthalmic antibiotic after 2-3 days may indicate the presence of resistant organisms, or another causative agent; use caution with systemic preparation in children <18 years of age due to association of other quinolones with transient arthropathy

Adverse Reactions

>10%: Gastrointestinal: Nausea

1% to 10%:

Cardiovascular: Chest pain

Central nervous system: Headache, insomnia, dizziness, fatigue, somnolence, sleep disorders, nervousness, pyrexia

Dermatologic: External genital pruritus in women, rash, pruritus

Gastrointestinal: Diarrhea, vomiting, GI distress, pain and cramps, abdominal cramps, flatulence, dysgeusia, dry mouth, decreased appetite

Genitourinary: Vaginitis

Neuromuscular & skeletal: Trunk pain

Ocular: Superinfection (ophthalmic), photophobia, lacrimation, dry eyes, stinging, visual disturbances

<1%:

Cardiovascular: Syncope, edema, hypertension, palpitations, vasodilation

Central nervous system: Anxiety, cognitive change, depression, dream abnormality, euphoria, hallucinations, vertigo, asthenia, chills, malaise, extremity pain

Gastrointestinal: Thirst, weight loss

Neuromuscular & skeletal: Paresthesia

Ocular: Photophobia

Otic: Decreased hearing acuity, tinnitus
Respiratory: Cough

Overdosage/Toxicology Symptoms of overdose include acute renal failure, seizures, nausea, vomiting; treatment includes GI decontamination, if possible, and supportive care; not removed by peritoneal or hemodialysis

Drug Interactions

Decreased effect: Decreased absorption with antacids containing aluminum, magnesium, and/or calcium (by up to 98% if given at the same time)

Increased toxicity/serum levels: Quinolones cause increased caffeine, warfarin, cyclosporine, and theophylline levels; azlocillin, cimetidine, probenecid increase quinolone levels

Mechanism of Action Ofloxacin, a fluorinated quinolone, is a pyridine carboxylic acid derivative which exerts a broad spectrum bactericidal effect. It inhibits DNA gyrase inhibitor, an essential bacterial enzyme that maintains the superhelical structure of DNA. DNA gyrase is required for DNA replication and transcription, DNA repair, recombination, and transposition within the bacteria.

Pharmacodynamics/Kinetics

Absorption: Well absorbed; administration with food causes only minor alterations in absorption

Distribution: V_d: 2.4-3.5 L/kg

Protein binding: 20%

Half-life, elimination 5-7.5 hours

Elimination: Primarily unchanged in urine

Usual Dosage

Children >1 year and Adults: Ophthalmic: Instill 1-2 drops in affected eye(s) every 2-4 hours for the first 2 days, then use 4 times daily for an additional 5 days

Adults: Oral, I.V.: 200-400 mg every 12 hours for 7-10 days for most infections or for 6 weeks for prostatitis

Dosing adjustment/interval in renal impairment:

Cl_{cr} 10-50 mL/minute: Administer 50% of normal dose or administer every 24 hours

Cl_{cr} <10 mL/minute: Administer 25% of normal dose or administer 50% of normal dose every 24 hours

Patient Information Report any skin rash or other allergic reactions; avoid excessive sunlight; do not take with food; do not take within 2 hours of any products including antacids which contain zinc, magnesium, or aluminum

Dosage Forms

Injection: 200 mg (50 mL); 400 mg (10 mL, 20 mL, 100 mL)

Solution, ophthalmic: 0.3% (5 mL)

Tablet: 200 mg, 300 mg, 400 mg

Ogen® see Estropipate on page 414

OGMT see Metyrosine on page 735

OKT3 see Muromonab-CD3 on page 761

Oleovitamin A see Vitamin A on page 1163

Oleum Ricini see Castor Oil on page 190

Olsalazine Sodium (ole sal' a zeen)

Brand Names Dipentum®

Use Maintenance of remission of ulcerative colitis in patients intolerant to sulfasalazine

Pregnancy Risk Factor C

Contraindications Hypersensitivity to salicylates

Warnings/Precautions Diarrhea is a common adverse effect of olsalazine; use with caution in patients with hypersensitivity to salicylates, sulfasalazine, or mesalamine

Adverse Reactions

>10%: Gastrointestinal: Diarrhea, cramps, abdominal pain

1% to 10%:

Central nervous system: Headache, fatigue, depression

Dermatologic: Rash, itching

Gastrointestinal: Nausea, dyspepsia, bloating, anorexia

Neuromuscular & skeletal: Arthralgia

<1%:

Central nervous system: Fever

Gastrointestinal: Bloody diarrhea

Hematologic: Blood dyscrasias

Hepatic: Hepatitis

Overdosage/Toxicology Decreased motor activity, diarrhea
(Continued)

Olsalazine Sodium *(Continued)*

Mechanism of Action The mechanism of action appears to be topical rather than systemic

Pharmacodynamics/Kinetics
Absorption: <3%; very little intact olsalazine is systemically absorbed
Protein binding: High
Metabolism: Mostly by colonic bacteria to the active drug, 5-aminosalicylic acid
Half-life, elimination: 56 minutes or 55 hours depending on the analysis used
Elimination: Primarily in feces

Usual Dosage Adults: Oral: 1 g/day in 2 divided doses

Test Interactions ↑ ALT, AST (S)

Patient Information Take with food in evenly divided doses; report any sign of allergic reaction including rash

Dosage Forms Capsule: 250 mg

Omeprazole *(oh me′ pray zol)*

Brand Names Prilosec™

Use Short-term (4-8 weeks) treatment of severe erosive esophagitis (grade 2 or above), diagnosed by endoscopy and short-term treatment of symptomatic gastroesophageal reflux disease (GERD) poorly responsive to customary medical treatment; pathological hypersecretory conditions; peptic ulcer disease
Unlabeled use: Gastric ulcer therapy and healing NSAID-induced ulcers

Pregnancy Risk Factor C

Contraindications Known hypersensitivity to omeprazole

Warnings/Precautions In long-term (2-year) studies in rats, omeprazole produced a dose-related increase in gastric carcinoid tumors. While available endoscopic evaluations and histologic examinations of biopsy specimens from human stomachs have not detected a risk from short-term exposure to omeprazole, further human data on the effect of sustained hypochlorhydria and hypergastrinemia are needed to rule out the possibility of an increased risk for the development of tumors in humans receiving long-term therapy. Bioavailability may be increased in the elderly.

Adverse Reactions
1% to 10%:
Cardiovascular: Angina, tachycardia, bradycardia, edema
Central nervous system: Headache (7%), dizziness, asthenia
Dermatologic: Rash, urticaria, pruritus, dry skin
Gastrointestinal: Diarrhea, nausea, abdominal pain, vomiting, constipation, anorexia, irritable colon, fecal discoloration, esophageal candidiasis, dry mouth, taste alterations
Genitourinary: Testicular pain, urinary tract infection, urinary frequency
Neuromuscular & skeletal: Back pain, asthenia occurred in more frequently than 1% of patients, muscle cramps, myalgia, joint pain, leg pain
Renal: Pyuria, proteinuria, hematuria, glycosuria
Respiratory: Cough
<1%:
Cardiovascular: Chest pain
Central nervous system: Fever, fatigue, malaise, apathy, somnolence, nervousness, anxiety, pain
Gastrointestinal: Abdominal swelling

Overdosage/Toxicology Symptoms of overdose include hypothermia, sedation, convulsions, decreased respiratory rate demonstrated in animals only; treatment is supportive; not dialyzable

Drug Interactions
Cytochrome P-450 1A2 enzyme inducer and cytochrome P-450 IIC enzyme inhibitor
Decreased effect: Decreased ketoconazole; decreased itraconazole
Increased toxicity: Diazepam → ↑ half-life; increased digoxin, increased phenytoin, increased warfarin

Stability Omeprazole stability is a function of pH; it is rapidly degraded in acidic media, but has acceptable stability under alkaline conditions. Prilosec™ is supplied as capsules for oral administration; each capsule contains 20 mg of omeprazole in the form of enteric coated granules to inhibit omeprazole degradation by gastric acidity; therefore, the manufacturer recommends against extemporaneously preparing it in an oral liquid form for administration via an NG tube.

Mechanism of Action Suppresses gastric acid secretion by inhibiting the parietal cell H+/K+ ATP pump

Pharmacodynamics/Kinetics
Onset of antisecretory action: Oral: Within 1 hour
Peak effect: 2 hours
Duration: 72 hours

Protein binding: 95%
Metabolism: Extensive in the liver
Half-life: 30-90 minutes

Usual Dosage Adults: Oral:
Active duodenal ulcer: 20 mg/day for 4-8 weeks

GERD or severe erosive esophagitis: 20 mg/day for 4-8 weeks

Pathological hypersecretory conditions: 60 mg once daily to start; doses up to 120 mg 3 times/day have been administered; administer daily doses >80 mg in divided doses

Helicobacter pylori: Combination therapy with bismuth subsalicylate, tetracycline, clarithromycin, and H₂ antagonist; or clarithromycin and omeprazole. Adult dose: Oral: 20 mg twice daily

Administration Administration via NG tube should be in an acidic juice

Patient Information Take before eating; do not chew, crush, or open capsule

Nursing Implications Capsule should be swallowed whole; not chewed, crushed, or opened

Dosage Forms Capsule: 20 mg

Omnipen® *see* Ampicillin *on page 73*

OMS® *see* Morphine Sulfate *on page 756*

Oncaspar® *see* Pegaspargase *on page 844*

Oncovin® *see* Vincristine Sulfate *on page 1159*

Ondansetron (on dan' se tron)

Related Information
Initial Doses in Selected Antiemetic Regimens *on page 1205*

Brand Names Zofran®

Use May be prescribed for patients who are refractory to or have severe adverse reactions to standard antiemetic therapy. Ondansetron may be prescribed for young patients (ie, <45 years of age who are more likely to develop extrapyramidal reactions to high-dose metoclopramide) who are to receive highly emetogenic chemotherapeutic agents as listed:

Agents with high emetogenic potential (>90%) (dose/m²):
Carmustine ≥200 mg
Cisplatin ≥75 mg
Cyclophosphamide ≥1000 mg
Cytarabine ≥1000 mg
Dacarbazine ≥500 mg
Ifosfamide ≥1000 mg
Lomustine ≥60 mg
Mechlorethamine
Pentostatin
Streptozocin

or two agents classified as having high or moderately high emetogenic potential as listed:

Agents with moderately high emetogenic potential (60% to 90%) (dose/m²):
Carmustine <200 mg
Cisplatin <75 mg
Cyclophosphamide 1000 mg
Cytarabine 250-1000 mg
Dacarbazine <500 mg
Doxorubicin ≥75 mg
Ifosfamide
Lomustine <60 mg
Methotrexate ≥250 mg
Mitomycin
Mitoxantrone
Procarbazine

Ondansetron should not be prescribed for chemotherapeutic agents with a low emetogenic potential (eg, bleomycin, busulfan, cyclophosphamide <1000 mg, etoposide, 5-fluorouracil, vinblastine, vincristine)

Pregnancy Risk Factor B

Contraindications Hypersensitivity to ondansetron or any component

Warnings/Precautions Ondansetron should be used on a scheduled basis, not as an "as needed" (PRN) basis, since data supports the use of this drug in the prevention of nausea and vomiting and not in the rescue of nausea and
(Continued)

817

Ondansetron *(Continued)*

vomiting. Ondansetron should only be used in the first 24-48 hours of receiving chemotherapy. Data does not support any increased efficacy of ondansetron in delayed nausea and vomiting.

Adverse Reactions

>10%:
  Central nervous system: Headache, fever
  Gastrointestinal: Constipation, diarrhea

1% to 10%:
  Central nervous system: Dizziness, weakness
  Gastrointestinal: Abdominal cramps, dry mouth

<1%:
  Cardiovascular: Tachycardia
  Central nervous system: Lightheadedness, seizures
  Dermatologic: Rash
  Endocrine & metabolic: Hypokalemia
  Hepatic: Transient elevations in serum levels of aminotransferases and bilirubin
  Respiratory: Bronchospasm, shortness of breath, wheezing

Drug Interactions

Decreased effect: Metabolized by the hepatic cytochrome P-450 enzymes; therefore, the drug's clearance and half-life may be changed with concomitant use of cytochrome P-450 inducers (eg, barbiturates, carbamazepine, rifampin, phenytoin, and phenylbutazone)

Increased toxicity: Inhibitors (eg, cimetidine, allopurinol, and disulfiram)

Stability Injection may be stored between 36°F and 86°F; stable when mixed in 5% dextrose or 0.9% sodium chloride for 48 hours at room temperature; does not need protection from light

Mechanism of Action Selective 5-HT$_3$ receptor antagonist, blocking serotonin, both peripherally on vagal nerve terminals and centrally in the chemoreceptor trigger zone

Pharmacodynamics/Kinetics

Plasma protein binding: 70% to 76%

Metabolism: Extensively by hydroxylation, followed by glucuronide or sulfate conjugation

Half-life:
  Children <15 years: 2-3 hours
  Adults: 4 hours

Elimination: In urine and feces; <10% of parent drug recovered unchanged in urine

Usual Dosage

Oral:
  Children 4-11 years: 4 mg 30 minutes before chemotherapy; repeat 4 and 8 hours after initial dose
  Children >11 years and Adults: 8 mg 30 minutes before chemotherapy; repeat 4 and 8 hours after initial dose or every 8 hours for a maximum of 48 hours

I.V.: Administer either three 0.15 mg/kg doses or a single 32 mg dose; with the 3-dose regimen, the initial dose is given 30 minutes prior to chemotherapy with subsequent doses administered 4 and 8 hours after the first dose. With the single-dose regimen 32 mg is infused over 15 minutes beginning 30 minutes before the start of emetogenic chemotherapy. Dosage should be calculated based on weight:
  Children: Pediatric dosing should follow the manufacturer's guidelines for 0.15 mg/kg/dose administered 30 minutes prior to chemotherapy, 4 and 8 hours after the first dose. While not as yet FDA-approved, literature supports the day's total dose administered as a single dose 30 minutes prior to chemotherapy.
  Adults:
    >80 kg: 12 mg IVPB
    45-80 kg: 8 mg IVPB
    <45 kg: 0.15 mg/kg/dose IVPB

Dosing in hepatic impairment: Maximum daily dose: 8 mg in cirrhotic patients with severe liver disease

Nursing Implications First dose should be given 30 minutes prior to beginning chemotherapy

Dosage Forms

Injection: 2 mg/mL (20 mL); 32 mg (single-dose vials)
Tablet: 4 mg, 8 mg

OP-CCK *see* Sincalide *on page 1007*

Opcon® *see* Naphazoline Hydrochloride *on page 775*

o,p′-DDD *see* Mitotane *on page 748*

Ophthacet® *see* Sodium Sulfacetamide *on page 1018*

Ophthaine® *see* Proparacaine Hydrochloride *on page 943*

Ophthalgan® *see* Glycerin *on page 506*

Ophthetic® *see* Proparacaine Hydrochloride *on page 943*

Ophthifluor® *see* Fluorescein Sodium *on page 470*

Ophthochlor® *see* Chloramphenicol *on page 219*

Opium and Belladonna *see* Belladonna and Opium *on page 117*

Opium Tincture (oh′ pee um)

Synonyms Deodorized Opium Tincture; DTO

Use Treatment of diarrhea or relief of pain

Restrictions C-II

Pregnancy Risk Factor B (D if used for prolonged periods or in high doses at term)

Contraindications Increased intracranial pressure, severe respiratory depression, severe liver or renal insufficiency, known hypersensitivity to morphine sulfate

Warnings/Precautions Opium shares the toxic potential of opiate agonists, and usual precautions of opiate agonist therapy should be observed; some preparations contain sulfites which may cause allergic reactions; infants <3 months of age are more susceptible to respiratory depression, use with caution and generally in reduced doses in this age group; this is **not** paregoric, dose accordingly

Adverse Reactions

>10%:
  Cardiovascular: Palpitations, hypotension, bradycardia
  Central nervous system: Weakness, drowsiness, dizziness

1% to 10%:
  Central nervous system: Restlessness, headache, malaise
  Genitourinary: Decreased urination
  Miscellaneous: Histamine release

<1%:
  Cardiovascular: Peripheral vasodilation
  Central nervous system: CNS depression, increased intracranial pressure, insomnia, mental depression
  Gastrointestinal: Nausea, vomiting, constipation, anorexia, stomach cramps
  Ocular: Miosis
  Respiratory: Respiratory depression
  Miscellaneous: Physical and psychological dependence, biliary or urinary tract spasm

Overdosage/Toxicology Primary attention should be directed to ensuring adequate respiratory exchange; opiate agonist-induced respiratory depression may be reversed with parenteral naloxone hydrochloride. Naloxone 2 mg I.V. (0.01 mg/kg for children) with repeat administration as necessary up to a total of 10 mg.

Drug Interactions

Decreased effect: Phenothiazines may antagonize the analgesic effect of opiate agonists

Increased toxicity: CNS depressants, MAO inhibitors, tricyclic antidepressants may potentiate the effects of opiate agonists; dextroamphetamine may enhance the analgesic effect of opiate agonists

Mechanism of Action Contains many narcotic alkaloids including morphine; its mechanism for gastric motility inhibition is primarily due to this morphine content; it results in a decrease in digestive secretions, an increase in GI muscle tone, and therefore a reduction in GI propulsion

Pharmacodynamics/Kinetics

Duration of effect: 4-5 hours
Absorption: Variable from GI tract
Metabolism: In the liver
Elimination: Urine

Usual Dosage Oral:

Children:
  Diarrhea: 0.005-0.01 mL/kg/dose every 3-4 hours for a maximum of 6 doses/24 hours
  Analgesia: 0.01-0.02 mL/kg/dose every 3-4 hours

Adults:
  Diarrhea: 0.3-1 mL/dose every 2-6 hours to maximum of 6 mL/24 hours
  Analgesia: 0.6-1.5 mL/dose every 3-4 hours

(Continued)

Opium Tincture *(Continued)*

Monitoring Parameters Observe patient for excessive sedation, respiratory depression, implement safety measures, assist with ambulation

Test Interactions ↑ aminotransferase [ALT (SGPT)/AST (SGOT)] (S)

Patient Information Avoid alcohol, may cause drowsiness, impair judgment, or coordination; may cause physical and psychological dependence with prolonged use

Dosage Forms Liquid: 10% [0.6 mL equivalent to morphine 6 mg]

Opticyl® *see* Tropicamide *on page 1134*

Optigene® [OTC] *see* Tetrahydrozoline Hydrochloride *on page 1071*

Optimine® *see* Azatadine Maleate *on page 105*

OptiPranolol® *see* Metipranolol Hydrochloride *on page 728*

OPV *see* Polio Vaccines *on page 898*

Orabase®-B [OTC] *see* Benzocaine *on page 121*

Orabase® HCA *see* Hydrocortisone *on page 546*

Orabase®-O [OTC] *see* Benzocaine *on page 121*

Oracit® *see* Sodium Citrate and Citric Acid *on page 1013*

Orajel® Brace-Aid Oral Anesthetic [OTC] *see* Benzocaine *on page 121*

Orajel® Brace-Aid Rinse [OTC] *see* Carbamide Peroxide *on page 179*

Orajel® Mouth-Aid [OTC] *see* Benzocaine *on page 121*

Orajel® Maximum Strength [OTC] *see* Benzocaine *on page 121*

Oraminic® II *see* Brompheniramine Maleate *on page 143*

Oramorph SR® *see* Morphine Sulfate *on page 756*

Orap™ *see* Pimozide *on page 885*

Orasept® [OTC] *see* Benzocaine *on page 121*

Orasol® [OTC] *see* Benzocaine *on page 121*

Orasone® *see* Prednisone *on page 921*

Oratect® [OTC] *see* Benzocaine *on page 121*

Orazinc® [OTC] *see* Zinc Supplements *on page 1176*

Orciprenaline Sulfate *see* Metaproterenol Sulfate *on page 697*

Oretic® *see* Hydrochlorothiazide *on page 542*

Oreton® Methyl *see* Methyltestosterone *on page 726*

ORG 946 *see* Rocuronium Bromide *on page 987*

Organidin® *see* Iodinated Glycerol *on page 587*

ORG NC 45 *see* Vecuronium *on page 1151*

Orimune® *see* Polio Vaccines *on page 898*

Orinase® *see* Tolbutamide *on page 1103*

ORLAAM® *see* Levomethadyl Acetate Hydrochloride *on page 627*

Ormazine *see* Chlorpromazine Hydrochloride *on page 230*

Ornidyl® *see* Eflornithine Hydrochloride *on page 383*

Orphenadrine Citrate *(or fen' a dreen)*

Brand Names Norflex™

Use Treatment of muscle spasm associated with acute painful musculoskeletal conditions; supportive therapy in tetanus

Pregnancy Risk Factor C

Contraindications Glaucoma, GI obstruction, cardiospasm, myasthenia gravis, hypersensitivity to orphenadrine or any component

Warnings/Precautions Use with caution in patients with CHF or cardiac arrhythmias; some products contain sulfites

Adverse Reactions

>10%:
  Central nervous system: Drowsiness, dizziness
  Ocular: Blurred vision
1% to 10%:
  Cardiovascular: Flushing of face, tachycardia
  Central nervous system: Weakness, fainting

Dermatologic: Skin rash
Gastrointestinal: Nausea, vomiting, constipation
Genitourinary: Decreased urination
Ocular: Nystagmus, increased intraocular pressure
Respiratory: Nasal congestion
<1%:
Central nervous system: Hallucinations
Hematologic: Aplastic anemia

Overdosage/Toxicology Symptoms of overdose include blurred vision, tachycardia, confusion, seizures, respiratory arrest, dysrhythmias. There is no specific treatment for an antihistamine overdose, however, most of its clinical toxicity is due to anticholinergic effects. Anticholinesterase inhibitors may be useful by reducing acetylcholinesterase. Anticholinesterase inhibitors include physostigmine, neostigmine, pyridostigmine and edrophonium. For anticholinergic overdose with severe life-threatening symptoms, physostigmine 1-2 mg (0.5 or 0.02 mg/kg for children) I.V., slowly may be given to reverse these effects. Lethal dose is 2-3 g; treatment is symptomatic.

Mechanism of Action Indirect skeletal muscle relaxant thought to work by central atropine-like effects; has some euphorogenic and analgesic properties

Pharmacodynamics/Kinetics
Peak effect: Oral: Within 2-4 hours
Duration: 4-6 hours
Protein binding: 20%
Metabolism: Extensive
Half-life: 14-16 hours
Elimination: Primarily in urine (8% as unchanged drug)

Usual Dosage Adults:
Oral: 100 mg twice daily
I.M., I.V.: 60 mg every 12 hours

Patient Information May cause drowsiness; swallow whole, do not crush or chew sustained release product; avoid alcohol, may impair coordination and judgment

Nursing Implications Do not crush sustained release drug product; raise bed rails, institute safety measures, assist with ambulation

Dosage Forms
Injection: 30 mg/mL (2 mL, 10 mL)
Tablet: 100 mg
Tablet, sustained release: 100 mg

Orthoclone® OKT3 *see* Muromonab-CD3 *on page 761*

Ortho® Dienestrol *see* Dienestrol *on page 333*

Ortho-Est® *see* Estropipate *on page 414*

Ortho-Novum™ *see* Ethinyl Estradiol and Norethindrone *on page 425*

Ortho-Novum™ 1/50 *see* Mestranol and Norethindrone *on page 695*

Or-Tyl® *see* Dicyclomine Hydrochloride *on page 330*

Orudis® *see* Ketoprofen *on page 611*

Oruvail® *see* Ketoprofen *on page 611*

Os-Cal® 250 [OTC] *see* Calcium Carbonate *on page 161*

Os-Cal® 500 [OTC] *see* Calcium Carbonate *on page 161*

Osmitrol® *see* Mannitol *on page 664*

Osmoglyn® *see* Glycerin *on page 506*

Otocort® *see* Neomycin, Polymyxin B, and Hydrocortisone *on page 781*

Otomycin-HPN® *see* Neomycin, Polymyxin B, and Hydrocortisone *on page 781*

Otosporin® *see* Neomycin, Polymyxin B, and Hydrocortisone *on page 781*

Otrivin® [OTC] *see* Xylometazoline Hydrochloride *on page 1171*

Ovcon® *see* Ethinyl Estradiol and Norethindrone *on page 425*

Ovral® *see* Ethinyl Estradiol and Norgestrel *on page 427*

Ovrette® *see* Norgestrel *on page 807*

O-V Staticin® *see* Nystatin *on page 811*

Oxacillin Sodium (ox a sill' in)

Brand Names Bactocill®; Prostaphlin®

Synonyms Isoxazolyl Penicillin; Methylphenyl

Use Treatment of susceptible bacterial infections such as osteomyelitis, septicemia, endocarditis, and CNS infections due to penicillinase-producing strains of *Staphylococcus*

Pregnancy Risk Factor B

Contraindications Hypersensitivity to oxacillin or other penicillins or any component

Warnings/Precautions Elimination rate will be slow in neonates; modify dosage in patients with renal impairment and in the elderly; use with caution in patients with cephalosporin hypersensitivity

Adverse Reactions

1% to 10%: Gastrointestinal: Nausea, diarrhea

<1%:

Central nervous system: Fever

Dermatologic: Rash

Gastrointestinal: Vomiting

Hematologic: Eosinophilia, leukopenia, neutropenia, thrombocytopenia, agranulocytosis, mild leukopenia

Hepatic: Hepatotoxicity, elevated AST

Renal: Hematuria, acute interstitial nephritis

Miscellaneous: Serum sickness-like reactions

Overdosage/Toxicology Symptoms of penicillin overdose include neuromuscular hypersensitivity (agitation, hallucinations, asterixis, encephalopathy, confusion, and seizures) and electrolyte imbalance with potassium or sodium salts, especially in renal failure; hemodialysis may be helpful to aid in the removal of the drug from the blood, otherwise most treatment is supportive or symptom directed

Drug Interactions

Decreased effect: Efficacy of oral contraceptives may be reduced

Increased effect: Disulfiram, probenecid → ↑ penicillin levels, increased effect of anticoagulants

Stability Reconstituted parenteral solution is stable for 3 days at room temperature and 7 days when refrigerated; for I.V. infusion in NS or D_5W, solution is stable for 6 hours at room temperature

Mechanism of Action Inhibits bacterial cell wall synthesis by binding to one or more of the penicillin binding proteins (PBPs); which in turn inhibits the final transpeptidation step of peptidoglycan synthesis in bacterial cell walls, thus inhibiting cell wall biosynthesis. Bacteria eventually lyse due to ongoing activity of cell wall autolytic enzymes (autolysins and murein hydrolases) while cell wall assembly is arrested.

Pharmacodynamics/Kinetics

Absorption: Oral: 35% to 67%

Distribution: Into bile, synovial and pleural fluids, bronchial secretions; also distributes to peritoneal and pericardial fluids; crosses the placenta and appears in breast milk; penetrates the blood-brain barrier only when meninges are inflamed

Metabolism: In the liver to active metabolites

Half-life:

Children 1 week to 2 years: 0.9-1.8 hours

Adults: 23-60 minutes (prolonged with reduced renal function and in neonates)

Time to peak serum concentration:

Oral: Within 2 hours

I.M.: Within 30-60 minutes

Elimination: By kidneys and to small degree the bile as parent drug and metabolites

Usual Dosage

Neonates: I.M., I.V.:

Postnatal age <7 days:

<2000 g: 25 mg/kg/dose every 12 hours

>2000 g: 25 mg/kg/dose every 8 hours

Postnatal age >7 days:

<1200 g: 25 mg/kg/dose every 12 hours

1200-2000 g: 30 mg/kg/dose every 8 hours

>2000 g: 37.5 mg/kg/dose every 6 hours

Infants and Children:

Oral: 50-100 mg/kg/day divided every 6 hours

I.M., I.V.: 150-200 mg/kg/day in divided doses every 6 hours; maximum dose: 12 g/day

Adults:
Oral: 500-1000 mg every 4-6 hours for at least 5 days
I.M., I.V.: 250 mg to 2 g/dose every 4-6 hours

Dosing adjustment in renal impairment: Cl_{cr} <10 mL/minute: Use lower range of the usual dosage
Not dialyzable (0% to 5%)

Administration Administer around-the-clock to promote less variation in peak and trough serum levels

Test Interactions May interfere with urinary glucose tests using cupric sulfate (Benedict's solution, Clinitest®); may inactivate aminoglycosides *in vitro*; false-positive urinary and serum proteins

Patient Information Take orally on an empty stomach 1 hour before meals or 2 hours after meals; take all medication, do not skip doses

Additional Information Sodium content of 1 g: 2.8-3.1 mEq

Dosage Forms
Capsule: 250 mg, 500 mg
Powder for injection: 250 mg, 500 mg, 1 g, 2 g, 4 g, 10 g
Powder for oral solution: 250 mg/5 mL (100 mL)

Oxaprozin (ox a proe' zin)

Brand Names Daypro™

Use Acute and long-term use in the management of signs and symptoms of osteoarthritis and rheumatoid arthritis

Pregnancy Risk Factor C

Contraindications Aspirin allergy, third trimester pregnancy or allergy to oxaprozin, history of GI disease, renal or hepatic dysfunction, bleeding disorders, cardiac failure, elderly, debilitated, nursing mothers

Adverse Reactions
>10%:
Central nervous system: Dizziness
Dermatologic: Skin rash
Gastrointestinal: Abdominal cramps, heartburn, indigestion, nausea
1% to 10%:
Cardiovascular: Angina pectoris, arrhythmia
Central nervous system: Dizziness, nervousness
Dermatologic: Skin rash, itching
Gastrointestinal: GI ulceration, vomiting
Genitourinary: Vaginal bleeding
Otic: Tinnitus
<1%:
Cardiovascular: Chest pain, congestive heart failure, hypertension, tachycardia
Central nervous system: Convulsions, forgetfulness, mental depression, drowsiness, nervousness, insomnia, weakness
Dermatologic: Hives, exfoliative dermatitis, erythema multiforme, Stevens-Johnson syndrome, angioedema
Gastrointestinal: Stomatitis
Genitourinary: Cystitis
Hematologic: Agranulocytosis, anemia, pancytopenia, leukopenia, thrombocytopenia
Hepatic: Hepatitis
Neuromuscular & skeletal: Peripheral neuropathy, trembling
Ocular: Blurred vision, change in vision
Otic: Decreased hearing
Renal: Interstitial nephritis, nephrotic syndrome, renal impairment
Respiratory: Shortness of breath, wheezing, laryngeal edema
Miscellaneous: Epistaxis, anaphylaxis, increased sweating

Overdosage/Toxicology Symptoms of overdose include acute renal failure, vomiting, drowsiness, leukocytes

Management of a nonsteroidal anti-inflammatory drug (NSAID) intoxication is primarily supportive and symptomatic. Fluid therapy is commonly effective in managing the hypotension that may occur following an acute NSAID overdose, except when this is due to an acute blood loss. Seizures tend to be very short-lived and often do not require drug treatment. Although, recurrent seizures should be treated with I.V. diazepam. Since many of the NSAID undergo entero-hepatic cycling, multiple doses of charcoal may be needed to reduce the potential for delayed toxicities.

Drug Interactions Increased toxicity: Aspirin, oral anticoagulants, diuretics

Mechanism of Action Inhibits prostaglandin synthesis by decreasing the activity of the enzyme, cyclo-oxygenase, which results in decreased formation of prostaglandin precursors
(Continued)

Oxaprozin (Continued)

Pharmacodynamics/Kinetics
Absorption: Almost completely
Protein binding: >99%
Half-life: 40-50 hours
Time to peak: 2-4 hours

Usual Dosage Adults: Oral (individualize dosage to lowest effective dose to minimize adverse effects):
Osteoarthritis: 600-1200 mg once daily
Rheumatoid arthritis: 1200 mg once daily
Maximum dose: 1800 mg/day or 26 mg/kg (whichever is lower) in divided doses

Monitoring Parameters Monitor blood, hepatic, renal, and ocular function
Dosage Forms Tablet: 600 mg

Oxazepam (ox a' ze pam)

Related Information
Benzodiazepines Comparison on page 1256

Brand Names Serax®

Use Treatment of anxiety and management of alcohol withdrawal; may also be used as an anticonvulsant in management of simple partial seizures

Restrictions C-IV

Pregnancy Risk Factor D

Contraindications Hypersensitivity to oxazepam or any component, cross-sensitivity with other benzodiazepines may exist

Warnings/Precautions Avoid using in patients with pre-existing CNS depression, severe uncontrolled pain, or narrow-angle glaucoma; use with caution in patients using other CNS depressants and in the elderly

Adverse Reactions
>10%:
Cardiovascular: Tachycardia, chest pain
Central nervous system: Drowsiness, fatigue, impaired coordination, lightheadedness, memory impairment, insomnia, anxiety, depression, headache
Dermatologic: Rash increased or decreased appetite
Endocrine & metabolic: Decreased libido
Gastrointestinal: Dry mouth, constipation, diarrhea, decreased salivation, nausea, vomiting
Neuromuscular & skeletal: Dysarthria
Ocular: Blurred vision
Miscellaneous: Sweating
1% to 10%:
Cardiovascular: Syncope, hypotension
Central nervous system: Confusion, nervousness, dizziness, akathisia
Dermatologic: Dermatitis
Gastrointestinal: Increased salivation, weight gain or loss
Neuromuscular & skeletal: Rigidity, tremor, muscle cramps
Ocular: Blurred vision
Otic: Tinnitus
Respiratory: Nasal congestion, hyperventilation
<1%:
Central nervous system: Reflex slowing
Endocrine & metabolic: Menstrual irregularities
Hematologic: Blood dyscrasias
Miscellaneous: Drug dependence

Overdosage/Toxicology Symptoms of overdose include somnolence, confusion, coma, hypoactive reflexes, dyspnea, hypotension, slurred speech, impaired coordination. Treatment for benzodiazepine overdose is supportive. Rarely is mechanical ventilation required. Flumazenil has been shown to selectively block the binding of benzodiazepines to CNS receptors, resulting in a reversal of benzodiazepine-induced CNS depression but not the respiratory depression due to toxicity.

Drug Interactions Increased toxicity with CNS depressants (eg, barbiturates, MAO inhibitors, TCAs, alcohol, narcotics, phenothiazines, and other sedative-hypnotics)

Mechanism of Action Benzodiazepine anxiolytic sedative that produces CNS depression at the subcortical level, except at high doses, whereby it works at the cortical level

Pharmacodynamics/Kinetics
Absorption: Oral: Almost completely
Protein binding: 86% to 99%
Metabolism: In the liver to inactive compounds (primarily as glucuronides)
Half-life: 2.8-5.7 hours

Time to peak serum concentration: Within 2-4 hours
Elimination: Excretion of unchanged drug (50%) and metabolites; excreted without need for liver metabolism
Usual Dosage Oral:
Children: 1 mg/kg/day has been administered

Adults:
Anxiety: 10-30 mg 3-4 times/day
Alcohol withdrawal: 15-30 mg 3-4 times/day
Hypnotic: 15-30 mg
Not dialyzable (0% to 5%)
Monitoring Parameters Respiratory and cardiovascular status
Reference Range Therapeutic: 0.2-1.4 µg/mL (SI: 0.7-4.9 µmol/L)
Patient Information Avoid alcohol and other CNS depressants; avoid activities needing good psychomotor coordination until CNS effects are known; drug may cause physical or psychological dependence; avoid abrupt discontinuation after prolonged use
Nursing Implications Provide safety measures (ie, side rails, night light, and call button); remove smoking materials from area; supervise ambulation
Dosage Forms
Capsule: 10 mg, 15 mg, 30 mg
Tablet: 15 mg

Oxiconazole Nitrate (ox i kon' a zole)
Brand Names Oxistat®
Use Treatment of tinea pedis (athlete's foot), tinea cruris (jock itch), and tinea corporis (ring worm)
Pregnancy Risk Factor B
Contraindications Hypersensitivity to this agent; not for ophthalmic use
Warnings/Precautions May cause irritation during therapy; if a sensitivity to oxiconazole occurs, therapy should be discontinued; avoid contact with eyes or vagina
Adverse Reactions 1% to 10%: Local: Itching, transient burning, local irritation, stinging, erythema, dryness
Mechanism of Action Inhibition of ergosterol synthesis. Effective for treatment of tinea pedis, tinea cruris, and tinea corporis. Active against *Trichophyton rubrum*, *Trichophyton mentagrophytes*, *Trichophyton violaceum*, *Microsporum canis*, *Microsporum audouini*, *Microsporum gypseum*, *Epidermophyton floccosum*, *Candida albicans*, and *Malassezia furfur*.
Pharmacodynamics/Kinetics
Absorption: In each layer of the dermis; very little is absorbed systemically after one topical dose
Distribution: To each layer of the dermis; excreted in breast milk
Elimination: <0.3% excreted in urine
Usual Dosage Children and Adults: Topical: Apply once to twice daily to affected areas for 2 weeks (tinea corporis/tinea cruris) to 1 month (tinea pedis)
Patient Information External use only; discontinue if sensitivity or chemical irritation occurs, contact physician if condition fails to improve in 3-4 days
Dosage Forms
Cream: 1% (15 g, 30 g, 60 g)
Lotion: 1% (30 mL)

Oxilapine Succinate *see Loxapine on page 653*

Oxistat® *see Oxiconazole Nitrate on this page*

Oxpentifylline *see Pentoxifylline on page 862*

Oxsoralen® *see Methoxsalen on page 716*

Oxsoralen-Ultra® *see Methoxsalen on page 716*

Oxtriphylline *see Theophylline/Aminophylline on page 1072*

Oxy-5® [OTC] *see Benzoyl Peroxide on page 122*

Oxy-10® [OTC] *see Benzoyl Peroxide on page 122*

Oxybutynin Chloride (ox i byoo' ti nin)
Brand Names Ditropan®
Use Antispasmodic for neurogenic bladder (urgency, frequency, urge incontinence) and uninhibited bladder
Pregnancy Risk Factor B
(Continued)

825

Oxybutynin Chloride *(Continued)*

Contraindications Glaucoma, myasthenia gravis, partial or complete GI obstruction, GU obstruction, ulcerative colitis, hypersensitivity to drug or specific component, intestinal atony, megacolon, toxic megacolon

Warnings/Precautions Use with caution in patients with urinary tract obstruction, angle-closure glaucoma, hyperthyroidism, reflux esophagitis, heart disease, hepatic or renal disease, prostatic hypertrophy, autonomic neuropathy, ulcerative colitis (may cause ileus and toxic megacolon), hypertension, hiatal hernia. Caution should be used in elderly due to anticholinergic activity (eg, confusion, constipation, blurred vision, and tachycardia).

Adverse Reactions
>10%:
Cardiovascular: Decreased sweating
Central nervous system: Drowsiness
Gastrointestinal: Dry mouth, constipation
1% to 10%:
Cardiovascular: Tachycardia, palpitations
Central nervous system: Drowsiness, weakness, dizziness, insomnia, fever, headache
Dermatologic: Rash
Endocrine & metabolic: Hot flushes, decreased flow of breast milk
Gastrointestinal: Nausea, vomiting
Genitourinary: Urinary hesitancy or retention, decreased sexual ability
Ocular: Blurred vision, mydriatic effect
<1%:
Ophthalmic: Increased intraocular pressure
Miscellaneous: Allergic reaction

Overdosage/Toxicology Symptoms of overdose include hypotension, circulatory failure, psychotic behavior, flushing, respiratory failure, paralysis, tremor, irritability, seizures, delirium, hallucinations, coma; symptomatic and supportive treatment; induce emesis or perform gastric lavage followed by charcoal and a cathartic; physostigmine may be required; treat hyperpyrexia with cooling techniques (ice bags, cold applications, alcohol sponges)

Drug Interactions
Increased toxicity:
Additive sedation with CNS depressants and alcohol
Additive anticholinergic effects with antihistamines and anticholinergic agents

Mechanism of Action Direct antispasmodic effect on smooth muscle, also inhibits the action of acetylcholine on smooth muscle (exhibits $\frac{1}{5}$ the anticholinergic activity of atropine, but is 4-10 times the antispasmodic activity); does not block effects at skeletal muscle or at autonomic ganglia; increases bladder capacity, decreases uninhibited contractions, and delays desire to void; therefore, decreases urgency and frequency

Pharmacodynamics/Kinetics
Onset of effect: Oral: 30-60 minutes
Peak effect: 3-6 hours
Duration: 6-10 hours
Absorption: Oral: Rapid and well absorbed
Metabolism: In the liver
Half-life: 1-2.3 hours
Time to peak serum concentration: Within 60 minutes
Elimination: In urine

Usual Dosage Oral:
Children:
1-5 years: 0.2 mg/kg/dose 2-4 times/day
>5 years: 5 mg twice daily, up to 5 mg 4 times/day maximum
Adults: 5 mg 2-3 times/day up to 5 mg 4 times/day maximum
Elderly: 2.5-5 mg twice daily; increase by 2.5 mg increments every 1-2 days

Note: Should be discontinued periodically to determine whether the patient can manage without the drug and to minimize resistance to the drug

Monitoring Parameters Incontinence episodes, postvoid residual (PVR)

Test Interactions May suppress the wheal and flare reactions to skin test antigens

Patient Information May impair ability to perform activities requiring mental alertness or physical coordination; alcohol or other sedating drugs may enhance drowsiness

Nursing Implications Raise bed rails, institute safety measures, assist with ambulation

Dosage Forms
Syrup: 5 mg/5 mL (473 mL)
Tablet: 5 mg

Oxycodone and Acetaminophen (ox i koe' done & a seet a min' fen)

Related Information
  Narcotic Agonist Comparison Charts *on page 1274-1275*
Brand Names Percocet®; Roxicet®; Tylox®
Synonyms Acetaminophen and Oxycodone
Use Management of moderate to severe pain
Restrictions C-II
Pregnancy Risk Factor C
Contraindications Hypersensitivity to oxycodone, acetaminophen or any component; severe respiratory depression, severe renal or liver insufficiency
Warnings/Precautions Use with caution in patients with hypersensitivity to other phenanthrene derivative opioid agonists (morphine, codeine, hydrocodone, hydromorphone, oxymorphone, levorphanol), asthma, COPD, severe liver or renal disease; some preparations may contain bisulfites which may cause allergies

Enhanced analgesia has been seen in elderly patients on therapeutic doses of narcotics; duration of action may be increased in the elderly; the elderly may be particularly susceptible to the CNS depressant and constipating effects of narcotics

Adverse Reactions
  >10%:
    Cardiovascular: Hypotension
    Central nervous system: Weakness, tiredness, drowsiness, dizziness
    Gastrointestinal: Nausea, vomiting
  1% to 10%:
    Central nervous system: Nervousness, headache, restlessness, malaise, confusion
    Gastrointestinal: Anorexia stomach cramps, dry mouth, constipation, biliary spasm
    Genitourinary: Ureteral spasms, decreased urination
    Local: Pain at injection site
    Respiratory: Troubled breathing, shortness of breath
  <1%:
    Central nervous system: Mental depression, hallucinations, paradoxical CNS stimulation
    Dermatologic: Skin rash, hives, increased intracranial pressure
    Gastrointestinal: Paralytic ileus
    Hematologic: Blood dyscrasias (neutropenia, pancytopenia, leukopenia)
    Hepatic: Hepatic necrosis with overdosage
    Renal: Renal injury with chronic use
    Miscellaneous: Physical and psychological dependence, hypersensitivity reactions (rare), histamine release

Overdosage/Toxicology Symptoms of overdose include hepatic necrosis, transient azotemia, renal tubular necrosis with acute toxicity, anemia, renal damage, and GI disturbances with chronic toxicity. Consult regional poison control center for additional information. Treatment of an overdose includes support of the patient's airway, establishment of an I.V. line and administration of naloxone 2 mg I.V. with repeat administration as necessary. Mucomyst® (acetylcysteine) 140 mg/kg orally (loading) followed by 70 mg/kg (maintenance) every 4 hours for 17 doses. Therapy should be initiated based upon acetaminophen levels that are suggestive of a high probability of hepatotoxic potential.
Drug Interactions
  Decreased effect: Phenothiazines may antagonize the analgesic effect of opiate agonists
  Increased toxicity: CNS depressants, tricyclic antidepressants may potentiate the effects of opiate agonists; dextroamphetamine may enhance the analgesic effect of opiate agonists
Mechanism of Action Inhibits the synthesis of prostaglandins in the central nervous system and peripherally blocks pain impulse generation; produces antipyresis from inhibition of hypothalamic heat-regulating center; binds to opiate receptors in the CNS, causing inhibition of ascending pain pathways, altering the perception of and response to pain; produces generalized CNS depression
Usual Dosage Oral (doses should be titrated to appropriate analgesic effects):
  Children: Oxycodone: 0.05-0.15 mg/kg/dose to 5 mg/dose (maximum) every 4-6 hours as needed

  Adults: 1-2 tablets every 4-6 hours as needed for pain
    Maximum daily dose of acetaminophen: 8 g/day, in alcoholics: 4 g/day

  Dosing adjustment in hepatic impairment: Dose should be reduced in patients with severe liver disease
(Continued)

Oxycodone and Acetaminophen *(Continued)*

Monitoring Parameters Pain relief, respiratory and mental status, blood pressure

Patient Information Do not exceed recommended dosage; do not take for more than 10 days without physician's advice; avoid alcohol, may cause drowsiness, impair judgment or coordination; may cause physical and psychological dependence with prolonged use

Nursing Implications Give with food, but high carbohydrate meal may retard absorption rate; observe patient for excessive sedation, respiratory depression; implement safety measures, assist with ambulation

Additional Information Oxycodone and acetaminophen: Oxycet®, Percocet®, Roxicet®, Tylox®

Dosage Forms
Capsule: Oxycodone hydrochloride 5 mg and acetaminophen 500 mg
Solution, oral: Oxycodone hydrochloride 5 mg and acetaminophen 325 mg per 5 mL (5 mL, 500 mL)
Tablet: Oxycodone hydrochloride 5 mg and acetaminophen 325 mg

Oxycodone and Aspirin *(as' pir in)*

Related Information
Narcotic Agonist Comparison Charts *on page 1274-1275*

Brand Names Codoxy®; Percodan®; Percodan®-Demi; Roxiprin®

Use Relief of moderate to moderately severe pain

Restrictions C-II

Pregnancy Risk Factor D

Contraindications Known hypersensitivity to oxycodone or aspirin; severe respiratory depression

Warnings/Precautions Use with caution in patients with hypersensitivity to other phenanthrene derivative opioid agonists (morphine, codeine, hydrocodone, hydromorphone, oxymorphone, levorphanol); children and teenagers should not be given aspirin products if chickenpox or flu symptoms are present; aspirin use has been associated with Reye's syndrome; severe liver or renal insufficiency, pre-existing CNS and depression

Adverse Reactions
>10%:
Cardiovascular: Hypotension heartburn, stomach pains, dyspepsia, epigastric discomfort
Central nervous system: Weakness, tiredness, drowsiness, dizziness
Gastrointestinal: Nausea, vomiting
1% to 10%:
Central nervous system: Nervousness, headache, restlessness, malaise
Dermatologic: Skin rash
Gastrointestinal: Anorexia, stomach cramps, dry mouth, constipation biliary spasm, gastrointestinal ulceration
Genitourinary: Ureteral spasms, decreased urination, confusion
Hematologic: Hemolytic anemia
Local: Pain at injection site
Respiratory: Troubled breathing, shortness of breath
Miscellaneous: Anaphylactic shock
<1%:
Central nervous system: Mental depression, hallucinations, paradoxical CNS stimulation, increased intracranial pressure, insomnia, nervousness, jitters
Dermatologic: Skin rash, hives
Gastrointestinal: Paralytic ileus
Hematologic: Occult bleeding, prolongation of bleeding time, leukopenia, thrombocytopenia, iron deficiency anemia
Hepatic: Hepatotoxicity
Renal: Impaired renal function
Respiratory: Bronchospasm
Miscellaneous: Physical and psychological dependence, histamine release

Overdosage/Toxicology Symptoms of overdose include CNS and respiratory depression, gastrointestinal cramping, constipation, tinnitus, headache, dizziness, confusion, metabolic acidosis, hyperpyrexia. Consult regional poison control center for additional information. Naloxone 2 mg I.V. (0.01 mg/kg for children) with repeat administration as necessary up to a total of 10 mg; see also Aspirin toxicology.

Drug Interactions
Decreased effect with phenothiazines
Increased effect/toxicity with CNS depressants, TCAs, dextroamphetamine

Mechanism of Action Binds to opiate receptors in the CNS, causing inhibition of ascending pain pathways, altering the perception of and response to pain;

produces generalized CNS depression; inhibits prostaglandin synthesis, acts on the hypothalamus heat-regulating center to reduce fever, blocks prostaglandin synthetase action which prevents formation of the platelet-aggregating substance thromboxane A_2

Usual Dosage Oral (based on oxycodone combined salts):

Children: 0.05-0.15 mg/kg/dose every 4-6 hours as needed; maximum: 5 mg/dose (1 tablet Percodan® or 2 tablets Percodan®-Demi/dose)

Adults: Percodan®: 1 tablet every 6 hours as needed for pain or Percodan®-Demi: 1-2 tablets every 6 hours as needed for pain

Dosing adjustment in hepatic impairment: Dose should be reduced in patients with severe liver disease

Monitoring Parameters Pain relief, respiratory and mental status, blood pressure

Patient Information Avoid alcohol, may cause drowsiness, impaired judgment or coordination; may cause physical and psychological dependence with prolonged use; watch for bleeding gums or any signs of GI bleeding; take with food or milk to minimize GI distress, notify physician if ringing in ears or persistent GI pain occurs

Nursing Implications Give with food, but high carbohydrate meal may retard absorption rate; observe patient for excessive sedation, respiratory depression; implement safety measures, assist with ambulation

Dosage Forms Tablet:

Percodan®: Oxycodone hydrochloride 4.5 mg, oxycodone terephthalate 0.38 mg, and aspirin 325 mg

Percodan®-Demi: Oxycodone hydrochloride 2.25 mg, oxycodone terephthalate 0.19 mg, and aspirin 325 mg

Oxydess® II see Dextroamphetamine Sulfate on page 319

Oxymetazoline Hydrochloride (ox i met az′ oh leen)

Brand Names Afrin® Nasal Solution [OTC]; Allerest® 12 Hours Nasal Solution [OTC]; Chlorphed®-LA Nasal Solution [OTC]; Dristan® Long Lasting Nasal Solution [OTC]; Duration® Nasal Solution [OTC]; Neo-Synephrine® 12 Hour Nasal Solution [OTC]; Nõstrilla®; Nõstrilla® Long-Acting Nasal Solution [OTC]; NTZ® Nasal Solution [OTC]; OcuClear® [OTC]; Sinarest® 12 Hour Nasal Solution; Vicks® Sinex® Long-Acting Nasal Solution [OTC]; 4-Way® Long-Acting Nasal Solution [OTC]

Use Symptomatic relief of nasal mucosal congestion and adjunctive therapy of middle ear infections, associated with acute or chronic rhinitis, the common cold, sinusitis, hay fever, or other allergies

Ophthalmic: Relief of redness of eye due to minor eye irritations

Pregnancy Risk Factor C

Contraindications Hypersensitivity to oxymetazoline or any component

Warnings/Precautions Rebound congestion may occur with extended use (>3 days); use with caution in the presence of hypertension, diabetes, hyperthyroidism, heart disease, coronary artery disease, cerebral arteriosclerosis, or long-standing bronchial asthma

Adverse Reactions

>10%:

Local: Transient burning, stinging

Respiratory: Dryness of the nasal mucosa, sneezing

1% to 10%:

Cardiovascular: Rebound congestion with prolonged use, hypertension, palpitations

Central nervous system: Nervousness, dizziness, insomnia, headache

Gastrointestinal: Nausea

Overdosage/Toxicology Symptoms of overdose include CNS depression, hypothermia, bradycardia, cardiovascular collapse, coma, apnea; following initiation of essential overdose management, toxic symptoms should be treated. Patient should be kept warm and monitored for alterations in vital functions. Seizures commonly respond to diazepam (5-10 mg I.V. bolus in adults every 15 minutes if needed up to a total of 30 mg; I.V. 0.25-0.4 mg/kg/dose up to a total of 10 mg for children) or to phenytoin or phenobarbital. Hypotension should be treated with fluids.

Drug Interactions Increased toxicity: MAO inhibitors

Mechanism of Action Stimulates alpha-adrenergic receptors in the arterioles of the nasal mucosa to produce vasoconstriction

Pharmacodynamics/Kinetics

Onset of effect: Intranasal: Within 5-10 minutes

Duration: 5-6 hours

(Continued)

Oxymetazoline Hydrochloride *(Continued)*

Metabolism: Metabolic fate is unknown

Usual Dosage Therapy should not exceed 3-5 days

Intranasal:

Children 2-5 years: 0.025% solution: Instill 2-3 drops in each nostril twice daily

Children ≥6 years and Adults: 0.05% solution: Instill 2-3 drops or 2-3 sprays into each nostril twice daily

Ophthalmic: Children ≥6 years and Adults: Instill 1-2 drops into affected eye(s) every 6-12 hours

Patient Information Should not be used for self-medication for longer than 3 days, if symptoms persist, drug should be discontinued and a physician consulted; notify physician of insomnia, tremor, or irregular heartbeat; burning, stinging, or drying of the nasal mucosa may occur

Dosage Forms Solution:

Nasal:

Drops: 0.05% drops (15 mL, 20 mL)

Drops, pediatric: 0.025% (20 mL)

Spray: 0.05% (15 mL, 30 mL)

Ophthalmic: 0.025% (15 mL, 30 mL)

Oxymetholone *(ox i meth' oh lone)*

Brand Names Anadrol®

Use Anemias caused by the administration of myelotoxic drugs

Restrictions C-III

Pregnancy Risk Factor X

Contraindications Carcinoma of breast or prostate, nephrosis, pregnancy, hypersensitivity to any component

Warnings/Precautions Anabolic steroids may cause peliosis hepatis, liver cell tumors, and blood lipid changes with increased risk of arteriosclerosis; monitor diabetic patients carefully; use with caution in elderly patients, they may be at greater risk for prostatic hypertrophy; use with caution in patients with cardiac, renal, or hepatic disease or epilepsy

Adverse Reactions

Male:

Postpubertal:

>10%:

Dermatologic: Acne

Endocrine & metabolic: Gynecomastia

Genitourinary: Bladder irritability, priapism

1% to 10%:

Central nervous system: Insomnia, chills

Endocrine & metabolic: Decreased libido

Gastrointestinal: Nausea, diarrhea

Genitourinary: Prostatic hypertrophy (elderly)

Hematologic: Iron deficiency anemia, suppression of clotting factors

Hepatic: Hepatic dysfunction

<1%:

Hepatic: Hepatic necrosis, hepatocellular carcinoma

Prepubertal:

>10%:

Dermatologic: Acne

Endocrine & metabolic: Virilism

1% to 10%:

Central nervous system: Chills, insomnia

Dermatologic: Hyperpigmentation

Gastrointestinal: Diarrhea, nausea

Hematologic: Iron deficiency anemia, suppression of clotting factors

<1%: Hepatic: Hepatic necrosis, hepatocellular carcinoma

Female:

>10%: Endocrine & metabolic: Virilism

1% to 10%:

Central nervous system: Chills, insomnia

Endocrine & metabolic: Hypercalcemia

Gastrointestinal: Nausea, diarrhea

Hematologic: Iron deficiency anemia, suppression of clotting factors

Hepatic: Hepatic dysfunction

<1%: Hepatic: Hepatic necrosis, hepatocellular carcinoma

Overdosage/Toxicology Abnormal liver function test

Drug Interactions Increased toxicity: Increased oral anticoagulants, insulin requirements may be decreased

Mechanism of Action Stimulates receptors in organs and tissues to promote growth and development of male sex organs and maintains secondary sex characteristics in androgen-deficient males

Pharmacodynamics/Kinetics
Half-life: 9 hours
Elimination: Primarily in urine

Usual Dosage Adults: Erythropoietic effects: Oral: 1-5 mg/kg/day in 1 daily dose; maximum: 100 mg/day; give for a minimum trial of 3-6 months because response may be delayed

Monitoring Parameters Liver function tests

Test Interactions Altered glucose tolerance tests, altered thyroid function tests, altered metyrapone tests

Dosage Forms Tablet: 50 mg

Oxymorphone Hydrochloride (ox i mor′ fone)

Related Information
Narcotic Agonist Comparison Charts *on page 1274-1275*

Brand Names Numorphan®

Use Management of moderate to severe pain and preoperatively as a sedative and a supplement to anesthesia

Restrictions C-II

Pregnancy Risk Factor B (D if used for prolonged periods or in high doses at term)

Contraindications Hypersensitivity to oxymorphone or any component, increased intracranial pressure; severe respiratory depression

Warnings/Precautions Some preparations contain sulfites which may cause allergic reactions; infants <3 months of age are more susceptible to respiratory depression, use with caution and generally in reduced doses in this age group; use with caution in patients with impaired respiratory function or severe hepatic dysfunction and in patients with hypersensitivity reactions to other phenanthrene derivative opioid agonists (codeine, hydrocodone, hydromorphone, levorphanol, oxycodone, oxymorphone)

Adverse Reactions
>10%:
  Cardiovascular: Hypotension
  Central nervous system: Weakness, tiredness, drowsiness, dizziness
  Gastrointestinal: Nausea, vomiting, constipation
  Miscellaneous: Histamine release
1% to 10%:
  Central nervous system: Nervousness, headache, restlessness, malaise, confusion
  Gastrointestinal: Anorexia, stomach cramps, dry mouth, biliary spasm
  Genitourinary: Decreased urination, ureteral spasms
  Local: Pain at injection site
  Respiratory: Troubled breathing, shortness of breath
<1%:
  Central nervous system: Mental depression, hallucinations, paradoxical CNS stimulation, increased intracranial pressure
  Dermatologic: Skin rash, hives
  Gastrointestinal: Paralytic ileus
  Miscellaneous: Histamine release, physical and psychological dependence

Overdosage/Toxicology Symptoms of overdose include respiratory depression, miosis, hypotension, bradycardia, apnea, pulmonary edema. Treatment of an overdose includes support of the patient's airway, establishment of an I.V. line and administration of naloxone 2 mg I.V. (0.01 mg/kg for children) with repeat administration as necessary up to a total of 10 mg.

Drug Interactions
Decreased effect with phenothiazines
Increased effect/toxicity with CNS depressants, TCAs, dextroamphetamine

Stability Refrigerate suppository

Mechanism of Action Oxymorphone hydrochloride (Numorphan®) is a potent narcotic analgesic with uses similar to those of morphine. The drug is a semisynthetic derivative of morphine (phenanthrene derivative) and is closely related to hydromorphone chemically (Dilaudid®).

Pharmacodynamics/Kinetics
Onset of analgesia:
  I.V., I.M., S.C.: Within 5-10 minutes
  Rectal: Within 15-30 minutes
Duration of analgesia: Parenteral, rectal: 3-4 hours
Metabolism: Conjugated with glucuronic acid
Elimination: In urine
(Continued)

Oxymorphone Hydrochloride *(Continued)*

Usual Dosage Adults:
    I.M., S.C.: 0.5 mg initially, 1-1.5 mg every 4-6 hours as needed
    I.V.: 0.5 mg initially
    Rectal: 5 mg every 4-6 hours
Monitoring Parameters Respiratory rate, heart rate, blood pressure, CNS activity
Patient Information Avoid alcohol, may cause drowsiness, impaired judgment or coordination; may cause physical and psychological dependence with prolonged use
Nursing Implications Observe patient for excessive sedation, respiratory depression, implement safety measures, assist with ambulation
Dosage Forms
    Injection: 1 mg (1 mL); 1.5 mg/mL (1 mL, 10 mL)
    Suppository, rectal: 5 mg

Oxytetracycline Hydrochloride (ox i tet ra sye' kleen)

Brand Names Terramycin® IV; Uri-Tet®
Use Treatment of susceptible bacterial infections; both gram-positive and gram-negative, as well as, *Rickettsia* and *Mycoplasma* organisms
Pregnancy Risk Factor D
Contraindications Hypersensitivity to tetracycline or any component
Warnings/Precautions Avoid in children ≤8 years of age, pregnant and nursing women; photosensitivity can occur with oxytetracycline
Adverse Reactions
  >10%: Miscellaneous: Discoloration of teeth and enamel hypoplasia (infants)
  1% to 10%:
    Dermatologic: Photosensitivity
    Gastrointestinal: Nausea, diarrhea
  <1%:
    Cardiovascular: Pericarditis
    Central nervous system: Increased intracranial pressure, bulging fontanels in infants, pseudotumor cerebri
    Dermatologic: Pruritus, exfoliative dermatitis, dermatologic effects
    Endocrine & metabolic: Diabetes insipidus syndrome
    Gastrointestinal: Vomiting, esophagitis, anorexia, abdominal cramps, antibiotic-associated pseudomembranous colitis, staphylococcal enterocolitis
    Hepatic: Hepatotoxicity
    Local: Thrombophlebitis,
    Neuromuscular & skeletal: Paresthesia
    Renal: Renal damage, acute renal failure, azotemia
    Miscellaneous: Superinfections, anaphylaxis, pigmentation of nails, hypersensitivity reactions, candidal superinfection
Overdosage/Toxicology Symptoms of overdose include nausea, anorexia, diarrhea; following GI decontamination, supportive care only
Drug Interactions
  Decreased effect with antacids containing aluminum, calcium or magnesium
  Iron and bismuth subsalicylate may decrease doxycycline bioavailability
  Barbiturates, phenytoin, and carbamazepine decrease doxycycline's half-life
  Increased effect of warfarin
Mechanism of Action Inhibits bacterial protein synthesis by binding with the 30S and possibly the 50S ribosomal subunit(s) of susceptible bacteria, cell wall synthesis is not affected
Pharmacodynamics/Kinetics
  Absorption:
    Oral: Adequate (~75%)
    I.M.: Poor
  Distribution: Crosses the placenta
  Metabolism: Small amounts in the liver
  Half-life: 8.5-9.6 hours (increases with renal impairment)
  Time to peak serum concentration: Within 2-4 hours
  Elimination: In urine, while much higher amounts can be found in bile
Usual Dosage
  Oral:
    Children: 40-50 mg/kg/day in divided doses every 6 hours (maximum: 2 g/24 hours)
    Adults: 250-500 mg/dose every 6 hours

  I.M.:
    Children >8 years: 15-25 mg/kg/day (maximum: 250 mg/dose) in divided doses every 8-12 hours

Adults: 250-500 mg every 24 hours or 300 mg/day divided every 8-12 hours

Dosing interval in renal impairment: Cl$_{cr}$ <10 mL/minute: Administer every 24 hours or avoid use if possible

Dosing adjustment/comments in hepatic impairment: Avoid use in patients with severe liver disease

Administration Injection for intramuscular use only; do not give with antacids, iron products, or dairy products; give 1 hour before or 2 hours after meals

Patient Information Avoid unnecessary exposure to sunlight; do not take with antacids, iron products, or dairy products; finish all medication; do not skip doses; take 1 hour before or 2 hours after meals

Dosage Forms
Capsule: 250 mg
Injection, with lidocaine 2%: 5% [50 mg/mL] (2 mL, 10 mL); 12.5% [125 mg/mL] (2 mL)

Oxytocin (ox i toe' sin)
Brand Names Pitocin®; Syntocinon®
Synonyms Pit
Use Induces labor at term; controls postpartum bleeding; nasal preparation used to promote milk letdown in lactating females
Pregnancy Risk Factor X
Contraindications Hypersensitivity to oxytocin or any component; significant cephalopelvic disproportion, unfavorable fetal positions, fetal distress, hypertonic or hyperactive uterus, contraindicated vaginal delivery, prolapse, total placenta previa, and vasa previa
Warnings/Precautions To be used for medical rather than elective induction of labor; may produce antidiuretic effect (ie, water intoxication and excess uterine contractions); high doses or hypersensitivity to oxytocin may cause uterine hypertonicity, spasm, tetanic contraction, or rupture of the uterus; severe water intoxication with convulsions, coma, and death is associated with a slow oxytocin infusion over 24 hours
Adverse Reactions
Fetal: <1%:
Cardiovascular: Bradycardia, arrhythmias, intracranial hemorrhage
Central nervous system: Brain damage
Hepatic: Neonatal jaundice
Respiratory: Hypoxia
Miscellaneous: Death
Maternal: <1%:
Cardiovascular: Cardiac arrhythmias, premature ventricular contractions, hypotension, tachycardia, arrhythmias
Central nervous system: Seizures, coma
Gastrointestinal: Nausea, vomiting
Hematologic: Postpartum hemorrhage, fatal afibrinogenemia, increased blood loss, pelvic hematoma
Miscellaneous: Death, increased uterine motility, anaphylactic reactions, SIADH with hyponatremia
Overdosage/Toxicology Symptoms of overdose include tetanic uterine contractions, impaired uterine blood flow, amniotic fluid embolism, uterine rupture, SIADH, seizures; treat SIADH via fluid restriction, diuresis, saline administration, and anticonvulsants, if needed
Stability Oxytocin should be stored at room temperature (15°C to 30°C) and protected from freezing; **incompatible** with norepinephrine, prochlorperazine
Mechanism of Action Produces the rhythmic uterine contractions characteristic to delivery and stimulates breast milk flow during nursing
Pharmacodynamics/Kinetics
Onset of uterine contractions: I.V.: Within 1 minute
Duration: <30 minutes
Metabolism: Rapid in the liver and plasma (by oxytocinase) and to a smaller degree the mammary gland
Half-life: 1-5 minutes
Elimination: Renal
Usual Dosage I.V. administration requires the use of an infusion pump
Adults:
Induction of labor: I.V.: 0.001-0.002 units/minute; increase by 0.001-0.002 units every 15-30 minutes until contraction pattern has been established; maximum dose should not exceed 20 milliunits/minute
Postpartum bleeding:
I.M.: Total dose of 10 units after delivery
(Continued)

Oxytocin *(Continued)*

I.V.: 10-40 units by I.V. infusion in 1000 mL of intravenous fluid at a rate sufficient to control uterine atony

Promotion of milk letdown: Intranasal: 1 spray or 3 drops in one or both nostrils 2-3 minutes before breast-feeding

Monitoring Parameters Fluid intake and output during administration; fetal monitoring

Additional Information Sodium chloride 0.9% (NS) and dextrose 5% in water (D_5W) have been recommended as diluents; dilute 10-40 units to 1 L in NS, LR, or D_5W

Dosage Forms
Injection: 10 units/mL (1 mL, 10 mL)
Solution, nasal: 40 units/mL (2 mL, 5 mL)

Paclitaxel *(pack li tax' el)*

Related Information
Cancer Chemotherapy Regimens *on page 1218-1241*

Brand Names Taxol®

Use Treatment of metastatic carcinoma of the ovary after failure of first-line or subsequent chemotherapy; treatment of metastatic breast cancer

Pregnancy Risk Factor D

Contraindications History of hypersensitivity to any component

Warnings/Precautions The FDA currently recommends that procedures for proper handling and disposal of antineoplastic agents be considered

All patients should be premedicated prior to Taxol® administration to prevent severe hypersensitivity reactions:

Current evidence indicates that prolongation of the infusion (to ≥6 hours) plus premedication may minimize this effect:

Dexamethasone 20 mg orally 14 and 7 hours before the infusion

Diphenhydramine 50 mg IVP 30 minutes before the infusion

Ranitidine 50 mg (or cimetidine 300 mg) IVPB 30 minutes before the infusion

Adverse Reactions

>10%:

Bone marrow suppression: Major dose-limiting (ie, more severe at doses of 200-250 mg/m²) toxicity

Dermatologic: Alopecia has been observed in almost all patients; loss of scalp hair occurs suddenly between day 14 and 21 and is reversible. Some patients experience a loss of all body hair. Local venous effects include erythema, tenderness, and discomfort during infusion and areas of extravasation include erythema, swelling, and induration. Necrotic changes and ulcers have not been reported even after extravasation of large volumes of infusate.

Myelosuppression: More frequent and more severe for patients who had received prior radiation therapy

Neutropenia: Dose related and generally rapidly reversible -

Nadir: Day 8

Recovery: Days 15-21

Thrombocytopenia: Less frequent and less pronounced than neutropenia - nadir at day 8 or 9 after administration

Hypersensitivity: Based on observations during early clinical trials, reactions were principally nonimmunologically mediated by the direct release of histamine or other vasoactive substances from mast cells and basophils

Neurotoxicity: Typically cumulative, with symptoms progressing after each treatment at both high and low doses. Patients with pre-existing neuropathies due to previous chemotherapy or coexisting medical illness (diabetes mellitus, alcoholism) appear to be predisposed to neurotoxicity. Neurotoxic effects such as sensory neuropathy, motor neuropathy, autonomic neuropathy, myopathy or myopathic effects, and central nervous system toxicity have been reported. Sensory neuropathy occurs invariably when the paclitaxel dose approaches 250 mg/m². Symptoms include numbness, tingling, and/or burning pain in the distal lower extremities, toes and/or fingers and begin as early as 24-72 hours after treatment with high single doses. Motor neuropathy occurs primarily at relatively high doses (250-275 mg/m²) and in those patients with diabetes mellitus who may be more predisposed to toxic neuropathies. Myopathy effects are commonly observed after treatment with moderate to high doses (ie, >200 mg/m²) administered over 6-24 hours. These symptoms generally occur 2-3 days after treatment and resolve within 5-6 days.

Miscellaneous: Hypersensitivity reactions, myalgia, abnormal liver function tests

1% to 10%:
 Cardiovascular: Bradycardia, severe cardiovascular events
 Gastrointestinal: Nausea and vomiting are not severe at any dose level
 Irritant chemotherapy
Drug Interactions Increased toxicity:
In phase I trials, myelosuppression was more profound when given after cisplatin than with alternative sequence; pharmacokinetic data demonstrates a decrease in clearance of ~33% when administered following cisplatin
Possibility of an inhibition of metabolism in patients treated with ketoconazole
Stability Vials must be stored under refrigeration 2°C to 8°C (36°F to 46°F) and protected from light. Dilute to a final concentration of 0.3-1.2 mg/mL in 0.9% sodium chloride injection, dextrose 5% in water, dextrose 5% in 0.9% sodium chloride, or dextrose 5% in Ringer's injection. These solutions are physically and chemically stable for up to 27 hours at ambient temperature (25°C) and room light; formulated in a vehicle known as Cremophor EL™ (polyoxyethylated castor oil). Cremophor EL™ has been found to leach the plasticizer DEHP from polyvinyl chloride infusion bags or administration sets. Taxol® solutions should be stored in glass bottles or polypropylene/polyolefin (Excel®) bags and administered through nonpolyvinyl chloride (ie, polyethylene-lined) administration sets; administer through I.V. tubing containing an in-line (0.22 micron) filter; administration through IVEX-2® filters (which incorporate short inlet and outlet polyvinyl chloride-coated tubing) has not resulted in significant leaching of DEHP.
Pharmacodynamics/Kinetics Administered by I.V. infusion and exhibits a biphasic decline in plasma concentrations
Distribution: Initial rapid decline represents distribution to the peripheral compartment and significant elimination of the drug; later phase is due to a relatively slow efflux of paclitaxel from the peripheral compartment; mean steady state: 42-162 L/m^2, indicating extensive extravascular distribution and/or tissue binding
Protein binding: 89% to 98% bound to human serum proteins at concentrations of 0.1-50 mcg/mL
Metabolism: In the liver in animals and evidence suggests hepatic metabolism in humans
Half-life, mean, terminal: 5.3-17.4 hours after 1- and 6-hour infusions at dosing levels of 15-275 mg/m^2
Elimination: Urinary recovery of unchanged drug: 1.3% to 12.6% following 1-, 6-, and 24-hour infusions of 15-275 mg/m^2
 Mean total body clearance range:
  After 1- and 6-hour infusions: 5.8-16.3 L/hour/m^2
  After 24-hour infusions: 14.2-17.2 L/hour/m^2
Usual Dosage Adults: I.V. infusion (refer to individual protocols):
Corticosteroids (dexamethasone), H_1 antagonists (Benadryl®), and H_2 antagonists (cimetidine, ranitidine), should be administered prior to paclitaxel administration to minimize potential for anaphylaxis
Ovarian carcinoma: 135-175 mg/m^2 over 3-24 hours• administered every 3 weeks
Metastatic breast cancer: Treatment is still undergoing investigation; most protocols have used doses of 200-250 mg/m^2 over 3-24 hours•

 •The results of an international study has demonstrated that a 3-hour infusion produces similar efficacy as a 24-hour infusion, but with less hematologic toxicity and less mucositis
Monitoring Parameters Monitor for hypersensitivity reactions
Reference Range Mean maximum serum concentrations: 435-802 ng/mL following 24-hour infusions of 200-275 mg/m^2 and were approximately 10% to 30% of those following 6-hour infusions of equivalent doses
Patient Information Alopecia occurs in almost all patients
Dosage Forms Injection: 30 mg/5 mL

2-PAM *see* Pralidoxime Chloride *on page 914*

Pamelor® *see* Nortriptyline Hydrochloride *on page 808*

Pamidronate Disodium *(pa mi droe' nate)*
Brand Names Aredia™
Use Treatment of hypercalcemia associated with malignancy
 Unlabeled use: Symptomatic treatment of Paget's disease and heterotopic ossification due to spinal cord injury or after total hip replacement, reduce severe bone pain in malignancy
Pregnancy Risk Factor C
Contraindications Previous hypersensitivity to pamidronate or other biphosphonates
(Continued)

Pamidronate Disodium *(Continued)*

Warnings/Precautions Use caution in patients with renal impairment as the potential nephrotoxic effects of pamidronate are not known; use caution in patients who are pregnant or in the breast-feeding period; leukopenia has been observed with oral pamidronate and monitoring of white blood cell counts is suggested; vein irritation and thrombophlebitis may occur with infusions. Has not been studied exclusively in the elderly; monitor serum electrolytes periodically since elderly are often receiving diuretics which can result in decreases in serum calcium, potassium, and magnesium.

Adverse Reactions
1% to 10%:
   Central nervous system: Malaise, fever, convulsions
   Endocrine & metabolic: Hypomagnesemia, hypocalcemia, hypokalemia, hypo-phosphatemia, fluid overload
   Gastrointestinal: GI symptoms, nausea, diarrhea, constipation, anorexia
   Hepatic: Abnormal hepatic function
   Neuromuscular & skeletal: Bone pain
   Respiratory: Dyspnea
<1%:
   Dermatologic: Skin rash, angioedema
   Hematologic: Leukopenia, occult blood in stools
   Neuromuscular & skeletal: Increased risk of fractures
   Renal: Nephrotoxicity
   Miscellaneous: Pain, hypersensitivity reactions, altered taste

Overdosage/Toxicology Symptoms of overdose include hypocalcemia, EKG changes, seizures, bleeding, paresthesia, carpopedal spasm, fever; treat hypocalcemia with I.V. calcium gluconate; general supportive care, fever, and hypotension can be treated with corticosteroids

Stability
Reconstitute by adding 10 mL of sterile water for injection to each 30 mg vial of lyophilized pamidronate disodium powder, the resulting solution will be 30 mg/10 mL
Pamidronate is **incompatible** with calcium-containing infusion solutions such as Ringer's injection; may be further diluted in 250-1000 mL of 0.45% or 0.9% sodium chloride or 5% dextrose; pamidronate [reconstituted solution and infusion solution] is stable at room temperature and under refrigeration (36°F to 46°F or 2°C to 8°C) for 24 hours

Mechanism of Action A biphosphonate which inhibits bone resorption via actions on osteoclasts or on osteoclast precursors. Does not appear to produce any significant effects on renal tubular calcium handling and is poorly absorbed following oral administration (high oral doses have been reported effective); therefore, I.V. therapy is preferred.

Pharmacodynamics/Kinetics
Onset of effect: 24-48 hours
Maximum effect: 5-7 days
Absorption: Poorly from the GI tract; pharmacokinetic studies are lacking
Half-life, unmetabolized: 2.5 hours
Distribution half-life: 1.6 hours
   Urinary (elimination) half-life: 2.5 hours
   Bone half-life: 300 days
Elimination: Biphasic; ~50% excreted unchanged in urine within 72 hours

Usual Dosage Drug must be diluted properly before administration and infused slowly (over at least 2 hours at a minimum rate of 7.5-15 mg/hour)

Adults: I.V.:
   Moderate cancer-related hypercalcemia (corrected serum calcium: 12-13 mg/dL): 60-90 mg given as a slow infusion over 2-24 hours
   Severe cancer-related hypercalcemia (corrected serum calcium: >13.5 mg/dL): 90 mg as a slow infusion over 2-24 hours
      A period of 7 days should elapse before the use of second course; repeat infusions every 2-3 weeks have been suggested, however, could be administered every 2-3 months according to the degree and of severity of hypercalcemia and/or the type of malignancy
   Paget's disease: 60 mg as a single 2- to 24-hour infusion

Monitoring Parameters Serum electrolytes, monitor for hypocalcemia for at least 2 weeks after therapy; serum calcium, phosphate, magnesium, creatinine; CBC with differential

Reference Range Calcium (total): Adults: 9.0-11.0 mg/dL (SI: 2.05-2.54 mmol/L), may slightly decrease with aging; Phosphorus: 2.5-4.5 mg/dL (SI: 0.81-1.45 mmol/L)

Patient Information Maintain adequate intake of calcium and vitamin D; report any fever, sore throat, or unusual bleeding to your physician

Dosage Forms Powder for injection, lyophilized: 30 mg, 60 mg, 90 mg

Pamine® *see* Methscopolamine Bromide *on page 717*

Pamprin IB® [OTC] *see* Ibuprofen *on page 561*

Panadol® [OTC] *see* Acetaminophen *on page 17*

Pancrease® *see* Pancrelipase *on this page*

Pancrease® MT *see* Pancrelipase *on this page*

Pancrelipase (pan kre li′ pase)

Brand Names Cotazym®; Cotazym-S®; Creon®; Creon® 25; Entolase®-HP; Festal®II [OTC]; Ilozyme®; Ku-Zyme HP®; Pancrease®; Pancrease® MT; Protilase®; Viokase®; Zymase®

Synonyms Lipancreatin

Use Replacement therapy in symptomatic treatment of malabsorption syndrome caused by pancreatic insufficiency

Pregnancy Risk Factor C

Contraindications Hypersensitivity to pancrelipase or any component, pork protein

Warnings/Precautions Pancrelipase is inactivated by acids; use microencapsulated products whenever possible, since these products permit better dissolution of enzymes in the duodenum and protect the enzyme preparations from acid degradation in the stomach

Adverse Reactions
1% to 10%: High doses:
Gastrointestinal: Nausea, cramps, constipation, diarrhea
Genitourinary: Hyperuricemia, hyperuricosuria
Ocular: Lacrimation
Respiratory: Sneezing, bronchospasm
<1%:
Dermatologic: Rash
Respiratory: Shortness of breath, bronchospasm
Miscellaneous: Irritation of the mouth

Overdosage/Toxicology Symptoms of overdose include diarrhea, other transient intestinal upset, hyperuricosuria, hyperuricemia

Drug Interactions
Decreased effect: Calcium carbonate, magnesium hydroxide
Increased effect: H_2 antagonists (eg, ranitidine, cimetidine)

Mechanism of Action Replaces endogenous pancreatic enzymes to assist in digestion of protein, starch and fats

Pancrelipase

Product	Dosage Form	Lipase USP Units	Amylase USP Units	Protease USP Units
Cotazym® Ku-Zyme® HP	Capsule	8000	30,000	30,000
Cotazym® -S	Capsule, enteric coated spheres	5000	20,000	20,000
Creon®		8000	30,000	13,000
Entolase® Pancrease® Protilase®	Capsule, delayed release	4000	20,000	25,000
Entolase HP®	enteric coated microbeads	8000	40,000	50,000
Festal® II	Tablet, delayed release	6000	30,000	20,000
Ilozyme®	Tablet	11,000	30,000	30,000
Pancrease® MT				
4	Capsule, enteric coated microtablets	4000	12,000	12,000
10		10,000	30,000	30,000
16		16,000	48,000	48,000
Viokase®	Powder	16,800 per 0.7 g	70,000 per 0.7 g	70,000 per 0.7 g
	Tablet	8000	30,000	30,000
Zymase®	Capsule, enteric coated spheres	12,000	24,000	24,000

(Continued)

Pancrelipase *(Continued)*

Pharmacodynamics/Kinetics
Absorption: Not absorbed, acts locally in GI tract

Elimination: In feces

Usual Dosage Oral:
Powder: Actual dose depends on the digestive requirements of the patient

Children <1 year: Start with $\frac{1}{8}$ teaspoonful with feedings

Adults: 0.7 g with meals

Enteric coated microspheres and microtablets: The following dosage recommendations are only an approximation for initial dosages. The actual dosage will depend on the digestive requirements of the individual patient.

Children:

<1 year: 2000 units of lipase with meals

1-6 years: 4000-8000 units of lipase with meals and 4000 units with snacks

7-12 years: 4000-12,000 units of lipase with meals and snacks

Adults: 4000-16,000 units of lipase with meals and with snacks or 1-3 tablets/capsules before or with meals and snacks; in severe deficiencies, dose may be increased to 8 tablets/capsules

Occluded feeding tubes: One tablet of Viokase® crushed with one 325 mg tablet of sodium bicarbonate (to activate the Viokase®) in 5 mL of water can be instilled into the nasogastric tube and clamped for 5 minutes; then, flushed with 50 mL of tap water

Patient Information Do not chew capsules, microspheres, or microtablets; take before or with meals; avoid inhaling powder dosage form

Dosage Forms See table.

Pancuronium Bromide *(pan kyoo roe' nee um)*

Related Information
Neuromuscular Blocking Agents Comparison Charts *on page 1276-1278*

Brand Names Pavulon®

Use Drug of choice for neuromuscular blockade except in patients with renal failure, hepatic failure, or cardiovascular instability

Produce skeletal muscle relaxation during surgery after induction of general anesthesia, increase pulmonary compliance during assisted respiration, facilitate endotracheal intubation, preferred muscle relaxant for neonatal cardiac patients, must provide artificial ventilation

Pregnancy Risk Factor C

Contraindications Hypersensitivity to pancuronium, bromide, or any component

Warnings/Precautions Ventilation must be supported during neuromuscular blockade. Electrolyte imbalance alters blockade. Use with caution in patients with myasthenia gravis or other neuromuscular diseases, pre-existing pulmonary, hepatic, renal disease, and in the elderly.

Adverse Reactions
1% to 10%:

Cardiovascular: Elevation in pulse rate, elevation in blood pressure, tachycardia, hypertension

Dermatologic: Rash, itching

Miscellaneous: Excessive salivation

<1%:

Cardiovascular: Skin flushing, edema

Dermatologic: Erythema, hypersensitivity reaction

Local: Burning sensation along the vein

Neuromuscular & skeletal: Profound muscle weakness

Respiratory: Wheezing, circulatory collapse, bronchospasm

Causes of prolonged neuromuscular blockade:

Excessive drug administration

Cumulative drug effect, decreased metabolism/excretion (hepatic and/or renal impairment)

Accumulation of active metabolites

Electrolyte imbalance (hypokalemia, hypocalcemia, hypermagnesemia, hypernatremia)

Hypothermia

Drug interactions

Increased sensitivity to muscle relaxants (eg, neuromuscular disorders such as myasthenia gravis or polymyositis)

Overdosage/Toxicology Symptoms of overdose include apnea, respiratory depression, cardiovascular collapse; pyridostigmine, neostigmine, or edrophonium in conjunction with atropine will usually antagonize the action of pancuronium

Drug Interactions
Increased toxicity: Magnesium sulfate, furosemide → can ↑ or ↓ neuromuscular blockade (dose-dependent)
Prolonged neuromuscular blockade:
Inhaled anesthetics
Local anesthetics
Calcium channel blockers
Antiarrhythmics (eg, quinidine or procainamide)
Antibiotics (eg, aminoglycosides, tetracyclines, vancomycin, clindamycin)
Immunosuppressants (eg, cyclosporine)
Stability Refrigerate; however, is stable for up to 6 months at room temperature; I.V. form is **incompatible** when mixed with diazepam at a Y-site injection
Mechanism of Action Blocks neural transmission at the myoneural junction by binding with cholinergic receptor sites
Pharmacodynamics/Kinetics
Peak effect: I.V.: Within 2-3 minutes
Duration: 40-60 minutes (dose dependent)
Metabolism: 30% to 45% in the liver
Half-life: 110 minutes
Elimination: In urine (55% to 70% as unchanged drug)
Usual Dosage I.V.: Based on ideal body weight in obese patients
Neonates <1 month:
Test dose: 0.02 mg/kg to measure responsiveness
Initial: 0.03 mg/kg/dose repeated twice at 5- to 10-minute intervals as needed; maintenance: 0.03-0.09 mg/kg/dose every 30 minutes to 4 hours as needed
Infants >1 month, Children, and Adults: Initial: 0.04-0.1 mg/kg; maintenance dose: 0.02-0.1 mg/kg/dose every 30 minutes to 3 hours as needed
Continuous I.V. infusions are not recommended due to case reports of prolonged paralysis

Dosing adjustment in renal impairment: Elimination half-life is doubled, plasma clearance is reduced and rate of recovery is sometimes much slower
Cl_{cr} 10-50 mL/minute: Administer 50% of normal dose
Cl_{cr} <10 mL/minute: Do not use

Dosing adjustment/comments in hepatic disease: Elimination half-life is doubled, plasma clearance is doubled, recovery time is prolonged, volume of distribution is increased (50%) and results in a slower onset, higher total dosage and prolongation of neuromuscular blockade

Patients with liver disease may develop slow resistance to nondepolarizing muscle relaxant; large doses may be required and problems may arise in antagonism
Monitoring Parameters Heart rate, blood pressure, assisted ventilation status; cardiac monitor, blood pressure monitor, and ventilator required
Dosage Forms Injection: 1 mg/mL (10 mL); 2 mg/mL (2 mL, 5 mL)

Panmycin® see Tetracycline on page 1069

PanOxyl®-AQ see Benzoyl Peroxide on page 122

PanOxyl® [OTC] see Benzoyl Peroxide on page 122

Panscol® see Salicylic Acid on page 991

Panthoderm® [OTC] see Dexpanthenol on page 317

Pantothenyl Alcohol see Dexpanthenol on page 317

Papaverine Hydrochloride (pa pav' er een)
Brand Names Cerespan®; Genabid®; Pavabid®; Pavagen®; Pavaspan®; Pavasull®; Pavatab®; Pavatine® Pavased®; Pavatym®; Paverolan®
Use
Oral: Relief of peripheral and cerebral ischemia associated with arterial spasm; smooth muscle relaxant
Parenteral: Various vascular spasms associated with muscle spasms as in myocardial infarction, angina, peripheral and pulmonary embolism, peripheral vascular disease, angiospastic states, and visceral spasm (ureteral, biliary, and GI colic); testing for impotence
Pregnancy Risk Factor C
Contraindications Complete atrioventricular block; Parkinson's disease
Warnings/Precautions Use with caution in patients with glaucoma; administer I.V. cautiously since apnea and arrhythmias may result; may, in large doses, depress cardiac conduction (eg, A-V node) leading to arrhythmias; may interfere with levodopa therapy of Parkinson's disease; hepatic hypersensitivity noted with jaundice, eosinophilia, and abnormal LFTs
(Continued)
839

Papaverine Hydrochloride *(Continued)*

Adverse Reactions
<1%:
Cardiovascular: Flushing of the face, tachycardias, hypotension, arrhythmias with rapid I.V. use
Central nervous system: Depression, dizziness, vertigo, drowsiness, sedation, lethargy, headache
Dermatologic: Pruritus
Gastrointestinal: Dry mouth, nausea, constipation
Hepatic: Hepatic hypersensitivity
Local: Thrombosis at the I.V. administration site
Respiratory: Apnea with rapid I.V. use
Miscellaneous: Sweating

Overdosage/Toxicology Symptoms of overdose include nausea, vomiting weakness, gastric distress, ataxia, hepatic dysfunction, drowsiness, nystagmus, hyperventilation, hypotension, hypokalemia; treatment is supportive with conventional therapy (ie, fluids, positioning and vasopressors for hypotension)

Drug Interactions
Decreased effect: Papaverine decreases the effects of levodopa
Increased toxicity: Additive effects with CNS depressants or morphine

Stability Protect from heat or freezing; refrigerate injection at 2°C to 8°C (35°F to 46°F); solutions should be clear to pale yellow; precipitates with lactated Ringer's

Mechanism of Action Smooth muscle spasmolytic producing a generalized smooth muscle relaxation including: vasodilatation, gastrointestinal sphincter relaxation, bronchiolar muscle relaxation, and potentially a depressed myocardium (with large doses); muscle relaxation may occur due to inhibition or cyclic nucleotide phosphodiesterase, increasing cyclic AMP; muscle relaxation is unrelated to nerve innervation; papaverine increases cerebral blood flow in normal subjects; oxygen uptake is unaltered

Pharmacodynamics/Kinetics
Onset of action: Oral: Rapid
Protein binding: 90%
Metabolism: Rapidly in the liver
Half-life: 0.5-1.5 hours
Elimination: Primarily as metabolites in urine

Usual Dosage
Children: I.M., I.V.: 1.5 mg/kg 4 times/day
Adults:
Oral: 100-300 mg 3-5 times/day
Oral, sustained release: 150-300 mg every 12 hours
I.M., I.V.: 30-120 mg every 3 hours as needed; for cardiac extrasystoles, give 2 doses 10 minutes apart I.V. or I.M.

Administration Rapid I.V. administration may result in arrhythmias and fatal apnea; administer no faster than over 1-2 minutes

Patient Information May cause dizziness, flushing, headache, constipation, caution when driving or performing tasks needing alertness

Nursing Implications Physically incompatible with Lactated Ringer's injection

Dosage Forms
Capsule, sustained release: 150 mg
Injection: 30 mg/mL (2 mL, 10 mL)
Tablet: 30 mg, 60 mg, 100 mg, 150 mg, 200 mg, 300 mg
Tablet, timed release: 200 mg
Topical gel (Pharmedic)

Parabromdylamine *see* Brompheniramine Maleate *on page 143*

Paracetamol *see* Acetaminophen *on page 17*

Paraflex® *see* Chlorzoxazone *on page 236*

Parafon Forte™ DSC *see* Chlorzoxazone *on page 236*

Paraplatin® *see* Carboplatin *on page 183*

Paregoric *(par e gor' ik)*
Synonyms Camphorated Tincture of Opium
Use Treatment of diarrhea or relief of pain; neonatal opiate withdrawal
Restrictions C-III
Pregnancy Risk Factor B (D when used long-term or in high doses)
Contraindications Hypersensitivity to opium or any component; diarrhea caused by poisoning until the toxic material has been removed
Warnings/Precautions Use with caution in patients with respiratory, hepatic or renal dysfunction, severe prostatic hypertrophy, or history of narcotic abuse; opium shares the toxic potential of opiate agonists, and usual precautions of

opiate agonist therapy should be observed; some preparations contain sulfites which may cause allergic reactions; infants <3 months of age are more susceptible to respiratory depression, use with caution and generally in reduced doses in this age group

Adverse Reactions

>10%:

Cardiovascular: Hypotension

Central nervous system: Weakness, drowsiness, dizziness

Gastrointestinal: Constipation

1% to 10%:

Central nervous system: Restlessness, headache, malaise

Genitourinary: Ureteral spasms, decreased urination

Miscellaneous: Histamine release

<1%:

Cardiovascular: Peripheral vasodilation

Central nervous system: Insomnia, CNS depression, mental depression, increased intracranial pressure

Gastrointestinal: Anorexia, stomach cramps, nausea, vomiting

Ocular: Miosis

Respiratory: Respiratory depression

Miscellaneous: Biliary or urinary tract spasm, physical and psychological dependence

Overdosage/Toxicology Symptoms of overdose include hypotension, drowsiness, seizures, respiratory depression. Naloxone 2 mg I.V. (0.01 mg/kg for children) with repeat administration as necessary up to a total of 10 mg.

Drug Interactions Increased effect/toxicity with CNS depressants (eg, alcohol, narcotics, benzodiazepines, TCAs, MAO inhibitors, phenothiazine)

Stability Store in light-resistant, tightly closed container

Mechanism of Action Increases smooth muscle tone in GI tract, decreases motility and peristalsis, diminishes digestive secretions

Pharmacodynamics/Kinetics In terms of opium

Metabolism: In the liver

Elimination: In urine, primarily as morphine glucuronide conjugates and as parent compound (morphine, codeine, papaverine, etc)

Usual Dosage Oral:

Neonatal opiate withdrawal: Instill 3-6 drops every 3-6 hours as needed, or initially 0.2 mL every 3 hours; increase dosage by approximately 0.05 mL every 3 hours until withdrawal symptoms are controlled; it is rare to exceed 0.7 mL/dose. Stabilize withdrawal symptoms for 3-5 days, then gradually decrease dosage over a 2- to 4-week period.

Children: 0.25-0.5 mL/kg 1-4 times/day

Adults: 5-10 mL 1-4 times/day

Test Interactions ↑ aminotransferase [ALT (SGPT)/AST (SGOT)] (S)

Patient Information Avoid alcohol, may cause drowsiness, impaired judgment or coordination; may cause physical and psychological dependence with prolonged use

Nursing Implications Observe patient for excessive sedation, respiratory depression, implement safety measures, assist with ambulation

Additional Information Contains morphine 0.4 mg/mL and alcohol 45%

Dosage Forms Liquid: 2 mg morphine equivalent/5 mL [equivalent to 20 mg opium powder] (5 mL, 60 mL, 473 mL, 4000 mL)

Parenteral Multiple Vitamin see Vitamin, Multiple on page 1166

Pargen Fortified® see Chlorzoxazone on page 236

Par Glycerol® see Iodinated Glycerol on page 587

Parlodel® see Bromocriptine Mesylate on page 142

Parnate® see Tranylcypromine Sulfate on page 1109

Paromomycin Sulfate (par oh moe mye' sin)

Brand Names Humatin®

Use Treatment of acute and chronic intestinal amebiasis; preoperatively to suppress intestinal flora; tapeworm infestations; rid bowel of nitrogen-forming bacteria in hepatic coma; treatment of Cryptosporidium diarrhea

Pregnancy Risk Factor C

Contraindications Intestinal obstruction, renal failure, known hypersensitivity to paromomycin or components

Warnings/Precautions Use with caution in patients with impaired renal function or possible or proven ulcerative bowel lesions

(Continued)

Paromomycin Sulfate (Continued)

Adverse Reactions
1% to 10%: Gastrointestinal: Diarrhea, abdominal cramps, nausea, vomiting, heartburn

<1%:
Central nervous system: Headache, vertigo
Dermatologic: Exanthema, rash, pruritus
Gastrointestinal: Steatorrhea, secondary enterocolitis
Hematologic: Eosinophilia
Otic: Ototoxicity

Overdosage/Toxicology
Symptoms of overdose include nausea, vomiting, diarrhea; following GI decontamination, if possible; care is supportive and symptomatic

Drug Interactions
Decreased effect of digoxin and methotrexate
Increased effect of oral anticoagulants

Mechanism of Action
Acts directly on ameba; has antibacterial activity against normal and pathogenic organisms in the GI tract; interferes with bacterial protein synthesis by binding to 30S ribosomal subunits

Pharmacodynamics/Kinetics
Absorption: Not absorbed via oral route
Elimination: 100% unchanged in feces

Usual Dosage
Oral:
Intestinal amebiasis: Children and Adults: 25-35 mg/kg/day in 3 divided doses for 5-10 days
Dientamoeba fragilis: Children and Adults: 25-30 mg/kg/day in 3 divided doses for 7 days
Cryptosporidium: Adults with AIDS: 1.5-2.25 g/day in 3-6 divided doses for 10-14 days (occasionally courses of up to 4-8 weeks may be needed)
Tapeworm (fish, dog, bovine, porcine):
Children: 11 mg/kg every 15 minutes for 4 doses
Adults: 1 g every 15 minutes for 4 doses
Hepatic coma: Adults: 4 g/day in 2-4 divided doses for 5-6 days
Dwarf tapeworm: Children and Adults: 45 mg/kg/dose every day for 5-7 days

Patient Information
Take full course of therapy; do not skip doses; notify physician if ringing in ears, hearing loss, or dizziness occurs

Dosage Forms
Capsule: 250 mg

Paroxetine (pa rox' e teen)

Related Information
Antidepressant Agents Comparison *on page 1250-1252*

Brand Names
Paxil™

Use
Treatment of depression; presently being investigated for obsessive-compulsive disorder

Pregnancy Risk Factor
B

Contraindications
Do not use within 14 days of MAO inhibitors

Warnings/Precautions
Use cautiously in patients with a history of seizures, mania, renal disease, cardiac disease, suicidal patients, children, or during breast-feeding in lactating women; avoid ECT

Adverse Reactions
>10%:
Central nervous system: Headache, asthenia, somnolence, dizziness, insomnia
Gastrointestinal: Nausea, dry mouth, constipation, diarrhea
Genitourinary: Ejaculatory disturbances
Miscellaneous: Sweating

1% to 10%:
Cardiovascular: Palpitations, vasodilation, postural hypotension
Central nervous system: Nervousness, anxiety
Endocrine & metabolic: Decreased libido
Gastrointestinal: Anorexia, flatulence, vomiting
Neuromuscular & skeletal: Tremor, paresthesia

<1%:
Cardiovascular: Bradycardia, hypotension
Central nervous system: Migraine, akinesia
Dermatologic: Alopecia
Endocrine & metabolic: Amenorrhea
Gastrointestinal: Gastritis,
Hematologic: Anemia, leukopenia
Neuromuscular & skeletal: Arthritis
Otic: Ear pain

Ocular: Eye pain
Respiratory: Asthma
Miscellaneous: Bruxism, thirst

Overdosage/Toxicology Symptoms of overdose include nausea, vomiting, drowsiness, sinus tachycardia, and dilated pupils. There are no specific antidotes, following attempts at decontamination, treatment is supportive and symptomatic; forced diuresis, dialysis, and hemoperfusion are unlikely to be beneficial.

Drug Interactions
Decreased effect: Phenobarbital, phenytoin
Increased toxicity: Alcohol, cimetidine, MAO inhibitors (hyperpyrexic crisis); increased effect/toxicity of TCAs, fluoxetine, sertraline, phenothiazines, class 1C antiarrhythmics, warfarin

Mechanism of Action Paroxetine is a selective serotonin reuptake inhibitor, chemically unrelated to tricyclic, tetracyclic, or other antidepressants; presumably, the inhibition of serotonin reuptake from brain synapse stimulated serotonin activity in the brain

Pharmacodynamics/Kinetics
Metabolism: Extensive following absorption by cytochrome P-450 enzymes
Half-life: 21 hours
Elimination: Metabolites are excreted in bile and urine

Usual Dosage Adults: Oral: 20 mg once daily (maximum: 50 mg/day), preferably in the morning; in elderly, debilitated, or patients with hepatic or renal impairment, start with 10 mg/day (maximum: 40 mg/day); adjust doses at 7-day intervals

Monitoring Parameters Hepatic and renal function tests, blood pressure, heart rate

Test Interactions ↑ LFTs

Dosage Forms Tablet: 20 mg, 30 mg

PAS see Aminosalicylate Sodium on page 57

Pathocil® see Dicloxacillin Sodium on page 329

Pavabid® see Papaverine Hydrochloride on page 839

Pavagen® see Papaverine Hydrochloride on page 839

Pavaspan® see Papaverine Hydrochloride on page 839

Pavasull® see Papaverine Hydrochloride on page 839

Pavatab® see Papaverine Hydrochloride on page 839

Pavatine® Pavased® see Papaverine Hydrochloride on page 839

Pavatym® see Papaverine Hydrochloride on page 839

Paverolan® see Papaverine Hydrochloride on page 839

Pavulon® see Pancuronium Bromide on page 838

Paxil™ see Paroxetine on previous page

PBZ® see Tripelennamine on page 1130

PBZ-SR® see Tripelennamine on page 1130

PCE® see Erythromycin on page 401

PediaCare® Oral see Pseudoephedrine on page 955

Pediaflor® see Fluoride on page 471

Pediapred® see Prednisolone on page 919

PediaProfen™ see Ibuprofen on page 561

Pediazole® see Erythromycin and Sulfisoxazole on page 403

PediOtic® see Neomycin, Polymyxin B, and Hydrocortisone on page 781

PedvaxHIB™ see Haemophilus b Conjugate Vaccine on page 521

Pegademase Bovine (peg a´ de mase)
Brand Names Adagen™
Use Enzyme replacement therapy for adenosine deaminase (ADA) deficiency in patients with severe combined immunodeficiency disease (SCID) who can not benefit from bone marrow transplant; not a cure for SCID, unlike bone marrow transplants, injections must be used the rest of the child's life, therefore is not really an alternative
Pregnancy Risk Factor C
Contraindications Hypersensitivity to pegademase bovine; not to be used as preparatory or support therapy for bone marrow transplantation
Warnings/Precautions Use with caution in patients with thrombocytopenia
(Continued)

Pegademase Bovine *(Continued)*

Adverse Reactions
<1%:
  Central nervous system: Headache
  Local: Pain at injection site

Drug Interactions Decreased effect: Vidarabine

Stability Refrigerate at 2°C to 8°C (36°F to 46°F); do not freeze

Mechanism of Action Adenosine deaminase is an enzyme that catalyzes the deamination of both adenosine and deoxyadenosine. Hereditary lack of adenosine deaminase activity results in severe combined immunodeficiency disease, a fatal disorder of infancy characterized by profound defects of both cellular and humoral immunity. It is estimated that 25% of patients with the autosomal recessive form of severe combined immunodeficiency lack adenosine deaminase.

Pharmacodynamics/Kinetics
Plasma adenosine deaminase activity generally normalizes after 2-3 weeks of weekly I.M. injections
Absorption: Rapid
Half-life: 48-72 hours

Usual Dosage Children: I.M.: Dose given every 7 days, 10 units/kg the first dose, 15 units/kg the second dose, and 20 units/kg the third dose; maintenance dose: 20 units/kg/week is recommended depending on patient's ADA level; maximum single dose: 30 units/kg

Patient Information Not a cure for SCID; unlike bone marrow transplants, injections must be used the rest of the child's life; frequent blood tests are necessary to monitor effect and adjust the dose as needed

Dosage Forms Injection: 250 units/mL (1.5 mL)

Pegaspargase *(peg a spare' a ji nase)*

Related Information
Cancer Chemotherapy Regimens *on page 1218-1241*

Brand Names Oncaspar®

Synonyms PEG-L-asparaginase

Use Patients with acute lymphoblastic leukemia (ALL) who require L-asparaginase in their treatment regimen, but have developed hypersensitivity to the native forms of L-asparaginase. Use as a single agent should only be undertaken when multi-agent chemotherapy is judged to be inappropriate for the patient.

Pregnancy Risk Factor C

Pregnancy/Breast Feeding Implications Based on limited reports in humans, the use of asparaginase does not seem to pose a major risk to the fetus when used in the 2nd and 3rd trimesters; or when exposure occurs prior to conception in either females or males. Because of the teratogenicity observed in animals and the lack of human data after 1st trimester exposure, asparaginase should be used cautiously, if at all, during this period.

Contraindications Pancreatitis or a history of pancreatitis; patients who have had significant hemorrhagic events associated with prior L-asparaginase therapy; previous serious allergic reactions, such as generalized urticaria, bronchospasm, laryngeal edema, hypotension, or other unacceptable adverse reactions to pegaspargase

Warnings/Precautions **The U.S. Food and Drug Administration (FDA) currently recommends that procedures for proper handling and disposal of antineoplastic agents be considered.**

Hypersensitivity reactions to pegaspargase, including life-threatening anaphylaxis, may occur during therapy, especially in patients with known hypersensitivity to the other forms of L-asparaginase. As a routine precaution, keep patients under observation for 1 hour with resuscitation equipment and other agents necessary to treat anaphylaxis (eg, epinephrine, oxygen, IV steroids) available.

Use caution when treating patients with pegaspargase in combination with hepatotoxic agents, especially when liver dysfunction is present.

Adverse Reactions
Overall, the adult patients had a somewhat higher incidence of L-asparaginase toxicities, except for hypersensitivity reactions, than the pediatric patients
>10%:
  Hypersensitivity: Acute or delayed, acute anaphylaxis, bronchospasm, dyspnea, urticaria, arthralgia, erythema, induration, edema, pain, tenderness, hives, swelling lip
  Pancreatic: Pancreatitis, (sometimes fulminant and fatal); increased serum amylase and lipase
  Hepatic: Elevations of AST, ALT and bilirubin (direct and indirect); jaundice, ascites and hypoalbuminemia, fatty changes in the liver; liver failure

>5%:

Allergic reactions: rash, erythema, edema, pain, fever, chills, urticaria, dyspnea or bronchospasm

Emetic potential: Mild (>5%)

Miscellaneous: ALT increase, fever, malaise

1% to 5%:

Cardiovascular: Hypotension, tachycardia, thrombosis

Central nervous system: Chills

Dermatologic: Lip edema, rash, urticaria

Gastrointestinal: Abdominal pain

Hematologic: Decreased anticoagulant effect, disseminated intravascular coagulation, decreased fibrinogen, hemolytic anemia, leukopenia, pancytopenia, thrombocytopenia, increased thromboplastin

Local: Injection site hypersensitivity

Myelosuppressive effects:

WBC: Mild

Platelets: Mild

Onset (days): 7

Nadir (days): 14

Recovery (days): 21

Respiratory: Dyspnea

Overdosage/Toxicology Symptoms of overdose include nausea, diarrhea

Drug Interactions

Decreased effect: Methotrexate: Asparaginase terminates methotrexate action by inhibition of protein synthesis and prevention of cell entry into the S phase

Increased toxicity:

Aspirin, dipyridamole, heparin, warfarin, NSAIDs: Imbalances in coagulation factors have been noted with the use of pegaspargase - use with caution

Vincristine and prednisone: An increased toxicity has been noticed when asparaginase is administered with VCR and prednisone

Cyclophosphamide (decreased metabolism)

Mercaptopurine (increased hepatotoxicity)

Vincristine (increased neuropathy)

Prednisone (increased hyperglycemia)

Stability

Avoid excessive agitation; do **not** shake

Refrigerate at 2°C to 8°C (36°F to 46°F).

Do not use of cloudy or if precipitate is present; do not use if stored at room temperature for >48 hours; do **not** freeze; do not use product if it is known to have been frozen

Single-use vial; discard unused portions

Mechanism of Action

Pegaspargase is a modified version of the enzyme L-asparaginase. The L-asparaginase used in the manufacture of pegaspargase is derived from *Escherichia coli*.

Some malignant cells (ie, lymphoblastic leukemia cells and those of lymphocyte derivation) must acquire the amino acid asparagine from surrounding fluid such as blood, whereas normal cells can synthesize their own asparagine. asparaginase is an enzyme that deaminates asparagine to aspartic acid and ammonia in the plasma and extracellular fluid and therefore deprives tumor cells of the amino acid for protein synthesis.

Pharmacodynamics/Kinetics

Distribution: V_d: 4-5 L/kg; 70% to 80% of plasma volume; does not penetrate the CSF

Metabolism: Systemically degraded, only trace amounts are found in the urine

Half-life: 5.73 days

Elimination: Clearance unaffected by age, renal function, or hepatic function; L-asparaginase was measurable for at least 15 days following initial treatment with pegaspargase

Usual Dosage

Dose must be individualized based upon clinical response and tolerance of the patient (refer to individual protocols)

I.M. administration is **preferred** over I.V. administration; I.M. administration may decrease the incidence of hepatotoxicity, coagulopathy, and GI and renal disorders

Children: I.M., I.V.:

Body surface area $\leq$0.6 m²: 82.5 IU/m² every 14 days

Body surface area $\geq$0.6 m²: 2500 IU/m² every 14 days

Adults: I.M., I.V.: 2500 IU/m² every 14 days

Administration Must only be given as a deep intramuscular injection into a large muscle; use two injection sites for I.M. doses >2 mL

I.M.: limit the volume of a single injection site to 2 mL. If the volume to be administered is >2 mL, use multiple injection sites

(Continued)

Pegaspargase *(Continued)*

I.V.: Administer over a period of 1-2 hours in 100 mL of 0.9% sodium chloride or dextrose 5% in water, through an infusion that is already running

Monitoring Parameters Vital signs during administration, CBC, urinalysis, amylase, liver enzymes, prothrombin time, renal function tests, urine dipstick for glucose, blood glucose

Patient Information

Inform patients of the possibility of hypersensitivity reactions, including immediate anaphylaxis

Instruct patients that the simultaneous use of pegaspargase with other drugs that may increase the risk of bleeding should be avoided

Patients should notify their physician of adverse reactions that occur

Nursing Implications Do not filter solution; appropriate agents for maintenance of an adequate airway and treatment of a hypersensitivity reaction (antihistamine, epinephrine, oxygen, I.V. corticosteroids) should be readily available. Be prepared to treat anaphylaxis at each administration; monitor for onset of abdominal pain and mental status changes.

Dosage Forms Injection: 750 IU/mL [preservative-free] vials

PEG-L-asparaginase *see* Pegaspargase *on page 844*

Pemoline *(pem' oh leen)*

Brand Names Cylert®

Synonyms Phenylisohydantoin; PIO

Use Treatment of attention deficit disorder with hyperactivity (ADDH); narcolepsy

Restrictions C-IV

Pregnancy Risk Factor B

Contraindications Liver disease; hypersensitivity to pemoline or any component; children <6 years of age; Tourette's syndrome, psychoses

Warnings/Precautions Use with caution in patients with renal dysfunction, hypertension, or a history of abuse

Adverse Reactions

>10%:

Central nervous system: Insomnia

Gastrointestinal: Anorexia, weight loss

1% to 10%:

Central nervous system: Dizziness, drowsiness, mental depression

Dermatologic: Skin rash

Gastrointestinal: Stomach pain, nausea

<1%:

Central nervous system: Seizures, precipitation of Tourette's syndrome, hallucination, headache, movement disorders

Dermatologic: Skin rashes

Endocrine & metabolic: Growth reaction

Gastrointestinal: Diarrhea

Hepatic: Increased liver enzymes (usually reversible upon discontinuation), hepatitis, jaundice

Overdosage/Toxicology Symptoms of overdose include tachycardia, hallucinations, agitation

There is no specific antidote for intoxication and the bulk of the treatment is supportive. Hyperactivity and agitation usually respond to reduced sensory input or benzodiazepines, however, with extreme agitation haloperidol (2-5 mg I.M. for adults) may be required. Hyperthermia is best treated with external cooling measures, or when severe or unresponsive, muscle paralysis with pancuronium may be needed.

Drug Interactions

Decreased effect of insulin

Increased effect/toxicity with CNS depressants, CNS stimulants, sympathomimetics

Mechanism of Action Blocks the reuptake mechanism of dopaminergic neurons, appears to act at the cerebral cortex and subcortical structures; CNS and respiratory stimulant with weak sympathomimetic effects; actions may be mediated via increase in CNS dopamine

Pharmacodynamics/Kinetics

Peak effect: 4 hours

Duration: 8 hours

Protein binding: 50%

Metabolism: Partially by the liver

Half-life:

Children: 7-8.6 hours

Adults: 12 hours

Time to peak serum concentration: Oral: Within 2-4 hours

Elimination: In urine; only negligible amounts can be detected in feces

Usual Dosage Children ≥6 years: Oral: Initial: 37.5 mg given once daily in the morning, increase by 18.75 mg/day at weekly intervals; usual effective dose range: 56.25-75 mg/day; maximum: 112.5 mg/day; dosage range: 0.5-3 mg/kg/24 hours; significant benefit may not be evident until third or fourth week of administration

Dosing adjustment/comments in renal impairment: Cl_{cr} <50 mL/minute: Avoid use

Monitoring Parameters Liver enzymes

Patient Information Avoid caffeine; avoid alcoholic beverages; last daily dose should be given several hours before retiring; do not abruptly discontinue; prolonged use may cause dependence

Nursing Implications Give medication in the morning

Dosage Forms

Tablet: 18.75 mg, 37.5 mg, 75 mg

Tablet, chewable: 37.5 mg

Penamp® see Ampicillin on page 73

Penecort® see Hydrocortisone on page 546

Penetrex™ see Enoxacin on page 386

Penicillamine (pen i sill' a meen)

Brand Names Cuprimine®; Depen®

Synonyms D-3-Mercaptovaline; β,β-Dimethylcysteine; D-Penicillamine

Use Treatment of Wilson's disease, cystinuria, adjunct in the treatment of rheumatoid arthritis; lead, mercury, copper, and possibly gold poisoning. **(Note:** Oral DMSA is preferable for lead or mercury poisoning); primary biliary cirrhosis; as adjunctive therapy following initial treatment with calcium EDTA or BAL.

Pregnancy Risk Factor D

Contraindications Hypersensitivity to penicillamine or components; renal insufficiency; patients with previous penicillamine-related aplastic anemia or agranulocytosis; concomitant administration with other hematopoietic-depressant drugs (eg, gold, immunosuppressants, antimalarials, phenylbutazone)

Warnings/Precautions Cross-sensitivity with penicillin is possible; therefore, should be used cautiously in patients with a history of penicillin allergy. Patients on penicillamine for Wilson's disease or cystinuria should receive pyridoxine supplementation 25 mg/day; once instituted for Wilson's disease or cystinuria, continue treatment on a daily basis; interruptions of even a few days have been followed by hypersensitivity with reinstitution of therapy. Penicillamine has been associated with fatalities due to agranulocytosis, aplastic anemia, thrombocytopenia, Goodpasture's syndrome, and myasthenia gravis; patients should be warned to report promptly any symptoms suggesting toxicity; approximately 33% of patients will experience an allergic reaction; since toxicity may be dose related, it is recommended not to exceed 750 mg/day in elderly.

Adverse Reactions

>10%:

Central nervous system: Fever

Dermatologic: Skin rash, hives, itching

Gastrointestinal: Hypogeusia

Neuromuscular & skeletal: Joint pain

1% to 10%:

Central nervous system: Fever, chills

Gastrointestinal: Weight gain

Genitourinary: Bloody or cloudy urine

Hematologic: Aplastic or hemolytic anemia, leukopenia, thrombocytopenia

Miscellaneous: Sore throat, white spots on lips or mouth, swelling of face, feet or lower legs

<1%:

Central nervous system: Weakness, tiredness

Dermatologic: Toxic epidermal necrolysis, pemphigus, increased friability of the skin

Gastrointestinal: Nausea, vomiting, anorexia, pancreatitis

Hepatic: Cholestatic jaundice, hepatitis

Neuromuscular & skeletal: Myasthenia gravis syndrome, arthralgia

Ocular: Optic neuritis

Otic: Tinnitus

Renal: Nephrotic syndrome

Respiratory: Coughing, wheezing

(Continued)

Penicillamine *(Continued)*

Miscellaneous: Iron deficiency, SLE-like syndrome, spitting of blood allergic reactions, lymphadenopathy

Overdosage/Toxicology Symptoms of overdose include nausea and vomiting; following GI decontamination, treatment is supportive

Drug Interactions

Decreased effect with iron and zinc salts, antacids (magnesium, calcium, aluminum) and food

Decreased effect/levels of digoxin

Increased effect of gold, antimalarials, immunosuppressants, phenylbutazone (hematologic, renal toxicity)

Stability Store in tight, well-closed containers

Mechanism of Action Chelates with lead, copper, mercury and other heavy metals to form stable, soluble complexes that are excreted in urine; depresses circulating IgM rheumatoid factor, depresses T-cell but not B-cell activity; combines with cystine to form a compound which is more soluble, thus cystine calculi are prevented

Pharmacodynamics/Kinetics

Absorption: Oral: 40% to 70%

Metabolism: Small amounts of hepatic metabolism

Protein binding: 80% bound to albumin

Half-life: 1.7-3.2 hours

Time to peak serum concentration: Within 2 hours

Elimination: Primarily (30% to 60%) in urine as unchanged drug

Usual Dosage Oral:

Rheumatoid arthritis:

Children: Initial: 3 mg/kg/day (≤250 mg/day) for 3 months, then 6 mg/kg/day (≤500 mg/day) in divided doses twice daily for 3 months to a maximum of 10 mg/kg/day in 3-4 divided doses

Adults: 125-250 mg/day, may increase dose at 1- to 3-month intervals up to 1-1.5 g/day

Wilson's disease (doses titrated to maintain urinary copper excretion >1 mg/day):

Infants <6 months: 250 mg/dose once daily

Children <12 years: 250 mg/dose 2-3 times/day

Adults: 250 mg 4 times/day

Cystinuria:

Children: 30 mg/kg/day in 4 divided doses

Adults: 1-4 g/day in divided doses every 6 hours

Lead poisoning (continue until blood lead level is <60 mcg/dL): Children and Adults: 25-35 mg/kg/d, administered in 3-4 divided doses; initiating treatment at 25% of this dose and gradually increasing to the full dose over 2-3 weeks may minimize adverse reactions

Primary biliary cirrhosis: 250 mg/day to start, increase by 250 mg every 2 weeks up to a maintenance dose of 1 g/day, usually given 250 mg 4 times/day

Arsenic poisoning: Children: 100 mg/kg/day in divided doses every 6 hours for 5 days; maximum: 1 g/day

Dosing adjustment/comments in renal impairment: Cl_{cr} <50 mL/minute: Avoid use

Monitoring Parameters Urinalysis, CBC with differential, platelet count, liver function tests; weekly measurements of urinary and blood concentration of the intoxicating metal is indicated (3 months has been tolerated)

CBC: WBC <3500/mm³, neutrophils <2000/mm³ or monocytes >500/mm³ indicate need to stop therapy immediately; quantitative 24-hour urine protein at 1- to 2-week intervals initially (first 2-3 months); urinalysis, LFTs occasionally; platelet counts <100,000/mm³ indicate need to stop therapy until numbers of platelets increase

Test Interactions Positive ANA

Patient Information Take at least 1 hour before a meal on an empty stomach; patients with cystinuria should drink copious amounts of water; notify physician if unusual bleeding or bruising, or persistent fever, sore throat, or fatigue occurs; report any unexplained cough, shortness of breath, or rash; loss of taste may occur; do not skip or miss doses or discontinue without notifying physician

Nursing Implications For patients who cannot swallow, contents of capsules may be administered in 15-30 mL of chilled puréed fruit or fruit juice; patients should be warned to report promptly any symptoms suggesting toxicity; give on an empty stomach (1 hour before meals and at bedtime)

Dosage Forms
  Capsule: 125 mg, 250 mg
  Tablet: 250 mg

Penicillin G Benzathine, Parenteral (pen i sill' in benz' a theen)

Brand Names Bicillin® L-A; Permapen®

Synonyms Benzathine Benzylpenicillin; Benzathine Penicillin G; Benzylpenicillin Benzathine

Use Active against some gram-positive organisms, few gram-negative organisms such as *Neisseria gonorrhoeae*, and some anaerobes and spirochetes; used only for the treatment of mild to moderately severe infections caused by organisms susceptible to low concentrations of penicillin G or for prophylaxis of infections caused by these organisms; used when patient cannot be kept in a hospital environment and neurosyphilis has been ruled out

The CDC and AAP do not currently recommend the use of penicillin G benzathine to treat congenital syphilis or neurosyphilis due to reported treatment failures and lack of published clinical data on its efficacy

Pregnancy Risk Factor B

Contraindications Known hypersensitivity to penicillin or any component

Warnings/Precautions Use with caution in patients with impaired renal function, seizure disorder, or history of hypersensitivity to other beta-lactams; CDC and AAP do not currently recommend the use of penicillin G benzathine to treat congenital syphilis or neurosyphilis due to reported treatment failures and lack of published clinical data on its efficacy

Adverse Reactions
  1% to 10%: Local: Local pain
  <1%:
    Central nervous system: Convulsions, confusion, drowsiness, fever
    Dermatologic: Rash
    Endocrine & metabolic: Electrolyte imbalance
    Hematologic: Hemolytic anemia, positive Coombs' reaction
    Local: Thrombophlebitis
    Neuromuscular & skeletal: Myoclonus
    Renal: Acute interstitial nephritis
    Miscellaneous: Jarisch-Herxheimer reaction, hypersensitivity reactions, anaphylaxis

Overdosage/Toxicology Symptoms of penicillin overdose include neuromuscular hypersensitivity (agitation, hallucinations, asterixis, encephalopathy, confusion, and seizures) and electrolyte imbalance with potassium or sodium salts, especially in renal failure; hemodialysis may be helpful to aid in the removal of the drug from the blood, otherwise most treatment is supportive or symptom directed

Drug Interactions
  Decreased effect: Tetracyclines → ↓ penicillin effectiveness
  Increased effect:
    Probenecid → ↑ penicillin levels
    Aminoglycosides → synergistic efficacy

Stability Store in refrigerator

Mechanism of Action Interferes with bacterial cell wall synthesis during active multiplication, causing cell wall death and resultant bactericidal activity against susceptible bacteria

Pharmacodynamics/Kinetics
  Absorption: I.M.: Slow
  Time to peak serum concentration: Within 12-24 hours; serum levels are usually detectable for 1-4 weeks depending on the dose; larger doses result in more sustained levels rather than higher levels

Usual Dosage I.M.: Give undiluted injection; higher doses result in more sustained rather than higher levels. Use a penicillin G benzathine-penicillin G procaine combination to achieve early peak levels in acute infections.

  Neonates >1200 g: 50,000 units/kg as a single dose
  Infants and Children:
    Group A streptococcal upper respiratory infection: 25,000-50,000 units/kg as a single dose; maximum: 1.2 million units
    Prophylaxis of recurrent rheumatic fever: 25,000-50,000 units/kg every 3-4 weeks; maximum: 1.2 million units/dose
    Early syphilis: 50,000 units/kg as a single injection; maximum: 2.4 million units
    Syphilis of more than 1-year duration: 50,000 units/kg every week for 3 doses; maximum: 2.4 million units/dose
(Continued)

ALPHABETICAL LISTING OF DRUGS

Penicillin G Benzathine, Parenteral *(Continued)*

Adults:

Group A streptococcal upper respiratory infection: 1.2 million units as a single dose

Prophylaxis of recurrent rheumatic fever: 1.2 million units every 3-4 weeks or 600,000 units twice monthly

Early syphilis: 2.4 million units as a single dose in 2 injection sites

Syphilis of more than 1-year duration: 2.4 million units in 2 injection sites once weekly for 3 doses

Not indicated as single drug therapy for neurosyphilis, but may be given 1 time/week for 3 weeks following I.V. treatment (refer to Penicillin G monograph for dosing)

Administration Administer by deep I.M. injection in the upper outer quadrant of the buttock do **not** give I.V., intra-arterially, or S.C.; in children <2 years of age, I.M. injections should be made into the midlateral muscle of the thigh, not the gluteal region; when doses are repeated, rotate the injection site

Test Interactions Positive Coombs' [direct], false-positive urinary and/or serum proteins; false-positive or negative urinary glucose using Clinitest®

Patient Information Report any rash

Dosage Forms Injection: 300,000 units/mL (10 mL); 600,000 units/mL (1 mL, 2 mL, 4 mL)

Penicillin G, Parenteral, Aqueous (pen i sill' in)

Brand Names Pfizerpen®

Synonyms Benzylpenicillin Potassium; Benzylpenicillin Sodium; Crystalline Penicillin; Penicillin G Potassium; Penicillin G Sodium

Use Active against some gram-positive organisms, generally not *Staphylococcus aureus*; some gram-negative such as *Neisseria gonorrhoeae*, and some anaerobes and spirochetes; although ceftriaxone is now the drug of choice for Lyme disease and gonorrhea

Pregnancy Risk Factor B

Contraindications Known hypersensitivity to penicillin or any component

Warnings/Precautions Avoid intravascular or intra-arterial administration or injection into or near major peripheral nerves or blood vessels since such injections may cause severe and/or permanent neurovascular damage; use with caution in patients with renal impairment (dosage reduction required), pre-existing seizure disorders, or with a history of hypersensitivity to cephalosporins

Adverse Reactions

<1%:

Central nervous system: Convulsions, confusion, drowsiness, fever

Dermatologic: Rash

Endocrine & metabolic: Electrolyte imbalance

Hematologic: Hemolytic anemia, positive Coombs' reaction

Local: Thrombophlebitis

Neuromuscular & skeletal: Myoclonus

Renal: Acute interstitial nephritis

Miscellaneous: Jarisch-Herxheimer reaction, hypersensitivity reactions, anaphylaxis

Overdosage/Toxicology Symptoms of penicillin overdose include neuromuscular hypersensitivity (agitation, hallucinations, asterixis, encephalopathy, confusion, and seizures) and electrolyte imbalance with potassium or sodium salts, especially in renal failure; hemodialysis may be helpful to aid in the removal of the drug from the blood, otherwise most treatment is supportive or symptom directed

Drug Interactions

Decreased effect: Tetracyclines → ↓ penicillin effectiveness

Increased effect:

Probenecid → ↑ penicillin levels

Aminoglycosides → synergistic efficacy

Stability

Penicillin G potassium is stable at room temperature

Reconstituted parenteral solution is stable for 7 days when refrigerated (2°C to 15°C)

Penicillin G potassium for I.V. infusion in NS or D₅W, solution is stable for 24 hours at room temperature

Incompatible with aminoglycosides; inactivated in acidic or alkaline solutions

Mechanism of Action Interferes with bacterial cell wall synthesis during active multiplication, causing cell wall death and resultant bactericidal activity against susceptible bacteria

850

Pharmacodynamics/Kinetics
Time to peak serum concentration:
  I.M.: Within 30 minutes
  I.V. Within 1 hour
Distribution: Crosses the placenta; appears in breast milk; penetration across the blood-brain barrier is poor, despite inflamed meninges
  Relative diffusion of antimicrobial agents from blood into cerebrospinal fluid (CSF): Good only with inflammation (exceeds usual MICs)
  Ratio of CSF to blood level (%):
    Normal meninges: <1
    Inflamed meninges: 3-5
Protein binding: 65%
Metabolism: In the liver (30%) to penicilloic acid
Half-life:
  Neonates:
    <6 days: 3.2-3.4 hours
    7-13 days: 1.2-2.2 hours
    >14 days: 0.9-1.9 hours
  Children and adults with normal renal function: 20-50 minutes
  End stage renal disease: 3.3-5.1 hours
Elimination: In urine
Usual Dosage I.M., I.V.:
Neonates:
  Postnatal age 0-4 weeks: <1200 g: 25,000 units/kg/dose every 12 hours; meningitis: 50,000 units/kg/dose every 12 hours
  Postnatal age <7 days:
    1200-2000 g: 25,000 units/kg/dose every 12 hours; meningitis: 50,000 units/kg/dose every 12 hours
    >2000 g: 25,000 units/kg/dose every 8 hours; meningitis: 50,000 units/kg/dose every 8 hours
  Postnatal age >7 days:
    1200-2000 g: 25,000 units/kg/dose every 8 hours; meningitis: 75,000 units/kg/dose every 8 hours
    >2000 g: 25,000 units/kg/dose every 6 hours; meningitis: 50,000 units/kg/dose every 6 hours
Infants and Children (sodium salt is preferred in children): 100,000-250,000 units/kg/day in divided doses every 4 hours; maximum: 4.8 million units/24 hours
  Severe infections: Up to 400,000 units/kg/day in divided doses every 4 hours; maximum dose: 24 million units/day
Adults: 2-24 million units/day in divided doses every 4 hours

Congenital syphilis:
  Newborns: 50,000 units/kg/day I.V. every 8-12 hours for 10-14 days
  Infants: 50,000 units/kg every 4-6 hours for 10-14 days

Disseminated gonococcal infections or gonococcus ophthalmia (if organism proven sensitive): 100,000 units/kg/day in 2 equal doses (4 equal doses/day for infants >1 week)

Gonococcal meningitis: 150,000 units/kg in 2 equal doses (4 doses/day for infants >1 week)

Dosing interval in renal impairment:
  Cl_{cr} 30-50 mL/minute: Administer every 6 hours
  Cl_{cr} 10-30 mL/minute: Administer every 8 hours
  Cl_{cr} <10 mL/minute: Administer every 12 hours
Moderately dialyzable (20% to 50%)
Administration Administer I.M. by deep injection in the upper outer quadrant of the buttock; administer injection around-the-clock to promote less variation in peak and trough levels; while I.M. route is preferred route of administration, large doses should be administered by continuous I.V. infusion; determine volume and rate of fluid administration required in a 24-hour period; add appropriate daily dosage to this fluid
Test Interactions False-positive or negative urinary glucose determination using Clinitest®; positive Coombs' [direct]; false-positive urinary and/or serum proteins
Patient Information Report any rash or shortness of breath
Nursing Implications Dosage modification required in patients with renal insufficiency
Additional Information
  Penicillin G potassium: 1.7 mEq of potassium and 0.3 mEq of sodium per 1 million units of penicillin G
  Penicillin G sodium: 2 mEq of sodium per 1 million units of penicillin G
(Continued)

Penicillin G, Parenteral, Aqueous *(Continued)*

Dosage Forms
Injection, as sodium: 5 million units
Injection:
  Frozen premixed, as potassium: 1 million units, 2 million units, 3 million units
  Powder, as potassium: 1 million units, 5 million units, 10 million units, 20 million units

Penicillin G Potassium *see* Penicillin G, Parenteral, Aqueous *on page 850*

Penicillin G Potassium, Oral (Withdrawn from Market)

Use Treatment of susceptible bacterial infections including most gram-positive organisms (except *Staphylococcus aureus*), some gram-negative organisms such as *Neisseria gonorrhoeae*, and some anaerobes and spirochetes

Pregnancy Risk Factor B

Contraindications Known hypersensitivity to penicillin or any component

Warnings/Precautions Use with caution in patients with renal impairment, history of hypersensitivity to cephalosporins

Adverse Reactions
<1%:
  Central nervous system: Convulsions, confusion, drowsiness, fever
  Dermatologic: Rash
  Endocrine & metabolic: Electrolyte imbalance
  Hematologic: Hemolytic anemia, positive Coombs' reaction
  Neuromuscular & skeletal: Myoclonus
  Renal: Acute interstitial nephritis
  Miscellaneous: Jarisch-Herxheimer reaction, hypersensitivity reactions, anaphylaxis

Overdosage/Toxicology Symptoms of penicillin overdose include neuromuscular hypersensitivity (agitation, hallucinations, asterixis, encephalopathy, confusion, and seizures) and electrolyte imbalance with potassium or sodium salts, especially in renal failure; hemodialysis may be helpful to aid in the removal of the drug from the blood, otherwise most treatment is supportive or symptom directed

Drug Interactions
Decreased effect: Tetracyclines → ↓ penicillin effectiveness
Increased effect:
  Probenecid → ↑ penicillin levels
  Aminoglycosides → synergistic efficacy

Stability Reconstituted oral solution is stable for 14 days when refrigerated

Mechanism of Action Inhibits bacterial cell wall synthesis by binding to one or more of the penicillin binding proteins (PBPs); which in turn inhibits the final transpeptidation step of peptidoglycan synthesis in bacterial cell walls, thus inhibiting cell wall biosynthesis. Bacteria eventually lyse due to ongoing activity of cell wall autolytic enzymes (autolysins and murein hydrolases) while cell wall assembly is arrested.

Pharmacodynamics/Kinetics
Absorption: Oral: <30%; acid labile
Distribution: Crosses the placenta; appears in breast milk; penetration across the blood-brain barrier is poor with uninflamed meninges
Protein binding: 65%
Metabolism: In the liver (30%) to penicilloic acid
Time to peak serum concentration: Oral: Within 0.5-1 hour
Elimination: Penicillin G and its metabolites are excreted in urine mainly by tubular secretion

Usual Dosage Oral:
Infants and Children: 25-50 mg/kg/day or 40,000-80,000 units/kg/day divided every 6-8 hours hours
Adults: 125-500 mg every 6-8 hours

Dosing interval in renal impairment:
Cl_{cr} 10-30 mL/minute: Administer every 8-12 hours
Cl_{cr} <10 mL/minute: Administer every 12-18 hours
Moderately dialyzable (20% to 50%)

Administration Administer on empty stomach 1 hour before or 2 hours after meals; give around-the-clock rather than 4 times/day to promote less variation in peak and trough serum levels

Test Interactions False-positive or negative urinary glucose determination using Clinitest®; positive Coombs' [direct]; false-positive urinary and/or serum proteins

Patient Information Take until gone, do not skip doses, notify physician if rash develops, take 1 hour before or 2 hours after meals

Additional Information Penicillin V potassium is preferred for oral therapy

Dosage Forms

Powder for oral solution, as potassium: 400,000 units/5 mL (100 mL, 200 mL); 400,000 units = 250 mg

Tablet, as potassium: 200,000 units, 250,000 units, 400,000 units, 500,000 units, 800,000 units; 400,000 units = 250 mg

Penicillin G Procaine (pen i sill' in proe' kane)

Brand Names Crysticillin® A.S.; Pfizerpen®-AS; Wycillin®

Synonyms APPG; Aqueous Procaine Penicillin G; Procaine Benzylpenicillin; Procaine Penicillin G

Use Moderately severe infections due to *Neisseria gonorrhoeae*, *Treponema pallidum* and other penicillin G-sensitive microorganisms that are susceptible to low but prolonged serum penicillin concentrations

Pregnancy Risk Factor B

Contraindications Known hypersensitivity to penicillin or any component; also contraindicated in patients hypersensitive to procaine

Warnings/Precautions May need to modify dosage in patients with severe renal impairment, seizure disorders, or history of hypersensitivity to cephalosporins; avoid I.V., intravascular, or intra-arterial administration of penicillin G procaine since severe and/or permanent neurovascular damage may occur

Adverse Reactions

>10%: Local: Pain at injection site

<1%:

Cardiovascular: Myocardial depression, vasodilation, conduction disturbances

Central nervous system: CNS stimulation, seizures, confusion, drowsiness

Hematologic: Hemolytic anemia, positive Coombs' reaction

Local: Sterile abscess at injection site

Neuromuscular & skeletal: Myoclonus

Renal: Interstitial nephritis

Miscellaneous: Pseudoanaphylactic reactions, Jarisch-Herxheimer reaction, hypersensitivity reactions

Overdosage/Toxicology Symptoms of penicillin overdose include neuromuscular hypersensitivity (agitation, hallucinations, asterixis, encephalopathy, confusion, and seizures) and electrolyte imbalance with potassium or sodium salts, especially in renal failure; hemodialysis may be helpful to aid in the removal of the drug from the blood, otherwise most treatment is supportive or symptom directed

Drug Interactions

Decreased effect: Tetracyclines → ↓ penicillin effectiveness

Increased effect:

Probenecid → ↑ penicillin levels

Aminoglycosides → synergistic efficacy

Stability Store in refrigerator

Mechanism of Action Inhibits bacterial cell wall synthesis by binding to one or more of the penicillin binding proteins (PBPs); which in turn inhibits the final transpeptidation step of peptidoglycan synthesis in bacterial cell walls, thus inhibiting cell wall biosynthesis. Bacteria eventually lyse due to ongoing activity of cell wall autolytic enzymes (autolysins and murein hydrolases) while cell wall assembly is arrested.

Pharmacodynamics/Kinetics

Absorption: I.M.: Slowly absorbed

Time to peak serum concentration: Within 1-4 hours; can persist within the therapeutic range for 15-24 hours

Distribution: Penetration across the blood-brain barrier is poor, despite inflamed meninges; appears in breast milk

Protein binding: 65%

Metabolism: ~30% of a dose is inactivated in the liver

Elimination: Renal clearance is delayed in neonates, young infants, and patients with impaired renal function; 60% to 90% of the drug is excreted unchanged via renal tubular excretion

Usual Dosage I.M.:

Neonates ≥1200 g: 50,000 units/kg/day given every 24 hours (avoid using in this age group since sterile abscesses and procaine toxicity occur more frequently with neonates than older patients)

Children: 25,000-50,000 units/kg/day in divided doses 1-2 times/day; not to exceed 4.8 million units/24 hours

Gonorrhea: 100,000 units/kg (maximum 4.8 million units) one time (in 2 injection sites) along with probenecid 25 mg/kg (maximum: 1 g orally) 30 minutes prior to procaine penicillin

(Continued)

853

Penicillin G Procaine *(Continued)*

Congenital syphilis: 50,000 units/kg/day for 10-14 days

Adults: 0.6-4.8 million units/day in divided doses every 12-24 hours

Uncomplicated gonorrhea: 1 g probenecid orally, then 4.8 million units procaine penicillin divided into 2 injection sites 30 minutes later

Endocarditis caused by susceptible viridans *Streptococcus* (when used in conjunction with an aminoglycoside): 1.2 million units every 6 hours for 2-4 weeks

Neurosyphilis: I.M.: 2-4 million units/day with 500 mg probenecid by mouth 4 times/day for 10-14 days; **penicillin G aqueous I.V. is the preferred agent**

Moderately dialyzable (20% to 50%)

Administration Procaine suspension for deep I.M. injection only; rotate the injection site avoid I.V., intravascular, or intra-arterial administration of penicillin G procaine since severe and/or permanent neurovascular damage may occur

Monitoring Parameters Periodic renal and hematologic function tests with prolonged therapy; fever, mental status, WBC count

Test Interactions Positive Coombs' [direct], false-positive urinary and/or serum proteins

Patient Information Notify physician if skin rash, itching, hives, or severe diarrhea occurs

Nursing Implications Renal and hematologic systems should be evaluated periodically during prolonged therapy; do not inject in gluteal muscle in children <2 years of age

Dosage Forms Injection, suspension: 300,000 units/mL (10 mL); 500,000 units/mL (1.2 mL); 600,000 units/mL (1 mL, 2 mL, 4 mL)

Penicillin G Sodium *see* Penicillin G, Parenteral, Aqueous *on page 850*

Penicillin V Potassium (pen i sill' in poe tass' y um)

Related Information

Antimicrobial Drugs of Choice *on page 1298-1302*

Brand Names Beepen-VK®; Betapen®-VK; Ledercillin® VK; Pen.Vee® K; Robicillin® VK; V-Cillin K®; Veetids®

Synonyms Pen VK; Phenoxymethyl Penicillin

Use Treatment of moderate to severe susceptible bacterial infections; no longer recommended for dental procedure prophylaxis; prophylaxis in rheumatic fever; infections caused by susceptible organisms involving the respiratory tract, otitis media, sinusitis, skin, and urinary tract

Pregnancy Risk Factor B

Contraindications Known hypersensitivity to penicillin or any component

Warnings/Precautions Use with caution in patients with severe renal impairment (modify dosage), history of seizures, or hypersensitivity to cephalosporins

Adverse Reactions

>10%: Gastrointestinal: Mild diarrhea, vomiting, nausea, oral candidiasis

<1%:

Central nervous system: Convulsions, fever

Hematologic: Hemolytic anemia, positive Coombs' reaction

Renal: Acute interstitial nephritis

Miscellaneous: Hypersensitivity reactions, anaphylaxis

Overdosage/Toxicology Symptoms of penicillin overdose include neuromuscular hypersensitivity (agitation, hallucinations, asterixis, encephalopathy, confusion, and seizures) and electrolyte imbalance with potassium or sodium salts, especially in renal failure; hemodialysis may be helpful to aid in the removal of the drug from the blood, otherwise most treatment is supportive or symptom directed

Drug Interactions

Decreased effect: Tetracyclines → ↓ penicillin effectiveness

Increased effect:

Probenecid → ↑ penicillin levels

Aminoglycosides → synergistic efficacy

Stability Refrigerate suspension after reconstitution; discard after 14 days

Mechanism of Action Inhibits bacterial cell wall synthesis by binding to one or more of the penicillin binding proteins (PBPs); which in turn inhibits the final transpeptidation step of peptidoglycan synthesis in bacterial cell walls, thus inhibiting cell wall biosynthesis. Bacteria eventually lyse due to ongoing activity of cell wall autolytic enzymes (autolysins and murein hydrolases) while cell wall assembly is arrested.

Pharmacodynamics/Kinetics

Absorption: Oral: 60% to 73% from GI tract

Distribution: Appears in breast milk

Plasma protein binding: 80%

Half-life: 0.5 hours; prolonged in patients with renal impairment

Time to peak serum concentration: Oral: Within 0.5-1 hour

Elimination: Penicillin V and its metabolites are excreted in urine mainly by tubular secretion

Usual Dosage Oral:

Systemic infections:

Children <12 years: 25-50 mg/kg/day in divided doses every 6-8 hours; maximum dose: 3 g/day

Children ≥12 years and Adults: 125-500 mg every 6-8 hours

Prophylaxis of pneumococcal infections:

Children <5 years: 125 mg twice daily

Children ≥5 years and Adults: 250 mg twice daily

Prophylaxis of recurrent rheumatic fever:

Children <5 years: 125 mg twice daily

Children ≥5 years and Adults: 250 mg twice daily

Dosing interval in renal impairment:

Cl_{cr} 10-50 mL/minute: Administer every 8-12 hours

Cl_{cr} <10 mL/minute: Administer every 12-16 hours

Administration Administer around-the-clock rather than 4 times/day to promote less variation in peak and trough serum levels; give on an empty stomach to increase oral absorption

Monitoring Parameters Periodic renal and hematologic function tests during prolonged therapy

Test Interactions False-positive or negative urinary glucose determination using Clinitest®; positive Coombs' [direct]; false-positive urinary and/or serum proteins

Patient Information Take on an empty stomach 1 hour before or 2 hours after meals, take until gone, do not skip doses, report any rash or shortness of breath; shake liquid well before use

Additional Information 0.7 mEq of potassium per 250 mg penicillin V; 250 mg equals 400,000 units of penicillin

Dosage Forms

Powder for oral solution: 125 mg/5 mL (3 mL, 100 mL, 150 mL, 200 mL); 250 mg/5 mL (100 mL, 150 mL, 200 mL)

Tablet: 125 mg, 250 mg, 500 mg

Penicilloyl-polylysine *see* Benzylpenicilloyl-polylysine *on page 125*

Pentaerythritol Tetranitrate (pen ta er ith′ ri tole te tra nye′ trate)

Brand Names Duotrate®; Peritrate®; Peritrate® SA

Synonyms PETN

Use Possibly effective for the prophylactic long-term management of angina pectoris. **Note:** Not indicated to abort acute anginal episodes.

Pregnancy Risk Factor C

Contraindications Known hypersensitivity to pentaerythritol tetranitrate or other nitrates; severe anemia, closed-angle glaucoma, postural hypotension, cerebral hemorrhage, head trauma

Warnings/Precautions Use with caution in patients with hypotension, hypovolemia, or increased intracranial pressure

Adverse Reactions

>10%:

Cardiovascular: Flushing, postural hypotension

Central nervous system: Headache, lightheadedness, dizziness

Neuromuscular & skeletal: Weakness

1% to 10%: Dermatologic: Drug rash, exfoliative dermatitis

<1%:

Gastrointestinal: Nausea, vomiting,

Hematologic: Methemoglobinemia (overdose)

Overdosage/Toxicology Symptoms of overdose include hypotension, throbbing headache, palpitations, bloody diarrhea, bradycardia, cyanosis, tissue hypoxia, metabolic acidosis, clonic convulsions, circulatory collapse. Formation of methemoglobinemia is dose-related and unusual in normal or moderate overdoses; treatment is supportive and symptomatic; hypotension is treated with fluids, positioning and alpha-adrenergic pressors if needed; treat methemoglobinemia with oxygen and methylene blue at a dose of 1-2 mg/kg I.V. slowly.

Mechanism of Action Stimulation of intracellular cyclic-GMP results in vascular smooth muscle relaxation of both arterial and venous vasculature. Increased (Continued)

Pentaerythritol Tetranitrate *(Continued)*

venous pooling decreases left ventricular pressure (preload) and arterial dilatation decreases arterial resistance (afterload). Therefore, this reduces cardiac oxygen demand by decreasing left ventricular pressure and systemic vascular resistance by dilating arteries. Additionally, coronary artery dilation improves collateral flow to ischemic regions; esophageal smooth muscle is relaxed via the same mechanism.

Pharmacodynamics/Kinetics
Onset of hemodynamic effect: Oral: Within 20-60 minutes
Duration: 4-5 hours, or up to 12 hours with the sustained release formulations
Metabolism: In the liver
Half-life: 10 minutes
Elimination: In urine and to a smaller degree in bile

Usual Dosage Adults: Oral: 10-20 mg 4 times/day up to 40 mg 4 times/day before or after meals and at bedtime; sustained release preparation 80 mg twice daily; use lowest recommended doses in elderly initially; titrations up to 240 mg/day are tolerated, however, headache may occur with increasing doses (reduce dose for a few days; if headache returns or is persistent, an analgesic can be used to treat symptoms)

Patient Information Keep tablets in original tightly closed container; do not chew or crush sustained release product; do not change brands without consulting your pharmacist or physician; any angina that persists for more than 20 minutes should be evaluated by a physician immediately

Dosage Forms
Capsule: sustained release: 15 mg, 30 mg
Tablet: 10 mg, 20 mg, 40 mg
Tablet, sustained release: 80 mg

Pentagastrin *(pen ta gas' trin)*

Brand Names Peptavlon®
Use Evaluate gastric acid secretory function in pernicious anemia, gastric carcinoma; in suspected duodenal ulcer or Zollinger-Ellison syndrome
Pregnancy Risk Factor C
Contraindications Known hypersensitivity to pentagastrin
Warnings/Precautions Use with caution in patients with pancreatic, hepatic or biliary tract disease
Adverse Reactions
>10%: Gastrointestinal: Abdominal pain, desire to defecate, nausea, vomiting
1% to 10%:
Cardiovascular: Flushing, tachycardia, palpitations, hypotension
Central nervous system: Dizziness, faintness, headache
Respiratory: Shortness of breath
<1%: Allergic reactions
Overdosage/Toxicology Symptoms of overdose include tachycardia, dizziness, abdominal pain, vomiting, drowsiness; symptomatic treatment
Stability Refrigerate
Mechanism of Action Excites the oxyntic cells of the stomach to secrete to their maximum capacity similar to the naturally occurring hormone, gastrin
Pharmacodynamics/Kinetics
Absorption: I.M., S.C.: Well absorbed
Metabolism: In the liver
Half-life: 1 minute
Elimination: In bile
Usual Dosage Adults:
I.M., S.C.: 6 mcg/kg
I.V. infusion: 0.1-12 mcg/kg/hour in 0.9% sodium chloride
Patient Information Fast from food and liquids overnight and do not take antacids on the morning of the test nor drugs that inhibit gastric secretion
Dosage Forms Injection: 0.25 mg/mL (2 mL)

Pentam-300® *see* Pentamidine Isethionate *on this page*

Pentamidine Isethionate *(pen tam' i deen eye se thi' o nate)*

Brand Names NebuPent™; Pentam-300®
Use Treatment and prevention of pneumonia caused by *Pneumocystis carinii*; treatment of trypanosomiasis
Pregnancy Risk Factor C
Contraindications Hypersensitivity to pentamidine isethionate or any component (inhalation and injection)

Warnings/Precautions Use with caution in patients with diabetes mellitus, renal or hepatic dysfunction; hypertension or hypotension; leukopenia, thrombocytopenia, asthma, hypo/hyperglycemia

Adverse Reactions
>10%:
  Cardiovascular: Chest pain
  Dermatologic: Skin rash
  Endocrine & metabolic: Hyperkalemia
  Local: Local reactions at injection site
  Respiratory: Wheezing, dyspnea, coughing, pharyngitis
1% to 10%: Gastrointestinal: Bitter or metallic taste
<1%:
  Cardiovascular: Hypotension, tachycardia
  Central nervous system: Dizziness, fever, fatigue
  Endocrine & metabolic: Hyperglycemia or hypoglycemia, hypocalcemia
  Gastrointestinal: Pancreatitis, vomiting
  Hematologic: Megaloblastic anemia, granulocytopenia, leukopenia, thrombocytopenia
  Renal: Renal insufficiency
  Respiratory: Extrapulmonary pneumocystosis, irritation of the airway
  Miscellaneous: Pneumothorax, Jarisch-Herxheimer-like reaction, mild renal or hepatic injury

Overdosage/Toxicology Symptoms of overdose include hypotension, hypoglycemia, cardiac arrhythmias; treatment is supportive

Stability Do not refrigerate due to the possibility of crystallization; do not use NS as a diluent, NS is **incompatible** with pentamidine; reconstituted solutions (60-100 mg/mL) are stable for 48 hours at room temperature and do not require light protection; diluted solutions (1-2.5 mg/mL) in D_5W are stable for at least 24 hours at room temperature

Mechanism of Action Interferes with RNA/DNA, phospholipids and protein synthesis, through inhibition of oxidative phosphorylation and/or interference with incorporation of nucleotides and nucleic acids into RNA and DNA, in protozoa

Pharmacodynamics/Kinetics
Absorption: I.M.: Well absorbed
Distribution: Systemic accumulation of pentamidine does not appear to occur following inhalation therapy
Half-life, terminal: 6.4-9.4 hours; may be prolonged in patients with severe renal impairment
Elimination: 33% to 66% excreted in urine as unchanged drug

Usual Dosage
Children:
  Treatment: I.M., I.V. (I.V. preferred): 4 mg/kg/day once daily for 10-14 days
  Prevention:
    I.M., I.V.: 4 mg/kg monthly or every 2 weeks
    Inhalation (aerosolized pentamidine in children ≥5 years): 300 mg/dose given every 3-4 weeks via Respirgard® II inhaler (8 mg/kg dose has also been used in children <5 years)
  Treatment of trypanosomiasis: I.V.: 4 mg/kg/day once daily for 10 days

Adults:
  Treatment: I.M., I.V. (I.V. preferred): 4 mg/kg/day once daily for 14 days
  Prevention: Inhalation: 300 mg every 4 weeks via Respirgard® II nebulizer

Not removed by hemo or peritoneal dialysis or continuous arterio-venous or veno-venous hemofiltration (CAVH/CAVHD); supplemental dosage is not necessary

Administration Infuse I.V. slowly over a period of at least 60 minutes or administer deep I.M.; patients receiving I.V. or I.M. pentamidine should be lying down and blood pressure should be monitored closely during administration of drug and several times thereafter until it is stable

Monitoring Parameters Liver function tests, renal function tests, blood glucose, serum potassium and calcium, EKG, blood pressure

Patient Information PCP pneumonia may still occur despite pentamidine use; notify physician of fever, shortness of breath, or coughing up blood; maintain adequate fluid intake

Nursing Implications Virtually indetectable amounts are transferred to healthcare personnel during aerosol administration; **do not use NS as a diluent**

Dosage Forms
Inhalation: 300 mg
Injection: 300 mg

Pentasa® *see* Mesalamine *on page 691*

Pentazocine (pen taz′ oh seen)

Related Information
Narcotic Agonist Comparison Charts *on page 1274-1275*

Brand Names Talwin®; Talwin® NX

Synonyms Pentazocine Hydrochloride; Pentazocine Lactate

Use Relief of moderate to severe pain; has also been used as a sedative prior to surgery and as a supplement to surgical anesthesia

Restrictions C-IV

Pregnancy Risk Factor B (D if used for prolonged periods or in high doses at term)

Contraindications Hypersensitivity to pentazocine or any component, increased intracranial pressure (unless the patient is mechanically ventilated)

Warnings/Precautions Use with caution in seizure-prone patients, acute myocardial infarction, patients undergoing biliary tract surgery, patients with renal and hepatic dysfunction, head trauma, increased intracranial pressure, and patients with a history of prior opioid dependence or abuse; pentazocine may precipitate opiate withdrawal symptoms in patients who have been receiving opiates regularly; injection contains sulfites which may cause allergic reaction

Adverse Reactions
>10%:
 Central nervous system: Euphoria, weakness, drowsiness
 Gastrointestinal: Nausea, vomiting
1% to 10%:
 Cardiovascular: Hypotension
 Central nervous system: Malaise, headache, restlessness, nightmares
 Dermatologic: Skin rash
 Gastrointestinal: Dry mouth
 Genitourinary: Ureteral spasm
 Ocular: Blurred vision
 Respiratory: Troubled breathing
<1%:
 Central nervous system: Insomnia, CNS depression, sedation, hallucinations, confusion, disorientation, seizures may occur in seizure-prone patients, increased intracranial pressure
 Cardiovascular: Palpitations, bradycardia, peripheral vasodilation
 Dermatologic: Pruritus
 Endocrine & metabolic: Antidiuretic hormone release
 Gastrointestinal: GI irritation, constipation
 Local: Tissue damage and irritation with I.M./S.C. use
 Ocular: Miosis
 Miscellaneous: Biliary or urinary tract spasm, histamine release physical and psychological dependence

Overdosage/Toxicology Symptoms of overdose include drowsiness, sedation, respiratory depression, coma. Naloxone 2 mg I.V. (0.01 mg/kg for children) with repeat administration as necessary up to a total of 10 mg.

Drug Interactions May potentiate or reduce analgesic effect of opiate agonist, (eg, morphine) depending on patients tolerance to opiates can precipitate withdrawal in narcotic addicts

Increased effect/toxicity with tripelennamine (can be lethal), CNS depressants (phenothiazines, tranquilizers, anxiolytics, sedatives, hypnotics, or alcohol)

Stability Store at room temperature, protect from heat and from freezing; I.V. form is **incompatible** with aminophylline, amobarbital (and all other I.V. barbiturates), glycopyrrolate (same syringe), heparin (same syringe), nafcillin (Y-site)

Mechanism of Action Binds to opiate receptors in the CNS, causing inhibition of ascending pain pathways, altering the perception of and response to pain; produces generalized CNS depression; partial agonist-antagonist

Pharmacodynamics/Kinetics
Onset of action:
 Oral, I.M., S.C.: Within 15-30 minutes
 I.V.: Within 2-3 minutes
Duration:
 Oral: 4-5 hours
 Parenteral: 2-3 hours
Protein binding: 60%
Metabolism: Large first-pass effect; metabolized in liver via oxidative and glucuronide conjugation pathways
Bioavailability, oral: ~20%; increased to 60% to 70% in patients with cirrhosis
Half-life: 2-3 hours; increased with decreased hepatic function
Elimination: Smaller amounts excreted unchanged in urine

Usual Dosage
Children: I.M., S.C.:
 5-8 years: 15 mg

8-14 years: 30 mg

Children >12 years and Adults: Oral: 50 mg every 3-4 hours; may increase to 100 mg/dose if needed, but should not exceed 600 mg/day

Adults:
I.M., S.C.: 30-60 mg every 3-4 hours, not to exceed total daily dose of 360 mg
I.V.: 30 mg every 3-4 hours

Dosing adjustment in renal impairment:
Cl_{cr} 10-50 mL/minute: Administer 75% of normal dose
Cl_{cr} <10 mL/minute: Administer 50% of normal dose

Dosing adjustment in hepatic impairment: Reduce dose or avoid use in patients with liver disease

Administration Rotate injection site for I.M., S.C. use; avoid intra-arterial injection

Monitoring Parameters Relief of pain, respiratory and mental status, blood pressure

Patient Information Avoid alcohol, may cause drowsiness, impaired judgment or coordination; may cause physical and psychological dependence with prolonged use; will cause withdrawal in patients currently dependent on narcotics

Nursing Implications Observe patient for excessive sedation, respiratory depression, implement safety measures, assist with ambulation; observe for narcotic withdrawal

Additional Information Pentazocine hydrochloride: Talwin® NX tablet (with naloxone); naloxone is used to prevent abuse by dissolving tablets in water and using as injection

Dosage Forms
Injection, as lactate: 30 mg/mL (1 mL, 1.5 mL, 2 mL, 10 mL)
Tablet: Pentazocine hydrochloride 50 mg and naloxone hydrochloride 0.5 mg

Pentazocine Hydrochloride see Pentazocine on page 857

Pentazocine Lactate see Pentazocine on page 857

Pentobarbital (pen toe bar' bi tal)
Brand Names Nembutal®
Synonyms Pentobarbital Sodium
Use Short-term treatment of insomnia; preoperative sedation; high-dose barbiturate coma for treatment of increased intracranial pressure or status epilepticus unresponsive to other therapy
Restrictions C-II (capsules, injection); C-III (suppositories)
Pregnancy Risk Factor D
Contraindications Marked liver function impairment or latent porphyria; hypersensitivity to barbiturates or any component
Warnings/Precautions Tolerance to hypnotic effect can occur; do not use for >2 weeks to treat insomnia; taper dose to prevent withdrawal; loading doses of 15-35 mg/kg (given over 1-2 hours) have been utilized in pediatric patients to induce pentobarbital coma, but these higher loading doses often cause hypotension requiring vasopressor therapy. Use of this agent as a hypnotic in the elderly is not recommended due to its long half-life and potential for physical and psychological dependence. Use with caution in patients with hypovolemic shock, congestive heart failure, hepatic impairment, respiratory dysfunction or depression, previous addiction to the sedative/hypnotic group, chronic or acute pain, renal dysfunction; tolerance or psychological and physical dependence may occur with prolonged use.
Adverse Reactions
Genitourinary: Oliguria
>10%:
Cardiovascular: Cardiac arrhythmias, bradycardia, hypotension, arterial spasm, and gangrene with inadvertent intra-arterial injection
Central nervous system: Drowsiness, lethargy, CNS excitation or depression, impaired judgment, "hangover" effect
Local: Pain at injection site, thrombophlebitis with I.V. use
1% to 10%:
Central nervous system: Confusion, mental depression, unusual excitement, nervousness, faint feeling, headache, insomnia, nightmares
Gastrointestinal: Nausea, vomiting, constipation
<1%:
Cardiovascular: Thrombophlebitis, hypotension
Central nervous system: Hallucinations
Dermatologic: Rash, exfoliative dermatitis, Stevens-Johnson syndrome
(Continued)

Pentobarbital *(Continued)*

    Endocrine & metabolic: Hypothermia
    Hematologic: Agranulocytosis, thrombocytopenia, megaloblastic anemia
    Respiratory: Laryngospasm, respiratory depression, apnea (especially with rapid I.V. use)

Overdosage/Toxicology Symptoms of overdose include unsteady gait, slurred speech, confusion, jaundice, hypothermia, hypotension, respiratory depression, coma

If hypotension occurs, administer I.V. fluids and place the patient in the Trendelenburg position. If unresponsive, an I.V. vasopressor (eg, dopamine, epinephrine) may be required. Forced alkaline diuresis is of no value in the treatment of intoxications with short-acting barbiturates. Charcoal hemoperfusion or hemodialysis may be useful in the harder to treat intoxications, especially in the presence of very high serum barbiturate levels when the patient is in a coma, shock, or renal failure.

Drug Interactions
    Decreased effect: Decreased chloramphenicol; decreased doxycycline effects
    Increased toxicity: Increased CNS depressants, cimetidine; → ↑ pentobarbital

Stability Protect from light; aqueous solutions are not stable, commercially available vehicle (containing propylene glycol) is more stable; low pH may cause precipitate; use only clear solution

Mechanism of Action Short-acting barbiturate with sedative, hypnotic, and anticonvulsant properties

Pharmacodynamics/Kinetics
    Onset of action:
        Oral, rectal: 15-60 minutes
        I.M.: Within 10-15 minutes
        I.V.: Within 1 minute
    Duration:
        Oral, rectal: 1-4 hours
        I.V.: 15 minutes
    Distribution: V_d:
        Children: 0.8 L/kg
        Adults: 1 L/kg
    Protein binding: 35% to 55%
    Metabolism: Extensively in liver via hydroxylation and oxidation pathways
    Half-life, terminal:
        Children: 25 hours
        Adults, normal: 22 hours; range: 35-50 hours
    Elimination: <1% excreted unchanged renally

Usual Dosage
    Children:
        Sedative: Oral: 2-6 mg/kg/day divided in 3 doses; maximum: 100 mg/day
        Hypnotic: I.M.: 2-6 mg/kg; maximum: 100 mg/dose
        Rectal:
            2 months to 1 year (10-20 lb): 30 mg
            1-4 years (20-40 lb): 30-60 mg
            5-12 years (40-80 lb): 60 mg
            12-14 years (80-110 lb): 60-120 mg
        or
            <4 years: 3-6 mg/kg/dose
            >4 years: 1.5-3 mg/kg/dose
        Preoperative/preprocedure sedation: ≥6 months:
            Oral, I.M., rectal: 2-6 mg/kg; maximum: 100 mg/dose
            I.V.: 1-3 mg/kg to a maximum of 100 mg until asleep
        Children 5-12 years: Conscious sedation prior to a procedure: I.V.: 2 mg/kg 5-10 minutes before procedures, may repeat one time

    Adolescents: Conscious sedation: Oral, I.V.: 100 mg prior to a procedure

    Adults:
        Hypnotic:
            Oral: 100-200 mg at bedtime or 20 mg 3-4 times/day for daytime sedation
            I.M.: 150-200 mg
            I.V.: Initial: 100 mg, may repeat every 1-3 minutes up to 200-500 mg total dose
        Rectal: 120-200 mg at bedtime
        Preoperative sedation: I.M.: 150-200 mg

    Children and Adults: Barbiturate coma in head injury patients: I.V.: Loading dose: 5-10 mg/kg given slowly over 1-2 hours; monitor blood pressure and respiratory rate; Maintenance infusion: Initial: 1 mg/kg/hour; may increase to 2-3 mg/kg/hour; maintain burst suppression on EEG

Dosing adjustment in hepatic impairment: Reduce dosage in patients with severe liver dysfunction

Administration Pentobarbital may be administered by deep I.M. or slow I.V. injection. I.M.: No more than 5 mL (250 mg) should be injected at any one site because of possible tissue irritation I.V. push doses can be given undiluted, but should be administered no faster than 50 mg/minute; parenteral solutions are highly alkaline; avoid extravasation; avoid rapid I.V. administration >50 mg/minute; avoid intra-arterial injection

Monitoring Parameters Respiratory status (for conscious sedation, includes pulse oximetry), cardiovascular status, CNS status; cardiac monitor and blood pressure monitor required

Reference Range
Therapeutic:
Hypnotic: 1-5 μg/mL (SI: 4-22 μmol/L)
Coma: 10-50 μg/mL (SI: 88-221 μmol/L)
Toxic: >10 μg/mL (SI: >44 μmol/L)

Test Interactions ↑ ammonia (B); ↓ bilirubin (S)

Patient Information Avoid the use of alcohol and other CNS depressants; avoid driving and other hazardous tasks; avoid abrupt discontinuation; may cause physical and psychological dependence; do not alter dose without notifying physician

Nursing Implications Avoid extravasation; institute safety measures to avoid injuries; has many incompatibilities when given I.V.

Additional Information Pentobarbital: Nembutal® elixir pentobarbital sodium: Nembutal® capsule, injection, and suppository
Sodium content of 1 mL injection: 5 mg (0.2 mEq)

Dosage Forms
Capsule, as sodium: 50 mg, 100 mg
Elixir: 18.2 mg/5 mL (473 mL, 4000 mL)
Injection, as sodium: 50 mg/mL (1 mL, 2 mL, 20 mL, 50 mL)
Suppository, rectal: 30 mg, 60 mg, 120 mg, 200 mg

Pentobarbital Sodium see Pentobarbital on page 859

Pentostatin (pen' toe stat in)

Brand Names Nipent™

Synonyms DCF; Deoxycoformycin; 2'-deoxycoformycin

Use Treatment of adult patients with alpha-interferon-refractory hairy cell leukemia; non-Hodgkin's lymphoma, cutaneous T-cell lymphoma

Pregnancy Risk Factor D

Contraindications Limited or severely compromised bone marrow reserves (white blood cell count <3000 cells/mm^3)

Warnings/Precautions The FDA currently recommends that procedures for proper handling and disposal of antineoplastic agents be considered. Pregnant women or women of childbearing age should be apprised of the potential risk to the fetus; use extreme caution in the presence of renal insufficiency; use with caution in patients with signs or symptoms of impaired hepatic function.

Adverse Reactions
>10%:
Central nervous system: Headache, neurologic disorder, fever, fatigue, chills
Dermatologic: Rash
Gastrointestinal: Vomiting, nausea, anorexia, diarrhea
Hematologic: Leukopenia, anemia, thrombocytopenia
Hepatic: Hepatic disorder, abnormal liver function tests
Neuromuscular & skeletal: Myalgia
Respiratory: Coughing
Miscellaneous: Pain, allergic reaction
1% to 10%:
Cardiovascular: Chest pain, arrhythmia, peripheral edema
Central nervous system: Anxiety, confusion, depression, dizziness, insomnia, lethargy, coma, seizures, asthenia, malaise
Dermatologic: Dry skin, eczema, pruritus, sweating
Gastrointestinal: Constipation, flatulence, stomatitis, weight loss
Hematologic: Myelosuppression
Hepatic: Liver dysfunction
Local: Thrombophlebitis
Neuromuscular & skeletal: Arthralgia, paresthesia
Ocular: Abnormal vision, eye pain, keratoconjunctivitis
Renal: Renal failure, hematuria, dysuria
Respiratory: Bronchitis, dyspnea, lung edema, pneumonia
Miscellaneous: Death, back pain, ear pain, opportunistic infections
(Continued)

Pentostatin *(Continued)*

Overdosage/Toxicology Symptoms of overdose include severe renal, hepatic, pulmonary, and CNS toxicity; supportive therapy

Drug Interactions Increased toxicity: Vidarabine, fludarabine, allopurinol

Stability Vials are stable under refrigeration at 2°C to 8°C; reconstituted vials, or further dilutions, may be stored at room temperature exposed to ambient light; diluted solutions are stable for 24 hours in D_5W or 48 hours in NS or lactated Ringer's at room temperature; infusion with 5% dextrose injection USP or 0.9% sodium chloride injection USP does not interact with PVC-containing administration sets or containers

Mechanism of Action An antimetabolite inhibiting adenosine deaminase (ADA), prevents ADA from controlling intracellular adenosine levels through the irreversible deamination of adenosine and deoxyadenosine. ADA is found to exhibit the highest activity in lymphoid tissue. Patients receiving pentostatin accumulate deoxyadenosine (dAdo) and deoxyadenosine 5′-triphosphate (dATP); accumulation of dATP results in cell death, probably through inhibiting DNA or RNA synthesis. Following a single dose, pentostatin has the ability to inhibit ADA for periods exceeding 1 week.

Pharmacodynamics/Kinetics

Distribution: I.V.: V_d: 36.1 L (20.1 L/m^2); distributes rapidly to body tissues and may obtain plasma concentrations ranging from 12-36 ng following doses of 250 mcg/kg for 4-5 days

Half-life, terminal: 5-15 hours

Elimination: ~50% to 96% is recovered in urine within 24 hours

Usual Dosage Refractory hairy cell leukemia: Adults (refer to individual protocols): 4 mg/m^2 every other week; I.V. bolus over ≥3-5 minutes in D_5W or NS at concentrations ≥2 mg/mL

Dosing interval in renal impairment:
Cl_{cr} <80 mL/minute: Use extreme caution
Cl_{cr} 50-60 mL/minute: 2 mg/m^2/dose

Dosage Forms Powder for injection: 10 mg/vial

Pentothal® Sodium *see* Thiopental Sodium *on page 1082*

Pentoxifylline (pen tox i′ fi leen)

Brand Names Trental®

Synonyms Oxpentifylline

Use Symptomatic management of peripheral vascular disease, mainly intermittent claudication

Unapproved use: AIDS patients with increased TNF, CVA, cerebrovascular diseases, diabetic atherosclerosis, diabetic neuropathy, gangrene, hemodialysis shunt thrombosis, vascular impotence, cerebral malaria, septic shock, sickle cell syndromes, and vasculitis

Pregnancy Risk Factor C

Contraindications Hypersensitivity to pentoxifylline or any component and other xanthine derivatives

Warnings/Precautions Use with caution in patients with renal impairment or chronic occlusive arterial disease of the limbs

Adverse Reactions

1% to 10%:
Central nervous system: Dizziness, headache
Gastrointestinal: Dyspepsia, nausea, vomiting

<1%:
Cardiovascular: Mild hypotension, angina
Central nervous system: Agitation
Ocular: Blurred vision
Otic: Earache

Overdosage/Toxicology Symptoms of overdose include hypotension, flushing, convulsions, deep sleep, agitation, bradycardia, A-V block. Treatment is supportive; seizures can be treated with diazepam 5-10 mg (0.25-0.4 mg/kg in children); arrhythmias respond to lidocaine.

Drug Interactions Increased effect/toxic potential with cimetidine (↑ levels) and other H_2 antagonists, warfarin; increased effect of antihypertensives

Mechanism of Action Mechanism of action remains unclear; is thought to reduce blood viscosity and improve blood flow by altering the rheology of red blood cells

Pharmacodynamics/Kinetics

Absorption: Oral: Well absorbed

Metabolism: Undergoes first-pass metabolism in the liver

Half-life:
  Parent drug: 24-48 minutes
  Metabolites: 60-96 minutes
Time to peak serum concentration: Within 2-4 hours
Elimination: Mainly in urine
Usual Dosage Adults: Oral: 400 mg 3 times/day with meals; may reduce to 400 mg twice daily if GI or CNS side effects occur
Test Interactions ↓ calcium (S), ↓ magnesium (S), false-positive theophylline levels
Patient Information Take with food or meals; if GI or CNS side effects continue, contact physician; while effects may be seen in 2-4 weeks, continue treatment for at least 8 weeks
Dosage Forms Tablet, controlled release: 400 mg

Pen.Vee® K *see* Penicillin V Potassium *on page 854*

Pen VK *see* Penicillin V Potassium *on page 854*

Pepcid® [OTC] *see* Famotidine *on page 440*

Peptavlon® *see* Pentagastrin *on page 856*

Pepto-Bismol® [OTC] *see* Bismuth *on page 134*

Pepto® Diarrhea Control [OTC *see* Loperamide Hydrochloride *on page 647*

Percocet® *see* Oxycodone and Acetaminophen *on page 826*

Percodan® *see* Oxycodone and Aspirin *on page 828*

Percodan®-Demi *see* Oxycodone and Aspirin *on page 828*

Perdiem® Plain [OTC] *see* Psyllium *on page 956*

Perfectoderm® [OTC] *see* Benzoyl Peroxide *on page 122*

Pergolide Mesylate (per' go lide)
Brand Names Permax®
Use Adjunctive treatment to levodopa/carbidopa in the management of Parkinson's Disease
Pregnancy Risk Factor B
Contraindications Known hypersensitivity to pergolide mesylate or other ergot derivatives
Warnings/Precautions Symptomatic hypotension occurs in 10% of patients; use with caution in patients with a history of cardiac arrhythmias, hallucinations, or mental illness
Adverse Reactions
>10%:
  Central nervous system: Dizziness, somnolence, insomnia, confusion, hallucinations, anxiety, dystonia
  Gastrointestinal: Nausea, constipation
  Neuromuscular & skeletal: Dyskinesia
  Respiratory: Rhinitis
1% to 10%:
  Central nervous system: Insomnia, abnormal vision, asthenia, chills
  Cardiovascular: Myocardial infarction, postural hypotension, syncope, arrhythmias, peripheral edema, vasodilation, palpitations, chest pain, dyspnea
  Gastrointestinal: Diarrhea, abdominal pain, vomiting, dry mouth, anorexia, weight gain
  Miscellaneous: Flu syndrome
Overdosage/Toxicology Symptoms of overdose include vomiting, hypotension, agitation, hallucinations, ventricular extrasystoles, possible seizures; data on overdose is limited; treatment is supportive and may require antiarrhythmias and/or neuroleptics for agitation; hypotension, when unresponsive to I.V. fluids or Trendelenburg positioning, often responds to norepinephrine infusions started at 0.1-0.2 mcg/kg/minute followed by a titrated infusion. If signs of CNS stimulation are present, a neuroleptic may be indicated; antiarrhythmics may be indicated, monitor EKG; activated charcoal is useful to prevent further absorption and to hasten elimination.
Drug Interactions
Decreased effect: Dopamine antagonists, metoclopramide
Increased toxicity: Highly plasma protein bound drugs
Mechanism of Action Pergolide is a semisynthetic ergot alkaloid similar to bromocriptine but stated to be more potent and longer-acting; it is a centrally-active dopamine agonist stimulating both D_1 and D_2 receptors
Pharmacodynamics/Kinetics
Absorption: Oral: Well absorbed
(Continued)

Pergolide Mesylate *(Continued)*

Protein binding: Plasma 90%

Metabolism: Extensive in the liver (on first-pass)

Elimination: ~50% excreted in urine and 50% in feces

Usual Dosage When adding pergolide to levodopa/carbidopa, the dose of the latter can usually and should be decreased. Patients no longer responsive to bromocriptine may benefit by being switched to pergolide.

Adults: Oral: Start with 0.05 mg/day for 2 days, then increase dosage by 0.1 or 0.15 mg/day every 3 days over next 12 days, increase dose by 0.25 mg/day every 3 days until optimal therapeutic dose is achieved, up to 5 mg/day maximum; usual dosage range: 2-3 mg/day in 3 divided doses

Monitoring Parameters Blood pressure (both sitting/supine and standing), symptoms of parkinsonism, dyskinesias, mental status

Patient Information Take with food or milk; rise slowly from sitting or lying down; report any confusion or change in mental status

Nursing Implications Monitor closely for orthostasis and other adverse effects; raise bed rails and institute safety measures; aid patient with ambulation, may cause postural hypotension and drowsiness

Dosage Forms Tablet: 0.05 mg, 0.25 mg, 1 mg

Pergonal® *see* Menotropins *on page 684*

Periactin® *see* Cyproheptadine Hydrochloride *on page 292*

Peridex® *see* Chlorhexidine Gluconate *on page 223*

Peritrate® *see* Pentaerythritol Tetranitrate *on page 855*

Peritrate® SA *see* Pentaerythritol Tetranitrate *on page 855*

Permapen® *see* Penicillin G Benzathine, Parenteral *on page 849*

Permax® *see* Pergolide Mesylate *on previous page*

Permethrin (per meth' rin)

Brand Names Elimite™; Nix™ [OTC]

Use Single application treatment of infestation with *Pediculus humanus capitis* (head louse) and its nits or *Sarcoptes scabiei* (scabies)

Pregnancy Risk Factor B

Contraindications Known hypersensitivity to pyrethyroid, pyrethrin, or chrysanthemums

Warnings/Precautions Treatment may temporarily exacerbate the symptoms of itching, redness, swelling; for external use only; use during pregnancy only if clearly needed

Adverse Reactions

1% to 10%:

Dermatologic: Pruritus, erythema, rash of the scalp, numbness or scalp discomfort,

Local: Burning, stinging, tingling, numbness or scalp discomfort, edema

Mechanism of Action Inhibits sodium ion influx through nerve cell membrane channels in parasites resulting in delayed repolarization and thus paralysis and death of the pest

Pharmacodynamics/Kinetics

Absorption: Topical: Minimal (<2%)

Metabolism: In the liver by ester hydrolysis to inactive metabolites

Elimination: In urine

Usual Dosage Topical: Children >2 months and Adults:

Head lice: After hair has been washed with shampoo, rinsed with water, and towel dried, apply a sufficient volume of topical liquid to saturate the hair and scalp. Leave on hair for 10 minutes before rinsing off with water; remove remaining nits; may repeat in 1 week if lice or nits still present.

Scabies: Apply cream from head to toe; leave on for 8-14 hours before washing off with water; for infants, also apply on the hairline, neck, scalp, temple, and forehead; may reapply in 1 week if live mites appear

Permethrin 5% cream was shown to be safe and effective when applied to an infant <1 month of age with neonatal scabies; time of application was limited to 6 hours before rinsing with soap and water

Patient Information Avoid contact with eyes and mucous membranes during application; shake well before using; notify physician if irritation persists; clothing and bedding should be washed in hot water or dry cleaned to kill the scabies mite

Dosage Forms

Cream: 5% (60 g)

Liquid, topical: 1% (60 mL)

Permitil® *see* Fluphenazine *on page 478*

Perphenazine (per fen′ a zeen)
Related Information
Antipsychotic Agents Comparison *on page 1255*
Brand Names Trilafon®
Use Management of manifestations of psychotic disorders, depressive neurosis, alcohol withdrawal, nausea and vomiting, nonpsychotic symptoms associated with dementia in elderly, Tourette's syndrome, Huntington's chorea, spasmodic torticollis and Reye's syndrome
Pregnancy Risk Factor C
Contraindications Hypersensitivity to perphenazine or any component, cross-sensitivity with other phenothiazines may exist; avoid use in patients with narrow-angle glaucoma, bone marrow depression, severe liver or cardiac disease; subcortical brain damage; circulatory collapse; severe hypotension or hypertension
Warnings/Precautions Safety in children <6 months of age has not been established; use with caution in patients with cardiovascular disease or seizures, bone marrow depression, severe liver or cardiac disease
Adverse Reactions
>10%:
  Cardiovascular: Hypotension, orthostatic hypotension
  Central nervous system: Pseudoparkinsonism, akathisia, dystonias, tardive dyskinesia (persistent), dizziness
  Gastrointestinal: Constipation
  Ocular: Pigmentary retinopathy
  Respiratory: Nasal congestion
  Miscellaneous: Decreased sweating
1% to 10%:
  Central nervous system: Dizziness
  Dermatologic: Increased sensitivity to sun, skin rash
  Endocrine & metabolic: Changes in menstrual cycle, changes in libido, pain in breasts
  Gastrointestinal: Weight gain, vomiting, stomach pain, nausea
  Genitourinary: Difficulty in urination, ejaculatory disturbances
  Neuromuscular & skeletal: Trembling of fingers
<1%:
  Central nervous system: Neuroleptic malignant syndrome (NMS)
  Dermatologic: Discoloration of skin (blue-gray), pigmentary retinopathy
  Endocrine & metabolic: Galactorrhea
  Genitourinary: Priapism
  Hematologic: Agranulocytosis, leukopenia
  Hepatic: Cholestatic jaundice, hepatotoxicity
  Ocular: Cornea and lens changes
  Miscellaneous: Impairment of temperature regulation, lowering of seizures threshold
Overdosage/Toxicology Symptoms of overdose include deep sleep, dystonia, agitation, coma, abnormal involuntary muscle movements, hypotension, arrhythmias

Following initiation of essential overdose management, toxic symptom treatment and supportive treatment should be initiated. Hypotension usually responds to I.V. fluids or Trendelenburg positioning. If unresponsive to these measures, the use of a parenteral inotrope may be required (eg, norepinephrine 0.1-0.2 mcg/kg/minute titrated to response). Seizures commonly respond to diazepam (I.V. 5-10 mg bolus in adults every 15 minutes if needed up to a total of 30 mg; I.V. 0.25-0.4 mg/kg/dose up to a total of 10 mg in children) or to phenytoin or phenobarbital. Extrapyramidal symptoms (eg, dystonic reactions) may be managed with diphenhydramine. When these reactions are unresponsive to diphenhydramine, benztropine mesylate may be effective.
Drug Interactions
Decreased effect: Anticholinergics, anticonvulsants; decreased effect of guanethidine, epinephrine
Increased toxicity: CNS depressants; increased effect/toxicity of anticonvulsants
Mechanism of Action Blocks postsynaptic mesolimbic dopaminergic receptors in the brain; exhibits a strong alpha-adrenergic blocking effect and depresses the release of hypothalamic and hypophyseal hormones
Pharmacodynamics/Kinetics
Absorption: Oral: Well absorbed
Distribution: Crosses the placenta
Metabolism: In the liver
Half-life: 9 hours
(Continued)

Perphenazine *(Continued)*

Time to peak serum concentration: Within 4-8 hours
Elimination: In urine and bile

Usual Dosage

Children:
  Psychoses: Oral:
    1-6 years: 4-6 mg/day in divided doses
    6-12 years: 6 mg/day in divided doses
    >12 years: 4-16 mg 2-4 times/day
    I.M.: 5 mg every 6 hours
  Nausea/vomiting: I.M.: 5 mg every 6 hours

Adults:
  Psychoses:
    Oral: 4-16 mg 2-4 times/day not to exceed 64 mg/day
    I.M.: 5 mg every 6 hours up to 15 mg/day in ambulatory patients and 30 mg/day in hospitalized patients
  Nausea/vomiting:
    Oral: 8-16 mg/day in divided doses up to 24 mg/day
    I.M.: 5-10 mg every 6 hours as necessary up to 15 mg/day in ambulatory patients and 30 mg/day in hospitalized patients
    I.V. (severe): 1 mg at 1- to 2-minute intervals up to a total of 5 mg

Not dialyzable (0% to 5%)

Dosing adjustment in hepatic impairment: Dosage reductions should be considered in patients with liver disease although no specific guidelines are available

Administration Dilute oral concentration to at least 2 oz with water, juice, or milk for I.V. use, injection should be diluted to at least 0.5 mg/mL with NS and given a a rate of 1 mg/minute; observe for tremor and abnormal movements or posturing

Reference Range 2-6 nmol/L

Test Interactions ↑ cholesterol (S), ↑ glucose; ↓ uric acid (S)

Patient Information May cause drowsiness, impair judgment and coordination report any feelings of restlessness or any involuntary movements; avoid alcohol and other CNS depressants; do not alter dose or discontinue without consulting physician

Nursing Implications Monitor for hypotension when administering I.M. or I.V during the first 3-5 days after initiating therapy or making a dosage adjustment

Dosage Forms

Concentrate, oral: 16 mg/5 mL (118 mL)
Injection: 5 mg/mL (1 mL)
Tablet: 2 mg, 4 mg, 8 mg, 16 mg

Persa-Gel® *see* Benzoyl Peroxide *on page 122*

Persantine® *see* Dipyridamole *on page 357*

Pertofrane® *see* Desipramine Hydrochloride *on page 309*

Pertussin® CS [OTC] *see* Dextromethorphan *on page 321*

Pertussin® ES [OTC] *see* Dextromethorphan *on page 321*

Pethidine Hydrochloride *see* Meperidine Hydrochloride *on page 684*

PETN *see* Pentaerythritol Tetranitrate *on page 855*

PFA *see* Foscarnet *on page 488*

Pfizerpen® *see* Penicillin G, Parenteral, Aqueous *on page 850*

Pfizerpen®-AS *see* Penicillin G Procaine *on page 853*

PGE₁ *see* Alprostadil *on page 45*

PGE₂ *see* Dinoprostone *on page 349*

Pharmaflur® *see* Fluoride *on page 471*

Phazyme® [OTC] *see* Simethicone *on page 1006*

Phenantoin *see* Mephenytoin *on page 686*

Phenaphen® With Codeine *see* Acetaminophen and Codeine *on page 19*

Phenazine® *see* Promethazine Hydrochloride *on page 939*

Phenazodine® *see* Phenazopyridine Hydrochloride *on this page*

Phenazopyridine Hydrochloride (fen az oh peer' i deen)

Brand Names Azo-Standard®; Baridium®; Eridium®; Geridium®; Phenazo-dine®; Pyridiate®; Pyridium®; Urodine®; Urogesic®

Synonyms Phenylazo Diamino Pyridine Hydrochloride

Use Symptomatic relief of urinary burning, itching, frequency and urgency in association with urinary tract infection or following urologic procedures

Pregnancy Risk Factor B

Contraindications Hypersensitivity to phenazopyridine or any component; kidney or liver disease

Warnings/Precautions Does not treat infection, acts only as an analgesic; drug should be discontinued if skin or sclera develop a yellow color; use with caution in patients with renal impairment. Use of this agent in the elderly is limited since accumulation of phenazopyridine can occur in patients with renal insufficiency. It should not be used in patients with a Cl_{cr} <50 mL/minute.

Adverse Reactions

1% to 10%:
Central nervous system: Headache, dizziness
Gastrointestinal: Stomach cramps
<1%:
Central nervous system: Vertigo
Dermatologic: Skin pigmentation, rash
Hematologic: Methemoglobinemia, hemolytic anemia
Hepatic: Hepatitis
Renal: Acute renal failure

Overdosage/Toxicology Symptoms of overdose include methemoglobinemia, hemolytic anemia, skin pigmentation, renal and hepatic impairment; antidote is methylene blue 1-2 mg/kg I.V. for methemoglobinemia

Mechanism of Action An azo dye which exerts local anesthetic or analgesic action on urinary tract mucosa through an unknown mechanism

Pharmacodynamics/Kinetics
Metabolism: In the liver and other tissues
Elimination: In urine (where it exerts its action); renal excretion (as unchanged drug) is rapid and accounts for 65% of the drug's elimination

Usual Dosage Oral:
Children: 12 mg/kg/day in 3 divided doses administered after meals for 2 days

Adults: 100-200 mg 3 times/day after meals for 2 days when used concomitantly with an antibacterial agent

Dosing interval in renal impairment:
Cl_{cr} 50-80 mL/minute: Administer every 8-16 hours
Cl_{cr} <50 mL/minute: Avoid use

Test Interactions Phenazopyridine may cause delayed reactions with glucose oxidase reagents (Clinistix®, Tes-Tape®); occasional false-positive tests occur with Tes-Tape®; cupric sulfate tests (Clinitest®) are not affected; interference may also occur with urine ketone tests (Acetest®, Ketostix®) and urinary protein tests; tests for urinary steroids and porphyrins may also occur

Patient Information Take after meals; tablets may color urine orange or red and may stain clothing

Dosage Forms Tablet: 100 mg, 200 mg

Phencen® *see* Promethazine Hydrochloride *on page 939*

Phenelzine Sulfate (fen' el zeen)

Related Information
Antidepressant Agents Comparison *on page 1250-1252*
Brand Names Nardil®
Use Symptomatic treatment of atypical, nonendogenous or neurotic depression

The MAO inhibitors are usually reserved for patients who do not tolerate or respond to the traditional "cyclic" or "second generation" antidepressants. The brain activity of monoamine oxidase increases with age and even more so in patients with Alzheimer's disease. Therefore, the MAO inhibitors may have an increased role in patients with Alzheimer's disease who are depressed. Phenelzine is less stimulating than tranylcypromine.

Pregnancy Risk Factor C

Contraindications Pheochromocytoma, hepatic or renal disease, cerebrovascular defect, cardiovascular disease, hypersensitivity to phenelzine or any component, do not use within 5 weeks of fluoxetine or 2 weeks of sertraline or paroxetine discontinuance

Warnings/Precautions Safety in children <16 years of age has not been established; use with caution in patients who are hyperactive, hyperexcitable, or who
(Continued)

Phenelzine Sulfate *(Continued)*

have glaucoma; avoid use of meperidine within 2 weeks of phenelzine use. Hypertensive crisis may occur with tyramine. See table for foods containing tyramine.

Tyramine-Containing Foods

Cheese/Dairy Products

American processed	Cheddar	Roquefort
Blue	Emmenthaler	Sour cream
Boursault	Gruyere	Stilton
Brick, natural	Mozzarella	Yogurt
Brie	Parmesan	
Camembert	Romano	

Meat/Fish

Beef or chicken liver, other meats, fish (unrefrigerated, fermented)	Fermented sausages (bologna, pepperoni, salami, summer sausage)	Caviar Dried fish (salted herring)
	Game meat	Herring, pickled, spoiled
Meats prepared with tenderizer		Shrimp paste

Alcoholic Beverages (Undistilled)

Beer and ale (imports, some nonalcoholic)	Red wine (especially Chianti)	Sherry

Fruit/Vegetables

Avocados (especially overripe)	Bananas	Soy sauce
	Figs, canned (overripe)	Miso soup
Yeast extracts (Marmite, etc)	Raisins	Bean curd

Foods Containing Other Vasopressors

Fava beans (overripe) — dopamine	Caffeine (eg, coffee, tea, colas) — caffeine	Chocolate — phenylethylamine Ginseng

The MAO inhibitors are effective and generally well tolerated by older patients. It is the potential interactions with tyramine or tryptophan-containing foods and other drugs, and their effects on blood pressure that have limited their use.

Adverse Reactions

>10%:
  Cardiovascular: Orthostatic hypotension
  Central nervous system: Drowsiness, weakness
  Endocrine & metabolic: Decreased sexual ability
  Neuromuscular & skeletal: Trembling
  Ocular: Blurred vision

1% to 10%:
  Cardiovascular: Tachycardia, peripheral edema
  Central nervous system: Nervousness, chills
  Gastrointestinal: Diarrhea, anorexia, dry mouth, constipation

<1%:
  Central nervous system: Parkinsonism syndrome
  Hematologic: Leukopenia
  Hepatic: Hepatitis

Overdosage/Toxicology Symptoms of overdose include tachycardia, palpitations, muscle twitching, seizures, insomnia, restlessness, transient hypertension, hypotension, drowsiness, hyperpyrexia, coma. Competent supportive care is the most important treatment for an overdose with a monoamine oxidase (MAO) inhibitor. Both hypertension or hypotension can occur with intoxication. Hypotension may respond to I.V. fluids or vasopressors and hypertension usually responds to an alpha-adrenergic blocker. While treating the hypertension, care is warranted to avoid sudden drops in blood pressure, since this may worsen the MAO inhibitor toxicity. Muscle irritability and seizures often respond to diazepam while hyperthermia is best treated antipyretics and cooling blankets. Cardiac arrhythmias are best treated with phenytoin or procainamide.

Drug Interactions

Increased effect/toxicity of barbiturates, psychotropics, rauwolfia alkaloids, CNS depressants

Increased toxicity with disulfiram (seizures), fluoxetine and other serotonin active agents (↑ cardiac effect), tricyclic antidepressants (↑ cardiovascular instability), meperidine (↑ cardiovascular instability), phenothiazine (hypertensive crisis), sympathomimetics (hypertensive crisis), levodopa (hypertensive crisis), tyramine-containing foods (↑ blood pressure), dextroamphetamine

Stability Protect from light

Mechanism of Action Thought to act by increasing endogenous concentrations of epinephrine, norepinephrine, dopamine and serotonin through inhibition of the enzyme (monoamine oxidase) responsible for the breakdown of these neurotransmitters

Pharmacodynamics/Kinetics
Onset of action: Within 2-4 weeks
Absorption: Oral: Well absorbed
Duration: May continue to have a therapeutic effect and interactions 2 weeks after discontinuing therapy
Elimination: In urine primarily as metabolites and unchanged drug

Usual Dosage Oral:
Adults: 15 mg 3 times/day; may increase to 60-90 mg/day during early phase of treatment, then reduce to dose for maintenance therapy slowly after maximum benefit is obtained; takes 2-4 weeks for a significant response to occur
Elderly: Initial: 7.5 mg/day; increase by 7.5-15 mg/day every 3-4 days as tolerated; usual therapeutic dose: 15-60 mg/day in 3-4 divided doses

Monitoring Parameters Blood pressure, heart rate, diet, weight, mood (if depressive symptoms)

Test Interactions ↓ glucose

Patient Information Avoid tyramine-containing foods: Red wine, cheese (except cottage, ricotta, and cream), smoked or pickled fish, beef or chicken liver, dried sausage, fava or broad bean pods, yeast vitamin supplements; do not begin any prescription or OTC medications without consulting your physician or pharmacist; may take as long as 3 weeks to see effects; report any severe headaches, irregular heartbeats, skin rash, insomnia, sedation, changes in strength; sensations of pain, burning, touch, or vibration; or any other unusual symptoms to your physician; avoid alcohol; get up slowly from chair or bed

Nursing Implications Watch for postural hypotension; monitor blood pressure carefully, especially at therapy onset or if other CNS drugs or cardiovascular drugs are added; check for dietary and drug restriction

Dosage Forms Tablet: 15 mg

Phenergan® see Promethazine Hydrochloride on page 939

Phenetron® see Chlorpheniramine Maleate on page 229

Phenobarbital (fee noe bar' bi tal)
Brand Names Barbita®; Luminal®; Solfoton®
Synonyms Phenobarbital Sodium; Phenobarbitone; Phenylethylmalonylurea
Use Management of generalized tonic-clonic (grand mal) and partial seizures; neonatal seizures; febrile seizures in children; sedation; may also be used for prevention and treatment of neonatal hyperbilirubinemia and lowering of bilirubin in chronic cholestasis
Restrictions C-IV
Pregnancy Risk Factor D
Contraindications Hypersensitivity to phenobarbital or any component; preexisting CNS depression, severe uncontrolled pain, porphyria, severe respiratory disease with dyspnea or obstruction
Warnings/Precautions Use with caution in patients with hypovolemic shock, congestive heart failure, hepatic impairment, respiratory dysfunction or depression, previous addiction to the sedative/hypnotic group, chronic or acute pain, renal dysfunction, and the elderly, due to its long half-life and risk of dependence, phenobarbital is not recommended as a sedative in the elderly; tolerance or psychological and physical dependence may occur with prolonged use. **Abrupt withdrawal in patients with epilepsy may precipitate status epilepticus.**
Adverse Reactions
>10%:
Cardiovascular: Hypotension, cardiac arrhythmias, bradycardia, arterial spasm, and gangrene with inadvertent intra-arterial injection
Central nervous system: Dizziness, lightheadedness, "hangover" effect, drowsiness, lethargy, CNS excitation or depression, impaired judgment
Local: Pain at injection site, thrombophlebitis with I.V. use
1% to 10%:
Central nervous system: Confusion, mental depression, unusual excitement, nervousness, faint feeling, headache, insomnia, nightmares
Gastrointestinal: Nausea, vomiting, constipation
(Continued)

Phenobarbital *(Continued)*

<1%:
Cardiovascular: Hypotension
Central nervous system: Hallucinations, hypothermia
Dermatologic: Exfoliative dermatitis, Stevens-Johnson syndrome, rash
Hematologic: Agranulocytosis, megaloblastic anemia, thrombocytopenia
Respiratory: Laryngospasm, respiratory depression, apnea (especially with rapid I.V. use)

Overdosage/Toxicology Symptoms of overdose include unsteady gait, slurred speech, confusion, jaundice, hypothermia, hypotension, respiratory depression, coma

If hypotension occurs, administer I.V. fluids and place the patient in the Trendelenburg position. If unresponsive, an I.V. vasopressor (eg, dopamine, epinephrine) may be required.

Repeated oral doses of activated charcoal significantly reduce the half-life of phenobarbital resulting from an enhancement of nonrenal elimination. The usual dose is 0.1-1 g/kg every 4-6 hours for 3-4 days unless the patient has no bowel movement causing the charcoal to remain in the GI tract. Assure adequate hydration and renal function. Urinary alkalinization with I.V. sodium bicarbonate also helps to enhance elimination. Hemodialysis or hemoperfusion is of uncertain value. Patients in stage IV coma due to high serum barbiturate levels may require charcoal hemoperfusion.

Drug Interactions
Decreased effect: Phenothiazines, haloperidol, quinidine, cyclosporine, tricyclic antidepressants, corticosteroids, theophylline, ethosuximide, warfarin, oral contraceptives, chloramphenicol, griseofulvin, doxycycline, beta-blockers
Increased toxicity: Propoxyphene, benzodiazepines, CNS depressants, valproic acid, methylphenidate, chloramphenicol

Stability Protect elixir from light; not stable in aqueous solutions; use only clear solutions; do not add to acidic solutions, precipitation may occur; I.V. form is **incompatible** with benzquinamide (in syringe), cephalothin, chlorpromazine, hydralazine, hydrocortisone, hydroxyzine, insulin, levorphanol, meperidine, methadone, morphine, norepinephrine, pentazocine, prochlorperazine, promazine, promethazine, ranitidine (in syringe), vancomycin

Mechanism of Action Interferes with transmission of impulses from the thalamus to the cortex of the brain resulting in an imbalance in central inhibitory and facilitatory mechanisms

Pharmacodynamics/Kinetics
Oral:
Onset of hypnosis: Within 20-60 minutes
Duration: 6-10 hours
I.V.:
Onset of action: Within 5 minutes
Peak effect: Within 30 minutes
Duration: 4-10 hours
Absorption: Oral: 70% to 90%
Protein binding: 20% to 45%, decreased in neonates
Metabolism: In the liver via hydroxylation and glucuronide conjugation
Half-life:
Neonates: 45-500 hours
Infants: 20-133 hours
Children: 37-73 hours
Adults: 53-140 hours
Time to peak serum concentration: Oral: Within 1-6 hours
Elimination: 20% to 50% excreted unchanged in urine

Usual Dosage
Children:
Sedation: Oral: 2 mg/kg 3 times/day
Hypnotic: I.M., I.V., S.C.: 3-5 mg/kg at bedtime
Preoperative sedation: Oral, I.M., I.V.: 1-3 mg/kg 1-1.5 hours before procedure

Anticonvulsant: Status epilepticus **Loading dose:** I.V.:
Neonates: 15-20 mg/kg in a single or divided dose
Infants and Children: 10-20 mg/kg in a single or divided dose; in select patients may give additional 5 mg/kg/dose every 15-30 minutes until seizure is controlled or a total dose of 40 mg/kg is reached
Adults: 300-800 mg initially followed by 120-240 mg/dose at 20-minute intervals until seizures are controlled or a total dose of 1-2 g

Anticonvulsant maintenance dose: Oral, I.V.:
Neonates: 2-4 mg/kg/day in 1-2 divided doses; assess serum concentrations; increase to 5 mg/kg/day if needed (usually by second week of therapy)

Infants: 5-8 mg/kg/day in 1-2 divided doses
Children:
  1-5 years: 6-8 mg/kg/day in 1-2 divided doses
  5-12 years: 4-6 mg/kg/day in 1-2 divided doses
Children >12 years and Adults: 1-3 mg/kg/day in divided doses or 50-100 mg 2-3 times/day

Adults:
  Sedation: Oral, I.M.: 30-120 mg/day in 2-3 divided doses
  Hypnotic: Oral, I.M., I.V., S.C.: 100-320 mg at bedtime
  Preoperative sedation: I.M.: 100-200 mg 1-1.5 hours before procedure

Dosing interval in renal impairment: Cl_{cr} <10 mL/minute: Administer every 12-16 hours
Moderately dialyzable (20% to 50%)

Dosing adjustment/comments in hepatic disease: Increased side effects may occur in severe liver disease; monitor plasma levels and adjust dose accordingly

Administration Avoid rapid I.V. administration >50 mg/minute; avoid intra-arterial injection

Monitoring Parameters Phenobarbital serum concentrations, mental status, CBC, LFTs, seizure activity

Reference Range
Therapeutic:
  Infants and children: 15-30 μg/mL (SI: 65-129 μmol/L)
  Adults: 20-40 μg/mL (SI: 86-172 μmol/L)
Toxic: >40 μg/mL (SI: >172 μmol/L)
Toxic concentration: Slowness, ataxia, nystagmus: 35-80 μg/mL (SI: 150-344 μmol/L)
Coma with reflexes: 65-117 μg/mL (SI: 279-502 μmol/L)
Coma without reflexes: >100 μg/mL (SI: >430 μmol/L)

Test Interactions ↑ ammonia (B); ↓ bilirubin (S), ↑ copper (S), assay interference of LDH, ↑ LFTs

Patient Information Avoid use of alcohol and other CNS depressants; avoid driving and other hazardous tasks; avoid abrupt discontinuation; may cause physical and psychological dependence; do not alter dose without notifying physician

Nursing Implications Parenteral solutions are highly alkaline; avoid extravasation; institute safety measures to avoid injuries; observe patient for excessive sedation and respiratory depression

Additional Information Injectable solutions contain propylene glycol
Sodium content of injection (65 mg, 1 mL): 6 mg (0.3 mEq)
Phenobarbital: Barbita®, Solfoton®
Phenobarbital sodium: Luminal®

Dosage Forms
Capsule: 16 mg
Elixir: 15 mg/5 mL (5 mL, 10 mL, 20 mL); 20 mg/5 mL (3.75 mL, 5 mL, 7.5 mL, 120 mL, 473 mL, 946 mL, 4000 mL)
Injection, as sodium: 30 mg/mL (1 mL); 60 mg/mL (1 mL); 65 mg/mL (1 mL); 130 mg/mL (1 mL)
Powder for injection: 120 mg
Tablet: 8 mg, 15 mg, 16 mg, 30 mg, 32 mg, 60 mg, 65 mg, 100 mg

Phenobarbital Sodium see Phenobarbital on page 869

Phenobarbitone see Phenobarbital on page 869

Phenoxybenzamine Hydrochloride (fen ox ee ben' za meen)
Brand Names Dibenzyline®
Use Symptomatic management of pheochromocytoma; treatment of hypertensive crisis caused by sympathomimetic amines
  Unlabeled use: Micturition problems associated with neurogenic bladder, functional outlet obstruction, and partial prostate obstruction
Pregnancy Risk Factor C
Contraindications Conditions in which a fall in blood pressure would be undesirable (eg, shock)
Warnings/Precautions Use with caution in patients with renal impairment, cerebral, or coronary arteriosclerosis, can exacerbate symptoms of respiratory tract infections. Because of the risk of adverse effects, avoid the use of this medication in the elderly if possible.
(Continued)

Phenoxybenzamine Hydrochloride *(Continued)*

Adverse Reactions
>10%:
  Cardiovascular: Postural hypotension, tachycardia, syncope
  Ocular: Miosis
  Respiratory: Nasal congestion
1% to 10%:
  Central nervous system: Lethargy, weakness, headache, confusion, tiredness, shock
  Gastrointestinal: Vomiting, nausea, diarrhea, dry mouth
  Genitourinary: Inhibition of ejaculation

Overdosage/Toxicology Symptoms of overdose include hypotension, tachycardia, lethargy, dizziness, shock; hypotension and shock should be treated with fluids and by placing the patient in the Trendelenburg position; only alpha-adrenergic pressors such as norepinephrine should be used; mixed agents such as epinephrine, may cause more hypotension

Drug Interactions
Decreased effect: Alpha agonists
Increased toxicity: Beta-blockers (hypotension, tachycardia)

Mechanism of Action Produces long-lasting noncompetitive alpha-adrenergic blockade of postganglionic synapses in exocrine glands and smooth muscle; relaxes urethra and increases opening of the bladder

Pharmacodynamics/Kinetics
Onset of action: Oral: Within 2 hours
Peak effect: Within 4-6 hours
Duration: Can continue for 4 or more days
Half-life: 24 hours
Elimination: Primarily in urine and feces

Usual Dosage Oral:
Children: Initial: 0.2 mg/kg (maximum: 10 mg) once daily, increase by 0.2 mg/kg increments; usual maintenance dose: 0.4-1.2 mg/kg/day every 6-8 hours, higher doses may be necessary
Adults: Initial: 10 mg twice daily, increase by 10 mg every other day until optimum dose is achieved; usual range: 20-40 mg 2-3 times/day

Monitoring Parameters Blood pressure, pulse, urine output, orthostasis

Patient Information Avoid alcoholic beverages; if dizziness occurs, avoid sudden changes in posture; may cause nasal congestion and constricted pupils; may inhibit ejaculation; avoid cough, cold or allergy medications containing sympathomimetics

Nursing Implications Monitor for orthostasis; assist with ambulation

Dosage Forms Capsule: 10 mg

Phenoxymethyl Penicillin *see* Penicillin V Potassium *on page 854*

Phentermine Hydrochloride *(fen' ter meen)*

Brand Names Adipex-P®; Fastin®; Ionamin®
Use Short-term adjunct in exogenous obesity
Restrictions C-IV
Pregnancy Risk Factor C
Contraindications Known hypersensitivity to phentermine
Warnings/Precautions Do not use in children <12 years of age; use with caution in patients with diabetes mellitus, cardiovascular disease, nephritis, angina pectoris, hypertension, glaucoma, patients with a history of drug abuse

Adverse Reactions
>10%:
  Cardiovascular: Hypertension
  Central nervous system: Euphoria, nervousness, insomnia
1% to 10%:
  Central nervous system: Confusion, mental depression, restlessness
  Gastrointestinal: Nausea, vomiting, constipation
  Endocrine & metabolic: Changes in libido
  Hematologic: Blood dyscrasias
  Neuromuscular & skeletal: Tremor
  Ocular: Blurred vision
<1%:
  Cardiovascular: Tachycardia, arrhythmias
  Central nervous system: Insomnia, restlessness, nervousness, depression, headache
  Dermatologic: Alopecia
  Gastrointestinal: Nausea, vomiting, diarrhea, abdominal cramps
  Neuromuscular & skeletal: Myalgia, tremor

Renal: Dysuria, polyuria
Respiratory: Dyspnea
Miscellaneous: Increased sweating

Overdosage/Toxicology Symptoms of overdose include hyperactivity, agitation, hyperthermia, hypertension, seizures. There is no specific antidote for phentermine intoxication and the bulk of the treatment is supportive. Hyperactivity and agitation usually respond to reduced sensory input, however with extreme agitation haloperidol (2-5 mg I.M. for adults) may be required. Hyperthermia is best treated with external cooling measures, or when severe or unresponsive, muscle paralysis with pancuronium may be needed. Hypertension is usually transient and generally does not require treatment unless severe. For diastolic blood pressures >110 mm Hg, a nitroprusside infusion should be initiated. Seizures usually respond to diazepam IVP and/or phenytoin maintenance regimens.

Drug Interactions
Decreased effect of guanethidine; decreased effect with CNS depressants
Increased effect/toxicity with MAO inhibitors (hypertensive crisis), sympathomimetics, CNS stimulants

Mechanism of Action Phentermine is structurally similar to dextroamphetamine and is comparable to dextroamphetamine as an appetite suppressant, but is generally associated with a lower incidence and severity of CNS side effects. Phentermine, like other anorexiants, stimulates the hypothalamus to result in decreased appetite; anorexiant effects are most likely mediated via norepinephrine and dopamine metabolism. However, other CNS effects or metabolic effects may be involved.

Pharmacodynamics/Kinetics
Absorption: Well absorbed; resin absorbed slower and produces more prolonged clinical effects
Half-life: 20 hours
Elimination: Primarily unchanged in urine

Usual Dosage Oral:
Children 3-15 years: 5-15 mg/day for 4 weeks

Adults: 8 mg 3 times/day 30 minutes before meals or food or 15-37.5 mg/day before breakfast or 10-14 hours before retiring

Monitoring Parameters CNS

Patient Information Take during day to avoid insomnia; do not discontinue abruptly, may cause physical and psychological dependence with prolonged use

Nursing Implications Dose should not be given in evening or at bedtime

Dosage Forms
Capsule: 15 mg, 18.75 mg, 30 mg, 37.5 mg
Capsule, resin complex: 15 mg, 30 mg
Tablet: 8 mg, 37.5 mg

Phentolamine Mesylate (fen tole' a meen)

Related Information
Extravasation Treatment of Other Drugs *on page 1209*

Brand Names Regitine®

Use Diagnosis of pheochromocytoma and treatment of hypertension associated with pheochromocytoma or other caused by excess sympathomimetic amines; as treatment of dermal necrosis after extravasation of drugs with alpha-adrenergic effects (norepinephrine, dopamine, epinephrine, dobutamine)

Pregnancy Risk Factor C

Contraindications Hypersensitivity to phentolamine or any component; renal impairment; coronary or cerebral arteriosclerosis

Warnings/Precautions Myocardial infarction, cerebrovascular spasm and cerebrovascular occlusion have occurred following administration; use with caution in patients with gastritis or peptic ulcer, tachycardia, or a history of cardiac arrhythmias

Adverse Reactions
>10%:
Cardiovascular: Hypotension, tachycardia, arrhythmias, nasal congestion, reflex tachycardia, anginal pain, orthostatic hypotension
Gastrointestinal: Nausea, vomiting, diarrhea, exacerbation of peptic ulcer, abdominal pain
1% to 10%:
Cardiovascular: Flushing of face
Central nervous system: Weakness, dizziness, fainting
Respiratory: Nasal stuffiness
<1%:
Cardiovascular: Myocardial infarction
Central nervous system: Severe headache
Miscellaneous: Exacerbation of peptic ulcer
(Continued)

873

Phentolamine Mesylate *(Continued)*

Overdosage/Toxicology Symptoms of overdose include tachycardia, shock, vomiting, dizziness. Hypotension and shock should be treated with fluids and by placing the patient in the Trendelenburg position; only alpha-adrenergic pressors such as norepinephrine should be used; mixed agents such as epinephrine, may cause more hypotension. Take care not to cause so much swelling of the extremity or digit that a compartment syndrome occurs.

Drug Interactions
Decreased effect: Epinephrine, ephedrine
Increased toxicity: Ethanol (disulfiram reaction)

Stability Reconstituted solution is stable for 48 hours at room temperature and 1 week when refrigerated

Mechanism of Action Competitively blocks alpha-adrenergic receptors to produce brief antagonism of circulating epinephrine and norepinephrine to reduce hypertension caused by alpha effects of these catecholamines; also has a positive inotropic and chronotropic effect on the heart

Pharmacodynamics/Kinetics
Onset of action:
I.M.: Within 15-20 minutes
I.V.: Immediate
Duration:
I.M.: 30-45 minutes
I.V.: 15-30 minutes
Metabolism: In the liver
Half-life: 19 minutes
Elimination: Urine (10% as unchanged drug)

Usual Dosage
Treatment of alpha-adrenergic drug extravasation: S.C.:
Children: 0.1-0.2 mg/kg diluted in 10 mL 0.9% sodium chloride infiltrated into area of extravasation within 12 hours
Adults: Infiltrate area with small amount of solution made by diluting 5-10 mg in 10 mL 0.9% sodium chloride within 12 hours of extravasation
If dose is effective, normal skin color should return to the blanched area within 1 hour

Diagnosis of pheochromocytoma: I.M., I.V.:
Children: 0.05-0.1 mg/kg/dose, maximum single dose: 5 mg
Adults: 5 mg

Surgery for pheochromocytoma: Hypertension: I.M., I.V.:
Children: 0.05-0.1 mg/kg/dose given 1-2 hours before procedure; repeat as needed every 2-4 hours until hypertension is controlled; maximum single dose: 5 mg
Adults: 5 mg given 1-2 hours before procedure and repeated as needed every 2-4 hours

Hypertensive crisis: Adults: 5-20 mg

Administration Infiltrate the area of dopamine extravasation with multiple small injections using only 27- or 30-gauge needles and changing the needle between each skin entry; take care not to cause so much swelling of the extremity or digit that a compartment syndrome occurs

Monitoring Parameters Blood pressure, heart rate

Test Interactions ↑ LFTs rarely

Nursing Implications Monitor patient for orthostasis; assist with ambulation

Dosage Forms Injection: 5 mg/mL (1 mL)

Phenylalanine Mustard *see* Melphalan *on page 681*

Phenylazo Diamino Pyridine Hydrochloride *see* Phenazopyridine Hydrochloride *on page 866*

Phenylephrine Hydrochloride *(fen ill ef' rin)*

Related Information
Adrenergic Agonists, Cardiovascular Comparison *on page 1242*
Extravasation Treatment of Other Drugs *on page 1209*

Brand Names AK-Dilate® Ophthalmic Solution; AK-Nefrin® Ophthalmic Solution; Alconefrin® Nasal Solution [OTC]; Doktors® Nasal Solution [OTC]; I-Phrine® Ophthalmic Solution; Isopto® Frin Ophthalmic Solution; Mydfrin® Ophthalmic Solution; Neo-Synephrine® Nasal Solution [OTC]; Neo-Synephrine® Ophthalmic Solution; Nostril® Nasal Solution [OTC]; Prefrin™ Ophthalmic Solution; Relief® Ophthalmic Solution; Rhinall® Nasal Solution [OTC]; Sinarest® Nasal Solution [OTC]; St. Joseph® Measured Dose Nasal Solution [OTC]; Vicks® Sinex® Nasal Solution [OTC]

Use Treatment of hypotension, vascular failure in shock; as a vasoconstrictor in regional analgesia; symptomatic relief of nasal and nasopharyngeal mucosal congestion; as a mydriatic in ophthalmic procedures and treatment of wide-angle glaucoma; supraventricular tachycardia

Pregnancy Risk Factor C

Contraindications Pheochromocytoma, severe hypertension, bradycardia, ventricular tachyarrhythmias; hypersensitivity to phenylephrine or any component; narrow-angle glaucoma (ophthalmic preparation), acute pancreatitis, hepatitis, peripheral or mesenteric vascular thrombosis, myocardial disease, severe coronary disease

Warnings/Precautions Injection may contain sulfites which may cause allergic reaction in some patients; do not use if solution turns brown or contains a precipitate; use with extreme caution in elderly patients, patients with hyperthyroidism, bradycardia, partial heart block, myocardial disease, or severe arteriosclerosis; infuse into large veins to help prevent extravasation which may cause severe necrosis; the 10% ophthalmic solution has caused increased blood pressure in elderly patients and its use should, therefore, be avoided

Adverse Reactions
Nasal:
>10%: Burning, rebound congestion, sneezing
1% to 10%: Stinging, dryness

Ophthalmic:
>10%: Transient stinging
1% to 10%:
Central nervous system: Headache, browache
Ocular: Blurred vision, photophobia, lacrimation

Systemic:
>10%: Neuromuscular & skeletal: Tremor
1% to 10%:
Cardiovascular: Peripheral vasoconstriction hypertension, angina, reflex bradycardia, arrhythmias
Central nervous system: Restlessness, excitability

Overdosage/Toxicology Symptoms of overdose include vomiting, hypertension, palpitations, paresthesia, ventricular extrasystoles. Treatment is supportive; in extreme cases, I.V. phentolamine may be used.

Drug Interactions
Decreased effect: With alpha- and beta-adrenergic blocking agents
Increased effect: With oxytocic drugs
Increased toxicity: With sympathomimetics, tachycardia or arrhythmias may occur; with MAO inhibitors, actions may be potentiated

Stability Is stable for 48 hours in 5% dextrose in water at pH 3.5-7.5; do not use brown colored solutions

Mechanism of Action Potent, direct-acting alpha-adrenergic stimulator with weak beta-adrenergic activity; causes vasoconstriction of the arterioles of the nasal mucosa and conjunctiva; activates the dilator muscle of the pupil to cause contraction; produces vasoconstriction of arterioles in the body; produces systemic arterial vasoconstriction

Pharmacodynamics/Kinetics
Onset of effect:
I.M., S.C.: Within 10-15 minutes
I.V.: Immediate
Duration:
I.M.: 30 minutes to 2 hours
I.V.: 15-30 minutes
S.C.: 1 hour
Metabolism: To phenolic conjugates; metabolized in liver and intestine by monoamine oxidase
Half-life: 2.5 hours
Elimination: Urine (90%)

Usual Dosage
Ophthalmic procedures:
Infants <1 year: Instill 1 drop of 2.5% 15-30 minutes before procedures
Children and Adults: Instill 1 drop of 2.5% or 10% solution, may repeat in 10-60 minutes as needed
Nasal decongestant: (therapy should not exceed 5 continuous days)
Children:
2-6 years: Instill 1 drop every 2-4 hours of 0.125% solution as needed
6-12 years: Instill 1-2 sprays or instill 1-2 drops every 4 hours of 0.25% solution as needed
Children >12 years and Adults: Instill 1-2 sprays or instill 1-2 drops every 4 hours of 0.25% to 0.5% solution as needed; 1% solution may be used in adult
(Continued)

Phenylephrine Hydrochloride *(Continued)*

in cases of extreme nasal congestion; do not use nasal solutions more than 3 days

Hypotension/shock:
Children:
I.M., S.C.: 0.1 mg/kg/dose every 1-2 hours as needed (maximum: 5 mg)
I.V. bolus: 5-20 mcg/kg/dose every 10-15 minutes as needed
I.V. infusion: 0.1-0.5 mcg/kg/minute
Adults:
I.M., S.C.: 2-5 mg/dose every 1-2 hours as needed (initial dose should not exceed 5 mg)
I.V. bolus: 0.1-0.5 mg/dose every 10-15 minutes as needed (initial dose should not exceed 0.5 mg)
I.V. infusion: 10 mg in 250 mL D_5W or NS (1:25,000 dilution) (40 mcg/mL); start at 100-180 mcg/minute (2-5 mL/minute; 50-90 drops/minute) initially; when blood pressure is stabilized, maintenance rate: 40-60 mcg/minute (20-30 drops/minute)

Paroxysmal supraventricular tachycardia: I.V.:
Children: 5-10 mcg/kg/dose over 20-30 seconds
Adults: 0.25-0.5 mg/dose over 20-30 seconds

Administration Concentration and rate of infusion can be calculated using the following formulas: Dilute 0.6 mg x weight (kg) to 100 mL; then the dose in mcg/kg/minute = 0.1 x the infusion rate in mL/hour

Monitoring Parameters Blood pressure, heart rate, arterial blood gases, central venous pressure

Patient Information Nasal decongestant should not be used for >3 days in a row, hereby reducing problems of rebound congestion; notify physician of insomnia, dizziness, tremor, or irregular heartbeat; if symptoms do not improve within 7 days or are accompanied by signs of infection, consult physician

Nursing Implications May cause necrosis or sloughing tissue if extravasation occurs during I.V. administration or S.C. administration

Extravasation: Use phentolamine as antidote; mix 5 mg with 9 mL of NS; inject a small amount of this dilution into extravasated area; blanching should reverse immediately. Monitor site; if blanching should recur, additional injections of phentolamine may be needed.

Dosage Forms
Jelly, nasal: 0.5% [5 mg/mL] (18.75 g)
Injection: 1% [10 mg/mL] (1 mL)
Solution:
Nasal:
Drops: 0.125% (15 mL, 30 mL); 0.16% (30 mL); 0.2% (30 mL); 0.25% (15 mL, 30 mL, 473 mL)
Spray: 0.25% (15 mL, 30 mL); 0.5% (15 mL, 30 mL); 1% (15 mL)
Ophthalmic: 0.12% (15 mL); 2.5% (2 mL, 3 mL, 5 mL, 15 mL); 10% (1 mL, 2 mL, 5 mL)

Phenylethylmalonylurea *see* Phenobarbital *on page 869*

Phenylisohydantoin *see* Pemoline *on page 846*

Phenylpropanolamine Hydrochloride *(fen ill proe pa nole' a meen)*

Brand Names Acutrim® Precision Release® [OTC]; Control® [OTC]; Dex-A-Diet® [OTC]; Dexatrim® [OTC]; Maigret-50; Prolamine® [OTC]; Propadrine; Propagest® [OTC]; Rhindecon®; Stay Trim® Diet Gum [OTC]; Westrim® LA [OTC]

Synonyms *dl*-Norephedrine Hydrochloride; PPA

Use Anorexiant; nasal decongestant

Pregnancy Risk Factor C

Contraindications Known hypersensitivity to drug

Warnings/Precautions Use with caution in patients with high blood pressure tachyarrhythmias, pheochromocytoma, bradycardia, cardiac disease, arteriosclerosis; do not use for more than 3 weeks for weight loss

Adverse Reactions
>10%: Cardiovascular: Hypertension, palpitations
1% to 10%:
Central nervous system: Insomnia, restlessness, dizziness
Gastrointestinal: Dry mouth, nausea
<1%:
Cardiovascular: Tightness in chest, bradycardia, arrhythmias angina
Central nervous system: Severe headache, anxiety, nervousness, restlessness

Genitourinary: Difficult urination

Overdosage/Toxicology Symptoms of overdose include vomiting, hypertension, palpitations, paresthesia, excitation, seizures. Treatment is supportive; diazepam 5-10 mg I.V. (0.25-0.4 mg/kg for children) may be used for excitation and seizures.

Drug Interactions
Decreased effect of antihypertensives
Increased effect/toxicity with MAO inhibitors (hypertensive crisis), beta-blockers (↑ pressor effects)

Mechanism of Action Releases tissue stores of epinephrine and thereby produces an alpha- and beta-adrenergic stimulation; this causes vasoconstriction and nasal mucosa blanching; also appears to depress central appetite centers

Pharmacodynamics/Kinetics
Absorption: Oral: Well absorbed
Metabolism: In the liver to norephedrine
Bioavailability: Close to 100%
Half-life: 4.6-6.6 hours
Elimination: In urine primarily as unchanged drug (80% to 90%)

Usual Dosage Oral:
Children: Decongestant:
2-6 years: 6.25 mg every 4 hours
6-12 years: 12.5 mg every 4 hours not to exceed 75 mg/day

Adults:
Decongestant: 25 mg every 4 hours or 50 mg every 8 hours, not to exceed 150 mg/day
Anorexic: 25 mg 3 times/day 30 minutes before meals or 75 mg (timed release) once daily in the morning
Precision release: 75 mg after breakfast

Monitoring Parameters Blood pressure, heart rate

Patient Information Should not be used more than 3 consecutive weeks for weight loss; contact physician for insomnia, tremor, or irregular heartbeat

Nursing Implications Give dose early in day to prevent insomnia; observe for signs of nervousness, excitability

Dosage Forms
Capsule: 37.5 mg
Capsule, timed release: 25 mg, 75 mg
Tablet: 25 mg
Tablet:
Precision release: 75 mg
Timed release: 75 mg

Phenytoin (fen' i toyn)
Brand Names Dilantin®; Diphenylan Sodium®
Synonyms Diphenylhydantoin; DPH; Phenytoin Sodium, Extended; Phenytoin Sodium, Prompt
Use Management of generalized tonic-clonic (grand mal), simple partial and complex partial seizures; prevention of seizures following head trauma/neurosurgery; ventricular arrhythmias, including those associated with digitalis intoxication, prolonged Q-T interval and surgical repair of congenital heart diseases in children; also used for epidermolysis bullosa
Pregnancy Risk Factor D
Contraindications Hypersensitivity to phenytoin, other hydantoins, or any component; heart block, sinus bradycardia
Warnings/Precautions May increase frequency of petit mal seizures; I.V. form may cause hypotension, skin necrosis at I.V. site; avoid I.V. administration in small veins; use with caution in patients with porphyria; discontinue if rash or lymphadenopathy occurs; use with caution in patients with hepatic dysfunction, sinus bradycardia, S-A block, A-V block, or hepatic impairment; elderly may have reduced hepatic clearance and low albumin levels, which will increase the free fraction of phenytoin in the serum and, therefore, the pharmacologic response
Adverse Reactions I.V. effects: Hypotension, bradycardia, cardiac arrhythmias, cardiovascular collapse (especially with rapid I.V. use), venous irritation and pain, thrombophlebitis
Effects not related to plasma phenytoin concentrations: Hypertrichosis, gingival hypertrophy, thickening of facial features, carbohydrate intolerance, folic acid deficiency, peripheral neuropathy, vitamin D deficiency, osteomalacia, systemic lupus erythematosus
Dose-related effects: Nystagmus, blurred vision, diplopia, ataxia, slurred speech, dizziness, drowsiness, lethargy, coma, rash, fever, nausea, vomiting, gum tenderness, confusion, mood changes, folic acid depletion, osteomalacia, hyperglycemia
(Continued)

Phenytoin (Continued)

Related to elevated concentrations:
>20 mcg/mL: Far lateral nystagmus
>30 mcg/mL: 45° lateral gaze nystagmus and ataxia
>40 mcg/mL: Decreased mentation
>100 mcg/mL: Death

>10%:
  Central nervous system: Psychiatric changes, slurred speech, dizziness, drowsiness
  Gastrointestinal: Constipation, nausea, vomiting, gingival hyperplasia
  Neuromuscular & skeletal: Trembling
1% to 10%:
  Central nervous system: Drowsiness, headache, insomnia
  Dermatologic: Skin rash
  Gastrointestinal: Anorexia, weight loss
  Hematologic: Leukopenia, increase in serum creatinine
  Hepatic: Hepatitis
<1%:
  Cardiovascular: Hypotension, bradycardia, cardiac arrhythmias, cardiovascular collapse
  Central nervous system: Confusion, fever, ataxia
  Local: Thrombophlebitis
  Neuromuscular & skeletal: Peripheral neuropathy, paresthesia
  Ocular: Diplopia, nystagmus, blurred vision
Rarely seen effects: SLE-like syndrome, lymphadenopathy, hepatitis, Stevens-Johnson syndrome, blood dyscrasias, dyskinesias, pseudolymphoma, lymphoma
  Miscellaneous: Venous irritation and pain

Overdosage/Toxicology Symptoms of overdose include unsteady gait, slurred speech, confusion, nausea, hypothermia, fever, hypotension, respiratory depression, coma. Treatment is supportive for hypotension; treat with I.V. fluids and place patient in Trendelenburg position; seizures may be controlled with diazepam 5-10 mg (0.25-0.4 mg/kg in children).

Drug Interactions Phenytoin is an inducer of cytochrome P-450 IIIA enzymes and is associated with many drug interactions

Decreased effect: Rifampin, cisplatin, vinblastine, bleomycin, folic acid, continuous NG feedings
Absorption is impaired when phenytoin suspension is given concurrently to patients who are receiving continuous nasogastric feedings, discontinuation of enteral feedings results in a marked increase in phenytoin concentrations. A method to resolve this interaction is to divide the daily dose of phenytoin and withhold the administration of nutritional supplements for 1-2 hours before and after each phenytoin dose.
Increased toxicity: Amiodarone decreases metabolism of phenytoin; disulfiram decreases metabolism of phenytoin; fluconazole, itraconazole decreases phenytoin serum concentrations; isoniazid may increase phenytoin serum concentrations
Increased effect/toxicity of valproic acid, ethosuximide, primidone, warfarin, oral contraceptives, corticosteroids, cyclosporine, theophylline, chloramphenicol, rifampin, doxycycline, quinidine, mexiletine, disopyramide, dopamine, nondepolarizing skeletal muscle relaxants

Stability
Phenytoin is stable as long as it remains free of haziness and precipitation
Use only clear solutions; parenteral solution may be used as long as there is no precipitate and it is not hazy, slightly yellowed solution may be used
Refrigeration may cause precipitate, sometimes the precipitate is resolved by allowing the solution to reach room temperature again
Drug may precipitate at a pH <11.5
May dilute with normal saline for I.V. infusion; stability is concentration dependent
Standard diluent: Dose/100 mL NS
Minimum volume: Concentration should be maintained at 1-10 mg/mL secondary to stability problems (stable for 4 hours)
Comments: Maximum rate of infusion: 50 mg/minute

IVPB dose should be administered via an in-line 0.22-5 micron filter because of high potential for precipitation I.V. form is highly **incompatible** with many drugs and solutions such as dextrose in water, some saline solutions, amikacin, bretylium, dobutamine, cephapirin, insulin, levorphanol, lidocaine, meperidine, metaraminol, morphine, norepinephrine, heparin, potassium chloride, vitamin B complex with C

Mechanism of Action Stabilizes neuronal membranes and decreases seizure activity by increasing efflux or decreasing influx of sodium ions across cell membranes in the motor cortex during generation of nerve impulses; prolongs effective refractory period and suppresses ventricular pacemaker automaticity, shortens action potential in the heart

Pharmacodynamics/Kinetics

Absorption: Oral: Slow

Distribution: V_d:

Neonates:

Premature: 1-1.2 L/kg

Full-term: 0.8-0.9 L/kg

Infants: 0.7-0.8 L/kg

Children: 0.7 L/kg

Adults: 0.6-0.7 L/kg

Protein binding:

Neonates: Up to 20% free

Infants: Up to 15% free

Adults: 90% to 95%

Others: Increased free fraction (decreased protein binding)

Patients with hyperbilirubinemia, hypoalbuminemia, uremia **(see table)**

Metabolism: Follows dose-dependent capacity-limited (Michaelis-Menten) pharmacokinetics with increased V_{max} in infants >6 months of age and children versus adults

Bioavailability: Dependent upon formulation administered

Time to peak serum concentration (dependent upon formulation administered):

Oral:

Extended-release capsule: Within 4-12 hours

Immediate release preparation: Within 2-3 hours

Elimination: Highly variable clearance dependent upon intrinsic hepatic function and dose administered; increased clearance and decreased serum concentrations with febrile illness; <5% excreted unchanged in urine; major metabolite (via oxidation) HPPA undergoes enterohepatic recycling and elimination in urine as glucuronides

Disease States Resulting in a Decrease in Serum Albumin Concentration	Disease States Resulting in an Apparent Decrease in Affinity of Phenytoin for Serum Albumin
Burns	Renal failure Cl_{cr} <25 mL/min (unbound fraction is increased 2-3 fold in uremia)
Hepatic cirrhosis	Jaundice (severe)
Nephrotic syndrome	Other drugs (displacers)
Pregnancy	Hyperbilirubinemia (total bilirubin >15 mg/dL)
Cystic fibrosis	

Usual Dosage

Status epilepticus: I.V.:

Neonates: Loading dose: 15-20 mg/kg in a single or divided dose; maintenance dose: Initial: 5 mg/kg/day in 2 divided doses; usual: 5-8 mg/kg/day in 2 divided doses; some patients may require dosing every 8 hours

Infants and Children: Loading dose: 15-20 mg/kg in a single or divided dose; maintenance dose: Initial: 5 mg/kg/day in 2 divided doses, usual doses:

6 months to 3 years: 8-10 mg/kg/day

4-6 years: 7.5-9 mg/kg/day

7-9 years: 7-8 mg/kg/day

10-16 years: 6-7 mg/kg/day, some patients may require every 8 hours dosing

Adults: Loading dose: 15-20 mg/kg in a single or divided dose, followed by 100-150 mg/dose at 30-minute intervals up to a maximum of 1500 mg/24 hours; maintenance dose: 300 mg/day or 5-6 mg/kg/day in 3 divided doses or 1-2 divided doses using extended release

Anticonvulsant: Children and Adults: Oral:

Loading dose: 15-20 mg/kg; based on phenytoin serum concentrations and recent dosing history; administer oral loading dose in 3 divided doses given every 2-4 hours to decrease GI adverse effects and to ensure complete oral absorption; maintenance dose: same as I.V.

Dosing adjustment/comments in renal impairment or hepatic disease: Safe in usual doses in mild liver disease; clearance may be substantially reduced in cirrhosis and plasma level monitoring with dose adjustment advisable. Free phenytoin levels should be monitored closely.

(Continued)

Phenytoin (Continued)

Administration

Phenytoin may be administered by IVP or IVPB administration

I.M. administration is not recommended due to erratic absorption, pain on injection and precipitation of drug at injection site

S.C. administration is not recommended because of the possibility of local tissue damage

The maximum rate of I.V. administration is 50 mg/minute; highly sensitive patients (eg, elderly, patients with pre-existing cardiovascular conditions) should receive phenytoin more slowly (eg, 20 mg/minute)

An in-line 0.22-5 micron filter is recommended for IVPB solutions due to the high potential for precipitation of the solution; avoid extravasation; following I.V. administration, NS should be injected through the same needle or I.V. catheter to prevent irritation

Monitoring Parameters
Blood pressure, vital signs (with I.V. use), plasma phenytoin level, CBC, liver function tests

Reference Range

Therapeutic range:

Total phenytoin: 10-20 µg/mL (children and adults), 8-15 µg/mL (neonates)

Concentrations of 5-10 µg/mL may be therapeutic for some patients but concentrations <5 µg/mL are not likely to be effective

50% of patients show decreased frequency of seizures at concentrations >10 µg/mL

86% of patients show decreased frequency of seizures at concentrations >15 µg/mL

Add another anticonvulsant if satisfactory therapeutic response is not achieved with a phenytoin concentration of 20 µg/mL

Free phenytoin: 1-2.5 µg/mL

Toxic: <30-50 µg/mL (SI: <120-200 µmol/L)

Lethal: >100 µg/mL (SI: >400 µmol/L)

Adjustment of Serum Concentration in Patients With Low Serum Albumin

Measured Total Phenytoin Concentration (mcg/mL)	Patient's Serum Albumin (g/dL)			
	3.5	3	2.5	2
	Adjusted Total Phenytoin Concentration (mcg/mL)*			
5	6	7	8	10
10	13	14	17	20
15	19	21	25	30

*Adjusted concentration = measured total concentration + [(0.2 x albumin) + 0.1].

Adjustment of Serum Concentration in Patients With Renal Failure (Cl_cr ≤10 mL/min) (Product Information from Parke-Davis)

Measured Total Phenytoin Concentration (mcg/mL)	Patient's Serum Albumin (g/dL)				
	4	3.5	3	2.5	2
	Adjusted Total Phenytoin Concentration (mcg/mL)*				
5	10	11	13	14	17
10	20	22	25	29	33
15	30	33	38	43	50

*Adjusted concentration = measured total concentration + [(0.1 x albumin) + 0.1].

Test Interactions
↑ glucose, alkaline phosphatase (S); ↓ thyroxine (S), calcium (S)

Patient Information
Shake oral suspension well prior to each dose; do not change brand or dosage form without consulting physician; do not skip doses, may cause drowsiness, dizziness, ataxia, loss of coordination or judgment; take with food; maintain good oral hygiene

Additional Information

Phenytoin: Dilantin® chewable tablet and oral suspension

Phenytoin sodium, extended: Dilantin® Kapseal®

Phenytoin sodium, prompt: Diphenylan Sodium® capsule

Sodium content of 1 g injection: 88 mg (3.8 mEq)

Dosage Forms

Capsule, as sodium:

Extended: 30 mg, 100 mg

Prompt: 30 mg, 100 mg
Injection, as sodium: 50 mg/mL (2 mL, 5 mL)
Suspension, oral: 30 mg/5 mL (5 mL, 240 mL); 125 mg/5 mL (5 mL, 240 mL)
Tablet, chewable: 50 mg

Phenytoin Sodium, Extended *see* Phenytoin *on page 877*

Phenytoin Sodium, Prompt *see* Phenytoin *on page 877*

Phicon® [OTC] *see* Pramoxine Hydrochloride *on page 915*

Phillips'® Milk of Magnesia [OTC] *see* Magnesium Hydroxide *on page 659*

pHisoHex® *see* Hexachlorophene *on page 535*

pHiso® Scrub *see* Hexachlorophene *on page 535*

Phos-Ex® *see* Calcium Acetate *on page 160*

Phos-Flur® *see* Fluoride *on page 471*

PhosLo® *see* Calcium Acetate *on page 160*

Phosphate, Potassium *see* Potassium Phosphate *on page 910*

Phospholine Iodide® *see* Echothiophate Iodide *on page 378*

Phosphonoformate *see* Foscarnet *on page 488*

Phosphonoformic Acid *see* Foscarnet *on page 488*

Phrenilin® *see* Butalbital Compound *on page 153*

Phrenilin Forte® *see* Butalbital Compound *on page 153*

***p*-Hydroxyampicillin** *see* Amoxicillin Trihydrate *on page 68*

Phyllocontin® *see* Theophylline/Aminophylline *on page 1072*

Phylloquinone *see* Phytonadione *on next page*

Physostigmine (fye zoe stig' meen)

Related Information
Glaucoma Drug Therapy Comparison *on page 1270*
Brand Names Antilirium®; Isopto® Eserine
Synonyms Eserine Salicylate
Use Reverse toxic CNS effects caused by anticholinergic drugs; used as miotic in treatment of glaucoma
Pregnancy Risk Factor C
Contraindications Hypersensitivity to physostigmine or any component; GI or GU obstruction; physostigmine therapy of drug intoxications should be used with extreme caution in patients with asthma, gangrene, severe cardiovascular disease, or mechanical obstruction of the GI tract or urogenital tract. In these patients, physostigmine should be used only to treat life-threatening conditions.
Warnings/Precautions Use with caution in patients with epilepsy, asthma, diabetes, gangrene, cardiovascular disease, bradycardia. Discontinue if excessive salivation or emesis, frequent urination or diarrhea occur. Reduce dosage if excessive sweating or nausea occurs. Administer I.V. slowly or at a controlled rate not faster than 1 mg/minute. Due to the possibility of hypersensitivity or overdose/cholinergic crisis, atropine should be readily available; ointment may delay corneal healing, may cause loss of dark adaptation; not intended as a first-line agent for anticholinergic toxicity or Parkinson's disease.
Adverse Reactions
Ophthalmic:
>10%:
Ocular: Lacrimation, marked miosis, blurred vision, eye pain
Miscellaneous: Sweating
1% to 10%:
Central nervous system: Headache, browache
Dermatologic: Burning, redness

Systemic:
>10%:
Gastrointestinal: Nausea, salivation, diarrhea, epigastric pain
Ocular: Lacrimation
Miscellaneous: Sweating
1% to 10%:
Cardiovascular: Palpitations, bradycardia
Central nervous system: Restlessness, nervousness, hallucinations, seizures
Genitourinary: Frequent urge to urinate
Neuromuscular & skeletal: Muscle twitching
(Continued)

881

Physostigmine *(Continued)*

Ocular: Miosis

Respiratory: Dyspnea, bronchospasm, respiratory paralysis, pulmonary edema

Overdosage/Toxicology Symptoms of overdose include muscle weakness, blurred vision, excessive sweating, tearing and salivation, nausea, vomiting, bronchospasm, seizures. If physostigmine is used in excess or in the absence of an anticholinergic overdose, patients may manifest signs of cholinergic toxicity. At this point a cholinergic agent (eg, atropine 0.015-0.05 mg/kg) may be necessary.

Drug Interactions Increased toxicity: Bethanechol, methacholine, succinylcholine → ↑ neuromuscular blockade with systemic administration

Stability Do not use solution if cloudy or dark brown

Mechanism of Action Inhibits destruction of acetylcholine by acetylcholinesterase which facilitates transmission of impulses across myoneural junction and prolongs the central and peripheral effects of acetylcholine

Pharmacodynamics/Kinetics

Onset of action:

Ophthalmic instillation: Within 2 minutes

Parenteral: Within 5 minutes

Absorption: I.M., ophthalmic, S.C.: Readily absorbed

Distribution: Crosses the blood-brain barrier readily and reverses both central and peripheral anticholinergic effects

Duration:

Ophthalmic: 12-48 hours

Parenteral: 0.5-5 hours

Metabolism: In the liver

Half-life: 15-40 minutes

Elimination: Via hydrolysis by cholinesterases

Usual Dosage

Children: Anticholinergic drug overdose: Reserve for life-threatening situations only: I.V.: 0.01-0.03 mg/kg/dose, (maximum: 0.5 mg/minute); may repeat after 5-10 minutes to a maximum total dose of 2 mg or until response occurs or adverse cholinergic effects occur

Adults: Anticholinergic drug overdose:

I.M., I.V., S.C.: 0.5-2 mg to start, repeat every 20 minutes until response occurs or adverse effect occurs

Repeat 1-4 mg every 30-60 minutes as life-threatening signs (arrhythmias, seizures, deep coma) recur; maximum I.V. rate: 1 mg/minute

Ophthalmic:

Ointment: Instill a small quantity to lower fornix up to 3 times/day

Solution: Instill 1-2 drops into eye(s) up to 4 times/day

Test Interactions ↑ aminotransferase [ALT (SGPT)/AST (SGOT)] (S), ↑ amylase (S)

Patient Information Burning or stinging may occur with application; may cause loss of dark adaptation; notify physician if abdominal cramps, sweating, salivation, or cramps occur

Dosage Forms

Injection, as salicylate: 1 mg/mL (2 mL)

Ointment, ophthalmic: 0.25% (3.5 g, 3.7 g)

Solution, ophthalmic: 0.25% (15 mL); 0.5% (2 mL, 15 mL)

Phytomenadione *see* Phytonadione *on this page*

Phytonadione *(fye toe na dye' one)*

Brand Names AquaMEPHYTON®; Konakion®; Mephyton®

Synonyms Methylphytyl Napthoquinone; Phylloquinone; Phytomenadione; Vitamin K$_1$

Use Prevention and treatment of hypoprothrombinemia caused by drug-induced or anticoagulant-induced vitamin K deficiency, hemorrhagic disease of the newborn; phytonadione is more effective and is preferred to other vitamin K preparations in the presence of impending hemorrhage; oral absorption depends on the presence of bile salts

Pregnancy Risk Factor C (X if used in 3rd trimester or near term)

Contraindications Hypersensitivity to phytonadione or any component

Warnings/Precautions Severe reactions resembling anaphylaxis or hypersensitivity have occurred rarely during or immediately after I.V. administration (even with proper dilution and rate of administration); restrict I.V. administration for emergency use only; ineffective in hereditary hypoprothrombinemia, hypoprothrombinemia caused by severe liver disease; severe hemolytic anemia has been reported rarely in neonates following large doses (10-20 mg) of phytonadione

Adverse Reactions

<1%:
Cardiovascular: Transient flushing reaction, rarely hypotension, cyanosis
Central nervous system: Rarely dizziness
Gastrointestinal: Dysgeusia, GI upset (oral)
Hematologic: Hemolysis in neonates and in patients with G-6-PD deficiency
Local: Tenderness at injection site
Respiratory: Dyspnea
Miscellaneous: Sweating, anaphylaxis, hypersensitivity reactions, pain

Drug Interactions Decreased effect: Warfarin sodium, dicumarol, anisindione effects antagonized by phytonadione

Stability Protect injection from light at all times; may be autoclaved

Mechanism of Action Promotes liver synthesis of clotting factors (II, VII, IX, X); however, the exact mechanism as to this stimulation is unknown. Menadiol is a water soluble form of vitamin K; phytonadione has a more rapid and prolonged effect than menadione; menadiol sodium diphosphate (K_4) is half as potent as menadione (K_3).

Pharmacodynamics/Kinetics

Onset of increased coagulation factors:
Oral: Within 6-12 hours
Parenteral: Within 1-2 hours; patient may become normal after 12-14 hours
Absorption: Oral: Absorbed from the intestines in the presence of bile
Metabolism: In the liver rapidly
Elimination: In bile and urine

Usual Dosage I.V. route should be restricted for emergency use only

Minimum daily requirement: Not well established
Infants: 1-5 mcg/kg/day
Adults: 0.03 mcg/kg/day
Hemorrhagic disease of the newborn:
Prophylaxis: I.M., S.C.: 0.5-1 mg within 1 hour of birth
Treatment: I.M., S.C.: 1-2 mg/dose/day
Oral anticoagulant overdose:
Infants: I.M., S.C.: 1-2 mg/dose every 4-8 hours
Children and Adults: Oral, I.M., I.V., S.C.: 2.5-10 mg/dose; rarely up to 25-50 mg has been used; may repeat in 6-8 hours if given by I.M., I.V., S.C. route; may repeat 12-48 hours after oral route
Vitamin K deficiency: Due to drugs, malabsorption or decreased synthesis of vitamin K
Infants and Children:
Oral: 2.5-5 mg/24 hours
I.M., I.V.: 1-2 mg/dose as a single dose
Adults:
Oral: 5-25 mg/24 hours
I.M., I.V.: 10 mg

Administration I.V. administration: Dilute in normal saline, D_5W or D_5NS and infuse slowly; rate of infusion should not exceed 1 mg/minute. **This route should be used only if administration by another route is not feasible.** The parenteral preparation has been administered orally to neonates. I.V. administration should not exceed 1 mg/minute; for I.V. infusion, dilute in PF (preservative free) D_5W or normal saline.

Monitoring Parameters PT

Additional Information Injection contains benzyl alcohol 0.9% as preservative

Dosage Forms

Injection:
Aqueous colloidal: 2 mg/mL (0.5 mL); 10 mg/mL (1 mL, 2.5 mL, 5 mL)
Aqueous (I.M. only): 2 mg/mL (0.5 mL); 10 mg/mL (1 mL)
Tablet: 5 mg

Pilagan® see Pilocarpine on this page

Pilocar® see Pilocarpine on this page

Pilocarpine (pye loe kar' peen)

Related Information

Glaucoma Drug Therapy Comparison on page 1270

Brand Names Adsorbocarpine®; Akarpine®; Isopto® Carpine; Ocu-Carpine®; Ocusert® Pilo; Ocusert Pilo-20®; Ocusert Pilo-40®; Pilagan®; Pilocar®; Pilopine HS®; Piloptic®; Pilostat®

Use Management of chronic simple glaucoma, chronic and acute angle-closure glaucoma; counter effects of cycloplegics

(Continued)

Pilocarpine *(Continued)*

Pregnancy Risk Factor C

Contraindications Acute inflammatory disease of anterior chamber, hypersensitivity to pilocarpine or any component

Warnings/Precautions Use with caution in patients with corneal abrasion, CHF, asthma, peptic ulcer, urinary tract obstruction, Parkinson's disease, or narrow-angle glaucoma

Adverse Reactions

>10%: Ocular: Blurred vision, miosis

1% to 10%:

Central nervous system: Headache

Genitourinary: Frequent urination

Local: Stinging, burning, lacrimation

Ocular: Ciliary spasm, retinal detachment, browache, photophobia, acute iritis, conjunctival and ciliary congestion early in therapy

Miscellaneous: Hypersensitivity reactions

<1%:

Cardiovascular: Hypertension, tachycardia

Gastrointestinal: Nausea, vomiting, diarrhea, salivation

Miscellaneous: Sweating

Overdosage/Toxicology Symptoms of overdose include bronchospasm, bradycardia, involuntary urination, vomiting, hypotension, tremors; atropine is the treatment of choice for intoxications manifesting with significant muscarinic symptoms. Atropine I.V. 2-4 mg every 3-60 minutes (or 0.04-0.08 mg I.V. every 5-60 minutes if needed for children) should be repeated to control symptoms and then continued as needed for 1-2 days following the acute ingestion. Epinephrine 0.1-1 mg S.C. may be useful in reversing severe cardiovascular or pulmonary sequel.

Stability Refrigerate gel; store solution at room temperature of 8°C to 30°C (46°F to 86°F) and protect from light

Mechanism of Action Directly stimulates cholinergic receptors in the eye causing miosis (by contraction of the iris sphincter), loss of accommodation (by constriction of ciliary muscle), and lowering of intraocular pressure (with decreased resistance to aqueous humor outflow)

Pharmacodynamics/Kinetics

Ophthalmic instillation:

Miosis:

Onset of effect: Within 10-30 minutes

Duration: 4-8 hours

Intraocular pressure reduction:

Onset of effect: 1 hour required

Duration: 4-12 hours

Ocusert® Pilo application:

Miosis: Onset of effect: 1.5-2 hours

Reduced intraocular pressure:

Onset: Within 1.5-2 hours; miosis within 10-30 minutes

Duration: ~1 week

Usual Dosage Ophthalmic: Adults:

Nitrate solution: Shake well before using; instill 1-2 drops 2-4 times/day

Hydrochloride solution:

Instill 1-2 drops up to 6 times/day; adjust the concentration and frequency as required to control elevated intraocular pressure

To counteract the mydriatic effects of sympathomimetic agents: Instill 1 drop of a 1% solution in the affected eye

Gel: Instill 0.5" ribbon into lower conjunctival sac once daily at bedtime

Ocular systems: Systems are labeled in terms of mean rate of release of pilocarpine over 7 days; begin with 20 mcg/hour at night and adjust based on response

Monitoring Parameters Intraocular pressure, funduscopic exam, visual field testing

Patient Information May sting on instillation; notify physician of sweating, urinary retention; usually causes difficulty in dark adaptation; advise patients to use caution while night driving or performing hazardous tasks in poor illumination; after topical instillation, finger pressure should be applied to lacrimal sac to decrease drainage into the nose and throat and minimize possible systemic absorption

Nursing Implications Usually causes difficulty in dark adaptation; advise patients to use caution while night driving or performing hazardous tasks in poor illumination; finger pressure should be applied to lacrimal sac for 1-2 minutes after instillation to decrease risk of absorption and systemic reactions. Assure the patient or a caregiver can adequately administer ophthalmic medication dosage form.

Additional Information
Ocusert® 20 mcg is approximately equivalent to 0.5% or 1% drops
Ocusert® 40 mcg is approximately equivalent to 2% or 3% drops
Dosage Forms See table.

Pilocarpine

Dosage Form	Strength %	1 mL	2 mL	15 mL	30 mL	3.5 g
Gel	4					x
Solution as hydrochloride	0.25			x		
	0.5			x	x	
	1	x	x	x	x	
	2	x	x	x	x	
	3			x	x	
	4	x	x	x	x	
	6			x	x	
	8		x			
	10			x		
Solution as nitrate	1			x		
	2			x		
	4			x		
Ocusert® Pilo-20: Releases 20 mcg/hour for 1 week						
Ocusert® Pilo-40: Releases 40 mcg/hour for 1 week						

Pilopine HS® *see* Pilocarpine *on page 883*

Piloptic® *see* Pilocarpine *on page 883*

Pilostat® *see* Pilocarpine *on page 883*

Pima® *see* Potassium Iodide *on page 909*

Pimaricin *see* Natamycin *on page 778*

Pimozide (pi' moe zide)
Brand Names Orap™
Use Suppression of severe motor and phonic tics in patients with Tourette's disorder
Pregnancy Risk Factor C
Contraindications Simple tics other than Tourette's, history of cardiac dysrhythmias, known hypersensitivity to pimozide
Adverse Reactions
>10%:
Cardiovascular: Tachycardia, orthostatic hypotension
Central nervous system: Akathisia, akinesia, extrapyramidal effects
Dermatologic: Skin rash
Endocrine & metabolic: Swelling of breasts
Gastrointestinal: Constipation, drowsiness, dry mouth
1% to 10%:
Cardiovascular: Swelling of face
Central nervous system: Tardive dyskinesia, mental depression
Gastrointestinal: Diarrhea, anorexia
<1%:
Central nervous system: Neuroleptic malignant syndrome (NMS)
Hematologic: Blood dyscrasias
Hepatic: Jaundice
Overdosage/Toxicology Symptoms of overdose include hypotension, respiratory depression, EKG abnormalities, extrapyramidal symptoms. Following attempts at decontamination, treatment is supportive and symptomatic. Seizures can be treated with diazepam, phenytoin, or phenobarbital.
Drug Interactions Increased effect/toxicity of alfentanil, CNS depressants, guanabenz (↑ sedation), MAO inhibitors
Mechanism of Action A potent centrally acting dopamine receptor antagonist resulting in its characteristic neuroleptic effects
Pharmacodynamics/Kinetics
Absorption: Oral: 50%
Protein binding: 99%
Metabolism: In the liver with significant first-pass decay
(Continued)

885

Pimozide *(Continued)*

Half-life: 50 hours
Time to peak serum concentration: Within 6-8 hours
Elimination: In urine

Usual Dosage Children >12 years and Adults: Oral: Initial: 1-2 mg/day, then increase dosage as needed every other day; range is usually 7-16 mg/day, maximum dose: 20 mg/day or 0.3 mg/kg/day should not be exceeded

Dosing adjustment in hepatic impairment: Reduction of dose is necessary in patients with liver disease

Test Interactions ↑ prolactin (S)

Patient Information Treatment with pimozide exposes the patient to serious risks; a decision to use pimozide chronically in Tourette's disorder is one that deserves full consideration by the patient (or patient's family) as well as by the treating physician. Because the goal of treatment is symptomatic improvement, the patient's view of the need for treatment and assessment of response are critical in evaluating the impact of therapy and weighing its benefits against the risks. Since the physician is the primary source of information about the use of a drug in any disease, it is recommended that the following information be discussed with patients and/or their families.

Dosage Forms Tablet: 2 mg

Pindolol *(pin' doe lole)*

Related Information

Beta-Blockers Comparison *on page 1257-1259*

Brand Names Visken®

Use Management of hypertension

Unlabeled use: Ventricular arrhythmias/tachycardia, antipsychotic-induced akathisia, situational anxiety; aggressive behavior associated with dementia

Pregnancy Risk Factor B

Contraindications Uncompensated congestive heart failure, cardiogenic shock, bradycardia or heart block, asthma, COPD; hypersensitivity to any component

Warnings/Precautions Use with caution in patients with inadequate myocardial function, undergoing anesthesia, bronchospastic disease, diabetes mellitus, hyperthyroidism, impaired hepatic function; abrupt withdrawal of the drug should be avoided (may exacerbate symptoms; discontinue over 1-2 weeks); do not use in pregnant or nursing women; may potentiate hypoglycemia in a diabetic patient and mask signs and symptoms

Adverse Reactions

>10%:
Central nervous system: Anxiety, dizziness, insomnia, weakness, tiredness
Endocrine & metabolic: Decreased sexual ability
Neuromuscular & skeletal: Joint pain
Miscellaneous: Back pain

1% to 10%:
Cardiovascular: Congestive heart failure, irregular heartbeat, reduced peripheral circulation,
Central nervous system: Hallucinations, nightmares, vivid dreams, numbness of extremities
Dermatologic: Skin rash, itching
Gastrointestinal: Diarrhea, nausea, vomiting, stomach discomfort
Respiratory: Breathing difficulty

<1%:
Cardiovascular: Bradycardia, chest pain
Central nervous system: Confusion, mental depression
Hematologic: Thrombocytopenia
Ocular: Dry eyes

Overdosage/Toxicology Symptoms of intoxication include cardiac disturbances, CNS toxicity, bronchospasm, hypoglycemia and hyperkalemia. The most common cardiac symptoms include hypotension and bradycardia; atrioventricular block, intraventricular conduction disturbances, cardiogenic shock, and systole may occur with severe overdose, especially with membrane-depressant drugs (eg, propranolol); CNS effects include convulsions, coma, and respiratory arrest is commonly seen with propranolol and other membrane-depressant and lipid-soluble drugs.

Treatment includes symptomatic treatment of seizures, hypotension, hyperkalemia and hypoglycemia; bradycardia and hypotension resistant to atropine, isoproterenol or pacing may respond to glucagon; wide QRS defects caused by the membrane-depressant poisoning may respond to hypertonic sodium bicarbonate; repeat-dose charcoal, hemoperfusion, or hemodialysis may be helpful in removal of only those beta-blockers with a small V_d, long half-life or low intrinsic clearance (acebutolol, atenolol, nadolol, sotalol).

Drug Interactions

Decreased effect of beta-blockers with aluminum salts, barbiturates, calcium salts, cholestyramine, colestipol, NSAIDs, penicillins (ampicillin), rifampin, salicylates and sulfinpyrazone due to decreased bioavailability and plasma levels

Beta-blockers may decrease the effect of sulfonylureas

Increased effect/toxicity of beta-blockers with calcium blockers (diltiazem, felo-dipine, nicardipine), contraceptives, flecainide, haloperidol (propranolol, hypo-tensive effects), H_2 antagonists (metoprolol, propranolol only by cimetidine, possibly ranitidine), hydralazine (metoprolol, propranolol), loop diuretics (propranolol, not atenolol), MAO inhibitors (metoprolol, nadolol, bradycardia), phenothiazines (propranolol), propafenone (metoprolol, propranolol), quinidine (in extensive metabolizers), ciprofloxacin, thyroid hormones (metoprolol, propranolol, when hypothyroid patient is converted to euthyroid state)

Beta-blockers may increase the effect/toxicity of flecainide, haloperidol (hypoten-sive effects), hydralazine, phenothiazines, acetaminophen, anticoagulants (propranolol, warfarin), benzodiazepines (not atenolol), clonidine (hypertensive crisis after or during withdrawal of either agent), epinephrine (initial hyperten-sive episode followed by bradycardia), nifedipine and verapamil lidocaine, ergots (peripheral ischemia), prazosin (postural hypotension)

Beta-blockers may affect the action or levels of ethanol, disopyramide, nondepo-larizing muscle relaxants and theophylline although the effects are difficult to predict

Mechanism of Action Blocks both beta$_1$- and beta$_2$-receptors and has mild intrinsic sympathomimetic activity; pindolol has negative inotropic and chrono-tropic effects and can significantly slow A-V nodal conduction

Pharmacodynamics/Kinetics

Absorption: Oral: Rapid, 50% to 95%

Protein binding: 50%

Metabolism: In the liver (60% to 65%) to conjugates

Half-life: 2.5-4 hours; increased with renal insufficiency, age, and cirrhosis

Time to peak serum concentration: Within 1-2 hours

Elimination: In urine (35% to 50% unchanged drug)

Usual Dosage

Adults: Initial: 5 mg twice daily, increase as necessary by 10 mg/day every 3-4 weeks; maximum daily dose: 60 mg

Elderly: Initial: 5 mg once daily, increase as necessary by 5 mg/day every 3-4 weeks

Dosing adjustment in renal and hepatic impairment: Reduction is necessary in severely impaired

Monitoring Parameters Blood pressure, standing and sitting/supine, pulse, respiratory function

Patient Information Adhere to dosage regimen; watch for postural hypotension; abrupt withdrawal of the drug should be avoided; take at the same time each day; may mask diabetes symptoms; do not discontinue medication abruptly; consult pharmacist or physician before taking over-the-counter cold preparations

Nursing Implications Evaluate blood pressure, apical and radial pulses; do not discontinue abruptly

Dosage Forms Tablet: 5 mg, 10 mg

Pink Bismuth® [OTC] see Bismuth on page 134

Pin-Rid® [OTC] see Pyrantel Pamoate on page 957

Pin-X® [OTC] see Pyrantel Pamoate on page 957

PIO see Pemoline on page 846

Pipecuronium Bromide (pi pe kure oh' nee um)

Related Information

Neuromuscular Blocking Agents Comparison Charts on page 1276-1278

Brand Names Arduan®

Use Adjunct to general anesthesia, to provide skeletal muscle relaxation during surgery and to provide skeletal muscle relaxation for endotracheal intubation; recommended only for procedures anticipated to last 90 minutes or longer

Pregnancy Risk Factor C

Contraindications Hypersensitivity to pipecuronium or bromide

Warnings/Precautions Use with caution in patients with renal impairment, obesity, cardiovascular disease, myasthenia gravis, myasthenic syndrome, and in the elderly

(Continued)

Pipecuronium Bromide *(Continued)*

Adverse Reactions
1% to 10%: Cardiovascular: Hypotension, bradycardia

<1%:
Cardiovascular: Atrial fibrillation, myocardial ischemia, thrombosis, hypertension, ventricular extrasystole
Central nervous system: CNS depression
Dermatologic: Urticaria
Endocrine & metabolic: Hypoglycemia, hyperkalemia
Neuromuscular & skeletal: Muscle atrophy
Renal: Anuria
Respiratory: Respiratory depression, dyspnea

Overdosage/Toxicology
Support ventilation by artificial means; paralysis including cessation of respiration

Drug Interactions
Increased effect with enflurane, halothane, isoflurane, ketorolac, quinidine, succinylcholine

Mechanism of Action
Pipecuronium bromide is a nondepolarizing neuromuscular blocking agent structurally related to pancuronium and vecuronium. Studies in adult patients have demonstrated that pipecuronium is ~20% to 50% more potent than pancuronium as a neuromuscular blocking agent. The neuromuscular effects and pharmacokinetics of pipecuronium appears to lack vagolytic or autonomic activity and produces minimal cardiovascular effects.

Pharmacodynamics/Kinetics
Onset of action: Effective neuromuscular blockade is generally observed within 2-3 minutes
Metabolism: In the liver primarily to 3-desacetyl-pipecuronium
Half-life, elimination: 2-2.5 hours
Elimination: Renally (40% unchanged drug)

Usual Dosage I.V.:
Children:
3 months to 1 year: Adult dosage
1-14 years: May be less sensitive to effects

Adults: Dose is individualized based on ideal body weight, ranges are 85-100 mcg/kg initially to a maintenance dose of 5-25 mcg/kg

Dosing adjustment in renal impairment:
Cl_{cr} 61-80 mL/minute: 70 mcg/kg
Cl_{cr} 41-60 mL/minute: 55 mcg/kg
Cl_{cr} <40 mL/minute: 50 mcg/kg
Extended duration should be expected

Administration
Not recommended for dilution into or administration from large volume I.V. solutions

Dosage Forms
Injection: 10 mg (10 mL)

Piperacillin Sodium *(pi per' a sill in)*

Related Information
Antimicrobial Drugs of Choice *on page 1298-1302*

Brand Names
Pipracil®

Use
Treatment of susceptible infections such as septicemia, acute and chronic respiratory tract infections, skin and soft tissue infections, and urinary tract infections due to susceptible strains of *Pseudomonas*, *Proteus*, and *Escherichia coli* and *Enterobacter*; normally used with other antibiotics (ie, aminoglycosides)

Pregnancy Risk Factor
B

Contraindications
Hypersensitivity to piperacillin or any component or penicillins

Warnings/Precautions
Dosage modification required in patients with impaired renal function; history of seizure activity; use with caution in patients with a history of beta-lactam allergy

Adverse Reactions
<1%:
Central nervous system: Convulsions, confusion, drowsiness, fever, Jarisch-Herxheimer reaction
Dermatologic: Rash
Endocrine & metabolic: Electrolyte imbalance
Hematologic: Hemolytic anemia, positive Coombs' reaction, abnormal platelet aggregation and prolonged prothrombin time (high doses)
Local: Thrombophlebitis
Neuromuscular: Myoclonus
Renal: Acute interstitial nephritis
Miscellaneous: Hypersensitivity reactions, anaphylaxis

Overdosage/Toxicology Symptoms of penicillin overdose include neuromuscular hypersensitivity (agitation, hallucinations, asterixis, encephalopathy, confusion, and seizures) and electrolyte imbalance with potassium or sodium salts, especially in renal failure; hemodialysis may be helpful to aid in the removal of the drug from the blood, otherwise most treatment is supportive or symptom directed

Drug Interactions

Decreased effect: Tetracyclines → ↓ penicillin effectiveness; aminoglycosides → physical inactivation of aminoglycosides in the presence of high concentrations of piperacillin and potential toxicity in patients with mild-moderate renal dysfunction

Increased effect:

Probenecid → ↑ penicillin levels

Neuromuscular blockers → ↑ duration of blockade

Aminoglycosides → synergistic efficacy

Stability Reconstituted solution is stable (I.V. infusion) in NS or D_5W for 24 hours at room temperature, 7 days when refrigerated or 4 weeks when frozen; after freezing, thawed solution is stable for 24 hours at room temperature or 48 hours when refrigerated; 40 g bulk vial should **not** be frozen after reconstitution; **incompatible** with aminoglycosides

Mechanism of Action Inhibits bacterial cell wall synthesis by binding to one or more of the penicillin binding proteins (PBPs); which in turn inhibits the final transpeptidation step of peptidoglycan synthesis in bacterial cell walls, thus inhibiting cell wall biosynthesis. Bacteria eventually lyse due to ongoing activity of cell wall autolytic enzymes (autolysins and murein hydrolases) while cell wall assembly is arrested.

Pharmacodynamics/Kinetics

Absorption: I.M.: 70% to 80%

Distribution: Crosses the placenta; distributes into milk at low concentrations

Protein binding: 22%

Half-life: Dose-dependent; prolonged with moderately severe renal or hepatic impairment:

Neonates:

1-5 days: 3.6 hours

>6 days: 2.1-2.7 hours

Children:

1-6 months: 0.79 hour

6 months to 12 years: 0.39-0.5 hour

Adults: 36-80 minutes

Time to peak serum concentration: I.M.: Within 30-50 minutes

Elimination: Principally in urine and partially in feces (via bile)

Usual Dosage

Neonates: I.M., I.V.: 100 mg/kg/dose every 12 hours

Infants and Children: I.M., I.V.: 200-300 mg/kg/day in divided doses every 4-6 hours; maximum dose: 24 g/day

Higher doses have been used in cystic fibrosis: 350-500 mg/kg/day in divided doses every 4 hours

Adults:

I.M.: 2-3 g/dose every 6-12 hours; maximum: 24 g/24 hours

I.V.: 3-4 g/dose every 4-6 hours; maximum: 24 g/24 hours

Dosing interval in renal impairment:

Cl_{cr} 10-50 mL/minute: Administer every 6-8 hours

Cl_{cr} <10 mL/minute: Administer every 8 hours

Moderately dialyzable (20% to 50%)

Administration Administer around-the-clock to promote less variation in peak and trough serum levels; give at least 1 hour apart from aminoglycosides

Test Interactions May interfere with urinary glucose tests using cupric sulfate (Benedict's solution, Clinitest®); may inactivate aminoglycosides *in vitro*; false-positive urinary and serum proteins, positive Coombs' test [direct]

Additional Information Sodium content of 1 g: 1.85 mEq

Dosage Forms Powder for injection: 2 g, 3 g, 4 g, 40 g

Piperacillin Sodium and Tazobactam Sodium (pi per< a sill in so' dee um & ta zoe bak' tam so' dee um)

Brand Names Zosyn™

Use

Treatment of infections of lower respiratory tract, urinary tract, skin and skin structures, gynecologic, bone and joint infections, and septicemia caused by susceptible organisms. Tazobactam expands activity of piperacillin to include

(Continued)

Piperacillin Sodium and Tazobactam Sodium
(Continued)

beta-lactamase producing strains of *S. aureus*, *H. influenzae*, Enterobacteria-ceae, *Pseudomonas*, *Klebsiella*, *Citrobacter*, *Serratia*, *Bacteroides*, and other gram-negative anaerobes.

Application to nosocomial infections may be limited by restricted activity against gram-negative organisms producing class I beta-lactamases and inactivity against methicillin-resistant *Staphylococcus aureus*

Pregnancy Risk Factor B

Pregnancy/Breast Feeding Implications Use by the breast feeding mother may result in diarrhea, candidiasis, or allergic response in the infant

Contraindications Hypersensitivity to penicillins, beta-lactamase inhibitors, or any component

Warnings/Precautions Due to sodium load and to the adverse effects of high serum concentrations of penicillins, dosage modification is required in patients with impaired or underdeveloped renal function; use with caution in patients with seizures or in patients with history of beta-lactam allergy; safety and efficacy have not been established in children <12 years of age

Adverse Reactions

>10%: Gastrointestinal: Diarrhea

1% to 10%:
Central nervous system: Insomnia, headache
Dermatologic: Rash, pruritus
Gastrointestinal: Constipation, nausea, vomiting, dyspepsia
Hematologic: Leukopenia
Miscellaneous: Serum sickness-like reaction

<1%:
Cardiovascular: Hypertension, hypotension, edema
Central nervous system: Dizziness, agitation, confusion
Gastrointestinal: Pseudomembranous colitis
Respiratory: Bronchospasm

Several laboratory abnormalities have rarely been associated with pipera-cillin/tazobactam including reversible eosinophilia, and neutropenia (associated most often with prolonged therapy), positive direct Coombs' test, prolonged PT and PTT, transient elevations of LFT, increases in creatinine

Overdosage/Toxicology Symptoms of penicillin overdose include neuromuscular hypersensitivity (agitation, hallucinations, asterixis, encephalopathy, confusion, and seizures) and electrolyte imbalance with potassium or sodium salts, especially in renal dysfunction; hemodialysis may be helpful to aid in the removal of the drug from the blood, otherwise most treatment is supportive or symptom directed

Drug Interactions

Decreased effect: Tetracyclines → ↓ penicillin effectiveness; aminoglycosides → physical inactivation of aminoglycosides in the presence of high concentrations of piperacillin and potential toxicity in patients with mild-moderate renal dysfunction

Increased effect:
Probenecid → ↑ penicillin levels
Neuromuscular blockers → ↑ duration of blockade
Aminoglycosides → synergistic efficacy

Stability Store at controlled room temperature; after reconstitution, solution is stable in NS or D₅W for 24 hours at room temperature and 7 days when refrigerated; use single dose vials immediately after reconstitution (discard unused portions after 24 hours at room temperature and 48 hours if refrigerated)

Mechanism of Action Piperacillin interferes with bacterial cell wall synthesis during active multiplication, causing cell wall death and resultant bactericidal activity against susceptible bacteria; tazobactam prevents degradation of piperacillin by binding to the active side on beta-lactamase; tazobactam inhibits many beta-lactamases, including staphylococcal penicillinase and Richmond and Sykes types II, III, IV, and V, including extended spectrum enzymes; it has only limited activity against class I beta-lactamases other than class Ic types

Pharmacodynamics/Kinetics Both AUC and peak concentrations are dose proportional

Distribution: Distributes well into lungs, intestinal mucosa, skin, muscle, uterus, ovary, prostate, gallbladder, and bile; penetration into CSF is low in subject with noninflamed meninges

Metabolism:
Piperacillin: 6% to 9%
Tazobactam: ~26%

Protein binding:
Piperacillin: ~26% to 33%
Tazobactam: 31% to 32%

Half-life:
Piperacillin: 1 hour
Metabolite: 1-1.5 hours
Tazobactam: 0.7-0.9 hour
Elimination: Both piperacillin and tazobactam are directly proportional to renal function
Piperacillin: 50% to 70% eliminated unchanged in urine, 10% to 20% excreted in bile
Tazobactam: Found in urine at 24 hours, with 26% as the inactive metabolite
Hemodialysis removes 30% to 40% of piperacillin and tazobactam; peritoneal dialysis removes 11% to 21% of tazobactam and 6% of piperacillin; hepatic impairment does not affect the kinetics of piperacillin or tazobactam significantly

Usual Dosage
Children <12 years: Not recommended due to lack of data
Children >12 years and Adults:
Severe infections: I.V.: Piperacillin/tazobactam 4/0.5 g every 8 hours or 3/0.375 g every 6 hours
Moderate infections: I.M.: Piperacillin/tazobactam 2/0.25 g every 6-1 hours; treatment should be continued for ≥7-10 days depending on severity of disease

Dosing interval in renal impairment:
Cl_{cr} >40 mL/minute: No change
Cl_{cr} 20-40 mL/minute: Administer 3/0.375 g every 6 hours
Cl_{cr} <20 mL/minute: Administer ≤3/0.375 g every 8 hours
Hemodialysis: Administer 2/0.25 g every 8 hours with an additional dose of 0.75 g after each dialysis

Administration Administer by I.V. infusion over 30 minutes; reconstitute with 5 mL of diluent per 1 g of piperacillin and then further dilute; compatible diluents include NS, SW, dextran 6%, D_5W, D_5W with potassium chloride 40 mEq, bacteriostatic saline and water; not compatible with lactated Ringer's solution

Monitoring Parameters LFTs, creatinine, BUN, CBC with differential, serum electrolytes, urinalysis, PT, PTT

Test Interactions Positive Coombs' [direct] test 3.8%, ALT, AST, bilirubin, and LDH

Nursing Implications Discontinue primary infusion, if possible, during infusion and administer aminoglycosides separately from Zosyn™

Dosage Forms Injection: Piperacillin sodium 2 g and tazobactam sodium 0.25 g; piperacillin sodium 3 g and tazobactam sodium 0.375 g; piperacillin sodium 4 g and tazobactam sodium 0.5 g (vials at an 8:1 ratio of piperacillin sodium/tazobactam sodium)

Piperazine Citrate (pi′ per a zeen)
Brand Names Vermizine®
Use Treatment of pinworm and roundworm infections (used as an alternative to first-line agents, mebendazole, or pyrantel pamoate)
Pregnancy Risk Factor B
Contraindications Seizure disorders, liver or kidney impairment, hypersensitivity to piperazine or any component
Warnings/Precautions Use with caution in patients with anemia or malnutrition; avoid prolonged use especially in children
Adverse Reactions
<1%:
Central nervous system: Dizziness, weakness, seizures, EEG changes, headache, vertigo
Gastrointestinal: Nausea, vomiting, diarrhea
Hematologic: Hemolytic anemia
Ocular: Visual impairment
Respiratory: Bronchospasms
Miscellaneous: Hypersensitivity reactions
Drug Interactions Pyrantel pamoate (antagonistic mode of action)
Mechanism of Action Causes muscle paralysis of the roundworm by blocking the effects of acetylcholine at the neuromuscular junction
Pharmacodynamics/Kinetics
Absorption: Well absorbed from GI tract
Time to peak serum concentration: 1 hour
Elimination: In urine as metabolites and unchanged drug
Usual Dosage Oral:
Pinworms: Children and Adults: 65 mg/kg/day (not to exceed 2.5 g/day) as a single daily dose for 7 days; in severe infections, repeat course after a 1-week interval
(Continued)

Piperazine Citrate *(Continued)*

Roundworms:
    Children: 75 mg/kg/day as a single daily dose for 2 days; maximum: 3.5 g/day
    Adults: 3.5 g/day for 2 days (in severe infections, repeat course, after a 1-week interval)

Monitoring Parameters Stool exam for worms and ova

Patient Information Take on empty stomach; if severe or persistent headache, loss of balance or coordination, dizziness, vomiting, diarrhea, or rash occurs, contact physician. If used for pinworm infections, all members of the family should be treated.

Nursing Implications Cure rates may be decreased with massive infections or in patients with hypermotility of the GI tract

Dosage Forms
    Syrup: 500 mg/5 mL (473 mL, 4000 mL)
    Tablet: 250 mg

Piperazine Estrone Sulfate *see* Estropipate *on page 414*

Pipobroman *(pi poe broe' man)*

Brand Names Vercyte®

Use Treat polycythemia vera; chronic myelocytic leukemia (in patients refractory to busulfan)

Pregnancy Risk Factor D

Contraindications Pre-existing bone marrow depression, hypersensitivity to any component

Warnings/Precautions The U.S. Food and Drug Administration (FDA) currently recommends that procedures for proper handling and disposal of antineoplastic agents be considered; bone marrow depression may not occur for 4 weeks

Adverse Reactions
1% to 10%:
    Dermatologic: Rash
    Gastrointestinal: Vomiting, diarrhea, nausea, abdominal cramps
    Hematologic: Leukopenia, thrombocytopenia, anemia

Overdosage/Toxicology Symptoms of overdose include severe marrow depression; supportive therapy is required

Mechanism of Action An alkylating agent considered to be cell-cycle nonspecific and capable of killing tumor cells in any phase of the cell cycle. Alkylating agents form covalent cross-links with DNA thereby resulting in cytotoxic, mutagenic, and carcinogenic effects. The end result of the alkylation process results in the misreading of the DNA code and the inhibition of DNA, RNA, and protein synthesis in rapidly proliferating tumor cells.

Usual Dosage Children >15 years and Adults: Oral:
    Polycythemia: 1 mg/kg/day for 30 days; may increase to 1.5-3 mg/kg until hematocrit reduced to 50% to 55%; maintenance: 0.1-0.2 mg/kg/day
    Myelocytic leukemia: 1.5-2.5 mg/kg/day until WBC drops to 10,000/mm^3 then start maintenance 7-175 mg/day; stop if WBC falls to <3000/mm^3 or platelets fall to <150,000/mm^3

Monitoring Parameters CBC, liver and renal function tests

Patient Information Notify physician if nausea, vomiting, diarrhea, or rash become severe or if unusual bleeding or bruising, sore throat, or fatigue occur; contraceptives are recommended during therapy

Dosage Forms Tablet: 25 mg

Pipracil® *see* Piperacillin Sodium *on page 888*

Pirbuterol Acetate *(peer byoo' ter ole)*

Brand Names Maxair™

Use Prevention and treatment of reversible bronchospasm including asthma

Pregnancy Risk Factor C

Contraindications Hypersensitivity to pirbuterol or albuterol

Warnings/Precautions Excessive use may result in tolerance; some adverse reactions may occur more frequently in children 2-5 years of age; use with caution in patients with hyperthyroidism, diabetes mellitus; cardiovascular disorders including coronary insufficiency or hypertension or sensitivity to sympathomimetic amines

Adverse Reactions
>10%:
    Central nervous system: Nervousness, restlessness
    Neuromuscular & skeletal: Trembling

1% to 10%:
    Central nervous system: Headache, dizziness
    Gastrointestinal: Taste changes, vomiting, nausea
<1%:
    Cardiovascular: Hypertension, arrhythmias, chest pain
    Central nervous system: Weakness, insomnia, numbness in hands
    Dermatologic: Bruising
    Gastrointestinal: Anorexia
    Respiratory: Paradoxical bronchospasm
Overdosage/Toxicology Symptoms of overdose include hypertension, tachycardia, angina, hypokalemia. In cases of overdose, supportive therapy should be instituted, and prudent use of a cardioselective beta-adrenergic blocker (eg, atenolol or metoprolol) should be considered, keeping in mind the potential for induction of bronchoconstriction in an asthmatic individual. Dialysis has not been shown to be of value in the treatment of an overdose with this agent.
Drug Interactions
    Decreased effect with beta-blockers
    Increased toxicity with other beta agonists, MAO inhibitors, TCAs
Mechanism of Action Pirbuterol is a beta$_2$-adrenergic agonist with a similar structure to albuterol, specifically a pyridine ring has been substituted for the benzene ring in albuterol. The increased beta$_2$ selectivity of pirbuterol results from the substitution of a tertiary butyl group on the nitrogen of the side chain, which additionally imparts resistance of pirbuterol to degradation by monoamine oxidase and provides a lengthened duration of action in comparison to the less selective previous beta-agonist agents.
Pharmacodynamics/Kinetics
    Peak therapeutic effect:
        Oral: 2-3 hours with peak serum concentration of 6.2-9.8 mcg/L
        Inhalation: 0.5-1 hour
    Half-life: 2-3 hours
    Metabolism: In the liver
    Elimination: 10% kidney excretion as unchanged drug
Usual Dosage Children >12 years and Adults: 2 inhalations every 4-6 hours for prevention; two inhalations at an interval of at least 1-3 minutes, followed by a third inhalation in treatment of bronchospasm, not to exceed 12 inhalations/day
Monitoring Parameters Respiratory rate, heart rate, and blood pressure
Patient Information Patient instructions are available with product. Do not exceed recommended dosage; rinse mouth with water following each inhalation to help with dry throat and mouth.
Nursing Implications Before using, the inhaler must be shaken well; assess lung sounds, pulse, and blood pressure before administration and during peak of medication; observe patient for wheezing after administration, if this occurs, call physician
Dosage Forms Aerosol, oral: 0.2 mg per actuation (25.6 g)

Piroxicam (peer ox' i kam)
Related Information
    Nonsteroidal Anti-Inflammatories Comparison on page 1280
Brand Names Feldene®
Use Management of inflammatory disorders; symptomatic treatment of acute and chronic rheumatoid arthritis, osteoarthritis, and ankylosing spondylitis; also used to treat sunburn
Pregnancy Risk Factor B (D if used in the 3rd trimester)
Contraindications Hypersensitivity to piroxicam, any component, aspirin or other nonsteroidal anti-inflammatory drugs (NSAIDs); active GI bleeding
Warnings/Precautions Use with caution in patients with impaired cardiac function, hypertension, impaired renal function, GI disease (bleeding or ulcers) and patients receiving anticoagulants; elderly have increased risk for adverse reactions to NSAIDs
Adverse Reactions
    >10%:
        Central nervous system: Dizziness
        Dermatologic: Skin rash
        Gastrointestinal: Abdominal cramps, heartburn, indigestion, nausea
    1% to 10%:
        Cardiovascular: Fluid retention
        Central nervous system: Headache, nervousness
        Dermatologic: Itching
        Gastrointestinal: Vomiting
        Otic: Ringing in ears
(Continued)

Piroxicam *(Continued)*

<1%:
- Cardiovascular: Congestive heart failure, hypertension, arrhythmias, tachycardia
- Central nervous system: Epistaxis, confusion, hallucinations, aseptic meningitis, mental depression, drowsiness, insomnia
- Dermatologic: Hives, erythema multiforme, toxic epidermal necrolysis, Stevens-Johnson syndrome, angioedema
- Endocrine & metabolic: Polydipsia, hot flushes
- Gastrointestinal: Gastritis, GI ulceration
- Genitourinary: Cystitis
- Hematologic: Agranulocytosis, anemia, hemolytic anemia, bone marrow depression, leukopenia, thrombocytopenia
- Hepatic: Hepatitis
- Neuromuscular & skeletal: Peripheral neuropathy
- Ocular: Toxic amblyopia, blurred vision, conjunctivitis, dry eyes
- Otic: Decreased hearing
- Renal: Polyuria, acute renal failure
- Respiratory: Allergic rhinitis, shortness of breath

Overdosage/Toxicology Symptoms of overdose include nausea, epigastric distress, CNS depression, leukocytosis, renal failure

Management of a nonsteroidal anti-inflammatory drug (NSAID) intoxication is primarily supportive and symptomatic

Fluid therapy is commonly effective in managing the hypotension that may occur following an acute NSAID overdose, except when this is due to an acute blood loss

Seizures tend to be very short-lived and often do not require drug treatment; although, recurrent seizures should be treated with I.V. diazepam

Since many of the NSAIDs undergo enterohepatic cycling, multiple doses of charcoal may be needed to reduce the potential for delayed toxicities

Drug Interactions

Decreased effect of diuretics, beta-blockers; decreased effect with aspirin, antacids, cholestyramine

Increased effect/toxicity of lithium, warfarin, methotrexate (controversial)

Mechanism of Action Inhibits prostaglandin synthesis, acts on the hypothalamus heat-regulating center to reduce fever, blocks prostaglandin synthetase action which prevents formation of the platelet-aggregating substance thromboxane A_2; decreases pain receptor sensitivity. Other proposed mechanisms of action for salicylate anti-inflammatory action are lysosomal stabilization, kinin and leukotriene production, alteration of chemotactic factors, and inhibition of neutrophil activation. This latter mechanism may be the most significant pharmacologic action to reduce inflammation.

Pharmacodynamics/Kinetics

Onset of analgesia: Oral: Within 1 hour
Peak effect: 3-5 hours
Protein binding: 99%
Metabolism: In the liver
Half-life: 45-50 hours
Elimination: As unchanged drug (5%) and metabolites primarily in urine and to a small degree in feces

Usual Dosage Oral:

Children: 0.2-0.3 mg/kg/day once daily; maximum dose: 15 mg/day

Adults: 10-20 mg/day once daily; although associated with increase in GI adverse effects, doses >20 mg/day have been used (ie, 30-40 mg/day)

Dosing adjustment in hepatic impairment: Reduction of dosage is necessary
Monitoring Parameters Occult blood loss, hemoglobin, hematocrit, and periodic renal and hepatic function tests; periodic ophthalmologic exams with chronic use
Test Interactions ↑ chloride (S), ↑ sodium (S), ↑ bleeding time
Patient Information Take with food, may cause drowsiness or dizziness
Dosage Forms Capsule: 10 mg, 20 mg

p-Isobutylhydratropic Acid *see* Ibuprofen *on page 561*

Pit *see* Oxytocin *on page 833*

Pitocin® *see* Oxytocin *on page 833*

Pitressin® *see* Vasopressin *on page 1149*

Placidyl® *see* Ethchlorvynol *on page 419*

Plague Vaccine (plaig vak seen')
Related Information
Vaccines *on page 1386-1388*

Use Selected travelers to countries reporting cases for whom avoidance of rodents and fleas is impossible; all laboratory and field personnel working with *Yersinia pestis* organisms possibly resistant to antimicrobials; those engaged in *Yersinia pestis* aerosol experiments or in field operations in areas with enzootic plague where regular exposure to potentially infected wild rodents, rabbits, or their fleas cannot be prevented. Prophylactic antibiotics may be indicated following definite exposure, whether or not the exposed persons have been vaccinated.

Pregnancy Risk Factor C

Contraindications Persons with known hypersensitivity to any of the vaccine constituents (see manufacturer's label); patients who have had severe local or systemic reactions to a previous dose; defer immunization in patients with a febrile illness until resolved

Warnings/Precautions Pregnancy, unless there is substantial and unavoidable risk of exposure

Adverse Reactions
1% to 10%:
Central nervous system: Malaise, fever, headache
Dermatologic: Local erythema
<1%:
Cardiovascular: Tachycardia
Gastrointestinal: Nausea, vomiting
Local: Sterile abscess

Drug Interactions Decreased effect with immunoglobulin, other live vaccine used within 1 month

Usual Dosage Three I.M. doses: First dose 1 mL, second dose (0.2 mL) 1 month later, third dose (0.2 mL) 5 months after the second dose; booster doses (0.2 mL) at 1- to 2-year intervals if exposure continues

Administration I.M. into deltoid muscle

Test Interactions Temporary suppression of tuberculosis skin test

Additional Information Federal law requires that the date of administration, the vaccine manufacturer, lot number of vaccine, and the administering person's name, title and address be entered into the patient's permanent medical record

Dosage Forms Injection: 2 mL, 20 mL

Plantago Seed *see* Psyllium *on page 956*

Plantain Seed *see* Psyllium *on page 956*

Plaquenil® *see* Hydroxychloroquine Sulfate *on page 552*

Plasbumin® *see* Albumin, Human *on page 32*

Platinol® *see* Cisplatin *on page 248*

Platinol®-AQ *see* Cisplatin *on page 248*

Plendil® *see* Felodipine *on page 442*

Plicamycin (plye kay mye' sin)
Related Information
Antiemetics for Chemotherapy Induced Nausea and Vomiting *on page 1202*
Cancer Chemotherapy Regimens *on page 1218-1241*

Brand Names Mithracin®

Synonyms Mithramycin

Use Malignant testicular tumors, in the treatment of hypercalcemia and hypercalciuria of malignancy not responsive to conventional treatment; Paget's disease

Pregnancy Risk Factor D

Contraindications Thrombocytopenia, bleeding diatheses, coagulation disorders; bone marrow function impairment; or hypocalcemia

Warnings/Precautions The U.S. Food and Drug Administration (FDA) currently recommends that procedures for proper handling and disposal of antineoplastic agents be considered. Use with caution in patients with hepatic or renal impairment; reduce dosage in patients with renal impairment; discontinue if bleeding or epistaxis occurs. Plicamycin may cause permanent sterility and may cause birth defects.

Adverse Reactions
>10%: Gastrointestinal: Nausea and vomiting occur in almost 100% of patients within the first 6 hours after treatment; incidence increases with rapid injection; stomatitis has also occurred; anorexia, diarrhea
1% to 10%:
Central nervous system: Headache, fever, mental depression, drowsiness, weakness
(Continued)

895

Plicamycin *(Continued)*

Myelosuppression: Mild leukopenia and thrombocytopenia

WBC: Moderate

Platelets: Moderate

Onset (days): 7-10

Nadir (days): 14

Recovery (days): 21

Clotting disorders: May also depress hepatic synthesis of clotting factors, leading to a form of coagulopathy; petechiae, increased prothrombin time, epistaxis, and thrombocytopenia may be seen and may require discontinuation of the drug

Endocrine & metabolic: Hypocalcemia

Extravasation: Is an irritant; may produce local tissue irritation or cellulitis if infiltrated; if extravasation occurs, follow hospital procedure, discontinue I.V., and apply ice for 24 hours

Irritant chemotherapy

Hepatic: Elevation in liver enzymes, hepatotoxicity

Renal: Nephrotoxicity, azotemia

Miscellaneous: Facial flushing, hemorrhagic diathesis

Overdosage/Toxicology Symptoms of overdose include bone marrow depression, bleeding syndrome, thrombocytopenia; supportive therapy. Treatment of hemorrhagic episodes should include transfusion of fresh whole blood or packed red blood cells and fresh frozen plasma, vitamin K, and corticosteroids.

Drug Interactions Increased toxicity: Calcitonin, etidronate, glucagon, → additive hypoglycemic effects

Stability Refrigeration is recommended for intact vials, but remains stable for up to 3 months unrefrigerated; drug is unstable at a pH <4; reconstituted solution is stable for 24 hours at room temperature and 48 hours when refrigerated

Mechanism of Action Potent osteoclast inhibitor; may inhibit parathyroid hormone effect on osteoclasts; inhibits bone resorption; forms a complex with DNA in the presence of magnesium or other divalent cations inhibiting DNA-directed RNA synthesis

Pharmacodynamics/Kinetics

Decreasing calcium levels:

Onset of action: Within 24 hours

Peak effect: 48-72 hours

Duration: 5-15 days

Distribution: Crosses blood-brain barrier in low concentrations

Protein binding: 0%

Half-life, plasma: 1 hour

Elimination: 90% of dose excreted in urine within the first 24 hours

Usual Dosage Adults (refer to individual protocols): I.V. (dose based on ideal body weight):

Testicular cancer: 25-30 mcg/kg/day for 8-10 days

Hypercalcemia: 15-25 mcg/kg/day for 3-4 days or 25 mcg/kg every 48-72 hours; additional courses of therapy may be given at intervals of 1 week or more if the initial course is unsuccessful

Paget's disease: 15 mcg/kg/day for 10 days

Dosing adjustment in renal impairment:

Cl_{cr} 10-50 mL/minute: Decrease dosage to 75% of normal dose

Cl_{cr} <10 mL/minute: Decrease dosage to 50% of normal dose

Dosing adjustment in hepatic impairment: Reduce dose to 12.5 mcg/kg/day

Administration For adults, the dose should be diluted in 1 L of D_5W or NS and administered as an I.V. infusion over 4-6 hours; bolus or short infusion over 30-60 minutes in 100-150 mL D_5W is an alternative method of administration

Monitoring Parameters Hepatic and renal function tests, CBC, platelet count, prothrombin time, serum electrolytes

Patient Information Any signs of infection, easy bruising or bleeding, shortness of breath, or painful or burning urination should be brought to physician's attention. Nausea, vomiting, or hair loss sometimes occur. The drug may cause permanent sterility and may cause birth defects. The drug may be excreted in breast milk, therefore, an alternative form of feeding your baby should be used.

Nursing Implications Rapid I.V. infusion has been associated with an increased incidence of nausea and vomiting; an antiemetic given prior to and during plicamycin infusion may be helpful. Avoid extravasation since plicamycin is a strong vesicant.

Dosage Forms Powder for injection: 2.5 mg

Pneumococcal Polysaccharide Vaccine, Polyvalent (new mo kock' al poly sack' a ride)

Related Information
Immunization Guidelines *on page 1389-1405*
Vaccines *on page 1386-1388*

Brand Names Pneumovax® 23; Pnu-Imune® 23

Use Children >2 years of age and adults who are at increased risk of pneumococcal disease and its complications because of underlying health conditions; older adults, including all those ≥65 years of age

Pregnancy Risk Factor C

Contraindications Active infections, Hodgkin's disease patients, <5 years of age, pregnancy, hypersensitivity to pneumococcal vaccine or any component; (children <5 years of age do not respond satisfactorily to the capsular types of 23 capsular pneumococcal vaccine; the safety of vaccine in pregnant women has not been evaluated; it should not be given during pregnancy unless the risk of infection is high)

Warnings/Precautions Epinephrine injection (1:1000) must be immediately available in the case of anaphylaxis; use caution in individuals who have had episodes of pneumococcal infection within the preceding 3 years (pre-existing pneumococcal antibodies may result in increased reactions to vaccine); may cause relapse in patients with stable idiopathic thrombocytopenia purpura

Adverse Reactions
>10%: Local: Induration and soreness at the injection site (2-3 days)
<1%:
Central nervous system: Guillain-Barré syndrome, low-grade fever
Dermatologic: Erythema, rash
Neuromuscular & skeletal: Paresthesias, myalgia, arthralgia
Miscellaneous: Anaphylaxis

Drug Interactions Decreased effect with immunosuppressive agents, immunoglobulin, other live vaccines within 1 month

Stability Refrigerate

Mechanism of Action Although there are more than 80 known pneumococcal capsular types, pneumococcal disease is mainly caused by only a few types of pneumococci. Pneumococcal vaccine contains capsular polysaccharides of 23 pneumococcal types which represent at least 98% of pneumococcal disease isolates in the United States and Europe. The pneumococcal vaccine with 23 pneumococcal capsular polysaccharide types became available in 1983. The 23 capsular pneumococcal vaccine contains purified capsular polysaccharides of pneumococcal types 1, 2, 3, 4, 5, 8, 9, 12, 14, 17, 19, 20, 22, 23, 26, 34, 43, 51, 56, 57, 67, 70 (American Classification). These are the main pneumococcal types associated with serious infections in the United States.

Usual Dosage Children >2 years and Adults: I.M., S.C.: 0.5 mL
Revaccination should be considered:
1) If ≥6 years since initial vaccination has elapsed, or
2) In patients who received 14-valent pneumococcal vaccine and are at highest risk (asplenic) for fatal infection or
3) at ≥6 years in patients with nephrotic syndrome, renal failure, or transplant recipients, or
4) 3-5 years in children with nephrotic syndrome, asplenia, or sickle cell disease

Administration Do not inject I.V., avoid intradermal, administer S.C. or I.M. (deltoid muscle or lateral midthigh)

Additional Information Federal law requires that the date of administration, the vaccine manufacturer, lot number of vaccine, and the administering person's name, title and address be entered into the patient's permanent medical record; inactivated bacteria vaccine

Dosage Forms Injection: 25 mcg each of 23 polysaccharide isolates/0.5 mL dose (0.5 mL, 1 mL, 5 mL)

Pneumovax® 23 *see* Pneumococcal Polysaccharide Vaccine, Polyvalent *on previous page*

Pnu-Imune® 23 *see* Pneumococcal Polysaccharide Vaccine, Polyvalent *on previous page*

Podocon-25® *see* Podophyllum Resin *on this page*

Podofin® *see* Podophyllum Resin *on this page*

Podophyllum Resin (pode oh fill' in)
Brand Names Podocon-25®; Podofin®
Synonyms Mandrake; May Apple
(Continued)

Podophyllum Resin *(Continued)*

Use Topical treatment of benign growths including external genital and perianal warts, papillomas, fibroids; compound benzoin tincture generally is used as the medium for topical application

Pregnancy Risk Factor X

Contraindications Not to be used on birthmarks, moles, or warts with hair growth; cervical, urethral, oral warts; not to be used by diabetic patient or patient with poor circulation; pregnant women

Warnings/Precautions Use of large amounts of drug should be avoided; avoid contact with the eyes as it can cause severe corneal damage; do not apply to moles, birthmarks, or unusual warts; to be applied by a physician only; for external use only; 25% solution should not be applied to or near mucous membranes

Adverse Reactions Local: Pain, swelling

1% to 10%:
Dermatologic: Pruritus
Gastrointestinal: Nausea, vomiting, abdominal pain, diarrhea

<1%:
Central nervous system: Confusion, lethargy, hallucinations
Genitourinary: Renal failure
Hematologic: Leukopenia, thrombocytopenia
Hepatic: Hepatotoxicity
Neuromuscular & skeletal: Peripheral neuropathy

Mechanism of Action Directly affects epithelial cell metabolism by arresting mitosis through binding to a protein subunit of spindle microtubules (tubulin)

Usual Dosage Topical:

Children and Adults: 10% to 25% solution in compound benzoin tincture; apply drug to dry surface, use 1 drop at a time allowing drying between drops until area is covered; total volume should be limited to <0.5 mL per treatment session

Condylomata acuminatum: 25% solution is applied daily; use a 10% solution when applied to or near mucous membranes

Verrucae: 25% solution is applied 3-5 times/day directly to the wart

Patient Information Notify physician if undue skin irritation develops; should be applied by a physician

Nursing Implications Shake well before using; solution should be washed off within 1-4 hours for genital and perianal warts and within 1-2 hours for accessible meatal warts; use protective occlusive dressing around warts to prevent contact with unaffected skin

Dosage Forms Liquid, topical: 25% in benzoin (15 mL)

Point-Two® *see* Fluoride *on page 471*

Poladex® *see* Dexchlorpheniramine Maleate *on page 316*

Polaramine® *see* Dexchlorpheniramine Maleate *on page 316*

Polargen® *see* Dexchlorpheniramine Maleate *on page 316*

Poliomyelitis Vaccine *see* Polio Vaccines *on this page*

Polio Vaccines *(poe' lee oh)*

Related Information
Immunization Guidelines *on page 1389-1405*
Vaccines *on page 1386-1388*

Brand Names IPOL™; Orimune®

Synonyms E-IPV; Enhanced-potency Inactivated Poliovirus Vaccine; OPV; Poliomyelitis Vaccine; Poliovirus Vaccine, Live, Trivalent; Sabin; Salk; TOPV

Use Oral: Prevention of poliomyelitis for infants (6-12 weeks of age) and all unimmunized children and adolescents through 18 years of age for routine prophylaxis. Persons traveling to areas where wild poliovirus is epidemic or endemic, and certain health personnel.

Although a protective immune response to E-IPV cannot be assured in the immunocompromised individual, E-IPV is recommended because the vaccine is safe and some protection may result from its administration.

Pregnancy Risk Factor C

Contraindications
Oral: Leukemia, lymphoma, or other generalized malignancies; diseases in which cellular immunity is absent or suppressed (hypogammaglobulinemia, agammaglobulinemia); immunosuppressive therapy; diarrhea; parenteral administration

Parenteral: Hypersensitivity to any component including neomycin, streptomycin, or polymyxin B; defer vaccination for persons with acute febrile illness until recovery

Warnings/Precautions Although there is no convincing evidence documenting adverse effects of either OPV or E-IPV on the pregnant woman or developing fetus, it is prudent on theoretical grounds to avoid vaccinating pregnant women. However, if immediate protection against poliomyelitis is needed, OPV is recommended. OPV should not be given to immunocompromised individuals or to persons with known or possibly immunocompromised family members; E-IPV is recommended in such situations.

Adverse Reactions All serious adverse reactions must be reported to the FDA

1% to 10%:
Dermatologic: Skin rash
Central nervous system: Fever >101.3°F
Local: Tenderness or pain at injection site

<1%:
Central nervous system: Tiredness, weakness, fussiness, sleepiness, crying, Guillain-Barré
Dermatologic: Reddening of skin, erythema
Gastrointestinal: Decreased appetite
Respiratory: Difficulty in breathing

Drug Interactions Decreased effect with immunosuppressive agents, immune globulin, other live vaccines within 1 month; may temporarily suppress tuberculin skin test sensitivity (4-6 weeks)

Usual Dosage
Oral:
Infants:
Primary series: 0.5 mL at 6-12 weeks of age, second dose 6-8 weeks after first dose, and third dose 8-12 months after second dose
Booster: All children who have received primary immunization series, should receive a single follow-up dose and all children who have not should complete primary series
Children (older) and Adults (adolescents through 18 years of age): Two 0.5 mL doses 6-8 weeks apart and a third dose of 0.5 mL 6-12 months after second dose

Subcutaneous: **Enhanced-potency inactivated poliovirus vaccine (E-IPV) is preferred for primary vaccination of adults**, two doses S.C. 4-8 weeks apart, a third dose 6-12 months after the second. For adults with a completed primary series and for whom a booster is indicated, either OPV or E-IPV can be given. If immediate protection is needed, either OPV or E-IPV is recommended.

Administration Do not administer I.V.

Additional Information Federal law requires that the date of administration, the vaccine manufacturer, lot number of vaccine, and the administering person's name, title and address be entered into the patient's permanent medical record

Dosage Forms
Injection (IPOL™, E-IPV, Enhanced-potency Inactivated Poliovirus Vaccine, Poliomyelitis Vaccine, Salk): Suspension of three types of poliovirus (Types 1, 2 and 3) grown in human diploid cell cultures (0.5 mL)
Solution, oral (Orimune®, OPV, Poliovirus Vaccine, Live, Trivalent, Sabin, TOPV): Mixture of type 1, 2, and 3 viruses in monkey kidney tissue (0.5 mL)

Poliovirus Vaccine, Live, Trivalent *see* Polio Vaccines *on previous page*

Polocaine® *see* Mepivacaine Hydrochloride *on page 688*

Polycillin® *see* Ampicillin *on page 73*

Polyestradiol Phosphate (pol ee ess tra dye′ ole)
Brand Names Estradurin®
Use Palliative treatment of advanced, inoperable carcinoma of the prostate
Pregnancy Risk Factor X
Contraindications Known or suspected estrogen-dependent neoplasm, carcinoma of the breast, active thromboembolic disorders, hypersensitivity to estrogens or any component
Warnings/Precautions Use with caution in patients with migraine, diabetes, cardiac, or renal impairment
Adverse Reactions
>10%:
Cardiovascular: Peripheral edema
Endocrine & metabolic: Enlargement of breasts (female and male), breast tenderness
(Continued)

Polyestradiol Phosphate *(Continued)*

Gastrointestinal: Nausea, anorexia, bloating

1% to 10%:

Central nervous system: Headache

Endocrine & metabolic: Increased libido (female), decrease libido (male)

Gastrointestinal: Vomiting, diarrhea

<1%:

Cardiovascular: Hypertension, thromboembolism, stroke, myocardial infarction, edema

Central nervous system: Depression, dizziness, anxiety

Dermatologic: Chloasma, melasma, rash

Endocrine: Breast tumors, amenorrhea, alterations in frequency and flow of menses, decreased glucose tolerance, increased triglycerides and LDL

Gastrointestinal: Nausea, GI distress

Hepatic: Cholestatic jaundice

Miscellaneous: Intolerance to contact lenses, increased susceptibility to *Candida* infection

Overdosage/Toxicology Toxicity is unlikely following single exposures of excessive doses; any treatment following emesis and charcoal administration should be supportive and symptomatic

Stability After reconstitution, solution is stable for 10 days at room temperature and protected from direct light

Mechanism of Action Estrogens exert their primary effects on the interphase DNA-protein complex (chromatin) by binding to a receptor (usually located in the cytoplasm of a target cell) and initiating translocation of the hormone-receptor complex to the nucleus

Pharmacodynamics/Kinetics

90% of injected dose leaves blood stream within 24 hours

Passive storage in reticuloendothelial system

Increasing the dose prolongs duration of action

Usual Dosage Adults: Deep I.M.: 40 mg every 2-4 weeks or less frequently; maximum dose: 80 mg

Dosage Forms Powder for injection: 40 mg

Polyethylene Glycol-Electrolyte Solution (pol ee eth' i leen)

Brand Names Colovage®; CoLyte®; GoLYTELY®; NuLytely®; OCL®

Synonyms Electrolyte Lavage Solution

Use Bowel cleansing prior to GI examination or following toxic ingestion

Pregnancy Risk Factor C

Contraindications Gastrointestinal obstruction, gastric retention, bowel perforation, toxic colitis, megacolon

Warnings/Precautions Safety and efficacy not established in children; do not add flavorings as additional ingredients before use; observe unconscious or semiconscious patients with impaired gag reflex or those who are otherwise prone to regurgitation or aspiration during administration; use with caution in ulcerative colitis, caution against the use of hot loop polypectomy

Adverse Reactions

>10%: Gastrointestinal: Nausea, abdominal fullness, bloating

1% to 10%: Gastrointestinal: Abdominal cramps, vomiting, anal irritation

<1%: Dermatologic: Skin rash

Drug Interactions Oral medications should not be administered within 1 hour of start of therapy

Stability Use within 48 hours of preparation; refrigerate reconstituted solution; tap water may be used for preparation of the solution; shake container vigorously several times to ensure dissolution of powder

Mechanism of Action Induces catharsis by strong electrolyte and osmotic effects

Pharmacodynamics/Kinetics Onset of effect: Oral: Within 1-2 hours

Usual Dosage The recommended dose for adults is 4 L of solution prior to gastrointestinal examination, as ingestion of this dose produces a satisfactory preparation in >95% of patients. Ideally the patient should fast for approximately 3-4 hours prior to administration, but in no case should solid food be given for at least 2 hours before the solution is given. The solution is usually administered orally, but may be given via nasogastric tube to patients who are unwilling or unable to drink the solution.

Children: Oral: 25-40 mL/kg/hour for 4-10 hours

Adults:

Oral: At a rate of 240 mL (8 oz) every 10 minutes, until 4 liters are consumed or the rectal effluent is clear; rapid drinking of each portion is preferred to drinking small amounts continuously

Nasogastric tube: At a rate of 20-30 mL/minute (1.2-1.8 L/hour); the first bowel movement should occur approximately 1 hour after the start of administration

Monitoring Parameters Electrolytes, serum glucose, BUN, urine osmolality

Patient Information Chilled solution is often more palatable

Nursing Implications Rapid drinking of each portion is preferred over small amounts continuously; first bowel movement should occur in 1 hour; chilled solution often more palatable; do not add flavorings as additional ingredients before use

Dosage Forms Powder, for oral solution: PEG 3350 236 g, sodium sulfate 22.74 g, sodium bicarbonate 6.74 g, sodium chloride 5.86 g and potassium chloride 2.97 g (2000 mL, 4000 mL, 4800 mL, 6000 mL)

Polyflex® see Chlorzoxazone on page 236

Polygam® see Immune Globulin, Intravenous on page 571

Polymox® see Amoxicillin Trihydrate on page 68

Polymyxin and Neomycin see Neomycin and Polymyxin B on page 780

Polymyxin B and Neomycin see Neomycin and Polymyxin B on page 780

Polymyxin B Sulfate (pol i mix' in)

Brand Names Aerosporin®

Use

Topical: Wound irrigation and bladder irrigation against *Pseudomonas aeruginosa*; used occasionally for gut decontamination

Parenteral use of polymyxin B has mainly been replaced by less toxic antibiotics; it is reserved for life-threatening infections caused by organisms resistant to the preferred drugs.

Pregnancy Risk Factor B

Contraindications Concurrent use of neuromuscular blockers

Warnings/Precautions Use with caution in patients with impaired renal function, (modify dosage) neurotoxic reactions are usually associated with high serum levels, found in patients with impaired renal function. Avoid concurrent or sequential use of other nephrotoxic and neurotoxic drugs, particularly bacitracin, colistin and the aminoglycosides. The drug's neurotoxicity can result in respiratory paralysis from neuromuscular blockade, especially when the drug is given soon after anesthesia or muscle relaxants. Polymyxin B sulfate is toxic when given parenterally; avoid parenteral use whenever possible.

Adverse Reactions

<1%:

Cardiovascular: Facial flushing

Central nervous system: Neurotoxicity (irritability, weakness, drowsiness, ataxia, perioral paresthesia, numbness of the extremities, and blurring of vision)

Dermatologic: Urticarial rash

Endocrine & metabolic: Hypocalcemia, hyponatremia, hypokalemia, hypochloremia

Neuromuscular & skeletal: Neuromuscular blockade

Renal: Nephrotoxicity

Respiratory: Respiratory arrest

Miscellaneous: Drug fever, anaphylactoid reaction, meningeal irritation with intrathecal administration

Overdosage/Toxicology Symptoms of overdose include respiratory paralysis, ototoxicity, nephrotoxicity; supportive care is indicated as treatment; ventilatory support may be necessary

Drug Interactions Increased/prolonged effect of neuromuscular blocking agents

Stability Parenteral solutions stable for 7 days when refrigerated; discard any unused portion after 72 hours. **Incompatible** with calcium, magnesium, cephalothin, chloramphenicol, heparin, penicillins; aqueous solutions remain stable for 6-12 months under refrigeration

Mechanism of Action Binds to phospholipids, alters permeability, and damages the bacterial cytoplasmic membrane permitting leakage of intracellular constituents

Pharmacodynamics/Kinetics

Absorption: Well absorbed from the peritoneum; minimal absorption from the GI tract (except in neonates) from mucous membranes or intact skin

(Continued)

Polymyxin B Sulfate *(Continued)*

Distribution: Minimal distribution into the CSF; crosses the placenta
Half-life: 4.5-6 hours, increased with reduced renal function
Time to peak serum concentration: I.M.: Within 2 hours
Elimination: Primarily as unchanged drug (>60%) in urine via glomerular filtration

Usual Dosage

Otic: 1-2 drops, 3-4 times/day; should be used sparingly to avoid accumulation of excess debris

Infants <2 years:
I.M.: 25,000-30,000 units/kg/day divided every 6 hours
I.V.: 30,000-45,000 units/kg/day by continuous I.V. infusion
Intrathecal: 20,000 units/day for 3-4 days, then 25,000 units every other day for at least 2 weeks

Children ≥2 years and Adults:
I.M.: 25,000-30,000 units/kg/day divided every 4-6 hours
I.V.: 15,000-25,000 units/kg/day divided every 12 hours or by continuous infusion
Intrathecal: 50,000 units/day for 3-4 days, then every other day for at least 2 weeks

Total daily dose should not exceed 2,000,000 units/day

Bladder irrigation: Continuous irrigant or rinse in the urinary bladder for up to 10 days using 20 mg (equal to 200,000 units) added to 1 L of normal saline; usually no more than 1 L of irrigant is used per day unless urine flow rate is high; administration rate is adjusted to patient's urine output

Topical irrigation or topical solution: 500,000 units/L of normal saline; topical irrigation should not exceed 2 million units/day in adults

Gut sterilization: Oral: 15,000-25,000 units/kg/day in divided doses every 6 hours

Clostridium difficile enteritis: Oral: 25,000 units every 6 hours for 10 days

Ophthalmic: A concentration of 0.1% to 0.25% is administered as 1-3 drops every hour, then increasing the interval as response indicates to 1-2 drops 4-6 times/day

Dosing adjustment/interval in renal impairment:
Cl_{cr} 50-20 mL/minute: Administer 75% to 100% of normal dose every 12 hours
Cl_{cr} 5-20 mL/minute: Administer 50% of normal dose every 12 hours
Cl_{cr} <5 mL/minute: Administer 15% of normal dose every 12 hours

Reference Range Serum concentrations >5 μg/mL are toxic in adults

Patient Information Report any dizziness or sensations of ringing in the ear, loss of hearing, or any muscle weakness

Nursing Implications Parenteral use is indicated only in life-threatening infections caused by organisms not susceptible to other agents

Additional Information 1 mg = 10,000 units

Dosage Forms
Injection: 500,000 units (20 mL)
Powder for solution, ophthalmic: 500,000 units (20-50 mL diluent)

Polymyxin E *see* Colistin Sulfate *on page 273*

Poly-Pred® *see* Neomycin, Polymyxin B, and Prednisolone *on page 782*

Polysporin® *see* Bacitracin and Polymyxin B *on page 112*

Polythiazide *(pol i thye′ a zide)*

Brand Names Renese®
Use Adjunctive therapy in treatment of edema and hypertension
Pregnancy Risk Factor D
Contraindications Anuria; hypersensitivity to polythiazide or any other sulfonamide derivatives
Warnings/Precautions Use with caution in renal disease, hepatic disease, gout, lupus erythematosus, diabetes mellitus; some products may contain tartrazine

Adverse Reactions
1% to 10%: Hypokalemia
<1%:
Cardiovascular: Hypotension
Central nervous system: Drowsiness
Dermatologic: Photosensitivity, rash
Endocrine & metabolic: Fluid and electrolyte imbalances (hypocalcemia, hypomagnesemia, hyponatremia), hyperglycemia
Gastrointestinal: Nausea, vomiting, anorexia
Genitourinary: Uremia

Hematologic: Rarely blood dyscrasias

Hepatic: Hepatitis

Renal: Prerenal azotemia, polyuria

Overdosage/Toxicology Symptoms of overdose include hypermotility, diuresis, lethargy; GI decontamination and supportive care

Drug Interactions Increased toxicity/levels of lithium

Mechanism of Action The diuretic mechanism of action of the thiazides is primarily inhibition of sodium, chloride, and water reabsorption in the renal distal tubules, thereby producing diuresis with a resultant reduction in plasma volume. The antihypertensive mechanism of action of the thiazides is unknown. It is known that doses of thiazides produce greater reductions in blood pressure than equivalent diuretic doses of loop diuretics (eg, furosemide). There has been speculation that the thiazides may have some influence on vascular tone mediated through sodium depletion, but this remains to be proven.

Pharmacodynamics/Kinetics

Onset of diuretic effect: Within ~2 hours

Duration: 24-48 hours

Usual Dosage Adults: Oral: 1-4 mg/day

Monitoring Parameters Blood pressure, fluids, weight loss, serum potassium

Test Interactions ↑ ammonia (B), ↑ amylase (S), ↑ calcium (S), ↑ chloride (S), ↑ cholesterol (S), ↑ glucose, ↑ uric acid (S); ↓ chloride (S), ↓ magnesium, ↓ potassium (S), ↓ sodium (S); tyramine and phentolamine tests, histamine tests for pheochromocytoma

Patient Information May be taken with food or milk; take early in day to avoid nocturia; take the last dose of multiple doses no later than 6 PM unless instructed otherwise. A few people who take this medication become more sensitive to sunlight and may experience skin rash, redness, itching, or severe sunburn, especially if sun block SPF ≥15 is not used on exposed skin areas.

Nursing Implications Assess weight, I & O reports daily to determine fluid loss; take blood pressure with patient lying down and standing

Dosage Forms Tablet: 1 mg, 2 mg, 4 mg

Poly-Vi-Flor® see Vitamin, Multiple on page 1166

Poly-Vi-Sol® [OTC] see Vitamin, Multiple on page 1166

Pondimin® see Fenfluramine Hydrochloride on page 444

Ponstel® see Mefenamic Acid on page 678

Pontocaine® see Tetracaine Hydrochloride on page 1068

Porcelana® [OTC] see Hydroquinone on page 551

Pork NPH Iletin® II [OTC] see Insulin Preparations on page 578

Pork Regular Iletin® II [OTC] see Insulin Preparations on page 578

Posture® [OTC] see Calcium Phosphate, Tribasic on page 171

Potasalan® see Potassium Chloride on page 906

Potassium Acetate (poe tass' y um as' i tate)

Use Potassium deficiency; to avoid chloride when high concentration of potassium is needed, source of bicarbonate

Pregnancy Risk Factor C

Contraindications Severe renal impairment, hyperkalemia

Warnings/Precautions Use with caution in patients with renal disease, hyperkalemia, cardiac disease, metabolic alkalosis; must be administered in patients with adequate urine flow

Adverse Reactions

>10%: Gastrointestinal: Diarrhea, nausea, stomach pain, flatulence, vomiting (oral)

1% to 10%:

Cardiovascular: Bradycardia

Endocrine & metabolic: Hyperkalemia

Respiratory: Difficult breathing, weakness

Local: Local tissue necrosis with extravasation

<1%:

Cardiovascular: Chest pain

Central nervous system: Mental confusion

Endocrine & metabolic: Alkalosis

Gastrointestinal: Abdominal pain

Local: Phlebitis

Neuromuscular & skeletal: Paresthesias, paralysis

Miscellaneous: Throat pain

(Continued)

Potassium Acetate *(Continued)*

Overdosage/Toxicology Symptoms of overdose include muscle weakness, paralysis, peaked T waves, flattened P waves, prolongation of chloride, QRS complex, ventricular arrhythmias. Removal of potassium can be accomplished by various means; removal through the GI tract with Kayexalate® administration; by way of the kidney through diuresis, mineralocorticoid administration or increased sodium intake; by hemodialysis or peritoneal dialysis; or by shifting potassium back into the cells by insulin and glucose infusion or administration of sodium bicarbonate; calcium chloride will reverse cardiac effects.

Drug Interactions Increased effect/levels with potassium-sparing diuretics, salt substitutes, ACE inhibitors

Mechanism of Action Potassium is the major cation of intracellular fluid and is essential for the conduction of nerve impulses in heart, brain, and skeletal muscle; contraction of cardiac, skeletal and smooth muscles; maintenance of normal renal function, acid-base balance, carbohydrate metabolism, and gastric secretion

Pharmacodynamics/Kinetics

Absorption: Absorbed well from upper GI tract

Distribution: Enters cells via active transport from extracellular fluid

Elimination: Largely by the kidneys, but also small amount via the skin and feces, with most intestinal potassium being reabsorbed

Usual Dosage I.V. doses should be incorporated into the patient's maintenance I.V. fluids, intermittent I.V. potassium administration should be reserved for severe depletion situations and requires EKG monitoring; doses listed as mEq of potassium

Treatment of hypokalemia: I.V.:

Children: 2-5 mEq/kg/day

Adults: 40-100 mEq/day

I.V. intermittent infusion (must be diluted prior to administration):

Children: 0.5-1 mEq/kg/dose (maximum: 30 mEq) to infuse at 0.3-0.5 mEq/kg/hour (maximum: 1 mEq/kg/hour)

Adults: 10-20 mEq/dose (maximum: 40 mEq/dose) to infuse over 2-3 hours (maximum: 40 mEq over 1 hour)

Administration Injections must be diluted for I.V. infusions

Nursing Implications Supplements usually not needed with adequate diet; EKG should be monitored continuously during the course of highly concentrate potassium solutions

Additional Information 1 mEq of acetate is equivalent to the alkalinizing effect of 1 mEq of bicarbonate

Dosage Forms Injection: 2 mEq/mL (20 mL, 50 mL, 100 mL); 4 mEq/mL (50 mL)

Potassium Acid Phosphate *(poe tass' y um as' id fos' fate)*

Brand Names K-Phos® Original

Use Acidifies urine and lowers urinary calcium concentration; reduces odor and rash caused by ammoniacal urine; increases the antibacterial activity of methenamine

Pregnancy Risk Factor C

Contraindications Severe renal impairment, hyperkalemia, hyperphosphatemia, and infected magnesium ammonium phosphate stones

Warnings/Precautions Use with caution in patients receiving other potassium supplementation and in patients with renal insufficiency, or severe tissue breakdown (eg, chemotherapy or hemodialysis)

Adverse Reactions

>10%: Gastrointestinal: Diarrhea, nausea, stomach pain, flatulence, vomiting

1% to 10%:

Cardiovascular: Bradycardia

Central nervous system: Weakness

Endocrine & metabolic: Hyperkalemia

Local: Local tissue necrosis with extravasation

Respiratory: Difficult breathing

<1%:

Cardiovascular: Chest pain, irregular heartbeat, edema

Central nervous system: Mental confusion, tetany, pain/weakness of extremities

Endocrine & metabolic: Hyperphosphatemia, hypocalcemia, alkalosis

Gastrointestinal: Abdominal pain, weight gain

Genitourinary: Decreased urine output

Local: Phlebitis

Neuromuscular & skeletal: Paresthesias, paralysis, bone/joint pain

Respiratory: Shortness of breath

Miscellaneous: Thirst, throat pain

Overdosage/Toxicology Symptoms of overdose include muscle weakness, paralysis, peaked T waves, flattened P waves, prolongation of QRS complex, ventricular arrhythmias. Removal of potassium can be accomplished by various means; removal through the GI tract with Kayexalate® administration; by way of the kidney through diuresis, mineralocorticoid administration or increased sodium intake; by hemodialysis or peritoneal dialysis; or by shifting potassium back into the cells by insulin and glucose infusion or sodium bicarbonate; calcium chloride will reverse cardiac effects.

Drug Interactions

Increased effect/levels with potassium-sparing diuretics, salt substitutes, salicylates, ACE inhibitors

Decreased effect with antacids containing magnesium, calcium or aluminum (bind phosphate and decreased its absorption)

Mechanism of Action The principal intracellular cation; involved in transmission of nerve impulses, muscle contractions, enzyme activity, and glucose utilization

Pharmacodynamics/Kinetics

Absorption: Absorbed well from upper GI tract

Distribution: Enters cells via active transport from extracellular fluid

Elimination: Largely by the kidneys, but also small amount via the skin and feces, with most intestinal potassium being reabsorbed

Usual Dosage Adults: Oral: 1000 mg dissolved in 6-8 oz of water 4 times/day with meals and at bedtime; for best results, soak tablets in water for 2-5 minutes, then stir and swallow

Monitoring Parameters Serum potassium, sodium, phosphate, calcium; serum salicylates (if taking salicylates)

Test Interactions ↓ ammonia (B)

Patient Information Dissolve tablets completely before drinking; avoid taking magnesium, calcium, or aluminum antacids at the same time; patients may pass old kidney stones when starting therapy; notify physician if experiencing nausea, vomiting, or abdominal pain

Dosage Forms Tablet, sodium free: 500 mg [potassium 3.67 mEq]

Potassium Bicarbonate and Potassium Citrate, Effervescent (poe tass' y um bye kar' bo nate & poe tass' y um cit' trate)

Brand Names Effer-K™; K-Ide®; Klor-con®/EF; K-Lyte®; K-Vescent®

Synonyms Potassium Citrate and Potassium Bicarbonate, Effervescent

Use Treatment or prevention of hypokalemia

Pregnancy Risk Factor C

Contraindications Severe renal impairment, hyperkalemia

Warnings/Precautions Use with caution in patients with renal disease, cardiac disease

Adverse Reactions

>10%: Gastrointestinal: Diarrhea, nausea, stomach pain, flatulence, vomiting

1% to 10%:

Cardiovascular: Bradycardia

Central nervous system: Weakness

Endocrine & metabolic: Hyperkalemia

Local: Local tissue necrosis with extravasation

Respiratory: Difficult breathing

<1%:

Cardiovascular: Chest pain

Central nervous system: Mental confusion

Endocrine & metabolic: Alkalosis

Gastrointestinal: Abdominal pain

Local: Phlebitis

Neuromuscular & skeletal: Paresthesias, paralysis

Miscellaneous: Throat pain

Overdosage/Toxicology Symptoms of overdose include muscle weakness, paralysis, peaked T waves, flattened P waves, prolongation of QRS complex, ventricular arrhythmias. Removal of potassium can be accomplished by various means; removal through the GI tract with Kayexalate® administration; by way of the kidney through diuresis, mineralocorticoid administration or increased sodium intake; by hemodialysis or peritoneal dialysis; or by shifting potassium back into the cells by insulin and glucose infusion or sodium bicarbonate; calcium chloride will reverse cardiac effects.

Drug Interactions Increased effect/levels with potassium-sparing diuretics, salt substitutes, ACE inhibitors

Mechanism of Action Needed for the conduction of nerve impulses in heart, brain, and skeletal muscle; contraction of cardiac, skeletal and smooth muscles; maintenance of normal renal function

(Continued)

Potassium Bicarbonate and Potassium Citrate, Effervescent *(Continued)*

Pharmacodynamics/Kinetics
Absorption: Absorbed well from upper GI tract
Distribution: Enters cells via active transport from extracellular fluid
Elimination: Largely by the kidneys, but also small amount via the skin and feces, with most intestinal potassium being reabsorbed

Usual Dosage Oral:
Children: 1-4 mEq/kg/24 hours in divided doses as required to maintain normal serum potassium

Adults:
Prevention: 16-24 mEq/day in 2-4 divided doses
Treatment: 40-100 mEq/day in 2-4 divided doses

Monitoring Parameters Serum potassium
Test Interactions ↓ ammonia (B)
Patient Information Dissolve completely in 3-8 oz cold water, juice, or other suitable beverage and drink slowly

Dosage Forms
Capsule, extended release: 8 mEq, 10 mEq
Powder for oral solution: 15 mEq/packet; 20 mEq/packet; 25 mEq/packet
Tablet, effervescent: 25 mEq, 50 mEq

Potassium Chloride (poe tass' y um klor' ide

Brand Names Cena-K®; Gen-K®; K*8®; Kaochlor® S-F; Kaon-CL®; Kato®; K-Dur®; K-Lor™; Klor-con®; Klorvess®; Klotrix®; K-Lyte/CL®; K-Tab®; Micro-K®; Potasalan®; Rum-K®; Slow-K®

Synonyms KCl

Use Treatment or prevention of hypokalemia

Pregnancy Risk Factor A

Contraindications Severe renal impairment, untreated Addison's disease, heat cramps, hyperkalemia, severe tissue trauma; solid oral dosage forms are contraindicated in patients in whom there is a structural, pathological, and/or pharmacologic cause for delay or arrest in passage through the GI tract; an oral liquid potassium preparation should be used in patients with esophageal compression or delayed gastric emptying time

Warnings/Precautions Use with caution in patients with cardiac disease, severe renal impairment, hyperkalemia

Adverse Reactions
>10%: Gastrointestinal: Diarrhea, nausea, stomach pain, flatulence, vomiting (oral)
1% to 10%:
Cardiovascular: Bradycardia
Central nervous system: Weakness
Endocrine & metabolic: Hyperkalemia
Local: Local tissue necrosis with extravasation, pain at the site of injection
Respiratory: Difficult breathing
<1%:
Cardiovascular: Chest pain, arrhythmias, heart block, hypotension
Central nervous system: Mental confusion
Endocrine & metabolic: Alkalosis
Gastrointestinal: Abdominal pain
Local: Phlebitis
Neuromuscular & skeletal: Paresthesias, paralysis
Miscellaneous: Throat pain

Overdosage/Toxicology Symptoms of overdose include muscle weakness, paralysis, peaked T waves, flattened P waves, prolongation of QRS complex, ventricular arrhythmias. Removal of potassium can be accomplished by various means; removal through the GI tract with Kayexalate® administration; by way of the kidney through diuresis, mineralocorticoid administration or increased sodium intake; by hemodialysis or peritoneal dialysis; or by shifting potassium back into the cells by insulin and glucose infusion or sodium bicarbonate; calcium chloride reverses cardiac effects.

Drug Interactions
Increased effect/levels with potassium-sparing diuretics, salt substitutes, ACE inhibitors
Increased effect of digitalis

Stability Store at room temperature, protect from freezing; use only clear solutions; use admixtures within 24 hours
Mechanism of Action Potassium is the major cation of intracellular fluid and is essential for the conduction of nerve impulses in heart, brain, and skeleta

muscle; contraction of cardiac, skeletal and smooth muscles; maintenance of normal renal function, acid-base balance, carbohydrate metabolism, and gastric secretion

Pharmacodynamics/Kinetics

Absorption: Absorbed well from upper GI tract

Distribution: Enters cells via active transport from extracellular fluid

Elimination: Largely by the kidneys, but also small amount via the skin and feces, with most intestinal potassium being reabsorbed

Usual Dosage I.V. doses should be incorporated into the patient's maintenance I.V. fluids; intermittent I.V. potassium administration should be reserved for severe depletion situations in patients undergoing EKG monitoring.

Normal daily requirements: Oral, I.V.:
Premature infants: 2-6 mEq/kg/24 hours
Term infants 0-24 hours: 0-2 mEq/kg/24 hours
Infants >24 hours: 1-2 mEq/kg/24 hours
Children: 2-3 mEq/kg/day
Adults: 40-80 mEq/day

Prevention during diuretic therapy: Oral:
Children: 1-2 mEq/kg/day in 1-2 divided doses
Adults: 20-40 mEq/day in 1-2 divided doses

Treatment of hypokalemia: Children:
Oral: 1-2 mEq/kg initially, then as needed based on frequently obtained lab values. If deficits are severe or ongoing losses are great, I.V. route should be considered.
I.V.: 1 mEq/kg over 1-2 hours initially, then repeated as needed based on frequently obtained lab values; severe depletion or ongoing losses may require >200% of normal limit needs
I.V. intermittent infusion: Dose should not exceed 1 mEq/kg/hour, or 40 mEq/hour; if it exceeds 0.5 mEq/kg/hour, physician should be at bedside and patient should have continuous EKG monitoring

Treatment of hypokalemia: Adults:
I.V. intermittent infusion: 10-20 mEq/hour, not to exceed 40 mEq/hour and 150 mEq/day. See table.

Potassium Dosage/Rate of Infusion Guidelines

Serum Potassium⁺	Maximum Infusion Rate	Maximum Concentration	Maximum 24-Hour Dose
>2.5 mEq/L	10 mEq/h	40 mEq/L	200 mEq
<2.5 mEq/L	40 mEq/h	80 mEq/L	400 mEq

Potassium >2.5 mEq/L:
Oral: 60-80 mEq/day plus additional amounts if needed
I.V.: 10 mEq over 1 hour with additional doses if needed
Potassium <2.5 mEq/L:
Oral: Up to 40-60 mEq initial dose, followed by further doses based on lab values; deficits at a plasma level of 2 mEq/L may be as high as 400-800 mEq of potassium
I.V.: Up to 40 mEq over 1 hour, with doses based on frequent lab monitoring; deficits at a plasma level of 2 mEq/L may be as high as 400-800 mEq of potassium

Administration Maximum concentration (peripheral line): 10 mEq/L; maximum concentration (central line): 30 mEq/100 mL; may not be given I.V. push or I.V. retrograde; oral liquid potassium supplements should be diluted with water or fruit juice during administration

Monitoring Parameters Serum potassium, glucose, chloride, pH, urine output (if indicated), cardiac monitor (if intermittent infusion or potassium infusion rates >0.25 mEq/kg/hour)

Patient Information Sustained release and wax matrix tablets should be swallowed whole, do not crush or chew; effervescent tablets must be dissolved in water before use; take with food; liquid and granules can be diluted or dissolved in water or juice

Nursing Implications Wax matrix tablets must be swallowed and not allowed to dissolve in mouth

Dosage Forms

Capsule, controlled release, micro encapsulated (Micro-K®): 600 mg [8 mEq]; 750 mg [10 mEq]

Injection: 1.5 mEq/mL, 2 mEq/mL, 3 mEq/mL

(Continued)

Potassium Chloride (Continued)

Liquid, oral: 10 mEq/15 mL, 15 mEq/15 mL, 20 mEq/15 mL, 30 mEq/15 mL, 40 mEq/15 mL, 45 mEq/15 mL

Powder, oral: 15 mEq, 20 mEq, 25 mEq packet

Tablet:

Effervescent, as potassium chloride: 25 mEq

Effervescent, as potassium bicarbonate: 20 mEq, 25 mEq, 50 mEq

Extended release (K⁺8®): 8 mEq

Sustained release, microcrystalloids (K-Dur®): 750 mg [10 mEq]; 1500 mg [20 mEq]

Wax matrix:

Kaon-Cl®: 500 mg [6.7 mEq]

Slow-K®: 600 mg [8 mEq]; 750 mg [10 mEq]

Potassium Citrate and Potassium Bicarbonate, Effervescent *see*
Potassium Bicarbonate and Potassium Citrate, Effervescent *on page 905*

Potassium Gluconate (poe tass' y um glue' coe nate)

Brand Names Kaon®; Kaylixir®; K-G® Elixir

Use Treatment or prevention of hypokalemia

Pregnancy Risk Factor A

Contraindications Severe renal impairment, untreated Addison's disease, heat cramps, hyperkalemia, severe tissue trauma; solid oral dosage forms are contra-indicated in patients in whom there is a structural, pathological, and/or pharmacologic cause for delay or arrest in passage through the GI tract; an oral liquid potassium preparation should be used in patients with esophageal compression or delayed gastric emptying time

Warnings/Precautions Use with caution in patients with cardiac disease, severe renal impairment, hyperkalemia; patients must be on a cardiac monitor during intermittent infusions

Adverse Reactions

>10%: Gastrointestinal: Diarrhea, nausea, stomach pain, flatulence, vomiting (oral)

1% to 10%:

Cardiovascular: Bradycardia

Endocrine & metabolic: Hyperkalemia

Neuromuscular & skeletal: Weakness

Respiratory: Difficult breathing

<1%:

Cardiovascular: Chest pain

Central nervous system: Mental confusion

Endocrine & metabolic: Alkalosis

Local: Phlebitis

Neuromuscular & skeletal: Paresthesias, paralysis

Miscellaneous: Throat pain

Overdosage/Toxicology Symptoms of overdose include muscle weakness, paralysis, peaked T waves, flattened P waves, prolongation of QRS complex, ventricular arrhythmias. Removal of potassium can be accomplished by various means; removal through the GI tract with Kayexalate® administration; by way of the kidney through diuresis, mineralocorticoid administration or increased sodium intake; by hemodialysis or peritoneal dialysis; or by shifting potassium back into the cells by insulin, glucose infusion, or sodium bicarbonate; calcium chloride reverses cardiac effects

Drug Interactions Increased effect/levels with potassium-sparing diuretics, salt substitutes, ACE inhibitors; Increased effect of digitalis

Stability Store at room temperature, protect from freezing; use only clear solutions

Mechanism of Action Potassium is the major cation of intracellular fluid and is essential for the conduction of nerve impulses in heart, brain, and skeletal muscle; contraction of cardiac, skeletal and smooth muscles; maintenance of normal renal function, acid-base balance, carbohydrate metabolism, and gastric secretion

Pharmacodynamics/Kinetics

Absorption: Absorbed well from upper GI tract

Distribution: Enters cells via active transport from extracellular fluid

Elimination: Largely by the kidneys, but also small amount via the skin and feces, with most intestinal potassium being reabsorbed

Usual Dosage Oral (doses listed as mEq of potassium):

Normal daily requirement:

Children: 2-3 mEq/kg/day

Adults: 40-80 mEq/day
Prevention of hypokalemia during diuretic therapy:
  Children: 1-2 mEq/kg/day in 1-2 divided doses
  Adults: 20-40 mEq/kg/day in 1-2 divided doses
Treatment of hypokalemia:
  Children: 2-5 mEq/kg/day in 2-4 divided doses
  Adults: 40-100 mEq/kg/day in 2-4 divided doses
Monitoring Parameters Serum potassium, chloride, glucose, pH, urine output (if indicated)
Test Interactions ↓ ammonia (B)
Patient Information Take with food, water, or fruit juice; swallow tablets whole; do not crush or chew
Nursing Implications Do not administer liquid full strength, must be diluted in 2-6 parts of water or juice
Additional Information 9.4 g potassium gluconate is approximately equal to 40 mEq potassium (4.3 mEq potassium/g salt)
Dosage Forms
Elixir: 20 mEq/15 mL (5 mL, 10 mL, 118 mL, 480 mL, 4000 mL)
Tablet: 500 mg, 595 mg

Potassium Iodide (poe tass' y um eye' oh dide)

Brand Names Iosat®; Pima®; Potassium Iodide Enseals®; SSKI®; Thyro-Block®
Synonyms KI; Lugol's Solution; Strong Iodine Solution
Use Facilitate bronchial drainage and cough; reduce thyroid vascularity prior to thyroidectomy and management of thyrotoxic crisis; block thyroidal uptake of radioactive isotopes of iodine in a radiation emergency
Pregnancy Risk Factor D
Contraindications Known hypersensitivity to iodine; hyperkalemia, pulmonary tuberculosis, pulmonary edema, bronchitis, impaired renal function
Warnings/Precautions Prolonged use can lead to hypothyroidism; cystic fibrosis patients have an exaggerated response; can cause acne flare-ups, can cause dermatitis, some preparations may contain sodium bisulfite (allergy); use with caution in patients with a history of thyroid disease, patients with renal failure, or GI obstruction
Adverse Reactions
1% to 10%:
  Central nervous system: Fever, headache
  Dermatologic: Urticaria, acne, angioedema
  Endocrine & metabolic: Goiter with hypothyroidism
  Gastrointestinal: Metallic taste, GI upset
  Hematologic: Cutaneous and mucosal hemorrhage, eosinophilia
  Neuromuscular & skeletal: Arthralgia
  Respiratory: Rhinitis
  Miscellaneous: Lymph node enlargement, soreness of teeth and gums
Overdosage/Toxicology Symptoms of overdose include angioedema, laryngeal edema in patients with hypersensitivity; muscle weakness, paralysis, peaked T waves, flattened P waves, prolongation of QRS complex, ventricular arrhythmias; removal of potassium can be accomplished by various means; removal through the GI tract with Kayexalate® administration; by way of the kidney through diuresis, mineralocorticoid administration or increased sodium intake; by hemodialysis or peritoneal dialysis; or by shifting potassium back into the cells by insulin and glucose infusion.
Drug Interactions Increased toxicity: Lithium → additive hypothyroid effects
Stability Store in tight, light-resistant containers at temperature <40°C; freezing should be avoided
Mechanism of Action Reduces viscosity of mucus by increasing respiratory tract secretions; inhibits secretion of thyroid hormone, fosters colloid accumulation in thyroid follicles
Pharmacodynamics/Kinetics
Onset of action: 24-48 hours
Peak effect: 10-15 days after continuous therapy
Elimination: In euthyroid patient, renal clearance rate is 2 times that of the thyroid
Usual Dosage Oral:
Adults: RDA: 130 mcg

Expectorant:
  Children: 60-250 mg every 6-8 hours; maximum single dose: 500 mg
  Adults: 300-650 mg 2-3 times/day
Preoperative thyroidectomy: Children and Adults: 50-250 mg (1-5 drops SSKI®) 3 times/day **or** 0.1-0.3 mL (3-5 drops) of strong iodine (Lugol's solution) 3 times/day; give for 10 days before surgery
(Continued)

Potassium Iodide *(Continued)*

Thyrotoxic crisis:
  Infants <1 year: 150-250 mg (3-5 drops SSKI®) 3 times/day
  Children and Adults: 300-500 mg (6-10 drops SSKI®) 3 times/day or 1 mL
    strong iodine (Lugol's solution) 3 times/day
Graves' disease in neonates: 1 drop of strong iodine (Lugol's solution) 3
  times/day
Sporotrichosis:
  Initial:
      Preschool: 50 mg/dose 3 times/day
      Children: 250 mg/dose 3 times/day
      Adults: 500 mg/dose 3 times/day
  Oral increase 50 mg/dose daily
  Maximum dose:
      Preschool: 500 mg/dose 3 times/day
      Children and Adults: 1-2 g/dose 3 times/day
      Continue treatment for 4-6 weeks after lesions have completely healed

Monitoring Parameters Thyroid function tests

Patient Information Take after meals with food or milk or dilute with a large
  quantity of water, fruit juice, milk, or broth; discontinue use if stomach pain, skin
  rash, metallic taste, or nausea and vomiting occurs

Nursing Implications Must be diluted before administration of 240 mL of water,
  fruit juice, milk, or broth

Additional Information 10 drops of SSKI® = potassium iodide 500 mg

Dosage Forms

Solution, oral:
  SSKI®: 1 g/mL (30 mL, 240 mL)
  Lugol's Solution, strong iodine: Potassium iodide 100 mg and iodine 50 mg per
    mL (120 mL, 473 mL, 4000 mL)
Syrup: 325 mg/5 mL (473 mL, 4000 mL)
Tablet: 130 mg

Potassium Iodide Enseals® *see* Potassium Iodide *on previous page*

Potassium Phosphate *(poe tass' y um fos' fate)*

Brand Names Neutra-Phos®-K

Synonyms Phosphate, Potassium

Use Treatment and prevention of hypophosphatemia or hypokalemia

Pregnancy Risk Factor C

Contraindications Hyperphosphatemia, hyperkalemia, hypocalcemia, hypomagnesemia, renal failure

Warnings/Precautions Use with caution in patients with renal insufficiency,
  cardiac disease, metabolic alkalosis; admixture of phosphate and calcium in I.V.
  fluids can result in calcium phosphate precipitation

Adverse Reactions

>10%: Gastrointestinal: Diarrhea, nausea, stomach pain, flatulence, vomiting
1% to 10%:
  Cardiovascular: Bradycardia
  Endocrine & metabolic: Hyperkalemia
  Neuromuscular & skeletal: Weakness
  Respiratory: Difficult breathing
<1%:
  Cardiovascular: Chest pain
  Central nervous system: Mental confusion
  Endocrine & metabolic: Alkalosis
  Gastrointestinal: Abdominal pain
  Local: Phlebitis
  Neuromuscular & skeletal: Paresthesias, paralysis
  Renal: Acute renal failure
  Miscellaneous: Throat pain

Overdosage/Toxicology Symptoms of overdose include muscle weakness,
  paralysis, peaked T waves, flattened P waves, prolongation of QRS complex,
  ventricular arrhythmias, tetany, calcium-phosphate precipitation. Removal of
  potassium can be accomplished by various means; removal through the GI tract
  with Kayexalate® administration; by way of the kidney through diuresis, mineralocorticoid administration or increased sodium intake; by hemodialysis or peritoneal dialysis; or by shifting potassium back into the cells by insulin, glucose
  infusion, or sodium bicarbonate; calcium chloride reverses cardiac effects.

Drug Interactions

Decreased effect/levels with aluminum and magnesium-containing antacids or
  sucralfate which can act as phosphate binders

Increased effect/levels with potassium-sparing diuretics, salt substitutes, or ACE-inhibitors; increased effect of digitalis

Stability Store at room temperature, protect from freezing; use only clear solutions; up to 10-15 mEq of calcium may be added per liter before precipitate may occur

Stability of parenteral admixture at room temperature (25°C): 24 hours

Phosphate salts may precipitate when mixed with calcium salts; solubility is improved in amino acid parenteral nutrition solutions; check with a pharmacist to determine compatibility

Usual Dosage I.V. doses should be incorporated into the patient's maintenance I.V. fluids; intermittent I.V. infusion should be reserved for severe depletion situations in patients undergoing continuous EKG monitoring. It is difficult to determine total body phosphorus deficit; the following dosages are empiric guidelines:

Normal requirements elemental phosphorus: Oral:
　0-6 months: 240 mg
　6-12 months: 360 mg
　1-10 years: 800 mg
　>10 years: 1200 mg
　Pregnancy lactation: Additional 400 mg/day

Adults RDA: 800 mg

Treatment: It is difficult to provide concrete guidelines for the treatment of severe hypophosphatemia because the extent of total body deficits and response to therapy are difficult to predict. Aggressive doses of phosphate may result in a transient serum elevation followed by redistribution into intracellular compartments or bone tissue. It is recommended that repletion of severe hypophosphatemia (<1 mg/dL in adults) be done I.V. because large doses of oral phosphate may cause diarrhea and intestinal absorption may be unreliable

Pediatric I.V. phosphate repletion:
　Neonates: 0.5 mmol/kg/dose up to 1-2 mmol/kg/day
　Children: 0.25-0.5 mmol/kg **administer over 4-6 hours and repeat if symptomatic hypophosphatemia persists**; to assess the need for further phosphate administration, obtain serum inorganic phosphate after administration of the first dose and base further doses on serum levels and clinical status

Adult I.V. phosphate repletion:
　Initial dose: 0.08 mmol/kg if recent uncomplicated hypophosphatemia
　Initial dose: 0.16 mmol/kg if prolonged hypophosphatemia with presumed total body deficits; increase dose by 25% to 50% if patient symptomatic with severe hypophosphatemia
　Do not exceed 0.24 mmol/kg/day; administer over 6 hours by I.V. infusion

With orders for I.V. phosphate, there is considerable confusion associated with the use of millimoles (mmol) versus milliequivalents (mEq) to express the phosphate requirement. Because inorganic phosphate exists as monobasic and dibasic anions, with the mixture of valences dependent on pH, ordering by mEq amounts is unreliable and may lead to large dosing errors. In addition, I.V. phosphate is available in the sodium and potassium salt; therefore, the content of these cations must be considered when ordering phosphate. The most reliable method of ordering I.V. phosphate is by millimoles, then specifying the potassium or sodium salt. For example, an order for 15 mmol of phosphate as potassium phosphate in one liter of normal saline would also provide 22 mEq of potassium.

Phosphate maintenance electrolyte requirement in parenteral nutrition: 2 mmol/kg/24 hours or 35 mmol/kcal/24 hours; maximum: 15-30 mmol/24 hours

Maintenance:
　I.V. solutions:
　　Children: 0.5-1.5 mmol/kg/24 hours I.V. or 2-3 mmol/kg/24 hours orally in divided doses
　　Adults: 15-30 mmol/24 hours I.V. or 50-150 mmol/24 hours orally in divided doses
　Oral:
　　Children <4 years: 1 capsule (250 mg phosphorus/8 mmol) 4 times/day; dilute as instructed
　　Children >4 years and Adults: 1-2 capsules (250-500 mg phosphorus/8-16 mmol) 4 times/day; dilute as instructed

Fleet® Phospho®-Soda: Laxative: Oral: Single dose
　Children: 5-15 mL

(Continued)

Potassium Phosphate *(Continued)*

Adults: 20-30 mL mixed with 120 mL cold water

Administration Injection must be diluted in appropriate I.V. solution and volume prior to administration and administered over a minimum of 4 hours

Monitoring Parameters Serum potassium, calcium, phosphate, sodium, cardiac monitor (when intermittent infusion or high-dose I.V. replacement needed)

Test Interactions ↓ ammonia (B)

Patient Information Do not swallow the capsule; empty contents of capsule into 75 mL (2.5 oz) of water before taking; take with food to reduce the risk of diarrhea

Nursing Implications Capsule must be emptied into 3-4 oz of water before administration

Dosage Forms See table.

	Elemental Phosphorous (mg)	Phosphate (mmol)	Sodium (mEq)	K (mEq)
Oral				
Whole cow's milk per mL		0.29	0.025	0.035
Neutra-Phos®				
capsule	250	8	7.1	7.1
powder concentrate per 75 mL				
Neutra-Phos® -K				
capsule	250	8		14.2
powder				
K-Phos® Neutral tablets	250	8	13	1.1
K-Phos® MF tablets	125.6	4	2.9	1.1
K-Phos® No. 2	250	8	5.8	2.3
K-Phos® Original tablets	114	3.6		3.7
Uro-KP-Neutral® tablets	250	8	10.8	1.3
Intravenous				
K phosphate per mL		3		4.4

Potassium Phosphate and Sodium Phosphate (poe tass' y um fos' fate & sow' dee um fos' fate)

Brand Names K-Phos® Neutral; Neutra-Phos®; Uro-KP-Neutral®

Synonyms Sodium Phosphate and Potassium Phosphate

Use Treatment of conditions associated with excessive renal phosphate loss or inadequate GI absorption of phosphate; to acidify the urine to lower calcium concentrations; to increase the antibacterial activity of methenamine; reduce odor and rash caused by ammonia in urine

Pregnancy Risk Factor C

Contraindications Addison's disease, hyperkalemia, hyperphosphatemia, infected urolithiasis or struvite stone formation, patients with severely impaired renal function

Warnings/Precautions Use with caution in patients with renal disease, hyperkalemia, cardiac disease and metabolic alkalosis

Adverse Reactions

>10%: Gastrointestinal: Diarrhea, nausea, stomach pain, flatulence, vomiting

1% to 10%:

Cardiovascular: Bradycardia

Endocrine & metabolic: Hyperkalemia

Neuromuscular & skeletal: Weakness

Respiratory: Difficult breathing

<1%:

Cardiovascular: Irregular heartbeat, shortness of breath, chest pain, edema

Central nervous system: Mental confusion, tetany

Endocrine & metabolic: Alkalosis

Genitourinary: Decreased urine output

Local: Phlebitis

Neuromuscular & skeletal: Paresthesias, paralysis, pain/weakness of extremities, bone/joint pain

Renal: Acute renal failure

Miscellaneous: Thirst, throat pain, weight gain

Overdosage/Toxicology Symptoms of overdose include muscle weakness, paralysis, peaked T waves, flattened P waves, prolongation of QRS complex, ventricular arrhythmias, tetany, calcium phosphate precipitation. Removal of potassium can be accomplished by various means; removal through the GI tract with Kayexalate® administration; by way of the kidney through diuresis, mineralocorticoid administration or increased sodium intake; by hemodialysis or peritoneal dialysis; or by shifting potassium back into the cells by insulin and glucose infusion; calcium chloride reverses cardiac effects.

Drug Interactions
Decreased effect/levels with aluminum and magnesium-containing antacids or sucralfate which can act as phosphate binders
Increased effect/levels with potassium-sparing diuretics or ACE-inhibitors; increased effect/levels of digitalis, salicylates

Usual Dosage All dosage forms to be mixed in 6-8 oz of water prior to administration
Children: 2-3 mmol phosphate/kg/24 hours given 4 times/day **or** 1 capsule 4 times/day
Adults: 1-2 capsules (250-500 mg phosphorus/8-16 mmol) 4 times/day after meals and at bedtime

Monitoring Parameters Serum potassium, sodium, calcium, phosphate, EKG

Patient Information Do not swallow, open capsule and dissolve in 6-8 oz of water; powder packets are to be mixed in 6-8 oz of water; tablets should be crushed and mixed in 6-8 oz of water

Nursing Implications Tablets may be crushed and stirred vigorously to speed dissolution

Dosage Forms See table in Potassium Phosphate monograph

Povidone-Iodine (poe' vi done)

Brand Names Betadine® [OTC]; Efodine® [OTC]; Iodex® Regular; Isodine® [OTC]

Use External antiseptic with broad microbicidal spectrum against bacteria, fungi, viruses, protozoa, and yeasts

Pregnancy Risk Factor D

Contraindications Hypersensitivity to iodine

Warnings/Precautions Highly toxic if ingested; sodium thiosulfate is the most effective chemical antidote; avoid contact with eyes

Adverse Reactions
1% to 10%:
Dermatologic: Rash, pruritus
Local: Local edema
<1%: Systemic absorption in extensive burns causing ioderma, metabolic acidosis, and renal impairment

Mechanism of Action Povidone-iodine is known to be a powerful broad spectrum germicidal agent effective against a wide range of bacteria, viruses, fungi, protozoa, and spores.

Pharmacodynamics/Kinetics Absorption: In normal individuals, topical application results in very little systemic absorption; with vaginal administration, however, absorption is rapid and serum concentrations of total iodine and inorganic iodide are increased significantly

Usual Dosage
Shampoo: Apply 2 tsp to hair and scalp, lather and rinse; repeat application 2 times/week until improvement is noted, then shampoo weekly
Topical: Apply as needed for treatment and prevention of susceptible microbial infections

Patient Information Do not swallow; avoid contact with eyes

Dosage Forms
Aerosol: 5% (88.7 mL, 90 mL)
Antiseptic gauze pads: 10% (3" x 9")
Cleanser:
Skin: 7.5% (30 mL, 118 mL)
Skin, foam: 7.5% (170 g)
Topical: 60 mL, 240 mL
Concentrate, whirlpool: 3,840 mL
Cream: 5% (14 g)
Douche (10%): 0.5 oz/packet (6 packets/box), 240 mL
Foam, topical (10%): 250 g
Gel:
Lubricating: 5% (5 g)
Vaginal (10%): 18 g, 90 g
Liquid: 473 mL
Mouthwash (8%): 177 mL
Ointment, topical: 10% (0.94 g, 3.8 g, 28 g, 30 g, 454 g); 1 g, 1.2 g, 2.7 g packets
(Continued)

Povidone-Iodine *(Continued)*

Perineal wash concentrate: 1% (240 mL); 10% (236 mL)
Scrub, surgical: 7.5% (15 mL, 473 mL, 946 mL)
Shampoo: 7.5% (118 mL)
Solution:
    Prep: 30 mL, 60 mL, 240 mL, 473 mL, 1000 mL, 4000 mL
    Swab aid: 1%
    Swabsticks: 4"
    Topical: 10% (15 mL, 30 mL, 120 mL, 237 mL, 473 mL, 480 mL, 1000 mL, 4000 mL)
Suppositories, vaginal: 10%

PPA *see* Phenylpropanolamine Hydrochloride *on page 876*

PPD *see* Tuberculin Purified Protein Derivative *on page 1135*

PPL *see* Benzylpenicilloyl-polylysine *on page 125*

Pralidoxime Chloride (pra li dox' eem)

Brand Names Protopam®
Synonyms 2-PAM; 2-Pyridine Aldoxime Methochloride
Use Reverse muscle paralysis with toxic exposure to organophosphate anticholinesterase pesticides and chemicals; control of overdose of drugs used to treat myasthenia gravis (ambenonium, neostigmine, pyridostigmine)
Pregnancy Risk Factor C
Contraindications Hypersensitivity to pralidoxime or any component; poisonings due to phosphorus, inorganic phosphates, or organic phosphates without anticholinesterase activity
Warnings/Precautions Use with caution in patients with myasthenia gravis; dosage modification required in patients with impaired renal function may not be effective for treating carbamate intoxication; use with caution in patients receiving theophylline, succinylcholine, phenothiazines, respiratory depressants (eg, narcotics, barbiturates)
Adverse Reactions
>10%: Local: Pain at injection site after I.M. administration
1% to 10%:
    Cardiovascular: Tachycardia, hypertension
    Central nervous system: Dizziness, weakness, headache, drowsiness
    Dermatologic: Rash
    Gastrointestinal: Nausea
    Neuromuscular & skeletal: Muscle rigidity
    Ocular: Blurred vision, diplopia
    Respiratory: Hyperventilation, laryngospasm
Overdosage/Toxicology Symptoms of overdose include blurred vision, nausea, tachycardia, dizziness; supportive therapy, mechanical ventilation may be required
Drug Interactions
Increased effect: Barbiturates (potentiated)
Increased toxicity: Avoid morphine, theophylline, succinylcholine, reserpine and phenothiazines in patients with organophosphate poisoning
Mechanism of Action Reactivates cholinesterase that had been inactivated by phosphorylation due to exposure to organophosphate pesticides by displacing the enzyme from its receptor sites; removes the phosphoryl group from the active site of the inactivated enzyme
Pharmacodynamics/Kinetics
Absorption: Slowly from GI tract
Metabolism: In the liver, not bound to plasma proteins
Half-life: 0.8-2.7 hours
Time to peak serum concentration: I.V.: Within 5-15 minutes
Elimination: 80% to 90% quickly excreted in urine, as metabolites and unchanged drug
Usual Dosage
Poisoning: I.M. (use in conjunction with atropine), I.V.:
    Children: 20-50 mg/kg/dose; repeat in 1-2 hours if muscle weakness has not been relieved, then at 10- to 12-hour intervals if cholinergic signs recur
    Adults: 1-2 g; repeat in 1-2 hours if muscle weakness has not been relieved, then at 10- to 12-hour intervals if cholinergic signs recur
Mild organophosphate poisoning: Oral: Initial: 1-3 g, repeat as needed in 5 hours

Dosing adjustment in renal impairment: Dose should be reduced
Administration Infuse over 15-30 minutes at a rate not to exceed 200 mg/minute; may give I.M. or S.C. if I.V. is not accessible; reconstitute with 20 mL sterile water (preservative free) resulting in 50 mg/mL solution; dilute in normal saline 20

mg/mL and infuse over 15-30 minutes; if a more rapid onset of effect is desired or in a fluid-restricted situation, the maximum concentration is 50 mg/mL; the maximum rate of infusion is over 5 minutes

Monitoring Parameters Heart rate, respiratory rate, blood pressure, continuous EKG; cardiac monitor and blood pressure monitor required for I.V. administration

Dosage Forms

Injection: 20 mL vial containing 1 g each pralidoxime chloride with one 20 mL ampul diluent, disposable syringe, needle, and alcohol swab

Injection: 300 mg/mL (2 mL)

Tablets: 500 mg

Pramet® FA see Vitamin, Multiple on page 1166

Pramilet® FA see Vitamin, Multiple on page 1166

Pramoxine Hydrochloride (pra mox' een)

Brand Names Itch-X® [OTC]; Phicon® [OTC]; Prax® [OTC]; Proctofoam® [OTC]; Tronolane® [OTC]; Tronothane® [OTC]

Use Temporary relief of pain and itching associated with anogenital pruritus or irritation; dermatosis, minor burns, or hemorrhoids

Pregnancy Risk Factor C

Contraindications Use in eyes or near nose, application over large areas, known hypersensitivity to pramoxine or any component

Warnings/Precautions Use with caution in patients with severe trauma to the local area

Adverse Reactions

1% to 10%:
Dermatologic: Angioedema
Local: Contact dermatitis, burning, stinging
<1%:
Cardiovascular: Edema
Dermatologic: Tenderness, urticaria
Genitourinary: Urethritis
Hematologic: Methemoglobinemia in infants

Mechanism of Action Pramoxine, like other anesthetics, decreases the neuronal membrane's permeability to sodium ions; both initiation and conduction of nerve impulses are blocked, thus depolarization of the neuron is inhibited

Pharmacodynamics/Kinetics

Onset of therapeutic effect: Within 2-5 minutes
Peak effect: 3-5 minutes
Duration: May last for several days

Usual Dosage Adults: Topical: Apply as directed, usually every 3-4 hours to affected area (maximum adult dose: 200 mg)

Patient Information Discontinue if rash appears or if condition worsens or does not improve in 3-4 days

Nursing Implications Apply sparingly, use the minimal effective dose

Dosage Forms

Cream: 0.5% (60 g); 1% (28.4 g, 30 g, 113.4 g, 454 g)
Gel: 1% (37.5 g)
Liquid: 1% (118 mL)
Lotion: 1% (15 mL, 120 mL, 240 mL)

Pravachol® see Pravastatin Sodium on this page

Pravastatin Sodium (pra' va stat in)

Related Information

Lipid-Lowering Agents on page 1273

Brand Names Pravachol®

Use Adjunct to diet for the reduction of elevated total and LDL-cholesterol levels in patients with hypercholesterolemia (Type IIa, IIb, and IIc)

Pregnancy Risk Factor X

Contraindications Previous hypersensitivity, active liver disease, or persistent, unexplained liver function enzyme elevations; specifically contraindicated in pregnant or lactating females

Warnings/Precautions May elevate aminotransferases; LFTs should be performed before and every 4-6 weeks during the first 12-15 months of therapy and periodically thereafter; can also cause myalgia and rhabdomyolysis; use with caution in patients who consume large quantities of alcohol or who have a history of liver disease

(Continued)

Pravastatin Sodium *(Continued)*

Adverse Reactions
1% to 10%:
  Central nervous system: Headache, dizziness
  Dermatologic: Rash
  Gastrointestinal: Flatulence, abdominal cramps, diarrhea, constipation, nausea, dyspepsia, heartburn
  Neuromuscular & skeletal: Myalgia
  Miscellaneous: Elevated creatine phosphokinase (CPK)
<1%:
  Central nervous system: Dizziness
  Gastrointestinal: Dysgeusia
  Ocular: Lenticular opacities, blurred vision

Overdosage/Toxicology Very little adverse events; treatment is symptomatic

Drug Interactions
  Increased effect with cholestyramine
  Increased effect/toxicity of oral anticoagulants
  Increased toxicity with gemfibrozil, clofibrate

Mechanism of Action Pravastatin is a competitive inhibitor of 3-hydroxy-3-methylglutaryl coenzyme A (HMG-CoA) reductase, which is the rate-limiting enzyme involved in *de novo* cholesterol synthesis.

Pharmacodynamics/Kinetics
  Absorption: Poor
  Metabolism: In the liver to at least two metabolites
  Bioavailability: 17%
  Half-life, elimination: ~2-3 hours
  Time to peak serum concentration: 1-1.5 hours
  Elimination: Up to 20% excreted in urine (8% unchanged)

Usual Dosage Adults: Oral: 10-20 mg once daily at bedtime, may increase to 40 mg/day at bedtime

Monitoring Parameters Creatinine phosphokinase due to possibility of myopathy

Patient Information Promptly report any unexplained muscle pain, tenderness or weakness, especially if accompanied by malaise or fever

Nursing Implications Liver enzyme elevations may be observed during therapy with pravastatin; diet, weight reduction, and exercise should be attempted prior to therapy with pravastatin

Dosage Forms Tablet: 10 mg, 20 mg, 40 mg

Prax® [OTC] *see* Pramoxine Hydrochloride *on previous page*

Prazepam (pra' ze pam)

Brand Names Centrax®

Use Treatment of anxiety and management of alcohol withdrawal; may also be used as an anticonvulsant in management of simple partial seizures

Restrictions C-IV

Pregnancy Risk Factor D

Contraindications Hypersensitivity to prazepam or any component, cross-sensitivity with other benzodiazepines

Warnings/Precautions Safety and efficacy in children <18 years of age have not been established; do not use in pregnant women; may cause drug dependency; avoid abrupt discontinuance in patients with prolonged therapy or seizure disorders; avoid using in patients with pre-existing CNS depression, severe uncontrolled pain, or narrow-angle glaucoma; use with caution in patients receiving other CNS depressants, in patients with hepatic dysfunction, and the elderly

Adverse Reactions
>10%:
  Cardiovascular: Tachycardia, chest pain
  Central nervous system: Drowsiness, fatigue, impaired coordination, lightheadedness, memory impairment, insomnia, anxiety, depression, headache
  Dermatologic: Rash
  Endocrine & metabolic: Decreased libido
  Gastrointestinal: Dry mouth, constipation, diarrhea, decreased salivation, nausea, vomiting, increased or decreased appetite
  Neuromuscular & skeletal: Dysarthria
  Ocular: Blurred vision
  Miscellaneous: Sweating
1% to 10%:
  Cardiovascular: Syncope, hypotension
  Central nervous system: Confusion, nervousness, dizziness, akathisia
  Dermatologic: Dermatitis

Gastrointestinal: Weight gain or loss, increased salivation
Neuromuscular & skeletal: Muscle cramps, rigidity, tremor
Ocular: Blurred vision
Otic: Tinnitus
Respiratory: Hyperventilation, nasal congestion
<1%:
Central nervous system: Reflex slowing
Endocrine & metabolic: Menstrual irregularities
Hematologic: Blood dyscrasias
Miscellaneous: Drug dependence
Overdosage/Toxicology Symptoms of overdose include somnolence, confusion, coma, hypoactive reflexes, dyspnea, hypotension, slurred speech, impaired coordination. Treatment for benzodiazepine overdose is supportive. Rarely is mechanical ventilation required. Flumazenil has been shown to selectively block the binding of benzodiazepines to CNS receptors, resulting in a reversal of benzodiazepine-induced CNS depression, but not respiratory depression.
Drug Interactions
Decreased effect of levodopa
Increased effect/toxicity with CNS depressants, disulfiram, cimetidine, anticonvulsants, digoxin
Mechanism of Action Benzodiazepine anxiolytic sedative that produces CNS depression at the subcortical level, except at high doses, whereby it works at the cortical level
Pharmacodynamics/Kinetics
Peak action: Within 6 hours
Duration: 48 hours
Metabolism: First-pass hepatic metabolism
Half-life:
Parent drug: 78 minutes
Desmethyldiazepam: 30-100 hours
Elimination: Renal excretion of unchanged drug and primarily N-desmethyldiazepam (active)
Usual Dosage Adults: Oral: 30 mg/day in divided doses, may increase gradually to a maximum of 60 mg/day
Monitoring Parameters Respiratory and cardiovascular status
Patient Information Avoid alcohol and other CNS depressants; avoid activities needing good psychomotor coordination until CNS effects are known; drug may cause physical or psychological dependence; avoid abrupt discontinuation after prolonged use
Nursing Implications Institute safety measures, remove smoking materials from area, supervise ambulation
Dosage Forms
Capsule: 5 mg, 10 mg, 20 mg
Tablet: 10 mg

Praziquantel (pray zi kwon' tel)
Brand Names Biltricide®
Use All stages of schistosomiasis caused by all *Schistosoma* species pathogenic to humans; clonorchiasis, opisthorchiasis, cysticercosis, and many intestinal tapeworms
Pregnancy Risk Factor B
Contraindications Ocular cysticercosis, known hypersensitivity to praziquantel
Warnings/Precautions Use caution in patients with severe hepatic disease; patients with cerebral cysticercosis require hospitalization
Adverse Reactions
1% to 10%:
Central nervous system: Dizziness, drowsiness, headache, malaise
Gastrointestinal: Abdominal pain, loss of appetite, nausea, vomiting
Miscellaneous: Sweating
<1%:
Central nervous system: CSF reaction syndrome in patients being treated for neurocysticercosis, fever
Dermatologic: Skin rash, hives, itching
Gastrointestinal: Diarrhea
Overdosage/Toxicology Symptoms of overdose include dizziness, drowsiness, headache, liver function impairment; treatment is supportive following GI decontamination; give fast-acting laxative
Mechanism of Action Increases the cell permeability to calcium in schistosomes, causing strong contractions and paralysis of worm musculature leading to detachment of suckers from the blood vessel walls and to dislodgment
(Continued)
917

Praziquantel *(Continued)*

Pharmacodynamics/Kinetics

Absorption: Oral: ~80%; CSF concentration is 14% to 20% of plasma concentration

Distribution: CSF concentration is 14% to 20% of plasma concentration; appears in breast milk

Protein binding: ~80%

Metabolism: Extensive first-pass metabolism

Half-life:
  Parent drug: 0.8-1.5 hours
  Metabolites: 4.5 hours

Time to peak serum concentration: Within 1-3 hours

Elimination: Urinary excretion (99% as metabolites)

Usual Dosage Children >4 years and Adults: Oral:

Schistosomiasis: 20 mg/kg/dose 2-3 times/day for 1 day at 4- to 6-hour intervals

Flukes: 25 mg/kg/dose every 8 hours for 1-2 days

Cysticercosis: 50 mg/kg/day divided every 8 hours for 14 days

Tapeworms: 10-20 mg/kg as a single dose (25 mg/kg for *Hymenolepis nana*)

Patient Information Do not chew tablets due to bitter taste; take with food; caution should be used when performing tasks requiring mental alertness, may impair judgment and coordination

Nursing Implications Tablets can be halved or quartered

Dosage Forms Tablet, tri-scored: 600 mg

Prazosin Hydrochloride (pra' zoe sin)

Brand Names Minipress®

Synonyms Furazosin

Use Treatment of hypertension, severe congestive heart failure (in conjunction with diuretics and cardiac glycosides); reduce mortality in stable postmyocardial patients with left ventricular dysfunction (ejection fraction ≤40%)

Unlabeled use: Symptoms of benign prostatic hypertrophy

Pregnancy Risk Factor C

Contraindications Hypersensitivity to prazosin or any component

Warnings/Precautions Marked orthostatic hypotension, syncope, and loss of consciousness may occur with first dose ("first dose phenomenon") occurs more often in patients receiving beta-blockers, diuretics, low sodium diets, or larger first doses (ie, >1 mg/dose in adults); avoid rapid increase in dose; use with caution in patients with renal impairment

Adverse Reactions

>10%:
  Cardiovascular: Orthostatic hypotension
  Central nervous system: Dizziness, lightheadedness, drowsiness, headache, malaise

1% to 10%:
  Cardiovascular: Edema, palpitations
  Central nervous system: Fatigue, nervousness
  Gastrointestinal: Dry mouth
  Genitourinary: Urinary incontinence

<1%:
  Cardiovascular: Angina
  Central nervous system: Nightmares, hypothermia
  Dermatologic: Rash
  Endocrine & metabolic: Sexual dysfunction
  Gastrointestinal: Nausea
  Genitourinary: Priapism, urinary frequency
  Respiratory: Dyspnea, nasal congestion

Overdosage/Toxicology Symptoms of overdose include hypotension, drowsiness; hypotension usually responds to I.V. fluids, Trendelenburg positioning or vasoconstrictors; treatment is otherwise supportive and symptomatic

Drug Interactions

Decreased effect (antihypertensive) with NSAIDs

Increased effect (hypotensive) with diuretics and antihypertensive medications (especially beta-blockers)

Mechanism of Action Competitively inhibits postsynaptic alpha-adrenergic receptors which results in vasodilation of veins and arterioles and a decrease in total peripheral resistance and blood pressure

Pharmacodynamics/Kinetics

Onset of hypotensive effect: Within 2 hours

Maximum decrease: 2-4 hours

Duration: 10-24 hours

Distribution: V_d: 0.5 L/kg (hypertensive adults)

Protein binding: 92% to 97%

Metabolism: Extensively in the liver

Bioavailability: Oral: 43% to 82%

Half-life: 2-4 hours; increased with congestive heart failure

Elimination: 6% to 10% excreted renally as unchanged drug

Usual Dosage Oral:

Children: Initial: 5 mcg/kg/dose (to assess hypotensive effects); usual dosing interval: every 6 hours; increase dosage gradually up to maximum of 25 mcg/kg/dose every 6 hours

Adults: Initial: 1 mg/dose 2-3 times/day; usual maintenance dose: 3-15 mg/day in divided doses 2-4 times/day; maximum daily dose: 20 mg

Monitoring Parameters Blood pressure, standing and sitting/supine

Test Interactions Increased urinary UMA 17%, norepinephrine metabolite 42%

Patient Information Rise from sitting/lying carefully; may cause dizziness; report if painful, persistent erection occurs; avoid alcohol

Nursing Implications Syncope may occur (usually within 90 minutes of the initial dose)

Dosage Forms Capsule: 1 mg, 2 mg, 5 mg

Predair® *see* Prednisolone *on this page*

Predaject® *see* Prednisolone *on this page*

Predalone T.B.A.® *see* Prednisolone *on this page*

Predcor® *see* Prednisolone *on this page*

Predcor-TBA® *see* Prednisolone *on this page*

Pred Forte® *see* Prednisolone *on this page*

Pred Mild® *see* Prednisolone *on this page*

Prednicarbate (pred' ni kar bate)

Brand Names Dermatop®

Use Relief of the inflammatory and pruritic manifestations of corticosteroid-responsive dermatoses (medium potency topical corticosteroid)

Contraindications Hypersensitivity to prednicarbate or any component; fungal, viral, or tubercular skin lesions, herpes simplex or zoster

Adverse Reactions

<10%:

Dermatologic: Acne, hypopigmentation, allergic dermatitis, maceration of the skin, skin atrophy

Endocrine & metabolic: HPA suppression, Cushing's syndrome, growth retardation

Local: Burning, itching, irritation, dryness, folliculitis, hypertrichosis

Miscellaneous: Secondary infection

Mechanism of Action Topical corticosteroids have anti-inflammatory, antipruritic, vasoconstrictive, and antiproliferative actions

Usual Dosage Adults: Topical: Apply a thin film to affected area twice daily

Monitoring Parameters Relief of symptoms

Patient Information Use only as prescribed and for no longer than the period prescribed; apply sparingly in a thin film and rub in lightly; avoid contact with eyes; notify physician if condition persists or worsens

Nursing Implications Use sparingly

Additional Information Has been shown that the atrophic activity of prednicarbate is many times less than agents with similar clinical potency, nevertheless, avoid prolonged use on the face

Dosage Forms Cream: 0.1% (15 g, 60 g)

Prednicen-M® *see* Prednisone *on page 921*

Prednisolone (pred niss' oh lone)

Related Information

Corticosteroids Comparisons *on page 1266-1268*

Brand Names AK-Pred®; Articulose-50®; Delta-Cortef®; Econopred®; Econopred® Plus; Hydeltrasol®; Hydeltra-T.B.A.®; Inflamase®; Inflamase® Mild; Key-Pred®; Key-Pred-SP®; Metreton®; Pediapred®; Predair®; Predaject®; Predalone T.B.A.®; Predcor®; Predcor-TBA®; Pred Forte®; Pred Mild®; Prelone®

Synonyms Deltahydrocortisone; Metacortandralone; Prednisolone Acetate; Prednisolone Acetate, Ophthalmic; Prednisolone Sodium Phosphate; Prednisolone Sodium Phosphate, Ophthalmic; Prednisolone Tebutate

(Continued)

919

Prednisolone *(Continued)*

Use Treatment of palpebral and bulbar conjunctivitis; corneal injury from chemical, radiation, thermal burns, or foreign body penetration; endocrine disorders, rheumatic disorders, collagen diseases, dermatologic diseases, allergic states, ophthalmic diseases, respiratory diseases, hematologic disorders, neoplastic diseases, edematous states, and gastrointestinal diseases; useful in patients with inability to activate prednisone (liver disease)

Pregnancy Risk Factor C

Contraindications Acute superficial herpes simplex keratitis; systemic fungal infections; varicella; hypersensitivity to prednisolone or any component

Warnings/Precautions Use with caution in patients with hyperthyroidism, cirrhosis, nonspecific ulcerative colitis, hypertension, osteoporosis, thromboembolic tendencies, CHF, convulsive disorders, myasthenia gravis, thrombophlebitis, peptic ulcer, diabetes; acute adrenal insufficiency may occur with abrupt withdrawal after long-term therapy or with stress; young pediatric patients may be more susceptible to adrenal axis suppression from topical therapy. Because of the risk of adverse effects, systemic corticosteroids should be used cautiously in the elderly, in the smallest possible dose, and for the shortest possible time.

Adverse Reactions

>10%:

Central nervous system: Insomnia, nervousness

Gastrointestinal: Increased appetite, indigestion

1% to 10%:

Central nervous system: Epistaxis

Dermatologic: Hirsutism

Endocrine & metabolic: Diabetes mellitus

Neuromuscular & skeletal: joint pain

Ocular: Cataracts, glaucoma

<1%:

Cardiovascular: Edema, hypertension

Central nervous system: Vertigo, seizures, psychoses, pseudotumor cerebri, headache, mood swings, delirium, hallucinations, euphoria

Dermatologic: Acne, skin atrophy, bruising, hyperpigmentation

Endocrine & metabolic: Cushing's syndrome, pituitary-adrenal axis suppression, growth suppression, glucose intolerance, hypokalemia, alkalosis, amenorrhea, sodium and water retention, hyperglycemia

Gastrointestinal: Abdominal distention, ulcerative esophagitis, pancreatitis, peptic ulcer, nausea, vomiting

Neuromuscular & skeletal: Muscle weakness, osteoporosis, fractures, muscle wasting

Miscellaneous: Hypersensitivity reactions

Overdosage/Toxicology When consumed in excessive quantities for prolonged periods, systemic hypercorticism and adrenal suppression may occur, in those cases discontinuation and withdrawal of the corticosteroid should be done judiciously.

Drug Interactions Decreased effect with barbiturates, phenytoin, rifampin; decreased effect of salicylates, vaccines, toxoids

Mechanism of Action Decreases inflammation by suppression of migration of polymorphonuclear leukocytes and reversal of increased capillary permeability; suppresses the immune system by reducing activity and volume of the lymphatic system

Pharmacodynamics/Kinetics

Protein binding: 65% to 91% (concentration dependent)

Metabolism: Primarily in the liver, but also metabolized in most tissues, to inactive compounds

Half-life: 3.6 hours

Biological: 18-36 hours

End stage renal disease: 3-5 hours

Elimination: In urine principally as glucuronides, sulfates, and unconjugated metabolites

Usual Dosage Dose depends upon condition being treated and response of patient; dosage for infants and children should be based on severity of the disease and response of the patient rather than on strict adherence to dosage indicated by age, weight, or body surface area. Consider alternate day therapy for long-term therapy. Discontinuation of long-term therapy requires gradual withdrawal by tapering the dose.

Children:

Acute asthma: Oral: 1-2 mg/kg/day in divided doses 1-2 times/day for 3-5 days

Anti-inflammatory or immunosuppressive dose: Oral, I.V., I.M. (sodium phosphate salt): 0.1-2 mg/kg/day in divided doses 1-4 times/day

Nephrotic syndrome: Oral:
Initial: 2 mg/kg/day (maximum: 80 mg/day) in divided doses 3-4 times/day until urine is protein free for 5 days (maximum: 28 days); if proteinuria persists, use 4 mg/kg/dose every other day for an additional 28 days
Maintenance: 2 mg/kg/dose (maximum: 80 mg/dose) every other morning for 28 days, then taper by 10 mg/dose at intervals of 2-3 weeks to 30 mg/dose, then by 5 mg/dose at intervals of 2-3 weeks until discontinued

Adults:
Oral, I.V., I.M. (sodium phosphate salt): 5-60 mg/day
I.M. (acetate salt): 4-60 mg/day
Rheumatoid arthritis: Oral: Initial: 5-7.5 mg/day, adjust dose as necessary
Multiple sclerosis (sodium phosphate): Oral: 200 mg/day for 1 week followed by 80 mg every other day for 1 month
Multiple sclerosis (acetate salt): I.M.: 200 mg/day for 1 week followed by 80 mg every other day for 1 month
Elderly: Use lowest effective adult dose

Slightly dialyzable (5% to 20%)

Intra-articular, intralesional, soft-tissue administration:
Tebutate salt: 4-40 mg/dose
Acetate salt: 4-100 mg/dose
Sodium phosphate salt: 2-30 mg/dose

Ophthalmic suspension/solution: Instill 1-2 drops into conjunctival sac every hour during day, every 2 hours at night until favorable response is obtained, then use 1 drop every 4 hours

Monitoring Parameters Blood pressure, blood glucose, electrolytes

Test Interactions Response to skin tests

Patient Information Notify surgeon or dentist before surgical repair; may cause GI upset; take oral formulation with food; notify physician if any sign of infection occurs; avoid abrupt withdrawal when on long-term therapy

Nursing Implications Give oral formulation with food or milk to decrease GI effects; do not give acetate or tebutate salt I.V.

Additional Information
Sodium phosphate injection: For I.V., I.M., intra-articular, intralesional, or soft tissue administration
Tebutate injection: For intra-articular, intralesional, or soft tissue administration only

Dosage Forms
Injection, as acetate (for I.M., intralesional, intra-articular, or soft tissue administration only): 25 mg/mL (10 mL, 30 mL); 50 mg/mL (30 mL)
Injection, as sodium phosphate (for I.M., I.V., intra-articular, intralesional, or soft tissue administration): 20 mg/mL (2 mL, 5 mL, 10 mL)
Injection, as tebutate (for intra-articular, intralesional, soft tissue administration only): 20 mg/mL (1 mL, 5 mL, 10 mL)
Liquid, oral, as sodium phosphate: 5 mg/5 mL (120 mL)
Solution, ophthalmic, as sodium phosphate: 0.125% (5 mL, 10 mL, 15 mL); 1% (5 mL, 10 mL, 15 mL)
Suspension, ophthalmic, as acetate: 0.12% (5 mL, 10 mL); 0.125% (5 mL, 10 mL, 15 mL); 1% (1 mL, 5 mL, 10 mL, 15 mL)
Syrup: 15 mg/5 mL (240 mL)
Tablet: 5 mg

Prednisolone Acetate see Prednisolone on page 919

Prednisolone Acetate, Ophthalmic see Prednisolone on page 919

Prednisolone Sodium Phosphate see Prednisolone on page 919

Prednisolone Sodium Phosphate, Ophthalmic see Prednisolone on page 919

Prednisolone Tebutate see Prednisolone on page 919

Prednisone (pred′ ni sone)
Related Information
Cancer Chemotherapy Regimens on page 1218-1241
Corticosteroids Comparisons on page 1266-1268
Brand Names Deltasone®; Liquid Pred®; Meticorten®; Orasone®; Prednicen-M®; Sterapred®
Synonyms Deltacortisone; Deltadehydrocortisone
Use Treatment of a variety of diseases including adrenocortical insufficiency, hypercalcemia, rheumatic and collagen disorders; dermatologic, ocular, respiratory, gastrointestinal, and neoplastic diseases; organ transplantation and a
(Continued)

Prednisone *(Continued)*

variety of diseases including those of hematologic, allergic, inflammatory, and autoimmune in origin; not available in injectable form, prednisolone must be used

Pregnancy Risk Factor B

Contraindications Serious infections, except septic shock or tuberculous meningitis; systemic fungal infections; hypersensitivity to prednisone or any component; varicella

Warnings/Precautions Use with caution in patients with hypothyroidism, cirrhosis, hypertension, congestive heart failure, ulcerative colitis, thromboembolic disorders, and patients with an increased risk for peptic ulcer disease; may retard bone growth; gradually taper dose to withdraw therapy. Because of the risk of adverse effects, systemic corticosteroids should be used cautiously in the elderly, in the smallest possible dose, and for the shortest possible time.

Adverse Reactions

>10%:
  Central nervous system: Insomnia, nervousness
  Gastrointestinal: Increased appetite, indigestion
1% to 10%:
  Central nervous system: Epistaxis
  Dermatologic: Hirsutism
  Endocrine & metabolic: Diabetes mellitus
  Neuromuscular & skeletal: Joint pain
  Ocular: Cataracts, glaucoma
<1%:
  Cardiovascular: Edema, hypertension
  Central nervous system: Vertigo, seizures, psychoses, pseudotumor cerebri, headache, mood swings, delirium, hallucinations, euphoria
  Dermatologic: Acne, skin atrophy, bruising, hyperpigmentation
  Endocrine & metabolic: Cushing's syndrome, pituitary-adrenal axis suppression, growth suppression, glucose intolerance, hypokalemia, alkalosis, amenorrhea, sodium and water retention, hyperglycemia
  Gastrointestinal: Abdominal distention, ulcerative esophagitis, pancreatitis, peptic ulcer, nausea, vomiting
  Neuromuscular & skeletal: Muscle weakness, osteoporosis, fractures, muscle wasting
  Miscellaneous: Hypersensitivity reactions

Overdosage/Toxicology When consumed in excessive quantities for prolonged periods, systemic hypercorticism and adrenal suppression may occur; in those cases, discontinuation and withdrawal of the corticosteroid should be done judiciously.

Drug Interactions Decreased effect with barbiturates, phenytoin, rifampin; decreased effect of salicylates, vaccines, toxoids

Mechanism of Action Decreases inflammation by suppression of migration of polymorphonuclear leukocytes and reversal of increased capillary permeability; suppresses the immune system by reducing activity and volume of the lymphatic system; suppresses adrenal function at high doses

Pharmacodynamics/Kinetics Refer to Prednisolone monograph for complete pharmacokinetic information
  Metabolism: Converted rapidly to prednisolone (active)
    Prednisone is inactive and must be metabolized to prednisolone which may be impaired in patients with impaired liver function
  Half-life: Normal renal function: 2.5-3.5 hours

Usual Dosage Dose depends upon condition being treated and response of patient; dosage for infants and children should be based on severity of the disease and response of the patient rather than on strict adherence to dosage indicated by age, weight, or body surface area. Consider alternate day therapy for long-term therapy. Discontinuation of long-term therapy requires gradual withdrawal by tapering the dose.

Children: Oral:
  Anti-inflammatory or immunosuppressive dose: 0.05-2 mg/kg/day divided 1-4 times/day
  Acute asthma: 1-2 mg/kg/day in divided doses 1-2 times/day for 3-5 days
  Alternatively (for 3-5 day "burst"):
    <1 year: 10 mg every 12 hours
    1-4 years: 20 mg every 12 hours
    5-13 years: 30 mg every 12 hours
    >13 years: 40 mg every 12 hours
  Asthma long-term therapy (alternative dosing by age):
    < 1 year: 10 mg every other day
    1-4 years: 20 mg every other day
    5-13 years: 30 mg every other day
    >13 years: 40 mg every other day

Severe refractory asthma: 5-10 mg/dose every day or 10-30 mg every other day

Nephrotic syndrome: Initial: 2 mg/kg/day (maximum: 80 mg/day) in divided doses 3-4 times/day until urine is protein free for 5 days (maximum: 28 days); if proteinuria persists, use 4 mg/kg/dose every other day (maximum: 120 mg/day) for an additional 28 days; maintenance: 2 mg/kg/dose (maximum: 80 mg/dose) every other day for 28 days; then taper over 4-6 weeks

Children and Adults: Physiologic replacement: 4-5 mg/m²/day

Adults: 5-60 mg/day in divided doses 1-4 times/day

Elderly: Use the lowest effective dose

Hemodialysis effects: Supplemental dose is not necessary

Monitoring Parameters Blood pressure, blood glucose, electrolytes

Test Interactions Response to skin tests

Patient Information Notify surgeon or dentist before surgical repair; may cause GI upset, take with food; notify physician if any sign of infection occurs; avoid abrupt withdrawal when on long-term therapy; do not discontinue or decrease drug without contacting physician, carry an identification card or bracelet advising that you are on steroids

Nursing Implications Give with meals to decrease GI upset; withdraw therapy with gradual tapering of dose

Dosage Forms

Solution, oral: Concentrate (30% alcohol): 5 mg/mL (30 mL); Nonconcentrate (5% alcohol): 5 mg/5 mL (5 mL, 500 mL)

Syrup: 5 mg/5 mL (120 mL, 240 mL)

Tablet: 1 mg, 2.5 mg, 5 mg, 10 mg, 20 mg, 50 mg

Prefrin™ Ophthalmic Solution see Phenylephrine Hydrochloride on page 874

Pregnenedione see Progesterone on page 936

Pregnyl® see Chorionic Gonadotropin on page 242

Prelone® see Prednisolone on page 919

Premarin® see Estrogens, Conjugated on page 410

Prenatal Vitamins see Vitamin, Multiple on page 1166

Prenavite® [OTC] see Vitamin, Multiple on page 1166

Pre-Par® see Ritodrine Hydrochloride on page 986

Pre-Pen® see Benzylpenicilloyl-polylysine on page 125

Prepidil® Gel see Dinoprostone on page 349

Pretz® [OTC] see Sodium Chloride on page 1012

Prevention of Bacterial Endocarditis see page 1285

Prevention of Malaria see page 1405

PreviDent® see Fluoride on page 471

Prilosec™ see Omeprazole on page 816

Primaclone see Primidone on next page

Primacor® see Milrinone Lactate on page 741

Primaquine and Chloroquine see Chloroquine and Primaquine on page 224

Primaquine Phosphate (prim' a kween)

Related Information

Prevention of Malaria on page 1405

Synonyms Prymaccone

Use Provides radical cure of *P. vivax* or *P. ovale* malaria after a clinical attack has been confirmed by blood smear or serologic titer and postexposure prophylaxis

Pregnancy Risk Factor C

Contraindications Acutely ill patients who have a tendency to develop granulocytopenia (rheumatoid arthritis, SLE); patients receiving other drugs capable of depressing the bone marrow; patients receiving quinacrine

Warnings/Precautions Use with caution in patients with G-6-PD deficiency, NADH methemoglobin reductase deficiency, acutely ill patients who have a tendency to develop granulocytopenia; patients receiving other drugs capable of depressing the bone marrow; do not exceed recommended dosage

Adverse Reactions

>10%:

Gastrointestinal: Abdominal pain, nausea, vomiting

Hematologic: Hemolytic anemia

(Continued)

923

Primaquine Phosphate (Continued)

1% to 10%: Hematologic: Methemoglobinemia

<1%:

Cardiovascular: Arrhythmias

Central nervous system: Headache

Dermatologic: Pruritus

Hematologic: Leukopenia, agranulocytosis, leukocytosis

Miscellaneous: Interference with visual accommodation

Overdosage/Toxicology Symptoms of acute overdose include abdominal cramps, vomiting, cyanosis, methemoglobinemia (possibly severe), leukopenia, acute hemolytic anemia (often significant), granulocytopenia; with chronic overdose, symptoms include ototoxicity and retinopathy; following GI decontamination, treatment is supportive (fluids, anticonvulsants, blood transfusions, methylene blue if methemoglobinemia severe - 1-2 mg/kg over several minutes)

Drug Interactions Increased toxicity/levels with quinacrine

Mechanism of Action Eliminates the primary tissue exoerythrocytic forms of *P. falciparum*; disrupts mitochondria and binds to DNA

Pharmacodynamics/Kinetics

Absorption: Oral: Well absorbed

Metabolism: Liver metabolism to carboxyprimaquine, an active metabolite

Half-life: 3.7-9.6 hours

Time to peak serum concentration: Within 1-2 hours

Elimination: Only a small amount of unchanged drug excreted in urine

Usual Dosage Oral:

Children: 0.3 mg base/kg/day once daily for 14 days (not to exceed 15 mg/day) or 0.9 mg base/kg once weekly for 8 weeks not to exceed 45 mg base/week

Adults: 15 mg/day (base) once daily for 14 days or 45 mg base once weekly for 8 weeks

Monitoring Parameters Periodic CBC, visual color check of urine, glucose, electrolytes; if hemolysis suspected - CBC, haptoglobin, peripheral smear, urinalysis dipstick for occult blood

Patient Information Take with meals to decrease adverse GI effects; drug has a bitter taste; notify physician if a darkening of urine occurs or if shortness of breath, weakness or skin discoloration (chocolate cyanosis) occurs; complete full course of therapy

Dosage Forms Tablet: 26.3 mg [15 mg base]

Primatene® Mist [OTC] *see* Epinephrine *on page 389*

Primaxin® *see* Imipenem/Cilastatin *on page 567*

Primidone (pri' mi done)

Brand Names Mysoline®

Synonyms Desoxyphenobarbital; Primaclone

Use Management of grand mal, complex partial, and focal seizures

Unlabeled use: Benign familial tremor (essential tremor)

Pregnancy Risk Factor D

Contraindications Hypersensitivity to primidone, phenobarbital, or any component; porphyria

Warnings/Precautions Use with caution in patients with renal or hepatic impairment, pulmonary insufficiency; abrupt withdrawal may precipitate status epilepticus

Adverse Reactions

>10%: Central nervous system: Drowsiness, vertigo, ataxia, lethargy, behavior change, sedation, headache

1% to 10%:

Gastrointestinal: Nausea, vomiting, anorexia

Genitourinary: Impotence

<1%:

Central nervous system: Behavior change

Dermatologic: Rash

Hematologic: Leukopenia, malignant lymphoma-like syndrome, megaloblastic anemia

Hepatic: Systemic lupus-like syndrome

Ocular: Diplopia, nystagmus

Overdosage/Toxicology Symptoms of overdose include unsteady gait, slurred speech, confusion, jaundice, hypothermia, fever, hypotension, coma, respiratory arrest; assure adequate hydration and renal function. Urinary alkalinization with I.V. sodium bicarbonate also helps to enhance elimination. Repeated oral doses of activated charcoal significantly reduces the half-life of primidone resulting from an enhancement of nonrenal elimination. The usual dose is 0.1-1 g/kg every 4-6 hours for 3-4 days unless the patient has no bowel movement causing the charcoal to remain in the GI tract. Hemodialysis or hemoperfusion is of uncertain value. Patients in stage IV coma due to high serum drug levels may require charcoal hemoperfusion.

Drug Interactions
Decreased effect: Primidone may decrease serum concentrations of ethosuximide, valproic acid, griseofulvin; phenytoin may decrease primidone serum concentrations
Increased toxicity: Methylphenidate may increase primidone serum concentrations; valproic acid may increase phenobarbital concentrations derived from primidone

Stability Protect from light

Mechanism of Action Decreases neuron excitability, raises seizure threshold similar to phenobarbital; primidone has two active metabolites, phenobarbital and phenylethylmalonamide (PEMA); PEMA may enhance the activity of phenobarbital

Pharmacodynamics/Kinetics
Distribution: V_d: 2-3 L/kg in adults
Protein binding: 99%
Metabolism: In the liver to phenobarbital (active) and phenylethylmalonamide (PEMA)
Bioavailability: 60% to 80%
Half-life (age dependent):
Primidone: 10-12 hours
PEMA: 16 hours
Phenobarbital: 52-118 hours
Time to peak serum concentration: Oral: Within 4 hours
Elimination: Urinary excretion of both active metabolites and unchanged primidone (15% to 25%)

Usual Dosage Oral:
Neonates: Loading dose: 15-25 mg/kg/dose as a single dose; 12-20 mg/kg/day in divided doses 2-4 times/day; start with lower dosage and titrate upward
Children <8 years: Initial: 50-125 mg/day given at bedtime; increase by 50-125 mg/day increments every 3-7 days; usual dose: 10-25 mg/kg/day in divided doses 3-4 times/day
Children >8 years and Adults: Initial: 125-250 mg/day at bedtime; increase by 125-250 mg/day every 3-7 days; usual dose: 750-1500 mg/day in divided doses 3-4 times/day with maximum dosage of 2 g/day

Dosing interval in renal impairment:
Cl_{cr} 50-80 mL/minute: Administer every 8 hours
Cl_{cr} 10-50 mL/minute: Administer every 8-12 hours
Cl_{cr} <10 mL/minute: Administer every 12-24 hours
Moderately dialyzable (20% to 50%)
Administer dose postdialysis or administer supplemental 30% dose

Monitoring Parameters Serum primidone and phenobarbital concentration, CBC, neurological status. Due to CNS effects, monitor closely when initiating drug in elderly. Monitor CBC at 6-month intervals to compare with baseline obtained at start of therapy. Since elderly metabolize phenobarbital at a slower rate than younger adults, it is suggested to measure both primidone and phenobarbital levels together.

Reference Range Therapeutic: Children <5 years: 7-10 µg/mL (SI: 32-46 µmol/L); Adults: 5-12 µg/mL (SI: 23-55 µmol/L); toxic effects rarely present with levels <10 µg/mL (SI: 46 µmol/L) if phenobarbital concentrations are low. Dosage of primidone is adjusted with reference mostly to the phenobarbital level; Toxic: >15 µg/mL (SI: >69 µmol/L)

Test Interactions ↑ alkaline phosphatase (S); ↓ calcium (S)

Patient Information May cause drowsiness, impair judgment and coordination; do not abruptly discontinue or change dosage without notifying physician; can take with food to avoid GI upset

Nursing Implications Observe patient for excessive sedation; institute safety measures

Dosage Forms
Suspension, oral: 250 mg/5 mL (240 mL)
Tablet: 50 mg, 250 mg

Principen® see Ampicillin on page 73

Prinivil® see Lisinopril on page 641

Priscoline® see Tolazoline Hydrochloride on page 1102

Privine® see Naphazoline Hydrochloride on page 775

Proaqua® see Benzthiazide on page 123

Probalan® see Probenecid on next page

Pro-Banthine® *see* Propantheline Bromide *on page 941*

Probenecid (proe ben' e sid)
Related Information
Antimicrobial Drugs of Choice *on page 1298-1302*
Brand Names Benemid®; Probalan®
Use Prevention of gouty arthritis; hyperuricemia; prolongation of beta-lactam effect (ie, serum levels)
Pregnancy Risk Factor B
Contraindications Hypersensitivity to probenecid or any component; high-dose aspirin therapy; moderate to severe renal impairment; children <2 years of age
Warnings/Precautions Use with caution in patients with peptic ulcer; use extreme caution in the use of probenecid with penicillin in patients with renal insufficiency; probenecid may not be effective in patients with a creatinine clearance <30 to 50 mL/minute; may cause exacerbation of acute gouty attack
Adverse Reactions
>10%:
  Central nervous system: Headache
  Gastrointestinal: Anorexia, nausea, vomiting
  Neuromuscular & skeletal: Gouty arthritis (acute)
1% to 10%:
  Central nervous system: Dizziness
  Cardiovascular: Flushing of face
  Dermatologic: Skin rash, itching
  Genitourinary: Painful urination
  Renal: Renal calculi
  Miscellaneous: Sore gums
<1%:
  Hematologic: Leukopenia, hemolytic anemia, aplastic anemia
  Hepatic: Hepatic necrosis
  Renal: Urate nephropathy, nephrotic syndrome
  Miscellaneous: Anaphylaxis
Overdosage/Toxicology Symptoms of overdose include nausea, vomiting, tonic-clonic seizures, coma; activated charcoal is especially effective at binding probenecid, for GI decontamination
Drug Interactions
Decreased effect:
  Salicylates (high dose) → ↓ uricosuria
  Decreased urinary levels of nitrofurantoin → ↓ efficacy
Increased toxicity:
  Increased methotrexate toxic potential
  Increased penicillin and cephalosporin (beta-lactam) serum levels
  Increased toxicity of acyclovir, thiopental, benzodiazepines, dapsone, sulfonylureas, zidovudine
Mechanism of Action Competitively inhibits the reabsorption of uric acid at the proximal convoluted tubule, thereby promoting its excretion and reducing serum uric acid levels; increases plasma levels of weak organic acids (penicillins, cephalosporins, or other beta-lactam antibiotics) by competitively inhibiting their renal tubular secretion
Pharmacodynamics/Kinetics
Onset of action: Effect on penicillin levels reached in about 2 hours
Absorption: Rapid and complete from GI tract
Metabolism: In the liver
Half-life: Normal renal function: 6-12 hours and is dose dependent
Time to peak serum concentration: 2-4 hours
Elimination: In urine
Usual Dosage Oral:
Children:
  <2 years: Not recommended
  2-14 years: Prolong penicillin serum levels: 25 mg/kg starting dose, then 40 mg/kg/day given 4 times/day
  Gonorrhea: <45 kg: 25 mg/kg x 1 (maximum: 1 g/dose) 30 minutes before penicillin, ampicillin or amoxicillin
Adults:
  Hyperuricemia with gout: 250 mg twice daily for one week; increase to 250-500 mg/day; may increase by 500 mg/month, if needed, to maximum of 2-3 g/day (dosages may be increased by 500 mg every 6 months if serum urate concentrations are controlled)
  Prolong penicillin serum levels: 500 mg 4 times/day
  Gonorrhea: 1 g 30 minutes before penicillin, ampicillin or amoxicillin

Dosing adjustment in renal impairment: Cl_{cr} <50 mL/minute: Avoid use

Monitoring Parameters Uric acid, renal function, CBC

Test Interactions False-positive glucosuria with Clinitest®

Patient Information Take with food or antacids; drink plenty of fluids to reduce the risk of uric acid stones; the frequency of acute gouty attacks may increase during the first 6-12 months of therapy; avoid taking large doses of aspirin or other salicylates

Dosage Forms Tablet: 500 mg

Probucol (proe′ byoo kole)

Related Information

Lipid-Lowering Agents *on page 1273*

Brand Names Lorelco®

Synonyms Biphenabid

Use Adjunct to dietary therapy to decrease elevated serum total and LDL cholesterol concentrations in primary hypercholesterolemia

Pregnancy Risk Factor B

Contraindications Ventricular arrhythmias, hypersensitivity to probucol or any component

Warnings/Precautions Avoid use in hypokalemia, hypomagnesemia, severe bradycardia due to intrinsic heart disease, recent or AMI, ischemia or inflammation, and those receiving other cardioactive drugs that prolong the Q-T; serious cardiovascular toxicity (arrhythmias associated with abnormally long Q-T intervals) have been reported; the manufacturer recommends that a baseline EKG be performed and at appropriate intervals during therapy; use with caution in patients with prolonged Q-T intervals

Adverse Reactions

>10%:

Cardiovascular: Q-T prolongation, serious arrhythmias

Gastrointestinal: Bloating, diarrhea, stomach pain, nausea, vomiting

1% to 10%: Central nervous system: Dizziness, headache, numbness of extremities

<1%:

Cardiovascular: Tachycardia

Hematologic: Anemia, Thrombocytopenia

Overdosage/Toxicology Symptoms of overdose include diarrhea, flatulence; probucol is not dialyzable; following GI decontamination, treatment is supportive

Drug Interactions Increased toxicity: Drugs that prolong the Q-T interval (eg, tricyclic antidepressants, some antiarrhythmic agents, phenothiazines) or with drugs that affect the atrial rate (eg, beta-adrenergic blocking agents) or that can cause A-V block (eg, digoxin)

Mechanism of Action Increases the fecal loss of bile acid-bound low density lipoprotein cholesterol, decreases the synthesis of cholesterol and inhibits enteral cholesterol absorption

Pharmacodynamics/Kinetics

Absorption: Very slowly and poorly absorbed (<10%)

Half-life, elimination: 20 days

Time to peak serum concentration: Oral: After ~3 months of continuous administration

Elimination: Primarily via bile in feces

Usual Dosage Oral:

Children:

<27 kg: 250 mg twice daily with meals

>27 kg: 500 mg twice daily with meals

Adults: 500 mg twice daily administered with the morning and evening meals

Monitoring Parameters EKG prior to therapy and monthly for 3 months; fractionated serum cholesterol

Patient Information Take with meals; notify physician if diarrhea, abdominal pain, nausea, or vomiting becomes severe or persist

Dosage Forms Tablet: 250 mg, 500 mg

Procainamide Hydrochloride (proe kane a′ mide)

Related Information

Antiarrhythmic Drugs *on page 1246-1248*

Brand Names Procan® SR; Promine®; Pronestyl®; Rhythmin®

Synonyms Procaine Amide Hydrochloride

Use Treatment of ventricular tachycardia, premature ventricular contractions, paroxysmal atrial tachycardia, and atrial fibrillation; to prevent recurrence of ventricular tachycardia, paroxysmal supraventricular tachycardia, atrial fibrillation or flutter

(Continued)

Procainamide Hydrochloride *(Continued)*

Pregnancy Risk Factor C

Contraindications Complete heart block; second or third degree heart block without pacemaker; "torsade de pointes"; hypersensitivity to the drug or procaine, or related drugs; myasthenia gravis; SLE

Warnings/Precautions Use with caution in patients with marked A-V conduction disturbances, bundle branch block or severe cardiac glycoside intoxication, ventricular arrhythmias with organic heart disease or coronary occlusion, supraventricular tachyarrhythmias unless adequate measures are taken to prevent marked increases in ventricular rates; may accumulate in patients with renal or hepatic dysfunction; some tablets contain tartrazine; injection may contain bisulfite (allergens). Long-term administration leads to the development of a positive antinuclear antibody test in 50% of patients which may result in a lupus erythematosus-like syndrome (in 20% to 30% of patients); discontinue procainamide with SLE symptoms and choose an alternative agent; elderly have reduced clearance and frequent drug interactions.

Adverse Reactions

>10%: SLE-like syndrome

1% to 10%:
Cardiovascular: Tachycardia, arrhythmias, A-V block, Q-T prolongation, widening QRS complex
Central nervous system: Dizziness, lightheadedness
Gastrointestinal: Diarrhea

<1%:
Cardiovascular: Hypotension
Central nervous system: Confusion, hallucinations, mental depression, confusion, disorientation, fever
Dermatologic: Rash
Gastrointestinal: Nausea, vomiting, GI complaints
Hematologic: Hemolytic anemia, agranulocytosis, neutropenia, thrombocytopenia, positive Coombs' test
Neuromuscular & skeletal: Arthralgia, myalgia
Respiratory: Pleural effusion
Miscellaneous: Drug fever

Overdosage/Toxicology Has a low toxic:therapeutic ratio and may easily produce fatal intoxication (acute toxic dose: 5 g in adults); symptoms of overdose include sinus bradycardia, sinus node arrest or asystole, PR, QRS or Q-T interval prolongation, torsade de pointes (polymorphous ventricular tachycardia) and depressed myocardial contractility, which along with alpha-adrenergic or ganglionic blockade, may result in hypotension and pulmonary edema; other effects are seizures, coma and respiratory arrest. Treatment is primarily symptomatic and effects usually respond to conventional therapies (fluids, positioning, vasopressors, anticonvulsants, antiarrhythmics). **Note:** Do not use other type 1a or 1c antiarrhythmic agents to treat ventricular tachycardia; sodium bicarbonate may treat wide QRS intervals or hypotension; markedly impaired conduction or high degree A-V block, unresponsive to bicarbonate, indicates consideration of a pacemaker is needed.

Drug Interactions
Increased plasma/NAPA concentrations with cimetidine, ranitidine, beta-blockers, and amiodarone
Increased effect of skeletal muscle relaxants, quinidine and lidocaine and neuromuscular blockers (succinylcholine)
Increased NAPA levels/toxicity with trimethoprim

Stability
Procainamide may be stored at room temperature up to 27°C; however, refrigeration retards oxidation, which causes color formation
The solution is initially colorless but may turn slightly yellow on standing. Injection of air into the vial causes the solution to darken. Solutions darker than a light amber should be discarded.
Minimum volume: 1 g/250 mL NS/D_5W
Stability of admixture at room temperature in D_5W or NS: 24 hours
Some information indicates that procainamide may be subject to greater decomposition in D_5W unless the admixture is refrigerated or the pH is adjusted. Procainamide is believed to form an association complex with dextrose - the bioavailability of procainamide in this complex is not known and the complex formation is reversible.

Mechanism of Action Decreases myocardial excitability and conduction velocity and may depress myocardial contractility, by increasing the electrical stimulation threshold of ventricle, HIS-Purkinje system and through direct cardiac effects

Pharmacodynamics/Kinetics
Onset of action: I.M. 10-30 minutes
Distribution: V_d:
Children: 2.2 L/kg

Adults: 2 L/kg

Congestive heart failure of shock: Decreased V_d

Protein binding: 15% to 20%

Metabolism: By acetylation in the liver to produce N-acetyl procainamide (NAPA) (active metabolite)

Bioavailability: Oral: 75% to 95%

Half-life:

Procainamide: (Dependent upon hepatic acetylator, phenotype, cardiac function, and renal function):

Children: 1.7 hours

Adults: 2.5-4.7 hours

Anephric: 11 hours

NAPA: (Dependent upon renal function):

Children: 6 hours

Adults: 6-8 hours

Anephric: 42 hours

Time to peak serum concentration:

Capsule: Within 45 minutes to 2.5 hours

I.M.: 15-60 minutes

Elimination: Urinary excretion (25% as NAPA)

Usual Dosage Must be titrated to patient's response

Children:

Oral: 15-50 mg/kg/24 hours divided every 3-6 hours; maximum: 4 g/24 hours

I.M.: 20-30 mg/kg/24 hours divided every 4-6 hours in divided doses; maximum: 4 g/24 hours

I.V. (infusion requires use of an infusion pump):

Load: 3-6 mg/kg/dose over 5 minutes not to exceed 100 mg/dose; may repeat every 5-10 minutes to maximum of 15 mg/kg/load

Maintenance as continuous I.V. infusion: 20-80 mcg/kg/minute; maximum: 2 g/24 hours

Adults:

Oral: 250-500 mg/dose every 3-6 hours or 500 mg to 1 g every 6 hours sustained release; usual dose: 50 mg/kg/24 hours; maximum: 4 g/24 hours

I.M.: 0.5-1 g every 4-8 hours until oral therapy is possible

I.V. (infusion requires use of an infusion pump): Loading dose: 15-18 mg/kg administered as slow infusion over 25-30 minutes or 100-200 mg/dose repeated every 5 minutes as needed to a total dose of 1 g; maintenance dose: 1-6 mg/minute by continuous infusion

Infusion rate: 2 g/250 mL D_5W/NS (I.V. infusion requires use of an infusion pump):

1 mg/minute: 7 mL/hour

2 mg/minute: 15 mL/hour

3 mg/minute: 21 mL/hour

4 mg/minute: 30 mL/hour

5 mg/minute: 38 mL/hour

6 mg/minute: 45 mL/hour

Refractory ventricular fibrillation: 30 mg/minute, up to a total of 17 mg/kg; I.V. maintenance infusion: 1-4 mg/minute; monitor levels and do not exceed 3 mg/minute for >24 hours in adults with renal failure

ACLS guidelines: I.V.: Infuse 20 mg/minute until arrhythmia is controlled, hypotension occurs, QRS complex widens by 50% of its original width, or total of 17 mg/kg is given

Dosing interval in renal impairment:

Cl_{cr} 10-50 mL/minute: Administer every 6-12 hours

Cl_{cr} <10 mL/minute: Administer every 8-24 hours

Dialysis:

Procainamide: **Moderately hemodialyzable (20% to 50%):** 200 mg supplemental dose posthemodialysis is recommended

N-acetylprocainamide: Not dialyzable (0% to 5%)

Procainamide/N-acetylprocainamide: Not peritoneal dialyzable (0% to 5%)

Procainamide/N-acetylprocainamide: Replace by blood level during continuous arterio-venous or veno-venous hemofiltration (CAVH/CAVHD)

Dosing adjustment in hepatic impairment: Reduce dose 50%

Administration Dilute I.V. with D_5W; maximum rate: 50 mg/minute; give around-the-clock rather than 4 times/day to promote less variation in peak and trough serum levels

Monitoring Parameters EKG, blood pressure, CBC with differential, platelet count; cardiac monitor and blood pressure monitor required during I.V. administration

(Continued)

Procainamide Hydrochloride *(Continued)*

Reference Range

Timing of serum samples: Draw trough just before next oral dose; draw 6-12 hours after I.V. infusion has started; half-life is 2.5-5 hours

Therapeutic levels: Procainamide: 4-10 µg/mL; NAPA 15-25 µg/mL; Combined: 10-30 µg/mL

Toxic concentration: Procainamide: >10-12 µg/mL

Patient Information Do not discontinue therapy unless instructed by physician; notify physician or pharmacist if soreness of mouth, throat or gums, unexplained fever, or symptoms of upper respiratory tract infection occur. Do not chew sustained release tablets; some sustained release tablets contain a wax core that slowly releases the drug; when this process is complete, the empty, nonabsorbable wax core is eliminated and may be visible in feces; some sustained release tablets may be broken in half.

Nursing Implications Do not crush sustained release drug product

Dosage Forms

Capsule: 250 mg, 375 mg, 500 mg

Injection: 100 mg/mL (10 mL); 500 mg/mL (2 mL)

Tablet: 250 mg, 375 mg, 500 mg

Tablet, sustained release: 250 mg, 500 mg, 750 mg, 1000 mg

Procaine Amide Hydrochloride *see* Procainamide Hydrochloride *on page 927*

Procaine Benzylpenicillin *see* Penicillin G Procaine *on page 853*

Procaine Hydrochloride *(proe' kane)*

Brand Names Novocain®

Use Produces spinal anesthesia and epidural and peripheral nerve block by injection and infiltration methods

Pregnancy Risk Factor C

Contraindications Known hypersensitivity to procaine, PABA, parabens, or other ester local anesthetics

Warnings/Precautions Patients with cardiac diseases, hyperthyroidism, or other endocrine diseases may be more susceptible to toxic effects of local anesthetics; some preparations contain metabisulfite

Adverse Reactions

1% to 10%: Local: Burning sensation at site of injection, pain, tissue irritation

<1%:

Central nervous system: Aseptic meningitis resulting in paralysis can occur, CNS stimulation followed by CNS depression, chills

Dermatologic: Skin discoloration

Gastrointestinal: Nausea, vomiting

Ocular: Miosis

Otic: Tinnitus

Miscellaneous: Anaphylactoid reaction

Overdosage/Toxicology Treatment is primarily symptomatic and supportive. Termination of anesthesia by pneumatic tourniquet inflation should be attempted when the agent is administered by infiltration or regional injection. Seizures commonly respond to diazepam, while hypotension responds to I.V. fluids and Trendelenburg positioning. Bradyarrhythmias (heart rate <60) can be treated with I.V., I.M., or S.C. atropine 15 mcg/kg. With the development of metabolic acidosis, I.V. sodium bicarbonate 0.5-2 mEq/kg and ventilatory assistance should be instituted.

Drug Interactions

Decreased effect of sulfonamides with the PABA metabolite of procaine, chloroprocaine, and tetracaine

Decreased/increased effect of vasopressors, ergot alkaloids, and MAO inhibitors on blood pressure when using anesthetic solutions with a vasoconstrictor

Mechanism of Action Blocks both the initiation and conduction of nerve impulses by decreasing the neuronal membrane's permeability to sodium ions, which results in inhibition of depolarization with resultant blockade of conduction

Pharmacodynamics/Kinetics

Onset of effect: Injection: Within 2-5 minutes

Duration: 0.5-1.5 hours (dependent upon patient, type of block, concentration, and method of anesthesia)

Metabolism: Rapidly hydrolyzed by plasma enzymes to para-aminobenzoic acid and diethylaminoethanol (80% conjugated before elimination)

Half-life: 7.7 minutes

Elimination: In urine as metabolites and some unchanged drug

Usual Dosage Dose varies with procedure, desired depth, and duration of anesthesia, desired muscle relaxation, vascularity of tissues, physical condition, and age of patient

Nursing Implications Prior to instillation of anesthetic agent, withdraw plunger to ensure needle is not in artery or vein; resuscitative equipment should be available when local anesthetics are administered

Dosage Forms Injection: 1% [10 mg/mL] (2 mL, 6 mL, 30 mL, 100 mL); 2% [20 mg/mL] (30 mL, 100 mL); 10% (2 mL)

Procaine Penicillin G *see Penicillin G Procaine on page 853*

Pro-Cal-Sof® [OTC] *see Docusate on page 362*

Procan® SR *see Procainamide Hydrochloride on page 927*

Procarbazine Hydrochloride (proe kar' ba zeen)

Related Information
Cancer Chemotherapy Regimens *on page 1218-1241*

Brand Names Matulane®

Synonyms Benzmethyzin; N-Methylhydrazine

Use Treatment of Hodgkin's disease, non-Hodgkin's lymphoma, brain tumor, bronchogenic carcinoma

Pregnancy Risk Factor D

Contraindications Hypersensitivity to procarbazine or any component, or pre-existing bone marrow aplasia, alcohol ingestion

Warnings/Precautions The U.S. Food and Drug Administration (FDA) currently recommends that procedures for proper handling and disposal of antineoplastic agents be considered. Use with caution in patients with pre-existing renal or hepatic impairment; modify dosage in patients with renal or hepatic impairment or marrow disorders; reduce dosage with serum creatinine >2 mg/dL or total bilirubin >3 mg/dL; procarbazine possesses MAO inhibitor activity. Procarbazine is a carcinogen which may cause acute leukemia; procarbazine may cause infertility.

Adverse Reactions
>10%:
  Central nervous system: Neuropathies, mental depression, manic reactions, hallucinations, dizziness, headache, nervousness, insomnia, nightmares, ataxia, disorientation, foot drop, decreased reflexes, confusion, seizure, CNS stimulation, weakness

  Emetic potential: Moderately high (60% to 90%)

  Endocrine & metabolic: Amenorrhea

  Gastrointestinal: Severe nausea and vomiting occur frequently and may be dose-limiting; anorexia, abdominal pain, stomatitis, dysphagia, diarrhea, and constipation; use a nonphenothiazine antiemetic, when possible

  Hematologic: Thrombocytopenia, hemolytic anemia

  Myelosuppressive: May be dose-limiting toxicity; procarbazine should be discontinued if leukocyte count is <4000 mL or platelet count <100,000 mL

    WBC: Moderate
    Platelets: Moderate
    Onset (days): 14
    Nadir (days): 21
    Recovery (days): 28

  Neuromuscular & skeletal: Paresthesia, tremor

  Ocular: Nystagmus

  Respiratory: Pleural effusion, cough

1% to 10%:
  Dermatologic: Alopecia, hyperpigmentation

  Gastrointestinal: Stomatitis, constipation, diarrhea, anorexia

  Hepatic: Hepatotoxicity

<1%:
  Cardiovascular: Orthostatic hypotension, hypertensive crisis

  Central nervous system: Nervousness, irritability, somnolence

  Dermatologic: Dermatitis, pruritus, hypersensitivity rash

  Hepatic: Jaundice

  Neuromuscular & skeletal: Arthralgia, myalgia

  Ocular: Diplopia, photophobia

  Respiratory: Pneumonitis, hoarseness

  Miscellaneous: Secondary malignancy, allergic reactions, disulfiram-like reaction of alcohol, flu-like syndrome

Overdosage/Toxicology Symptoms of overdose include arthralgia, alopecia, paresthesia, bone marrow depression, hallucinations, nausea, vomiting, diarrhea, seizures, coma; treatment is supportive, adverse effects such as marrow toxicity may begin as late as 2 weeks after exposure

(Continued)

931

Procarbazine Hydrochloride (Continued)

Drug Interactions Increased toxicity:

Procarbazine exhibits weak monoamine oxidase (MAO) inhibitor activity; foods containing high amounts of tyramine should, therefore, be avoided (ie, beer, yogurt, yeast, wine, cheese, pickled herring, chicken liver, and bananas). When a MAO inhibitor is given with food high in tyramine, a hypertensive crisis, intracranial bleeding, and headache have been reported.

Sympathomimetic amines (epinephrine and amphetamines) and antidepressants (tricyclics) should be used cautiously with procarbazine.

Barbiturates, narcotics, phenothiazines, and other CNS depressants can cause somnolence, ataxia, and other symptoms of CNS depression

Alcohol has caused a disulfiram-like reaction with procarbazine; may result in headache, respiratory difficulties, nausea, vomiting, sweating, thirst, hypotension, and flushing

Stability Protect from light

Mechanism of Action Mechanism of action is not clear, methylating of nucleic acids; inhibits DNA, RNA, and protein synthesis; may damage DNA directly and suppresses mitosis; metabolic activation required by host

Pharmacodynamics/Kinetics

Absorption: Oral: Rapid and complete

Distribution: Crosses the blood-brain barrier and distributes into CSF

Metabolism: In the liver and kidney

Half-life: 1 hour

Elimination: In urine and through respiratory tract (<5% as unchanged drug) and 70% as metabolites

Usual Dosage Refer to individual protocols

Oral (dose based on patients ideal weight if the patients has abnormal fluid retention):

Children: 50-100 mg/m^2/day once daily; doses as high as 100-200 mg/m^2/day once daily have been used for neuroblastoma and medulloblastoma

BMT aplastic anemia conditioning regimen: 12.5 mg/kg/dose every other day for 4 doses

MOPP/IC-MOPP regimens: 100 mg/m^2/day for 14 days and repeated every 4 weeks

Adults: Initial: 2-4 mg/kg/day in single or divided doses for 7 days then increase dose to 4-6 mg/kg/day until response is obtained or leukocyte count decreased <4000/mm^3 or the platelet count decreased <100,000/mm^3; maintenance: 1-2 mg/kg/day

In MOPP, 100 mg/m^2/day on days 1-14 of a 28-day cycle

Dosing in renal/hepatic impairment: Use with caution, may result in increased toxicity

Monitoring Parameters CBC with differential, platelet and reticulocyte count, urinalysis, liver function test, renal function test.

Patient Information Avoid food with high tyramine content; obtain a list from your physician or pharmacist; do not take any new prescription or OTC drug without consulting your physician or pharmacist; avoid alcohol and alcohol containing products including topicals; notify physician of persistent fever, sore throat, bleeding, or bruising; may impair judgment and coordination; avoid prolonged exposure to sunlight

Dosage Forms Capsule: 50 mg

Procardia® see Nifedipine on page 794

Procardia XL® see Nifedipine on page 794

Procetofene see Fenofibrate on page 444

Prochlorperazine (proe klor per' a zeen)

Related Information

Initial Doses in Selected Antiemetic Regimens on page 1205

Brand Names Compazine®

Synonyms Prochlorperazine Edisylate; Prochlorperazine Maleate

Use Management of nausea and vomiting; acute and chronic psychosis

Pregnancy Risk Factor C

Contraindications Hypersensitivity to prochlorperazine or any component; cross-sensitivity with other phenothiazines may exist; avoid use in patients with narrow-angle glaucoma; bone marrow depression; severe liver or cardiac disease

Warnings/Precautions Injection contains sulfites which may cause allergic reactions; may impair ability to perform hazardous tasks requiring mental alertness or physical coordination; some products contain tartrazine dye, avoid use in sensitive individuals

Tardive dyskinesia: Prevalence rate may be 40% in elderly; development of the syndrome and the irreversible nature are proportional to duration and total cumulative dose over time. May be reversible if diagnosed early in therapy.

High incidence of extrapyramidal reactions, especially in children or the elderly, so reserve use in children <5 years of age to those who are unresponsive to other antiemetics; incidence of extrapyramidal reactions is increased with acute illnesses such as chicken pox, measles, CNS infections, gastroenteritis, and dehydration

Drug-induced **Parkinson's syndrome** occurs often. **Akathisia** is the most common extrapyramidal reaction in elderly.

Increased confusion, memory loss, psychotic behavior, and agitation frequently occur as a consequence of anticholinergic effects

Lowers seizure threshold, use cautiously in patients with seizure history

Orthostatic hypotension is due to alpha-receptor blockade, the elderly are at greater risk for orthostatic hypotension

Antipsychotic associated sedation in nonpsychotic patients is extremely unpleasant due to feelings of depersonalization, derealization, and dysphoria

Life-threatening arrhythmias have occurred at therapeutic doses of antipsychotics

Adverse Reactions Incidence of extrapyramidal reactions are higher with prochlorperazine than chlorpromazine

Central nervous system: Sedation, drowsiness, restlessness, anxiety, extrapyramidal reactions, parkinsonian signs and symptoms, seizures

Dermatologic: Photosensitivity, hyperpigmentation, pruritus, rash

Endocrine & metabolic: Amenorrhea, galactorrhea, gynecomastia

Gastrointestinal: Weight gain, GI upset

Miscellaneous: Anaphylactoid reactions, altered central temperature regulation

>10%:
  Cardiovascular: Hypotension (especially with I.V. use), orthostatic hypotension, tachycardia, arrhythmias
  Central nervous system: Pseudoparkinsonism, akathisia, tardive dyskinesia (persistent), decreased sweating, dizziness, dystonias
  Gastrointestinal: Dry mouth, constipation
  Genitourinary: Urinary retention
  Ocular: Pigmentary retinopathy, blurred vision
  Respiratory: Nasal congestion

1% to 10%:
  Central nervous system: Dizziness, trembling of fingers
  Dermatologic: Increased sensitivity to sun, skin rash
  Endocrine & metabolic: Changes in menstrual cycle pain in breasts, changes in libido
  Gastrointestinal: Weight gain, nausea, vomiting, stomach pain
  Genitourinary: Difficulty in urination, ejaculatory disturbances

<1%:
  Central nervous system: Neuroleptic malignant syndrome (NMS)
  Dermatologic: Discoloration of skin (blue-gray)
  Endocrine & metabolic: Galactorrhea
  Genitourinary: Priapism
  Hematologic: Agranulocytosis, leukopenia, thrombocytopenia
  Hepatic: Cholestatic jaundice, hepatotoxicity
  Ocular: Cornea and lens changes, pigmentary retinopathy
  Miscellaneous: Impairment of temperature regulation lowering of seizures threshold

Overdosage/Toxicology Symptoms of overdose include deep sleep, coma, extrapyramidal symptoms, abnormal involuntary muscle movements, hypotension

Following initiation of essential overdose management, toxic symptom treatment and supportive treatment should be initiated. Hypotension usually responds to I.V. fluids or Trendelenburg positioning. If unresponsive to these measures, the use of a parenteral inotrope may be required (eg, norepinephrine 0.1-0.2 mcg/kg/minute titrated to response). Seizures commonly respond to diazepam (I.V. 5-10 mg bolus in adults every 15 minutes if needed up to a total of 30 mg; I.V. 0.25-0.4 mg/kg/dose up to a total of 10 mg in children) or to phenytoin or phenobarbital. Critical cardiac arrhythmias often respond to I.V. phenytoin (15 mg/kg up to 1 g), while other antiarrhythmics can be used. Extrapyramidal symptoms (eg, dystonic reactions) may require management with diphenhydramine 1-2 mg/kg (adults) up to a maximum of 50 mg I.M. or I.V. slow push followed by a maintenance dose for 48-72 hours. When these reactions are unresponsive to diphenhydramine, benztropine mesylate I.V. 1-2 mg (adults) may be effective. These agents are generally effective within 2-5 minutes.

Drug Interactions Increased toxicity: Additive effects with other CNS depressants; anticonvulsants; epinephrine may cause hypotension

(Continued)

Prochlorperazine (Continued)

Stability Protect from light; clear or slightly yellow solutions may be used; **incompatible** when mixed with aminophylline, amphotericin B, ampicillin, calcium salts, cephalothin, foscarnet (Y-site), furosemide, hydrocortisone, hydromorphone, methohexital, midazolam, penicillin G, pentobarbital, phenobarbital, thiopental

Mechanism of Action Blocks postsynaptic mesolimbic dopaminergic D_1 and D_2 receptors in the brain, including the medullary chemoreceptor trigger zone; exhibits a strong alpha-adrenergic and anticholinergic blocking effect and depresses the release of hypothalamic and hypophyseal hormones; believed to depress the reticular activating system, thus affecting basal metabolism, body temperature, wakefulness, vasomotor tone and emesis

Pharmacodynamics/Kinetics
Onset of effect:
Oral: Within 30-40 minutes
I.M.: Within 10-20 minutes
Rectal: Within 60 minutes
Duration: Persists longest with I.M. and oral extended-release doses (12 hours); shortest following rectal and immediate release oral administration (3-4 hours)
Distribution: Crosses the placenta; appears in breast milk
Metabolism: Hepatic
Half-life: 23 hours
Elimination: Primarily by hepatic metabolism

Usual Dosage
Antiemetic: Children:
Oral, rectal:
>10 kg: 0.4 mg/kg/24 hours in 3-4 divided doses; **or**
9-14 kg: 2.5 mg every 12-24 hours as needed; maximum: 7.5 mg/day
14-18 kg: 2.5 mg every 8-12 hours as needed; maximum: 10 mg/day
18-39 kg: 2.5 mg every 8 hours or 5 mg every 12 hours as needed; maximum: 15 mg/day
I.M.: 0.1-0.15 mg/kg/dose; usual: 0.13 mg/kg/dose; change to oral as soon as possible
I.V.: Not recommended in children <10 kg or <2 years

Antiemetic: Adults:
Oral: 5-10 mg 3-4 times/day; usual maximum: 40 mg/day
I.M.: 5-10 mg every 3-4 hours; usual maximum: 40 mg/day
I.V.: 2.5-10 mg; maximum 10 mg/dose or 40 mg/day; may repeat dose every 3-4 hours as needed
Rectal: 25 mg twice daily

Antipsychotic:
Children 2-12 years:
Oral, rectal: 2.5 mg 2-3 times/day; increase dosage as needed to maximum daily dose of 20 mg for 2-5 years and 25 mg for 6-12 years
I.M.: 0.13 mg/kg/dose; change to oral as soon as possible
Adults:
Oral: 5-10 mg 3-4 times/day; doses up to 150 mg/day may be required in some patients for treatment of severe disturbances
I.M.: 10-20 mg every 4-6 hours may be required in some patients for treatment of severe disturbances; change to oral as soon as possible

Dementia behavior (nonpsychotic): Elderly: Initial: 2.5-5 mg 1-2 times/day; increase dose at 4- to 7-day intervals by 2.5-5 mg/day; increase dosing intervals (twice daily, 3 times/day, etc) as necessary to control response or side effects; maximum daily dose should probably not exceed 75 mg in elderly; gradual increases (titration) may prevent some side effects or decrease their severity

Not dialyzable (0% to 5%)

Administration Prochlorperazine may be administered I.M. or I.V.
I.M. should be administered into the upper outer quadrant of the buttock
I.V. may be administered IVP or IVPB
IVP should be administered at a concentration of 1 mg/mL at a rate of 1 mg/minute

Test Interactions False-positives for phenylketonuria, urinary amylase, uroporphyrins, urobilinogen

Patient Information May cause drowsiness, impair judgment and coordination; may cause photosensitivity; avoid excessive sunlight; notify physician of involuntary movements or feelings of restlessness

Nursing Implications Avoid skin contact with oral solution or injection, contact dermatitis has occurred; observe for extrapyramidal symptoms

Additional Information
Prochlorperazine: Compazine® suppository

Prochlorperazine edisylate: Compazine® oral solution and injection
Prochlorperazine maleate: Compazine® capsule and tablet
Dosage Forms
Capsule, sustained action, as maleate: 10 mg, 15 mg, 30 mg
Injection, as edisylate: 5 mg/mL (2 mL, 10 mL)
Suppository, rectal: 2.5 mg, 5 mg, 25 mg (12/box)
Syrup, as edisylate: 5 mg/5 mL (120 mL)
Tablet, as maleate: 5 mg, 10 mg, 25 mg

Prochlorperazine Edisylate *see* Prochlorperazine *on page 932*

Prochlorperazine Maleate *see* Prochlorperazine *on page 932*

ProCrit® *see* Epoetin Alfa *on page 392*

Proctocort™ *see* Hydrocortisone *on page 546*

ProctoCream-HC™ *see* Hydrocortisone *on page 546*

Proctofene *see* Fenofibrate *on page 444*

Proctofoam® [OTC] *see* Pramoxine Hydrochloride *on page 915*

Procyclidine Hydrochloride (proe sye′ kli deen)
Brand Names Kemadrin®
Use Relieves symptoms of parkinsonian syndrome and drug-induced extrapyramidal symptoms
Pregnancy Risk Factor C
Contraindications Angle-closure glaucoma; safe use in children not established
Warnings/Precautions Use with caution in hot weather or during exercise. Elderly patients frequently develop increased sensitivity and require strict dosage regulation - side effects may be more severe in elderly patients with atherosclerotic changes. Use with caution in patients with tachycardia, cardiac arrhythmias, hypertension, hypotension, prostatic hypertrophy (especially in the elderly) or any tendency toward urinary retention, liver or kidney disorders and obstructive disease of the GI or GU tract. When given in large doses or to susceptible patients, may cause weakness and inability to move particular muscle groups.
Adverse Reactions
>10%:
Gastrointestinal: Constipation
Miscellaneous: Decreased sweating, dry mouth, nose, throat, or skin
1% to 10%: Decreased flow of breast milk, difficulty in swallowing, increased sensitivity to light
<1%:
Cardiovascular: Orthostatic hypotension, ventricular fibrillation, tachycardia, palpitations
Central nervous system: Confusion, drowsiness, headache, loss of memory, weakness, tiredness, ataxia
Dermatologic: Skin rash
Gastrointestinal: Bloated feeling, nausea, vomiting
Genitourinary: Difficult urination
Ocular: Increased intraocular pain, blurred vision
Overdosage/Toxicology Symptoms of overdose include disorientation, hallucinations, delusions, blurred vision, dysphagia, absent bowel sounds, hyperthermia, hypertension, urinary retention. Anticholinergic toxicity is caused by strong binding of the drug to cholinergic receptors. Anticholinesterase inhibitors reduce acetylcholinesterase, the enzyme that breaks down acetylcholine and thereby allows acetylcholine to accumulate and compete for receptor binding with the offending anticholinergic. For anticholinergic overdose with severe life-threatening symptoms, physostigmine 1-2 mg (0.5 or 0.02 mg/kg for children) S.C. or I.V., slowly may be given to reverse these effects.
Drug Interactions
Decreased effect of psychotropics
Increased toxicity with phenothiazines, meperidine, TCAs
Mechanism of Action Thought to act by blocking excess acetylcholine at cerebral synapses; many of its effects are due to its pharmacologic similarities with atropine
Pharmacodynamics/Kinetics
Onset of effect: Oral: Within 30-40 minutes
Duration: 4-6 hours
Usual Dosage Adults: Oral: 2.5 mg 3 times/day after meals; if tolerated, gradually increase dose, maximum of 20 mg/day if necessary

Dosing adjustment in hepatic impairment: Decrease dose to a twice daily dosing regimen
(Continued)

Procyclidine Hydrochloride (Continued)

Patient Information Take after meals; do not discontinue drug abruptly; notify physician if adverse GI effects, fever or heat intolerance occurs; may cause drowsiness; avoid alcohol; adequate fluid intake or sugar free gum or hard candy may help dry mouth; adequate fluid and exercise may help constipation

Dosage Forms Tablet: 5 mg

Profasi® HP *see* Chorionic Gonadotropin *on page 242*

Profenal® *see* Suprofen *on page 1050*

Profilate® OSD *see* Antihemophilic Factor (Human) *on page 80*

Profilate® SD *see* Antihemophilic Factor (Human) *on page 80*

Profilnine® Heat-Treated *see* Factor IX Complex (Human) *on page 438*

Progestaject® *see* Progesterone *on this page*

Progesterone (proe jess' ter one)

Brand Names Gesterol®; Progestaject®

Synonyms Pregnenedione; Progestin

Use Endometrial carcinoma or renal carcinoma as well as secondary amenorrhea or abnormal uterine bleeding due to hormonal imbalance

Pregnancy Risk Factor X

Contraindications Pregnancy, thrombophlebitis, undiagnosed vaginal bleeding, hypersensitivity to progesterone or any component, carcinoma of the breast, cerebral apoplexy

Warnings/Precautions Use with caution in patients with impaired liver function, depression, diabetes, and epilepsy; use of any progestin during the first 4 months of pregnancy is not recommended; monitor closely for loss of vision, proptosis, diplopia, migraine, and signs and symptoms of embolic disorders. Not a progestin of choice in the elderly for hormonal cycling.

Adverse Reactions

>10%:
  Cardiovascular: Edema
  Central nervous system: Weakness
  Endocrine & metabolic: Breakthrough bleeding, spotting, changes in menstrual flow, amenorrhea
  Gastrointestinal: Anorexia
  Local: Pain at injection site

1% to 10%:
  Cardiovascular: Embolism, central thrombosis
  Central nervous system: Mental depression, fever, insomnia
  Dermatologic: Melasma or chloasma, allergic rash with or without pruritus
  Endocrine: Changes in cervical erosion and secretions, weight gain or loss, increased breast tenderness
  Hepatic: Cholestatic jaundice
  Local: Thrombophlebitis

Overdosage/Toxicology Toxicity is unlikely following single exposures of excessive doses; supportive treatment is adequate in most cases

Drug Interactions Decreased effect: Aminoglutethimide may decrease effect by increasing hepatic metabolism

Mechanism of Action Natural steroid hormone that induces secretory changes in the endometrium, promotes mammary gland development, relaxes uterine smooth muscle, blocks follicular maturation and ovulation, and maintains pregnancy

Pharmacodynamics/Kinetics

Duration of action: ~24 hours
Absorption: Rapid after injection but inactivated by the liver when taken orally
Half-life: 5 minutes
Elimination: In urine

Usual Dosage Adults: Female: I.M.:
  Amenorrhea: 5-10 mg/day for 6-8 days usually beginning 8-10 days before anticipated start of menstruation
  Abnormal uterine bleeding: 5-10 mg/day for 6-8 days

Monitoring Parameters Before starting therapy, a physical exam including the breasts and pelvis are recommended, also a PAP smear; signs or symptoms of depression, glucose in diabetics

Test Interactions Thyroid function, metyrapone, liver function, coagulation tests, endocrine function tests

Patient Information Take this medicine only as directed; do not take more of it and do not take it for a longer period of time; if you suspect you may have become pregnant, stop taking this medicine; notify physician if sudden loss of vision or migraine headache occur; may cause photosensitivity, wear protective clothing or sunscreen

Nursing Implications Patients should receive a copy of the patient labeling for the drug; administer deep I.M. only; monitor patient closely for loss of vision, sudden onset of proptosis, diplopia, migraine, and signs and symptoms of embolic disorders

Dosage Forms Injection, in oil: 50 mg/mL (10 mL)

Progestin see Progesterone *on previous page*

Proglycem® see Diazoxide *on page 326*

Prograf® see Tacrolimus *on page 1053*

ProHIBiT® see Haemophilus b Conjugate Vaccine *on page 521*

Prolamine® [OTC] see Phenylpropanolamine Hydrochloride *on page 876*

Prolastin® see Alpha₁-Proteinase Inhibitor (Human) *on page 43*

Proleukin® see Aldesleukin *on page 35*

Prolixin® see Fluphenazine *on page 478*

Prolixin Decanoate® see Fluphenazine *on page 478*

Prolixin Enanthate® see Fluphenazine *on page 478*

Proloprim® see Trimethoprim *on page 1127*

Promazine Hydrochloride (proe′ ma zeen)

Related Information

Antipsychotic Agents Comparison *on page 1255*

Brand Names Sparine®

Use Management of manifestations of psychotic disorders; depressive neurosis; alcohol withdrawal; nausea and vomiting; nonpsychotic symptoms associated with dementia in elderly, Tourette's syndrome; Huntington's chorea; spasmodic torticollis and Reye's syndrome

Pregnancy Risk Factor C

Contraindications Hypersensitivity to promazine or any component; severe CNS depression, cross-sensitivity to other phenothiazines may exist; avoid use in patients with narrow-angle glaucoma, blood dyscrasias, severe liver or cardiac disease; subcortical brain damage; circulatory collapse; severe hypotension or hypertension

Warnings/Precautions

Tardive dyskinesia: Prevalence rate may be 40% in elderly; development of the syndrome and the irreversible nature are proportional to duration and total cumulative dose over time. May be reversible if diagnosed early in therapy.

Extrapyramidal reactions are more common in elderly with up to 50% developing these reactions after 60 years of age. These reactions may be more common in dementia patients.

Drug-induced **Parkinson's syndrome** occurs often. **Akathisia** is the most common extrapyramidal reaction in elderly.

Increased confusion, memory loss, psychotic behavior, and agitation frequently occur as a consequence of anticholinergic effects

Orthostatic hypotension is due to alpha-receptor blockade, the elderly are at greater risk for orthostatic hypotension

Antipsychotic associated sedation in nonpsychotic patients is extremely unpleasant due to feelings of depersonalization, derealization, and dysphoria

Life-threatening arrhythmias have occurred at therapeutic doses of antipsychotics; use with caution in patients with narrow-angle glaucoma, severe liver disease or severe cardiac disease

Adverse Reactions

>10%:

Cardiovascular: Hypotension, orthostatic hypotension

Central nervous system: Pseudoparkinsonism, akathisia, dystonias, tardive dyskinesia (persistent), dizziness

Gastrointestinal: Constipation

Ocular: Pigmentary retinopathy

Respiratory: Nasal congestion

Miscellaneous: Decreased sweating

1% to 10%:

Central nervous system: Dizziness

Dermatologic: Increased sensitivity to sun, skin rash

Endocrine & metabolic: Changes in menstrual cycle, changes in libido, pain in breasts

(Continued)

Promazine Hydrochloride *(Continued)*

Gastrointestinal: Weight gain, nausea, vomiting, stomach pain
Genitourinary: Difficulty in urination, ejaculatory disturbances
Neuromuscular & skeletal: Trembling of fingers
<1%:
Central nervous system: Neuroleptic malignant syndrome (NMS)
Dermatologic: Discoloration of skin (blue-gray), pigmentary retinopathy
Endocrine & metabolic: Galactorrhea
Genitourinary: Priapism
Hematologic: Agranulocytosis, leukopenia
Hepatic: Cholestatic jaundice, hepatotoxicity
Ocular: Cornea and lens changes
Miscellaneous: Impairment of temperature regulation, lowering of seizures threshold

Overdosage/Toxicology Symptoms of overdose include deep sleep, coma, extrapyramidal symptoms, abnormal involuntary muscle movements, hypotension

Following initiation of essential overdose management, toxic symptom treatment and supportive treatment should be initiated. Hypotension usually responds to I.V. fluids or Trendelenburg positioning. If unresponsive to these measures, the use of a parenteral inotrope may be required (eg, norepinephrine 0.1-0.2 mcg/kg/minute titrated to response). Seizures commonly respond to diazepam (I.V. 5-10 mg bolus in adults every 15 minutes if needed up to a total of 30 mg; I.V. 0.25-0.4 mg/kg/dose up to a total of 10 mg in children) or to phenytoin or phenobarbital. Critical cardiac arrhythmias often respond to I.V. phenytoin (15 mg/kg up to 1 g), while other antiarrhythmics can be used. Neuroleptics often cause extrapyramidal symptoms (eg, dystonic reactions) requiring management with diphenhydramine 1-2 mg/kg (adults) up to a maximum of 50 mg I.M. or I.V. slow push followed by a maintenance dose for 48-72 hours. When these reactions are unresponsive to diphenhydramine, benztropine mesylate I.V. 1-2 mg (adults) may be effective. These agents are generally effective within 2-5 minutes.

Stability Protect all dosage forms from light, clear or slightly yellow solutions may be used; should be dispensed in amber or opaque vials/bottles. Solutions may be diluted or mixed with fruit juices or other liquids, but must be administered immediately after mixing

Injection: **Incompatible** when mixed with aminophylline, dimenhydrinate, methohexital, nafcillin, penicillin G, pentobarbital, phenobarbital, sodium bicarbonate, thiopental

Mechanism of Action Blocks postsynaptic mesolimbic dopaminergic D_1 and D_2 receptors in the brain; exhibits a strong alpha-adrenergic blocking and anticholinergic effect, depresses the release of hypothalamic and hypophyseal hormones; believed to depress the reticular activating system thus affecting basal metabolism, body temperature, wakefulness, vasomotor tone, and emesis

Pharmacodynamics/Kinetics The specific pharmacokinetics of promazine are poorly established but probably resemble those of other phenothiazines.

Absorption: Phenothiazines are only partially absorbed; great variability in plasma levels resulting from a given dose
Metabolism: Extensively in the liver
Half-life: Most phenothiazines have long half-lives in the range of 24 hours or more

Usual Dosage Oral, I.M.:
Children >12 years: Antipsychotic: 10-25 mg every 4-6 hours

Adults:
Psychosis: 10-200 mg every 4-6 hours not to exceed 1000 mg/day
Antiemetic: 25-50 mg every 4-6 hours as needed

Not dialyzable (0% to 5%)
Administration I.M. injections should be deep injections; if giving I.V., dilute to at least 25 mg/mL and give slowly
Test Interactions ↑ cholesterol (S), ↑ glucose; ↓ uric acid (S)
Patient Information May cause drowsiness, impair judgment and coordination; may cause photosensitivity; avoid excessive sunlight; notify physician of involuntary movements or feelings of restlessness
Nursing Implications Watch for hypotension
Dosage Forms
Injection: 25 mg/mL (10 mL); 50 mg/mL (1 mL, 2 mL, 10 mL)
Tablet: 25 mg, 50 mg, 100 mg

Prometa® *see* Metaproterenol Sulfate *on page 697*

Prometh® *see* Promethazine Hydrochloride *on this page*

Promethazine Hydrochloride (proe meth' a zeen)

Brand Names Anergan®; Phenazine®; Phencen®; Phenergan®; Prometh®; Prorex®; V-Gan®

Use Symptomatic treatment of various allergic conditions, antiemetic, motion sickness, and as a sedative

Pregnancy Risk Factor C

Contraindications Hypersensitivity to promethazine or any component; narrowangle glaucoma

Warnings/Precautions Do not give S.C. or intra-arterially, necrotic lesions may occur; injection may contain sulfites which may cause allergic reactions in some patients; use with caution in patients with cardiovascular disease, impaired liver function, asthma, sleep apnea, seizures. Rapid I.V. administration may produce a transient fall in blood pressure, rate of administration should not exceed 25 mg/minute; slow I.V. administration may produce a slightly elevated blood pressure. Because promethazine is a phenothiazine (and can, therefore, cause side effects such as extrapyramidal symptoms), it is not considered an antihistamine of choice in the elderly.

Adverse Reactions
Hematologic: Thrombocytopenia
Hepatic: Jaundice

>10%:
Central nervous system: Slight to moderate drowsiness
Respiratory: Thickening of bronchial secretions
1% to 10%:
Central nervous system: Headache, fatigue, nervousness, dizziness
Gastrointestinal: Dry mouth, abdominal pain, nausea, diarrhea, appetite increase, weight increase
Neuromuscular & skeletal: Arthralgia
Respiratory: Pharyngitis
<1%:
Cardiovascular: Tachycardia, bradycardia, palpitations, hypotension
Central nervous system: Sedation (pronounced), confusion, excitation, extrapyramidal reactions with high doses, dystonia, faintness with I.V. administration, depression, dizziness, insomnia, sedation (pronounced)
Dermatologic: Photosensitivity, allergic reactions, rash, angioedema
Genitourinary: Urinary retention
Hepatic: Hepatitis
Neuromuscular & skeletal: Tremor, paresthesia, myalgia
Ocular: Blurred vision
Respiratory: Irregular respiration, bronchospasm
Miscellaneous: Epistaxis

Overdosage/Toxicology Symptoms of overdose include CNS depression, respiratory depression, possible CNS stimulation, dry mouth, fixed and dilated pupils, hypotension

Following initiation of essential overdose management, toxic symptom treatment and supportive treatment should be initiated. Hypotension usually responds to I.V. fluids or Trendelenburg positioning. If unresponsive to these measures, norepinephrine 0.1-0.2 mcg/kg/minute titrated to response may be tried. Seizures commonly respond to diazepam (I.V. 5-10 mg bolus in adults every 15 minutes if needed up to a total of 30 mg; I.V. 0.25-0.4 mg/kg/dose up to a total of 10 mg in children) or to phenytoin or phenobarbital. Critical cardiac arrhythmias often respond to I.V. phenytoin (15 mg/kg up to 1 g), while other antiarrhythmics can be used. Neuroleptics often cause extrapyramidal symptoms (eg, dystonic reactions) requiring management with diphenhydramine 1-2 mg/kg (adults) up to a maximum of 50 mg I.M. or I.V. slow push followed by a maintenance dose for 48-72 hours. When these reactions are unresponsive to diphenhydramine, benztropine mesylate I.V. 1-2 mg (adults) may be effective. These agents are generally effective within 2-5 minutes.

Drug Interactions Increased toxicity: Epinephrine should not be used together with promethazine since blood pressure may decrease further; additive effects with other CNS depressants

Stability Protect from light and from freezing; **compatible** (when comixed in the same syringe) with atropine, chlorpromazine, diphenhydramine, droperidol, fentanyl, glycopyrrolate, hydromorphone, hydroxyzine hydrochloride, meperidine, midazolam, nalbuphine, pentazocine, prochlorperazine, scopolamine; **incompatible** when mixed with aminophylline, cefoperazone (Y-site), chloramphenicol, dimenhydrinate (same syringe), foscarnet (Y-site), furosemide, heparin, hydrocortisone, methohexital, penicillin G, pentobarbital, phenobarbital, thiopental

(Continued)

Promethazine Hydrochloride (Continued)

Mechanism of Action Blocks postsynaptic mesolimbic dopaminergic receptors in the brain; exhibits a strong alpha-adrenergic blocking effect and depresses the release of hypothalamic and hypophyseal hormones; competes with histamine for the H_1-receptor; reduces stimuli to the brainstem reticular system

Pharmacodynamics/Kinetics
Onset of effect: I.V.: Within 20 minutes (3-5 minutes with I.V. injection)
Duration: 2-6 hours
Metabolism: In the liver
Elimination: Principally as inactive metabolites in urine and in feces

Usual Dosage
Children:
Antihistamine: Oral, rectal: 0.1 mg/kg/dose every 6 hours during the day and 0.5 mg/kg/dose at bedtime as needed
Antiemetic: Oral, I.M., I.V., rectal: 0.25-1 mg/kg 4-6 times/day as needed
Motion sickness: Oral, rectal: 0.5 mg/kg/dose 30 minutes to 1 hour before departure, then every 12 hours as needed
Sedation: Oral, I.M., I.V., rectal: 0.5-1 mg/kg/dose every 6 hours as needed

Adults:
Antihistamine (including allergic reactions to blood or plasma):
Oral, rectal: 12.5 mg 3 times/day and 25 mg at bedtime
I.M., I.V.: 25 mg, may repeat in 2 hours when necessary; switch to oral route as soon as feasible
Antiemetic: Oral, I.M., I.V., rectal: 12.5-25 mg every 4 hours as needed
Motion sickness: Oral, rectal: 25 mg 30-60 minutes before departure, then every 12 hours as needed
Sedation: Oral, I.M., I.V., rectal: 25-50 mg/dose

Not dialyzable (0% to 5%)

Administration Avoid I.V. use; if necessary, may dilute to a maximum concentration of 25 mg/mL and infuse at a maximum rate of 25 mg/minute; rapid I.V. administration may produce a transient fall in blood pressure

Test Interactions Alters the flare response in intradermal allergen tests

Patient Information May cause drowsiness, impair judgment and coordination; may cause photosensitivity; avoid excessive sunlight; notify physician of involuntary movements or feelings of restlessness

Dosage Forms
Injection: 25 mg/mL (1 mL, 10 mL); 50 mg/mL (1 mL, 10 mL)
Suppository, rectal: 12.5 mg, 25 mg, 50 mg
Syrup: 6.25 mg/5 mL (5 mL, 120 mL, 240 mL, 480 mL, 4000 mL); 25 mg/5 mL (120 mL, 480 mL, 4000 mL)
Tablet: 12.5 mg, 25 mg, 50 mg

Promine® see Procainamide Hydrochloride on page 927

Promit® see Dextran 1 on page 319

Pronestyl® see Procainamide Hydrochloride on page 927

Propadrine see Phenylpropanolamine Hydrochloride on page 876

Propafenone Hydrochloride (proe pa feen' one)

Related Information
Antiarrhythmic Drugs on page 1246-1248
Brand Names Rythmol®
Use Life-threatening ventricular arrhythmias
Unlabeled use: Supraventricular tachycardias, including those patients with Wolff-Parkinson-White syndrome
Pregnancy Risk Factor C
Contraindications Hypersensitivity to propafenone or any component; uncontrolled congestive heart failure; bronchospastic disorders; cardiogenic shock; conduction disorders (A-V block, sick-sinus syndrome), bradycardia
Warnings/Precautions Until evidence to the contrary, propafenone should be considered acceptable only for the treatment of life-threatening arrhythmias; propafenone may cause new or worsened arrhythmias, worsen CHF, decrease A-V conduction and alter pacemaker thresholds; use with caution in patients with recent myocardial infarction, congestive heart failure, hepatic or renal dysfunction; elderly may be at greater risk for toxicity
Adverse Reactions
>10%:
Central nervous system: Dizziness, drowsiness
Gastrointestinal: Dry mouth

1% to 10%:

    Cardiovascular: A-V block (first and second degree), cardiac conduction disturbances, palpitations, congestive heart failure, angina, bradycardia

    Central nervous system: Dizziness, headache, anxiety, loss of balance

    Gastrointestinal: Altered taste, constipation, nausea, vomiting, abdominal pain, dyspepsia, anorexia, flatulence, diarrhea

    Ocular: Blurred vision

    Respiratory: Dyspnea

<1%:

    Cardiovascular: New or worsened arrhythmias (proarrhythmic effect), bundle branch block

    Central nervous system: Abnormal speech, vision, or dreams, numbness

    Hematologic: Leukopenia, thrombocytopenia, agranulocytosis

    Neuromuscular & skeletal: Paresthesias

Overdosage/Toxicology Has a narrow therapeutic index and severe toxicity may occur slightly above the therapeutic range, especially if combined with other antiarrhythmic drugs. Acute single ingestion of twice the daily therapeutic dose is life-threatening. Symptoms of overdose include increases in P-R, QRS, Q-T intervals and amplitude of the T wave, A-V block, bradycardia, hypotension, ventricular arrhythmias (monomorphic or polymorphic ventricular tachycardia), and asystole; other symptoms include dizziness, blurred vision, headache, and GI upset. Treatment is supportive, using conventional treatment (fluids, positioning, anticonvulsants, antiarrhythmics). **Note:** Type 1a antiarrhythmic agents should not be used to treat cardiotoxicity caused by type 1c drugs; sodium bicarbonate may reverse QRS prolongation, bradycardia and hypotension; ventricular pacing may be needed; hemodialysis only of possible benefit for tocainide or flecainide overdose in patients with renal failure.

Drug Interactions

Decreased levels with rifampin

Increased levels with cimetidine, quinidine, and beta-blockers

Increased effect/levels of warfarin, beta-blockers metabolized by the liver, local anesthetics, cyclosporine, and digoxin (**Note:** Reduce dose of digoxin by 25%)

Mechanism of Action Propafenone is a 1C antiarrhythmic agent which possesses local anesthetic properties, blocks the fast inward sodium current, and slows the rate of increase of the action potential. prolongs conduction and refractoriness in all areas of the myocardium, with a slightly more pronounced effect on intraventricular conduction; it prolongs effective refractory period, reduces spontaneous automaticity and exhibits some beta-blockade activity.

Pharmacodynamics/Kinetics

Absorption: Well absorbed

Metabolism: Two genetically determined metabolism groups exist: fast or slow metabolizers; 10% of Caucasians are slow metabolizers

Half-life after a single dose (100-300 mg): 2-8 hours; half-life after chronic dosing ranges from 10-32 hours

Time to peak: Peak levels occur in 2 hours with a 150 mg dose and 3 hours after a 300 mg dose; this agent exhibits nonlinear pharmacokinetics; when dose is increased from 300 mg to 900 mg/day, serum concentrations increase tenfold; this nonlinearity is thought to be due to saturable first-pass hepatic enzyme metabolism

Usual Dosage Adults: Oral: 150 mg every 8 hours, increase at 3- to 4-day intervals up to 300 mg every 8 hours. **Note:** Patients who exhibit significant widening of QRS complex or second or third degree A-V block may need dose reduction.

Dosing adjustment in hepatic impairment: Reduction is necessary

Monitoring Parameters EKG, blood pressure, pulse (particularly at initiation of therapy)

Patient Information Take dose the same way each day, either with or without food; do not double the next dose if present dose is missed; do not discontinue drug or change dose without advice of physician; report any severe or persistent fatigue, sore throat, or any unusual bleeding or bruising; may cause drowsiness and impair coordination and judgment

Nursing Implications Patients should be on a cardiac monitor during initiation of therapy or when dosage is increased; monitor heart sounds and pulses for rate, rhythm and quality

Dosage Forms Tablet: 150 mg, 300 mg

Propagest® [OTC] *see* Phenylpropanolamine Hydrochloride *on page 876*

Propantheline Bromide (proe pan' the leen)

Brand Names Pro-Banthine®

Use Adjunctive treatment of peptic ulcer, irritable bowel syndrome, pancreatitis, ureteral and urinary bladder spasm; reduce duodenal motility during diagnostic radiologic procedures

Pregnancy Risk Factor C

Contraindications Narrow-angle glaucoma, known hypersensitivity to propantheline; ulcerative colitis; toxic megacolon; obstructive disease of the GI or urinary tract

Warnings/Precautions Use with caution in patients with hyperthyroidism, hepatic, cardiac, or renal disease, hypertension, GI infections, or other endocrine diseases

Adverse Reactions

>10%:

Gastrointestinal: Constipation

Miscellaneous: Decreased sweating, dry mouth, skin, nose, or throat

1% to 10%: Difficulty in swallowing

<1%:

Dermatologic: Rash

Cardiovascular: Tachycardia

Central nervous system: Confusion, headache, loss of memory, weakness, tiredness, drowsiness, nervousness, insomnia

Gastrointestinal: Bloated feeling, nausea, vomiting

Genitourinary: Urinary retention

Ocular: Increased intraocular pressure, blurred vision

Overdosage/Toxicology Symptoms of overdose include CNS disturbances, flushing, respiratory failure, paralysis, coma, urinary retention, hyperthermia. Anticholinergic toxicity is caused by strong binding of the drug to cholinergic receptors. For anticholinergic overdose with severe life-threatening symptoms, physostigmine 1-2 mg (0.5 or 0.02 mg/kg for children) S.C. or I.V., slowly may be given to reverse these effects.

Drug Interactions

Decreased effect with antacids (↓ absorption); decreased effect of sustained release dosage forms (↓ absorption)

Increased effect/toxicity with anticholinergics, disopyramide, narcotic analgesics, bretylium, type I antiarrhythmics, antihistamines, phenothiazines, TCAs, corticosteroids (↑ IOP), CNS depressants (sedation), adenosine, amiodarone, beta-blockers, amoxapine

Mechanism of Action Competitively blocks the action of acetylcholine at postganglionic parasympathetic receptor sites

Pharmacodynamics/Kinetics

Onset of effect: Oral: Within 30-45 minutes

Duration: 4-6 hours

Metabolism: In the liver and GI tract

Elimination: In urine, bile, and other body fluids

Usual Dosage Oral:

Antisecretory:

Children: 1-2 mg/kg/day in 3-4 divided doses

Adults: 15 mg 3 times/day before meals or food and 30 mg at bedtime

Elderly: 7.5 mg 3 times/day before meals and at bedtime

Antispasmodic:

Children: 2-3 mg/kg/day in divided doses every 4-6 hours and at bedtime

Adults: 15 mg 3 times/day before meals or food and 30 mg at bedtime

Patient Information Take 30 minutes before meals and at bedtime. Maintain good oral hygiene habits, because lack of saliva may increase chance of cavities. Observe caution while driving or performing other tasks requiring alertness, as may cause drowsiness, dizziness, or blurred vision. Notify physician if skin rash, flushing, or eye pain occurs; or if difficulty in urinating, constipation, or sensitivity to light becomes severe or persists.

Nursing Implications Give before meals so that the drug's peak effect occurs at the proper time (peak inhibition of gastric acid secretion occurs at 1 and 3 hours after dosing in fasting subjects and approximately 2 hours in nonfasting subjects. This correlates well with the time food is no longer in the stomach offering a buffering effect).

Dosage Forms Tablet: 7.5 mg, 15 mg

Proparacaine and Fluorescein (proe par' a kane with flure' e seen)

Brand Names Fluoracaine®; I-Parescein®

Use Anesthesia for tonometry, gonioscopy; suture removal from cornea; removal of corneal foreign body; cataract extraction, glaucoma surgery

Pregnancy Risk Factor C

Contraindications Known hypersensitivity to proparacaine or fluorescein or any component or ester-type local anesthetics

Warnings/Precautions Use with caution in patients with cardiac disease, hyperthyroidism; for topical ophthalmic use only; prolonged use not recommended

Adverse Reactions

1% to 10%: Local: Burning, stinging of eye

<1%: Local: Allergic contact dermatitis, irritation, sensitization, keratitis, iritis, erosion of the corneal epithelium, conjunctival congestion and hemorrhage, corneal opacification

Stability Store in tight, light-resistant containers

Mechanism of Action Prevents initiation and transmission of impulse at the nerve cell membrane by decreasing ion permeability through stabilizing

Pharmacodynamics/Kinetics

Onset of action: Within 20 seconds of instillation

Duration: 15-20 minutes

Usual Dosage

Ophthalmic surgery: Children and Adults: Instill 1 drop in each eye every 5-10 minutes for 5-7 doses

Tonometry, gonioscopy, suture removal: Adults: Instill 1-2 drops in each eye just prior to procedure

Patient Information May slow wound healing; use sparingly, avoid touching or rubbing the eye until anesthesia has worn off

Nursing Implications Do not use if discolored; protect eye from irritating chemicals, foreign bodies, and blink reflex; use eye patch if necessary

Dosage Forms Solution: Proparacaine hydrochloride 0.5% and fluorescein sodium 0.25% (2 mL, 5 mL)

Proparacaine Hydrochloride (proe par' a kane)

Brand Names AK-Taine®; Alcaine®; I-Paracaine®; Ophthaine®; Ophthetic®

Synonyms Proxymetacaine

Use Anesthesia for tonometry, gonioscopy; suture removal from cornea; removal of corneal foreign body; cataract extraction, glaucoma surgery; short operative procedure involving the cornea and conjunctiva

Pregnancy Risk Factor C

Contraindications Known hypersensitivity to proparacaine

Warnings/Precautions Use with caution in patients with cardiac disease, hyperthyroidism; for typical ophthalmic use only; prolonged use not recommended

Adverse Reactions

1% to 10%: Local: Burning, stinging, redness

<1%:

Cardiovascular: Arrhythmias

Central nervous system: CNS depression

Dermatologic: Allergic contact dermatitis, irritation, sensitization

Ocular: Lacrimation, keratitis, iritis, erosion of the corneal epithelium, conjunctival congestion and hemorrhage, corneal opacification, blurred vision

Miscellaneous: Increased sweating

Drug Interactions Increased effect of phenylephrine, tropicamide

Stability Store in tight, light-resistant containers

Mechanism of Action Prevents initiation and transmission of impulse at the nerve cell membrane by decreasing ion permeability through stabilizing

Pharmacodynamics/Kinetics

Onset of action: Within 20 seconds of instillation

Duration: 15-20 minutes

Usual Dosage Children and Adults:

Ophthalmic surgery: Instill 1 drop of 0.5% solution in eye every 5-10 minutes for 5-7 doses

Tonometry, gonioscopy, suture removal: Instill 1-2 drops of 0.5% solution in eye just prior to procedure

Patient Information May slow wound healing; use sparingly, avoid touching or rubbing the eye until anesthesia has worn off

Nursing Implications Do not use if discolored; protect eye from irritating chemicals, foreign bodies, and blink reflex; use eye patch if necessary

Dosage Forms Ophthalmic, solution: 0.5% (2 mL, 15 mL)

Propine® *see* Dipivefrin *on page 356*

Proplex® SX-T *see* Factor IX Complex (Human) *on page 438*

Proplex® T *see* Factor IX Complex (Human) *on page 438*

Propofol (proe' po fole)

Brand Names Diprivan®

Use Induction or maintenance of anesthesia for inpatient or outpatient surgery; may be used (for patients >18 years of age who are intubated and mechanically ventilated) as an alternative to benzodiazepines for the treatment of agitation in the intensive care unit; pain should be treated with analgesic agents, propofol must be titrated separately from the analgesic agent; has demonstrated antiemetic properties in the postoperative setting

Pregnancy Risk Factor B

Contraindications

Absolute contraindications:

Patients with a hypersensitivity to propofol

Patients with a hypersensitivity to propofol's emulsion which contains soybean oil, egg phosphatide, and glycerol or any of the components

Patients who are not intubated or mechanically ventilated

Patients who are pregnant or nursing: Propofol is not recommended for obstetrics, including cesarian section deliveries. Propofol crosses the placenta and, therefore, may be associated with neonatal depression.

Relative contraindications:

Pediatric Intensive Care Unit patients: Safety and efficacy of propofol is not established

Patients with severe cardiac disease (ejection fraction <50%) or respiratory disease - propofol may have more profound adverse cardiovascular responses

Patients with a history of epilepsy or seizures

Patients with increased intracranial pressure or impaired cerebral circulation - substantial decreases in mean arterial pressure and subsequent decreases in cerebral perfusion pressure may occur

Patients with hyperlipidemia as evidenced by increased serum triglyceride levels or serum turbidity

Patients who are hypotensive, hypovolemic, or hemodynamically unstable

Warnings/Precautions Use slower rate of induction in the elderly; transient local pain may occur during I.V. injection; perioperative myoclonia has occurred; do not administer with blood or blood products through the same I.V. catheter; not for obstetrics, including cesarean section deliveries. Safety and effectiveness has not been established in children. Abrupt discontinuation prior to weaning or daily wake up assessments should be avoided. Abrupt discontinuation can result in rapid awakening, anxiety, agitation, and resistance to mechanical ventilation. Use slower rate of induction in the elderly; transient local pain may occur during I.V. injection; perioperative myoclonia has occurred; not for use in neurosurgical anesthesia.

Adverse Reactions

>10%:

Cardiovascular: Hypotension, intravenous propofol produces a dose-related degree of hypotension and decrease in systemic vascular resistance which is not associated with a significant increase in heart rate or decrease in cardiac output

Local: Pain at injection site occurs at an incidence of 28.5% when administered into smaller veins of hand versus 6% when administered into antecubital veins

Respiratory: Apnea (incidence occurs in 50% to 84% of patients and may be dependent on premedication, speed of administration, dose and presence of hyperventilation and hyperoxia)

1% to 10%:

Anaphylaxis: Several cases of anaphylactic reactions have been reported with propofol

Central nervous system: Dizziness, twitching, fever, headache; although propofol has demonstrated anticonvulsant activity, several cases of propofol-induced seizures with opisthotonos have occurred

Gastrointestinal: Nausea, vomiting, abdominal cramps

Respiratory: Cough, apnea

Miscellaneous: Hiccups

Overdosage/Toxicology Symptoms of overdose include hypotension, bradycardia, cardiovascular collapse; treatment is symptomatic and supportive; hypotension usually responds to I.V. fluids and/or Trendelenburg positioning; parenteral inotropes may be needed

Drug Interactions

Increased toxicity:

Neuromuscular blockers:

Atracurium: Anaphylactoid reactions (including bronchospasm) have been reported in patients who have received concomitant atracurium and propofol

Vecuronium: Propofol may potentiate the neuromuscular blockade of vecuronium

Central nervous system depressants: Additive CNS depression and respiratory depression may necessitate dosage reduction when used with: Anesthetics, benzodiazepines, opiates, ethanol, narcotics, phenothiazines

Decreased effect: Theophylline: May antagonize the effect of propofol, requiring dosage increases

Stability

Do not use if there is evidence of separation of phases of emulsion

Store at room temperature 4°C to 22°C (40°F to 72°F), refrigeration is not recommended; protect from light

Propofol may be further diluted in dextrose 5% in water to a concentration ≥2 mg/mL and is stable for 8 hours at room temperature

Y-site **compatible** with D_5LR, D_5NS, D_5W, LR, lidocaine

Soybean fat emulsion is used as a vehicle for propofol. This soybean fat emulsion contains no preservatives. **Strict aseptic technique must be maintained in handling because this vehicle is capable of supporting rapid bacterial growth.**

Mechanism of Action Propofol is a hindered phenolic compound with intravenous general anesthetic properties. The drug is unrelated to any of the currently used barbiturate, opioid, benzodiazepine, arylcyclohexylamine, or imidazole intravenous anesthetic agents.

Pharmacodynamics/Kinetics

Onset of anesthesia: Within 9-51 seconds (average 30 seconds) after bolus infusion (dose dependent)

Duration: 3-10 minutes depending on the dose and the rate of administration

Distribution: V_d: 2-6 mcg/mL during anesthesia; 1-2 mcg/mL upon awakening; large volume of distribution; highly lipophilic

Protein binding: 97% to 99%

Half-life, elimination (biphasic):
Initial: 40 minutes
Terminal: 1-3 days

Metabolism: In the liver to water-soluble sulfate and glucuronide conjugates; total body clearance exceeds liver blood flow

Elimination: ~88% of a propofol dose is recovered in the urine as metabolites (40% as glucuronide metabolite) and <2% of a propofol dose is excreted in the feces

Usual Dosage Dosage must be individualized based on total body weight and titrated to the desired clinical effect; however, as a general guideline:

No pediatric dose has been established; however, induction for children 1-12 years 2-2.8 mg/kg has been used

Induction: I.V.:
Adults ≤55 years, and/or ASA I or II patients: 2-2.5 mg/kg of body weight (approximately 40 mg every 10 seconds until onset of induction)
Elderly, debilitated, hypovolemic, and/or ASA III or IV patients: 1-1.5 mg/kg of body weight (approximately 20 mg every 10 seconds until onset of induction)

Maintenance: I.V. infusion:
Adults ≤55 years, and/or ASA I or II patients: 0.1-0.2 mg/kg of body weight/minute (6-12 mg/kg of body weight/hour)
Elderly, debilitated, hypovolemic, and/or ASA III or IV patients: 0.05-0.1 mg/kg of body weight/minute (3-6 mg/kg of body weight/hour)

I.V. intermittent: 25-50 mg increments, as needed

ICU sedation: Rapid bolus injection should be avoided. Bolus injection can result in hypotension, oxyhemoglobin desaturation, apnea, airway obstruction, and oxygen desaturation. The preferred route of administration is slow infusion. Doses are based on individual need and titrated to response.
Recommended starting dose: 1-3 mg/kg/hour
Adjustments in dose can occur at 3- to 5-minute intervals. An 80% reduction in dose should be considered in elderly, debilitated, and ASA II or IV patients. Once sedation is established, the dose should be decreased for the maintenance infusion period and adjusted to response. The dose required for maintenance is 1.5-4.5 mg/kg/hour or 25-75 mcg/kg/minute. An alternative, but less preferred method of administration is intermittent slow I.V. bolus injection of 10-20 mg, administered over 3-5 minutes.

Monitoring Parameters Cardiac monitor, blood pressure monitor, and ventilator required; serum triglyceride levels should be obtained prior to initiation of therapy (ICU setting) and every 3-7 days, thereafter

Vital signs: Blood pressure, heart rate, cardiac output, pulmonary capillary wedge pressure should be monitored

(Continued)

Propofol (Continued)

Test Interactions ↓ cholesterol (S); ↑ porphyrin (U); ↓ cortisol (S), but does not appear to inhibit adrenal responsiveness to ACTH

Nursing Implications Changes urine color to green; abrupt discontinuation of infusion may result in rapid awakening of the patient associated with anxiety, agitation, and resistance to mechanical ventilation, making weaning from mechanical ventilation difficult; use a light level of sedation throughout the weaning process until 10-15 minutes before extubation; titrate the infusion rate so the patient awakens slowly. Tubing and any unused portions of propofol vials should be discarded after 12 hours.

Dosage Forms Injection: 10 mg/mL (20 mL, 50 mL, 100 mL)

Propoxyphene (proe pox' i feen)

Related Information

Narcotic Agonist Comparison Charts *on page 1274-1275*

Brand Names Darvon®; Darvon-N®; Dolene®

Synonyms Dextropropoxyphene; Propoxyphene Hydrochloride; Propoxyphene Napsylate

Use Management of mild to moderate pain

Restrictions C-IV

Pregnancy Risk Factor C (D if used for prolonged periods)

Contraindications Hypersensitivity to propoxyphene or any component

Warnings/Precautions Give with caution in patients dependent on opiates, substitution may result in acute opiate withdrawal symptoms, use with caution in patients with severe renal or hepatic dysfunction; when given in excessive doses, either alone or in combination with other CNS depressants or propoxyphene products, propoxyphene is a major cause of drug-related deaths; **do not exceed recommended dosage**

Adverse Reactions

Hepatic: Increased liver enzymes

>10%:

Cardiovascular: Hypotension

Central nervous system: Dizziness, lightheadedness, weakness, sedation, paradoxical excitement and insomnia, tiredness, drowsiness

Gastrointestinal: GI upset, nausea, vomiting, constipation

Miscellaneous: Histamine release

1% to 10%:

Central nervous system: Nervousness, headache, restlessness, malaise, confusion

Gastrointestinal: Anorexia, stomach cramps, dry mouth, biliary spasm

Genitourinary: Decreased urination, ureteral spasms

Local: Pain at injection site

Respiratory: Troubled breathing, shortness of breath

<1%:

Central nervous system: Mental depression hallucinations, paradoxical CNS stimulation, increased intracranial pressure

Dermatologic: Rash, hives

Gastrointestinal: Paralytic ileus

Miscellaneous: Psychologic and physical dependence with prolonged use, histamine release

Overdosage/Toxicology Symptoms of overdose include CNS, respiratory depression, hypotension, pulmonary edema, seizures

Treatment of an overdose includes support of the patient's airway; establishment of an I.V. line and administration of naloxone 2 mg I.V. (0.01 mg/kg for children) with repeat administration as necessary up to a total of 10 mg; emesis is not indicated as overdose may cause seizures; charcoal is very effective (>95%) at binding propoxyphene

Drug Interactions

Decreased effect with charcoal, cigarette smoking

Increased toxicity: CNS depressants may potentiate pharmacologic effects; propoxyphene may inhibit the metabolism and increase the serum concentrations of carbamazepine, phenobarbital, MAO inhibitors, tricyclic antidepressants, and warfarin

Mechanism of Action Binds to opiate receptors in the CNS, causing inhibition of ascending pain pathways, altering the perception of and response to pain; produces generalized CNS depression

Pharmacodynamics/Kinetics

Onset of effect: Oral: Within 0.5-1 hour

Duration: 4-6 hours

Metabolism: First-pass effect; metabolized in the liver to an active metabolite (norpropoxyphene) and inactive metabolites

Bioavailability: Oral: 30% to 70%

Half-life: Adults:
  Parent drug: 8-24 hours (mean: ~15 hours)
  Norpropoxyphene: 34 hours

Elimination: 20% to 25% excreted in urine

Usual Dosage Oral:

Children: Doses for children are not well established; doses of the hydrochloride of 2-3 mg/kg/d divided every 6 hours have been used

Adults:
  Hydrochloride: 65 mg every 3-4 hours as needed for pain; maximum: 390 mg/day
  Napsylate: 100 mg every 4 hours as needed for pain; maximum: 600 mg/day

Dosing comments in renal impairment: Cl_{cr} <10 mL/minute: Avoid use

Not dialyzable (0% to 5%)

Dosing adjustment in hepatic impairment: Reduced doses should be used

Monitoring Parameters Pain relief, respiratory and mental status, blood pressure

Reference Range

Therapeutic: Ranges published vary between laboratories and may not correlate with clinical effect

Therapeutic concentration: 0.1-0.4 µg/mL (SI: 0.3-1.2 µmol/L)

Toxic: >0.5 µg/mL (SI: >1.5 µmol/L)

Test Interactions False-positive methadone test, ↓ glucose (S), ↑ LFTs, ↓ 17-OHCS (U)

Patient Information May cause drowsiness, dizziness, or blurring of vision; avoid alcohol and other sedatives; may take with food; can impair judgment and coordination

Additional Information 100 mg of napsylate = 65 mg of hydrochloride

Propoxyphene hydrochloride: Darvon®

Propoxyphene napsylate: Darvon-N®

Dosage Forms

Capsule, as hydrochloride: 32 mg, 65 mg

Suspension, oral, as napsylate: 50 mg/5 mL (480 mL)

Tablet, as napsylate: 100 mg

Propoxyphene Hydrochloride see Propoxyphene on previous page

Propoxyphene Napsylate see Propoxyphene on previous page

Propranolol Hydrochloride (proe pran' oh lole)

Related Information

Antiarrhythmic Drugs on page 1246-1248

Beta-Blockers Comparison on page 1257-1259

Brand Names Betachron E-R®; Inderal®; Inderal® LA

Use Management of hypertension, angina pectoris, pheochromocytoma, essential tremor, tetralogy of Fallot cyanotic spells, and arrhythmias (such as atrial fibrillation and flutter, A-V nodal re-entrant tachycardias, and catecholamine-induced arrhythmias); prevention of myocardial infarction, migraine headache; symptomatic treatment of hypertrophic subaortic stenosis

Unlabeled use: Tremor due to Parkinson's disease, alcohol withdrawal, aggressive behavior, antipsychotic-induced akathisia, esophageal varices bleeding, anxiety, schizophrenia, acute panic, and gastric bleeding in portal hypertension

Pregnancy Risk Factor C

Contraindications Uncompensated congestive heart failure, cardiogenic shock, bradycardia or heart block, pulmonary edema, severe hyperactive airway disease or chronic obstructive lung disease, Raynaud's disease, hypersensitivity to beta-blockers

Warnings/Precautions Safety and efficacy in children have not been established; administer very cautiously to patients with CHF, asthma, diabetes mellitus, hyperthyroidism. Abrupt withdrawal of the drug should be avoided, drug should be discontinued over 1-2 weeks; do not use in pregnant or nursing women; may potentiate hypoglycemia in a diabetic patient and mask signs and symptoms.

Adverse Reactions

>10%:
  Cardiovascular: Bradycardia
  Central nervous system: Mental depression
  Endocrine & metabolic: Decreased sexual ability

(Continued)

Propranolol Hydrochloride *(Continued)*

1% to 10%:
Cardiovascular: Congestive heart failure, reduced peripheral circulation
Central nervous system: Confusion, hallucinations, dizziness, insomnia, weakness, tiredness
Dermatologic: Skin rash
Gastrointestinal: Diarrhea, nausea, vomiting, stomach discomfort
Respiratory: Wheezing

<1%:
Cardiovascular: Chest pain, hypotension, impaired myocardial contractility, worsening of A-V conduction disturbances
Central nervous system: Nightmares, vivid dreams, lethargy
Dermatologic: Red, scaling, or crusted skin
Endocrine & metabolic: Hypoglycemia, hyperglycemia
Gastrointestinal: GI distress
Hematologic: Leukopenia, thrombocytopenia, agranulocytosis
Respiratory: Bronchospasm
Miscellaneous: Cold extremities

Overdosage/Toxicology Symptoms of intoxication include cardiac disturbances, CNS toxicity, bronchospasm, hypoglycemia and hyperkalemia. The most common cardiac symptoms include hypotension and bradycardia; atrioventricular block, intraventricular conduction disturbances, cardiogenic shock, and systole may occur with severe overdose, especially with membrane-depressant drugs (eg, propranolol); CNS effects include convulsions, coma, and respiratory arrest is commonly seen with propranolol and other membrane-depressant and lipid-soluble drugs.

Treatment includes symptomatic treatment of seizures, hypotension, hyperkalemia and hypoglycemia; bradycardia and hypotension resistant to atropine, isoproterenol or pacing may respond to glucagon; wide QRS defects caused by the membrane-depressant poisoning may respond to hypertonic sodium bicarbonate; repeat-dose charcoal, hemoperfusion, or hemodialysis may be helpful in removal of only those beta-blockers with a small V_d, long half-life or low intrinsic clearance (acebutolol, atenolol, nadolol, sotalol)

Drug Interactions
Decreased effect of beta-blockers with aluminum salts, barbiturates, calcium salts, cholestyramine, colestipol, NSAIDs, penicillins (ampicillin), rifampin, salicylates and sulfinpyrazone due to decreased bioavailability and plasma levels

Beta-blockers may decrease the effect of sulfonylureas

Increased effect/toxicity of beta-blockers with calcium blockers (diltiazem, felodipine, nicardipine), contraceptives, flecainide, haloperidol (propranolol, hypotensive effects), H_2 antagonists (metoprolol, propranolol only by cimetidine, possibly ranitidine), hydralazine (metoprolol, propranolol), loop diuretics (propranolol, not atenolol), MAO inhibitors (metoprolol, nadolol, bradycardia), phenothiazines (propranolol), propafenone (metoprolol, propranolol), quinidine (in extensive metabolizers), ciprofloxacin, thyroid hormones (metoprolol, propranolol, when hypothyroid patient is converted to euthyroid state)

Beta-blockers may increase the effect/toxicity of flecainide, haloperidol (hypotensive effects), hydralazine, phenothiazines, acetaminophen, anticoagulants (propranolol, warfarin), benzodiazepines (not atenolol), clonidine (hypertensive crisis after or during withdrawal of either agent), epinephrine (initial hypertensive episode followed by bradycardia), nifedipine and verapamil lidocaine, ergots (peripheral ischemia), prazosin (postural hypotension)

Beta-blockers may affect the action or levels of ethanol, disopyramide, nondepolarizing muscle relaxants and theophylline although the effects are difficult to predict

Stability Compatible in saline, **incompatible** with HCO_3^-; protect injection from light; solutions have maximum stability at pH of 3 and decompose rapidly in alkaline pH; propranolol is stable for 24 hours at room temperature in D_5W or NS

Mechanism of Action Nonselective beta-adrenergic blocker (class II antiarrhythmic); competitively blocks response to beta$_1$- and beta$_2$-adrenergic stimulation which results in decreases in heart rate, myocardial contractility, blood pressure, and myocardial oxygen demand

Pharmacodynamics/Kinetics
Onset of beta blockade: Oral: Within 1-2 hours
Duration: ~6 hours
Distribution: V_d: 3.9 L/kg in adults; crosses the placenta; small amounts appear in breast milk
Protein binding:
Newborns: 68%
Adults: 93%

Metabolism: Extensive first-pass effect; metabolized in the liver to active and inactive compounds

Bioavailability: 30% to 40%; oral bioavailability may be increased in Down syndrome children

Half-life:

Neonates and Infants: Possible increased half-life

Children: 3.9-6.4 hours

Adults: 4-6 hours

Elimination: Primarily in urine (96% to 99%)

Usual Dosage

Tachyarrhythmias:

Oral:

Children: Initial: 0.5-1 mg/kg/day in divided doses every 6-8 hours; titrate dosage upward every 3-7 days; usual dose: 2-4 mg/kg/day; higher doses may be needed; do not exceed 16 mg/kg/day or 60 mg/day

Adults: 10-30 mg/dose every 6-8 hours

Elderly: Initial: 10 mg twice daily; increase dosage every 3-7 days; usual dosage range: 10-320 mg given in 2 divided doses

I.V.:

Children: 0.01-0.1 mg/kg slow IVP over 10 minutes; maximum dose: 1 mg

Adults: 1 mg/dose slow IVP; repeat every 5 minutes up to a total of 5 mg

Hypertension: Oral:

Children: Initial: 0.5-1 mg/kg/day in divided doses every 6-12 hours; increase gradually every 3-7 days; maximum: 2 mg/kg/24 hours

Adults: Initial: 40 mg twice daily; increase dosage every 3-7 days; usual dose: ≤320 mg divided in 2-3 doses/day; maximum daily dose: 640 mg

Migraine headache prophylaxis: Oral:

Children: 0.6-1.5 mg/kg/day **or**

≤35 kg: 10-20 mg 3 times/day

>35 kg: 20-40 mg 3 times/day

Adults: Initial: 80 mg/day divided every 6-8 hours; increase by 20-40 mg/dose every 3-4 weeks to a maximum of 160-240 mg/day given in divided doses every 6-8 hours; if satisfactory response not achieved within 6 weeks of starting therapy, drug should be withdrawn gradually over several weeks

Tetralogy spells: Children:

Oral: 1-2 mg/kg/day every 6 hours as needed, may increase by 1 mg/kg/day to a maximum of 5 mg/kg/day, or if refractory may increase slowly to a maximum of 10-15 mg/kg/day

I.V.: 0.15-0.25 mg/kg/dose slow IVP; may repeat in 15 minutes

Thyrotoxicosis:

Neonates: Oral: 2 mg/kg/day in divided doses every 6-12 hours; occasionally higher doses may be required

Adolescents and Adults: Oral: 10-40 mg/dose every 6 hours

Adults: I.V.: 1-3 mg/dose slow IVP as a single dose

Adults: Oral:

Angina: 80-320 mg/day in doses divided 2-4 times/day

Pheochromocytoma: 30-60 mg/day in divided doses

Myocardial infarction prophylaxis: 180-240 mg/day in 3-4 divided doses

Hypertrophic subaortic stenosis: 20-40 mg 3-4 times/day

Essential tremor: 40 mg twice daily initially; maintenance doses: usually 120-320 mg/day

Dosing adjustment in renal impairment:

Cl_{cr} 31-40 mL/minute: Administer every 24-36 hours or administer 50% of normal dose

Cl_{cr} 10-30 mL/minute: Administer every 24-48 hours or administer 50% of normal dose

Cl_{cr} <10 mL/minute: Administer every 40-60 hours or administer 25% of normal dose

Not dialyzable (0% to 5%); supplemental dose is not necessary

Peritoneal dialysis effects: Supplemental dose is not necessary

Dosing adjustment/comments in hepatic disease: Marked slowing of heart rate may occur in cirrhosis with conventional doses; low initial dose and regular heart rate monitoring

Administration I.V. administration should not exceed 1 mg/minute; I.V. dose much smaller than oral dose

Monitoring Parameters Blood pressure, EKG, heart rate, CNS and cardiac effects

Reference Range Therapeutic: 50-100 ng/mL (SI: 190-390 nmol/L) at end of dose interval

Test Interactions ↑ thyroxine (S)

Patient Information Do not discontinue abruptly; notify physician if CHF symptoms become worse or side effects develop; take at the same time each day; (Continued)

Propranolol Hydrochloride *(Continued)*

may mask diabetes symptoms; consult pharmacist or physician before taking with other adrenergic drugs (eg, cold medications); use with caution while driving or performing tasks requiring alertness

Nursing Implications Patient's therapeutic response may be evaluated by looking at blood pressure, apical and radial pulses, fluid I & O, daily weight, respirations, and circulation in extremities before and during therapy

Dosage Forms

Capsule, sustained action: 60 mg, 80 mg, 120 mg, 160 mg

Injection: 1 mg/mL (1 mL)

Solution, oral (strawberry-mint flavor): 4 mg/mL (5 mL, 500 mL); 8 mg/mL (5 mL, 500 mL)

Solution, oral, concentrate: 80 mg/mL (30 mL)

Tablet: 10 mg, 20 mg, 40 mg, 60 mg, 80 mg, 90 mg

Propulsid® *see* Cisapride *on page 247*

2-Propylpentanoic Acid *see* Valproic Acid and Derivatives *on page 1143*

Propylthiouracil *(proe pill thye oh yoor' a sill)*

Synonyms PTU

Use Palliative treatment of hyperthyroidism as an adjunct to ameliorate hyperthyroidism in preparation for surgical treatment or radioactive iodine therapy and in the management of thyrotoxic crisis. The use of antithyroid thioamides is as effective in elderly as they are in younger adults; however, the expense, potential adverse effects, and inconvenience (compliance, monitoring) make them undesirable. The use of radioiodine, due to ease of administration and less concern for long-term side effects and reproduction problems, makes it a more appropriate therapy.

Pregnancy Risk Factor D

Contraindications Hypersensitivity to propylthiouracil or any component

Warnings/Precautions Use with caution in patients >40 years of age because PTU may cause hypoprothrombinemia and bleeding, use with extreme caution in patients receiving other drugs known to cause agranulocytosis; may cause agranulocytosis, thyroid hyperplasia, thyroid carcinoma (usage >1 year)

Adverse Reactions

>10%:

Central nervous system: Fever

Dermatologic: Skin rash

Hematologic: Leukopenia

1% to 10%:

Central nervous system: Dizziness

Gastrointestinal: Nausea, vomiting, loss of taste, stomach pain

Hematologic: Agranulocytosis

Miscellaneous: SLE-like syndrome

<1%:

Cardiovascular: Edema, cutaneous vasculitis

Central nervous system: Drowsiness, neuritis, vertigo, headache

Dermatologic: Rash, urticaria, pruritus, exfoliative dermatitis, hair loss

Gastrointestinal: Constipation, weight gain

Hematologic: Agranulocytosis, thrombocytopenia, bleeding, aplastic anemia

Hepatic: Cholestatic jaundice, hepatitis

Neuromuscular & skeletal: Arthralgia, paresthesia

Renal: Nephritis

Miscellaneous: Swollen salivary glands, goiter

Overdosage/Toxicology Symptoms of overdose include nausea, vomiting, arthralgia, pancytopenia, epigastric distress, headache, fever, CNS stimulation or depression; treatment is supportive in nature only; monitor bone marrow response, forced diuresis, peritoneal and hemodialysis, as well as charcoal hemoperfusion

Drug Interactions Increased effect: Increased anticoagulant activity

Mechanism of Action Inhibits the synthesis of thyroid hormones by blocking the oxidation of iodine in the thyroid gland; blocks synthesis of thyroxine and tri-iodothyronine

Pharmacodynamics/Kinetics

Onset of action: For significant therapeutic effects 24-36 hours are required

Peak effect: Remissions of hyperthyroidism do not usually occur before 4 months of continued therapy

Protein binding: 75% to 80%

Metabolism: Hepatic

Half-life: 1.5-5 hours

End stage renal disease: 8.5 hours
Time to peak serum concentration: Oral: Within 1 hour; persists for 2-3 hours
Elimination: 35% in urine
Usual Dosage Oral: Administer in 3 equally divided doses at approximately 8-hour intervals. Adjust dosage to maintain T_3, T_4, and TSH levels in normal range; elevated T_3 may be sole indicator of inadequate treatment. Elevated TSH indicates excessive antithyroid treatment.

Neonates: 5-10 mg/kg/day in divided doses every 8 hours
Children: Initial: 5-7 mg/kg/day in divided doses every 8 hours **or**
 6-10 years: 50-150 mg/day
 >10 years: 150-300 mg/day
 Maintenance: $1/3$ to $2/3$ of the initial dose in divided doses every 8-12 hours. This usually begins after 2 months on an effective initial dose.
Adults: Initial: 300-450 mg/day in divided doses every 8 hours (severe hyperthyroidism may require 600-1200 mg/day); maintenance: 100-150 mg/day in divided doses every 8-12 hours
Elderly: Use lower dose recommendations; initial dose: 150-300 mg/day

Dosing adjustment in renal impairment:
 Cl_{cr} 10-50 mL/minute: Administer at 75% of normal dose
 Cl_{cr} <10 mL/minute: Administer at 50% of normal dose
Monitoring Parameters CBC with differential, prothrombin time, liver function tests, thyroid function tests (T_4, T_3, TSH); periodic blood counts are recommended chronic therapy
Reference Range See table.

Laboratory Ranges

	Normal Values
Total T_4	5-12 µg/dL
Serum T_3	90-185 ng/dL
Free thyroxine index (FT_4 I)	6-10.5
TSH	0.5-4.0 µIU/mL

Patient Information Do not exceed prescribed dosage; take at regular intervals around-the-clock; notify physician or pharmacist if fever, sore throat, unusual bleeding or bruising, headache, or general malaise occurs
Additional Information The use of antithyroid thioamides is as effective in elderly as in younger adults; however, the expense, potential adverse effects, and inconvenience (compliance, monitoring) make them undesirable. The use of radioiodine, due to ease of administration and less concern for long-term side effects and reproduction problems, makes it a more appropriate therapy.
Dosage Forms Tablet: 50 mg

2-Propylvaleric Acid see Valproic Acid and Derivatives on page 1143

Prorex® see Promethazine Hydrochloride on page 939

Proscar® see Finasteride on page 456

Pro-Sof® [OTC] see Docusate on page 362

ProSom™ see Estazolam on page 406

Prostaglandin E₁ see Alprostadil on page 45

Prostaglandin E₂ see Dinoprostone on page 349

Prostaphlin® see Oxacillin Sodium on page 821

ProStep® see Nicotine on page 792

Prostigmin® see Neostigmine on page 784

Prostin/15M® see Carboprost Tromethamine on page 184

Prostin E₂® see Dinoprostone on page 349

Prostin VR Pediatric® see Alprostadil on page 45

Protamine Sulfate (proe′ ta meen)
Use Treatment of heparin overdosage; neutralize heparin during surgery or dialysis procedures
Pregnancy Risk Factor C
Contraindications Hypersensitivity to protamine or any component
Warnings/Precautions May not be totally effective in some patients following cardiac surgery despite adequate doses; may cause hypersensitivity reaction in
(Continued)

Protamine Sulfate *(Continued)*

patients with a history of allergy to fish (have epinephrine 1:1000 available) and in patients sensitized to protamine (via protamine zinc insulin); too rapid administration can cause severe hypotensive and anaphylactoid-like reactions. Heparin rebound associated with anticoagulation and bleeding has been reported to occur occasionally; symptoms typically occur 8-9 hours after protamine administration, but may occur as long as 18 hours later.

Adverse Reactions

>10%:

Cardiovascular: Sudden fall in blood pressure, bradycardia

Respiratory: Dyspnea

1% to 10%: Hemorrhage

<1%:

Cardiovascular: Hypotension, flushing

Central nervous system: Lassitude

Gastrointestinal: Nausea, vomiting

Respiratory: Pulmonary hypertension

Miscellaneous: Hypersensitivity reactions

Overdosage/Toxicology Symptoms of overdose include hypertension; may cause hemorrhage; doses exceeding 100 mg may cause paradox anticoagulation

Stability Refrigerate, avoid freezing; remains stable for at least 2 weeks at room temperature; **incompatible** with cephalosporins and penicillins

Mechanism of Action Combines with strongly acidic heparin to form a stable complex (salt) neutralizing the anticoagulant activity of both drugs

Pharmacodynamics/Kinetics Onset of effect: I.V. injection: Heparin neutralization occurs within 5 minutes

Usual Dosage Protamine dosage is determined by the dosage of heparin; 1 mg of protamine neutralizes 90 USP units of heparin (lung) and 115 USP units of heparin (intestinal); maximum dose: 50 mg

In the situation of heparin overdosage, since blood heparin concentrations decrease rapidly **after** administration, adjust the protamine dosage depending upon the duration of time since heparin administration as follows:

Time Elapsed	Dose of Protamine (mg) to Neutralize 100 units of Heparin
Immediate	1-1.5
30-60 min	0.5-0.75
>2 h	0.25-0.375

If heparin administered by deep S.C. injection, use 1-1.5 mg protamine per 100 units heparin; this may be done by a portion of the dose (eg, 25-50 mg) given slowly I.V. followed by the remaining portion as a continuous infusion over 8-16 hours (the expected absorption time of the S.C. heparin dose)

Administration For I.V. use only; incompatible with cephalosporins and penicillins; administer slow IVP (50 mg over 10 minutes); rapid I.V. infusion causes hypotension; reconstitute vial with 5 mL sterile water; if using protamine in neonates, reconstitute with preservative-free sterile water for injection; resulting solution equals 10 mg/mL; inject without further dilution over 1-3 minutes; maximum of 50 mg in any 10-minute period

Monitoring Parameters Coagulation test, APTT or ACT, cardiac monitor and blood pressure monitor required during administration

Dosage Forms Injection: 10 mg/mL (5 mL, 10 mL, 25 mL)

Protilase® *see* Pancrelipase *on page 837*

Protirelin *(proe tye' re lin)*

Brand Names Relefact® TRH; Thypinone®

Synonyms Lopremone; Thyrotropin Releasing Hormone; TRH

Use Adjunct in the diagnostic assessment of thyroid function and an adjunct to other diagnostic procedures in patients with pituitary or hypothalamic dysfunction; also causes release of prolactin from the pituitary and is used to detect defective control of prolactin secretion.

Pregnancy Risk Factor C

Contraindications Hypersensitivity to protirelin additives

Warnings/Precautions Monitor blood pressure frequently during and 15 minutes after administration; use with caution in patients predisposed to seizures

Adverse Reactions
>10%:
Central nervous system: Lightheadedness, headache
Endocrine & metabolic: Flushing of face
Gastrointestinal: Nausea, dry mouth
Genitourinary: Urge to urinate
1% to 10%:
Central nervous system: Anxiety, sweating, tingling
Endocrine & metabolic: Breast enlargement, leaking in lactating women
Gastrointestinal: Bad taste in mouth, abdominal discomfort
<1%:
Cardiovascular: Severe hypotension, hypertension
Ophthalmic: Temporary loss of vision

Drug Interactions Decreased effect: Aspirin, levodopa, thyroid hormones, adrenocorticoid drugs

Mechanism of Action Increase release of thyroid stimulating hormone from the anterior pituitary

Pharmacodynamics/Kinetics
Peak TSH levels: 20-30 minutes
Duration: TSH returns to baseline after ~3 hours
Half-life, mean plasma: 5 minutes

Usual Dosage I.V.:
Infants and Children <6 years: Experience limited, but doses of 7 mcg/kg have been administered
Children 6-16 years: 7 mcg/kg to a maximum dose of 500 mcg
Adults: 500 mcg (range 200-500 mcg)

Administration Administer I.V. bolus over 15-30 seconds with patient remaining in supine position; monitor blood pressure frequently during and 15 minutes after administration

Monitoring Parameters Blood pressure, prolactin, TSH, T_4 and T_3

Reference Range TSH test results vary with the laboratory; therefore, be familiar with the TSH assay method used and the normal range for the laboratory performing the assay. See table.

Characterization Based on Serum TSH Levels at Baseline and 30 Minutes After Protirelin

Thyroid Function	Baseline Serum TSH (µIU/mL)	Change of Serum TSH (µIU/mL) at 30 min
Euthyroidism (normal thyroid function)	10 or less (usually 6 or less; 20% have <1.5)	2 or more (usually 6-30)
Hyperthyroidism	10 or less (usually 4 or less)	<2
Primary hypothyroidism (thyroidal)	More than 10 (usually 15-200)	2 or more (usually 20 or more)
Secondary hypothyroidism (pituitary)	10 or less (usually 6 or less)	<2 (59%) 2-50 (41%)
Tertiary hypothyroidism (hypothalamic)	10 or less (often <2)	2 or more

Test Interactions Elevated serum lipids

Dosage Forms Injection: 500 mcg/mL (1 mL)

Protopam® see Pralidoxime Chloride *on page 914*

Protostat® see Metronidazole *on page 733*

Protriptyline Hydrochloride (proe trip' ti leen)
Related Information
Antidepressant Agents Comparison *on page 1250-1252*
Brand Names Vivactil®
Use Treatment of various forms of depression, often in conjunction with psychotherapy
Pregnancy Risk Factor C
Contraindications Narrow-angle glaucoma, hypersensitivity to protriptyline or any component
(Continued)

Protriptyline Hydrochloride (Continued)

Warnings/Precautions Use with caution in patients with cardiac conduction disturbances, history of hyperthyroid, seizure disorders, or decreased renal function; safe use of tricyclic antidepressants in children <12 years of age has not been established; protriptyline should not be abruptly discontinued in patients receiving high doses for prolonged periods

Adverse Reactions

>10%:

    Central nervous system: Dizziness, drowsiness, headache, weakness

    Gastrointestinal: Dry mouth, constipation, unpleasant taste, weight gain, increased appetite, nausea

1% to 10%:

    Cardiovascular: Arrhythmias, hypotension

    Central nervous system: Confusion, delirium, hallucinations, nervousness, restlessness, parkinsonian syndrome

    Gastrointestinal: Diarrhea, heartburn

    Genitourinary: Difficult urination, insomnia

    Neuromuscular & skeletal: Fine muscle tremors, sexual function impairment

    Ocular: Blurred vision, eye pain

    Miscellaneous: Excessive sweating

<1%:

    Central nervous system: Anxiety, seizures

    Dermatologic: Alopecia, photosensitivity

    Endocrine & metabolic: Breast enlargement, galactorrhea, SIADH

    Genitourinary: Testicular swelling

    Hematologic: Agranulocytosis, leukopenia, eosinophilia

    Hepatic: Cholestatic jaundice, increased liver enzymes

    Ocular: Increased intraocular pressure

    Otic: Tinnitus

    Miscellaneous: Trouble with gums, decreased lower esophageal sphincter tone may cause GE reflux, allergic reactions

Overdosage/Toxicology Symptoms of overdose include confusion, hallucinations, urinary retention, hypotension, tachycardia, seizures, hyperthermia

Following initiation of essential overdose management, toxic symptoms should be treated

Ventricular arrhythmias often respond to systemic alkalinization (sodium bicarbonate 0.5-2 mEq/kg I.V.). Arrhythmias unresponsive to this therapy may respond to lidocaine 1 mg/kg I.V. followed by a titrated infusion. Physostigmine (1-2 mg I.V. slowly for adults or 0.5 mg I.V. slowly for children) may be indicated in reversing cardiac arrhythmias that are life-threatening.

Seizures usually respond to diazepam I.V. boluses (5-10 mg for adults up to 30 mg or 0.25-0.4 mg/kg/dose for children up to 10 mg/dose). If seizures are unresponsive or recur, phenytoin or phenobarbital may be required.

Drug Interactions

Decreased effect of guanethidine; decreased effect with barbiturates, carbamazepine, phenytoin

Increased toxicity of alcohol, MAO inhibitors, sympathomimetics, CNS depressants, anticholinergics (paralytic ileus and hyperpyrexia); increased toxicity with MAO inhibitors (hyperpyretic crisis, convulsions, and death), cimetidine (↑ drug levels)

Mechanism of Action Increases the synaptic concentration of serotonin and/or norepinephrine in the central nervous system by inhibition of their reuptake by the presynaptic neuronal membrane

Pharmacodynamics/Kinetics

Maximum antidepressant effect: 2 weeks of continuous therapy is commonly required

Distribution: Crosses the placenta

Protein binding: 92%

Metabolism: Undergoes first-pass metabolism (10% to 25%); extensively metabolized in the liver by N-oxidation, hydroxylation and glucuronidation

Half-life: 54-92 hours, averaging 74 hours

Time to peak serum concentration: Oral: Within 24-30 hours

Elimination: In urine

Usual Dosage Oral:

Adolescents: 15-20 mg/day

Adults: 15-60 mg in 3-4 divided doses

Elderly: 15-20 mg/day

Reference Range Therapeutic: 70-250 ng/mL (SI: 266-950 nmol/L); Toxic: >500 ng/mL (SI: >1900 nmol/L)

Test Interactions ↑ glucose

Patient Information Avoid unnecessary exposure to sunlight; do not discontinue abruptly; take dose in morning to avoid insomnia

Nursing Implications Offer patient sugarless hard candy or gum for dry mouth
Dosage Forms Tablet: 5 mg, 10 mg

Protropin® see Human Growth Hormone on page 538

Provatene® [OTC] see Beta-Carotene on page 129

Proventil® see Albuterol on page 33

Provera® see Medroxyprogesterone Acetate on page 677

Provocholine® see Methacholine Chloride on page 702

Proxigel® [OTC] see Carbamide Peroxide on page 179

Proxymetacaine see Proparacaine Hydrochloride on page 943

Prozac® see Fluoxetine Hydrochloride on page 476

PRP-D see Haemophilus b Conjugate Vaccine on page 521

Prudent Vancomycin Use see page 1297

Prymaccone see Primaquine Phosphate on page 923

Pseudoephedrine (soo doe e fed' rin)
Brand Names Afrinol® [OTC]; Cenafed® [OTC]; Decofed® Syrup [OTC]; Drix-oral® Non-Drowsy [OTC]; Efidac/24® [OTC]; Neofed® [OTC]; Novafed®; Pedia-Care® Oral; Sudafed® [OTC]; Sudafed® 12 Hour [OTC]; Sufedrin® [OTC]
Synonyms d-Isoephedrine Hydrochloride; Pseudoephedrine Hydrochloride; Pseudoephedrine Sulfate
Use Temporary symptomatic relief of nasal congestion due to common cold, upper respiratory allergies, and sinusitis; also promotes nasal or sinus drainage
Pregnancy Risk Factor C
Contraindications Hypersensitivity to pseudoephedrine or any component; MAO inhibitor therapy
Warnings/Precautions Use with caution in patients >60 years of age; administer with caution to patients with hypertension, hyperthyroidism, diabetes mellitus, cardiovascular disease, ischemic heart disease, increased intraocular pressure, or prostatic hypertrophy. Elderly patients are more likely to experience adverse reactions to sympathomimetics. Overdosage may cause hallucinations, seizures, CNS depression, and death.
Adverse Reactions
>10%:
  Cardiovascular: Tachycardia, palpitations, arrhythmias
  Central nervous system: Nervousness, transient stimulation, insomnia, excita-bility, dizziness, drowsiness, headache
  Neuromuscular & skeletal: Tremor
1% to 10%: Central nervous system: Dizziness, headache, diaphoresis, weakness
<1%:
  Central nervous system: Convulsions, hallucinations
  Gastrointestinal: Nausea, vomiting
  Genitourinary: Difficult urination
  Respiratory: Shortness of breath, troubled breathing
Overdosage/Toxicology Symptoms of overdose include seizures, nausea, vomiting, cardiac arrhythmias, hypertension, agitation

There is no specific antidote for pseudoephedrine intoxication; the bulk treatment is supportive. Hyperactivity and agitation usually respond to reduced sensory input; however, with extreme agitation, haloperidol (2-5 mg I.M. for adults) may be required. Hyperthermia is best treated with external cooling measures; or when severe or unresponsive, muscle paralysis with pancuronium may be needed. Hypertension is usually transient and generally does not require treatment unless severe. For diastolic blood pressures >110 mm Hg, a nitroprusside infusion should be initiated. Seizures usually respond to diazepam I.V. and/or phenytoin maintenance regimens.
Drug Interactions
Decreased effect of methyldopa, reserpine
Increased toxicity: MAO inhibitors → ↑ blood pressure effects of pseudoephedrine; propranolol, sympathomimetic agents → ↑ toxicity
Mechanism of Action Directly stimulates alpha-adrenergic receptors of respiratory mucosa causing vasoconstriction; directly stimulates beta-adrenergic receptors causing bronchial dilation, increased heart rate and contractility
Pharmacodynamics/Kinetics
Onset of decongestant effect: Oral: 15-30 minutes
Duration: 4-6 hours (up to 12 hours with extended release formulation administration)
Metabolism: Partially in the liver
(Continued)
955

Pseudoephedrine *(Continued)*

Half-life: 9-16 hours
Elimination: 70% to 90% of dose excreted in urine as unchanged drug and 1% to
6% as norpseudoephedrine (active); renal elimination is dependent on urine
pH and flow rate; alkaline urine decreases renal elimination of pseudoephedrine

Usual Dosage Oral:

Children:
<2 years: 4 mg/kg/day in divided doses every 6 hours
2-5 years: 15 mg every 6 hours; maximum: 60 mg/24 hours
6-12 years: 30 mg every 6 hours; maximum: 120 mg/24 hours

Adults: 30-60 mg every 4-6 hours, sustained release: 120 mg every 12 hours;
maximum: 240 mg/24 hours

Dosing adjustment in renal impairment: Reduce dose

Test Interactions Interferes with urine detection of amphetamine (false-positive)

Patient Information Do not exceed recommended dosage and do not use for
more than 3-5 days; may cause wakefulness or nervousness; take last dose 4-6
hours before bedtime; do not crush sustained release product; consult pharmacist or physician before using

Nursing Implications Do not crush extended release drug product; elderly
patients should be counseled about the proper use of over-the-counter cough
and cold preparations

Additional Information
Pseudoephedrine hydrochloride: Cenafed® syrup [OTC], Decofed® syrup
[OTC], Neofed® [OTC], Novafed®, Sudafed® [OTC], Sudafed® 12 Hour
[OTC], Sudafed® tablet [OTC], Sufedrin® [OTC]
Pseudoephedrine sulfate: Afrinol® [OTC]

Dosage Forms
Capsule: 60 mg
Capsule, timed release, as hydrochloride: 120 mg
Drops, oral, as hydrochloride: 7.5 mg/0.8 mL (15 mL)
Liquid, as hydrochloride: 15 mg/5 mL (120 mL); 30 mg/5 mL (120 mL, 240 mL,
473 mL)
Tablet, as hydrochloride: 30 mg, 60 mg
Tablet:
Timed release, as hydrochloride: 120 mg
Extended release, as sulfate: 120 mg, 240 mg

Pseudoephedrine and Acrivastine *see* Acrivastine and Pseudoephedrine *on page 27*

Pseudoephedrine and Triprolidine *see* Triprolidine and Pseudoephedrine *on page 1131*

Pseudoephedrine Hydrochloride *see* Pseudoephedrine *on previous page*

Pseudoephedrine Sulfate *see* Pseudoephedrine *on previous page*

Pseudomonic Acid A *see* Mupirocin *on page 760*

Psorcon™ *see* Diflorasone Diacetate *on page 335*

P&S® [OTC] *see* Salicylic Acid *on page 991*

Psyllium *(sill′ i yum)*

Related Information
Laxatives, Classification and Properties *on page 1272*

Brand Names Effer-Syllium® [OTC]; Fiberall® Powder [OTC]; Fiberall® Wafer
[OTC]; Hydrocil® [OTC]; Konsyl-D® [OTC]; Konsyl® [OTC]; Metamucil® [OTC];
Metamucil® Instant Mix [OTC]; Modane® Bulk [OTC]; Perdiem® Plain [OTC];
Reguloid® [OTC]; Serutan® [OTC]; Siblin® [OTC]; Syllact® [OTC]; V-Lax®
[OTC]

Synonyms Plantago Seed; Plantain Seed; Psyllium Hydrophilic Mucilloid

Use Treatment of chronic atonic or spastic constipation and in constipation associated with rectal disorders; management of irritable bowel syndrome

Pregnancy Risk Factor C

Contraindications Fecal impaction, GI obstruction, hypersensitivity to psyllium
or any component

Warnings/Precautions May contain aspartame which is metabolized in the GI
tract to phenylalanine which is contraindicated in individuals with phenylketonuria; use with caution in patients with esophageal strictures, ulcers, stenosis, or
intestinal adhesions; elderly may have insufficient fluid intake which may predispose them to fecal impaction and bowel obstruction.

Adverse Reactions

1% to 10%:

Gastrointestinal: Esophageal or bowel obstruction, diarrhea, constipation, abdominal cramps

Respiratory: Bronchospasm, anaphylaxis upon inhalation in susceptible individuals, rhinoconjunctivitis

Overdosage/Toxicology Symptoms of overdose include abdominal pain, diarrhea, constipation

Drug Interactions Decreased effect of warfarin, digitalis, potassium-sparing diuretics, salicylates, tetracyclines, nitrofurantoin

Mechanism of Action Adsorbs water in the intestine to form a viscous liquid which promotes peristalsis and reduces transit time

Pharmacodynamics/Kinetics

Onset of action: 12-24 hour, but full effect may take 2-3 days

Peak effect: May take 2-3 days

Absorption: Oral: Generally not absorbed following administration, small amounts of grain extracts present in the preparation have been reportedly absorbed following colonic hydrolysis

Usual Dosage Oral (administer at least 3 hours before or after drugs):

Children 6-11 years: (Approximately ½ adult dosage) ½ to 1 rounded teaspoonful in 4 oz glass of liquid 1-3 times/day

Adults: 1-2 rounded teaspoonfuls or 1-2 packets or 1-2 wafers in 8 oz glass of liquid 1-3 times/day

Patient Information Must be mixed in a glass of water or juice; drink a full glass of liquid with each dose; do not use for longer than 1 week without the advice of a physician

Nursing Implications Inhalation of psyllium dust may cause sensitivity to psyllium (runny nose, watery eyes, wheezing)

Additional Information 3.4 g psyllium hydrophilic mucilloid per 7 g powder is equivalent to a rounded teaspoonful or one packet

Sodium content of Metamucil® Instant Mix (orange): 6 mg (0.27 mEq)

Dosage Forms

Granules: 4.03 g per rounded teaspoon (100 g, 250 g); 2.5 g per rounded teaspoon

Powder: Psyllium 50% and dextrose 50% (6.5 g, 325 g, 420 g, 480 g, 500 g)

Powder:

Effervescent: 3 g/dose (270 g, 480 g); 3.4 g/dose (single-dose packets)

Psyllium hydrophilic: 3.4 g per rounded teaspoon (210 g, 300 g, 420 g, 630 g)

Squares, chewable: 1.7 g, 3.4 g

Wafers: 3.4 g

Psyllium Hydrophilic Mucilloid see Psyllium on previous page

Pteroylglutamic Acid see Folic Acid on page 487

PTU see Propylthiouracil on page 950

Pulmozyme® see Dornase Alfa on page 365

Purge® [OTC] see Castor Oil on page 190

Purinethol® see Mercaptopurine on page 690

Pyonto® [OTC] see Pyrethrins on page 959

Pyrantel Pamoate (pi ran' tel pam' oh ate

Brand Names Antiminth® [OTC]; Pin-Rid® [OTC]; Pin-X® [OTC]; Reese's® Pinworm Medicine [OTC]

Use Treatment of roundworm, pinworm, and hookworm infestations, and trichostrongyliasis

Pregnancy Risk Factor C

Contraindications Known hypersensitivity to pyrantel pamoate

Warnings/Precautions Use with caution in patients with liver impairment, anemia, malnutrition, or pregnancy

Adverse Reactions

1% to 10%: Gastrointestinal: Anorexia, nausea, vomiting, abdominal cramps, diarrhea

<1%:

Central nervous system: Dizziness, weakness, drowsiness, insomnia, headache

Dermatologic: Rash

Hematologic: Elevated liver enzymes

Gastrointestinal: Tenesmus

Overdosage/Toxicology Symptoms of overdose include anorexia, nausea, vomiting, cramps, diarrhea, ataxia; treatment is supportive following GI decontamination

(Continued)

957

Pyrantel Pamoate *(Continued)*

Drug Interactions Decreased effect with piperazine

Stability Protect from light

Mechanism of Action Causes the release of acetylcholine and inhibits cholinesterase; acts as a depolarizing neuromuscular blocker, paralyzing the helminths

Pharmacodynamics/Kinetics

Absorption: Oral: Poor

Metabolism: Undergoes partial hepatic metabolism

Time to peak serum concentration: Within 1-3 hours

Elimination: In feces (50% as unchanged drug) and urine (7% as unchanged drug)

Usual Dosage Children and Adults (purgation is not required prior to use): Oral: Roundworm, pinworm, or trichostrongyliasis: 11 mg/kg administered as a single dose; maximum dose: 1 g. **(Note:** For pinworm infection, dosage should be repeated in 2 weeks and all family members should be treated).

Hookworm: 11 mg/kg administered once daily for 3 days

Monitoring Parameters Stool for presence of eggs, worms, and occult blood, serum AST and ALT

Patient Information May mix drug with milk or fruit juice; strict hygiene is essential to prevent reinfection

Nursing Implications Shake well before pouring to assure accurate dosage; protect from light

Dosage Forms

Capsule: 180 mg

Liquid: 50 mg/mL (30 mL); 144 mg/mL (30 mL)

Suspension, oral (caramel-currant flavor): 50 mg/mL (60 mL)

Pyrazinamide *(peer a zin' a mide)*

Related Information

Recommendations of the Advisory Council on the Elimination of Tuberculosis *on page 1303-1304*

Synonyms Pyrazinoic Acid Amide

Use Adjunctive treatment of tuberculosis in combination with other antituberculosis agents

Pregnancy Risk Factor C

Contraindications Severe hepatic damage; hypersensitivity to pyrazinamide or any component; acute gout

Warnings/Precautions Administer with at least one other effective agent for tuberculosis; use with caution in patients with renal failure, chronic gout, diabetes mellitus, or porphyria. Pyrazinamide is used in the 2-month intensive treatment phase of a 6-month treatment plan.

Adverse Reactions

1% to 10%:

Central nervous system: Malaise

Gastrointestinal: Nausea, vomiting, anorexia

Neuromuscular & skeletal: Arthralgia, myalgia

<1%:

Central nervous system: Fever

Dermatologic: Skin rash, itching, acne, photosensitivity

Hematologic: Porphyria, thrombocytopenia

Hepatic: Hepatotoxicity

Neuromuscular & skeletal: Gout

Renal: Dysuria, interstitial nephritis

Overdosage/Toxicology Symptoms of overdose include gout, gastric upset, hepatic damage (mild); treatment following GI decontamination is supportive

Mechanism of Action Converted to pyrazinoic acid in susceptible strains of *Mycobacterium* which lowers the pH of the environment

Pharmacodynamics/Kinetics Bacteriostatic or bactericidal depending on the drug's concentration at the site of infection

Absorption: Oral: Well absorbed

Distribution: Widely distributed into body tissues and fluids including the liver, lung, and CSF

Relative diffusion of antimicrobial agents from blood into cerebrospinal fluid (CSF): Adequate with or without inflammation (exceeds usual MICs)

Ratio of CSF to blood level (%):

Inflamed meninges: 100

Protein binding: 50%

Metabolism: In the liver

Half-life: 9-10 hours, increased with reduced renal or hepatic function

End stage renal disease: 9 hours

Time to peak serum concentration: Within 2 hours

Elimination: In urine (4% as unchanged drug)

Usual Dosage Oral (calculate dose on ideal body weight rather than total body weight): **Note:** A four-drug regimen (isoniazid, rifampin, pyrazinamide, and either streptomycin or ethambutol) is preferred for the initial, empiric treatment of TB. When the drug susceptibility results are available, the regimen should be altered as appropriate.

Patients with TB and without HIV infection:

OPTION 1:

Isoniazid resistance rate <4%: Administer daily isoniazid, rifampin, and pyrazinamide for 8 weeks followed by isoniazid and rifampin daily or directly observed therapy (DOT) 2-3 times/week for 16 weeks

If isoniazid resistance rate is not documented, ethambutol or streptomycin should also be administered until susceptibility to isoniazid or rifampin is demonstrated. Continue treatment for at least 6 months or 3 months beyond culture conversion.

OPTION 2: Administer daily isoniazid, rifampin, pyrazinamide, and either strep-tomycin or ethambutol for 2 weeks followed by DOT 2 times/week administration of the same drugs for 6 weeks, and subsequently, with isoniazid and rifampin DOT 2 times/week administration for 16 weeks

OPTION 3: Administer isoniazid, rifampin, pyrazinamide, and either etham-butol or streptomycin by DOT 3 times/week for 6 months

Patients with TB and with HIV infection:

Administer any of the above OPTIONS 1, 2 or 3, however, treatment should be continued for a total of 9 months and at least 6 months beyond culture conversion

Note: Some experts recommend that the duration of therapy should be extended to 9 months for patients with disseminated disease, miliary disease, disease involving the bones or joints, or tuberculosis lymphadenitis

Children and Adults:

Daily therapy: 15-30 mg/kg/day (maximum: 2 g/day)

Directly observed therapy (DOT): Twice weekly: 50-70 mg/kg (maximum: 4 g)

DOT: 3 times/week: 50-70 mg/kg (maximum: 3 g)

Elderly: Start with a lower daily dose (15 mg/kg) and increase as tolerated

Dosing adjustment in renal impairment: Cl_{cr} <50 mL/minute: Avoid use or reduce dose to 12-20 mg/kg/day

Avoid use in hemo- and peritoneal dialysis as well as continuous arterio-venous or veno-venous hemofiltration (CAVH/CAVHD)

Dosing adjustment in hepatic impairment: Reduce dose

Monitoring Parameters Periodic liver function tests, serum uric acid, sputum culture, chest x-ray 2-3 months into treatment and at completion

Test Interactions Reacts with Acetest® and Ketostix® to produce pinkish-brown color

Patient Information Notify physician if fever, loss of appetite, malaise, nausea, vomiting, darkened urine, pale stools occur; do not stop taking without consulting a physician

Dosage Forms Tablet: 500 mg

Pyrazinoic Acid Amide *see* Pyrazinamide *on previous page*

Pyrethrins (pye ree' thrins)

Brand Names A-200™ Pyrinate [OTC]; Barc™ [OTC]; Blue® [OTC]; Control-L™ [OTC]; End Lice® [OTC]; Pyonto® [OTC]; Pyrinyl II® [OTC]; RID® [OTC]; Tisit® [OTC]

Use Treatment of *Pediculus humanus* infestations (head lice, body lice, pubic lice and their eggs)

Pregnancy Risk Factor C

Contraindications Known hypersensitivity to pyrethrins, ragweed, or chrysanthe-mums

Warnings/Precautions For external use only; do not use in eyelashes or eyebrows

Adverse Reactions 1% to 10%: Local: Pruritus, burning, stinging, irritation with repeat use

Mechanism of Action Pyrethrins are derived from flowers that belong to the chrysanthemum family. The mechanism of action on the neuronal membranes of lice is similar to that of DDT. Piperonyl butoxide is usually added to pyrethrin to enhance the product's activity by decreasing the metabolism of pyrethrins in arthropods.

(Continued)

Pyrethrins *(Continued)*

Pharmacodynamics/Kinetics
Onset of action: ~30 minutes
Absorption: Topical into the system is minimal
Metabolism: By ester hydrolysis and hydroxylation

Usual Dosage Application of pyrethrins: Topical:
Apply enough solution to completely wet infested area, including hair
Allow to remain on area for 10 minutes
Wash and rinse with large amounts of warm water
Use fine-toothed comb to remove lice and eggs from hair
Shampoo hair to restore body and luster
Treatment may be repeated if necessary once in a 24-hour period
Repeat treatment in 7-10 days to kill newly hatched lice

Patient Information For external use only; avoid touching eyes, mouth, or other mucous membranes; contact physician if irritation occurs or if condition does not improve in 2-3 days

Dosage Forms
Gel, topical: 0.3% (30 g)
Liquid, topical: 0.18% (60 mL); 0.2% (60 mL, 120 mL); 0.3% (60 mL, 118 mL, 120 mL, 177 mL, 237 mL, 240 mL)
Shampoo: 0.3% (59 mL, 60 mL, 118 mL, 120 mL, 240 mL); 0.33% (60 mL, 120 mL)

Pyribenzamine® *see* Tripelennamine *on page 1130*

Pyridiate® *see* Phenazopyridine Hydrochloride *on page 866*

2-Pyridine Aldoxime Methochloride *see* Pralidoxime Chloride *on page 914*

Pyridium® *see* Phenazopyridine Hydrochloride *on page 866*

Pyridostigmine Bromide *(peer id oh stig' meen)*

Brand Names Mestinon®; Regonol®

Use Symptomatic treatment of myasthenia gravis; also used as an antidote for nondepolarizing neuromuscular blockers; not a cure; patient may develop resistance to the drug

Pregnancy Risk Factor C

Contraindications Hypersensitivity to pyridostigmine, bromides, or any component; GI or GU obstruction

Warnings/Precautions Use with caution in patients with epilepsy, asthma, bradycardia, hyperthyroidism, cardiac arrhythmias, or peptic ulcer; adequate facilities should be available for cardiopulmonary resuscitation when testing and adjusting dose for myasthenia gravis; have atropine and epinephrine ready to treat hypersensitivity reactions; overdosage may result in cholinergic crisis, this must be distinguished from myasthenic crisis; anticholinesterase insensitivity can develop for brief or prolonged periods

Adverse Reactions
>10%:
Gastrointestinal: Diarrhea, nausea, stomach cramps
Miscellaneous: Increased sweating and mouth watering
1% to 10%:
Genitourinary: Urge to urinate
Ocular: Small pupils, lacrimation
Respiratory: Increased bronchial secretions
<1%:
Cardiovascular: Bradycardia, A-V block
Central nervous system: Seizures, headache, dysphoria, drowsiness, weakness
Local: Thrombophlebitis
Neuromuscular & skeletal: Muscle spasms
Ocular: Miosis, diplopia
Respiratory: Laryngospasm, respiratory paralysis
Miscellaneous: Hypersensitivity, hyper-reactive cholinergic responses

Overdosage/Toxicology Symptoms of overdose include muscle weakness, blurred vision, excessive sweating, tearing and salivation, nausea, vomiting, diarrhea, hypertension, bradycardia, paralysis. Atropine is the treatment of choice for intoxications manifesting with significant muscarinic symptoms. Atropine I.V. 2-4 mg every 3-60 minutes (or 0.04-0.08 mg I.V. every 5-60 minutes if needed for children) should be repeated to control symptoms and then continued as needed for 1-2 days following the acute ingestion.

Drug Interactions
Increased effect of depolarizing neuromuscular blockers (succinylcholine)

Increased toxicity with edrophonium

Stability Protect from light

Mechanism of Action Inhibits destruction of acetylcholine by acetylcholinesterase which facilitates transmission of impulses across myoneural junction

Pharmacodynamics/Kinetics

Onset of action:

Oral, I.M.: Within 15-30 minutes

I.V. injection: Within 2-5 minutes

Absorption: Oral: Very poor (10% to 20%) from GI tract

Metabolism: In the liver

Usual Dosage Normally, sustained release dosage form is used at bedtime for patients who complain of morning weakness

Myasthenia gravis:

Oral:

Children: 7 mg/kg/day in 5-6 divided doses

Adults: Initial: 60 mg 3 times/day with maintenance dose ranging from 60 mg to 1.5 g/day; sustained release formulation should be dosed at least every 6 hours (usually 12-24 hours)

I.M., I.V.:

Children: 0.05-0.15 mg/kg/dose (maximum single dose: 10 mg)

Adults: 2 mg every 2-3 hours or 1/30th of oral dose

Reversal of nondepolarizing neuromuscular blocker: I.M., I.V.:

Children: 0.1-0.25 mg/kg/dose preceded by atropine

Adults: 10-20 mg preceded by atropine

Test Interactions ↑ aminotransferase [ALT (SGPT)/AST (SGOT)] (S), ↑ amylase (S)

Patient Information Side effects are generally due to exaggerated pharmacologic effects; most common side effects are salivation and muscle fasciculations; notify physician if nausea, vomiting, muscle weakness, severe abdominal pain, or difficulty breathing occurs

Nursing Implications Do not crush sustained release drug product; observe for cholinergic reactions, particularly when administered I.V.

Dosage Forms

Injection: 5 mg/mL (2 mL, 5 mL)

Syrup (raspberry flavor): 60 mg/5 mL (480 mL)

Tablet: 60 mg

Tablet, sustained release: 180 mg

Pyridoxine Hydrochloride (peer i dox' een)

Brand Names Beesix®; Nestrex®

Synonyms Vitamin B₆

Use Prevents and treats vitamin B₆ deficiency, pyridoxine-dependent seizures in infants, adjunct to treatment of acute toxicity from isoniazid, cycloserine, or hydralazine overdose

Pregnancy Risk Factor A (C if dose exceeds RDA recommendation)

Contraindications Hypersensitivity to pyridoxine or any component

Warnings/Precautions Dependence and withdrawal may occur with doses >200 mg/day

Adverse Reactions

<1%:

Central nervous system: Sensory neuropathy, seizures have occurred following I.V. administration of very large doses, headache

Gastrointestinal: Nausea

Endocrine & metabolic: Decreased serum folic acid secretions

Neuromuscular & skeletal: Paresthesia

Miscellaneous: Allergic reactions have been reported, increased AST

Overdosage/Toxicology Ataxia, sensory neuropathy with doses of 50 mg to 2 g daily over prolonged periods

Drug Interactions Decreased serum levels of levodopa, phenobarbital, and phenytoin

Stability Protect from light

Mechanism of Action Precursor to pyridoxal, which functions in the metabolism of proteins, carbohydrates, and fats; pyridoxal also aids in the release of liver and muscle-stored glycogen and in the synthesis of GABA (within the central nervous system) and heme

Pharmacodynamics/Kinetics

Absorption: Enteral, parenteral: Well absorbed from GI tract

Metabolism: Metabolized in 4-pyridoxic acid (active form), and other metabolites

Half-life: 15-20 days

(Continued)

961

Pyridoxine Hydrochloride *(Continued)*

Usual Dosage
Recommended daily allowance (RDA):
Children:
1-3 years: 0.9 mg
4-6 years: 1.3 mg
7-10 years: 1.6 mg
Adults:
Male: 1.7-2.0 mg
Female: 1.4-1.6 mg
Pyridoxine-dependent Infants:
Oral: 2-100 mg/day
I.M., I.V., S.C.: 10-100 mg
Dietary deficiency: Oral:
Children: 5-25 mg/24 hours for 3 weeks, then 1.5-2.5 mg/day in multiple vitamin product
Adults: 10-20 mg/day for 3 weeks
Drug-induced neuritis (eg, isoniazid, hydralazine, penicillamine, cycloserine): Oral:
Children:
Treatment: 10-50 mg/24 hours
Prophylaxis: 1-2 mg/kg/24 hours
Adults:
Treatment: 100-200 mg/24 hours
Prophylaxis: 25-100 mg/24 hours
Treatment of seizures and/or coma from acute isoniazid toxicity, a dose of pyridoxine hydrochloride equal to the amount of INH ingested can be given I.M./I.V. in divided doses together with other anticonvulsants; if the amount INH ingested is not known, administer 5 g I.V. pyridoxine
Treatment of acute hydralazine toxicity, a pyridoxine dose of 25 mg/kg in divided doses I.M./I.V. has been used

Reference Range Over 50 ng/mL (SI: 243 nmol/L) (varies considerably with method). A broad range is ~25-80 ng/mL (SI: 122-389 nmol/L). HPLC method for pyridoxal phosphate has normal range of 3.5-18 ng/mL (SI: 17-88 nmol/L).

Test Interactions Urobilinogen

Patient Information Dietary sources of pyridoxine include red meats, bananas, potatoes, yeast, lima beans, whole grain cereals; do not exceed recommended doses

Nursing Implications Burning may occur at the injection site after I.M. or S.C. administration; seizures have occurred following I.V. administration of very large doses

Dosage Forms
Injection: 100 mg/mL (10 mL, 30 mL)
Tablet: 25 mg, 50 mg, 100 mg
Tablet, extended release: 100 mg

Pyrimethamine *(peer i meth' a meen)*

Related Information
Prevention of Malaria *on page 1405*

Brand Names Daraprim®

Use Prophylaxis of malaria due to susceptible strains of plasmodia; used in conjunction with quinine and sulfadiazine for the treatment of uncomplicated attacks of chloroquine-resistant *P. falciparum* malaria; used in conjunction with fast-acting schizonticide to initiate transmission control and suppression cure; synergistic combination with sulfonamide in treatment of toxoplasmosis

Pregnancy Risk Factor C

Contraindications Megaloblastic anemia secondary to folate deficiency; known hypersensitivity to pyrimethamine, chloroguanide; resistant malaria; patients with seizure disorders

Warnings/Precautions When used for more than 3-4 days, it may be advisable to give leucovorin to prevent hematologic complications; monitor CBC and platelet counts every 2 weeks; use with caution in patients with impaired renal or hepatic function or with possible G-6-PD

Adverse Reactions
1% to 10%:
Gastrointestinal: Anorexia, abdominal cramps, vomiting
Hematologic: Megaloblastic anemia, leukopenia, thrombocytopenia, agranulocytosis
<1%:
Central nervous system: Insomnia, lightheadedness, fever, malaise, seizures, depression

Dermatologic: Skin rash, dermatitis, abnormal skin pigmentation
Gastrointestinal: Diarrhea dry mouth, atrophic glossitis
Hematologic: Pulmonary eosinophilia

Overdosage/Toxicology Symptoms of overdose include megaloblastic anemia, leukopenia, thrombocytopenia, anorexia, CNS stimulation, seizures, nausea, vomiting, hematemesis; following GI decontamination, leucovorin should be administered in a dosage of 5-15 mg/day I.M., I.V., or oral for 5-7 days or as required to reverse symptoms of folic acid deficiency; diazepam 0.1-0.25 mg/kg can be used to treat seizures

Drug Interactions
Decreased effect: Pyrimethamine effectiveness decreased by acid
Increased effect: Sulfonamides (synergy), methotrexate, TMP/SMX

Stability Pyrimethamine tablets may be crushed to prepare oral suspensions of the drug in water, cherry syrup, or sucrose-containing solutions at a concentration of 1 mg/mL; stable at room temperature for 5-7 days

Mechanism of Action Inhibits parasitic dihydrofolate reductase, resulting in inhibition of vital tetrahydrofolic acid synthesis

Pharmacodynamics/Kinetics
Absorption: Oral: Well absorbed
Distribution: V_d: 2.9 L/kg in adults; appears in breast milk
Protein binding: 80%
Half-life: 80-95 hours
Time to peak serum concentration: Within 1.5-8 hours

Usual Dosage
Malaria chemoprophylaxis (for areas where chloroquine-resistant *P. falciparum* exists): Begin prophylaxis 2 weeks before entering endemic area:
Children: 0.5 mg/kg once weekly; not to exceed 25 mg/dose
or
Children:
<4 years: 6.25 mg once weekly
4-10 years: 12.5 mg once weekly
Children >10 years and Adults: 25 mg once weekly
Dosage should be continued for all age groups for at least 6-10 weeks after leaving endemic areas
Chloroquine-resistant *P. falciparum* malaria (when used in conjunction with quinine and sulfadiazine):
Children:
<10 kg: 6.25 mg/day once daily for 3 days
10-20 kg: 12.5 mg/day once daily for 3 days
20-40 kg: 25 mg/day once daily for 3 days
Adults: 25 mg twice daily for 3 days
Toxoplasmosis:
Infants for congenital toxoplasmosis: Oral: 1 mg/kg once daily for 6 months with sulfadiazine then every other month with sulfa, alternating with spiramycin.
Children: Loading dose: 2 mg/kg/day divided into 2 equal daily doses for 1-3 days (maximum: 100 mg/day) followed by 1 mg/kg/day divided into 2 doses for 4 weeks; maximum: 25 mg/day
With sulfadiazine or trisulfapyrimidines: 2 mg/kg/day divided every 12 hours for 3 days followed by 1 mg/kg/day once daily or divided twice daily for 4 weeks given with trisulfapyrimidines or sulfadiazine
Adults: 50-75 mg/day together with 1-4 g of a sulfonamide for 1-3 weeks depending on patient's tolerance and response, then reduce dose by 50% and continue for 4-5 weeks **or** 25-50 mg/day for 3-4 weeks

Monitoring Parameters CBC, including platelet counts twice weekly

Patient Information Take with meals to minimize vomiting; begin malaria prophylaxis at least 1-2 weeks prior to departure; discontinue at first sign of skin rash; notify physician if persistent fever, sore throat, bleeding or bruising occurs; regular blood work may be necessary in patients taking high doses

Dosage Forms Tablet: 25 mg

Pyrinyl II® [OTC] *see Pyrethrins* *on page 959*

Quazepam (kway' ze pam)
Related Information
Benzodiazepines Comparison *on page 1256*
Brand Names Doral®
Use Treatment of insomnia; more likely than triazolam to cause daytime sedation and fatigue; is classified as a long-acting benzodiazepine hypnotic (like flurazepam - Dalmane®), this long duration of action may prevent withdrawal symptoms when therapy is discontinued
Restrictions C-IV
(Continued)

Quazepam *(Continued)*

Pregnancy Risk Factor X

Contraindications Narrow-angle glaucoma, pregnancy, known hypersensitivity to quazepam

Warnings/Precautions Safety and efficacy in children <18 years of age have not been established; do not use in pregnant women; may cause drug dependency; avoid abrupt discontinuance in patients with prolonged therapy or seizure disorders; avoid using in patients with pre-existing CNS depression, severe uncontrolled pain, or narrow-angle glaucoma; use with caution in patients receiving other CNS depressants, in patients with hepatic dysfunction, and the elderly

Adverse Reactions

>10%:
  Cardiovascular: Tachycardia, chest pain
  Central nervous system: Drowsiness, fatigue, impaired coordination, lightheadedness, memory impairment, insomnia, anxiety, depression, headache
  Dermatologic: Rash
  Endocrine & metabolic: Decreased libido
  Gastrointestinal: Dry mouth, constipation, diarrhea, decreased salivation, nausea, vomiting, increased or decreased appetite
  Neuromuscular & skeletal: Dysarthria
  Ocular: Blurred vision
  Miscellaneous: Sweating

1% to 10%:
  Cardiovascular: Syncope, hypotension
  Central nervous system: Confusion, nervousness, dizziness, akathisia
  Dermatologic: Dermatitis
  Gastrointestinal: Increased salivation, weight gain or loss
  Neuromuscular & skeletal: Rigidity, tremor, muscle cramps
  Otic: Tinnitus
  Respiratory: Nasal congestion, hyperventilation

<1%:
  Endocrine & metabolic: Menstrual irregularities
  Hematologic: Blood dyscrasias
  Miscellaneous: Drug dependence, reflex slowing

Overdosage/Toxicology Symptoms of overdose include somnolence, confusion, coma, hypoactive reflexes, dyspnea, hypotension, slurred speech, impaired coordination

Treatment for benzodiazepine overdose is supportive; rarely is mechanical ventilation required; has been shown to selectively block the binding of benzodiazepines to CNS receptors, resulting in a reversal of benzodiazepine-induced CNS depression, but not respiratory depression

Drug Interactions Increased effect/toxicity with CNS depressants (narcotics, alcohol, MAO inhibitors, TCAs, anesthetics, barbiturates, phenothiazines)

Mechanism of Action Depresses all levels of the CNS, including the limbic and reticular formation, probably through the increased action of gamma-aminobutyric acid (GABA), which is a major inhibitory neurotransmitter in the brain

Pharmacodynamics/Kinetics
  Absorption: Oral: Rapid
  Protein binding: 95%
  Metabolism: In the liver to at least one active compound
  Half-life:
    Parent drug: 25-41 hours
    Active metabolite: 40-114 hours

Usual Dosage Adults: Oral: Initial: 15 mg at bedtime, in some patients the dose may be reduced to 7.5 mg after a few nights

Dosing adjustment in hepatic impairment: Dose reduction may be necessary

Monitoring Parameters Respiratory and cardiovascular status

Patient Information Avoid alcohol and other CNS depressants; avoid activities needing good psychomotor coordination until CNS effects are known; drug may cause physical or psychological dependence; avoid abrupt discontinuation after prolonged use

Nursing Implications Institute safety measures, remove smoking materials from area, supervise ambulation

Dosage Forms Tablet: 7.5 mg, 15 mg

Quelicin® *see* Succinylcholine Chloride *on page 1035*

Questran® *see* Cholestyramine Resin *on page 237*

Questran® **Light** *see* Cholestyramine Resin *on page 237*

Quibron®-T *see* Theophylline/Aminophylline *on page 1072*

Quibron®-T/SR *see* Theophylline/Aminophylline *on page 1072*

Quiess® *see* Hydroxyzine *on page 556*

Quinaglute® Dura-Tabs® *see* Quinidine *on page 968*

Quinalan® *see* Quinidine *on page 968*

Quinalbarbitone Sodium *see* Secobarbital Sodium *on page 999*

Quinamm® *see* Quinine Sulfate *on page 970*

Quinapril Hydrochloride (kwin' a pril)

Related Information

Angiotensin-Converting Enzyme Inhibitors, Comparative Pharmacokinetics *on page 1244*

Angiotensin-Converting Enzyme Inhibitors, Comparisons of Indications and Adult Dosages *on page 1243*

Brand Names Accupril®

Use Management of hypertension and treatment of congestive heart failure; increase circulation in Raynaud's phenomenon; idiopathic edema

Unlabeled use: Hypertensive crisis, diabetic nephropathy, rheumatoid arthritis, diagnosis of anatomic renal artery stenosis, hypertension secondary to scleroderma renal crisis, diagnosis of aldosteronism, idiopathic edema, Bartter's syndrome, postmyocardial infarction for prevention of ventricular failure

Pregnancy Risk Factor D

Contraindications Hypersensitivity to quinapril or history of angioedema induced by other ACE inhibitors

Warnings/Precautions Use with caution in patients with renal insufficiency, autoimmune disease, renal artery stenosis; excessive hypotension may be more likely in volume-depleted patients, the elderly, and following the first dose (first dose phenomenon); quinapril should be discontinued if laryngeal stridor or angioedema of the face, tongue, or glottis is observed

Adverse Reactions

1% to 10%:

Cardiovascular: Hypotension

Central nervous system: Dizziness, headache, fatigue

Gastrointestinal: Diarrhea

Renal: Increased BUN and serum creatinine

Respiratory: Upper respiratory symptoms, cough

<1%:

Cardiovascular: Chest discomfort, flushing, myocardial infarction, angina pectoris, orthostatic hypotension, rhythm disturbances, tachycardia, peripheral edema, vasculitis, palpitations, syncope

Central nervous system: Fever, malaise, depression, somnolence, insomnia

Dermatologic: Urticaria, pruritus, angioedema

Endocrine & metabolic: Gout

Gastrointestinal: Pancreatitis, abdominal pain, anorexia, constipation, flatulence, dry mouth

Drug-Drug Interactions With ACEIs

Precipitant Drug	Drug (Category) and Effect	Description
Antacids	ACEIs: decreased	Decreased bioavailability of ACEIs. May be more likely with captopril. Separate administration times by 1-2 hours.
NSAIDs (indomethacin)	ACEIs: decreased	Reduced hypotensive effects of ACEIs. More prominent in low renin or volume dependent hypertensive patients.
Phenothiazines	ACEIs: increased	Pharmacologic effects of ACEIs may be increased.
ACEIs	Allopurinol: increased	Higher risk of hypersensitivity reaction possible when given concurrently. Three case reports of Stevens-Johnson syndrome with captopril.
ACEIs	Digoxin: increased	Increased plasma digoxin levels.
ACEIs	Lithium: increased	Increased serum lithium levels and symptoms of toxicity may occur.
ACEIs	Potassium preps/potassium-sparing diuretics increased	Coadministration may result in elevated potassium levels.

(Continued)

Quinapril Hydrochloride *(Continued)*

Hematologic: Neutropenia, bone marrow depression
Hepatic: Hepatitis
Neuromuscular & skeletal: Joint pain, shoulder pain
Ocular: Blurred vision
Respiratory: Bronchitis, sinusitis, pharyngeal pain
Miscellaneous: Diaphoresis

Overdosage/Toxicology Mild hypotension has been the only toxic effect seen with acute overdose. Bradycardia may also occur; hyperkalemia occurs even with therapeutic doses, especially in patients with renal insufficiency and those taking NSAIDs. Following initiation of essential overdose management, toxic symptom treatment and supportive treatment should be initiated. Hypotension usually responds to I.V. fluids or Trendelenburg positioning.

Drug Interactions See table.

Stability Store at room temperature; unstable in aqueous solutions; to prepare solution for oral administration, mix prior to administration and use within 10 minutes

Mechanism of Action Competitive inhibitor of angiotensin-converting enzyme (ACE); prevents conversion of angiotensin I to angiotensin II, a potent vasoconstrictor; results in lower levels of angiotensin II which causes an increase in plasma renin activity and a reduction in aldosterone secretion; a CNS mechanism may also be involved in hypotensive effect as angiotensin II increases adrenergic outflow from CNS; vasoactive kallikreins may be decreased in conversion to active hormones by ACE inhibitors, thus reducing blood pressure

Pharmacodynamics/Kinetics

Metabolism: Rapidly hydrolyzed to quinaprilat, the active metabolite
Half-life, elimination:
  Quinapril: 0.8 hours
  Quinaprilat: 2 hours
Time to peak serum concentration:
  Quinapril: 1 hour
  Quinaprilat: ~2 hours
Elimination: 50% to 60% of quinapril excreted in urine primarily as quinaprilat

Usual Dosage

Adults: Oral: Initial: 10 mg once daily, adjust according to blood pressure response at peak and trough blood levels; in general, the normal dosage range is 20-80 mg/day
Elderly: Initial: 2.5-5 mg/day; increase dosage at increments of 2.5-5 mg at 1- to 2-week intervals

Dosing adjustment in renal impairment:
Cl_{cr} >60 mL/minute: Administer 10 mg/day
Cl_{cr} 30-60 mL/minute: 5 mg/day
Cl_{cr} 10-30 mL/minute: 2.5 mg/day

Dosing comments in hepatic impairment: In patients with alcoholic cirrhosis, hydrolysis of quinapril to quinaprilat is impaired; however, the subsequent elimination of quinaprilat is unaltered

Patient Information Do not discontinue medication without advice of physician; notify physician if sore throat, swelling, palpitations, cough, chest pains, difficulty swallowing, swelling of face, eyes, tongue, lips; hoarseness, sweating, vomiting, or diarrhea occurs; may cause dizziness, lightheadedness during first few days; may also cause changes in taste perception

Nursing Implications May cause depression in some patients; discontinue if angioedema of the face, extremities, lips, tongue, or glottis occurs; watch for hypotensive effects within 1-3 hours of first dose or new higher dose

Dosage Forms Tablet: 5 mg, 10 mg, 20 mg, 40 mg

Quinestrol *(kwin ess′ trole)*

Brand Names Estrovis®

Use Atrophic vaginitis; hypogonadism; primary ovarian failure; vasomotor symptoms of menopause; prostatic carcinoma; osteoporosis prophylactic

Pregnancy Risk Factor X

Contraindications Thrombophlebitis, undiagnosed vaginal bleeding, hypersensitivity to quinestrol or any component, known or suspected pregnancy, carcinoma of the breast, estrogen-dependent tumor

Warnings/Precautions Use with caution in patients with asthma, seizure disorders, migraine, cardiac, renal or hepatic impairment, cerebrovascular disorders or history of breast cancer, past or present thromboembolic disease, smokers >35 years of age; may cause serious bleeding in women sterilized by endometriosis

Adverse Reactions
>10%:
Cardiovascular: Peripheral edema
Endocrine & metabolic: Enlargement of breasts (female and male), breast tenderness
Gastrointestinal: Nausea, anorexia, bloating
1% to 10%:
Central nervous system: Headache
Endocrine & metabolic: Increased libido (female), decreased libido (male)
Gastrointestinal: Vomiting, diarrhea
<1%:
Cardiovascular: Hypertension, thromboembolism, stroke, myocardial infarction, edema
Central nervous system: Depression, dizziness, anxiety
Dermatologic: Chloasma, melasma, rash
Endocrine: Breast tumors, amenorrhea, alterations in frequency and flow of menses, decreased glucose tolerance, increased triglycerides and LDL
Gastrointestinal: Nausea, GI distress
Hepatic: Cholestatic jaundice
Miscellaneous: Intolerance to contact lenses, increased susceptibility to *Candida* infection

Overdosage/Toxicology Symptoms of overdose include fluid retention, jaundice, thrombophlebitis, nausea; toxicity is unlikely following single exposures of excessive doses, any treatment following emesis and charcoal administration should be supportive and symptomatic

Drug Interactions
Decreased effect: Anticoagulants, barbiturates, rifampin
Increased toxicity: Corticosteroids

Mechanism of Action Increases the synthesis of DNA, RNA, and various proteins in target tissues; reduces the release of gonadotropin-releasing hormone from the hypothalamus; reduces FSH and LH release from the pituitary

Pharmacodynamics/Kinetics
Onset of therapeutic effect: Commonly within 3 days of treatment
Duration: Can persist for as long as 4 months
Distribution: Stored in body fat, slowly released over several days
Metabolism: By the liver to form ethinyl estradiol, cyclopentanol, and other metabolites (including ethinyl estradiol byproducts)
Half-life: 120 hours
Elimination: Primarily in urine; secondarily in bile

Usual Dosage Adults: Female: Oral: 100 mcg once daily for 7 days; followed by 100 mcg/week beginning 2 weeks after inception of treatment; may increase to 200 mcg/week if necessary

Dosing comments in hepatic impairment: Administer with caution

Test Interactions Thyroid function tests, coagulation tests, glucose tolerance tests, metyrapone tests, triglyceride tests

Patient Information Patients should inform their physicians if signs or symptoms of any of the following occur: Thromboembolic or thrombotic disorders including sudden severe headache or vomiting, disturbance of vision or speech, loss of vision, numbness or weakness in an extremity, sharp or crushing chest pain, calf pain, shortness of breath, severe abdominal pain or mass, mental depression or unusual bleeding; patients should discontinue taking the medication if they suspect they are pregnant or become pregnant.

Nursing Implications Monitor blood pressure for increase caused by sodium and water retention

Dosage Forms Tablet: 100 mcg

Quinethazone (kwin eth' a zone)

Brand Names Hydromox®

Use Adjunctive therapy in treatment of edema and hypertension

Pregnancy Risk Factor D

Contraindications Anuria; hypersensitivity to sulfonamide-derived drugs

Warnings/Precautions Use with caution in renal disease, hepatic disease, gout, lupus erythematosus, diabetes mellitus; some products may contain tartrazine

Adverse Reactions
1% to 10%: Endocrine & metabolic: Hypokalemia
<1%:
Cardiovascular: Hypotension
Central nervous system: Drowsiness
Dermatologic: Photosensitivity, rash
Endocrine & metabolic: Fluid and electrolyte imbalances (hypocalcemia, hypomagnesemia, hyponatremia), hyperglycemia

(Continued)

Quinethazone *(Continued)*

Gastrointestinal: Nausea, vomiting, anorexia

Genitourinary: Uremia

Hematologic: Aplastic anemia, hemolytic anemia, leukopenia, agranulocytosis, thrombocytopenia

Hepatic: Hepatitis

Renal: Prerenal azotemia, polyuria

Overdosage/Toxicology Symptoms of overdose include hypermotility, diuresis, lethargy, confusion, muscle weakness; following GI decontamination, therapy is supportive with I.V. fluids, electrolytes, and I.V. pressors if needed

Drug Interactions

Decreased effect of oral hypoglycemics; decreased absorption with cholestyramine and colestipol

Increased effect with furosemide and other loop diuretics

Increased toxicity/levels of lithium

Mechanism of Action Quinethazone is a quinazoline derivative which increases the renal excretion of sodium and chloride and an accompanying volume of water due to inhibition of the tubular mechanism of electrolyte reabsorption.

Pharmacodynamics/Kinetics

Onset of action: 2 hours

Duration: 18-24 hours

Usual Dosage Adults: Oral: 50-100 mg once daily up to a maximum of 200 mg/day

Patient Information May be taken with food or milk; take early in day to avoid nocturia; take the last dose of multiple doses no later than 6 PM unless instructed otherwise. A few people who take this medication become more sensitive to sunlight and may experience skin rash, redness, itching, or severe sunburn, especially if sun block SPF ≥15 is not used on exposed skin areas.

Nursing Implications Assess weight, I & O reports daily to determine fluid loss; take blood pressure with patient lying down and standing

Dosage Forms Tablet: 50 mg

Quinidex® Extentabs® *see* Quinidine *on this page*

Quinidine *(kwin' i deen)*

Related Information

Antiarrhythmic Drugs *on page 1246-1248*

Brand Names Cardioquin®; Quinaglute® Dura-Tabs®; Quinalan®; Quinidex® Extentabs®; Quinora®

Synonyms Quinidine Gluconate; Quinidine Polygalacturonate; Quinidine Sulfate

Use Prophylaxis after cardioversion of atrial fibrillation and/or flutter to maintain normal sinus rhythm; also used to prevent reoccurrence of paroxysmal supraventricular tachycardia, paroxysmal A-V junctional rhythm, paroxysmal ventricular tachycardia, paroxysmal atrial fibrillation, and atrial or ventricular premature contractions; also has activity against *Plasmodium falciparum* malaria

Pregnancy Risk Factor C

Contraindications Patients with complete A-V block with an A-V junctional or idioventricular pacemaker; patients with intraventricular conduction defects (marked widening of QRS complex); patients with cardiac-glycoside induced A-V conduction disorders; hypersensitivity to the drug or cinchona derivatives

Warnings/Precautions Use with caution in patients with myocardial depression, sick-sinus syndrome, incomplete A-V block, hepatic and/or renal insufficiency, myasthenia gravis; hemolysis may occur in patients with G-6-PD (glucose-6-phosphate dehydrogenase) deficiency; quinidine-induced hepatotoxicity, including granulomatous hepatitis can occur, increased serum AST and alkaline phosphatase concentrations, and jaundice may occur; use with caution in nursing women and elderly

Adverse Reactions

>10%: Gastrointestinal: Bitter taste, diarrhea, anorexia, nausea, vomiting, stomach cramping

1% to 10%:

Cardiovascular: Hypotension, syncope

Central nervous system: Lightheadedness, severe headache

Dermatologic: Skin rash

Ocular: Blurred vision

Otic: Tinnitus

Respiratory: Wheezing

<1%:

Cardiovascular: Tachycardia, heart block, ventricular fibrillation, vascular collapse

Central nervous system: Confusion, delirium, fever

Dermatologic: Angioedema
Gastrointestinal: Vertigo
Hematologic: Anemia, thrombocytopenic purpura, blood dyscrasias
Otic: Impaired hearing
Respiratory: Respiratory depression

Overdosage/Toxicology Has a low toxic:therapeutic ratio and may easily produce fatal intoxication (acute toxic dose: 1 g in adults); symptoms of overdose include sinus bradycardia, sinus node arrest or asystole, PR, QRS or Q-T interval prolongation, torsade de pointes (polymorphous ventricular tachycardia) and depressed myocardial contractility, which along with alpha-adrenergic or ganglionic blockade, may result in hypotension and pulmonary edema; other effects are anticholinergic (dry mouth, dilated pupils, and delirium) as well as seizures, coma and respiratory arrest. Treatment is primarily symptomatic and effects usually respond to conventional therapies (fluids, positioning, vasopressors, anticonvulsants, antiarrhythmics). **Note:** Do not use other type 1a or 1c antiarrhythmic agents to treat ventricular tachycardia; sodium bicarbonate may treat wide QRS intervals or hypotension; markedly impaired conduction or high degree A-V block, unresponsive to bicarbonate, indicates consideration of a pacemaker is needed.

Drug Interactions
Decreased effect: Phenobarbital, phenytoin, and rifampin may decrease quinidine serum concentrations
Increased toxicity:
Quinidine potentiates nondepolarizing and depolarizing muscle relaxants; quinidine may increase plasma concentration of digoxin, closely monitor digoxin concentrations, digoxin dosage may need to be reduced (by one-half) when quinidine is initiated, new steady-state digoxin plasma concentrations occur in 5-7 days; quinidine may enhance coumarin anticoagulants
Beta-blockers + quinidine → ↑ bradycardia
Verapamil, amiodarone, alkalinizing agents, and cimetidine may increase quinidine serum concentrations

Stability Do not use discolored parenteral solution

Mechanism of Action Class 1A antiarrhythmic agent; depresses phase O of the action potential; decreases myocardial excitability and conduction velocity, and myocardial contractility by decreasing sodium influx during depolarization and potassium efflux in repolarization; also reduces calcium transport across cell membrane

Pharmacodynamics/Kinetics
Distribution: V_d: Adults: 2-3.5 L/kg, decreased with congestive heart failure, malaria; increased with cirrhosis; crosses the placenta; appears in breast milk
Protein binding:
Newborns: 60% to 70%; decreased protein binding with cyanotic congenital heart disease, cirrhosis, or acute myocardial infarction
Adults: 80% to 90%
Metabolism: Extensively in the liver (50% to 90%) to inactive compounds
Bioavailability:
Sulfate: 80%
Gluconate: 70%
Plasma half-life:
Children: 2.5-6.7 hours
Adults: 6-8 hours; increased half-life with elderly, cirrhosis, and congestive heart failure
Elimination: In urine (15% to 25% as unchanged drug)

Usual Dosage Dosage expressed in terms of the salt: 267 mg of quinidine gluconate = 200 mg of quinidine sulfate

Children: Test dose for idiosyncratic reaction (sulfate, oral or gluconate, I.M.): 2 mg/kg or 60 mg/m²
Oral (quinidine sulfate): 15-60 mg/kg/day in 4-5 divided doses or 6 mg/kg every 4-6 hours; usual 30 mg/kg/day or 900 mg/m²/day given in 5 daily doses
I.V. **not** recommended (quinidine gluconate): 2-10 mg/kg/dose given at a rate ≤10 mg/minute every 3-6 hours as needed

Adults: Test dose: Oral, I.M.: 200 mg administered several hours before full dosage (to determine possibility of idiosyncratic reaction)
Oral:
Sulfate: 100-600 mg/dose every 4-6 hours; begin at 200 mg/dose and titrate to desired effect (maximum daily dose: 3-4 g)
Gluconate: 324-972 mg every 8-12 hours
I.M.: 400 mg/dose every 4-6 hours
I.V.: 200-400 mg/dose diluted and given at a rate ≤10 mg/minute

Dosing adjustment in renal impairment: Cl_{cr} <10 mL/minute: Administer 75% of normal dose
(Continued)

Quinidine (Continued)

Slightly hemodialyzable (5% to 20%); 200 mg supplemental dose posthemodialysis is recommended; not dialyzable (0% to 5%) by peritoneal dialysis

Dosing adjustment/comments in hepatic impairment: Larger loading dose may be indicated, reduce maintenance doses by 50% and monitor serum levels closely

Administration When injecting I.M., aspirate carefully to avoid injection into a vessel; give around-the-clock to promote less variation in peak and trough serum levels; maximum I.V. infusion rate: 10 mg/minute

Monitoring Parameters Cardiac monitor required during I.V. administration; CBC, liver and renal function tests, should be routinely performed during long-term administration

Reference Range Therapeutic: 2-5 µg/mL (SI: 6.2-15.4 µmol/L). Patient dependent therapeutic response occurs at levels of 3-6 µg/mL (SI: 9.2-18.5 µmol/L). Optimal therapeutic level is method dependent; >6 µg/mL (SI: >18 µmol/L).

Patient Information Do not crush sustained release preparations. Patients should notify their physician if rash, fever, unusual bleeding or bruising, ringing in the ears, visual disturbances, or syncope occurs; seek emergency help if palpitations occur.

Nursing Implications Do not crush sustained release drug product

Additional Information
Quinidine gluconate: Duraquin®, Quinaglute® Dura-Tabs®, Quinalan®, Quina-time®
Quinidine polygalacturonate: Cardioquin®
Quinidine sulfate: Cin-Quin®, Quinidex® Extentabs®, Quinora®

Dosage Forms
Injection, as gluconate: 80 mg/mL (10 mL)
Tablet, as polygalacturonate: 275 mg
Tablet, as sulfate: 200 mg, 300 mg
Tablet:
Sustained action, as sulfate: 300 mg
Sustained release, as gluconate: 324 mg

Quinidine Gluconate see Quinidine on page 968

Quinidine Polygalacturonate see Quinidine on page 968

Quinidine Sulfate see Quinidine on page 968

Quinine Sulfate (kwye' nine)

Brand Names Formula Q® [OTC]; Legatrin® [OTC]; M-KYA® [OTC]; Quinamm®; Quiphile®; Q-vel®

Use Suppression or treatment of chloroquine-resistant *P. falciparum* malaria; treatment of *Babesia microti* infection; prevention and treatment of nocturnal recumbency leg muscle cramps

Pregnancy Risk Factor D

Contraindications Tinnitus, optic neuritis, G-6-PD deficiency, hypersensitivity to quinine or any component, history of black water fever, and thrombocytopenia with quinine or quinidine

Warnings/Precautions Use with caution in patients with cardiac arrhythmias (quinine has quinidine-like activity) and in patients with myasthenia gravis

Adverse Reactions
>10%:
Central nervous system: Severe headache
Gastrointestinal: Nausea, vomiting, diarrhea
Ocular: Blurred vision
Otic: Tinnitus
<1%:
Cardiovascular: Flushing of the skin, anginal symptoms
Central nervous system: Fever
Dermatologic: Rash, pruritus
Endocrine & metabolic: Hypoglycemia
Gastrointestinal: Epigastric pain
Hematologic: Hemolysis, thrombocytopenia
Hepatic: Hepatitis
Ocular: Nightblindness, diplopia, optic atrophy
Otic: Impaired hearing
Miscellaneous: Hypersensitivity reactions

Overdosage/Toxicology Symptoms of mild toxicity include nausea, vomiting, and cinchonism; sever intoxication may cause ataxia, obtundation, convulsions, coma, and respirator arrest; with massive intoxication quinidine-like cardiotoxicity (hypotension, QRS and Q-T interval prolongation, A-V block, and ventricular arrhythmias) may be fatal; retinal toxicity occurs 9-10 hours after ingestion (blurred vision, impaired color perception, constriction of visual fields and blindness); other toxic effects include hypokalemia, hypoglycemia, hemolysis and congenital malformations when taken during pregnancy. Treatment includes symptomatic therapy with conventional agents (anticonvulsants, fluids, positioning, vasoconstrictors, antiarrhythmias). **Note:** Avoid type 1a and 1c antiarrhythmic drugs; treat cardiotoxicity with sodium bicarbonate; dialysis and hemoperfusion procedures are ineffective in enhancing elimination.

Drug Interactions

Decreased effect: Phenobarbital, phenytoin, and rifampin may decrease quinine serum concentrations

Increased toxicity:

Beta-blockers + quinine → ↑ bradycardia

Quinine may enhance coumarin anticoagulants; quinine potentiates nondepolarizing and depolarizing muscle relaxants; quinine may increase plasma concentration of digoxin, closely monitor digoxin concentrations, digoxin dosage may need to be reduced (by one-half) when quinine is initiated, new steady-state digoxin plasma concentrations occur in 5-7 days

Verapamil, amiodarone, alkalinizing agents, and cimetidine may increase quinine serum concentrations

Stability Protect from light

Mechanism of Action Depresses oxygen uptake and carbohydrate metabolism; intercalates into DNA, disrupting the parasite's replication and transcription; affects calcium distribution within muscle fibers and decreases the excitability of the motor end-plate region; cardiovascular effects similar to quinidine

Pharmacodynamics/Kinetics

Absorption: Oral: Readily absorbed mainly from the upper small intestine

Protein binding: 70% to 95%

Metabolism: Primarily in the liver

Half-life:

Children: 6-12 hours

Adults: 8-14 hours

Time to peak serum concentration: Within 1-3 hours

Elimination: In bile and saliva with <5% excreted unchanged in urine

Usual Dosage Oral:

Children:

Treatment of chloroquine-resistant malaria: 25 mg/kg/day in divided doses every 8 hours for 3-7 days in conjunction with another agent

Babesiosis: 25 mg/kg/day, (up to a maximum of 650 mg/dose) divided every 8 hours for 7 days

Adults:

Treatment of chloroquine-resistant malaria: 650 mg every 8 hours for 3-7 days in conjunction with another agent

Suppression of malaria: 325 mg twice daily and continued for 6 weeks after exposure

Babesiosis: 650 mg every 6-8 hours for 7 days

Leg cramps: 200-300 mg at bedtime

Dosing interval/adjustment in renal impairment:

Cl_{cr} 10-50 mL/minute: Administer every 8-12 hours or 75% of normal dose

Cl_{cr} <10 mL/minute: Administer every 24 hours or 30% to 50% of normal dose

Not removed by hemo- or peritoneal dialysis or continuous arterio-venous or veno-venous hemofiltration (CAVH/CAVHD); dose for Cl_{cr} <10 mL/minute

Reference Range Toxic: >10 µg/mL

Test Interactions Positive Coombs' [direct]

Patient Information Do not crush sustained release preparations. Avoid use of aluminum-containing antacids because of drug absorption problems; swallow dose whole to avoid bitter taste; may cause night blindness. Patients should notify their physician if rash, fever, unusual bleeding or bruising, ringing in the ears, visual disturbances, or syncope occur; seek emergency help if palpitations occur.

Dosage Forms

Capsule: 64.8 mg, 65 mg, 200 mg, 300 mg, 325 mg

Tablet: 162.5 mg, 260 mg

Quinora® *see* Quinidine *on page 968*

Quiphile® *see* Quinine Sulfate *on previous page*

Q-vel® *see* Quinine Sulfate *on previous page*

Rabies Immune Globulin, Human (ray' beez)

Related Information
Immunization Guidelines *on page 1389-1405*
Vaccines *on page 1386-1388*

Brand Names Hyperab®; Imogam®

Synonyms RIG

Use Part of postexposure prophylaxis of persons with rabies exposure who lack a history or pre-exposure or postexposure prophylaxis with rabies vaccine or a recently documented neutralizing antibody response to previous rabies vaccination; although it is preferable to give RIG with the first dose of vaccine, it can be given up to 8 days after vaccination

Pregnancy Risk Factor C

Contraindications Inadvertent I.V. administration; allergy to thimerosal or any component

Warnings/Precautions Use with caution in individuals with thrombocytopenia, bleeding disorders, or prior allergic reactions to immune globulins

Adverse Reactions
1% to 10%:
Central nervous system: Fever (mild)
Local: Soreness at injection site
<1%:
Dermatologic: Urticaria, angioedema
Neuromuscular & skeletal: Stiffness, soreness of muscles
Miscellaneous: Anaphylactic shock

Drug Interactions
Decreased effect: Live vaccines, corticosteroids, immunosuppressive agents; should not be administered within 3 months

Stability Refrigerate

Mechanism of Action Rabies immune globulin is a solution of globulins dried from the plasma or serum of selected adult human donors who have been immunized with rabies vaccine and have developed high titers of rabies antibody. It generally contains 10% to 18% of protein of which not less than 80% is monomeric immunoglobulin G.

Usual Dosage Children and Adults: I.M.: 20 units/kg in a single dose (RIG should always be administered in conjunction with rabies vaccine (HDCV)); infiltrate ½ of the dose locally around the wound; give the remainder I.M.

Administration Intramuscular injection only; injection should be made into the deltoid muscle or anterolateral aspect of the thigh

Nursing Implications Severe adverse reactions can occur if patient receives RIG I.V.

Dosage Forms Injection: 150 units/mL (2 mL, 10 mL)

Rabies Virus Vaccine (ray' beez)

Related Information
Immunization Guidelines *on page 1389-1405*
Vaccines *on page 1386-1388*

Brand Names Imovax® Rabies I.D. Vaccine; Imovax® Rabies Vaccine

Synonyms HDCV; Human Diploid Cell Cultures Rabies Vaccine; Human Diploid Cell Cultures Rabies Vaccine (Intradermal use)

Use Veterinarians, animal handlers, certain laboratory workers, and persons living in or visiting countries for longer than 1 month where rabies is a constant threat.

Complete pre-exposure prophylaxis does not eliminate the need for additional therapy with rabies vaccine after a rabies exposure. The Food and Drug Administration has not approved the I.D. use of rabies vaccine for postexposure prophylaxis. Recommendations for I.D. use of HDCV are currently being discussed. The decision for postexposure rabies vaccination depends on the species of biting animal, the circumstances of biting incident, and the type of exposure (bite, saliva contamination of wound, and so on). The type of and schedule for postexposure prophylaxis depends upon the person's previous rabies vaccination status or the result of a previous or current serologic test for rabies antibody. For postexposure prophylaxis, rabies vaccine should always be administered I.M., **not** I.D.

Pregnancy Risk Factor C

Contraindications Developing febrile illness (during pre-exposure therapy only); allergy to neomycin, gentamicin, or amphotericin B

Warnings/Precautions Rabies vaccine is available only in I.M. form; cannot be given intradermally

Adverse Reactions

>10%:

Central nervous system: Dizziness, malaise, encephalomyelitis, transverse myelitis, fever

Dermatologic: Itching, pain, local discomfort, swelling, erythema

Gastrointestinal: Nausea, headache, abdominal pain

Neuromuscular & skeletal: Neuroparalytic reactions, muscle aches

Drug Interactions Decreased effect with immunosuppressive agents, corticosteroids, antimalarial drugs (ie, chloroquine); persons on these drugs should receive RIG (3 doses/1 mL each) by the I.M. route

Stability Refrigerate; reconstituted vaccine should be used immediately

Mechanism of Action Rabies vaccine is an inactivated virus vaccine which promotes immunity by inducing an active immune response. The production of specific antibodies requires about 7-10 days to develop. Rabies immune globulin or antirabies serum, equine (ARS) is given in conjunction with rabies vaccine to provide immune protection until an antibody response can occur.

Usual Dosage

Pre-exposure prophylaxis: Two 1 mL doses I.M. 1 week apart, third dose 3 weeks after second. If exposure continues, booster doses can be given every 2 years, or an antibody titer determined and a booster dose given if the titer is inadequate.

Postexposure prophylaxis: All postexposure treatment should begin with immediate cleansing of the wound with soap and water

Persons not previously immunized as above: Rabies immune globulin 20 units/kg body weight, half infiltrated at bite site if possible, remainder I.M.; and 5 doses of rabies vaccine, 1 mL I.M., one each on days 0, 3, 7, 14, 28

Persons who have previously received postexposure prophylaxis with rabies vaccine, received a recommended I.M. pre-exposure series of rabies vaccine or have a previously documented rabies antibody titer considered adequate: Two doses of rabies vaccine, 1 mL I.M., one each on days 0 and 3

Reference Range Antibody titers ≥115 as determined by rapid fluorescent-focus inhibition test are indicative of adequate response; collect titers on day 28 postexposure

Additional Information Federal law requires that the date of administration, the vaccine manufacturer, lot number of vaccine, and the administering person's name, title and address be entered into the patient's permanent medical record

Dosage Forms Injection:

I.M. (HDCV): Rabies antigen 2.5 units/mL (1 mL)

Intradermal: Rabies antigen 0.25 units/mL (1 mL)

Racemic Amphetamine Sulfate *see* Amphetamine Sulfate *on page 69*

Racemic Epinephrine *see* Epinephrine *on page 389*

Ramipril (ra mi′ prill)

Related Information

Angiotensin-Converting Enzyme Inhibitors, Comparative Pharmacokinetics *on page 1244*

Angiotensin-Converting Enzyme Inhibitors, Comparisons of Indications and Adult Dosages *on page 1243*

Brand Names Altace™

Use Treatment of hypertension, alone or in combination with thiazide diuretics

Unlabeled use: Congestive heart failure

Pregnancy Risk Factor D

Contraindications Hypersensitivity to ramipril or ramiprilat, or any other angiotensin-converting enzyme inhibitors

Warnings/Precautions Use with caution and modify dosage in patients with renal impairment (decrease dosage) (especially renal artery stenosis), severe congestive heart failure, or with coadministered diuretic; severe hypotension may occur in the elderly and patients who are sodium and/or volume depleted, initiate lower doses and monitor closely when starting therapy in these patients; should be discontinued if laryngeal stridor or angioedema of the face, tongue, or glottis is observed

Adverse Reactions

1% to 10%:

Cardiovascular: Tachycardia, chest pain, palpitations,

Central nervous system: Insomnia, headache, dizziness, fatigue, malaise,

Dermatologic: Rash, pruritus, alopecia

Gastrointestinal: Dysgeusia, abdominal pain, vomiting, nausea, diarrhea, anorexia, constipation, loss of taste perception

Neuromuscular & skeletal: Paresthesia

(Continued)

973

Ramipril *(Continued)*

    Renal: Oliguria

    Respiratory: Transient cough

  <1%:

    Cardiovascular: Hypotension

    Dermatologic: Angioedema

    Endocrine & metabolic: Hyperkalemia

    Hematologic: Neutropenia, agranulocytosis,

    Renal: Proteinuria; increased BUN, serum creatinine

Overdosage/Toxicology Mild hypotension has been the only toxic effect seen with acute overdose. Bradycardia may also occur; hyperkalemia occurs even with therapeutic doses, especially in patients with renal insufficiency and those taking NSAIDs. Following initiation of essential overdose management, toxic symptom treatment and supportive treatment should be initiated. Hypotension usually responds to I.V. fluids or Trendelenburg positioning.

Drug Interactions See table.

Drug-Drug Interactions With ACEIs

Precipitant Drug	Drug (Category) and Effect	Description
Antacids	ACEIs: decreased	Decreased bioavailability of ACEIs. May be more likely with captopril. Separate administration times by 1-2 hours.
NSAIDs (indomethacin)	ACEIs: decreased	Reduced hypotensive effects of ACEIs. More prominent in low renin or volume dependent hypertensive patients.
Phenothiazines	ACEIs: increased	Pharmacologic effects of ACEIs may be increased.
ACEIs	Allopurinol: increased	Higher risk of hypersensitivity reaction possible when given concurrently. Three case reports of Stevens-Johnson syndrome with captopril.
ACEIs	Digoxin: increased	Increased plasma digoxin levels.
ACEIs	Lithium: increased	Increased serum lithium levels and symptoms of toxicity may occur.
ACEIs	Potassium preps/potassium-sparing diuretics increased	Coadministration may result in elevated potassium levels.

Mechanism of Action Ramipril is an angiotensin-converting enzyme (ACE) inhibitor which prevents the formation of angiotensin II from angiotensin I and exhibits pharmacologic effects that are similar to captopril. Ramipril must undergo enzymatic saponification by esterases in the liver to its biologically active metabolite, ramiprilat. The pharmacodynamic effects of ramipril result from the high-affinity, competitive, reversible binding of ramiprilat to angiotensin-converting enzyme thus preventing the formation of the potent vasoconstrictor angiotensin II. This isomerized enzyme-inhibitor complex has a slow rate of dissociation, which results in high potency and a long duration of action; a CNS mechanism may also be involved in the hypotensive effect as angiotensin II increases adrenergic outflow from CNS; vasoactive kallikreins may be decreased in conversion to active hormones by ACE inhibitors, thus reducing blood pressure

Pharmacodynamics/Kinetics

  Absorption: Well absorbed from GI tract (50% to 60%)

  Distribution: Plasma levels decline in a triphasic fashion; rapid decline is a distribution phase to peripheral compartment, plasma protein and tissue ACE (half-life 2-4 hours); 2nd phase is an apparent elimination phase representing the clearance of free ramiprilat (half-life: 9-18 hours); and final phase is the terminal elimination phase representing the equilibrium phase between tissue binding and dissociation (half-life: >50 hours)

  Metabolism: Hepatic to the active form, ramiprilat

  Half-life: Ramiprilat: >50 hours

  Time to peak serum concentration: ~1 hour

  Elimination: Ramipril and its metabolites are eliminated primarily through the kidneys (60%) and feces (40%)

Usual Dosage Adults: Oral: 2.5-5 mg once daily, maximum: 20 mg/day

  Dosing adjustment in renal impairment:

    Cl_{cr} 10-50 mL/minute: Administer 50% to 75% of normal dose

Cl$_{cr}$ <40 mL/minute: Patients should be started on 1.25 mg/day and titrated up to 5 mg/day maximum

Cl$_{cr}$ <10 mL/minute: Administer 25% to 50% of normal dose

Test Interactions Increases BUN, creatinine, potassium, positive Coombs' [direct]; decreases cholesterol (S); may cause false-positive results in urine acetone determinations using sodium nitroprusside reagent

Patient Information Notify physician if vomiting, diarrhea, excessive perspiration, or dehydration should occur; also if swelling of face, lips, tongue, or difficulty in breathing occurs or if persistent cough develops

Nursing Implications May cause depression in some patients; discontinue if angioedema of the face, extremities, lips, tongue, or glottis occurs; watch for hypotensive effects within 1-3 hours of first dose or new higher dose

Dosage Forms Capsule: 1.25 mg, 2.5 mg, 5 mg, 10 mg

Ranitidine Hydrochloride (ra nye' te deen)

Brand Names Zantac®

Use Short-term treatment of active duodenal ulcers and benign gastric ulcers; long-term prophylaxis of duodenal ulcer and gastric hypersecretory states, gastroesophageal reflux, recurrent postoperative ulcer, upper GI bleeding, prevention of acid-aspiration pneumonitis during surgery, and prevention of stress-induced ulcers; causes fewer interactions than cimetidine

Pregnancy Risk Factor B

Contraindications Hypersensitivity to ranitidine or any component

Warnings/Precautions Use with caution in children <12 years of age; use with caution in patients with liver and renal impairment; dosage modification required in patients with renal impairment; long-term therapy may cause vitamin B$_{12}$ deficiency

Adverse Reactions

Endocrine & metabolic: Gynecomastia

Hepatic: Hepatitis

Neuromuscular & skeletal: Arthralgias

1% to 10%:

Central nervous system: Dizziness, sedation, malaise, headache, drowsiness

Dermatologic: Rash

Gastrointestinal: Constipation, nausea, vomiting, diarrhea

<1%:

Cardiovascular: Bradycardia, tachycardia

Central nervous system: Fever, confusion

Hematologic: Thrombocytopenia, neutropenia, agranulocytosis

Respiratory: Bronchospasm

Overdosage/Toxicology Symptoms of overdose include muscular tremors, vomiting, rapid respiration, renal failure, CNS depression; treatment is primarily symptomatic and supportive

Drug Interactions

Decreased effect: Variable effects on warfarin; antacids may decrease absorption of ranitidine; ketoconazole and itraconazole absorptions are decreased; may produce altered serum levels of procainamide and ferrous sulfate; decreased effect of nondepolarizing muscle relaxants, cefpodoxime, cyanocobalamin (decreased absorption), diazepam, oxaprozin

Decreased toxicity of atropine

Increased toxicity of cyclosporine (increased serum creatinine), gentamicin (neuromuscular blockade), glipizide, glyburide, midazolam (increased concentrations), metoprolol, pentoxifylline, phenytoin, quinidine

Stability

Ranitidine injection should be stored at 4°C to 30°C and protected from light; injection solution is a clear, colorless to yellow solution; slight darkening does not affect potency

Stability at room temperature:

Prepared bags: 2 days

Premixed bags: Manufacturer expiration dating and out of overwrap stability: 15 days

Stability of prepared bags at refrigeration temperature (4°C): 10 days

Solution for I.V. infusion in NS or D$_5$W is stable for 30 days when frozen; I.V. form is **incompatible** with amphotericin B, clindamycin, diazepam (same syringe), hetastarch (Y-line), hydroxyzine (same syringe), midazolam (same syringe), pentobarbital (same syringe), phenobarbital (same syringe)

Mechanism of Action Competitive inhibition of histamine at H$_2$-receptors of the gastric parietal cells, which inhibits gastric acid secretion, gastric volume and hydrogen ion concentration reduced

Pharmacodynamics/Kinetics

Absorption: Oral: 50% to 60%

(Continued)

Ranitidine Hydrochloride *(Continued)*

Distribution: Minimally penetrates the blood-brain barrier; appears in breast milk

Protein binding: 15%

Metabolism: In the liver (<10%)

Half-life:

Children 3.5-16 years: 1.8-2 hours

Adults: 2-2.5 hours

End stage renal disease: 6-9 hours

Time to peak serum concentration: Oral: Within 1-3 hours and persisting for 8 hours

Elimination: Primarily in urine (35% as unchanged drug) and in feces

Usual Dosage Giving oral dose at 6 PM may be better than 10 PM bedtime, the highest acid production usually starts at approximately 7 PM, thus giving at 6 PM controls acid secretion better

Children:

Oral: 1.25-2.5 mg/kg/dose every 12 hours; maximum: 300 mg/day

I.M., I.V.: 0.75-1.5 mg/kg/dose every 6-8 hours, maximum daily dose: 400 mg

Continuous infusion: 0.1-0.25 mg/kg/hour (preferred for stress ulcer prophylaxis in patients with concurrent maintenance I.V.s or TPNs)

Adults:

Short-term treatment of ulceration: 150 mg/dose twice daily or 300 mg at bedtime

Prophylaxis of recurrent duodenal ulcer: Oral: 150 mg at bedtime

Gastric hypersecretory conditions:

Oral: 150 mg twice daily, up to 6 g/day

I.M., I.V.: 50 mg/dose every 6-8 hours (dose not to exceed 400 mg/day)

I.V.: 50 mg/dose IVPB every 6-8 hours (dose not to exceed 400 mg/day)

or

Continuous I.V. infusion: Initial: 50 mg IVPB, followed by 6.25 mg/hour titrated to gastric pH >4.0 for prophylaxis or >7.0 for treatment; **continuous I.V. infusion is preferred in patients with active bleeding**

Gastric hypersecretory conditions: Doses up to 2.5 mg/kg/hour (220 mg/hour) have been used

Dosing adjustment in renal impairment:

Cl_{cr} 10-50 mL/minute: Administer at 75% of normal dose or administer every 18-24 hours

Cl_{cr} <10 mL/minute: Administer at 50% of normal dose or administer every 18-24 hours

Slightly dialyzable (5% to 20%)

Dosing adjustment/comments in hepatic disease: Unchanged

Administration Ranitidine injection may be administered I.M. or I.V.

I.M.: Injection is given undiluted

I.V. must be diluted and may be administered IVP or IVPB or continuous I.V. infusion

IVP: Ranitidine (usually 50 mg) should be diluted to a total of 20 mL with NS or D_5W and administered over at least 5 minutes

IVPB: administer over 15-20 minutes

Continuous I.V. infusion: Administer at 6.25 mg/hour and titrate dosage based on gastric pH by continuous infusion over 24 hours

Monitoring Parameters AST, ALT, serum creatinine; when used to prevent stress-related GI bleeding, measure the intragastric pH and try to maintain pH >4; signs and symptoms of peptic ulcer disease, occult blood with GI bleeding, monitor renal function to correct dose; monitor for side effects

Test Interactions False-positive urine protein using Multistix®, gastric acid secretion test, skin test allergen extracts, serum creatinine and serum transaminase concentrations, urine protein test

Patient Information It may take several days before this medicine begins to relieve stomach pain; antacids may be taken with ranitidine unless your physician has told you not to use them; wait 30-60 minutes between taking the antacid and ranitidine; may cause drowsiness, impair judgment, or coordination

Nursing Implications I.M. solution does not need to be diluted before use; monitor creatinine clearance for renal impairment; observe caution in patients with renal function impairment and hepatic function impairment

Dosage Forms

Infusion, preservative free, in NaCl 0.45%: 1 mg/mL (50 mL)

Injection: 25 mg/mL (2 mL, 10 mL, 40 mL)

Syrup (peppermint flavor): 15 mg/mL (473 mL)

Tablet: 150 mg, 300 mg

Rea-Lo® [OTC] *see* Urea *on page 1139*

Recombinant Human Deoxyribonuclease *see* Dornase Alfa *on page 365*

Recombivax HB® *see* Hepatitis B Vaccine *on page 533*

Recommendations of the Advisory Council on the Elimination of Tuberculosis *see page 1303*

Redisol® *see* Cyanocobalamin *on page 282*

Reese's® Pinworm Medicine [OTC] *see* Pyrantel Pamoate *on page 957*

Regitine® *see* Phentolamine Mesylate *on page 873*

Reglan® *see* Metoclopramide *on page 728*

Regonol® *see* Pyridostigmine Bromide *on page 960*

Regular Concentrated Iletin® II *see* Insulin Preparations *on page 578*

Regular Iletin® I [OTC] *see* Insulin Preparations *on page 578*

Regular Insulin [OTC] *see* Insulin Preparations *on page 578*

Regular Purified Pork Insulin [OTC] *see* Insulin Preparations *on page 578*

Regulax SS® [OTC] *see* Docusate *on page 362*

Reguloid® [OTC] *see* Psyllium *on page 956*

Regutol® [OTC] *see* Docusate *on page 362*

Rela® *see* Carisoprodol *on page 185*

Relafen® *see* Nabumetone *on page 764*

Relaxadon® *see* Hyoscyamine, Atropine, Scopolamine, and Phenobarbital *on page 557*

Relefact® TRH *see* Protirelin *on page 952*

Relief® Ophthalmic Solution *see* Phenylephrine Hydrochloride *on page 874*

Renese® *see* Polythiazide *on page 902*

Repan® *see* Butalbital Compound *on page 153*

Reposans-10® *see* Chlordiazepoxide *on page 221*

Resectisol® *see* Mannitol *on page 664*

Reserpine (re ser' peen)

Brand Names Serpalan®; Serpasil®

Use Management of mild to moderate hypertension

  Unlabeled use: Management of tardive dyskinesia

Pregnancy Risk Factor C

Contraindications Any ulcerative condition, mental depression, hypersensitivity to reserpine or any component

Warnings/Precautions Discontinue reserpine 7 days before electroshock therapy; use with caution in patients with impaired renal function or peptic ulcer disease, gallstones, and the elderly; at high doses, significant mental depression may occur; some products may contain tartrazine

Adverse Reactions

>10%:

  Central nervous system: Dizziness

  Gastrointestinal: Anorexia, diarrhea, dry mouth, nausea, vomiting

  Respiratory: Nasal congestion

1% to 10%:

  Cardiovascular: Peripheral edema, arrhythmias, bradycardia, chest pain

  Central nervous system: Headache

  Genitourinary: Impotence

  Miscellaneous: Black stools, bloody vomit

<1%:

  Cardiovascular: Hypotension

  Central nervous system: Drowsiness, fatigue, mental depression, parkinsonism

  Dermatologic: Skin rash

  Gastrointestinal: Increased gastric acid secretion

  Genitourinary: Urination difficulty

  Neuromuscular & skeletal: Trembling of hands/fingers

  Miscellaneous: Sodium and water retention

Overdosage/Toxicology Symptoms of overdose include hypotension, bradycardia, CNS depression, sedation, coma, hypothermia, miosis, tremors, diarrhea,

(Continued)

Reserpine *(Continued)*

vomiting. Hypotension usually responds to I.V. fluids or Trendelenburg positioning. If unresponsive to these measures, the use of a parenteral inotrope may be required (eg, norepinephrine 0.1-0.2 mcg/kg/minute titrated to response). Anticholinergic agents may be useful in reducing the parkinsonian effects and bradycardia.

Drug Interactions

Decreased effect of indirect-acting sympathomimetics

Increased effect/toxicity of MAO inhibitors, direct-acting sympathomimetics, and tricyclic antidepressants

Stability Protect oral dosage forms from light

Mechanism of Action Reduces blood pressure via depletion of sympathetic biogenic amines (norepinephrine and dopamine); this also commonly results in sedative effects

Pharmacodynamics/Kinetics

Onset of antihypertensive effect: Within 3-6 days

Duration: 2-6 weeks

Absorption: Oral: ~40%

Distribution: Crosses the placenta; appears in breast milk

Protein binding: 96%

Metabolism: Extensively in the liver, >90%

Half-life: 50-100 hours

Elimination: Principal excretion in feces (30% to 60%) and small amounts in urine (10%)

Usual Dosage Oral (full antihypertensive effects may take as long as 3 weeks):

Children: 0.01-0.02 mg/kg/24 hours divided every 12 hours; maximum dose: 0.25 mg/day

Adults: 0.1-0.25 mg/day in 1-2 doses; initial: 0.5 mg/day for 1-2 weeks; maintenance: reduce to 0.1-0.25 mg/day

Elderly: Initial: 0.05 mg once daily, increasing by 0.05 mg every week as necessary

Dosing adjustment in renal impairment: Cl_{cr} <10 mL/minute: Avoid use

Not removed by hemo or peritoneal dialysis; supplemental dose is not necessary

Monitoring Parameters Blood pressure, standing and sitting/supine

Test Interactions ↓ catecholamines (U)

Patient Information Take with food or milk; impotency is reversible; notify physician if a weight gain of more than 5 lb has taken place during therapy; may cause drowsiness, may impair judgment and coordination

Nursing Implications Observe for mental depression and alert family members to report any symptoms

Dosage Forms Tablet: 0.1 mg, 0.25 mg, 1 mg

Respbid® *see* Theophylline/Aminophylline *on page 1072*

Restoril® *see* Temazepam *on page 1056*

Retin-A™ *see* Tretinoin *on page 1112*

Retinoic Acid *see* Tretinoin *on page 1112*

Retrovir® *see* Zidovudine *on page 1173*

Reversol® *see* Edrophonium Chloride *on page 381*

Rēv-Eyes™ *see* Dapiprazole Hydrochloride *on page 302*

R-Gen® *see* Iodinated Glycerol *on page 587*

R-Gene® *see* Arginine Hydrochloride *on page 87*

rGM-CSF *see* Sargramostim *on page 994*

Rheaban® [OTC] *see* Attapulgite *on page 102*

Rheomacrodex® *see* Dextran *on page 318*

Rhesonativ® *see* Rho(D) Immune Globulin *on this page*

Rheumatrex® *see* Methotrexate *on page 711*

Rhinall® Nasal Solution [OTC] *see* Phenylephrine Hydrochloride *on page 874*

Rhindecon® *see* Phenylpropanolamine Hydrochloride *on page 876*

Rhinocort™ *see* Budesonide *on page 145*

Rhinosyn-DMX® [OTC] *see* Guaifenesin and Dextromethorphan *on page 517*

Rho(D) Immune Globulin

Brand Names Gamulin® Rh; HypRho®-D; HypRho®-D Mini-Dose; MICRhoGAM™; Mini-Gamulin® Rh; Rhesonativ®; RhoGAM™

Use Prevention of isoimmunization in Rh-negative individuals exposed to Rh-positive blood during delivery of an Rh-positive infant, as a result of an abortion, following amniocentesis or abdominal trauma, or following a transfusion accident; prevention of hemolytic disease of the newborn if there is a subsequent pregnancy with an Rh-positive fetus

Pregnancy Risk Factor C

Contraindications Rh₀(D)-positive patient; known hypersensitivity to immune globulins or to thimerosal; transfusion of Rh₀(D)-positive blood in previous 3 months; prior sensitization to Rh₀(D)

Warnings/Precautions Use with caution in patients with thrombocytopenia or bleeding disorders, patients with IgA deficiency; do not inject I.V.; do not administer to neonates

Adverse Reactions

<1%:

Central nervous system: Lethargy

Gastrointestinal: Splenomegaly

Hepatic: Elevated bilirubin

Local: Pain at the injection site

Neuromuscular & skeletal: Myalgia

Miscellaneous: Temperature elevation

Stability Reconstituted solution should be refrigerated and will remain stable for 30 days; solution that have been frozen should be discarded

Mechanism of Action Suppresses the immune response and antibody formation of Rh-negative individuals to Rh-positive red blood cells

Pharmacodynamics/Kinetics

Distribution: Appears in breast milk; however, not absorbed by the nursing infant

Half-life: 23-26 days

Usual Dosage Adults (administered I.M. to mothers **not** to infant) I.M.:

Obstetrical usage: 1 vial (300 mcg) prevents maternal sensitization if fetal packed red blood cell volume that has entered the circulation is <15 mL; if it is more, give additional vials. The number of vials = RBC volume of the calculated fetomaternal hemorrhage divided by 15 mL

Postpartum prophylaxis: 300 mcg within 72 hours of delivery

Antepartum prophylaxis: 300 mcg at approximately 26-28 weeks gestation; followed by 300 mcg within 72 hours of delivery if infant is Rh-positive

Following miscarriage, abortion, or termination of ectopic pregnancy at up to 13 weeks of gestation: 50 mcg ideally within 3 hours, but may be given up to 72 hours after; if pregnancy has been terminated at 13 or more weeks of gestation, administer 300 mcg

Administration Give I.M. in deltoid muscle; do **not** give I.V.; the total volume can be given in divided doses at different sites at one time or may be divided and given at intervals, provided the total dosage is given within 72 hours of the fetomaternal hemorrhage or transfusion.

Patient Information Acetaminophen may be taken to ease minor discomfort after vaccination

Dosage Forms

Injection: Each package contains one single dose 300 mcg of Rh₀ (D) immune globulin

Injection, microdose: Each package contains one single dose of microdose, 50 mcg of Rh₀ (D) immune globulin

RhoGAM™ see Rho(D) Immune Globulin *on previous page*

rHuEPO-α see Epoetin Alfa *on page 392*

Rhulicaine® [OTC] see Benzocaine *on page 121*

Rhythmin® see Procainamide Hydrochloride *on page 927*

Ribavirin (rye ba vye′ rin)

Related Information

Antimicrobial Drugs of Choice *on page 1298-1302*

Brand Names Virazole®

Synonyms RTCA; Tribavirin

Use Treatment of patients with respiratory syncytial virus (RSV) infections; may also be used in other viral infections including influenza A and B and adenovirus; specially indicated for treatment of severe lower respiratory tract RSV infections

(Continued)

Ribavirin *(Continued)*

in patients with an underlying compromising condition (prematurity, bronchopulmonary dysplasia and other chronic lung conditions, congenital heart disease, immunodeficiency, immunosuppression), and recent transplant recipients

Pregnancy Risk Factor X

Contraindications Females of childbearing age

Warnings/Precautions Use with caution in patients requiring assisted ventilation because precipitation of the drug in the respiratory equipment may interfere with safe and effective patient ventilation; monitor carefully in patients with COPD and asthma for deterioration of respiratory function. Ribavirin is potentially mutagenic, tumor-promoting, and gonadotoxic.

Adverse Reactions
1% to 10%:
Central nervous system: Fatigue, headache, insomnia
Gastrointestinal: Nausea, anorexia
Hematologic: Anemia
<1%:
Cardiovascular: Hypotension, cardiac arrest, digitalis toxicity
Dermatologic: Rash, skin irritation
Ocular: Conjunctivitis
Respiratory: Mild bronchospasm, worsening of respiratory function, apnea

Drug Interactions Decreased effect of zidovudine

Stability Do not use any water containing an antimicrobial agent to reconstitute drug; reconstituted solution is stable for 24 hours at room temperature

Mechanism of Action Inhibits replication of RNA and DNA viruses; inhibits influenza virus RNA polymerase activity and inhibits the initiation and elongation of RNA fragments resulting in inhibition of viral protein synthesis

Pharmacodynamics/Kinetics
Absorption: Absorbed systemically from the respiratory tract following nasal and oral inhalation; absorption is dependent upon respiratory factors and method of drug delivery; maximal absorption occurs with the use of the aerosol generator via an endotracheal tube; highest concentrations are found in the respiratory tract and erythrocytes
Metabolism: Occurs intracellularly and may be necessary for drug action
Half-life, plasma:
Children: 6.5-11 hours
Adults: 24 hours, much longer in the erythrocyte (16-40 days), which can be used as a marker for intracellular metabolism
Time to peak serum concentration: Inhalation: Within 60-90 minutes
Elimination: Hepatic metabolism is major route of elimination with 40% of the drug cleared renally as unchanged drug and metabolites

Usual Dosage Infants, Children, and Adults:
Aerosol inhalation: Use with Viratek® small particle aerosol generator (SPAG-2) at a concentration of 20 mg/mL (6 g reconstituted with 300 mL of sterile water without preservatives)
Aerosol only: 12-18 hours/day for 3 days, up to 7 days in length

Monitoring Parameters Respiratory function, CBC, reticulocyte count, I & O

Nursing Implications Keep accurate I & O record, discard solutions placed in the SPAG-2 unit at least every 24 hours and before adding additional fluid; healthcare workers who are pregnant or who may become pregnant should be advised of the potential risks of exposure and counseled about risk reduction strategies including alternate job responsibilities; ribavirin may adsorb to contact lenses

Dosage Forms Powder for aerosol: 6 g (100 mL)

Riboflavin *(rye' boe flay vin)*

Brand Names Riobin®

Synonyms Lactoflavin; Vitamin B_2; Vitamin G

Use Prevent riboflavin deficiency and treat ariboflavinosis

Pregnancy Risk Factor A (C if dose exceeds RDA recommendation)

Warnings/Precautions Riboflavin deficiency often occurs in the presence of other B vitamin deficiencies

Drug Interactions Decreased absorption with probenecid

Mechanism of Action Component of flavoprotein enzymes that work together, which are necessary for normal tissue respiration; also needed for activation of pyridoxine and conversion of tryptophan to niacin

Pharmacodynamics/Kinetics
Absorption: Readily via GI tract, however, food increases extent of GI absorption; GI absorption is decreased in patients with hepatitis, cirrhosis, or biliary obstruction
Metabolism: Metabolic fate unknown

Half-life, biologic: 66-84 minutes

Elimination: 9% excreted unchanged in urine

Usual Dosage Oral:

Riboflavin deficiency:

Children: 2.5-10 mg/day in divided doses

Adults: 5-30 mg/day in divided doses

Recommended daily allowance:

Children: 0.4-1.8 mg

Adults: 1.2-1.7 mg

Test Interactions Large doses may interfere with urinalysis based on spectrometry; may cause false elevations in fluorometric determinations of catecholamines and urobilinogen

Patient Information Take with food; large doses may cause bright yellow or orange urine

Additional Information Dietary sources of riboflavin include liver, kidney, dairy products, green vegetables, eggs, whole grain cereals, yeast, mushroom

Dosage Forms Tablet: 25 mg, 50 mg, 100 mg

Rid-A-Pain® [OTC] *see* Benzocaine *on page 121*

Ridaura® *see* Auranofin *on page 103*

RID® [OTC] *see* Pyrethrins *on page 959*

Rifabutin (rif a bu′ tin)

Related Information

Antimicrobial Drugs of Choice *on page 1298-1302*

Brand Names Mycobutin®

Synonyms Ansamycin

Use Adjunctive therapy for the prevention of disseminated *Mycobacterium avium* complex (MAC) in patients with advanced HIV infection

Pregnancy Risk Factor B

Contraindications Hypersensitivity to rifabutin or any other rifamycins; rifabutin is contraindicated in patients with a WBC <1000/mm^3 or a platelet count <50,000 mm^3

Warnings/Precautions Rifabutin as a single agent must not be administered to patients with active tuberculosis since its use may lead to the development of tuberculosis that is resistant to both rifabutin and rifampin; rifabutin should be discontinued in patients with AST >500 IU/L or if total bilirubin is >3 mg/dL. Use with caution in patients with liver impairment; modification of dosage should be considered in patients with renal impairment.

Adverse Reactions

>10%:

Dermatologic: Rash

Hematologic: Neutropenia, leukopenia

Miscellaneous: Discolored urine

1% to 10%:

Central nervous system: Headache

Gastrointestinal: Vomiting, nausea, abdominal pain, diarrhea, anorexia, flatulence, eructation

Hematologic: Anemia, thrombocytopenia

Neuromuscular & skeletal: Myalgia

<1%:

Cardiovascular: Chest pain

Central nervous system: Fever, insomnia

Gastrointestinal: Dyspepsia, flatulence, nausea, vomiting, taste perversion

Overdosage/Toxicology Symptoms of overdose include nausea, vomiting, hepatotoxicity, lethargy, CNS depression; treatment is supportive; hemodialysis will remove rifabutin, its effect on outcome is unknown

Drug Interactions Decreased plasma concentration (due to induction of liver enzymes) of verapamil, methadone, digoxin, cyclosporine, corticosteroids, oral anticoagulants, theophylline, barbiturates, chloramphenicol, ketoconazole, oral contraceptives, quinidine, halothane

Mechanism of Action Inhibits DNA-dependent RNA polymerase at the beta subunit which prevents chain initiation

Pharmacodynamics/Kinetics

Absorption: Oral: Readily absorbed 53%

Distribution: V$_d$: 9.32 L/kg; distributes to body tissues including the lungs, liver, spleen, eyes, and kidneys

Protein binding: 85%

Metabolism: To active and inactive metabolites

Bioavailability: Absolute, 20% in HIV patients

Half life, terminal: 45 hours (range: 16-69 hours)

(Continued)

Rifabutin *(Continued)*

Peak serum level: Within 2-4 hours

Elimination: Renal and biliary clearance of unchanged drugs is 10%; 30% excreted in feces; 53% in urine as metabolites

Usual Dosage Oral:

Children: Efficacy and safety of rifabutin have not been established in children; a limited number of HIV-positive children with MAC have been given rifabutin for MAC prophylaxis; doses of 5 mg/kg/day have been useful

Adults: 300 mg once daily; for patients who experience gastrointestinal upset, rifabutin can be administered 150 mg twice daily with food

Monitoring Parameters Periodic liver function tests, CBC with differential, platelet count

Patient Information May discolor urine, tears, sweat, or other body fluids to a red-orange color; take 1 hour before or 2 hours after a meal on an empty stomach; soft contact lenses may be permanently stained; report to physician any severe or persistent flu-like symptoms, nausea, vomiting, dark urine or pale stools, or unusual bleeding or bruising; can be taken with meals or sprinkled on applesauce

Nursing Implications Administer with meals

Dosage Forms Capsule: 150 mg

Rifadin® *see* Rifampin *on this page*

Rifampicin *see* Rifampin *on this page*

Rifampin *(rif′ am pin)*

Related Information

Antimicrobial Drugs of Choice *on page 1298-1302*

Recommendations of the Advisory Council on the Elimination of Tuberculosis *on page 1303-1304*

Brand Names Rifadin®; Rimactane®

Synonyms Rifampicin

Use Management of active tuberculosis; eliminate meningococci from asymptomatic carriers; prophylaxis of *Haemophilus influenzae* type b infection; used in combination with other anti-infectives in the treatment of staphylococcal infections

Pregnancy Risk Factor C

Contraindications Hypersensitivity to rifampin or any component

Warnings/Precautions Use with caution in patients with liver impairment; modification of dosage should be considered in patients with severe liver impairment; use with caution in patients with porphyria; monitor closely if intermittent therapy is used; hypersensitivity reactions and thrombocytopenia occur more frequently in this setting

Adverse Reactions

1% to 10%:

Gastrointestinal: Diarrhea, stomach cramps

Miscellaneous: Discoloration of urine, feces, saliva, sputum, sweat, and tears (reddish orange); fungal overgrowth

<1%:

Central nervous system: Drowsiness, fatigue, ataxia, confusion, fever, headache

Dermatologic: Rash, pruritus

Gastrointestinal: Nausea, vomiting, stomatitis

Hematologic: Eosinophilia, blood dyscrasias (leukopenia, thrombocytopenia)

Hepatic: Hepatitis

Local: Irritation at the I.V. site

Renal: Renal failure

Miscellaneous: Flu-like syndrome

Overdosage/Toxicology Symptoms of overdose include nausea, vomiting, hepatotoxicity, lethargy, CNS depression; treatment is supportive

Drug Interactions Inducer of both Cytochrome P-450 3A and cytochrome P-450 2D6

Decreased effect: Rifampin induces liver enzymes which may decrease the plasma concentration of verapamil, methadone, digoxin, cyclosporine, corticosteroids, oral anticoagulants, theophylline, barbiturates, chloramphenicol, ketoconazole, oral contraceptives, quinidine, halothane, ketoconazole

Stability

Rifampin powder is reddish brown. Intact vials should be stored at room temperature and protected from excessive heat and light.

Reconstituted vials are stable for 24 hours at room temperature

Stability of parenteral admixture at room temperature (25°C) is 4 hours

Comments: Do not use sodium chloride as a diluent, rifampin has a reduced stability in NS

Mechanism of Action Inhibits bacterial RNA synthesis by binding to the beta subunit of DNA-dependent RNA polymerase, blocking RNA transcription

Pharmacodynamics/Kinetics

Absorption: Oral: Well absorbed

Time to peak serum concentration: Oral: 2-4 hours and persisting for up to 24 hours; food may delay or slightly reduce

Distribution: Crosses the blood-brain barrier well

Relative diffusion of antimicrobial agents from blood into cerebrospinal fluid (CSF): Adequate with or without inflammation (exceeds usual MICs)

Ratio of CSF to blood level (%):

Inflamed meninges: 25

Protein binding: 80%

Metabolism: Highly lipophilic; metabolized in the liver, undergoes enterohepatic recycling

Half-life: 3-4 hours, prolonged with hepatic impairment

End stage renal disease: 1.8-11 hours

Elimination: Undergoes enterohepatic recycling; principally excreted unchanged in the feces (60% to 65%) and urine (~30%); excreted unchanged: 15% to 30%; plasma rifampin concentrations are not significantly affected by hemodialysis or peritoneal dialysis

Usual Dosage I.V. infusion dose is the same as for the oral route

Tuberculosis therapy: Oral:

Note: A four-drug regimen (isoniazid, rifampin, pyrazinamide, and either streptomycin or ethambutol) is preferred for the initial, empiric treatment of TB. When the drug susceptibility results are available, the regimen should be altered as appropriate.

Patients with TB and without HIV infection:

OPTION 1:

Isoniazid resistance rate <4%: Administer daily isoniazid, rifampin, and pyrazinamide for 8 weeks followed by isoniazid and rifampin daily or directly observed therapy (DOT) 2-3 times/week for 16 weeks

If isoniazid resistance rate is not documented, ethambutol or streptomycin should also be administered until susceptibility to isoniazid or rifampin is demonstrated. Continue treatment for at least 6 months or 3 months beyond culture conversion.

OPTION 2: Administer daily isoniazid, rifampin, pyrazinamide, and either streptomycin or ethambutol for 2 weeks followed by DOT 2 times/week administration of the same drugs for 6 weeks, and subsequently, with isoniazid and rifampin DOT 2 times/week administration for 16 weeks

OPTION 3: Administer isoniazid, rifampin, pyrazinamide, and either ethambutol or streptomycin by DOT 3 times/week for 6 months

Patients with TB and with HIV infection:

Administer any of the above OPTIONS 1, 2 or 3, however, treatment should be continued for a total of 9 months and at least 6 months beyond culture conversion

Note: Some experts recommend that the duration of therapy should be extended to 9 months for patients with disseminated disease, miliary disease, disease involving the bones or joints, or tuberculosis lymphadenitis

Infants and Children <12 years of age: Oral:

Daily therapy: 10-20 mg/kg/day in divided doses every 12-24 hours (maximum: 600 mg/day)

Directly observed therapy (DOT): Twice weekly: 10-20 mg/kg (maximum: 600 mg)

DOT: 3 times/week: 10-20 mg/kg (maximum: 600 mg)

Adults: Oral:

Daily therapy: 10 mg/kg/day (maximum: 600 mg/day)

Directly observed therapy (DOT): Twice weekly: 10 mg/kg (maximum: 600 mg)

DOT: Three times weekly: 10 mg/kg (maximum: 600 mg)

H. influenzae prophylaxis: Oral:

Neonates <1 month: 10 mg/kg/day every 24 hours for 4 days

Infants and Children: 20 mg/kg/day every 24 hours for 4 days, not to exceed 600 mg/dose

Adults: 600 mg every 24 hours for 4 days

Meningococcal prophylaxis: Oral:

<1 month: 10 mg/kg/day in divided doses every 12 hours for 2 days

Infants and Children: 20 mg/kg/day in divided doses every 12 hours for 2 days

Adults: 600 mg every 12 hours for 2 days

(Continued)

Rifampin *(Continued)*

Nasal carriers of *Staphylococcus aureus*: Oral:
Children: 15 mg/kg/day divided every 12 hours for 5-10 days in combination with other antibiotics
Adults: 600 mg/day for 5-10 days in combination with other antibiotics

Synergy for *Staphylococcus aureus* infections: Oral: Adults: 300-600 mg twice daily with other antibiotics

Dosing adjustment in hepatic impairment: Dose reductions are necessary to reduce hepatotoxicity

Monitoring Parameters Periodic monitoring of liver function (AST, ALT), CBC; hepatic status and mental status, sputum culture, chest x-ray 2-3 months into treatment

Test Interactions Positive Coombs' reaction [direct], inhibit standard assay's ability to measure serum folate and B$_{12}$

Patient Information May discolor urine, tears, sweat, or other body fluids to a red-orange color; take 1 hour before or 2 hours after a meal on an empty stomach; soft contact lenses may be permanently stained; report to physician any severe or persistent flu-like symptoms, nausea, vomiting, dark urine or pale stools, or unusual bleeding or bruising

Nursing Implications Give on an empty stomach (ie, 1 hour prior to, or 2 hours after meals) to increase total absorption

Dosage Forms
Capsule: 150 mg, 300 mg
Injection: 600 mg

Extemporaneous Preparations Rifampin oral suspension can be compounded with simple syrup or wild cherry syrup at a concentration of 10 mg/mL; the suspension is stable for 4 weeks at room temperature or in a refrigerator when stored in a glass amber prescription bottle. However, there are some experts who do not recommend using rifampin syrup formulated from capsules due to conflicting reports indicating that the product is unstable (30% of labeled potency after preparation).

rIFN-A *see* Interferon Alfa-2a *on page 581*

rIFN-α2 *see* Interferon Alfa-2b *on page 583*

RIG *see* Rabies Immune Globulin, Human *on page 971*

Rimactane® *see* Rifampin *on page 982*

Rimantadine Hydrochloride (ri man' ti deen)

Brand Names Flumadine®

Use Prophylaxis (adults and children >1 year) and treatment (adults) of influenza A viral infection

Pregnancy Risk Factor C

Pregnancy/Breast Feeding Implications Embryotoxic in high dose rat studies; avoid use in nursing mothers due to potential adverse effect in infants; rimantadine is concentrated in milk

Contraindications Hypersensitivity to drugs of the adamantine class, including rimantadine and amantadine

Warnings/Precautions Use with caution in patients with renal and hepatic dysfunction; avoid use, if possible, in patients with recurrent and eczematoid dermatitis, uncontrolled psychosis, or severe psychoneurosis. An increase in seizure incidence may occur in patients with seizure disorders; discontinue drug if seizures occur; consider the development of resistance during rimantadine treatment of the index case as likely if failure of rimantadine prophylaxis among family contact occurs and if index case is a child; viruses exhibit cross-resistance between amantadine and rimantadine.

Adverse Reactions
1% to 10%:
Cardiovascular: Orthostatic hypotension, edema
Central nervous system: Dizziness, confusion, headache, insomnia, difficulty in concentrating, anxiety, restlessness, irritability, hallucinations; incidence of CNS side effects may be less than that associated with amantadine
Gastrointestinal: Nausea, vomiting, dry mouth, abdominal pain, anorexia
Genitourinary: Urinary retention

Overdosage/Toxicology Agitation, hallucinations, ventricular cardiac arrhythmias (torsade de pointes and PVCs), slurred speech, anticholinergic effects (dry mouth, urinary retention and mydriasis), ataxia, tremor, myoclonus, seizures and death have been reported with amantadine, a related drug; treatment is symptomatic (do not use physostigmine); tachyarrhythmias may be treated with beta-blockers such as propranolol; dialysis is not recommended except possibly in renal failure

Drug Interactions
Acetaminophen: Reduction in AUC and peak concentration of rimantadine
Aspirin: Peak plasma and AUC concentrations of rimantadine are reduced
Cimetidine: Rimantadine clearance is decreased (~16%)

Mechanism of Action Exerts its inhibitory effect on three antigenic subtypes of influenza A virus (H1N1, H2N2, H3N2) early in the viral replicative cycle, possibly inhibiting the uncoating process; it has no activity against influenza B virus and is 2- to 8-fold more active than amantadine

Pharmacodynamics/Kinetics
Absorption: Tablet and syrup formulations are equally absorbed; T_{max}: 6 hours
Metabolism: Extensive in the liver
Half-life: 25.4 hours (increased in elderly)
Elimination: <25% of dose excreted in urine as unchanged drug; hemodialysis does not contribute to the clearance of rimantadine; no data exist establishing a correlation between plasma concentration and antiviral effect

Usual Dosage Oral:
Prophylaxis:
Children <10 years: 5 mg/kg give once daily; maximum: 150 mg
Children >10 years and Adults: 100 mg twice daily; decrease to 100 mg/day in elderly or in patients with severe hepatic or renal impairment (Cl_{cr} ≤10 mL/minute)
Treatment: Adults: 100 mg twice daily; decrease to 100 mg/day in elderly or in patients with severe hepatic or renal impairment (Cl_{cr} ≤10 mL/minute)

Administration Initiation of aramantadine within 48 hours of the onset of influenza A illness halves the duration of illness and significantly reduces the duration of viral shedding and increased peripheral airways resistance; continue therapy for 5-7 days after symptoms begin

Monitoring Parameters Monitor for CNS or GI effects in elderly or patients with renal or hepatic impairment

Dosage Forms
Syrup: 50 mg/5 mL (60 mL, 240 mL, 480 mL)
Tablet: 100 mg

Riobin® see Riboflavin on page 980

Risperdal® see Risperidone on this page

Risperidone (ris per' i done)

Related Information
Antipsychotic Agents Comparison on page 1255

Brand Names Risperdal®

Use Management of psychotic disorders (eg, schizophrenia); nonpsychotic symptoms associated with dementia in elderly

Contraindications Known hypersensitivity to any component of the product

Adverse Reactions
1% to 10%:
Anticholinergic: Dry mouth (problem for denture user), urinary retention, constipation, adynamic ileus, overflow incontinence, blurred vision
Cardiovascular: Hypotension (especially orthostatic), tachycardia, arrhythmias, abnormal T waves with prolonged ventricular repolarization; EKG changes, syncope
Central nervous system: Sedation (occurs at daily doses ≥20 mg/day), headache, dizziness, restlessness, anxiety, extrapyramidal reactions, dystonic reactions, pseudoparkinson signs and symptoms, tardive dyskinesia, neuroleptic malignant syndrome, altered central temperature regulation
Dermatologic: Photosensitivity (rare)
Endocrine & metabolic: Amenorrhea, galactorrhea, gynecomastia
Gastrointestinal: Constipation, adynamic ileus, GI upset, dry mouth (problem for denture user), nausea and anorexia, weight gain
Genitourinary: Urinary retention, overflow incontinence, priapism, sexual dysfunction (up to 60%)
Hematologic: Agranulocytosis, leukopenia (usually in patients with large doses for prolonged periods)
Hepatic: Cholestatic jaundice
Ocular: Blurred vision, retinal pigmentation, decreased visual acuity (may be irreversible)
<1%: Seizures

Drug Interactions
Increased toxicity: Quinidine, warfarin
May antagonize effects of levodopa; carbamazepine decreases risperidone serum concentrations; clozapine decreases clearance of risperidone
(Continued)

Risperidone (Continued)

Mechanism of Action Risperidone is a benzisoxazole derivative, mixed serotonin-dopamine antagonist; binds to 5-HT$_2$ receptors in the CNS and in the periphery with a very high affinity; binds to dopamine-D$_2$ receptors with less affinity. The binding affinity to the dopamine-D$_2$ receptor is 20 times lower than the 5-HT$_2$ affinity. The addition of serotonin antagonism to dopamine antagonism (classic neuroleptic mechanism) is thought to improve negative symptoms of psychoses and reduce the incidence of extrapyramidal side effects.

Pharmacodynamics/Kinetics
Absorption: Oral: Rapid
Metabolism: Extensive by cytochrome P-450
Protein binding: Plasma: 90%
Half-life: 24 hours (risperidone and its active metabolite)
Time to peak: Peak plasma concentrations within 1 hour

Usual Dosage
Recommended starting dose: 1 mg twice daily; slowly increase to the optimum range of 4-8 mg/day; daily dosages >10 mg does not appear to confer any additional benefit, and the incidence of extrapyramidal reactions is higher than with lower doses

Dosing adjustment in renal, hepatic impairment, and elderly: Starting dose of 0.5 mg twice daily is advisable
Nursing Implications Monitor and observe for extrapyramidal effects, orthostatic blood pressure changes for 3-5 days after starting or increasing dose
Dosage Forms Tablet: 1 mg, 2 mg, 3 mg, 4 mg

Ritalin® see Methylphenidate Hydrochloride on page 722

Ritalin-SR® see Methylphenidate Hydrochloride on page 722

Ritodrine Hydrochloride (ri' toe dreen)

Brand Names Pre-Par®; Yutopar®
Use Inhibits uterine contraction in preterm labor
Pregnancy Risk Factor B
Contraindications Do not use before 20th week of pregnancy, cardiac arrhythmias, pheochromocytoma
Warnings/Precautions Monitor hydration status and blood glucose concentrations; fatal maternal pulmonary edema has been reported, sometimes after delivery; fluid overload must be avoided, hydration levels should be monitored closely; if pulmonary edema occurs, the drug should be discontinued; use with caution in patients with moderate pre-eclampsia, diabetes, or migraine; some products may contain sulfites; maternal deaths have been reported in patients treated with ritodrine and concurrent corticosteroids (pulmonary edema)
Adverse Reactions
>10%:
Cardiovascular: Increases in maternal and fetal heart rates and maternal hypertension, palpitations
Endocrine & metabolic: Temporary hyperglycemia
Gastrointestinal: Nausea, vomiting
Neuromuscular & skeletal: Tremor
1% to 10%:
Cardiovascular: Chest pain
Central nervous system: Nervousness, anxiety, restlessness
<1%:
Hepatic: Impaired liver function
Miscellaneous: Anaphylactic shock, ketoacidosis
Overdosage/Toxicology Symptoms of overdose include tachycardia, palpitations, hypotension, nervousness, nausea, vomiting, tremor; use an appropriate beta-blocker as an antidote
Drug Interactions
Decreased effect with beta-blockers
Increased effect/toxicity with meperidine, sympathomimetics, diazoxide, magnesium, betamethasone (pulmonary edema), potassium-depleting diuretics, general anesthetics
Stability Stable for 48 hours at room temperature after dilution in 500 mL of NS, D$_5$W, or LR I.V. solutions
Mechanism of Action Tocolysis due to its uterine beta$_2$-adrenergic receptor stimulating effects; this agent's beta$_2$ effects can also cause bronchial relaxation and vascular smooth muscle stimulation
Pharmacodynamics/Kinetics
Absorption: Oral: Rapid
Distribution: Crosses the placenta

Protein binding: 32%

Metabolism: In the liver

Half-life: 15 hours

Time to peak serum concentration: Within 0.5-1 hour

Elimination: In urine as unchanged drug and inactive conjugates

Usual Dosage Adults:

I.V.: 50-100 mcg/minute; increase by 50 mcg/minute every 10 minutes; continue for 12 hours after contractions have stopped

Oral: Start 30 minutes before stopping I.V. infusion; 10 mg every 2 hours for 24 hours, then 10-20 mg every 4-6 hours up to 120 mg/day

Removed by hemodialysis

Administration Monitor amount of I.V. fluid administered to prevent fluid overload; place patient in left lateral recumbent position to reduce risk of hypotension; use microdrip chamber or I.V. pump to control infusion rate

Monitoring Parameters Hematocrit, serum potassium, glucose, colloidal osmotic pressure, heart rate, and uterine contractions

Patient Information Remain in bed during infusion

Dosage Forms

Injection: 10 mg/mL (5 mL); 15 mg/mL (10 mL)

Tablet: 10 mg

Rocuronium Bromide (roe kyoor oh' nee um)

Related Information

Neuromuscular Blocking Agents Comparison Charts on page 1276-1278

Brand Names Zemuron®

Synonyms ORG 946

Use Inpatient and outpatient use as an adjunct to general anesthesia to facilitate both rapid-sequence and routine tracheal intubation, and to provide skeletal muscle relaxation during surgery or mechanical ventilation

Pregnancy Risk Factor B

Contraindications Known hypersensitivity to rocuronium or vecuronium

Warnings/Precautions Use with caution in patients with cardiovascular or pulmonary disease, hepatic impairment, neuromuscular disease, myasthenia gravis, dehydration (may alter neuromuscular blocking effects); respiratory acidosis, hypomagnesemia, hypokalemia, or hypocalcemia (may enhance actions) and the elderly; ventilation must be supported during neuromuscular blockade

Adverse Reactions

>1%: Cardiovascular: Transient hypotension and hypertension

<1%:

Cardiovascular: Arrhythmias, abnormal EKG, tachycardia, edema

Dermatologic: Rash, injection site pruritus

Gastrointestinal: Nausea, vomiting

Respiratory: Bronchospasm, wheezing, rhonchi

Miscellaneous: Hiccups

(Continued)

Rocuronium Bromide *(Continued)*

Overdosage/Toxicology Symptoms of overdose include prolonged skeletal muscle block, muscle weakness and apnea; treatment is maintenance of a patent airway and controlled ventilation until recovery of normal neuromuscular block is observed, further recovery may be facilitated by administering an anticholinesterase agent (eg, neostigmine, edrophonium, or pyridostigmine) with atropine, to antagonize the skeletal muscle relaxation; support of the cardiovascular system with fluids and pressors may be necessary

Drug Interactions

Decreased effect: Chronic carbamazepine or phenytoin can shorten the duration of neuromuscular blockade; phenylephrine can severely inhibit neuromuscular blockade

Increased effect: Infusion requirements are reduced 35% to 40% during anesthesia with enflurane or isoflurane

Increased toxicity: Aminoglycosides, vancomycin, tetracyclines, bacitracin

Stability Store under refrigeration (2°C to 8°C), do not freeze; when stored at room temperature, it is stable for 30 days; unlike vecuronium, it is stable in 0.9% sodium chloride and 5% dextrose in water, this mixture should be used within 24 hours of preparation

Mechanism of Action Blocks acetylcholine from binding to receptors on motor endplate inhibiting depolarization

Pharmacodynamics/Kinetics

Onset: Good intubation conditions within 1-2 minutes; maximum neuromuscular blockade within 4 minutes

Duration: ~30 minutes (with standard doses, increases with higher doses)

Metabolism: Undergoes minimal hepatic metabolism

Elimination: Primarily through hepatic uptake and biliary excretion

Usual Dosage

Children:

Initial: 0.6 mg/kg under halothane anesthesia produce excellent to good intubating conditions within 1 minute and will provide a median time of 41 minutes of clinical relaxation in children 3 months to 1 year of age, and 27 minutes in children 1-12 years

Maintenance: 0.075-0.125 mg/kg administered upon return of T_1 to 25% of control provides clinical relaxation for 7-10 minutes

Adults:

Tracheal intubation: I.V.:

Initial: 0.6 mg/kg is expected to provide approximately 31 minutes of clinical relaxation under opioid/nitrous oxide/oxygen anesthesia with neuromuscular block sufficient for intubation attained in 1-2 minutes; lower doses (0.45 mg/kg) may be used to provide 22 minutes of clinical relaxation with median time to neuromuscular block of 1-3 minutes; maximum blockade is achieved in <4 minutes

Maximum: 0.9-1.2 mg/kg may be given during surgery under opioid/nitrous oxide/oxygen anesthesia without adverse cardiovascular effects and is expected to provide 58-67 minutes of clinical relaxation; neuromuscular blockade sufficient for intubation is achieved in <2 minutes with maximum blockade in <3 minutes

Maintenance: 0.1, 0.15, and 0.2 mg/kg administered at 25% recovery of control T_1 (defined as 3 twitches of train-of-four) provides a median of 12, 17, and 24 minutes of clinical duration under anesthesia

Rapid sequence intubation: 0.6-1.2 mg/kg in appropriately premedicated and anesthetized patients with excellent or good intubating conditions within 2 minutes

Continuous infusion: Initial: 0.01-0.012 mg/kg/minute only after early evidence of spontaneous recovery of neuromuscular function is evident

Dosing adjustment in hepatic impairment: Reductions are necessary in patients with liver disease

Administration Administer I.V. only

Monitoring Parameters Peripheral nerve stimulator measuring twitch response, heart rate, blood pressure, assisted ventilation status

Nursing Implications Concurrent sedation and analgesia are needed

Additional Information Dose based on actual body weight

Dosage Forms Injection: 10 mg/mL

Roferon-A® *see* Interferon Alfa-2a *on page 581*

Rogaine® *see* Minoxidil *on page 744*

Rolaids® **Calcium Rich [OTC]** *see* Calcium Carbonate *on page 161*

Romazicon™ *see* Flumazenil *on page 466*

Rondec® Drops *see* Carbinoxamine and Pseudoephedrine *on page 181*

Rondec® Filmtab® *see* Carbinoxamine and Pseudoephedrine *on page 181*

Rondec® Syrup *see* Carbinoxamine and Pseudoephedrine *on page 181*

Rondec-TR® *see* Carbinoxamine and Pseudoephedrine *on page 181*

Rowasa® *see* Mesalamine *on page 691*

Roxanol™ *see* Morphine Sulfate *on page 756*

Roxanol SR™ *see* Morphine Sulfate *on page 756*

Roxicet® *see* Oxycodone and Acetaminophen *on page 826*

Roxiprin® *see* Oxycodone and Aspirin *on page 828*

RTCA *see* Ribavirin *on page 979*

Rubella and Measles Vaccines, Combined *see* Measles and Rubella Vaccines, Combined *on page 667*

Rubella and Mumps Vaccines, Combined (rue bell' a)
Related Information
Immunization Guidelines *on page 1389-1405*
Brand Names Biavax®_{II}
Use Promote active immunity to rubella and mumps by inducing production of antibodies
Pregnancy Risk Factor X
Contraindications Known hypersensitivity to neomycin, eggs; children <1 year, pregnant women, primary immunodeficient patients, patients receiving immunosuppressant drugs except corticosteroids
Warnings/Precautions Women planning on becoming pregnant in the next 3 months should not be vaccinated
Adverse Reactions
1% to 10%:
Central nervous system: Febrile seizures, fever
Local: Soreness, burning, stinging, allergic reactions
Drug Interactions Immune globulin, whole blood
Stability Refrigerate, discard unused portion within 8 hours, protect from light
Usual Dosage Children >12 months and Adults: 1 vial in outer aspect of the upper arm; children vaccinated before 12 months of age should be revaccinated
Administration Administer S.C. only
Test Interactions Temporary suppression of TB skin test
Patient Information
Mumps vaccine: A little swelling of the glands in the cheeks and under the jaw that lasts for a few days; this could happen from 1-2 weeks after getting the mumps vaccine; this happens rarely
Rubella vaccine: Swelling of the lymph glands in the neck or a rash that lasts 1-2 days; this could happen 1-2 weeks after getting the rubella vaccine in about 1/7 children who get the vaccine
Mild pain or stiffness in the joints that may last up to 3 days; this could happen from 1-3 weeks after getting the shot. this problem happens to about 1/100 children who get the shot and 25/100 adults who get the shot. Women have this problem more than men and it may happen in up to 40 women out of every 100. Rarely, pain or stiffness can last for months or longer and can come and go.
Painful swelling of the joints (arthritis) happens to <1/100 children who get the rubella vaccine. About 10/100 adults can also have this problem, which usually lasts a few days to a week. Rarely, this swelling has been reported to last longer, or to come and go. Damage to the joints is very rare.
Pain or numbness, or "pins and needles" feeling in the hands and feet that lasts for a short time; this happens rarely
Nursing Implications Children immunized before 12 months of age should be reimmunized
Additional Information Federal law requires that the date of administration, the vaccine manufacturer, lot number of vaccine, and the administering person's name, title and address be entered into the patient's permanent medical record
Dosage Forms Injection (mixture of 2 viruses):
1. Wistar RA 27/3 strain of rubella virus
2. Jeryl Lynn (B level) mumps strain grown cell cultures of chick embryo

Rubella, Measles and Mumps Vaccines, Combined *see* Measles, Mumps, and Rubella Vaccines, Combined *on page 668*

Rubella Virus Vaccine, Live (rue bell' a)

Related Information
Immunization Guidelines *on page 1389-1405*
Vaccines *on page 1386-1388*

Brand Names Meruvax® II

Synonyms German Measles Vaccine

Use All adults, both male and female, lacking documentation of live vaccine on or after first birthday, or laboratory evidence of immunity (particularly women of childbearing age and young adults who work in or congregate in hospitals, colleges, and on military bases) should be vaccinated. Susceptible travelers should be vaccinated.

Pregnancy Risk Factor X

Warnings/Precautions Pregnancy, immunocompromised persons, history of anaphylactic reaction following receipt of neomycin; do not administer with other live vaccines

Adverse Reactions

>10%:
  Dermatologic: Local tenderness and erythema, urticaria, rash
  Neuromuscular & skeletal: Arthralgias

1% to 10%:
  Central nervous system: Malaise, fever, headache
  Miscellaneous: Lymphadenopathy, sore throat

<1%:
  Ocular: Optic neuritis
  Miscellaneous: Hypersensitivity, allergic reactions to the vaccine

Drug Interactions Decreased effect when immune globulin is given within 3 months and with concurrent use of corticosteroids and other immunosuppressant agents

Stability Refrigerate, discard reconstituted vaccine after 8 hours; store at 2°C to 8°C (36°F to 46°F); ship vaccine at 10°C; may use dry ice, protect from light

Mechanism of Action Rubella vaccine is a live attenuated vaccine that contains the Wistar Institute RA 27/3 strain, which is adapted to and propagated in human diploid cell culture. It is the only strain of rubella vaccine marketed in the U.S. Antibody titers after immunization last 6 years without significant decline; 90% of those vaccinated have protection for at least 15 years.

Pharmacodynamics/Kinetics

Onset of effect: Antibodies to the vaccine are detectable within 2-4 weeks following immunization

Duration: Protection against both clinical rubella and asymptomatic viremia is probably life-long. Vaccine-induced antibody levels have been shown to persist for at least 10 years without substantial decline. If the present pattern continues, it will provide a basis for the expectation that immunity following vaccination will be permanent. However, continued surveillance will be required to demonstrate this point.

Usual Dosage Children ≥12 months and Adults: S.C.: 0.5 mL in outer aspect of upper arm; children vaccinated before 12 months of age should be revaccinated

Test Interactions May depress tuberculin skin test sensitivity

Patient Information

Swelling of the lymph glands in the neck or a rash that lasts 1-2 days; this could happen 1-2 weeks after getting the rubella vaccine in about 1/7 children who get the vaccine

Mild pain or stiffness in the joints that may last up to 3 days; this could happen from 1-3 weeks after getting the shot. This problem happens to about 1/100 children who get the shot and 25/100 adults who get the shot. Women have this problem more than men and it may happen in up to 40 women out of every 100. Rarely, pain or stiffness can last for months or longer and can come and go.

Painful swelling of the joints (arthritis) happens to <1/100 children who get the rubella vaccine. About 10/100 adults can also have this problem, which usually lasts a few days to a week. Rarely, this swelling has been reported to last longer, or to come and go. Damage to the joints is very rare.

Pain or numbness, or "pins and needles" feeling in the hands and feet that lasts for a short time; this happens rarely

Nursing Implications Reconstituted vaccine should be used within 8 hours; S.C. injection only

Additional Information Live virus vaccine: Federal law requires that the date of administration, the vaccine manufacturer, lot number of vaccine, and the administering person's name, title and address be entered into the patient's permanent record

Women who are pregnant when vaccinated or who become pregnant within 3 months of vaccination should be counseled on the theoretical risks to the fetus. The risk of rubella-associated malformations in these women is so small as to be negligible. MMR is the vaccine of choice if recipients are likely to be susceptible to measles or mumps as well as to rubella.

Dosage Forms Injection, single dose: 1000 $TCID_{50}$ (Wistar RA 27/3 Strain)

Rubeola vaccine *see* Measles Virus Vaccine, Live *on page 670*

Rubex® *see* Doxorubicin Hydrochloride *on page 370*

Rubidomycin Hydrochloride *see* Daunorubicin Hydrochloride *on page 304*

Rubramin-PC® *see* Cyanocobalamin *on page 282*

Rufen® *see* Ibuprofen *on page 561*

Rum-K® *see* Potassium Chloride *on page 906*

Ru-Vert-M® *see* Meclizine Hydrochloride *on page 674*

Rythmol® *see* Propafenone Hydrochloride *on page 940*

Sabin *see* Polio Vaccines *on page 898*

Safe Tussin 30 Liquid® [OTC] *see* Guaifenesin and Dextromethorphan *on page 517*

Salacid® *see* Salicylic Acid *on this page*

SalAc® [OTC] *see* Salicylic Acid *on this page*

Salbutamol *see* Albuterol *on page 33*

Saleto-200® [OTC] *see* Ibuprofen *on page 561*

Saleto-400® *see* Ibuprofen *on page 561*

Salflex® *see* Salsalate *on page 993*

Salgesic® *see* Salsalate *on page 993*

Salicylazosulfapyridine *see* Sulfasalazine *on page 1043*

Salicylic Acid (sal i sill' ik)

Brand Names ClearAway®; Compound W® [OTC]; Hydrisalic™; Ionil® [OTC]; Keralyt®; Panscol®; P&S® [OTC]; SalAc® [OTC]; Salacid®; Saligel™; Trans-Ver-Sal®

Use Topically for its keratolytic effect in controlling seborrheic dermatitis or psoriasis of body and scalp, dandruff, and other scaling dermatoses; also used to remove warts, corns, and calluses

Pregnancy Risk Factor C

Contraindications Hypersensitivity to salicylic acid or any components; children <2 years of age

Warnings/Precautions Should not be used systemically, severe irritating effect on GI mucosa; use with caution in areas of ischemia; prolonged use over large areas, especially in children, may result in salicylate toxicity; do not apply on irritated, reddened, or infected skin; for external use only; avoid contact with eyes, face, and other mucous membranes

Adverse Reactions

>10%: Local: Burning and irritation at site of exposure on normal tissue

1% to 10%:

Central nervous system: Dizziness, mental confusion, headache,

Otic: Tinnitus

Respiratory: Hyperventilation

Overdosage/Toxicology Signs and symptoms of salicylate toxicity include nausea, vomiting, dizziness, tinnitus, loss of hearing, lethargy, diarrhea, psychic disturbances

Mechanism of Action Produces desquamation of hyperkeratotic epithelium via dissolution of the intercellular cement which causes the cornified tissue to swell, soften, macerate, and desquamate. Salicylic acid is keratolytic at concentrations of 3% to 6%; it becomes destructive to tissue at concentrations >6%. Concentrations of 6% to 60% are used to remove corns and warts and in the treatment of psoriasis and other hyperkeratotic disorders.

Pharmacodynamics/Kinetics

Absorption: Absorbed percutaneously, but systemic toxicity is unlikely with normal use

Time to peak serum concentration: Topical: Within 5 hours of application with occlusion

Elimination: Salicyluric acid (52%), salicylate glucuronides (42%), and salicylic acid (6%) are major metabolites identified in urine after percutaneous absorption

Usual Dosage

Lotion, cream, gel: Apply a thin layer to affected area once or twice daily

(Continued)

Salicylic Acid (Continued)

Plaster: Cut to size that covers the corn or callus, apply and leave in place for 48 hours; do not exceed 5 applications over a 14-day period

Solution: Apply a thin layer directly to wart using brush applicator once daily as directed for 1 week or until wart is removed

Patient Information When applying in concentrations >10%, protect surrounding tissue with petrolatum; do not use on open skin, avoid contact with eyes, mouth, and other mucous membranes

Nursing Implications For warts: Before applying product, soak area in warm water for 5 minutes; dry area thoroughly, then apply medication

Dosage Forms

Cream: 10% (60 g); 60% (56.7 g)

Disc: 40%

Gel: 6% (30 g); 12% (8 g); 17% (7.5 g, 15 g); 26% (8 g)

Liquid: 12% (10 mL); 17% (9.3 mL, 13.5 mL, 15 mL); 16.7% (15 mL); 20% (15 mL); 26% (10 mL)

Lotion: 3% (120 mL)

Ointment: 3% (90 g); 25% (60 g, 454 g); 60% (60 g, 454 g)

Patch, transdermal: 15%, 21%, 40%

Plaster: 40%, 50%

Shampoo: 2% (120 mL, 240 mL); 4% (120 mL)

Solution: 13.6% (9.3 mL), 17% (15 mL), 26% (15 mL)

Salicylsalicylic Acid see Salsalate on next page

Saligel™ see Salicylic Acid on previous page

Saline® [OTC] see Sodium Chloride on page 1012

Salk see Polio Vaccines on page 898

Salmeterol Xinafoate (sal me' te role)

Brand Names Serevent®

Use Maintenance treatment of asthma and in prevention of bronchospasm in patients >12 years of age with reversible obstructive airway disease, including patients with symptoms of nocturnal asthma, who require regular treatment with inhaled, short-acting beta$_2$ agonists; prevention of exercise-induced bronchospasm

Pregnancy Risk Factor C

Contraindications Hypersensitivity to salmeterol, adrenergic amines or any ingredients; need for acute bronchodilation

Warnings/Precautions Salmeterol is not meant to relieve acute asthmatic symptoms. Acute episodes should be treated with short-acting beta$_2$ agonist. Do not increase the frequency of salmeterol. Cardiovascular effects are not common with salmeterol when used in recommended doses. All beta agonists may cause elevation in blood pressure, heart rate, and result in excitement (CNS). Use with caution in patients with prostatic hypertrophy, diabetes, cardiovascular disorders, convulsive disorders, thyrotoxicosis, or others who are sensitive to the effects of sympathomimetic amines. Paroxysmal bronchospasm (which can be fatal) has been reported with this and other inhaled agents. If this occurs, discontinue treatment. The elderly may be at greater risk of cardiovascular side effects; safety and efficacy have not been established in children <12 years of age.

Adverse Reactions

>10%:

Central nervous system: Headache

Respiratory: Pharyngitis

1% to 10%:

Cardiovascular: Tachycardia, palpitations, elevation or depression of blood pressure, cardiac arrhythmias

Central nervous system: Nervousness, CNS stimulation, hyperactivity, insomnia, malaise, dizziness

Gastrointestinal: GI upset, diarrhea, nausea

Neuromuscular & skeletal: Tremors (may be more common in the elderly), myalgias, back pain, joint pain

Respiratory: Upper respiratory infection, cough, bronchitis

<1%: Immediate hypersensitivity reactions (rash, urticaria, bronchospasm)

Overdosage/Toxicology

Decontamination: Lavage/activated charcoal

Supportive therapy: Beta-blockers can be used for hyperadrenergic signs (use with caution in patients with bronchospasm)

Prudent use of a cardioselective beta-adrenergic blocker (eg, atenolol or metoprolol); keep in mind the potential for induction of bronchoconstriction in an asthmatic. Dialysis has not been shown to be of value in the treatment of an overdose with this agent.

Drug Interactions
Increased effect: Beta-adrenergic blockers (eg, propranolol)
Decreased toxicity (cardiovascular): MAO inhibitors, tricyclic antidepressants

Stability Store cannister with nozzle down; protect from freezing temperature and direct sunlight The therapeutic effect may decrease when the canister is cold therefore the canister should remain at room temperature. Do not store at temperatures >120°F.

Mechanism of Action Relaxes bronchial smooth muscle by selective action on beta$_2$-receptors with little effect on heart rate; because salmeterol acts locally in the lung, therapeutic effect is not predicted by plasma levels

Pharmacodynamics/Kinetics
Onset of action: 5-20 minutes (average 10 minutes)
Peak effect: 2-4 hours
Duration: 12 hours
Protein binding: 94% to 98%
Metabolism: Hydroxylated in liver
Half-life: 3-4 hours

Usual Dosage
Inhalation: 42 mcg (2 puffs) twice daily (12 hours apart) for maintenance and prevention of symptoms of asthma

Prevention of exercise-induced asthma: 42 mcg (2 puffs) 30-60 minutes prior to exercise; additional doses should not be used for 12 hours

Monitoring Parameters Pulmonary function tests, blood pressure, pulse, CNS stimulation

Patient Information Do not use to treat acute symptoms; do not exceed the prescribed dose of salmeterol; do not stop using inhaled or oral corticosteroids without medical advise even if you "feel better"; shake well before using. Avoid spraying in eyes, remove the canister and rinse the plastic case and cap under warm water and dry daily. Store canister with nozzle end down.

Nursing Implications Not to be used for the relief of acute attacks; monitor lung sounds, pulse, blood pressure. Before using, the inhaler must be shaken well; observe for wheezing after administration; if this occurs, call physician.

Dosage Forms Aerosol, oral: 21 mcg/spray [60 inhalations] (6.5 g), [120 inhalations] (13 g)

Salsalate (sal' sa late)

Brand Names Argesic®-SA; Artha-G®; Disalcid®; Mono-Gesic®; Salflex®; Salgesic®; Salsitab®

Synonyms Disalicylic Acid; Salicylsalicylic Acid

Use Treatment of minor pain or fever; arthritis

Pregnancy Risk Factor C

Contraindications GI ulcer or bleeding, known hypersensitivity to salsalate

Warnings/Precautions Use with caution in patients with platelet and bleeding disorders, renal dysfunction, erosive gastritis, or peptic ulcer disease, previous nonreaction does not guarantee future safe taking of medication; do not use aspirin in children <16 years of age for chickenpox or flu symptoms due to the association with Reye's syndrome

Adverse Reactions
>10%: Gastrointestinal: Nausea, heartburn, stomach pains, dyspepsia, epigastric discomfort
1% to 10%:
Central nervous system: Weakness, tiredness
Dermatologic: Skin rash
Gastrointestinal: Gastrointestinal ulceration
Hematologic: Hemolytic anemia
Respiratory: Troubled breathing
Miscellaneous: Anaphylactic shock
<1%:
Central nervous system: Insomnia, nervousness, jitters
Hematologic: Leukopenia, thrombocytopenia, iron deficiency anemia, does not appear to inhibit platelet aggregation, occult bleeding
Hepatic: Hepatotoxicity, hepatotoxicity
Renal: Impaired renal function
Respiratory: Bronchospasm

Overdosage/Toxicology Symptoms of overdose include respiratory alkalosis, hyperpnea, tachypnea, tinnitus, headache, hyperpyrexia, metabolic acidosis, hypoglycemia, coma. The "Done" nomogram is very helpful for estimating the severity of aspirin poisoning and directing treatment using serum salicylate levels. Treatment can also be based upon symptomatology.
(Continued)

Salsalate *(Continued)*

Salicylates

Toxic Symptoms	Treatment
Overdose	Induce emesis with ipecac, and/or lavage with saline, followed with activated charcoal
Dehydration	I.V. fluids with KCl (no D_5W only)
Metabolic acidosis (must be treated)	Sodium bicarbonate
Hyperthermia	Cooling blankets or sponge baths
Coagulopathy/hemorrhage	Vitamin K I.V.
Hypoglycemia (with coma, seizures, or change in mental status)	Dextrose 25 g I.V.
Seizures	Diazepam 5-10 mg I.V.

Drug Interactions
Decreased effect with urinary alkalinizers, antacids, corticosteroids; decreased effect of uricosurics, spironolactone
Increased effect/toxicity of oral anticoagulants, hypoglycemics, methotrexate

Mechanism of Action Inhibits prostaglandin synthesis, acts on the hypothalamus heat-regulating center to reduce fever, blocks prostaglandin synthetase action which prevents formation of the platelet-aggregating substance thromboxane A_2

Pharmacodynamics/Kinetics
Onset of action: Therapeutic effects occur within 3-4 days of continuous dosing
Absorption: Oral: Completely from the small intestine
Metabolism: Hydrolyzed in the liver to 2 moles of salicylic acid (active)
Half-life: 7-8 hours
Elimination: Almost totally excreted renally

Usual Dosage Adults: Oral: 3 g/day in 2-3 divided doses
Dosing comments in renal impairment: In patients with end stage renal disease undergoing hemodialysis: 750 mg twice daily with an additional 500 mg after dialysis

Test Interactions False-negative results for glucose oxidase urinary glucose tests (Clinistix®); false-positives using the cupric sulfate method (Clinitest®); also, interferes with Gerhardt test, VMA determination; 5-HIAA, xylose tolerance test and T_3 and T_4

Patient Information Do not self-medicate with other drug products containing aspirin; use antacids to relieve upset stomach; watch for bleeding gums or any signs of GI bleeding; take with food or milk to minimize GI distress, notify physician if ringing in ears or persistent GI pain occurs

Dosage Forms
Capsule: 500 mg
Tablet: 500 mg, 750 mg

Salsitab® *see* Salsalate *on previous page*

Salt *see* Sodium Chloride *on page 1012*

Salt Poor Albumin *see* Albumin, Human *on page 32*

Saluron® *see* Hydroflumethiazide *on page 549*

Sandimmune® *see* Cyclosporine *on page 290*

Sandoglobulin® *see* Immune Globulin, Intravenous *on page 571*

Sandostatin® *see* Octreotide Acetate *on page 812*

Sani-Supp® [OTC] *see* Glycerin *on page 506*

Sansert® *see* Methysergide Maleate *on page 727*

Santyl® *see* Collagenase *on page 273*

Sargramostim *(sar gram' oh stim)*
Related Information
Filgrastim *on page 454*
Brand Names Leukine™
Synonyms GM-CSF; Granulocyte-Macrophage Colony Stimulating Factor; rGM-CSF
Use
Myeloid reconstitution after autologous bone marrow transplantation: (FDA-labeled indication)

Non-Hodgkin's lymphoma (NHL)

Acute lymphoblastic leukemia (ALL)

Hodgkin's lymphoma

Bone marrow transplantation failure or engraftment delay (FDA-labeled indication): Patients who have undergone allogeneic or autologous BMT in whom engraftment is delayed or has failed. Survival benefit is relatively greater in those patients demonstrating one or more of the following characteristics:

Autologous BMT failure or engraftment delay

No previous total body irradiation

Malignancy other than leukemia

Multiple organ failure score ≤2

Unlabeled uses:

Increase WBC counts in patients with myelodysplastic syndromes and in AIDS patients receiving zidovudine

Decrease nadir of leukopenia secondary to myelosuppressive chemotherapy and decrease myelosuppression in preleukemic patients.

Correct neutropenia in aplastic anemia patients.

Decrease transplantation-associated organ system damage, especially in the liver and kidney

Pregnancy Risk Factor C

Pregnancy/Breast Feeding Implications Animal reproduction studies have not been conducted. It is not known whether sargramostim can cause fetal harm when administered to a pregnant woman or can affect reproductive capability. Sargramostim should be given to a pregnant woman only if clearly needed.

Contraindications GM-CSF is contraindicated in the following instances:

Patients with excessive myeloid blasts (>30%) in the bone marrow or peripheral blood

Patients with known hypersensitivity to GM-CSF, yeast-derived products, or any known component of the product

Warnings/Precautions Do **not** administer 24 hours prior to or after chemotherapy or 12 hours prior to or after radiation therapy; use with caution in patients with pre-existing cardiac problems, hypoxia, fluid retention, pulmonary infiltrates or CHF, renal or hepatic impairment; rapid increase in peripheral blood counts; if ANC >20,000/mm³, or platelets >500,000/mm³ decrease dose by 50% or discontinue drug (counts will fall to normal within 3-7 days after discontinuing drug); growth factor potential: caution with myeloid malignancies. Precaution should be exercised in the usage of GM-CSF in any malignancy with myeloid characteristics. GM-CSF can potentially act as a growth factor for any tumor type, particularly myeloid malignancies. Tumors of nonhematopoietic origin may have surface receptors for GM-CSF.

Adverse Reactions

>10%:

"First-dose" effects: Fever, hypotension, tachycardia, rigors, flushing, nausea, vomiting, dyspnea

Dermatologic: Alopecia

Endocrine & metabolic: Polydipsia

Gastrointestinal: Nausea, vomiting, diarrhea, stomatitis, GI hemorrhage, mucositis

Neuromuscular & skeletal: Bone pain, myalgia

Miscellaneous: Neutropenic fever

1% to 10%:

Cardiovascular: Peripheral edema

Central nervous system: Malaise, fever, headache

Dermatologic: Rash, pain at injection site

Gastrointestinal: Anorexia, sore throat, stomatitis, constipation

Hematologic: Leukocytosis

Neuromuscular & skeletal: Rigors

Respiratory: Dyspnea, asthenia, cough, chest pain, capillary leak syndrome

Miscellaneous: Fluid retention

<1%:

Cardiovascular: Hypotension, flushing, pericardial effusion, transient supraventricular arrhythmias, pericarditis

Hepatic: Elevation in liver function tests

Local: Thrombophlebitis

Miscellaneous: Anaphylactic reactions

Overdosage/Toxicology Symptoms of overdose include dyspnea, malaise, nausea, fever, headache, chills; discontinue drug, wait for levels to fall, monitor CBC, respiratory symptoms, fluid status; increase WBC; discontinue drug and wait for levels to fall; monitor for pulmonary edema; toxicity of GM-CSF is dose-dependent. Severe reactions such as capillary leak syndrome are seen at higher doses (>15 mcg/kg/day).

Drug Interactions Increased toxicity: Lithium, corticosteroids may potentiate myeloproliferative effects

(Continued)

Sargramostim *(Continued)*

Stability

Sargramostim is available as a sterile, white, preservative-free, lyophilized powder

Sargramostim should be stored at 2°C to 8°C (36°F to 46°F)

Vials should not be frozen or shaken

Sargramostim is stable after dilution in 1 mL of bacteriostatic or nonbacteriostatic sterile water for injection for 30 days at 2°C to 8°C or 25°C

Sargramostim may also be further diluted in 0.9% sodium chloride to a concentration ≥10 mcg/mL for I.V. infusion administration

This diluted solution is stable for 48 hours at room temperature and refrigeration

If the final concentration of sargramostim is <10 mcg/mL, human albumin should be added to the saline prior to the addition of sargramostim to prevent absorption of the components to the delivery system

It is recommended that 1 mg of human albumin/1 mL of 0.9% sodium chloride (eg, 1 mL of 5% human albumin/50 mL of 0.9% sodium chloride) be added

Standard diluent: Dose ≥250 mcg/25 mL NS

Incompatible with dextrose-containing solutions

Mechanism of Action Stimulates proliferation, differentiation and functional activity of neutrophils, eosinophils, monocytes, and macrophages; see table.

Proliferation/Differentiation	G-CSF (Filgrastim)	GM-CSF (Sargramostim)
Neutrophils	Yes	Yes
Eosinophils	No	Yes
Macrophages	No	Yes
Neutrophil migration	Enhanced	Inhibited

Pharmacodynamics/Kinetics

Onset of action: Increase in WBC in 7-14 days

Duration: WBC will return to baseline within 1 week after discontinuing drug

Half-life: 2 hours

Time to peak serum concentration: S.C.: Within 1-2 hours

Usual Dosage

Children and Adults: I.V. infusion over ≥2 hours or S.C.

Bone marrow transplantation failure or engraftment delay: I.V.: 250 mcg/m²/day for 14 days. The dose can be repeated after 7 days off therapy if engraftment has not occurred. If engraftment still has not occurred, a third course of 500 mcg/m²/day for 14 days may be tried after another 7 days off therapy. If there is still no engraftment, it is unlikely that further dose escalation be beneficial.

Myeloid reconstitution after autologous bone marrow transplant: I.V.: 250 mcg/m²/day to begin 2-4 hours after the marrow infusion on day 0 of autologous bone marrow transplant or ≥24 hours after chemotherapy or 12 hours after last dose of radiotherapy. If significant adverse effects or "first dose" reaction is seen at this dose, discontinue the drug until toxicity resolves, then restart at a reduced dose of 125 mcg/m²/day.

Length of therapy: Bone marrow transplant patients: GM-CSF should be administered daily for up to 30 days or until the ANC has reached 1000/mm³ for 3 consecutive days following the expected chemotherapy-induced neutrophil-nadir

Cancer chemotherapy recovery: I.V.: 3-15 mcg/kg/day for 14-21 days; maximum daily dose is 15 mcg/kg/day due to dose-related adverse effects; **discontinue therapy** if the ANC count is >20,000/mm³

Excessive blood counts return to normal or baseline levels within 3-7 days following cessation of therapy

Administration Administer by S.C. (undiluted) or I.V. infusion; I.V. infusion should be over at least 2 hours; **incompatible with dextrose-containing solutions**

Monitoring Parameters

To avoid potential complications of excessive leukocytosis (WBC >50,000 cells/mm³, ANC >20,000 cells/mm³) a CBC with differential is recommended twice per week during therapy. Sargramostim therapy should be interrupted or the dose reduced by half if the ANC is >20,000 cells/mm³.

Monitoring of renal and hepatic function in patients displaying renal or hepatic dysfunction prior to initiation of treatment is recommended at least biweekly during sargramostim administration

Body weight and hydration status should be carefully monitored during sargramostim administration

Reference Range Excessive leukocytosis: ANC >20,000/mm³ or WBC >50,000 cells/mm³

Patient Information May cause bone pain and first dose reaction

Nursing Implications Can premedicate with analgesics and antipyretics; control bone pain with non-narcotic analgesics; do not shake solution; when administering GM-CSF subcutaneously, rotate injection sites

Additional Information
Reimbursement Hotline (Prokine™): 1-800-445-4774
Professional Services (Hoechst-Roussel): 1-800-445-4774
Reimbursement Hotline (Leukine™): 1-800-321-4669
Professional Services (IMMUNEX): 1-800-334-6273

Dosage Forms Injection: 250 mcg, 500 mcg

Scabene® *see* Lindane *on page 636*

Scalpicin® *see* Hydrocortisone *on page 546*

Sclavo-PPD Solution® *see* Tuberculin Purified Protein Derivative *on page 1135*

Scleromate™ *see* Morrhuate Sodium *on page 759*

Scopolamine (skoe pol' a meen)

Related Information
Cycloplegic Mydriatics Comparison *on page 1269*

Brand Names Isopto® Hyoscine; Transderm Scop®

Synonyms Hyoscine; Scopolamine Hydrobromide

Use Preoperative medication to produce amnesia and decrease salivation and respiratory secretions to produce cycloplegia and mydriasis; treatment of iridocyclitis, prevention of nausea and vomiting by motion; produces more CNS depression, mydriasis, and cycloplegia but less effective in preventing reflex bradycardia and effecting the intestines than atropine

Pregnancy Risk Factor C

Contraindications Hypersensitivity to scopolamine or any component; narrow-angle glaucoma; acute hemorrhage, gastrointestinal or genitourinary obstruction, thyrotoxicosis, tachycardia secondary to cardiac insufficiency, paralytic ileus

Warnings/Precautions Use with caution with hepatic or renal impairment since adverse CNS effects occur more often in these patients; use with caution in infants and children since they may be more susceptible to adverse effects of scopolamine; use with caution in patients with GI obstruction; anticholinergic agents are not well tolerated in the elderly and their use should be avoided when possible

Adverse Reactions
Ophthalmic:
>10%: Ocular: Blurred vision, photophobia
1% to 10%:
Ocular: Local irritation, increased intraocular pressure
Respiratory: Congestion
<1%:
Cardiovascular: Vascular congestion, edema
Central nervous system: Drowsiness
Dermatologic: Eczematoid dermatitis
Ocular: Follicular conjunctivitis
Miscellaneous: Exudate
Systemic:
>10%:
Gastrointestinal: Constipation
Local: Irritation at injection site
Miscellaneous: Decreased sweating, dry mouth, nose, throat, or skin
1% to 10%: Decreased flow of breast milk, difficulty in swallowing, increased sensitivity to light
<1%:
Cardiovascular: Orthostatic hypotension
Central nervous system: Confusion, drowsiness, headache, loss of memory, ataxia, weakness, tiredness
Dermatologic: Skin rash
Gastrointestinal: Bloated feeling, nausea, vomiting
Genitourinary: Difficult urination
Ocular: Increased intraocular pain, blurred vision, ventricular fibrillation, tachycardia, palpitations
Note: Systemic adverse effects have been reported following ophthalmic administration

Overdosage/Toxicology Symptoms of overdose include dilated pupils, flushed skin, tachycardia, hypertension, EKG abnormalities, CNS manifestations
(Continued)

997

Scopolamine *(Continued)*

resemble acute psychosis; CNS depression, circulatory collapse, respiratory failure, and death can occur. Pure scopolamine intoxication is extremely rare. However, for a scopolamine overdose with severe life-threatening symptoms, physostigmine 1-2 mg (0.5 or 0.02 mg/kg for children) S.C. or I.V. slowly should be given to reverse the toxic effects.

Drug Interactions

Decreased effect of acetaminophen, levodopa, ketoconazole, digoxin, riboflavin, potassium chloride in wax matrix preparations

Increased toxicity: Additive adverse effects with other anticholinergic agents; GI absorption of the following drugs may be affected: acetaminophen, levodopa, ketoconazole, digoxin, riboflavin, potassium chloride wax-matrix preparations

Stability Avoid acid solutions, because hydrolysis occurs at pH <3; **physically compatible** when mixed in the same syringe with atropine, butorphanol, chlorpromazine, dimenhydrinate, diphenhydramine, droperidol, fentanyl, glycopyrrolate, hydromorphone, hydroxyzine, meperidine, metoclopramide, morphine, pentazocine, pentobarbital, perphenazine, prochlorperazine, promazine, promethazine, or thiopental

Mechanism of Action Blocks the action of acetylcholine at parasympathetic sites in smooth muscle, secretory glands and the CNS; increases cardiac output, dries secretions, antagonizes histamine and serotonin

Pharmacodynamics/Kinetics

Onset of effect:
Oral, I.M.: 0.5-1 hour
I.V.: 10 minutes
Duration of effect:
Oral, I.M.: 4-6 hours
I.V.: 2 hours
Peak effect: 20-60 minutes; it may take 3-7 days for full recovery
Absorption: Well absorbed by all routes of administration
Protein binding: Reversibly bound to plasma proteins
Metabolism: In the liver
Elimination: In urine

Usual Dosage

Preoperatively:
Children: I.M., S.C.: 6 mcg/kg/dose (maximum: 0.3 mg/dose) or 0.2 mg/m^2 may be repeated every 6-8 hours **or** alternatively:
4-7 months: 0.1 mg
7 months to 3 years: 0.15 mg
3-8 years: 0.2 mg
8-12 years: 0.3 mg
Adults: I.M., I.V., S.C.: 0.3-0.65 mg; may be repeated every 4-6 hours

Motion sickness: Transdermal: Children >12 years and Adults: Apply 1 disc behind the ear at least 4 hours prior to exposure and every 3 days as needed; effective if applied as soon as 2-3 hours before anticipated need, best if 12 hours before

Ophthalmic:
Refraction:
Children: Instill 1 drop of 0.25% to eye(s) twice daily for 2 days before procedure
Adults: Instill 1-2 drops of 0.25% to eye(s) 1 hour before procedure
Iridocyclitis:
Children: Instill 1 drop of 0.25% to eye(s) up to 3 times/day
Adults: Instill 1-2 drops of 0.25% to eye(s) up to 4 times/day

Administration I.V.: Dilute with an equal volume of sterile water and give by direct I.V. injection over 2-3 minutes

Patient Information Report any changes of vision; wait 5 minutes after instilling ophthalmic preparation before using any other drops, do not blink excessively, after instilling ophthalmic preparation, apply pressure to the side of the nose near the eye to minimize systemic absorption; put patch on day before traveling; once applied, do not remove the patch for 3 full days; may cause drowsiness, dizziness, and blurred vision; may impair coordination and judgment; report to physician any CNS effects; apply patch behind ear

Nursing Implications Topical disc is programmed to deliver *in vivo* 0.5 mg over 3 days; wash hands before and after applying the disc to avoid drug contact with eyes

Dosage Forms

Disc, transdermal: 1.5 mg/disc (4's)
Injection, as hydrobromide: 0.3 mg/mL (1 mL); 0.4 mg/mL (0.5 mL, 1 mL); 0.86 mg/mL (0.5 mL); 1 mg/mL (1 mL)
Solution, ophthalmic, as hydrobromide: 0.25% (5 mL, 15 mL)

Scopolamine Hydrobromide *see* Scopolamine *on page 997*

Scot-Tussin DM® Cough Chasers [OTC] *see* Dextromethorphan *on page 321*

Scot-Tussin® [OTC] *see* Guaifenesin *on page 515*

Sebaquin® [OTC] *see* Iodoquinol *on page 588*

Sebizon® *see* Sodium Sulfacetamide *on page 1018*

Secobarbital Sodium (see koe bar' bi tal)

Brand Names Seconal™

Synonyms Quinalbarbitone Sodium

Use Short-term treatment of insomnia and as preanesthetic agent

Restrictions C-II

Pregnancy Risk Factor D

Contraindications CNS depression, uncontrolled pain, hypersensitivity to secobarbital or any component

Warnings/Precautions Use with caution in patients with hypovolemic shock, congestive heart failure, hepatic impairment, respiratory dysfunction or depression, previous addiction to the sedative/hypnotic group, chronic or acute pain, renal dysfunction, and the elderly; tolerance or psychological and physical dependence may occur with prolonged use, pregnancy with toxemia or bleeding

Adverse Reactions

>10%:

Central nervous system: Dizziness, lightheadedness, drowsiness, "hangover" effect

Local: Pain at injection site

1% to 10%:

Central nervous system: Confusion, mental depression, unusual excitement, nervousness, faint feeling, headache, insomnia, nightmares

Gastrointestinal: Constipation, nausea, vomiting

<1%:

Cardiovascular: Hypotension

Central nervous system: Hallucinations

Dermatologic: Skin rash, exfoliative dermatitis, Stevens-Johnson syndrome

Hematologic: Megaloblastic anemia, thrombocytopenia, agranulocytosis

Local: Thrombophlebitis

Respiratory: Respiratory depression

Overdosage/Toxicology Symptoms of overdose include unsteady gait, slurred speech, confusion, jaundice, hypothermia, fever, hypotension, respiratory depression, coma

If hypotension occurs, administer I.V. fluids and place the patient in the Trendelenburg position. If unresponsive, an I.V. vasopressor (eg, dopamine, epinephrine) may be required. Charcoal hemoperfusion or hemodialysis may be useful in the harder to treat intoxications, especially in the presence of very high serum barbiturate levels when the patient is in shock, coma, or renal failure. Forced alkaline diuresis is of no value in the treatment of intoxications with short-acting barbiturates.

Drug Interactions

Decreased effect of betamethasone and other corticosteroids, TCAs, chloramphenicol, estrogens, cyclophosphamide, oral anticoagulants, doxycycline, theophylline

Increased effect/toxicity with CNS depressants, chloramphenicol, chlorpropamide

Stability Do not shake vial during reconstitution, rotate ampul; aqueous solutions are not stable, reconstitute with aqueous polyethylene glycol; aqueous (sterile water) solutions should be used within 30 minutes; do not use bacteriostatic water for injection or lactated Ringer's. I.V. form is **incompatible** when mixed with benzquinamide (in syringe), cimetidine (same syringe), codeine, erythromycin, glycopyrrolate (same syringe), hydrocortisone, insulin, levorphanol, methadone, norepinephrine, pentazocine, phenytoin, sodium bicarbonate, tetracycline, vancomycin

Mechanism of Action Interferes with transmission of impulses from the thalamus to the cortex of the brain resulting in an imbalance in central inhibitory and facilitatory mechanisms

Pharmacodynamics/Kinetics

Onset of hypnosis:

Oral: Within 1-3 minutes

I.V. injection: Within 15-30 minutes

Duration: ~15 minutes

Absorption: Oral: Well absorbed (90%)

(Continued)

Secobarbital Sodium *(Continued)*

Distribution: Crosses the placenta; appears in breast milk

Protein binding: 45% to 60%

Metabolism: In the liver

Half-life: 25 hours

Time to peak serum concentration: Within 2-4 hours

Elimination: Renally as inactive metabolites and small amounts as unchanged drug

Usual Dosage

Children:

Hypnotic: I.M.: 3-5 mg/kg/dose; maximum: 100 mg/dose

Preoperative sedation:

Oral: 50-100 mg 1-2 hours before procedure

Rectal: 5 mg/kg **or** <6 months: 30-60 mg; 6 months to 3 years: 60 mg; >3 years: 60-120 mg

Sedation: Oral: 6 mg/kg/day divided every 8 hours

Adults:

Hypnotic:

Oral, I.M.: 100-200 mg/dose

I.V.: 50-250 mg/dose

Preoperative sedation: Oral: 100-300 mg 1-2 hours before procedure

Sedation: Oral: 20-40 mg/dose 2-3 times/day

Slightly dialyzable (5% to 20%)

Administration I.V.: Give undiluted or diluted with sterile water for injection, normal saline, or Ringer's injection; maximum infusion rate: 50 mg/15 seconds; avoid intra-arterial injection

Reference Range Therapeutic: 1-2 µg/mL (SI: 4.2-8.4 µmol/L); Toxic: >5 µg/mL (SI: >21 µmol/L)

Patient Information Avoid the use of alcohol and other CNS depressants; avoid driving and other hazardous tasks; avoid abrupt discontinuation; may cause physical and psychological dependence; do not alter dose without notifying physician

Dosage Forms

Capsule: 100 mg

Injection: 50 mg/mL (2 mL)

Injection, rectal: 50 mg/mL (20 mL)

Tablet: 100 mg

Seconal™ *see* Secobarbital Sodium *on previous page*

Secran® *see* Vitamin, Multiple *on page 1166*

Secretin *(see' cre tin)*

Brand Names Secretin-Ferring; Secretin-Kabi

Use Diagnosis of Zollinger-Ellison syndrome, chronic pancreatic dysfunction, and some hepatobiliary disease such as obstructive jaundice resulting from cancer or stones in the biliary tract

Contraindications Do not give to patients with acute pancreatitis

Warnings/Precautions Patients with a history of hypersensitivity, allergy, or asthma should receive a test dose of 0.1-1 CU; use with caution in patients who are highly nervous or have an excessive gag reflex; an exaggerated response may be seen in patients with severe hepatic disease

Adverse Reactions <1%: Fainting, venous spasm, hypersensitivity reactions

Stability Unstable; should be used immediately after reconstitution, store in freezer (-20°C) or store at 25°C for up to 3 weeks

Mechanism of Action Hormone normally secreted by duodenal mucosa and upper jejunal mucosa which increases the volume and bicarbonate content of pancreatic juice; stimulates the flow of hepatic bile with a high bicarbonate concentration, stimulates gastrin release in patients with Zollinger-Ellison syndrome

Pharmacodynamics/Kinetics

Inactivated by proteolytic enzymes if administered orally

Peak output of pancreatic secretions: Within 30 minutes

Duration of action: At least 2 hours

Metabolism: Metabolic fate is thought to be enzymatic inactivation in blood

Usual Dosage Potency of secretin is expressed in terms of clinical units (CU).

I.V.:

Pancreatic function: 1 CU/kg slow I.V. injection over 1 minute

Zollinger-Ellison: 2 CU/kg slow I.V. injection over 1 minute

Administration Reconstitute with 7.5 mL of normal saline; **do not shake**; use immediately by direct I.V. injection slowly over 1 minute

Monitoring Parameters Duodenal fluid volume and bicarbonate content; serum gastrin (Zollinger-Ellison syndrome)

Reference Range Normal adult response: Gastric volume: 175-295 mL/hour, gastric bicarbonate concentration of 94-134 mEq/L and bicarbonate output of 0.295-0.577 mEq/kg/hour

Patient Information Patients should fast 12-15 hours before test

Dosage Forms Powder for injection: 75 CU (10 mL)

Secretin-Ferring *see* Secretin *on previous page*

Secretin-Kabi *see* Secretin *on previous page*

Sectral® *see* Acebutolol Hydrochloride *on page 16*

Sedapap-10® *see* Butalbital Compound *on page 153*

Seldane® *see* Terfenadine *on page 1061*

Selegiline Hydrochloride (seh ledge' ah leen)

Brand Names Eldepryl®

Synonyms Deprenyl; L-Deprenyl

Use Adjunct in the management of parkinsonian patients in which levodopa/carbidopa therapy is deteriorating

Unlabeled use: Early Parkinson's disease

Investigational use: Alzheimer's disease

Selegiline is also being studied in Alzheimer's disease. Small studies have shown some improvement in behavioral and cognitive performance in patients, however, further study is needed.

Pregnancy Risk Factor C

Contraindications Known hypersensitivity to selegiline, concomitant use of meperidine

Warnings/Precautions Increased risk of nonselective MAO inhibition occurs with doses >10 mg/day; is a monoamine oxidase inhibitor type "B", there should **not** be a problem with tyramine-containing products as long as the typical doses are employed

Adverse Reactions

>10%:

Central nervous system: Mood changes, dyskinesias, dizziness

Gastrointestinal: Nausea, vomiting, dry mouth, abdominal pain

1% to 10%:

Cardiovascular: Orthostatic hypotension, arrhythmias, hypertension

Central nervous system: Hallucinations, confusion, depression, insomnia, agitation, loss of balance

Neuromuscular & skeletal: Increased involuntary movements, bradykinesia, muscle twitches

Miscellaneous: Bruxism

Overdosage/Toxicology Symptoms of overdose include tachycardia, palpitations, muscle twitching, seizures; competent supportive care is the most important treatment; both hypertension or hypotension can occur with intoxication. Hypotension may respond to I.V. fluids or vasopressors, and hypertension usually responds to an alpha-adrenergic blocker. While treating the hypertension, care is warranted to avoid sudden drops in blood pressure, since this may worsen the MAO inhibitor toxicity. Muscle irritability and seizures often respond to diazepam, while hyperthermia is best treated antipyretics and cooling blankets. Cardiac arrhythmias are best treated with phenytoin or procainamide.

Drug Interactions

Increased toxicity

Meperidine in combination with selegiline has caused agitation, delirium, and death; it may be prudent to avoid other opioids as well

Fluoxetine increases pressor effect

Mechanism of Action Potent monoamine oxidase (MAO) type-B inhibitor; MAO-B plays a major role in the metabolism of dopamine; selegiline may also increase dopaminergic activity by interfering with dopamine reuptake at the synapse

Pharmacodynamics/Kinetics

Onset of therapeutic effects: Within 1 hour

Duration: 24-72 hours

Half-life: 9 minutes

Metabolism: In the liver to amphetamine and methamphetamine

Usual Dosage Oral:

Adults: 5 mg twice daily with breakfast and lunch or 10 mg in the morning

Elderly: Initial: 5 mg in the morning, may increase to a total of 10 mg/day

(Continued)

Selegiline Hydrochloride *(Continued)*

Monitoring Parameters Blood pressure, symptoms of parkinsonism

Patient Information Do not exceed daily doses of 10 mg; report to physician any involuntary movements or CNS agitation; explain the tyramine reaction to patients and tell them to report severe headaches or other unusual symptoms to physician

Nursing Implications Monoamine oxidase inhibitor type "B"; there should **not** be a problem with tyramine-containing products as long as the typical doses are employed

Dosage Forms Tablet: 5 mg

Selenium *(se lee' nee um)*

Brand Names Sele-Pak®; Selepen®

Use Trace metal supplement

Pregnancy Risk Factor C

Contraindications Known hypersensitivity to selenium or any component

Adverse Reactions

1% to 10%:

Central nervous system: Lethargy

Dermatologic: Hair loss or discoloration

Gastrointestinal: Vomiting following long-term use on damaged skin; abdominal pain, garlic breath

Local: Irritation

Neuromuscular & skeletal: Tremor

Miscellaneous: Sweating

Overdosage/Toxicology Nausea, vomiting, diarrhea

Mechanism of Action Part of glutathione peroxidase which protects cell components from oxidative damage due to peroxidases produced in cellular metabolism

Pharmacodynamics/Kinetics Elimination: Urine, feces, lungs, skin

Usual Dosage I.V. in TPN solutions:

Children: 3 mcg/kg/day

Adults:

Metabolically stable: 20-40 mcg/day

Deficiency from prolonged TPN support: 100 mcg/day for 24 and 21 days

Dosage Forms Injection: 40 mcg/mL (10 mL, 30 mL)

Selenium Sulfide *(se lee' nee um)*

Brand Names Exsel®; Selsun®; Selsun Blue® [OTC]

Use Treatment of itching and flaking of the scalp associated with dandruff, to control scalp seborrheic dermatitis; treatment of tinea versicolor

Pregnancy Risk Factor C

Contraindications Known hypersensitivity to selenium or any component

Warnings/Precautions Do not use on damaged skin to avoid any systemic toxicity; avoid topical use in very young children; safety of topical in infants has not been established

Adverse Reactions

>10%: Dermatologic: Unusual dryness or oiliness of scalp

1% to 10%:

Central nervous system: Lethargy

Dermatologic: Hair loss or discoloration

Gastrointestinal: Vomiting following long-term use on damaged skin, abdominal pain, garlic breath, local irritation

Neuromuscular & skeletal: Tremor

Miscellaneous: Sweating

Overdosage/Toxicology Nausea, vomiting, diarrhea

Mechanism of Action May block the enzymes involved in growth of epithelial tissue

Pharmacodynamics/Kinetics

Absorption: Topical: Not absorbed through intact skin, but can be absorbed through damaged skin

Elimination: Urine, feces, lungs, skin

Usual Dosage Topical:

Dandruff, seborrhea: Massage 5-10 mL into wet scalp, leave on scalp 2-3 minutes, rinse thoroughly, and repeat application; shampoo twice weekly for 2 weeks initially, then use once every 1-4 weeks as indicated depending upon control

Tinea versicolor: Apply the 2.5% lotion to affected area and lather with small amounts of water; leave on skin for 10 minutes, then rinse thoroughly; apply every day for 7 days

Patient Information Topical formulations are for external use only; notify physician if condition persists or worsens; avoid contact with eyes; thoroughly rinse after application

Dosage Forms Lotion, shampoo; 1% (120 mL, 210 mL, 240 mL, 330 mL); 2.5% (120 mL)

Sele-Pak® *see* Selenium *on previous page*

Selepen® *see* Selenium *on previous page*

Selestoject® *see* Betamethasone *on page 129*

Selsun® *see* Selenium Sulfide *on previous page*

Selsun Blue® [OTC] *see* Selenium Sulfide *on previous page*

Semprex-D® *see* Acrivastine and Pseudoephedrine *on page 27*

Sensorcaine® *see* Bupivacaine Hydrochloride *on page 147*

Septa® Ointment [OTC] *see* Bacitracin, Neomycin, and Polymyxin B *on page 113*

Septisol® *see* Hexachlorophene *on page 535*

Septra® *see* Co-trimoxazole *on page 278*

Septra® DS *see* Co-trimoxazole *on page 278*

Serax® *see* Oxazepam *on page 824*

Serentil® *see* Mesoridazine Besylate *on page 693*

Serevent® *see* Salmeterol Xinafoate *on page 992*

Seromycin® Pulvules® *see* Cycloserine *on page 289*

Serophene® *see* Clomiphene Citrate *on page 259*

Serpalan® *see* Reserpine *on page 977*

Serpasil® *see* Reserpine *on page 977*

Sertraline Hydrochloride (ser' tra leen)

Related Information
Antidepressant Agents Comparison *on page 1250-1252*

Brand Names Zoloft™

Use Treatment of major depression; also being studied for use in obesity and obsessive-compulsive disorder

Pregnancy Risk Factor B

Contraindications Hypersensitivity to sertraline or any component

Warnings/Precautions Do not use in combination with monoamine oxidase inhibitor or within 14 days of discontinuing treatment or initiating treatment with a monoamine oxidase inhibitor due to the risk of serotonin syndrome; use with caution in patients with pre-existing seizure disorders, patients in whom weight loss is undesirable, patients with recent myocardial infarction, unstable heart disease, hepatic or renal impairment, patients taking other psychotropic medications, agitated or hyperactive patients as drug may produce or activate mania or hypomania; because the risk of suicide is inherent in depression, patient should be closely monitored until depressive symptoms remit and prescriptions should be written for minimum quantities to reduce the risk of overdose

Adverse Reactions
1% to 10%: In clinical trials, dizziness and nausea were two most frequent side effects that led to discontinuation of therapy
Cardiovascular: Palpitations
Central nervous system: Insomnia, agitation, dizziness, headache, somnolence, nervousness, fatigue
Dermatologic: Dermatological reactions, sweating
Gastrointestinal: Dry mouth, diarrhea or loose stools, nausea, constipation
Genitourinary: Sexual dysfunction in men, micturition disorders
Neuromuscular & skeletal: Pain, tremors
Ocular: Visual difficulty
Otic: Tinnitus

Overdosage/Toxicology Symptoms of overdose include serious toxicity has not yet been reported, monitor cardiovascular, gastrointestinal, and hepatic functions. Establish and maintain an airway, ensure adequate oxygenation and ventilation. Activated charcoal with 70% sorbitol may be as or more effective than emesis or lavage. Monitoring of cardiac and vital signs is recommended along with general symptomatic and supportive measures. There is no specific antidote for sertraline. Treatment should be aimed at first decontamination, then symptomatic and supportive care; forced diuresis, dialysis, hemoperfusion and exchange transfusion are unlikely to enhance elimination due to sertraline's large volume of distribution.
(Continued)

Sertraline Hydrochloride (Continued)

Drug Interactions

All serotonin reuptake inhibitors are capable of inhibiting cytochrome P-450 IID6 isoenzyme enzyme system. The drugs metabolized by this system include desipramine, dextromethorphan, encainide, haloperidol, imipramine, metoprolol, perphenazine, propafenone, and thioridazine

Increased toxicity:

MAO inhibitors and possibly with lithium or tricyclic antidepressants → **serotonin syndrome** serotonergic hyperstimulation with the following clinical features: mental status changes, restlessness, myoclonus, hyperreflexia, diaphoresis, diarrhea, shivering, and tremor

May decrease metabolism/plasma clearance of some drugs (diazepam, tolbutamide) to result in increased duration and pharmacological effects

May displace highly plasma protein bound drugs from binding sites (eg, warfarin) to result in increased effect

Mechanism of Action Antidepressant with selective inhibitory effects on presynaptic serotonin (5-HT) reuptake

Pharmacodynamics/Kinetics

Absorption: Slow

Protein binding: High

Metabolism: Extensive

Half-life:

Parent: 24 hours

Metabolites: 66 hours

Elimination: In both urine and feces

Usual Dosage Oral:

Adults: Start with 50 mg/day in the morning and increase by 50 mg/day increments every 2-3 days if tolerated to 100 mg/day; additional increases may be necessary; maximum dose: 200 mg/day. If somnolence is noted, give at bedtime.

Elderly: Start treatment with 25 mg/day in the morning and increase by 25 mg/day increments every 2-3 days if tolerated to 75-100 mg/day; additional increases may be necessary; maximum dose: 200 mg/day

Not removed by hemodialysis

Dosage comments in hepatic impairment: Sertraline is extensively metabolized by the liver; caution should be used in patients with hepatic impairment

Test Interactions Minor ↑ triglycerides (S), ↑ LFTs, ↓ uric acid (S)

Patient Information If you are currently on another antidepressant drug, please notify your physician. Although sertraline has not been shown to increase the effects of alcohol, it is recommended that you refrain from drinking while on this medication. If you are pregnant or intend becoming pregnant while on this drug, please alert your physician to this fact. You may experience some weight loss, but it is usually minimal.

Dosage Forms Tablet: 50 mg, 100 mg

Serutan® [OTC] see Psyllium on page 956

Serzone® see Nefazodone on page 778

Siblin® [OTC] see Psyllium on page 956

Silain® [OTC] see Simethicone on page 1006

Silvadene® see Silver Sulfadiazine on next page

Silver Nitrate

Brand Names Dey-Drop® Ophthalmic Solution

Synonyms AgNO$_3$

Use Prevention of gonococcal ophthalmia neonatorum; cauterization of wounds and sluggish ulcers, removal of granulation tissue and warts; aseptic prophylaxis of burns

Pregnancy Risk Factor C

Contraindications Not for use on broken skin or cuts; hypersensitivity to silver nitrate or any component

Warnings/Precautions Do not use applicator sticks on the eyes; repeated applications of the ophthalmic solution into the eye can cause cauterization of the cornea and blindness

Adverse Reactions

>10%:

Dermatologic: Burning and skin irritation

Ocular: Chemical conjunctivitis

1% to 10%:
    Dermatologic: Staining of the skin
    Hematologic: Methemoglobinemia
    Ocular: Cauterization of the cornea, blindness

Overdosage/Toxicology Symptoms of overdose include pain and burning of mouth, salivation, vomiting, diarrhea, shock, coma, convulsions, death; blackening of skin and mucous membranes; absorbed nitrate can cause methemoglobinemia. Fatal dose is as low as 2 g; administer sodium chloride in water (10 g/L) to cause precipitation of silver.

Drug Interactions Decreased effect: Sulfacetamide preparations are incompatible

Stability Must be stored in a dry place; exposure to light causes silver to oxidize and turn brown, dipping in water causes oxidized film to readily dissolve

Mechanism of Action Free silver ions precipitate bacterial proteins by combining with chloride in tissue forming silver chloride; coagulates cellular protein to form an eschar; silver ions or salts or colloidal silver preparations can inhibit the growth of both gram-positive and gram-negative bacteria. This germicidal action is attributed to the precipitation of bacterial proteins by liberated silver ions. Silver nitrate coagulates cellular protein to form an eschar, and this mode of action is the postulated mechanism for control of benign hematuria, rhinitis, and recurrent pneumothorax.

Pharmacodynamics/Kinetics
    Absorption: Because silver ions readily combine with protein, there is minimal GI and cutaneous absorption of the 0.5% and 1% preparations
    Elimination: Although the highest amounts of silver noted on autopsy have been in the kidneys, excretion in urine is minimal

Usual Dosage
    Neonates: Ophthalmic: Instill 2 drops immediately after birth (no later than 1 hour after delivery) into conjunctival sac of each eye as a single dose, allow to sit for ≥30 seconds; do not irrigate eyes following instillation of eye drops

    Children and Adults:
        Ointment: Apply in an apertured pad on affected area or lesion for approximately 5 days
        Sticks: Apply to mucous membranes and other moist skin surfaces only on area to be treated 2-3 times/week for 2-3 weeks
        Topical solution: Apply a cotton applicator dipped in solution on the affected area 2-3 times/week for 2-3 weeks

Monitoring Parameters With prolonged use, monitor methemoglobin levels

Patient Information Discontinue topical preparation if redness or irritation develop

Nursing Implications Silver nitrate solutions stain skin and utensils

Additional Information Applicators are **not** for ophthalmic use

Dosage Forms
    Applicator sticks: 75% with potassium nitrate 25% (6")
    Ointment: 10% (30 g)
    Solution:
        Ophthalmic: 1% (wax ampuls)
        Topical: 10% (30 mL); 25% (30 mL); 50% (30 mL)

Silver Sulfadiazine (sul fa dye´ a zeen)

Brand Names Silvadene®; SSD™; SSD-AF™; Thermazene™

Use Prevention and treatment of infection in second and third degree burns

Pregnancy Risk Factor C

Contraindications Hypersensitivity to silver sulfadiazine or any component; premature infants or neonates <2 months of age because sulfonamides compete with bilirubin for protein binding sites which may displace bilirubin and cause kernicterus

Warnings/Precautions Use with caution in patients with G-6-PD deficiency, renal impairment, or history of allergy to other sulfonamides; sulfadiazine may accumulate in patients with impaired hepatic or renal function; use of analgesic might be needed before application; systemic absorption is significant and adverse reactions may be due to sulfa component

Adverse Reactions
    >10%: Local: Pain, burning
    1% to 10%:
        Dermatologic: Itching, rash, erythema multiforme, skin discoloration
        Genitourinary: Interstitial nephritis
        Hematologic: Hemolytic anemia, leukopenia, agranulocytosis, aplastic anemia
        Hepatic: Hepatitis
        Sensitivity reactions: Allergic reactions may be related to sulfa component
    <1%: Ocular: Photosensitivity
(Continued)

Silver Sulfadiazine *(Continued)*

Drug Interactions Decreased effect: Topical proteolytic enzymes are inactivated

Stability Discard if cream is darkened (reacts with heavy metals resulting in release of silver)

Mechanism of Action Acts upon the bacterial cell wall and cell membrane. Bactericidal for many gram-negative and gram-positive bacteria and is effective against yeast. Active against *Pseudomonas aeruginosa*, *Pseudomonas maltophilia*, *Enterobacter* species, *Klebsiella* species, *Serratia* species, *Escherichia coli*, *Proteus mirabilis*, *Morganella morganii*, *Providencia rettgeri*, *Proteus vulgaris*, *Providencia* species, *Citrobacter* species, *Acinetobacter calcoaceticus*, *Staphylococcus aureus*, *Staphylococcus epidermidis*, *Enterococcus* species, *Candida albicans*, *Corynebacterium diphtheriae*, and *Clostridium perfringens*

Pharmacodynamics/Kinetics

Absorption: Significant percutaneous absorption of sulfadiazine can occur especially when applied to extensive burns

Half-life: 10 hours and is prolonged in patients with renal insufficiency

Time to peak serum concentration: Within 3-11 days of continuous therapy

Elimination: ~50% excreted unchanged in urine

Usual Dosage Children and Adults: Topical: Apply once or twice daily with a sterile-gloved hand; apply to a thickness of $^1/_{16}$"; burned area should be covered with cream at all times

Monitoring Parameters Serum electrolytes, urinalysis, renal function tests, CBC in patients with extensive burns on long-term treatment

Patient Information For external use only; bathe daily to aid in debridement (if not contraindicated); apply liberally to burned areas; for external use only; notify physician if condition persists or worsens

Nursing Implications Evaluate the development of granulation

Additional Information Contains methylparaben and propylene glycol

Dosage Forms Cream, topical: 1% [10 mg/g] (20 g, 25 g, 50 g, 85 g, 400 g, 1000 g)

Simethicone *(sye meth' i kone)*

Brand Names Flatulex® [OTC]; Gas Relief® [OTC]; Gas-X® [OTC]; Mylanta® Gas [OTC]; Mylicon® [OTC]; Phazyme® [OTC]; Silain® [OTC]

Synonyms Activated Dimethicone; Activated Methylpolysiloxane

Use Relieves flatulence and functional gastric bloating, and postoperative gas pains

Pregnancy Risk Factor C

Contraindications Hypersensitivity to drug or components

Warnings/Precautions Not recommended for the treatment of infant colic; do not exceed recommended dosing guidelines

Overdosage/Toxicology Nontoxic orally

Stability Protect from light

Mechanism of Action Decreases the surface tension of gas bubbles thereby disperses and prevents gas pockets in the GI system

Pharmacodynamics/Kinetics Elimination: In feces

Usual Dosage Oral:

Infants: 20 mg 4 times/day

Children <12 years: 40 mg 4 times/day

Children >12 years and Adults: 40-120 mg after meals and at bedtime as needed, not to exceed 500 mg/day

Test Interactions False-negative gastric guaiac

Patient Information Some tablets may be chewed thoroughly before swallowing, follow with a glass of water

Nursing Implications Shake suspension before using; mix with water, infant formula, or other liquids

Dosage Forms

Capsule: 125 mg

Drops, oral: 40 mg/0.6 mL (15 mL, 30 mL)

Tablet: 50 mg, 60 mg, 95 mg

Tablet, chewable: 40 mg, 80 mg, 125 mg

Simron® [OTC] *see* Ferrous Gluconate *on page 451*

Simvastatin *(sim' va stat in)*

Related Information

Lipid-Lowering Agents *on page 1273*

Brand Names Zocor™

Use Adjunct to dietary therapy to decrease elevated serum total and LDL cholesterol concentrations in primary hypercholesterolemia

Pregnancy Risk Factor X

Contraindications Previous hypersensitivity to simvastatin or lovastatin or other HMG-CoA reductase inhibitors; active liver disease or unexplained elevations of serum transaminases; pregnancy and lactation

Adverse Reactions
1% to 10%:
Central nervous system: Headache, dizziness,
Dermatologic: Rash
Gastrointestinal: Flatulence, abdominal cramps, diarrhea, constipation, nausea, dyspepsia, heartburn
Neuromuscular & skeletal: Myalgia
Renal: Elevated creatine phosphokinase (CPK)
<1%:
Central nervous system: Dizziness
Gastrointestinal: Dysgeusia
Ocular: Lenticular opacities, blurred vision

Overdosage/Toxicology Very few adverse events; treatment is symptomatic

Drug Interactions
Increased effect of warfarin, erythromycin, niacin
Increased toxicity of cyclosporin, gemfibrozil

Stability Tablets should be stored in well closed containers at temperatures between 5°C to 30°C (41°F to 86°F)

Mechanism of Action Simvastatin is a methylated derivative of lovastatin that acts by competitively inhibiting 3 hydroxy 3 methylglutaryl coenzyme A reductase (HMB CoA reductase), the enzyme that catalyzes the rate-limiting step in cholesterol biosynthesis

Pharmacodynamics/Kinetics
Absorption: Oral: Although 85% is absorbed following administration, <5% reaches the general circulation due to an extensive first-pass effect
Time to peak concentrations: 1.3-2.4 hours
Protein binding: ~95%
Elimination: 13% excreted in urine and 60% in feces; the elimination half-life is unknown
In patients with severe renal insufficiency, high systemic levels may occur

Usual Dosage Adults: Oral: Start with 5-10 mg/day as a single bedtime dose; if LDL is ≤90 mg/dL start with 5 mg; if LDL >100 mg/dL, start with 10 mg/day; increase every 4 weeks as needed; maximum dose: 40 mg/day

Dosing adjustment/comments in renal impairment: Recommended starting dose: 5 mg; patient should be closely monitored

Monitoring Parameters Creatine phosphokinase levels due to possibility of myopathy; serum cholesterol (total and fractionated)

Patient Information Promptly report any unexplained muscle pain, tenderness or weakness, especially if accompanied by malaise or fever; follow prescribed diet; take with meals

Nursing Implications Liver enzyme elevations may be observed during simvastatin therapy; combination therapy with other hypolipidemic agents may be required to achieve optimal reductions of LDL cholesterol; diet, weight reduction, and exercise should be attempted to control hypercholesterolemia before the institution of simvastatin therapy

Dosage Forms Tablet: 5 mg, 10 mg, 20 mg, 40 mg

Sinarest® 12 Hour Nasal Solution see Oxymetazoline Hydrochloride on page 829

Sinarest® Nasal Solution [OTC] see Phenylephrine Hydrochloride on page 874

Sincalide (sin' ka lide)
Brand Names Kinevac®
Synonyms C8-CCK; OP-CCK
Use Postevacuation cholecystography; gallbladder bile sampling; stimulate pancreatic secretion for analysis
Pregnancy Risk Factor B
Contraindications Hypersensitivity to sincalide or any component
Warnings/Precautions Use with caution in patients with small gallbladder stones
Adverse Reactions
1% to 10%:
Cardiovascular: Flushing
(Continued)

Sincalide *(Continued)*

Central nervous system: Dizziness

Gastrointestinal: Nausea, abdominal pain, urge to defecate

Stability Reconstituted solution may be kept at room temperature for 24 hours

Mechanism of Action Stimulates contraction of the gallbladder and simultaneous relaxation of the sphincter of Oddi, inhibits gastric emptying, and increases intestinal motility. Graded doses have been shown to produce graded decreases in small intestinal transit time, thought to be mediated by acetylcholine.

Pharmacodynamics/Kinetics

Onset of action: Contraction of the gallbladder occurs within 5-15 minutes

Duration: ~1 hour

Usual Dosage Adults: I.V.:

Contraction of gallbladder: 0.02 mcg/kg over 30 seconds to 1 minute, may repeat in 15 minutes a 0.04 mcg/kg dose

Pancreatic function: 0.02 mcg/kg over 30 minutes administered after secretin

Dosage Forms Injection: 5 mcg

Sinemet® *see* Levodopa and Carbidopa *on page 625*

Sinequan® *see* Doxepin Hydrochloride *on page 369*

Sinumist®-SR Capsulets® *see* Guaifenesin *on page 515*

Sinusol-B® *see* Brompheniramine Maleate *on page 143*

Skelaxin® *see* Metaxalone *on page 700*

Skelex® *see* Chlorzoxazone *on page 236*

Skin Test Antigens, Multiple

Brand Names Multitest CMI®

Use Detection of nonresponsiveness to antigens by means of delayed hypersensitivity skin testing

Pregnancy Risk Factor C

Contraindications Infected or inflamed skin, known hypersensitivity to skin test antigens; do not apply at sites involving acneiform, infected or inflamed skin; although severe systemic reactions are rare to diphtheria and tetanus antigens, persons known to have a history of systemic reactions should be tested with this test only after the test heads containing these antigens have been removed

Warnings/Precautions Epinephrine should be available is case of severe reactions. Safety and effectiveness in children <17 years of age have not been established; discard applicator after use, do not reuse.

Adverse Reactions 1% to 10%: Local irritation

Drug Interactions Decreased effect: Drugs or procedures that suppress immunity such as corticosteroids, chemotherapeutic agents, antilymphocyte globulin and irradiation, may possibly cause a loss of reactivity

Stability Keep in refrigerator at 2°C to 8°C (35°F to 46°F)

Usual Dosage Select only test sites that permit sufficient surface area and subcutaneous tissue to allow adequate penetration of all eight points, avoid hairy areas

Press loaded unit into the skin with sufficient pressure to puncture the skin and allow adequate penetration of all points, maintain firm contact for at least 5 seconds, during application the device should not be "rocked" back and forth and side to side without removing any of the test heads from the skin sites

If adequate pressure is applied it will be possible to observe:

1. The puncture marks of the nine tines on each of the eight test heads
2. An imprint of the circular platform surrounding each test head
3. Residual antigen and glycerin at each of the eight sites

If any of the above three criteria are not fully followed, the test results may not be reliable

Reading should be done in good light, read the test sites at both 24 and 48 hours, the largest reaction recorded from the two readings at each test site should be used; if two readings are not possible, a single 48 hour is recommended

A positive reaction from any of the seven delayed hypersensitivity skin test antigens is **induration ≥2 mm** providing there is no induration at the negative control site; the size of the induration reactions with this test may be smaller than those obtained with other intradermal procedures

Nursing Implications Patients should be informed of the types of test site reactions that may be expected. Remove tests from refrigeration approximately 1 hour before use; select only test sites that permit sufficient surface area and subcutaneous tissue to allow adequate penetration of all points on all eight test heads; avoid hairy areas when possible because interpretation of reactions will be more difficult

Additional Information Contains disposable plastic applicator consisting of eight sterile test heads preloaded with the following seven delayed hypersensitivity skin test antigens and glycerin negative control for percutaneous administration

Test Head No. 1 = Tetanus toxoid antigen
Test Head No. 2 = Diphtheria toxoid antigen
Test Head No. 3 = *Streptococcus* antigen
Test Head No. 4 = Tuberculin, old
Test Head No. 5 = Glycerin negative control
Test Head No. 6 = *Candida* antigen
Test Head No. 7 = *Trichophyton* antigen
Test Head No. 8 = *Proteus* antigen

Dosage Forms Individual carton containing one preloaded skin test antigen for cellular hypersensitivity

Skin Testing for Delayed Hypersensitivity *see page 1325*

Sleep-eze 3® [OTC] *see* Diphenhydramine Hydrochloride *on page 351*

Slim-Mint® [OTC] *see* Benzocaine *on page 121*

Slo-bid™ *see* Theophylline/Aminophylline *on page 1072*

Slo-Niacin® [OTC] *see* Niacin *on page 788*

Slo-Phyllin® *see* Theophylline/Aminophylline *on page 1072*

Slo-Salt® [OTC] *see* Sodium Chloride *on page 1012*

Slow FE® [OTC] *see* Ferrous Sulfate *on page 452*

Slow-K® *see* Potassium Chloride *on page 906*

Smallpox Vaccine

Use There are no indications for the use of smallpox vaccine in the general civilian population. Laboratory workers involved with Orthopoxvirus or in the production and testing of smallpox vaccines should receive regular smallpox vaccinations. For advice on vaccine administration and contraindications, contact the Division of Immunization, CDC, Atlanta, GA 30333 (404-639-3356).

SMX-TMP *see* Co-trimoxazole *on page 278*

Sodium 2-Mercaptoethane Sulfonate *see* Mesna *on page 692*

Sodium Acetate (sow' dee um as' i tate)

Use Sodium source in large volume I.V. fluids to prevent or correct hyponatremia in patients with restricted intake; used to counter acidosis through conversion to bicarbonate

Pregnancy Risk Factor C

Contraindications Alkalosis, hypocalcemia, low sodium diets, edema, cirrhosis

Warnings/Precautions Avoid extravasation, use with caution in patients with hepatic failure

Adverse Reactions
1% to 10%:
Cardiovascular: Thrombosis, hypervolemia
Endocrine & metabolic: Hypernatremia, dilution of serum electrolytes, overhydration, hypokalemia, metabolic alkalosis, hypocalcemia
Gastrointestinal: Gastric distension, flatulence
Local: Chemical cellulitis at injection site (extravasation), phlebitis
Respiratory: Pulmonary edema
Miscellaneous: Congestive conditions

Stability Protect from light, heat, and from freezing; **incompatible** with acids, acidic salts, alkaloid salts, calcium salts, catecholamines, atropine

Usual Dosage Sodium acetate is metabolized to bicarbonate on an equimolar basis outside the liver; administer in large volume I.V. fluids as a sodium source. Refer to Sodium Bicarbonate monograph.

Maintenance electrolyte requirements of sodium in parenteral nutrition solutions:
Daily requirements: 3-4 mEq/kg/24 hours or 25-40 mEq/1000 kcal/24 hours
Maximum: 100-150 mEq/24 hours

Additional Information Sodium and acetate content of 1 g: 7.3 mEq

Dosage Forms Injection: 2 mEq/mL (20 mL, 50 mL); 4 mEq/mL (50 mL)

Sodium Acid Carbonate *see* Sodium Bicarbonate *on next page*

Sodium Ascorbate (a skor′ bate)
Brand Names Cenolate®
Use Prevention and treatment of scurvy and to acidify urine
Pregnancy Risk Factor C
Contraindications Large doses during pregnancy
Warnings/Precautions Use with caution in diabetics, patients with renal calculi, and those on sodium-restricted diets
Adverse Reactions
1% to 10%:
    Cardiovascular: Hypotension with rapid I.V. administration
    Gastrointestinal: Diarrhea
    Local: Soreness at injection site
    Miscellaneous: Precipitation of cystine, oxalate or urate renal stones
Overdosage/Toxicology Symptoms of overdose include diarrhea, precipitation of cystine, oxalate or urate stones; supportive care only following GI decontamination
Pharmacodynamics/Kinetics
Therapeutic serum levels: 0.4-1.5 mg/dL
Time to peak serum concentration: Oral: Within 2-3 hours
Elimination: Without supplementation, 75 mg of ascorbic acid is excreted in urine daily, increasing to 400 mg within 24 hours with the administration of 1 g/day; hemodialysis and peritoneal dialysis remove significant amounts of the drug and supplementation is suggested following dialysis periods
Usual Dosage Oral, I.V.:
Children:
    Scurvy: 100-300 mg/day in divided doses for at least 2 weeks
    Urinary acidification: 500 mg every 6-8 hours
    Dietary supplement: 35-45 mg/day

Adults:
    Scurvy: 100-250 mg 1-2 times/day for at least 2 weeks
    Urinary acidification: 4-12 g/day in divided doses
    Dietary supplement: 50-60 mg/day
    Prevention and treatment of cold: 1-3 g/day
Test Interactions May result in false-positive stool occult blood if given within 72 hours; large doses may cause false-negative urine glucose determination
Patient Information Do not exceed recommended daily allowance
Dosage Forms
Crystals: 1020 mg per 1/4 teaspoonful [ascorbic acid 900 mg]
Injection: 250 mg/mL [ascorbic acid 222 mg/mL] (30 mL); 562.5 mg/mL [ascorbic acid 500 mg/mL] (1 mL, 2 mL)
Tablet: 585 mg [ascorbic acid 500 mg]

Sodium Bicarbonate (sow′ dee um bye kar′ bo nate)
Brand Names Neut®
Synonyms Baking Soda; $NaHCO_3$; Sodium Acid Carbonate; Sodium Hydrogen Carbonate
Use Management of metabolic acidosis; gastric hyperacidity; as an alkalinization agent for the urine; treatment and hyperkalemia
Pregnancy Risk Factor C
Contraindications Alkalosis, hypernatremia, severe pulmonary edema, hypocalcemia, unknown abdominal pain
Warnings/Precautions Rapid administration in neonates and children <2 years of age has led to hypernatremia, decreased CSF pressure and intracranial hemorrhage. **Use of I.V. $NaHCO_3$ should be reserved for documented metabolic acidosis and for hyperkalemia-induced cardiac arrest.** Routine use in cardiac arrest is not recommended. Avoid extravasation, tissue necrosis can occur due to the hypertonicity of $NaHCO_3$. May cause sodium retention especially if renal function is impaired; not to be used in treatment of peptic ulcer; use with caution in patients with CHF, edema, cirrhosis, or renal failure. Not the antacid of choice for the elderly because of sodium content and potential for systemic alkalosis.
Adverse Reactions
>10%: Gastrointestinal: Belching, gastric distension, flatulence
1% to 10%:
    Cardiovascular: Edema, cerebral hemorrhage, aggravation of congestive heart failure
    Central nervous system: Tetany, intracranial acidosis
    Endocrine & metabolic: Metabolic alkalosis, hypernatremia, hypokalemia, hypocalcemia, hyperosmolality
    Respiratory: Pulmonary edema

Miscellaneous: Increased affinity of hemoglobin for oxygen-reduced pH in myocardial tissue necrosis when extravasated

Overdosage/Toxicology Symptoms of overdose include hypocalcemia, hypokalemia, hypernatremia, seizures; seizures can be treated with diazepam 0.1-0.25 mg/kg; hypernatremia is resolved through the use of diuretics and free water replacement

Drug Interactions

Decreased effect/levels of lithium, chlorpropamide, salicylates due to urinary alkalinization

Increased toxicity/levels of amphetamines, ephedrine, pseudoephedrine, flecainide, quinidine, quinine due to urinary alkalinization

Stability Store injection at room temperature; protect from heat and from freezing; use only clear solutions; Advise patient of milk-alkali syndrome if use is long-term; observe for extravasation when giving I.V.; **incompatible** with acids, acidic salts, alkaloid salts, calcium salts, catecholamines, atropine

Mechanism of Action Dissociates to provide bicarbonate ion which neutralizes hydrogen ion concentration and raises blood and urinary pH

Pharmacodynamics/Kinetics

Oral:
Onset of action: Rapid
Duration: 8-10 minutes

I.V.:
Onset of action: 15 minutes
Duration: 1-2 hours

Absorption: Oral: Well absorbed

Elimination: Reabsorbed by kidney and <1% is excreted by urine

Usual Dosage

Cardiac arrest: **Routine use of $NaHCO_3$ is not recommended and should be given only after adequate alveolar ventilation has been established and effective cardiac compressions are provided**

Infants and Children: I.V.: 0.5-1 mEq/kg/dose repeated every 10 minutes or as indicated by arterial blood gases; rate of infusion should not exceed 10 mEq/minute; neonates and children <2 years of age should receive 4.2% (0.5 mEq/mL) solution

Adults: I.V.: Initial: 1 mEq/kg/dose one time; maintenance: 0.5 mEq/kg/dose every 10 minutes or as indicated by arterial blood gases

Metabolic acidosis: Dosage should be based on the following formula if blood gases and pH measurements are available:

Infants and Children:
$HCO_3^-(mEq) = 0.3$ x weight (kg) x base deficit (mEq/L) **or**
$HCO_3^-(mEq) = 0.5$ x weight (kg) x [24 - serum HCO_3^- (mEq/L)]

Adults:
$HCO_3^-(mEq) = 0.2$ x weight (kg) x base deficit (mEq/L) **or**
$HCO_3^-(mEq) = 0.5$ x weight (kg) x [24 - serum HCO_3^- (mEq/L)]

If acid-base status is not available: Dose for older Children and Adults: 2-5 mEq/kg I.V. infusion over 4-8 hours; subsequent doses should be based on patient's acid-base status

Chronic renal failure: Oral: Initiate when plasma HCO_3^- <15 mEq/L
Children: 1-3 mEq/kg/day
Adults: Start with 20-36 mEq/day in divided doses, titrate to bicarbonate level of 18-20 mEq/L

Renal tubular acidosis: Oral:
Distal:
Children: 2-3 mEq/kg/day
Adults: 0.5-2 mEq/kg/day in 4-5 divided doses
Proximal: Children: Initial: 5-10 mEq/kg/day; maintenance: Increase as required to maintain serum bicarbonate in the normal range

Urine alkalinization: Oral:
Children: 1-10 mEq (84-840 mg)/kg/day in divided doses every 4-6 hours; dose should be titrated to desired urinary pH
Adults: Initial: 48 mEq (4 g), then 12-24 mEq (1-2 g) every 4 hours; dose should be titrated to desired urinary pH; doses up to 16 g/day (200 mEq) in patients <60 years and 8 g (100 mEq) in patients >60 years

Antacid: Adults: Oral: 325 mg to 2 g 1-4 times/day

Patient Information Avoid chronic use as an antacid (<2 weeks)

Nursing Implications Advise patient of milk-alkali syndrome if use is long-term; observe for extravasation when giving I.V.

Additional Information

Sodium content of injection 50 mL, 8.4% = 1150 mg = 50 mEq; each 6 mg of $NaHCO_3$ contains 12 mEq sodium; 1 mEq $NaHCO_3$ = 84 mg

Each 84 mg of sodium bicarbonate provides 1 mEq of sodium and bicarbonate ions; each gram of sodium bicarbonate provides 12 mEq of sodium and bicarbonate ions

(Continued)

Sodium Bicarbonate *(Continued)*

Dosage Forms

Injection: 4% [40 mg/mL = 2.4 mEq/5 mL] (5 mL); 4.2% [42 mg/mL = 5 mEq/10 mL] (10 mL); 7.5% [75 mg/mL = 8.92 mEq/10 mL] (10 mL, 50 mL); 8.4% [84 mg/mL = 10 mEq/10 mL] (10 mL, 50 mL)

Powder: 120 g, 480 g

Tablet: 300 mg [3.6 mEq]; 325 mg [3.8 mEq]; 520 mg [6.3 mEq]; 600 mg [7.3 mEq]; 650 mg [7.6 mEq]

Sodium Chloride *(sow' dee um klor' ide)*

Brand Names Adsorbonac® [OTC] Ophthalmic; Ayr® [OTC]; HuMIST® [OTC]; Muro 128® Ophthalmic [OTC]; NāSal™ [OTC]; Ocean Nasal Mist [OTC]; Pretz® [OTC]; Saline® [OTC]; Slo-Salt® [OTC]

Synonyms NaCl; Normal Saline; Salt

Use Prevention of muscle cramps and heat prostration; restoration of sodium ion in hyponatremia; induce abortion; restore moisture to nasal membranes; GU irrigant; reduction of corneal edema; source of electrolytes and water for expansion of the extracellular fluid compartment

Pregnancy Risk Factor C

Contraindications Hypertonic uterus, hypernatremia, fluid retention

Warnings/Precautions Use with caution in patients with congestive heart failure, renal insufficiency, liver cirrhosis, hypertension, edema; sodium toxicity is almost exclusively related to how fast a sodium deficit is corrected; both rate and magnitude are extremely important

Adverse Reactions

1% to 10%:

Cardiovascular: Thrombosis, hypervolemia

Endocrine & metabolic: Hypernatremia, dilution of serum electrolytes, overhydration, hypokalemia

Local: Phlebitis

Respiratory: Pulmonary edema

Miscellaneous: Congestive conditions, extravasation

Overdosage/Toxicology Symptoms of overdose include nausea, vomiting, diarrhea, abdominal cramps, hypocalcemia, hypokalemia, hypernatremia; hypernatremia is resolved through the use of diuretics and free water replacement

Drug Interactions Decreased levels of lithium

Stability Store injection at room temperature; protect from heat and from freezing; use only clear solutions

Mechanism of Action Principal extracellular cation; functions in fluid and electrolyte balance, osmotic pressure control, and water distribution

Pharmacodynamics/Kinetics

Absorption: Oral, I.V.: Rapid

Distribution: Widely distributed

Elimination: Mainly in urine but also in sweat, tears, and saliva

Usual Dosage

Newborn electrolyte requirement:

Premature: 2-8 mEq/kg/24 hours

Term:

0-48 hours: 0-2 mEq/kg/24 hours

>48 hours: 1-4 mEq/kg/24 hours

Children: I.V.: Hypertonic solutions (>0.9%) should only be used for the initial treatment of acute serious symptomatic hyponatremia; maintenance: 3-4 mEq/kg/day; maximum: 100-150 mEq/day; dosage varies widely depending on clinical condition

Replacement: Determined by laboratory determinations mEq

Sodium deficiency (mEq/kg) = [% dehydration (L/kg)/100 x 70 (mEq/L) = [0.6 (L/kg) x (140 - serum sodium) (mEq/L)]

Nasal: Use as often as needed

Adults:

GU irrigant: 1-3 L/day by intermittent irrigation

Heat cramps: Oral: 0.5-1 g with full glass of water, up to 4.8 g/day

Replacement I.V.: Determined by laboratory determinations mEq

Sodium deficiency (mEq/kg) = [% dehydration (L/kg)/100 x 70 (mEq/L)] + [0.6 (L/kg) x (140 - serum sodium) (mEq/L)]

To correct acute, serious hyponatremia: mEq sodium = (desired sodium (mEq/L) - actual sodium (mEq/L) x 0.6 x wt (kg)); for acute correction use 125 mEq/L as the desired serum sodium; acutely correct serum sodium in 5 mEq/L/dose increments; more gradual correction in increments of 10 mEq/L/day is indicated in the asymptomatic patient

Chloride maintenance electrolyte requirement in parenteral nutrition: 2-4 mEq/kg/24 hours or 25-40 mEq/1000 kcals/24 hours; maximum: 100-150 mEq/24 hours

Sodium maintenance electrolyte requirement in parenteral nutrition: 3-4 mEq/kg/24 hours or 25-40 mEq/1000 kcals/24 hours; maximum: 100-150 mEq/24 hours. See table.

Approximate Deficits of Water and Electrolytes in Moderately Severe Dehydration

Condition	Water (mL/kg)	Sodium (mEq/kg)
Fasting and thirsting	100-200	5-7
Diarrhea		
isonatremic	100-120	8-10
hypernatremic	100-120	2-4
hyponatremic	100-120	10-12
Pyloric stenosis	100-120	8-10
Diabetic acidosis		

*A **negative** deficit indicates total body **excess** prior to treatment.

Adapted from Vaughan VC III, McKay RJ Jr, and Behrman RE, eds, *Nelson Textbook of Pediatrics*, 11th ed, WB Saunders Co, 1979.

Ophthalmic:
  Ointment: Apply once daily or more often
  Solution: Instill 1-2 drops into affected eye(s) every 3-4 hours
  Abortifacient: 20% (250 mL) administered by transabdominal intra-amniotic instillation

Monitoring Parameters Serum sodium, potassium, chloride, and bicarbonate levels; I & O, weight

Reference Range Serum/plasma sodium levels:
  Neonates:
  Full-term: 133-142 mEq/L
  Premature: 132-140 mEq/L
  Children ≥2 months to Adults: 135-145 mEq/L

Patient Information Blurred vision is common with ophthalmic ointment; may sting eyes when first applied

Nursing Implications Bacteriostatic NS should not be used for diluting or reconstituting drugs for administration in neonates; I.V. infusion of 3% or 5% sodium chloride should not exceed 100 mL/hour and should be administered in a central line only

Dosage Forms
  Drops, nasal: 0.9% with dropper
  Injection: 0.2% (3 mL); 0.45% (3 mL, 5 mL, 500 mL, 1000 mL); 0.9% (1 mL, 2 mL, 3 mL, 4 mL, 5 mL, 10 mL, 20 mL, 25 mL, 30 mL, 50 mL, 100 mL, 130 mL, 150 mL, 250 mL, 500 mL, 1000 mL); 3% (500 mL); 5% (500 mL); 20% (250 mL); 23.4% (30 mL, 100 mL)
  Injection:
    Admixtures: 50 mEq (20 mL); 100 mEq (40 mL); 625 mEq (250 mL)
    Bacteriostatic: 0.9% (30 mL)
    Concentrated: 14.6% (20 mL, 40 mL, 200 mL); 23.4% (10 mL, 20 mL, 30 mL)
  Irrigation: 0.45% (500 mL, 1000 mL, 1500 mL); 0.9% (250 mL, 500 mL, 1000 mL, 1500 mL, 2000 mL, 3000 mL, 4000 mL)
  Ointment, ophthalmic (Muro 128®): 5% (3.5 g)
  Solution:
    Irrigation: 0.9% (1000 mL, 2000 mL)
    Nasal: 0.4% (15 mL, 50 mL); 0.6% (15 mL); 0.65% (20 mL, 45 mL, 50 mL)
    Ophthalmic (Adsorbonac®): 2% (15 mL); 5% (15 mL, 30 mL)
  Tablet: 650 mg, 1 g, 2.25
  Tablet:
    Enteric coated: 1 g
    Slow release: 600 mg

Sodium Citrate and Citric Acid (sow' dee um cit' trate & si' trik as' id)

Brand Names Bicitra®; Oracit®

Synonyms Modified Shohl's Solution

Use Treatment of metabolic acidosis; alkalinizing agent in conditions where long-term maintenance of an alkaline urine is desirable
(Continued)

Sodium Citrate and Citric Acid *(Continued)*

Pregnancy Risk Factor C

Contraindications Severe renal insufficiency, sodium-restricted diet

Warnings/Precautions Conversion to bicarbonate may be impaired in patients with hepatic failure, in shock, or who are severely ill

Adverse Reactions

1% to 10%:

Central nervous system: Tetany

Endocrine & metabolic: Metabolic alkalosis, hyperkalemia

Gastrointestinal: Diarrhea, nausea, vomiting

Overdosage/Toxicology Symptoms of overdose include hypokalemia, hypernatremia, tetany, seizures; hypernatremia is resolved through the use of diuretics and free water replacement

Drug Interactions

Decreased effect/levels of lithium, chlorpropamide, salicylates due to urinary alkalinization

Increased toxicity/levels of amphetamines, ephedrine, pseudoephedrine, flecainide, quinidine, quinine due to urinary alkalinization

Usual Dosage Oral:

Infants and Children: 2-3 mEq/kg/day in divided doses 3-4 times/day **or** 5-15 mL with water after meals and at bedtime

Adults: 15-30 mL with water after meals and at bedtime

Patient Information Palatability is improved by chilling solution, dilute each dose with 1-3 oz of water and follow with additional water; take after meals to prevent saline laxative effect

Nursing Implications May be ordered as modified Shohl's solution; dilute with 30-90 mL of chilled water to enhance taste; give after meals

Additional Information 1 mL of Bicitra® contains 1 mEq of sodium and the equivalent of 1 mEq of bicarbonate

Dosage Forms Solution, oral:

Bicitra®: Sodium citrate 500 mg and citric acid 334 mg per 5 mL (15 mL unit dose, 480 mL)

Oracit®: Sodium citrate 490 mg and citric acid 640 mg per 5 mL

Polycitra®: Sodium citrate 500 mg and citric acid 334 mg with potassium citrate 550 mg per 5 mL

Sodium Edetate *see* Edetate Disodium *on page 381*

Sodium Etidronate *see* Etidronate Disodium *on page 432*

Sodium Fluoride *see* Fluoride *on page 471*

Sodium Hyaluronate *(hye al yoor on' nate)*

Brand Names Amvisc®; Healon®

Synonyms Hyaluronic Acid

Use Surgical aid in cataract extraction, intraocular implantation, corneal transplant, glaucoma filtration, and retinal attachment surgery

Pregnancy Risk Factor C

Contraindications Hypersensitivity to hyaluronate

Warnings/Precautions Do not overfill the anterior chamber; carefully monitor intraocular pressure; risk of hypersensitivity exists

Adverse Reactions 1% to 10%: Ocular: Postoperative inflammatory reactions (iritis, hypopyon), corneal edema, corneal decompensation, transient postoperative increase in IOP

Stability Store in refrigerator (2°C to 8°C); do not freeze

Mechanism of Action Functions as a tissue lubricant and is thought to play an important role in modulating the interactions between adjacent tissues. Sodium hyaluronate is a polysaccharide which is distributed widely in the extracellular matrix of connective tissue in man. (Vitreous and aqueous humor of the eye, synovial fluid, skin, and umbilical cord.) Sodium hyaluronate forms a viscoelastic solution in water (at physiological pH and ionic strength) which makes it suitable for aqueous and vitreous humor in ophthalmic surgery.

Pharmacodynamics/Kinetics

Absorption: Following intravitreous injection, diffusion occurs slowly

Elimination: By way of the Canal of Schlemm

Usual Dosage Depends upon procedure (slowly introduce a sufficient quantity into eye)

Monitoring Parameters Intraocular pressure

Dosage Forms Injection, intraocular: 10 mg/mL (0.25 mL, 0.4 mL, 0.5 mL, 0.75 mL, 0.8 mL, 2 mL, 4 mL); 16 mg/mL (0.25 mL, 0.5 mL, 8 mL)

Sodium Hyaluronate-Chrondroitin Sulfate *see* Chondroitin Sulfate-Sodium Hyaluronate *on page 241*

Sodium Hydrogen Carbonate *see* Sodium Bicarbonate *on page 1010*

Sodium Hypochlorite Solution (hye poe klor' ite)
Synonyms Dakin's Solution; Modified Dakin's Solution
Use Treatment of athlete's foot (0.5%); wound irrigation (0.5%); disinfect utensils and equipment (5%)
Pregnancy Risk Factor C
Contraindications Hypersensitivity
Warnings/Precautions For external use only; avoid eye or mucous membrane contact; do not use on open wounds
Adverse Reactions 1% to 10%: Dissolves blood clots, delays clotting, irritating to skin
Stability Use prepared solution within 7 days
Usual Dosage Topical irrigation
Patient Information External use only
Nursing Implications Dakin's solution may hinder wound healing
Dosage Forms
Solution: 5% (4000 mL)
Solution (modified Dakin's solution):
Full strength: 0.5% (1000 mL)
Half strength: 0.25% (1000 mL)
Quarter strength: 0.125% (1000 mL)

Sodium *L*-Triiodothyronine *see* Liothyronine Sodium *on page 637*

Sodium Methicillin *see* Methicillin Sodium *on page 707*

Sodium Nafcillin *see* Nafcillin Sodium *on page 768*

Sodium Nitroferricyanide *see* Nitroprusside Sodium *on page 801*

Sodium Nitroprusside *see* Nitroprusside Sodium *on page 801*

Sodium P.A.S. *see* Aminosalicylate Sodium *on page 57*

Sodium Phosphate and Potassium Phosphate *see* Potassium Phosphate and Sodium Phosphate *on page 912*

Sodium Phosphates (sow' dee um fos' fates)
Related Information
Laxatives, Classification and Properties *on page 1272*
Brand Names Fleet® Enema [OTC]; Fleet® Phospho®-Soda [OTC]
Use Short-term treatment of constipation, evacuation of the colon for rectal and bowel exams; source of sodium and phosphorus; treatment and prevention of hypophosphatemia
Pregnancy Risk Factor C
Contraindications Hyperphosphatemia, hypernatremia, hypocalcemia, renal failure, congestive heart failure, abdominal pain, fecal impaction
Warnings/Precautions Use with caution in patients with renal insufficiency, CHF, sodium restriction, cirrhosis; phosphate salts may precipitate in the presence of calcium; prolonged and/or excessive use of laxative may result in dependence; risks of rapid I.V. infusion include hypocalcemia, hypotension, muscular irritability, calcium deposits, renal function deterioration, and hyperkalemia
Adverse Reactions
1% to 10%:
Cardiovascular: Edema, hypotension
Endocrine & metabolic: Hyperphosphatemia, hypocalcemia, hypernatremia, calcium phosphate precipitation
Gastrointestinal: Nausea, vomiting, diarrhea
Renal: Acute renal failure
Overdosage/Toxicology Symptoms of overdose include tetany, convulsions and neuroexcitability, secondary to the hypocalcemia associated with hyperphosphatemia or hypernatremia; aluminum hydroxide may be administered to adults in doses of 60-200 mL/day; 8-24 capsules (or tablets)/day

The dose should be tailored to the patient (aluminum forms an insoluble compound with the phosphate which is excreted in the stool); hypernatremia is treated with loop diuretics and free water replacement; seizures may require diazepam 0.1-0.25 mg/kg; tetany should be treated with I.V. calcium salts
Drug Interactions Do not give with magnesium- and aluminum-containing antacids or sucralfate which can bind with phosphate
(Continued)

Sodium Phosphates *(Continued)*

Stability Phosphate salts may precipitate when mixed with calcium salts; solubility is improved in amino acid parenteral nutrition solutions; check with a pharmacist to determine compatibility

Mechanism of Action As a laxative, exerts osmotic effect in the small intestine by drawing water into the lumen of the gut, producing distention and promoting peristalsis and evacuation of the bowel; phosphorous participates in bone deposition, calcium metabolism, utilization of B complex vitamins, and as a buffer in acid-base equilibrium

Pharmacodynamics/Kinetics

Onset of action:
  Cathartic: 3-6 hours
  Rectal: 2-5 minutes
Absorption: Oral: ~1% to 20%
Elimination:
  Oral phosphate: In feces
  I.V. phosphate: In urine with over 80% of dose reabsorbed by the kidney

Usual Dosage

Normal requirements elemental phosphorus: Oral:
  0-6 months: 240 mg
  6-12 months: 360 mg
  1-10 years: 800 mg
  >10 years: 1200 mg
Pregnancy lactation: Additional 400 mg/day
Adults RDA: 800 mg

I.V. doses should be incorporated into the patient's maintenance I.V. fluids whenever possible; intermittent I.V. infusion should be reserved for severe depletion situations and requires continuous EKG monitoring. It is difficult to determine total body phosphorus deficit due to redistribution into intracellular compartment or bone tissue; (it is recommended that repletion of severe hypophosphatemia (<1 mg/dL in adults) be done via I.V. route since large dose of oral phosphate may cause diarrhea and intestinal absorption may be unreliable). The following dosages are empiric guidelines. **Note:** Doses listed as mmol of phosphate.

Severe hypophosphatemia: I.V.:
  Children:
    Low dose: 0.08 mmol/kg over 6 hours; use if recent losses and uncomplicated
    Intermediate dose: 0.16-0.24 mmol/kg over 4-6 hours; use if phosphorus level 0.5-1 mg/dL
    High dose: 0.36 mmol/kg over 6 hours; use if serum phosphorus <0.5 mg/dL
  Adults: 0.15-0.3 mmol/kg/dose over 12 hours, may repeat as needed to achieve desired serum level
  Maintenance:
    Children: 0.5-1.5 mmol/kg/24 hours I.V. or 2-3 mmol/kg/24 hours orally in divided doses
    Adults: 50-70 mmol/24 hours I.V. or 50-150 mmol/24 hours orally in divided doses **or**

Children <4 years: Oral: 1 capsule (250 mg/8 mmol phosphorus) 4 times/day; dilute as instructed
Children >4 years and Adults: Oral: 1-2 capsules (250-500 mg/8-16 mmol phosphorus) 4 times/day; dilute as instructed
Phosphate maintenance electrolyte requirement in parenteral nutrition: 2 mmol/kg/24 hours or 35 mmol/kcal/24 hours; maximum: 15-30 mmol/24 hours

Laxative (Fleet®): Rectal:
  Children 2-12 years: Contents of one 2.25 oz pediatric enema, may repeat
  Children ≥12 years and Adults: Contents of one 4.5 oz enema as a single dose, may repeat

Laxative (Fleet® Phospho®-Soda): Oral:
  Children 5-9 years: 5 mL as a single dose
  Children 10-12 years: 10 mL as a single dose
  Children ≥12 years and Adults: 20-30 mL as a single dose

Administration Rate of I.V. infusion should not exceed 0.05 mmol/kg/hour; risks of rapid I.V. infusion include hypocalcemia, hypotension, muscular irritability, calcium deposits, renal function deterioration, and hyperkalemia

With orders for I.V. phosphate, there is considerable confusion associated with the use of millimoles versus milliequivalents to express the phosphate requirement. Because inorganic phosphate exists as monobasic and dibasic anions, with the mixture of valences dependent on pH, ordering by mEq amounts is unreliable and may lead to large dosing errors. In addition, I.V. phosphate is available in the sodium and potassium salt, therefore, the content of these cations must be considered when ordering phosphate. The most reliable method of ordering I.V. phosphate is by millimoles, then specifying the potassium or sodium salt.

Contents of one packet should be diluted in 75 mL water before administration; maintain adequate fluid intake

Monitoring Parameters Serum sodium, phosphorus, calcium, renal function, EKG monitor if severe hypophosphatemia

Reference Range Phosphorous serum levels; it should be noted that serum levels do not accurately reflect intracellular phosphorous levels or extent of total body depletion

Newborns: 4.2-9 mg/dL
Children:
    1-2 years: 3.8-6.2 mg/dL
    3-15 years: 3.6-5.6 mg/dL
Adults: 3-4.5 mg/dL

Patient Information May cause diarrhea with the oral preparation; excessive or prolonged use as a laxative may cause dependence

Dosage Forms
Enema: Sodium phosphate 6 g and sodium biphosphate 16 g/100 mL (67.5 mL pediatric enema unit, 135 mL adult enema unit)
Injection: 3 mmol phosphate, 4 mEq sodium/mL (5 mL, 10 mL, 15 mL, 30 mL, 50 mL)
Solution, oral: Sodium phosphate 18 g and sodium biphosphate 48 g/100 mL (45 mL, 90 mL, 273 mL)
See table.

	Phosphate (mmol)	Sodium (mEq)	Potassium (mEq)
Oral			
Whole cow's milk	0.29/mL	0.025/mL	0.035/mL
Fleet® Phospho® -Soda	4.15/mL	4.8/mL	None
Intravenous			
Sodium phosphate	3/mL	4/mL	None

Sodium Polystyrene Sulfonate (pol ee stye' reen)

Brand Names Kayexalate®; SPS®

Use Treatment of hyperkalemia

Pregnancy Risk Factor C

Contraindications Hypernatremia, hypersensitivity to any component

Warnings/Precautions Use with caution in patients with severe congestive heart failure, hypertension, edema, or renal failure; avoid using the commercially available liquid product in neonates due to the preservative content; large oral doses may cause fecal impaction (especially in elderly); enema will reduce the serum potassium faster than oral administration, but the oral route will result in a greater reduction over several hours.

Adverse Reactions
>10%: Gastrointestinal: Constipation, loss of appetite, nausea, vomiting
1% to 10%:
    Endocrine & metabolic: Hypokalemia, hypocalcemia, hypomagnesemia
    Miscellaneous: Fecal impaction, sodium retention

Overdosage/Toxicology Symptoms of overdose include hypokalemia including cardiac dysrhythmias, confusion, irritability, EKG changes, muscle weakness, gastrointestinal effects; treatment is supportive, limited to management of fluid and electrolytes

Mechanism of Action Removes potassium by exchanging sodium ions for potassium ions in the intestine before the resin is passed from the body; exchange capacity is 1 mEq/g *in vivo*, and *in vitro* capacity is 3.1 mEq/g, therefore, a wide range of exchange capacity exists such that close monitoring of serum electrolytes is necessary

Pharmacodynamics/Kinetics
Onset of action: Within 2-24 hours
Absorption: Remains in GI tract
Elimination: Completely in feces (primarily as potassium polystyrene sulfonate)
(Continued)

Sodium Polystyrene Sulfonate *(Continued)*

Usual Dosage
Children:
Oral: 1 g/kg/dose every 6 hours
Rectal: 1 g/kg/dose every 2-6 hours (In small children and infants, employ lower doses by using the practical exchange ratio of 1 mEq K+/g of resin as the basis for calculation)

Adults:
Oral: 15 g (60 mL) 1-4 times/day
Rectal: 30-50 g every 6 hours

Monitoring Parameters Serum electrolytes (potassium, sodium, calcium, magnesium), EKG

Reference Range Serum potassium: Adults: 3.5-5.2 mEq/L

Patient Information Mix well in full glass of liquid prior to drinking

Nursing Implications Administer oral (or NG) as ~25% sorbitol solution, never mix in orange juice; enema route is less effective than oral administration; retain enema in colon for at least 30-60 minutes and for several hours, if possible; chilling the oral mixture will increase palatability; enema should be followed by irrigation with normal saline to prevent necrosis

Additional Information 1 g of resin binds approximately 1 mEq of potassium; sodium content of 1 g: 31 mg (1.3 mEq)

Dosage Forms Oral or rectal:
Powder for suspension: 454 g
Suspension: 1.25 g/5 mL with sorbitol 33% and alcohol 0.3% (60 mL, 120 mL, 200 mL, 500 mL)

Sodium Sulamyd® *see* Sodium Sulfacetamide *on this page*

Sodium Sulfacetamide *(sul fa see' ta mide)*

Brand Names AK-Sulf®; Bleph®-10; Cetamide®; Ophthacet®; Sebizon®; Sodium Sulamyd®; Sulf-10®; Sulfair®; Sulten-10®

Synonyms Sulfacetamide Sodium

Use Treatment and prophylaxis of conjunctivitis due to susceptible organisms; corneal ulcers; adjunctive treatment with systemic sulfonamides for therapy of trachoma; topical application in scaling dermatosis (seborrheic); bacterial infections of the skin

Pregnancy Risk Factor C

Contraindications Hypersensitivity to sulfacetamide or any component, sulfonamides; infants <2 months of age

Warnings/Precautions Inactivated by purulent exudates containing PABA; use with caution in severe dry eye; ointment may retard corneal epithelial healing; sulfite in some products may cause hypersensitivity reactions; cross-sensitivity may occur with previous exposure to other sulfonamides given by other routes

Adverse Reactions
1% to 10%: Local: Irritation, stinging, burning
<1%:
Central nervous system: Headache
Dermatologic: Stevens-Johnson syndrome, exfoliative dermatitis, toxic epidermal necrolysis
Ocular: Blurred vision, browache
Sensitivity reactions: Hypersensitivity reactions

Drug Interactions Decreased effect: Silver, gentamicin (antagonism)

Stability Protect from light; discolored solution should not be used; **incompatible** with silver and zinc sulfate; sulfacetamide is inactivated by blood or purulent exudates

Mechanism of Action Interferes with bacterial growth by inhibiting bacterial folic acid synthesis through competitive antagonism of PABA

Pharmacodynamics/Kinetics
Half-life: 7-13 hours
Elimination: When absorbed, excreted primarily in urine as unchanged drug

Usual Dosage
Children >2 months and Adults: Ophthalmic:
Ointment: Apply to lower conjunctival sac 1-4 times/day and at bedtime
Solution: Instill 1-3 drops several times daily up to every 2-3 hours in lower conjunctival sac during waking hours and less frequently at night
Seborrheic dermatitis: Children >12 years and Adults: Topical: Apply at bedtime and allow to remain overnight; in severe cases, may apply twice daily
Secondary cutaneous bacterial infections: Children >12 years and Adults: Topically: Apply 2-4 times/day until infection clears

Monitoring Parameters Response to therapy

Patient Information Eye drops will burn upon instillation; wait at least 10 minutes before using another eye preparation; may sting eyes when first applied; do not touch container to eye, ointment will cause blurred vision; notify physician if condition does not improve in 3-4 days; may cause sensitivity to sunlight

Nursing Implications Assess whether patient can adequately instill drops or ointment

Dosage Forms
Lotion, topical: 10% (85 g)
Ointment, ophthalmic: 10% (3.5 g)
Solution, ophthalmic: 10% (1 mL, 2 mL, 5 mL, 15 mL); 15% (2 mL, 5 mL, 15 mL); 30% (5 mL, 15 mL)

Sodium Sulfacetamide and Prednisolone Acetate (sul fa see' ta mide & pred niss' oh lone)

Brand Names Blephamide®; Cetapred®; Metimyd®; Vasocidin®

Use Steroid-responsive inflammatory ocular conditions where infection is present or there is a risk of infection; ophthalmic suspension may be used as an otic preparation

Pregnancy Risk Factor C

Contraindications Mycobacteria infections, fungal infections, herpes simplex keratitis, hypersensitivity to sulfacetamide, prednisolone or any component, infants <2 months of age

Warnings/Precautions Inactivated by purulent exudates containing PABA; use with caution in severe dry eyes; ointment may retard corneal epithelial healing; sulfite in some products may cause hypersensitivity reactions

Adverse Reactions
1% to 10%: Local burning, stinging
<1%:
Central nervous system: Vertigo, seizures, psychoses, pseudotumor cerebri, headache
Dermatologic: Stevens-Johnson syndrome, skin atrophy
Endocrine & metabolic: Cushing's syndrome, pituitary-adrenal axis suppression, growth suppression
Gastrointestinal: Peptic ulcer, nausea, vomiting
Neuromuscular & skeletal: Muscle weakness, osteoporosis, fractures
Ocular: Cataracts, glaucoma

Drug Interactions Decreased effect: Silver, gentamicin, vaccines, toxoids

Mechanism of Action Interferes with bacterial growth by inhibiting bacterial folic acid synthesis through competitive antagonism of PABA; decreases inflammation by suppression of migration of polymorphonuclear leukocytes and reversal of increased capillary permeability; suppresses the immune system by reducing activity and volume of the lymphatic system

Pharmacodynamics/Kinetics Refer to Sodium Sulfacetamide and Prednisolone Acetate monographs

Usual Dosage Children >2 months and Adults: Ophthalmic:
Ointment: Apply to lower conjunctival sac 1-4 times/day
Solution: Instill 1-3 drops every 2-3 hours while awake

Patient Information Eye drops will burn upon instillation; wait at least 10 minutes before using another eye preparation; may sting eyes when first applied; do not touch container to eye; ointment will cause blurred vision; notify physician if condition does not improve in 3-4 days; may cause sensitivity to sunlight

Nursing Implications Shake ophthalmic suspension before using; assess whether patient can adequately instill drops or ointment

Dosage Forms Ophthalmic:
Ointment:
Blephamide®: Sodium sulfacetamide 10% and prednisolone acetate 0.2% (3.5 g)
Cetapred®: Sodium sulfacetamide 10% and prednisolone acetate 0.25% (3.5 g)
Metimyd®: Sodium sulfacetamide 10% and prednisolone acetate 0.5% (3.5 g)
Suspension:
Blephamide®: Sodium sulfacetamide 10% and prednisolone acetate 0.2% (2.5 mL, 5 mL, 10 mL)
Isopto® Cetapred®: Sodium sulfacetamide 10% and prednisolone acetate 0.25% (5 mL, 15 mL)
Optimyd®: Sodium sulfacetamide 10% and prednisolone sodium phosphate 0.5% (5 mL)
Vasocidin®: Sodium sulfacetamide 10% and prednisolone acetate 0.25% (5 mL, 10 mL)

Sodium Tetradecyl Sulfate (tetra deck' il)

Brand Names Sotradecol®

Use Treatment of small, uncomplicated varicose veins of the lower extremities; endoscopic sclerotherapy in the management of bleeding esophageal varices

Pregnancy Risk Factor C

Contraindications Arterial disease, thrombophlebitis, hypersensitivity to sodium tetradecyl or any component, valvular or deep vein incompetence, phlebitis, migraines, cellulitis, acute infections

Warnings/Precautions Buerger's disease, peripheral arteriosclerosis, avoid extravasation

Adverse Reactions

1% to 10%:

  Central nervous system: Headache

  Dermatologic: Urticaria, mucosal lesions

  Gastrointestinal: Nausea, vomiting

  Local: Discoloration at the site of injection, pain, ulceration at the site, sloughing and tissue necrosis following extravasation

  Respiratory: Pulmonary edema

<1%:

  Dermatologic: Hives

  Gastrointestinal: Esophageal perforation

  Respiratory: Asthma

Stability Store at controlled room temperature in a well-closed container; protect from light

Mechanism of Action Acts by irritation of the vein intimal endothelium

Usual Dosage I.V.: Test dose: 0.5 mL given several hours prior to administration of larger dose; 0.5-2 mL in each vein, maximum: 10 mL per treatment session; 3% solution reserved for large varices

Patient Information Notify physician if chest pain, shortness of breath, or heat, pain, or tenderness in lower extremities

Nursing Implications Observe for signs and symptoms of embolism

Dosage Forms Injection: 1% [10 mg/mL] (2 mL); 3% [30 mg/mL] (2 mL)

Sodium Thiosulfate (thye oh sul' fate)

Brand Names Tinver® Lotion

Use

Parenteral: Used alone or with sodium nitrite or amyl nitrite in cyanide poisoning or arsenic poisoning; reduce the risk of nephrotoxicity associated with cisplatin therapy

Topical: Treatment of tinea versicolor

Pregnancy Risk Factor C

Contraindications Hypersensitivity to any component

Warnings/Precautions Safety in pregnancy has not been established; discontinue topical use if irritation or sensitivity occurs; rapid I.V. infusion has caused transient hypotension and EKG changes in dogs; can increase risk of thiocyanate intoxication

Adverse Reactions

1% to 10%:

  Cardiovascular: Hypotension

  Central nervous system: Coma, CNS depression secondary to thiocyanate intoxication, psychosis, confusion, weakness

  Dermatologic: Contact dermatitis, local irritation

  Otic: Tinnitus

Mechanism of Action

Cyanide toxicity: Increases the rate of detoxification of cyanide by the enzyme rhodanese by providing an extra sulfur

Cisplatin toxicity: Complexes with cisplatin to form a compound that is nontoxic to either normal or cancerous cells

Pharmacodynamics/Kinetics

Half-life: 0.65 hour

Elimination: 28.5% excreted unchanged in urine

Usual Dosage

Cyanide and nitroprusside antidote: I.V.:

  Children <25 kg: 50 mg/kg after receiving 4.5-10 mg/kg sodium nitrite; a half dose of each may be repeated if necessary

  Children >25 kg and Adults: 12.5 g after 300 mg of sodium nitrite; a half dose of each may be repeated if necessary

Cyanide poisoning: I.V.: Dose should be based on determination as with nitrite at rate of 2.5-5 mL/minute to maximum of 50 mL. See table.

Variation of Sodium Nitrite and Sodium Thiosulfate Dose With Hemoglobin Concentration*

Hemoglobin (g/dL)	Initial Dose Sodium Nitrite (mg/kg)	Initial Dose Sodium Nitrite 33% (mL/kg)	Initial Dose Sodium Thiosulfate 25% (mL/kg)
7	5.8	0.19	0.95
8	6.6	0.22	1.10
9	7.5	0.25	1.25
10	8.3	0.27	1.35
11	9.1	0.30	1.50
12	10.0	0.33	1.65
13	10.8	0.36	1.80
14	11.6	0.39	1.95

*Adapted from Berlin DM Jr, 'The Treatment of Cyanide Poisoning in Children,' *Pediatrics*, 1970, 46:793.

Cisplatin rescue should be given before or during cisplatin administration: I.V. infusion (in sterile water): 12 g/m² over 6 hours or 9 g/m² I.V. push followed by 1.2 g/m² continuous infusion for 6 hours

Arsenic poisoning: I.V.: 1 mL first day, 2 mL second day, 3 mL third day, 4 mL fourth day, 5 mL on alternate days thereafter

Children and Adults: Topical: 20% to 25% solution: Apply a thin layer to affected areas twice daily

Administration I.V.: Inject slowly, over at least 10 minutes; rapid administration may cause hypotension

Monitoring Parameters Monitor for signs of thiocyanate toxicity

Patient Information Avoid topical application near the eyes, mouth, or other mucous membranes; notify physician if condition worsens or burning or irritation occurs; shake well before using

Dosage Forms
Injection: 100 mg/mL (10 mL); 250 mg/mL (50 mL)
Lotion: 25% with salicylic acid 1% and isopropyl alcohol 10% (120 mL, 180 mL)

Sodol® *see* Carisoprodol *on page 185*

Sofarin® *see* Warfarin Sodium *on page 1168*

Solaquin Forte® *see* Hydroquinone *on page 551*

Solaquin® [OTC] *see* Hydroquinone *on page 551*

Solarcaine® [OTC] *see* Benzocaine *on page 121*

Solatene® *see* Beta-Carotene *on page 129*

Solfoton® *see* Phenobarbital *on page 869*

Solganal® *see* Aurothioglucose *on page 104*

Soluble Fluorescein *see* Fluorescein Sodium *on page 470*

Solu-Cortef® *see* Hydrocortisone *on page 546*

Solu-Medrol® *see* Methylprednisolone *on page 724*

Solurex L.A.® *see* Dexamethasone *on page 314*

Soma® *see* Carisoprodol *on page 185*

Soma® Compound *see* Carisoprodol *on page 185*

Somatrem *see* Human Growth Hormone *on page 538*

Somatropin *see* Human Growth Hormone *on page 538*

Sominex® [OTC] *see* Diphenhydramine Hydrochloride *on page 351*

Somnos® *see* Chloral Hydrate *on page 217*

Soothe® [OTC] *see* Tetrahydrozoline Hydrochloride *on page 1071*

Soprodol® *see* Carisoprodol *on page 185*

Sorbitol (sor' bi tole)

Use Genitourinary irrigant in transurethral prostatic resection or other transurethral resection or other transurethral surgical procedures; diuretic; humectant; sweetening agent; hyperosmotic laxative; facilitate the passage of sodium polystyrene sulfonate through the intestinal tract
(Continued)

Sorbitol *(Continued)*

Contraindications Anuria

Warnings/Precautions Use with caution in patients with severe cardiopulmonary or renal impairment and in patients unable to metabolize sorbitol

Adverse Reactions
1% to 10%:
Cardiovascular: Edema
Endocrine & metabolic: Fluid and electrolyte losses, lactic acidosis
Gastrointestinal: Diarrhea, nausea, vomiting, abdominal discomfort, dry mouth

Overdosage/Toxicology Symptoms of overdose include nausea, diarrhea, fluid and electrolyte loss; treatment is supportive to ensure fluid and electrolyte balance

Mechanism of Action A polyalcoholic sugar with osmotic cathartic actions

Pharmacodynamics/Kinetics
Onset of action: About 0.25-1 hour
Absorption: Oral, rectal: Poor
Metabolism: Mainly in the liver to fructose

Usual Dosage Hyperosmotic laxative (as single dose, at infrequent intervals):
Children 2-11 years:
Oral: 2 mL/kg (as 70% solution)
Rectal enema: 30-60 mL as 25% to 30% solution

Children >12 years and Adults:
Oral: 30-150 mL (as 70% solution)
Rectal enema: 120 mL as 25% to 30% solution
Adjunct to sodium polystyrene sulfonate: 15 mL as 70% solution orally until diarrhea occurs (10-20 mL/2 hours) or 20-100 mL as an oral vehicle for the sodium polystyrene sulfonate resin

When administered with charcoal:
Oral:
Children: 4.3 mL/kg of 35% sorbitol with 1 g/kg of activated charcoal
Adults: 4.3 mL/kg of 70% sorbitol with 1 g/kg of activated charcoal every 4 hours until first stool containing charcoal is passed
Topical: 3% to 3.3% as transurethral surgical procedure irrigation

Nursing Implications Do not use unless solution is clear

Dosage Forms
Solution: 70%
Solution, genitourinary irrigation: 3% (1500 mL, 3000 mL); 3.3% (2000 mL)

Sorbitrate® *see* Isosorbide Dinitrate *on page 599*

Soridol® *see* Carisoprodol *on page 185*

Sotalol Hydrochloride *(soe' ta lole)*

Related Information
Antiarrhythmic Drugs *on page 1246-1248*
Beta-Blockers Comparison *on page 1257-1259*

Brand Names Betapace®

Use Treatment of documented ventricular arrhythmias, such as sustained ventricular tachycardia, that in the judgment of the physician are life-threatening
Unlabeled use: Supraventricular arrhythmias

Pregnancy Risk Factor B

Pregnancy/Breast Feeding Implications Sotalol should be used during pregnancy only if the potential benefit outweighs the potential risk

Contraindications Bronchial asthma, sinus bradycardia, second and third degree A-V block (unless a functioning pacemaker is present), congenital or acquired long Q-T syndromes, cardiogenic shock, uncontrolled congestive heart failure, and previous evidence of hypersensitivity to sotalol

Warnings/Precautions Use with caution in patients with congestive heart failure, peripheral vascular disease, hypokalemia, hypomagnesemia, renal dysfunction, sick-sinus syndrome; abrupt withdrawal may result in return of life-threatening arrhythmias; sotalol can provoke new or worsening ventricular arrhythmias

Adverse Reactions
>10%:
Cardiovascular: Bradycardia
Central nervous system: Mental depression
Endocrine & metabolic: Decreased sexual ability
1% to 10%:
Cardiovascular: Congestive heart failure

    Central nervous system: Mental confusion, hallucinations, reduced peripheral circulation, anxiety, dizziness, drowsiness, nightmares, insomnia, weakness, tiredness

    Dermatologic: Itching

    Gastrointestinal: Constipation, diarrhea, nausea, vomiting, stomach discomfort

    Respiratory: Breathing difficulties

<1%:

    Cardiovascular: Chest pain, hypotension (especially with higher doses), Raynaud's phenomena

    Dermatologic: Skin rash; red, crusted skin, skin necrosis after extravasation

    Hematologic: Leukopenia

    Local: Phlebitis

    Miscellaneous: Diaphoresis, cold extremities

Overdosage/Toxicology Symptoms of intoxication include cardiac disturbances, CNS toxicity, bronchospasm, hypoglycemia and hyperkalemia. The most common cardiac symptoms include hypotension and bradycardia; atrioventricular block, intraventricular conduction disturbances, cardiogenic shock, and systole may occur with severe overdose, especially with membrane-depressant drugs (eg, propranolol); CNS effects include convulsions, coma, and respiratory arrest is commonly seen with propranolol and other membrane-depressant and lipid-soluble drugs.

Treatment includes symptomatic treatment of seizures, hypotension, hyperkalemia and hypoglycemia; bradycardia and hypotension resistant to atropine, isoproterenol or pacing may respond to glucagon; wide QRS defects caused by the membrane-depressant poisoning may respond to hypertonic sodium bicarbonate; repeat-dose charcoal, hemoperfusion, or hemodialysis may be helpful in removal of only those beta-blockers with a small V_d, long half-life or low intrinsic clearance (acebutolol, atenolol, nadolol, sotalol)

Drug Interactions

Decreased effect of beta-blockers with aluminum salts, barbiturates, calcium salts, cholestyramine, colestipol, NSAIDs, penicillins (ampicillin), rifampin, salicylates and sulfinpyrazone due to decreased bioavailability and plasma levels

Beta-blockers may decrease the effect of sulfonylureas

Increased effect/toxicity of beta-blockers with calcium blockers (diltiazem, felodipine, nicardipine), contraceptives, flecainide, haloperidol (propranolol, hypotensive effects), H_2 antagonists (metoprolol, propranolol only by cimetidine, possibly ranitidine), hydralazine (metoprolol, propranolol), loop diuretics (propranolol, not atenolol), MAO inhibitors (metoprolol, nadolol, bradycardia), phenothiazines (propranolol), propafenone (metoprolol, propranolol), quinidine (in extensive metabolizers), ciprofloxacin, thyroid hormones (metoprolol, propranolol, when hypothyroid patient is converted to euthyroid state)

Beta-blockers may increase the effect/toxicity of flecainide, haloperidol (hypotensive effects), hydralazine, phenothiazines, acetaminophen, anticoagulants (propranolol, warfarin), benzodiazepines (not atenolol), clonidine (hypertensive crisis after or during withdrawal of either agent), epinephrine (initial hypertensive episode followed by bradycardia), nifedipine and verapamil lidocaine, ergots (peripheral ischemia), prazosin (postural hypotension)

Beta-blockers may affect the action or levels of ethanol, disopyramide, nondepolarizing muscle relaxants and theophylline although the effects are difficult to predict

Mechanism of Action

Beta-blocker which contains both beta-adrenoreceptor-blocking (Vaughan Williams Class II) and cardiac action potential duration prolongation (Vaughan Williams Class III) properties

Class II effects: Increased sinus cycle length, slowed heart rate, decreased A-V nodal conduction, and increased A-V nodal refractoriness

Class III effects: Prolongation of the atrial and ventricular monophasic action potentials, and effective refractory prolongation of atrial muscle, ventricular muscle, and atrioventricular accessory pathways in both the antegrade and retrograde directions

Sotalol is a racemic mixture of d- and l-sotalol; both isomers have similar Class III antiarrhythmic effects while the l-isomer is responsible for virtually all of the beta-blocking activity

Sotalol has both beta$_1$- and beta$_2$-receptor blocking activity

The beta-blocking effect of sotalol is a noncardioselective [half maximal at about 80 mg/day and maximal at doses of 320-640 mg/day]. Significant beta blockade occurs at oral doses as low as 25 mg/day.

The Class III effects are seen only at oral doses ≥160 mg/day

Pharmacodynamics/Kinetics

Onset of action: Rapid, 1-2 hours

Peak effect: 2.5-4 hours

Absorption: Decreased 20% to 30% by meals compared to fasting

(Continued)

Sotalol Hydrochloride *(Continued)*

Bioavailability: 90% to 100%

Distribution: Low lipid solubility

Sotalol is excreted in the milk of laboratory animals and is reported to be present in human milk

Metabolism: Sotalol is **not** metabolized

Protein binding: Not protein bound

Half-life: 12 hours

Elimination: Unchanged through kidney

Serum concentrations have not been systematically evaluated: Concentration-effect curves for the beta-blocking and antiarrhythmic agents of sotalol are different

Serum levels of 340-3,440 ng/mL have showed a 70% to 100% reduction in PVBs

Average serum concentrations associated with significant Q-T prolongation were 2,550 ng/mL

Average serum concentrations associated with maximum heart reduction by 50% was 804 ng/mL

Usual Dosage Sotalol should be initiated and doses increased in a hospital with facilities for cardiac rhythm monitoring and assessment. Proarrhythmic events can occur after initiation of therapy and with each upward dosage adjustment.

Children (oral): The safety and efficacy of sotalol in children have not been established

Supraventricular arrhythmias: 2-4 mg/kg/24 hours was given in 2 equal doses every 12 hours to 18 infants (≤2 months of age). All infants, except one with chaotic atrial tachycardia, were successful controlled with sotalol. Ten infants discontinued therapy between the ages of 7-18 months when it was no longer necessary. Median duration of treatment was 12.8 months.

Adults (oral):

Initial: 80 mg twice daily

Dose may be increased (gradually allowing 2-3 days between dosing increments in order to attain steady-state plasma concentrations and to allow monitoring of Q-T intervals) to 240-320 mg/day

Most patients respond to a total daily dose of 160-320 mg/day in 2-3 divided doses

Some patients, with life-threatening refractory ventricular arrhythmias, may require doses as high as 480-640 mg/day; however, these doses should only be prescribed when the potential benefit outweighs the increased of adverse events

Elderly patients: Age does not significantly alter the pharmacokinetics of sotalol, but impaired renal function in elderly patients can increase the terminal half-life, resulting in increased drug accumulation

Dosing adjustment in renal impairment:

Cl_{cr} >60 mL/minute: Administer every 12 hours

Cl_{cr} 30-60 mL/minute: Administer every 24 hours

Cl_{cr} 10-30 mL/minute: Administer every 36-48 hours

Cl_{cr} <10 mL/minute: Individualize dose

Hemodialysis would be expected to reduce sotalol plasma concentrations because sotalol is not bound to plasma proteins and does not undergo extensive metabolism; administer dose postdialysis or administer supplemental 80 mg dose; peritoneal dialysis does not remove sotalol; supplemental dose is not necessary

Monitoring Parameters Serum magnesium, potassium, EKG

Patient Information Seek emergency help if palpitations occur; do not discontinue abruptly or change dose without notifying physician; take on an empty stomach

Nursing Implications Initiation of therapy and dose escalation should be done in a hospital with cardiac monitoring; lidocaine and other resuscitative measures should be available

Dosage Forms Tablet: 80 mg, 160 mg, 240 mg

Sotradecol® *see* Sodium Tetradecyl Sulfate *on page 1019*

Soyacal® *see* Fat Emulsion *on page 441*

SPA *see* Albumin, Human *on page 32*

Spancap® No. 1 *see* Dextroamphetamine Sulfate *on page 319*

Span-FF® [OTC] *see* Ferrous Fumarate *on page 450*

Sparine® *see* Promazine Hydrochloride *on page 937*

Spaslin® *see* Hyoscyamine, Atropine, Scopolamine, and Phenobarbital *on page 557*

Spasmoject® *see* Dicyclomine Hydrochloride *on page 330*

Spasmolin® *see* Hyoscyamine, Atropine, Scopolamine, and Phenobarbital *on page 557*

Spasmophen® *see* Hyoscyamine, Atropine, Scopolamine, and Phenobarbital *on page 557*

Spasquid® *see* Hyoscyamine, Atropine, Scopolamine, and Phenobarbital *on page 557*

Spectam® *see* Spectinomycin Hydrochloride *on this page*

Spectazole™ *see* Econazole Nitrate *on page 379*

Spectinomycin Hydrochloride (spek ti noe mye′ sin)

Related Information
Antimicrobial Drugs of Choice *on page 1298-1302*

Brand Names Spectam®; Trobicin®

Use Treatment of uncomplicated gonorrhea (ineffective against syphilis)

Pregnancy Risk Factor B

Contraindications Hypersensitivity to spectinomycin or any component

Warnings/Precautions Since spectinomycin is ineffective in the treatment of syphilis and may mask symptoms, all patients should be tested for syphilis at the time of diagnosis and 3 months later

Adverse Reactions
<1%:
 Central nervous system: Dizziness, headache, chills
 Dermatologic: Urticaria, rash, pruritus
 Gastrointestinal: Nausea, vomiting
 Local: Pain at injection site

Stability Use reconstituted solutions within 24 hours; reconstitute with supplied diluent only

Mechanism of Action A bacteriostatic antibiotic that selectively binds to the 30s subunits of ribosomes, and thereby inhibiting bacterial protein synthesis

Pharmacodynamics/Kinetics
Duration of action: Up to 8 hours
Distribution: V_d: 0.2 L/kg
Half-life: 1.7 hours
Time to peak serum concentration: Within 1 hour
Elimination: Almost entirely as unchanged drug in urine (70% to 100%)

Usual Dosage I.M.:
Children:
 <45 kg: 40 mg/kg/dose 1 time
 ≥45 kg: See adult dose
Children >8 years who are allergic to PCNS/cephalosporins may be treated with oral tetracycline
Adults:
 Uncomplicated urethral endocervical or rectal gonorrhea: 2 g deep I.M. or 4 g where antibiotic resistance is prevalent 1 time; 4 g (10 mL) dose should be given as two 5 mL injections, followed by doxycycline 100 mg twice daily for 7 days
 Disseminated gonococcal infection: 2 g every 12 hours
50% removed by hemodialysis

Administration For I.M. use only

Dosage Forms Injection: 2 g, 4 g

Spec-T® [OTC] *see* Benzocaine *on page 121*

Spironolactone (speer on oh lak′ tone)

Brand Names Aldactone®

Use Management of edema associated with excessive aldosterone excretion; hypertension; primary hyperaldosteronism; hypokalemia; treatment of hirsutism; cirrhosis of liver accompanied by edema or ascites

Pregnancy Risk Factor D

Contraindications Hypersensitivity to spironolactone or any component, hyperkalemia, renal failure, anuria, patients receiving other potassium-sparing diuretics or potassium supplements

Warnings/Precautions Use with caution in patients with dehydration, hepatic disease, hyponatremia, renal sufficiency; it is recommended the drug may be (Continued)

Spironolactone *(Continued)*

discontinued several days prior to adrenal vein catheterization; shown to be tumorigenic in toxicity studies using rats at 25-250 times the usual human dose

Adverse Reactions

1% to 10%:

Cardiovascular: Hypotension, edema, bradycardia, congestive heart failure

Central nervous system: Constipation, dizziness, fatigue, headache

Dermatologic: Rash

Gastrointestinal: Nausea

Respiratory: Dyspnea

<1%:

Cardiovascular: Flushing

Endocrine & metabolic: Hyperkalemia, dehydration, hyponatremia, gynecomastia, hyperchloremia, metabolic acidosis, postmenopausal bleeding

Genitourinary: Inability to achieve or maintain an erection

Overdosage/Toxicology Symptoms of overdose include drowsiness, confusion, clinical signs of dehydration and electrolyte imbalance, hyperkalemia; ingestion of large amounts of potassium-sparing diuretics, may result in life-threatening hyperkalemia. This can be treated with I.V. glucose, with concurrent regular insulin; sodium bicarbonate may also be used as a temporary measure. If needed, Kayexalate® oral or rectal solutions in sorbitol may also be used.

Drug Interactions Increased toxicity: Potassium, potassium-sparing diuretics, indomethacin, angiotensin-converting enzymes inhibitors may increase serum potassium levels

Stability Protect from light

Mechanism of Action Competes with aldosterone for receptor sites in the distal renal tubules, increasing sodium chloride and water excretion while conserving potassium and hydrogen ions; may block the effect of aldosterone on arteriolar smooth muscle as well

Pharmacodynamics/Kinetics

Protein binding: 91% to 98%

Metabolism: In the liver to multiple metabolites, including canrenone (active)

Half-life: 78-84 minutes

Time to peak serum concentration: Within 1-3 hours (primarily as the active metabolite)

Elimination: Urinary and biliary excretion

Usual Dosage Administration with food increases absorption. To reduce delay in onset of effect, a loading dose of 2 or 3 times the daily dose may be administered on the first day of therapy. Oral:

Neonates: 0.5-1 mg/kg/dose every 8 hours

Children:

Diuretic, hypertension: 1.5-3.5 mg/kg/day in divided doses every 6-24 hours

Diagnosis of primary aldosteronism: 125-375 mg/m^2/day in divided doses

Vaso-occlusive disease: 7.5 mg/kg/day in divided doses twice daily (not FDA approved)

Adults:

Edema, hypertension, hypokalemia: 25-200 mg/day in 1-2 divided doses

Diagnosis of primary aldosteronism: 100-400 mg/day in 1-2 divided doses

Elderly: Initial: 25-50 mg/day in 1-2 divided doses, increasing by 25-50 mg every 5 days as needed

Dosing interval in renal impairment:

Cl$_{cr}$ 10-50 mL/minute: Administer every 12-24 hours

Cl$_{cr}$ <10 mL/minute: Avoid use

Monitoring Parameters Blood pressure, serum electrolytes (potassium, sodium), renal function, I & O ratios and daily weight throughout therapy

Test Interactions May cause false elevation in serum digoxin concentrations measured by RIA

Patient Information Avoid hazardous activity such as driving, until response to drug is known; take with meals or milk; avoid excessive ingestion of foods high in potassium or use of salt substitutes

Nursing Implications Diuretic effect may be delayed 2-3 days and maximum hypertensive may be delayed 2-3 weeks; monitor I & O ratios and daily weight throughout therapy

Dosage Forms Tablet: 25 mg, 50 mg, 100 mg

Sporanox® *see* Itraconazole *on page 605*

SPS® *see* Sodium Polystyrene Sulfonate *on page 1017*

S-P-T *see* Thyroid *on page 1088*

SSD™ *see* Silver Sulfadiazine *on page 1005*

SSD-AF™ *see* Silver Sulfadiazine *on page 1005*

SSKI® *see* Potassium Iodide *on page 909*

Stadol® *see* Butorphanol Tartrate *on page 155*

Stadol® NS *see* Butorphanol Tartrate *on page 155*

Stagesic® *see* Hydrocodone and Acetaminophen *on page 543*

Stannous Fluoride *see* Fluoride *on page 471*

Stanozolol (stan oh′ zoe lole)

Brand Names Winstrol®

Use Prophylactic use against hereditary angioedema

Restrictions C-III

Pregnancy Risk Factor X

Contraindications Nephrosis, carcinoma of breast or prostate, pregnancy, hypersensitivity to any component

Warnings/Precautions May stunt bone growth in children; anabolic steroids may cause peliosis hepatis, liver cell tumors, and blood lipid changes with increased risk of arteriosclerosis; monitor diabetic patients carefully; use with caution in elderly patients, they may be at greater risk for prostatic hypertrophy; use with caution in patients with cardiac, renal, or hepatic disease or epilepsy

Adverse Reactions

Male:

Postpubertal:

>10%:

Dermatologic: Acne

Endocrine & metabolic: Bladder irritability, priapism, gynecomastia

1% to 10%:

Central nervous system: Insomnia

Endocrine & metabolic: Decreased libido, hepatic dysfunction, chills, prostatic hypertrophy (elderly)

Gastrointestinal: Nausea, diarrhea

Hematologic: Iron deficiency anemia, suppression of clotting factors

<1%: Hepatic: Hepatic necrosis, hepatocellular carcinoma

Prepubertal:

>10%:

Dermatologic: Acne

Endocrine & metabolic: Virilism

1% to 10%:

Central nervous system: Chills, insomnia, factors

Dermatologic: Hyperpigmentation

Gastrointestinal: Diarrhea, nausea

Hematologic: Iron deficiency anemia, suppression of clotting

<1%: Hepatic: Hepatic necrosis, hepatocellular carcinoma

Female:

>10%: Endocrine & metabolic: Virilism

1% to 10%:

Central nervous system: Chills, insomnia

Endocrine & metabolic: Hypercalcemia

Gastrointestinal: Nausea, diarrhea

Hematologic: Iron deficiency anemia, suppression of clotting factors

Hepatic: Hepatic dysfunction

<1%: Hepatic: Hepatic necrosis, hepatocellular carcinoma

Drug Interactions Increased toxicity: ACTH, adrenal steroids → ↑ risk of edema and acne; stanozolol enhances the hypoprothrombinemic effects of oral anticoagulants; enhances the hypoglycemic effects of insulin and sulfonylureas (oral hypoglycemics)

Mechanism of Action Synthetic testosterone derivative with similar androgenic and anabolic actions

Pharmacodynamics/Kinetics

Metabolism: In an analogous fashion to testosterone

Elimination: In an analogous fashion to testosterone

Usual Dosage

Children: Acute attacks:

<6 years: 1 mg/day

6-12 years: 2 mg/day

Adults: Oral: Initial: 2 mg 3 times/day, may then reduce to a maintenance dose of 2 mg/day or 2 mg every other day after 1-3 months

Dosing adjustment in hepatic impairment: Avoid use in patients with severe liver dysfunction

(Continued)

Stanozolol *(Continued)*

Patient Information High protein, high caloric diet is suggested, restrict salt intake; glucose tolerance may be altered in diabetics
Dosage Forms Tablet: 2 mg

Staphcillin® *see* Methicillin Sodium *on page 707*

Statrol® *see* Neomycin and Polymyxin B *on page 780*

Stavudine *(stav' yoo deen)*

Brand Names Zerit®
Synonyms d4T
Use For the treatment of adults with advanced HIV infection who are intolerant to approved therapies with proven clinical benefit or who have experienced significant clinical or immunologic deterioration while receiving these therapies, or for whom such therapies are contraindicated
Contraindications Hypersensitivity to stavudine
Warnings/Precautions Use with caution in patients who demonstrate previous hypersensitivity to zidovudine, didanosine, zalcitabine, pre-existing bone marrow suppression, or renal insufficiency, peripheral neuropathy, folic acid or vitamin B^{12} deficiency. Peripheral neuropathy may be the dose limiting side effect.
Adverse Reactions
>10%: Neuromuscular & skeletal: Peripheral neuropathy
1% to 10%:
Central nervous system: Headache, chills/fever abdominal or back pain, malaise, asthenia, insomnia, anxiety, depression
Gastrointestinal: Nausea, vomiting, diarrhea, pancreatitis
Neuromuscular & skeletal: Myalgia
Mechanism of Action Inhibits reverse transcriptase of the human immunodeficiency virus (HIV)
Pharmacodynamics/Kinetics
Distribution: V_d: 0.5 L/kg
Peak serum level: 1 hour after administration
Bioavailability: 86.4%
Half-life: 1-1.6 hours
Elimination: Renal (40%)
Usual Dosage
Adults: Oral:
≥60 kg: 40 mg every 12 hours
<60 kg: 30 mg every 12 hours
Dose may be cut in half if symptoms of peripheral neuropathy occur

Dosing adjustment in renal impairment:
Cl_{cr} >50 mL/minute: ≥60 kg: 40 mg every 12 hours
Cl_{cr} >50 mL/minute: <60 kg: 30 mg every 12 hours
Cl_{cr} 26-50 mL/minute: ≥60 kg: 20 mg every 12 hours
Cl_{cr} 26-50 mL/minute: <60 kg: 15 mg every 12 hours
Cl_{cr} 10-25 mL/minute: ≥60 kg: 20 mg every 24 hours
Cl_{cr} 10-25 mL/minute: <60 kg: 15 mg every 24 hours
Monitoring Parameters Monitor liver function tests and signs and symptoms of peripheral neuropathy.
Patient Information Contact physician at first signs or symptoms of peripheral neuropathy
Dosage Forms Capsule: 15 mg, 20 mg, 30 mg, 40 mg

Stay Trim® Diet Gum [OTC] *see* Phenylpropanolamine Hydrochloride *on page 876*

S-T Cort® *see* Hydrocortisone *on page 546*

Stelazine® *see* Trifluoperazine Hydrochloride *on page 1121*

Sterapred® *see* Prednisone *on page 921*

Stilbestrol *see* Diethylstilbestrol *on page 334*

Stilphostrol® *see* Diethylstilbestrol *on page 334*

Stimate™ *see* Desmopressin Acetate *on page 311*

St. Joseph® Cough Suppressant [OTC] *see* Dextromethorphan *on page 321*

St. Joseph® Measured Dose Nasal Solution [OTC] *see* Phenylephrine Hydrochloride *on page 874*

Stop® [OTC] *see* Fluoride *on page 471*

Streptase® *see* Streptokinase *on this page*

Streptokinase (strep toe kye' nase)

Brand Names Kabikinase®; Streptase®

Use Thrombolytic agent used in treatment of recent severe or massive deep vein thrombosis, pulmonary emboli, myocardial infarction, and occluded arteriovenous cannulas

Pregnancy Risk Factor C

Contraindications Hypersensitivity to streptokinase or any component; recent streptococcal infection within the last 6 months; any internal bleeding; brain carcinoma; pregnancy; cerebrovascular accident or transient ischemic attack, gastrointestinal bleeding, trauma or surgery, prolonged external cardiac massage, intracranial or intraspinal surgery or trauma within 1 month; arteriovenous malformation or aneurysm; bleeding diathesis; severe hepatic or renal disease; subacute bacterial endocarditis; pericarditis; hemostatic defects; suspected aortic dissection, severe uncontrolled hypertension (BP systolic ≥180 mm Hg, BP diastolic ≥110 mm Hg)

Warnings/Precautions Avoid I.M. injections; use with caution in patients with a history of cardiac arrhythmias, major surgery within last 10 days, GI bleeding, recent trauma, or severe hypertension; antibodies to streptokinase remain for 3-6 months after initial dose, use another thrombolytic enzyme (ie, alteplase) if thrombolytic therapy is indicated in patients with prior streptokinase therapy

Adverse Reactions

>10%:

    Cardiovascular: Hypotension, arrhythmias, trauma arrhythmias

    Dermatologic: Angioneurotic edema

    Hematologic: Surface bleeding, internal bleeding, cerebral hemorrhage

    Respiratory: Bronchospasm

    Miscellaneous: Periorbital swelling, anaphylaxis

<1%:

    Cardiovascular: Flushing

    Central nervous system: Headache, chills, sweating, fever

    Dermatologic: Rash, itching

    Gastrointestinal: Nausea, vomiting

    Hematologic: Anemia, eye hemorrhage

    Neuromuscular & skeletal: Musculoskeletal pain

    Respiratory: Bronchospasm

    Miscellaneous: Epistaxis

Overdosage/Toxicology Symptoms of overdose include epistaxis, bleeding gums, hematoma, spontaneous ecchymoses, oozing at catheter site. If uncontrollable bleeding occurs, discontinue infusion; whole blood or blood products may be used to reverse bleeding.

Drug Interactions

Decreased effect: Antifibrinolytic agents (aminocaproic acid) → ↓ effectiveness

Increased toxicity: Anticoagulants, antiplatelet agents → ↑ risk of bleeding

Stability

Streptokinase, a white lyophilized powder, may have a slight yellow color in solution due to the presence of albumin; intact vials should be stored at room temperature; reconstituted solutions should be refrigerated and are stable for 24 hours

Stability of parenteral admixture at room temperature (25°C): 8 hours; at refrigeration (4°C): 24 hours

Mechanism of Action Activates the conversion of plasminogen to plasmin by forming a complex, exposing plasminogen-activating site, and cleaving a peptide bond that converts plasminogen to plasmin; plasmin degrades fibrin, fibrinogen and other procoagulant proteins into soluble fragments; effective both outside and within the formed thrombus/embolus

Pharmacodynamics/Kinetics

Onset of action: Activation of plasminogen occurs almost immediately

Duration: Fibrinolytic effects last only a few hours, while anticoagulant effects can persist for 12-24 hours

Half-life: 83 minutes

Elimination: By circulating antibodies and via the reticuloendothelial system

Usual Dosage I.V.:

Children: Safety and efficacy not established; limited studies have used 3500-4000 units/kg over 30 minutes followed by 1000-1500 units/kg/hour

    Clotted catheter: 25,000 units, clamp for 2 hours then aspirate contents and flush with normal saline

Adults: Antibodies to streptokinase remain for at least 3-6 months after initial dose: Administration requires the use of an infusion pump

(Continued)

Streptokinase *(Continued)*

An intradermal skin test of 100 IU has been suggested to predict allergic response to streptokinase. If a positive reaction is not seen after 15-20 minutes, a therapeutic dose may be administered.

Guidelines for acute myocardial infarction (AMI): 1.5 million units over 60 minutes
Administration:

Dilute two 750,000 unit vials of streptokinase with 5 mL dextrose 5% in water (D_5W) each, gently swirl to dissolve

Add this dose of the 1.5 million units to 150 mL D_5W

This should be infused over 60 minutes; an in-line filter ≥0.45 micron should be used

Monitor for the first few hours for signs of anaphylaxis or allergic reaction. **Infusion should be slowed if lowering of 25 mm Hg in blood pressure or terminated if asthmatic symptoms appear.**

Begin heparin 5000-10,000 unit bolus followed by 1000 units/hour approximately 3-4 hours after completion of streptokinase infusion or when PTT is <100 seconds

Guidelines for acute pulmonary embolism (APE): 3 million unit dose over 24 hours
Administration:

Dilute four 750,000 unit vials of streptokinase with 5 mL dextrose 5% in water (D_5W) each, gently swirl to dissolve

Add this dose of 3 million units to 250 mL D_5W, an in-line filter ≥0.45 micron should be used

Administer 250,000 units (23 mL) over 30 minutes followed by 100,000 units/hour (9 mL/hour) for 24 hours

Monitor for the first few hours for signs of anaphylaxis or allergic reaction. **Infusion should be slowed if blood pressure is lowered by 25 mm Hg or if asthmatic symptoms appear.**

Begin heparin 1000 units/hour about 3-4 hours after completion of streptokinase infusion or when PTT is <100 seconds

Monitor PT, PTT, and fibrinogen levels during therapy

Thromboses: 250,000 units to start, then 100,000 units/hour for 24-72 hours depending on location

Cannula occlusion: 250,000 units into cannula, clamp for 2 hours, then aspirate contents and flush with normal saline

Administration Avoid I.M. injections

Monitoring Parameters Blood pressure, PT, APTT, platelet count, hematocrit, fibrinogen concentration, signs of bleeding

Reference Range

Partial thromboplastin time (PTT) activated: 20.4-33.2 seconds

Prothrombin time (PT): 10.9-13.7 seconds (same as control)

Fibrinogen: 200-400 mg/dL

Nursing Implications For I.V. or intracoronary use only; monitor for bleeding every 15 minutes for the first hour of therapy; do not mix with other drugs

Dosage Forms Powder for injection: 250,000 units (5 mL, 6.5 mL); 600,000 units (5 mL); 750,000 units (6 mL, 6.5 mL); 1,500,000 units (6.5 mL, 50 mL)

Streptomycin Sulfate *(strep toe mye' sin)*

Related Information

Antimicrobial Drugs of Choice *on page 1298-1302*

Recommendations of the Advisory Council on the Elimination of Tuberculosis *on page 1303-1304*

Use Combination therapy of active tuberculosis; used in combination with other agents for treatment of streptococcal or enterococcal endocarditis, mycobacterial infections, plague, tularemia, and brucellosis. Streptomycin is indicated for persons from endemic areas of drug-resistant *Mycobacterium tuberculosis* or who are HIV infected.

Pregnancy Risk Factor D

Contraindications Hypersensitivity to streptomycin, aminoglycosides, or any component

Warnings/Precautions Use with caution in patients with pre-existing vertigo, tinnitus, hearing loss, neuromuscular disorders, or renal impairment; modify dosage in patients with renal impairment; aminoglycosides are associated with nephrotoxicity or ototoxicity; the ototoxicity may be proportional to the amount of drug given and the duration of treatment; tinnitus or vertigo are indications of vestibular injury and impending hearing damage; renal damage is usually reversible

Adverse Reactions

1% to 10%:

Neuromuscular & skeletal: Neuromuscular blockade

Otic: Ototoxicity (auditory), ototoxicity (vestibular)

Renal: Nephrotoxicity

<1%:

Cardiovascular: Hypotension

Central nervous system: Drug fever, headache, drowsiness, weakness

Dermatologic: Skin rash

Gastrointestinal: Nausea, vomiting

Hematologic: Eosinophilia, anemia

Neuromuscular & skeletal: Paresthesia, tremor, arthralgia

Respiratory: Difficulty in breathing

Overdosage/Toxicology Symptoms of overdose include ototoxicity, nephrotoxicity, and neuromuscular toxicity; the treatment of choice following a single acute overdose appears to be the maintenance of good urine output of at least 3 mL/kg/hour. Dialysis is of questionable value in the enhancement of aminoglycoside elimination. If required, hemodialysis is preferred over peritoneal dialysis in patients with normal renal function. Careful hydration may be all that is required to promote diuresis and therefore the enhancement of the drug's elimination. Chelation with penicillins is experimental.

Drug Interactions

Increased/prolonged effect: Depolarizing and nondepolarizing neuromuscular blocking agents

Increased toxicity: Concurrent use of amphotericin, loop diuretics may increase nephrotoxicity

Stability Depending upon manufacturer, reconstituted solution remains stable for 2-4 weeks when refrigerated and 24 hours at room temperature; exposure to light causes darkening of solution without apparent loss of potency

Mechanism of Action Inhibits bacterial protein synthesis by binding directly to the 30S ribosomal subunits causing faulty peptide sequence to form in the protein chain

Pharmacodynamics/Kinetics

Absorption: Oral: Absorbed poorly; usually given parenterally

Time to peak serum concentration: Within 1 hour

Distribution: To extracellular fluid including serum, abscesses, ascitic, pericardial, pleural, synovial, lymphatic, and peritoneal fluids; crosses the placenta and small amounts appear in breast milk

V_d:

Neonates: <1 week, <1500 g: Up to 0.68 L/kg; ≥1 week, >1500 g: Up to 0.58 L/kg

Children: 0.2-0.4 L/kg

Adults: 0.26 L/kg (range, 0.20-0.40 L/kg)

Cystic fibrosis patients: 0.30-0.39 L/kg

Protein binding: 34%

Metabolism: None

Half-life:

Newborns: 4-10 hours

Adults: 2-4.7 hours, prolonged with renal impairment

Elimination: Almost completely (90%) excreted as unchanged drug in urine, with small amounts (1%) excreted in the bile, saliva, sweat and tears

Usual Dosage Intramuscular (may also be given intravenous piggyback):

Tuberculosis therapy: **Note:** A four-drug regimen (isoniazid, rifampin, pyrazinamide and either streptomycin or ethambutol) is preferred for the initial, empiric treatment of TB. When the drug susceptibility results are available, the regimen should be altered as appropriate.

Patients with TB and without HIV infection:

OPTION 1:

Isoniazid resistance rate <4%: Administer daily isoniazid, rifampin, and pyrazinamide for 8 weeks followed by isoniazid and rifampin daily or directly observed therapy (DOT) 2-3 times/week for 16 weeks

If isoniazid resistance rate is not documented, ethambutol or streptomycin should also be administered until susceptibility to isoniazid or rifampin is demonstrated. Continue treatment for at least 6 months or 3 months beyond culture conversion.

OPTION 2: Administer daily isoniazid, rifampin, pyrazinamide, and either streptomycin or ethambutol for 2 weeks followed by DOT 2 times/week administration of the same drugs for 6 weeks, and subsequently, with isoniazid and rifampin DOT 2 times/week administration for 16 weeks

OPTION 3: Administer isoniazid, rifampin, pyrazinamide, and either ethambutol or streptomycin by DOT 3 times/week for 6 months

(Continued)

Streptomycin Sulfate *(Continued)*

Patients with TB and with HIV infection: Administer any of the above OPTIONS 1, 2 or 3, however, treatment should be continued for a total of 9 months and at least 6 months beyond culture conversion

Note: Some experts recommend that the duration of therapy should be extended to 9 months for patients with disseminated disease, miliary disease, disease involving the bones or joints, or tuberculosis lymphadenitis

Children:
    Daily therapy: 20-30 mg/kg/day (maximum: 1 g/day)
    Directly observed therapy (DOT): Twice weekly: 25-30 mg/kg (maximum: 1.5 g)
    DOT: 3 times/week: 25-30 mg/kg (maximum: 1 g)
Adults:
    Daily therapy: 15 mg/kg/day (maximum: 1 g)
    Directly observed therapy (DOT): Twice weekly: 25-30 mg/kg (maximum: 1.5 g)
    DOT: 3 times/week: 25-30 mg/kg (maximum: 1 g)
    Enterococcal endocarditis: 1 g every 12 hours for 2 weeks, 500 mg every 12 hours for 4 weeks in combination with penicillin
    Streptococcal endocarditis: 1 g every 12 hours for 1 week, 500 mg every 12 hours for 1 week
    Tularemia: 1-2 g/day in divided doses for 7-10 days or until patient is afebrile for 5-7 days
    Plague: 2-4 g/day in divided doses until the patient is afebrile for at least 3 days
Elderly: 10 mg/kg/day, not to exceed 750 mg/day; dosing interval should be adjusted for renal function; some authors suggest not to give more than 5 days/week or give as 20-25 mg/kg/dose twice weekly

Dosing interval in renal impairment:
    Cl_{cr} 10-50 mL/minute: Administer every 24-72 hours
    Cl_{cr} <10 mL/minute: Administer every 72-96 hours
    Removed by hemo and peritoneal dialysis: Administer dose postdialysis

Administration Inject deep I.M. into large muscle mass; I.V. administration is not recommended

Monitoring Parameters Hearing (audiogram), BUN, creatinine; serum concentration of the drug should be monitored; eighth cranial nerve damage is usually preceded by high-pitched tinnitus, roaring noises, sense of fullness in ears, or impaired hearing and may persist for weeks after drug is discontinued

Reference Range
    Therapeutic: Peak: 15-40 µg/mL; Trough: <5 µg/mL
    Toxic: Peak: >50 µg/mL; Trough: >10 µg/mL

Test Interactions False-positive urine glucose with Benedict's solution

Patient Information Report any unusual symptoms of hearing loss, dizziness, roaring noises, or fullness in ears

Dosage Forms Injection: 400 mg/mL (2.5 mL)

Streptozocin *(strep toe zoe' sin)*

Related Information
    Antiemetics for Chemotherapy Induced Nausea and Vomiting *on page 1202*
    Cancer Chemotherapy Regimens *on page 1218-1241*

Brand Names Zanosar®

Use Treat metastatic islet cell carcinoma of the pancreas, carcinoid tumor and syndrome, Hodgkin's disease, palliative treatment of colorectal cancer

Pregnancy Risk Factor C

Warnings/Precautions The U.S. Food and Drug Administration (FDA) currently recommends that procedures for proper handling and disposal of antineoplastic agents be considered. Renal toxicity is dose-related and cumulative and may be severe or fatal; other major toxicities include liver dysfunction, diarrhea, nausea, and vomiting.

Adverse Reactions
>10%:
    Gastrointestinal: Nausea and vomiting in all patients usually 1-4 hours after infusion; diarrhea in 10% of patients; increased LFTs and hypoalbuminemia
    Emetic potential: High (>90%)
    Renal: Renal dysfunction occurs in 65% of patients; proteinuria, decreased Cl_{cr}, increased BUN, hypophosphatemia, and renal tubular acidosis; be careful with patients on other nephrotoxic agents; nephrotoxicity (25% to 75% of patients)
1% to 10%:
    Gastrointestinal: Diarrhea
    Hypoglycemia: Seen in 6% of patients; may be prevented with the administration of nicotinamide

Local: Pain at injection site

<1%:

Central nervous system: Confusion, lethargy, depression

Hematologic: Leukopenia, thrombocytopenia

Hepatic: Liver dysfunction

Myelosuppressive:

WBC: Mild

Platelets: Mild

Onset (days): 7

Nadir (days): 14

Recovery (days): 21

Secondary malignancy

Overdosage/Toxicology Symptoms of overdose include bone marrow depression, nausea, vomiting; treatment of bone marrow suppression is supportive

Drug Interactions

Decreased effect: Phenytoin results in negation of streptozocin cytotoxicity

Increased toxicity: Doxorubicin prolongs half-life and thus prolonged leukopenia and thrombocytopenia

Stability Refrigerate vials; solution is stable 48 hours at room temperature and 96 hours with refrigeration; may be diluted in D_5W or sodium chloride; protect from light

Mechanism of Action Interferes with the normal function of DNA by alkylation and cross-linking the strands of DNA, and by possible protein modification

Pharmacodynamics/Kinetics

Distribution: Concentrates in the liver, intestine, pancreas, and kidney

Metabolism: Rapidly metabolized and disappears from serum in 4 hours

Half-life: 35-40 minutes

Elimination: Majority (60% to 70%) excreted in the urine as metabolites, and smaller amounts eliminated in bile (1%) and in expired air (5%)

Usual Dosage I.V. (refer to individual protocols): Children and Adults: 500 mg/m^2 for 5 days every 4-6 weeks until optimal benefit or toxicity occurs or may be given in single dose 1000 mg/m^2 at weekly intervals for 2 doses, then increased to 1500 mg/m^2; usual course of therapy: 4-6 weeks

Dosing adjustment in renal impairment:

Cl_{cr} 10-50 mL/minute: Administer 75% of dose

Cl_{cr} <10 mL/minute: Administer 50% of dose

Dosing adjustment in hepatic impairment: Dose should be decreased in patients with severe liver disease

Administration Slow I.V. infusion in ≥100 mL D_5W or NS over 30-60 minutes; may be administered by rapid I.V. push

Monitoring Parameters Monitor renal function closely

Patient Information Avoid aspirin; use electric shaver; any signs of infection, easy bruising or bleeding, shortness of breath, or painful or burning urination should be brought to physician's attention. Nausea, vomiting or hair loss sometimes occur. The drug may cause permanent sterility and may cause birth defects. The drug may be excreted in breast milk, therefore, an alternative form of feeding your baby should be used.

Nursing Implications Wear gloves when preparing and administering; avoid extravasation

Dosage Forms Injection: 1 g

Stresstabs® 600 Advanced Formula Tablets [OTC] *see* Vitamin, Multiple *on page 1166*

Strong Iodine Solution *see* Potassium Iodide *on page 909*

Strontium-89 Chloride (stron' shee um)

Brand Names Metastron®

Use Relief of bone pain in patients with skeletal metastases

Pregnancy Risk Factor D

Contraindications Patients with a history of hypersensitivity to any strontium-containing compounds, or any other component; pregnancy, lactation

Warnings/Precautions Use caution in patients with bone marrow compromise; incontinent patients may require urinary catheterization. Body fluids may remain radioactive up to one week after injection. Not indicated for use in patients with cancer not involving bone and should be used with caution in patients whose platelet counts fall <60,000 or whose white blood cell counts fall <2400. A small number of patients have experienced a transient increase in bone pain at 36-72 hours post-dose; this reaction is generally mild and self-limiting. It should be handled cautiously, in a similar manner to other radioactive drugs. Appropriate safety measures to minimize radiation to personnel should be instituted.

(Continued)

Strontium-89 Chloride *(Continued)*

Adverse Reactions Most severe reactions of marrow toxicity can be managed by conventional means

Dermatologic: Flushing (most common after rapid injection)

Hematologic: Thrombocytopenia, leukopenia

Neuromuscular & skeletal: An increase in bone pain may occur (10% to 20% of patients)

Miscellaneous: Fever and chills (rare)

Stability Store vial and its contents inside its transportation container at room temperature

Usual Dosage Adults: I.V.: 148 megabecquerel (4 millicurie) administered by slow I.V. injection over 1-2 minutes or 1.5-2.2 megabecquerel (40-60 microcurie)/kg; repeated doses are generally not recommended at intervals <90 days; measure the patient dose by a suitable radioactivity calibration system immediately prior to administration

Monitoring Parameters Routine blood tests

Patient Information Eat and drink normally, there is no need to avoid alcohol or caffeine unless already advised to do so; may be advised to take analgesics until Metastron® begins to become effective; the effect lasts for several months, if pain returns before that, notify medical personnel

Nursing Implications During the first week after injection, strontium-89 will be present in the blood and urine, therefore, the following common sense precautions should be instituted:

1. Where a normal toilet is available, use in preference to a urinal, flush the toilet twice
2. Wipe away any spilled urine with a tissue and flush it away
3. Have patient wash hands after using the toilet
4. Immediately wash any linen or clothes that become stained with blood or urine
5. Wash away any spilled blood if a cut occurs

Dosage Forms Injection: 10.9-22.6 mg/mL [148 megabecquerel, 4 millicurie] (10 mL)

Stuartnatal® 1 + 1 *see* Vitamin, Multiple *on page 1166*

Stuart Prenatal® [OTC] *see* Vitamin, Multiple *on page 1166*

Sublimaze® *see* Fentanyl *on page 446*

Succimer *(sux' sim mer)*

Brand Names Chemet®

Use Treatment of lead poisoning in children with blood levels >45 mcg/dL. It is not indicated for prophylaxis of lead poisoning in a lead-containing environment. Following oral administration, succimer is generally well tolerated and produces a linear dose-dependent reduction in serum lead concentrations. This agent appears to offer advantages over existing lead chelating agents.

Pregnancy Risk Factor C

Contraindications Known hypersensitivity to succimer

Warnings/Precautions Caution in patients with renal or hepatic impairment; adequate hydration should be maintained during therapy

Adverse Reactions

>10%:

Gastrointestinal: Nausea, vomiting, diarrhea, appetite loss, hemorrhoidal symptoms, metallic taste

Miscellaneous: Back pain, fever

1% to 10%:

Central nervous system: Drowsiness, dizziness

Dermatologic: Rash

Endocrine & metabolic: Serum cholesterol

Hematologic: Alkaline phosphatase

Hepatic: Elevated AST, ALT

Respiratory: Sore throat, nasal congestion, cough

Miscellaneous: Flu-like symptoms

<1%: Cardiovascular: Arrhythmias

Overdosage/Toxicology Anorexia, vomiting, nephritis, hepatotoxicity, renal tubular necrosis, GI bleeding

Drug Interactions Not recommended for concomitant administration with edetate calcium disodium or penicillinamine

Mechanism of Action Succimer is an analog of dimercaprol. It forms water soluble chelates with heavy metals which are subsequently excreted renally. Initial data have shown encouraging results in the treatment of mercury and arsenic poisoning. Succimer binds heavy metals; however, the chemical form of these chelates is not known.

Pharmacodynamics/Kinetics
Absorption: Rapid but incomplete
Metabolism: Rapidly and extensively to mixed succimer cysteine disulfides
Half-life, elimination: 2 days
Time to peak serum concentration: ~1-2 hours
Elimination: ~25% in urine with peak urinary excretion occurring between 2-4 hours after dosing; of the total amount of succimer eliminated in urine, 90% is eliminated as mixed succimer-cysteine disulfide conjugates; 10% is excreted unchanged; fecal excretion of succimer probably represents unabsorbed drug

Usual Dosage Children and Adults: Oral: 10 mg/kg/dose every 8 hours for an additional 5 days followed by 10 mg/kg/dose every 12 hours for 14 days

Dosing adjustment in renal/hepatic impairment: Administer with caution and monitor closely

Concomitant iron therapy has been reported in a small number of children without the formation of a toxic complex with iron (as seen with dimercaprol); courses of therapy may be repeated if indicated by weekly monitoring of blood lead levels; lead levels should be stabilized <15 mg/dL; 2 weeks between courses is recommended unless more timely treatment is indicated by lead levels

Monitoring Parameters Blood lead levels, serum aminotransferases

Test Interactions False-positive ketones (U) using nitroprusside methods, falsely elevated serum CPK; falsely decreased uric acid measurement

Patient Information Maintain adequate fluid intake; notify physician if rash occurs; capsules may be opened and contents sprinkled on food or put on a spoon

Nursing Implications Adequately hydrate patients; rapid rebound of serum lead levels can occur; monitor closely

Dosage Forms Capsule: 100 mg

Succinylcholine Chloride (suk sin ill koe' leen)

Related Information
Neuromuscular Blocking Agents Comparison Charts *on page 1276-1278*

Brand Names Anectine® Chloride; Anectine® Flo-Pack®; Quelicin®; Sucostrin®

Synonyms Suxamethonium Chloride

Use Produces skeletal muscle relaxation in procedures of short duration such as endotracheal intubation or endoscopic exams

Pregnancy Risk Factor C

Contraindications Malignant hyperthermia, myopathies associated with elevated serum creatine phosphokinase (CPK) values, narrow-angle glaucoma, hyperkalemia, penetrating eye injuries, disorders of plasma pseudocholinesterase, hypersensitivity to succinylcholine or any component

Warnings/Precautions Use in pediatrics and adolescents; use with caution in patients with pre-existing hyperkalemia, paraplegia, extensive or severe burns, extensive denervation of skeletal muscle because of disease or injury to the CNS or with degenerative or dystrophic neuromuscular disease; may increase vagal tone

Adverse Reactions
>10%:
Ocular: Increased intraocular pressure
Miscellaneous: Postoperative stiffness
1% to 10%:
Cardiovascular: Bradycardia, hypotension, cardiac arrhythmias, tachycardia
Gastrointestinal: Intragastric pressure, salivation
<1%:
Cardiovascular: Hypertension
Dermatologic: Rash, itching, erythema
Endocrine & metabolic: Hyperkalemia
Hematologic: Myoglobinuria
Neuromuscular & skeletal: Muscle pain
Respiratory: Apnea, bronchospasm, circulatory collapse
Miscellaneous: Malignant hyperthermia

Causes of prolonged neuromuscular blockade:
Excessive drug administration
Cumulative drug effect, decreased metabolism/excretion (hepatic and/or renal impairment)
Accumulation of active metabolites
Electrolyte imbalance (hypokalemia, hypocalcemia, hypermagnesemia, hypernatremia)
Hypothermia
(Continued)

Succinylcholine Chloride *(Continued)*

Drug interactions

Increased sensitivity to muscle relaxants (eg, neuromuscular disorders such as myasthenia gravis or polymyositis)

Overdosage/Toxicology Symptoms of overdose include respiratory paralysis, cardiac arrest; bradyarrhythmias can often be treated with atropine 0.1 mg (infants); do not treat with anticholinesterase drugs (eg, neostigmine, physostigmine) since this may worsen its toxicity by interfering with its metabolism

Drug Interactions

Increased toxicity: Anticholinesterase drugs (neostigmine, physostigmine, or pyridostigmine) in combination with succinylcholine can cause cardiorespiratory collapse; cyclophosphamide, oral contraceptives, lidocaine, thiotepa, pancuronium, and procaine enhance and prolong the effects of succinylcholine

Prolonged neuromuscular blockade:

Inhaled anesthetics

Local anesthetics

Calcium channel blockers

Antiarrhythmics (eg, quinidine or procainamide)

Antibiotics (eg, aminoglycosides, tetracyclines, vancomycin, clindamycin)

Immunosuppressants (eg, cyclosporine)

Stability

Refrigerate (2°C to 8°C/36°F to 46°F); however, remains stable for 14 days unrefrigerated

Stability of parenteral admixture at refrigeration temperature (4°C): 24 hours in D_5W or NS

I.V. form is **incompatible** when mixed with sodium bicarbonate, pentobarbital, thiopental

Mechanism of Action Acts similar to acetylcholine, produces depolarization of the motor endplate at the myoneural junction which causes sustained flaccid skeletal muscle paralysis produced by state of accommodation that developes in adjacent excitable muscle membranes

Pharmacodynamics/Kinetics

Onset of effect:

I.M.: 2-3 minutes

I.V.: Complete muscular relaxation occurs within 30-60 seconds of injection

Duration:

I.M.: 10-30 minutes

I.V.: 4-6 minutes with single administration

Metabolism: Rapidly hydrolyzed by plasma pseudocholinesterase

Usual Dosage I.M., I.V.:

Neonates and small Children: Intermittent: Initial: 2 mg/kg/dose one time; maintenance: 0.3-0.6 mg/kg/dose at intervals of 5-10 minutes as necessary

Older Children and Adolescents: Intermittent: Initial: 1 mg/kg/dose one time; maintenance: 0.3-0.6 mg/kg every 5-10 minutes as needed

Adults: 0.6 mg/kg (range: 0.3-1.1 mg/kg) over 10-30 seconds, up to 150 mg total dose

Maintenance: 0.04-0.07 mg/kg every 5-10 minutes as needed

Continuous infusion: 2.5 mg/minute (or 0.5-10 mg/minute); dilute to concentration of 1-2 mg/mL in D_5W or NS

Note: Pretreatment with atropine may reduce occurrence of bradycardia

Dosing adjustment in hepatic impairment: Dose should be decreased in patients with severe liver disease

Administration I.M. injections should be made deeply, preferably high into deltoid muscle

Monitoring Parameters Cardiac monitor, blood pressure monitor, and ventilator required during administration; temperature, serum potassium and calcium, assisted ventilator status

Test Interactions ↑ potassium (S)

Dosage Forms

Injection: 20 mg/mL (10 mL); 50 mg/mL (10 mL); 100 mg/mL (5 mL, 10 mL, 20 mL)

Powder for injection: 100 mg, 500 mg, 1 g

Sucostrin® *see* Succinylcholine Chloride *on previous page*

Sucralfate (soo kral' fate)

Brand Names Carafate®

Synonyms Aluminum Sucrose Sulfate, Basic

Use Short-term management of duodenal ulcers

Unlabeled uses: Gastric ulcers; maintenance of duodenal ulcers; suspension may be used topically for treatment of stomatitis due to cancer chemotherapy and other causes of esophageal and gastric erosions; GERD, esophagitis, treatment of NSAID mucosal damage, prevention of stress ulcers, postschlerotherapy for esophageal variceal bleeding.

Pregnancy Risk Factor B

Contraindications Hypersensitivity to sucralfate or any component

Warnings/Precautions Successful therapy with sucralfate should not be expected to alter the post-healing frequency of recurrence or the severity of duodenal ulceration; use with caution in patients with chronic renal failure who have an impaired excretion of absorbed aluminum; may decrease gastric emptying. Because of the potential for sucralfate to alter the absorption of some drugs, separate administration (2 hours before or after) should be considered when alterations in bioavailability are believed to be critical; do not give antacids within 30 minutes of administration

Adverse Reactions

1% to 10%: Constipation

<1%:

Central nervous system: Dizziness, sleepiness, vertigo

Dermatologic: Rash, pruritus

Gastrointestinal: Diarrhea, nausea, gastric discomfort, indigestion, dry mouth

Neuromuscular & skeletal: Back pain

Overdosage/Toxicology Toxicity is minimal, may cause constipation

Drug Interactions Decreased effect:

Digoxin, phenytoin, theophylline, ciprofloxacin, itraconazole; because of the potential for sucralfate to alter the absorption of some drugs, separate administration (2 hours before or after) should be considered when alterations in bioavailability are believed to be critical

Antacids/cimetidine/ranitidine: Do not administer concomitantly - sucralfate requires gastric acid for it's mechanism of action (ie, to form a gel in the stomach as a protective barrier)

Stability Shake well and refrigerate suspension

Mechanism of Action Forms a complex by binding with positively charged proteins in exudates, forming a viscous paste-like, adhesive substance, when combined with gastric acid adheres to the damaged mucosal area. This selectively forms a protective coating that protects the lining against peptic acid, pepsin, and bile salts.

Pharmacodynamics/Kinetics

Onset of action: Paste formation and ulcer adhesion occur within 1-2 hours

Duration: Up to 6 hours

Absorption: Oral: <5%

Distribution: Acts locally at ulcer sites; unbound in the GI tract to aluminum and sucrose octasulfate

Metabolism: Not metabolized

Elimination: Small absorbed amounts are excreted in urine as unchanged compounds

Usual Dosage Oral:

Children: Dose not established, doses of 40-80 mg/kg/day divided every 6 hours have been used

Stomatitis: 2.5-5 mL (1 g/15 mL suspension), swish and spit or swish and swallow 4 times/day

Adults:

Stress ulcer prophylaxis: 1 g 4 times/day

Stress ulcer treatment: 1 g every 4 hours

Duodenal ulcer:

Treatment: 1 g 4 times/day, 1 hour before meals or food and at bedtime for 4-8 weeks, or alternatively 2 g twice daily; treatment is recommended for 4-8 weeks in adults, the elderly will require 12 weeks

Maintenance: Prophylaxis: 1 g twice daily

Stomatitis: 1 g/15 mL suspension, swish and spit or swish and swallow 4 times/day

Dosage comment in renal impairment: Aluminum salt is minimally absorbed (<5%), however, may accumulate in renal failure

Patient Information Take before meals or on an empty stomach; do not take antacids 30 minutes before or after taking sucralfate

Nursing Implications Monitor for constipation; give 2 hours before or after administration of other oral drugs

Dosage Forms Tablet: 1 g

(Continued)

Sucralfate *(Continued)*

Extemporaneous Preparations 100 mL of sucralfate suspension (200 mg/mL) may be prepared by crushing 20 sucralfate (1 g) tablets and mixing with a sufficient quantity of water to bring the volume to 100 mL; sorbitol can replace a portion of the water if desired; the suspension is stable for 14 days when refrigerated

Sucrets® Cough Calmers [OTC] *see* Dextromethorphan *on page 321*

Sudafed® 12 Hour [OTC] *see* Pseudoephedrine *on page 955*

Sudafed® [OTC] *see* Pseudoephedrine *on page 955*

Sufedrin® [OTC] *see* Pseudoephedrine *on page 955*

Sufenta® *see* Sufentanil Citrate *on this page*

Sufentanil Citrate *(soo fen' ta nil)*

Related Information
Narcotic Agonist Comparison Charts *on page 1274-1275*

Brand Names Sufenta®

Use Analgesic supplement in maintenance of balanced general anesthesia

Restrictions C-II

Pregnancy Risk Factor C

Contraindications Hypersensitivity to sufentanil or any component

Warnings/Precautions Sufentanil can cause severely compromised respiratory depression; use with caution in patients with head injuries, hepatic or renal impairment or with pulmonary disease; sufentanil shares the toxic potential of opiate agonists, precaution of opiate agonist therapy should be observed; rapid I.V. infusion may result in skeletal muscle and chest wall rigidity → impaired ventilation → respiratory distress/arrest; inject slowly over 3-5 minutes; nondepolarizing skeletal muscle relaxant may be required

Adverse Reactions
>10%:
Cardiovascular: Bradycardia, hypotension
Central nervous system: Drowsiness
Gastrointestinal: Nausea, vomiting
Respiratory: Respiratory depression
1% to 10%:
Cardiovascular: Cardiac arrhythmias, orthostatic hypotension
Central nervous system: Confusion, CNS depression
Gastrointestinal: Biliary spasm
Ocular: Blurred vision
<1%:
Cardiovascular: Bronchospasm, circulatory depression
Central nervous system: Convulsions, dysesthesia, paradoxical CNS excitation or delirium; mental depression, dizziness
Dermatologic: Skin rash, hives, itching
Respiratory: Laryngospasm
Miscellaneous: Cold, clammy skin; biliary or urinary tract spasm, physical and psychological dependence with prolonged use

Overdosage/Toxicology Naloxone 2 mg I.V. (0.01 mg/kg for children) with repeat administration as necessary up to a total of 10 mg; supportive care includes establishment of respiratory change; naloxone may be used to treat respiratory depression; muscular rigidity may also respond to opiate antagonist therapy or to neuromuscular blocking agents

Drug Interactions Increased effect/toxicity with CNS depressants, beta-blockers

Mechanism of Action Binds with stereospecific receptors at many sites within the CNS, increases pain threshold, alters pain reception, inhibits ascending pain pathways; ultra short-acting narcotic

Pharmacodynamics/Kinetics
Onset of action: 1-3 minutes
Duration: Dose dependent
Metabolism: Primarily by the liver

Usual Dosage
Children <12 years: 10-25 mcg/kg with 100% O_2, maintenance: 25-50 mcg as needed

Adults: Dose should be based on body weight. **Note:** In obese patients (ie, >20% above ideal body weight), use lean body weight to determine dosage.
1-2 mcg/kg with NO_2/O_2 for endotracheal intubation; maintenance: 10-25 mcg as needed
2-8 mcg/kg with NO_2/O_2 more complicated major surgical procedures; maintenance: 10-50 mcg as needed

8-30 mcg/kg with 100% O_2 and muscle relaxant produces sleep; at doses ≥8 mcg/kg maintains a deep level of anesthesia; maintenance: 10-50 mcg as needed

Nursing Implications Patient may develop rebound respiratory depression post-operatively

Dosage Forms Injection: 50 mcg/mL (1 mL, 2 mL, 5 mL)

Sulbactam and Ampicillin see Ampicillin Sodium and Sulbactam Sodium on page 74

Sulconazole Nitrate (sul kon' a zole)
Brand Names Exelderm®
Use Treatment of superficial fungal infections of the skin, including tinea cruris (jock itch), tinea corporis (ringworm), tinea versicolor, and possibly tinea pedis (athlete's foot - cream only)
Pregnancy Risk Factor C
Contraindications Known hypersensitivity to sulconazole
Warnings/Precautions Use with caution in nursing mothers; for external use only
Adverse Reactions 1% to 10%: Local: Itching, burning, stinging, redness
Mechanism of Action Substituted imidazole derivative which inhibits metabolic reactions necessary for the synthesis of ergosterol, an essential membrane component. The end result is usually fungistatic; however, sulconazole may act as a fungicide in Candida albicans and parapsilosis during certain growth phases.
Pharmacodynamics/Kinetics
Absorption: Topical: About 8.7% absorbed percutaneously
Elimination: Mostly in urine
Usual Dosage Adults: Topical: Apply a small amount to the affected area and gently massage once or twice daily for 3 weeks (tinea cruris, tinea corporis, tinea versicolor) to 4 weeks (tinea pedis).
Patient Information For external use only; avoid contact with eyes; if burning or irritation develops, notify physician
Dosage Forms
Cream: 1% (15 g, 30 g, 60 g)
Solution, topical: 1% (30 mL)

Sulf-10® see Sodium Sulfacetamide on page 1018

Sulfabenzamide, Sulfacetamide, and Sulfathiazole (sul fa benz' a mide)
Brand Names Gyne-Sulf®; Sultrin™; Trysul®; Vagilia®; V.V.S.®
Synonyms Triple Sulfa
Use Treatment of Haemophilus vaginalis vaginitis
Pregnancy Risk Factor C
Contraindications Hypersensitivity to sulfabenzamide, sulfacetamide, sulfathiazole or any component, renal dysfunction
Warnings/Precautions Associated with Stevens-Johnson syndrome; if local irritation or systemic toxicity develops, discontinue therapy
Adverse Reactions
>10%: Dermatologic: Local irritation, pruritus, urticaria
<1%: Dermatologic: Allergic reactions, Stevens-Johnson syndrome
Mechanism of Action Interferes with microbial folic acid synthesis and growth via inhibition of para-aminobenzoic acid metabolism
Pharmacodynamics/Kinetics
Absorption: Absorption from the vagina is variable and unreliable
Metabolism: Primarily by acetylation
Elimination: By glomerular filtration into urine
Usual Dosage Adults:
Cream: Insert one applicatorful in vagina twice daily for 4-6 days; dosage may then be decreased to ½ to ¼ of an applicatorful twice daily
Tablet: Insert one intravaginally twice daily for 10 days
Patient Information Complete full course of therapy; notify physician if burning, irritation, or signs of a systemic allergic reaction occur
Dosage Forms
Cream, vaginal: Sulfabenzamide 3.7%, sulfacetamide 2.86%, and sulfathiazole 3.42% (78 g with applicator, 90 g, 120 g)
Tablet, vaginal: Sulfabenzamide 184 mg, sulfacetamide 143.75 mg, and sulfathiazole 172.5 mg (20 tablets/box with vaginal applicator)

Sulfacetamide Sodium *see* Sodium Sulfacetamide *on page 1018*

Sulfadiazine (sul fa dye′ a zeen)
Brand Names Microsulfon®
Use Treatment of urinary tract infections and nocardiosis, rheumatic fever prophylaxis; adjunctive treatment in toxoplasmosis; uncomplicated attack of malaria
Pregnancy Risk Factor B (D at term)
Contraindications Porphyria, hypersensitivity to any sulfa drug or any component, pregnancy at term, children <2 months of age unless indicated for the treatment of congenital toxoplasmosis, sunscreens containing PABA
Warnings/Precautions Use with caution in patients with impaired hepatic function or impaired renal function, G-6-PD deficiency; dosage modification required in patients with renal impairment; fluid intake should be maintained ≥1500 mL/day, or give sodium bicarbonate to keep urine alkaline; more likely to cause crystalluria because it is less soluble than other sulfonamides
Adverse Reactions
>10%:
Central nervous system: Fever, dizziness, headache
Dermatologic: Itching, skin rash, photosensitivity
Gastrointestinal: Anorexia, nausea, vomiting, diarrhea
1% to 10%:
Dermatologic: Lyell's syndrome, Stevens-Johnson syndrome
Hematologic: Granulocytopenia, leukopenia, thrombocytopenia, aplastic anemia, hemolytic anemia
Hepatic: Hepatitis
<1%:
Endocrine & metabolic: Thyroid function disturbance
Hematologic: Hematuria
Hepatic: Jaundice
Renal: Interstitial nephritis, acute nephropathy, crystalluria
Miscellaneous: Serum sickness-like reactions
Overdosage/Toxicology Symptoms of overdose include drowsiness, dizziness, anorexia, abdominal pain, nausea, vomiting, hemolytic anemia, acidosis, jaundice, fever, agranulocytosis; doses of as little as 2-5 g/day may produce toxicity; the aniline radical is responsible for hematologic toxicity; high volume diuresis may aid in elimination and prevention of renal failure
Drug Interactions Decreased effect with PABA or PABA metabolites of drugs (eg, procaine, proparacaine, tetracaine, sunscreens); decreased effect of oral anticoagulants and oral hypoglycemic agents
Stability Tablets may be crushed to prepare oral suspension of the drug in water or with a sucrose-containing solution; aqueous suspension with concentrations of 100 mg/mL should be stored in the refrigerator and used within 7 days
Mechanism of Action Interferes with bacterial growth by inhibiting bacterial folic acid synthesis through competitive antagonism of PABA
Pharmacodynamics/Kinetics
Absorption: Oral: Well absorbed
Distribution: Throughout body tissues and fluids including pleural, peritoneal, synovial, and ocular fluids; distributed throughout total body water; readily diffused into CSF; appears in breast milk
Metabolism: By N-acetylation
Half-life: 10 hours
Time to peak serum concentration: Within 3-6 hours
Elimination: In urine as metabolites (15% to 40%) and as unchanged drug (43% to 60%)
Usual Dosage Oral:
Congenital toxoplasmosis:
Newborns and Children <2 months: 100 mg/kg/day divided every 6 hours in conjunction with pyrimethamine 1 mg/kg/day once daily and supplemental folinic acid 5 mg every 3 days for 6 months
Children >2 months: 25-50 mg/kg/dose 4 times/day

Toxoplasmosis:
Children: 120-150 mg/kg/day, maximum dose: 6 g/day; divided every 6 hours in conjunction with pyrimethamine 2 mg/kg/day divided every 12 hours for 3 days followed by 1 mg/kg/day once daily (maximum: 25 mg/day) with supplemental folinic acid
Adults: 2-8 g/day divided every 6 hours in conjunction with pyrimethamine 25 mg/day and with supplemental folinic acid
Administration Administer around-the-clock rather than 4 times/day to promote less variation in peak and trough serum levels
Monitoring Parameters Monitor urine output

Patient Information Drink plenty of fluids; take on an empty stomach; avoid prolonged exposure to sunlight or wear protective clothing and sunscreen; notify physician if rash, difficulty breathing, severe or persistent fever, or sore throat occurs

Nursing Implications Maintain adequate hydration

Dosage Forms Tablet: 500 mg

Sulfadoxine and Pyrimethamine (sul fa dox' een)

Brand Names Fansidar®

Use Treatment of *Plasmodium falciparum* malaria in patients in whom chloroquine resistance is suspected; malaria prophylaxis for travelers to areas where chloroquine-resistant malaria is endemic

Pregnancy Risk Factor C

Contraindications Known hypersensitivity to any sulfa drug, pyrimethamine, or any component; porphyria, megaloblastic anemia due to folate deficiency, severe renal insufficiency; children <2 months of age due to competition with bilirubin for protein binding sites, pregnancy at term or during breast-feeding

Warnings/Precautions Use with caution in patients with renal or hepatic impairment, patients with possible folate deficiency, and patients with seizure disorders, increased adverse reactions are seen in patients also receiving chloroquine; fatalities associated with sulfonamides, although rare, have occurred due to severe reactions including Stevens-Johnson syndrome, toxic epidermal necrolysis, hepatic necrosis, agranulocytosis, aplastic anemia and other blood dyscrasias; discontinue use at first sign of rash or any sign of dermatologic reaction; hemolysis occurs in patients with G-6-PD deficiency (reversed by leucovorin)

Adverse Reactions

>10%:

　Central nervous system: Ataxia, seizures, headache

　Dermatologic: Photosensitivity

　Gastrointestinal: Atrophic glossitis, vomiting, gastritis

　Hematologic: Megaloblastic anemia, leukopenia, thrombocytopenia, pancytopenia

　Neuromuscular & skeletal: Tremors

　Miscellaneous: Hypersensitivity

1% to 10%:

　Dermatologic: Stevens-Johnson syndrome

　Hepatic: Hepatitis

<1%:

　Dermatologic: Erythema multiforme, toxic epidermal necrolysis, rash

　Endocrine & metabolic: Thyroid function dysfunction

　Gastrointestinal: Anorexia, glossitis

　Hepatic: Hepatic necrosis

　Renal: Crystalluria

　Respiratory: Respiratory failure

Overdosage/Toxicology Symptoms of overdose include anorexia, vomiting, CNS stimulation including seizures, megaloblastic anemia, leukopenia, thrombocytopenia, crystalluria; doses of as little as 2-5 g/day may produce toxicity; the aniline radical is responsible for hematologic toxicity; following GI contamination, leucovorin should be administered (3-9 mg/day for 3 days or as required) to reverse symptoms of folic acid deficiency; high volume diuresis may aid in elimination and prevention of renal failure; diazepam can be used to control seizures

Drug Interactions

Decreased effect with PABA or PABA metabolites of local anesthetics

Increased toxicity with methotrexate, other sulfonamides, co-trimoxazole

Mechanism of Action Sulfadoxine interferes with bacterial folic acid synthesis and growth via competitive inhibition of para-aminiobenzoic acid; pyrimethamine inhibits microbial dihydrofolate reductase, resulting in inhibition of tetrahydrofolic acid synthesis

Pharmacodynamics/Kinetics

Absorption: Oral: Well absorbed

Distribution:

　Pyrimethamine: Widely distributed; mainly concentrated in blood cells, kidneys, lungs, liver, and spleen

　Sulfadoxine: Well distributed like other sulfonamides

Metabolism:

　Pyrimethamine: Hepatic

　Sulfadoxine: None

Half-life:

　Pyrimethamine: 80-95 hours

　Sulfadoxine: 5-8 days

(Continued)

Sulfadoxine and Pyrimethamine *(Continued)*

Time to peak serum concentration: Within 2-8 hours

Elimination: In urine as parent compounds and several unidentified metabolites

Usual Dosage Children and Adults: Oral:

Treatment of acute attack of malaria: A single dose of the following number of Fansidar® tablets is used in sequence with quinine or alone:

2-11 months: $\frac{1}{4}$ tablet

1-3 years: $\frac{1}{2}$ tablet

4-8 years: 1 tablet

9-14 years: 2 tablets

>14 years: 2-3 tablets

Malaria prophylaxis:

The first dose of Fansidar® should be taken 1-2 days before departure to an endemic area (CDC recommends that therapy be initiated 1-2 weeks before such travel), administration should be continued during the stay and for 4-6 weeks after return. Dose = pyrimethamine 0.5 mg/kg/dose and sulfadoxine 10 mg/kg/dose up to a maximum of 25 mg pyrimethamine and 500 mg sulfadoxine/dose weekly.

2-11 months: $\frac{1}{8}$ tablet weekly **or** $\frac{1}{4}$ tablet once every 2 weeks

1-3 years: $\frac{1}{4}$ tablet once weekly **or** $\frac{1}{2}$ tablet once every 2 weeks

4-8 years: $\frac{1}{2}$ tablet once weekly **or** 1 tablet once every 2 weeks

9-14 years: $\frac{3}{4}$ tablet once weekly **or** $1\frac{1}{2}$ tablets once every 2 weeks

>14 years: 1 tablet once weekly **or** 2 tablets once every 2 weeks

Monitoring Parameters CBC and platelet count, and urinalysis should be performed periodically

Patient Information Begin therapy for malaria prophylaxis at least 2 days before departure; drink plenty of fluids; avoid prolonged exposure to the sun; notify physician if rash, sore throat, pallor, shortness of breath, or glossitis occurs

Dosage Forms Tablet: Sulfadoxine 500 mg and pyrimethamine 25 mg

Sulfair® *see* Sodium Sulfacetamide *on page 1018*

Sulfalax® [OTC] *see* Docusate *on page 362*

Sulfamethoprim® *see* Co-trimoxazole *on page 278*

Sulfamethoxazole *(sul fa meth ox' a zole)*

Related Information

Antimicrobial Drugs of Choice *on page 1298-1302*

Brand Names Gantanol®; Urobak®

Use Treatment of urinary tract infections, nocardiosis, toxoplasmosis, acute otitis media, and acute exacerbations of chronic bronchitis due to susceptible organisms

Pregnancy Risk Factor B (D at term)

Contraindications Porphyria, hypersensitivity to any sulfa drug or any component, pregnancy during third trimester, children <2 months of age unless indicated for the treatment of congenital toxoplasmosis, sunscreens containing PABA

Warnings/Precautions Maintain adequate fluid intake to prevent crystalluria; use with caution in patients with renal or hepatic impairment, and patients with G-6-PD deficiency; should not be used for group A beta-hemolytic streptococcal infections

Adverse Reactions

>10%:

Central nervous system: Fever, dizziness, headache

Dermatologic: Itching, skin rash, photosensitivity

Gastrointestinal: Anorexia, nausea, vomiting, diarrhea

1% to 10%:

Dermatologic: Lyell's syndrome, Stevens-Johnson syndrome

Hematologic: Granulocytopenia, leukopenia, thrombocytopenia, aplastic anemia, hemolytic anemia

Hepatic: Hepatitis

<1%:

Cardiovascular: Vasculitis

Endocrine & metabolic: Thyroid function disturbance

Hepatic: Jaundice

Renal: Crystalluria, hematuria, acute nephropathy, interstitial nephritis

Miscellaneous: Serum sickness-like reactions

Overdosage/Toxicology Symptoms of overdose include drowsiness, dizziness, anorexia, abdominal pain, nausea, vomiting, hemolytic anemia, acidosis, jaundice, fever, agranulocytosis; the aniline radical is responsible for hematologic toxicity; high volume diuresis may aid in elimination and prevention of renal failure

Drug Interactions
Decreased effect with PABA or PABA metabolites of drugs (ie, procaine, proparacaine, tetracaine)
Increased effect of oral anticoagulants, oral hypoglycemic agents, and methotrexate

Stability Protect from light

Mechanism of Action Interferes with bacterial growth by inhibiting bacterial folic acid synthesis through competitive antagonism of PABA

Pharmacodynamics/Kinetics
Absorption: Oral: 90%
Distribution: Crosses the placenta; readily enters the CSF
Protein binding: 70%
Metabolism: Primarily in the liver, with 10% to 20% as the N-acetylated form in the plasma
Half-life: 9-12 hours, prolonged with renal impairment
Time to peak serum concentration: Within 3-4 hours
Elimination: Unchanged drug (20%) and its metabolites are excreted in urine

Usual Dosage Oral:
Children >2 months: 50-60 mg/kg as single dose followed by 50-60 mg/kg/day divided every 12 hours; maximum: 3 g/24 hours or 75 mg/kg/day
Adults: 2 g stat, 1 g 2-3 times/day; maximum: 3 g/24 hours

Dosing adjustment/interval in renal impairment:
Cl_{cr} 10-50 mL/minute: Administer every 18 hours
Cl_{cr} <10 mL/minute: Administer every 24 hours
Moderately dialyzable (20% to 50%)

Administration Administer around-the-clock to promote less variation in peak and trough serum levels

Monitoring Parameters Monitor urine output

Patient Information Drink plenty of fluids; avoid prolonged exposure to sunlight or wear protective clothing; avoid aspirin and vitamin C products, notify physician if rash, unusual bleeding, difficulty breathing, severe or persistent fever, or sore throat occurs

Nursing Implications Maintain adequate hydration

Dosage Forms
Suspension, oral (cherry flavor): 500 mg/5 mL (480 mL)
Tablet: 500 mg

Sulfamethoxazole and Trimethoprim see Co-trimoxazole on
page 278

Sulfamylon® see Mafenide Acetate on page 657

Sulfanilamide (sul fa nill' a mide)
Brand Names AVC™ Cream; AVC™ Suppository; Vagitrol®
Use Treatment of vulvovaginitis caused by Candida albicans
Pregnancy Risk Factor B (D at term)
Contraindications Hypersensitivity to sulfanilamide, aminacrine, allantoin or any component
Adverse Reactions
1% to 10%:
Dermatologic: Itching, skin rash, burning, irritation, exfoliative dermatitis, Stevens-Johnson syndrome
Gastrointestinal: Nausea, vomiting
Hematologic: Agranulocytosis, hemolytic anemia in patients with severe G-6-PD deficiency
Hepatic: Kernicterus, hepatic toxicity
Renal: Crystalluria
<1%: Irritation of penis of sexual partner
Mechanism of Action Interferes with microbial folic acid synthesis and growth via inhibition of para-aminiobenzoic acid metabolism
Usual Dosage Adults: Female: Insert one applicatorful intravaginally once or twice daily continued through 1 complete menstrual cycle or insert one suppository intravaginally once or twice daily for 30 days
Patient Information Avoid excessive exposure to sunlight; complete full course of therapy; notify physician if burning or irritation become severe or persist or if allergic symptoms occur
Dosage Forms
Cream, vaginal (AVC™, Vagitrol®): 15% [150 mg/g] (120 g with applicator)
Suppository, vaginal (AVC™): 1.05 g (16s)

Sulfasalazine (sul fa sal' a zeen)

Brand Names Azulfidine®; Azulfidine® EN-tabs®

Synonyms Salicylazosulfapyridine

Use Management of ulcerative colitis

Pregnancy Risk Factor B (D at term)

Contraindications Hypersensitivity to sulfasalazine, sulfa drugs, or any component; porphyria, GI or GU obstruction; hypersensitivity to salicylates; children <2 years of age

Warnings/Precautions Use with caution in patients with renal impairment; impaired hepatic function or urinary obstruction, blood dysosmias, severe allergies or asthma, or G-6-PD deficiency; may cause folate deficiency (consider providing 1 mg/day folate supplement)

Adverse Reactions
>10%:
  Central nervous system: Fever, dizziness, headache
  Dermatologic: Itching, skin rash, photosensitivity
  Gastrointestinal: Anorexia, nausea, vomiting, diarrhea
  Genitourinary: Reversible oligospermia
1% to 10%:
  Dermatologic: Lyell's syndrome, Stevens-Johnson syndrome
  Hematologic: Granulocytopenia, leukopenia, thrombocytopenia, aplastic anemia, hemolytic anemia
  Hepatic: Hepatitis
<1%:
  Endocrine & metabolic: Thyroid function disturbance
  Hepatic: Jaundice
  Renal: Interstitial nephritis, acute nephropathy, crystalluria, hematuria
  Miscellaneous: Serum sickness-like reactions

Overdosage/Toxicology Symptoms of overdose include drowsiness, dizziness, anorexia, abdominal pain, nausea, vomiting, hemolytic anemia, acidosis, jaundice, fever, agranulocytosis; the aniline radical is responsible for hematologic toxicity; high volume diuresis may aid in elimination and prevention of renal failure

Drug Interactions
  Decreased effect with iron, digoxin and PABA or PABA metabolites of drugs (ie, procaine, proparacaine, tetracaine)
  Decreased effect of oral anticoagulants, methotrexate, and oral hypoglycemic agents

Stability Protect from light; shake suspension well

Mechanism of Action Acts locally in the colon to decrease the inflammatory response and systemically interferes with secretion by inhibiting prostaglandin synthesis

Pharmacodynamics/Kinetics
  Absorption: 10% to 15% of dose is absorbed as unchanged drug from the small intestine
  Distribution: Small amounts appear in feces and breast milk
  Metabolism: Following absorption, both components are metabolized in the liver; split into sulfapyridine and 5-aminosalicylic acid (5-ASA) in the colon
  Half-life: 5.7-10 hours
  Elimination: Primary excretion in urine (as unchanged drug, components, and acetylated metabolites)

Usual Dosage Oral:
  Children >2 years: 40-60 mg/kg/day in 3-6 divided doses, not to exceed 6 g/day; maintenance dose: 20-30 mg/kg/day in 4 divided doses; not to exceed 2 g/day

  Adults: 1 g 3-4 times/day, 2 g/day maintenance in divided doses; not to exceed 6 g/day

  Dosing interval in renal impairment:
    Cl_{cr} 10-30 mL/minute: Administer twice daily
    Cl_{cr} <10 mL/minute: Administer once daily
  Dosing adjustment in hepatic impairment: Avoid use

Patient Information Maintain adequate fluid intake; take after meals; may cause orange-yellow discoloration of urine and skin; take after meals or with food; do not take with antacids; may permanently stain soft contact lenses yellow; avoid prolonged exposure to sunlight; shake well before using

Nursing Implications GI intolerance is common during the first few days of therapy (give with meals); drug commonly imparts an orange-yellow discoloration to urine and skin

Dosage Forms
  Suspension, oral: 250 mg/5 mL (473 mL)
  Tablet: 500 mg
  Tablet, enteric coated: 500 mg

Sulfatrim® see Co-trimoxazole on page 278

Sulfatrim® DS see Co-trimoxazole on page 278

Sulfinpyrazone (sul fin peer' a zone)

Brand Names Anturane®

Use Treatment of chronic gouty arthritis and intermittent gouty arthritis

    Unlabeled use: To decrease the incidence of sudden death postmyocardial infarction

Pregnancy Risk Factor C

Contraindications Active peptic ulcers, hypersensitivity to sulfinpyrazone, phenylbutazone, or other pyrazoles, GI inflammation, blood dyscrasias

Warnings/Precautions Safety and efficacy not established in children <18 years of age, use with caution in patients with impaired renal function and urolithiasis

Adverse Reactions

  >10%: Gastrointestinal: Nausea, vomiting, stomach pain

  1% to 10%: Dermatologic: Dermatitis, skin rash

  <1%:

    Cardiovascular: Flushing

    Central nervous system: Dizziness, headache

    Dermatologic: Rash

    Hematologic: Anemia, leukopenia, increased bleeding time (decreased platelet aggregation)

    Hepatic: Hepatic necrosis

    Genitourinary: Urinary frequency, uric acid stones

    Renal: Nephrotic syndrome

Overdosage/Toxicology Symptoms of overdose include nausea, vomiting, ataxia, respiratory depression, seizures; following GI decontamination, treatment is supportive only

Drug Interactions

  Decreased effect/levels of theophylline, verapamil; decreased uricosuric activity with salicylates, niacins

  Increased effect of oral hypoglycemics and anticoagulants

  Risk of acetaminophen hepatotoxicity is increased, but therapeutic effects may be reduced

Mechanism of Action Acts by increasing the urinary excretion of uric acid, thereby decreasing blood urate levels; this effect is therapeutically useful in treating patients with acute intermittent gout, chronic tophaceous gout, and acts to promote resorption of tophi; also has antithrombic and platelet inhibitory effects

Pharmacodynamics/Kinetics

  Absorption: Complete and rapid

  Metabolism: Hepatic to two active metabolites

  Half-life, elimination: 2.7-6 hours

  Time to peak serum concentration: 1.6 hours

  Elimination: Renal excretion with 22% to 50% as unchanged drug

Usual Dosage Adults: Oral: 100-200 mg twice daily; maximum daily dose: 800 mg

  Dosing adjustment in renal impairment: Cl_{cr} <50 mL/minute: Avoid use

Monitoring Parameters Serum and urinary uric acid, CBC

Test Interactions ↓ uric acid (S)

Patient Information Take with food or antacids; drink plenty of fluids; avoid aspirin and other salicylate products

Dosage Forms

  Capsule: 200 mg

  Tablet: 100 mg

Sulfisoxazole (sul fi sox' a zole)

Related Information

  Antimicrobial Drugs of Choice on page 1298-1302

Brand Names Gantrisin®

Synonyms Sulfisoxazole Acetyl; Sulphafurazole

Use Treatment of urinary tract infections, otitis media, *Chlamydia*; nocardiosis; treatment of acute pelvic inflammatory disease in prepubertal children; often used in combination with trimethoprim

Pregnancy Risk Factor B (D at term)

Contraindications Hypersensitivity to any sulfa drug or any component, porphyria, pregnancy during third trimester, infants <2 months of age (sulfas compete with bilirubin for protein binding sites), patients with urinary obstruction, sunscreens containing PABA

(Continued)

Sulfisoxazole *(Continued)*

Warnings/Precautions Use with caution in patients with G-6-PD deficiency (hemolysis may occur), hepatic or renal impairment; dosage modification required in patients with renal impairment; risk of crystalluria should be considered in patients with impaired renal function

Adverse Reactions
>10%:
Central nervous system: Fever, dizziness, headache
Dermatologic: Itching, skin rash, photosensitivity
Gastrointestinal: Anorexia, nausea, vomiting, diarrhea
1% to 10%:
Dermatologic: Lyell's syndrome, Stevens-Johnson syndrome
Hematologic: Granulocytopenia, leukopenia, thrombocytopenia, aplastic anemia, hemolytic anemia
Hepatic: Hepatitis
<1%:
Endocrine & metabolic: Thyroid function disturbance
Hepatic: Jaundice
Renal: Interstitial nephritis, acute nephropathy, crystalluria, hematuria
Miscellaneous: Serum sickness-like reactions

Overdosage/Toxicology Symptoms of overdose include drowsiness, dizziness, anorexia, abdominal pain, nausea, vomiting, hemolytic anemia, acidosis, jaundice, fever, agranulocytosis; doses of as little as 2-5 g/day may produce toxicity; the aniline radical is responsible for hematologic toxicity; high volume diuresis may aid in elimination and prevention of renal failure

Drug Interactions
Decreased effect with PABA or PABA metabolites of drugs (ie, procaine, proparacaine, tetracaine), thiopental
Increased effect of oral anticoagulants, methotrexate and oral hypoglycemic agents

Stability Protect from light

Mechanism of Action Interferes with bacterial growth by inhibiting bacterial folic acid synthesis through competitive antagonism of PABA

Pharmacodynamics/Kinetics
Absorption: Sulfisoxazole acetyl is hydrolyzed in the GI tract to sulfisoxazole which is readily absorbed
Distribution: Crosses the placenta; excreted into breast milk
Relative diffusion of antimicrobial agents from blood into cerebrospinal fluid (CSF): Adequate with or without inflammation (exceeds usual MICs); routine alkalinization of urine is normally not required; not for use in patients <2 months of age
Ratio of CSF to blood level (%):
Normal meninges: 50-80
Inflamed meninges: 80+
Protein binding: 85% to 88%
Metabolized: In the liver by acetylation and glucuronide conjugation to inactive compounds
Half-life: 4-7 hours, prolonged with renal impairment
Time to peak serum concentration: Within 2-3 hours
Elimination: Primarily in urine (95% within 24 hours), 40% to 60% as unchanged drug

Usual Dosage
Oral (not for use in patients <2 months of age):
Children >2 months: 75 mg/kg stat, followed by 120-150 mg/kg/day in divided doses every 4-6 hours; not to exceed 6 g/day
Pelvic inflammatory disease: 100 mg/kg/day in divided doses every 6 hours; used in combination with ceftriaxone
Chlamydia trachomatis: 100 mg/kg/day in divided doses every 6 hours
Adults: 2-4 g stat, 4-8 g/day in divided doses every 4-6 hours
Pelvic inflammatory disease: 500 mg every 6 hours for 21 days; used in combination with ceftriaxone
Chlamydia trachomatis: 500 mg every 6 hours for 10 days
Elderly: 2 g stat, then 2-8 g/day in divided doses every 6 hours
Ophthalmic: Children and Adults:
Solution: Instill 1-2 drops to affected eye every 2-3 hours
Ointment: Apply small amount to affected eye 1-3 times/day and at bedtime

Dosing interval in renal impairment:
Cl_{cr} 10-50 mL/minutes: Administer every 8-12 hours
Cl_{cr} <10 mL/minute: Administer every 12-24 hours
>50% removed by hemodialysis

Administration Administer around-the-clock to promote less variation in peak and trough serum levels

Monitoring Parameters CBC, urinalysis, renal function tests, temperature

Test Interactions False-positive protein in urine; false-positive urine glucose with Clinitest®

Patient Information Take with a glass of water on an empty stomach; avoid prolonged exposure to sunlight; report to physician any sore throat, mouth sores, rash, unusual bleeding, or fever; complete full course of therapy

Nursing Implications Maintain adequate fluid intake; obtain specimen for culture prior to first dose, if possible

Additional Information
Sulfisoxazole: Gantrisin® tablet
Sulfisoxazole acetyl: Gantrisin® pediatric syrup/suspension

Dosage Forms
Ointment, ophthalmic, as diolamine: 4% [40 mg/mL] (3.75 g)
Solution, ophthalmic, as diolamine: 4% [40 mg/mL] (15 mL)
Suspension, oral, pediatric, as acetyl (raspberry flavor): 500 mg/5 mL (480 mL)
Syrup, as acetyl (chocolate flavor): 500 mg/5 mL (480 mL)
Tablet: 500 mg

Sulfisoxazole Acetyl see Sulfisoxazole on page 1045

Sulfisoxazole and Erythromycin see Erythromycin and Sulfisoxazole on page 403

Sulfisoxazole and Phenazopyridine (sul fi sox′ zole)

Brand Names Azo Gantrisin®

Use Treatment of urinary tract infections and nocardiosis

Pregnancy Risk Factor B (D at term)

Contraindications Porphyria, hypersensitivity to any sulfa drug or any component, pregnancy at term, children <2 months of age unless indicated for the treatment of congenital toxoplasmosis, sunscreens containing PABA

Warnings/Precautions Use with caution in patients with G-6-PD deficiency (hemolysis may occur), hepatic or renal impairment; dosage modification required in patients with renal impairment; risk of crystalluria should be considered in patients with impaired renal function; drug should be discontinued if skin or sclera develop a yellow color

Adverse Reactions
>10%:
Central nervous system: Fever, dizziness, headache
Dermatologic: Itching, skin rash, photosensitivity
Gastrointestinal: Anorexia, nausea, vomiting, diarrhea
1% to 10%:
Dermatologic: Lyell's syndrome, Stevens-Johnson syndrome
Hematologic: Granulocytopenia, leukopenia, thrombocytopenia, aplastic anemia, hemolytic anemia
Hepatic: Hepatitis
<1%:
Endocrine & metabolic: Thyroid function disturbance
Hepatic: Jaundice
Renal: Crystalluria, hematuria, acute nephropathy, interstitial nephritis
Miscellaneous: Serum sickness-like reactions

Overdosage/Toxicology Symptoms of overdose include methemoglobinemia, skin pigmentation, renal and hepatic impairment, drowsiness, dizziness, anorexia, abdominal pain, nausea, vomiting, hemolytic anemia, acidosis, jaundice, fever, agranulocytosis; the aniline radical is responsible for hematologic toxicity; high volume diuresis may aid in elimination and prevention of renal failure; methylene blue 1-2 mg/kg I.V. or 100-200 mg ascorbic acid should reduce methemoglobinemia

Drug Interactions
Decreased effect with PABA or PABA metabolites of drugs (ie, procaine, proparacaine, tetracaine), thiopental
Increased effect of oral anticoagulants, methotrexate and oral hypoglycemic agents

Mechanism of Action Interferes with bacterial growth by inhibiting bacterial folic acid synthesis through competitive antagonism of PABA; phenazopyridine exerts local anesthetic or analgesic action on urinary tract mucosa through an unknown mechanism

Pharmacodynamics/Kinetics
Absorption: Sulfisoxazole acetyl is hydrolyzed in the GI tract to sulfisoxazole which is readily absorbed
Distribution: Crosses the placenta; excreted into breast milk
Protein binding: 85% to 88%
(Continued)

Sulfisoxazole and Phenazopyridine *(Continued)*

Metabolized: In the liver and other tissues by acetylation and glucuronide conjugation to inactive compounds

Half-life: 4-7 hours, prolonged with renal impairment

Time to peak serum concentration: Within 2-3 hours

Elimination: Primarily in urine (95% within 24 hours) where it exerts its action, 40% to 60% as unchanged drug; excretion (as unchanged drug) is rapid and accounts for 65% of the drug's elimination

Usual Dosage Adults: Oral: 4-6 tablets to start, then 2 tablets 4 times/day for 2 days, then continue with sulfisoxazole only

Dosing adjustment/comments in renal impairment: Cl_{cr} <50 mL/minute: Avoid use of phenazopyridine

Administration Administer around-the-clock rather than 4 times/day to promote less variation in peak and trough serum levels

Monitoring Parameters Monitor urine output

Test Interactions Urine tests which depend on spectrometry or color reactions, ↑ creatinine

Patient Information Take with meals, may cause reddish-orange discoloration of urine; staining of contact lenses has also been reported; drink plenty of fluids; take on an empty stomach; avoid prolonged exposure to sunlight or wear protective clothing and sunscreen; notify physician if rash, difficulty breathing, severe or persistent fever, or sore throat occurs

Nursing Implications Maintain adequate hydration

Dosage Forms Tablet: Sulfisoxazole 500 mg and phenazopyridine 50 mg

Sulfoxaprim® *see Co-trimoxazole on page 278*

Sulfoxaprim® DS *see Co-trimoxazole on page 278*

Sulindac *(sul in' dak)*

Related Information

Nonsteroidal Anti-Inflammatories Comparison *on page 1280*

Brand Names Clinoril®

Use Management of inflammatory disease, rheumatoid disorders; acute gouty arthritis; structurally similar to indomethacin but acts like aspirin; safest NSAID for use in mild renal impairment

Pregnancy Risk Factor B (D at term)

Contraindications Hypersensitivity to sulindac, any component, aspirin or other nonsteroidal anti-inflammatory drugs (NSAIDs)

Warnings/Precautions Used with caution in patients with peptic ulcer disease, GI bleeding, bleeding abnormalities, impaired renal or hepatic function, congestive heart failure, hypertension, and patients receiving anticoagulants

Adverse Reactions

>10%:

Central nervous system: Dizziness

Dermatologic: Skin rash

Gastrointestinal: Abdominal cramps, heartburn, indigestion, nausea

1% to 10%:

Cardiovascular: Fluid retention

Central nervous system: Headache, nervousness

Dermatologic: Itching

Gastrointestinal: Vomiting

Otic: Ringing in ears

<1%:

Cardiovascular: Congestive heart failure, hypertension, arrhythmias tachycardia

Central nervous system: Epistaxis, confusion, hallucinations, aseptic meningitis, mental depression, drowsiness, insomnia

Dermatologic: Hives, erythema multiforme, toxic epidermal necrolysis, Stevens-Johnson syndrome, angioedema

Endocrine & metabolic: Polydipsia, hot flushes

Gastrointestinal: Gastritis, GI ulceration

Genitourinary: Cystitis

Hematologic: Agranulocytosis, anemia, hemolytic anemia, bone marrow depression, leukopenia, thrombocytopenia

Hepatic: Hepatitis

Neuromuscular & skeletal: Peripheral neuropathy

Ocular: Toxic amblyopia, blurred vision, conjunctivitis, dry eyes

Otic: Decreased hearing

Renal: Polyuria, acute renal failure

Respiratory: Allergic rhinitis, shortness of breath

Overdosage/Toxicology Symptoms of overdose include dizziness, vomiting, nausea, abdominal pain, hypotension, coma, stupor, metabolic acidosis, leukocytosis, renal failure

Management of a nonsteroidal anti-inflammatory drug (NSAID) intoxication is primarily supportive and symptomatic. Fluid therapy is commonly effective in managing the hypotension that may occur following an acute NSAID overdose, except when this is due to an acute blood loss. Seizures tend to be very short-lived and often do not require drug treatment; although, recurrent seizures should be treated with I.V. diazepam.

Drug Interactions
Decreased effect of diuretics, beta-blockers, hydralazine, captopril
Increased toxicity with probenecid, NSAIDs; increased toxicity of digoxin, methotrexate, lithium, aminoglycosides antibiotics (reported in neonates), cyclosporine (↑ nephrotoxicity), potassium-sparing diuretics (hyperkalemia)

Mechanism of Action Inhibits prostaglandin synthesis by decreasing the activity of the enzyme, cyclo-oxygenase, which results in decreased formation of prostaglandin precursors

Pharmacodynamics/Kinetics
Absorption: 90%
Metabolism: Sulindac is a prodrug and, therefore, requires metabolic activation; requires hepatic metabolism to sulfide metabolite (active) for therapeutic effects; also metabolized in the liver to sulfone metabolites (inactive)
Half-life:
Parent drug: 7 hours
Active metabolite: 18 hours
Elimination: Principally in urine (50%) with some biliary excretion (25%)

Usual Dosage Maximum therapeutic response may not be realized for up to 3 weeks. Oral:

Children: Dose not established
Adults: 150-200 mg twice daily or 300-400 mg once daily; not to exceed 400 mg/day

Dosing adjustment in hepatic impairment: Dose reduction is necessary

Monitoring Parameters Liver enzymes, BUN, serum creatinine, CBC, blood pressure

Test Interactions ↑ chloride (S), ↑ sodium (S), ↑ bleeding time

Patient Information Take with food or milk; inform dentist or surgeon because of prolonged bleeding time; do not take aspirin; may cause dizziness, drowsiness, impair coordination and judgment

Nursing Implications Observe for edema and fluid retention; monitor blood pressure

Dosage Forms Tablet: 150 mg, 200 mg

Extemporaneous Preparations A suspension of sulindac can be prepared by triturating 1000 mg sulindac (5 x 200 mg tablets) with 50 mg of kelco and 400 mg of Veegum® until a powder mixture is formed; then add 30 mL of sorbitol 35% (prepared from 70% sorbitol) to form a slurry; finally add a sufficient quantity of 35% sorbitol to make a final volume of 100 mL; the final suspension is 10 mg/mL and is stable for 7 days

Sulphafurazole *see* Sulfisoxazole *on page 1045*

Sulten-10® *see* Sodium Sulfacetamide *on page 1018*

Sultrin™ *see* Sulfabenzamide, Sulfacetamide, and Sulfathiazole *on page 1039*

Sumatriptan Succinate (soo′ ma trip tan)
Brand Names Imitrex®
Use Acute treatment of migraine with or without aura
Unlabeled use: Cluster headaches
Pregnancy Risk Factor C
Contraindications
Intravenous administration
Use in patients with ischemic heart disease or Prinzmetal angina, patients with signs or symptoms of ischemic heart disease, uncontrolled HTN.
Use with ergotamine derivatives
Hypersensitivity to any component
Management of hemiplegic or basilar migraine
Warnings/Precautions
Sumatriptan is indicated only in patient populations with a clear diagnosis of migraine
(Continued)

Sumatriptan Succinate *(Continued)*

Use with caution in elderly, patients with hepatic or renal impairment; may cause mild, transient elevation of blood pressure; may cause coronary vasospasm

Adverse Reactions
>10%:
   Central nervous system: Tingling, dizziness
   Endocrine & metabolic: Hot flushes
   Local: Injection site reaction
1% to 10%:
   Cardiovascular: Tightness in chest
   Central nervous system: Weakness, burning sensation, drowsiness, headache, numbness, neck pain
   Gastrointestinal: Abdominal discomfort, sweating
   Neuromuscular & skeletal: Myalgia
   Miscellaneous: Mouth discomfort, jaw discomfort
<1%:
   Dermatologic: Skin rashes
   Endocrine & metabolic: Polydipsia, dehydration, dysmenorrhea
   Renal: Dysuria, renal calculus
   Respiratory: Dyspnea
   Miscellaneous: Thirst, hiccups

Drug Interactions Increased toxicity: Ergot-containing drugs

Stability Store at 2°C to 20°C (36°F to 86°F); protect from light

Mechanism of Action Selective agonist for serotonin (5HT-$_{1-D}$ receptor) in cranial arteries to cause vasoconstriction and reduces sterile inflammation associated with antidromic neuronal transmission correlating with relief of migraine

Pharmacodynamics/Kinetics After S.C. administration:
Distribution: V_d: 50 L
Protein binding: 14% to 21%
Bioavailability: 97%
Half-life:
   Distribution: 15 minutes
   Terminal: 115 minutes
Time to peak serum concentration: 5-20 minutes
Elimination: In urine unchanged (22%), excreted as indole acetic acid metabolite (38%)

Usual Dosage Adults: S.C.: 6 mg; a second injection may be administered at least 1 hour after the initial dose, but not more than 2 injections in a 24-hour period

Administration Do not administer I.V.; may cause coronary vasospasm

Patient Information If pain or tightness in chest or throat occurs, notify physician; females should avoid pregnancy; pain at injection site lasts <1 hour

Nursing Implications If pain or tightness in chest occurs, notify physician; females should avoid pregnancy; pain at injection site lasts <1 hour

Dosage Forms Injection: 12 mg/mL (0.5 mL, 2 mL)

Sumycin® *see* Tetracycline *on page 1069*

SuperChar® [OTC] *see* Charcoal *on page 214*

Suplical® [OTC] *see* Calcium Carbonate *on page 161*

Supprelin™ *see* Histrelin *on page 536*

Suppress® [OTC] *see* Dextromethorphan *on page 321*

Suprax® *see* Cefixime *on page 195*

Suprofen *(soo proe′ fen)*

Brand Names Profenal®

Use Inhibition of intraoperative miosis

Pregnancy Risk Factor C

Contraindications Previous hypersensitivity or intolerance to suprofen; epithelial herpes simplex keratitis; history of hypersensitivity reactions to aspirin or other nonsteroidal anti-inflammatory agents

Warnings/Precautions Use with caution in patients sensitive to acetylsalicylic acid and other NSAIDs; some systemic absorption occurs; use with caution in patients with bleeding tendencies; perform ophthalmic evaluation for those who develop eye complaints during therapy (blurred vision, diminished vision, changes in color vision, retinal changes)

Adverse Reactions
1% to 10%: Topical: Transient burning or stinging, redness, iritis
<1%:
   Systemic: Chemosis, photophobia

Topical: Discomfort, pain, punctate epithelial staining

Overdosage/Toxicology Not usually a problem; if accidental oral ingestion, dilute with fluids

Drug Interactions Decreased effect: When used concurrently with suprofen, acetylcholine chloride and carbachol may be ineffective

Mechanism of Action Inhibits prostaglandin synthesis, acts on the hypothalamus heat-regulating center to reduce fever, blocks prostaglandin synthetase action which prevents formation of the platelet-aggregating substance thromboxane A_2; decreases pain receptor sensitivity.

Pharmacodynamics/Kinetics

Protein binding: 99%

Metabolism: Occurs in the liver to one major inactive metabolite

Half-life, elimination: 2-4 hours

Time to peak serum concentration: ~1 hour

Elimination: <15% excreted unchanged in urine in 48 hours

Usual Dosage Adults: On day of surgery, instill 2 drops in conjunctival sac at 3, 2, and 1 hour prior to surgery; or 2 drops in sac every 4 hours, while awake, the day preceding surgery

Patient Information Avoid aspirin and aspirin-containing products while taking this medication; get instructions on administration of eye drops

Nursing Implications In elderly, remove contact lenses before administering; assess ability to self-administer

Dosage Forms Solution, ophthalmic: 1% (2.5 mL)

Surfak® [OTC] see Docusate on page 362

Surmontil® see Trimipramine Maleate on page 1128

Survanta® see Beractant on page 128

Susano® see Hyoscyamine, Atropine, Scopolamine, and Phenobarbital on page 557

Sus-Phrine® see Epinephrine on page 389

Sustaire® see Theophylline/Aminophylline on page 1072

Sutilains (soo′ ti lains)

Brand Names Travase®

Use Promote debridement of necrotic debris, as an adjunct in the treatment of second and third degree burns, decubitus ulcers

Pregnancy Risk Factor B

Contraindications Wounds communicating with major body cavities; wounds with exposed nerves; fungating neoplastic ulcers; hypersensitivity to sutilains

Warnings/Precautions Should not be applied to more than 10% to 15% of the burned area at one time; safety and efficacy have not been established in children; a topical anti-infective agent should be used with sutilains; avoid contact with eyes

Adverse Reactions

1% to 10%:

Central nervous system: Pain

Dermatologic: Transient dermatitis

Hematologic: Bleeding

Neuromuscular & skeletal: Paresthesia

Drug Interactions Decreased effect: Benzalkonium chloride, hexachlorophene, iodine, thimerosal, and silver nitrate decrease its activity

Stability Store in the refrigerator; activity is greatest at pH 6-6.8

Mechanism of Action Enzymatically converts denatured proteins (necrotic soft tissue, hemoglobin and purulent exudate) to peptides and amino acids

Pharmacodynamics/Kinetics

Onset of action: Within 1 hour

Duration: 8-12 hours

Peak effect: May take 7 days for maximal effect to be achieved for burns or wounds and up to 14 days in decubital and peripheral vascular ulcers

Usual Dosage Children and Adults: Topical: Thoroughly cleanse and irrigate wound then apply ointment in a thin layer extending 1/4" to 1/2" beyond the tissue being debrided; apply loose moist dressing; repeat 3-4 times/day

Patient Information If severe or persistent pain or bleeding occurs, discontinue use

Nursing Implications Avoid contact with the eyes; cleanse area with water or saline solution before applying drug; action is adversely affected by presence of detergents, rinse area completely

Dosage Forms Ointment: 82,000 casein units/g (14.2 g)

Suxamethonium Chloride see Succinylcholine Chloride on page 1035

Syllact® [OTC] *see* Psyllium *on page 956*

Symadine® *see* Amantadine Hydrochloride *on page 49*

Symmetrel® *see* Amantadine Hydrochloride *on page 49*

Synacort® *see* Hydrocortisone *on page 546*

Synacthen *see* Cosyntropin *on page 278*

Synalar® *see* Fluocinolone Acetonide *on page 469*

Synalar-HP® *see* Fluocinolone Acetonide *on page 469*

Synalgos®-DC *see* Dihydrocodeine Compound *on page 342*

Synalgos® [OTC] *see* Aspirin *on page 92*

Synarel® *see* Nafarelin Acetate *on page 767*

Synemol® *see* Fluocinolone Acetonide *on page 469*

Synthetic Lung Surfactant *see* Colfosceril Palmitate *on page 272*

Synthroid® *see* Levothyroxine Sodium *on page 629*

Syntocinon® *see* Oxytocin *on page 833*

Syprine® *see* Trientine Hydrochloride *on page 1120*

Syracol-CF® [OTC] *see* Guaifenesin and Dextromethorphan *on page 517*

Sytobex® *see* Cyanocobalamin *on page 282*

T₃ Sodium *see* Liothyronine Sodium *on page 637*

T₃/T₄ Liotrix *see* Liotrix *on page 639*

T₄ *see* Levothyroxine Sodium *on page 629*

Tac™-3 *see* Triamcinolone *on page 1112*

TACE® *see* Chlorotrianisene *on page 228*

Tacrine Hydrochloride (tak' reen)

Brand Names Cognex®

Synonyms Tetrahydroaminoacrine; THA

Use Treatment of mild to moderate dementia of the Alzheimer's type

Pregnancy Risk Factor C

Contraindications Patients previously treated with the drug who developed jaundice and in those who are hypersensitive to tacrine or acridine derivatives

Warnings/Precautions The use of tacrine has been associated with elevations in serum transaminases; serum transaminases (specifically ALT) must be monitored throughout therapy; use extreme caution in patients with current evidence of a history of abnormal liver function tests; use caution in patients with bladder outlet obstruction, asthma, and sick-sinus syndrome (tacrine may cause bradycardia). Also, patients with cardiovascular disease, asthma, or peptic ulcer should use cautiously.

Overdosage/Toxicology General supportive measures; can cause a cholinergic crisis characterized by severe nausea, vomiting, salivation, sweating, bradycardia, hypotension, collapse, and convulsions; increased muscle weakness is a possibility and may result in death if respiratory muscles are involved

Tertiary anticholinergics, such as atropine, may be used as an antidote for overdosage. I.V. atropine sulfate titrated to effect is recommended; initial dose of 1-2 mg I.V. with subsequent doses based upon clinical response. Atypical

Dose Adjustment Based Upon Transaminase Elevations

ALT	Regimen
≤3 x ULN*	Continue titration
>3 to ≤5 x ULN	Decrease dose by 40 mg/day, resume when ALT returns to normal
>5 x ULN	Stop treatment, may rechallenge upon return of ALT to normal

*ULN = upper limit of normal.

increases in blood pressure and heart rate have been reported with other cholinomimetics when coadministered with quaternary anticholinergics such as glycopyrrolate.

Drug Interactions Increased effect of theophylline, cimetidine, succinylcholine, cholinesterase inhibitors, or cholinergic agonists

Usual Dosage Adults: Initial: 10 mg 4 times/day; may increase by 40 mg/day adjusted every 6 weeks; maximum: 160 mg/day; best administered separate from meal times; see table.

Patients with clinical jaundice confirmed by elevated total bilirubin (>3 mg/dL) should not be rechallenged with tacrine

Monitoring Parameters ALT (SGPT) levels and other liver enzymes weekly for at least the first 18 weeks, then monitor once every 3 months

Reference Range In clinical trials, serum concentrations >20 ng/mL were associated with a much higher risk of development of symptomatic adverse effects

Patient Information Effect of tacrine therapy is thought to depend upon its administration at regular intervals, as directed; possibility of adverse effects such as those occurring in close temporal association with the initiation of treatment or an increase in dose (ie, nausea, vomiting, loose stools, diarrhea) and those with a delayed onset (ie, rash, jaundice, changes in the color of stool); inform physician of the emergence of new events or any increase in the severity of existing adverse effects; abrupt discontinuation of the drug or a large reduction in total daily dose (80 mg/day or more) may cause a decline in cognitive function and behavioral disturbances; unsupervised increases in the dose may also have serious consequences; do not change dose without consulting physician

Dosage Forms Capsule: 10 mg, 20 mg, 30 mg, 40 mg

Tacrolimus (ta kroe' li mus)

Brand Names Prograf®

Synonyms FK506

Use Potent immunosuppressive drug used in liver, kidney, heart, lung, or small bowel transplant recipients

Pregnancy Risk Factor C

Pregnancy/Breast Feeding Implications Because FK-506 does cross into breast milk, breast feeding is not advised while therapy is ongoing

Contraindications Hypersensitivity to tacrolimus or any component (eg, hydrogenated castor oil, used in the parenteral dosage formulation)

Warnings/Precautions Increased susceptibility to infection and the possible development of lymphoma may occur after administration of tacrolimus; it should not be administered simultaneously with cyclosporine; since the pharmacokinetics show great inter and intrapatient variability over time, monitoring of serum concentrations (trough for oral therapy) is essential to prevent organ rejection and reduce drug-related toxicity

Adverse Reactions

>10%:

Cardiovascular: Hypertension

Central nervous system: Headache, insomnia, abdominal/back pain, fever, asthenia

Dermatologic: Pruritus

Endocrine & metabolic: Hypo-/hyperkalemia, hyperglycemia, hypomagnesemia

Gastrointestinal: Diarrhea, nausea, anorexia, vomiting

Hematologic: Anemia, leukocytosis

Hepatic: LFT abnormalities, ascites

Neuromuscular & skeletal: Tremors, paresthesias

Renal: Nephrotoxicity, elevated creatinine and BUN

Respiratory: Peripheral edema, pleural effusion, atelectasis, dyspnea

1% to 10%:

Dermatologic: Rash

Gastrointestinal: Constipation

Genitourinary: Urinary tract infection

Hematologic: Thrombocytopenia

Renal: Oliguria

Drug Interactions

Antacids: Tacrolimus absorption impaired (separate administration by at least 2 hours)

Nephrotoxic antibiotics potentially increase tacrolimus associated nephrotoxicity

Amphotericin B potentially increases tacrolimus associated nephrotoxicity

Agents which may increase tacrolimus plasma concentrations and consequently effect and toxicity include erythromycin, clarithromycin, clotrimazole, fluconazole, itraconazole, ketoconazole, diltiazem, nicardipine, verapamil, bromocriptine, cimetidine, danazol, metoclopramide, methylprednisolone, cyclosporine (synergistic immunosuppression)

(Continued)

Tacrolimus *(Continued)*

Agents which may decrease tacrolimus plasma concentrations and consequently effect include rifampin, rifabutin, phenytoin, phenobarbital, and carbamazepine

Stability 24 hours in dextrose 5% solutions or normal saline; tacrolimus is completely available from plastic syringes, glass, or polyolefin containers, however, polyvinyl-containing sets (eg, Venoset®, Accuset®) adsorb significant amounts of the drug, and their use may lead to a lower dose being delivered to the patient; adsorption of the drug to PVC tubing may become clinically significant with use of low concentrations

Mechanism of Action Suppressed humoral immunity (inhibits T-lymphocyte activation); produced by the fungus streptomyces tsukubaensis

Pharmacodynamics/Kinetics

Absorption: Better in small bowel patients with a closed stoma; unlike cyclosporine, clamping of the jT-tube in liver transplant patients does not alter trough concentrations or AUC; food within 15 minutes of administration decreases absorption (27%); T_{max}: 0.5-4 hours

Distribution: V_d: 17 L/kg; crosses placenta (placental plasma concentrations are 4 times greater than maternal plasma); breast milk concentrations = plasma concentrations

Protein binding, plasma: 77% (primarily alpha$_1$-glycoprotein); blood:plasma = >4:1

Metabolism: >99% metabolized in liver; 9 less active metabolites

Bioavailability, oral: 5% to 67% (average 30%)

Half-life, elimination: 12 hours (range: 4-40 hours, twice as fast in children)

Elimination: <1% in urine as unchanged drug; elimination from the body is primarily via bile; clearance: 43 mL/kg/minute

Usual Dosage

Children:

I.V. continuous infusion: 0.1 mg/kg/day

Oral: 0.3 mg/kg/day

Adults:

I.V. continuous infusion: Initial (at least 6 hours after transplantation): 0.05-0.1 mg/kg/day

Oral (within 2-3 days): 0.15-0.3 mg/kg/day in divided doses every 12 hours; give 8-12 hours after discontinuation of the I.V. infusion; may gradually adjust (decrease) maintenance dose via pharmacokinetic monitoring

Dosing adjustment in renal impairment: Administer the lowest value of the recommended I.V./oral doses, adjusting downward if needed; delay therapy for ≥48 hours in patients with postoperative oliguria

Not dialyzable

Dosing adjustment in hepatic impairment: Moderate-severe hepatic dysfunction may result in decreased clearance and accumulation of active metabolites; adjust doses per pharmacokinetic monitoring and clinical evaluation

Administration Administer by I.V. continuous infusion only (use infusion pump); dilute with 0.9% sodium chloride of D$_5$W to a concentration of 0.004-0.02 mg/mL prior to administration; use only glass or polyethylene containers for storage; do not mix with acyclovir or ganciclovir due to chemical degradation of tacrolimus (use different ports in multilumen lines); do not alter dose with concurrent T-tube clamping

Monitoring Parameters Renal function, hepatic function, serum electrolytes, glucose and blood pressure, hypersensitivity indicators, neurological responses, and other clinical parameters; since the pharmacokinetics show great inter- and intrapatient variability over time, monitoring of serum concentrations (trough for oral therapy) has proven helpful to prevent organ rejection and reduce drug-related toxicity; measure 3 times/week for first few weeks, then gradually decrease frequency as patient stabilizes

Reference Range Trough levels: 0.5-2 ng/mL (ELISA, plasma, extracted at 37°C) for all transplant procedures (liver, heart, lung, kidney, small bowel) whole blood measurements produce concentration 5-40 times higher than those in serum due to high binding to RBCs (therapeutic range: 5-10 ng/mL, although levels >20 ng/mL may be desirable for short periods to prevent rejection)

Patient Information Separate administration with antacids by at least 2 hours

Nursing Implications For I.V. administration, tacrolimus is dispensed in a 50 mL glass container with no overfill; it is intended to be infused over 12 hours; polyolefin administration sets should be used

Additional Information Each mL of injection contains polyoxyl 60 hydrogenated castor oil (HCO-60), 200 mg and dehydrated alcohol, USP, 80% v/v

Dosage Forms

Capsule: 1 mg, 5 mg

Injection, with alcohol and surfactant: 5 mg/mL (1 mL)

Tagamet® *see* Cimetidine *on page 244*

Talwin® *see* Pentazocine *on page 857*

Talwin® NX *see* Pentazocine *on page 857*

Tambocor™ *see* Flecainide Acetate *on page 458*

Tamoxifen Citrate (ta mox′ i fen)
Related Information
Cancer Chemotherapy Regimens *on page 1218-1241*
Brand Names Nolvadex®
Use Palliative or adjunctive treatment of advanced breast cancer
Unlabeled use: Treatment of mastalgia, gynecomastia, male breast cancer, and pancreatic carcinoma. Studies have shown tamoxifen to be effective in the treatment of primary breast cancer in elderly women. Comparative studies with other antineoplastic agents in elderly women with breast cancer had more favorable survival rates with tamoxifen. Initiation of hormone therapy rather than chemotherapy is justified for elderly patients with metastatic breast cancer who are responsive.
Pregnancy Risk Factor D
Contraindications Hypersensitivity to tamoxifen
Warnings/Precautions Use with caution in patients with leukopenia, thrombocytopenia, or hyperlipidemias; ovulation may be induced; "hot flashes" may be countered by Bellergal-S® tablets; decreased visual acuity, retinopathy and corneal changes have been reported with use for more than 1 year at doses above recommended; hypercalcemia in patients with bone metastasis; hepatocellular carcinomas have been reported in animal studies; endometrial hyperplasia and polyps have occurred
Adverse Reactions
>10%:
Gastrointestinal: Little to mild nausea (10%), vomiting, weight gain

General: Flushing, increased bone and tumor pain and local disease flare shortly after starting therapy; this will subside rapidly, but patients should be aware of this since many may discontinue the drug due to the side effects; skin rash, hepatotoxicity

Myelosuppressive: Transient thrombocytopenia occurs in ~24% of patients receiving 10-20 mg/day; platelet counts return to normal within several weeks in spite of continued administration; leukopenia has also been reported and does resolve during continued therapy; anemia has also been reported
WBC: Rare
Platelets: None

1% to 10%:
Central nervous system: Lightheadedness, depression, dizziness, headache, lassitude, mental confusion, weakness

Dermatologic: Rash

Endocrine & metabolic: Hypercalcemia may occur in patients with bone metastases; galactorrhea and vitamin deficiency, menstrual irregularities

Genitourinary: Vaginal bleeding or discharge, endometriosis, priapism, possible endometrial cancer

Ocular: Ophthalmologic effects (visual acuity changes, cataracts, or retinopathy), corneal opacities

Thromboembolism: Tamoxifen has been associated with the occurrence of venous thrombosis and pulmonary embolism; arterial thrombosis has also been described in a few case reports
Overdosage/Toxicology Symptoms of overdose include hypercalcemia, edema; general supportive care
Drug Interactions
Increased toxicity:
Allopurinol results in exacerbation of allopurinol-induced hepatotoxicity

Cyclosporine may result in increased cyclosporine serum levels

Warfarin results in significant enhancement of the anticoagulant effects of warfarin; has been speculated that a decrease in antitumor effect of tamoxifen may also occur due to alterations in the percentage of active tamoxifen metabolites
Mechanism of Action Competitively binds to estrogen receptors on tumors and other tissue targets, producing a nuclear complex that decreases DNA synthesis and inhibits estrogen effects; nonsteroidal agent with potent antiestrogenic properties which compete with estrogen for binding sites in breast and other tissues; cells accumulate in the G_0 and G_1 phases; therefore, tamoxifen is cytostatic rather than cytocidal.
Pharmacodynamics/Kinetics
Absorption: Well absorbed from GI tract

Time to peak serum concentration: Oral: Within 4-7 hours
(Continued)

Tamoxifen Citrate *(Continued)*

Distribution: High concentrations found in uterus, endometrial and breast tissue

Metabolism: In the liver

Half-life: 7 days

Elimination: Undergoes enterohepatic recycling; excreted in feces with only small amounts appearing in urine

Usual Dosage Adults: Oral (refer to individual protocols): 10-20 mg twice daily in the morning and evening; high-dose therapy is under investigation

Monitoring Parameters Monitor WBC and platelet counts, tumor

Test Interactions T_4 elevations (no clinical evidence of hyperthyroidism)

Patient Information Report any vomiting that occurs after taking dose; patients should be advised to notify their physician of vaginal bleeding, weakness, mental confusion; increased bone and tumor pain and local disease flare may occur with start of therapy

Nursing Implications Increase of bone pain usually indicates a good therapeutic response

Dosage Forms Tablet: 10 mg

Tanac® [OTC] *see* Benzocaine *on page 121*

Tao® *see* Troleandomycin *on page 1133*

Tapazole® *see* Methimazole *on page 708*

Taractan® *see* Chlorprothixene *on page 233*

TAT *see* Tetanus Antitoxin *on page 1065*

Tavist® *see* Clemastine Fumarate *on page 253*

Taxol® *see* Paclitaxel *on page 834*

Tazicef® *see* Ceftazidime *on page 204*

Tazidime® *see* Ceftazidime *on page 204*

TCN *see* Tetracycline *on page 1069*

Td *see* Diphtheria and Tetanus Toxoid *on page 353*

Tebamide® *see* Trimethobenzamide Hydrochloride *on page 1126*

Tega-Cert® [OTC] *see* Dimenhydrinate *on page 347*

Tegison® *see* Etretinate *on page 436*

Tegopen® *see* Cloxacillin Sodium *on page 266*

Tegretol® *see* Carbamazepine *on page 177*

Tegrin®-HC *see* Hydrocortisone *on page 546*

Telachlor® *see* Chlorpheniramine Maleate *on page 229*

Teladar® *see* Betamethasone *on page 129*

Teldrin® [OTC] *see* Chlorpheniramine Maleate *on page 229*

Teline® *see* Tetracycline *on page 1069*

Temaril® *see* Trimeprazine Tartrate *on page 1124*

Temazepam *(te maz' e pam)*

Related Information

Benzodiazepines Comparison *on page 1256*

Brand Names Restoril®

Use Treatment of anxiety and as an adjunct in the treatment of depression; also may be used in the management of panic attacks; transient insomnia and sleep latency

Restrictions C-IV

Pregnancy Risk Factor X

Contraindications Hypersensitivity to temazepam or any component, severe uncontrolled pain, pre-existing CNS depression, or narrow-angle glaucoma; not to be used in pregnancy or lactation

Warnings/Precautions Safety and efficacy in children <18 years of age have not been established; do not use in pregnant women; may cause drug dependency; avoid abrupt discontinuance in patients with prolonged therapy or seizure disorders; use with caution in patients receiving other CNS depressants, in patients with hepatic dysfunction, and the elderly

Adverse Reactions

>10%:

Cardiovascular: Tachycardia, chest pain

Central nervous system: Drowsiness, fatigue, impaired coordination, lightheadedness, memory impairment, insomnia, anxiety, depression, headache

Dermatologic: Rash

Endocrine & metabolic: Decreased libido

Gastrointestinal: Dry mouth, constipation, diarrhea, decreased salivation, nausea, vomiting, increased or decreased appetite

Neuromuscular & skeletal: Dysarthria

Ocular: Blurred vision

Miscellaneous: Sweating

1% to 10%:

Cardiovascular: Syncope, hypotension

Central nervous system: Confusion, nervousness, dizziness, akathisia

Dermatologic: Dermatitis

Gastrointestinal: Increased salivation

Neuromuscular & skeletal: Rigidity, tremor, muscle cramps

Otic: Tinnitus

Respiratory: Nasal congestion, hyperventilation weight gain or loss

<1%:

Central nervous system: Reflex slowing

Endocrine & metabolic: Menstrual irregularities

Hematologic: Blood dyscrasias

Miscellaneous: Drug dependence

Overdosage/Toxicology Symptoms of overdose include somnolence, confusion, coma, hypoactive reflexes, dyspnea, hypotension, slurred speech, impaired coordination. Treatment for benzodiazepine overdose is supportive. Rarely is mechanical ventilation required. Flumazenil has been shown to selectively block the binding of benzodiazepines to CNS receptors, resulting in a reversal of benzodiazepine-induced CNS depression.

Drug Interactions Increased effect of CNS depressants

Mechanism of Action Benzodiazepine anxiolytic sedative that produces CNS depression at the subcortical level, except at high doses, whereby it works at the cortical level; causes minimal change in REM sleep patterns

Pharmacodynamics/Kinetics

Protein binding: 96%

Metabolism: In the liver

Half-life: 9.5-12.4 hours

Time to peak serum concentration: Within 2-3 hours

Elimination: 80% to 90% excreted in urine as inactive metabolites

Usual Dosage Adults: Oral: 15-30 mg at bedtime; 15 mg in elderly or debilitated patients

Monitoring Parameters Respiratory and cardiovascular status

Reference Range Therapeutic: 26 ng/mL after 24 hours

Patient Information Avoid alcohol and other CNS depressants; avoid activities needing good psychomotor coordination until CNS effects are known; drug may cause physical or psychological dependence; avoid abrupt discontinuation after prolonged use

Nursing Implications Provide safety measures (ie, side rails, night light, and call button); remove smoking materials from area; supervise ambulation

Dosage Forms Capsule: 15 mg, 30 mg

Temovate® see Clobetasol Propionate on page 256

Tempra® [OTC] see Acetaminophen on page 17

Tenex® see Guanfacine Hydrochloride on page 520

Teniposide (ten i poe' side)

Related Information

Extravasation Management of Chemotherapeutic Agents on page 1207-1208

Brand Names Vumon

Synonyms EPT; VM-26

Use Treatment of acute lymphocytic leukemia, small cell lung cancer

Pregnancy Risk Factor D

Contraindications Hypersensitivity to teniposide or Cremophor EL (polyoxyethylated castor oil) any component

Warnings/Precautions The U.S. Food and Drug Administration (FDA) currently recommends that procedures for proper handling and disposal of antineoplastic agents be considered. Administer I.V. infusions over a period of at least 30-60 minutes, must be diluted, do not give IVP. Teniposide contains benzyl alcohol, which has been associated with a fatal "gasping" syndrome in premature infants.

Adverse Reactions

>10%:

Gastrointestinal: Mucositis, nausea, vomiting, diarrhea

Hematologic: Myelosuppression, leukopenia, neutropenia, thrombocytopenia

Miscellaneous: Infection

(Continued)

Teniposide *(Continued)*

1% to 10%:
  Cardiovascular: Hypotension
  Dermatologic: Alopecia, rash
  Miscellaneous: Hypersensitivity, fever, hemorrhage
<1%:
  Endocrine & metabolic: Metabolic abnormalities
  Hepatic: Hepatic dysfunction
  Neuromuscular & skeletal: Peripheral neurotoxicity
  Renal: Renal dysfunction

Overdosage/Toxicology Symptoms of overdose include bone marrow depression, leukopenia, thrombocytopenia, nausea, vomiting; treatment is supportive

Drug Interactions Increased toxicity:
  Methotrexate: Alteration of MTX transport has been found as a slow efflux of MTX and its polyglutamated form out of the cell, leading to intercellular accumulation of MTX
  Sodium salicylate, sulfamethizole, tolbutamide: displace teniposide from protein-binding sites - could cause substantial increases in free drug levels, resulting in potentiation of toxicity

Stability Store ampuls in refrigerator at 2°C to 8°C (36°F to 46°F); reconstituted solutions are stable at room temperature for up to 24 hours after preparation. Teniposide must be diluted with either D_5W or 0.9% sodium chloride solutions to a final concentration of 0.1, 0.2, 0.4 or 1 mg/mL. In order to prevent extraction of the plasticizer DEHP, **solutions should be prepared in non-DEHP-containing containers such as glass or polyolefin containers.** The use of polyvinylchloride (PVC) containers is not recommended. Administer 1 mg/mL solutions within 4 hours of preparation to reduce the potential for precipitation. Precipitation may occur at any concentration. **incompatible** with heparin

Mechanism of Action Inhibits mitotic activity; inhibits cells from entering mitosis

Pharmacodynamics/Kinetics
  Distribution: V_d: 0.28 L/kg; distributed mainly into liver, kidneys, small intestine, and adrenals; crosses blood-brain barrier to a limited extent
  V_d: 3-11 L (children); 8-44 L (adults)
  Protein binding: 99.4%
  Metabolism: Extensively in the liver
  Half-life: 5 hours
  Elimination: In urine (21% as unchanged drug); renal (44%) and fecal (≤10%)

Usual Dosage I.V.:
  Children: 130 mg/m² /week, increasing to 150 mg/m² after 3 weeks and up to 180 mg/m² after 6 weeks
  Adults: 50-180 mg/m² once or twice weekly for 4-6 weeks or 20-60 mg/m² /day for 5 days
  Acute lymphoblastic leukemia (ALL): 165 mg/m² twice weekly for 8-9 doses **or** 250 mg/m² weekly for 4-8 weeks
  Small cell lung cancer: 80-90 mg/m² /day for 5 days

  Dosage adjustment in renal/hepatic impairment: Data is insufficient, but dose adjustments may be necessary in patient with significant renal or hepatic impairment

  Dosage adjustment in Down syndrome patients: Reduce initial dosing; give the first course at half the usual dose. Patients with both Down syndrome and leukemia may be especially sensitive to myelosuppressive chemotherapy.

Administration Do not use in-line filter during I.V. infusion; slow I.V. infusion over ≥30 minutes

  Tenoposide must be diluted with either D_5W or 0.9% sodium chloride solutions to a final concentration of 0.1, 0.2, 0.4, or 1 mg/mL. In order to prevent extraction of the plasticizer DEHP, solutions should be prepared in non-DEHP-containing containers such as glass or polyolefin containers. **The use of polyvinylchloride (PVC) containers is not recommended.**

Patient Information Hair should grow back after treatment

Nursing Implications Monitor blood pressure during infusion; observe for chemical phlebitis at injection site

Additional Information May be available only through investigational protocols

Dosage Forms Injection: 10 mg/mL (5 mL)

Tenormin® *see* Atenolol *on page 96*

Tensilon® *see* Edrophonium Chloride *on page 381*

Tenuate® *see* Diethylpropion Hydrochloride *on page 333*

Tenuate® Dospan® *see* Diethylpropion Hydrochloride *on page 333*

Tepanil® *see* Diethylpropion Hydrochloride *on page 333*

Terazol® *see* Terconazole *on page 1061*

Terazosin (ter ay' zoe sin)

Brand Names Hytrin®

Use Management of mild to moderate hypertension; considered a step 2 drug in stepped approach to hypertension; benign prostate hypertrophy

Pregnancy Risk Factor C

Contraindications Hypersensitivity to terazosin, other alpha-adrenergic antagonists, or any component

Warnings/Precautions Marked orthostatic hypotension, syncope, and loss of consciousness may occur with first dose ("first dose phenomenon"). This reaction is more likely to occur in patients receiving beta-blockers, diuretics, low sodium diets, or first doses >1 mg/dose in adults; avoid rapid increase in dose; use with caution in patients with renal impairment.

Adverse Reactions

>10%:

Cardiovascular: Orthostatic hypotension

Central nervous system: Dizziness, lightheadedness, drowsiness, headache, malaise

1% to 10%:

Cardiovascular: Edema, palpitations

Central nervous system: Fatigue, nervousness

Genitourinary: Urinary incontinence, dry mouth

<1%:

Cardiovascular: Angina

Central nervous system: Nightmares, drowsiness, hypothermia

Dermatologic: Rash

Endocrine & metabolic: Sexual dysfunction

Gastrointestinal: Nausea, urinary frequency

Genitourinary: Priapism

Respiratory: Dyspnea, nasal congestion

Overdosage/Toxicology Symptoms of overdose include hypotension, drowsiness, shock; hypotension usually responds to I.V. fluids or Trendelenburg positioning; if unresponsive to these measures, the use of a parenteral vasoconstrictor may be required; treatment is primarily supportive and symptomatic

Drug Interactions

Decreased antihypertensive response with NSAIDs

Increased hypotensive effect with diuretics and antihypertensive medications (especially beta-blockers)

Mechanism of Action Alpha$_1$-specific blocking agent with minimal alpha$_2$ effects; this allows peripheral postsynaptic blockade, with the resultant decrease in arterial tone, while preserving the negative feedback loop which is mediated by the peripheral presynaptic alpha$_2$-receptors; terazosin relaxes the smooth muscle of the bladder neck, thus reducing bladder outlet obstruction

Pharmacodynamics/Kinetics

Absorption: Oral: Rapid

Protein binding: 90% to 95%

Metabolism: Extensively in the liver

Half-life: 9.2-12 hours

Time to peak serum concentration: Within 1 hour

Elimination: Principally in feces (60%) and in urine (40%)

Usual Dosage Adults: Oral:

Hypertension: Initial: 1 mg at bedtime; slowly increase dose to achieve desired blood pressure, up to 20 mg/day; usual dose: 1-5 mg/day

Benign prostatic hypertrophy: Initial: 1 mg at bedtime, increasing as needed; most patients require 10 mg day; if no response after 4-6 weeks of 10 mg/day, may increase to 20 mg/day

Monitoring Parameters Blood pressure, standing and sitting/supine, urinary symptoms

Patient Information Report any gain of body weigh or painful, persistent erection; fainting sometimes occurs after the first dose; rise slowly from prolonged sitting or standing

Dosage Forms Tablet: 1 mg, 2 mg, 5 mg, 10 mg

Terbinafine (ter' bin a feen)

Brand Names Lamisil®

Use Topical antifungal for the treatment of tinea pedis (athlete's foot), tinea cruris (jock itch), and tinea corporis (ring worm)

Unlabeled use: Cutaneous candidiasis and pityriasis versicolor

(Continued)

Terbinafine *(Continued)*

Pregnancy Risk Factor B

Contraindications Hypersensitivity to terbinafine or any component

Warnings/Precautions For external use only

Adverse Reactions 1% to 10%: Local: Pruritus, contact dermatitis, irritation, stinging

Stability Store at 5°C to 30°C/41°F to 86°F

Mechanism of Action Synthetic alkylamine derivative which inhibits squalene epoxidases which is a key enzyme in sterol biosynthesis in fungi to result in a deficiency in ergosterol within fungal cell wall and result in fungal cell death

Pharmacodynamics/Kinetics
Absorption: Topical: Limited
Elimination: ~75% of cutaneously absorbed drug excreted in urine; 3.5% of administered dose recovered in urine and feces

Usual Dosage Adults: Topical:
Athlete's foot: Apply to affected area twice daily for at least 1 week, not to exceed 4 weeks
Ringworm and jock itch: Apply to affected area once or twice daily for at least 1 week, not to exceed 4 weeks

Patient Information For external use only; not for oral, ophthalmic, or intravaginal use; if irritation or sensitivity occurs, discontinue use and notify physician

Dosage Forms Cream: 1% (15 g, 30 g)

Terbutaline Sulfate (ter byoo' ta leen)

Brand Names Brethaire®; Brethine®; Bricanyl®

Use Bronchodilator in reversible airway obstruction and bronchial asthma

Pregnancy Risk Factor B

Contraindications Hypersensitivity to terbutaline or any component, cardiac arrhythmias associated with tachycardia, tachycardia caused by digitalis intoxication

Warnings/Precautions Excessive or prolonged use may lead to tolerance; paradoxical bronchoconstriction may occur with excessive use; if it occurs, discontinue terbutaline immediately

Adverse Reactions
>10%: Central nervous system: Nervousness, restlessness, trembling
1% to 10%:
Cardiovascular: Tachycardia, hypertension
Central nervous system: Dizziness, drowsiness, headache, weakness, insomnia
Gastrointestinal: Dry mouth, nausea, vomiting, bad taste in mouth
Neuromuscular & skeletal: Muscle cramps
Miscellaneous: Diaphoresis
<1%:
Cardiovascular: Chest pain, arrhythmias
Respiratory: Paradoxical bronchospasm

Overdosage/Toxicology Symptoms of overdose include seizures, nausea, vomiting, tachycardia, cardiac dysrhythmias, hypokalemia. In cases of overdose, supportive therapy should be instituted; prudent use of a cardioselective beta-adrenergic blocker (eg, atenolol or metoprolol) should be considered, keeping in mind the potential for induction of bronchoconstriction in an asthmatic individual. Dialysis has not been shown to be of value in the treatment of an overdose with this agent.

Drug Interactions
Decreased effect with beta-blockers
Increased toxicity with MAO inhibitors, TCAs

Stability Store injection at room temperature; protect from heat, light, and from freezing; use only clear solutions

Mechanism of Action Relaxes bronchial smooth muscle by action on beta$_2$ receptors with less effect on heart rate

Pharmacodynamics/Kinetics
Onset of action:
Oral: 30-45 minutes
S.C.: Within 6-15 minutes
Protein binding: 25%
Metabolism: In the liver to inactive sulfate conjugates
Bioavailability: S.C. doses are more bioavailable than oral
Half-life: 11-16 hours
Elimination: In urine

Usual Dosage

Children <12 years:

Oral: Initial: 0.05 mg/kg/dose 3 times/day, increased gradually as required; maximum: 0.15 mg/kg/dose 3-4 times/day or a total of 5 mg/24 hours

S.C.: 0.005-0.01 mg/kg/dose to a maximum of 0.3 mg/dose every 15-20 minutes for 3 doses

Nebulization: 0.1-0.3 mg/kg/dose up to a maximum of 10 mg/dose every 4-6 hours

Inhalation: 1-2 inhalations every 4-6 hours

Children >12 years and Adults:

Oral:

12-15 years: 2.5 mg every 6 hours 3 times/day; not to exceed 7.5 mg in 24 hours

>15 years: 5 mg/dose every 6 hours 3 times/day; if side effects occur, reduce dose to 2.5 mg every 6 hours; not to exceed 15 mg in 24 hours

S.C.: 0.25 mg/dose repeated in 15-30 minutes for one time only; a total dose of 0.5 mg should not be exceeded within a 4-hour period

Nebulization: 0.1-0.3 mg/kg/dose every 4-6 hours

Inhalation: 2 inhalations every 4-6 hours; wait 1 minute between inhalations

Dosing adjustment/comments in renal impairment:

Cl_{cr} 10-50 mL/minute: Administer at 50% of normal dose

Cl_{cr} <10 mL/minute: Avoid use

Administration Injection with S.C. use; in oral administration give around-the-clock to promote less variation in peak and trough serum levels

Monitoring Parameters Serum potassium, heart rate, blood pressure, respiratory rate

Patient Information Precede administration of aerosol adrenocorticoid by 15 minutes; report any decreased effectiveness of drug; do not exceed recommended dose or frequency; may take last dose at 6 PM to avoid insomnia

Dosage Forms

Aerosol, oral: 0.2 mg/actuation (10.5 g)

Injection: 1 mg/mL (1 mL)

Tablet: 2.5 mg, 5 mg

Terconazole (ter kone´ a zole)

Brand Names Terazol®

Synonyms Triaconazole

Use Local treatment of vulvovaginal candidiasis

Pregnancy Risk Factor C

Contraindications Known hypersensitivity to terconazole or components of the vaginal cream or suppository

Warnings/Precautions Should be discontinued if sensitization or irritation occurs. Microbiological studies (KOH smear and/or cultures) should be repeated in patients not responding to terconazole in order to confirm the diagnosis and rule out other other pathogens.

Adverse Reactions 1% to 10%: Genitourinary: Vulvar/vaginal burning

Stability Room temperature (13°C to 30°C/59°F to 86°F)

Mechanism of Action Triazole ketal antifungal agent; involves inhibition of fungal cytochrome P-450. Specifically, terconazole inhibits cytochrome P-450-dependent 14-alpha-demethylase which results in accumulation of membrane disturbing 14-alpha-demethylsterols and ergosterol depletion.

Pharmacodynamics/Kinetics Absorption: Extent of systemic absorption after vaginal administration may be dependent on the presence of a uterus; 5% to 8% in women who had a hysterectomy versus 12% to 16% in nonhysterectomy women

Usual Dosage Adults: Female: Insert 1 applicatorful intravaginally at bedtime for 7 consecutive days

Patient Information Insert high into vagina; complete full course of therapy; contact physician if itching or burning occurs

Nursing Implications Watch for local irritation; assist patient in administration, if necessary; assess patient's ability to self-administer, may be difficult in patients with arthritis or limited range of motion

Dosage Forms

Cream, vaginal: 0.4% (45 g); 0.8% (20 g)

Suppository, vaginal: 80 mg (3s)

Terfenadine (ter fen' a deen)

Brand Names Seldane®

Use Perennial and seasonal allergic rhinitis and other allergic symptoms including urticaria; has drying effect in patients with asthma

Pregnancy Risk Factor C

Contraindications Hypersensitivity to terfenadine or any component

Warnings/Precautions Safety and efficacy in children <12 years of age have not been established; use with caution in patients with a history of cardiac conduction disturbances or cardiac arrhythmias, or those receiving antiarrhythmic medication

Adverse Reactions

1% to 10%:
   Central nervous system: Headache, fatigue, nervousness, dizziness
   Gastrointestinal: Appetite increase, weight increase, nausea, diarrhea, abdominal pain, dry mouth
   Neuromuscular & skeletal: Arthralgia
   Respiratory: Pharyngitis

<1%:
   Cardiovascular: Edema, palpitations, hypotension, torsade de pointes
   Central nervous system: Depression, epistaxis, slight drowsiness, sedation, dizziness, paradoxical excitement, insomnia
   Dermatologic: Angioedema, photosensitivity, rash
   Genitourinary: Urinary retention
   Hepatic: Hepatitis
   Neuromuscular & skeletal: Myalgia, paresthesia, tremor
   Ocular: Blurred vision
   Respiratory: Bronchospasm, thickening of bronchial secretions

Overdosage/Toxicology Symptoms of overdose include nausea, confusion, sedation, prolonged Q-T interval, torsade de pointes. Lidocaine has been used successfully to treat cardiac arrhythmias; avoid type I antiarrhythmics, torsade may respond to I.V. magnesium.

Drug Interactions Serious cardiac events have occurred with elevated terfenadine levels

Increased effect with pseudoephedrine

Increased toxicity with ketoconazole, itraconazole, fluconazole, metronidazole, miconazole, erythromycin, troleandomycin, azithromycin, clarithromycin, cimetidine, bepridil, psychotropics, probucol, astemizole, carbamazepine

Stability Keep away from direct sunlight

Mechanism of Action Competes with histamine for H_1-receptor sites on effector cells in the gastrointestinal tract, blood vessels, and respiratory tract; binds to lung receptors significantly greater than it binds to cerebellar receptors, resulting in a reduced sedative potential

Pharmacodynamics/Kinetics

Duration of antihistaminic effect: Up to 12 hours
Metabolism: Extensive first-pass metabolism; metabolized in the liver
Half-life: 16-22 hours
Time to peak serum concentration: Within 1-2 hours
Elimination: Primarily in feces and secondarily in urine

Usual Dosage Oral:

Children:
   3-6 years: 15 mg twice daily
   6-12 years: 30 mg twice daily
Children >12 years and Adults: 60 mg twice daily

Monitoring Parameters Relief of symptoms

Test Interactions Antigen skin testing procedures

Patient Information Drink plenty of water; may cause dry mouth, sedation, drowsiness, can impair judgment and coordination

Nursing Implications Patient on medications that prolong the Q-T interval should be on a cardiac monitor when starting this drug

Dosage Forms Tablet: 60 mg

Terramycin® IV see Oxytetracycline Hydrochloride on page 832

Tesanone® see Testosterone on next page

Teslac® see Testolactone on this page

TESPA see Thiotepa on page 1086

Tessalon® Perles see Benzonatate on page 122

Testex® see Testosterone on next page

Testoderm® see Testosterone on next page

Testolactone (tess toe lak' tone)

Brand Names Teslac®

Use Palliative treatment of advanced disseminated breast carcinoma

Restrictions C-III

Pregnancy Risk Factor C

Contraindications In men for the treatment of breast cancer; known hypersensitivity to testolactone

Warnings/Precautions The U.S. Food and Drug Administration (FDA) currently recommends that procedures for proper handling and disposal of antineoplastic agents be considered. Use with caution in hepatic, renal, or cardiac disease; prolonged use may cause drug-induced hepatic disease; history or porphyria.

Adverse Reactions

1% to 10%:

Cardiovascular: Edema

Dermatologic: Maculopapular rash

Endocrine & metabolic: Hypercalcemia,

Gastrointestinal: Anorexia, diarrhea, nausea, swelling of tongue

Neuromuscular & skeletal: Paresthesias, peripheral neuropathies

Overdosage/Toxicology Increased toxicity: ↑ effects of oral anticoagulants

Mechanism of Action Testolactone is a synthetic testosterone derivative without significant androgen activity. The drug inhibits steroid aromatase activity, thereby blocking the production of estradiol and estrone from androgen precursors such as testosterone and androstenedione. Unfortunately, the enzymatic block provided by testolactone is transient and is usually limited to a period of 3 months.

Pharmacodynamics/Kinetics

Absorption: Oral: Absorbed well

Metabolism: In the liver

Elimination: In urine

Usual Dosage Adults: Female: Oral: 250 mg 4 times/day for at least 3 months; desired response may take as long as 3 months

Monitoring Parameters Plasma calcium levels

Test Interactions Plasma estradiol concentrations by RIA

Patient Information Passive exercises should be maintained throughout therapy to keep patient mobile; notify physician if numbness of fingers, toes, or face occurs

Dosage Forms Tablet: 50 mg

Testosterone (tess toss' ter one)

Brand Names Andro®; Andro-Cyp®; Andro-L.A.®; Andronate®; Andropository®; Andryl®; Delatest®; Delatestryl®; Depotest®; Depo®-Testosterone; Duratest®; Durathate®; Everone®; Histerone®; Tesanone®; Testex®; Testoderm®; Testrin® P.A.

Synonyms Aqueous Testosterone; Testosterone Cypionate; Testosterone Enanthate; Testosterone Propionate

Use Androgen replacement therapy in the treatment of delayed male puberty; postpartum breast pain and engorgement; inoperable breast cancer; male hypogonadism

Restrictions C-III

Pregnancy Risk Factor X

Contraindications Severe renal or cardiac disease, benign prostatic hypertrophy with obstruction, undiagnosed genital bleeding, males with carcinoma of the breast or prostate; hypersensitivity to testosterone or any component

Warnings/Precautions Perform radiographic examination of the hand and wrist every 6 months to determine the rate of bone maturation; may accelerate bone maturation without producing compensating gain in linear growth; has both androgenic and anabolic activity, the anabolic action may enhance hypoglycemia

Adverse Reactions

>10%:

Dermatologic: Acne

Endocrine & metabolic: Menstrual problems (amenorrhea), virilism, breast soreness

Genitourinary: Epididymitis, priapism, bladder irritability

1% to 10%:

Cardiovascular: Flushing, edema

Central nervous system: Excitation, aggressive behavior, sleeplessness, anxiety, mental depression, headache

Endocrine & metabolic: Prostatic hypertrophy, prostatic carcinoma, hirsutism (increase in pubic hair growth), impotence, testicular atrophy

Gastrointestinal: Nausea, vomiting, GI irritation

Hepatic: Hepatic dysfunction

(Continued)

Testosterone *(Continued)*

<1%:

Endocrine & metabolic: Gynecomastia, hypercalcemia, leukopenia, suppression of clotting factors, polycythemia, hypoglycemia

Hepatic: Cholestatic hepatitis, hepatic necrosis

Miscellaneous: Hypersensitivity reactions

Drug Interactions Increased toxicity: Effects of oral anticoagulants may be enhanced

Mechanism of Action Principal endogenous androgen responsible for promoting the growth and development of the male sex organs and maintaining secondary sex characteristics in androgen-deficient males

Pharmacodynamics/Kinetics

Duration of effect: Based upon the route of administration and which testosterone ester is used; the cypionate and enanthate esters have the longest duration, up to 2-4 weeks after I.M. administration

Distribution: Crosses the placenta; appears in breast milk

Protein binding: 98% (to transcortin and albumin)

Metabolism: In the liver

Half-life: 10-100 minutes

Elimination: In urine (90%) and feces via bile (6%)

Usual Dosage

Delayed puberty: Males: Children: I.M.: 40-50 mg/m²/dose (cypionate or enanthate) monthly for 6 months

Male hypogonadism: I.M.: 50-400 mg every 2-4 weeks

Initiation of pubertal growth: 40-50 mg/m²/dose (cypionate or enanthate) monthly until the growth rate falls to prepubertal levels (~5 cm/year)

During terminal growth phase: 100 mg/m²/dose (cypionate or enanthate) monthly until growth ceases

Maintenance virilizing dose: 100 mg/m²/dose (cypionate or enanthate) twice monthly or 50-400 mg/dose every 2-4 weeks

Inoperable breast cancer: Adults: I.M.: 200-400 mg every 2-4 weeks

Hypogonadism: Males: Adults:

I.M.:

Testosterone or testosterone propionate: 10-25 mg 2-3 times/week

Testosterone cypionate or enanthate: 50-400 mg every 2-4 weeks

Postpubertal cryptorchism: Testosterone or testosterone propionate: 10-25 mg 2-3 times/week

Topical: Initial: 6 mg/day system applied daily applied on scrotal skin. If scrotal area is inadequate, start with a 4 mg/day system. Transdermal system should be worn for 22-24 hours. Determine total serum testosterone after 3-4 weeks of daily application. If patients have not achieved desired results after 6-8 weeks of therapy, another form of testosterone replacement therapy should be considered.

Dosing adjustment/comments in hepatic disease: Reduce dose

Monitoring Parameters Periodic liver function tests, radiologic examination of wrist and hand every 6 months (when using in prepubertal children)

Reference Range Testosterone, urine: Male: 100-1500 ng/24 hours; Female: 100-500 ng/24 hours

Test Interactions May cause a decrease in creatinine and creatine excretion and an increase in the excretion of 17-ketosteroids, thyroid function tests

Patient Information Virilization may occur in female patients; report menstrual irregularities; male patients report persistent penile erections; all patients should report persistent GI distress, diarrhea, or jaundice

Nursing Implications Warm injection to room temperature and shaking vial will help redissolve crystals that have formed after storage; administer by deep I.M. injection into the upper outer quadrant of the gluteus maximus. Transdermal system should be applied on clean, dry, scrotal skin. Dry-shave scrotal hair for optimal skin contact. Do not use chemical depilatories.

Additional Information

Testosterone (aqueous): Andro®, Histerone®, Tesanone®

Testosterone cypionate: Andro-Cyp®, Andronate®, Depotest®, Depo®-Testosterone, Duratest®

Testosterone enanthate: Andro-L.A.®, Andropository®, Delatestryl®, Durathate®, Everone®, Testrin® P.A.

Testosterone propionate: Testex®

Dosage Forms

Injection:

Aqueous suspension: 25 mg/mL (10 mL); 50 mg/mL (10 mL, 30 mL); 100 mg/mL (10 mL)

In oil, as cypionate: 100 mg/mL (10 mL); 200 mg/mL (1 mL, 10 mL)

In oil, as enanthate: 100 mg/mL (10 mL); 200 mg/mL (1 mL, 5 mL, 10 mL)

In oil, as propionate: 100 mg/mL (10 mL)

Transdermal system:
4 mg/hour (40 cm²): total testosterone content = 10 mg
6 mg/hour (60 cm²): total testosterone content = 15 mg

Testosterone Cypionate see Testosterone on page 1063

Testosterone Enanthate see Testosterone on page 1063

Testosterone Propionate see Testosterone on page 1063

Testred® see Methyltestosterone on page 726

Testrin® P.A. see Testosterone on page 1063

Tetanus and Diphtheria Toxoid see Diphtheria and Tetanus Toxoid on page 353

Tetanus Antitoxin (tet' n us)
Synonyms TAT
Use Tetanus prophylaxis or treatment of active tetanus only when tetanus immune globulin (TIG) is not available; tetanus immune globulin (Hyper-Tet®) is the preferred tetanus immunoglobulin for the treatment of active tetanus; may be given concomitantly with tetanus toxoid adsorbed when immediate treatment is required, but active immunization is desirable
Pregnancy Risk Factor D
Contraindications Patients sensitive to equine-derived preparations
Warnings/Precautions Tetanus antitoxin is not the same as tetanus immune globulin; sensitivity testing should be conducted in all individuals regardless of clinical history; have epinephrine 1:1000 available
Adverse Reactions Dermatologic: Skin eruptions, erythema, urticaria, serum sickness may develop up to several weeks after injection in 10% of patients, local pain, numbness, joint pain, anaphylaxis
Stability Refrigerate, do not freeze
Mechanism of Action Provides passive immunization; solution of concentrated globulins containing antitoxic antibodies obtained from horse serum after immunization against tetanus toxin
Usual Dosage
Prophylaxis: I.M., S.C.:
Children <30 kg: 1500 units
Children and Adults ≥30 kg: 3000-5000 units
Treatment: Children and Adults: Inject 10,000-40,000 units into wound; give 40,000-100,000 units I.V.
Nursing Implications All patients should have sensitivity testing prior to starting therapy with tetanus antitoxin
Dosage Forms Injection, equine: Not less than 400 units/mL (12.5 mL, 50 mL)

Tetanus Immune Globulin, Human (tet' a nus)
Related Information
Immunization Guidelines on page 1389-1405
Vaccines on page 1386-1388
Brand Names Hyper-Tet®
Synonyms TIG
Use Passive immunization against tetanus; tetanus immune globulin is preferred over tetanus antitoxin for treatment of active tetanus; part of the management of an unclean, nonminor wound in a person whose history of previous receipt of tetanus toxoid is unknown or who has received less than three doses of tetanus toxoid
Pregnancy Risk Factor C
Contraindications Hypersensitivity to tetanus immune globulin, thimerosal, or any immune globulin product or component; patients with IgA deficiency; I.V. administration
Warnings/Precautions Have epinephrine 1:1000 available for anaphylactic reactions; do not give I.V.
Adverse Reactions
>10%: Local: Pain, tenderness, erythema at injection site
1% to 10%:
Central nervous system: Fever (mild)
Dermatologic: Hives, angioedema
Neuromuscular & skeletal: Muscle stiffness
Miscellaneous: Anaphylaxis reaction
<1%: Sensitization to repeated injections
Drug Interactions Never administer tetanus toxoid and TIG in same syringe (toxoid will be neutralized); toxoid may be given at a separate site
(Continued)

Tetanus Immune Globulin, Human *(Continued)*

Stability Refrigerate at 2°C to 8°C (36°F to 46°F)

Mechanism of Action Passive immunity toward tetanus

Pharmacodynamics/Kinetics Absorption: Well absorbed

Usual Dosage I.M.:

Prophylaxis of tetanus:

Children: 4 units/kg; some recommend administering 250 units to small children

Adults: 250 units

Treatment of tetanus:

Children: 500-3000 units; some should infiltrate locally around the wound

Adults: 3000-6000 units

Administration Do not administer I.V.; I.M. use only

Additional Information Tetanus immune globulin (TIG) must not contain <50 units/mL. Protein makes up 10% to 18% of TIG preparations. The great majority of this (≥90%) is IgG. TIG has almost no color or odor and it is a sterile, nonpyrogenic, concentrated preparation of immunoglobulins that has been derived from the plasma of adults hyperimmunized with tetanus toxoid. The pooled material from which the immunoglobulin is derived may be from fewer than 1000 donors. This plasma has been shown to be free of hepatitis B surface antigen.

Dosage Forms Injection: 250 units/mL

Tetanus Toxoid, Adsorbed *(tet′ a nus)*

Related Information

Immunization Guidelines *on page 1389-1405*

Skin Testing for Delayed Hypersensitivity *on page 1325-1327*

Vaccines *on page 1386-1388*

Use Active immunity against tetanus; tetanus is a rare disease in the U.S. with <100 cases annually; 66% of cases occur in persons >50 years of age; protective tetanus and diphtheria antibodies decline with age; it is estimated that <50% of elderly are protected

Elderly are at risk because:

Many lack proper immunization maintenance

Higher case fatality ratio

Immunizations are not available from childhood

Indications for vaccination:

Primary series with combined tetanus-diphtheria (Td) should be given to all elderly lacking a clean history of vaccination

Boosters should be given at 10-year intervals; earlier for wounds

Elderly are more likely to require tetanus immune globulin with infection of tetanus due to lower antibody titer

Pregnancy Risk Factor C

Contraindications Hypersensitivity to tetanus toxoid or any component; neurological signs or symptoms after prior administration; acute respiratory infections or other active infections

Warnings/Precautions Not equivalent to tetanus toxoid fluid; the tetanus toxoid adsorbed is the preferred toxoid for immunization; avoid injection into a blood vessel; have epinephrine (1:100) available

Adverse Reactions

>10%: Local: Induration/redness at injection site

1% to 10%:

Central nervous system: Chills, fever

Local: Sterile abscess at injection site

Miscellaneous: Allergic reaction

<1%:

Central nervous system: Fever >103°F, malaise, neurological disturbances

Local: Blistering at injection site

Miscellaneous: Arthus-type hypersensitivity reactions

Drug Interactions If primary immunization is started in individuals receiving an immunosuppressive agent or corticosteroids, serologic testing may be needed to ensure adequate antibody response

Stability Refrigerate, do not freeze

Mechanism of Action Tetanus toxoid preparations contain the toxin produced by virulent tetanus bacilli (detoxified growth products of *Clostridium tetani*). The toxin has been modified by treatment with formaldehyde so that is has lost toxicity but still retains ability to act as antigen and produce active immunity.

Pharmacodynamics/Kinetics Duration of immunization following primary immunization: ~12 years

Usual Dosage Adults: I.M.:
Primary immunization: 0.5 mL; repeat 0.5 mL at 4-8 weeks after first dose and at 6-12 months after second dose
Routine booster doses are recommended only every 5-10 years
Routine wound management: See table.

Tetanus Prophylaxis in Wound Management

Number of Prior Tetanus Toxoid Doses	Clean, Minor Wounds		All Other Wounds	
	Td*	TIG†	Td*	TIG†
Unknown or <3	Yes	No	Yes	Yes
≥3‡	No#	No	No¶	No

Adapted from Report of the Committee on Infectious Diseases, American Academy of Pediatrics, Elk Grove Village, IL: © American Academy of Pediatrics, 1986.

*Adult tetanus and diphtheria toxoids; use pediatric preparations (DT or DTP) if the patient is less than 7 years old.

†Tetanus immune globulin.

‡If only three doses of fluid tetanus toxoid have been received, a fourth dose of toxoid, preferably an adsorbed toxoid, should be given.

#Yes, if more than 10 years since last dose.

¶Yes, if more than 5 years since last dose.

Administration Inject intramuscularly in the area of the vastus lateralis (midthigh laterally) or deltoid

Patient Information A nodule may be palpable at the injection site for a few weeks. DT, Td and T vaccines cause few problems; they may cause mild fever or soreness, swelling, and redness where the shot was given. These problems usually last 1-2 days, but this does not happen nearly as often as with DTP vaccine. Sometimes, adults who get these vaccines can have a lot of soreness and swelling where the shot was given.

Dosage Forms Injection, adsorbed:
Tetanus 5 Lf units per 0.5 mL dose (0.5 mL, 5 mL)
Tetanus 10 Lf units per 2.5 mL dose (5 mL)

Tetanus Toxoid, Fluid (tet′ a nus)
Related Information
Immunization Guidelines *on page 1389-1405*
Skin Testing for Delayed Hypersensitivity *on page 1325-1327*
Vaccines *on page 1386-1388*

Synonyms Tetanus Toxoid Plain

Use Active immunization against tetanus in adults and children

Pregnancy Risk Factor C

Contraindications Prior hypersensitivity reactions, neurological signs or symptoms after prior administrations

Warnings/Precautions For primary immunization, tetanus toxoid, adsorbed is preferred; in concomitant administration of immunosuppressive therapy, allergic reactions may occur; epinephrine 1:1000 must be available; use in pediatrics should be deferred until >1 year of age when a history of a CNS disorder is present

Adverse Reactions
>10%: Local: Induration/redness at injection site
1% to 10%:
Central nervous system: chills, fever
Local: Sterile abscess at injection site
Miscellaneous: Allergic reaction
<1%:
Central nervous system: Fever >103°F, malaise, neurological disturbances
Local: Blistering at injection site
Miscellaneous: Arthus-type hypersensitivity reactions

Drug Interactions If primary immunization is started in individuals receiving an immunosuppressive agent or corticosteroids, serologic testing may be needed to ensure adequate antibody response

Stability Refrigerate

Mechanism of Action Tetanus toxoid preparations contain the toxin produced by virulent tetanus bacilli (detoxified growth products of *Clostridium tetani*). The toxin has been modified by treatment with formaldehyde so that is has lost toxicity but still retains ability to act as antigen and produce active immunity.

Pharmacodynamics/Kinetics Duration of immunization following primary immunization: ~12 years

Usual Dosage Adults:
(Continued)

Tetanus Toxoid, Fluid *(Continued)*

Primary immunization: Inject 3 doses of 0.5 mL I.M. or S.C. at 4- to 8-week intervals with fourth dose given only 6-12 months after third dose
Booster doses: I.M., S.C.: 0.5 mL every 10 years
Anergy testing: Intradermal: 0.1 mL
Administration Must not be used I.V.
Patient Information A nodule may be palpable at the injection site for a few weeks
Dosage Forms Injection, fluid:
Tetanus 4 Lf units per 0.5 mL dose (7.5 mL)
Tetanus 5 Lf units per 0.5 mL dose (0.5 mL, 7.5 mL)

Tetanus Toxoid Plain *see* Tetanus Toxoid, Fluid *on previous page*

Tetracaine Hydrochloride (tet′ ra kane)

Brand Names Pontocaine®
Synonyms Amethocaine Hydrochloride
Use Spinal anesthesia; local anesthesia in the eye for various diagnostic and examination purposes; topically applied to nose and throat for various diagnostic procedures; **approximately 10 times more potent than procaine**
Pregnancy Risk Factor C
Contraindications Hypersensitivity to tetracaine or any component; ophthalmic secondary bacterial infection, patients with liver disease, CNS disease, meningitis (if used for epidural or spinal anesthesia), myasthenia gravis
Warnings/Precautions No pediatric dosage recommendations; ophthalmic preparations may delay wound healing; use with caution in patients with cardiac disease and hyperthyroidism
Adverse Reactions
1% to 10%: Dermatologic: Contact dermatitis, burning, stinging, angioedema
<1%:
Dermatologic: Tenderness, urticaria
Genitourinary: Urethritis
Hematologic: Methemoglobinemia in infants
Overdosage/Toxicology Treatment is primarily symptomatic and supportive. Termination of anesthesia by pneumatic tourniquet inflation should be attempted when the agent is administered by infiltration or regional injection. Seizures commonly respond to diazepam, while hypotension responds to I.V. fluids and Trendelenburg positioning. Bradyarrhythmias (when the heart rate is <60) can be treated with I.V., I.M., or S.C. atropine 15 mcg/kg. With the development of metabolic acidosis, I.V. sodium bicarbonate 0.5-2 mEq/kg and ventilatory assistance should be instituted.
Drug Interactions Decreased effect: Aminosalicylic acid, sulfonamide effect may be antagonized
Stability Store solution in the refrigerator
Mechanism of Action Blocks both the initiation and conduction of nerve impulses by decreasing the neuronal membrane's permeability to sodium ions, which results in inhibition of depolarization with resultant blockade of conduction
Pharmacodynamics/Kinetics
Onset of anesthetic effect:
Ophthalmic instillation: Within 60 seconds
Topical or spinal injection: Within 3-8 minutes after applied to mucous membranes or when saddle block administered for spinal anesthesia
Duration of action: Topical: 1.5-3 hours
Metabolism: By the liver
Elimination: Renal
Usual Dosage Maximum adult dose: 50 mg
Children: Safety and efficacy have not been established

Adults:
Ophthalmic (not for prolonged use):
Ointment: Apply ½" to 1" to lower conjunctival fornix
Solution: Instill 1-2 drops
Spinal anesthesia:
High, medium, low, and saddle blocks: 0.2% to 0.3% solution
Prolonged (2-3 hours): 1% solution
Subarachnoid injection: 5-20 mg
Saddle block: 2-5 mg; a 1% solution should be diluted with equal volume of CSF before administration
Topical mucous membranes (2% solution): Apply as needed; dose should not exceed 20 mg
Topical for skin: Ointment/cream: Apply to affected areas as needed

Patient Information Report any rashes; keep refrigerated; may cause transient burning or stinging of eyes upon instillation; do not touch or rub eye until anesthesia (if ophthalmic) has worn off

Nursing Implications Store the solutions in the refrigerator; before injection, withdraw syringe plunger to make sure injection is not into vein or artery

Dosage Forms
Cream: 1% (28 g)
Injection: 1% [10 mg/mL] (2 mL)
Injection, with dextrose 6%: 0.2% [2 mg/mL] (2 mL); 0.3% [3 mg/mL] (5 mL)
Ointment:
   Ophthalmic: 0.5% [5 mg/mL] (3.75 g)
   Topical: 0.5% [5 mg/mL] (28 g)
Solution:
   Ophthalmic: 0.5% [5 mg/mL] (1 mL, 2 mL, 15 mL, 59 mL)
   Topical: 2% [20 mg/mL] (30 mL, 118 mL)

Tetraclear® [OTC] see Tetrahydrozoline Hydrochloride on page 1071

Tetracosactide see Cosyntropin on page 278

Tetracycline (tet ra sye′ kleen)

Brand Names Achromycin®; Achromycin® V; Ala-Tet®; Nor-tet®; Panmycin®; Robitet®; Sumycin®; Teline®; Tetracyn®; Tetralan®; Topicycline®

Synonyms TCN; Tetracycline Hydrochloride

Use Treatment of susceptible bacterial infections of both gram-positive and gram-negative organisms; also some unusual organisms including *Mycoplasma, Chlamydia,* and *Rickettsia;* may also be used for acne, exacerbations of chronic bronchitis, and treatment of gonorrhea and syphilis in patients that are allergic to penicillin

Pregnancy Risk Factor D; B (topical)

Contraindications Hypersensitivity to tetracycline or any component; do not administer to children ≤8 years of age

Warnings/Precautions Use of tetracyclines during tooth development may cause permanent discoloration of the teeth and enamel, hypoplasia and retardation of skeletal development and bone growth with risk being the greatest for children <4 years and those receiving high doses; use with caution in patients with renal or hepatic impairment and in pregnancy; dosage modification required in patients with renal impairment; pseudotumor cerebri has been reported with tetracycline use; outdated drug can cause nephropathy.

Adverse Reactions
>10%: Discoloration of teeth and enamel hypoplasia (infants)
1% to 10%:
   Dermatologic: Photosensitivity
   Gastrointestinal: Nausea, diarrhea
<1%:
   Cardiovascular: Pericarditis
   Central nervous system: Increased intracranial pressure, bulging fontanels in infants, pseudotumor cerebri
   Dermatologic: Dermatologic effects, pruritus, pigmentation of nails, exfoliative dermatitis
   Endocrine & metabolic: Diabetes insipidus syndrome
   Gastrointestinal: Vomiting, esophagitis, anorexia, abdominal cramps, antibiotic-associated pseudomembranous colitis, staphylococcal enterocolitis
   Hepatic: Hepatotoxicity
   Local: Thrombophlebitis
   Neuromuscular & skeletal: Paresthesia
   Renal: Acute renal failure, azotemia, renal damage
   Miscellaneous: Superinfections, anaphylaxis, hypersensitivity reactions, candidal superinfection

Overdosage/Toxicology Symptoms of overdose include nausea, anorexia, diarrhea; following GI decontamination, supportive care only

Drug Interactions
Decreased effect: Dairy products; calcium, magnesium or aluminum-containing antacids, iron, zinc, sodium bicarbonate, methoxyflurane, penicillins, cimetidine → ↓ tetracycline absorption
Increased toxicity: Methoxyflurane anesthesia when concurrent with tetracycline may cause fatal nephrotoxicity; warfarin with tetracyclines → increased anticoagulation

Stability Outdated tetracyclines have caused a Fanconi-like syndrome; protect oral dosage forms from light

Mechanism of Action Inhibits bacterial protein synthesis by binding with the 30S and possibly the 50S ribosomal subunit(s) of susceptible bacteria; may also cause alterations in the cytoplasmic membrane
(Continued)

Tetracycline *(Continued)*

Pharmacodynamics/Kinetics

Absorption: Oral: 75%

Distribution: Small amount appears in bile

Relative diffusion of antimicrobial agents from blood into cerebrospinal fluid (CSF): Good only with inflammation (exceeds usual MICs)

Ratio of CSF to blood level (%): Inflamed meninges: 25

Protein binding: 20% to 60%

Half-life:

Normal renal function: 8-11 hours

End stage renal disease: 57-108 hours

Time to peak serum concentration: Oral: Within 2-4 hours

Elimination: Primary route is the kidney, with 60% of a dose excreted as unchanged drug in the urine

Usual Dosage

Children >8 years:

Oral: 25-50 mg/kg/day in divided doses every 6 hours; not to exceed 3 g/day

Ophthalmic:

Suspension: Instill 1-2 drops 2-4 times/day or more often as needed

Ointment: Instill every 2-12 hours

Adults:

Oral: 250-500 mg/dose every 6 hours

Ophthalmic:

Suspension: Instill 1-2 drops 2-4 times/day or more often as needed

Ointment: Instill every 2-12 hours

Children >8 years and Adults: Topical: Apply to affected areas 1-4 times/day

Helicobacter pylori: Clinically effective treatment regimens include triple therapy with amoxicillin or tetracycline, metronidazole, and bismuth subsalicylate; amoxicillin, metronidazole, and H_2 receptor antagonist; or double therapy with amoxicillin and omeprazole. Adult dose: 850 mg 3 times/day to 500 mg 4 times/day

Dosing interval in renal impairment:

Cl_{cr} 50-80 mL/minute: Administer every 8-12 hours

Cl_{cr} 10-50 mL/minute: Administer every 12-24 hours

Cl_{cr} <10 mL/minute: Administer every 24 hours

Slightly dialyzable (5% to 20%) via hemo- and peritoneal dialysis nor via continuous arterio-venous or veno-venous hemofiltration (CAVH/CAVHD); no supplemental dosage necessary

Dosing adjustment in hepatic impairment: Avoid use or maximum dose is 1 g/day

Administration Oral should be given on an empty stomach (ie, 1 hour prior to, or 2 hours after meals) to increase total absorption. Administer at least 1-2 hours prior to, or 4 hours after antacid because aluminum and magnesium cations may chelate with tetracycline and reduce its total absorption. Administer around-the-clock rather than 4 times/day to promote less variation in peak and trough serum levels.

Monitoring Parameters Renal, hepatic, and hematologic function test, temperature, WBC, cultures and sensitivity, appetite, mental status

Test Interactions False-negative urine glucose with Clinistix®

Patient Information Take 1 hour before or 2 hours after meals with adequate amounts of fluid; avoid prolonged exposure to sunlight or sunlamps; avoid taking antacids, iron, or dairy products within 2 hours of taking tetracyclines; report persistent nausea, vomiting, yellow coloring of skin or eyes, dark urine, or pale stools; ophthalmic may cause transient burning or itching; topical is for external use only and may stain skin yellow

Additional Information

Tetracycline: Achromycin® V oral suspension, Sumycin® syrup, Tetralan® syrup

Tetracycline hydrochloride: Achromycin® injection, Achromycin® V capsule, Nor-tet® capsule, Panmycin® capsule, Robitet® capsule, Sumycin® capsule and tablet, Teline® capsule, Tetracyn® capsule, Tetralan® capsule

Dosage Forms

Capsule: 100 mg, 250 mg, 500 mg

Ointment:

Ophthalmic: 1% [10 mg/mL] (3.5 g)

Topical: 3% [30 mg/mL] (14.2 g, 30 g)

Solution, topical: 2.2 mg/mL (70 mL)

Suspension:

Ophthalmic: 1% [10 mg/mL] (0.5 mL, 1 mL, 4 mL)

Oral: 125 mg/5 mL (60 mL, 480 mL)

Tablet: 250 mg, 500 mg

Tetracycline Hydrochloride *see* Tetracycline *on page 1069*

Tetracyn® *see* Tetracycline *on page 1069*

Tetrahydroaminoacrine *see* Tacrine Hydrochloride *on page 1052*

Tetrahydrocannabinol, THC *see* Dronabinol *on page 374*

Tetrahydrozoline Hydrochloride (tet ra hye drozz' a leen)

Brand Names Collyrium Fresh® [OTC]; Eye-Zine® [OTC]; Murine® Plus [OTC]; Ocu-Drop® [OTC]; Optigene® [OTC]; Soothe® [OTC]; Tetraclear® [OTC]; Tetra-Ide® [OTC]; Tyzine®; Visine® [OTC]; Visine A.C.® [OTC]

Synonyms Tetryzoline

Use Symptomatic relief of nasal congestion and conjunctival congestion

Pregnancy Risk Factor C

Contraindications Narrow-angle glaucoma, patients receiving MAO inhibitors, known hypersensitivity to tetrahydrozoline

Warnings/Precautions Do not use in children <2 years of age; excessive use may cause rebound congestion or chemical rhinitis; use with caution in patients with hypertension, diabetes, cardiovascular or coronary artery disease; discontinue use prior to the use of anesthetics which sensitize the myocardium to the systemic effects of sympathomimetics

Adverse Reactions
>10%: Local: Transient stinging, sneezing
1% to 10%:
Cardiovascular: Tachycardia, palpitations, increased blood pressure, heart rate
Central nervous system: Headache
Neuromuscular & skeletal: Tremor
Ocular: Blurred vision

Overdosage/Toxicology Symptoms of overdose include CNS depression, hypothermia, bradycardia, cardiovascular collapse, coma; following initiation of essential overdose management, toxic symptoms should be treated. The patient should be kept warm and monitored for alterations in vital functions. Seizures commonly respond to diazepam (5-10 mg I.V. bolus in adults every 15 minutes if needed up to a total of 30 mg; I.V. 0.25-0.4 mg/kg/dose up to a total of 10 mg for children) or to phenytoin or phenobarbital; apnea will respond to naloxone.

Drug Interactions Increased toxicity: MAO inhibitors can cause an exaggerated adrenergic response if taken concurrently or within 21 days of discontinuing MAO inhibitor; beta-blockers can cause hypertensive episodes and increased risk of intracranial hemorrhage; anesthetics

Mechanism of Action Stimulates alpha-adrenergic receptors in the arterioles of the conjunctiva and the nasal mucosa to produce vasoconstriction

Pharmacodynamics/Kinetics
Onset of decongestant effect: Intranasal: Within 4-8 hours
Duration: Ophthalmic vasoconstriction: 2-3 hours
Absorption: Topical: Systemic absorption sometimes occurs

Usual Dosage
Nasal congestion: Intranasal:
Children 2-6 years: Instill 2-3 drops of 0.05% solution every 4-6 hours as needed, no more frequent than every 3 hours
Children >6 years and Adults: Instill 2-4 drops or 3-4 sprays of 0.1% solution every 3-4 hours as needed, no more frequent than every 3 hours

Conjunctival congestion: Ophthalmic: Adults: Instill 1-2 drops in each eye 2-4 times/day

Monitoring Parameters Blood pressure, heart rate, symptom response

Patient Information Remove contact lenses before using in eye, do not use for more than 72 hours unless directed to do so; consult physician if changes in vision or visual acuity occur; do not exceed recommended dosage

Nursing Implications Do not use for >3-4 days without direct physician supervision

Dosage Forms Solution:
Nasal: 0.05% (15 mL), 0.1% (15 mL spray, 30 mL drops)
Ophthalmic: 0.05% (15 mL, 22.5 mL, 30 mL)

Tetra-Ide® [OTC] *see* Tetrahydrozoline Hydrochloride *on this page*

Tetralan® *see* Tetracycline *on page 1069*

Tetramune® *see* Diphtheria, Tetanus Toxoids, Whole-Cell Pertussis Vaccine, and Haemophilus b Conjugate Vaccine *on page 355*

Tetryzoline *see* Tetrahydrozoline Hydrochloride *on this page*

Texacort™ *see* Hydrocortisone *on page 546*

TG *see* Thioguanine *on page 1081*

6-TG see Thioguanine on page 1081

T-Gen® see Trimethobenzamide Hydrochloride on page 1126

T-Gesic® see Hydrocodone and Acetaminophen on page 543

THA see Tacrine Hydrochloride on page 1052

Thalitone® see Chlorthalidone on page 235

THAM® see Tromethamine on page 1134

THAM-E® see Tromethamine on page 1134

Theelin® see Estrone on page 413

Theo-24® see Theophylline/Aminophylline on this page

Theobid® see Theophylline/Aminophylline on this page

Theochron® see Theophylline/Aminophylline on this page

Theoclear® L.A. see Theophylline/Aminophylline on this page

Theo-Dur® see Theophylline/Aminophylline on this page

Theodur-Sprinkle® see Theophylline/Aminophylline on this page

Theolair™ see Theophylline/Aminophylline on this page

Theon® see Theophylline/Aminophylline on this page

Theophylline see Theophylline/Aminophylline on this page

Theophylline/Aminophylline (am in off' i lin)/(thee off' i lin)

Brand Names Aerolate®; Aerolate III®; Aerolate JR®; Aerolate SR®; Aminophyllin™; Aquaphyllin®; Asmalix®; Bronkodyl®; Choledyl®; Constant-T®; Duraphyl™; Elixophyllin®; Elixophyllin® SR; LaBID®; Phyllocontin®; Quibron®-T; Quibron®-T/SR; Respbid®; Slo-bid™; Slo-Phyllin®; Sustaire®; Theo-24®; Theobid®; Theochron®; Theoclear® L.A.; Theo-Dur®; Theodur-Sprinkle®; Theolair™; Theon®; Theospan®-SR; Theovent®; Truphylline®

Synonyms Aminophylline; Choline Theophyllinate; Oxtriphylline; Theophylline; Theophylline Ethylenediamine

Use Bronchodilator in reversible airway obstruction due to asthma, chronic bronchitis, and emphysema; for neonatal apnea/bradycardia

Pregnancy Risk Factor C

Contraindications Uncontrolled arrhythmias, hyperthyroidism, peptic ulcers, uncontrolled seizure disorders, hypersensitivity to xanthines or any component

Warnings/Precautions Use with caution in patients with peptic ulcer, hyperthyroidism, hypertension, tachyarrhythmias, and patients with compromised cardiac function; do not inject I.V. solution faster than 25 mg/minute; elderly, acutely ill, and patients with severe respiratory problems, pulmonary edema, or liver dysfunction are at greater risk of toxicity because of reduced drug clearance
Although there is a great intersubject variability for half-lives of methylxanthines (2-10 hours), elderly as a group have slower hepatic clearance. Therefore, use lower initial doses and monitor closely for response and adverse reactions. Additionally, elderly are at greater risk for toxicity due to concomitant disease (eg, CHF, arrhythmias), and drug use (eg, cimetidine, ciprofloxacin, etc).

Adverse Reactions See table.

Theophylline Serum Levels (mcg/mL)*	Adverse Reactions
15-25	GI upset, diarrhea, N/V, abdominal pain, nervousness, headache, insomnia, agitation, dizziness, muscle cramp, tremor
25-35	Tachycardia, occasional PVC
>35	Ventricular tachycardia, frequent PVC, seizure

*Adverse effects do not necessarily occur according to serum levels.
Arrhythmia and seizure can occur without seeing the other adverse effects.

Uncommon at serum theophylline concentrations ≤20 mcg/mL
1% to 10%:
Cardiovascular: Tachycardia
Central nervous system: Nervousness, restlessness
Gastrointestinal: Nausea, vomiting,
<1%:
Allergic reactions
Central nervous system: Insomnia, irritability, seizures
Dermatologic: Skin rash
Gastrointestinal: Gastric irritation
Neuromuscular & skeletal: Tremor

Overdosage/Toxicology Symptoms of overdose include nausea, vomiting, insomnia, irritability, tachycardia, seizures, tonic-clonic seizures, insomnia, circulatory failure. If seizures have not occurred, induce vomiting; ipecac syrup is preferred. Do not induce emesis in the presence of impaired consciousness. Repeated doses of charcoal have been shown to be effective in enhancing the total body clearance of theophylline. Do not repeat charcoal doses if an ileus is present. Charcoal hemoperfusion may be considered if the serum theophylline levels exceed 40 mcg/mL, the patient is unable to tolerate repeat oral charcoal administrations, or if severe toxic symptoms are present. Clearance with hemoperfusion is better than clearance from hemodialysis. Administer a cathartic, especially if sustained release agents were used. Phenobarbital administered prophylactically may prevent seizures.

Drug Interactions Decreased effect/increased toxicity: Changes in diet may affect the elimination of theophylline; charcoal-broiled foods may increase elimination, reducing half-life by 50%; see table for factors affecting serum levels.

Factors Reported to Affect Theophylline Serum Levels

Decreased Theophylline Level	Increased Theophylline Level
Smoking (cigarettes, marijuana)	Hepatic cirrhosis
High protein/low carbohydrate diet	Cor pulmonale
Charcoal	CHF
Phenytoin	Fever/viral illness
Phenobarbital	Propranolol
Carbamazepine	Allopurinol (>600 mg/d)
Rifampin	Erythromycin
I.V. isoproterenol	Cimetidine
Aminoglutethimide	Troleandomycin
Barbiturates	Ciprofloxacin
Hydantoins	Oral contraceptives
Ketoconazole	Beta blockers
Sulfinpyrazone	Calcium channel blockers
Isoniazide	Corticosteroids
Loop diuretics	Disulfiram
Sympathomimetics	Ephedrine
	Influenza virus vaccine
	Interferon
	Macrolides
	Mexiletine
	Quinolones
	Thiabendazole
	Thyroid hormones
	Carbamazepine
	Isoniazid
	Loop diuretics

Stability

Theophylline injection should be stored at room temperature and protected from freezing

Stability of parenteral admixture at room temperature (25°C): manufacturer expiration dating; out of overwrap stability: 30 days

Standard diluent: 400 mg theophylline/500 mL D_5W (premixed); 800 mg theophylline/1000 mL D_5W (premixed)

Aminophylline injection [content = 80% theophylline] should be stored at room temperature and protected from freezing and light

Stability of parenteral admixture at room temperature (25°C): 24 hours

Standard diluent: 250 mg aminophylline/100 mL D_5W ; 500 mg aminophylline/100 mL D_5W

Mechanism of Action Causes bronchodilatation, diuresis, CNS and cardiac stimulation, and gastric acid secretion by blocking phosphodiesterase which increases tissue concentrations of cyclic adenine monophosphate (cAMP) which in turn promotes catecholamine stimulation of lipolysis, glycogenolysis, and gluconeogenesis and induces release of epinephrine from adrenal medulla cells

Pharmacodynamics/Kinetics

Absorption: Oral:

Oxtriphylline [64% theophylline]: Depends on the formulation and ranges from 75%-100%

Theophylline: Up to 100% absorbed depending upon formulation used

Distribution: V_d: 0.45 L/kg; distributes into breast milk (approximates serum concentration); crosses the placenta

(Continued)

Theophylline/Aminophylline (Continued)

Aminophylline

Patient Group	Approximate Half-Life (h)
Neonates	
Premature	30
Normal newborn	24
Infants	
4-52 weeks	4-30
Children/Adolescents	
1-9 years	2-10 (4 avg)
9-16 years	4-16
Adults	
Nonsmoker	4-16 (8.7 avg)
Smoker	4.4
Cardiac compromised, liver failure	20-30

Dosage Form	Time to Peak	Dosing Interval
Uncoated tablet/syrup	2 h	6 h
Enteric coated tablet	5 h	12 h
Chewable tablet	1-1.5 h	6 h
Extended release	4-7 h	12 h
Intravenous	<30 min	

Metabolism: In the liver by demethylation and oxidation

Half-life: Highly variable and dependent upon age, liver function, cardiac function, lung disease, and smoking history

Elimination: In urine; adults excrete 10% in urine as unchanged drug; neonates excrete a greater percentage of the dose unchanged in urine (up to 50%)

Usual Dosage Use ideal body weight for obese patients

Apnea of prematurity: Neonates: Oral, I.V.: Loading dose: 4 mg/kg (theophylline); 5 mg/kg (aminophylline)

There appears to be a delay in theophylline elimination in infants <1 year of age, especially neonates; both the initial dose and maintenance dosage should be conservative

Approximate I.V. Theophylline Dosage for Treatment of Acute Bronchospasm

Group	Dosage for next 12 h*	Dosage after 12 h*
Infants 6 wk to 6 mo	0.5 mg/kg/h	
Children 6 mo to 1 y	0.6-0.7 mg/kg/h	
Children 1-9 y	0.95 mg/kg/h (1.2 mg/kg/h)	0.79 mg/kg/h (1 mg/kg/h)
Children 9-16 y and young adult smokers	0.79 mg/kg/h (1 mg/kg/h)	0.63 mg/kg/h (0.8 mg/kg/h)
Healthy, nonsmoking adults	0.55 mg/kg/h (0.7 mg/kg/h)	0.39 mg/kg/h (0.5 mg/kg/h)
Older patients and patients with cor pulmonale	0.47 mg/kg/h (0.6 mg/kg/h)	0.24 mg/kg/h (0.3 mg/kg/h)
Patients with congestive heart failure or liver failure	0.39 mg/kg/h (0.5 mg/kg/h)	0.08-0.16 mg/kg/h (0.1-0.2 mg/kg/h)

*Equivalent hydrous aminophylline dosage indicated in parentheses.

Initial: Maintenance infusion rates: I.V.:
Neonates:
≤24 days: 0.08 mg/kg/hour theophylline
>24 days: 0.12 mg/kg/hour theophylline
Infants (6-52 weeks): 0.008 (age in weeks) + 0.21 mg/kg/hour theophylline
Children:
6 weeks to 6 months: 0.5 mg/kg/hour
6 months to 1 year: 0.6-0.7 mg/kg/hour

Bolus dosing determination: Approximate I.V. maintenance dosages are based upon continuous infusions: Bolus dosing (often used in children <6 months of age) may be determined by multiplying the hourly infusion rate by 24 hours and dividing by the desired number of doses/day.

Treatment of acute bronchospasm: Children >1 year and Adults: I.V.: Loading dose (in patients not currently receiving aminophylline or theophylline): 6 mg/kg (based on aminophylline) given I.V. over 20-30 minutes; administration rate should not exceed 25 mg/minute (aminophylline). See table.

Dosage should be adjusted according to serum level measurements during the first 12- to 24-hour period.

Maintenance Dose for Acute Symptoms

Population Group	Oral Theophylline (mg/kg/day)	I.V. Aminophylline
Premature infant or newborn - 6 wk (for apnea/bradycardia)	4	5 mg/kg/day
6 wk - 6 mo	10	12 mg/kg/day or continuous I.V. infusion*
Infants 6 mo-1 y	12-18	15 mg/kg/day or continuous I.V. infusion*
Children 1-9 y	20-24	1 mg/kg/hour
Children 9-12 y, and adolescent daily smokers of cigarettes or marijuana, and otherwise healthy adult smokers <50 y	16	0.9 mg/kg/hour
Adolescents 12-16 y (nonsmokers)	13	0.7 mg/kg/hour
Otherwise healthy nonsmoking adults (including elderly patients)	10 (not to exceed 900 mg/day)	0.5 mg/kg/hour
Cardiac decompensation, cor pulmonale and/or liver dysfunction	5 (not to exceed 400 mg/day)	0.25 mg/kg/hour

*For continuous I.V. infusion divide total daily dose by 24 = mg/kg/hour.

Oral theophylline: Treatment of acute bronchospasm: Initial dosage recommendation: Loading dose (to achieve a serum level of about 10 mcg/mL; loading doses should be given using a rapidly absorbed oral product **not** a sustained release product):

If no theophylline has been administered in the previous 24 hours: 4-6 mg/kg theophylline

If theophylline has been administered in the previous 24 hours, administer ½ the loading dose or 2-3 mg/kg theophylline can be given in emergencies when serum levels are not available

On the average, for every 1 mg/kg theophylline given, blood levels will rise 2 mcg/mL. Ideally, defer the loading dose if a serum theophylline concentration can be obtained rapidly. However, if this is not possible, exercise clinical judgment. If the patient is not experiencing theophylline toxicity, this is unlikely to result in dangerous adverse effects.

These recommendations, based on mean clearance rates for age or risk factors, were calculated to achieve a serum level of 10 mcg/mL (5 mcg/mL for newborns with apnea/bradycardia). In newborns and infants, a fast-release oral product can be used. The total daily dose can be divided every 12 hours in newborns and every 6-8 hours in infants. In children and healthy adults, a slow-release product can be used. The total daily dose can be divided every 8-12 hours.

(Continued)

Theophylline/Aminophylline *(Continued)*
Oral Theophylline Dosage for Bronchial Asthma*

Age	Initial 3 Days	Second 3 Days	Steady-State Maintenance
<1 y	0.2 x (age in weeks) + 5		0.3 x (age in weeks) + 8
1-9 y	16 up to a maximum of 400 mg/24 h	20	22
9-12 y	16 up to a maximum of 400 mg/24 h	16 up to a maximum of 600 mg/24 h	20 up to a maximum of 800 mg/24 h
12-16 y	16 up to a maximum of 400 mg/24 h	16 up to a maximum of 600 mg/24 h	18 up to a maximum of 900 mg/24 h
Adults	400 mg/24 h	600 mg/24 h	900 mg/24 h

*Dose in mg/kg/24 hours of theophylline.

Increasing dose: The dosage may be increased in approximately 25% increments at 2- to 3-day intervals so long as the drug is tolerated or until the maximum dose is reached

Maintenance dose:

These recommendations, based on mean clearance rates for age or risk factors, were calculated to achieve a serum level of 10 mcg/mL (5 mcg/mL for newborns with apnea/bradycardia). In newborns and infants, a fast-release oral product can be used. The total daily dose can be divided every 12 hours in newborns and every 6-8 hours in infants. In children and healthy adults, a slow-release product can be used. The total daily dose can be divided every 8-12 hours.

Dose should be further adjusted based on serum levels.

Oxtriphylline: Oral:
Children 1-9 years: 6.2 mg/kg/dose every 6 hours
Children 9-16 years and Adult smokers: 4.7 mg/kg/dose every 6 hours
Adult nonsmokers: 4.7 mg/kg/dose every 8 hours

Aminophylline: Rectal: Adults: 250-500 mg 3 times/day; avoid using suppositories due to erratic, unreliable absorption

Dosing adjustment/comments in hepatic disease: Higher incidence of toxic effects including seizures in cirrhosis; plasma levels should be monitored closely during long-term administration in cirrhosis and during acute hepatitis, with dose adjustment as necessary.
Administer dose posthemodialysis or administer supplemental 50% dose
Peritoneal dialysis effects: Supplemental dose is not necessary

Administration Administer oral and I.V. administration around-the-clock to promote less variation in peak and trough serum levels; theophylline injection may be administered by continuous I.V. infusion (requires an infusion pump) or IVPB; maximum rate of I.V. administration of theophylline is 20-25 mg per minute

Monitoring Parameters Heart rate, CNS effects (insomnia, irritability); respiratory rate (COPD patients often have resting controlled respiratory rates in low 20s), serum theophylline level, arterial or capillary blood gases (if applicable)

Reference Range
Saliva levels are approximately equal to 60% of plasma levels
Sample size: 0.5-1 mL (red top)
Therapeutic levels: 10-20 µg/mL
Neonatal apnea 6-13 µg/mL
Pregnancy: 3-12 µg/mL
Toxic concentration: >20 µg/mL
Timing of serum samples: If toxicity is suspected, draw a level any time during a continuous I.V. infusion, or 2 hours after an oral dose; if lack of therapeutic is effected, draw a trough immediately before the next oral dose; see table.

Test Interactions May elevate uric acid levels

Patient Information Oral preparations should be taken with a full glass of water; capsule forms may be opened and sprinkled on soft foods; do not chew beads; notify physician if nausea, vomiting, severe GI pain, restlessness, or irregular heartbeat occurs; do not drink or eat large quantities of caffeine-containing beverages or food (colas, coffee, chocolate); remain in bed for 15-20 minutes after inserting suppository; do not chew or crush enteric coated or sustained

Dosage Adjustment After Serum Theophylline Measurement

Serum Theophylline		Guidelines
Within normal limits	10-20 mcg/mL	Maintain dosage if tolerated. Recheck serum theophylline concentration at 6-12 mo intervals.*
Too high	20-25 mcg/mL	Decrease doses by about 10%. Recheck serum theophylline concentration after 3 d and then at 6-12 mo intervals.*
	25-30 mcg/mL	Skip next dose and decrease subsequent doses by about 25%. Recheck serum theophylline.
	>30 mcg/mL	Skip next 2 doses and decrease subsequent doses by 50%. Recheck serum theophylline.
Too low	7.5-10 mcg/mL	Increase dose by about 25%.† Recheck serum theophylline concentration after 3 d and then at 6-12 mo intervals.*
	5-7.5 mcg/mL	Increase dose by about 25% to the nearest dose increment† and recheck serum theophylline for guidance in further dosage adjustment (another increase will probably be needed, but this provides a safety check).

From Weinberger M and Hendeles L, 'Practical Guide to Using Theophylline,' *J Resp Dis*, 1981, 2:12-27.

*Finer adjustments in dosage may be needed for some patients.

†Dividing the daily dose into 3 doses administered at 8-hour intervals may be indicated if symptoms occur repeatedly at the end of a dosing interval.

Guidelines for Drawing Theophylline Serum Levels

Dosage Form	Time to Draw Level
I.V. bolus	30 min after end of 30 min infusion
I.V. continuous infusion	12-24 h after initiation of infusion
P.O. liquid, fast-release tab	Peak: 1 h postdose after at least 1 day of therapy Trough: Just before a dose after at least one day of therapy
P.O. slow-release product	Peak: 4 h postdose after at least 1 day of therapy Trough: Just before a dose after at least one day of therapy

Salt	% Theophylline Content
Theophylline anhydrous (eg, most oral solids)	100%
Theophylline monohydrate (eg, oral solutions)	91%
Aminophylline (theophylline) (eg, injection)	80% (79% to 86%)
Oxtriphylline (choline theophylline) (eg, Choledyl®)	64%

Theophylline/Aminophylline *(Continued)*

release products; take at regular intervals; notify physician if insomnia, nervousness, irritability, palpitations, seizures occur; do not change brands or doses without consulting physician

Nursing Implications Do not crush sustained release drug products; do not crush enteric coated drug product; encourage patient to drink adequate fluids (2 L/day) to decrease mucous viscosity

Additional Information See table for theophylline content.

Dosage Forms

Aminophylline (79% theophylline):

Injection: 25 mg/mL (10 mL, 20 mL); 250 mg (equivalent to 187 mg theophylline) per 10 mL; 500 mg (equivalent to 394 mg theophylline) per 20 mL

Liquid, oral: 105 mg (equivalent to 90 mg theophylline) per 5 mL (240 mL, 500 mL)

Suppository, rectal: 250 mg (equivalent to 198 mg theophylline); 500 mg (equivalent to 395 mg theophylline)

Tablet: 100 mg (equivalent to 79 mg theophylline); 200 mg (equivalent to 158 mg theophylline)

Tablet, controlled release: 225 mg (equivalent to 178 mg theophylline)

Oxtriphylline (64% theophylline):

Elixir: 100 mg (equivalent to 64 mg theophylline)/5 mL (5 mL, 10 mL, 473 mL)

Syrup: 50 mg (equivalent to 32 mg theophylline)/5 mL (473 mL)

Tablet: 100 mg (equivalent to 64 mg theophylline); 200 mg (equivalent to 127 mg theophylline)

Tablet, sustained release: 400 mg (equivalent to 254 mg theophylline); 600 mg (equivalent to 382 mg theophylline)

Theophylline:

Capsule:

Immediate release: 100 mg, 200 mg

Sustained release (8-12 hours): 50 mg, 60 mg, 65 mg, 75 mg, 100 mg, 125 mg, 130 mg, 200 mg, 250 mg, 260 mg, 300 mg

Timed release (12 hours): 50 mg, 75 mg, 125 mg, 130 mg, 200 mg, 250 mg, 260 mg

Timed release (24 hours): 100 mg, 200 mg, 300 mg

Injection: Theophylline in 5% dextrose: 200 mg/container (50 mL, 100 mL); 400 mg/container (100 mL, 250 mL, 500 mL, 1000 mL); 800 mg/container (250 mL, 500 mL, 1000 mL)

Elixir, oral: 80 mg/15 mL (15 mL, 30 mL, 500 mL, 4000 mL)

Solution, oral: 80 mg/15 mL (15 mL, 18.75 mL, 30 mL, 120 mL, 500 mL, 4000 mL); 150 mg/15 mL (480 mL)

Syrup, oral: 80 mg/15 mL (5 mL, 15 mL, 30 mL, 120 mL, 500 mL, 4000 mL); 150 mg/15 mL (480 mL)

Tablet:

Immediate release: 100 mg, 125 mg, 200 mg, 250 mg, 300 mg

Timed release (8-12 hours): 100 mg, 200 mg, 250 mg, 300 mg, 500 mg

Timed release (8-24 hours): 100 mg, 200 mg, 300 mg, 450 mg

Timed release (12-24 hours): 100 mg, 200 mg, 300 mg

Timed release (24 hours): 400 mg

Theophylline Ethylenediamine *see* Theophylline/Aminophylline *on page 1072*

Theospan®-SR *see* Theophylline/Aminophylline *on page 1072*

Theovent® *see* Theophylline/Aminophylline *on page 1072*

Therabid® [OTC] *see* Vitamin, Multiple *on page 1166*

TheraCys™ *see* Bacillus Calmette-Guérin *on page 110*

Thera-Flur® *see* Fluoride *on page 471*

Thera-Flur-N® *see* Fluoride *on page 471*

Theragran® Hematinic® *see* Vitamin, Multiple *on page 1166*

Theragran-M® [OTC] *see* Vitamin, Multiple *on page 1166*

Theragran® [OTC] *see* Vitamin, Multiple *on page 1166*

Theragran® Liquid [OTC] *see* Vitamin, Multiple *on page 1166*

Theralax® [OTC] *see* Bisacodyl *on page 134*

Therapeutic Multivitamins *see* Vitamin, Multiple *on page 1166*

Thermazene™ *see* Silver Sulfadiazine *on page 1005*

Thiabendazole (thye a ben' da zole)

Brand Names Mintezol®

Synonyms Tiabendazole

Use Treatment of strongyloidiasis, cutaneous larva migrans, visceral larva migrans, dracunculiasis, trichinosis, and mixed helminthic infections

Pregnancy Risk Factor C

Contraindications Known hypersensitivity to thiabendazole

Warnings/Precautions Use with caution in patients with renal or hepatic impairment, malnutrition or anemia, or dehydration

Adverse Reactions

>10%:

Central nervous system: Numbness, seizures, hallucinations, delirium, dizziness, drowsiness, headache

Gastrointestinal: Anorexia, diarrhea, nausea, vomiting

Otic: Tinnitus

Miscellaneous: Drying of mucous membranes

1% to 10%: Dermatologic: Skin rash, Stevens-Johnson syndrome

<1%:

Central nervous system: Chills

Genitourinary: Malodor of urine

Hematologic: Leukopenia

Hepatic: Hepatotoxicity

Ocular: Blurred or yellow vision

Renal: Nephrotoxicity

Miscellaneous: Lymphadenopathy, hypersensitivity reactions

Overdosage/Toxicology Symptoms of overdose include altered mental status, visual problems; supportive care only following GI decontamination

Drug Interactions Increased levels of theophylline and other xanthines

Mechanism of Action Inhibits helminth-specific mitochondrial fumarate reductase

Pharmacodynamics/Kinetics

Absorption: Rapid and nearly complete

Metabolism: Rapid

Time to peak serum concentration: Within 1-2 hours

Elimination: In feces (5%) and urine (87%), primarily as conjugated metabolites

Usual Dosage Purgation is not required prior to use; drinking of fruit juice aids in expulsion of worms by removing the mucous to which the intestinal tapeworms attach themselves

Children and Adults: Oral: 50 mg/kg/day divided every 12 hours; maximum dose: 3 g/day

Strongyloidiasis: For 2 consecutive days

Cutaneous larva migrans: For 2-5 consecutive days

Visceral larva migrans: For 5-7 consecutive days

Trichinosis: For 2-4 consecutive days

Dracunculosis: 50-75 mg/kg/day divided every 12 hours for 3 days

Dosing comments in renal/hepatic impairment: Use with caution

Test Interactions ↑ glucose

Patient Information Take after meals, chew chewable tablet well; may decrease alertness, avoid driving or operating machinery; drinking of fruit juice aids in expulsion of worms by removing the mucous to which the intestinal tapeworms attach themselves

Nursing Implications Purgation is not required prior to use; pinworm infections are easily transmitted, all close family members should be treated

Dosage Forms

Suspension, oral: 500 mg/5 mL (120 mL)

Tablet, chewable (orange flavor): 500 mg

Thiamazole see Methimazole on page 708

Thiamine Hydrochloride (thye' a min)

Brand Names Betalin®S; Biamine®

Synonyms Aneurine Hydrochloride; Thiaminium Chloride Hydrochloride; Vitamin B_1

Use Treatment of thiamine deficiency including beriberi, Wernicke's encephalopathy syndrome, and peripheral neuritis associated with pellagra, alcoholic patients with altered sensorium; various genetic metabolic disorders

Pregnancy Risk Factor A (C if dose exceeds RDA recommendation)

Contraindications Hypersensitivity to thiamine or any component

(Continued)

Thiamine Hydrochloride *(Continued)*

Warnings/Precautions Use with caution with parenteral route (especially I.V.) of administration

Adverse Reactions

<1%:
Cardiovascular: Cardiovascular collapse and death
Central nervous system: Warmth, tingling
Dermatologic: Rash, angioedema

Stability Protect oral dosage forms from light; **incompatible** with alkaline or neutral solutions and with oxidizing or reducing agents

Mechanism of Action An essential coenzyme in carbohydrate metabolism by combining with adenosine triphosphate to form thiamine pyrophosphate

Pharmacodynamics/Kinetics

Absorption:
Oral: Adequate
I.M.: Rapid and complete
Elimination: Renally as unchanged drug, and as pyrimidine after body storage sites become saturated

Usual Dosage

Recommended daily allowance:
<6 months: 0.3 mg
6 months to 1 year: 0.4 mg
1-3 years: 0.7 mg
4-6 years: 0.9 mg
7-10 years: 1 mg
11-14 years: 1.1-1.3 mg
>14 years: 1-1.5 mg
Thiamine deficiency (beriberi):
Children: 10-25 mg/dose I.M. or I.V. daily (if critically ill), or 10-50 mg/dose orally every day for 2 weeks, then 5-10 mg/dose orally daily for 1 month
Adults: 5-30 mg/dose I.M. or I.V. 3 times/day (if critically ill); then orally 5-30 mg/day in single or divided doses 3 times/day for 1 month
Wernicke's encephalopathy: Adults: Initial: 100 mg I.V., then 50-100 mg/day I.M. or I.V. until consuming a regular, balanced diet
Dietary supplement (depends on caloric or carbohydrate content of the diet):
Infants: 0.3-0.5 mg/day
Children: 0.5-1 mg/day
Adults: 1-2 mg/day
Note: The above doses can be found in multivitamin preparations
Metabolic disorders: Oral: Adults: 10-20 mg/day (dosages up to 4 g/day in divided doses have been used)

Administration Parenteral form may be administered by I.M. or slow I.V. injection

Reference Range Therapeutic: 1.6-4 mg/dL

Test Interactions False-positive for uric acid using the phosphotungstate method and for urobilinogen using the Ehrlich's reagent; large doses may interfere with the spectrophotometric determination of serum theophylline concentration

Patient Information Dietary sources include legumes, pork, beef, whole grains, yeast, fresh vegetables; a deficiency state can occur in as little 3 weeks following total dietary absence

Nursing Implications Single vitamin deficiency is rare; look for other deficiencies

Additional Information Dietary sources include legumes, pork, beef, whole grains, yeast, fresh vegetables; a deficiency state can occur in as little 3 weeks following total dietary absence

Dosage Forms

Injection: 100 mg/mL (1 mL, 2 mL, 10 mL, 30 mL)
Tablet: 50 mg, 100 mg, 250 mg, 500 mg
Tablet, enteric coated: 20 mg

Thiaminium Chloride Hydrochloride *see* Thiamine Hydrochloride *on previous page*

Thiethylperazine Maleate *(thye eth il per' a zeen)*

Brand Names Torecan®

Use Relief of nausea and vomiting
Unlabeled use: Treatment of vertigo

Pregnancy Risk Factor X

Contraindications Comatose states, hypersensitivity to thiethylperazine or any component; pregnancy, cross-sensitivity to other phenothiazines may exist

Warnings/Precautions Reduce or discontinue if extrapyramidal effects occur; safety and efficacy in children <12 years of age have not been established; postural hypotension may occur after I.M. injection; the injectable form contains sulfite which may cause allergic reactions in some patients; use caution in patients with narrow-angle glaucoma

Adverse Reactions
>10%:
 Central nervous system: Drowsiness, dizziness
 Miscellaneous: Dry mouth and nose
1% to 10%:
 Cardiovascular: Tachycardia, orthostatic hypotension
 Central nervous system: Confusion, convulsions, extrapyramidal effects, tardive dyskinesia, fever, headache
 Hematologic: Agranulocytosis
 Hepatic: Cholestatic jaundice
 Otic: Tinnitus

Overdosage/Toxicology Symptoms of overdose include deep sleep, coma, extrapyramidal symptoms, abnormal involuntary muscle movements, hypotension

Following initiation of essential overdose management, toxic symptom treatment and supportive treatment should be initiated. Hypotension usually responds to I.V. fluids or Trendelenburg positioning. If unresponsive to these measures, use of a parenteral inotrope may be required (eg, norepinephrine 0.1-0.2 mcg/kg/minute titrated to response); avoid epinephrine for thiethylperazine-induced hypotension. Seizures commonly respond to diazepam (I.V. 5-10 mg bolus in adults every 15 minutes if needed up to a total of 30 mg; I.V. 0.25-0.4 mg/kg/dose up to a total of 10 mg in children) or to phenytoin or phenobarbital. Critical cardiac arrhythmias often respond to I.V. phenytoin (15 mg/kg up to 1 g), while other antiarrhythmics can be used. Neuroleptics often cause extrapyramidal symptoms (eg, dystonic reactions) requiring management with diphenhydramine 1-2 mg/kg (adults) up to a maximum of 50 mg I.M. or I.V. slow push followed by a maintenance dose for 48-72 hours. When these reactions are unresponsive to diphenhydramine, benztropine mesylate I.V. 1-2 mg (adults) may be effective. These agents are generally effective within 2-5 minutes.

Drug Interactions Increased effect/toxicity with CNS depressants (eg, anesthetics, opiates, tranquilizers, alcohol), lithium, atropine, epinephrine, MAO inhibitors, TCAs

Mechanism of Action Blocks postsynaptic mesolimbic dopaminergic receptors in the brain; exhibits a strong alpha-adrenergic blocking effect and depresses the release of hypothalamic and hypophyseal hormones; acts directly on chemoreceptor trigger zone and vomiting center

Pharmacodynamics/Kinetics
Onset of antiemetic effect: Within 30 minutes
Duration of action: ~4 hours

Usual Dosage Children >12 years and Adults:
Oral, I.M., rectal: 10 mg 1-3 times/day as needed
I.V. and S.C. routes of administration are not recommended

Not dialyzable (0% to 5%)
Dosing comments in hepatic impairment: Use with caution

Administration Inject I.M. deeply into large muscle mass, patient should be lying down and remain so for at least 1 hour after administration

Patient Information May cause drowsiness, impair judgment and coordination; may cause photosensitivity; avoid excessive sunlight; notify physician of involuntary movements or feelings of restlessness

Nursing Implications Assist with ambulation, observe for extrapyramidal symptoms

Dosage Forms
Injection: 5 mg/mL (2 mL)
Suppository, rectal: 10 mg
Tablet: 10 mg

Thioguanine (thye oh gwah' neen)

Related Information
 Cancer Chemotherapy Regimens *on page 1218-1241*
Synonyms 2-Amino-6-Mercaptopurine; TG; 6-TG; 6-Thioguanine; Tioguanine
Use Remission induction in acute myelogenous (nonlymphocytic) leukemia; treatment of chronic myelogenous leukemia and granulocytic leukemia
Pregnancy Risk Factor D
Contraindications History of previous therapy resistance with either thioguanine or mercaptopurine (there is usually complete cross resistance between these two); hypersensitivity to thioguanine or any component
Warnings/Precautions The U.S. Food and Drug Administration (FDA) currently recommends that procedures for proper handling and disposal of antineoplastic
(Continued)

Thioguanine *(Continued)*

agents be considered. Use with caution and reduce dose of thioguanine in patients with renal or hepatic impairment; thioguanine is potentially carcinogenic and teratogenic; myelosuppression may be delayed.

Adverse Reactions

>10%:

Myelosuppressive:

WBC: Moderate

Platelets: Moderate

Onset (days): 7-10

Nadir (days): 14

Recovery (days): 21

1% to 10%:

Dermatologic: Skin rash

Gastrointestinal: Mild nausea or vomiting, anorexia, stomatitis, diarrhea

Emetic potential: Low (<10%)

Miscellaneous: Hyperuricemia, unsteady gait

<1%:

Central nervous system: Neurotoxicity

Dermatologic: Photosensitivity

Gastrointestinal: Stomatitis

Hepatic: Hepatitis, jaundice, veno-occlusive hepatic disease

Overdosage/Toxicology Symptoms of overdose include bone marrow depression, nausea, vomiting, malaise, hypertension, sweating; treatment is supportive; dialysis is not useful

Drug Interactions

Increased toxicity:

Allopurinol can be used in full doses with 6 TG unlike 6-MP

Busulfan → hepatotoxicity and esophageal varices

Mechanism of Action Purine analog that is incorporated into DNA and RNA resulting in the blockage of synthesis and metabolism of purine nucleotides

Pharmacodynamics/Kinetics

Absorption: Oral: 30%

Distribution: Crosses placenta

Metabolism: Rapidly and extensively in the liver to 2-amino-6-methylthioguanine (active) and inactive compounds

Half-life, terminal: 11 hours

Time to peak serum concentration: Within 8 hours

Elimination: In urine

Usual Dosage Total daily dose can be given at one time; offers little advantage over mercaptopurine; is sometimes ordered as 6-thioguanine, with 6 being part of the drug name and not some kind of units or strength.

Oral (refer to individual protocols):

Infants <3 years: Combination drug therapy for acute nonlymphocytic leukemia: 3.3 mg/kg/day in divided doses twice daily for 4 days

Children and Adults: 2-3 mg/kg/day calculated to nearest 20 mg or 75-200 mg/m²/day in 1-2 divided doses for 5-7 days or until remission is attained

Dosing comments in renal or hepatic impairment: Reduce dose

Monitoring Parameters CBC with differential and platelet count, liver function tests, serum uric acid

Patient Information Avoid exposure to persons with infections. Drink plenty of fluids while taking the drug. May cause diarrhea, fever and weakness. Notify physician if these become pronounced. Notify physician if fever, chills, nausea, vomiting, sore throat, unusual bleeding or bruising, yellow discoloration of the skin or eyes, swelling of the feet or legs, or abdominal, joint, or flank pain occurs. Any signs of infection, easy bruising or bleeding, shortness of breath, or painful or burning urination should be brought to physician's attention. Hair loss sometimes occur. The drug may cause permanent sterility and may cause birth defects. The drug may be excreted in breast milk, therefore, an alternative form of feeding your baby should be used.

Dosage Forms Tablet, scored: 40 mg

6-Thioguanine *see* Thioguanine *on previous page*

Thiopental Sodium *(thye oh pen' tal)*

Brand Names Pentothal® Sodium

Use Induction of anesthesia; adjunct for intubation in head injury patients; control of convulsive states; treatment of elevated intracranial pressure

Restrictions C-III

Pregnancy Risk Factor C

Contraindications Porphyria (variegate or acute intermittent); known hypersensitivity to thiopental or other barbiturates

Warnings/Precautions Use with caution in patients with asthma, unstable aneurysms, severe cardiovascular disease, hepatic or renal disease, laryngospasm or bronchospasms which can occur; hypotension; extravasation or intra-arterial injection causes necrosis due to pH of 10.6, ensure patient has intravenous access

Adverse Reactions
>10%: Local: Pain on I.M. injection
1% to 10%: Gastrointestinal: Cramping, diarrhea, rectal bleeding
<1%:
Cardiovascular: Hypotension, peripheral vascular collapse, myocardial depression, cardiac arrhythmias
Central nervous system: Radial nerve palsy, seizures, headache, emergence delirium, prolonged somnolence and recovery, anxiety
Dermatologic: Erythema, pruritus, urticaria
Gastrointestinal: Nausea, vomiting, emesis
Hematologic: Hemolytic anemia
Local: Thrombophlebitis
Neuromuscular & skeletal: Tremor, involuntary muscle movement, twitching, rigidity
Respiratory: Respiratory depression, coughing, circulatory depression, rhinitis, apnea, laryngospasm, bronchospasm, sneezing, dyspnea
Miscellaneous: Hiccups, anaphylactic reactions

Overdosage/Toxicology Symptoms of overdose include respiratory depression, hypotension, shock; hypotension should respond to I.V. fluids and placement of patient in Trendelenburg position; if necessary, pressors such as norepinephrine may be used; patient may require ventilatory support

Drug Interactions Increased toxicity with CNS depressants (especially narcotic analgesics and phenothiazines), salicylates, sulfisoxazole

Stability Reconstituted solutions remain stable for 3 days at room temperature and 7 days when refrigerated; solutions are alkaline and **incompatible** with drugs with acidic pH, such as succinylcholine, atropine sulfate, etc. I.V. form is **incompatible** when mixed with amikacin, codeine, dimenhydrinate, diphenhydramine, hydromorphone, insulin, levorphanol, meperidine, metaraminol, morphine, norepinephrine, penicillin G, prochlorperazine, succinylcholine, tetracycline, benzquinamide, chlorpromazine, glycopyrrolate

Mechanism of Action Interferes with transmission of impulses from the thalamus to the cortex of the brain resulting in an imbalance in central inhibitory and facilitatory mechanisms

Pharmacodynamics/Kinetics
Onset of action: I.V.: Anesthesia occurs in 30-60 seconds
Duration: 5-30 minutes
Distribution: V_d: 1.4 L/kg
Protein binding: 72% to 86%
Metabolism: In the liver primarily to inactive metabolites but pentobarbital is also formed
Half-life: 3-11.5 hours, decreased in children vs adults

Usual Dosage I.V.:
Induction anesthesia:
Neonates: 3-4 mg/kg
Infants: 5-8 mg/kg
Children 1-12 years: 5-6 mg/kg
Adults: 3-5 mg/kg

Maintenance anesthesia:
Children: 1 mg/kg as needed
Adults: 25-100 mg as needed

Increased intracranial pressure: Children and Adults: 1.5-5 mg/kg/dose; repeat as needed to control intracranial pressure

Seizures:
Children: 2-3 mg/kg/dose, repeat as needed
Adults: 75-250 mg/dose, repeat as needed

Rectal administration: (Patient should be NPO for no less than 3 hours prior to administration)
Suggested initial doses of thiopental rectal suspension are:
<3 months: 15 mg/kg/dose
>3 months: 25 mg/kg/dose
Note: The age of a premature infant should be adjusted to reflect the age that the infant would have been if full-term (eg, an infant, now age 4
(Continued)

Thiopental Sodium *(Continued)*

months, who was 2 months premature should be considered to be a 2-month old infant).

Doses should be rounded downward to the nearest 50 mg increment to allow for accurate measurement of the dose

Inactive or debilitated patients and patients recently medicated with other sedatives, (eg, chloral hydrate, meperidine, chlorpromazine, and promethazine), may require smaller doses than usual

If the patient is not sedated within 15-20 minutes, a single repeat dose of thiopental can be given. The single repeat doses are:
<3 months: <7.5 mg/kg/dose
>3 months: 15 mg/kg/dose
Adults weighing >90 kg should not receive >3 g as a total dose (initial plus repeat doses)
Children weighing >34 kg should not receive >1 g as a total dose (initial plus repeat doses)
Neither adults nor children should receive more than one course of thiopental rectal suspension (initial dose plus repeat dose) per 24-hour period

Dosing adjustment in renal impairment: Cl_{cr} <10 mL/minute: Administer at 75% of normal dose

Note: Accumulation may occur with chronic dosing due to lipid solubility; prolonged recovery may result from redistribution of thiopental from fat stores
Monitoring Parameters Respiratory rate, heart rate, blood pressure
Reference Range Therapeutic: Hypnotic: 1-5 µg/mL (SI: 4.1-20.7 µmol/L); Coma: 30-100 µg/mL (SI: 124-413 µmol/L); Anesthesia: 7-130 µg/mL (SI: 29-536 µmol/L); Toxic: >10 µg/mL (SI: >41 µmol/L)
Test Interactions ↑ potassium (S)
Nursing Implications Monitor vital signs every 3-5 minutes; monitor for respiratory distress; place patient in Sim's position if vomiting, to prevent from aspirating vomitus; avoid extravasation, necrosis may occur
Additional Information Sodium content of 1 g (injection) : 86.8 mg (3.8 mEq)
Dosage Forms
Injection: 250 mg, 400 mg, 500 mg, 1 g, 2.5 g, 5 g
Suspension, rectal: 400 mg/g (2 g)

Thiophosphoramide *see* Thiotepa *on page 1086*

Thioridazine *(thye oh rid' a zeen)*
Related Information
Antipsychotic Agents Comparison *on page 1255*
Brand Names Mellaril®; Mellaril-S®
Synonyms Thioridazine Hydrochloride
Use Management of manifestations of psychotic disorders; depressive neurosis; alcohol withdrawal; dementia in elderly; behavioral problems in children
Pregnancy Risk Factor C
Contraindications Severe CNS depression, hypersensitivity to thioridazine or any component; cross-sensitivity to other phenothiazines may exist
Warnings/Precautions Oral formulations may cause stomach upset; may cause thermoregulatory changes; use caution in patients with narrow-angle glaucoma, severe liver or cardiac disease; doses of 1 g/day frequently cause pigmentary retinopathy
Adverse Reactions
>10%:
Central nervous system: Pseudoparkinsonism, akathisia, dystonias, tardive dyskinesia (persistent), dizziness
Cardiovascular: Hypotension, orthostatic hypotension
Gastrointestinal: Constipation
Ocular: Pigmentary retinopathy
Respiratory: Basal congestion
Miscellaneous: Decreased sweating
1% to 10%:
Dermatologic: Increased sensitivity to sun, skin rash
Endocrine & metabolic: Changes in menstrual cycle, changes in libido, pain in breasts
Gastrointestinal: Weight gain, nausea, vomiting, stomach pain
Genitourinary: Difficulty in urination, ejaculatory disturbances
Neuromuscular & skeletal: Trembling of fingers
<1%:
Central nervous system: Neuroleptic malignant syndrome (NMS),

Dermatologic: Discoloration of skin (blue-gray)
Endocrine & metabolic: Galactorrhea
Genitourinary: Priapism
Hematologic: Agranulocytosis, leukopenia
Hepatic: Cholestatic jaundice, hepatotoxicity
Ocular: Cornea and lens changes, pigmentary retinopathy
Miscellaneous: Impairment of temperature regulation, lowering of seizures threshold

Overdosage/Toxicology Symptoms of overdose include deep sleep, coma, extrapyramidal symptoms, abnormal involuntary muscle movements, hypotension, arrhythmias

Following initiation of essential overdose management, toxic symptom treatment and supportive treatment should be initiated. Hypotension usually responds to I.V. fluids or Trendelenburg positioning. If unresponsive to these measures, the use of a parenteral inotrope may be required (eg, norepinephrine 0.1-0.2 mcg/kg/minute titrated to response); do not use epinephrine. Seizures commonly respond to diazepam (I.V. 5-10 mg bolus in adults every 15 minutes if needed up to a total of 30 mg; I.V. 0.25-0.4 mg/kg/dose up to a total of 10 mg in children) or to phenytoin or phenobarbital. Neuroleptics often cause extrapyramidal symptoms (eg, dystonic reactions) requiring management with diphenhydramine 1-2 mg/kg (adults) up to a maximum of 50 mg I.M. or I.V. slow push followed by a maintenance dose for 48-72 hours. When these reactions are unresponsive to diphenhydramine, benztropine mesylate I.V. 1-2 mg (adults) may be effective. These agents are generally effective within 2-5 minutes.

Drug Interactions
Decreased effect with anticholinergics
Decreased effect of guanethidine
Increased toxicity with CNS depressants, epinephrine (hypotension), lithium (rare), TCA (cardiotoxicity), propranolol, pindolol

Stability Protect all dosage forms from light
Mechanism of Action Blocks postsynaptic mesolimbic dopaminergic receptors in the brain; exhibits a strong alpha-adrenergic blocking effect and depresses the release of hypothalamic and hypophyseal hormones

Pharmacodynamics/Kinetics
Duration of action: 4-5 days
Half-life: 21-25 hours
Time to peak serum concentration: Within 1 hour

Usual Dosage Oral:
Children >2 years: Range: 0.5-3 mg/kg/day in 2-3 divided doses; usual: 1 mg/kg/day; maximum: 3 mg/kg/day
Behavior problems: Initial: 10 mg 2-3 times/day, increase gradually
Severe psychoses: Initial: 25 mg 2-3 times/day, increase gradually

Adults:
Psychoses: Initial: 50-100 mg 3 times/day with gradual increments as needed and tolerated; maximum: 800 mg/day in 2-4 divided doses; if >65 years, initial dose: 10 mg 3 times/day
Depressive disorders, dementia: Initial: 25 mg 3 times/day; maintenance dose: 20-200 mg/day

Not dialyzable (0% to 5%)
Administration Dilute oral concentrate with water or juice before administration
Monitoring Parameters For patients on prolonged therapy: CBC, ophthalmologic exam, blood pressure, liver function tests
Reference Range Therapeutic: 1.0-1.5 µg/mL (SI: 2.7-4.1 µmol/L); Toxic: >10 µg/mL (SI: >27 µmol/L)
Test Interactions False-positives for phenylketonuria, urinary amylase, uroporphyrins, urobilinogen
Patient Information Oral concentrate must be diluted in 2-4 oz of liquid (water, fruit juice, carbonated drinks, milk, or pudding); do not take antacid within 1 hour of taking drug; avoid excess sun exposure; may cause drowsiness, restlessness, avoid alcohol and other CNS depressants; do not alter dosage or discontinue without consulting physician; yearly eye exams are necessary; might discolor urine (pink or reddish brown)
Nursing Implications Avoid skin contact with oral suspension or solution; may cause contact dermatitis
Additional Information
Thioridazine: Mellaril-S® oral suspension
Thioridazine hydrochloride: Mellaril® oral solution and tablet
Dosage Forms
Concentrate, oral: 30 mg/mL (120 mL); 100 mg/mL (3.4 mL, 120 mL)
Suspension, oral: 25 mg/5 mL (480 mL); 100 mg/5 mL (480 mL)
Tablet: 10 mg, 15 mg, 25 mg, 50 mg, 100 mg, 150 mg, 200 mg

Thioridazine Hydrochloride *see* Thioridazine *on page 1084*

Thiotepa (thye oh tep' a)
Related Information
Cancer Chemotherapy Regimens *on page 1218-1241*
Synonyms TESPA; Thiophosphoramide; Triethylenethiophosphoramide; TSPA
Use Treatment of superficial tumors of the bladder; palliative treatment of adenocarcinoma of breast or ovary; lymphomas and sarcomas; controlling intracavitary effusions caused by metastatic tumors
I.T. use: CNS leukemia/lymphoma
Pregnancy Risk Factor D
Contraindications Hypersensitivity to thiotepa or any component; severe myelosuppression with leukocyte count <3000/mm^3 or platelet count <150,000/mm^3
Warnings/Precautions The U.S. Food and Drug Administration (FDA) currently recommends that procedures for proper handling and disposal of antineoplastic agents be considered. The drug is potentially mutagenic, carcinogenic, and teratogenic. Reduce dosage in patients with hepatic, renal, or bone marrow damage.
Adverse Reactions
>10%:
   Hematopoietic: Dose-limiting toxicity which is dose-related and cumulative; moderate to severe leukopenia and severe thrombocytopenia have occurred. Anemia and pancytopenia may become fatal, so careful hematologic monitoring is required; intravesical administration may cause bone marrow suppression as well.
   Local: Pain at injection site
   Myelosuppressive:
      WBC: Moderate
      Platelets: Severe
      Onset (days): 7-10
      Nadir (days): 14
      Recovery (days): 28
1% to 10%:
   Central nervous system: Dizziness, fever, headache
   Dermatologic: Alopecia, rash, pruritus
   Gastrointestinal: Anorexia, nausea and vomiting rarely occur
   Emetic potential: Low (<10%)
   Renal: Hyperuricemia, hematuria, hemorrhagic cystitis
   Miscellaneous: Tightness of the throat, allergic reactions
<1%:
   Carcinogenesis: Like other alkylating agents, this drug is carcinogenic
   Gastrointestinal: Stomatitis
   Miscellaneous: Anaphylaxis
Overdosage/Toxicology Symptoms of overdose include nausea, vomiting, precipitation of uric acid in kidney tubules, bone marrow suppression; therapy is supportive only
Drug Interactions
Increased toxicity:
   Other alkylating agents or irradiation concomitantly with thiotepa intensifies toxicity rather than enhancing therapeutic response
   Prolonged muscular paralysis and respiratory depression may occur when neuromuscular blocking agents are administered
   Succinylcholine and other neuromuscular blocking agents' action can be prolonged due to thiotepa inhibiting plasma pseudocholinesterase
Stability Refrigerate, protect from light; **compatible** with D$_5$W, 0.9% sodium chloride, D$_5$NS, or lactated Ringer's
Mechanism of Action Alkylating agent that reacts with DNA phosphate groups to produce cross-linking of DNA strands leading to inhibition of DNA, RNA, and protein synthesis; mechanism of action has not been explored as thoroughly as the other alkylating agents, it is presumed that the azridine rings open and react as nitrogen mustard; reactivity is enhanced at a lower pH
Pharmacodynamics/Kinetics
Absorption: Following intracavitary instillation, the drug is unreliably absorbed (10% to 100%) through the bladder mucosa; variable I.M. absorption
Metabolism: Extensively in the liver
Half-life, terminal: 109 minutes with dose-dependent clearance
Elimination: As metabolites and unchanged drug in urine
Usual Dosage Dosing must be based on the clinical and hematologic response of the patient (refer to individual protocols)

Children: Sarcomas: I.V.: 25-65 mg/m^2 as a single dose every 21 days
Adults:
   I.M., I.V., S.C.: 30-60 mg/m^2 once per week

I.V. doses of 0.3-0.4 mg/kg by rapid I.V. administration every 1-4 weeks, or 0.2 mg/kg or 6-8 mg/m^2/day for 4-5 days every 2-4 weeks

High-dose therapy for bone marrow transplant:

    I.M. doses of 15-30 mg in various schedules have been given

    I.V.: 500 mg/m^2 up to 900 mg/m^2

Dosing comments/adjustment in renal impairment: Use with extreme caution, reduced dose is probably warranted

Intracavitary: 0.6-0.8 mg/kg

Intrapericardial dose: Usually 15-30 mg

Intrathecal: Doses of 1-10 mg/m^2 administered 1-2 times/week in concentrations of 1 mg/mL diluted with preservative-free sterile water for injection. Dilutions of 1-5 mg/mL in lactated Ringer's have also been administered.

Intravesical: Used for treatment of carcinoma of the bladder; patients should be dehydrated for 8-12 hours prior to treatment; instill 60 mg (in 30-60 mL of sterile water) into the bladder and retain for a minimum of 2 hours. Patient should be positioned every 15 minutes for maximal area exposure. Instillations usually once a week for 4 weeks. Monitor for bone marrow suppression.

Intratumor: Use a 22-gauge needle to inject thiotepa directly into the tumor. Initial dose: 0.6-0.8 mg/kg (diluted to 10 mg/mL) are used every 1-4 weeks; maintenance dose: 0.07-0.8 mg/kg are administered at 1- to 4-week intervals

Ophthalmic: 0.05% solution in LR has been instilled into the eye every 3 hours for 6-8 weeks for the prevention of pterygium recurrence

Administration Can be administered slow IVP over 5 minutes at a concentration not to exceed 10 mg/mL or I.V. infusion at a final concentration for administration of 1 mg/mL

Monitoring Parameters CBC with differential and platelet count, uric acid, urinalysis

Patient Information Any signs of infection, easy bruising or bleeding, shortness of breath, or painful or burning urination should be brought to physician's attention. Nausea, vomiting, or hair loss sometimes occur. The drug may cause permanent sterility and may cause birth defects. The drug may be excreted in breast milk, therefore, an alternative form of feeding your baby should be used.

Nursing Implications A 1 mg/mL solution is considered isotonic; not a vesicant

Dosage Forms Powder for injection: 15 mg

Thiothixene (thye oh thix' een)

Related Information

Antipsychotic Agents Comparison *on page 1255*

Brand Names Navane®

Synonyms Tiotixene

Use Management of psychotic disorders

Pregnancy Risk Factor C

Contraindications Hypersensitivity to thiothixene or any component; cross-sensitivity with other phenothiazines may exist, lactation

Warnings/Precautions Watch for hypotension when administering I.M. or I.V.; safety in children <6 months of age has not been established; use with caution in patients with narrow-angle glaucoma, bone marrow depression, severe liver or cardiac disease, seizures

Adverse Reactions

>10%:

    Cardiovascular: Hypotension, orthostatic hypotension

    Central nervous system: Pseudoparkinsonism, akathisia, dystonias, tardive dyskinesia (persistent), dizziness

    Gastrointestinal: Constipation

    Ocular: Pigmentary retinopathy

    Respiratory: Nasal congestion

    Miscellaneous: Decreased sweating

1% to 10%:

    Dermatologic: Increased sensitivity to sun, skin rash

    Endocrine & metabolic: Changes in menstrual cycle, changes in libido, pain in breasts

    Gastrointestinal: Weight gain, nausea, vomiting, stomach pain

    Genitourinary: Difficulty in urination, ejaculatory disturbances

    Neuromuscular & skeletal: Trembling of fingers

<1%:

    Central nervous system: Neuroleptic malignant syndrome (NMS)

    Endocrine & metabolic: Galactorrhea

    Dermatologic: Discoloration of skin (blue-gray)

    Genitourinary: Priapism

    Hematologic: Agranulocytosis, leukopenia

(Continued)

Thiothixene *(Continued)*

Hepatic: Cholestatic jaundice, hepatotoxicity
Ocular: Cornea and lens changes, pigmentary retinopathy
Miscellaneous: Impairment of temperature regulation, lowering of seizures threshold

Overdosage/Toxicology Symptoms of overdose include muscle twitching, drowsiness, dizziness, rigidity, tremor, hypotension, cardiac arrhythmias

Following initiation of essential overdose management, toxic symptom treatment and supportive treatment should be initiated. Hypotension usually responds to I.V. fluids or Trendelenburg positioning. If unresponsive to these measures, the use of a parenteral inotrope may be required (eg, norepinephrine 0.1-0.2 mcg/kg/minute titrated to response). Seizures commonly respond to diazepam (I.V. 5-10 mg bolus in adults every 15 minutes if needed up to a total of 30 mg; I.V. 0.25-0.4 mg/kg/dose up to a total of 10 mg in children) or to phenytoin or phenobarbital. Neuroleptics often cause extrapyramidal symptoms (eg, dystonic reactions) requiring management with diphenhydramine 1-2 mg/kg (adults) up to a maximum of 50 mg I.M. or I.V. slow push followed by a maintenance dose for 48-72 hours. When these reactions are unresponsive to diphenhydramine, benztropine mesylate I.V. 1-2 mg (adults) may be effective. These agents are generally effective within 2-5 minutes.

Drug Interactions
Decreased effect of guanethidine
Increased toxicity with CNS depressants, anticholinergics, alcohol

Stability Refrigerate

Mechanism of Action Elicits antipsychotic activity by postsynaptic blockade of CNS dopamine receptors resulting in inhibition of dopamine-mediated effects; also has alpha-adrenergic blocking activity

Pharmacodynamics/Kinetics
Metabolism: Extensive in the liver
Half-life: >24 hours with chronic use

Usual Dosage
Children <12 years: Oral: 0.25 mg/kg/24 hours in divided doses (dose not well established)

Children >12 years and Adults: Mild to moderate psychosis:
Oral: 2 mg 3 times/day, up to 20-30 mg/day; more severe psychosis: Initial: 5 mg 2 times/day, may increase gradually, if necessary; maximum: 60 mg/day
I.M.: 4 mg 2-4 times/day, increase dose gradually; usual: 16-20 mg/day; maximum: 30 mg/day; change to oral dose as soon as able

Not dialyzable (0% to 5%)

Monitoring Parameters Liver function tests; for patients on prolonged therapy: CBC, ophthalmologic exam

Test Interactions ↑ cholesterol (S), ↑ glucose; ↓ uric acid (S); may cause false-positive pregnancy test

Patient Information May cause drowsiness, restlessness, avoid alcohol and other CNS depressants; do not alter dosage or discontinue without consulting physician

Nursing Implications Observe for extrapyramidal effects; concentrate should be mixed in juice before administration

Dosage Forms
Capsule: 1 mg, 2 mg, 5 mg, 10 mg, 20 mg
Concentrate, oral, as hydrochloride: 5 mg/mL (30 mL, 120 mL)
Injection, as hydrochloride: 2 mg/mL (2 mL)
Powder for injection, as hydrochloride: 5 mg/mL (2 mL)

Thorazine® *see* Chlorpromazine Hydrochloride *on page 230*

Thrombate III™ *see* Antithrombin III *on page 83*

Thypinone® *see* Protirelin *on page 952*

Thyrar® *see* Thyroid *on this page*

Thyro-Block® *see* Potassium Iodide *on page 909*

Thyroid *(thye′ roid)*

Brand Names Armour® Thyroid; S-P-T; Thyrar®; Thyroid Strong®
Synonyms Desiccated Thyroid; Thyroid Extract
Use Replacement or supplemental therapy in hypothyroidism; pituitary TSH suppressants (thyroid nodules, thyroiditis, multinodular goiter, thyroid cancer), thyrotoxicosis, diagnostic suppression tests
Pregnancy Risk Factor A

Contraindications Recent myocardial infarction or thyrotoxicosis uncomplicated by hypothyroidism uncorrected adrenal insufficiency, hypersensitivity to beef or pork or any constituent

Warnings/Precautions Ineffective for weight reduction; high doses may produce serious or even life-threatening toxic effects particularly when used with some anorectic drugs; use cautiously in patients with pre-existing cardiovascular disease (angina, CHD), elderly since they may be more likely to have compromised cardiovascular function. Chronic hypothyroidism predisposes patients to coronary artery disease. Desiccated thyroid contains variable amounts of T_3, T_4, and other tri-iodothyronine compounds which are more likely to cause cardiac signs and symptoms due to fluctuating levels; should avoid use in elderly for this reason; drug of choice is levothyroxine in the minds of many clinicians.

Adverse Reactions

<1%:

Cardiovascular: Palpitations, tachycardia, cardiac arrhythmias, chest pain

Central nervous system: Nervousness, headache, insomnia, fever, clumsiness

Dermatologic: Hair loss

Endocrine & metabolic: Changes in menstrual cycle, shortness of breath

Gastrointestinal: Weight loss, increased appetite, diarrhea, abdominal cramps, vomiting, constipation

Neuromuscular & skeletal: Excessive bone loss with overtreatment (excess thyroid replacement), tremor, hand tremors, muscle aches

Miscellaneous: Heat intolerance, sweating

Overdosage/Toxicology

Chronic excessive use results in signs and symptoms of hyperthyroidism, weight loss, nervousness, sweating, tachycardia, insomnia, heat intolerance, palpitations, vomiting, psychosis, fever, seizures, angina, arrhythmias, and CHF in those predisposed

Reduce dose or temporarily discontinue therapy; normal hypothalamic-pituitary-thyroid axis will return to normal in 6-8 weeks; serum T_4 levels do not correlate well with toxicity

In massive acute ingestion, reduce GI absorption, give general supportive care; treat CHF with digitalis glycosides; excessive adrenergic activity (tachycardia) require propranolol 1-3 mg I.V. over 10 minutes or 80-160 mg orally/day; fever may be treated with acetaminophen

Drug Interactions

Decreased effect:

Thyroid hormones increase the therapeutic need for oral hypoglycemics or insulin

Cholestyramine can bind thyroid and reduce its absorption

Increased toxicity: Thyroid may potentiate the hypoprothrombinemic effect of oral anticoagulants

Mechanism of Action The primary active compound is T_3 (tri-iodothyronine), which may be converted from T_4 (thyroxine) and then circulates throughout the body to influence growth and maturation of various tissues; exact mechanism of action is unknown; however, it is believed the thyroid hormone exerts its many metabolic effects through control of DNA transcription and protein synthesis; involved in normal metabolism, growth, and development; promotes gluconeogenesis, increases utilization and mobilization of glycogen stores and stimulates protein synthesis, increases basal metabolic rate

Pharmacodynamics/Kinetics

Absorption: T_4 is 48% to 79% absorbed; T_3 is 95% absorbed; desiccated thyroid contains thyroxine, liothyronine, and iodine (primarily bound); following absorption thyroxine is largely converted to liothyronine

Protein binding: 99% (bound to albumin, thyroxine-binding globulin, and thyroxin-binding prealbumin)

Metabolism: Liothyronine is metabolized in the liver, kidneys, and other tissues to inactive compounds

Recommended Pediatric Dosage for Congenital Hypothyroidism

Age	Daily Dose (mg)	Daily Dose/kg (mg)
0-6 mo	15-30	4.8-6
6-12 mo	30-45	3.6-4.8
1-5 y	45-60	3-3.6
6-12 y	60-90	2.4-3
>12 y	>90	1.2-1.8

(Continued)

Thyroid *(Continued)*

Half-life:
Liothyronine: 1-2 days
Thyroxine: 6-7 days
Elimination: In urine as conjugated forms

Usual Dosage Oral:

Children: See table.

Adults: Initial: 15-30 mg; increase with 15 mg increments every 2-4 weeks; use 15 mg in patients with cardiovascular disease or myxedema. Maintenance dose: Usually 60-120 mg/day; monitor TSH and clinical symptoms.

Thyroid cancer: Requires larger amounts than replacement therapy

Monitoring Parameters T_4, TSH, heart rate, blood pressure, clinical signs of hypo- and hyperthyroidism; TSH is the most reliable guide for evaluating adequacy of thyroid replacement dosage. TSH may be elevated during the first few months of thyroid replacement despite patients being clinically euthyroid. In cases where T_4 remains low and TSH is within normal limits, an evaluation of "free" (unbound) T_4 is needed to evaluate further increase in dosage.

Reference Range

TSH 0.4-10 (for those ≥80 years) million IU/L

T_4: 4-12 μg/dL (51-154 mmol:/L)

T_3 (RIA) (total T_3): 80-230 ng/dL (1.2-3.5 mmol/L)

T_4 free (free T_4): 0.7-1.8 ng/dL (9-23 pmol/L)

Test Interactions Many drugs may have effects on thyroid function tests; para-aminosalicylic acid, aminoglutethimide, amiodarone, barbiturates, carbamazepine, chloral hydrate, clofibrate, colestipol, corticosteroids, danazol, diazepam, estrogens, ethionamide, fluorouracil, I.V. heparin, insulin, lithium, methadone, methimazole, mitotane, nitroprusside, oxyphenbutazone, phenylbutazone, PTU, perphenazine, phenytoin, propranolol, salicylates, sulfonylureas, and thiazides

Patient Information Do not change brands, dose, or discontinue without physician's knowledge; report immediately to physician any chest pain, increased pulse, palpitations, heat intolerances, excessive sweating; replacement therapy will be for life; take as a single daily dose

Nursing Implications Monitor pulse rate and blood pressure

Additional Information

Equivalent levothyroxine dose: Thyroid USP 60 mg = levothyroxine 0.05-0.06 mg; liothyronine 15-37.5 mcg; liotrix 60 mg

Thyroid Strong® is 50% stronger than thyroid U.S.P.: each grain is equivalent to 1.5 grains of thyroid U.S.P.

Thyrar®: Bovine thyroid

S-P-T®: Pork thyroid suspended in soybean oil

Dosage Forms

Capsule, Thyroid U.S.P: 60 mg, 120 mg, 180 mg, 300 mg

Tablet, Thyroid U.S.P.: 15 mg, 30 mg, 60 mg, 90 mg, 120 mg, 180 mg, 240 mg, 300 mg

Tablet, Thyroid Strong®: 30 mg, 60 mg, 120 mg, 180 mg

Thyroid Extract *see Thyroid on page 1088*

Thyroid Stimulating Hormone *see Thyrotropin on this page*

Thyroid Strong® *see Thyroid on page 1088*

Thyrolar® *see Liotrix on page 639*

Thyrotropic Hormone *see Thyrotropin on this page*

Thyrotropin *(thye roe troe' pin)*

Brand Names Thytropar®

Synonyms Thyroid Stimulating Hormone; Thyrotropic Hormone; TSH

Use Diagnostic aid to differentiate thyroid failure; diagnosis of decreased thyroid reserve, to differentiate between primary and secondary hypothyroidism and between primary hypothyroidism and euthyroidism in patients receiving thyroid replacement

Pregnancy Risk Factor C

Contraindications Coronary thrombosis, untreated Addison's disease, hypersensitivity to thyrotropin or any component

Warnings/Precautions Use with caution in patients with angina pectoris or cardiac failure, patients with hypopituitarism, adrenal cortical suppression as may be seen with corticosteroid therapy; may cause thyroid hyperplasia

Adverse Reactions

<1%:

Cardiovascular: Tachycardia

Central nervous system: Fever, headache

Endocrine & metabolic: Menstrual irregularities

Gastrointestinal: Nausea, vomiting, increased bowel motility
Sensitivity reactions: Anaphylaxis with repeated administration

Overdosage/Toxicology Symptoms of overdose include weight loss, nervousness, sweating, tachycardia, insomnia, heat intolerance, menstrual irregularities, headache, angina pectoris, CHF; acute massive overdose may require cardiac glycosides for CHF; fever should be controlled with the help of acetaminophen; antiadrenergic agents, particularly propranolol 1-3 mg I.V. every 6 hours or 80-160 mg/day, can be used to treat increased sympathetic activity

Stability Refrigerate at 2°C to 8°C (36°F to 46°F) after reconstitution; use within 2 weeks

Mechanism of Action Stimulates formation and secretion of thyroid hormone, increases uptake of iodine by thyroid gland

Pharmacodynamics/Kinetics
Half-life: 35 minutes, dependent upon thyroid state
Elimination: Rapidly by the kidney in the urine

Usual Dosage Adults: I.M., S.C.: 10 units/day for 1-3 days; follow by a radioiodine study 24 hours past last injection, no response in thyroid failure, substantial response in pituitary failure

Dosage Forms Injection: 10 units

Thyrotropin Releasing Hormone see Protirelin on page 952

Thytropar® see Thyrotropin on previous page

Tiabendazole see Thiabendazole on page 1078

Ticar® see Ticarcillin Disodium on next page

Ticarcillin and Clavulanic Acid (tye kar sill' in & klav yoo lan' ick as' id)

Related Information
Antimicrobial Drugs of Choice on page 1298-1302

Brand Names Timentin®

Synonyms Ticarcillin Disodium and Clavulanate Potassium

Use Treatment of infections of lower respiratory tract, urinary tract, skin and skin structures, bone and joint, and septicemia caused by susceptible organisms. Clavulanate expands activity of ticarcillin to include beta-lactamase producing strains of S. aureus, H. influenzae, Enterobacteriaceae, Klebsiella, Citrobacter, and Serratia

Pregnancy Risk Factor B

Contraindications Known hypersensitivity to ticarcillin, clavulanate, or any penicillin

Warnings/Precautions Not approved for use in children <12 years of age; use with caution and modify dosage in patients with renal impairment; serious and occasionally fatal hypersensitivity (anaphylactoid) reactions have been reported in patients on penicillin therapy. These reactions are more likely to occur in individuals with a history of cephalosporin hypersensitivity and/or a history of sensitivity to multiple allergens. There have been reports of individuals with a history of cephalosporin hypersensitivity who have experienced severe reactions when treated with penicillins.

Adverse Reactions
<1%:
Central nervous system: Convulsions, confusion, drowsiness, fever, Jarisch-Herxheimer reaction
Dermatologic: Rash
Endocrine & metabolic: Electrolyte imbalance
Hematologic: Hemolytic anemia, positive Coombs' reaction
Local: Thrombophlebitis
Neuromuscular & skeletal: Myoclonus
Renal: Acute interstitial nephritis
Miscellaneous: Hypersensitivity reactions, anaphylaxis

Overdosage/Toxicology Symptoms of overdose include neuromuscular hypersensitivity and seizures; hemodialysis may be helpful to aid in the removal of the drug from the blood, otherwise most treatment is supportive or symptom directed

Drug Interactions
Decreased effect: Tetracyclines → ↓ penicillin effectiveness; aminoglycosides → physical inactivation of aminoglycosides in the presence of high concentrations of ticarcillin and potential toxicity in patients with mild-moderate renal dysfunction
Increased effect:
Probenecid → ↑ penicillin levels
Neuromuscular blockers → ↑ duration of blockade
Aminoglycosides → synergistic efficacy
(Continued)

Ticarcillin and Clavulanic Acid *(Continued)*

Stability Reconstituted solution is stable for 6 hours at room temperature and 72 hours when refrigerated; for I.V. infusion in NS is stable for 24 hours at room temperature, 7 days when refrigerated, or 30 days when frozen; darkening of drug indicates loss of potency of clavulanate potassium; **incompatible** with sodium bicarbonate, aminoglycosides

Mechanism of Action Ticarcillin interferes with bacterial cell wall synthesis during active multiplication, causing cell wall death and resultant bactericidal activity against susceptible bacteria; clavulanic acid prevents degradation of ticarcillin by binding to the active site on beta-lactamase

Pharmacodynamics/Kinetics

Distribution: Low concentrations of ticarcillin distribute into the CSF and increase when meninges are inflamed

Protein binding:
Ticarcillin: 45% to 65%
Clavulanic acid: 9% to 30% removed by hemodialysis

Metabolism: Clavulanic acid is metabolized in the liver

Half-life:
Clavulanate: 66-90 minutes
Ticarcillin: 66-72 minutes in patients with normal renal function; clavulanic acid does not affect the clearance of ticarcillin

Elimination: 45% excreted unchanged in urine, whereas 60% to 90% of ticarcillin excreted unchanged in urine

Usual Dosage I.V.:

Children: 200-300 mg of ticarcillin component/kg/day in divided doses every 4-6 hours

Adults: 3.1 g (ticarcillin 3 g plus clavulanic acid 0.1 g) every 4-6 hours; maximum: 18-24 g/day

Urinary tract infections: 3.1 g every 6-8 hours

Dosing interval in renal impairment:
Cl_{cr} 10-30 mL/minute: Administer every 8 hours
Cl_{cr} <10 mL/minute: Administer every 12 hours

Dosing interval in hepatic impairment: Cl_{cr} <10 mL/hour: Administer every 24 hours

Administration Infuse over 30 minutes; administer 1 hour apart from aminoglycosides; give around-the-clock

Test Interactions Positive Coombs' test, false-positive urinary proteins

Nursing Implications Draw sample for culture and sensitivity prior to first dose if possible

Additional Information
Sodium content of 1 g: 4.75 mEq
Potassium content of 1 g: 0.15 mEq

Dosage Forms
Infusion, premixed (frozen): Ticarcillin disodium 3 g and clavulanic acid 0.1 g (100 mL)
Powder for injection: Ticarcillin disodium 3 g and clavulanic acid 0.1 g (3.1 g, 31 g)

Ticarcillin Disodium *(tye kar sill' in)*

Related Information

Antimicrobial Drugs of Choice *on page 1298-1302*

Brand Names Ticar®

Use Treatment of susceptible infections such as septicemia, acute and chronic respiratory tract infections, skin and soft tissue infections, and urinary tract infections due to susceptible strains of *Pseudomonas*, *Proteus*, and *Escherichia coli* and *Enterobacter*, normally used with other antibiotics (ie, aminoglycosides)

Pregnancy Risk Factor B

Contraindications Hypersensitivity to ticarcillin or any component or penicillins

Warnings/Precautions Due to sodium load and adverse effects (anemia, neuropsychological changes), use with caution and modify dosage in patients with renal impairment; serious and occasionally severe or fatal hypersensitivity (anaphylactoid) reactions have been reported in patients on penicillin therapy (especially with a history of beta-lactam hypersensitivity and/or a history of sensitivity to multiple allergens); use with caution in patients with seizures

Adverse Reactions
<1%:
Central nervous system: Convulsions, confusion, drowsiness, fever, Jarisch-Herxheimer reaction
Dermatologic: Rash
Endocrine & metabolic: Electrolyte imbalance

Hematologic: Hemolytic anemia, positive Coombs' reaction
Local: Thrombophlebitis
Neuromuscular & skeletal: Myoclonus
Renal: Acute interstitial nephritis
Miscellaneous: Hypersensitivity reactions, anaphylaxis

Overdosage/Toxicology Symptoms of penicillin overdose include neuromuscular hypersensitivity (agitation, hallucinations, asterixis, encephalopathy, confusion, and seizures) and electrolyte imbalance with potassium or sodium salts, especially in renal failure; hemodialysis may be helpful to aid in the removal of the drug from the blood, otherwise most treatment is supportive or symptom directed

Drug Interactions

Decreased effect: Tetracyclines → ↓ penicillin effectiveness; aminoglycosides → physical inactivation of aminoglycosides in the presence of high concentrations of ticarcillin and potential toxicity in patients with mild-moderate renal dysfunction

Increased effect:
Probenecid → ↑ penicillin levels
Neuromuscular blockers → ↑ duration of blockade
Aminoglycosides → synergistic efficacy

Stability Reconstituted solution is stable for 72 hours at room temperature and 14 days when refrigerated or 30 days when frozen; for I.V. infusion in NS or D_5W; **incompatible** with aminoglycosides

Mechanism of Action Interferes with bacterial cell wall synthesis during active multiplication, causing cell wall death and resultant bactericidal activity against susceptible bacteria

Pharmacodynamics/Kinetics

Absorption: I.M.: 86%

Distribution: V_d: Neonates: 0.42-0.76 L/kg; distributed into milk at low concentrations; attains high concentrations in bile; minimal concentrations attained in CSF with uninflamed meninges

Protein binding: 45% to 65%

Half-life, adults: 1-1.3 hours, prolonged with renal impairment and/or hepatic impairment
Neonates:
    <1 week: 3.5-5.6 hours
    1-8 weeks: 1.3-2.2 hours
Children 5-13 years: 0.9 hours

Peak serum levels: I.M.: Within 30-75 minutes

Elimination: Almost entirely in urine as unchanged drug and its metabolites with small amounts excreted in feces (3.5%)

Usual Dosage Ticarcillin is generally given I.M. only for the treatment of uncomplicated urinary tract infections

Neonates: I.V.:
Postnatal age ≤7 days:
    ≤2000 g: 150 mg/kg/day in divided doses every 12 hours
    >2000 g: 225 mg/kg/day in divided doses every 8 hours
Postnatal age >7 days:
    <1200 g: 150 mg/kg/day in divided doses every 12 hours
    1200-2000 g: 225 mg/kg/day in divided doses every 8 hours
    >2000 g: 300 mg/kg/day in divided doses every 6 hours
Infants and Children: I.V.: Serious Infections: 200-300 mg/kg/day in divided doses every 4-6 hours; doses as high as 400 mg/kg/day divided every 4 hours have been used in acute pulmonary exacerbations of cystic fibrosis
Maximum dose: 24 g/day
Urinary tract infections: I.M., I.V.: 50-100 mg/kg/day in divided doses every 6-8 hours
Adults: I.V.: 1-4 g every 4-6 hours

Dosing interval in renal impairment:
Cl_{cr} 10-30 mL/minute: Administer every 8 hours
Cl_{cr} <10 mL/minute: Administer every 12 hours

Administration Administer around-the-clock; administer 1 hour apart from aminoglycosides

Monitoring Parameters Serum electrolytes, bleeding time, and periodic tests of renal, hepatic, and hematologic function

Test Interactions False-positive urinary or serum protein, positive Coombs' test

Nursing Implications Draw sample for culture and sensitivity before administering first dose, if possible

Additional Information Sodium content of 1 g: 5.2-6.5 mEq

Dosage Forms Powder for injection: 1 g, 3 g, 6 g, 20 g, 30 g

Ticarcillin Disodium and Clavulanate Potassium *see* Ticarcillin and Clavulanic Acid *on page 1091*

TICE® BCG *see* Bacillus Calmette-Guérin *on page 110*

Ticlid® *see* Ticlopidine Hydrochloride *on this page*

Ticlopidine Hydrochloride (tye kloe' pi deen)
Brand Names Ticlid®

Use Platelet aggregation inhibitor that reduces the risk of thrombotic stroke in patients who have had a stroke or stroke precursors

   Unlabeled use: Protection of aortocoronary bypass grafts, diabetic microangiopathy, ischemic heart disease, prevention of postoperative DVT, reduction of graft loss following renal transplant

Pregnancy Risk Factor B

Contraindications Hypersensitivity to ticlopidine; active bleeding disorders; neutropenia or thrombocytopenia; severe liver impairment

Warnings/Precautions Patients predisposed to bleeding such as those with gastric or duodenal ulcers; patients with underlying hematologic disorders; patients receiving oral anticoagulant therapy or nonsteroidal anti-inflammatory agents (including aspirin); liver disease; patients undergoing lumbar puncture or surgical procedure. Ticlopidine should be discontinued if the absolute neutrophil count falls to <1200/mm^3 or if the platelet count falls to <80,000/mm^3. If possible, ticlopidine should be discontinued 10-14 days prior to surgery. Use caution when phenytoin or propranolol is used concurrently.

Adverse Reactions
   1% to 10%: Dermatologic: Skin rash
   <1%:
      Central nervous system: Epistaxis
      Dermatologic: Ecchymosis
      Gastrointestinal: Diarrhea, nausea, vomiting, GI pain
      Hematologic: Neutropenia, thrombocytopenia
      Hepatic: Increased liver function tests
      Otic: Tinnitus
      Renal: Hematuria

Overdosage/Toxicology Symptoms of overdose include ataxia, seizures, vomiting, abdominal pain, hematologic abnormalities; specific treatments are lacking; after decontamination, treatment is symptomatic and supportive

Drug Interactions
   Decreased effect with antacids (↓ absorption), corticosteroids; decreased effect of digoxin, cyclosporine
   Increased effect/toxicity of aspirin, anticoagulants, antipyrine, theophylline, cimetidine (↑ levels), NSAIDs

Mechanism of Action Ticlopidine is an inhibitor of platelet function with a mechanism which is different from other antiplatelet drugs. The drug significantly increases bleeding time. This effect may not be solely related to ticlopidine's effect on platelets. The prolongation of the bleeding time caused by ticlopidine is further increased by the addition of aspirin in *ex vivo* experiments. Although many metabolites of ticlopidine have been found, none have been shown to account for *in vivo* activity.

Pharmacodynamics/Kinetics
   Onset of action: Within 6 hours
   Peak: Achieved after 3-5 days of oral therapy; serum levels do not correlate with clinical antiplatelet activity
   Metabolism: Extensively in the liver and has at least one active metabolite
   Half-life, elimination: 24 hours

Usual Dosage Adults: Oral: 1 tablet twice daily with food

Monitoring Parameters Bleeding times, CBC and platelet count

Test Interactions ↑ cholesterol (S), ↑ alkaline phosphatase, ↑ transaminases (S)

Dosage Forms Tablet: 250 mg

Ticon® *see* Trimethobenzamide Hydrochloride *on page 1126*

TIG *see* Tetanus Immune Globulin, Human *on page 1065*

Tigan® *see* Trimethobenzamide Hydrochloride *on page 1126*

Tiject® *see* Trimethobenzamide Hydrochloride *on page 1126*

Timentin® *see* Ticarcillin and Clavulanic Acid *on page 1091*

Timolol Maleate (tye' moe lole)
Related Information
   Beta-Blockers Comparison *on page 1257-1259*

Glaucoma Drug Therapy Comparison *on page 1270*

Brand Names Blocadren®; Timoptic®

Use Ophthalmic dosage form used to treat elevated intraocular pressure such as glaucoma or ocular hypertension; orally for treatment of hypertension and angina and reduce mortality following myocardial infarction and prophylaxis of migraine

Pregnancy Risk Factor C

Contraindications Uncompensated congestive heart failure, cardiogenic shock, bradycardia or heart block, severe chronic obstructive pulmonary disease, asthma, hypersensitivity to beta-blockers

Warnings/Precautions Some products contain sulfites which can cause allergic reactions; tachyphylaxis may develop; use with a miotic in angle-closure glaucoma; use with caution in patients with decreased renal or hepatic function (dosage adjustment required); severe CNS, cardiovascular and respiratory adverse effects have been seen following ophthalmic use; patients with a history of asthma, congestive heart failure, or bradycardia appear to be at a higher risk

Adverse Reactions
Ophthalmic:
1% to 10%:
Dermatologic: Alopecia
Ocular: Burning, stinging of eyes
<1%:
Dermatologic: Skin rash
Ocular: Blepharitis, conjunctivitis, keratitis, vision disturbances
Oral:
>10%: Endocrine & metabolic: Decreased sexual ability
1% to 10%:
Cardiovascular: Bradycardia, breathing difficulty, irregular heartbeat, reduced peripheral circulation
Central nervous system: Dizziness, itching, tiredness, weakness
<1%:
Cardiovascular: Chest pain, congestive heart failure
Central nervous system: Hallucinations, mental depression, anxiety, nightmares
Dermatologic: Skin rash
Gastrointestinal: Diarrhea, nausea, vomiting, stomach discomfort
Neuromuscular & skeletal: Numbness in toes and fingers
Ocular: Dry sore eyes

Overdosage/Toxicology Symptoms of intoxication include cardiac disturbances, CNS toxicity, bronchospasm, hypoglycemia and hyperkalemia. The most common cardiac symptoms include hypotension and bradycardia; atrioventricular block, intraventricular conduction disturbances, cardiogenic shock, and systole may occur with severe overdose, especially with membrane-depressant drugs (eg, propranolol); CNS effects include convulsions, coma, and respiratory arrest is commonly seen with propranolol and other membrane-depressant and lipid-soluble drugs.

Treatment includes symptomatic treatment of seizures, hypotension, hyperkalemia and hypoglycemia; bradycardia and hypotension resistant to atropine, isoproterenol or pacing may respond to glucagon; wide QRS defects caused by the membrane-depressant poisoning may respond to hypertonic sodium bicarbonate; repeat-dose charcoal, hemoperfusion, or hemodialysis may be helpful in removal of only those beta-blockers with a small V_d, long half-life or low intrinsic clearance (acebutolol, atenolol, nadolol, sotalol).

Drug Interactions
Decreased effect of beta-blockers with aluminum salts, barbiturates, calcium salts, cholestyramine, colestipol, NSAIDs, penicillins (ampicillin), rifampin, salicylates and sulfinpyrazone due to decreased bioavailability and plasma levels
Beta-blockers may decrease the effect of sulfonylureas
Increased effect/toxicity of beta-blockers with calcium blockers (diltiazem, felodipine, nicardipine), contraceptives, flecainide, haloperidol (propranolol, hypotensive effects), H_2 antagonists (metoprolol, propranolol only by cimetidine, possibly ranitidine), hydralazine (metoprolol, propranolol), loop diuretics (propranolol, not atenolol), MAO inhibitors (metoprolol, nadolol, bradycardia), phenothiazines (propranolol), propafenone (metoprolol, propranolol), quinidine (in extensive metabolizers), ciprofloxacin, thyroid hormones (metoprolol, propranolol, when hypothyroid patient is converted to euthyroid state)
Beta-blockers may increase the effect/toxicity of flecainide, haloperidol (hypotensive effects), hydralazine, phenothiazines, acetaminophen, anticoagulants (propranolol, warfarin), benzodiazepines (not atenolol), clonidine (hypertensive crisis after or during withdrawal of either agent), epinephrine (initial hypertensive episode followed by bradycardia), nifedipine and verapamil lidocaine, ergots (peripheral ischemia), prazosin (postural hypotension)
(Continued)

Timolol Maleate *(Continued)*

Beta-blockers may affect the action or levels of ethanol, disopyramide, nondepolarizing muscle relaxants and theophylline although the effects are difficult to predict

Mechanism of Action Blocks both beta$_1$- and beta$_2$-adrenergic receptors, reduces intraocular pressure by reducing aqueous humor production or possibly outflow; reduces blood pressure by blocking adrenergic receptors and decreasing sympathetic outflow, produces a negative chronotropic and inotropic activity through an unknown mechanism

Pharmacodynamics/Kinetics

Onset of hypotensive effect: Oral: Within 15-45 minutes

Peak effect: Within 0.5-2.5 hours

Duration of action: ~4 hours; intraocular effects persist for 24 hours after ophthalmic instillation

Protein binding: 60%

Metabolism: Extensive first-pass effect; extensively metabolized in the liver

Half-life: 2-2.7 hours; prolonged with reduced renal function

Elimination: Urinary excretion (15% to 20% as unchanged drug)

Usual Dosage

Children and Adults: Ophthalmic: Initial: 0.25% solution, instill 1 drop twice daily; increase to 0.5% solution if response not adequate; decrease to 1 drop/day if controlled; do not exceed 1 drop twice daily of 0.5% solution

Adults: Oral:

Hypertension: Initial: 10 mg twice daily, increase gradually every 7 days, usual dosage: 20-40 mg/day in 2 divided doses; maximum: 60 mg/day

Prevention of myocardial infarction: 10 mg twice daily initiated within 1-4 weeks after infarction

Migraine headache: Initial: 10 mg twice daily, increase to maximum of 30 mg/day

Patient Information Apply gentle pressure to lacrimal sac during and immediately following instillation (1 minute) to avoid systemic absorption; stop drug if breathing difficulty occurs

Nursing Implications Monitor for systemic effect of beta blockade even when administering ophthalmic product

Dosage Forms

Solution, ophthalmic (Timoptic®): 0.25% (2.5 mL, 5 mL, 10 mL, 15 mL); 0.5% (2.5 mL, 5 mL, 10 mL, 15 mL)

Solution, ophthalmic, preservative free, single use (Timoptic® OcuDose®): 0.25%, 0.5%

Tablet (Blocadren®): 5 mg, 10 mg, 20 mg

Timoptic® *see* Timolol Maleate *on page 1094*

Tinactin® [OTC] *see* Tolnaftate *on page 1106*

Tindal® *see* Acetophenazine Maleate *on page 24*

Tine Test *see* Tuberculin Purified Protein Derivative *on page 1135*

Tinver® Lotion *see* Sodium Thiosulfate *on page 1020*

Tioconazole *(tye oh kone' a zole)*

Brand Names Vagistat®

Use Local treatment of vulvovaginal candidiasis

Pregnancy Risk Factor C

Contraindications Known hypersensitivity to tioconazole

Warnings/Precautions Not effective when applied to the scalp

Adverse Reactions

1% to 10%: Genitourinary: Vulvar/vaginal burning

<1%: Genitourinary: Vulvar itching, soreness, swelling, or discharge; urinary frequency

Mechanism of Action A 1-substituted imidazole derivative with a broad antifungal spectrum against a wide variety of dermatophytes and yeasts, usually at a concentration ≤6.25 mg/L; has been demonstrated to be at least as active *in vitro* as other imidazole antifungals. *In vitro*, tioconazole has been demonstrated 2-4 times as potent as miconazole against common dermal pathogens including *Trichophyton mentagrophytes*, *T. rubrum*, *T. erinacei*, *T. tonsurans*, *Microsporum canis*, *Microsporum gypseum*, and *Candida albicans*. Both agents appear to be similarly effective against *Epidermophyton floccosum*.

Pharmacodynamics/Kinetics

Absorption: Intravaginal: Following application small amounts of drug are absorbed systemically (25%) within 2-8 hours

Half-life: 21-24 hours

Elimination: Into urine and feces in approximate equal amounts

Usual Dosage Adults: Vaginal: Insert 1 applicatorful in vagina, just prior to bedtime, as a single dose

Patient Information Insert high into vagina; contact physician if itching or burning continues

Dosage Forms Cream, vaginal: 6.5% with applicator (4.6 g)

Tioguanine *see* Thioguanine *on page 1081*

Tiotixene *see* Thiothixene *on page 1087*

Tisit® [OTC] *see* Pyrethrins *on page 959*

Tissue Plasminogen Activator, Recombinant *see* Alteplase *on page 46*

Titralac® [OTC] *see* Calcium Carbonate *on page 161*

TMP *see* Trimethoprim *on page 1127*

TMP-SMX *see* Co-trimoxazole *on page 278*

TobraDex® *see* Tobramycin and Dexamethasone *on page 1100*

Tobramycin (toe bra mye' sin)

Related Information
Antimicrobial Drugs of Choice *on page 1298-1302*

Brand Names Nebcin®; Tobrex®

Use Treatment of documented or suspected *Pseudomonas aeruginosa* infection; infection with a nonpseudomonal enteric bacillus which is more sensitive to tobramycin than gentamicin based on susceptibility tests; empiric therapy in cystic fibrosis and immunocompromised patients; topically used to treat superficial ophthalmic infections caused by susceptible bacteria

Pregnancy Risk Factor C

Contraindications Hypersensitivity to tobramycin or other aminoglycosides or components

Warnings/Precautions Use with caution in patients with renal impairment (dosage modification required), pre-existing auditory or vestibular impairment, and in patients with neuromuscular disorders; aminoglycosides are associated with nephrotoxicity or ototoxicity; the ototoxicity may be proportional to the amount of drug given and the duration of treatment; tinnitus or vertigo are indications of vestibular injury and impending hearing loss; renal damage is usually reversible

Adverse Reactions
1% to 10%:
  Renal: Nephrotoxicity
  Neuromuscular & skeletal: Neurotoxicity (neuromuscular blockade)
  Otic: Ototoxicity (auditory), ototoxicity (vestibular)
<1%:
  Cardiovascular: Hypotension
  Central nervous system: Drug fever, headache, drowsiness, weakness
  Dermatologic: Skin rash
  Gastrointestinal: Nausea, vomiting,
  Hematologic: Eosinophilia anemia,
  Neuromuscular & skeletal: Paresthesia, tremor, arthralgia
  Ocular: Lacrimation, itching, edema of the eyelid, keratitis
  Respiratory: Difficulty in breathing

Overdosage/Toxicology Symptoms of overdose include ototoxicity, nephrotoxicity, and neuromuscular toxicity; the treatment of choice following a single acute overdose appears to be the maintenance of good urine output of at least 3 mL/kg/hour. Dialysis is of questionable value in the enhancement of aminoglycoside elimination. If required, hemodialysis is preferred over peritoneal dialysis in patients with normal renal function. Careful hydration may be all that is required to promote diuresis and therefore the enhancement of the drug's elimination. Chelation with penicillins is investigational.

Drug Interactions
Increased effect: Extended spectrum penicillins (synergistic)
Increased toxicity:
  Neuromuscular blockers increase neuromuscular blockade
  Amphotericin B, cephalosporins, loop diuretics → ↑ risk of nephrotoxicity

Stability
Tobramycin is stable at room temperature both as the clear, colorless solution and as the dry powder; reconstituted solutions remain stable for 24 hours at room temperature and 96 hours when refrigerated
Stability of parenteral admixture at room temperature (25°C) and at refrigeration temperature (4°C): 48 hours
(Continued)

1097

Tobramycin (Continued)

Standard diluent: Dose/100 mL NS
Minimum volume: 50 mL NS
Incompatible with penicillins
Mechanism of Action Interferes with bacterial protein synthesis by binding to 30S and 50S ribosomal subunits resulting in a defective bacterial cell membrane
Pharmacodynamics/Kinetics
Absorption: I.M.: Rapid and complete
Time to peak serum concentration:
I.M.: Within 30-60 minutes
I.V.: Within 30 minutes
Distribution: Crosses the placenta
V_d: 0.2-0.3 L/kg; Pediatric patients: 0.2-0.7 L/kg; see table.

Aminoglycoside Penetration Into Various Tissues

Site	Extent of Distribution
Eye	Poor
CNS	Poor (<25%)
Pleural	Excellent
Bronchial secretions	Poor
Sputum	Fair (10%-50%)
Pulmonary tissue	Excellent
Ascitic fluid	Variable (43%-132%)
Peritoneal fluid	Poor
Bile	Variable (25%-90%)
Bile with obstruction	Poor
Synovial fluid	Excellent
Bone	Poor
Prostate	Poor
Urine	Excellent
Renal tissue	Excellent

Relative diffusion of antimicrobial agents from blood into cerebrospinal fluid (CSF): Minimal even with inflammation
Ratio of CSF to blood level (%):
Normal meninges: Nil
Inflamed meninges: 14-23
Protein binding: <30%
Half-life:
Neonates:
≤1200 g: 11 hours
>1200 g: 2-9 hours
Adults: 2-3 hours, directly dependent upon glomerular filtration rate
Adults with impaired renal function: 5-70 hours
Elimination: With normal renal function, about 90% to 95% of a dose is excreted in the urine within 24 hours
Usual Dosage Individualization is critical because of the low therapeutic index
Use of ideal body weight (IBW) for determining the mg/kg/dose appears to be more accurate than dosing on the basis of total body weight (TBW)
In morbid obesity, dosage requirement may best be estimated using a dosing weight of IBW + 0.4 (TBW - IBW)
Initial and periodic peak and trough plasma drug levels should be determined particularly in critically ill patients with serious infections or in disease states known to significantly alter aminoglycoside pharmacokinetics (eg, cystic fibrosis, burns, or major surgery); 2-3 serum level measurements should be obtained after the initial dose to measure the half-life in order to determine the frequency of subsequent doses

Once daily dosing: Higher peak serum drug concentration to MIC ratios, demonstrated aminoglycoside postantibiotic effect, decreased renal cortex drug uptake, and improved cost-time efficiency are supportive reasons for the use of once daily dosing regimens for aminoglycosides. Current research indicates these regimens to be as effective for nonlife-threatening infections, with no higher incidence of nephrotoxicity, than those requiring multiple daily doses. Doses are determined by calculating the entire day's dose via usual multiple dose calculation techniques and administering this quantity as a single dose. Doses are then adjusted to maintain mean serum concentrations above the MIC(s) of the causative organism(s). (Example: 4.5-6 mg/kg as a single dose adjusted to achieve an average serum level of 3-4 mcg/mL). Further research is needed for universal recommendation in all patient populations and gram-negative disease.

Neonates: I.M., I.V.:
  0-4 weeks, <1200 g: 2.5 mg/kg/dose every 18-24 hours
  Postnatal age ≤7 days:
    1200-2000 g: 2.5 mg/kg/dose every 12-18 hours
    >2000 g: 2.5 mg/kg/dose every 12 hours
  Postnatal age >7 days:
    1200-2000 g: 2.5 mg/kg/dose every 12-18 hours
    >2000 g: 2.5 mg/kg/dose every 8 hours
  Infants and Children <5 years: I.M., I.V.: 2.5 mg/kg/dose every 8 hours
  Children >5 years: 1.5-2.5 mg/kg/dose every 8 hours
  Note: Some patients may require larger or more frequent doses if serum levels document the need (ie, cystic fibrosis or febrile granulocytopenic patients).
Adults: I.M., I.V.:
  Severe life-threatening infections: 2-2.5 mg/kg/dose
  Urinary tract infection: 1.5 mg/kg/dose
  Synergy (for gram-positive infections): 1 mg/kg/dose
Children and Adults: Ophthalmic: Instill 1-2 drops of solution every 4 hours; apply ointment 2-3 times/day; for severe infections apply ointment every 3-4 hours, or solution 2 drops every 30-60 minutes initially, then reduce to less frequent intervals

Dosing interval in renal impairment:
  Cl$_{cr}$ ≥60 mL/minute: Administer every 8 hours
  Cl$_{cr}$ 40-60 mL/minute: Administer every 12 hours
  Cl$_{cr}$ 20-40 mL/minute: Administer every 24 hours
  Cl$_{cr}$ 10-20 mL/minute: Administer every 48 hours
  Cl$_{cr}$ <10 mL/minute: Administer every 72 hours
Dialyzable; 30% removal of aminoglycosides occurs during 4 hours of HD - administer dose after dialysis and follow levels
Continuous arterio-venous or veno-venous hemofiltration (CAVH/CAVHD): Dose as for Cl$_{cr}$ of 10-15 mL/minute and follow levels
  Administration in CAPD fluid:
    Gram-negative infection: 4-8 mg/L (4-8 mcg/mL) of CAPD fluid
    Gram-positive infection (ie, synergy): 3-4 mg/L (3-4 mcg/mL) of CAPD fluid
  Administration IVPB/I.M.: Dose as for Cl$_{cr}$ <10 mL/minute and follow levels

Dosing adjustment/comments in hepatic disease: Monitor plasma concentrations
Monitoring Parameters Urinalysis, urine output, BUN, serum creatinine, peak and trough plasma tobramycin levels; be alert to ototoxicity; hearing should be tested before and during treatment
Reference Range
  Timing of serum samples: Draw peak 30 minutes after 30-minute infusion has been completed or 1 hour following I.M. injection or beginning of infusion; draw trough immediately before next dose
  Therapeutic levels:
    Peak:
      Serious infections: 6-8 µg/mL (SI: 12-17 mg/L)
      Life-threatening infections: 8-10 µg/mL (SI: 17-21 mg/L)
      Urinary tract infections: 4-6 µg/mL (SI: 7-12 mg/L)
      Synergy against gram-positive organisms: 3-5 µg/mL
    Trough:
      Serious infections: 0.5-1 µg/mL
      Life-threatening infections: 1-2 µg/mL
      Monitor serum creatinine and urine output; obtain drug levels after the third dose unless otherwise directed
Test Interactions ↑ protein, ↓ magnesium, ↑ BUN, AST, GPT, alk phos, creatinine, ↓ potassium, sodium, calcium (S)
Patient Information Report symptoms of superinfection; for eye drops - no other eye drops 5-10 minutes before or after tobramycin; report any dizziness or sensations of ringing or fullness in ears
Nursing Implications Eye solutions: Allow 5 minutes between application of "multiple-drop" therapy; obtain drug levels after the third dose; peak levels are drawn 30 minutes after the end of a 30-minute infusion or 1 hour after initiation of infusion or I.M. injection; the trough is drawn just before the next dose; give penicillins or cephalosporins at least 1 hour apart from tobramycin
Dosage Forms
Injection, as sulfate: 10 mg/mL (2 mL); 40 mg/mL (1.5 mL, 2 mL)
Ointment, ophthalmic: 0.3% [3 mg/mL] (3.5 g)
Powder for injection: 40 mg/mL (1.2 g vials)
(Continued)

Tobramycin *(Continued)*

Solution, ophthalmic: 0.3% [3 mg/mL] (5 mL)

Tobramycin and Dexamethasone *(toe bra mye' sin)*

Brand Names TobraDex®

Synonyms Dexamethasone and Tobramycin

Use Treatment of external ocular infection caused by susceptible gram-negative bacteria and steroid responsive inflammatory conditions of the palpebral and bulbar conjunctiva, lid, cornea, and anterior segment of the globe

Pregnancy Risk Factor B

Contraindications Known hypersensitivity to tobramycin or dexamethasone, most viral diseases of the cornea, fungal diseases, use after uncomplicated removal of a corneal foreign body

Adverse Reactions 1% to 10%: Ocular: Allergic contact dermatitis, delayed wound healing, lacrimation, itching, edema of eyelid, keratitis, increased intraocular pressure, glaucoma, cataract formation

Overdosage/Toxicology Symptoms of overdose include punctate keratitis, erythema, increased lacrimation, edema, lid itching; flush eye with copious amounts of fluid at low pressure for 15 minutes

Drug Interactions Refer to individual monographs for Dexamethasone and Tobramycin

Mechanism of Action Refer to individual monographs for Dexamethasone and Tobramycin

Pharmacodynamics/Kinetics

Absorption: Absorbed into the aqueous humor

Time to peak serum concentration: 1-2 hours after instillation in the cornea and aqueous humor

Usual Dosage Children and Adults: Ophthalmic: Instill 1-2 drops of solution every 4 hours; apply ointment 2-3 times/day; for severe infections apply ointment every 3-4 hours, or solution 2 drops every 30-60 minutes initially, then reduce to less frequent intervals

Patient Information Shake well before using, do not touch dropper to eye, apply light finger pressure on lacrimal sac for 1 minute following instillation; notify physician if condition fails to improve or worsens

Dosage Forms

Ointment, ophthalmic: Tobramycin 0.3% and dexamethasone 0.1% (3.5 g)

Suspension, ophthalmic: Tobramycin 0.3% and dexamethasone 0.1% (2.5 mL, 5 mL)

Tobrex® *see* Tobramycin *on page 1097*

Tocainide Hydrochloride *(toe kay' nide)*

Related Information

Antiarrhythmic Drugs *on page 1246-1248*

Brand Names Tonocard®

Use Suppress and prevent symptomatic life-threatening ventricular arrhythmias

Unlabeled use: Trigeminal neuralgia

Pregnancy Risk Factor C

Contraindications Second or third degree A-V block without a pacemaker, hypersensitivity to tocainide, amide-type anesthetics, or any component

Warnings/Precautions May exacerbate some arrhythmias (ie, atrial fibrillation/flutter); use with caution in CHF patients; administer with caution in patients with pre-existing bone marrow failure, cytopenia, severe renal or hepatic disease

Adverse Reactions

>10%:

Central nervous system: Nervousness, confusion, ataxia

Gastrointestinal: Nausea, dizziness, anorexia

Neuromuscular & skeletal: Tremor

1% to 10%:

Cardiovascular: Hypotension, tachycardia

Central nervous system: Ataxia,

Dermatologic: Skin rash

Gastrointestinal: Vomiting, diarrhea

Neuromuscular & skeletal: Arthralgia, myalgia, paresthesia

Ocular: Blurred vision

<1%:

Cardiovascular: Bradycardia, palpitations

Hematologic: Agranulocytosis, anemia, leukopenia, neutropenia

Respiratory: Respiratory arrest

Miscellaneous: Sweating

Overdosage/Toxicology Has a narrow therapeutic index and severe toxicity may occur slightly above the therapeutic range, especially with other antiarrhythmic drugs; and acute ingestion of twice the daily therapeutic dose is potentially life-threatening; symptoms of overdose includes sedation, confusion, coma, seizures, respiratory arrest and cardiac toxicity (sinus arrest, A-V block, asystole, and hypotension); the QRS and Q-T intervals are usually normal, although they may be prolonged after massive overdose; other effects include dizziness, paresthesias, tremor, ataxia, and GI disturbance. Treatment is supportive, using conventional therapies (fluids, positioning, vasopressors, antiarrhythmics, anticonvulsants); sodium bicarbonate may reverse the QRS prolongation (if present), bradyarrhythmias, and hypotension; enhanced elimination with dialysis, hemoperfusion or repeat charcoal is not effective.

Drug Interactions
Decreased plasma levels: Phenobarbital, phenytoin, rifampin, and other hepatic enzyme inducers, cimetidine and drugs which make the urine acidic
Increased effect of tocainide, allopurinol
Increased toxicity/levels of caffeine and theophylline

Mechanism of Action Class 1B antiarrhythmic agent; suppresses automaticity of conduction tissue, by increasing electrical stimulation threshold of ventricle, HIS-Purkinje system, and spontaneous depolarization of the ventricles during diastole by a direct action on the tissues; blocks both the initiation and conduction of nerve impulses by decreasing the neuronal membrane's permeability to sodium ions, which results in inhibition of depolarization with resultant blockade of conduction

Pharmacodynamics/Kinetics
Absorption: Oral: Extensive, 99% to 100%
Distribution: V_d: 1.62-3.2 L/kg
Protein binding: 10% to 20%
Metabolism: In the liver to inactive metabolites; first-pass effect is negligible
Half-life: 11-14 hours, prolonged with renal and hepatic impairment with half-life increased to 23-27 hours
Time to peak: Peak serum levels occur within 30-160 minutes
Elimination: In urine (40% to 50% as unchanged drug)

Usual Dosage Adults: Oral: 1200-1800 mg/day in 3 divided doses, up to 2400 mg/day

Dosing adjustment in renal impairment: Cl_{cr} <30 mL/minute: Administer 50% of normal dose or 600 mg once daily
Moderately dialyzable (20% to 50%)

Dosing adjustment in hepatic impairment: Maximum daily dose: 1200 mg

Reference Range Therapeutic: 5-12 µg/mL (SI: 22-52 µmol/L)

Patient Information Report any unusual bleeding, fever, sore throat, or any breathing difficulties; do not discontinue or alter dose without notifying physician; may cause drowsiness, dizziness, impair judgment, and coordination

Nursing Implications Monitor for tremor; titration of dosing and initiation of therapy require cardiac monitoring

Dosage Forms Tablet: 400 mg, 600 mg

Tofranil® *see* Imipramine *on page 568*

Tofranil-PM® *see* Imipramine *on page 568*

Tolazamide (tole az' a mide)

Related Information
Hypoglycemic Agents Comparison *on page 1271*

Brand Names Tolinase®

Use Adjunct to diet for the management of mild to moderately severe, stable, noninsulin-dependent (type II) diabetes mellitus

Pregnancy Risk Factor D

Contraindications Type I diabetes therapy (IDDM), hypersensitivity to sulfonylureas, diabetes complicated by ketoacidosis

Warnings/Precautions False-positive response has been reported in patients with liver disease, idiopathic hypoglycemia of infancy, severe malnutrition, acute pancreatitis, renal dysfunction. Transferring a patient from one sulfonylurea to another does not require a priming dose; doses >1000 mg/day normally do not improve diabetic control. Has not been studied in older patients; however, except for drug interactions, it appears to have a safe profile and decline in renal function does not affect its pharmacokinetics. How "tightly" an elderly patient's blood glucose should be controlled is controversial; however, a fasting blood sugar <150 mg/dL is now an acceptable end point. Such a decision should be based on the patient's functional and cognitive status, how well they recognize
(Continued)

Tolazamide *(Continued)*

hypoglycemic or hyperglycemic symptoms, and how to respond to them and their other disease states.

Adverse Reactions
>10%:
Central nervous system: Headache, dizziness
Gastrointestinal: Anorexia, nausea, vomiting, diarrhea, constipation, heartburn, epigastric fullness
1% to 10%: Dermatologic: Rash, urticaria, hives, photosensitivity
<1%:
Endocrine & metabolic: Hypoglycemia
Hematologic: Aplastic anemia, hemolytic anemia, bone marrow depression, thrombocytopenia, agranulocytosis
Hepatic: Cholestatic jaundice
Renal: Diuretic effect

Overdosage/Toxicology Symptoms of overdose include low blood sugar, tingling of lips and tongue, nausea, yawning, confusion, agitation, tachycardia, sweating, convulsions, stupor, and coma; intoxications with sulfonylureas can cause hypoglycemia and are best managed with glucose administration (oral for milder hypoglycemia or by injection in more severe forms)

Drug Interactions Increased toxicity: Monitor patient closely; large number of drugs interact with sulfonylureas including salicylates, anticoagulants, H_2 antagonists, TCA, MAO inhibitors, beta-blockers, thiazides

Mechanism of Action Stimulates insulin release from the pancreatic beta cells; reduces glucose output from the liver; insulin sensitivity is increased at peripheral target sites

Pharmacodynamics/Kinetics
Onset of action: Oral: Within 4-6 hours
Duration: 10-24 hours
Protein binding: >98% ionic/nonionic
Metabolism: Extensively in the liver to one active and three inactive metabolites
Half-life: 7 hours
Elimination: Renal

Usual Dosage Oral (doses >1000 mg/day normally do not improve diabetic control):

Adults: Initial: 100 mg/day, increase at 2- to 4-week intervals; maximum dose: 1000 mg; give as a single or twice daily dose
Conversion from insulin → tolazamide
10 units day = 100 mg/day
20-40 units/day = 250 mg/day
>40 units/day = 250 mg/day and 50% of insulin dose
Doses >500 mg/day should be given in 2 divided doses

Dosing comments in hepatic impairment: Initial and maintenance doses should be conservative

Monitoring Parameters Signs and symptoms of hypoglycemia, (fatigue, sweating, numbness of extremities); urine for glucose and ketones; fasting blood glucose; hemoglobin A_{1c} or fructosamine

Reference Range Fasting blood glucose: Adults: 80-140 mg/dL; Elderly: 100-180 mg/dL

Patient Information Tablets may be crushed; take drug at the same time each day; avoid alcohol; recognize signs and symptoms of hyper- and hypoglycemia; report any persistent or severe sore throat, fever, malaise, unusual bleeding, or bruising; can take with food; do not skip meals; carry a quick sugar source; medical alert bracelet

Nursing Implications Patients who are anorexic or NPO may need to have their dose held to avoid hypoglycemia

Dosage Forms Tablet: 100 mg, 250 mg, 500 mg

Tolazoline Hydrochloride *(tole az′ oh leen)*

Brand Names Priscoline®
Synonyms Benzazoline Hydrochloride
Use Treatment of persistent pulmonary vasoconstriction and hypertension of the newborn (persistent fetal circulation), peripheral vasospastic disorders
Pregnancy Risk Factor C
Contraindications Hypersensitivity to tolazoline; known or suspected coronary artery disease
Warnings/Precautions Stimulates gastric secretion and may activate stress ulcers; therefore, use with caution in patients with gastritis, peptic ulcer; use with caution in patients with mitral stenosis

Adverse Reactions

>10%:
  Cardiovascular: Hypotension,
  Endocrine & metabolic: Hypochloremic alkalosis
  Gastrointestinal: GI bleeding, abdominal pain
  Hematologic: Thrombocytopenia
  Local: Burning at injection site
  Renal: Acute renal failure, oliguria
1% to 10%:
  Cardiovascular: Peripheral vasodilation, tachycardia
  Gastrointestinal: Nausea, diarrhea
  Neuromuscular & skeletal: Increased pilomotor activity
<1%:
  Cardiovascular: Hypertension, tachycardia, arrhythmias
  Hematologic: Increased agranulocytosis, pancytopenia
  Ocular: Mydriasis
  Respiratory: Pulmonary hemorrhage
  Miscellaneous: Increased secretions

Overdosage/Toxicology Symptoms of overdose include hypotension, shock, flushing; I.V. fluids and Trendelenburg position for hypotension; if pressors are required, use direct-acting alpha agonists (norepinephrine)

Drug Interactions
  Decreased effect (vasopressor) of epinephrine followed by a rebound increase in blood pressure
  Increased toxicity: Disulfiram reaction may possibly be seen with concomitant ethanol use

Stability Compatible in D_5W, $D_{10}W$, and saline solutions

Mechanism of Action Competitively blocks alpha-adrenergic receptors to produce brief antagonism of circulating epinephrine and norepinephrine; reduces hypertension caused by catecholamines and causes vascular smooth muscle relaxation (direct action); results in peripheral vasodilation and decreased peripheral resistance

Pharmacodynamics/Kinetics
  Half-life: Neonates: 3-10 hours, increased half-life with decreased renal function, oliguria
  Time to peak serum concentration: Within 30 minutes
  Elimination: Excreted rapidly in urine primarily as unchanged drug

Usual Dosage
  Neonates: Initial: I.V.: 1-2 mg/kg over 10-15 minutes via scalp vein or upper extremity; maintenance: 1-2 mg/kg/hour; use lower maintenance doses in patients with decreased renal function. Also used in neonates for acute vasospasm "cath toes" at 0.25 mg/kg/hour (no load); maximum dose: 6-8 mg/kg/hour

  Dosing interval in renal impairment in newborns: Urine output <0.9 mL/kg/hour: Decrease dose to 0.08 mg/kg/hour for every 1 mg/kg of loading dose

  Adults: Peripheral vasospastic disorder: I.M., I.V., S.C.: 10-50 mg 4 times/day

Monitoring Parameters Vital signs, blood gases, cardiac monitor

Patient Information Side effects decrease with continued therapy; avoid alcohol

Nursing Implications Dilute in D_5W; monitor blood pressure for hypotension; observe limbs for change in color; do not mix with any other drug in syringe or bag

Dosage Forms Injection: 25 mg/mL (4 mL)

Tolbutamide (tole byoo' ta mide)

Related Information
  Hypoglycemic Agents Comparison on page 1271

Brand Names Orinase®

Use Adjunct to diet for the management of mild to moderately severe, stable, noninsulin-dependent (type II) diabetes mellitus

Pregnancy Risk Factor D

Contraindications Diabetes complicated by ketoacidosis, therapy of IDDM, hypersensitivity to sulfonylureas

Warnings/Precautions False-positive response has been reported in patients with liver disease, idiopathic hypoglycemia of infancy, severe malnutrition, acute pancreatitis. Because of its low potency and short duration, it is a useful agent in the elderly if drug interactions can be avoided. How "tightly" an elderly patient's blood glucose should be controlled is controversial; however, a fasting blood sugar <150 mg/dL is now an acceptable end point. Such a decision should be based on the patient's functional and cognitive status, how well they recognize (Continued)

Tolbutamide *(Continued)*

hypoglycemic or hyperglycemic symptoms, and how to respond to them and their other disease states.

Adverse Reactions
>10%:
  Central nervous system: Headache, dizziness
  Gastrointestinal: Constipation, diarrhea, heartburn, anorexia, epigastric fullness
1% to 10%: Dermatologic: Skin rash, hives, photosensitivity
<1%:
  Endocrine & metabolic: SIADH
  Hematologic: Thrombocytopenia, agranulocytosis, hypoglycemia, leukopenia, aplastic anemia, hemolytic anemia, bone marrow depression
  Hepatic: Cholestatic jaundice
  Local: Thrombophlebitis
  Otic: Tinnitus
  Miscellaneous: Venospasm, disulfiram-type reactions, hypersensitivity reaction

Overdosage/Toxicology Symptoms of overdose include low blood sugar, tingling of lips and tongue, nausea, yawning, confusion, agitation, tachycardia, sweating, convulsions, stupor, and coma; I.V. glucose (12.5-25 g), epinephrine for anaphylaxis

Drug Interactions Increased toxicity: Phenylbutazone may potentiate hypoglycemic effect; chloramphenicol $\rightarrow$ $\uparrow$ half-life of tolbutamide

Stability Use parenteral formulation within 1 hour following reconstitution

Mechanism of Action A sulfonylurea hypoglycemic agent; its ability to lower elevated blood glucose levels in patients with functional pancreatic beta cells is similar to the other sulfonylurea agents; stimulates synthesis and release of endogenous insulin from pancreatic islet tissue. The hypoglycemic effect is attributed to an increased sensitivity of insulin receptors and improved peripheral utilization of insulin. Suppression of glucagon secretion may also contribute to the hypoglycemic effects of tolbutamide.

Pharmacodynamics/Kinetics
Peak hypoglycemic action:
  Oral: 1-3 hours
  I.V.: 30 minutes
Duration:
  Oral: 6-24 hours
  I.V.: 3 hours
Time to peak serum concentration: 3-5 hours
Absorption: Oral: Rapid
Distribution: V_d: 6-10 L
Protein binding: 95% to 97% (principally to albumin) ionic/nonionic
Metabolism/Elimination: Hepatic metabolism to hydroxymethyltolbutamide (mildly active) and carboxytolbutamide (inactive) both rapidly excreted renally, less 2% excreted in the urine unchanged; metabolism does not appear to be affected by age
Increased plasma concentrations and volume of distribution secondary to decreased albumin concentrations and less protein binding have been reported.
Half-life:
  Plasma: 4-25 hours
  Elimination: 4-9 hours

Usual Dosage Divided doses may increase gastrointestinal side effects
Adults:
  Oral: Initial: 500-1000 mg 1-3 times/day; usual dose should not be more than 2 g/day
  I.V. bolus: 1 g over 2-3 minutes

Elderly: Oral: Initial: 250 mg 1-3 times/day; usual: 500-2000 mg; maximum: 3 g/day

  Dosing adjustment in hepatic impairment: Dose reduction is necessary
  Not dialyzable (0% to 5%)

Monitoring Parameters Fasting blood glucose, hemoglobin A_{1c} or fructosamine

Reference Range Fasting blood glucose: Adults: 80-140 mg/dL; Elderly: 100-180 mg/dL

Patient Information Tablets may be crushed; take drug at the same time each day; avoid alcohol; recognize signs and symptoms of hyper- and hypoglycemia; report any persistent or severe sore throat, fever, malaise, unusual bleeding, or bruising; can take with food

Nursing Implications Patients who are anorexic or NPO may need to have their dose held to avoid hypoglycemia

Additional Information Sodium content of 1 g vial: 3.5 mEq

Dosage Forms
  Injection, diagnostic, as sodium: 1 g (20 mL)
  Tablet: 250 mg, 500 mg

Tolectin® *see* Tolmetin Sodium *on this page*

Tolinase® *see* Tolazamide *on page 1101*

Tolmetin Sodium (tole′ met in)
  Related Information
    Nonsteroidal Anti-Inflammatories Comparison *on page 1280*
  Brand Names Tolectin®
  Use Treatment of rheumatoid arthritis and osteoarthritis, juvenile rheumatoid arthritis
  Pregnancy Risk Factor C (D at term)
  Contraindications Known hypersensitivity to tolmetin or any component, aspirin, or other nonsteroidal anti-inflammatory drugs (NSAIDs)
  Warnings/Precautions Use with caution in patients with upper GI disease, impaired renal function, congestive heart failure, hypertension, and patients receiving anticoagulants; if GI upset occurs with tolmetin, take with antacids other than sodium bicarbonate
  Adverse Reactions
    >10%:
      Dermatologic: Skin rash, dizziness
      Gastrointestinal: Abdominal cramps, heartburn, indigestion, nausea
    1% to 10%:
      Cardiovascular: Fluid retention
      Central nervous system: Headache, nervousness
      Dermatologic: Itching
      Gastrointestinal: Vomiting
      Otic: Ringing in ears
    <1%:
      Cardiovascular: Congestive heart failure, hypertension, arrhythmias, tachycardia
      Central nervous system: Epistaxis, confusion, hallucinations, aseptic meningitis, mental depression, drowsiness, insomnia
      Dermatologic: Hives, erythema multiforme, toxic epidermal necrolysis, Stevens-Johnson syndrome, angioedema
      Endocrine & metabolism: Polydipsia, hot flushes
      Gastrointestinal: Gastritis, GI ulceration
      Genitourinary: Cystitis
      Hematologic: Agranulocytosis, anemia, hemolytic anemia, bone marrow depression, leukopenia, thrombocytopenia
      Hepatic: Hepatitis
      Neuromuscular & skeletal: Peripheral neuropathy
      Ocular: Toxic amblyopia, blurred vision, conjunctivitis, dry eyes
      Otic: Decreased hearing
      Renal: Polyuria, acute renal failure
      Respiratory: Allergic rhinitis, shortness of breath
  Overdosage/Toxicology Symptoms of overdose include lethargy, mental confusion, dizziness, leukocytosis, renal failure

  Management of a nonsteroidal anti-inflammatory drug (NSAID) intoxication is primarily supportive and symptomatic. Fluid therapy is commonly effective in managing the hypotension that may occur following an acute NSAID overdose, except when this is due to an acute blood loss. Seizures tend to be very short-lived and often do not require drug treatment; although, recurrent seizures should be treated with I.V. diazepam. Since many of the NSAID undergo enterohepatic cycling, multiple doses of charcoal may be needed to reduce the potential for delayed toxicities.
  Drug Interactions
    Decreased effect with aspirin; decreased effect of thiazides, furosemide
    Increased toxicity of digoxin, methotrexate, cyclosporine, lithium, insulin, sulfonylureas, potassium-sparing diuretics, aspirin
  Mechanism of Action Inhibits prostaglandin synthesis by decreasing the activity of the enzyme, cyclo-oxygenase, which results in decreased formation of prostaglandin precursors
  Pharmacodynamics/Kinetics
    Absorption: Oral: Well absorbed
    Bioavailability: Food/milk decreases total bioavailability by 16%
    Time to peak serum concentration: Within 30-60 minutes
  Usual Dosage Oral:
    (Continued)

Tolmetin Sodium *(Continued)*

Children ≥2 years:
 Anti-inflammatory: Initial: 20 mg/kg/day in 3 divided doses, then 15-30 mg/kg/day in 3 divided doses
 Analgesic: 5-7 mg/kg/dose every 6-8 hours

Adults: 400 mg 3 times/day; usual dose: 600 mg to 1.8 g/day; maximum: 2 g/day
Monitoring Parameters Occult blood loss, CBC, liver enzymes, BUN, serum creatinine, periodic liver function test
Test Interactions ↑ protein, ↑ bleeding time
Patient Information Take with food, milk, or water; may cause drowsiness, impair judgment or coordination
Additional Information Sodium content of 200 mg: 0.8 mEq
Dosage Forms
 Capsule: 400 mg
 Tablet: 200 mg, 600 mg

Tolnaftate *(tole naf' tate)*
Brand Names Aftate® [OTC]; Footwork® [OTC]; Fungatin® [OTC]; Genaspor® [OTC]; NP-27® [OTC]; Tinactin® [OTC]; Zeasorb-AF® [OTC]
Use Treatment of tinea pedis, tinea cruris, tinea corporis, tinea manuum, tinea versicolor infections
Pregnancy Risk Factor C
Contraindications Known hypersensitivity to tolnaftate; nail and scalp infections
Warnings/Precautions Cream is not recommended for nail or scalp infections; keep from eyes; if no improvement within 4 weeks, treatment should be discontinued. Usually not effective alone for the treatment of infections involving hair follicles or nails.
Adverse Reactions 1% to 10%: Dermatologic: Pruritus, contact dermatitis, irritation, stinging
Mechanism of Action Distorts the hyphae and stunts mycelial growth in susceptible fungi
Pharmacodynamics/Kinetics Onset of action: Response may be seen 24-72 hours after initiation of therapy
Usual Dosage Children and Adults: Topical: Wash and dry affected area; apply 1-3 drops of solution or a small amount of cream or powder and rub into the affected areas 2-3 times/day for 2-4 weeks
Monitoring Parameters Resolution of skin infection
Patient Information Avoid contact with the eyes; apply to clean dry area; consult the physician if a skin irritation develops or if the skin infection worsens or does not improve after 10 days of therapy; does not stain skin or clothing
Nursing Implications Itching, burning, and soreness are usually relieved within 24-72 hours
Dosage Forms
 Aerosol, topical:
  Liquid: 1% (59.2 mL, 90 mL, 118.3 mL, 120 mL)
  Powder: 1% (90 g, 100 g, 105 g, 150 g)
 Cream: 1% (15 g, 30 g)
 Gel, topical: 1% (15 g)
 Powder, topical: 1% (45 g, 56.7 g, 67.5 g, 70.9 g, 90 g)
 Solution, topical: 1% (10 mL, 15 mL)

Tolu-Sed® DM [OTC] *see* Guaifenesin and Dextromethorphan *on page 517*

Tonocard® *see* Tocainide Hydrochloride *on page 1100*

Topicort® *see* Desoximetasone *on page 313*

Topicort®-LP *see* Desoximetasone *on page 313*

Topicycline® *see* Tetracycline *on page 1069*

Toprol XL® *see* Metoprolol Tartrate *on page 731*

TOPV *see* Polio Vaccines *on page 898*

Toradol® *see* Ketorolac Tromethamine *on page 612*

Torecan® *see* Thiethylperazine Maleate *on page 1080*

Tornalate® *see* Bitolterol Mesylate *on page 137*

Torsemide *(tore' se mide)*
Related Information
 Diuretics, Loop Comparison *on page 1269*

Brand Names Demadex®

Use Management of edema associated with congestive heart failure and hepatic or renal disease; used alone or in combination with antihypertensives in treatment of hypertension; I.V. form is indicated when rapid onset is desired

Pregnancy Risk Factor B

Pregnancy/Breast Feeding Implications A decrease in fetal weight, an increase in fetal resorption, and delayed fetal ossification has occurred in animal studies

Contraindications Anuria; hypersensitivity to torsemide or any component, or other sulfonylureas; safety in children <18 years has not been established

Warnings/Precautions Excessive diuresis may result in dehydration, acute hypotensive or thromboembolic episodes and cardiovascular collapse; rapid injection, renal impairment, or excessively large doses may result in ototoxicity; SLE may be exacerbated; sudden alterations in electrolyte balance may precipitate hepatic encephalopathy and coma in patients with hepatic cirrhosis and ascites; monitor carefully for signs of fluid or electrolyte imbalances, especially hypokalemia in patients at risk for such (eg, digitalis therapy, history of ventricular arrhythmias, elderly, etc), hyperuricemia, hypomagnesemia, or hypocalcemia; use caution with exposure to ultraviolet light.

Adverse Reactions
>10%: Cardiovascular: Orthostatic hypotension
1% to 10%:
  Central nervous system: Headache, dizziness, vertigo
  Dermatologic: Photosensitivity, urticaria
  Endocrine & metabolic: Electrolyte imbalance, dehydration, hyperuricemia
  Gastrointestinal: Diarrhea, loss of appetite, stomach cramps or pain, pancreatitis
  Ocular: Blurred vision
<1%:
  Dermatologic: Skin rash
  Endocrine & metabolic: Gout
  Gastrointestinal: Pancreatitis, nausea
  Hepatic: Hepatic dysfunction
  Hematologic: Agranulocytosis, leukopenia, anemia, thrombocytopenia
  Local: Redness at injection site
  Otic: Ototoxicity
  Renal: Nephrocalcinosis, prerenal azotemia, interstitial nephritis

Overdosage/Toxicology Symptoms include electrolyte depletion, volume depletion, hypotension, dehydration, circulatory collapse; electrolyte depletion may be manifested by weakness, dizziness, mental confusion, anorexia, lethargy, vomiting, and cramps; following GI decontamination, treatment is supportive; hypotension responds to fluids and Trendelenburg position

Drug Interactions
  Aminoglycosides: Ototoxicity may be increased; anticoagulant activity is enhanced
  Beta-blockers: Plasma concentrations of beta blockers may be increased
  Cisplatin: Ototoxicity may be increased
  Digitalis: Arrhythmias may occur with diuretic-induced electrolyte disturbances
  Lithium: Plasma concentrations of lithium may be increased
  NSAIDs: Torsemide efficacy may be decreased
  Probenecid: Torsemide action may be reduced
  Salicylates: Diuretic action may be impaired in patients with cirrhosis and ascites
  Sulfonylureas: Glucose tolerance may be decreased
  Thiazides: Synergistic effects may result

Mechanism of Action Inhibits reabsorption of sodium and chloride in the ascending loop of Henle and distal renal tubule, interfering with the chloride-binding cotransport system, thus causing increased excretion of water, sodium, chloride, magnesium, and calcium; does not alter GFR, renal plasma flow, or acid-base balance

Pharmacodynamics/Kinetics
  Onset of diuresis: 30-60 minutes
  Peak effect: 1-4 hours
  Duration: ~6 hours
  Absorption: Oral: Rapid
  Protein binding: Plasma: ~97% to 99%
  Metabolism: Hepatic by cytochrome P-450, 80%
  Bioavailability: 80% to 90%
  Half-life: 2-4; 7-8 hours in cirrhosis (dose modification appears unnecessary)
  Elimination: 20% eliminated unchanged in urine; hemodialysis does not accelerate removal

Usual Dosage Adults: Oral, I.V.:
  Congestive heart failure: 10-20 mg once daily; may increase gradually for chronic treatment by doubling dose until the diuretic response is apparent (for acute
(Continued)

1107

Torsemide *(Continued)*

treatment, I.V. dose may be repeated every 2 hours with double the dose as needed)

Chronic renal failure: 20 mg once daily; increase as described above

Hepatic cirrhosis: 5-10 mg once daily with an aldosterone antagonist or a potassium-sparing diuretic; increase as described above

Hypertension: 5 mg once daily; increase to 10 mg after 4-6 weeks if an adequate hypotensive response is not apparent; if still not effective, an additional antihypertensive agent may be added

Administration I.V. injections should be given over ≥2 minutes; the oral form may be given regardless of meal times; patients may be switched from the I.V. form to the oral and vice-versa with no change in dose; no dosage adjustment is needed in the elderly or patients with hepatic impairment

Monitoring Parameters Renal function, electrolytes, and fluid status (weight and I & O), blood pressure

Patient Information May be taken with food or milk; rise slowly from a lying or sitting position to minimize dizziness, lightheadedness or fainting; also use extra care when exercising, standing for long periods of time, and during hot weather; take dose in the morning or early in the evening to prevent nocturia; use caution with exposure to ultraviolet light

Additional Information 10-20 mg torsemide is approximately equivalent to furosemide 40 mg or bumetanide 1 mg

Dosage Forms

Injection: 10 mg/mL (2 mL, 5 mL)

Tablet: 5 mg, 10 mg, 20 mg, 100 mg

Totacillin® *see* Ampicillin *on page 73*

t-PA *see* Alteplase *on page 46*

Tracrium® *see* Atracurium Besylate *on page 99*

Tramadol Hydrochloride (tra′ ma dole)

Brand Names Ultram®

Use Relief of moderate to moderately severe pain

Pregnancy Risk Factor C

Contraindications Previous hypersensitivity to tramadol or any components; concurrent use of monoamine oxidase inhibitors; acute alcohol intoxication; concurrent use of centrally acting analgesics, opioids, or psychotropic drugs

Warnings/Precautions Elderly patients and patients with chronic respiratory disorders may be at greater risk of adverse events; liver disease; patients with myxedema, hypothyroidism, or hypoadrenalism should use tramadol with caution and at reduced dosages; not recommended during pregnancy or in nursing mothers

Adverse Reactions

>1%:

Central nervous system: Dizziness, headache, somnolence, stimulation, asthenia, restlessness

Gastrointestinal: Nausea, diarrhea, constipation, vomiting, dyspepsia

Miscellaneous: Sweating

<1%:

Cardiovascular: Palpitations

Respiratory: Respiratory depression

Overdosage/Toxicology Symptoms of overdose include CNS and respiratory depression, gastrointestinal cramping, constipation; naloxone 2 mg I.V. (0.01 mg/kg children) with repeat administration as needed up to 18 mg

Drug Interactions

Decreased effects: Carbamazepine (decreases half-life by 33% to 50%)

Increased toxicity: Monoamine oxidase inhibitors (seizures); quinidine (inhibits cytochrome P450IID6, thereby increases tramadol serum concentrations); cimetidine (tramadol half-life increased 20% to 25%)

Mechanism of Action Binds to μ-opiate receptors in the CNS causing inhibition of ascending pain pathways, altering the perception of and response to pain; also inhibits the reuptake of norepinephrine and serotonin, which also modifies the ascending pain pathway

Usual Dosage Oral: Adults: 50-100 mg every 4-6 hours, not to exceed 400 mg/day

Monitoring Parameters Monitor patient for pain, respiratory rate, and look for signs of tolerance and, therefore, abuse potential; monitor blood pressure and pulse rate, especially in patients on higher doses

Reference Range 100-300 ng/mL; however, serum level monitoring is not required

Patient Information Avoid driving or operating machinery until the effect of drug wears off; tramadol has not been fully evaluated for its abuse potential, report cravings to your physician immediately

Dosage Forms Tablet: 50 mg

Trandate® *see* Labetalol Hydrochloride *on page 614*

Tranexamic Acid (tran ex am' ik)
Brand Names Cyklokapron®
Use Short-term use (2-8 days) in hemophilia patients during and following tooth extraction to reduce or prevent hemorrhage, has also been used as an alternative to aminocaproic acid for subarachnoid hemorrhage
Pregnancy Risk Factor B
Contraindications Acquired defective color vision, active intravascular clotting
Warnings/Precautions Dosage modification required in patients with renal impairment; ophthalmic exam before and during therapy required if patient is treated beyond several days; caution in patients with cardiovascular, renal, or cerebrovascular disease; when used for subarachnoid hemorrhage, ischemic complications may occur
Adverse Reactions
>10%: Gastrointestinal: Nausea, diarrhea, vomiting
1% to 10%:
Cardiovascular: Hypotension, thrombosis
Ocular: Blurred vision
<1%: Endocrine & metabolic: Unusual menstrual discomfort
Stability Incompatible with solutions containing penicillin
Mechanism of Action Forms a reversible complex that displaces plasminogen from fibrin resulting in inhibition of fibrinolysis; it also inhibits the proteolytic activity of plasmin
Pharmacodynamics/Kinetics
Half-life: 2-10 hours
Elimination: Primarily as unchanged drug (>90%) in urine
Usual Dosage Children and Adults: I.V.: 10 mg/kg immediately before surgery, then 25 mg/kg/dose orally 3-4 times/day for 2-8 days

Alternatively:
Oral: 25 mg/kg 3-4 times/day beginning 1 day prior to surgery
I.V.: 10 mg/kg 3-4 times/day in patients who are unable to take oral

Dosing adjustment/interval in renal impairment:
Cl_{cr} 50-80 mL/minute: Administer 50% of normal dose or 10 mg/kg twice daily I.V. or 15 mg/kg twice daily orally
Cl_{cr} 10-50 mL/minute: Administer 25% of normal dose or 10 mg/kg/day I.V. or 15 mg/kg/day orally
Cl_{cr} <10 mL/minute: Administer 10% of normal dose or 10 mg/kg/dose every 48 hours I.V. or 15 mg/kg/dose every 48 hours orally
Administration Use plastic syringe only for I.V. push
Reference Range 5-10 µg/mL is required to decrease fibrinolysis
Patient Information Report any signs of bleeding or myopathy, changes in vision; GI upset usually disappears when dose is reduced
Nursing Implications Dosage modification required in patients with renal impairment
Dosage Forms
Injection: 100 mg/mL (10 mL)
Tablet: 500 mg

Transamine Sulphate *see* Tranylcypromine Sulfate *on this page*
Transdermal-NTG® *see* Nitroglycerin *on page 799*
Transderm-Nitro® *see* Nitroglycerin *on page 799*
Transderm Scop® *see* Scopolamine *on page 997*
***trans*-Retinoic Acid** *see* Tretinoin *on page 1112*
Trans-Ver-Sal® *see* Salicylic Acid *on page 991*
Tranxene® *see* Clorazepate Dipotassium *on page 263*

Tranylcypromine Sulfate (tran ill sip' roe meen)
Related Information
Antidepressant Agents Comparison *on page 1250-1252*
Brand Names Parnate®
Synonyms Transamine Sulphate
(Continued)

Tranylcypromine Sulfate *(Continued)*

Use Symptomatic treatment of depressed patients refractory to or intolerant to tricyclic antidepressants or electroconvulsive therapy; has a more rapid onset of therapeutic effect than other MAO inhibitors, but causes more severe hypertensive reactions

Pregnancy Risk Factor C

Contraindications Uncontrolled hypertension, known hypersensitivity to tranylcypromine, pheochromocytoma, cardiovascular disease, severe renal or hepatic impairment, pheochromocytoma

Warnings/Precautions Safety in children <16 years of age has not been established; use with caution in patients who are hyperactive, hyperexcitable, or who have glaucoma, suicidal tendencies, diabetes, elderly

Adverse Reactions

1% to 10%: Cardiovascular: Orthostatic hypotension

<1%:

Cardiovascular: Edema, hypertensive crises

Central nervous system: Drowsiness, hyperexcitability, headache

Dermatologic: Skin rash, photosensitivity

Gastrointestinal: Dry mouth, constipation

Genitourinary: Urinary retention

Hepatic: Hepatitis

Ocular: Blurred vision

Overdosage/Toxicology Symptoms of overdose include tachycardia, palpitations, muscle twitching, seizures, insomnia, transient hypotension, hypertension, hyperpyrexia, coma. Competent supportive care is the most important treatment for an overdose with a monoamine oxidase (MAO) inhibitor. Both hypertension or hypotension can occur with intoxication. Hypotension may respond to I.V. fluids or vasopressors, and hypertension usually responds to an alpha-adrenergic blocker. While treating the hypertension, care is warranted to avoid sudden drops in blood pressure, since this may worsen the MAO inhibitor toxicity. Muscle irritability and seizures often respond to diazepam, while hyperthermia is best treated antipyretics and cooling blankets. Cardiac arrhythmias are best treated with phenytoin or procainamide.

Drug Interactions

Decreased effect of antihypertensives

Increased toxicity with disulfiram (seizures), fluoxetine and other serotonin-active agents (eg, paroxetine, sertraline), TCAs (cardiovascular instability), meperidine (cardiovascular instability), phenothiazine (hypertensive crisis), sympathomimetics (hypertensive crisis), sumatriptan (hypothetical), CNS depressants, levodopa (hypertensive crisis), tyramine-containing foods (eg, aged foods), dextroamphetamine (psychosis)

Mechanism of Action Inhibits the enzymes monoamine oxidase A and B which are responsible for the intraneuronal metabolism of norepinephrine and serotonin and increasing their availability to postsynaptic neurons; decreased firing rate of the locus ceruleus, reducing norepinephrine concentration in the brain; agonist effects of serotonin

Pharmacodynamics/Kinetics

Onset of action: 2-3 weeks are required of continued dosing to obtain full therapeutic effect

Half-life: 90-190 minutes

Time to peak serum concentration: Within 2 hours

Elimination: In urine

Usual Dosage Adults: Oral: 10 mg twice daily, increase by 10 mg increments at 1- to 3-week intervals; maximum: 60 mg/day

Dosing comments in hepatic impairment: Use with care and monitor plasma levels and patient response closely

Monitoring Parameters Blood pressure, blood glucose

Test Interactions ↓ glucose

Patient Information Tablets may be crushed; avoid alcohol; do not discontinue abruptly; avoid foods high in tyramine (eg, aged cheeses, Chianti wine, raisins, liver, bananas, chocolate, yogurt, sour cream); discuss list of drugs and foods to avoid with pharmacist or physician; arise slowly from prolonged sitting or lying

Nursing Implications Assist with ambulation during initiation of therapy; monitor blood pressure closely, patients should be cautioned against eating foods high in tyramine or tryptophan (cheese, wine, beer, pickled herring, dry sausage)

Dosage Forms Tablet: 10 mg

Trasylol® *see Aprotinin on page 85*

Travase® *see Sutilains on page 1051*

Trazodone (traz' oh done)
Related Information
Antidepressant Agents Comparison *on page 1250-1252*
Brand Names Desyrel®
Use Treatment of depression
Pregnancy Risk Factor C
Contraindications Hypersensitivity to trazodone or any component
Warnings/Precautions
Safety and efficacy in children <18 years of age have not been established; monitor closely and use with extreme caution in patients with cardiac disease or arrhythmias. Very sedating, but little anticholinergic effects; therapeutic effects may take up to 4 weeks to occur; therapy is normally maintained for several months after optimum response is reached to prevent recurrence of depression.
Adverse Reactions
>10%:
  Central nervous system: Dizziness, dry mouth, headache, confusion
  Gastrointestinal: Nausea, bad taste in mouth
  Neuromuscular & skeletal: Muscle tremors
1% to 10%:
  Central nervous system: Weakness
  Gastrointestinal: Diarrhea, constipation
  Ocular: Blurred vision
<1%:
  Cardiovascular: Hypotension, tachycardia, bradycardia
  Central nervous system: Agitation, seizures, extrapyramidal reactions
  Dermatologic: Skin rash
  Genitourinary: Prolonged priapism, urinary retention
  Hepatic: Hepatitis
Overdosage/Toxicology
Symptoms of overdose include drowsiness, vomiting, hypotension, tachycardia, incontinence, coma, priapism

Following initiation of essential overdose management, toxic symptoms should be treated. Ventricular arrhythmias often respond to lidocaine 1.5 mg/kg bolus followed by 2 mg/minute infusion with concurrent systemic alkalinization (sodium bicarbonate 0.5-2 mEq/kg I.V.). Seizures usually respond to diazepam I.V. boluses (5-10 mg for adults up to 30 mg or 0.25-0.4 mg/kg/dose for children up to 10 mg/dose). If seizures are unresponsive or recur, phenytoin or phenobarbital may be required. Hypotension is best treated by I.V. fluids and by placing the patient in the Trendelenburg position.
Drug Interactions
Decreased effect: Clonidine, methyldopa, anticoagulants
Increased toxicity: Fluoxetine; increased effect/toxicity of phenytoin, CNS depressants, MAO inhibitors; digoxin serum levels increase
Mechanism of Action
Inhibits reuptake of serotonin and norepinephrine by the presynaptic neuronal membrane and desensitization of adenyl cyclase, down regulation of beta-adrenergic receptors, and down regulation of serotonin receptors
Pharmacodynamics/Kinetics
Onset of effect: Therapeutic effects take 1-3 weeks to appear
Protein binding: 85% to 95%
Metabolism: In the liver
Half-life: 4-7.5 hours, 2 compartment kinetics
Time to peak serum concentration: Within 30-100 minutes, prolonged in the presence of food (up to 2.5 hours)
Elimination: Primarily in urine and secondarily in feces
Usual Dosage
Oral: Therapeutic effects may take up to 4 weeks to occur; therapy is normally maintained for several months after optimum response is reached to prevent recurrence of depression

Children 6-18 years: Initial: 1.5-2 mg/kg/day in divided doses; increase gradually every 3-4 days as needed; maximum: 6 mg/kg/day in 3 divided doses
Adolescents: Initial: 25-50 mg/day; increase to 100-150 mg/day in divided doses
Adults: Initial: 150 mg/day in 3 divided doses (may increase by 50 mg/day every 3-7 days); maximum: 600 mg/day
Elderly: 25-50 mg at bedtime with 25-50 mg/day dose increase every 3 days for inpatients and weekly for outpatients, if tolerated; usual dose: 75-150 mg/day
Reference Range
Plasma levels do not always correlate with clinical effectiveness
Therapeutic: 0.5-2.5 µg/mL
Potentially toxic: >2.5 µg/mL
Toxic: >4 µg/mL
(Continued)

Trazodone *(Continued)*

Patient Information Take shortly after a meal or light snack, can be given as bedtime dose if drowsiness occurs; avoid alcohol; be aware of possible photosensitivity reaction; report any prolonged or painful erection

Nursing Implications Dosing after meals may decrease lightheadedness and postural hypotension; use side rails on bed if administered to the elderly; observe patient's activity and compare with admission level; assist with ambulation; sitting and standing blood pressure and pulse

Dosage Forms Tablet: 50 mg, 100 mg, 150 mg, 300 mg

Trecator®-SC *see* Ethionamide *on page 429*

Trendar® [OTC] *see* Ibuprofen *on page 561*

Trental® *see* Pentoxifylline *on page 862*

Tretinoin *(tret′ i noyn)*

Brand Names Retin-A™

Synonyms Retinoic Acid; *trans*-Retinoic Acid; Vitamin A Acid

Use Treatment of acne vulgaris, photodamaged skin, and some skin cancers

Pregnancy Risk Factor C

Pregnancy/Breast Feeding Implications Oral tretinoin is teratogenic and fetotoxic in rats at doses 1000 and 500 times the topical human dose, respectively; however, tretinoin does not appear to be teratogenic when used topically since it is rapidly metabolized by the skin

Contraindications Hypersensitivity to tretinoin or any component; sunburn

Warnings/Precautions Use with caution in patients with eczema; avoid excessive exposure to sunlight and sunlamps; avoid contact with abraded skin, mucous membranes, eyes, mouth, angles of the nose

Adverse Reactions

1% to 10%:

Cardiovascular: Edema

Dermatologic: Excessive dryness, erythema, scaling of the skin, hyperpigmentation or hypopigmentation, photosensitivity, initial acne flare-up

Local: Stinging, blistering

Overdosage/Toxicology Toxic signs of an overdose commonly respond to drug discontinuation, and generally return to normal spontaneously within a few days to weeks; when confronted with signs of increased intracranial pressure, treatment with mannitol (0.25 g/kg I.V. up to 1 g/kg/dose repeated every 5 minutes as needed), dexamethasone (1.5 mg/kg I.V. load followed with 0.375 mg/kg every 6 hours for 5 days), and/or hyperventilation should be employed

Drug Interactions Increased toxicity: Sulfur, benzoyl peroxide, salicylic acid, resorcinol (potentiates adverse reactions seen with tretinoin)

Mechanism of Action Keratinocytes in the sebaceous follicle become less adherent which allows for easy removal; decreases microcomedone formation

Pharmacodynamics/Kinetics

Absorption: Topical: Minimum absorption occurs

Metabolism: Of the small amount absorbed, metabolism occurs in the liver

Elimination: In bile and urine

Usual Dosage Children >12 years and Adults: Topical: Apply once daily before retiring; if stinging or irritation develops, decrease frequency of application. Relapses normally occur within 3-6 weeks after stopping medication.

Patient Information Thoroughly wash hands after applying; avoid hydration of skin immediately before application; minimize exposure to sunlight; avoid washing face more frequently than 2-3 times/day; if severe irritation occurs, discontinue medication temporarily and adjust dose when irritation subsides; avoid using topical preparations with high alcoholic content during treatment period; do not exceed prescribed dose

Nursing Implications Observe for signs of hypersensitivity, blistering, excessive dryness; do not apply to mucous membranes

Dosage Forms

Cream: 0.025% (20 g, 45 g); 0.05% (20 g, 45 g); 0.1% (20 g, 45 g)

Gel, topical: 0.01% (15 g, 45 g); 0.025% (15 g, 45 g)

Liquid, topical: 0.05% (28 mL)

Trexan™ *see* Naltrexone Hydrochloride *on page 773*

TRH *see* Protirelin *on page 952*

Triacetyloleandomycin *see* Troleandomycin *on page 1133*

Triaconazole *see* Terconazole *on page 1061*

Triam-A® *see* Triamcinolone *on this page*

Triamcinolone (trye am sin' oh lone)

Related Information

Corticosteroids Comparisons *on page 1266-1268*

Brand Names Amcort®; Aristocort® Forte; Aristocort® Intralesional Suspension; Aristocort® Tablet; Aristospan®; Atolone®; Azmacort™; Cenocort®; Cenocort® Forte; Flutex®; Kenacort® Syrup; Kenacort® Tablet; Kenalog® Injection; Nasacort®; Tac™-3; Triam-A®; Triamolone®; Tri-Kort®; Trilog®; Trilone®; Trisoject®

Synonyms Triamcinolone Acetonide, Aerosol; Triamcinolone Acetonide, Parenteral; Triamcinolone Diacetate, Oral; Triamcinolone Diacetate, Parenteral; Triamcinolone Hexacetonide; Triamcinolone, Oral

Use

Inhalation: Control of bronchial asthma and related bronchospastic conditions.

Systemic: Adrenocortical insufficiency, rheumatic disorders, allergic states, respiratory diseases, systemic lupus erythematosus, and other diseases requiring anti-inflammatory or immunosuppressive effects

Topical: Inflammatory dermatoses responsive to steroids

Pregnancy Risk Factor C

Contraindications Known hypersensitivity to triamcinolone; systemic fungal infections; serious infections (except septic shock or tuberculous meningitis); primary treatment of status asthmaticus

Warnings/Precautions Because of the risk of adverse effects, systemic corticosteroids should be used cautiously in the elderly, in the smallest possible dose, and for the shortest possible time. Azmacort™ (metered dose inhaler) comes with its own spacer device attached and may be easier to use in older patients. Use with caution in patients with hypothyroidism, cirrhosis, nonspecific ulcerative colitis, and patients at increased risk for peptic ulcer disease; do not use occlusive dressings on weeping or exudative lesions, and general caution with occlusive dressings should be observed; discontinue if skin irritation or contact dermatitis should occur; do not use in patients with decreased skin circulation; avoid the use of high potency steroids on the face. Fatalities have occurred due to adrenal insufficiency in asthmatic patients during and after transfer from systemic corticosteroids to aerosol steroids; several months may be required for recovery from this syndrome; during this period, aerosol steroids do **not** provide the increased systemic steroid requirement needed to treat patients having trauma, surgery, or infections; avoid using higher than recommended dose.

Adverse Reactions

>10%:

Central nervous system: Insomnia, nervousness

Gastrointestinal: Increased appetite, indigestion

1% to 10%:

Ocular: Cataracts

Endocrine & metabolic: Diabetes mellitus hirsutism, joint pain, epistaxis

<1%:

Central nervous system: Fatigue, seizures, mood swings, headache, delirium, hallucinations, euphoria

Dermatologic: Itching, hypertrichosis, skin atrophy, hyperpigmentation, hypopigmentation, acne

Endocrine & metabolic: Amenorrhea, sodium and water retention, Cushing's syndrome, hyperglycemia, bone growth suppression

Gastrointestinal: Oral candidiasis, dry throat, dry mouth, peptic ulcer, abdominal distention, ulcerative esophagitis, pancreatitis

Local: Burning

Neuromuscular & skeletal: Osteoporosis, muscle wasting

Respiratory: Hoarseness, wheezing, cough

Miscellaneous: Bruising, hypersensitivity reactions

Overdosage/Toxicology When consumed in excessive quantities, systemic hypercorticism and adrenal suppression may occur, in those cases discontinuation and withdrawal of the corticosteroid should be done judiciously

Drug Interactions

Decreased effect: Barbiturates, phenytoin, rifampin increased metabolism of triamcinolone; vaccine and toxoid effects may be reduced

Increased toxicity: Salicylates → ↑ risk of GI ulceration

Mechanism of Action Decreases inflammation by suppression of migration of polymorphonuclear leukocytes and reversal of increased capillary permeability; suppresses the immune system by reducing activity and volume of the lymphatic system; suppresses adrenal function at high doses

Pharmacodynamics/Kinetics

Duration of action: Oral: 8-12 hours

Absorption: Topical: Systemic absorption may occur

Time to peak: I.M.: Within 8-10 hours

Half-life, biologic: 18-36 hours

(Continued)

Triamcinolone *(Continued)*

Usual Dosage In general, single I.M. dose of 4-7 times oral dose will control patient from 4-7 days up to 3-4 weeks.

Children 6-12 years:
  Oral inhalation: 1-2 inhalations 3-4 times/day, not to exceed 12 inhalations/day
  I.M. (acetonide or hexacetonide): 0.03-0.2 mg/kg at 1- to 7-day intervals
  Intra-articular, intrabursal, or tendon-sheath injection: 2.5-15 mg, repeated as needed

Children >12 years and Adults:
  Intranasal: 2 sprays in each nostril once daily; may increase after 4-7 days up to 4 sprays once daily or 1 spray 4 times/day in each nostril
  Topical: Apply a thin film 2-3 times/day
  Oral: 4-48 mg/day
  I.M.: Acetonide or hexacetonide: 60 mg (of 40 mg/mL), additional 20-100 mg doses (usual: 40-80 mg) may be given when signs and symptoms recur, best at 6-week intervals to minimize HPA suppression
  Oral inhalation: 2 inhalations 3-4 times/day, not to exceed 16 inhalations/day
  Intra-articular (hexacetonide): 2-20 mg every 3-4 weeks as hexacetonide salt
  Intralesional (use 10 mg/mL) (diacetate or acetonide): 1 mg/injection site, may be repeated one or more times/week depending upon patients response; maximum; 30 mg at any one time; may use multiple injections if they are more than 1 cm apart
  Intra-articular, intrasynovial, and soft-tissue injection (use 10 mg/mL or 40 mg/mL) (diacetate or acetonide): 2.5-40 mg depending upon location, size of joints, and degree of inflammation; repeat when signs and symptoms recur
  Sublesional (as acetonide): Up to 1 mg per injection site and may be repeated one or more times weekly; multiple sites may be injected if they are 1 cm or more apart, not to exceed 30 mg
  See table.

Triamcinolone Dosing

	Acetonide	Diacetate	Hexacetonide
Intrasynovial	2.5-40 mg	5-40 mg	
Intralesional	2.5-40 mg	5-48 mg	Up to 0.5 mg per square inch of affected area
Sublesional	1-30 mg		
Systemic I.M.	2.5-60 mg/d	~40 mg/wk	20-100 mg
Intra-articular		5-40 mg	2-20 average
large joints	5-15 mg		10-20 mg
small joints	2.5-5 mg		2-6 mg
Tendon sheaths	10-40 mg		
Intradermal	1 mg/site		

Patient Information
  Inhaler: Rinse mouth and throat after use to prevent candidiasis
  Topical: Apply sparingly to affected area, rub in until drug disappears, do not use on open skin
  Report any change in body weight; do not discontinue or decrease the drug without contacting your physician; carry an identification card or bracelet advising that you are on steroids; may take with meals to decrease GI upset

Nursing Implications Once daily doses should be given in the morning; evaluate clinical response and mental status; may mask signs and symptoms of infection; inject I.M. dose deep in large muscle mass, avoid deltoid; avoid S.C. dose; a thin film is effective topically and avoid topical application on the face; do not occlude area unless directed

Additional Information 16 mg triamcinolone is equivalent to 100 mg cortisone (no mineralocorticoid activity)

Dosage Forms
  Aerosol:
    Oral inhalation: 100 mcg/metered spray (20 g)
    Topical, as acetonide: 0.2 mg/2 second spray (23 g, 63 g)
  Cream, as acetonide: 0.025% (15 g, 30 g, 60 g, 80 g, 120 g, 240 g); 0.1% (15 g, 20 g, 30 g, 60 g, 80 g, 90 g, 120 g, 240 g); 0.5% (15 g, 20 g, 30 g, 120 g, 240 g)
  Injection, as acetonide: 3 mg/mL (5 mL); 10 mg/mL (5 mL); 40 mg/mL (1 mL, 5 mL, 10 mL)
  Injection, as diacetate: 25 mg/mL (5 mL); 40 mg/mL (1 mL, 5 mL)
  Injection, as hexacetonide: 5 mg/mL (5 mL); 20 mg/mL (1 mL, 5 mL)
  Lotion, as acetonide: 0.025% (60 mL); 0.1% (15 mL, 60 mL)

Ointment, topical, as acetonide: 0.025% (15 g, 28 g, 30 g, 57 g, 80 g, 113 g, 240 g); 0.1% (15 g, 28 g, 57 g, 60 g, 80 g, 113 g, 240 g, 454 g); 0.5% (15 g, 28 g, 57 g, 113 g, 240 g)

Spray, intranasal acetonide: 55 mcg per actuation (100 sprays/canister) (15 mg canister)

Syrup: 4 mg/5 mL (120 mL)

Tablet: 1 mg, 2 mg, 4 mg, 8 mg

Triamcinolone Acetonide, Aerosol *see* Triamcinolone *on page 1112*

Triamcinolone Acetonide, Parenteral *see* Triamcinolone *on page 1112*

Triamcinolone and Nystatin *see* Nystatin and Triamcinolone *on page 812*

Triamcinolone Diacetate, Oral *see* Triamcinolone *on page 1112*

Triamcinolone Diacetate, Parenteral *see* Triamcinolone *on page 1112*

Triamcinolone Hexacetonide *see* Triamcinolone *on page 1112*

Triamcinolone, Oral *see* Triamcinolone *on page 1112*

Triamolone® *see* Triamcinolone *on page 1112*

Triamterene (trye am' ter een)

Brand Names Dyrenium®

Use Alone or in combination with other diuretics to treat edema and hypertension; decreases potassium excretion caused by kaliuretic diuretics

Pregnancy Risk Factor D

Contraindications Hyperkalemia, renal impairment, hypersensitivity to triamterene or any component; do not give to patients receiving spironolactone or amiloride

Warnings/Precautions Use with caution in patients with severe hepatic encephalopathy, patients with diabetes, renal dysfunction, a history of renal stones, or those receiving potassium supplements or ACE inhibitors

Adverse Reactions

1% to 10%:
  Cardiovascular: Hypotension, edema, congestive heart failure, bradycardia
  Central nervous system: Dizziness, headache, fatigue
  Dermatologic: Rash
  Gastrointestinal: Constipation, nausea
  Respiratory: Dyspnea

<1%:
  Cardiovascular: Flushing
  Endocrine & metabolic: Hyperkalemia, dehydration, hyponatremia, gynecomastia, hyperchloremic, metabolic acidosis, postmenopausal bleeding
  Genitourinary: Inability to achieve or maintain an erection

Overdosage/Toxicology Symptoms of overdose include drowsiness, confusion, clinical signs of dehydration, electrolyte imbalance, and hypotension; ingestion of large amounts of potassium-sparing diuretics, may result in life-threatening hyperkalemia. This can be treated with I.V. glucose, with concurrent regular insulin, I.V. sodium bicarbonate. If needed, Kayexalate® oral or rectal solutions in sorbitol may also be used.

Drug Interactions Increased risk of hyperkalemia if given together with amiloride, spironolactone, angiotensin-converting enzyme (ACE) inhibitors
  Increased toxicity of amantadine (possibly by decreasing its renal excretion)

Mechanism of Action Competes with aldosterone for receptor sites in the distal renal tubules, increasing sodium, chloride, and water excretion while conserving potassium and hydrogen ions; may block the effect of aldosterone on arteriolar smooth muscle as well

Pharmacodynamics/Kinetics
  Onset of action: Diuresis occurs within 2-4 hours
  Duration: 7-9 hours
  Absorption: Oral: Unreliable

Usual Dosage Oral:
  Children: 2-4 mg/kg/day in 1-2 divided doses; maximum: 300 mg/day
  Adults: 100-300 mg/day in 1-2 divided doses; maximum dose: 300 mg/day

Dosing comments in renal impairment: Cl_{cr} <10 mL/minute: Avoid use

Dosing adjustment in hepatic impairment: Dose reduction is recommended in patients with cirrhosis

Monitoring Parameters Blood pressure, serum electrolytes, renal function, weight, I & O

Test Interactions Interferes with fluorometric assay of quinidine

(Continued)

Triamterene *(Continued)*

Patient Information Take in the morning; take the last dose of multiple doses no later than 6 PM unless instructed otherwise; take after meals; notify physician if weakness, headache or nausea occurs; avoid excessive ingestion of food high in potassium or use of salt substitute; may increase blood glucose; may impart a blue fluorescence color to urine

Nursing Implications Observe for hyperkalemia; assess weight and I & O daily to determine weight loss; if ordered once daily, dose should be given in the morning

Dosage Forms Capsule: 50 mg, 100 mg

Triamterene and Hydrochlorothiazide *(trye am' ter een & hye droe klor oh thye' a zide)*

Brand Names Dyazide®; Maxzide®

Use Management of mild to moderate hypertension; treatment of edema in congestive heart failure and nephrotic syndrome

Pregnancy Risk Factor C

Contraindications Anuria, hyperkalemia, renal or hepatic failure, hypersensitivity to hydrochlorothiazide, triamterene or any component; concurrent use of potassium supplements

Warnings/Precautions This fixed combination is not indicated for initial therapy of hypertension; therapy requires titration to the individual patient, if dosage so determined represents this fixed combination, its use may be more convenient; safety and efficacy in children have not been established; avoid interchanging brands of drug.

Serum potassium concentrations do not necessarily indicate the true body potassium concentration. A rise in plasma pH or an increase in the circulating levels of insulin or epinephrine may cause a decrease in plasma potassium concentration and an increase in the intracellular potassium concentration. The efficacy of hydrochlorothiazide is limited in patients with Cl_{cr} <30 mL/minute.

Adverse Reactions

1% to 10%: Gastrointestinal: Loss of appetite, nausea, vomiting, stomach cramps, diarrhea, upset stomach

<1%:

Central nervous system: Dizziness, fatigue

Dermatologic: Purpura

Endocrine & metabolic: Electrolyte disturbances

Hematologic: Aplastic anemia, agranulocytosis, hemolytic anemia, leukopenia, thrombocytopenia, megaloblastic anemia

Neuromuscular & skeletal: Muscle cramps

Ocular: Xanthopsia, transient blurred vision

Respiratory: Allergic pneumonitis, pulmonary edema, respiratory distress

Miscellaneous: Bright orange tongue, burning of tongue, cracked corners of mouth

Overdosage/Toxicology

Triamterene: Symptoms of overdose include drowsiness, confusion, clinical signs of dehydration, electrolyte imbalance, and hypotension; ingestion of large amounts of potassium-sparing diuretics, may result in life-threatening hyperkalemia. This can be treated with I.V. glucose with concurrent regular insulin, I.V. sodium bicarbonate and, if needed, Kayexalate® oral or rectal solutions in sorbitol may also be used.

Hydrochlorothiazide: Symptoms of overdose include hypermotility, diuresis, lethargy, confusion, muscle weakness; following GI decontamination, therapy is supportive with I.V. fluids, electrolytes, and I.V. pressors if needed

Drug Interactions

Hydrochlorothiazide:

Decreased effect of oral hypoglycemics; decreased absorption with cholestyramine and colestipol

Increased effect with furosemide and other loop diuretics

Increased toxicity/levels of lithium

Triamterene:

Increased risk of hyperkalemia if given together with amiloride, spironolactone, angiotensin-converting enzyme (ACE) inhibitors

Increased toxicity of amantadine (possibly by decreasing its renal excretion)

Usual Dosage Oral:

Adults: 1-2 capsules twice daily after meals

Elderly: Initial: 1 capsule/day or every other day

Monitoring Parameters Blood pressure, serum electrolytes, BUN, creatinine, liver function tests

Test Interactions Serum creatinine and BUN, bentiromide test, fluorescent measurement of quinidine

Patient Information May be taken with food or milk; take early in day to avoid nocturia; take the last dose of multiple doses no later than 6 PM unless instructed otherwise. A few people who take this medication become more sensitive to sunlight and may experience skin rash, redness, itching, or severe sunburn, especially if sun block SPF ≥15 is not used on exposed skin areas. May increase blood glucose levels in diabetics. Notify physician if weakness, headache, joint swelling, or nausea becomes severe or persistent; may increase blood glucose and may impart a blue fluorescent color to urine.

Nursing Implications Assess weight, I & O reports daily to determine fluid loss; take blood pressure with patient lying down and standing; observe for hyperkalemia; if ordered once daily, dose should be given in the morning

Additional Information Dyazide® and Maxzide® are not bioequivalent. *One product should not be substituted for the other.* Retitration and appropriate changes in dosage may be necessary if patients are to be transferred from one dosage form to the other.

Dosage Forms
Capsule (Dyazide®): Hydrochlorothiazide 25 mg and triamterene 50 mg
Tablet:
Maxzide®-25: Hydrochlorothiazide 25 mg and triamterene 37.5 mg
Maxzide®: Hydrochlorothiazide 50 mg and triamterene 75 mg

Triapin® *see* Butalbital Compound *on page 153*

Triazolam (trye ay' zoe lam)

Related Information
Benzodiazepines Comparison *on page 1256*
Brand Names Halcion®
Use Short-term treatment of insomnia
Restrictions C-IV
Pregnancy Risk Factor X
Contraindications Hypersensitivity to triazolam, or any component, cross-sensitivity with other benzodiazepines may occur; severe uncontrolled pain; preexisting CNS depression; narrow-angle glaucoma; not to be used in pregnancy or lactation
Warnings/Precautions May cause drug dependency; avoid abrupt discontinuance in patients with prolonged therapy or seizure disorders; not considered a drug of choice in the elderly
Adverse Reactions
>10%:
  Cardiovascular: Tachycardia, chest pain
  Central nervous system: Drowsiness, fatigue, impaired coordination, lightheadedness, memory impairment, insomnia, anxiety, depression, headache
  Dermatologic: Rash
  Endocrine & metabolic: Decreased libido
  Gastrointestinal: Dry mouth, decreased salivation, constipation, nausea, vomiting, diarrhea, increased or decreased appetite
  Neuromuscular & skeletal: Dysarthria
  Ocular: Blurred vision
  Miscellaneous: Sweating
1% to 10%:
  Cardiovascular: Syncope, hypotension
  Central nervous system: Confusion, nervousness, dizziness, akathisia
  Dermatologic: Dermatitis
  Gastrointestinal: Weight gain or loss, increased salivation, muscle cramps
  Neuromuscular & skeletal: Rigidity, tremor
  Otic: Tinnitus
  Respiratory: Nasal congestion, hyperventilation
<1%:
  Central nervous system: Reflex slowing
  Endocrine & metabolic: Menstrual irregularities
  Hematologic: Blood dyscrasias
  Miscellaneous: Drug dependence
Overdosage/Toxicology Symptoms of overdose include somnolence, confusion, coma, diminished reflexes, dyspnea, and hypotension. Treatment for benzodiazepine overdose is supportive. Rarely is mechanical ventilation required. Flumazenil has been shown to selectively block the binding of benzodiazepines to CNS receptors, resulting in a reversal of benzodiazepine-induced CNS depression but not always respiratory depression.
Drug Interactions
Decreased effect with phenytoin, phenobarbital
(Continued)

Triazolam *(Continued)*

Increased effect/toxicity with CNS depressants, cimetidine, erythromycin

Mechanism of Action Depresses all levels of the CNS, including the limbic and reticular formation, probably through the increased action of gamma-aminobutyric acid (GABA), which is a major inhibitory neurotransmitter in the brain

Pharmacodynamics/Kinetics
Onset of hypnotic effect: Within 15-30 minutes
Duration: 6-7 hours
Distribution: V_d: 0.8-1.8 L/kg
Protein binding: 89%
Metabolism: Extensively in the liver
Half-life: 1.7-5 hours
Elimination: In urine as unchanged drug and metabolites

Usual Dosage Onset of action is rapid, patient should be in bed when taking medication. Oral:
Children <18 years: Dosage not established
Adults: 0.125-0.25 mg at bedtime

Dosing adjustment/comments in hepatic impairment: Reduce dose or avoid use in cirrhosis
Monitoring Parameters Respiratory and cardiovascular status
Patient Information Avoid alcohol and other CNS depressants; avoid activities needing good psychomotor coordination until CNS effects are known; drug may cause physical or psychological dependence; avoid abrupt discontinuation after prolonged use
Nursing Implications Patients may require assistance with ambulation; lower doses in the elderly are usually effective; institute safety measures
Dosage Forms Tablet: 0.125 mg, 0.25 mg

Triban® see Trimethobenzamide Hydrochloride *on page 1126*

Tribavirin see Ribavirin *on page 979*

Trichlormethiazide (trye klor meth eye' a zide)

Brand Names Metahydrin®; Naqua®
Use Management of mild to moderate hypertension; treatment of edema in congestive heart failure and nephrotic syndrome
Pregnancy Risk Factor D
Contraindications Hypersensitivity to trichlormethiazide, other thiazides and sulfonamides, or any component
Warnings/Precautions Use with caution in renal disease, hepatic disease, gout, lupus erythematosus, diabetes mellitus; some products may contain tartrazine
Adverse Reactions
1% to 10%: Hypokalemia
<1%:
Cardiovascular: Hypotension
Dermatologic: photosensitivity
Endocrine & metabolic: Fluid and electrolyte imbalances (hypocalcemia, hypomagnesemia, hyponatremia); hyperglycemia
Hematologic: Rarely blood dyscrasias
Renal: Prerenal azotemia
Overdosage/Toxicology Symptoms of overdose include hypermotility, diuresis, lethargy, confusion, muscle weakness; following GI decontamination, therapy is supportive with I.V. fluids, electrolytes, and I.V. pressors if needed
Drug Interactions
Decreased effect of oral hypoglycemics; decreased absorption with cholestyramine and colestipol
Increased effect with furosemide and other loop diuretics
Increased toxicity/levels of lithium
Mechanism of Action The diuretic mechanism of action of the thiazides is primarily inhibition of sodium, chloride, and water reabsorption in the renal distal tubules, thereby producing diuresis with a resultant reduction in plasma volume. The antihypertensive mechanism of action of the thiazides is unknown. It is known that doses of thiazides produce greater reduction in blood pressure than equivalent diuretic doses of loop diuretics. There has been speculation that the thiazides may have some influence on vascular tone mediated through sodium depletion, but this remains to be proven.
Pharmacodynamics/Kinetics
Onset of of diuretic effect: Within 2 hours
Peak: 4 hours
Duration: 12-24 hours
Usual Dosage Oral:

Children >6 months: 0.07 mg/kg/24 hours or 2 mg/m²/24 hours
Adults: 1-4 mg/day

Dosing adjustment in renal impairment: Reduced dosage is necessary

Test Interactions ↑ ammonia (B), ↑ amylase (S), ↑ calcium (S), ↑ chloride (S), ↑ cholesterol (S), ↑ glucose, ↑ uric acid (S); ↓ chloride (S), ↓ magnesium, ↓ potassium (S), ↓ sodium (S)

Patient Information May be taken with food or milk; take early in day to avoid nocturia; take the last dose of multiple doses no later than 6 PM unless instructed otherwise. A few people who take this medication become more sensitive to sunlight and may experience skin rash, redness, itching, or severe sunburn, especially if sun block SPF ≥15 is not used on exposed skin areas.

Nursing Implications Assess weight, I & O reports daily to determine fluid loss; take blood pressure with patient lying down and standing

Dosage Forms Tablet: 2 mg, 4 mg

Trichloroacetaldehyde Monohydrate *see* Chloral Hydrate *on page 217*

Trichophyton **Skin Test** (try ko fi′ ton)

Related Information

Skin Testing for Delayed Hypersensitivity *on page 1325-1327*

Brand Names Dermatophytin®

Use Assess cell-mediated immunity; screen for detection of nonresponsiveness to antigens in immunocompromised individuals

Pregnancy Risk Factor C

Contraindications Hypersensitivity to *Trichophyton* as therapy

Warnings/Precautions Systemic reactions can occur if too high a concentration is used; have epinephrine available; do not administer I.V.; observe patient for 15 minutes for an immediate systemic allergic reaction; use with caution in patients with coccidial erythema nodosum; a dilution of 1:10,000 should be used for initial skin test; resuscitative equipment should be available. Scratch or prick test first; test intradermally only to those antigens giving negative or questionable reactions on scratch or prick testing

Adverse Reactions 1% to 10%: Dermatologic: Severe erythema, induration, necrosis, ulceration

Drug Interactions

Decreased effect: Corticosteroids and other immunosuppressive agents may inhibit the immune response to the skin test

Increased toxicity: Patients on nonselective beta-blockers may be more reactive to allergens given for testing or treatment and may be unresponsive to the usual doses of epinephrine used to treat allergic reactions

Stability Refrigerate at 2°C to 8°C (36°F to 46°F)

Usual Dosage

Cleanse the rubber stopper of the vial with liquid antiseptic before withdrawing extract. A sterile tuberculin syringe with 26-gauge, short bevel needle should be used for the injection. The anterior surface of the upper and lower arm is preferable for testing. Cleanse the skin with soap and water or wash with alcohol or other antiseptic. Introduce the needle between the superficial layers of the skin and inject 0.02 mL of the extract.

The intradermal strength supplied is usually safe for testing patients presenting negative scratch test reactions. It is recommended a 1:10 dilution of the stock intradermal strength be used in preliminary testing of patients not previously screened by scratch tests.

The reactions can be read in from 10-30 minutes. A positive reaction is one showing erythema twice as large as the control. Pseudopod formation indicates a definite positive reaction. For uniformity in reporting reactions, see the recommended system in the table.

Trichophyton **Skin Test**

Grade	Erythema (mm)	Papule or Wheal (mm)
0	<5	
±	5-10	5-10
1+	11-20	5-10
2+	21-30	5-10
3+	31-40	10-15 (or with pseudopods)
4+	>40	>15 (or with many pseudopods)

(Continued)

Trichophyton Skin Test *(Continued)*

0.1 mL of the 1:30 V/V concentration intradermally, examine reaction site in 24-48 hours; induration ≥5 mm in diameter is a positive reaction

Administration Administer by intradermal injection into flexor surface of forearm using a tuberculin syringe with a ⅜" to ½" 26- or 27-gauge needle; do not administer I.V.

Patient Information Test must be read at 24-48 hours or 48-72 hours

Dosage Forms Injection:
Diluted: 1:30 V/V (5 mL)
Undiluted: 5 mL

Tridesilon® *see* Desonide *on page 312*

Tridil® *see* Nitroglycerin *on page 799*

Trientine Hydrochloride (trye' en teen)

Brand Names Syprine®

Use Treatment of Wilson's disease in patients intolerant to penicillamine

Pregnancy Risk Factor C

Contraindications Rheumatoid arthritis, biliary cirrhosis, cystinuria, known hypersensitivity to trientine

Warnings/Precautions May cause iron deficiency anemia; monitor closely; use with caution in patients with reactive airway disease

Adverse Reactions
1% to 10%: Hematologic: Anemia, iron deficiency
<1%:
Central nervous system: Malaise
Gastrointestinal: Heartburn, epigastric pain
Local: Tenderness, thickening and fissuring of skin
Neuromuscular & skeletal: Muscle cramps
Miscellaneous: SLE

Overdosage/Toxicology Overdosage is unknown; a single 30 g ingestion resulted in no toxicity; following GI decontamination, treatment is supportive

Drug Interactions Decreased effect with iron and possibly other mineral supplements

Mechanism of Action Trientine hydrochloride is an oral chelating agent structurally dissimilar from penicillamine and other available chelating agents; an effective oral chelator of copper used to induce adequate cupriuresis

Usual Dosage Oral (administer on an empty stomach):
Children <12 years: 500-750 mg/day in divided doses 2-4 times/day; maximum: 1.5 g/day
Adults: 750-1250 mg/day in divided doses 2-4 times/day; maximum dose: 2 g/day

Patient Information Take 1 hour before or 2 hours after meals and at least 1 hour apart from any drug, food, or milk; do not chew capsule, swallow whole followed by a full glass of water; notify physician of any fever or skin changes; any skin exposed to the contents of a capsule should be promptly washed with water

Dosage Forms Capsule: 250 mg

Triethanolamine Polypeptide Oleate-Condensate (trye eth a nole' a meen)

Brand Names Cerumenex®

Use Removal of ear wax (cerumen)

Pregnancy Risk Factor C

Contraindications Perforated tympanic membrane or otitis media, hypersensitivity to product or any component

Warnings/Precautions Avoid undue exposure to peridural skin during administration and the flushing out of ear canal; discontinue if sensitization or irritation occurs

Adverse Reactions <1%: Dermatologic: Mild erythema and pruritus, severe eczematoid reactions, localized dermatitis

Mechanism of Action Emulsifies and disperses accumulated cerumen

Pharmacodynamics/Kinetics Onset of effect: Produces slight disintegration of very hard ear wax by 24 hours

Usual Dosage Children and Adults: Otic: Fill ear canal, insert cotton plug; allow to remain 15-30 minutes; flush ear with lukewarm water as a single treatment; if a second application is needed for unusually hard impactions, repeat the procedure

Monitoring Parameters Evaluate hearing before and after instillation of medication

Patient Information For external use in the ear only; warm to body temperature before using to improve effect; avoid touching dropper to any surface; hold ear lobe up and back; lie on your side or tilt the affected ear up for ease of administration; fill ear canal, let stand for 15-30 minutes, then flush

Nursing Implications Warm solution to body temperature before using; avoid undue exposure of the drug to the periauricular skin

Dosage Forms Solution, otic: 6 mL, 12 mL

Triethylenethiophosphoramide see Thiotepa on page 1086

Trifed® [OTC] see Triprolidine and Pseudoephedrine on page 1131

Trifluoperazine Hydrochloride (trye floo oh per′ a zeen)
Related Information
Antipsychotic Agents Comparison on page 1255
Brand Names Stelazine®
Use Treatment of psychoses and management of nonpsychotic anxiety
Pregnancy Risk Factor C
Contraindications Hypersensitivity to trifluoperazine or any component, cross-sensitivity with other phenothiazines may exist, coma, circulatory collapse, history of blood dyscrasias
Warnings/Precautions Safety in children <6 months of age has not been established; use with caution in patients with cardiovascular disease, seizures, hepatic dysfunction, narrow-angle glaucoma, or bone marrow depression; watch for hypotension when administering I.M. or I.V.; use with caution in patients with myasthenia gravis or Parkinson's disease
Adverse Reactions
>10%:
  Cardiovascular: Hypotension, orthostatic hypotension
  Central nervous system: Pseudoparkinsonism, akathisia, dystonias, tardive dyskinesia (persistent), dizziness
  Gastrointestinal: Constipation
  Ocular: Pigmentary retinopathy
  Respiratory: Nasal congestion
  Miscellaneous: Decreased sweating
1% to 10%:
  Central nervous system: Dizziness
  Genitourinary: Difficulty in urination, ejaculatory disturbances
  Dermatologic: Increased sensitivity to sun, skin rash
  Endocrine & metabolic: Changes in menstrual cycle, changes in libido, pain in breasts
  Gastrointestinal: Weight gain, nausea, vomiting, stomach pain
  Neuromuscular & skeletal: Trembling of fingers
<1%:
  Central nervous system: Neuroleptic malignant syndrome (NMS),
  Dermatologic: Discoloration of skin (blue-gray)
  Endocrine & metabolic: Galactorrhea
  Genitourinary: Priapism
  Hematologic: Agranulocytosis, leukopenia,
  Hepatic: Cholestatic jaundice, hepatotoxicity
  Ocular: Cornea and lens changes, pigmentary retinopathy
  Miscellaneous: Impairment of temperature regulation, lowering of seizures threshold
Overdosage/Toxicology Symptoms of overdose include deep sleep, coma, extrapyramidal symptoms, abnormal involuntary muscle movements, hypo- or hypertension, cardiac arrhythmias

Following initiation of essential overdose management, toxic symptom treatment and supportive treatment should be initiated. Hypotension usually responds to I.V. fluids or Trendelenburg positioning. If unresponsive to these measures, the use of a parenteral inotrope may be required (eg, norepinephrine 0.1-0.2 mcg/kg/minute titrated to response). Seizures commonly respond to diazepam (I.V. 5-10 mg bolus in adults every 15 minutes if needed up to a total of 30 mg; I.V. 0.25-0.4 mg/kg/dose up to a total of 10 mg in children) or to phenytoin or phenobarbital. Neuroleptics often cause extrapyramidal symptoms (eg, dystonic reactions) requiring management with diphenhydramine 1-2 mg/kg (adults) up to a maximum of 50 mg I.M. or I.V. slow push followed by a maintenance dose for 48-72 hours. When these reactions are unresponsive to diphenhydramine, benztropine mesylate I.V. 1-2 mg (adults) may be effective. These agents are generally effective within 2-5 minutes. Cardiac arrhythmias are treated with lidocaine 1-2 mg/kg bolus followed by a maintenance infusion.
(Continued)

Trifluoperazine Hydrochloride *(Continued)*

Drug Interactions
Decreased effect of anticonvulsants (↑ requirements), guanethidine, anticoagulants; decreased effect with anticholinergics

Increased effect/toxicity with CNS depressants, metrizamide (↑ seizures), propranolol, lithium (rare encephalopathy)

Stability Store injection at room temperature; protect from heat and from freezing; use only clear or slightly yellow solutions

Mechanism of Action Blocks postsynaptic mesolimbic dopaminergic receptors in the brain; exhibits a strong alpha-adrenergic blocking effect and depresses the release of hypothalamic and hypophyseal hormones

Pharmacodynamics/Kinetics
Metabolism: Extensive in the liver

Half-life: >24 hours with chronic use

Usual Dosage
Children 6-12 years: Psychoses:

Oral: Hospitalized or well supervised patients: Initial: 1 mg 1-2 times/day, gradually increase until symptoms are controlled or adverse effects become troublesome; maximum: 15 mg/day

I.M.: 1 mg twice daily

Adults:

Psychoses:

Outpatients: Oral: 1-2 mg twice daily

Hospitalized or well supervised patients: Initial: 2-5 mg twice daily with optimum response in the 15-20 mg/day range; do not exceed 40 mg/day

I.M.: 1-2 mg every 4-6 hours as needed up to 10 mg/24 hours maximum

Nonpsychotic anxiety: Oral: 1-2 mg twice daily; maximum: 6 mg/day; therapy for anxiety should not exceed 12 weeks; do not exceed 6 mg/day for longer than 12 weeks when treating anxiety; agitation, jitteriness, or insomnia may be confused with original neurotic or psychotic symptoms

Not dialyzable (0% to 5%)

Administration Give I.M. injection deep in upper outer quadrant of buttock

Reference Range Therapeutic response and blood levels have not been established

Test Interactions ↑ cholesterol (S), ↑ glucose; ↓ uric acid (S)

Patient Information This drug usually requires several weeks for a full therapeutic response to be seen. Avoid excessive exposure to sunlight tanning lamps; concentrate must be diluted in 2-4 oz of liquid (water, carbonated drinks, fruit juices, tomato juice, milk, or pudding); wash hands if undiluted concentrate is spilled on skin to prevent contact dermatosis

Nursing Implications Watch for hypotension when administering I.M. or I.V.; observe for extrapyramidal effects

Dosage Forms
Concentrate, oral: 10 mg/mL (60 mL)

Injection: 2 mg/mL (10 mL)

Tablet: 1 mg, 2 mg, 5 mg, 10 mg

Trifluorothymidine *see* Trifluridine *on this page*

Trifluridine *(trye flure′ i deen)*

Related Information
Antimicrobial Drugs of Choice *on page 1298-1302*

Brand Names Viroptic®

Synonyms F_3T; Trifluorothymidine

Use Treatment of primary keratoconjunctivitis and recurrent epithelial keratitis caused by herpes simplex virus types I and II

Pregnancy Risk Factor C

Contraindications Known hypersensitivity to trifluridine or any component

Warnings/Precautions Mild local irritation of conjunctival and cornea may occur when instilled but usually transient effects

Adverse Reactions
1% to 10%: Ocular: Burning, stinging

<1%: Ocular: Palpebral edema, epithelial keratopathy, keratitis, stromal edema, increased intraocular pressure, hyperemia, hypersensitivity reactions

Stability Refrigerate at 2°C to 8°C (36°F to 46°F); storage at room temperature may result in a solution altered pH which could result in ocular discomfort upon administration and/or decreased potency

Mechanism of Action Interferes with viral replication by incorporating into viral DNA in place of thymidine, inhibiting thymidylate synthetase resulting in the formation of defective proteins

Pharmacodynamics/Kinetics Absorption: Ophthalmic instillation: Systemic absorption is negligible, while corneal penetration is adequate

Usual Dosage Adults: Instill 1 drop into affected eye every 2 hours while awake, to a maximum of 9 drops/day, until re-epithelialization of corneal ulcer occurs; then use 1 drop every 4 hours for another 7 days; do **not** exceed 21 days of treatment; if improvement has not taken place in 7-14 days, consider another form of therapy

Patient Information Notify physician if improvement is not seen after 7 days, condition worsens, or if irritation occurs; do not discontinue without notifying the physician, do not exceed recommended dosage

Dosage Forms Solution, ophthalmic: 1% (7.5 mL)

Trihexy® see Trihexyphenidyl Hydrochloride on this page

Trihexyphenidyl Hydrochloride (trye hex ee fen' i dill)

Brand Names Artane®; Trihexy®

Synonyms Benzhexol Hydrochloride

Use Adjunctive treatment of Parkinson's disease; also used in treatment of drug-induced extrapyramidal effects and acute dystonic reactions

Pregnancy Risk Factor C

Contraindications Hypersensitivity to trihexyphenidyl or any component, patients with narrow-angle glaucoma; pyloric or duodenal obstruction, stenosing peptic ulcers; bladder neck obstructions; achalasia; myasthenia gravis

Warnings/Precautions Use with caution in hot weather or during exercise. Elderly patients require strict dosage regulation. Use with caution in patients with tachycardia, cardiac arrhythmias, hypertension, hypotension, prostatic hypertrophy or any tendency toward urinary retention, liver or kidney disorders, and obstructive disease of the GI or GU tract. May exacerbate mental symptoms when used to treat extrapyramidal reactions When given in large doses or to susceptible patients, may cause weakness.

Adverse Reactions

>10%:

  Gastrointestinal: Constipation

  Miscellaneous: Decreased sweating, dry mouth, nose, throat, or skin

1% to 10%: Decreased flow of breast milk, difficulty in swallowing, increased sensitivity to light

<1%:

  Cardiovascular: Orthostatic hypotension, ventricular fibrillation, tachycardia, palpitations

  Central nervous system: Confusion, drowsiness, headache, loss of memory, weakness, tiredness, ataxia

  Dermatologic: Skin rash

  Gastrointestinal: Bloated feeling, nausea, vomiting

  Genitourinary: Difficult urination

  Ocular: Increased intraocular pain, blurred vision

Overdosage/Toxicology Symptoms of overdose include blurred vision, urinary retention, tachycardia. Anticholinergic toxicity is caused by strong binding of the drug to cholinergic receptors. Anticholinesterase inhibitors reduce acetylcholinesterase; for anticholinergic overdose with severe life-threatening symptoms, physostigmine 1-2 mg (0.5 or 0.02 mg/kg for children) S.C. or I.V., slowly may be given to reverse these effects

Drug Interactions

Decreased effect of levodopa (↑↓)

Increased toxicity with narcotic analgesics, phenothiazines, TCAs, quinidine, levodopa (↑↓), anticholinergics

Mechanism of Action Thought to act by blocking excess acetylcholine at cerebral synapses; many of its effects are due to its pharmacologic similarities with atropine

Pharmacodynamics/Kinetics

Peak effect: Within 1 hour

Half-life: 3.3-4.1 hours

Time to peak serum concentration: Within 1-1.5 hours

Elimination: Primarily in urine

Usual Dosage Adults: Oral: Initial: 1-2 mg/day, increase by 2 mg increments at intervals of 3-5 days; usual dose: 5-15 mg/day in 3-4 divided doses

Monitoring Parameters IOP monitoring and gonioscopic evaluations should be performed periodically

Patient Information Take after meals or with food if GI upset occurs; do not discontinue drug abruptly; notify physician if adverse GI effects, rapid or pounding heartbeat, confusion, eye pain, rash, fever or heat intolerance occurs. Observe caution when performing hazardous tasks or those that require alertness such as driving, as may cause drowsiness. Avoid alcohol and other CNS

(Continued)

Trihexyphenidyl Hydrochloride (Continued)

depressants. May cause dry mouth - adequate fluid intake or hard sugar free candy may relieve. Difficult urination or constipation may occur - notify physician if effects persist; may increase susceptibility to heat stroke.

Nursing Implications Tolerated best if given in 3 daily doses and with food; high doses may be divided into 4 doses, at meal times and at bedtime; patients may be switched to sustained-action capsules when stabilized on conventional dosage forms

Dosage Forms

Capsule, sustained release: 5 mg

Elixir: 2 mg/5 mL (480 mL)

Tablet: 2 mg, 5 mg

Tri-Kort® see Triamcinolone on page 1112

Trilafon® see Perphenazine on page 865

Tri-Levlen® see Ethinyl Estradiol and Levonorgestrel on page 423

Trilisate® see Choline Magnesium Salicylate on page 238

Trilog® see Triamcinolone on page 1112

Trilone® see Triamcinolone on page 1112

Trimazide® see Trimethobenzamide Hydrochloride on page 1126

Trimeprazine Tartrate (trye mep' ra zeen)

Brand Names Temaril®

Synonyms Alimenazine Tartrate

Use Perennial and seasonal allergic rhinitis and other allergic symptoms including urticaria

Pregnancy Risk Factor C

Contraindications Hypersensitivity to trimeprazine or any component

Warnings/Precautions Use with caution in patients with history of narrow-angle glaucoma, bladder neck obstruction, symptomatic prostate hypertrophy, asthmatic attacks, sleep apnea, and stenosing peptic ulcer

Adverse Reactions

>10%:

Central nervous system: Slight to moderate drowsiness

Respiratory: Thickening of bronchial secretions

1% to 10%:

Central nervous system: Headache, fatigue, nervousness, dizziness

Gastrointestinal: Appetite increase, weight increase nausea, diarrhea, abdominal pain, dry mouth

Neuromuscular & skeletal: Arthralgia

Respiratory: Pharyngitis

<1%:

Cardiovascular: Edema, hypotension, palpitations

Central nervous system: Depression, sedation, dizziness, paradoxical excitement, insomnia

Dermatologic: Angioedema, photosensitivity, rash

Genitourinary: Urinary retention

Hepatic: Hepatitis

Neuromuscular & skeletal: Myalgia, paresthesia, tremor

Ocular: Blurred vision

Respiratory: Bronchospasm

Miscellaneous: Epistaxis

Overdosage/Toxicology Symptoms of overdose include deep sleep, coma, extrapyramidal symptoms, abnormal involuntary muscle movements, hypo- or hypertension. There is no specific treatment for an antihistamine overdose, however, most of its clinical toxicity is due to anticholinergic effects. For anticholinergic overdose with severe life-threatening symptoms, physostigmine 1-2 mg (0.5 or 0.02 mg/kg for children) I.V., slowly may be given to reverse these effects.

Drug Interactions Increased effect/toxicity with CNS depressants, alcohol, MAO inhibitors (avoid concomitant use), oral contraceptives, progesterone, reserpine nylidrin

Mechanism of Action Blocks postsynaptic mesolimbic dopaminergic receptors in the brain, exhibits a strong alpha-adrenergic blocking effect and depresses the release of hypothalamic and hypophyseal hormones; competes with histamine for the H_1-receptor; reduces stimuli to the brainstem reticular system

Pharmacodynamics/Kinetics

Absorption: Well absorbed

Metabolism: Extensively hepatically metabolized largely to n-desalkyl metabolites

Bioavailability: Tablet: ~70%; the sustained release capsules give closely comparable serum and urinary levels

Half-life, elimination: 4.78 hours mean

Time to peak serum concentration:

Syrup: 3.5 hours

Tablet: 4.5 hours

Usual Dosage Oral:

Children:

6 months to 3 years: 1.25 mg at bedtime or 3 times/day if needed

>3 years: 2.5 mg at bedtime or 3 times/day if needed

>6 years: Sustained release: 5 mg/day

Adults: 2.5 mg 4 times/day (5 mg every 12-hour sustained release)

Not dialyzable (0% to 5%)

Patient Information May cause drowsiness, impair judgment and coordination; sugarless candy or gum can help with dry mouth; report urinary retention or involuntary movements to physician; do not chew or break sustained release capsule

Nursing Implications Raise bed rails, institute safety measures, observe for extrapyramidal reactions

Dosage Forms

Capsule, extended release: 5 mg

Syrup: 2.5 mg/5 mL

Tablet: 2.5 mg

Trimetaphan Camsilate see Trimethaphan Camsylate on this page

Trimethaphan Camphorsulfonate see Trimethaphan Camsylate on this page

Trimethaphan Camsylate (trye meth' a fan)

Brand Names Arfonad®

Synonyms Trimetaphan Camsilate; Trimethaphan Camphorsulfonate

Use Immediate and temporary reduction of blood pressure in patients with hypertensive emergencies; controlled hypotension during surgery

Pregnancy Risk Factor C

Contraindications Hypersensitivity to trimethaphan camsylate or any component; hypovolemia or shock; anemia; respiratory insufficiency

Warnings/Precautions Use with caution in patients with arteriosclerosis, cardiac, hepatic and renal dysfunction, diabetes mellitus, or Addison's disease. Pupillary dilation does not necessarily indicate anoxia or the depth of anesthesia since the drug appears to have a specific effect on the pupil.

Adverse Reactions

1% to 10%:

Cardiovascular: Hypotension (especially orthostatic), tachycardia

Central nervous system: Restlessness, weakness

Dermatologic: Itching, urticaria

Gastrointestinal: Anorexia, nausea, vomiting, dry mouth, adynamic ileus

Genitourinary: Urinary retention

Ocular: Mydriasis, cycloplegia

Respiratory: Apnea, respiratory arrest

Miscellaneous: Sodium and water retention

Overdosage/Toxicology Symptoms of overdose include hypotension; hypotension usually responds to I.V. fluids or Trendelenburg positioning. If unresponsive to these measures, the use of a parenteral vasoconstrictor may be needed. Bethanechol has proven useful in treating the drug-induced urinary retention.

Drug Interactions

Increased effect:

Anesthetics, procainamide, diuretics, and other hypotensive agents may increase hypotensive effects of trimethaphan

Effects of tubocurarine and succinylcholine may be prolonged by trimethaphan

Stability Refrigerate; however, is stable for up to 14 days at room temperature; solution should be freshly prepared and any unused portion discarded

Mechanism of Action Blocks transmission in both adrenergic and cholinergic ganglia by blocking stimulation from presynaptic receptors to postsynaptic receptors mediated by acetylcholine; possesses direct peripheral vasodilatory activity and is a weak histamine releaser

Pharmacodynamics/Kinetics

Onset of action: Immediate

Peak effect: 5 minutes

Duration: 10-30 minutes

Metabolism: Primarily by postganglionic pseudocholinesterase

(Continued)

Trimethaphan Camsylate *(Continued)*

Elimination: Urinary excretion

Usual Dosage Administration requires the use of an infusion pump

Severe hypertension and hypertensive emergencies: I.V.:

Children: 50-150 mcg/kg/minute; dilute 150 mg x weight (kg) to 250 mL in D_5W then dose in mcg/kg/minute = 10 x infusion rate in mL/hour

Adults: Initial rate: 0.5-1 mg/minute; titrate dose to the desired effect

Hypertension due to acute dissecting aneurysms: Initial rate: 1-2 mg/minute, adjusting as needed to keep systolic blood pressure of 100-120 mm Hg

Controlled hypotension during surgery: Initial rate: 3-4 mg/minute adjusted to maintain blood pressure at a desirable level; usual dosage needed 0.3-6 mg/minute

Monitoring Parameters Blood pressure and heart rate; cardiac monitor and blood pressure monitor required during administration

Nursing Implications Must be diluted; usually mixed as 1 mg/mL concentration in 5% dextrose; solution should be freshly prepared and any unused portion discarded; discontinue drug before wound closure

Dosage Forms Injection: 50 mg/mL (10 mL)

Trimethobenzamide Hydrochloride (trye meth oh ben' za mide)

Brand Names Arrestin®; Tebamide®; T-Gen®; Ticon®; Tigan®; Tiject®; Triban®; Trimazide®

Use Control of nausea and vomiting (especially for long-term antiemetic therapy); less effective than phenothiazines but may be associated with fewer side effects

Pregnancy Risk Factor C

Contraindications Hypersensitivity to trimethobenzamide, benzocaine, or any component; injection contraindicated in children and suppositories are contraindicated in premature infants or neonates

Warnings/Precautions May mask emesis due to Reye's syndrome or mimic CNS effects of Reye's syndrome in patients with emesis of other etiologies; use in patients with acute vomiting should be avoided

Adverse Reactions

>10%: Central nervous system: Drowsiness

1% to 10%:

Cardiovascular: Hypotension

Central nervous system: Dizziness, headache

Gastrointestinal: Diarrhea

Neuromuscular & skeletal: Muscle cramps

<1%:

Central nervous system: Mental depression, convulsions, opisthotonus

Dermatologic: Hypersensitivity skin reactions

Hematologic: Blood dyscrasias

Hepatic: Hepatic impairment

Overdosage/Toxicology Symptoms of overdose include hypotension, seizures, CNS depression, cardiac arrhythmias, disorientation, confusion

Following initiation of essential overdose management, toxic symptom treatment and supportive treatment should be initiated. Hypotension usually responds to I.V. fluids or Trendelenburg positioning. If unresponsive to these measures, the use of a parenteral inotrope may be required (eg, norepinephrine 0.1-0.2 mcg/kg/minute titrated to response). Seizures commonly respond to diazepam (I.V. 5-10 mg bolus in adults every 15 minutes, if needed, up to a total of 30 mg; I.V. 0.25-0.4 mg/kg/dose up to a total of 10 mg in children) or to phenytoin or phenobarbital. Critical cardiac arrhythmias often respond to lidocaine 1-2 mg/kg bolus followed by a maintenance infusion. Extrapyramidal symptoms (eg, dystonic reactions) may be managed with diphenhydramine 1-2 mg/kg (adults) up to a maximum of 50 mg I.M. or I.V. slow push followed by a maintenance dose for 48-72 hours. When these reactions are unresponsive to diphenhydramine, benztropine mesylate I.V. 1-2 mg (adults) may be effective. These agents are generally effective within 2-5 minutes.

Drug Interactions Antagonism of oral anticoagulants may occur

Stability Store injection at room temperature; protect from heat and from freezing; use only clear solutions

Mechanism of Action Acts centrally to inhibit the medullary chemoreceptor trigger zone

Pharmacodynamics/Kinetics

Onset of antiemetic effect:

Oral: Within 10-40 minutes

I.M.: Within 15-35 minutes

Duration: 3-4 hours

Absorption: Rectal: ~60%

Usual Dosage Rectal use is contraindicated in neonates and premature infants

Children:

Rectal: <14 kg: 100 mg 3-4 times/day

Oral, rectal: 14-40 kg: 100-200 mg 3-4 times/day

Adults:

Oral: 250 mg 3-4 times/day

I.M., rectal: 200 mg 3-4 times/day

Patient Information May cause drowsiness, impair judgment and coordination; report any restlessness or involuntary movements to physician

Nursing Implications Use only clear solution; observe for extrapyramidal and anticholinergic effects

Dosage Forms

Capsule: 100 mg, 250 mg

Injection: 100 mg/mL (2 mL, 20 mL)

Suppository, rectal: 100 mg, 200 mg

Trimethoprim (trye meth' oh prim)

Brand Names Proloprim®; Trimpex®

Synonyms TMP

Use Treatment of urinary tract infections; acute otitis media in children; acute exacerbations of chronic bronchitis in adults; in combination with other agents for treatment of toxoplasmosis, *Pneumocystis carinii*

Pregnancy Risk Factor C

Contraindications Hypersensitivity to trimethoprim or any component, megaloblastic anemia due to folate deficiency

Warnings/Precautions Use with caution in patients with impaired renal or hepatic function or with possible folate deficiency

Adverse Reactions

>10%: Dermatologic: Rash, pruritus

1% to 10%: Hematologic: Megaloblastic anemia

<1%:

Central nervous system: Fever

Dermatologic: Exfoliative dermatitis

Gastrointestinal: Nausea, vomiting, epigastric distress

Hepatic: Cholestatic jaundice

Hematologic: Thrombocytopenia, neutropenia, leukopenia

Miscellaneous: Increased LFTS, BUN, and serum creatinine

Overdosage/Toxicology Symptoms of acute toxicity includes: nausea, vomiting, confusion, dizziness; chronic overdose results in bone marrow depression; treatment of acute overdose is supportive following GI decontamination; treatment of chronic overdose is use of oral leucovorin 5-15 mg/day

Drug Interactions Increased effect/toxicity/levels of phenytoin

Mechanism of Action Inhibits folic acid reduction to tetrahydrofolate, and thereby inhibits microbial growth

Pharmacodynamics/Kinetics

Absorption: Oral: Readily and extensive

Protein binding: 42% to 46%

Metabolism: Partially in the liver

Half-life: 8-14 hours, prolonged with renal impairment

Time to peak serum concentration: Within 1-4 hours

Elimination: Significantly in urine (60% to 80% as unchanged drug)

Usual Dosage Oral:

Children: 4 mg/kg/day in divided doses every 12 hours

Adults: 100 mg every 12 hours or 200 mg every 24 hours

Dosing interval in renal impairment:

Cl_{cr} 15-30 mL/minute: Administer 100 mg every 18 hours or 50 mg every 12 hours

Cl_{cr} <15 mL/minute: Administer 100 mg every 24 hours or avoid use

Moderately dialyzable (20% to 50%)

Reference Range Therapeutic: Peak: 5-15 mg/L; Trough: 2-8 mg/L

Patient Information Take with milk or food; report any skin rash, persistent or severe fatigue, fever, sore throat, or unusual bleeding or bruising; complete full course of therapy

Dosage Forms Tablet: 100 mg, 200 mg

Trimethoprim and Sulfamethoxazole *see* Co-trimoxazole *on page 278*

Trimethylpsoralen *see* Trioxsalen *on page 1130*

Trimetrexate Glucuronate (tri me trex' ate)

Brand Names Neutrexin™

Use Alternative therapy for the treatment of moderate-to-severe *Pneumocystis carinii* pneumonia (PCP) in immunocompromised patients, including patients with acquired immunodeficiency syndrome (AIDS), who are intolerant of, or are refractory to, co-trimoxazole therapy or for whom co-trimoxazole and pentamidine are contraindicated (concurrent folinic acid (leucovorin) must always be administered)

Contraindications Previous hypersensitivity to trimetrexate or methotrexate, severe existing myelosuppression

Warnings/Precautions Must be administered with concurrent leucovorin to avoid potentially serious or life-threatening toxicities; leucovorin therapy must extend for 72 hours past the last dose of trimetrexate; use with caution in patients with mild myelosuppression, severe hepatic or renal dysfunction, hypoproteinemia, hypoalbuminemia, or previous extensive myelosuppressive therapies

Adverse Reactions

1% to 10%:

Central nervous system: Seizures, fever

Dermatologic: Rash

Gastrointestinal: Stomatitis, nausea, vomiting

Hematologic: Neutropenia, thrombocytopenia, anemia

Hepatic: Elevated liver function tests

Neuromuscular & skeletal: Peripheral neuropathy

Miscellaneous: Increased serum creatinine, flu-like illness, hypersensitivity reactions

Drug Interactions

Decreased effect of pneumococcal vaccine

Increased toxicity (infection rates) of yellow fever vaccine

Stability Reconstituted I.V. solution is stable for 24 hours at room temperature or 7 days when refrigerated; intact vials should be refrigerated at 2°C to 8°C

Mechanism of Action Exerts an antimicrobial effect through potent inhibition of the enzyme dihydrofolate reductase (DHFR)

Pharmacodynamics/Kinetics

Distribution: V_d: 0.62 L/kg

Metabolism: Extensive in the liver

Half-life: 15-17 hours

Usual Dosage Adults: I.V.: 45 mg/m² once daily over 60 minutes for 21 days; it is necessary to reduce the dose in patients with liver dysfunction, although no specific recommendations exist

Administration Reconstituted solution should be filtered (0.22 µM) prior to further dilution; final solution should be clear, hue will range from colorless to pale yellow; trimetrexate forms a precipitate instantly upon contact with chloride ion or leucovorin, therefore it should not be added to solutions containing sodium chloride or other anions; trimetrexate and leucovorin solutions **must** be administered separately; intravenous lines should be flushed with at least 10 mL of D_5W between trimetrexate and leucovorin

Monitoring Parameters Check and record patient's temperature daily; absolute neutrophil counts (ANC), platelet count, renal function tests (serum creatinine, BUN), hepatic function tests (ALT, AST, alkaline phosphatase)

Patient Information Report promptly any fever, rash, flu-like symptoms, numbness or tingling in the extremities, nausea, vomiting, abdominal pain, mouth sores, increased bruising or bleeding, black tarry stools

Nursing Implications Notify primary physician if there is:

Fever ≥103°F

Generalized rash

Seizures

Bleeding from any site

Uncontrolled nausea/vomiting

Laboratory abnormalities which warrant dose modification

Any other clinical adverse event or laboratory abnormality occurring in therapy which is judged as serious for that patient or which causes unexplained effects or concern

Initiate "Bleeding Precautions" for platelet counts ≤50,000/mm³

Initiate "Infection Control Measures" for absolute neutrophil counts (ANC) ≤1000/mm³

Additional Information Not a vesicant; methotrexate derivative

Dosage Forms Injection: 25 mg

Trimipramine Maleate (trye mi' pra meen)

Related Information

Antidepressant Agents Comparison *on page 1250-1252*

Brand Names Surmontil®

Use Treatment of various forms of depression, often in conjunction with psychotherapy

Pregnancy Risk Factor C

Contraindications Narrow-angle glaucoma; avoid use during pregnancy and lactation

Warnings/Precautions Use with caution in patients with cardiovascular disease, conduction disturbances, seizure disorders, urinary retention, hyperthyroidism or those receiving thyroid replacement; avoid use during lactation; use with caution in pregnancy; do not discontinue abruptly in patients receiving chronic high-dose therapy

Adverse Reactions

>10%:

Central nervous system: Dizziness, drowsiness, headache

Gastrointestinal: Dry mouth, constipation, increased appetite, nausea, weakness, unpleasant taste, weight gain

1% to 10%:

Cardiovascular: Arrhythmias, hypotension

Central nervous system: Confusion, delirium, hallucinations, nervousness, restlessness, parkinsonian syndrome, insomnia

Endocrine & metabolic: Sexual function impairment

Gastrointestinal: Diarrhea, heartburn

Genitourinary: Difficult urination

Neuromuscular & skeletal: Fine muscle tremors

Ocular: Blurred vision, eye pain

Miscellaneous: Excessive sweating

<1%:

Central nervous system: Anxiety, seizures

Dermatologic: Alopecia, allergic reactions, photosensitivity

Endocrine & metabolic: Breast enlargement, galactorrhea, SIADH

Genitourinary: Testicular swelling

Hematologic: Agranulocytosis, leukopenia, eosinophilia

Hepatic: Cholestatic jaundice, increased liver enzymes

Ocular: Increased intraocular pressure

Otic: Tinnitus

Miscellaneous: Trouble with gums, decreased lower esophageal sphincter tone may cause GE reflux

Overdosage/Toxicology Symptoms of overdose include agitation, confusion, hallucinations, urinary retention, hypothermia, hypotension, tachycardia, cardiac arrhythmias

Following initiation of essential overdose management, toxic symptoms should be treated. Ventricular arrhythmias and EKG changes (QRS widening) often respond to systemic alkalinization (sodium bicarbonate 0.5-2 mEq/kg I.V.). Arrhythmias unresponsive to this therapy may respond to lidocaine 1 mg/kg I.V. followed by a titrated infusion. Physostigmine (1-2 mg I.V. slowly for adults or 0.5 mg I.V. slowly for children) may be indicated in reversing cardiac arrhythmias that are life-threatening. Seizures usually respond to diazepam I.V. boluses (5-10 mg for adults up to 30 mg or 0.25-0.4 mg/kg/dose for children up to 10 mg/dose). If seizures are unresponsive or recur, phenytoin or phenobarbital may be required.

Drug Interactions

Decreased effect of guanethidine, clonidine; decreased effect with barbiturates, carbamazepine, phenytoin

Increased effect/toxicity with MAO inhibitors (hyperpyretic crises), CNS depressants, alcohol (CNS depression), methylphenidate (↑ levels), cimetidine (↓ clearance), anticholinergics

Mechanism of Action Increases the synaptic concentration of serotonin and/or norepinephrine in the central nervous system by inhibition of their reuptake by the presynaptic neuronal membrane

Pharmacodynamics/Kinetics

Therapeutic plasma levels: Oral: Occurs within 6 hours

Protein binding: 95%

Metabolism: Undergoes significant first-pass metabolism; metabolized in the liver

Half-life: 20-26 hours

Elimination: In urine

Usual Dosage Adults: Oral: 50-150 mg/day as a single bedtime dose up to a maximum of 200 mg/day outpatient and 300 mg/day inpatient

Monitoring Parameters Blood pressure and pulse rate prior to and during initial therapy; evaluate mental status; monitor weight

Test Interactions ↑ glucose

Patient Information Avoid unnecessary exposure to sunlight; avoid alcohol ingestion; do not discontinue medication abruptly; may cause urine to turn blue-(Continued)

Trimipramine Maleate *(Continued)*

green; may cause drowsiness; can use sugarless gum or hard candy for dry mouth; full effect may not occur for 4-6 weeks

Nursing Implications May increase appetite; may cause drowsiness, raise bed rails, institute safety precautions

Dosage Forms Capsule: 25 mg, 50 mg, 100 mg

Trimox® *see* Amoxicillin Trihydrate *on page 68*

Trimpex® *see* Trimethoprim *on page 1127*

Tri-Norinyl® *see* Ethinyl Estradiol and Norethindrone *on page 425*

Triofed® [OTC] *see* Triprolidine and Pseudoephedrine *on next page*

Triostat™ *see* Liothyronine Sodium *on page 637*

Trioxsalen *(trye ox' sa len)*

Brand Names Trisoralen®

Synonyms Trimethylpsoralen

Use In conjunction with controlled exposure to ultraviolet light or sunlight for repigmentation of idiopathic vitiligo; increasing tolerance to sunlight with albinism; enhance pigmentation

Pregnancy Risk Factor C

Contraindications Hypersensitivity to psoralens, melanoma, a history of melanoma, or other diseases associated with photosensitivity; porphyria, acute lupus erythematosus; patients <12 years of age

Warnings/Precautions Serious burns from UVA or sunlight can occur if dosage or exposure schedules are exceeded; patients must wear protective eye wear to prevent cataracts; use with caution in patients with severe hepatic or cardiovascular disease

Adverse Reactions

>10%:

Dermatologic: Itching

Gastrointestinal: Nausea

1% to 10%:

Central nervous system: Dizziness, headache, mental depression, insomnia, nervousness

Dermatologic: Severe burns from excessive sunlight or ultraviolet exposure

Gastrointestinal: Gastric discomfort

Mechanism of Action Psoralens are thought to form covalent bonds with pyrimidine bases in DNA which inhibit the synthesis of DNA. This reaction involves excitation of the trioxsalen molecule by radiation in the long-wave ultraviolet light (UVA) resulting in transference of energy to the trioxsalen molecule producing an excited state. Binding of trioxsalen to DNA occurs only in the presence of ultraviolet light. The increase in skin pigmentation produced by trioxsalen and UVA radiation involves multiple changes in melanocytes and interaction between melanocytes and keratinocytes. In general, melanogenesis is stimulated but the size and distribution of melanocytes is unchanged.

Pharmacodynamics/Kinetics

Peak photosensitivity: 2 hours

Duration: Skin sensitivity to light remains for 8-12 hours

Absorption: Rapid

Half-life, elimination: ~2 hours

Usual Dosage Children >12 years and Adults: Oral: 10 mg/day as a single dose, 2-4 hours before controlled exposure to UVA (for 15-35 minutes) or sunlight; do not continue for longer than 14 days

Patient Information To minimize gastric discomfort, tablets may be taken with milk or after a meal; wear sunglasses during exposure and a light-screening lipstick; do not exceed dose or exposure duration

Dosage Forms Tablet: 5 mg

Tripedia® *see* Diphtheria and Tetanus Toxoids and Acellular Pertussis Vaccine *on page 354*

Tripelennamine *(tri pel enn' a meen)*

Brand Names PBZ®; PBZ-SR®

Synonyms Pyribenzamine®; Tripelennamine Citrate; Tripelennamine Hydrochloride

Use Perennial and seasonal allergic rhinitis and other allergic symptoms including urticaria

Pregnancy Risk Factor B

Contraindications Hypersensitivity to tripelennamine or any component

Warnings/Precautions Use with caution in patients with narrow-angle glaucoma, bladder neck obstruction, symptomatic prostate hypertrophy, asthmatic attacks, and stenosing peptic ulcer

Adverse Reactions
>10%:
  Central nervous system: Slight to moderate drowsiness
  Respiratory: Thickening of bronchial secretions
1% to 10%:
  Central nervous system: Headache, fatigue, nervousness, dizziness
  Gastrointestinal: Appetite increase, weight increase, nausea, diarrhea, abdominal pain, dry mouth
  Neuromuscular & skeletal: Arthralgia
  Respiratory: Pharyngitis
<1%:
  Cardiovascular: Edema, palpitations, hypotension
  Central nervous system: Depression, epistaxis, sedation, paradoxical excitement, insomnia
  Dermatologic: Angioedema, photosensitivity, rash
  Genitourinary: Urinary retention
  Hepatic: Hepatitis
  Neuromuscular & skeletal: Myalgia, paresthesia, tremor
  Ocular: Blurred vision
  Respiratory: Bronchospasm

Overdosage/Toxicology Symptoms of overdose include CNS stimulation or depression; flushed skin, mydriasis, ataxia, athetosis, dry mouth; there is no specific treatment for an antihistamine overdose, however, most of its clinical toxicity is due to anticholinergic effects. For anticholinergic overdose with severe life-threatening symptoms, physostigmine 1-2 mg (0.5 or 0.02 mg/kg for children) I.V., slowly may be given to reverse these effects.

Drug Interactions Increased effect/toxicity with alcohol, CNS depressants, MAO inhibitors

Mechanism of Action Competes with histamine for H_1-receptor sites on effector cells in the gastrointestinal tract, blood vessels, and respiratory tract

Pharmacodynamics/Kinetics
Onset of antihistaminic effect: Within 15-30 minutes
Duration: 4-6 hours (up to 8 hours with PBZ-SR®)
Metabolism: Almost completely in the liver
Elimination: In urine

Usual Dosage Oral:
Infants and Children: 5 mg/kg/day in 4-6 divided doses, up to 300 mg/day maximum
Adults: 25-50 mg every 4-6 hours, extended release tablets 100 mg morning and evening up to 100 mg every 8 hours

Patient Information Do not crush extended release tablets; urinary hesitancy can be reduced if patient voids just prior to taking drug; may cause drowsiness; swallow whole, do not crush or chew sustained release product; avoid alcohol, may impair coordination and judgment

Nursing Implications Raise bed rails, institute safety measures, assist with ambulation

Dosage Forms
Elixir, as citrate: 37.5 mg/5 mL (473 mL)
Tablet, as hydrochloride: 25 mg, 50 mg
Tablet, extended release, as hydrochloride: 100 mg

Tripelennamine Citrate *see* Tripelennamine *on previous page*

Tripelennamine Hydrochloride *see* Tripelennamine *on previous page*

Triphasil® *see* Ethinyl Estradiol and Levonorgestrel *on page 423*

Triple Antibiotic® *see* Bacitracin, Neomycin, and Polymyxin B *on page 113*

Triple Sulfa *see* Sulfabenzamide, Sulfacetamide, and Sulfathiazole *on page 1039*

Triposed® [OTC] *see* Triprolidine and Pseudoephedrine *on this page*

Triprolidine and Pseudoephedrine (trye proe' li deen)
Related Information
Pseudoephedrine *on page 955*
Brand Names Actagen® [OTC]; Actifed® [OTC]; Allerfrin® [OTC]; Allerphed® [OTC]; Aprodine® [OTC]; Cenafed® Plus [OTC]; Genac® [OTC]; Trifed® [OTC]; Triofed® [OTC]; Triposed® [OTC]
(Continued)

Triprolidine and Pseudoephedrine *(Continued)*

Synonyms Pseudoephedrine and Triprolidine

Use Temporary relief of nasal congestion, decongest sinus openings, running nose, sneezing, itching of nose or throat and itchy, watery eyes due to common cold, hay fever, or other upper respiratory allergies

Pregnancy Risk Factor C

Contraindications MAO therapy, hypertension, coronary artery disease, hypersensitivity to pseudoephedrine or any component

Warnings/Precautions Use with caution in patients >60 years of age; use with caution in patients with high blood pressure, heart disease, diabetes, asthma, or thyroid disease

Adverse Reactions

>10%:

Cardiovascular: Tachycardia

Central nervous system: Slight to moderate drowsiness, nervousness, insomnia, transient stimulation

Respiratory: Thickening of bronchial secretions

1% to 10%:

Central nervous system: Headache, fatigue, weakness, dizziness

Gastrointestinal: Appetite increase, weight increase, nausea, diarrhea, abdominal pain, dry mouth,

Genitourinary: Difficult urination

Neuromuscular & skeletal: Arthralgia

Renal: Dysuria

Respiratory: Pharyngitis

Miscellaneous: Diaphoresis

<1%:

Central nervous system: Depression, epistaxis, hallucinations, convulsions, paradoxical excitement, sedation

Cardiovascular: Edema, palpitations, hypotension

Dermatologic: Angioedema, rash, photosensitivity

Genitourinary: Urinary retention

Hepatic: Hepatitis

Neuromuscular & skeletal: Myalgia, paresthesia, tremor

Ocular: Blurred vision

Respiratory: Bronchospasm, shortness of breath, troubled breathing

Overdosage/Toxicology Symptoms of overdose include hallucinations, CNS depression, seizures, death

There is no specific antidote for pseudoephedrine intoxication and the bulk of the treatment is supportive. Hyperactivity and agitation usually respond to reduced sensory input, however with extreme agitation haloperidol (2-5 mg I.M. for adults) may be required. Hyperthermia is best treated with external cooling measures, or when severe or unresponsive, muscle paralysis with pancuronium may be needed. Hypertension is usually transient and generally does not require treatment unless severe. For diastolic blood pressures >110 mm Hg, a nitroprusside infusion should be initiated. Seizures usually respond to diazepam I.V. and/or phenytoin maintenance regimens.

Drug Interactions

Decreased effect of guanethidine, reserpine, methyldopa

Increased toxicity with MAO inhibitors (hypertensive crisis), sympathomimetics, CNS depressants, alcohol (sedation)

Mechanism of Action Refer to Pseudoephedrine monograph

Triprolidine is a member of the propylamine (alkylamine) chemical class of H_1-antagonist antihistamines. As such, it is considered to be relatively less sedating than traditional antihistamines of the ethanolamine, phenothiazine, and ethylenediamine classes of antihistamines. Triprolidine has a shorter half-life and duration of action than most of the other alkylamine antihistamines. Like all H_1-antagonist antihistamines, the mechanism of action of triprolidine is believed to involve competitive blockade of H_1-receptor sites resulting in the inability of histamine to combine with its receptor sites and exert its usual effects on target cells. Antihistamines do not interrupt any effects of histamine which have already occurred. Therefore, these agents are used more successfully in the prevention rather than the treatment of histamine-induced reactions.

Usual Dosage Oral:

Children:

Syrup:

4 months to 2 years: 1.25 mL 3-4 times/day

2-4 years: 2.5 mL 3-4 times/day

4-6 years: 3.75 mL 3-4 times/day

6-12 years: 5 mL every 4-6 hours; do not exceed 4 doses in 24 hours

Tablet: 1/2 every 4-6 hours; do not exceed 4 doses in 24 hours

Children >12 years and Adults:
  Syrup: 10 mL every 4-6 hours; do not exceed 4 doses in 24 hours
  Tablet: 1 every 4-6 hours; do not exceed 4 doses in 24 hours
Test Interactions ↑ amylase, lipase
Dosage Forms
  Capsule: Triprolidine hydrochloride 2.5 mg and pseudoephedrine hydrochloride 60 mg
  Capsule, extended release: Triprolidine hydrochloride 5 mg and pseudoephedrine hydrochloride 120 mg
  Syrup: Triprolidine hydrochloride 1.25 mg and pseudoephedrine hydrochloride 30 mg per 5 mL
  Tablet: Triprolidine hydrochloride 2.5 mg and pseudoephedrine hydrochloride 60 mg

TripTone® Caplets® [OTC] see Dimenhydrinate on page 347

Tris Buffer see Tromethamine on next page

Tris(hydroxymethyl)aminomethane see Tromethamine on next page

Trisoject® see Triamcinolone on page 1112

Trisoralen® see Trioxsalen on page 1130

Tri-Statin® II see Nystatin and Triamcinolone on page 812

Trisulfam® see Co-trimoxazole on page 278

Tri-Vi-Flor® see Vitamin, Multiple on page 1166

Trobicin® see Spectinomycin Hydrochloride on page 1025

Trocal® [OTC] see Dextromethorphan on page 321

Troleandomycin (troe lee an doe mye' sin)
Brand Names Tao®
Synonyms Triacetyloleandomycin
Use Adjunct in the treatment of corticosteroid-dependent asthma due to its steroid-sparing properties; antibiotic with spectrum of activity similar to erythromycin
Pregnancy Risk Factor C
Contraindications Hypersensitivity to troleandomycin, other macrolides, or any component
Warnings/Precautions Use with caution in patients with impaired hepatic function; chronic hepatitis may occur in patients with long or repetitive courses
Adverse Reactions
  >10%: Gastrointestinal: Abdominal cramping and discomfort
  1% to 10%:
    Dermatologic: Urticaria, skin rashes
    Gastrointestinal: Nausea, vomiting, diarrhea
  <1%:
    Dermatologic: Rectal burning
    Hepatic: Cholestatic jaundice
Overdosage/Toxicology Symptoms of overdose include nausea, vomiting, diarrhea, hearing loss; following GI decontamination, treatment is supportive
Drug Interactions Increased effect/toxicity/levels of carbamazepine, ergot alkaloids, methylprednisolone, theophylline, and triazolam
Mechanism of Action Decreases methylprednisolone clearance from a linear first order decline to a nonlinear decline in plasma concentration. Tao® also has an undefined action independent of its effects on steroid elimination. Inhibits RNA-dependent protein synthesis at the chain elongation step; binds to the 50S ribosomal subunit resulting in blockage of transpeptidation.
Pharmacodynamics/Kinetics
  Time to peak serum concentration: Within 2 hours
  Elimination: 10% to 25% of dose excreted in urine as active drug; also excreted in feces via bile
Usual Dosage Oral:
  Children 7-13 years: 25-40 mg/kg/day divided every 6 hours (125-250 mg every 6 hours)
    Adjunct in corticosteroid-dependent asthma: 14 mg/kg/day in divided doses every 6-12 hours not to exceed 250 mg every 6 hours; dose is tapered to once daily then alternate day dosing
  Children >13 years and adults: 250-500 mg 4 times/day
Administration Administer around-the-clock instead of 4 times/day
Monitoring Parameters Hepatic function tests
Patient Information Complete full course of therapy; notify physician if persistent or severe abdominal pain, nausea, vomiting, jaundice, darkened urine, or fever occurs
(Continued)

Troleandomycin *(Continued)*
Dosage Forms Capsule: 250 mg

Tromethamine *(troe meth' a meen)*
Brand Names THAM®; THAM-E®

Synonyms Tris Buffer; Tris(hydroxymethyl)aminomethane

Use Correction of metabolic acidosis associated with cardiac bypass surgery or cardiac arrest; to correct excess acidity of stored blood that is preserved with acid citrate dextrose; to prime the pump-oxygenator during cardiac bypass surgery; indicated in infants needing alkalinization after receiving maximum sodium bicarbonate (8-10 mEq/kg/24 hours); (advantage of THAM® is that it alkalinizes without increasing pCO_2 and sodium)

Pregnancy Risk Factor C

Contraindications Uremia or anuria; chronic respiratory acidosis

Warnings/Precautions Reduce dose and monitor pH carefully in renal impairment; drug should not be given for a period of longer than 24 hours unless for a life-threatening situation

Adverse Reactions
1% to 10%: Local: Tissue irritation, necrosis with extravasation, venospasm
<1%:
Endocrine & metabolic: Hyperosmolality of serum, hyperkalemia, hypoglycemia
Hematologic: Increased blood coagulation time
Hepatic: Liver cell destruction from direct contact with THAM®
Respiratory: Apnea, respiratory depression

Overdosage/Toxicology Symptoms of overdose include alkalosis, hypokalemia, respiratory depression, hypoglycemia; supportive therapy is required to correct electrolyte, osmolality, and abnormalities

Mechanism of Action Acts as a proton acceptor, which combines with hydrogen ions to form bicarbonate buffer, to correct acidosis

Pharmacodynamics/Kinetics
Absorption: 30% of dose is not ionized
Elimination: Rapidly eliminated by kidneys (>75% in 3 hours)

Usual Dosage Dose depends on buffer base deficit; when deficit is known: tromethamine (mL of 0.3 M solution) = body weight (kg) x base deficit (mEq/L); when base deficit is not known: 3-6 mL/kg/dose I.V. (1-2 mEq/kg/dose)

Metabolic acidosis with cardiac arrest:
I.V.: 3.5-6 mL/kg (1-2 mEq/kg/dose) into large peripheral vein; 500-1000 mL if needed in adults
I.V. continuous drip: Infuse slowly by syringe pump over 3-6 hours

Excess acidity of acid citrate dextrose priming blood: 14-70 mL of 0.3 molar solution added to each 500 mL of blood

Dosing comments in renal impairment: Use with caution and monitor for hyperkalemia and EKG

Administration May give undiluted; infuse into as large a vein as possible; not effective if given orally

Monitoring Parameters Serum electrolytes, arterial blood gases, serum pH, blood sugar, EKG monitoring, renal function tests

Reference Range Blood pH: 7.35-7.45

Nursing Implications If extravasation occurs, aspirate as much fluid as possible, then infiltrate area with procaine 1% to which hyaluronidase has been added

Additional Information 1 mM = 120 mg = 3.3 mL = 1 mEq of THAM®

Dosage Forms
Injection: 36 mg/mL (500 mL)
Powder for injection: 240 mg/mL (150 mL)

Tronolane® [OTC] *see* Pramoxine Hydrochloride *on page 915*

Tronothane® [OTC] *see* Pramoxine Hydrochloride *on page 915*

Tropicacyl® *see* Tropicamide *on this page*

Tropicamide *(troe pik' a mide)*
Related Information
Cycloplegic Mydriatics Comparison *on page 1269*
Brand Names Mydriacyl®; Opticyl®; Tropicacyl®
Synonyms Bistropamide

Use Short-acting mydriatic used in diagnostic procedures; as well as preoperatively and postoperatively; treatment of some cases of acute iritis, iridocyclitis, and keratitis

Pregnancy Risk Factor C

Contraindications Glaucoma, hypersensitivity to tropicamide or any component

Warnings/Precautions Use with caution in infants and children since tropicamide may cause potentially dangerous CNS disturbances; tropicamide may cause an increase in intraocular pressure

Adverse Reactions
1% to 10%:
Cardiovascular: Tachycardia, vascular congestion, edema
Central nervous system: Parasympathetic stimulations, drowsiness, headache
Dermatologic: Eczematoid dermatitis
Gastrointestinal: Dryness of the mouth
Local: Transient stinging
Ocular: Blurred vision, photophobia with or without corneal staining, increased intraocular pressure, follicular conjunctivitis

Overdosage/Toxicology Symptoms of overdose include blurred vision, urinary retention, tachycardia, cardiorespiratory collapse. Antidote is physostigmine, pilocarpine; anticholinergic toxicity is caused by strong binding of the drug to cholinergic receptors. For anticholinergic overdose with severe life-threatening symptoms, physostigmine 1-2 mg (0.5 or 0.02 mg/kg for children) S.C. or I.V., slowly may be given to reverse systemic effects.

Stability Store in tightly closed containers

Mechanism of Action Prevents the sphincter muscle of the iris and the muscle of the ciliary body from responding to cholinergic stimulation

Pharmacodynamics/Kinetics
Onset of mydriasis: ~20-40 minutes
Duration: ~6-7 hours
Onset of cycloplegia: Within 30 minutes
Duration: <6 hours

Usual Dosage Children and Adults (individuals with heavily pigmented eyes may require larger doses):
Cycloplegia: Instill 1-2 drops (1%); may repeat in 5 minutes
Exam must be performed within 30 minutes after the repeat dose; if the patient is not examined within 20-30 minutes, instill an additional drop
Mydriasis: Instill 1-2 drops (0.5%) 15-20 minutes before exam; may repeat every 30 minutes as needed

Monitoring Parameters Ophthalmic exam

Patient Information If irritation persists or increases, discontinue use, may cause blurred vision and increased light sensitivity

Nursing Implications Finger pressure should be applied on the lacrimal sac for 1-2 minutes following topical instillation of the solution

Dosage Forms Solution, ophthalmic: 0.5% (2 mL, 15 mL); 1% (2 mL, 3 mL, 15 mL)

Truphylline® *see* Theophylline/Aminophylline *on page 1072*

Trysul® *see* Sulfabenzamide, Sulfacetamide, and Sulfathiazole *on page 1039*

TSH *see* Thyrotropin *on page 1090*

TSPA *see* Thiotepa *on page 1086*

TST *see* Tuberculin Purified Protein Derivative *on this page*

Tuberculin Purified Protein Derivative (too ber' kyoo lin)

Related Information
Skin Testing for Delayed Hypersensitivity *on page 1325-1327*

Brand Names Aplisol®; Sclavo-PPD Solution®; Tubersol®

Synonyms Mantoux; PPD; Tine Test; TST; Tuberculin Skin Test

Use Skin test in diagnosis of tuberculosis, cell-mediated immunodeficiencies

Pregnancy Risk Factor C

Contraindications 250 TU strength should not be used for initial testing

Warnings/Precautions Do not give I.V. or S.C.; epinephrine (1:1000) should be available to treat possible allergic reactions

Adverse Reactions
1% to 10%:
Dermatologic: Ulceration, necrosis
Local: Vesiculation, pain

Drug Interactions Decreased effect: Reaction may be suppressed in patients receiving systemic corticosteroids, aminocaproic acid, or within 4-6 weeks following immunization with live or inactivated viral vaccines
(Continued)

Tuberculin Purified Protein Derivative *(Continued)*

Stability Refrigerate

Mechanism of Action Tuberculosis results in individuals becoming sensitized to certain antigenic components of the *M. tuberculosis* organism. Culture extracts called tuberculins are contained in tuberculin skin test preparations. Upon intracutaneous injection of these culture extracts, a classic delayed (cellular) hypersensitivity reaction occurs. This reaction is characteristic of a delayed course (peak occurs >24 hours after injection, induration of the skin secondary to cell infiltration, and occasional vesiculation and necrosis). Delayed hypersensitivity reactions to tuberculin may indicate infection with a variety of nontuberculosis mycobacteria, or vaccination with the live attenuated mycobacterial strain of *M. bovis* vaccine, BCG, in addition to previous natural infection with *M. tuberculosis*.

Pharmacodynamics/Kinetics
Onset of action: Delayed hypersensitivity reactions to tuberculin usually occur within 5-6 hours following injection
Peak effect: Become maximal at 48-72 hours
Duration: Reactions subside over a few days

Usual Dosage Children and Adults: Intradermal: 0.1 mL about 4" below elbow; use ¼" to ½" or 26- or 27-gauge needle; significant reactions are ≥5 mm in diameter
Interpretation of induration of tuberculin skin test injections: Positive: ≥10 mm; inconclusive: 5-9 mm; negative: <5 mm
Interpretation of induration of Tine test injections: Positive: >2 mm and vesiculation present; inconclusive: <2 mm (give patient Mantoux test of 5 TU/0.1 mL - base decisions on results of Mantoux test); negative: <2 mm or erythema of any size (no need for retesting unless person is a contact of a patient with tuberculosis or there is clinical evidence suggestive of the disease)

Patient Information Return to physician for reaction interpretation at 48-72 hours

Nursing Implications Test dose: 0.1 mL intracutaneously; store in refrigerator; examine site at 48-72 hours after administration; whenever tuberculin is administered, a record should be made of the administration technique (Mantoux method, disposable multiple-puncture device), tuberculin used (OT or PPD), manufacturer and lot number of tuberculin used, date of administration, date of test reading, and the size of the reaction in millimeters (mm).

Dosage Forms Injection:
First test strength: 1 TU/0.1 mL (1 mL)
Intermediate test strength: 5 TU/0.1 mL (1 mL, 5 mL, 10 mL)
Second test strength: 250 TU/0.1 mL (1 mL)
Tine: 5 TU each test

Tuberculin Skin Test *see* Tuberculin Purified Protein Derivative *on previous page*

Tubersol® *see* Tuberculin Purified Protein Derivative *on previous page*

Tubocurarine Chloride *(too boe kyoor ar' een)*

Related Information
Neuromuscular Blocking Agents Comparison Charts *on page 1276-1278*

Synonyms *d*-Tubocurarine Chloride

Use Adjunct to anesthesia to induce skeletal muscle relaxation

Pregnancy Risk Factor C

Contraindications Hypersensitivity to tubocurarine or any component; patients in whom histamine release is a definite hazard

Warnings/Precautions Use with caution in patients with renal impairment, respiratory depression, impaired hepatic or endocrine function, myasthenia gravis, and the elderly; ventilation must be supported during neuromuscular blockade; rapid administration may cause histamine release resulting in respiratory depression and bronchospasm

Adverse Reactions
1% to 10%: Cardiovascular: Hypotension
<1%:
Cardiovascular Edema, circulatory collapse, cardiac arrhythmias, increased heart rate or bradycardia
Dermatologic: Skin rash, itching, skin flushing, erythema
Gastrointestinal: Increased salivation, decreased GI motility
Respiratory: Bronchospasm
Miscellaneous: Hypersensitivity reactions, allergic reactions

Overdosage/Toxicology Symptoms of overdose include prolonged skeletal muscle weakness and apnea, cardiovascular collapse. Use neostigmine, edrophonium or pyridostigmine with atropine to antagonize skeletal muscle relaxation; support of ventilation and the cardiovascular system through mechanical means, fluids, and pressors may be necessary.

Drug Interactions Increased effect/toxicity with aminoglycosides, ketamine, magnesium sulfate, verapamil, quinidine, clindamycin, furosemide

Stability Refrigerate; **incompatible** with barbiturates

Mechanism of Action Blocks acetylcholine from binding to receptors on motor endplate inhibiting depolarization

Pharmacodynamics/Kinetics Elimination: ~33% to 75% of parenteral dose is excreted unchanged in urine in 24 hours; ~10% excreted in bile

Usual Dosage I.V.:

Neonates <1 month: 0.3 mg/kg as a single dose; maintenance: 0.15 mg/kg/dose as needed to maintain paralysis

Children and Adults: 0.2-0.4 mg/kg as a single dose; maintenance: 0.04-0.2 mg/kg/dose as needed to maintain paralysis

Alternative adult dose: 6-9 mg once daily, then 3-4.5 mg as needed to maintain paralysis

Dosing adjustment/comments in renal impairment: May accumulate with multiple doses and reductions in subsequent doses is recommended

Cl_{cr} 50-80 mL/minute: Administer 75% of normal dose

Cl_{cr} 10-50 mL/minute: Administer 50% of normal dose

Cl_{cr} <10 mL/minute: Avoid use

Dosing comments in hepatic impairment: Larger doses may be necessary

Administration May also give I.M.; administer I.V. undiluted over 60-90 seconds and flush I.V. cannula with NS or D_5W

Monitoring Parameters Mean arterial pressure, heart rate, respiratory status, serum potassium

Dosage Forms Injection: 3 mg/mL [3 units/mL] (5 mL, 10 mL, 20 mL)

Tums® [OTC] *see* Calcium Carbonate *on page 161*

Tuss-DM® [OTC] *see* Guaifenesin and Dextromethorphan *on page 517*

Tussigon® *see* Hydrocodone and Homatropine *on page 545*

Tusstat® *see* Diphenhydramine Hydrochloride *on page 351*

Twilite® [OTC] *see* Diphenhydramine Hydrochloride *on page 351*

Two-Dyne® *see* Butalbital Compound *on page 153*

Tylenol® [OTC] *see* Acetaminophen *on page 17*

Tylenol® With Codeine *see* Acetaminophen and Codeine *on page 19*

Tylox® *see* Oxycodone and Acetaminophen *on page 826*

Typhoid Vaccine (tye' foid)

Related Information

Immunization Guidelines *on page 1389-1405*

Vaccines *on page 1386-1388*

Brand Names Vivotif Berna™

Synonyms Typhoid Vaccine Live Oral Ty21a

Use

Parenteral: Promotes active immunity to typhoid fever for patients intimately exposed to a typhoid carrier or foreign travel to a typhoid fever endemic area

Oral: For immunization of children >6 years and adults who expect intimate exposure of or household contact with typhoid fever, travelers to areas of world with risk of exposure to typhoid fever, and workers in microbiology laboratories with expected frequent contact with *S. typhi*

Typhoid vaccine: Live, attenuated TY21a typhoid vaccine should not be administered to immunocompromised persons, including those known to be infected with HIV. Parenteral inactivated vaccine is a theoretically safer alternative for this group.

Pregnancy Risk Factor C

Contraindications Acute respiratory or other active infections, previous sensitivity to typhoid vaccine, congenital or acquired immunodeficient state, acute febrile illness, acute GI illness, other active infection, persistent diarrhea or vomiting

Warnings/Precautions Postpone use in presence of acute infection; use during pregnancy only when clearly needed, immune deficiency conditions; not all recipients of typhoid vaccine will be fully protected against typhoid fever. Travelers should take all necessary precautions to avoid contact or ingestion of potentially contaminated food or water sources. Unless a complete immunization schedule is followed, an optimum immune response may not be achieved.

(Continued)

Typhoid Vaccine *(Continued)*

Adverse Reactions

Oral:

1% to 10%:

Dermatologic: Skin rash

Gastrointestinal: Abdominal discomfort, stomach cramps, diarrhea, nausea, vomiting

<1%: Anaphylactic reaction

Injection: >10%:

Dermatologic: Local tenderness, erythema, induration

Neuromuscular & skeletal: Myalgia

Drug Interactions Simultaneous administration with other vaccines which cause local or systemic adverse effects should be avoided

Decreased effect with concurrent use of sulfonamides or other antibiotics

Stability Refrigerate, do not freeze; potency is not harmed if mistakenly placed in freezer; however, remove from freezer as soon as possible and place in refrigerator; can still be used if exposed to temperature ≤80°F

Mechanism of Action Virulent strains of *Salmonella typhi* cause disease by penetrating the intestinal mucosa and entering the systemic circulation via the lymphatic vasculature. One possible mechanism of conferring immunity may be the provocation of a local immune response in the intestinal tract induced by oral ingesting of a live strain with subsequent aborted infection. The ability of *Salmonella typhi* to produce clinical disease (and to elicit an immune response) is dependent on the bacteria having a complete lipopolysaccharide. The live attenuate Ty21a strain lacks the enzyme UDP-4-galactose epimerase so that lipopolysaccharide is only synthesized under conditions that induce bacterial autolysis. Thus, the strain remains avirulent despite the production of sufficient lipopolysaccharide to evoke a protective immune response. Despite low levels of lipopolysaccharide synthesis, cells lyse before gaining a virulent phenotype due to the intracellular accumulation of metabolic intermediates.

Pharmacodynamics/Kinetics

Oral:

Onset of immunity to *Salmonella typhi*: Within about 1 week

Duration: ~5 years

Parenteral: Duration of immunity: ~3 years

Usual Dosage

S.C.:

Children 6 months to 10 years: 0.25 mL; repeat in ≥4 weeks (total immunization is 2 doses)

Children >10 years and Adults: 0.5 mL; repeat dose in ≥4 weeks (total immunization is 2 doses)

Booster: 0.25 mL every 3 years for children 6 months to 10 years and 0.5 mL every 3 years for children >10 years and adults

Oral: Adults:

Primary immunization: 1 capsule on alternate days (day 1, 3, 5, and 7)

Booster immunization: Repeat full course of primary immunization every 5 years

Patient Information Oral capsule should be taken 1 hour before a meal with cold or lukewarm drink, do not chew, swallow whole; systemic adverse effects may persist for 1-2 days. Take all 4 doses exactly as directed on alternate days to obtain a maximal response.

Nursing Implications The doses of vaccine are different between S.C. and intradermal; S.C. injection only should be used

Additional Information Inactivated bacteria vaccine; federal law requires that the date of administration, the vaccine manufacturer, lot number of vaccine, and the administering person's name, title and address be entered into the patient's permanent medical record

Dosage Forms

Capsule, enteric coated: Viable *S. typhi* Ty21a Colony-forming units 2-6 x 10^9 and nonviable *S. typhi* Ty21a Colony-forming units 50 x 10^9 with sucrose, ascorbic acid, amino acid mixture, lactose and magnesium stearate

Injection: 1.5 mL

Typhoid Vaccine Live Oral Ty21a *see* Typhoid Vaccine *on previous page*

Tyzine® *see* Tetrahydrozoline Hydrochloride *on page 1071*

U-Cort™ Cortifoam® *see* Hydrocortisone *on page 546*

Ultracef® *see* Cefadroxil Monohydrate *on page 192*

Ultralente® U [OTC] *see* Insulin Preparations *on page 578*

Ultram® *see* Tramadol Hydrochloride *on page 1108*

Ultra Mide® *see* Urea *on next page*

Ultravate™ *see* Halobetasol Propionate *on page 524*

Unasyn® *see* Ampicillin Sodium and Sulbactam Sodium *on page 74*

Unguentine® [OTC] *see* Benzocaine *on page 121*

Unicap® [OTC] *see* Vitamin, Multiple *on page 1166*

Unipen® *see* Nafcillin Sodium *on page 768*

Uni-Pro® [OTC] *see* Ibuprofen *on page 561*

Uni-Tussin® [OTC] *see* Guaifenesin *on page 515*

Uni-tussin® DM [OTC] *see* Guaifenesin and Dextromethorphan *on page 517*

Unna's Boot *see* Zinc Gelatin *on page 1175*

Unna's Paste *see* Zinc Gelatin *on page 1175*

Urabeth® *see* Bethanechol Chloride *on page 132*

Uracil Mustard (yoor´ a sill)

Use Palliative treatment in symptomatic chronic lymphocytic leukemia; non-Hodgkin's lymphomas, chronic myelocytic leukemia, mycosis fungoides, thrombocytosis, polycythemia vera, ovarian carcinoma

Pregnancy Risk Factor X

Contraindications Severe leukopenia, thrombocytopenia, aplastic anemia; in patients whose bone marrow is infiltrated with malignant cells; hypersensitivity to any component

Warnings/Precautions The U.S. Food and Drug Administration (FDA) currently recommends that procedures for proper handling and disposal of antineoplastic agents be considered. Impaired kidney or liver function. The drug should be discontinued if intractable vomiting or diarrhea, precipitous falls in leukocyte or platelet count, or myocardial ischemia occurs. Use with caution in patients who have had high-dose pelvic radiation or previous use of alkylating agents. Patient should be hospitalized during initial course of therapy; may impair fertility in men and women; use with caution in patients with pre-existing marrow depression.

Adverse Reactions
>10%:
  Gastrointestinal: Nausea, vomiting, diarrhea
  Myelosuppressive: Leukopenia and thrombocytopenia nadir: 2-4 weeks, anemia
1% to 10%:
  Central nervous system: Mental depression, nervousness
  Dermatologic: Hyperpigmentation, alopecia
  Renal: Hyperuricemia
<1%:
  Dermatologic: Pruritus
  Gastrointestinal: Stomatitis, hepatotoxicity

Overdosage/Toxicology Symptoms of overdose include diarrhea, vomiting, severe marrow depression; no specific antidote to marrow toxicity is available

Mechanism of Action Polyfunctional alkylating agent. The basic reaction of uracil mustard, like that of any alkylating agent, is the replacement of the hydrogen in a reacting chemical with an alkyl group; cell cycle-phase nonspecific antineoplastic agent; exact site of drug action within the cell is not known, but the nucleoproteins of the cell nucleus are believed to be involved.

Pharmacodynamics/Kinetics
Absorption: Oral
Elimination: <1% detected in urine

Usual Dosage Oral (do not administer until 2-3 weeks after maximum effect of any previous x-ray or cytotoxic drug therapy of the bone marrow is obtained):

Children: 0.3 mg/kg in a single weekly dose for 4 weeks
Adults: 0.15 mg/kg in a single weekly dose for 4 weeks
  Thrombocytosis: 1-2 mg/day for 14 days

Patient Information Notify physician of persistent or severe nausea, diarrhea, fever, sore throat, chills, bleeding, or bruising

Dosage Forms Capsule: 1 mg

Urea (yoor ee´ a)

Brand Names Amino-Cerv™ Vaginal Cream; Aquacare® [OTC]; Carmol® [OTC]; Nutraplus® [OTC]; Rea-Lo® [OTC]; Ultra Mide®; Ureacin®-20 [OTC]; Ureacin®-40; Ureaphil®

Synonyms Carbamide
(Continued)

Urea *(Continued)*

Use Reduces intracranial pressure and intraocular pressure; topically promotes hydration and removal of excess keratin in hyperkeratotic conditions and dry skin; mild cervicitis

Pregnancy Risk Factor C

Contraindications Severely impaired renal function, hepatic failure; active intracranial bleeding, sickle cell anemia, topical use in viral skin disease

Warnings/Precautions Urea should not be used near the eyes; use with caution if applied to face, broken, or inflamed skin; use with caution in patients with mild hepatic or renal impairment

Adverse Reactions
>10%: Gastrointestinal: Nausea, vomiting
1% to 10%:
  Central nervous system: Headache
  Local: Transient stinging, local irritation, tissue necrosis from extravasation of I.V. preparation
<1%: Endocrine & metabolic: Electrolyte imbalance

Overdosage/Toxicology Increased BUN, decreased renal function; treatment is supportive

Drug Interactions Decreased effect/toxicity/levels of lithium

Mechanism of Action Elevates plasma osmolality by inhibiting tubular reabsorption of water, thus enhancing the flow of water into extracellular fluid

Pharmacodynamics/Kinetics
Onset of therapeutic effect: I.V.: Maximum effects within 1-2 hours
Duration: 3-6 hours (diuresis can continue for up to 10 hours)
Distribution: Crosses the placenta; appears in breast milk
Half-life: 1 hour
Elimination: Excreted unchanged in urine

Usual Dosage
Children: I.V. slow infusion:
  <2 years: 0.1-0.5 g/kg
  >2 years: 0.5-1.5 g/kg

Adults:
  I.V. infusion: 1-1.5 g/kg by slow infusion (1-2½ hours); maximum: 120 g/24 hours
  Topical: Apply 1-3 times/day
  Vaginal: Insert 1 applicatorful in vagina at bedtime for 2-4 weeks

Patient Information Moisturizing effect is enhanced by applying to the skin while it is still moist after washing or bathing; for external use only

Nursing Implications Do not infuse into leg veins; injection dosage form may be used orally, mix with carbonated beverages, jelly or jam, to mask unpleasant flavor

Dosage Forms
Cream:
  Topical: 2% [20 mg/mL] (75 g); 10% [100 mg/mL] (75 g, 90 g, 454 g); 20% [200 mg/mL] (45 g, 75 g, 90 g, 454 g); 30% [300 mg/mL] (60 g, 454 g); 40% (30 g)
  Vaginal: 8.34% [83.4 mg/g] (82.5 g)
Injection: 40 g/150 mL
Lotion: 2% (240 mL); 10% (180 mL, 240 mL, 480 mL); 15% (120 mL, 480 mL); 25% (180 mL)

Ureacin®-20 [OTC] *see* Urea *on previous page*

Ureacin®-40 *see* Urea *on previous page*

Urea Peroxide *see* Carbamide Peroxide *on page 179*

Ureaphil® *see* Urea *on previous page*

Urecholine® *see* Bethanechol Chloride *on page 132*

Urex® *see* Methenamine *on page 706*

Urised® *see* Methenamine *on page 706*

Urispas® *see* Flavoxate *on page 457*

Uri-Tet® *see* Oxytetracycline Hydrochloride *on page 832*

Urobak® *see* Sulfamethoxazole *on page 1042*

Urodine® *see* Phenazopyridine Hydrochloride *on page 866*

Urofollitropin *(yoor oh fol li troe' pin)*

Brand Names Metrodin®

Use Induction of ovulation in patients with polycystic ovarian disease and to stimulate the development of multiple oocytes

Pregnancy Risk Factor X

Contraindications Prior hypersensitivity to the drug; high levels of both LH and FSH indicating primary ovarian failure; uncontrolled thyroid or adrenal dysfunction; organic intracranial lesion such as a pituitary tumor; presence of any cause of infertility other than anovulation, unless the patient is a candidate for *in vitro* fertilization; abnormal bleeding of undetermined nature; ovarian cysts or enlargement not due to polycystic ovarian disease; pregnancy; may cause fetal harm when administered to pregnant women

Warnings/Precautions Use lowest dose possible to avoid abnormal ovarian enlargement; if hyperstimulation occurs, discontinue use and hospitalize patient; use with caution in patients with a history of thromboembolism

Adverse Reactions
>10%:
Endocrine & metabolic: Ovarian enlargement
Local: Swelling at injection site, pain
1% to 10%:
Cardiovascular: Arterial thromboembolism
Central nervous system: Fever, chills
Dermatologic: Rash
Gastrointestinal: Nausea, vomiting, abdominal pain, diarrhea
Miscellaneous: Hyperstimulation syndrome

Overdosage/Toxicology Symptoms of overdose include possible hyperstimulation and multiple gestations; supportive care to maintain fluid and electrolyte imbalance may be needed

Stability Protect from light; refrigerate at 3°C to 25°C (37°F to 77°F)

Mechanism of Action Preparation of follicle-stimulating hormone 75 IU with <1 IU of luteinizing hormone (LH) which is isolated from the urine of postmenopausal women. Follicle-stimulating hormone plays a role in the development of follicles. Elevated FSH levels early in the normal menstrual cycle are thought to play a significant role in recruiting a cohort of follicles for maturation. A single follicle is enriched with FSH receptors and becomes dominant over the rest of the recruited follicles. The increased number of FSH receptors allows it to grow despite declining FSH levels. This dominant follicle secretes low levels of estrogen and inhibin which further reduces pituitary FSH output. The ovarian stroma, under the influence of luteinizing hormone, produces androgens which the dominant follicle uses as precursors for estrogens.

Pharmacodynamics/Kinetics
Half-life, elimination: 3.9 hours and 70.4 hours (FSH has two half-lives)
Elimination:
Renal clearance: 0.75 mL/minute
Metabolic: 17.2 mL/minute

Usual Dosage Adults: Female: I.M.: 75 units/day for 7-12 days, used with hCG may repeat course of treatment 2 more times

Dosage Forms Injection: 0.83 mg [75 units FSH activity] (2 mL)

Urogesic® *see* Phenazopyridine Hydrochloride *on page 866*

Urokinase (yoor oh kin' ase)
Brand Names Abbokinase®
Use Thrombolytic agent used in treatment of recent severe or massive deep vein thrombosis, pulmonary emboli, myocardial infarction, and occluded arteriovenous cannulas; more expensive than streptokinase; not useful on thrombi over 1 week old

Pregnancy Risk Factor B

Contraindications Hypersensitivity to urokinase or any component; active internal bleeding; CVA (within 2 months); brain carcinoma, bacterial endocarditis, anticoagulant therapy, intracranial or intraspinal surgery, surgery or trauma within past 10 days

Warnings/Precautions Use with caution in patients with severe hypertension, recent L.P., patients receiving I.M. administration of medications, patients with trauma or surgery in the last 10 days

Adverse Reactions
>10%:
Cardiovascular: Hypotension, arrhythmias
Central nervous system: Angioneurotic edema
Endocrine & metabolic: Periorbital swelling
Hematologic: Bleeding at sites of percutaneous trauma
Respiratory: Bronchospasm
Miscellaneous: Anaphylaxis
<1%:
Central nervous system: Epistaxis, headache, chills
Dermatologic: Rash
(Continued)

Urokinase (Continued)

Gastrointestinal: Nausea, vomiting
Hematologic: Anemia
Ocular: Eye hemorrhage
Respiratory: Bronchospasm
Miscellaneous: Sweating

Overdosage/Toxicology Symptoms of overdose include epistaxis, bleeding gums, hematoma, spontaneous ecchymoses, oozing at catheter site. In case of overdose, stop infusion, reverse bleeding with blood products that contain clotting factors.

Drug Interactions Increased toxicity (↑ bleeding) with anticoagulants, antiplatelet drugs, aspirin, indomethacin, dextran

Stability Store in refrigerator; reconstitute by gently rolling and tilting; do not shake; contains no preservatives, should not be reconstituted until immediately before using, discard unused portion; stable at room temperature for 24 hours after reconstitution

Mechanism of Action Promotes thrombolysis by directly activating plasminogen to plasmin, which degrades fibrin, fibrinogen, and other procoagulant plasma proteins

Pharmacodynamics/Kinetics

Onset of action: I.V.: Fibrinolysis occurs rapidly

Duration: 4 or more hours

Half-life: 10-20 minutes

Elimination: Cleared by the liver with a small amount excreted in urine and bile

Usual Dosage

Children and Adults: Deep vein thrombosis: I.V.: Loading: 4400 units/kg over 10 minutes, then 4400 units/kg/hour for 12 hours

Adults:

Myocardial infarction: Intracoronary: 750,000 units over 2 hours (6000 units/minute over up to 2 hours)

Occluded I.V. catheters:

5000 units (use only Abbokinase® Open Cath) in each lumen over 1-2 minutes, leave in lumen for 1-4 hours, then aspirate; may repeat with 10,000 units in each lumen if 5000 units fails to clear the catheter; **do not infuse into the patient**; volume to instill into catheter is equal to the volume of the catheter

I.V. infusion: 200 units/kg/hour in each lumen for 12-48 hours at a rate of at least 20 mL/hour

Dialysis patients: 5000 units is administered in each lumen over 1-2 minutes; leave urokinase in lumen for 1-2 days, then aspirate

Clot lysis (large vessel thrombi): Loading: I.V.: 4400 units/kg over 10 minutes, increase to 6000 units/kg/hour; maintenance: 4400-6000 units/kg/hour adjusted to achieve clot lysis or patency of affected vessel; doses up to 50,000 units/kg/hour have been used. **Note:** Therapy should be initiated as soon as possible after diagnosis of thrombi and continued until clot is dissolved (usually 24-72 hours).

Acute pulmonary embolism: Three treatment alternatives: 3 million unit dosage

Alternative 1: 12-hour infusion: 4400 units/kg (2000 units/lb) bolus over 10 minutes followed by 4400 units/kg/hour (2000 units/lb); begin heparin 1000 units/hour approximately 3-4 hours after completion of urokinase infusion or when PTT is <100 seconds

Alternative 2: 2-hour infusion: 1 million unit bolus over 10 minutes followed by 2 million units over 110 minutes; begin heparin 1000 units/hour approximately 3-4 hours after completion of urokinase infusion or when PTT is <100 seconds

Alternative 3: Bolus dose only: 15,000 units/kg over 10 minutes; begin heparin 1000 units/hour approximately 3-4 hours after completion of urokinase infusion or when PTT is <100 seconds

Administration Use 0.22 or 0.45 micron filter during I.V. therapy

Monitoring Parameters CBC, reticulocyte count, platelet count, DIC panel (fibrinogen, plasminogen, FDP, D-dimer, PT, PTT), thrombosis panel (AT-III, protein C), urinalysis, ACT

Dosage Forms

Powder for injection: 250,000 units (5 mL)

Powder for injection, catheter clear: 5000 units (1 mL)

Uro-KP-Neutral® see Potassium Phosphate and Sodium Phosphate on page 912

Urolene Blue® see Methylene Blue on page 721

Uroplus® DS see Co-trimoxazole on page 278

Uroplus® SS *see* Co-trimoxazole *on page 278*

Ursodeoxycholic Acid *see* Ursodiol *on this page*

Ursodiol (er' soe dye ole)

Brand Names Actigall™

Synonyms Ursodeoxycholic Acid

Use Gallbladder stone dissolution

Pregnancy Risk Factor B

Contraindications Not to be used with cholesterol, radiopaque, bile pigment stones, or stones >20 mm in diameter; allergy to bile acids

Warnings/Precautions Gallbladder stone dissolution may take several months of therapy; complete dissolution may not occur and recurrence of stones within 5 years has been observed in 50% of patients; use with caution in patients with a nonvisualizing gallbladder and those with chronic liver disease; not recommended for children

Adverse Reactions

1% to 10%: Gastrointestinal: Diarrhea

<1%:

Central nervous system: Fatigue, headache

Dermatologic: Pruritus, rash

Gastrointestinal: Nausea, vomiting, dyspepsia, metallic taste, abdominal pain, biliary pain, constipation

Overdosage/Toxicology Symptoms of overdose include diarrhea; no specific therapy for diarrhea and for overdose

Drug Interactions Decreased effect with aluminum-containing antacids, cholestyramine, colestipol, clofibrate, oral contraceptives (estrogens)

Mechanism of Action Decreases the cholesterol content of bile and bile stones by reducing the secretion of cholesterol from the liver and the fractional reabsorption of cholesterol by the intestines

Pharmacodynamics/Kinetics

Metabolism: Undergoes extensive enterohepatic recycling; following hepatic conjugation and biliary secretion, the drug is hydrolyzed to active ursodiol, where it is recycled or transformed to lithocholic acid by colonic microbial flora

Half-life: 100 hours

Elimination: In feces via bile

Usual Dosage Adults: Oral: 8-10 mg/kg/day in 2-3 divided doses; use beyond 24 months is not established; obtain ultrasound images at 6-month intervals for the first year of therapy; 30% of patients have stone recurrence after dissolution

Monitoring Parameters ALT, AST, sonogram

Patient Information Frequent blood work necessary to follow drug effects; report any persistent nausea, vomiting, abdominal pain

Dosage Forms Capsule: 300 mg

Urticort® *see* Betamethasone *on page 129*

Utimox® *see* Amoxicillin Trihydrate *on page 68*

Vaccines *see page 1386*

Vagilia® *see* Sulfabenzamide, Sulfacetamide, and Sulfathiazole *on page 1039*

Vagistat® *see* Tioconazole *on page 1096*

Vagitrol® *see* Sulfanilamide *on page 1043*

Valadol® [OTC] *see* Acetaminophen *on page 17*

Valdrene® *see* Diphenhydramine Hydrochloride *on page 351*

Valergen® *see* Estradiol *on page 407*

Valisone® *see* Betamethasone *on page 129*

Valium® *see* Diazepam *on page 324*

Valpin® 50 *see* Anisotropine Methylbromide *on page 78*

Valproate Semisodium *see* Valproic Acid and Derivatives *on this page*

Valproate Sodium *see* Valproic Acid and Derivatives *on this page*

Valproic Acid *see* Valproic Acid and Derivatives *on this page*

Valproic Acid and Derivatives (val proe' ik)

Brand Names Depakene®; Depakote®

Synonyms Dipropylacetic Acid; Divalproex Sodium; DPA; 2-Propylpentanoic Acid; 2-Propylvaleric Acid; Valproate Semisodium; Valproate Sodium; Valproic Acid

Use Management of simple and complex absence seizures; mixed seizure types; myoclonic and generalized tonic-clonic (grand mal) seizures; may be effective in partial seizures and infantile spasms

Pregnancy Risk Factor D

Contraindications Hypersensitivity to valproic acid or derivatives or any component; hepatic dysfunction

Warnings/Precautions Hepatic failure resulting in fatalities has occurred in patients; children <2 years of age are at considerable risk; monitor patients closely for appearance of malaise, weakness, facial edema, anorexia, jaundice, and vomiting; may cause severe thrombocytopenia, bleeding; hepatotoxicity has been reported after 3 days to 6 months of therapy; tremors may indicate overdosage; use with caution in patients receiving other anticonvulsants

Adverse Reactions

1% to 10%:

Endocrine & metabolic: Change in menstrual cycle

Gastrointestinal: Abdominal cramps, anorexia, diarrhea, nausea, vomiting, weight gain

<1%:

Central nervous system: Drowsiness, ataxia, irritability, confusion, restlessness, hyperactivity, headache

Dermatologic: Alopecia, erythema multiforme

Endocrine & metabolic: Hyperammonemia

Gastrointestinal: Pancreatitis

Hematologic: Thrombocytopenia, prolongation of bleeding time

Hepatic: Transient increased liver enzymes, liver failure

Neuromuscular & skeletal: Tremor, malaise

Ocular: Nystagmus, spots before eyes

Overdosage/Toxicology Symptoms of overdose include coma, deep sleep, motor restlessness, visual hallucinations; supportive treatment is necessary; naloxone has been used to reverse CNS depressant effects, but may block action of other anticonvulsants

Drug Interactions

Decreased effect of phenytoin, clonazepam, diazepam; decreased effect with phenobarbital, primidone, phenytoin, carbamazepine

Increased effect/toxicity with CNS depressants, alcohol, aspirin (bleeding), warfarin (bleeding)

Mechanism of Action Causes increased availability of gamma-aminobutyric acid (GABA), an inhibitory neurotransmitter, to brain neurons or may enhance the action of GABA or mimic its action at postsynaptic receptor sites

Pharmacodynamics/Kinetics

Protein binding: 80% to 90% (dose dependent)

Metabolism: Extensively in the liver

Half-life (increased in neonates and patients with liver disease):

Children: 4-14 hours

Adults: 8-17 hours

Time to peak serum concentration: Within 1-4 hours; 3-5 hours after divalproex (enteric coated)

Elimination: 2% to 3% excreted unchanged in urine

Usual Dosage Children and Adults:

Oral: Initial: 10-15 mg/kg/day in 1-3 divided doses; increase by 5-10 mg/kg/day at weekly intervals until therapeutic levels are achieved; maintenance: 30-60 mg/kg/day in 2-3 divided doses

Children receiving more than 1 anticonvulsant (ie, polytherapy) may require doses up to 100 mg/kg/day in 3-4 divided doses

Rectal: Dilute syrup 1:1 with water for use as a retention enema; loading dose: 17-20 mg/kg one time; maintenance: 10-15 mg/kg/dose every 8 hours

Not dialyzable (0% to 5%)

Dosing adjustment/comments in hepatic impairment: Reduce dose

Monitoring Parameters Liver enzymes, CBC with platelets

Reference Range Therapeutic: 50-100 µg/mL (SI: 350-690 µmol/L); Toxic: >200 µg/mL (SI: >1390 µmol/L). Seizure control may improve at levels >100 µg/mL (SI: 690 µmol/L), but toxicity may occur at levels of 100-150 µg/mL (SI: 690-1040 µmol/L).

Test Interactions False-positive result for urine ketones

Patient Information Take with food or milk; do not chew, break, or crush the tablet or capsule; do not administer with carbonated drinks; report any sore throat, fever or fatigue, bleeding or bruising that is severe or that persists; may cause drowsiness, impair judgment or coordination

Nursing Implications Do not crush enteric coated drug product or capsules

Additional Information Sodium content of valproate sodium syrup (5 mL): 23 mg (1 mEq)

Divalproex sodium: Depakote®
Valproate sodium: Depakene® syrup
Valproic acid: Depakene® capsule

Dosage Forms

Capsule, sprinkle, as divalproex sodium (Depakote® Sprinkle®): 125 mg
Capsule, as valproic acid (Depakene®): 250 mg
Syrup, as sodium valproate (Depakene®): 250 mg/5 mL (5 mL, 50 mL, 480 mL)
Tablet, delayed release, as divalproex sodium (Depakote®): 125 mg, 250 mg, 500 mg

Valrelease® *see* Diazepam *on page 324*

Vamate® *see* Hydroxyzine *on page 556*

Vancenase® *see* Beclomethasone Dipropionate *on page 115*

Vancenase® AQ *see* Beclomethasone Dipropionate *on page 115*

Vanceril® *see* Beclomethasone Dipropionate *on page 115*

Vancocin® *see* Vancomycin Hydrochloride *on this page*

Vancoled® *see* Vancomycin Hydrochloride *on this page*

Vancomycin Hydrochloride (van koe mye' sin)

Related Information

Antimicrobial Drugs of Choice *on page 1298-1302*
Prevention of Bacterial Endocarditis *on page 1285-1288*
Prudent Vancomycin Use *on page 1297*

Brand Names Lyphocin®; Vancocin®; Vancoled®

Use Treatment of patients with the following infections or conditions:

Infections due to documented or suspected methicillin-resistant *S. aureus* or beta-lactam resistant coagulase negative *Staphylococcus*

Serious or life-threatening infections (ie, endocarditis, meningitis) due to documented or suspected staphylococcal or streptococcal infections in patients who are allergic to penicillins and/or cephalosporins

Empiric therapy of infections associated with gram-positive organisms; used orally for staphylococcal enterocolitis or for antibiotic-associated pseudomembranous colitis produced by *C. difficile*

Pregnancy Risk Factor C

Contraindications Hypersensitivity to vancomycin or any component; avoid in patients with previous severe hearing loss

Warnings/Precautions Use with caution in patients with renal impairment or those receiving other nephrotoxic or ototoxic drugs; dosage modification required in patients with impaired renal function (especially elderly)

Adverse Reactions

Oral:
>10%: Gastrointestinal: Bitter taste, nausea, vomiting
1% to 10%:
Central nervous system: Chills
Hematologic: Eosinophilia
Miscellaneous: Drug fever
<1%:
Cardiovascular: Vasculitis
Hematologic: Thrombocytopenia
Otic: Ototoxicity
Renal: Renal failure, interstitial nephritis

Parenteral:
>10%: Cardiovascular: Hypotension accompanied by flushing and erythematous rash on face and upper body (red neck or red man syndrome)
1% to 10%:
Central nervous system: Chills
Hematologic: Eosinophilia
Miscellaneous: Drug fever
<1%:
Cardiovascular: Vasculitis
Otic: Ototoxicity
Hematologic: Thrombocytopenia
Renal: Renal failure

(Continued)

Vancomycin Hydrochloride *(Continued)*

Overdosage/Toxicology Symptoms of overdose include ototoxicity, nephrotoxicity; there is no specific therapy for an overdosage with vancomycin. Care is symptomatic and supportive in nature. Peritoneal filtration and hemofiltration (not dialysis) have been shown to reduce the serum concentration of vancomycin; high flux dialysis may remove up to 25%.

Drug Interactions Increased toxicity: Anesthetic agents

Stability

Vancomycin reconstituted intravenous solutions are stable for 14 days at room temperature or refrigeration

Stability of parenteral admixture at room temperature (25°C) or refrigeration temperature (4°C): 7 days

Standard diluent: 500 mg/150 mL D_5W; 750 mg/250 mL D_5W; 1 g/250 mL D_5W

Minimum volume: Maximum concentration is 5 mg/mL to minimize thrombophlebitis

Incompatible with heparin, phenobarbital

After the oral solution is reconstituted, it should be refrigerated and used within 2 weeks

Mechanism of Action Inhibits bacterial cell wall synthesis by blocking glycopeptide polymerization through binding tightly to D-alanyl-D-alanine portion of cell wall precursor

Pharmacodynamics/Kinetics

Absorption:

Oral: Poor

I.M.: Erratic

Intraperitoneal: Can result in 38% absorption systemically

Distribution: Widely distributed in body tissues and fluids except for CSF

Relative diffusion of antimicrobial agents from blood into cerebrospinal fluid (CSF): Good only with inflammation (exceeds usual MICs)

Ratio of CSF to blood level (%):

Normal meninges: Nil

Inflamed meninges: 20-30

Protein binding: 10%

Half-life (biphasic): Terminal:

Newborns: 6-10 hours

Infants and Children 3 months to 4 years: 4 hours

Children >3 years: 2.2-3 hours

Adults: 5-11 hours, prolonged significantly with reduced renal function

End stage renal disease: 200-250 hours

Time to peak serum concentration: I.V.: Within 45-65 minutes

Elimination: As unchanged drug in the urine via glomerular filtration (80% to 90%); oral doses are excreted primarily in the feces

Usual Dosage Initial dosage recommendation: I.V.:

Neonates:

Postnatal age ≤7 days:

    <1200 g: 15 mg/kg/dose every 24 hours

    1200-2000 g: 15 mg/kg/dose every 12-18 hours

    >2000 g: 15 mg/kg/dose every 12 hours

Postnatal age >7 days:

    <1200 g: 15 mg/kg/dose every 24 hours

    1200-2000 g: 15 mg/kg/dose every 8-12 hours

    >2000 g: 15 mg/kg/dose every 8 hours

Infants >1 month and Children: 10 mg/kg/dose every 6 hours

Infants >1 month and Children with staphylococcal central nervous system infection: 10 mg/kg/dose every 6 hours

Adults (select dosage based on weight):

<60 kg: 750 mg

60-100 kg: 1 g

100-120 kg: 1.25 g

>120 kg: 1.5 g

Dosing interval in renal impairment:

Cl_{cr} >90 mL/minute: Administer every 12 hours

Cl_{cr} 40-90 mL/minute: Administer every 24 hours

Cl_{cr} 30-40 mL/minute: Administer every 48 hours

Cl_{cr} 20-30 mL/minute: Administer every 72 hours

Cl_{cr} 10-20 mL/minute: Administer every 96 hours

Cl_{cr} <10 mL/minute: Administer every 5-7 days

Not dialyzable (0% to 5%)

Removal of vancomycin by dialysis:

Hemodialysis: Generally not removed; exception minimal-moderate removal by some of the newer high-flux filters

Continuous ambulatory peritoneal dialysis (CAPD): Not significantly removed; administration via CAPD fluid: 15-30 mg/L (15-30 mcg/mL) of CAPD fluid

Continuous arteriovenous hemofiltration: Dose similar to Cl$_{cr}$ of approximately 10-15 mL/minute

Dosing adjustments/comments in hepatic impairment: Reduce dose by 60%

Antibiotic lock technique (for catheter infections): 2 mg/mL in SWI/NS or D$_5$W; instill 3-5 mL into catheter port as a flush solution instead of heparin lock (**Note:** Do not mix with any other solutions)

Intrathecal: Vancomycin is available as a powder for injection and may be diluted to 1-5 mg/mL concentration in preservative-free 0.9% sodium chloride for administration into the CSF

Neonates: 5-10 mg/day

Children: 5-20 mg/day

Adults: 20 mg/day

Oral: Pseudomembranous colitis produced by *C. difficile*:

Neonates: 10 mg/kg/day in divided doses every 6-8 hours

Children: 40 mg/kg/day in divided doses every 6-8 hours, added to fluids

Adults: 125 mg 4 times/day

Monitoring Parameters Periodic renal function tests, urinalysis, serum vancomycin concentrations, WBC, audiogram

Reference Range

Timing of serum samples: Draw peak 1 hour after 1-hour infusion has completed; draw trough just before next dose

Therapeutic levels: Peak: 25-40 µg/mL; Trough: 5-12 µg/mL

Toxic: >80-100 µg/mL (SI: >80-100 mg/L)

Patient Information Report pain at infusion site, dizziness, fullness or ringing in ears with I.V. use; nausea or vomiting with oral use; complete full course of therapy

Nursing Implications Obtain drug levels after the third dose unless otherwise directed; peaks are drawn 1 hour after the completion of a 1- to 2-hour infusion; troughs are obtained just before the next dose; slow I.V. infusion rate if maculopapular rash appears on face, neck, trunk, and upper extremities (Red man reaction)

Dosage Forms

Capsule: 125 mg, 250 mg

Powder for oral solution: 1 g, 10 g

Powder for injection: 500 mg, 1 g, 2 g, 5 g, 10 g

Vanoxide® [OTC] *see* Benzoyl Peroxide *on page 122*

Vantin® *see* Cefpodoxime Proxetil *on page 202*

Vapo-Iso® *see* Isoproterenol *on page 597*

Vaponefrin® *see* Epinephrine *on page 389*

Varicella Virus Vaccine (veer i sel' a)

Related Information

Immunization Guidelines *on page 1389-1405*

Brand Names Varivax®

Synonyms Chicken Pox Vaccine

Use Vaccination against varicella in individuals ≥12 months of age; postmarketing surveillance studies are ongoing to evaluate the need and timing for booster vaccination

Pregnancy Risk Factor C

Pregnancy/Breast Feeding Implications Varivax® should not be administered to pregnant females and pregnancy should be avoided for 3 months following vaccination; use during breast feeding should be avoided

Contraindications Hypersensitivity to any component of the vaccine, including gelatin; a history of anaphylactoid reaction to neomycin; individuals with blood dyscrasias, leukemia, lymphomas, or other malignant neoplasms affecting the bone marrow or lymphatic systems; those receiving immunosuppressive therapy; primary and acquired immunodeficiency states; a family history of congenital or hereditary immunodeficiency; active untreated tuberculosis; febrile illness; pregnancy; I.V. injection

Warnings/Precautions Children and adolescents with acute lymphoblastic leukemia in remission can receive the vaccine under an investigational protocol (215-283-0897); no clinical data are available or efficacy in children <12 months of age

Adverse Reactions

1% to 10%:

Central nervous system: Pain, fever, irritability/nervousness, fatigue, disturbed sleep, headache, malaise, chills

(Continued)

1147

Varicella Virus Vaccine *(Continued)*

Dermatologic: Redness, rash, pruritus, generalized varicella-like rash,

Gastrointestinal: Diarrhea, loss of appetite, vomiting, abdominal pain, nausea, chills

Local: Hematoma, induration and stiffness at the injection site

Neuromuscular & skeletal: Myalgia, arthralgia

Otic: Otitis

Respiratory: Upper respiratory illness, cough

Miscellaneous: Lymphadenopathy, allergic reactions

<1%:

Central nervous system: Febrile seizures (casuality not established)

Respiratory: Pneumonitis

Drug Interactions Clinical studies show that Varivax® can be administered concomitantly with MMR and limited data indicate that DTP and Pedvax® HIB may also be administered together (using separate sites and syringes); see Precautions

Stability Store in freezer (-15°C), store diluent separately at room temperature or in refrigerator; discard if reconstituted vaccine is not used within 30 minutes

Mechanism of Action As a live, attenuated vaccine, varicella virus vaccine offers active immunity to disease caused by the varicella-zoster virus

Pharmacodynamics/Kinetics

Onset of action: Approximately 4-6 weeks postvaccination

Duration: Lowest breakthrough rates (0.2% to 2.9%) exist in the first 2 years following postvaccination, with slightly higher rates in the third through the fifth year

Usual Dosage S.C.:

Children 12 months to 12 years: 0.5 mL

Children 12 years to Adults: 2 doses of 0.5 mL separated by 4-8 weeks

Administration Inject S.C. into the outer aspect of the upper arm, if possible

Monitoring Parameters Rash, fever

Patient Information Report any adverse reactions to the health care provider or Vaccine Adverse Event Reporting System (1-800-822-7967); avoid pregnancy for 3 months following vaccination; avoid salicylates for 5 weeks after vaccination; avoid close association with susceptible high risk individuals following vaccination

Nursing Implications Obtain the previous immunization history (including allergic reactions) to previous vaccines; do not inject into a blood vessel; use the supplied diluent only for reconstitution; inject immediately after reconstitution

Additional Information Minimum potency level: 1350 plaque forming units (PFU)/0.5 mL

Dosage Forms Injection, lyophilized powder, preservative free: 0.5 mL (single-dose vials)

Varicella-Zoster Immune Globulin (Human) (veer i sel′ a- zos′ ter)

Related Information

Immunization Guidelines *on page 1389-1405*

Vaccines *on page 1386-1388*

Synonyms VZIG

Use Passive immunization of susceptible immunodeficient patients after exposure to varicella; most effective if begun within 72 hours of exposure; there is no evidence VZIG modifies established varicella-zoster infections.

Restrict administration to those patients meeting the following criteria:

Neoplastic disease (eg, leukemia or lymphoma)

Congenital or acquired immunodeficiency

Immunosuppressive therapy with steroids, antimetabolites or other immunosuppressive treatment regimens

Newborn of mother who had onset of chickenpox within 5 days before delivery or within 48 hours after delivery

Premature (≥28 weeks gestation) whose mother has no history of chickenpox

Premature (<28 weeks gestation or ≤1000 g VZIG) regardless of maternal history

One of the following types of exposure to chickenpox or zoster patient(s) may warrant administration:

Continuous household contact

Playmate contact (>1 hour play indoors)

Hospital contact (in same 2-4 bedroom or adjacent beds in a large ward or prolonged face-to-face contact with an infectious staff member or patient)

Susceptible to varicella-zoster

Age <15 years; administer to immunocompromised adolescents and adults and to other older patients on an individual basis

An acceptable alternative to VZIG prophylaxis is to treat varicella, if it occurs, with high-dose I.V. acyclovir

Age is the most important risk factor for reactivation of varicella zoster; persons <50 years of age have incidence of 2.5 cases per 1000, whereas those 60-79 have 6.5 cases per 1000 and those >80 years have 10 cases per 1000

Pregnancy Risk Factor C

Contraindications Not for prophylactic use in immunodeficient patients with history of varicella, unless patient's immunosuppression is associated with bone marrow transplantation; **not** recommended for nonimmunodeficient patients, including pregnant women, because the severity of chickenpox is much less than in immunosuppressed patients; allergic response to gamma globulin or anti-immunoglobulin; sensitivity to thimerosal; persons with IgA deficiency; do not administer to patients with thrombocytopenia or coagulopathies

Warnings/Precautions VZIG is not indicated for prophylaxis or therapy of normal adults who are exposed to or who develop varicella; it is not indicated for treatment of herpes zoster. Do not inject I.V.

Adverse Reactions

1% to 10%: Local discomfort at the site of injection (pain, redness, swelling)

<1%:

Central nervous system: Malaise, headache

Dermatologic: Rash, angioedema

Gastrointestinal: GI symptoms

Respiratory: Respiratory symptom

Miscellaneous: Anaphylactic shock

Drug Interactions Decreased effect: Live virus vaccines (do not administer within 3 months of immune globulin administration)

Stability Refrigerate at 2°C to 8°C (36°F to 46°F)

Mechanism of Action The exact mechanism has not been clarified but the antibodies in varicella-zoster immune globulin most likely neutralize the varicella-zoster virus and prevent its pathological actions

Usual Dosage High risk susceptible patients who are exposed again more than 3 weeks after a prior dose of VZIG should receive another full dose; there is no evidence VZIG modifies established varicella-zoster infections.

I.M.: Administer by deep injection in the gluteal muscle or in another large muscle mass. Inject 125 units/10 kg (22 lb); maximum dose: 625 units (5 vials); minimum dose: 125 units; do not give fractional doses. Do not inject I.V. See table.

VZIG Dose Based on Weight

Weight of Patient		Dose	
kg	lb	Units	No. of Vials
0-10	0-22	125	1
10.1-20	22.1-44	250	2
20.1-30	44.1-66	375	3
30.1-40	66.1-88	500	4
>40	>88	625	5

Administration Do not inject I.V.; administer deep I.M. into the gluteal muscle or other large muscle mass. For patients ≤10 kg, administer 1.25 mL at a single site; for patients >10 kg, give no more than 2.5 mL at a single site. Administer entire contents of each vial

Dosage Forms Injection: 125 units of antibody in single dose vials

Varivax® see Varicella Virus Vaccine on page 1147

Vascor® see Bepridil Hydrochloride on page 126

Vasocidin® see Sodium Sulfacetamide and Prednisolone Acetate on page 1019

VasoClear® [OTC] see Naphazoline Hydrochloride on page 775

Vasocon Regular® see Naphazoline Hydrochloride on page 775

Vasodilan® see Isoxsuprine Hydrochloride on page 603

Vasopressin (vay soe press' in)

Brand Names Pitressin®

Synonyms ADH; Antidiuretic Hormone; 8-Arginine Vasopressin; Vasopressin Tannate

(Continued)

Vasopressin (Continued)

Use Treatment of diabetes insipidus; prevention and treatment of postoperative abdominal distention; differential diagnosis of diabetes insipidus

Unlabeled use: Adjunct in the treatment of GI hemorrhage and esophageal varices

Pregnancy Risk Factor B

Contraindications Hypersensitivity to vasopressin or any component

Warnings/Precautions Use with caution in patients with seizure disorders, migraine, asthma, vascular disease, renal disease, cardiac disease, chronic nephritis with nitrogen retention, goiter with cardiac complications, arteriosclerosis, I.V. infiltration may lead to severe vasoconstriction and localized tissue necrosis; also gangrene of extremities, tongue, and ischemic colitis

Adverse Reactions

1% to 10%:

Cardiovascular: Increased blood pressure, bradycardia, arrhythmias, venous thrombosis, vasoconstriction with higher doses, angina

Central nervous system: Pounding in the head, fever

Dermatologic: Urticaria

Gastrointestinal: Vertigo, flatulence, abdominal cramps, nausea, vomiting

Neuromuscular & skeletal: Tremor

Miscellaneous: Sweating, circumoral pallor

<1%:

Cardiovascular: Myocardial infarction

Miscellaneous: Allergic reaction, water intoxication

Overdosage/Toxicology Symptoms of overdose include drowsiness, weight gain, confusion, listlessness, water intoxication; water intoxication requires withdrawal of the drug; severe intoxication may require osmotic diuresis and loop diuretics

Drug Interactions

Decreased effect: Lithium, epinephrine, demeclocycline, heparin, and alcohol block antidiuretic activity to varying degrees

Increased effect: Chlorpropamide, phenformin, urea and fludrocortisone potentiate antidiuretic response

Stability Store injection at room temperature; protect from heat and from freezing; use only clear solutions

Mechanism of Action Increases cyclic adenosine monophosphate (cAMP) which increases water permeability at the renal tubule resulting in decreased urine volume and increased osmolality; causes peristalsis by directly stimulating the smooth muscle in the GI tract

Pharmacodynamics/Kinetics

Nasal:

Onset of action: 1 hour

Duration: 3-8 hours

Parenteral: Duration of action: I.M., S.C.: 2-8 hours

Absorption: Destroyed by trypsin in GI tract, must be administered parenterally or intranasally

Nasal:

Metabolism: In the liver, kidneys

Half-life: 15 minutes

Elimination: In urine

Parenteral:

Metabolism: Most of dose metabolized by liver and kidneys

Half-life: 10-20 minutes

Elimination: 5% of S.C. dose (aqueous) excreted unchanged in urine after 4 hours

Usual Dosage

Diabetes insipidus (highly variable dosage; titrated based on serum and urine sodium and osmolality in addition to fluid balance and urine output):

Children: I.M., S.C.: 2.5-10 units 2-4 times/day as needed

Adults:

I.M., S.C.: 5-10 units 2-4 times/day as needed (dosage range 5-60 units/day)

Intranasal: Administer on cotton pledget or nasal spray

Abdominal distention: Adults: I.M.: 5 mg stat, 10 mg every 3-4 hours

GI hemorrhage: Children and Adults: Continuous I.V. infusion: 0.5 milliunit/kg/hour (0.0005 unit/kg/hour); double dosage as needed every 30 minutes to a maximum of 10 milliunits/kg/hour

Children: 0.01 units/kg/minute; continue at same dosage (if bleeding stops) for 12 hours, then taper off over 24-48 hours

Adults: I.V.: Initial: 0.2-0.4 unit/minute, then titrate dose as needed; if bleeding stops, continue at same dose for 12 hours, taper off over 24-48 hours

Dosing adjustment in hepatic impairment: Some patients respond to much lower doses with cirrhosis

Administration I.V. infusion administration requires the use of an infusion pump and should be administered in a peripheral line to minimize adverse reactions on coronary arteries; dilute aqueous in NS or D_5W to 0.1-1 unit/mL

Infusion rates:
100 units (aqueous) in 500 mL D_5W rate
0.1 unit/minute: 30 mL/hour
0.2 units/minute: 60 mL/hour
0.3 units/minute: 90 mL/hour
0.4 units/minute: 120 mL/hour
0.5 units/minute: 150 mL/hour
0.6 units/minute: 180 mL/hour

Monitoring Parameters Serum and urine sodium, urine output, fluid input and output, urine specific gravity, urine and serum osmolality

Reference Range Plasma: 0-2 pg/mL (SI: 0-2 ng/L) if osmolality <285 mOsm/L; 2-12 pg/mL (SI: 2-12 ng/L) if osmolality >290 mOsm/L

Patient Information Side effects such as abdominal cramps and nausea may be reduced by drinking a glass of water with each dose

Nursing Implications Watch for signs of I.V. infiltration and gangrene; elderly patients should be cautioned not to increase their fluid intake beyond that sufficient to satisfy their thirst in order to avoid water intoxication and hyponatremia; under experimental conditions, the elderly have shown to have a decreased responsiveness to vasopressin with respect to its effects on water homeostasis

Dosage Forms Injection, aqueous: 20 pressor units/mL (0.5 mL, 1 mL)

Vasopressin Tannate *see Vasopressin on page 1149*

Vasotec® *see Enalapril on page 384*

Vasoxyl® *see Methoxamine Hydrochloride on page 716*

V-Cillin K® *see Penicillin V Potassium on page 854*

VCR *see Vincristine Sulfate on page 1159*

Vecuronium (ve kyoo' roe ni um)
Related Information
Neuromuscular Blocking Agents Comparison Charts *on page 1276-1278*
Brand Names Norcuron®
Synonyms ORG NC 45
Use Adjunct to anesthesia, to facilitate intubation, and provide skeletal muscle relaxation during surgery or mechanical ventilation
Pregnancy Risk Factor C
Contraindications Known hypersensitivity to vecuronium
Warnings/Precautions Use with caution in patients with hepatic impairment, neuromuscular disease, myasthenia gravis, and the elderly; ventilation must be supported during neuromuscular blockade
Adverse Reactions
<1%:
Cardiovascular: Tachycardia, flushing, edema, hypotension, circulatory collapse, bradycardia
Dermatologic: Rash, itching
Miscellaneous: Hypersensitivity reaction
Overdosage/Toxicology Symptoms of overdose include prolonged skeletal muscle weakness and apnea cardiovascular collapse; use neostigmine, edrophonium, or pyridostigmine with atropine to antagonize skeletal muscle relaxation; support of ventilation and the cardiovascular system through mechanical means, fluids, and pressors may be necessary
Drug Interactions Increased toxicity/effect with aminoglycosides, ketamine, magnesium sulfate, verapamil, quinidine, clindamycin, furosemide
Stability Stable for 5 days at room temperature when reconstituted with bacteriostatic water; stable for 24 hours at room temperature when reconstituted with preservative-free sterile water (avoid preservatives in neonates); do not mix with alkaline drugs
Mechanism of Action Blocks acetylcholine from binding to receptors on motor endplate inhibiting depolarization
Pharmacodynamics/Kinetics
Good intubation conditions within 2.5-3 minutes; maximum neuromuscular blockade within 3-5 minutes
(Continued)

Vecuronium (Continued)

Elimination: Vecuronium bromide and its metabolite(s) appear to be excreted principally in feces via biliary eliminations; the drug and its metabolite(s) are also excreted in urine

Usual Dosage I.V. (do not administer I.M.):

Infants >7 weeks to 1 year: Initial: 0.08-0.1 mg/kg/dose; maintenance: 0.05-0.1 mg/kg/every hour as needed

Children >1 year and Adults: Initial: 0.08-0.1 mg/kg/dose; maintenance: 0.05-0.1 mg/kg/every hour as needed; may be administered with caution as a continuous infusion at 0.075 mg/kg/hour (concern has been raised of drug-induced myopathies in ICU setting)

Note: Children (1-10 years) may require slightly higher initial doses and slightly more frequent supplementation

Dosing adjustment in hepatic impairment: Dose reductions are necessary in patients with liver disease

Administration Give undiluted I.V. injection as a single bolus

Monitoring Parameters Blood pressure, heart rate

Dosage Forms Powder for injection: 10 mg (5 mL, 10 mL)

Veetids® see Penicillin V Potassium on page 854

Velban® see Vinblastine Sulfate on page 1157

Velosef® see Cephradine on page 213

Velosulin® Human [OTC] see Insulin Preparations on page 578

Velsar® see Vinblastine Sulfate on page 1157

Veltane® see Brompheniramine Maleate on page 143

Venlafaxine (ven' la fax een)

Related Information

Antidepressant Agents Comparison on page 1250-1252

Brand Names Effexor®

Use Treatment of depression in adults

Unapproved use: Obsessive-compulsive disorder

Pregnancy Risk Factor C

Contraindications Do not use concomitantly with MAO inhibitors, contraindicated in patients with hypersensitivity to venlafaxine or other components

Warnings/Precautions Venlafaxine is associated with sustained increases in blood pressure (10-15 mm Hg SDBP); venlafaxine may actuate mania or hypomania and seizures. Concurrent therapy with a monoamine oxidase inhibitor may result in serious or fatal reactions; at least 14 days should elapse between treatment with an MAO inhibitor and venlafaxine. Patients with cardiovascular disorders or a recent myocardial infarction probably should only receive venlafaxine if the benefits of therapy outweigh the risks.

Adverse Reactions

≥10%:

Central nervous system: Headache, somnolence, dizziness, insomnia, nervousness

Gastrointestinal: Nausea, dry mouth, constipation

Genitourinary: Abnormal ejaculation

Neuromuscular & skeletal: Weakness, neck pain

Miscellaneous: Sweating

1% to 10%:

Cardiovascular: Palpitations, hypertension, sinus tachycardia

Central nervous system: Anxiety, asthenia

Gastrointestinal: Weight loss, anorexia, vomiting, diarrhea, dysphagia

Genitourinary: Impotence

Neuromuscular & skeletal: Tremor

Ocular: Blurred vision

<1%: Ear pain, seizures

Overdosage/Toxicology

Symptoms of overdose include somnolence and occasionally tachycardia; most overdoses resolve with only supportive treatment

Use of activated charcoal, inductions of emesis, or gastric lavage should be considered for acute ingestion; forced diuresis, dialysis, and hemoperfusion not effective due to large volume of distribution

Drug Interactions Increased toxicity: Cimetidine MAO inhibitors (hyperpyrexic crisis); TCAs, fluoxetine, setraline, phenothiazine, class 1C antiarrhythmics, warfarin; venlafaxine is a weak inhibitor of cytochrome P-450-2D6, which is responsible for metabolizing antipsychotics, antiarrhythmics, TCAs, and beta-blockers. Therefore, interactions with these agents are possible, however, less likely than with more potent enzyme inhibitors.

Mechanism of Action Venlafaxine and its active metabolite o-desmethylvenlafaxine (ODV) are potent inhibitors of neuronal serotonin and norepinephrine reuptake and weak inhibitors of dopamine reuptake; causes beta-receptor down regulation and reduces adenylcyclase coupled beta-adrenergic systems in the brain

Pharmacodynamics/Kinetics

Absorption: Oral: 92% to 100%

Protein binding: Bound to human plasma 27% to 30%; steady-state achieved within 3 days of multiple dose therapy

Metabolism: In the liver by cytochrome P-450 enzyme system to active metabolite, O-desmethyel-venlafaxine (ODV)

Half-life: 3-7 hours (venlafaxine) and 11-13 hours (ODV)

Time to peak: 1-2 hours

Elimination: Primarily by renal route

Usual Dosage Adults: Oral: 75 mg/day, administered in 2 or 3 divided doses, taken with food; dose may be increased in 75 mg/day increments at intervals of at least 4 days, up to 225-375 mg/day

Dosing adjustment in renal impairment: Cl_{cr} 10-70 mL/minute: Decrease dose by 25%; decrease total daily dose by 50% if dialysis patients; dialysis patients should receive dosing after completion of dialysis

Dosing adjustment in moderate hepatic impairment: Reduce total dosage by 25%

Monitoring Parameters Blood pressure should be regularly monitored, especially in patients with a high baseline blood pressure

Reference Range Peak serum level of 163 ng/mL (325 ng/mL of ODV metabolite) obtained after a 150 mg oral dose

Test Interactions ↑ thyroid, ↑ uric acid, ↑ glucose, ↑ potassium, ↑ SGOT, ↑ cholesterol (S)

Patient Information Avoid use of alcohol; use caution when operating hazardous machinery; if a rash or shortness of breath occurs while using venlafaxine, contact physician immediately

Nursing Implications Causes mean increase in heart rate of 4 beats/minute; may be taken without regard to food; tapering to minimize symptoms of discontinuation is recommended when the drug is discontinued; tapering should be over a 2-week period if the patient has received it longer than 6 weeks

Dosage Forms Tablet: 25 mg, 37.5 mg, 50 mg, 75 mg, 100 mg

Venoglobulin®-I *see* Immune Globulin, Intravenous *on page 571*

Ventolin® *see* Albuterol *on page 33*

VePesid® *see* Etoposide *on page 434*

Verapamil Hydrochloride (ver ap' a mill)

Related Information

Antiarrhythmic Drugs *on page 1246-1248*

Calcium Channel Blockers Cardiovascular Adverse Reactions *on page 1262*

Calcium Channel Blockers Central Nervous System Adverse Reactions *on page 1264*

Calcium Channel Blockers Comparative Actions *on page 1260*

Calcium Channel Blockers Comparative Pharmacokinetics *on page 1261*

Calcium Channel Blockers FDA-Approved Indications *on page 1263*

Calcium Channel Blockers Gastrointestinal and Miscellaneous Adverse Reactions *on page 1265*

Brand Names Calan®; Isoptin®; Verelan®

Synonyms Iproveratril Hydrochloride

Use Orally used for treatment of angina pectoris (vasospastic, chronic stable, unstable) and hypertension; I.V. for supraventricular tachyarrhythmias (PSVT, atrial fibrillation, atrial flutter)

Pregnancy Risk Factor C

Pregnancy/Breast Feeding Implications Use in pregnancy only when clearly needed and when the benefits outweigh the potential hazard to the fetus

Contraindications Sinus bradycardia; advanced heart block; ventricular tachycardia; cardiogenic shock; hypersensitivity to verapamil or any component; atrial fibrillation or flutter associated with accessory conduction pathways

Warnings/Precautions Use with caution in sick-sinus syndrome, severe left ventricular dysfunction, hepatic or renal impairment, hypertrophic cardiomyopathy (especially obstructive), abrupt withdrawal may cause increased duration (Continued)

Verapamil Hydrochloride *(Continued)*

and frequency of chest pain; avoid I.V. use in neonates and young infants due to severe apnea, bradycardia, or hypotensive reactions; elderly may experience more constipation and hypotension. Monitor EKG and blood pressure closely in patients receiving I.V. therapy particularly in patients with supraventricular tachycardia.

Adverse Reactions

1% to 10%:

Cardiovascular: Bradycardia; first, second, or third degree A-V block; congestive heart failure, hypotension, peripheral edema

Central nervous system: Dizziness, lightheadedness, nausea, tiredness, weakness

Dermatologic: Skin rash

Gastrointestinal: Constipation

<1%:

Cardiovascular: Chest pain, hypotension (excessive), tachycardia, flushing

Endocrine & metabolic: Galactorrhea

Gastrointestinal: Gingival hyperplasia

Overdosage/Toxicology The primary cardiac symptoms of calcium blocker overdose includes hypotension and bradycardia. The hypotension is caused by peripheral vasodilation, myocardial depression, and bradycardia. Bradycardia results from sinus bradycardia, second- or third-degree atrioventricular block, or sinus arrest with junctional rhythm. Intraventricular conduction is usually not affected so QRS duration is normal (verapamil does prolong the P-R interval and bepridil prolongs the Q-T and may cause ventricular arrhythmias, including torsade de pointes).

The noncardiac symptoms include confusion, stupor, nausea, vomiting, metabolic acidosis and hyperglycemia. Following initial gastric decontamination, if possible, repeated calcium administration may promptly reverse the depressed cardiac contractility (but not sinus node depression or peripheral vasodilation); glucagon, epinephrine, and amrinone may treat refractory hypotension; glucagon and epinephrine also increase the heart rate (outside the U.S., 4-aminopyridine may be available as an antidote); dialysis and hemoperfusion are not effective in enhancing elimination although repeat-dose activated charcoal may serve as an adjunct with sustained-release preparations.

Drug Interactions

Increased toxicity/effect/levels:

H_2 blockers → ↑ bioavailability of verapamil

Beta-blockers → ↑ cardiac depressant effects on A-V conduction

Carbamazepine → ↑ carbamazepine levels

Cyclosporine → ↑ cyclosporine levels

Fentanyl → ↑ hypotension

Digitalis → ↑ digitalis levels

Quinidine → ↑ quinidine levels (hypotension, bradycardia)

Theophylline → ↑ pharmacologic actions of theophylline

Stability Store injection at room temperature; protect from heat and from freezing; use only clear solutions; **compatible** in solutions of pH of 3-6, but may precipitate in solutions having a pH ≥6

Mechanism of Action Inhibits calcium ion from entering the "slow channels" or select voltage-sensitive areas of vascular smooth muscle and myocardium during depolarization; produces a relaxation of coronary vascular smooth muscle and coronary vasodilation; increases myocardial oxygen delivery in patients with vasospastic angina; slows automaticity and conduction of A-V node.

Pharmacodynamics/Kinetics

Oral (nonsustained tablets):

Peak effect: 2 hours

Duration: 6-8 hours

I.V.:

Peak effect: 1-5 minutes

Duration: 10-20 minutes

Protein binding: 90%

Metabolism: In the liver; extensive first-pass effect

Bioavailability: Oral: 20% to 30%

Half-life:

Infants: 4.4-6.9 hours

Adults: Single dose: 2-8 hours, increased up to 12 hours with multiple dosing; increased half-life with hepatic cirrhosis

Elimination: 70% of dose excreted in urine (3% to 4% as unchanged drug) and 16% in feces

Usual Dosage

Children: SVT:

I.V.:

<1 year: 0.1-0.2 mg/kg over 2 minutes; repeat every 30 minutes as needed

1-16 years: 0.1-0.3 mg/kg over 2 minutes; maximum: 5 mg/dose, may repeat dose in 15 minutes if adequate response not achieved; maximum for second dose: 10 mg/dose

Oral (dose not well established):

1-5 years: 4-8 mg/kg/day in 3 divided doses **or** 40-80 mg every 8 hours

>5 years: 80 mg every 6-8 hours

Adults:

SVT: I.V.: 5-10 mg (approximately 0.075-0.15 mg/kg), second dose of 10 mg (~0.15 mg/kg) may be given 15-30 minutes after the initial dose if patient tolerates, but does not respond to initial dose

Angina: Oral: Initial dose: 80-120 mg twice daily (elderly or small stature: 40 mg twice daily); range: 240-480 mg/day in 3-4 divided doses

Hypertension: Usual dose is 80 mg 3 times/day or 240 mg/day (sustained release); range 240-480 mg/day (no evidence of additional benefit in doses >360 mg/day)

Dosing adjustment in renal impairment: Cl_{cr} <10 mL/minute: Administer at 50% to 75% of normal dose

Not dialyzable (0% to 5 %) via hemo or peritoneal dialysis; supplemental dose is not necessary

Dosing adjustment/comments in hepatic disease: Reduce dose in cirrhosis, reduce dose to 20% to 50% of normal and monitor EKG

Administration Administer around-the-clock to promote less variation in peak and trough serum levels; I.V. rate of infusion is over 2 minutes

Monitoring Parameters Monitor blood pressure closely

Reference Range Therapeutic: 50-200 ng/mL (SI: 100-410 nmol/L) for parent; under normal conditions norverapamil concentration is the same as parent drug. Toxic: >90 µg/mL

Patient Information Sustained release products should be taken with food and not crushed; limit caffeine intake; notify physician if angina pain is not reduced when taking this drug, or if irregular heartbeat or shortness of breath occurs

Nursing Implications Do not crush sustained release drug product

Dosage Forms

Capsule, sustained release: 120 mg, 180 mg, 240 mg

Injection: 2.5 mg/mL (2 mL, 4 mL)

Tablet: 40 mg, 80 mg, 120 mg

Tablet, sustained release: 120 mg, 180 mg, 240 mg

Vicon Forte® *see* Vitamin, Multiple *on page 1166*

Vicon® Plus [OTC] *see* Vitamin, Multiple *on page 1166*

Vidarabine (vye dare' a been)

Related Information
Antimicrobial Drugs of Choice *on page 1298-1302*

Brand Names Vira-A®

Synonyms Adenine Arabinoside; Ara-A; Arabinofuranosyladenine

Use Treatment of acute keratoconjunctivitis and epithelial keratitis due to herpes simplex virus; herpes simplex encephalitis; neonatal herpes simplex virus infections; herpes zoster in immunosuppressed patients; herpes simplex conjunctivitis

Pregnancy Risk Factor C

Contraindications Hypersensitivity to vidarabine or any component

Warnings/Precautions Vidarabine must be administered slow I.V. to neonates; administration requires dilution in large fluid volumes; use with caution in patients at risk of fluid overload (cerebral edema) and in patients with impaired renal function; reduce dosage in patients with severe renal insufficiency

Adverse Reactions
1% to 10%:
Gastrointestinal: Nausea, vomiting, anorexia, diarrhea, weight loss
Hepatic: Elevated bilirubin and AST
<1%:
Cardiovascular: Thrombophlebitis
Central nervous system: Weakness, ataxia, disorientation, depression, agitation, pain, stromal edema
Dermatologic: Rash
Endocrine & metabolic: Hypokalemia, SIADH
Hematologic: Decreased WBC and platelets
Ocular: Burning, lacrimation, keratitis, photophobia, foreign body sensation, uveitis
Neuromuscular & skeletal: Myoclonus

Overdosage/Toxicology Symptoms of overdose include bone marrow depression, thrombocytopenia, leukopenia with doses >20 mg/kg/day; treatment is supportive only

Drug Interactions Increased toxicity with allopurinol

Stability Do **not** refrigerate diluted I.V. solution; constituted solutions remain stable for 2 weeks at room temperature; however, should be diluted just prior to administration and used within 48 hours
Stability of parenteral admixture at room temperature (25°C): 2 days

Mechanism of Action Inhibits viral DNA synthesis by blocking DNA polymerase

Pharmacodynamics/Kinetics
Absorption: Oral, I.M., S.C.: Poor
Distribution: Crosses into the CNS
Protein binding: 20% to 30% (vidarabine) and 0% to 3% (ara-hypoxanthine)
Metabolism: Following administration rapidly deaminated to ara-hypoxanthine (active)
Half-life:
Infants: 2.4-3.1 hours
Children: 2.8 hours
Adults: 1.5 hours
Ara-hypoxanthine: Normal renal function: 3.3 hours
Elimination: In urine as unchanged drug (1% to 3%) and the active metabolite (40% to 53%)

Usual Dosage
Neonates: I.V.: 15-30 mg/kg/day as an 18- to 24-hour infusion for 10-14 days
Children and Adults:
I.V.: 15 mg/kg/day as a 12-hour or longer infusion for 10 days
Ophthalmic: Keratoconjunctivitis: Instill ½" of ointment in lower conjunctival sac 5 times/day every 3 hours while awake until complete re-epithelialization has occurred, then twice daily for an additional 7 days

Dosing adjustment in renal impairment: Cl$_{cr}$ <10 mL/minute: Administer 75% of normal dose

Administration Do not give I.M. or S.C.; administer I.V. solution through an in-line 0.22 or 0.45 micron filter; administer by slow I.V. infusion over 12-24 hours

Patient Information Do not use eye make-up when on this medication for ophthalmic infection; use sunglasses if photophobic reaction occurs; may cause blurred vision; notify physician if improvement not seen after 7 days or if condition worsens

Dosage Forms
Injection, suspension: 200 mg/mL [base 187.4 mg] (5 mL)

Ointment, ophthalmic, as monohydrate: 3% [30 mg/mL = 28 mg/mL base] (3.5 g)

Vi-Daylin/F® *see* Vitamin, Multiple *on page 1166*

Vi-Daylin® [OTC] *see* Vitamin, Multiple *on page 1166*

Videx® *see* Didanosine *on page 331*

Vinblastine Sulfate (vin blas' teen)
Related Information
Cancer Chemotherapy Regimens *on page 1218-1241*
Extravasation Management of Chemotherapeutic Agents *on page 1207-1208*
Brand Names Alkaban-AQ®; Velban®; Velsar®
Synonyms Vincaleukoblastine; VLB
Use Treatment of Hodgkin's and non-Hodgkin's lymphoma, testicular, lung, head and neck, breast, and renal carcinomas, Kaposi's sarcoma, histiocytosis, choriocarcinoma, and idiopathic thrombocytopenic purpura
Pregnancy Risk Factor D
Contraindications For I.V. use only; **I.T. use may result in death**; severe bone marrow suppression or presence of bacterial infection not under control prior to initiation of therapy
Warnings/Precautions The U.S. Food and Drug Administration (FDA) currently recommends that procedures for proper handling and disposal of antineoplastic agents be considered. Avoid extravasation; dosage modification required in patients with impaired liver function and neurotoxicity. Using small amounts of drug daily for long periods may increase neurotoxicity and is therefore not advised. For I.V. use only. **Intrathecal administration may result in death.** Use with caution in patients with cachexia or ulcerated skin; monitor closely for shortness of breath or bronchospasm in patients receiving mitomycin C.
Adverse Reactions
>10%:
Dermatologic: Alopecia
Emetic potential: Moderate (30% to 60%)
Gastrointestinal: Nausea and vomiting are most common and are easily controlled with standard antiemetics; constipation, diarrhea, stomatitis, abdominal cramps, anorexia, metallic taste
Hematologic: May cause severe bone marrow depression and is the dose-limiting toxicity of VLB (unlike vincristine); severe granulocytopenia and thrombocytopenia may occur following the administration of VLB and nadir 7-10 days after treatment
Myelosuppressive:
WBC: Moderate - severe
Platelets: Moderate - severe
Onset (days): 4-7
Nadir (days): 4-10
Recovery (days): 17
1% to 10%:
Cardiovascular: Tachycardia, orthostatic hypotension
Central nervous system: Depression, malaise, headache, paresthesias, depression, seizures
Dermatologic: Rash, photosensitivity, alopecia, dermatitis
Extravasation: VLB is a vesicant and can cause tissue irritation and necrosis if infiltrated; if extravasation occurs, follow institutional policy, which may include hyaluronidase and hot compresses
Gastrointestinal: Constipation, abdominal pain, paralytic ileus, stomatitis
Neuromuscular & skeletal: Jaw pain, muscle pain, paresthesia
Renal: Urinary retention, hyperuricemia
Respiratory: Bronchospasm
Vesicant chemotherapy
<1%:
Gastrointestinal: Hemorrhagic colitis
Neurologic: VLB rarely produces neurotoxicity at clinical doses; however, neurotoxicity may be seen, especially at high doses; if it occurs, symptoms are similar to VCR toxicity (ie, peripheral neuropathy, loss of deep tendon reflexes, headache, weakness, urinary retention, and GI symptoms)
Overdosage/Toxicology Symptoms of overdose include bone marrow depression, mental depression, paresthesia, loss of deep reflexes, neurotoxicity; there are no antidotes for vinblastine. Treatment is supportive and symptomatic, including fluid restriction or hypertonic saline (3% sodium chloride) for drug-induced secretion of inappropriate antidiuretic hormone (SIADH), diazepam or phenytoin for seizures, laxatives for constipation, and antiemetics for toxic emesis.
(Continued)

Vinblastine Sulfate *(Continued)*

Drug Interactions

Decreased effect:

Phenytoin plasma levels may be reduced with concomitant combination chemotherapy with vinblastine

Alpha-interferon enhances interferon toxicity; phenytoin may reduce plasma levels

Increased toxicity:

Previous or simultaneous use with mitomycin-C has resulted in acute shortness of breath and severe bronchospasm within minutes or several hours after *Vinca* alkaloid injection and may occur up to 2 weeks after the dose of mitomycin

Mitomycin-C in combination with administration of VLB may cause acute shortness of breath and severe bronchospasm, onset may be within minutes or several hours after VLB injection

Stability Refrigerate; however, is stable for up to 1-3 months (depending on manufacturer) at room temperature; constituted solutions remain stable for 30 days when refrigerated; protect from light, must be dispersed in amber bag. **Compatible** with doxorubicin, metoclopramide, dacarbazine, bleomycin

Mechanism of Action VLB binds to tubulin and inhibits microtubule formation, therefore, arresting the cell at metaphase by disrupting the formation of the mitotic spindle; it is specific for the M and S phases; binds to microtubular protein of the mitotic spindle causing metaphase arrest

Pharmacodynamics/Kinetics

Absorption: Not reliably absorbed from the GI tract and must be given I.V.

Distribution: V_d: 27.3 L/kg; binds extensively to tissues; does not penetrate CNS or other fatty tissues; distributes to the liver

Protein binding: 99% rapidly

Metabolism: Hepatic metabolism to an active metabolite

Half-life (biphasic):

Initial 0.164 hours

Terminal: 25 hours

Elimination: Biliary excretion (95%); <1% eliminated unchanged in urine

Usual Dosage Refer to individual protocols. Varies depending upon clinical and hematological response. Give at intervals of at least 7 days and only after leukocyte count has returned to at least 4000/mm³; maintenance therapy should be titrated according to leukocyte count. Dosage should be reduced in patients with recent exposure to radiation therapy or chemotherapy; single doses in these patients should not exceed 5.5 mg/m².

Children and Adults: I.V.: 4-12 mg/m² every 7-10 days **or** 5-day continuous infusion of 1.4-1.8 mg/m²/day **or** 0.1-0.5 mg/kg/week

Not removed by hemodialysis

Dosing adjustment in hepatic impairment:

Serum bilirubin 1.5-3.0 mg/dL or AST 60-180 units: Administer 50% of normal dose

Serum bilirubin 3.0-5.0 mg/dL: Administer 25% of dose

Serum bilirubin >5.0 mg/dL or AST >180 units: Omit dose

Administration May be administered IVP or into a free flowing I.V. over a 1-minute period at a concentration for administration of 1 mg/mL

Monitoring Parameters CBC with differential and platelet count, serum uric acid, hepatic function tests

Patient Information Hair may be lost during treatment but will regrow to its pretreatment extent even with continued treatment; report any bleeding; examine mouth daily and report soreness to a physician; jaw pain or pain in the organs containing tumor tissue; avoid constipation. Any signs of infection, easy bruising or bleeding, shortness of breath, or painful or burning urination should be brought to physician's attention. Nausea, vomiting or hair loss sometimes occur. The drug may cause permanent sterility and may cause birth defects. The drug may be excreted in breast milk, therefore, an alternative form of feeding your baby should be used.

Nursing Implications Monitor for life-threatening bronchospasm (most likely to occur if patient is also taking mitomycin). Maintain adequate hydration; allopurinol may be given to prevent uric acid nephropathy; may cause sloughing upon extravasation

Extravasation treatment: Inject 3-5 mL of hyaluronidase (10 units/mL) S.C. clockwise into the infiltrated area using a 25-gauge needle; change the needle with each injection; apply heat immediately for 1 hour, repeat 4 times/day for 3-5 days (application of cold and injection of hydrocortisone is contraindicated)

Dosage Forms

Injection: 1 mg/mL (10 mL)

Powder for injection: 10 mg

Vincaleukoblastine *see* Vinblastine Sulfate *on page 1157*

Vincasar® PFS *see* Vincristine Sulfate *on this page*

Vincristine Sulfate (vin kris' teen)
Related Information
Cancer Chemotherapy Regimens *on page 1218-1241*
Extravasation Management of Chemotherapeutic Agents *on page 1207-1208*
Brand Names Oncovin®; Vincasar® PFS
Synonyms LCR; Leurocristine; VCR
Use Treatment of leukemias, Hodgkin's disease, neuroblastoma, malignant lymphomas, Wilms' tumor, and rhabdomyosarcoma
Pregnancy Risk Factor D
Contraindications Hypersensitivity to vincristine or any component; **for I.V. use only, fatal if given intrathecally**; patients with demyelinating form of Charcot-Marie-Tooth syndrome
Warnings/Precautions The U.S. Food and Drug Administration (FDA) currently recommends that procedures for proper handling and disposal of antineoplastic agents be considered. Dosage modification required in patients with impaired hepatic function or who have pre-existing neuromuscular disease; avoid extravasation; use with caution in the elderly; avoid eye contamination; observe closely for shortness of breath, bronchospasm, especially in patients treated with mitomycin C. For I.V. use only; **intrathecal administration results in death**; give allopurinol to prevent uric acid nephropathy; not to be used with radiation.
Adverse Reactions
>10%:
　Dermatologic: Alopecia occurs in 20% to 70% of patients
　Extravasation: VCR is a vesicant and can cause tissue irritation and necrosis if infiltrated; if extravasation occurs, follow institutional policy, which may include hyaluronidase and hot compresses
　Vesicant chemotherapy
1% to 10%:
　Emetic potential: Low (<10%)
　Gastrointestinal: Constipation and possible paralytic ileus secondary to neurologic toxicity; oral ulceration, abdominal cramps, anorexia, metallic taste
　Neurologic: Alterations in mental status such as depression, confusion, or insomnia; constipation, paralytic ileus, and urinary tract disturbances may occur. All patients should be on a prophylactic bowel management regimen. Cranial nerve palsies, headaches, jaw pain, optic atrophy with blindness have been reported. Intrathecal administration of VCR has uniformly caused death; VCR should **never** be administered by this route. Neurologic effects of VCR may be additive with those of other neurotoxic agents and spinal cord irradiation.
　Peripheral neuropathy: Frequently the dose-limiting toxicity of VCR. Most frequent in patients >40 years of age; occurs usually after an average of 3 weekly doses, but may occur after just one dose. Manifested as loss of the deep tendon reflexes in the lower extremities, numbness, tingling, pain, paresthesias of the fingers and toes (stocking glove sensation), and "foot drop" or "wrist drop"
　SIADH: Rarely occurs, but may be related to the neurologic toxicity; may cause symptomatic hyponatremia with seizures; the increase in serum ADH concentration usually subsides within 2-3 days after onset
　Miscellaneous: Rash, photophobia, headache, weight loss, fever, hypertension, hypotension
1% to 10%:
　Cardiovascular: Orthostatic hypotension
　Central nervous system: Numbness, weakness, motor difficulties, seizures, CNS depression, cranial nerve paralysis
　Endocrine & metabolic: Hyperuricemia, SIADH
　Gastrointestinal: Bloating, nausea, vomiting, weight loss, diarrhea
　Local: Phlebitis
　Neuromuscular & skeletal: Jaw pain, leg pain, myalgia, cramping
<1%:
　Gastrointestinal: Stomatitis
　Myelosuppressive: Occasionally mild leukopenia and thrombocytopenia may occur
　　WBC: Rare
　　Platelets: Rare
　　Onset (days): 7
　　Nadir (days): 10
　　Recovery (days): 21
(Continued)

Vincristine Sulfate *(Continued)*

Overdosage/Toxicology Symptoms of overdose include bone marrow depression, mental depression, paresthesia, loss of deep reflexes, alopecia, nausea, severe symptoms may occur with 3-4 mg/m^2; there are no antidotes for vincristine. Treatment is supportive and symptomatic, including fluid restriction or hypertonic saline (3% sodium chloride) for drug-induced secretion of inappropriate antidiuretic hormone (SIADH), diazepam or phenytoin for seizures, laxatives for constipation, and antiemetics for toxic emesis. The use of pyridoxine, leucovorin factor, cyanocobalamin or thiamine have been used with little success for drug-induced peripheral neuropathy.

Drug Interactions

Decreased effect: Phenytoin levels may decrease with combination chemotherapy

Increased toxicity:

Digoxin plasma levels and renal excretion may decrease with combination chemotherapy including vincristine

Vincristine should be given 12-24 hours before asparaginase to minimize toxicity (may reduce the hepatic clearance of vincristine)

Acute pulmonary reactions may occur with mitomycin-C. Previous or simultaneous use with mitomycin-C has resulted in acute shortness of breath and severe bronchospasm within minutes or several hours after *Vinca* alkaloid injection and may occur up to 2 weeks after the dose of mitomycin.

Stability Refrigerate; however, is stable for up to 1 month at room temperature; drug may be administered IVP or IVPB and is **compatible** with D$_5$W; should be protected from light. **Compatible** with doxorubicin, bleomycin, cytarabine, fluorouracil, methotrexate, metoclopramide.

Mechanism of Action Binds to microtubular protein of the mitotic spindle causing metaphase arrest; cell-cycle phase specific in the M and S phases

Pharmacodynamics/Kinetics

Absorption: Oral: Poor

Distribution: Poor penetration into the CSF; rapidly removed from the blood stream and tightly bound to tissues; penetrates blood-brain barrier poorly

Protein binding: 75%

Metabolism: Extensively in the liver

Half-life: Terminal: 24 hours

Elimination: Primarily in the bile (~80%); <1% excreted unchanged in urine

Usual Dosage Refer to individual protocols as dosages vary with protocol used. Adjustments are made depending upon clinical and hematological response and upon adverse reactions

Children: I.V. (maximum single dose: 2 mg): ≤10 kg or BSA <1 m^2: 0.05 mg/kg once weekly; 2 mg/m^2; may repeat every week

Adults: I.V.: 0.4-1.4 mg/m^2 (up to 2 mg maximum); may repeat every week

Dosing adjustment in hepatic impairment:

Serum bilirubin 1.5-3.0 mg/dL or AST 60-180 units: Administer 50% of normal dose

Serum bilirubin 3.0-5.0 mg/dL: Administer 25% of dose

Serum bilirubin >5.0 mg/dL or AST >180 units: Omit dose

The average total dose per course of treatment should be around 2-2.5 mg; some recommend capping the dose at 2 mg maximum to reduce toxicity; however, it is felt that this measure can reduce the efficacy of the drug

Administration Vincristine is administered IVP or into a free flowing I.V. over a period of 1 minute at a concentration for administration of 1 mg/mL

Monitoring Parameters Serum electrolytes (sodium), hepatic function tests, neurologic examination, CBC, serum uric acid

Patient Information Maintain adequate fluid intake; rinse mouth with water 3-4 times/day, brush teeth with soft brush and floss with waxed floss; loss of hair occurs in approximately 70% of patients; report any nerve effects to physician; stool softener should be used for constipation prophylaxis; report to physician any persistent or severe fever, sore throat, bleeding, or bruising; shortness of breath

Nursing Implications Maintain adequate hydration; allopurinol may be given to prevent uric acid nephropathy; observe for life-threatening bronchospasm after administration; use of rectal thermometer or rectal tubing should be avoided to prevent injury to rectal mucosa

Extravasation treatment: Inject 3-5 mL of hyaluronidase (10 units/mL) S.C. clockwise into the infiltrated area using a 25-gauge needle; change the needle with each injection; apply heat immediately for 1 hour, repeat 4 times/day for 3-5 days (application of cold and injection of hydrocortisone is contraindicated)

Dosage Forms Injection: 1 mg/mL (1 mL, 2 mL, 5 mL)

Vinorelbine Tartrate (vi nor' el been)

Related Information

Cancer Chemotherapy Regimens *on page 1218-1241*

Brand Names Navelbine®

Use Treatment of nonsmall cell lung cancer (as a single agent or in combination with cisplatin)

> **Unlabeled use:** Breast cancer, ovarian carcinoma (cisplatin-resistant), Hodgkin's disease

Pregnancy Risk Factor D

Contraindications For I.V. use only; **I.T. use may result in death**; severe bone marrow suppression (granulocyte counts <1000 cells/mm^3) or presence of bacterial infection not under control prior to initiation of therapy

Warnings/Precautions The U.S. Food and Drug Administration (FDA) currently recommends that procedures for proper handling and disposal of antineoplastic agents be considered. Avoid extravasation; dosage modification required in patients with impaired liver function and neurotoxicity. Frequently monitor patients for myelosuppression both during and after therapy. Granulocytopenia is dose-limiting. **Intrathecal administration may result in death.** Use with caution in patients with cachexia or ulcerated skin.

Adverse Reactions

>10%:

Dermatologic: Alopecia (12%)

Gastrointestinal: Nausea and vomiting are most common and are easily controlled with standard antiemetics; constipation, diarrhea, stomatitis, abdominal cramps, anorexia, metallic taste

Emetic potential: Moderate (30% to 60%)

Hematologic: May cause severe bone marrow depression and is the dose-limiting toxicity of vinorelbine; severe granulocytopenia may occur following the administration of vinorelbine.

Myelosuppressive:

WBC: Moderate - severe

Onset (days): 4-7

Nadir (days): 7-10

Recovery (days): 14-21

1% to 10%:

Central nervous system: Fatigue

Extravasation: Vesicant and can cause tissue irritation and necrosis if infiltrated; if extravasation occurs, follow institutional policy, which may include hyaluronidase and hot compresses

Vesicant chemotherapy

Neuromuscular & skeletal: Mild-moderate peripheral neuropathy manifested by paresthesia and hyperesthesia, loss of deep tendon reflexes; myalgia, arthralgia, jaw pain

<1%:

Gastrointestinal: Hemorrhagic colitis

Neuromuscular & skeletal: Severe peripheral neuropathy (generally reversible)

Overdosage/Toxicology Symptoms of overdose include bone marrow depression, mental depression, paresthesia, loss of deep reflexes, neurotoxicity. There are no antidotes for vinorelbine. Treatment is supportive and symptomatic, including fluid restriction or hypertonic saline (3% sodium chloride) for drug-induced secretion of inappropriate antidiuretic hormone (SIADH), diazepam or phenytoin for seizures, laxatives for constipation, and antiemetics for toxic emesis.

Drug Interactions

Increased toxicity:

Previous or simultaneous use with mitomycin-C has resulted in acute shortness of breath and severe bronchospasm within minutes or several hours after *Vinca* alkaloid injection and may occur up to 2 weeks after the dose of mitomycin

Cisplatin: Incidence of granulocytopenia is significantly higher than with single-agent vinorelbine

Stability Store unopened vials under refrigeration (2°C to 8°C/36°F to 46°F) and protect from light; unopened vials are stable at temperatures of up to 25°C/77°F for up to 72 hours; do not freeze. Dilutions of vinorelbine in 75-125 mL of D$_5$W, 0.45% NaCl, 0.9% NaCl, Ringer's injection or lactated Ringer's injection are stable for 24 hours when stored in polyvinyl chloride bags at 5°C to 30°C/41°F to 86°F under normal room light.

Mechanism of Action Semisynthetic vinca alkaloid which binds to tubulin and inhibits microtubule formation, therefore, arresting the cell at metaphase by disrupting the formation of the mitotic spindle; it is specific for the M and S phases; binds to microtubular protein of the mitotic spindle causing metaphase arrest

(Continued)

Vinorelbine Tartrate *(Continued)*

Pharmacodynamics/Kinetics

Absorption: Not reliably absorbed from the GI tract and must be given I.V.

Distribution: V_d: 25.4-40.1 L/kg; binds extensively to human platelets and lymphocytes (79.6% to 91.2%)

Metabolism: Extensive hepatic metabolism to an active metabolite (deacetylvinorelbine)

Half-life (triphasic):

Terminal: 27.7-43.6 hours

Mean plasma clearance: 0.97-1.26 L/hour/kg

Elimination: Feces (46%) and urine (18%)

Usual Dosage Varies depending upon clinical and hematological response (refer to individual protocols)

Adults: I.V.: 30 mg/m² every 7 days

Dosage adjustment in hematologal toxicity (based on granulocyte counts):

Granulocytes ≥1500 cells/mm³ on day of treatment: Administer 30 mg/m²

Granulocytes 1000-1499 cells/mm³ on day of treatment: Administer 15 mg/m²

Granulocytes <1000 cells/mm³ on day of treatment: Do not administer. Repeat granulocyte count in one week; if 3 consecutive doses are held because granulocyte count is <1000 cells/mm³, discontinue vinorelbine

For patients who, during treatment, have experienced fever or sepsis while granulocytopenic or had 2 consecutive weekly doses held due to granulocytopenia, subsequent doses of vinorelbine should be:

22.5 mg/m² for granulocytes ≥1,500 cells/mm³

11.25 mg/m² for granulocytes 1000-1499 cells/mm³

Dosage adjustment in renal impairment: No dose adjustments are required. If moderate or severe neurotoxicity develops, discontinue vinorelbine. Adjust the dosage according to hematologic toxicity or hepatic insufficiency, whichever results in the lower dose.

Dosing adjustment in hepatic impairment:

Serum bilirubin ≤2 mg/dL: Administer 30 mg/m²

Serum bilirubin 2.1-3 mg/dL: Administer 15 mg/m²

Serum bilirubin >3 mg/dL: Administer 7.5 mg/m²

Dosing adjustment in patients with concurrent hematologic toxicity and hepatic impairment: Administer the lower doses determined from the above recommendations

Administration Must administer intravenously; avoid extravasation

Monitoring Parameters CBC with differential and platelet count, serum uric acid, hepatic function tests

Patient Information Hair may be lost during treatment but will regrow to its pretreatment extent even with continued treatment; report any bleeding; examine mouth daily and report soreness to a physician; jaw pain or pain in the organs containing tumor tissue; avoid constipation. Any signs of infection, easy bruising or bleeding, shortness of breath, or painful or burning urination should be brought to physician's attention. Nausea, vomiting or hair loss sometimes occur. The drug may cause permanent sterility and may cause birth defects. The drug may be excreted in breast milk, therefore, an alternative form of feeding your baby should be used.

Nursing Implications Monitor for life-threatening bronchospasm (most likely to occur if patient is also taking mitomycin). Maintain adequate hydration; allopurinol may be given to prevent uric acid nephropathy; may cause sloughing upon extravasation

Extravasation treatment: Inject 3-5 mL of hyaluronidase (10 units/mL) S.C. clockwise into the infiltrated area using a 25-gauge needle; change the needle with each injection; apply heat immediately for 1 hour, repeat 4 times/day for 3-5 days (application of cold and injection of hydrocortisone is contraindicated).

Dosage Forms Injection: 10 mg/mL (1 mL, 5 mL)

Vioform® [OTC] *see* Iodochlorhydroxyquin *on page 588*

Viokase® *see* Pancrelipase *on page 837*

Viosterol *see* Ergocalciferol *on page 396*

Vira-A® *see* Vidarabine *on page 1156*

Virazole® *see* Ribavirin *on page 979*

Virilon® *see* Methyltestosterone *on page 726*

Viroptic® *see* Trifluridine *on page 1122*

Viscoat® *see* Chondroitin Sulfate-Sodium Hyaluronate *on page 241*

Visine A.C.® **[OTC]** *see* Tetrahydrozoline Hydrochloride *on page 1071*

Visine® **[OTC]** *see* Tetrahydrozoline Hydrochloride *on page 1071*

Visken® *see* Pindolol *on page 886*

Vistacon-50® *see* Hydroxyzine *on page 556*

Vistaject-25® *see* Hydroxyzine *on page 556*

Vistaject-50® *see* Hydroxyzine *on page 556*

Vistaquel® *see* Hydroxyzine *on page 556*

Vistaril® *see* Hydroxyzine *on page 556*

Vistazine® *see* Hydroxyzine *on page 556*

Vita-C® **[OTC]** *see* Ascorbic Acid *on page 88*

Vitamin A (vye' ta min)
Brand Names Aquasol A® [OTC]
Synonyms Oleovitamin A
Use Treatment and prevention of vitamin A deficiency
Pregnancy Risk Factor A (X if dose exceeds RDA recommendation)
Contraindications Hypervitaminosis A, hypersensitivity to vitamin A or any component
Warnings/Precautions Evaluate other sources of vitamin A while receiving this product; patients receiving >25,000 units/day should be closely monitored for toxicity
Adverse Reactions
  1% to 10%:
    Central nervous system: Irritability, vertigo, lethargy, malaise, fever, headache
    Dermatologic: Drying or cracking of skin
    Endocrine & metabolic: Hypercalcemia
    Gastrointestinal: Weight loss
    Ocular: Visual changes
    Miscellaneous: Hypervitaminosis A
Overdosage/Toxicology Symptoms of chronic overdose (adults: 25,000 IU/day for 2-3 weeks) include increased intracranial pressure (headache, altered mental status, blurred vision), bulging fontanelles in infants, jaundice, ascites, cutaneous desquamation; symptoms of acute overdose (12,000 IU/kg) include nausea, vomiting, and diarrhea; toxic signs of an overdose commonly respond to drug discontinuation and generally return to normal spontaneously within a few days to weeks. When confronted with signs of increased intracranial pressure, treatment with dexamethasone (1.5 mg/kg I.V. load followed with 0.375 mg/kg every 6 hours for 5 days), and/or hyperventilation may be employed; forced diuresis, dialysis, and hemoperfusion are of no clinical benefit.
Drug Interactions
  Decreased effect: Cholestyramine decreases absorption of vitamin A; neomycin and mineral oil may also interfere with vitamin A absorption
  Increased toxicity: Retinoids may have additive adverse effects
Stability Protect from light
Mechanism of Action Needed for bone development, growth, visual adaptation to darkness, testicular and ovarian function, and as a cofactor in many biochemical processes
Pharmacodynamics/Kinetics
  Absorption: Vitamin A in dosages **not** exceeding physiologic replacement is well absorbed after oral administration; water miscible preparations are absorbed more rapidly than oil preparations; large oral doses, conditions of fat malabsorption, low protein intake, or hepatic or pancreatic disease reduces oral absorption
  Distribution: Following oral absorption, large amounts concentrate for storage in the liver; appears in breast milk
  Metabolism: Conjugated with glucuronide, undergoes enterohepatic circulation
  Elimination: In feces via biliary elimination
Usual Dosage
  RDA:
    <1 year: 375 mcg
    1-3 years: 400 mc
    4-6 years: 500 mcg•
    7-10 years: 700 mcg•
    >10 years: 800-1000 mcg•
    Male: 1000 mcg
    Female: 800 mcg
(Continued)

Vitamin A *(Continued)*

•mcg retinol equivalent (0.3 mcg retinol = 1 unit vitamin A)

Vitamin A supplementation in measles (recommendation of the World Health Organization): Children: Oral: Give as a single dose; repeat the next day and at 4 weeks for children with ophthalmologic evidence of vitamin A deficiency:

6 months to 1 year: 100,000 units

>1 year: 200,000 units

Note: Use of vitamin A in measles is recommended only for patients 6 months to 2 years of age hospitalized with measles and its complications **or** patients >6 months of age who have any of the following risk factors and who are not already receiving vitamin A: immunodeficiency, ophthalmologic evidence of vitamin A deficiency including night blindness, Bitot's spots or evidence of xerophthalmia, impaired intestinal absorption, moderate to severe malnutrition including that associated with eating disorders, or recent immigration from areas where high mortality rates from measles have been observed

Note: Monitor patients closely; dosages >25,000 units/kg have been associated with toxicity

Severe deficiency with xerophthalmia: Oral:

Children 1-8 years: 5000-10,000 units/kg/day for 5 days or until recovery occurs

Children >8 years and Adults: 500,000 units/day for 3 days, then 50,000 units/day for 14 days, then 10,000-20,000 units/day for 2 months

Deficiency (without corneal changes): Oral:

Infants <1 year: 100,000 units every 4-6 months

Children 1-8 years: 200,000 units every 4-6 months

Children >8 years and Adults: 100,000 units/day for 3 days then 50,000 units/day for 14 days

Malabsorption syndrome (prophylaxis): Children >8 years and Adults: Oral: 10,000-50,000 units/day of water miscible product

Dietary supplement: Oral:

Infants up to 6 months: 1500 units/day

Children:

6 months to 3 years: 1500-2000 units/day

4-6 years: 2500 units/day

7-10 years: 3300-3500 units/day

Children >10 years and Adults: 4000-5000 units/day

Reference Range 1 RE = 1 retinol equivalent; 1 RE = 1 µg retinol or 6 mg beta-carotene; Normal levels of Vitamin A in serum = 80-300 IU/mL

Patient Information Avoid use of mineral oil when taking drug; take with food; notify physician if nausea, vomiting, anorexia, malaise, drying or cracking of skin or lips, irritability, headache, or loss of hair occurs

Nursing Implications Do not give by I.V. push; patients receiving >25,000 units/day should be closely monitored for toxicity

Additional Information 1 mg equals 3333 units

Dosage Forms

Capsule: 10,000 units, 25,000 units, 50,000 units

Drops, oral (water miscible): 5000 units/0.1 mL (30 mL)

Injection: 50,000 units/mL (2 mL)

Vitamin A Acid *see* Tretinoin *on page 1112*

Vitamin B₁ *see* Thiamine Hydrochloride *on page 1079*

Vitamin B₂ *see* Riboflavin *on page 980*

Vitamin B₃ *see* Niacin *on page 788*

Vitamin B₃ *see* Niacinamide *on page 789*

Vitamin B₆ *see* Pyridoxine Hydrochloride *on page 961*

Vitamin B₁₂ *see* Cyanocobalamin *on page 282*

Vitamin B₁₂ *see* Hydroxocobalamin *on page 552*

Vitamin C *see* Ascorbic Acid *on page 88*

Vitamin D₂ *see* Ergocalciferol *on page 396*

Vitamin E

Brand Names Amino-Opti-E® [OTC]; Aquasol E® [OTC]; E-Complex-600® [OTC]; E-Vitamin® [OTC]; Vita-Plus® E Softgels® [OTC]; Vitec® [OTC]; Vite E® Creme [OTC]

Synonyms *d*-Alpha Tocopherol; *dl*-Alpha Tocopherol

Use Prevention and treatment hemolytic anemia secondary to vitamin E deficiency, dietary supplement

Pregnancy Risk Factor A (C if dose exceeds RDA recommendation)

Contraindications Hypersensitivity to drug or any components

Warnings/Precautions May induce vitamin K deficiency; necrotizing enterocolitis has been associated with oral administration of large dosages (eg, >200 units/day) of a hyperosmolar vitamin E preparation in low birth weight infants

Adverse Reactions

<1%:

Central nervous system: Weakness, headache

Dermatologic: Contact dermatitis with topical preparation

Gastrointestinal: Nausea, diarrhea, intestinal cramps

Ocular: Blurred vision

Miscellaneous: Gonadal dysfunction

Drug Interactions

Decreased absorption with mineral oil

Delayed absorption of iron

Increased effect of oral anticoagulants

Stability Protect from light

Mechanism of Action Prevents oxidation of vitamin A and C; protects polyunsaturated fatty acids in membranes from attack by free radicals and protects red blood cells against hemolysis

Pharmacodynamics/Kinetics

Absorption: Oral: Depends upon the presence of bile; absorption is reduced in conditions of malabsorption, in low birth weight premature infants, and as dosage increases; water miscible preparations are better absorbed than oil preparations

Distribution: Distributes to all body tissues, especially adipose tissue, where it is stored

Metabolism: In the liver to glucuronides

Elimination: In feces and bile

Usual Dosage One unit of vitamin E = 1 mg dl-alpha-tocopherol acetate. Oral:

Vitamin E deficiency:

Neonates, premature, low birthweight: 25-50 units/day results in normal levels within 1 week

Children (with malabsorption syndrome): 1 unit/kg/day of water miscible vitamin E (to raise plasma tocopherol concentrations to the normal range within 2 months and to maintain normal plasma concentrations)

Adults: 60-75 units/day

Prevention of vitamin E deficiency:

Neonates:

Low birthweight: 5 units/day

Full term: 5 units/L of formula ingested

Adults: 30 units/day

Prevention of retinopathy of prematurity or BPD secondary to O_2 therapy: (American Academy of Pediatrics considers this use investigational and routine use is not recommended):

Retinopathy prophylaxis: 15-30 units/kg/day to maintain plasma levels between 1.5-2 mcg/mL (may need as high as 100 units/kg/day)

Cystic fibrosis, beta-thalassemia, sickle cell anemia may require higher daily maintenance doses:

Cystic fibrosis: 100-400 units/day

Beta-thalassemia: 750 units/day

Sickle cell: 450 units/day

Recommended daily allowance:

Premature infants ≤3 months: 17 mg (25 units)

Infants:

≤6 months: 3 mg (4.5 units)

6-12 months: 4 mg (6 units)

Children:

1-3 years: 6 mg (9 units)

4-10 years: 7 mg (10.5 units)

Children >11 years and Adults:

Male: 10 mg (15 units)

Female: 8 mg (12 units)

Topical: Apply a thin layer over affected area

Reference Range Therapeutic: 0.8-1.5 mg/dL (SI: 19-35 μmol/L), some method variation

Patient Information Drops can be placed directly in the mouth or mixed with cereal, fruit juice, or other food; take only the prescribed dose. Vitamin E toxicity appears as blurred vision, diarrhea, dizziness, flu-like symptoms, nausea, headache; swallow capsules whole, do not crush or chew

Dosage Forms

Capsule: 100 units, 200 units, 330 mg, 400 units, 500 units, 600 units, 1000 units

Capsule, water miscible: 73.5 mg, 147 mg, 165 mg, 330 mg, 400 units

(Continued)

Vitamin E *(Continued)*

Cream: 50 mg/g (15 g, 30 g, 60 g, 75 g, 120 g, 454 g)
Drops, oral: 50 mg/mL (12 mL, 30 mL)
Liquid, topical: 10 mL, 15 mL, 30 mL, 60 mL
Lotion: 120 mL
Oil: 15 mL, 30 mL, 60 mL
Ointment, topical: 30 mg/g (45 g, 60 g)
Tablet: 200 units, 400 units

Vitamin G *see* Riboflavin *on page 980*

Vitamin K₁ *see* Phytonadione *on page 882*

Vitamin, Multiple

Brand Names Adeflor®; Allbee® With C; Becotin® Pulvules®; Berocca®; Cefol® Filmtab®; Chromagen® OB [OTC]; Eldercaps® [OTC]; Filibon® [OTC]; Florvite®; Iberet-Folic-500®; LKV-Drops® [OTC]; Mega-B® [OTC]; Multi Vit® Drops [OTC]; M.V.I.®; M.V.I.®-12; M.V.I.® Concentrate; M.V.I.® Pediatric; Natabec® [OTC]; Natabec® FA [OTC]; Natabec® Rx; Natalins® [OTC]; Natalins® Rx; NeoVadrin® [OTC]; Nephrocaps® [OTC]; Niferex®-PN; Poly-Vi-Flor®; Poly-Vi-Sol® [OTC]; Pramet® FA; Pramilet® FA; Prenavite® [OTC]; Secran®; Stresstabs® 600 Advanced Formula Tablets [OTC]; Stuartnatal® 1 + 1; Stuart Prenatal® [OTC]; Therabid® [OTC]; Theragran® [OTC]; Theragran® Hema-tinic®; Theragran® Liquid [OTC]; Theragran-M® [OTC]; Tri-Vi-Flor®; Unicap® [OTC]; Vicon Forte®; Vicon® Plus [OTC]; Vi-Daylin® [OTC]; Vi-Daylin/F®

Synonyms B Complex; B Complex With C; Children's Vitamins; Hexavitamin; Multiple Vitamins; Multivitamins/Fluoride; Parenteral Multiple Vitamin; Prenatal Vitamins; Therapeutic Multivitamins; Vitamin, Multiple, Prenatal; Vitamin, Multiple, Therapeutic; Vitamin, Multiple With Iron

Use Dietary supplement

Pregnancy Risk Factor A (C if used in doses above RDA recommendation)

Contraindications Hypersensitivity to product components

Warnings/Precautions RDA values are not requirements, but are recommended daily intakes of certain essential nutrients; periodic dental exams should be performed to check for dental fluorosis; use with caution in patients with severe renal or liver failure

Adverse Reactions 1% to 10%: Hypervitaminosis; refer to individual vitamin entries for individual reactions

Usual Dosage

Infants 1.5-3 kg: I.V.: 3.25 mL/24 hours (M.V.I.® Pediatric)

Children:
Oral:
≤2 years: Drops: 1 mL/day (premature infants may get 0.5-1 mL/day)
>2 years: Chew 1 tablet/day
≥4 years: 5 mL/day liquid
I.V.: >3 kg and <11 years: 5 mL/24 hours (M.V.I.® Pediatric)

Adults:
Oral: 1 tablet/day or 5 mL/day liquid
I.V.: >11 years: 5 mL of vials 1 and 2 (M.V.I.®-12)/one TPN bag/day
I.V. solutions: 10 mL/24 hours (M.V.I.®-12)

Reference Range Recommended daily allowances are published by Food and Nutrition Board, National Research Council - National Academy of Sciences and are revised periodically. RDA quantities apply only to healthy persons and are not intended to cover therapeutic nutrition requirements in disease or other abnormal states (ie, metabolic disorders, weight reduction, chronic disease, drug therapy).

Patient Information Take only amount prescribed

Nursing Implications Doses may be higher for burn or cystic fibrosis patients

Dosage Forms See table on next page.

Vitamin, Multiple, Prenatal *see* Vitamin, Multiple *on this page*

Vitamin, Multiple, Therapeutic *see* Vitamin, Multiple *on this page*

Vitamin, Multiple With Iron *see* Vitamin, Multiple *on this page*

Vita-Plus® E Softgels® [OTC] *see* Vitamin E *on page 1164*

Vitec® [OTC] *see* Vitamin E *on page 1164*

Vite E® Creme [OTC] *see* Vitamin E *on page 1164*

Vivactil® *see* Protriptyline Hydrochloride *on page 953*

Vivotif Berna™ *see* Typhoid Vaccine *on page 1137*

Multivitamin Products Available

Product	Content Given Per	A IU	D IU	E IU	C mg	FA mg	B₁ mg	B₂ mg	B₃ mg	B₆ mg	B₁₂ mcg	Other
Drops/Liquid												
Theragran®	5 mL liquid	10,000	400		200		10	10	100	4.1	5	B₅ 21.4 mg
Vi-Daylin®	1 mL drops	1500	400	4.1	35		0.5	0.6	8	0.4	1.5	Alcohol <0.5%
Vi-Daylin® Iron	1 mL	1500.	400	4.1	35		0.5	0.6	8	0.4		Fe 10 mg
Capsules/Tablets												
Allbee® with C	Tablet				300		15	10.2		5		Niacinamide 50 mg, pantothenic acid 10 mg
Vitamin B Complex	Tablet					400 mcg	1.5	1.7		2	6	Niacinamide 20 mg
Hexavitamin	Cap/Tab	5000	400		75		2	3	20			
Iberet® -Folic - 500	Tablet				500	0.8	6	6	30	5	25	B₅ 10, Fe 105 mg
Stuartnatal 1+1	Tablet	4000	400	11	120	1	1.5	3	20	10	12	Cu, Zn 25 mg, Fe 65 mg, Ca 200 mg
Theragran® M	Tablet	5000	400	30	90	0.4	3	3.4	30	3	9	Cl, Cr, I, K, B₅ 10, Mg, Mn, Mo, P, Se, Zn 15 mg, biotin 35 mcg, beta-carotene 1250 IU
Vi-Daylin®	Tablet	2500	400	15	60	0.3	1.05	1.2	13.5	1.05	4.5	
Injectables												
M.V.I.-12 injection	5 mL	3300	200	10	100	0.4	3	3.6	40	4	5	B₅ 15 mg, biotin 60 mcg
M.V.I.-12 unit vial	20 mL											
M.V.I. pediatric powder	5 mL	2300	400	7	80	0.14	1.2	1.4	17	1	1	B₅ 5 mg, biotin 20 mcg, vitamin K 200 mcg

Warfarin Sodium (war' far in)

Brand Names Coumadin®; Sofarin®

Use Prophylaxis and treatment of venous thrombosis, pulmonary embolism and thromboembolic disorders; atrial fibrillation with risk of embolism and as an adjunct in the prophylaxis of systemic embolism after myocardial infarction
Unlabeled use: Prevention of recurrent transient ischemic attacks and to reduce risk of recurrent myocardial infarction

Pregnancy Risk Factor D

Contraindications Hypersensitivity to warfarin or any component; severe liver or kidney disease; open wounds; uncontrolled bleeding; GI ulcers; neurosurgical procedures; malignant hypertension, pregnancy

Warnings/Precautions

Do not switch brands once desired therapeutic response has been achieved

Use with caution in patients with active tuberculosis or diabetes

Concomitant use with vitamin K may decrease anticoagulant effect; monitor carefully

Concomitant use with NSAIDs or aspirin may cause severe GI irritation and also increase the risk of bleeding due to impaired platelet function

Salicylates may further increase warfarin's effect by displacing it from plasma protein binding sites

Patients with protein C or S deficiency are at increased risk of skin necrosis syndrome

Before committing an elderly patient to long-term anticoagulation therapy, their risk for bleeding complications secondary to falls, drug interactions, living situation, and cognitive status should be considered. The risk for bleeding complications decreases with the duration of therapy and may increase with advancing age.

If a patient is to undergo an invasive surgical procedure (dental to actual minor/major surgery), warfarin should be stopped 3 days before the scheduled surgery date and the INR/PT should be checked prior to the procedure

Adverse Reactions

1% to 10%:

Dermatologic: Skin lesions, alopecia, skin necrosis

Gastrointestinal: Anorexia, nausea, vomiting, stomach cramps, diarrhea

Hematologic: Hemorrhage, leukopenia, unrecognized bleeding sites (eg, colon cancer) may be uncovered by anticoagulation

Respiratory: Hemoptysis

<1%:

Dermatologic: Skin rash

Gastrointestinal: Anorexia

Hematologic: Agranulocytosis

Hepatic: Hepatotoxicity

Renal: Renal damage

Miscellaneous: Mouth ulcers, fever, discolored toes (blue or purple)

Overdosage/Toxicology

Symptoms of overdose include internal or external hemorrhage, hematuria. Avoid emesis and lavage to avoid the possible trauma and incidental bleeding.

Symptoms of overdose include internal or external hemorrhage, hematuria. Avoid emesis and lavage to avoid the possible trauma and incidental bleeding. When overdose occurs, the drug should be immediately discontinued and vitamin K₁ (phytonadione) may be administered 1-5 mg I.V. for children or up to 25 mg I.V. for adults. When hemorrhaging occurs, fresh frozen plasma transfusions can help control bleeding by replacing clotting factors. In urgent bleeding, prothrombin complex concentrates may be needed.

See table.

INR	Patient Situation	Action
>3 and ≤6	No bleeding or need for rapid reversal (ie, no need for surgery)	Omit next few warfarin doses and restart at lower dose when INR ≤3.0
>6 and <10.0	No bleeding but in need of rapid reversal for surgery	Stop warfarin and give phytonadione 0.5-1 mg IV; Repeat 0.5 mg phytonadione I.V. if INR >3 after 24 hours; restart warfarin at a lower dose
>10.0 and <20.0	No bleeding	Stop warfarin, give phytonadione 3-5 mg I.V; check INR every 6-12 hours; repeat phytonadione if needed; reassess need and dose of warfarin
>20.0	Serious bleeding or warfarin overdose	Stop warfarin, give phytonadione 10 mg I.V., check INR every 6 hours, if needed, repeat phytonadione every 12 hours and give plasma transfusion or factor concentrate; consider giving heparin if warfarin still indicated

Drug Interactions See tables.

Decreased Anticoagulant Effects

Induction of Enzymes		Increased Procoagulant Factors	Decreased Drug Absorption	Other
Barbiturates Carbamazepine Glutethimide Griseofulvin	Nafcillin Phenytoin Rifampin	Estrogens Oral contraceptives Vitamin K (including nutritional supplements)	Aluminum hydroxide Cholestyramine* Colestipol*	Ethchlorvynol Griseofulvin Spironolactone† Sucralfate

Decreased anticoagulant effect may occur when these drugs are administered with oral anticoagulants.

*Cholestyramine and colestipol may increase the anticoagulant effect by binding vitamin K in the gut; yet, the decreased drug absorption appears to be of more concern.

†Diuretic-induced hemoconcentration with subsequent concentration of clotting factors has been reported to decrease the effects of oral anticoagulants.

Enhanced Anticoagulant Effects

Decrease Vitamin K	Displace Anticoagulant	Inhibit Metabolism	Other
Oral antibiotics Can ↑ or ↓ an INR Check an INR 3 days after a patient begins antibiotics to see the INR value and adjust the warfarin dose accordingly	Chloral hydrate Clofibrate Diazoxide Ethacrynic acid Miconazole Nalidixic acid Phenylbutazone Salicylates Sulfonamides Sulfonylureas Triclofos	Alcohol (acute ingestion)* Allopurinol Amiodarone Chloramphenicol Chlorpropamide Cimetidine Co-trimoxazole Disulfiram Methylphenidate Metronidazole Phenylbutazone Phenytoin Propoxyphene Sulfinpyrazone Sulfonamides Tolbutamide	Acetaminophen Anabolic steroids Clofibrate Danazol Erythromycin Gemfibrozil Glucagon Influenza vaccine Ketoconazole Propranolol Ranitidine Sulindac Thyroid drugs

*The hypoprothrombinemic effect of oral anticoagulants has been reported to be both increased and decreased during chronic and excessive alcohol ingestion. Data are insufficient to predict the direction of this interaction in alcoholic patients.

Warfarin Sodium *(Continued)*

Increased Bleeding Tendency

Inhibit Platelet Aggregation	Inhibit Procoagulant Factors	Ulcerogenic Drugs
Cephalosporins	Antimetabolites	Adrenal corticosteroids
Dipyridamole	Quinidine	Indomethacin
Indomethacin	Quinine	Oxyphenbutazone
Oxyphenbutazone	Salicylates	Phenylbutazone
Penicillin, parenteral		Potassium products
Phenylbutazone		Salicylates
Salicylates		
Sulfinpyrazone		

Use of these agents with oral anticoagulants may increase the chances of hemorrhage.

Stability Protect from light; injection is stable for 4 hours at room temperature after reconstitution with 2.7 mL of sterile water

Mechanism of Action Interferes with hepatic synthesis of vitamin K-dependent coagulation factors (II, VII, IX, X)

Pharmacodynamics/Kinetics

Onset of anticoagulation effect: Oral: Within 36-72 hours

Peak effect: Within 5-7 days

Absorption: Oral: Rapid

Metabolism: In the liver

Half-life: 42 hours, highly variable among individuals

Usual Dosage

Oral:

Infants and Children: 0.05-0.34 mg/kg/day; infants <12 months of age may require doses at or near the high end of this range; consistent anticoagulation may be difficult to maintain in children <5 years of age

Adults: 5-15 mg/day for 2-5 days, then adjust dose according to results of prothrombin time; usual maintenance dose ranges from 2-10 mg/day

I.V. (administer as a slow bolus injection): 2-5 mg/day

Dosing adjustment/comments in hepatic disease: Monitor effect at usual doses; the response to oral anticoagulants may be markedly enhanced in obstructive jaundice (due to reduced vitamin K absorption) and also in hepatitis and cirrhosis (due to decreased production of vitamin K-dependent clotting factors); prothrombin index should be closely monitored

Administration Administer as a slow bolus injection over 1-2 minutes; avoid all I.M. injections

Monitoring Parameters Prothrombin time, hematocrit, INR

Reference Range

Therapeutic: 2-5 µg/mL (SI: 6.5-16.2 µmol/L)

Prothrombin time should be 1½ to 2 times the control or INR should be ↑ 2 to 3 times based upon indication

Normal prothrombin time: 10-13 seconds

Test Interactions Warfarin ↑ PTT

Patient Information Do not take with food; report any signs of bleeding; avoid hazardous activities; use soft tooth brush; urine may turn red/orange; carry Medi-Alert® ID identifying drug usage; be sure of other drugs and foods to avoid report any bleeding to physician at once; notify physician if urine turns dark brown or if red or tar black stools occur

Dosage Forms

Powder for injection, lyophilized: 5 mg vial

Tablet: 1 mg, 2 mg, 2.5 mg, 4 mg, 5 mg, 7.5 mg, 10 mg

4-Way® Long-Acting Nasal Solution [OTC] *see* Oxymetazoline Hydrochloride *on page 829*

Wehamine® *see* Dimenhydrinate *on page 347*

Wellbutrin® *see* Bupropion *on page 149*

Wellcovorin® *see* Leucovorin Calcium *on page 619*

Westcort® *see* Hydrocortisone *on page 546*

Westrim® LA [OTC] *see* Phenylpropanolamine Hydrochloride *on page 876*

White Mineral Oil *see* Mineral Oil *on page 743*

Wigraine® *see* Ergotamine *on page 399*

Winstrol® *see* Stanozolol *on page 1027*

Wyamycin® S *see* Erythromycin *on page 401*

Wycillin® *see* Penicillin G Procaine *on page 853*

Wydase® *see* Hyaluronidase *on page 539*

Wymox® *see* Amoxicillin Trihydrate *on page 68*

Wytensin® *see* Guanabenz Acetate *on page 517*

Xanax® *see* Alprazolam *on page 44*

Xylocaine® *see* Lidocaine Hydrochloride *on page 633*

Xylocaine® With Epinephrine *see* Lidocaine and Epinephrine *on page 631*

Xylometazoline Hydrochloride (zye loe met az' oh leen)

Brand Names Otrivin® [OTC]
Use Symptomatic relief of nasal and nasopharyngeal mucosal congestion
Pregnancy Risk Factor C
Contraindications Known hypersensitivity to xylometazoline hydrochloride, narrow-angle glaucoma, patients receiving MAO inhibitors
Warnings/Precautions Do not use in children <2 years of age; excessive use may cause rebound congestion or chemical rhinitis; use with caution in patients with hypertension, diabetes, cardiovascular or coronary artery disease
Adverse Reactions
  1% to 10%:
    Cardiovascular: Palpitations
    Central nervous system: Drowsiness, dizziness, seizures, headache
    Ocular: Blurred vision, ocular irritation, photophobia
    Miscellaneous: Sweating
Overdosage/Toxicology Symptoms of overdose include CNS depression, hypothermia, bradycardia, cardiovascular collapse, coma, respiratory depression, apnea; following initiation of essential overdose management, toxic symptoms should be treated. The patient should be kept warm and monitored for alterations in vital functions. Seizures commonly respond to diazepam (5-10 mg I.V. bolus in adults every 15 minutes if needed up to a total of 30 mg; I.V. 0.25-0.4 mg/kg/dose up to a total of 1 mg for children) or to phenytoin or phenobarbital. Apnea will respond to naloxone.
Mechanism of Action Stimulates alpha-adrenergic receptors in the arterioles of the conjunctiva and the nasal mucosa to produce vasoconstriction
Pharmacodynamics/Kinetics
  Onset of action: Intranasal: Local vasoconstriction occurs within 5-10 minutes
  Duration: 5-6 hours
Usual Dosage
  Children 2-12 years: Instill 2-3 drops (0.05%) in each nostril every 8-10 hours
  Children >12 years and Adults: Instill 2-3 drops or sprays (0.1%) in each nostril every 8-10 hours
Patient Information Do not exceed recommended dosage; do not use for more than 4 consecutive days
Dosage Forms Solution: 0.05% [0.5 mg/mL] (25 mL); 0.1% [1 mg/mL] (20 mL spray, 25 mL drops)

Yellow Fever Vaccine

Related Information
  Immunization Guidelines *on page 1389-1405*
  Vaccines *on page 1386-1388*
Brand Names YF-VAX®
  (Continued)

Yellow Fever Vaccine *(Continued)*

Use Selected persons traveling or living in areas where yellow fever infection exists.

Some countries require a valid international Certification of Vaccination showing receipt of vaccine; if a pregnant woman is to be vaccinated only to satisfy an international requirement, efforts should be made to obtain a waiver letter.

Pregnancy Risk Factor D

Contraindications Sensitivity to egg or chick embryo protein; pregnant women, children <6 months of age unless in high risk area

Adverse Reactions
>10%: Central nervous system: Fever, malaise
1% to 10%:
    Central nervous system: Headache
    Neuromuscular & skeletal: Myalgia
<1%: Encephalitis in very young infants (rare), anaphylaxis

Drug Interactions Administer yellow fever vaccine at least 1 month apart from other live virus vaccines; defer vaccination for 3 weeks following blood, plasma, or immune globulin

Stability Yellow fever vaccine is shipped with dry ice; do not use vaccine unless shipping case contains some dry ice on arrival; maintain vaccine continuously at a temperature between 0°C to 5°C (32°F to 41°F)

Usual Dosage One dose S.C. 10 days to 10 years before travel, booster every 10 years

Patient Information Immunity develops by the tenth day and **WHO** requires revaccination every 10 years to maintain travelers' vaccination certificates

Nursing Implications Sterilize and discard all unused rehydrated vaccine and containers after 1 hour; avoid vigorous shaking

Additional Information Federal law requires that the date of administration, the vaccine manufacturer, lot number of vaccine, and the administering person's name, title and address be entered into the patient's permanent medical record

Dosage Forms Injection: Not less than 5.04 Log_{10} Plaque Forming Units (PFU) per 0.5 mL

YF-VAX® *see* Yellow Fever Vaccine *on previous page*

Yodoxin® *see* Iodoquinol *on page 588*

Yutopar® *see* Ritodrine Hydrochloride *on page 986*

Zalcitabine (zal site' a been)

Brand Names Hivid®

Synonyms ddC; Dideoxycytidine

Use FDA approved: Treatment of HIV infections only in combination with zidovudine in adult patients with advanced HIV disease demonstrating a significant clinical or immunologic deterioration

Pregnancy Risk Factor C

Contraindications Hypersensitivity to the drug or any component of the product

Warnings/Precautions Approved for use only in combination with zidovudine; warnings and precautions associated with zidovudine should be observed; careful monitoring of pancreatic enzymes and liver function tests in patients with a history of pancreatitis, increased amylase, those on parenteral nutrition or with a history of ethanol abuse. Use with caution in patients on digitalis, CHF, renal failure, hyperphosphatemia.

Adverse Reactions
>10%: Oral ulcers
1% to 10%:
    Cardiovascular: Chest pain
    Central nervous system: Headache, dizziness, myalgia, foot pain, fatigue
    Dermatologic: Rash, pruritus
    Gastrointestinal: Nausea, dysphagia, anorexia, abdominal pain, vomiting, diarrhea, weight decrease
    Respiratory: Pharyngitis
<1%:
    Cardiovascular: Edema, hypertension, palpitations, syncope, atrial fibrillation, tachycardia, heart racing
    Central nervous system: Night sweats, fever, pain, malaise, asthenia
    Endocrine & metabolic: Hyperglycemia, hypocalcemia
    Gastrointestinal: Constipation, pancreatitis
    Hepatic: Jaundice, hepatitis
    Neuromuscular & skeletal: Myositis, peripheral neuropathy
    Miscellaneous: Epistaxis

Overdosage/Toxicology Symptoms of overdose include delayed peripheral neurotoxicity; following oral decontamination, treatment is supportive

Drug Interactions Increased toxicity:

Amphotericin, foscarnet, and aminoglycosides may potentiate the risk of developing peripheral neuropathy or other toxicities associated with zalcitabine by interfering with the renal elimination of zalcitabine

Other drugs associated with peripheral neuropathy include chloramphenicol, cisplatin, dapsone, disulfiram, ethionamide, glutethimide, gold hydralazine, iodoquinol, isoniazid, metronidazole, nitrofurantoin, phenytoin, ribavirin, and vincristine

Concomitant use of zalcitabine with didanosine is not recommended

Stability Tablets should be stored in tightly closed bottles at 59°F to 86°F

Mechanism of Action

Purine nucleoside analogue, zalcitabine or 2',3'-dideoxycitidine (ddC) has been found to have *in vitro* activity and is reported to be successful against HIV in short term clinical trials

Intracellularly, ddc is converted to active metabolite ddCTP; lack the presence of the 3'-hydroxyl group necessary for phosphodiester linkages during DNA replication. As a result viral replication is prematurely terminated. ddCTP acts as a competitor for binding sites on the HIV-RNA dependent DNA polymerase (reverse transcriptase) to further contribute to inhibition of viral replication.

Pharmacodynamics/Kinetics

Absorption: Food decreases absorption by 39%

Distribution: CSF levels are 20% of serum levels

Protein binding: Minimal, 1% to 2%

Metabolism: Intracellularly to active triphosphoralated agent; no significant hepatic metabolism

Bioavailability: >80%

Half-life: 2.9 hours

Elimination: Renal, >70% unchanged

Usual Dosage Safety and efficacy in children <13 years of age have not been established

Adults: Oral (dosed in combination with zidovudine): Daily dose: 0.75 mg every 8 hours, given together with 200 mg of zidovudine (ie, total daily dose: 2.25 mg of zalcitabine and 600 mg of zidovudine)

Dosing adjustment in renal impairment: Since renal excretion appears to be the major route of elimination, zalcitabine's elimination may be prolonged in patients with poor renal function

Cl_{cr} 10-40 mL/minute: Daily dose may be adjusted to 0.75 mg every 12 hours

Cl_{cr} <10 mL/minute: Further reduce dose to 0.75 mg every 24 hours

Hemodialysis reduces plasma levels by 50%

Dosing in hepatic impairment: Zalcitabine could possible exacerbate existing liver dysfunction in patients with a previous history of liver disease or alcohol abuse. An increase in liver function tests was observed in patients on zalcitabine therapy; caution should be exercised in patients with hepatic impairment.

Monitoring Parameters Renal function, CD4 counts, CBC, serum amylase, triglyceride, calcium (see zidovudine monograph)

Patient Information Zalcitabine is not a cure; if numbness or tingling occurs, or if persistent, severe abdominal pain, nausea, or vomiting occur, notify physician. Women of childbearing age should use effective contraception while on zalcitabine; take on an empty stomach; take in combination with zidovudine.

Dosage Forms Tablet: 0.375 mg, 0.75 mg

Zidovudine (zye doe' vue deen)

Related Information

Antimicrobial Drugs of Choice *on page 1298-1302*

Brand Names Retrovir®

Synonyms Azidothymidine; AZT; Compound S

Use Management of patients with HIV infections who have had at least one episode of *Pneumocystis carinii* pneumonia or who have CD4 cell counts ≤500/mm³; patients who have HIV-related symptoms or who are asymptomatic with abnormal laboratory values indicating HIV-related immunosuppression; does not reduce risk of transmitting HIV infections

Pregnancy Risk Factor C

Contraindications Life-threatening hypersensitivity to zidovudine or any component

Warnings/Precautions Use with caution in patients with impaired renal or hepatic function; reduce dosage or interrupt therapy in patients with anemia and/or granulocytopenia and myopathy; often associated with hematologic toxicity including granulocytopenia, thrombocytopenia, and severe anemia requiring transfusions; zidovudine has been shown to be carcinogenic in rats and mice

Adverse Reactions

>10%:

Central nervous system: Severe headache, insomnia

Gastrointestinal: Nausea

Hematologic: Anemia, leukopenia, neutropenia

1% to 10%:

Dermatologic: Rash, hyperpigmentation of nails (bluish-brown)

Hematologic: Changes in platelet count

<1%:

Central nervous system: Weakness, neurotoxicity, confusion, mania, seizures

Gastrointestinal: Anorexia

Hematologic: Bone marrow depression, granulocytopenia, thrombocytopenia, pancytopenia

Hepatic: Hepatotoxicity, cholestatic jaundice

Local: Tenderness

Ocular: Myopathy

Overdosage/Toxicology Symptoms of overdose include nausea, vomiting, ataxia, granulocytopenia; erythropoietin, thymidine, and cyanocobalamin have been used experimentally to treat zidovudine-induced hematopoietic toxicity, yet none are presently specified as the agent of choice. Treatment is supportive.

Drug Interactions Increased toxicity: Coadministration with drugs that are nephrotoxic (amphotericin B), cytotoxic (flucytosine, vincristine, vinblastine, doxorubicin, interferon), inhibit glucuronidation or excretion (acetaminophen, cimetidine, indomethacin, lorazepam, probenecid, aspirin), or interfere with RBC/WBC number or function (acyclovir, ganciclovir, pentamidine, dapsone)

Mechanism of Action Zidovudine is a thymidine analog which interferes with the HIV viral RNA dependent DNA polymerase resulting in inhibition of viral replication

Pharmacodynamics/Kinetics

Absorption: Oral: Well absorbed (66% to 70%)

Distribution: Significant penetration into the CSF; crosses the placenta

Relative diffusion of antimicrobial agents from blood into cerebrospinal fluid (CSF): Adequate with or without inflammation (exceeds usual MICs)

Ratio of CSF to blood level (%): Normal meninges: ~60

Protein binding: 25% to 38%

Metabolism: Extensive first-pass metabolism; metabolized in the liver via glucuronidation to inactive metabolites

Half-life: Terminal: 60 minutes

Time to peak serum concentration: Within 30-90 minutes

Elimination: Urinary excretion (63% to 95%); following oral administration, 72% to 74% of the drug is excreted in the urine as metabolites and 14% to 18% as unchanged drug

Usual Dosage

Prevention of maternal-fetal HIV transmission: Neonatal (oral): 2 mg/kg/dose every 6 hours for 6 weeks beginning 8-12 hours after birth

Asymptomatic/symptomatic HIV infection:

Children 3 months to 12 years (oral): 90-180 mg/m²/dose every 6 hours; maximum: 200 mg every 6 hours

Children 3 months to 12 years (I.V.): 1-2 mg/kg/dose [infused over 1 hour] administered every 4 hours around-the-clock (6 doses/day)

Adults:

Asymptomatic HIV infection (oral): 100 mg every 4 hours while awake (500 mg/day)

Symptomatic HIV infection (oral): Initial: 200 mg every 4 hours (1200 mg/day), then after 1 month, 100 mg every 4 hours (600 mg/day)

Symptomatic HIV infection (I.V.): 1-2 mg/kg/dose [infused over 1 hour] administered every 4 hours around-the-clock (6 doses/day)

Patients should receive I.V. therapy only until oral therapy can be administered

The I.V. dosage of 1 mg/kg every 4 hours is approximately equivalent to 100 mg every 4 hours orally

Prevention of maternal-fetal HIV transmission: HIV-infected pregnant women:

Antepartum, beginning at 14 weeks gestational age or later (oral): 100 mg 5 times daily every 4 hours while awake

Intrapartum (I.V.): 2 mg/kg intravenous loading dose, followed by 1 mg/kg/hour until delivery

Dosing interval in renal impairment: Cl_{cr} <10 mL/minute: Administer 100 mg every 4 hours

At least partially removed by hemo and peritoneal dialysis; administer dose after hemodialysis or administer 100 mg supplemental dose; during CAPD, dose as for Cl_{cr} <10 mL/minute; during continuous arterio-venous or veno-venous hemofiltration (CAVH/CAVHD), administer 100 mg every 4 hours

Dosing adjustment in hepatic impairment: Reduce dose by 50% or double dosing interval in patients with cirrhosis

Dosage adjustment in anemia/granulocytopenia:

Significant anemia (hemoglobin <7.5 g/dL or reduction >25% of baseline) or significant granulocytopenia (granulocyte count <750/mm^3 or reduction >50% from baseline) may require a dose interruption until evidence of marrow recovery is observed

For less severe anemia or granulocytopenia, dose reduction may be adequate

Administration Administer around-the-clock to promote less variation in peak and trough serum levels

Monitoring Parameters Monitor CBC and platelet count at least every 2 weeks, MCV, serum creatinine kinase, CD4 cell count; observe for appearance of opportunistic infections

Patient Information Take 30 minutes before or 1 hour after a meal with a glass of water; take zidovudine exactly as prescribed; take around-the-clock; limit acetaminophen-containing analgesics; report all side effects to you physician

Dosage Forms

Capsule: 100 mg

Injection: 10 mg/mL (20 mL)

Syrup (strawberry flavor): 50 mg/5 mL (240 mL)

ZilaDent® [OTC] see Benzocaine on page 121

Zinacef® see Cefuroxime on page 208

Zinca-Pak® see Zinc Supplements on next page

Zincate® see Zinc Supplements on next page

Zinc Chloride see Zinc Supplements on next page

Zinc Gelatin

Brand Names Gelucast®

Synonyms Dome Paste Bandage; Unna's Boot; Unna's Paste; Zinc Gelatin Boot

Use As a protectant and to support varicosities and similar lesions of the lower limbs

Contraindications Hypersensitivity to any component

Adverse Reactions 1% to 10%: Irritation

Usual Dosage Apply externally as an occlusive boot

Nursing Implications After a period of about 2 weeks, the dressing is removed by soaking in warm water

Dosage Forms Bandage: 3" x 10 yards, 4" x 10 yards

Zinc Gelatin Boot see Zinc Gelatin on this page

Zinc Gluconate see Zinc Supplements on next page

Zinc Oxide

Synonyms Base Ointment; Lassar's Zinc Paste

Use Protective coating for mild skin irritations and abrasions, soothing and protective ointment to promote healing of chapped skin, diaper rash

Contraindications Hypersensitivity to any component

Warnings/Precautions Do not use in eyes; for external use only

(Continued)

Zinc Oxide *(Continued)*

Adverse Reactions 1% to 10%: Local: Skin sensitivity, irritation

Stability Avoid prolonged storage at temperatures >30°C

Mechanism of Action Mild astringent with weak antiseptic properties

Usual Dosage Infants, Children, and Adults: Topical: Apply as required for affected areas several times daily

Patient Information If irritation develops, discontinue use and consult a physician; paste is easily removed with mineral oil; for external use only; do not use in the eyes

Dosage Forms

Ointment, topical: 20% in white ointment (480 g)

Paste, topical: 25% in white petrolatum (480 g)

Zinc Oxide, Cod Liver Oil, and Talc

Brand Names Desitin® [OTC]

Use Relief of diaper rash, superficial wounds and burns, and other minor skin irritations

Contraindications Hypersensitivity to any component

Adverse Reactions 1% to 10%: Skin sensitivity, irritation

Usual Dosage Topical: Apply thin layer as needed

Patient Information If condition persists, or if rash, irritation or sensitivity develops, discontinue and contact physician; for external use only

Dosage Forms Ointment, topical: Zinc oxide, cod liver oil and talc in a petrolatum and lanolin base (30 g, 60 g, 120 g, 240 g, 270 g)

Zinc Sulfate *see* Zinc Supplements *on this page*

Zinc Supplements

Brand Names Eye-Sed® [OTC]; Orazinc® [OTC]; Verazinc® [OTC]; Zinca-Pak®; Zincate®

Synonyms Zinc Chloride; Zinc Gluconate; Zinc Sulfate

Use Cofactor for replacement therapy to different enzymes helps maintain normal growth rates, normal skin hydration and senses of taste and smell; zinc supplement (oral and parenteral); may improve wound healing in those who are deficient. May be useful to promote wound healing in patients with pressure sores.

Pregnancy Risk Factor C

Contraindications Hypersensitivity to any component

Warnings/Precautions Do not take undiluted by direct injection into a peripheral vein because of potential for phlebitis, tissue irritation, and potential to increase renal loss of minerals from a bolus injection; administration of zinc in absence of copper may decrease plasma levels; excessive dose may increase HDL and impair immune system function

Adverse Reactions

<1%:

Cardiovascular: Hypotension

Gastrointestinal: Indigestion, nausea, vomiting

Hematologic: Neutropenia, leukopenia

Hepatic: Jaundice

Respiratory: Pulmonary edema

Overdosage/Toxicology Symptoms of overdose include hypotension, pulmonary edema, diarrhea, vomiting, oliguria, nausea, gastric ulcers, restlessness, dizziness, profuse sweating, decreased consciousness, blurred vision, tachycardia, hypothermia, hyperamylasemia, jaundice; this agent is corrosive and emesis or gastric lavage should be avoided, instead dilute rapidly with milk or water. Calcium disodium edetate or dimercaprol can be very effective at binding zinc. Supportive care should always be instituted.

Drug Interactions Decreased effect: Decreased penicillamine, decreased tetracycline effect reduced, iron decreased uptake of zinc, bran products, dairy products reduce absorption of zinc

Mechanism of Action Provides for normal growth and tissue repair, is a cofactor for more than 70 enzymes; ophthalmic astringent and weak antiseptic due to precipitation of protein and clearing mucus from outer surface of the eye

Pharmacodynamics/Kinetics

Absorption: Poor from gastrointestinal tract (20% to 30%)

Elimination: In feces with only traces appearing in urine

Usual Dosage Clinical response may not occur for up to 6-8 weeks

Zinc sulfate:

RDA: Oral:

Birth to 6 months: 3 mg elemental zinc/day

6-12 months: 5 mg elemental zinc/day

1-10 years: 10 mg elemental zinc/day (44 mg zinc sulfate)

≥11 years: 15 mg elemental zinc/day (65 mg zinc sulfate)

Zinc deficiency: Oral:

Infants and Children: 0.5-1 mg elemental zinc/kg/day divided 1-3 times/day; somewhat larger quantities may be needed if there is impaired intestinal absorption or an excessive loss of zinc

Adults: 110-220 mg zinc sulfate (25-50 mg elemental zinc)/dose 3 times/day

Parenteral: TPN: I.V. infusion (chloride or sulfate):

Supplemental to I.V. solutions (clinical response may not occur for up to 6-8 weeks):

Premature Infants <1500 g, up to 3 kg: 300 mcg/kg/day

Full-term Infants and Children ≤5 years: 100 mcg/kg/day

or

Premature Infants: 400 mcg/kg/day

Term <3 months: 250 mcg/kg/day

Term >3 months: 100 mcg/kg/day

Children: 50 mcg/kg/day

Adults:

Stable with fluid loss from small bowel: 12.2 mg zinc/liter TPN or 17.1 mg zinc/kg (added to 1000 mL I.V. fluids) of stool or ileostomy output

Metabolically stable: 2.5-4 mg/day, add 2 mg/day for acute catabolic states

Monitoring Parameters Patients on TPN therapy should have periodic serum copper and serum zinc levels, skin integrity

Reference Range

Serum: 50-150 µg/dL (<20 µg/dL as solid test with dermatitis followed by alopecia)

Therapeutic: 66-110 µg/dL (SI: 10-16.8 µmol/L)

Patient Information Take with food if GI upset occurs, but avoid foods high in calcium, phosphorous, or phytate; do not exceed recommended dose; if irritation persists or continues with ophthalmic use, notify physician

Nursing Implications Give oral formulation with food if GI upset occurs; avoid foods high in calcium or phosphorus; do not give undiluted by direct injection into a peripheral vein because of potential for phlebitis, tissue irritation, and potential to increase renal loss of minerals from a bolus injection

Dosage Forms

Zinc carbonate, complex: Liquid: 15 mg/mL (30 mL)

Zinc chloride: Injection: 1 mg/mL (10 mL)

Zinc gluconate (14.3% zinc): Tablet: 10 mg (elemental zinc 1.4 mg), 15 mg (elemental zinc 2 mg), 50 mg (elemental zinc 7 mg), 78 mg (elemental zinc 11 mg)

Zinc sulfate (23% zinc):

Capsule: 110 mg (elemental zinc 25 mg), 220 mg (elemental zinc 50 mg)

Injection: 1 mg/mL (10 mL, 30 mL); 4 mg/mL (10 mL); 5 mg/mL (5 mL, 10 mL)

Tablet: 66 mg (elemental zinc 15 mg), 110 mg (elemental zinc 25 mg), 200 mg (elemental zinc 45 mg)

Zithromax™ see Azithromycin on page 107

Zocor™ see Simvastatin on page 1006

Zofran® see Ondansetron on page 817

Zoladex® see Goserelin Acetate on page 511

Zolicef® see Cefazolin Sodium on page 194

Zoloft™ see Sertraline Hydrochloride on page 1003

Zolpidem Tartrate (zole pi′ dem)

Brand Names Ambien™

Use Short-term treatment of insomnia

Restrictions C-IV

Pregnancy Risk Factor B

Contraindications Lactation

Warnings/Precautions Closely monitor elderly or debilitated patients for impaired cognitive or motor performance; not recommended for use in children <18 years of age

Adverse Reactions

1% to 10%:

Central nervous system: Headache, drowsiness, dizziness

Gastrointestinal: Nausea, diarrhea

Neuromuscular & skeletal: Myalgia

(Continued)

Zolpidem Tartrate *(Continued)*

<1%:
  Central nervous system: Amnesia, confusion
  Gastrointestinal: Vomiting
  Neuromuscular & skeletal: Falls, tremor

Overdosage/Toxicology Symptoms of overdose include coma and hypotension. Treatment for overdose is supportive. Rarely is mechanical ventilation required. Flumazenil has been shown to selectively block binding to CNS receptors, resulting in a reversal of CNS depression but not always respiratory depression.

Drug Interactions Increased effect/toxicity with alcohol, CNS depressants

Mechanism of Action Structurally dissimilar to benzodiazepine, however, has much or all of its actions explained by its effects on benzodiazepine (BZD) receptors, especially the omega-1 receptor; retains hypnotic and much of the anxiolytic properties of the BZD, but has reduced effects on skeletal muscle and seizure threshold.

Pharmacodynamics/Kinetics
  Onset of action: 30 minutes
  Duration: 6-8 hours
  Absorption: Rapid
  Distribution: Very low amounts secreted into breast milk
  Protein binding: 92%
  Metabolism: Hepatic to inactive metabolites
  Half-life: 2-2.6 hours, in cirrhosis increased to 9.9 hours

Usual Dosage Duration of therapy should be limited to 7-10 days
  Adults: Oral: 10 mg immediately before bedtime; maximum dose: 10 mg
  Elderly: 5 mg immediately before bedtime

  Not dialyzable
  Dosing adjustment in hepatic impairment: Decrease dose to 5 mg
Monitoring Parameters Respiratory, cardiac and mental status
Reference Range 80-150 ng/mL
Patient Information Avoid alcohol and other CNS depressants while taking this medication; for fastest onset, take on an empty stomach; may cause drowsiness
Nursing Implications Patients may require assistance with ambulation; lower doses in the elderly are usually effective; institute safety measures
Dosage Forms Tablet: 5 mg, 10 mg

Zolyse® *see* Chymotrypsin, Alpha *on page 243*

ZORprin® *see* Aspirin *on page 92*

Zostrix®-HP [OTC] *see* Capsaicin *on page 173*

Zostrix® [OTC] *see* Capsaicin *on page 173*

Zosyn™ *see* Piperacillin Sodium and Tazobactam Sodium *on page 889*

Zovirax® *see* Acyclovir *on page 28*

Zydone® *see* Hydrocodone and Acetaminophen *on page 543*

Zyloprim® *see* Allopurinol *on page 41*

Zymase® *see* Pancrelipase *on page 837*

Zymenol® [OTC] *see* Mineral Oil *on page 743*

APPENDIX

ABBREVIATIONS COMMONLY USED IN MEDICAL ORDERS

Abbreviation	From	Meaning
aa, aa	ana	of each
ac	ante cibum	before meals or food
ad	ad	to, up to
a.d.	aurio dextra	right ear
ad lib	ad libitum	at pleasure
AM	ante meridiem	morning
amp		ampul
amt		amount
aq	aqua	water
a.s.	aurio sinister	left ear
ASAP		as soon as possible
a.u.	aures utrae	each ear
bid	bis in die	twice daily
bm		bowel movement
bp		blood pressure
BSA		body surface area
c̄	cum	with
cal		calorie
cap	capsula	capsule
cm		centimeter
comp	compositus	compound
cont		continue
d	dies	day
d/c		discontinue
disp	dispensa	dispense
elix	elixir	elixir
ex aq		in water
FDA		Food and Drug Administration
g	gramma	gram
gr	granum	grain
gtt	gutta	a drop
h	hora	hour
hs	hora somni	at bedtime
I.M.		intramuscular
I.V.		intravenous
kcal		kilocalorie
kg		kilogram
L		liter
μg		microgram
mEq		milliequivalent
mg		milligram
mL		milliliter
mm		millimeter
NF		National Formulary
no.	numerus	number
noc	nocturnal	in the night
non rep	non repetatur	do not repeat, no refills
NPO		nothing by mouth
o.d.	oculus dexter	right eye
o.s.	oculus sinister	left eye
o.u.	oculo uterque	each eye
pc	post cibos	after meals
per		through or by
PM	post meridiem	afternoon or evening
P.O.	per os	by mouth
P.R.	per rectum	rectally
prn	pro re nata	as needed
q		every
qd		every day
qh	quiaque hora	every hour
qid	quater in die	four times a day
qod		every other day
qs	quantum sufficiat	a sufficient quantity
qs ad		a sufficient quantity to make
qty		quantity

(continued)

Abbreviation	From	Meaning
Rx	recipe	take, a recipe
rep	repetatur	let it be repeated
$\overline{s}$	sine	without
S.C.		subcutaneous
sig	signa	label, or let it be printed
sol	solutio	solution
$\overline{ss}$	semis	one-half
stat	statim	at once, immediately
supp	suppositorium	suppository
syr	syrupus	syrup
tab	tabella	tablet
tal		such
tid	ter in die	three times a day
tr, tinct	tincture	tincture
tsp		teaspoonful
ung	unguentum	ointment
USAN		United States Adopted Names
USP		United States Pharmacopeia
u.d., ut dict	ut dictum	as directed
v.o.		verbal order
w.a.		while awake
x3		3 times
x4		4 times

MILLIMOLE AND MILLIEQUIVALENT CALCULATIONS

Definitions

mole = gram molecular weight of a substance (aka molar weight)

millimole (mM) = milligram molecular weight of a substance (a millimole is 1/1000 of a mole)

equivalent weight = gram weight of a substance which will combine with or replace one gram (one mole) of hydrogen; an equivalent weight can be determined by dividing the molar weight of a substance by its ionic valence

milliequivalent (mEq) = milligram weight of a substance which will combine with or replace one milligram (one millimole) of hydrogen (a milliequivalent is 1/1000 of an equivalent)

Calculations

moles $= \dfrac{\text{weight of a substance (grams)}}{\text{molecular weight of that substance (grams)}}$

millimoles $= \dfrac{\text{weight of a substance (milligrams)}}{\text{molecular weight of that substance (milligrams)}}$

equivalents = moles x valence of ion

milliequivalents = millimoles x valence of ion

moles $= \dfrac{\text{equivalents}}{\text{valence of ion}}$

millimoles $= \dfrac{\text{milliequivalents}}{\text{valence of ion}}$

millimoles = moles x 1000

milliequivalents = equivalents x 1000

Note: Use of equivalents and milliequivalents is valid only for those substances which have fixed ionic valences (eg, sodium, potassium, calcium, chlorine, magnesium bromine, etc). For substances with variable ionic valences (eg, phosphorous), a reliable equivalent value cannot be determined. In these instances, one should calculate millimoles (which are fixed and reliable) rather than milliequivalents.

MILLIEQUIVALENT CONVERSIONS

To convert mg/100 mL to mEq/L the following formula may be used:

$$\frac{(mg/100\ mL) \times 10 \times valence}{atomic\ weight} = mEq/L$$

To convert mEq/L to mg/100 mL the following formula may be used:

$$\frac{(mEq/L) \times atomic\ weight}{10 \times valence} = mg/100\ mL$$

To convert mEq/L to volume percent of a gas the following formula may be used:

$$\frac{(mEq/L) \times 22.4}{10} = volume\ percent$$

Valences and Atomic Weights of Selected Ions

Substance	Electrolyte	Valence	Molecular Wt
Calcium	Ca^{++}	2	40
Chloride	Cl^-	1	35.5
Magnesium	Mg^{++}	2	24
Phosphate	HPO_4^{--} (80%)	1.8	96*
pH = 7.4	$H_2PO_4^-$ (20%)	1.8	96*
Potassium	K^+	1	39
Sodium	Na^+	1	23
Sulfate	SO_4^{--}	2	96*

*The molecular weight of phosphorus only is 31, and sulfur only is 32.

Approximate Milliequivalents — Weights of Selected Ions

Salt	mEq/g Salt	Mg Salt/mEq
Calcium carbonate ($CaCO_3$)	20	50
Calcium chloride ($CaCl_2 - 2H_2O$)	14	73
Calcium gluconate (Ca gluconate$_2$ – 1H_2O)	4	224
Calcium lactate (Ca lactate$_2$ – 5H_2O)	6	154
Magnesium sulfate ($MgSO_4$)	16	60
Magnesium sulfate ($MgSO_4$ – 7H_2O)	8	123
Potassium acetate (K acetate)	10	98
Potassium chloride (KCl)	13	75
Potassium citrate (K_3 citrate – 1H_2O)	9	108
Potassium iodide (KI)	6	166
Sodium bicarbonate ($NaHCO_3$)	12	84
Sodium chloride (NaCl)	17	58
Sodium citrate (Na_3 citrate – 2H_2O)	10	98
Sodium iodine (NaI)	7	150
Sodium lactate (Na lactate)	9	112

CORRECTED SODIUM

Corrected Na^+ = measured Na^+ + $[1.5 \times (\frac{glucose - 150}{100})]$

Note: Do not correct for glucose <150.

WATER DEFICIT

Water deficit = $0.6 \times$ body wt $[1 - (\frac{140}{Na^+})]$

Note: Body weight is estimated weight in kg when fully hydrated; **Na^+** is serum or plasma sodium. Use corrected Na^+ if necessary. Consult medical references for recommendations for replacement of deficit.

TOTAL SERUM CALCIUM CORRECTED FOR ALBUMIN LEVEL

[(Normal albumin – patient's albumin) $\times$ 0.8] + patient's measured total calcium

ACID-BASE EQUATION

H^+ (in mEq/L) = $\frac{24 \times P_aCO_2}{HCO_3^-}$

Aa GRADIENT

Aa Gradient $[(713)(F_iO_2 - (\frac{P_aCO_2}{0.8})] - P_aO_2$

Aa gradient	=	alveolar-arterial oxygen gradient
F_iO_2	=	inspired oxygen (expressed as a fraction)
P_aCO_2	=	arterial partial pressure carbon dioxide (mm Hg)
P_aO_2	=	arterial partial pressure oxygen (mm Hg)

OSMOLALITY

Definition: The summed concentrations of all osmotically active solute particles.

Predicted serum osmolality =
    2 Na^+ + glucose (mg/dL) / 18 + BUN (mg/dL) / 2.8

The normal range of serum osmolality is 285-295 mOsm/L.

Differential diagnosis of increased serum osmolal gap (>10 mOsm/L)

    Medications and toxins
        Alcohols (ethanol, methanol, isopropanol, glycerol, ethylene glycol)
        Mannitol
        Paraldehyde

Calculated Osm

Osmolal gap = measured Osm – calculated Osm

0 to +10:	Normal
>10:	Abnormal
<0:	Probable lab or calculation error

BICARBONATE DEFICIT

HCO_3^- deficit = (0.4 x wt in kg) x (HCO_3^- desired – HCO_3^- measured)

Note: In clinical practice, the calculated quantity may differ markedly from the actual amount of bicarbonate needed or that which may be safely administered.

RETICULOCYTE INDEX

$$\frac{\% \text{ retic}}{2} \times \frac{\text{patient's Hct}}{\text{normal Hct}} \quad \text{or} \quad \frac{\% \text{ retic}}{2} \times \frac{\text{patient's Hgb}}{\text{normal Hgb}}$$

Normal index: 1.0
Good marrow response: 2.0-6.0

ANION GAP

Definition: The difference in concentration between unmeasured cation and anion equivalents in serum.

Anion gap = $Na^+ - Cl^- - HCO_3^-$
(The normal anion gap is 10-14 mEq/L.)

Differential Diagnosis of Increased Anion Gap
Organic anions
Lactate (sepsis, hypovolemia, large tumor burden)
Pyruvate
Uremia
Ketoacidosis (β-hydroxybutyrate and acetoacetate)
Amino acids and their metabolites
Other organic acids (eg, formate from methanol, glycolate from ethylene glycol)

Inorganic anions
Hyperphosphatemia
Sulfates
Nitrates

Medications and toxins
Penicillins and cephalosporins
Salicylates (including aspirin)
Cyanide
Carbon monoxide

Differential Diagnosis of Decreased Anion Gap
Organic cations
Hypergammaglobulinemia

Inorganic cations
Hyperkalemia
Hypercalcemia
Hypermagnesemia

Medications and toxins
Lithium

Hypoalbuminemia

APOTHECARY/METRIC EQUIVALENTS

Liquid Measures

Basic equivalent: 1 fluid ounce = 30 mL

Examples:

1 gallon . . . . . . 3800 mL	4 fluid ounces . . 120 mL
1 quart . . . . . . .960 mL	15 minims . . . . .1 mL
1 pint . . . . .480 mL	10 minims . . . . . . .0.6 mL
8 fluid ounces . . .240 mL	

1 gallon . . . . . . .128 fluid ounces	
1 quart . . . . 32 fluid ounces	
1 pint . . . . 16 fluid ounces	

Approximate Household Equivalents

1 teaspoonful . . . . 5 mL   1 tablespoonful . . . 15 mL

Weights

Basic equivalents:

1 ounce = 30 g   15 grains = 1 g

Examples:

4 ounces . . . . . .120 g	1 grain . . . . 60 mg
2 ounces . . . . . . 60 g	1/100 grain . . . . 600 µg
10 grains . . . . . .600 mg	1/150 grain . . . . 400 µg
7 ½ grains . . .500 mg	1/200 grain . . . . 300 µg
16 ounces . . . . 1 pound	

Metric Conversions

Basic equivalents:

1 g . . . . 1000 mg   1 mg . . . . .1000 µg

Examples:

5 g . . . . 5000 mg	5 mg . . . . .5000 µg
0.5 g . . . . .500 mg	0.5 mg . . . . 500 µg
0.05 g . . . . 50 mg	0.05 mg . . . . 50 µg

Exact Equivalents

1 gram (g) = 15.43 grains	0.1 mg = 1/600 gr
1 milliliter (mL) = 16.23 minims	0.12 mg = 1/500 gr
1 minim (♏) = 0.06 milliliter	0.15 mg = 1/400 gr
1 grain (gr) = 64.8 milligrams	0.2 mg = 1/300 gr
1 ounce (ʒ) = 31.1 grams	0.5 mg = 1/120 gr
1 ounce (oz) = 28.35 grams	0.8 mg = 1/80 gr
1 pound (lb) = 453.6 grams	1 mg = 1/65 gr
1 kilogram (kg) = 2.2 pounds	

Solids*

¼ grain = 15 mg
½ grain = 30 mg
1½ grain = 100 mg
5 grains = 300 mg
10 grains = 600 mg

*Use exact equivalents for compounding and calculations requiring a high degree of accuracy.

POUNDS/KILOGRAMS CONVERSION

1 pound = 0.45359 kilograms
1 kilogram = 2.2 pounds

lb	=	kg	lb	=	kg	lb	=	kg
1		0.45	70		31.75	140		63.50
5		2.27	75		34.02	145		65.77
10		4.54	80		36.29	150		68.04
15		6.80	85		38.56	155		70.31
20		9.07	90		40.82	160		72.58
25		11.34	95		43.09	165		74.84
30		13.61	100		45.36	170		77.11
35		15.88	105		47.63	175		79.38
40		18.14	110		49.90	180		81.65
45		20.41	115		52.16	185		83.92
50		22.68	120		54.43	190		86.18
55		24.95	125		56.70	195		88.45
60		27.22	130		58.91	200		90.72
65		29.48	135		61.24			

TEMPERATURE CONVERSION

Centigrade to Fahrenheit = (°C x 9/5) + 32 = °F
Fahrenheit to Centigrade = (°F - 32) x 5/9 = °C

°C	=	°F	°C	=	°F	°C	=	°F
100.0		212.0	39.0		102.2	36.8		98.2
50.0		122.0	38.8		101.8	36.6		97.9
41.0		105.8	38.6		101.5	36.4		97.5
40.8		105.4	38.4		101.1	36.2		97.2
40.6		105.1	38.2		100.8	36.0		96.8
40.4		104.7	38.0		100.4	35.8		96.4
40.2		104.4	37.8		100.1	35.6		96.1
40.0		104.0	37.6		99.7	35.4		95.7
39.8		103.6	37.4		99.3	35.2		95.4
39.6		103.3	37.2		99.0	35.0		95.0
39.4		102.9	37.0		98.6	0		32.0
39.2		102.6						

BODY SURFACE AREA OF ADULTS AND CHILDREN

Calculating Body Surface Area

In a child of average size, find weight and corresponding surface area on the boxed scale to the left. Or, for adults or children, use the nomogram to the right. Lay a straightedge on the correct height and weight points for the child, then read the intersecting point on the surface area scale.

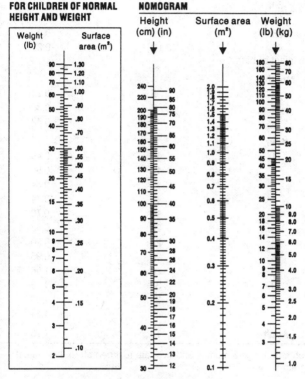

BODY SURFACE AREA FORMULA
(Adult and Pediatric)

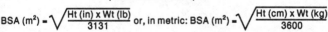

$$\text{BSA (m}^2) = \sqrt{\frac{\text{Ht (in)} \times \text{Wt (lb)}}{3131}} \quad \text{or, in metric: BSA (m}^2) = \sqrt{\frac{\text{Ht (cm)} \times \text{Wt (kg)}}{3600}}$$

References:
1. Mosteller RD, "Simplified Calculation of Body Surface Area", *N Engl J Med*, 1987, 317:1098.
2. Lam TK, Leung DT, (Letter to the Editor), *N Engl J Med*, 1988, 318:1130.

AVERAGE WEIGHTS AND SURFACE AREAS

**Average Weight and Surface Area of Preterm
Infants, Term Infants and Children**

Age	Average Weight (kg)*	Approximate Surface Area (m^2)
Weeks Gestation		
26	0.9-1	0.1
30	1.3-1.5	0.12
32	1.6-2	0.15
38	2.9-3	0.2
40	3.1-4	0.25
(term infant at birth)		
Months		
3	5	0.29
6	7	0.38
9	8	0.42
Year		
1	10	0.49
2	12	0.55
3	15	0.64
4	17	0.74
5	18	0.76
6	20	0.82
7	23	0.90
8	25	0.95
9	28	1.06
10	33	1.18
11	35	1.23
12	40	1.34
Adult	70	1.73

*Weights from age 3 months and over are rounded off to the nearest kilogram.

PEDIATRIC DOSAGE ESTIMATIONS

Dosage Estimations Based on Weight:

Augsberger's rule:

$$\frac{(1.5 \times \text{weight in kg} + 10)}{\% \text{ of adult dose}} = \text{child's approximate dose}$$

Clark's rule:

$$\frac{\text{weight (in pounds)}}{150} \times \text{adult dose} = \text{child's approximate dose}$$

Dosage Estimations Based on Age:

Augsberger's rule:

$$\frac{(4 \times \text{age in years} + 20)}{\% \text{ of adult dose}} = \text{child's approximate dose}$$

Bastedo's rule:

$$\frac{\text{age in years} + 3}{30} \times \text{adult dose} = \text{child's approximate dose}$$

Cowling's rule:

$$\frac{\text{age at next birthday (in years)}}{24} \times \text{adult dose} = \text{child's approximate dose}$$

Dilling's rule:

$$\frac{\text{age (in years)}}{20} \times \text{adult dose} = \text{child's approximate dose}$$

Fried's rule for infants (younger than 1 year):

$$\frac{\text{age (in months)}}{150} \times \text{adult dose} = \text{infant's approximate dose}$$

Young's rule:

$$\frac{\text{age (in years)}}{\text{age} + 12} \times \text{adult dose} = \text{child's approximate dose}$$

IDEAL BODY WEIGHT CALCULATION

Adults (18 years and older)

IBW (male)   = 50 + (2.3 x height in inches over 5 feet)
IBW (female) = 45.5 + (2.3 x height in inches over 5 feet)
*IBW is in kg.

Children
a. 1-18 years

$$IBW = \frac{(height^2 \times 1.65)}{1000}$$

*IBW is in kg.
Height is in cm.

b. 5 feet and taller

IBW (male)   = 39 + (2.27 x height in inches over 5 feet)
IBW (female) = 42.2 + (2.27 x height in inches over 5 feet)
*IBW is in kg.

LIVER DISEASE, PUGH'S MODIFICATION OF CHILD'S CLASSIFICATION FOR SEVERITY

Parameter	Points for Increasing Abnormality		
	1	2	3
Encephalopathy	None	1 or 2	3 or 4
Ascites	Absent	Slight	Moderate
Bilirubin (mg/dL)	<2.9	2.9-5.8	>5.8
Albumin (g/dL)	>3.5	2.8-3.5	<2.8
Prothrombin time (seconds over control)	1-4	4-6	>6

Scores: **Mild hepatic impairment** = <6 points.
Moderate hepatic impairment = 6-10 points.
Severe hepatic impairment = >10 points.

LIVER DISEASE, CONSIDERATIONS FOR DRUG DOSE ADJUSTMENT

Extent of Change in Drug Dose	Conditions or Requirements to Be Satisfied
No or minor change	Mild liver disease
	Extensive elimination of drug by kidneys and no renal dysfunction
	Elimination by pathways of metabolism spared by liver disease
	Drug is enzyme-limited and given acutely
	Drug is flow/enzyme-sensitive and only given acutely by I.V. route
	No alteration in drug sensitivity
Decrease in dose up to 25%	Elimination by the liver does not exceed 40% of the dose; no renal dysfunction
	Drug is flow-limited and given by I.V. route, with no large change in protein binding
	Drug is flow/enzyme-limited and given acutely by oral route
	Drug has a large therapeutic ratio
>25% decrease in dose	Drug metabolism is affected by liver disease; drug administered chronically
	Drug has a narrow therapeutic range; protein binding altered significantly
	Drug is flow-limited and given orally
	Drug is eliminated by kidneys and renal function severely affected
	Altered sensitivity to drug due to liver disease

Reference: Arns PA, Wedlund PJ, and Branch RA, "Adjustment of Medications in Liver Failure," *The Pharmacologic Approach to the Critically Ill Patient*, 2nd ed, Chernow B, ed, Baltimore, MD: Williams & Wilkins, 1988, 85-111.

CREATININE CLEARANCE ESTIMATING METHODS IN PATIENTS WITH STABLE RENAL FUNCTION

The following formulas provide an acceptable estimate of the patient's creatinine clearance except when:

a. patient's serum creatinine is changing rapidly (either up or down)

b. patients are markedly emaciated

In these situations (a and b above), certain assumptions have to be made.

a. In patients with rapidly rising serum creatinines (ie, >0.5-0.7 mg/dL/day), it is best to assume that the patient's creatinine clearance is probably <10 mL/minute.

b. In emaciated patients, although their actual creatinine clearance is less than their calculated creatinine clearance (because of decreased creatinine production), it is not possible to easily predict how much less.

Adults (18 years and older)

Method 1: (Cockroft DW and Gault MH, *Nephron*, 1976, 16:31-41)

Estimated creatinine clearance (Cl_{cr}):
(mL/min)

$$\text{Male} = \frac{(140 - age)\ IBW\ (kg)}{72 \times S_{cr}}$$

$$\text{Female} = \text{Estimated } Cl_{cr} \text{ male} \times 0.85$$

Note: The use of the patient's ideal body weight (IBW) is recommended for the above formula except when the patient's actual body weight is less than ideal. Use of the IBW is especially important in obese patients.

Method 2: (Jelliffe RW, *Ann Intern Med*, 1973, 79:604)

Estimated creatinine clearance (Cl_{cr}):
(mL/min/1.73 m^2)

$$\text{Male} = \frac{98 - 0.8\ (age - 20)}{S_{cr}}$$

$$\text{Female} = \text{Estimated } Cl_{cr} \text{ male} \times 0.90$$

Children (1-18 years)

Method 1: (Traub SL, Johnson CE, *Am J Hosp Pharm*, 1980, 37:195-201)

$$Cl_{cr} = \frac{0.48 \times (height)}{S_{cr}}$$

where

Cl_{cr} = creatinine clearance in mL/min/1.73 m^2
S_{cr} = serum creatinine in mg/dL
Height = in cm

Method 2: Nomogram (Traub SL and Johnson CE, *Am J Hosp Pharm*, 1980, 37:195-201)

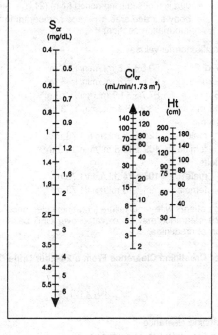

The nomogram below is for rapid evaluation of endogenous creatinine clearance (Cl_{cr}) in pediatric patients (aged 1-18 years).

To predict Cl_{cr}, connect the child's S_{cr} (serum creatinine) and Ht (height) with a ruler and read the Cl_{cr} where the ruler intersects the center line.

S_{cr}
(mg/dL)

Cl_{cr}
(mL/min/1.73 m²)

Ht
(cm)

RENAL FUNCTION TESTS

Endogenous creatinine clearance vs age (timed collection)

Creatinine clearance (mL/min/1.73 m^2) = (Cr_uV/Cr_sT) (1.73/A)

where:

Cr_u	=	urine creatinine concentration (mg/dL)
V	=	total urine volume collected during sampling period (mL)
Cr_s	=	serum creatinine concentration (mg/dL)
T	=	duration of sampling period (min) (24 h = 1440 min)
A	=	body surface area (m^2) (see nomogram in Calculation Information section)

Age-specific normal values

5-7 d	50.6 ± 5.8 mL/min/1.73 m^2
1-2 mo	64.6 ± 5.8 mL/min/1.73 m^2
5-8 mo	87.7 ± 11.9 mL/min/1.73 m^2
9-12 mo	86.9 ± 8.4 mL/min/1.73 m^2
≥18 mo	
male	124 ± 26 mL/min/1.73 m^2
female	109 ± 13.5 mL/min/1.73 m^2
Adults	
male	105 ± 14 mL/min/1.73 m^2
female	95 ± 18 mL/min/1.73 m^2

Note: In patients with renal failure (creatinine clearance <25 mL/min), creatinine clearance may be elevated over GFR because of tubular secretion of creatinine.

Calculation of Creatinine Clearance From a 24-Hour Urine Collection

Equation 1:

$$Cl_{cr} = \frac{(U) \times (V)}{P}$$

Cl_{cr}	=	creatinine clearance
U	=	urine concentration of creatinine
V	=	total urine volume in the collection
P	=	plasma creatinine concentration

Equation 2:

$$Cl_{cr} = \frac{(\text{total urine volume}) \times (\text{urine Cr concentration}) \times 100}{(\text{serum creatinine}) \times (\text{time of urine collection in minutes})}$$

Occasionally, a patient will have a 12- or 24-hour urine collection done for direct calculation of creatinine clearance. Although a urine collection for 24 hours is best, it is difficult to do since many urine collections occur for a much shorter period. A 24-hour urine collection is the desired duration of urine collection because the urine excretion of creatinine is diurnal and thus the measured creatinine clearance will vary throughout the day as the creatinine in the urine varies. When the urine collection is less than 24 hours, the total excreted creatinine will be affected by the time of the day during which the collection is performed. A 24-hour urine collection is sufficient to be able to accurately average the diurnal creatinine excretion variations. If a patient has 24 hours of urine collected for creatinine clearance, equation 1 can be used for calculating the creatinine clearance. To use equation 1 to calculate the creatinine clearance, it will be necessary to know the duration of urine collection, the urine collection volume, the urine creatinine concentration, and the serum creatinine value that reflects the urine collection period. In most cases, a serum creatinine concentration is drawn anytime during the day, but it is best to have the value drawn half way through the collection period.

Amylase/Creatinine Clearance Ratio*

$$\frac{Amylase_u \times creatinine_p}{Amylase_p \times creatinine_u} \times 100$$

u = urine; p = plasma.

Serum BUN/Serum Creatinine Ratio

Serum BUN (mg/dL:serum creatinine (mg/dL)

Normal BUN:creatinine ratio is 10-15.

BUN:creatinine ratio >20 suggests prerenal azotemia (also seen with high urea-generation states such as GI bleeding).

BUN:creatinine ratio <5 may be seen with disorders affecting urea biosynthesis such as urea cycle enzyme deficiencies and with hepatitis.

Fractional Sodium Excretion

Fractional sodium secretion (FENa) = $Na_uCr_s / Na_sCr_u \times 100\%$

where:

Na_u = urine sodium (mEq/L)
Na_s = serum sodium (mEq/L)
Cr_u = urine creatinine (mg/dL)
Cr_s = serum creatinine (mg/dL)

FENa <1% suggests prerenal failure
FENa >2% suggest intrinsic renal failure
(for newborns, normal FENa is approximately 2.5%)

Note: Disease states associated with a falsely elevated FENa include severe volume depletion (>10%), early acute tubular necrosis and volume depletion in chronic renal disease. Disorders associated with a lowered FENa include acute glomerulonephritis, hemoglobinuric or myoglobinuric renal failure, nonoliguric acute tubular necrosis and acute urinary tract obstruction. In addition, FENa may be <1% in patients with acute renal failure **and** a second condition predisposing to sodium retention (eg, burns, congestive heart failure, nephrotic syndrome).

Urine Calcium/Urine Creatinine Ratio (spot sample)

Urine calcium (mg/dL): urine creatinine (mg/dL)

Normal values <0.21 (mean values 0.08 males, 0.06 females)

Premature infants show wide variability of calcium: creatinine ratio, and tend to have lower thresholds for calcium loss than older children. Prematures without nephrolithiasis had mean Ca:Cr ratio of 0.75 ± 0.76. Infants with nephrolithiasis had mean Ca:Cr ratio of 1.32 ± 1.03 (Jacinto, et al, *Pediatrics*, vol 81, p 31).

Urine Protein/Urine Creatinine Ratio (spot sample)

P_u/Cr_u	Total Protein Excretion (mg/m²/d)
0.1	80
1	800
10	8000

where:

P_u = urine protein concentration (mg/dL)
Cr_u = urine creatinine concentration (mg/dL)

ANTIEMETICS FOR CHEMOTHERAPY INDUCED NAUSEA AND VOMITING

Basic Principles of Antiemetic Therapy

1. Rule out other causes of nausea and vomiting before prescribing antiemetics.

2. Evaluate the relative emetic potential of antineoplastic drugs and choose antiemetics accordingly.

3. Treat delayed nausea and vomiting with **scheduled antiemetics** for a period of several days.

4. **Combination antiemetic regimens** provide greater protection against chemotherapy induced emesis than do single agents.

5. Head off trouble before it starts by initiating an aggressive antiemetic regimen before giving highly emetogenic chemotherapy.

Time Course of Nausea and Vomiting

Drug	Onset (h)	Duration (h)
Azacitidine	1-3	3-4
Carboplatin	2-6	1-48
Carmustine	2-6	4-6
Cisplatin	1-4	12-96
Cyclophosphamide	6-8	8-24
Cytarabine	1-3	3-8
Dacarbazine	1-2	2-4
Dactinomycin	2-5	4-24
Daunorubicin	1-3	4-24
Doxorubicin	1-3	4-24
Ifosfamide	2-3	12-72
Lomustine	2-6	4-6
Mechlorethamine	1-3	2-8
Mitomycin	1-2	3-4
Plicamycin	4-6	4-24
Streptozocin	1-3	1-12

Emetogenic Potential of Single Chemotherapeutic Agents

Class I
Low (<10%)

Chlorambucil
Cyclophosphamide (oral)
Busulfan (oral)

Thioguanine (oral)
Thiotepa <60 mg
Vincristine

Class II
Moderately Low (10% to 30%)

Busulfan 1 mg/kg (oral)
Bleomycin
Cytarabine ≤20 mg
Doxorubicin ≤20 mg

Etoposide
Fluorouracil <1000 mg
Methotrexate <100 mg
Thiotepa >200 mg

Class III
Moderate (30% to 60%)

Azacitidine
Carboplatin
Cyclophosphamide <1 g
Doxorubicin <75 mg or >20 mg
Fluorouracil ≥1000 mg
Methotrexate <250 mg or
    ≥100 mg

Mitoxantrone
Paclitaxel
Teniposide
Vinblastine
Vinorelbine

Class IV
Moderately High (60% to 90%)

Carmustine <200 mg
Cisplatin <75 mg
Cyclophosphamide 1 g
Cytarabine 250 mg - 1 g
Dacarbazine <500 mg
Doxorubicin ≥75 mg

Ifosfamide
Lomustine <60 mg
Methotrexate ≥250 mg
Mitomycin
Procarbazine

Class V
High (>90%)

Carmustine ≥200 mg
Cisplatin ≥75 mg
Cyclophosphamide >1 g
Cytarabine >1 g
Dacarbazine ≥500 mg

Lomustine ≥60 mg
Mechlorethamine
Pentostatin
Streptozocin

Types of Antiemetic Drugs*

Anticholinergic drugs
    Scopolamine (Transderm-Scop®)
Antihistamines
    Diphenhydramine (Benadryl®)
Benzodiazepines
    Alprazolam (Xanax®)
    Lorazepam (Ativan®)
Butyrophenones
    Domperidone (Motilium®)
    Droperidol (Inapsine®)
    Haloperidol (Haldol®)
Cannabinoids
    Dronabinol (Marinol®)
    Nabilone (Cesamet®)
Corticosteroids
    Dexamethasone (Decadron®)
    Methylprednisolone (Medrol®)
Phenothiazines
    Chlorpromazine (Thorazine®)
    Perphenazine (Trilafon®)
    Prochlorperazine (Compazine®)
    Promethazine (Phenergan®)
    Thiethylperazine (Torecan®)
Serotonin antagonists
    Dolasetron (investigational)
    Granisetron (Kytril®)
    Ondansetron (Zofran®)
    Tropisetron (Navoban®) (investigational)
Substituted benzamides
    Alizapride (Plitican®) (investigational)
    Cisapride (Propulsid®)
    Metoclopramide (Reglan®)
    Trimethobenzamide (Tigan®)

Potency of Antiemetic Drugs

Potency	Type of Antiemetic Drug
Active against highly emetogenic chemotherapy	Serotonin antagonist Substituted benzamide (high dose)
Active against mildly or moderately emetogenic chemotherapy	Butyrophenone Cannabinoid Corticosteroid Phenothiazine
Minimally active	Anticholinergic agent Antihistamine Benzodiazepine

Initial Doses in Selected Antiemetic Regimens*

Antiemetic Regimen	Adult Dose	Pediatric Dose
For moderately emetogenic chemotherapy		
Dexamethasone	I.V.: 10-20 mg	I.V.: 10 mg/m^2/dose for the first dose, then 5 mg/m^2/dose q6h as needed
Dronabinol	P.O.: 10 mg	P.O.: 5 mg/m^2 starting 6-8 hours before chemotherapy and q4-6h after; to be continued for 12 hours after therapy discontinuation
Ondansetron	P.O.: 8 mg or I.V.: 10 mg	P.O.: 4-12 y: 4 mg 30 minutes before treatment; repeat 4 and 8 hours after initial dose >12 y: As adults I.V.: 10 mg/m^2/dose for the first dose, then 5 mg/m^2/dose q6h as needed
Prochlorperazine	P.O.: 5-10 mg, I.V.: 5-10 mg, or 25 mg by rectal suppository	P.O./P.R.: 0.4 mg/kg/24 hours in 3-4 divided doses I.M.: 0.1-0.15 mg/kg/dose
For highly emetogenic chemotherapy†		
Dexamethasone	I.V.: 20 mg	I.V.: 20 mg/m^2/dose for the first dose, then 5-10 mg/m^2/dose q6h as needed
Diphenhydramine	I.V.: 25-50 mg q2h x 2	I.V.: ≤50 mg/m^2 q2h x 2
Lorazepam	I.V.: 1-2 mg	I.V.: 2-15 y: 0.05 mg/kg (≤2 mg/dose) prior to chemotherapy
Metoclopramide	I.V.: 3 mg/kg of body weight q2h x 2	I.V.: 1-2 mg/kg 30 minutes before chemotherapy q2-4h
Ondansetron	I.V.: 32 mg (in divided doses)	I.V.: 0.45 mg/kg as single dose 30 minutes prior to chemotherapy or 0.15 mg/kg 30 minutes before and 0.15 mg/kg at 4 and 8 hours after treatment

*Antiemetic regimens for moderately emetogenic chemotherapy consist of single drugs; regimens for highly emetogenic chemotherapy consist of drugs given in combination (denoted by brackets).

†Use combination therapy.

Reference: Adapted with revisions from *N Engl J Med*, 1993, 329;1790-6.

Combinations of Antiemetic Drugs Resulting in Decreased Toxicity of the Primary Drug

Primary Antiemetic Drug	Effective Secondary Drug
Phenothiazine	Antihistamine
Butyrophenone	Antihistamine
Substituted benzamide	Antihistamine Corticosteroid Benzodiazepine
Cannabinoid	Phenothiazine

Combinations of Antiemetic Drugs Resulting in Improved Efficacy of the Primary Antiemetic Drug

Primary Antiemetic Drug	Effective Secondary Drug
Serotonin antagonist	Corticosteroid Phenothiazine Butyrophenone
Substituted benzamide	Corticosteroid Corticosteroid with anticholinergic drug
Phenothiazine	Corticosteroid
Butyrophenone	Corticosteroid
Cannabinoid	Corticosteroid
Corticosteroid	Benzodiazepine

EXTRAVASATION MANAGEMENT OF CHEMOTHERAPEUTIC AGENTS

Risk Factors for Extravasation

- Vascular disease
- Elderly patients
- Vascular obstruction
- Vascular ischemia
- Prior radiation
- Small vessel diameter
- Venous spasms
- Traumatic catheter or needle insertion
- Decreased lymphatic drainage in mastectomy patients

Purpose

To minimize harm caused to the patient by the extravasation of vesicant chemotherapeutic agents through prompt detection and treatment.

Procedure

1. Stop administration of the chemotherapeutic agent.

2. Leave the needle in place.

3. Aspirate any residual drug and blood in the I.V. tubing, needle, and suspected extravasation site.

4. For all drugs except mechlorethamine (nitrogen mustard), remove the needle.

5. Apply cold pack if the extravasated drug is amsacrine, doxorubicin, daunorubicin, or mechlorethamine. Apply a hot pack if the extravasated drug is etoposide, teniposide, navelbine, vinblastine, vincristine, or vindesine. Refer to individual drug in Alphabetical Listing of Drugs for appropriate management.

6. Notify the physician who ordered the chemotherapy of the suspected extravasation. Institute the attached recommended interventions unless countermanded by the physician.

7. Document the date, time, needle size and type, insertion site, drug sequence, drug administration technique, approximate amount of drug extravasated, management, patient complaints, appearance of site, physician notification, and follow-up measures.

8. The extravasation site should be evaluated by the physician as soon as possible after the extravasation and periodically thereafter as indicated by symptoms.

9. For inpatients, assess the site every day for pain, erythema, induration, or skin breakdown. For outpatients, contact the patient daily for 3 days for assessment of the site, and weekly thereafter until the problem is resolved.

10. The plastic surgery service should be consulted by the physician if pain and/or tissue breakdown occur.

Amsacrine/Daunorubicin/Doxorubicin

1. Apply cold pack immediately for 1 hour; repeat qid for 3-5 days.[1,2]

2. Dimethyl sulfoxide (DMSO) 50% to 99% (w/v) solution: Apply 1.5 mL to site every 6 hours for 14 days; allow to air dry, do not cover.[3]

3. Injection of sodium bicarbonate is contraindicated.[4]

4. Injection of hydrocortisone is of doubtful benefit.[4,5]

Mechlorethamine (nitrogen mustard)

1. Mix 4 mL of 10% sodium thiosulfate with 6 mL of sterile water for injection.

2. Inject 4 mL of this solution into the existing I.V. line.

3. Remove the needle.

4. Inject 2-3 mL of the solution subcutaneously clockwise into the infiltrated area using a 25-gauge needle. Change the needle with each new injection.

5. Apply ice immediately for 6-12 hours.

Mitomycin

1. Data is not currently available regarding potential antidotes and the application of heat or cold.

2. The site should be observed closely. These injuries frequently cause necrosis. A plastic surgery consult may be required.

3. Dimethyl sulfoxide (DMSO) 50% to 99% (w/v) solution: Apply 1.5 mL to site every 6 hours for 14 days; allow to air dry, do not cover.[3]

Etoposide/Teniposide/Navelbine/Vinblastine/Vincristine/Vindesine[6]

1. Inject 3-5 mL of hyaluronidase (150 units/mL) subcutaneously clockwise into the infiltrated area using a 25-gauge needle. Change the needle with each injection.

2. Apply heat immediately for 1 hour; repeat qid for 3-5 days.

3. Application of cold is contraindicated.

4. Injection of hydrocortisone is contraindicated.

[1] Dorr RT, Alberts DS, and Stone A, "Cold Protection and Heat Enhancement of Doxorubicin Skin Toxicity in the Mouse," *Cancer Treat Rep*, 1985, 69:431-7.

[2] Larson D, "What Is the Appropriate Management of Tissue Extravasation by Antitumor Agents?" *Plastic & Reconstr Surg*, 1985, 75:397-402.

[3] Oliver IW, Aisner J, Hament A, et al, "A Prospective Study of Topical Dimethyl Sulfoxide for Treating Anthracycline Extravasation," *J Clin Onc*, 1988, 6:1732-5.

[4] Dorr RT, Alberts DS, and Chen HS, "Limited Role of Corticosteroids in Ameliorating Experimental Doxorubicin Skin Toxicity in the Mouse," *Canc Chemother and Pharmacol*, 1980, 5:17-20.

[5] Coleman JJ, Walker AP, and Didolkar MS, "Treatment of Adriamycin Induced Skin Ulcers: A Prospective Controlled Study," *J of Surg Oncol*, 1983, 22:129-35.

[6] Dorr RT and Alberts DS, "Vinca Alkaloid Skin Toxicity Antidote and Drug Disposition Studies in the Mouse," *JNCI*, 1985, 74:113-20.

EXTRAVASATION TREATMENT OF OTHER DRUGS

Medication Extravasated	Cold/Warm Pack	Antidote
Vasopressors		
Dobutamine	None	Phentolamine (Regitine®)
Dopamine		Mix 5 mg with 9 mL of NS
Epinephrine		Inject a small amount of this
Norepinephrine		dilution into extravasated area.
Phenylephrine		Blanching should reverse immediately. Monitor site. If blanching should recur, additional injections of phentolamine may be needed.
I.V. Fluids and Other Medications		
Aminophylline	Cold	Hyaluronidase (Wydase®)
Calcium		1. Add 1 mL NS to 150-unit vial to make 150 units/mL concentration
Dextrose 10%		
Nafcillin		
Parenteral nutrition prep		2. Mix 0.1 mL of above with 0.9 mL NS in 1 mL syringe to make final concentration = 15 units/mL
Potassium		
Radiocontrast media		
		3. Inject 5 injections of 0.2 mL each with a 25-gauge needle into area of extravasation

TOXICITIES OF CHEMOTHERAPEUTIC AGENTS

Drug	Radiation-Recall Reactions	Ocular Toxicity	Pulmonary Toxicity	Cardio-toxicity	Hepato-toxicity	Cumulative Myelosuppression	Peripheral Neuropathy	CNS Depression
Allopurinol								
Altretamine		x					x	
Ara-C								x
Azathioprine					x			
BCNU (carmustine)			x		x			
Bleomycin	x		x			x		
Busulfan		x	x		x			
Carboplatin								
CCNU (lomustine)					x	x	x	
Chlorambucil		x	x		x			
Cisplatin		x			x		x	
Corticosteroids		x						
Cyclophosphamide		x	x	x*	x			
Cytarabine		x	x					
Dactinomycin	x		x		x			
Daunomycin				x†				
2'-Deoxycoformycin		x						
Doxorubicin	x	x	x	x†	x			
Etoposide	x		x		x			
Fludarabine			x					
Fluorouracil		x		x‡	x			x
G-CSF			x					
Hydroxyurea	x							
Idarubicin				x†				
Ifosfamide			x					x

(continued)

Drug	Radiation-Recall Reactions	Ocular Toxicity	Pulmonary Toxicity	Cardio-toxicity	Hepato-toxicity	Cumulative Myelosuppression	Peripheral Neuropathy	CNS Depression
Interferon		x	x					
L-asparaginase					x			x
Melphalan			x			x		
Mercaptopurine					x			
Methotrexate	x	x	x					
Methyl-CCNU (semustine)			x			x		
Mithramycin		x						
Mitomycin-C		x	x			x		
Mitotane		x						
Mitoxantrone				x†				
Nitrogen mustard		x						
Nitrosoureas		x						
Procarbazine			x			x		x
Streptozocin					x			
Tamoxifen		x	x					
Taxol®			x				x	
Teniposide			x					
Trimetrexate	x							
Vinblastine	x	x	x		x		x	
Vincristine	x	x	x				x	

Adapted from Patterson W and Perry MC, "Chemotherapeutic Toxicities: A Comprehensive Overview," *Contemporary Oncology*, 1993, 3(7):58-61.
G-CSF = granulocyte-colony stimulating factor.
*At high dose.
†Dose-related.
‡Idiosyncratic.

CANCER PAIN MANAGEMENT
(Adapted from the Agency for Healthcare Policy and Research,
Publication No. 94-0593, March, 1994)

Recommended Clinical Approach

A   **Ask** about pain regularly.
    Assess pain systematically.

B   **Believe** the patient and family in their reports of pain and what
    relieves it.

C   **Choose** pain control options appropriate for the patient, family,
    and setting.

D   **Deliver** interventions in a timely, logical, coordinated fashion.

E   **Empower** patients and their families.
    Enable patients to control their course to the greatest extent
    possible.

WHO Three-Step Analgesic Ladder

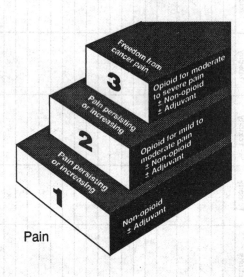

Continuing Pain Management

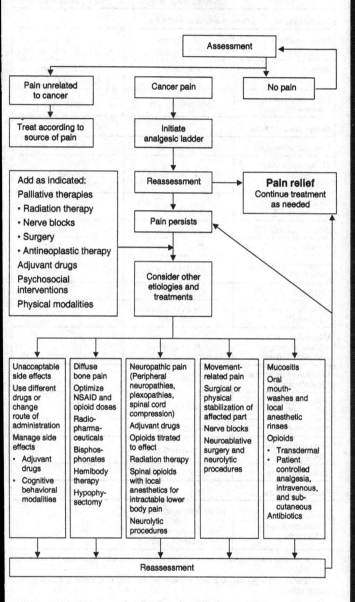

Table 1. Dosing Data for Acetaminophen and NSAIDs

Drug	Usual Dose for Adults >50 kg Body Weight	Usual Dose for Adults* <50 kg Body Weight
Acetaminophen and Over-the-Counter NSAIDs		
Acetaminophen†	650 mg q4h 975 mg q6h	10-15 mg/kg q4h 15-20 mg/kg q4h (rectal)
Aspirin‡	650 mg q4h 975 mg q6h	10-15 mg/kg q4h 15-20 mg/kg q4h (rectal)
Ibuprofen (Motrin®, others)	400-600 mg q6h	10 mg/kg q6-8h
Prescription NSAIDs		
Carprofen (Rimadyl®)	100 mg tid	
Choline magnesium trisalicylate§ (Trilisate®)	1000-1500 mg tid	25 mg/kg tid
Choline salicylate (Arthropan®)§	870 mg q3-4h	
Diflunisal (Dolobid®)¶	500 mg q12h	
Etodolac (Lodine®)	200-400 mg q6-8h	
Fenoprofen calcium (Nalfon®)	300-600 mg q6h	
Ketoprofen (Orudis®)	25-60 mg q6-8h	
Ketorolac tromethamine# (Toradol®)	10 mg q4-6h to a maximum of 40 mg/d	
Magnesium salicylate (Doan's®, Magan®, Mobidin®, others)	650 mg q4h	
Meclofenamate sodium (Meclomen®)•	50-100 mg q6h	
Mefenamic acid (Ponstel®)	250 mg q6h	
Naproxen (Naprosyn®)	250-275 mg q6-8h	5 mg/kg q8h
Naproxen sodium (Anaprox®)	275 mg q6-8h	
Sodium salicylate	325-650 mg q3-4h	
Parental NSAIDs		
Ketorolac tromethamine#,♦ (Toradol®)	60 mg initially, then 30 mg q6h Intramuscular dose not to exceed 5 days	

*Acetaminophen and NSAID dosages for adults weighing <50 kg should be adjusted for weight.

†Acetaminophen lacks the peripheral anti-inflammatory and antiplatelet activities of the other NSAIDs.

‡The standard against which other NSAIDs are compared. May inhibit platelet aggregation for ≥1 week and may cause bleeding.

§May have minimal antiplatelet activity.

¶Administration with antacids may decrease absorption.

#For short-term use only.

•Coombs'-positive autoimmune hemolytic anemia has been associated with prolonged use.

♦Has the same GI toxicities as oral NSAIDs.

Note: Only the above NSAIDs have FDA approval for use as simple analgesics, but clinical experience has been gained with other drugs as well.

Table 2. Dose Equivalents for Opioid Analgesics in Opioid-Naive Adults ≥50 kg*

Drug	Approximate Equianalgesic Dose		Usual Starting Dose for Moderate to Severe Pain	
	Oral	Parenteral	Oral	Parenteral
Opioid Agonist†				
Hydromorphone‡ (Dilaudid®)	7.5 mg q3-4h	1.5 mg q3-4h	6 mg q3-4h	1.5 mg q3-4h
Levorphanol (Levo-Dromoran®)	4 mg q6-8h	2 mg q6-8h	4 mg q6-8h	2 mg q6-8h
Meperidine (Demerol®)	300 mg q2-3h	100 mg q3h	NR	100 mg q3h
Methadone (Dolophine®, others)	20 mg q6-8h	10 mg q6-8h	20 mg q6-8h	10 mg q6-8h
Morphine‡	30 mg q3-4h (repeat around-the-clock dosing) 60 mg q3-4h (single dose or intermittent dosing)	10 mg q3-4h	30 mg q3-4h	10 mg q3-4h
Morphine, controlled-release‡, (MS Contin®, Oramorph®)	90-120 mg q12h	NA	90-120 mg q12h	NA
Oxymorphone‡ (Numorphan®)	NA	1 mg q3-4h	NA	1 mg q3-4h
Combination Opioid/NSAID Preparations				
Codeine (with aspirin or acetaminophen)	180-200 mg q3-4h	130 mg q3-4h	60 mg q3-4h	60 mg q2h (I.M./S.C.)
Hydrocodone (in Lorcet®, Lortab®, Vicodin®, others)	30 mg q3-4h	NA	10 mg q3-4h	NA
Oxycodone (Roxicodone®, also in Percocet®, Percodan®, Tylox®, others)	30 mg q3-4h	NA	10 mg q3-4h	NA

*Caution: Recommended doses do not apply for adult patients with body weight <50 kg. For recommended starting doses for adults <50 kg body weight, see Table 3.

†Caution: Recommended doses do not apply to patients with renal or hepatic insufficiency or other conditions affecting drug metabolism and kinetics.

‡Caution: For morphine, hydromorphone, and oxymorphone, rectal administration is an alternate route for patients unable to take oral medications. Equianalgesic doses may differ from oral and parenteral ...

Table 3. Dose Equivalents for Opioid Analgesics in Opioid-Naive Adults <50 kg

Drug	Approximate Equianalgesic Dose		Usual Starting Dose for Moderate to Severe Pain	
	Oral	Parenteral	Oral	Parenteral
Opioid Agonist*				
Hydromorphone† (Dilaudid®)	7.5 mg q3-4h	1.5 mg q3-4h	0.06 mg/kg q3-4h	0.015 mg/kg q3-4h
Levorphanol (Levo-Dromoran®)	4 mg q6-8h	2 mg q6-8h	0.04 mg/kg q6-8h	0.02 mg/kg q6-8h
Meperidine (Demerol®)	300 mg q2-3h	100 mg q3h	NR	0.75 mg/kg q2-3h
Methadone (Dolophine®, others)	20 mg q6-8h	10 mg q6-8h	0.2 mg/kg q6-8h	0.1 mg/kg q6-8h
Morphine†	30 mg q3-4h (repeat around-the-clock dosing) 60 mg q3-4h (single dose or intermittent dosing)	10 mg q3-4h	0.3 mg/kg q3-4h	0.1 mg/kg q3-4h
Morphine, controlled-release†,§ (MS Contin®, Oramorph®)	90-120 mg q12h	NA	NA	NA
Combination Opioid/NSAID Preparations				
Codeine (with aspirin or acetaminophen)	180-200 mg q3-4h	130 mg q3-4h	0.5-1 mg/kg q3-4h	NR
Hydrocodone (in Lorcet®, Lortab®, Vicodin®, others)	30 mg q3-4h	NA	0.2 mg/kg q3-4h	NA
Oxycodone (Roxicodone®, also in Percocet®, Percodan®, Tylox®, others)	30 mg q3-4h	NA	0.2 mg/kg q3-4h	NA

*Caution: Recommended doses do not apply to patients with renal or hepatic insufficiency or other conditions affecting drug metabolism and kinetics.

†Caution: For morphine, hydromorphone, and oxymorphone, rectal administration is an alternate route for patients unable to take oral medications. Equianalgesic doses may differ from oral and parenteral doses because of pharmacokinetic differences. **Note:** A short-acting opioid should normally be used for initial therapy of moderate to severe pain.

§Transdermal fentanyl (Duragesic®) is an alternative option. Transdermal fentanyl dosage is not calculated as equianalgesic to a single morphine dosage. See the package insert for dosing calculations. Doses above 25 mcg/h should not be used in opioid-naive patients.

Table 4. Drugs and Routes of Administration Not Recommended for Treatment of Cancer Pain

Class	Drug	Rationale for Not Recommending
Antagonist	Naloxone Naltrexone	May precipitate withdrawal. Limit use to treatment of life-threatening respiratory depression.
Anxiolytics alone	Benzodiazepine (eg, alprazolam)	Analgesic properties not demonstrated except for some instances of neuropathic pain. Added sedation from anxiolytics may limit opioid dosing.
Combination preparations	Brompton's cocktail	No evidence of analgesic benefit to using Brompton's cocktail over single opioid analgesics.
	DPT (meperidine, promethazine, and chlorpromazine)	Efficacy is poor compared with that of other analgesics. High incidence of adverse effects.
Opioid agonist-antagonists	Pentazocine Butorphanol Nalbuphine	Risk of precipitating withdrawal in opioid-dependent patients. Analgesic ceiling. Possible production of unpleasant psychomimetic effects (eg, dysphoria, hallucinations).
Opioids	Meperidine	Short (2-3 hour) duration. Repeated administration may lead to CNS toxicity (tremor, confusion, or seizures). High oral doses required to relieve severe pain, and these increase the risk of CNS toxicity.
Partial agonist	Buprenorphine	Analgesic ceiling. Can precipitate withdrawal.
Sedative/hypnotic drugs alone	Barbiturates Benzodiazepine	Analgesic properties not demonstrated. Added sedation from sedative/hypnotic drugs limits opioid dosing.
Miscellaneous	Cannabinoids	Side effects of dysphoria, drowsiness, hypotension, and bradycardia preclude its routine use as an analgesic.
	Cocaine	Has demonstrated no efficacy as an analgesic or coanalgesic in combination with opioids.

Routes of Administration	Rationale for Not Recommending
Intramuscular (I.M.)	Painful. Absorption unreliable. Should not be used for children or patients prone to develop dependent edema or in patients with thrombocytopenia.
Transnasal	The only drug approved by the FDA for transnasal administration at this time is butorphanol, an agonist-antagonist drug, which generally is not recommended. (See opioid agonist-antagonists above.)

CANCER CHEMOTHERAPY REGIMENS

ADULT REGIMENS

Breast Cancer

AC

Doxorubicin (Adriamycin®, I.V., 45 mg/m², day 1
Cyclophosphamide, I.V., 500 mg/m², day 1

Repeat cycle every 21 days

ACe

Doxorubicin (Adriamycin®, I.V., 40 mg/m², day 1
Cyclophosphamide, P.O., 200 mg/m²/d, days 1-3 or 3-6

Repeat cycle every 21-28 days

CAF

Cyclophosphamide, P.O., 100 mg/m², days 1-14
Doxorubicin (Adriamycin®, I.V., 30 mg/m², days 1 & 8
Fluorouracil, I.V., 400-500 mg/m², days 1 & 8

Repeat cycle every 28 days

or

Cyclophosphamide, I.V., 500 mg/m², day 1
Doxorubicin (Adriamycin®, I.V., 50 mg/m², day 1
Fluorouracil, I.V., 500 mg/m², day 1

Repeat cycle every 21 days

or Dose Intensification of CAF*

Cyclophosphamide, I.V., 600 mg/m², day 1
Doxorubicin (Adriamycin®, I.V., 60 mg/m², day 1
Fluorouracil, I.V., 600 mg/m², day 1
G-CSF, I.V./S.C., 5 mcg/kg/dose

Repeat cycle every 21 days

*Preliminary data presented at ASCO (March, 1992) suggests better response with dose intensification.

CFM

Cyclophosphamide, I.V., 500 mg/m², day 1
Fluorouracil, I.V., 500 mg/m², day 1
Mitoxantrone, I.V., 10 mg/m², day 1

Repeat cycle every 21 days

CFPT

Cyclophosphamide, I.V., 150 mg/m², days 1-5
Fluorouracil, I.V., 300 mg/m², days 1-5
Prednisone, P.O., 10 mg tid, days 1-7
Tamoxifen, P.O., 10 mg bid, days 1-42

Repeat cycle every 42 days

CMF

Cyclophosphamide, P.O., 100 mg/m², days 1-14
Methotrexate, I.V., 40-60 mg/m², days 1 & 8
Fluorouracil, I.V., 400-600 mg/m², days 1 & 8

Repeat cycle every 28 days

or

Cyclophosphamide, I.V., 600 mg/m², days 1 & 8
Methotrexate, I.V., 40-60 mg/m², days 1 & 8
Fluorouracil, I.V., 400-600 mg/m², days 1 & 8

Repeat cycle every 28 days

Breast Cancer *(continued)*

CMFP

Cyclophosphamide, P.O., 100 mg/m², days 1-14
Methotrexate, I.V., 40-60 mg/m², days 1 & 8
Fluorouracil, I.V., 600-700 mg/m², days 1 & 8
Prednisone, P.O., 40 mg (first 3 cycles only), days 1-14

Repeat cycle every 28 days

CMFVP (Cooper's)

Cyclophosphamide, P.O., 2-2.5 mg/kg/d for 9 months
Methotrexate, I.V., 0.7 mg/kg/wk for 8 weeks then every other week for 7 months
Fluorouracil, I.V., 12 mg/kg/wk for 8 weeks then every other week for 7 months
Vincristine, I.V., 0.035 mg/kg (max 2 mg/wk) for 5 weeks then once monthly
Prednisone, P.O., 0.75 mg/kg/d, taper over next 40 days, discontinue, days 1-10
or
Cyclophosphamide, I.V., 400 mg/m², day 1
Methotrexate, I.V., 30 mg/m², days 1 & 8
Fluorouracil, I.V., 400 mg/m², days 1 & 8
Vincristine, I.V., 1 mg, days 1 & 8
Prednisone, P.O., 20 mg qid, days 1-7

Repeat cycle every 28 days

FAC

Fluorouracil, I.V., 500 mg/m², days 1 & 8
Doxorubicin (Adriamycin®), I.V., 50 mg/m², day 1
Cyclophosphamide, I.V., 500 mg/m², day 1

Repeat cycle every 21 days

IMF

Ifosfamide, I.V., 1.5 g/m², days 1 & 8
Mesna, I.V., 20% of ifosfamide dose, give immediately before and 4 and 8 hours after ifosfamide infusion, days 1 & 8
Methotrexate, I.V., 40 mg/m², days 1 & 8
Fluorouracil, I.V., 600 mg/m², days 1 & 8

Repeat cycle every 28 days

NFL

Mitoxantrone (Novantrone®), I.V., 12 mg/m², day 1
Fluorouracil, I.V., 350 mg/m², days 1-3, given after leucovorin calcium
Leucovorin calcium, I.V., 300 mg/m², days 1-3
or
Mitoxantrone (Novantrone®), I.V., 10 mg/m², day 1
Fluorouracil, I.V., 1000 mg/m² continuous infusion, given after leucovorin calcium, days 1-3
Leucovorin calcium, I.V., 100 mg/m², days 1-3

Repeat cycle every 21 days

VATH

Vinblastine, I.V., 4.5 mg/m², day 1
Doxorubicin (Adriamycin®), I.V., 45 mg/m², day 1
Thiotepa, I.V., 12 mg/m², day 1
Fluoxymesterone (Halotestin®), P.O., 30 mg qd, days 1-21

Repeat cycle every 21 days

Breast Cancer *(continued)*

Single-Agent Regimens

Doxorubicin, I.V., 60 mg/m^2, every 3 weeks

or

Doxorubicin, I.V., 20 mg/m^2, every week

or

Doxorubicin, I.V., 20 mg/m^2 continuous infusion, days 1-3, every 3 weeks

Mitomycin C, I.V., 8-10 mg/m^2, every 6-8 weeks

Paclitaxel, I.V., 175 mg/m^2 over 3-24 h, every 21 d
Patient must be premedicated with:
Dexamethasone 20 mg P.O., 12 and 6 h prior
Diphenhydramine 50 mg I.V., 30 min prior
Cimetidine 300 mg I.V., or ranitidine 50 mg I.V., 30 min prior

Vinblastine, I.V., 12 mg/m^2, every 3-4 weeks

Colon Cancer

F-CL
Fluorouracil, I.V., 375 mg/m^2, days 1-5
Calcium leucovorin, I.V., 200 mg/m^2, days 1-5

Repeat cycle every 28 days

or

Fluorouracil, I.V., 500 mg/m^2 weekly 1 h after initiating the calcium leucovorin
infusion for 6 weeks
Calcium leucovorin, I.V., 500 mg/m^2, over 2 h, weekly for 6 weeks

Two-week break, then repeat cycle

FLe
Fluorouracil, I.V., 450 mg/m^2 for 5 days, then, after a pause of 4 weeks, 450
mg/m^2, weekly for 48 weeks
Levamisole, P.O., 50 mg tid for 3 days, repeated every 2 weeks for 1 year

FMV
Fluorouracil, I.V., 10 mg/kg/d, days 1-5
Methyl-CCNU, P.O., 175 mg/m^2, day 1
Vincristine, I.V., 1 mg/m^2 (max 2 mg), day 1

Repeat cycle every 35 days

FU/LV
Fluorouracil, I.V., 370-400 mg/m^2/d, days 1-5
Leucovorin calcium, I.V., 200 mg/m^2/d, commence infusion 15 min prior to
fluorouracil infusion, days 1-5

Repeat cycle every 21 days

or

Fluorouracil, I.V., 1000 mg/m^2/d by continuous infusion, days 1-4
Leucovorin calcium, I.V., 200 mg/m^2/d, days 1-4

Repeat cycle every 28 days

Weekly 5FU/LV
Fluorouracil, I.V., 600 mg/m^2 over 1 h given after leucovorin, repeat weekly x 6
then 2-week rest period = 1 cycle, days 1, 8, 15, 22, 29, 36
Leucovorin calcium, I.V., 500 mg/m^2 over 2 h, days 1, 8, 15, 22, 29, 36

Repeat cycle every 56 days

5FU/LDLF
Fluorouracil, I.V., 370 mg/m^2/d, days 1-5
Leucovorin calcium, I.V., 20-25 mg/m^2/d, days 1-5

Repeat cycle every 28 days

Gastric Cancer

EAP

Etoposide, I.V., 120 mg/m^2, days 4, 5, 6
Doxorubicin (Adriamycin®), I.V., 20 mg/m^2, days 1, 7
Cisplatin (Platinol®), I.V., 40 mg/m^2, days 2, 8

Repeat cycle every 21 days

ELF

Etoposide, I.V., 120 mg/m^2, days 1-3
Leucovorin calcium, I.V., 300 mg/m^2, days 1-3
Fluorouracil, I.V., 500 mg/m^2, days 1-3

Repeat cycle every 21-28 days

FAM

Fluorouracil, I.V., 600 mg/m^2, days 1, 8, 29, & 36
Doxorubicin (Adriamycin®), I.V., 30 mg/m^2, days 1 & 29
Mitomycin C, I.V., 10 mg/m^2, day 1

Repeat cycle every 56 days

FAME

Fluorouracil, I.V., 350 mg/m^2, days 1-5, 36-40
Doxorubicin (Adriamycin®), I.V., 40 mg/m^2, days 1 & 36
Methyl-CCNU, P.O., 150 mg/m^2, day 1

Repeat cycle every 70 days

FAMTX

Methotrexate, IVPB, 1500 mg/m^2, day 1
Fluorouracil, IVPB, 1500 mg/m^2 1 h after methotrexate, day 1
Leucovorin calcium, P.O., 15 mg/m^2 q6h x 48 h 24 h after methotrexate, day 2
Doxorubicin (Adriamycin®), IVPB, 30 mg/m^2, day 15

Repeat cycle every 28 days

FCE

Fluorouracil, I.V., 900 mg/m^2/d continuous infusion, days 1-5
Cisplatin, I.V., 20 mg/m^2, days 1-5
Etoposide, I.V., 90 mg/m^2, days 1, 3, & 5

Repeat cycle every 21 days

PFL

Cisplatin (Platinol®), I.V., 25 mg/m^2 continuous infusion, days 1-5
Fluorouracil, I.V., 800 mg/m^2 continuous infusion, days 2-5
Leucovorin calcium, I.V., 500 mg/m^2 continuous infusion, days 1-5

Repeat cycle every 28 days

Genitourinary Cancer

Bladder

CAP

Cyclophosphamide, I.V., 400 mg/m^2, day 1
Doxorubicin (Adriamycin®), I.V., 40 mg/m^2, day 1
Cisplatin (Platinol®), I.V., 60 mg/m^2, day 1

Repeat cycle every 21 days

CISCA

Cisplatin, I.V., 70-100 mg/m^2, day 2
Cyclophosphamide, I.V., 650 mg/m^2, day 1
Doxorubicin (Adriamycin®), I.V., 50 mg/m^2, day 1

Repeat cycle every 21-28 days

Genitourinary Cancer — Bladder *(continued)*

CMV

Cisplatin, I.V., 100 mg/m^2 over 4 h start 12 h after MTX, day 2
Methotrexate, I.V., 30 mg/m^2, days 1 & 8
Vinblastine, I.V., 4 mg/m^2, days 1 & 8

Repeat cycle every 21 days

m-PFL

Methotrexate, I.V., 60 mg/m^2, day 1
Cisplatin (Platinol®), I.V., 25 mg/m^2 continuous infusion, days 2-6
Fluorouracil, I.V., 800 mg/m^2 continuous infusion, days 2-6
Leucovorin calcium, I.V., 500 mg/m^2 continuous infusion, days 2-6

Repeat cycle every 28 days for 4 cycles

MVAC

Methotrexate, I.V., 30 mg/m^2, days 1, 15, 22
Vinblastine, I.V., 3 mg/m^2, days 2, 15, 22
Doxorubicin (Adriamycin®), I.V., 30 mg/m^2, day 2
Cisplatin, I.V., 70 mg/m^2, day 2

Repeat cycle every 28 days

Prostate

FL

Flutamide, P.O., 250 mg tid, days 1-28
Leuprolide acetate, S.C., 1 mg qd, days 1-28

Repeat cycle every 28 days

or

Flutamide, P.O., 250 mg tid, days 1-28
Leuprolide acetate depot, I.M., 7.5 mg, day 1

Repeat cycle every 28 days

FZ

Flutamide, P.O., 250 mg tid
Goserelin acetate (Zoladex®), S.C., 3.6 mg implant, every 28 days

L-VAM

Leuprolide acetate, S.C., 1 mg qd, days 1-28
Vinblastine, I.V., 1.5 mg/m^2/d continuous infusion, days 2-7
Doxorubicin (Adriamycin®), I.V., 50 mg/m^2 continuous infusion, day 1
Mitomycin C, I.V., 10 mg/m^2, day 2

Repeat cycle every 28 days

Testicular, Induction, Good Risk

BEP

Bleomycin, I.V., 30 units, days 2, 9, 16
Etoposide, I.V., 100 mg/m^2, days 1-5
Cisplatin (Platinol®), I.V., 20 mg/m^2, days 1-5

Repeat cycle every 21 days

PE

Cisplatin (Platinol®), I.V., 20 mg/m^2, days 1-5
Etoposide, I.V., 100 mg/m^2, days 1-5

Repeat cycle every 21 days

PVB

Cisplatin (Platinol®), I.V., 20 mg/m^2, days 1-5
Vinblastine, I.V., 6 mg/m^2, days 1, 2
Bleomycin, I.V., 30 units, weekly

Repeat cycle every 21-28 days

Genitourinary Cancer *(continued)*

Testicular, Induction, Poor Risk

VIP

Etoposide (VePesid®), I.V., 75 mg/m², days 1-5
Ifosfamide, I.V., 1.2 g/m², days 1-5
Cisplatin (Platinol®), I.V., 20 mg/m², days 1-5
Mesna, I.V., 120 mg/m² then 1200 mg/m²/d continuous infusion, days 1-5

Repeat cycle every 21 days

VIP (Einhorn)

Vinblastine, I.V., 0.11 mg/kg, days 1-2
Ifosfamide, I.V., 1200 mg/m², days 1-5
Cisplatin (Platinol®), I.V., 20 mg/m², days 1-5
Mesna, I.V., 120 mg/m², then 1200 mg/m²/d continuous infusion, days 1-5

Repeat cycle every 21 days

Testicular, Induction, Salvage

VAB VI

Vinblastine, I.V., 4 mg/m², day 1
Dactinomycin (Actinomycin D), I.V., 1 mg/m², day 1
Bleomycin, I.V., 30 units push day 1, then 20 units/m²/d continuous infusion, days 1-3
Cisplatin, I.V., 120 mg/m², day 4
Cyclophosphamide, I.V., 600 mg/m², day 1

Repeat cycle every 21 days

VBP (PVB)

Vinblastine, I.V., 6 mg/m², days 1 & 2
Bleomycin, I.V., 30 units, days 1, 8, 15, (22)
Cisplatin (Platinol®), I.V., 20 mg/m², days 1-5

Repeat cycle every 21-28 days

Gestational Trophoblastic Cancer

DMC

Dactinomycin, I.V., 0.37 mg/m², days 1-5
Methotrexate, I.V., 11 mg/m², days 1-5
Cyclophosphamide, I.V., 110 mg/m², days 1-5

Repeat cycle every 21 days

Head and Neck Cancer

CAP

Cyclophosphamide, I.V., 500 mg/m², day 1
Doxorubicin (Adriamycin®), I.V., 50 mg/m², day 1
Cisplatin (Platinol®), I.V., 50 mg/m², day 1

Repeat cycle every 28 days

CF

Cisplatin, I.V., 100 mg/m², day 1
Fluorouracil, I.V., 1000 mg/m²/d continuous infusion, days 1-5

Repeat cycle every 21-28 days

CF

Carboplatin, I.V., 400 mg/m², day 1
Fluorouracil, I.V., 1000 mg/m²/d continuous infusion, days 1-5

Repeat cycle every 21-28 days

Head and Neck Cancer *(continued)*

COB

Cisplatin, I.V., 100 mg/m², day 1
Vincristine (Oncovin®), I.V., 1 mg/m², days 2 & 5
Bleomycin, I.V., 30 units/d continuous infusion, days 2-5

Repeat cycle every 21 days

5-FU HURT

Hydroxyurea, P.O., 1000 mg q12h x 11 doses; start PM of admission, give 2 hours prior to radiation therapy, days 0-5
Fluorouracil, I.V., 800 mg/m²/d continuous infusion, start AM after admission, days 1-5
Paclitaxel, I.V., 5-25 mg/m²/d continuous infusion, start AM after admission; dose escalation study — refer to protocol, days 1-5
G-CSF, S.C., 5 mcg/kg/d, days 6-12, start ≥12 hours after completion of 5-FU infusion

5-7 cycles may be administered

MAP

Mitomycin C, I.V., 8 mg/m², day 1
Doxorubicin (Adriamycin®), I.V., 40 mg/m², day 1
Cisplatin (Platinol®), I.V., 60 mg/m², day 1

Repeat cycle every 28 days

MBC (MBD)

Methotrexate, I.M./I.V., 40 mg/m², days 1 & 15
Bleomycin, I.M./I.V., 10 units, days 1, 8, 15
Cisplatin, I.V., 50 mg/m², day 4

Repeat cycle every 21 days

MF

Methotrexate, I.V., 125-250 mg/m², day 1
Fluorouracil, I.V., 600 mg/m² beginning 1 h after methotrexate, day 1
Leucovorin calcium, I.V./P.O., 10 mg/m² q6h x 5 doses beginning 24 h after methotrexate

Repeat cycle every 7 days

PFL

Cisplatin (Platinol®), I.V., 100 mg/m², day 1
Fluorouracil, I.V., 600-800 mg/m²/d continuous infusion, days 1-5
Leucovorin calcium, I.V., 200-300 mg/m²/d, days 1-5

Repeat cycle every 21 days

PFL+IFN

Cisplatin (Platinol®), I.V., 100 mg/m², day 1
Fluorouracil, I.V., 640 mg/m²/d continuous infusion, days 1-5
Leucovorin calcium, P.O., 100 mg q4h, days 1-5
Interferon alfa-2b, S.C., 2 x 10⁶ units/m², days 1-6

Wayne State

Cisplatin (Platinol®), I.V., 100 mg/m² over 30 minutes, day 1
Fluorouracil, I.V., 1000 mg/m² continuous infusion, days 1-4 (or 5)

Repeat cycle every 21 days

Single-Agent Regimens

Carboplatin, I.V., 300-400 mg/m², over 2 hours every 21-28 days
Methotrexate, I.V., 40 mg/m², every week, escalating day 14 by 5 mg/m²/wk as tolerated
Cisplatin I.V., 100 mg/m², every 28 days divided into 1, 2, or 4 equal doses per month

Leukemias

Acute Lymphoblastic, Induction

DVP

Daunorubicin, I.V., 45 mg/m^2, days 1, 2, 3, 14
Vincristine, I.V., 2 mg/m^2 (max 2 mg), days 1, 8, 15, 22
Prednisone, P.O., 45 mg/m^2, days 1-28 (35)

DVPA

Daunorubicin, I.V., 50 mg/m^2, days 1-3
Vincristine, I.V., 2 mg, days 1, 8, 15, 22
Prednisone, P.O., 60 mg/m^2, days 1-28
Asparaginase, I.M., 6000 units/m^2, days 17-28

VAD

Vincristine, I.V., 0.4 mg continuous infusion, days 1-4
Doxorubicin (Adriamycin®), I.V., 12 mg/m^2 continuous infusion, days 1-4
Dexamethasone, P.O., 40 mg, days 1-4, 9-12, 17-20

VP

Vincristine, I.V., 2 mg/m^2/wk for 4-6 weeks (max 2 mg)
Prednisone, P.O., 60 mg/m^2/d in divided doses for 4 weeks, taper weeks 5-7

VP-L-Asparaginase

Vincristine, I.V., 2 mg/m^2/wk for 4-6 wk (max 2 mg)
Prednisone, P.O., 60 mg/m^2/d for 4-6 wk, then taper
L-asparaginase, I.V., 10,000 units/m^2/d

no known acronym

Cyclophosphamide, I.V., 1200 mg/m^2, day 1
Daunorubicin, I.V., 45 mg/m^2, days 1-3
Prednisone, P.O., 60 mg/m^2, days 1-21
Vincristine, I.V., 2 mg/m^2, weekly
L-asparaginase, I.V., 6000 units/m^2, 3 times/wk

or

Pegaspargase, I.M./I.V., 2500 units/m^2, every 14 days if patient develops hypersensitivity to native L-asparaginase

Acute Lymphoblastic, Maintenance

MM

Mercaptopurine, P.O., 50-75 mg/m^2, days 1-7
Methotrexate, P.O./I.V., 20 mg/m^2, day 1

Repeat cycle every 7 days

MMC (MTX + MP + CTX)*

Methotrexate, I.V., 20 mg/m^2/wk
Mercaptopurine, P.O., 50 mg/m^2/d
Cyclophosphamide, I.V., 200 mg/m^2/wk

*Continue all 3 drugs until relapse of disease or after 3 years of remission.

Acute Lymphoblastic, Relapse

AVDP

Asparaginase, I.V., 15,000 units/m^2, days 1-5, 8-12, 15-19, 22-26
Vincristine, I.V., 2 mg/m^2 (max 2 mg), days 8, 15, 22
Daunorubicin, I.V., 30-60 mg/m^2, days 8, 15, 22
Prednisone, P.O., 40 mg/m^2, days 8-12, 15-19, 22-26

Acute Myeloid Leukemia

5+2

Induction
Cytarabine (Ara-C), I.V., 100-200 mg/m^2 continuous infusion, days 1-5
Daunorubicin, I.V., 45 mg/m^2, days 1-2

7+3

Induction
Cytarabine, I.V., 100-200 mg/m^2/d continuous infusion, days 1-7
Daunorubicin, I.V., 45 mg/m^2/d, days 1-3

Modified 7+3 (considerations in elderly patients)
Cytarabine, I.V., 100 mg/m^2/d continuous infusion, days 1-7
Daunorubicin, I.V., 30 mg/m^2/d, days 1-3

D-3+7

Induction
Daunorubicin, I.V., 45 mg/m^2, days 1-3
Cytarabine (Ara-C), I.V., 100-200 mg/m^2 continuous infusion, days 1-7

DAT/DCT

Induction
Daunorubicin, I.V., 60 mg/m^2/d, days 1-3
Cytarabine (Ara-C), I.V., 200 mg/m^2/d continuous infusion, days 1-5
Thioguanine, P.O., 100 mg/m^2 q12h, days 1-5

Modified DAT (considerations in elderly patients)
Daunorubicin, I.V., 50 mg/m^2/d, day 1
Cytarabine (Ara-C), S.C., 100 mg/m^2/d q12h, days 1-5
Thioguanine, P.O., 100 mg/m^2 q12h, days 1-5

HDAC

Induction
Cytarabine, I.V., 3 g/m^2 I.V. over 2-3 h q12h x 12 doses, days 1-6

Modified (considerations in elderly patients)
Cytarabine, I.V., 2 g/m^2 I.V. over 2-3 h q12h x 12 doses, days 1-6

HiDAC

Consolidation
Cytarabine (Ara-C), I.V., 3000 mg/m^2 q12h, days 1-6
or
Cytarabine (Ara-C), I.V., 3000 mg/m^2 q12h, days 1, 3, 5

I-3+7

Induction
Idarubicin, I.V., 12 mg/m^2, days 1-3
Cytarabine (Ara-C), I.V., 100 mg/m^2 continuous infusion, days 1-7

IC

Induction
Idarubicin (Idamycin®), I.V., 12 mg/m^2/d, days 1-3
Cytarabine, I.V., 100-200 mg/m^2/d continuous infusion, days 1-7

LDAC

Considerations in Elderly Patients
Cytarabine, S.C., 10 mg/m^2 bid, days 10-21

Leukemias — Acute Myeloid Leukemia *(continued)*
MC

Induction
Mitoxantrone, I.V., 12 mg/m²/d, days 1-3
Cytarabine, I.V., 100-200 mg/m²/d continuous infusion, days 1-7

Consolidation
Mitoxantrone, I.V., 12 mg/m², days 1-2
Cytarabine (Ara-C), I.V., 100 mg/m² continuous infusion, days 1-5

Repeat cycle every 28 days

MV

Induction
Mitoxantrone, I.V., 10 mg/m²/d, days 1-5
Etoposide (VePesid®), I.V., 100 mg/m²/d, days 1-3

Acute Nonlymphoblastic, Consolidation

CD
Cytarabine, I.V., 3000 mg/m² q12h, days 1-6
Daunorubicin, I.V., 30 mg/m²/d, days 7-9

Chronic Lymphocytic Leukemia

CHL + PRED
Chlorambucil, P.O., 0.4 mg/kg/d for 1 day every other week
Prednisone, P.O., 100 mg/d for 2 days every other week; adjust dosage according to blood counts every 2 weeks prior to therapy; increase initial dose of 0.4 mg/kg by 0.1 mg/kg every 2 weeks until toxicity or disease control is achieved

CVP
Cyclophosphamide, P.O., 400 mg/m²/d, days 1-5
Vincristine (Oncovin®), I.V., 1.4 mg/m² (max 2 mg), day 1
Prednisone, P.O., 100 mg/m², days 1-5

Repeat cycle every 21 days

Fludarabine, I.V., 25-30 mg/m² over 30 min, days 1-5

Repeat cycle every 28 days

Cladribine (2-CdA) for fludarabine resistant, I.V., 0.1 mg/kg/d continuous infusion, days 1-7

Repeat cycle every 28 days

Lung Cancer

Small Cell

ACE/CAE
Doxorubicin (Adriamycin®), I.V., 45 mg/m², day 1
Cyclophosphamide, I.V., 1000 mg/m², day 1
Etoposide, I.V., 50 mg/m²/d, days 1-5

Repeat cycle every 21 days

CAV
Cyclophosphamide, I.V., 1000 mg/m², day 1
Doxorubicin (Adriamycin®), I.V., 50 mg/m², day 1
Vincristine, I.V., 1.4 mg/m² (max 2 mg), day 1

Repeat cycle every 3 weeks

Lung Cancer — Small Cell *(continued)*

CAVE
Cyclophosphamide, I.V., 750 mg/m^2, day 1
Doxorubicin (Adriamycin®), I.V., 50 mg/m^2, day 1
Vincristine, I.V., 1.4 mg/m^2 (max 2 mg), day 1
Etoposide, I.V., 60-100 mg/m^2, days 1-3

Repeat cycle every 3 weeks

CHOR*
Cyclophosphamide, I.V., 750 mg/m^2/d, days 1 & 22
Doxorubicin (Adriamycin®), I.V., 50 mg/m^2/d, days 1 & 22
Vincristine, I.V., 1 mg, days 1, 8, 15, 22
Radiation, total dose 3000 rad, 10 daily fractions over 2 weeks beginning with
    day 36, days 1, 8, 15, 22

CMC-High Dose*
Cyclophosphamide, I.V., 1000 mg/m^2/d, days 1 & 29
Methotrexate, I.V., 15 mg/m^2/d twice weekly for 6 weeks, days 1 & 29
Lomustine (CCNU), P.O., 100 mg/m^2, day 1

*If disease responds, proceed to maintenance therapy.

CODE
Cisplatin, I.V., 25 mg/m^2, every week for 9 weeks
Vincristine (Oncovin®), I.V., 1 mg/m^2, weeks 1, 2, 4, 6, 8
Doxorubicin, I.V., 25 mg/m^2, weeks 1, 3, 5, 7, 9
Etoposide, I.V., 80 mg/m^2, weeks 1, 3, 5, 7, 9

COPE
Cyclophosphamide, I.V., 750 mg/m^2, day 1
Vincristine (Oncovin®), I.V., 1.4 mg/m^2 (max 2 mg), day 3
Cisplatin (Platinol®), I.V., 20 mg/m^2, days 1-3
Etoposide, I.V., 100 mg/m^2, days 1-3

Repeat cycle every 21 days

EC
Etoposide, I.V., 60-100 mg/m^2, days 1-3
Carboplatin, I.V., 400 mg/m^2, day 1

Repeat cycle every 28 days

EP
Etoposide, I.V., 75-100 mg/m^2, days 1-3
Cisplatin (Platinol®), I.V., 75-100 mg/m^2, day 1

Repeat cycle every 21-28 days

MICE (ICE)
Mesna uroprotection, I.V. at 20% of ifosfamide doses given immediately before
    and at 4 and 8 hours after ifosfamide infusion
Ifosfamide, I.V., 2000 mg/m^2, days 1-3
Carboplatin, I.V., 300-350 mg/m^2, day 1
Etoposide, I.V., 60-100 mg/m^2, day 1

PE
Cisplatin (Platinol®), I.V., 50 mg/m^2, day 1
Etoposide, I.V., 60 mg/m^2, days 1-5

Repeat cycle every 21-28 days

or

Cisplatin (Platinol®), I.V., 75 mg/m^2, day 2
Etoposide, I.V., 125 mg/m^2, days 1, 3, & 5

Repeat cycle every 28 days

or

Cisplatin (Platinol®), I.V., 100 mg/m^2, day 1
Etoposide, I.V., 100 mg/m^2, days 1-3

Repeat cycle every 28 days

Lung Cancer — Small Cell *(continued)*

POCC
Procarbazine, P.O., 100 mg/m^2/d, days 1-14
Vincristine (Oncovin®), I.V., 2 mg/d (max 2 mg), days 1 & 8
Cyclophosphamide, I.V., 600 mg/m^2/d, days 1 & 8
Lomustine (CCNU), P.O., 60 mg/m^2, day 1

Repeat cycle every 28 days

VAC (CAV) (Induction)
Vincristine, I.V., 2 mg/m^2, day 1
Doxorubicin (Adriamycin®), I.V., 50 mg/m^2, day 1
Cyclophosphamide, I.V., 750 mg/m^2, day 1

Repeat cycle every 21 days x 4 cycles

VC
Etoposide (VePesid®), I.V., 100-200 mg/m^2, days 1-3
Carboplatin, I.V., 50-125 mg/m^2, days 1-3

Repeat cycle every 28 days

Single-Agent Regimen
Etoposide, P.O., 160 mg/m^2, days 1-5

Repeat cycle every 28 days

Nonsmall Cell

CAMP
Cyclophosphamide, I.V., 300 mg/m^2, days 1 & 8
Doxorubicin (Adriamycin®), I.V., 20 mg/m^2, days 1 & 8
Methotrexate, I.V., 15 mg/m^2, days 1 & 8
Procarbazine, P.O., 100 mg/m^2, days 1-10

Repeat cycle every 28 days

CAP
Cyclophosphamide, I.V., 400 mg/m^2, day 1
Doxorubicin (Adriamycin®), I.V., 40 mg/m^2, day 1
Cisplatin (Platinol®), I.V., 60 mg/m^2, day 1

Repeat cycle every 28 days

CV
Cisplatin, I.V., 60-80 mg/m^2, day 1
Etoposide (VePesid®), I.V., 120 mg/m^2, days 4, 6, & 8

Repeat cycle every 21-28 days

CVI
Carboplatin, I.V., 300 mg/m^2, day 1
Etoposide (VePesid®), I.V., 60-100 mg/m^2, day 1
Ifosfamide, I.V., 1.5 g/m^2, days 1, 3 & 5
Mesna, I.V., 20% of ifosfamide dose, given immediately before and 4 and 8
hours after ifosfamide infusion, days 1, 3 & 5

Repeat cycle every 28 days

EP
Etoposide, I.V., 75-100 mg/m^2, days 1-3
Cisplatin (Platinol®), I.V., 75-100 mg/m^2, day 1

Repeat cycle every 21-28 days

FAM
Fluorouracil, I.V., 600 mg/m^2, days 1, 8, 28, & 36
Doxorubicin (Adriamycin®), I.V., 30 mg/m^2, days 1 & 28
Mitomycin C, I.V., 10 mg/m^2, day 1

Repeat cycle every 56 days

Lung Cancer — Nonsmall Cell *(continued)*

FOMi*
Fluorouracil, I.V., 300 mg/m^2/d, days 1-4
Vincristine (Oncovin®), I.V., 2 mg, day 1
Mitomycin C, I.V., 10 mg/m^2, day 1

*Repeat at 3-week intervals for 3 courses; thereafter, every 6 weeks.

FOMi/CAP
Fluorouracil, I.V., 300 mg/m^2, days 1-4
Vincristine, I.V., 2 mg, day 1
Mitomycin C, I.V., 10 mg/m^2, day 1
Cyclophosphamide, I.V., 400 mg/m^2, day 28
Doxorubicin (Adriamycin®), I.V., 40 mg/m^2, day 28
Cisplatin, I.V., 40 mg/m^2, day 28

Repeat cycle every 56 days

MACC
Methotrexate, I.V., 40 mg/m^2, day 1
Doxorubicin (Adriamycin®), I.V., 40 mg/m^2, day 1
Cyclophosphamide, I.V., 400 mg/m^2, day 1
Lomustine, P.O., 30 mg/m^2, day 1

Repeat cycle every 21 days

MICE (ICE)
Mesna uroprotection, I.V. at 20% of ifosfamide doses given immediately before
and at 4 and 8 hours after ifosfamide infusion
Ifosfamide, I.V., 2000 mg/m^2, days 1-3
Carboplatin, I.V., 300-350 mg/m^2, day 1
Etoposide, I.V., 60-100 mg/m^2, day 1

MVP
Mitomycin, I.V., 8 mg/m^2, days 1, 29, 71
Vinblastine, I.V., 4.5 mg/m^2, days 15, 22, 29, then every 2 weeks
Cisplatin (Platinol®), I.V., 120 mg/m^2, days 1, 29, then every 6 weeks

PFL
Cisplatin (Platinol®), I.V., 25 mg/m^2, days 1-5
Fluorouracil, I.V., 800 mg/m^2 continuous infusion, days 2-5
Leucovorin calcium, I.V., 500 mg/m^2 continuous infusion, days 1-5

Repeat cycle every 28 days

Single-Agent Regimen

Vinorelbine (Navelbine®), I.V., 30 mg/m^2, every week

Lymphoma

Hodgkin's

ABVD
Doxorubicin (Adriamycin®), I.V., 25 mg/m^2, days 1 & 15
Bleomycin, I.V., 10 units/m^2, days 1 & 15
Vinblastine, I.V., 6 mg/m^2, days 1 & 15
Dacarbazine, I.V., 150 mg/m^2, days 1-5

Repeat cycle every 28 days

or

Dacarbazine, I.V., 375 mg/m^2, days 1 & 15

ChIVPP
Chlorambucil, P.O., 6 mg/m^2, days 1-14 (max 10 mg/d)
Vinblastine, I.V., 6 mg/m^2, days 1-8 (max 10 mg dose)
Procarbazine, P.O., 50 mg/m^2, days 1-14 (max 150 mg/d)
Prednisone, P.O., 40 mg/m^2, days 1-14 (25 mg/m^2 for children)

Lymphoma — Hodgkin's *(continued)*

CVPP

Lomustine (CCNU), P.O., 75 mg/m^2, day 1
Vinblastine, I.V., 4 mg/m^2, days 1, 8
Procarbazine, P.O., 100 mg/m^2, days 1-14
Prednisone, P.O., 30 mg/m^2, days 1-14 (cycles 1 & 4 only)

Repeat cycle every 28 days

DHAP

Dexamethasone, P.O./I.V., 40 mg, days 1-4
Cytarabine (Ara-C), I.V., 2 g/m^2, q12h for 2 doses, day 2
Cisplatin (Platinol®), I.V., 100 mg/m^2 continuous infusion, day 1

Repeat cycle every 3-4 weeks

EVA

Etoposide, I.V., 100 mg/m^2, days 1-3
Vinblastine, I.V., 6 mg/m^2, day 1
Doxorubicin (Adriamycin®), I.V., 50 mg/m^2, day 1

Repeat cycle every 28 days

MOPP

Mechlorethamine, I.V., 6 mg/m^2, days 1 & 8
Vincristine (Oncovin®), I.V., 1.4 mg/m^2 (max 2.5 mg), days 1 & 8
Procarbazine, P.O., 100 mg/m^2, days 1-14
Prednisone, P.O., 40 mg/m^2 (cycles 1 & 4 only), days 1-14

Repeat cycle every 28 days

MOPP/ABV Hybrid

Mechlorethamine, I.V., 6 mg/m^2, day 1
Vincristine (Oncovin®), I.V., 1.4 mg/m^2 (max 2 mg), day 1
Procarbazine, P.O., 100 mg/m^2, days 1-7
Prednisone, P.O., 40 mg/m^2, days 1-14
Doxorubicin (Adriamycin®), I.V., 35 mg/m^2, day 8
Bleomycin, I.V., 10 units/m^2, day 8
Vinblastine, I.V., 6 mg/m^2, day 8

Repeat cycle every 28 days

MVPP

Mechlorethamine, I.V., 6 mg/m^2, days 1 & 8
Vinblastine, I.V., 6 mg/m^2, days 1 & 8
Procarbazine, P.O., 100 mg/m^2, days 1-14
Prednisone, P.O., 40 mg/m^2, days 1-14

Repeat cycle every 42 days

NOVP

Mitoxantrone (Novantrone®), I.V., 10 mg/m^2, day 1
Vincristine (Oncovin®), I.V., 2 mg, day 8
Vinblastine, I.V., 6 mg/m^2, day 1
Prednisone, P.O., 100 mg/m^2, days 1-5

Repeat cycle every 21 days

Stanford V

Mechlorethamine, I.V., 6 mg/m^2, weeks 1, 5, 9
Doxorubicin, I.V., 25 mg/m^2, weeks 1, 3, 5, 7, 9, 11
Vinblastine, I.V., 6 mg/m^2, weeks 1, 3, 5, 7, 9, 11
Vincristine, I.V., 1.4 mg/m^2, weeks 2, 4, 6, 8, 10, 12
Bleomycin, I.V., 5 units/m^2, weeks 2, 4, 6, 8, 10, 12
Etoposide, I.V., 60 mg/m^2 x 2, weeks 3, 7, 11
Prednisone, P.O., 40 mg/m^2, daily, dose tapered over the last 15 days

Non-Hodgkin's

BACOP

Bleomycin, I.V., 5 units/m^2, days 15 & 22
Doxorubicin (Adriamycin®), I.V., 25 mg/m^2, days 1 & 8
Cyclophosphamide, I.V., 650 mg/m^2, days 1 & 8
Vincristine (Oncovin®), I.V., 1.4 mg/m^2 (max 2 mg), days 1 & 8
Prednisone, P.O., 60 mg/m^2, days 15-28

Repeat cycle every 28 days

CHOP

Cyclophosphamide, I.V., 750 mg/m^2, day 1
Doxorubicin (Hydroxydaunomycin), I.V., 50 mg/m^2, day 1
Vincristine (Oncovin®), I.V., 1.4 mg/m^2 (max 2 mg), day 1
Prednisone, P.O., 100 mg/m^2, days 1-5

Repeat cycle every 21 days

CHOP-Bleo

Cyclophosphamide, I.V., 750 mg/m^2, day 1
Doxorubicin (Hydroxydaunomycin), I.V., 50 mg/m^2, day 1
Vincristine (Oncovin®), I.V., 2 mg, days 1 & 5
Prednisone, P.O., 100 mg, days 1-5
Bleomycin, I.V., 15 units, days 1 & 5

Repeat cycle every 21-28 days

COMLA

Cyclophosphamide, I.V., 1500 mg/m^2, day 1
Vincristine (Oncovin®), I.V., 1.4 mg/m^2 (max 2.5 mg), days 1, 8, 15
Methotrexate, I.V., 120 mg/m^2, days 22, 29, 36, 43, 50, 57, 64, 71
Leucovorin calcium rescue, P.O., 25 mg/m^2, q6h for 4 doses, beginning 24
    hours after each methotrexate dose
Cytarabine (Ara-C), I.V., 300 mg/m^2, days 22, 29, 36, 43, 50, 57, 64, 71

Repeat cycle every 21 days

COP

Cyclophosphamide, I.V., 800-1000 mg/m^2, day 1
Vincristine (Oncovin®), I.V., 1.4 mg/m^2 (max 2 mg), day 1
Prednisone, P.O., 60 mg/m^2, days 1-5

Repeat cycle every 21 days

COP-BLAM

Cyclophosphamide, I.V., 400 mg/m^2, day 1
Vincristine (Oncovin®), I.V., 1 mg/m^2, day 1
Prednisone, P.O., 40 mg/m^2, days 1-10
Bleomycin, I.V., 15 mg, day 14
Doxorubicin (Adriamycin®), I.V., 40 mg/m^2, day 1
Procarbazine (Matulane®), P.O., 100 mg/m^2, days 1-10

COPP (or 'C" MOPP)

Cyclophosphamide, I.V., 400-650 mg/m^2, days 1 & 8
Vincristine (Oncovin®), I.V., 1.4-1.5 mg/m^2 (max 2 mg), days 1 & 8
Procarbazine, P.O., 100 mg/m^2, days 1-14
Prednisone, P.O., 40 mg/m^2, days 1-14

Repeat cycle every 28 days

CVP

Cyclophosphamide, P.O., 400 mg/m^2, days 1-5
Vincristine, I.V., 1.4 mg/m^2 (max 2 mg), day 1
Prednisone, P.O., 100 mg/m^2, days 1-5

Repeat cycle every 21 days

Lymphoma — Non-Hodgkin's *(continued)*

DHAP
Dexamethasone (Decadron®), I.V., 10 mg q6h, days 1-4
Cytarabine (Ara-C), I.V., 2 g/m^2 q12h x 2 doses, day 2
Cisplatin (Platinol®), I.V., 100 mg/m^2 continuous infusion, day 1

Repeat cycle every 21-28 days

ESHAP
Etoposide, I.V., 60 mg/m^2, days 1-4
Cisplatin, I.V., 25 mg/m^2 continuous infusion, days 1-4
Cytarabine (Ara-C), I.V., 2 g/m^2, immediately following completion of etoposide and cisplatin therapy
Methylprednisolone, I.V., 500 mg/d, days 1-4

Repeat cycle every 21-28 days

IMVP-16
Ifosfamide, I.V., 4 g/m^2 continuous infusion over 24 h, day 1
Mesna, I.V., 800 mg/m^2 bolus prior to ifosfamide, then 4 g/m^2 continuous infusion over 12 hours concurrent w/ifosfamide; then 2.4 g/m^2 continuous infusion over 12 hours after ifosfamide infusion, day 1
Methotrexate, I.V., 30 mg/m^2, days 3 & 10
Etoposide (VePesid®), I.V., 100 mg/m^2, days 1-3

Repeat cycle every 21-28 days

MACOP-B
Methotrexate, I.V., 100 mg/m^2 weeks 2, 6, 10
Doxorubicin (Adriamycin®), I.V., 50 mg/m^2 weeks 1, 3, 5, 7, 9, 11
Cyclophosphamide, I.V., 350 mg/m^2 weeks 1, 3, 5, 7, 9, 11
Vincristine (Oncovin®), I.V., 1.4 mg/m^2 (max 2 mg) weeks 2, 4, 8, 10, 12
Bleomycin, I.V., 10 units/m^2, weeks 4, 8, 12
Prednisone, P.O., 75 mg/d tapered over 15 d, days 1-15
Leucovorin calcium, P.O., 15 mg q6h x 6 doses 24 h after methotrexate, weeks 2, 6, 10

m-BACOD
Methotrexate, I.V., 200 mg/m^2, days 8 & 15
Leucovorin calcium, P.O., 10 mg/m^2 q6h x 8 doses beginning 24 h after each methotrexate dose, days 8 & 15
Bleomycin, I.V., 4 units/m^2, day 1
Doxorubicin (Adriamycin®), I.V., 45 mg/m^2, day 1
Cyclophosphamide, I.V., 600 mg/m^2, day 1
Vincristine (Oncovin®), I.V., 1 mg/m^2, day 1
Dexamethasone, P.O., 6 mg/m^2, days 1-5

Repeat cycle every 21 days

m-BACOS
Methotrexate, I.V., 1 g/m^2, day 2
Bleomycin, I.V., 10 units/m^2, day 1
Doxorubicin (Adriamycin®), I.V., 50 mg/m^2 continuous infusion, day 1
Cyclophosphamide, I.V., 750 mg/m^2, day 1
Vincristine (Oncovin®), I.V., 1.4 mg/m^2 (max 2 mg), day 1
Leucovorin calcium rescue, P.O., 15 mg q6h for 8 doses, starting 24 hours after methotrexate
Methylprednisolone, I.V., 500 mg, days 1-3

Repeat cycle every 21-25 days

MINE
Mesna, I.V., 1.33 g/m^2/d concurrent with ifosfamide dose, then 500 mg P.O. 4 hours after each ifosfamide infusion, days 1-3
Ifosfamide, I.V., 1.33 g/m^2/d, days 1-3
Mitoxantrone (Novantrone®), I.V., 8 mg/m^2, day 1
Etoposide, I.V., 65 mg/m^2/d, days 1-3

Repeat cycle every 28 days

CANCER CHEMOTHERAPY

Lymphoma — Non-Hodgkin's *(continued)*
Pro-MACE
    Prednisone, P.O., 60 mg/m^2, days 1-14
    Methotrexate, I.V., 1.5 g/m^2, day 14
    Leucovorin calcium, I.V., 50 mg/m^2 q6h x 5 doses beginning 24 h after metho-
        trexate dose, day 14
    Doxorubicin (Adriamycin®), I.V., 25 mg/m^2, days 1 & 8
    Cyclophosphamide, I.V., 650 mg/m^2, days 1 & 8
    Etoposide, I.V., 120 mg/m^2, days 1 & 8

            Repeat cycle every 28 days

Pro-MACE-CytaBOM
    Prednisone, P.O., 60 mg/m^2, days 1-14
    Doxorubicin (Adriamycin®), I.V., 25 mg/m^2, day 1
    Cyclophosphamide, I.V., 650 mg/m^2, day 1
    Etoposide, I.V., 120 mg/m^2, day 1
    Cytarabine, I.V., 300 mg/m^2, day 8
    Bleomycin, I.V., 5 units/m^2, day 8
    Vincristine (Oncovin®), I.V., 1.4 mg/m^2 (max 2 mg), day 8
    Methotrexate, I.V., 120 mg/m^2, day 8
    Leucovorin calcium, P.O., 25 mg/m^2 q6h x 4 doses, day 9

            Repeat cycle every 21 days

Malignant Melanoma

BCDT
    Carmustine (BCNU), I.V., 150 mg/m^2, day 1
    Cisplatin, I.V., 25 mg/m^2, days 1-3, 21-23
    Dacarbazine, I.V., 220 mg/m^2, days 1-3, 21-23
    Tamoxifen, P.O., 10 mg bid, days 1-42

BHD
    Carmustine (BCNU), I.V., 100-150 mg/m^2, day 1

            Repeat cycle every 42 days

    Hydroxyurea, P.O., 1480 mg/m^2, days 1-5
    Dacarbazine, I.V., 100-150 mg/m^2, days 1-5

            Repeat cycle every 21 days

DTIC-ACTD
    Dacarbazine, I.V., 750 mg/m^2, day 1
    Dactinomycin, I.V., 1 mg/m^2, day 1

            Repeat cycle every 28 days

VBC
    Vinblastine, I.V., 6 mg/m^2, days 1 & 2
    Bleomycin, I.V., 15 units/m^2/d continuous infusion, days 1-5
    Cisplatin, I.V., 50 mg/m^2, day 5

            Repeat cycle every 28 days

VDP
    Vinblastine, I.V., 5 mg/m^2, days 1 & 2
    Dacarbazine, I.V., 150 mg/m^2, days 1-5
    Cisplatin (Platinol®), I.V., 75 mg/m^2, day 5

            Repeat cycle every 21-28 days

Multiple Myeloma

AC (DC)
    Doxorubicin (Adriamycin®), I.V., 30 mg/m^2, day 1
    Carmustine, I.V., 30 mg/m^2, day 1

            Repeat cycle every 21-28 days

Multiple Myeloma *(continued)*

BCP

Carmustine (BCNU), I.V., 75 mg/m^2, day 1
Cyclophosphamide, I.V., 400 mg/m^2, day 1
Prednisone, P.O., 75 mg, days 1-7

Repeat cycle every 28 days

EDAP

Etoposide, I.V., 100-200 mg/m^2, days 1-4
Dexamethasone, P.O./I.V., 40 mg/m^2, days 1-5
Cytarabine (Ara-C), 1000 mg, day 5
Cisplatin (Platinol®), I.V., 20 mg continuous infusion, days 1-4

MeCP

Methyl-CCNU, P.O., 100 mg/m^2, day 1

Repeat cycle every 56 days

Cyclophosphamide, I.V., 600 mg/m^2, day 1
Prednisone, P.O., 40 mg/m^2/d, days 1-7

Repeat cycle every 28 days

MP

Melphalan, P.O., 8 mg/m^2, days 1-4
Prednisone, P.O., 40 mg/m^2/d, days 1-7

Repeat cycle every 28 days

M-2

Vincristine, I.V., 0.03 mg/kg (max 2 mg), day 1
Carmustine, I.V., 0.5 mg/kg, day 1
Cyclophosphamide, I.V., 10 mg/kg, day 1
Melphalan, P.O., 0.25 mg/kg, days 1-4
Prednisone, P.O., 1 mg/kg/d, then taper next 14 days, days 1-7

Repeat cycle every 35 days

VAD

Vincristine, I.V., 0.4 mg/d continuous infusion, days 1-4
Doxorubicin (Adriamycin®), I.V., 9-10 mg/m^2/d continuous infusion, days 1-4
Dexamethasone, P.O., 40 mg, days 1-4, 9-12, 17-20

Repeat cycle every 25-35 days

VBAP

Vincristine, I.V., 1 mg, day 1
Carmustine (BCNU), I.V., 30 mg/m^2, day 1
Doxorubicin (Adriamycin®), I.V., 30 mg/m^2, day 1
Prednisone, P.O., 100 mg, days 1-4

Repeat cycle every 21 days

VCAP

Vincristine, I.V., 1 mg, day 1
Cyclophosphamide, P.O., 100 mg/m^2, days 1-4
Doxorubicin (Adriamycin®), I.V., 25 mg/m^2, day 2
Prednisone, P.O., 60 mg/m^2, days 1-4

Repeat cycle every 28 days

Single-Agent Regimens

DEX

Dexamethasone, 20 mg/m^2 every morning for 4 days beginning on days 1, 9, and 17, every 14 days for 3 cycles

Interferon alfa-2b, S.C., 3 million units 3 times/week for maintenance therapy in patients with significant response to initial chemotherapy treatment

Ovarian Cancer

Epithelial

CC

    Carboplatin, I.V., 300 mg/m^2, day 1
    Cyclophosphamide, I.V., 600 mg/m^2, day 1

Repeat cycle every 28 days

CDC

    Carboplatin, I.V., 300 mg/m^2, day 1
    Doxorubicin, I.V., 40 mg/m^2, day 1
    Cyclophosphamide, I.V., 500 mg/m^2, day 1

Repeat cycle every 28 days

CHAP

    Cyclophosphamide, I.V., 300-500 mg/m^2, day 1
    Hexamethylmelamine, P.O., 150 mg/m^2, days 1-7
    Doxorubicin (Adriamycin®), I.V., 30-50 mg/m^2, day 1
    Cisplatin (Platinol®), I.V., 50 mg/m^2, day 1

Repeat cycle every 28 days

CP

    Cyclophosphamide, I.V., 600 mg/m^2, day 1
    Cisplatin (Platinol®), I.V., 75-100 mg/m^2, day 1

Repeat cycle every 21 days

PAC (CAP)

    Cisplatin (Platinol®), I.V., 50 mg/m^2, day 1
    Doxorubicin (Adriamycin®), I.V., 50 mg/m^2, day 1
    Cyclophosphamide, I.V., 750 mg/m^2, day 1

Repeat cycle every 21 days x 8 cycles

PT

    Cisplatin (Platinol®), I.V., 75 mg/m^2 (after Taxol®), day 1
    Taxol®, I.V., 135 mg/m^2, day 1

Repeat cycle every 21 days

Single-Agent Regimen

    Paclitaxel, I.V., 135 mg/m^2 continuous infusion, over 24 hours
        Patient must be premedicated with:
        Dexamethasone 20 mg P.O., 12 and 6 h prior
        Diphenhydramine 50 mg I.V., 30 min prior
        Cimetidine 300 mg I.V., or ranitidine 50 mg I.V., 30 min prior

Germ Cell

BEP

    Bleomycin, I.V., 30 units, days 2, 9, 16
    Etoposide, I.V., 100 mg/m^2, days 1-5
    Cisplatin (Platinol®), I.V., 20 mg/m^2, days 1-5

VAC

    Vincristine, I.V., 1.2-1.5 mg/m^2 (max 2 mg) weekly for 10-12 weeks, or every 2
        weeks for 12 doses
    Dactinomycin (Actinomycin D), I.V., 0.3-0.4 mg/m^2, days 1-5
    Cyclophosphamide, I.V., 150 mg/m^2, days 1-5

Repeat every 28 days

Pancreatic Cancer

FAM

Fluorouracil, I.V., 600 mg/m^2/wk, weeks 1, 2, 5, 6, 9
Doxorubicin (Adriamycin®), I.V., 30 mg/m^2/wk, weeks 1, 5, 9
Mitomycin C, I.V., 10 mg/m^2/wk, weeks 1, 9

FMS (SMF)

Fluorouracil, I.V., 600 mg/m^2, days 1, 8, 29 & 36
Mitomycin C, I.V., 10 mg/m^2, day 1
Streptozocin, I.V., 1 g/m^2, days 1, 8, 29 & 36

Repeat cycle every 56 days

SD

Streptozocin, I.V., 500 mg/m^2, days 1-5
Doxorubicin, I.V., 50 mg/m^2, days 1 & 22

Repeat cycle every 42 days

Renal Cancer

Single-Agent Regimens

Aldesleukin (rIL-2), various dosing regimens — please refer to the literature

Interferon alfa-2b, various dosing regimens — please refer to the literature

Floxuridine, S.C., 0.1 mg/kg, days 1-14

Repeat cycle every 21 days

Vinblastine, I.V., 1.2 mg/m^2 continuous infusion, days 1-4

Sarcoma

Bony Sarcoma

AC

Doxorubicin (Adriamycin®), I.V., 75-90 mg/m^2 96-h continuous infusion
Cisplatin, I.A./I.V., 90-120 mg/m^2, 6 days

Repeat cycle every 28 days

CYVADIC

Cyclophosphamide, I.V., 600 mg/m^2, day 1
Vincristine, I.V., 1.4 mg/m^2 (max 2 mg) weekly x 6 weeks, then on day 1 of
   future cycles
Doxorubicin (Adriamycin®), I.V., 15 mg/m^2/d continuous infusion, days 1-4
Dacarbazine (DTIC), I.V., 250 mg/m^2/d continuous infusion, days 1-4

Repeat cycle every 21-28 days

HDMTX

Methotrexate, I.V., 8-12 g/m^2
Leucovorin calcium, I.V./P.O., 15-25 mg q6h for at least 10 doses beginning 24
   h after methotrexate dose; courses repeated weekly for 2-4 weeks, alternating with various cancer chemotherapy combination regimens

IMAC

Ifosfamide, I.V., 1.2 g/m^2/d continuous infusion, days 1-5
Mesna, I.V., 400 mg/m^2 bolus prior to ifosfamide infusion day 1, then 1.2 g/m^2/d
   continuous infusion days 1-5 concurrent with ifosfamide, then 600 mg/m^2
   continuous infusion over 12 hours after ifosfamide infusion, days 1-5
Doxorubicin (Adriamycin®), I.V., 15 mg/m^2/d continuous infusion, days 2-5
Cisplatin, I.V./I.A., 120 mg/m^2 continuous infusion over 24 hours, day 7

Repeat cycle every 28 days

Sarcoma — Bony Sarcoma *(continued)*

VAIE

Vincristine, I.V., 1.5 mg/m^2/d, days 1 & 5
Doxorubicin (Adriamycin®), I.V., 20 mg/m^2/d continuous infusion, days 1-4
Ifosfamide, I.V., 1800 mg/m^2/d, days 1-5
Etoposide, I.V., 50 mg/m^2/d, days 1-5

Repeat cycle every 21 days

VADRIAC — High Dose

Vincristine, I.V., 1.5 mg/m^2/d, days 1 & 5
Cyclophosphamide, I.V., 2.1 g/m^2/d, days 1 & 2
Doxorubicin (Adriamycin®), I.V., 25 mg/m^2/d continuous infusion, days 1-3

Repeat cycle every 21 days

Soft-Tissue Sarcoma

CYADIC

Cyclophosphamide, I.V., 600 mg/m^2, day 1
Doxorubicin (Adriamycin®), I.V., 15 mg/m^2/d continuous infusion, days 1-4
Dacarbazine (DTIC), I.V., 250 mg/m^2/d continuous infusion, days 1-4

Repeat cycle every 21-28 days

CYVADIC

Cyclophosphamide, I.V., 500 mg/m^2, day 1
Vincristine, I.V., 1.4 mg/m^2 (max 2 mg), days 1 & 5
Doxorubicin (Adriamycin®), I.V., 50 mg/m^2, day 1
Dacarbazine (DTIC), I.V., 250 mg/m^2, days 1-5

Repeat cycle every 21 days

ICE

Ifosfamide, I.V., 2000 mg/m^2, days 1-3
Carboplatin, I.V., 300-600 mg/m^2, day 3
Etoposide, I.V., 100 mg/m^2, days 1-3

ID

Ifosfamide, I.V., 5 g/m^2 continuous infusion over 24 hours, day 1
Mesna, I.V., 1 g/m^2 bolus prior to ifosfamide infusion, then 4 g/m^2 continuous
    infusion over 32 hours, day 1
Doxorubicin, I.V., 40 mg/m^2, day 1

Repeat cycle every 21 days

MAID

Mesna, I.V., 500 mg/m^2 bolus 15 min prior to ifosfamide infusion, then q3h x 3,
    days 1-3
Doxorubicin (Adriamycin®), I.V., 20 mg/m^2 continuous infusion over 24 h, days
    1-3
Ifosfamide, I.V., 2500 mg/m^2 over 1 h, days 1-3
Dacarbazine*, I.V., 300 mg/m^2 continuous infusion over 24 h, days 1-3

Repeat cycle every 28 days

*Adriamycin and dacarbazine may be mixed in the same bag.

VAC

Vincristine, I.V., 2 mg/m^2 (max 2 mg) per week on weeks 1-12
Dactinomycin, I.V., 0.015 mg/kg (max 0.5 mg) every 3 months for 5-6 courses,
    days 1-5
Cyclophosphamide, P.O., 2.5 mg/kg/d for 2 years

PEDIATRIC REGIMENS

ALL, Induction

DVP

    Daunorubicin, I.V., 25 mg/m^2, days 1, 8
    Vincristine, I.V., 1.5 mg/m^2 days 1, 8, 15, 22
    Prednisone, P.O., 40 mg/m^2, days 1-29

PVDA

    Prednisone, P.O., 40 mg/m^2, days 1-29
    Vincristine, I.V., 1.5 mg/m^2, days 1, 8, 15, 22
    Daunorubicin, I.V., 25 mg/m^2, days 1, 8
    Asparaginase, I.M., 10,000 units/m^2, days 2, 4, 6, 8, 10, 12, 15, 17, 19

VPA

    Vincristine, I.V., 1.5 mg/m^2, days 1, 8, 15, 22
    Daunorubicin, I.V., 25 mg/m^2, days 1, 8
    Asparaginase, I.M., 10,000 units/m^2, days 2, 4, 6, 8, 10, 12, 15, 17, 19

AML, Induction

DA

    Daunorubicin, I.V., 45-60 mg/m^2 continuous infusion, days 1-3
    Cytarabine (Ara-C), I.V., 100 mg/m^2, q12h for 5-7 days

DAT

    Daunorubicin, I.V., 45 mg/m^2 continuous infusion, days 1-3
    Cytarabine (Ara-C), I.V., 100 mg/m^2 continuous infusion, days 1-7
    Thioguanine, P.O., 100 mg/m^2, days 1-7

DAV

    Daunorubicin, I.V., 30 mg/m^2 continuous infusion, days 1-3
    Cytarabine (Ara-C), I.V., 250 mg/m^2 continuous infusion, days 1-5
    Etoposide (VePesid®), I.V., 200 mg/m^2 continuous infusion, days 5-7

VAPA

    Vincristine, I.V., 1.5 mg/m^2, days 1, 5
    Doxorubicin (Adriamycin®), I.V., 30 mg/m^2 continuous infusion, days 1, 2, 3
    Prednisone, P.O., 40 mg/m^2, days 1-5
    Cytarabine (Ara-C), I.V., 100 mg/m^2 continuous infusion, days 1-7

Brain Tumors

CDDP/VP

    Cisplatin, I.V., 90 mg/m^2, day 1
    Etoposide, I.V., 150 mg/m^2, days 2, 3

MOP

    Mechlorethamine (nitrogen mustard), I.V., 6 mg/m^2, days 1, 8
    Vincristine (Oncovin®), I.V., 1.4 mg/m^2, days 1, 8
    Procarbazine, P.O., 100 mg/m^2, days 1-14

PCV

    Procarbazine, P.O., 60 mg/m^2, days 18-21
    Methyl-CCNU, P.O., 110 mg/m^2, day 1
    Vincristine, I.V., 1.4 mg/m^2, days 8-29

For calculating pediatric doses of chemotherapy agents, as a general rule 1 m^2 corresponds to about 30 kg of ideal body weight. **For children weighing <15 kg or with surface area <0.6 m^2,** the dose per m^2 of an agent listed herein should be divided by 30 and multiplied by the weight of the child (in kg) to obtain the correct dose.

Brain Tumors *(continued)*

POC

Prednisone, P.O., 40 mg/m^2, days 1-14
Methyl-CCNU, P.O., 100 mg/m^2, day 2
Vincristine, I.V., 1.5 mg/m^2, days 1, 8, 15

Repeat cycle every 6 weeks

"8 in 1"

Methylprednisolone, I.V., 300 mg/m^2, day 1
Vincristine, I.V., 1.5 mg/m^2, day 1
Methyl-CCNU, P.O., 75 mg/m^2, day 1
Procarbazine, P.O., 75 mg/m^2/d, day 1
Hydroxyurea, P.O., 1500 or 3000 mg/m^2, day 1
Cisplatin, I.V., 60 or 90 mg/m^2, day 1
Cytarabine, I.V., 300 mg/m^2, day 1
Cyclophosphamide, I.V., 300 mg/m^2 **or**
    dacarbazine (DTIC), I.V., 150 mg/m^2, day 1

Hodgkin's Lymphoma

ABVD

Doxorubicin (Adriamycin®), I.V., 25 mg/m^2, days 1, 15
Bleomycin, I.V., 10 units/m^2, days 1-15
Vinblastine, I.V., 6 mg/m^2, days 1, 15
Dacarbazine (DTIC), I.V., 375 mg/m^2, days 1, 15

Repeat cycle every 28 days

COMP

Cyclophosphamide, I.V., 500 mg/m^2, days 1-8
Vincristine (Oncovin®), I.V., 1.4 mg/m^2, days 1, 8
Methotrexate, I.V., 40 mg/m^2, days 1, 2
Prednisone, P.O., 40 mg/m^2, days 1-15

COPP

Cyclophosphamide, I.V., 500 mg/m^2, days 1-8
Vincristine (Oncovin®), I.V., 1.4 mg/m^2, days 1, 8
Procarbazine, P.O., 100 mg/m^2, days 1-15
Prednisone, P.O., 40 mg/m^2, days 1-15

MOPP

Mechlorethamine (nitrogen mustard), I.V., 6 mg/m^2, days 1, 8
Vincristine (Oncovin®), I.V., 1.4 mg/m^2, days 1, 8
Procarbazine, P.O., 100 mg/m^2, days 1-15
Prednisone, P.O., 40 mg/m^2, days 1-15

Repeat cycle every 28 days

OPA

Vincristine (Oncovin®), I.V., 1.5 mg/m^2, days 1, 8, 15
Prednisone, P.O., 60 mg/m^2, days 1-15
Doxorubicin (Adriamycin®), I.V., 40 mg/m^2, days 1, 15

OPPA

Vincristine (Oncovin®), I.V., 1.5 mg/m^2, days 1, 8, 15
Procarbazine, P.O., 100 mg/m^2, days 1-15
Prednisone, P.O., 60 mg/m^2, days 1-15
Doxorubicin (Adriamycin®), I.V., 40 mg/m^2, days 1, 15

Repeat cycle every 28 days

For calculating pediatric doses of chemotherapy agents, as a general rule 1 m^2 corresponds to about 30 kg of ideal body weight. **For children weighing <15 kg or with surface area <0.6 m^2** the dose per m^2 of an agent listed herein should be divided by 30 and multiplied by the weight of the child (in kg) to obtain the correct dose.

Osteosarcoma

HDMTX

    Methotrexate, I.V., 12 g/m^2, weekly for 2-12 weeks

    Leucovorin calcium rescue, P.O./I.V., 15 mg/m^2 q6h for 10 doses beginning 30
        hours after the beginning of the 4-hour methotrexate infusion

    (serum methotrexate levels must be monitored)

MTXCP-PDAdr

    Methotrexate, I.V., 12 g/m^2, weekly for 2-12 weeks

    Leucovorin calcium rescue, P.O./I.V., 15 mg/m^2 q6h for 10 doses beginning 30
        hours after the beginning of the 4-hour methotrexate infusion

    (serum methotrexate levels must be monitored)

    Cisplatin (Platinol®), I.V., 100 mg/m^2, day 1

    Doxorubicin (Adriamycin®), I.V., 37.5 mg/m^2, days 2, 3

MTXCP-PDAdrI

    Methotrexate, I.V., 12 g/m^2, weekly for 2-12 weeks

    Leucovorin calcium rescue, P.O./I.V., 15 mg/m^2 q6h for 10 doses beginning 30
        hours after the beginning of the 4-hour methotrexate infusion

    (serum methotrexate levels must be monitored)

    Cisplatin (Platinol®), I.V., 100 mg/m^2, day 1

    Doxorubicin (Adriamycin®), I.V., 37.5 mg/m^2, days 2, 3

    Ifosfamide, I.V., 1.6 mg/m^2, days 1-5

Sarcomas (Bony and Soft-Tissue)

ICE

    Ifosfamide, I.V., 2 g/m^2, days 2, 3, 4

    Carboplatin, I.V., 300-600 mg/m^2, day 1

    Etoposide, I.V., 100 mg/m^2, days 2, 3, 4

VAC + Adr

    Vincristine, I.V., 1.5 mg/m^2 (max 2 mg)

    Dactinomycin, I.V., 0.5-1.5 mg/m^2, days 1-5, every other week

    Cyclophosphamide, I.V., 500-1500 mg/m^2

    Doxorubicin (Adriamycin®), I.V., 35-60 mg/m^2

VACAdr-IfoVP

    Vincristine, I.V., 1.5 mg/m^2 (max 2 mg), weekly

    Dactinomycin, I.V., 1.5 mg/m^2 (max 2 mg), every other week

    Doxorubicin (Adriamycin®), I.V., 60 mg/m^2 continuous infusion over 24 hours

    Cyclophosphamide, I.V., 1-1.5 g/m^2

    Ifosfamide, I.V., 1.6-2 g/m^2, days 1-5

    Etoposide, I.V., 150 mg/m^2, days 1-5

VAdrC

    Vincristine, I.V., 1.5 mg/m^2 (max 2 mg)

    Doxorubicin (Adriamycin®), I.V., 35-60 mg/m^2

    Cyclophosphamide, I.V., 500-1500 mg/m^2

Wilms' Tumor

VAD

    Vincristine, I.V., 1.5 mg/m^2, every other week

    Dactinomycin, I.V., 0.4 mg/m^2, every other week
        alternating with doxorubicin, I.V., 25 mg/m^2, every other week

                         Repeat for a total of 6 months

VAD2

    Vincristine, I.V., 1.5 mg/m^2

    Dactinomycin, I.V., 0.15 mg/kg, days 1-5

    Doxorubicin, I.V., 20 mg/m^2, days 1-3

ADRENERGIC AGONISTS, CARDIOVASCULAR COMPARISON

Drug	Hemodynamic Effects			
	CO	TPR	Mean BP	Renal Perfusion
Amrinone	↑	↓	<->	↑
Dobutamine	↑	↓	↑	<->
Dopamine	↑	+/-*	<->/↑*	↑*
Epinephrine	↑	↓	↑	↓
Isoproterenol	↑	↓	↓	+/-†
Metaraminol	↓	↑	↑	↓
Milrinone	↑	↓	<->	↑
Norepinephrine	<->/↓	↑	↑	↓
Phenylephrine	↓	↑	↑	↓

↑ = increase ↓ = decrease, <-> = no change, * = dose dependent.

† In patients with cardiogenic or septic shock, renal perfusion commonly increases; however, in the normal patient, renal perfusion may be reduced with isoproterenol.

Drug	Hemodynamic Effects			
	α_1	β_1	β_2	Dopamine
Dobutamine (Dobutrex®)	+	+ + + +	+ +	0
Dopamine (Intropin®)	+ + + +	+ + + +	+ +	+ +
Epinephrine (Adrenalin®)	+ + + +	+ + + +	+ +	0
Isoproterenol (Isuprel®)	0	+ + + +	+ + + +	0
Norepinephrine (Levophed®)	+ + + +	+ + + +	0	0

ANGIOTENSIN-CONVERTING ENZYME INHIBITORS

Comparisons of Indications and Adult Dosages

Drug	Hypertension	CHF	Renal Dysfunction	Dialyzable	Tablet Strengths (mg)
Benazepril	20-80 mg qd qd-bid Maximum: 80 mg qd	Not FDA approved	Cl_{cr} <30 mL/min: 5 mg/day initially Maximum: 40 mg qd	Yes	5, 10, 20, 40
Captopril	25-150 mg qd bid-tid Maximum: 450 mg qd	6.25-100 mg tid Maximum: 450 mg qd	Unspecified dosage reduction	Yes	12.5, 25, 50, 100
Enalapril	5-40 mg qd qd-bid Maximum: 40 mg qd	2.5-20 mg bid Maximum: 20 mg bid	Cl_{cr} 30-80 mL/mL: 5 mg/day initially Cl_{cr} <30 mL/mL: 2.5 mg/day initially	Yes	2.5, 5, 10, 20
(Enalaprilat*)	(1.25 mg q6h)	(Not FDA approved)	(Cl_{cr} <30 mL/min: 0.625 mg)	(Yes)	(2.5 mg/2 mL vial)
Fosinopril	10-40 mg qd Maximum: 80 mg qd	Not FDA approved	No dosage reduction necessary	Not well dialyzed	10, 20
Lisinopril	10-40 mg qd Maximum: 80 mg qd	5-40 mg qd	Cl_{cr} 10-30 mL/min: 5 mg/day initially Cl_{cr} <10 mL/min: 2.5 mg/day initially	Yes	5, 10, 20, 40
Quinapril	10-80 mg qd qd-bid	5-20 mg bid	Cl_{cr} 30-60 mL/min: 5 mg/day initially Cl_{cr} <10 mL/min: 2.5 mg qd initially	Not well dialyzed	5, 10, 20, 40
Ramipril	2.5-20 mg qd qd-bid	Not FDA approved	Cl_{cr} <40 mL/min: 1.25 mg/day Maximum: 5 mg qd	Unknown	1.25, 2.5, 5, 10

*Enalaprilat is the only available ACEI in a parenteral formulation.
Dosage is based on 70 kg adult with normal hepatic and renal function.

ANGIOTENSIN-CONVERTING ENZYME INHIBITORS

Comparative Pharmacokinetics

Drug	Prodrug	Lipid Solubility	Absorption (%)	Serum $t_{1/2}$ (h)	Serum Protein Binding (%)	Elimination	Onset of Hypotensive Action (h)	Peak Hypotensive Effects (h)	Duration of Hypotensive Effects (h)
Benazepril	Yes	No data	37		>95	Primarily renal some biliary	1	2-4	>20 mg/d 24
Benazeprilat				10-12					
Captopril	No	Not very lipophilic	75	<2	25-30	Metabolism to disulfide, then renally	0.25	1-1.5	Dose related
Enalapril	Yes	Lipophilic	60 (53-73)	1.3	<50	Renal	1	4-6	24 (18-30)
Enalaprilat				11					
Fosinopril	Yes	Very lipophilic	36		>95	Renal 50 hepatic 50	1	2-6	24
Fosinoprilat				12					
Lisinopril	No	Very hydrophilic	25 (6-60)	12	0	Renal	1	6	24 (18-30)
Quinapril	Yes	No data	60	0.8	97	Renal 61 hepatic 37	1	2	24
Quinaprilat				2					
Ramipril	Yes	Somewhat lipophilic	50-60	1-2	73	Renal	1-2	3-6	≥24 (24-60)
Ramiprilat				13-17	56				

ANTACID DRUG INTERACTIONS

Drug	Antacid				
	Al Salts	Ca Salts	Mg Salts	NaHCO₃	Mg/Al
Allopurinol	↓				
Anorexiants				↑	
Benzodiazepines	↑		↓	↓	↓
Calcitriol			x*		x*
Captopril					↓
Cimetidine					↓
Corticosteroids	↓		↓		↓
Dicumarol			↑		
Diflunisal	↓				
Digoxin	↓		↓		
Flecainide				↑	
Iron	↓	↓	↓	↓	↓
Isoniazid	↓				
Ketoconazole				↓	↓
Levodopa					↑
Lithium				↓	
Nitrofurantoin			↓		
Penicillamine	↓		↓		↓
Phenothiazines	↓		↓		↓
Phenytoin		↓			↓
Quinidine		↑	↑		↑
Quinolones					↓
Ranitidine	↓				↓
Salicylates		↓		↓	↓
Sodium polystyrene sulfonate	x†		x†		x†
Sulfonylureas				↑	
Sympathomimetics				↑	
Tetracyclines	↓	↓	↓	↓	↓
Tolmetin				x‡	
Valproic acid					↑

Pharmacologic effect increased (↑) or decreased (↓) by antacids.

*Concomitant use in patients on chronic renal dialysis may lead to hypermagnesemia.

†Concomitant use may cause metabolic alkalosis in patients with renal failure.

‡Concomitant use not recommended by manufacturer.

ANTIARRHYTHMIC DRUGS

Effects of Long-Term Antiarrhythmic Therapy on Mortality in Placebo-Controlled, Randomized Trials

Effect	Therapy
Increases mortality	Encainide
	Flecainide
	Moricizine (short-term)
Reduces mortality	β-Adrenergic antagonists (propranolol, timolol, metoprolol)
May reduce mortality; adequate data not available	Amiodarone*
	Disopyramide†
	Mexiletine†
	Moricizine (long-term)†
	Procainamide
	Propafenone
	Quinidine†
	Sotalol
	Tocainide
	Implanted cardioverter-defibrillators

From *N Engl J Med*, 1994, 331:785-91.

*A trend toward decreased mortality was found in small trials; large trials are under way.

†Some data indicate a trend toward increased mortality.

Vaughan Williams Classification of Antiarrhythmic Drugs Based on Cardiac Effects

Type	Drug(s)	Conduction Velocity*	Refractory Period	Automaticity
Ia	Disopyramide Procainamide Quinidine	↓	↑	↓
Ib	Lidocaine Mexiletine Moricizine† Tocainide	0/↓	↓	↓
Ic	Encainide Flecainide Indecainide Propafenone‡	↓↓	0	↓
II	Beta-Blockers	↓	↑	↓
III	Amiodarone Bretylium Sotalol‡	0	↑↑	0
IV	Diltiazem Verapamil§	↓	↑	↓

*Variables for normal tissue models in ventricular tissue.

†Also has type Ia actions to decrease conduction velocity more than most type Ib.

‡Also has type II, beta-blocking action.

§Variables for SA and AV nodal tissue only.

Vaughan Williams Classification of Antiarrhythmic Agents and Their Indications/Adverse Effects

Type	Drug(s)	Indication	Route of Administration	Adverse Effects
Ia	Disopyramide	AF, VT	P.O.	Anticholinergic effects, CHF
	Procainamide	AF, VT, WPW	P.O./I.V.	GI, CNS, lupus fever, hematological, anticholinergic effects
	Quinidine	AF, PSVT VT, WPW	P.O./I.V.	Hypotension, GI, thrombocytopenia, cinchonism
Ib	Lidocaine	VT, VF, PVC	I.V.	CNS, GI, blood dyscrasia
	Mexiletine	VT	P.O.	GI, CNS
	Tocainide	VT	P.O.	GI, CNS, pulmonary, agranulocytosis
Ic	Encainide	VT	P.O.	GI, CNS
	Flecainide	VT	P.O.	CHF, GI, CNS, blurred vision
	Propafenone	VT	P.O.	GI, blurred vision, dizziness
	Moricizine	VT	P.O.	Dizziness, nausea, rash, seizures
II	Esmolol	ST, SVT	I.V.	CHF, CNS, lupus-like syndrome, hypotension, bradycardia, bronchospasm
	Propranolol	SVT, VT, PVC, digoxin toxicity	P.O./I.V.	CHF, bradycardia, hypotension, CNS, fatigue
III	Amiodarone	VT	P.O.	CNS, GI, thyroid, pulmonary fibrosis, liver, corneal deposits
	Bretylium	VT, VF	I.V.	GI, orthostatic hypotension, CNS
	Sotalol	VT	P.O.	Bradycardia, hypotension, CHF, CNS, fatigue
IV	Diltiazem	AF, PSVT	P.O./I.V.	Hypotension, GI, liver
	Verapamil	AF, PSVT	P.O./I.V.	Hypotension, CHF, bradycardia, vertigo, constipation
Miscellaneous	Adenosine	SVT, PSVT	I.V.	Flushing, dizziness, bradycardia, syncope
	Digoxin	AF, PSVT	P.O./I.V.	GI, CNS, arrhythmias
	Magnesium	VT, VF	I.V.	Hypotension, CNS hypothermia, myocardial depression

AF = atrial fibrillation, PSVT = paroxysmal supraventricular tachycardia,
VT = ventricular tachycardia, WPW = Wolf-Parkinson-White arrhythmias,
VF = ventricular fibrillation, SVT = supraventricular tachycardia.

Comparative Pharmacokinetic Properties of Antiarrhythmic Agents

Type	Drug(s)	Bioavailability (%)	Primary Route of Elimination	Volume of Distribution (L/kg)	Protein Binding (%)	Half-Life	Therapeutic Range (mcg/mL)
Ia	Disopyramide	70-95	Hepatic/Renal	0.8-2	50-80	4-8 h	2-6
	Procainamide	75-95	Hepatic/Renal	1.5-3	10-20	2.5-5 h	4-15
	Quinidine	70-80	Hepatic	2-3.5	80-90	5-9 h	2-6
Ib	Lidocaine	20-40	Hepatic	1-2	65-75	60-180 min	1.5-5
	Mexiletine	80-95	Hepatic	5-12	60-75	6-12 h	0.75-2
	Tocainide	90-95	Hepatic	1.5-3	10-30	12-15 h	4-10
Ic	Encainide*	85-95 / 20-30	Hepatic/Renal	2.5-4	70-80	8-11 h / 1-3 h	—
	Flecainide	90-95	Hepatic/Renal	8-10	35-45	1-6 h	—
	Propafenone*	11-39	Hepatic	2.5-4	85-95	12-32 h / 2-10 h	—
	Moricizine	34-38	Hepatic	6-11	10-30	12-15 h	4-10
II	Esmolol			Refer to Beta-Blocker Comparison Chart			
	Propranolol			Refer to Beta-Blocker Comparison Chart			
III	Amiodarone	22-28	Hepatic	70-150	95-97	15-100 d	1-2.5
	Bretylium	15-20	Renal	4-8	Negligible	5-10 h	0.5-2
	Sotalol	90-95	Renal	1.6-2.4	Negligible	12-15 h	—
IV	Diltiazem	80-90	Hepatic/Renal	1.7	77-85	4-6 h	0.05-0.2
	Verapamil	20-40	Hepatic	1.5-5	95-99	4-12 h	>50 ng/mL

*Top numbers reflect **poor** metabolizers and **bottom numbers** reflect **extensive** metabolizers.

ANTICONVULSANTS BY SEIZURE TYPE

Seizure Type	Age	Commonly Used	Alternatives
Primarily generalized tonic-clonic seizures	1-12 mo	Carbamazepine* Phenytoin Phenobarbital	Valproate
	1-6 y	Carbamazepine* Phenytoin Phenobarbital	Valproate
	6-11 y	Carbamazepine	Valproate Phenytoin Phenobarbital Lamotrigine†
Primarily generalized tonic-clonic seizures with absence or with myoclonic seizures	1 mo - 18 y	Valproate	Phenytoin‡ Phenobarbital‡ Carbamazepine‡
Absence seizures	Any age	Ethosuximide	Valproate Clonazepam Diamox Lamotrigine†
Myoclonic seizures	Any age	Valproate Clonazepam	Phenytoin† Phenobarbital†
Tonic and atonic seizures	Any age	Valproate	Phenytoin† Clonazepam Phenobarbital†
Partial seizures	1-12 mo	Phenobarbital	Carbamazepine Phenytoin
	1-6 y	Carbamazepine*	Phenytoin Phenobarbital Valproate† Lamotrigine Gabapentin
	6-18 y	Carbamazepine	Phenytoin Phenobarbital Valproate†
Infantile spasms		Corticotropin (ACTH)	Prednisone† Valproate† Clonazepam† Diazepam†

*Not FDA approved for children younger than 6 years of age.
†Not FDA approved for this indication.
‡Phenytoin, phenobarbital, carbamazepine will not treat absence seizures. Addition of another anticonvulsant (ie, ethosuximide) would be needed.

ANTIDEPRESSANT AGENTS COMPARISON

Comparison of Usual Dosage, Mechanism of Action, and Adverse Effects of Antidepressants

Drug	Usual Dosage (mg/d)	Reuptake Inhibition		Adverse Effects					
		N	S	ACH	Drowsiness	Orthostatic Hypotension	Cardiac Arrhythmias	GI Distress	Weight Gain
First-Generation Antidepressants									
Tricyclic Antidepressants									
Amitriptyline (Elavil®, Endep®)	100–300	Moderate	High	4+	4+	4+	3+	0	4+
Clomipramine† (Anafranil®)	100–250	Moderate	High	4+	4+	2+	3+	1+	4+
Desipramine (Norpramin®, Pertofrane®)	100–300	High	Low	1+	2+	2+	2+	0	1+
Doxepin (Adapin®, Sinequan®)	100–300	Low	Moderate	3+	4+	2+	2+	0	4+
Imipramine (Janimine®, Tofranil®)	100–300	Moderate	Moderate	3+	3+	4+	3+	1+	4+
Nortriptyline (Aventyl®, Pamelor®)	50–200	Moderate	Low	2+	2+	1+	2+	0	1+
Protriptyline (Vivactil®)	15–60	Moderate	Low	2+	1+	2+	3+	0	0
Trimipramine (Surmontil®)	100–300	Low	Low	4+	4+	3+	3+	0	4+
Monoamine Oxidase Inhibitors									
Phenelzine (Nardil®)	15–90	—	—	2+	2+	2+	1+	1+	3+
Tranylcypromine (Parnate®)	10–40	—	—	2+	1+	2+	1+	1+	2+

(continued)

| Drug | Usual Dosage (mg/d) | Reuptake Inhibition | | Adverse Effects | | | | | |
		N	S	ACH	Drowsiness	Orthostatic Hypotension	Cardiac Arrhythmias	GI Distress	Weight Gain
Second-Generation Antidepressants *Older Second-Generation Antidepressants*									
Amoxapine (Asendin®)	100–400	Moderate	Low	2+	2+	2+	2+	0	2+
Maprotiline (Ludiomil®)	100–225	Moderate	Low	2+	3+	2+	2+	0	2+
Nefazodone (Serzone®)	300–600	Very low	High	1+	2+	2+	1+	1+	2+
Trazodone (Desyrel®)	150–500	Very low	Moderate	0	4+	3+	1+	1+	2+
Newer Second-Generation Antidepressants									
Bupropion (Wellbutrin®)	300–450‡	Very low§	Very low§	0	0	0	1+	1+	0
Third-Generation Antidepressants *Selective Serotonin Reuptake Inhibitors*									
Fluoxetine (Prozac®)	10–40	Very low	High	0	0	0	0	3+¶	0
Paroxetine (Paxil®)	20–50	Very low	Very high	1+	1+	0	0	3+¶	1+
Sertraline (Zoloft®)	50–150	Very low	Very high	0	0	0	0	3+¶	0
Serotonin/Norepinephrine Reuptake Inhibitors									
Venlafaxine# (Effexor®)	75–375	Very high	Very high	1+	1+	0	1+	3+¶	0

Key: N = norepinephrine; S = serotonin; ACH = anticholinergic effects (dry mouth, blurred vision, urinary retention, constipation).
0 – 4+ = absent or rare – relatively common.
†Not approved by FDA for depression.
‡Not to exceed 150 mg/dose to minimize seizure risk.
§Norepinephrine and serotonin reuptake inhibition is minimal, but inhibits dopamine reuptake.
¶Nausea is usually mild and transient.
#Comparative studies evaluating the adverse effects of venlafaxine in relation to other antidepressants have not been performed.

ANTIDEPRESSANTS, COMPARISONS OF THE SEROTONIN REUPTAKE INHIBITORS

Comparison of Pharmacokinetic Parameters of SSRIs

Parameter	Fluoxetine	Paroxetine	Sertraline
Time of peak plasma concentration from initial dose (h)	4-8	3-8	6-10
Elimination half-life (h)	24-48	15-20	26
Protein binding (%)	95	95	97
Time to reach steady-state plasma concentration (d)	14-28	4-14	7-10
Volume of distribution (L/kg)	25	13	20
Plasma clearance (L/h/kg)	0.29	0.76	NA
Active metabolites	Norfluoxetine	None	Desmethylsertraline

NA = not available.

Comparison of Pharmacokinetic Properties of SSRIs Which Contribute to Drug Interactions

Drug	Half-Life (h)	Protein Binding (%)	Inhibition of CYP2D6
Fluoxetine	24-48	95	Yes
Norfluoxetine (fluoxetine metabolite)	168	NA	Yes
Paroxetine	15-20	95	Yes
Sertraline	26	97	NA
Desmethylsertraline (sertraline metabolite)	62-104	NA	NA

NA = not available.

ANTIFUNGAL AGENTS

Activities of Various Agents Against Specific Fungi

Fungus	Itraconazole	Amphotericin B	Ketoconazole	Fluconazole
Aspergillus	x	x	—	?
Blastomyces	x	x	x	?
Candida	x	x	x	x
Chromomycosis	x	—	—	?
Coccidioides	x	x	x	x
Cryptococcus	x	x	x	x
Histoplasma	x	x	x	x
Sporothrix	x	x	—	?

Pharmacokinetic Properties of Systemically Active Agents

Characteristic	Imidazoles		Triazoles			Amphotericin B	Flucytosine
	Miconazole	Ketoconazole	Itraconazole	Fluconazole			
Absorption							
Relative bioavailability (T)	NA	75	99.8 (40)	ND (85)		<10	75–90
C_{max} (mcg/mL)	1–3.7	3–6.5	0.63	1.4		1.7	70–120
T_{max} (h)	1	2.6	4	1–4		NA	<2
AUC (mcg × h/mL)	ND	12.9 (13.6)	1.9 (0.7)	42		ND	ND
Distribution							
Protein binding (%)	91–93	99	99.8	11		90–95	2–4
CSF/serum concentration (%)	<10	<10	<10	>60		<10	<60
Excretion							
Beta half-life (h)	2.1	8.1	17	22		1–15 days	2.5–6
Active drug in urine (%)	1	2	<1	64		40	80

Parameters are estimated from the administration of currently recommended doses to normal volunteers for imidazoles and triazoles.
Relative bioavailability was obtained with meals. Values in parentheses represent date obtained in fasting state.
Excretion (beta half-life) of ketoconazole and itraconazole are dose-dependent.
AUC = area under the curve; C_{max} = maximum concentration at steady-state; CSF = cerebrospinal fluid
NA = not applicable; ND = no data; T_{max} = time of maximum concentration

ANTIPSYCHOTIC AGENTS COMPARISON

Antipsychotic Agent	Equivalent Dosages (approx) (mg)	Usual Adult Daily Maintenance Dose (mg)	Sedation (Incidence)	Extrapyramidal Side Effects	Anticholinergic Side Effects	Cardiovascular Side Effects
Chlorpromazine	100	200–1000	High	Moderate	Moderate	Moderate/high
Clozapine	50	50–400	High	Low	High	High
Fluphenazine	2	5–40	Low	High	Low	Low
Haloperidol	2	5–40	Low	High	Low	Low
Loxapine	10	25–100	Moderate	High	Low	Low
Mesoridazine	50	30–400	High	Low	High	Moderate
Molindone	15	25–100	Low	High	Low	Low
Perphenazine	10	16–48	Low	High	Low	Low
Promazine	200	40–1200	Moderate	Moderate	High	Moderate
Risperidone	2	4–6	Moderate	Low	Low	Low/moderate
Thioridazine	100	200–800	High	Low	High	Moderate/high
Thiothixene	5	5–40	Low	Moderate	Low	Low/moderate
Trifluoperazine	5	10–40	Low	High	Low	Low

BENZODIAZEPINES COMPARISON

Agent	Peak Blood Levels (oral) (h)	Protein Binding (%)	Volume of Distribution (L/kg)	Major Active Metabolite	Half-Life (parent) (h)	Half-Life (metabolite) (h)	Adult Oral Dosage Range
Anxiolytic							
Alprazolam (Xanax®)	1–2	80	1.1	No	12–15	—	0.75–4 mg/d
Chlordiazepoxide (Librium®)	2–4	90–98	0.3	Yes	5–30	24–96	15–100 mg/d
Diazepam (Valium®)	0.5–2	96	1.1	Yes	20–80	50–100	4–40 mg/d
Lorazepam (Ativan®)	1–6	88–92	1.3	No	10–20	—	2–4 mg/d
Oxazepam (Serax®)	2–4	86–96	0.6–2	No	5–20	—	30–120 mg/d
Sedative/Hypnotic							
Estazolam (ProSom™)	2	93	—	No	10–24	—	1–2 mg
Flurazepam (Dalmane®)	0.5–2	97	—	Yes	Not significant	40–114	15–60 mg
Quazepam (Doral®)	2	>95	5	Yes	25–41	28–114	7.5–15 mg
Temazepam (Restoril®)	2–3	96	1.4	No	10–40	—	15–30 mg
Triazolam (Halcion®)	1	89–94	0.8–1.3	No	2.3	—	0.125–0.25 mg
Miscellaneous							
Clonazepam (Klonopin®)	1–2	86	1.8–4	No	18–50	—	1.5–20 mg/d
Clorazepate (Tranxene®)	1–2	80–95	—	Yes	Not significant	50–100	15–60 mg
Midazolam (Versed®)	0.4–0.7‡	>95	0.8–6.6	No	2–5	—	NA

† = significant metabolite.
‡ = I.V. only.
NA = not available.

BETA-BLOCKERS COMPARISON

Agent	Adrenergic Receptor Blocking Activity	Lipid Solubility	Protein Bound (%)	Half-life (h)	Bioavailability (%)	Primary (Secondary) Route of Elimination	Indications	Usual Dosage
Acebutolol (Sectral®)	beta₁	Low	15–25	3–4	40 7-fold‡	Hepatic (renal)	Hypertension Arrhythmias	P.O.: 400–1200 mg/d
Atenolol (Tenormin®)	beta₁	Low	<5–10	6–9†	50–60 4-fold‡	Renal (hepatic)	Hypertension Angina pectoris Acute MI	P.O. 50–200 mg/d I.V.: 5 mg x 2 doses
Betaxolol (Kerlone®)	beta₁	Low	50–55	14–22	84–94	Hepatic (renal)	Hypertension	P.O.: 10–20 mg/d
Bisoprolol (Zebeta®)	beta₁	Low	26–33	9–12	80	Renal (hepatic)	Hypertension	P.O.: 2.5–5 mg
Esmolol (Brevibloc®)	beta₁	Low	55	0.15	NA 5-fold‡	Red blood cell	Supraventricular tachycardia Sinus tachycardia	I.V. infusion: 25–300 mcg/kg/min
Labetalol (Trandate® Normodyne®)	alpha₁ beta₁ beta₂	Moderate	50	5.5–8	18–30 10-fold‡	Renal (hepatic)	Hypertension	P.O.: 200–2400 mg/d I.V.: 20–80 mg at 10-min intervals up to a maximum of 300 mg **or** continuous infusion of 2 mg/min
Metoprolol (Lopressor®)	beta₁	Moderate	10–12	3–7	50 10-fold‡	Hepatic (renal)	Hypertension Angina pectoris Acute MI	P.O.: 100–450 mg/d I.V.: Post-MI 15 mg Angina: 15 mg then 2–5 mg/hour Arrhythmias: 0.2 mg/kg

Note: All beta₁ selective agents will inhibit beta₂ receptors at higher doses.
†Half-life increased to 16–27 h in creatinine clearances of 15–35 mL/min and >27 h in Cl$_{cr}$ <15 mL/min.
‡Interpatient variations in plasma levels.

(continued)

Agent	Adrenergic Receptor Blocking Activity	Lipid Solubility	Protein Bound (%)	Half-life (h)	Bioavailability (%)	Primary (Secondary) Route of Elimination	Indications	Usual Dosage
Nadolol (Corgard®)	beta₁ beta₂	Low	25–30	20–24	30 5–8-fold‡	Renal	Hypertension Angina pectoris	P.O.: 40–320 mg/d
Pindolol (Visken®)	beta₁ beta₂	Moderate	57	3–4†	90 4-fold‡	Hepatic (renal)	Hypertension	P.O.: 20–60 mg/d
Propranolol (Inderal® various)	beta₁ beta₂	High	90	3–5	30 20-fold‡	Hepatic	Hypertension Angina pectoris Arrhythmias Hypertrophic subaortic stenosis Prophylaxis (post-MI)	P.O.: 40–480 mg/d I.V.: Reflex tachycardia 1–10 mg P.O.: 180–240 mg/d
Propranolol long-acting (Inderal-LA®)	beta₁ beta₂	High	90	9–18	30 20-fold‡	Hepatic		
Timolol (Blocadren®)	beta₁ beta₂	Low to moderate	<10	4	75 7-fold‡	Hepatic (renal)	Hypertension Prophylaxis (post-MI)	P.O.: 20–60 mg/d P.O.: 20 mg/d

Dosage is based on 70 kg adult with normal hepatic and renal function.
Note: All beta₁ selective agents will inhibit beta₂ receptors at higher doses.
†Half-life variable: 7–15 hours.
‡Interpatient variations in plasma levels.

Selected Properties of Beta-Adrenergic Blocking Drugs

Drug	Relative Beta₁ Selectivity	Beta-Blockade Potency Ratio*	ISA	MSA
Acebutolol	+	0.3	+	+
Atenolol	+	1	–	–
Betaxolol	++	1	–	+
Bisoprolol	+		–	–
Esmolol	+	0.02	–	–
Metoprolol	+	1	–	–
Nadolol	–	2-9	–	–
Pindolol	–	6	++	+
Propranolol	–	1	–	++
Sotalol	–	0.3	–	–
Timolol	–	6	–	–

*Propranolol = 1

ISA = intrinsic sympathomimetic activity, MSA = membrane stabilizing activity.

CALCIUM CHANNEL BLOCKERS COMPARISON

Calcium Channel Blockers Comparative Actions

Agent	A-V Conduction Node	SA Node Automaticity	Contractility	Heart Rate	Cardiac Output	Peripheral Vascular Resistance
DIHYDROPYRIDINES						
Nifedipine (Procardia®)	NE	0	0-SD*	0-SI	MI	PD
Amlodipine (Norvasc®)	0	0	0-SI	NE	SI	PD
Felodipine (Plendil®)	0	0	0-SI	0-SI	SI	PD
Isradipine (DynaCirc®)	0	0	0-SI	NE	SI	PD
Nicardipine (Cardene®)	0-SI	0	0-SI	0-SI	MI	PD
Nimodipine (Nimotop®)	NA	NA	NA	NA	NA	NA
PHENYLALKYLAMINES						
Verapamil (Calan®, Isoptin®)	NE	MD	MD	SE	SE	MD
BENZOTHIAZEPINES						
Diltiazem (Cardizem®)	NE	SD	SD	SD	SE	SD
MISCELLANEOUS						
Bepridil (Vascor®)	NE	SD	SD	SD	0	SD

*Drug may worsen symptomos of congestive heart failure due to systolic dysfunction (ejection fraction <40%).
MD = moderate decrease, MI = moderate increase, NA = not available, NE = negligible effect, PD = pronounced decrease, SD = slight decrease, SE = slight effect (increase or decrease), SI = slight increase.

Calcium Channel Blockers Comparative Pharmacokinetics

Agent	Bioavailability (%)	Protein Binding (%)	Onset (min)	Peak (h)	Half-Life (h)	Volume of Distribution	Route of Metabolism	Route of Excretion
DIHYDROPYRIDINES								
Nifedipine (prototype) (Adalat®, Procardia®Procardia XL®)	Immediate/ sustained release 45-70/86	92-98	20	Immediate/ sustained release 0.5/6	2-5	ND	Liver, inactive metabolites	60%-80% urine, feces, bile
Amlodipine (Norvasc®)	52-88	97	6 h	6-9	33.8	21 L/kg	Liver, inactive metabolites, not a significant first-pass metabolism/presystemic metabolism	Bile, gut wall
Felodipine (Plendil®)	10-25	>99	3-5 h	2.5-5	10-36	10.3 L/kg	Liver, inactive metabolites, extensive metabolism by several pathways including cytochrome P-450, extensive first-pass metabolism/presystemic metabolism	70% urine, 10% feces
Isradipine (DynaCirc®)	15-24	97	120	0.5-2.5	8	2.9 L/kg	Liver, inactive metabolites, extensive first-pass metabolism	90% urine, 10% feces
Nicardipine (Cardene®)	35	>95	20	0.5-2	2-4	ND	Liver, saturable first-pass metabolism	60% urine, 35% feces
Nimodipine (Nimotop®)	13	>95	ND	≤1	1-2	0.43 L/kg	Liver, inactive metabolites, high first-pass metabolism	Urine
PHENYLALKYLAMINES								
Verapamil (prototype) (Calan®/Calan® SR, Isoptin®/Isoptin® SR, Verelan®)	20-35	83-92	30	1-2.2	3-7	4.5-7 L/kg	Liver	70% urine, 16% feces
BENZOTHIAZEPINES								
Diltiazem (prototype) (Cardizem®/Cardizem® CD, Dilacor® XR)	40-67	70-80	30-60	Immediate/ sustained release 2-3/6-11	Immediate/ sustained release 3.5-6/5-7	ND	Liver, drugs which inhibit/induce hepatic microsomal enzymes may alter disposition	Urine
MISCELLANEOUS								
Bepridil (Vascor®)	59	>99	60	2-3	24	ND	Liver	70% urine, 22% feces

Calcium Channel Blockers Cardiovascular Adverse Effects

Agent	Cardiovascular Adverse Reactions (%)						
	Edema	Hypotension	Palpitations	Syncope	CHF	MI	Tachycardia
DIHYDROPYRIDINES							
Nifedipine (prototype) (Adalat®, Procardia®/Procardia XL®)	10-30	≤1-5	≤2-7	≤1	2-6.7	4-6.7	≤1
Amlodipine (Norvasc®)	9-33	NR	≤2	NR	NR	NR	Negative
Felodipine (Plendil®)	22.3	≤1.5	1.8	≤1.5	NR	≤1.5	≤1.5
Isradipine (DynaCirc®)	7.2	≤1	4	≤1	≤1	≤1	1.5
Nicardipine (Cardene®)	7.1-8	<0.4	3.3-4.1	0.8	NR	<0.4	0.8-3.4
Nimodipine (Nimotop®)	0.2-1.2	1.2-8.1	≤1	NR	NR	NR	1
PHENYLALKYLAMINES							
Verapamil (prototype) (Calan®/Calan® SR, Isoptin®/Isoptin® SR, Verelan®)	2.1	2.5	<1	NR	1.8	0.8-1.2	1.4
BENZOTHIAZEPINES							
Diltiazem (prototype) (Cardizem®/Cardizem® CD, Dilacor® XR)	2.4-9	1	<1	NR	<1	0.6-7.6	1.5-6
MISCELLANEOUS							
Bepridil (Vascor®)	≤2	NR	0-6.5	NR	NR	NR	≤2

NR = not reported

Calcium Channel Blockers FDA-Approved Indications

Agent	Hypertension	Subarachnoid Hemorrhage	Arrhythmias	Angina
DIHYDROPYRIDINES				
Nifedipine (prototype) (Adalat®, Procardia®/Procardia XL®)	X Sustained release only			Vasospastic and chronic stable
Amlodipine (Norvasc®)	X			Vasospastic and chronic stable
Felodipine (Plendil®)	X			
Isradipine (DynaCirc®)	X			
Nicardipine (Cardene®)	X			Chronic stable
Nimodipine (Nimotop®)		X		
PHENYLALKYLAMINES				
Verapamil (prototype) (Calan®/Calan® SR, Isoptin®/Isoptin® SR, Verelan®)	X		X I.V. — supraventricular arrhythmias	Unstable, vasospastic, and chronic stable
BENZOTHIAZEPINES				
Diltiazem (prototype) (Cardizem®/Cardizem® CD, Dilacor® XR)	X Sustained release only			Vasospastic and chronic stable
MISCELLANEOUS				
Bepridil (Vascor®)				Chronic stable

Calcium Channel Blockers Central Nervous System Adverse Reactions

Agent	Central Nervous System Reactions (%)						
	Dizzy/Lightheaded	Headache	Weakness	Malaise	Nervousness	Asthenia
DIHYDROPYRIDINES							
Nifedipine (prototype) (Adalat®, Procardia®/Procardia XL®)	4.1-27	10-23	≤2-12	≤1	NR	NR
Amlodipine (Norvasc®)	3	8.1	NR	4	NR	NR
Felodipine (Plendil®)	5.8	18.6	NR	NR	NR	NR
Isradipine (DynaCirc®)	7.3	13.7	1.2	NR	NR	NR
Nicardipine (Cardene®)	4-6.9	6.4-8.2	0.6	0.6	NR	NR
Nimodipine (Nimotop®)	<1	1.4-4.1	NR	NR	NR	NR
PHENYLALKYLAMINES							
Verapamil (prototype) (Calan®/Calan® SR, Isoptin®/Isoptin® SR, Verelan®)	3.5	2.2	NR	NR	NR	1.7
BENZOTHIAZEPINES							
Diltiazem (prototype) (Cardizem®/Cardizem® CD, Dilacor® XR)	1.5-7	2.1-12	NR	NR	<1	2.8-5
MISCELLANEOUS							
Bepridil (Vascor®)	11.6-27	6.9-13.6	NR	NR	7.4-11.6	6.5-14

NR = not reported.

Calcium Channel Blockers Gastrointestinal and Miscellaneous Adverse Effects

Agent	Gastrointestinal Effects (%)				Miscellaneous Effects (%)					
	Nausea	Diarrhea	Constipation	Abdominal Discomfort	Rash	Flushing	Muscle Cramps	Cough	Shortness of Breath
DIHYDROPYRIDINES									
Nifedipine (prototype) (Adalat®, Procardia®/Procardia XL®)	3.3-11	NR	≤3.3	NR	≤3	<3-25	≤2-8	6	NR
Amlodipine (Norvasc®)	3	NR	NR	NR	NR	2.4	NR	NR	NR
Felodipine (Plendil®)	1.9	NR	1.6	NR	1.5	6.4	≤1.9	2.9	NR
Isradipine (DynaCirc®)	1.8	NR	≤1	NR	1.5	2.6	NR	≤1	NR
Nicardipine (Cardene®)	1.9-2.2	NR	0.6	NR	0.4-1.2	5.6-9.7	NR	NR	NR
Nimodipine (Nimotop®)	0.6-1.4	NR	NR	NR	0.6-2.4	1-2.1	0.2-1.4	NR	NR
PHENYLALKYLAMINES									
Verapamil (prototype) (Calan®/Calan® SR, Isoptin®/Isoptin® SR, Verelan®)	2.7	<1	7.3	<1	1.2	NR	NR	NR	1.4
BENZOTHIAZEPINES									
Diltiazem (prototype) (Cardizem®/Cardizem® CD, Dilacor® XR)	1.6-1.9	<1	1.6	1.3	1-1.5	NR	NR	NR	<1
MISCELLANEOUS									
Bepridil (Vascor®)	7-26	0-10.9	2.8	3-6.8	≤2	NR	NR	NR	0-8.7

NR = not reported.

CORTICOSTEROIDS, SYSTEMIC EQUIVALENCIES COMPARISON

Glucocorticoid	Approximate Equivalent Dose (mg)	Routes of Administration	Relative Anti-inflammatory Potency	Relative Mineralocorticoid Potency	Half-life Plasma (min)	Half-life Biologic (h)
Short-Acting						
Cortisone	25	P.O., I.M.	0.8	2	30	8-12
Hydrocortisone	20	I.M., I.V.	1	2	80-118	
Intermediate-Acting						
Prednisone	5	P.O.	4	1	60	18-36
Prednisolone	5	P.O., I.M., I.V., intra-articular, intradermal, soft tissue injection	4	1	115-212	
Triamcinolone	4	P.O., I.M., intra-articular, intradermal, intrasynovial, soft tissue injection	5	0	200+	
Methylprednisolone	4	P.O., I.M., I.V.	5	0	78-188	
Long-Acting						
Dexamethasone	0.75	P.O., I.M., I.V., intra-articular, intradermal, soft tissue injection	25-30	0	110-210	36-54
Betamethasone	0.6-0.75	P.O., I.M., intra-articular, intradermal, intrasynovial, soft tissue injection	25	0	300+	

CORTICOSTEROIDS, INHALED COMPARISON

Agent	Relative Binding Affinity*	Relative Blanching Potency†	Inhaled Dose (mcg/puff)
Beclomethasone diproprionate‡	0.4	600	50
Beclomethasone monoproprionate‡	13.5	450	—
Flunisolide	1.8	330	250
Triamcinolone	3.6	330	100

*Values are for binding affinity to human glucocorticoid receptors *in vitro*, relative to that of dexamethasone.

†Blanching potency on human skin indicates topical potency, relative to that of dexamethasone.

‡Beclomethasone diproprionate is converted n the liver to the more active beclomethasone monoproprionate.

Reference: Barnes PJ, "Inhaled Glucocorticoids for Asthma," *N Engl J Med*, 1995, 332:868-75.

CORTICOSTEROIDS, TOPICAL COMPARISON

Steroid		Vehicle
Lowest Potency (may be ineffective for some indications)		
0.1%	Betamethasone	Cream
0.2%	Betamethasone (Celestone®)	Cream
0.05%	Desonide	Cream
0.04%	Dexamethasone (Hexadrol®)*	Cream
0.1%	Dexamethasone (Decadron® Phosphate, Decaderm®)*	Cream, gel
1%	Hydrocortisone	Cream, ointment, lotion
2.5%	Hydrocortisone	Cream, ointment
0.25%	Methylprednisolone acetate (Medrol®)	Ointment
1%	Methylprednisolone acetate (Medrol®)	Ointment
0.5%	Prednisolone (Meti-Derm®)	Cream
Low Potency		
0.01%	Betamethasone valerate (Valisone®, reduced strength)	Cream
0.1%	Clocortolone (Cloderm®)	Cream
0.03%	Flumethasone pivalate (Locorten®)	Cream
0.01%	Fluocinolone acetonide (Synalar®)*	Cream, solution
0.025%	Fluorometholone (Oxylone®)	Cream
0.025%	Flurandrenolide (Cordran®, Cordran® SP)*	Cream, ointment
0.2%	Hydrocortisone valerate (Westcort®)	Cream
0.025%	Triamcinolone acetonide (Kenalog®)*	Cream, ointment
Intermediate Potency		
0.025%	Betamethasone benzoate	Cream, gel, lotion
0.1%	Betamethasone valerate (Valisone®)*	Cream, ointment, lotion
0.05%	Desonide (Tridesilon®)	Cream, ointment
0.05%	Desoximetasone (Topicort® LP)	Cream
0.025%	Fluocinolone acetonide*	Cream, ointment
0.05%	Flurandrenolide (Cordran®, Cordran® SP)*	Cream, ointment, lotion
0.025%	Halcinonide (Halog®)	Cream, ointment
0.1%	Triamcinolone acetonide (Kenalog®)*	Cream, ointment
High Potency		
0.1%	Amcinonide (Cyclocort®)	Cream, ointment
0.05%	Betamethasone dipropionate (Diprosone®)	Cream, ointment, lotion
0.05%	Clobetasol dipropionate	Cream, ointment
0.25%	Desoximetasone (Topicort®)	Cream
0.05%	Diflorasone diacetate (Florone®, Maxiflor®)	Cream, ointment
0.2%	Fluocinolone (Synalar-HP®)	Cream
0.05%	Fluocinonide (Lidex®)*	Cream, ointment
0.1%	Halcinonide (Halog®)	Cream, ointment, solution
0.5%	Triamcinolone acetonide*	Cream, ointment

*Fluorinated.

CYCLOPLEGIC MYDRIATICS COMPARISON

Agent	Peak Mydriasis	Peak Cycloplegia	Time to Recovery
Atropine	30-40 min	1-3 h	> 14 d
Cyclopentolate	25-75 min	25-75 min	24 h
Homatropine	30-90 min	30-90 min	6 h-4 d
Scopolamine	20-30 min	30 min-1 h	5-7 d
Tropicamide	20-40 min	20-35 min	1-6 h

DIURETICS, LOOP COMPARISON

Agent	Equivalent Potency	Usual Dose	Oral Bioavailability %	Duration of Action (h)
Bumetanide				
P.O.	1	0.5-2 mg qd	72-95	4
I.V. injection	1	0.5-1 mg qd	—	2-3
Ethacrynic acid				
P.O.	0.6-0.75	50-100 mg qd-bid	90-100	6-12
I.V. injection	0.6-0.75	50 mg IVPB*	—	2
Furosemide				
P.O.	40	20-80 mg bid	60-70	6-8
I.V. injection	40	20-40 mg qd-tid*	—	2
Torsemide				
P.O.	10-20	5-10 mg qd	80-90	6
I.V. injection	10-20	10-20 mg qd	—	6

Dosage is based on 70 kg adult with normal hepatic and renal function.

*Repeat doses may be required based upon response to initial doses.

GLAUCOMA DRUG THERAPY COMPARISON

	Ophthalmic Agent	Reduces Aqueous Humor Production	Increases Aqueous Humor Outflow	Average Duration of Action	Strengths Available
Miotics	Cholinesterase Inhibitors				
	Demecarium	No data	Significant	7 d	0.125–0.25%
	Echothiophate	No data	Significant	2 wk	0.03–0.25%
	Isoflurophate	No data	Significant	2 wk	0.025%
	Physostigmine	No data	Significant	24 h	0.25%
	Direct Acting				
	Acetylcholine	Some activity	Significant	14 min	Injection 1%
	Carbachol	Some activity	Significant	8 h	0.75–3%
	Pilocarpine	Some activity	Significant	5 h	0.5% 1% 2% 3% 4%
Mydriatics	Sympathomimetics				
	Dipivefrin	Significant	Moderate	12 h	0.1%
	Epinephrine	Significant	Moderate	18 h	0.25–2%
	Beta blockers				
	Betaxolol	Significant	Some activity	12 h	0.5%
	Levobunolol	Significant	Some activity	18 h	0.5%
	Metipranolol	Significant	Some activity	18 h	0.3%
	Timolol	Significant	Some activity	18 h	0.25% 0.5%
Miscellaneous	Carbonic Anhydrase Inhibitors				
	Acetazolamide	Significant	No data	10 h	250 mg tab 500 mg cap
	Methazolamide	Significant	No data	14 h	50 mg

All miotic drugs significantly affect accommodation.

HYPOGLYCEMIC AGENTS COMPARISON

Sulfonylureas	Equivalent Dose	Usual Regimen	Duration of Action (h)	Onset of Action (h)	Half-Life (h)	Metabolism/Elimination
Acetohexamide	500 mg	qd-bid	10-14	1	5	Metabolized in liver; metabolized potency ≥ parent compound; renally eliminated
Chlorpropamide	250 mg	qd	72	1	35	Metabolized in liver; excreted unchanged in the urine also
Glipizide	5 mg	qd-bid	10-24	1	3-7	Metabolized in liver to inactive metabolites; renally eliminated
Glyburide	5 mg	qd-bid	18-24	1.5	2-4	Metabolized in liver; 50% of metabolites eliminated in urine, 50% in the feces
Tolazamide	250 mg	qd-bid	10-14	4-6	7	Metabolized in liver; metabolite less active than parent compound; renally eliminated
Tolbutamide	1 g	bid-tid	6-12	1	5.6	Metabolized in liver to inactive metabolites that are excreted renally

Dosage is based on 70 kg adult with normal hepatic and renal function.

LAXATIVES, CLASSIFICATION AND PROPERTIES

Laxative	Onset of Action	Site of Action	Mechanism of Action
Saline			
Magnesium Citrate (Citroma®)	0.5-3 h	Small and large intestine	Attract/retain water in intestinal lumen increasing intraluminal pressure; cholecystokinin release
Magnesium Hydroxide (Milk of Magnesia)			
Sodium Phosphate/ Biphosphate Enema (Fleet® Enema)	2-15 min	Colon	
Irritant/Stimulant			
Senna (Senokot®)	6-10 h	Colon	Direct action on intestinal mucosa; stimulate myenteric plexus; alter water and electrolyte secretion
Bisacodyl Tab (Dulcolax®)			
Bisacodyl Supp (Dulcolax®)	0.25-1 h		
Castor Oil	2-6 h	Small intestine	
Cascara Aromatic Fluid Extract	6-10 h	Colon	
Bulk-Producing			
Methylcellulose	12-24 h (up to 72 h)	Small and large intestine	Holds water in stool; mechanical distention; malt soup extract reduces fecal pH
Psyllium (Metamucil®)			
Malt Soup Extract (Maltsupex®)			
Lubricant			
Mineral Oil	6-8 h	Colon	Lubricates intestine; retards colonic absorption of fecal water
Surfactants/Stool Softener			
Docusate (Colace®)	24-72 h	Small and large intestine	Detergent activity; facilitates admixture of fat and water to soften stool
Miscellaneous and Combination Laxatives			
Glycerin Supp	0.25-0.5 h	Colon	Local irritation; hyperosmotic action
Lactulose (Cephulac®)	24-48 h	Colon	Delivers osmotically active molecules to colon
Docusate/Casanthranol (Peri-Colace®)	8-12 h	Small and large intestine	Casanthranol – mild stimulant; docusate – stool softener

LIPID-LOWERING AGENTS

Effects on Lipoproteins

Drug	Total Cholesterol (%)	LDL-C (%)	HDL-C (%)	TG (%)
Bile-acid resins	↓20-25	↓20-35	→	↑5-20
Fibric acid derivatives	↓10	↓10 (↑)	↑10-25	↓40-55
HMG-CoA RI	↓15-35	↓20-40	↑2-15	↓7-25
Nicotinic acid	↓25	↓20	↑20	↓40
Probucol	↓10-15	↓<10	↓30	→

Comparative Dosages of Agents Used to Treated Hyperlipidemia

Antilipemic Agent*	Usual Daily Dose	Average Dosing Interval
HMG-CoA Reductase Inhibitors		
Fluvastatin	20-40 mg	hs
Lovastatin	20-40 mg	hs
Pravastatin	20-40 mg	hs
Simvastatin	10-20 mg	hs
Fibric Acid Derivatives		
Clofibrate	2000 mg	qid
Gemfibrozil	1200 mg	bid
Miscellaneous Agents		
Niacin	6 g	tid
Probucol	1 g	bid
Bile Acid Sequestrants		
Colestipol	30 g	bid
Cholestyramine	24 g	tid-qid

Dosage is based on 70 kg adult with normal hepatic and renal function.

NARCOTIC AGONIST CHARTS

Comparative Pharmacokinetics

Drug	Onset (min)	Peak (h)	Duration (h)	t ½ (h)	Average Dosing Interval (h)		Equianalgesic Doses* (mg)	
							I.M.	P.O.
Alfentanil	Immediate	ND	ND	1–2	—	—	ND	NA
Buprenorphine	15	1	4–8	2–3			0.4	—
Butorphanol	I.M.: 30–60 I.V.: 4–5	0.5–1	3–5	2.5–3.5	3	(3–6)	2	—
Codeine	P.O.: 30–60 I.M.: 10–30	0.5–1	4–6	3–4	3	(3–6)	120	200
Fentanyl	I.M.: 7–15 I.V.: Immediate	ND	1–2	1.5–6	1	(0.5–2)	0.1	NA
Hydrocodone	ND	ND	4–8	3.3–4.4	6	(4–8)	ND	ND
Hydromorphone	P.O.: 15–30	0.5–1	4–6	2–4	4	(3–6)	1.5	7.5
Levorphanol	P.O.: 10–60	0.5–1	4–8	12–16	6	(6–24)	2	4
Meperidine	P.O./I.M./S.C.: 10–15 I.V.: ≤5	0.5–1	2–4	3–4	3	(2–4)	75	300
Methadone	P.O.: 30–60 I.V.: 10–20	0.5–1	4–6 (acute) >8 (chronic)	15–30	8	(6–12)	10	20
Morphine	P.O.: 15–60 I.V.: ≤5	P.O./I.M./S.C.: 0.5–1 I.V.: 0.3	3–6	2–4	4	(3–6)	10	60# (acute) 30 (chronic)
Nalbuphine	I.M.: 30 I.V.: 1–3	1	3–6	5		—	10	—
Naloxone†	2–5	0.5–2	0.5–1	0.5–1.5		—	—	—
Oxycodone	P.O.: 10–15	0.5–1	4–6	3–4	4	(3–6)	NA	30
Oxymorphone	5–15	0.5–1	3–6				1	10‡
Pentazocine	15–20	0.25–1	3–4	2–3	3	(3–6)		
Propoxyphene	P.O.: 30–60	2–2.5	4–6	3.5–15	6	(4–8)	ND	130§–200¶
Sufentanil	1.3–3	ND	ND	2.5–3	—	—	0.02	NA

ND = no data available.   NA = not applicable.
*Based on acute, short–term use. Chronic administration may alter pharmacokinetics and decrease the oral parenteral dose ratio. The morphine oral–parenteral ratio decreases to ~1.5–2.5:1 upon chronic dosing.
#Extensive survey data suggest that the relative potency of I.M.:P.O. morphine of 1:6 changes to 1:2–3 with chronic dosing.
†Narcotic antagonist.
‡Rectal.
§HCl salt.
¶Napsylate salt.

Comparative Pharmacology

Drug	Analgesic	Antitussive	Constipation	Respiratory Depression	Sedation	Emesis
Phenanthrenes						
Codeine	+	+++	+	+	+	+
Hydrocodone	+	+++		+		
Hydromorphone	++	+++	+	++	+	+
Levorphanol	++	++	++	++	++	+
Morphine	++	+++	++	++	++	++
Oxycodone	++	+++	++	++	++	++
Oxymorphone	++	+	++	+++		+++
Phenylpiperidines						
Alfentanil	++					
Fentanyl	++			+		+
Meperidine	++	+	+	++	+	
Sufentanil	+++					
Diphenylheptanes						
Methadone	++	++	++	++	+	+
Propoxyphene	+			+	+	+
Agonist/Antagonist						
Buprenorphine	++	N/A	+++	+++	++	++
Butorphanol	++	N/A	+++	+++	++	+
Dezocine	++		+	++	+	++
Nalbuphine	++	N/A	+++	+++	++	++
Pentazocine	++	N/A	+	++	++ or stimu-lation	++

NEUROMUSCULAR BLOCKING AGENTS

Comparative Neuromuscular Blocking Dosages*

Agent	Comparative Dosages (mcg/kg)	Recommended Bolus Dose	Recommended I.V. Infusion Rates
Short-Acting Agents			
Mivacurium (Mivacron®)	80-90	150 mcg/kg	1-15 mcg/kg/min
Rocuronium (Zemuron®)	300	0.6-1.2 mg/kg	10-40 mcg/kg/min
Succinylcholine	300	25-75 mg (1-2 mg/kg)	2.5 mg/min
Intermediate-Acting Agents			
Atracurium (Tracrium®)	225	400-500 mcg/kg	2-15 mcg/kg/min
Pancuronium (Pavulon®)	60	40-100 mcg/kg	50-100 mcg/kg/h
Vecuronium (Norcuron®)	50-60	80-100 mcg/kg	0.8-1.2 mcg/kg/min
Long-Acting Agents			
Doxacurium (Nuromax®)	25-30	50 mcg/kg	Not applicable
Pipecuronium (Arduan®)	45	50-100 mcg/kg	Not applicable
Tubocurarine	500	100-600 mcg/kg	Not applicable

*Dosages in a 70 kg adult patient with normal renal and hepatic function.

Comparative Pharmacokinetic Parameters for Neuromuscular Blocking Agents in Adult Patients With Normal Renal and Hepatic Function

Agent	Volume of Distribution (central compartment)	Onset of Action	Duration of Action	Half-Life	Body Clearance
Short-Acting Agents		*1-2 min*	*10-20 min*		
Mivacurium (Mivacron®)	0.15-0.25 L/kg	2 min	17 min	16.9 min	3.3 L/kg/h 55 mL/kg/min
Rocuronium (Zemuron®)	0.22-0.25 L/kg	0.7-1 min	31-67 min	84-90 min	2.7 L/kg/min
Succinylcholine	Unknown	1-1.5 min	5-10 min	Unknown	Unknown
Intermediate-Acting Agents		*2-3 min*	*40-60 min*		
Atracurium (Tracrium®)	0.16-0.18 L/kg (0.04-0.06 L/kg)	2 min	30 min	20-21 min	5.3-6.1 mL/kg/min
Pancuronium (Pavulon®)	0.26-0.28 L/kg (0.05-0.12 L/kg)	1-5.2 min	60 min	114-140 min	1.8-1.9 mL/kg/min
Vecuronium (Norcuron®)	0.19-0.25 L/kg (0.05-0.11 L/kg)	1.5 min	30 min	58-80 min	3.0-5.2 mL/kg/min
Long-Acting Agents		*4-6 min*	*90-180 min*		
Doxacurium (Nuromax®)	0.22 ± 0.11 L/kg	6 min	83 min	99 ± 54 min	2.67 ± 0.09 mL/kg/min
Pipecuronium (Arduan®)	0.31 ± 0.1 L/kg	3-5 min	70 min	137 ± 68 min	2.3 ± 0.04 mL/kg/min
Tubocurarine	0.22-0.39 L/kg	6 min	80 min	3.9 h	Unknown

Causes of Prolonged Neuromuscular Blockade

Excessive drug administration

"Cumulative" drug effect
(eg, vecuronium and pancuronium)

Decreased metabolism/excretion
(eg, renal and/or hepatic dysfunction)

Accumulation of active metabolites

Electrolyte imbalances
(eg, hypokalemia or hypocalcemia or hypermagnesemia or hypernatremia)

Hypothermia

Drug interactions
Inhaled anesthetics
Local anesthetics
Calcium channel blockers
Antiarrhythmics
(eg, quinidine or procainamide)
Antibiotics
(eg, aminoglycosides or tetracyclines or vancomycin or clindamycin)
Immunosuppressives
(eg, cyclosporine)

Increased sensitivity to muscle relaxants
(eg, neuromuscular disorders such as myasthenia gravis or polymyositis)

NITRATES COMPARISON

Nitrates	Dosage Form	Onset (min)	Duration
Nitroglycerin	I.V.	1-2	3-5 min
	Sublingual	1-3	30-60 min
	Translingual spray	2	30-60 min
	Oral, sustained release	40	4-8 h
	Topical ointment	20-60	2-12 h
	Transdermal	40-60	18-24 h
Isosorbide dinitrate	Sublingual and chewable	2-5	1-2 h
	Oral	20-40	4-6 h
	Oral, sustained release	Slow	8-12 h
Isosorbide mononitrate	Oral	60-120	5-12 h

Adapted from Corwin S and Reiffel JA, "Nitrate Therapy for Angina Pectoris," *Arch Intern Med*, 1985, 145:538-43 and Franciosa JA, "Nitroglycerin and Nitrates in Congestive Heart Failure," *Heart and Lung*, 1980, 9(5):873-82.

*Hemodynamic and antianginal tolerance often develops within 24-48 h of continuous nitrate administration.

NONSTEROIDAL ANTI-INFLAMMATORY AGENTS, COMPARATIVE DOSAGES, AND PHARMACOKINETICS

Drug	Maximum Recommended Daily Dose (mg)	Time to Peak Levels (h)†	Half-life (h)
Propionic Acids			
Fenoprofen (Nalfon®)	3200	1-2	2-3
Flurbiprofen (Ansaid®)	300	1.5	5.7
Ibuprofen	3200	1-2	1.8-2.5
Ketoprofen (Orudis®)	300	0.5-2	2-4
Naproxen (Naprosyn®)	1500	2-4	12-15
Naproxen sodium (Anaprox®)	1375	1-2	12-13
Acetic Acids			
Diclofenac sodium delayed release (Voltaren®)	225	2-3	1-2
Diclofenac potassium immediate release (Cataflam®)	200	1	1-2
Etodolac (Lodine®)	1200	1-2	7.3
Indomethacin (Indocin®)	200	1-2	4.5
Indomethacin SR	150	2-4	4.5-6
Ketorolac (Toradol®)	I.M.: 120‡ P.O.: 40	0.5-1	3.8-8.6
Sulindac (Clinoril®)	400	2-4	7.8 (16.4)§
Tolmetin (Tolectin®)	2000	0.5-1	1-1.5
Fenamates (Anthranilic Acids)			
Meclofenamate (Meclomen®)	400	0.5-1	2 (3.3)¶
Mefenamic acid (Ponstel®)	1000	2-4	2-4
Nonacidic Agent			
Nabumetone (Relafen®)	2000	3-6	24
Oxicam			
Piroxicam (Feldene®)	20	3-5	30-86

Dosage is based on **70 kg adult with normal hepatic and renal function.**
†Food decreases the rate of absorption and may delay the time to peak levels.
‡150 mg on the first day.
§Half-life of active sulfide metabolite.
¶Half-life with multiple doses.

PENICILLINS

Classification of Penicillins

Classification	Compounds
Benzylpenicillin, penicillin G and its long-acting formulations	Benzylpenicillin Benzathine penicillin Procaine penicillin
Orally absorbed penicillins similar to benzylpenicillin	Phonoxymethylpenicillin (penicillin V)
Staphylococcal β-lactamase-resistant penicillins	Isoxazolyl penicillins Dicloxacillin, oxacillin Methicillin Nafcillin
Extended spectrum penicillins	Aminopenicillins Ampicillin, amoxicillin

Penicillins active against *Pseudomonas aeruginosa*	Acylureidopenicillins
	    Azlocillin, mezlocillin, piperacillin
	Carboxypenicillins
	    Carbenicillin, carbenicillin esters
	Ticarcillin

Choice of Penicillin for the Treatment of Infections Caused by Various Organisms

Organism	Penicillin
GRAM-POSITIVE ORGANISMS	
Gram-Positive Cocci	
Penicillinase-producing *Staphylococcus aureus*	Dicloxacillin, nafcillin
Nonpenicillinase-producing *Staphylococcus aureus*	Benzylpenicillin
Penicillinase-producing coagulase-negative staphylococci	Dicloxacillin, nafcillin
Nonpenicillinase-producing coagulase negative staphylococci	Benzylpenicillin
Streptococcus viridans	Benzylpenicillin
Group A,B,C, and G streptococci	Benzylpenicillin
Streptococcus bovis	Benzylpenicillin
Streptococcus pneumoniae	Benzylpenicillin
Enterococcus faecalis	Ampicillin ± gentamicin
Gram-Positive Bacilli	
Bacillus anthracis	Benzylpenicillin
Clostridium tetani	Benzylpenicillin
Clostridium perfringens	Benzylpenicillin
Listeria monocytogenes	Ampicillin ± gentamicin
GRAM-NEGATIVE ORGANISMS	
Gram-Negative Bacilli	
Nonpenicillinase producing *Bacteroides* species (except *B. fragilis* and some *B. melaninogenicus*)	Benzylpenicillin
Citrobacter species	Ticarcillin, ureidopenicillin
Escherichia coli	Ampicillin, ticarcillin, ureidopenicillin
Eikenella corrodens	Ampicillin
*Klebsiella pneumoniae**	Ureidopenicillin
Proteus mirabilis	Ampicillin
Proteus vulgaris	Ureidopenicillin, ticarcillin
*Pseudomonas aeruginosa**	Ureidopenicillin + aminoglycoside
Providencia species	Ureidopenicillin, ticarcillin
Enterobacter species*	Ureidopenicillin
Salmonella species (nontyphi)	Ampicillin, ticarcillin
*Serratia marcescens**	Ureidopenicillin (± aminoglycoside)
Spirillum minus	Benzylpenicillin
Streptobacillus moniliformis	Benzylpenicillin
Gram-Negative Cocci	
Nonpenicillinase producing *Neisseria gonorrhoeae*	Benzylpenicillin
Neisseria meningitidis	Benzylpenicillin
Haemophilus influenzae (β-lactamase-negative)	Ampicillin
Haemophilus influenzae (β-lactamase-positive)	Amoxicillin + clavulanic acid
Moraxella catarrhalis	Amoxicillin + clavulanic acid

*For some strains resistant to a penicillin, a third or fourth generation cephalosporin or an aminoglycoside should be used.

SEDATIVE AGENTS IN THE INTENSIVE CARE UNIT

Comparative Pharmacokinetics of Sedative Agents

Drug	Onset (min)	Peak (min)	Half-Life (h)	Equianalgesic Doses (mg)	Comments
Benzodiazepines					
Diazepam	1-5	3-4	20-80 h parent compound 50-100 h active metabolite	2-5 mg	Metabolized in liver to active metabolites which accumulate in the presence of hepatic failure. Long half-life and metabolites can lead to accumulation with repeated doses which limits usefulness as a continuous infusion. Poor stability as a continuous infusion.
Lorazepam	1-5	15-20	10-20 h parent compound metabolized to in liver to no active metabolites	1-2 mg	Drug of choice in presence of liver disease. Concentration limitation of 40 mg/1000 mL of D_5W due to precipitation in solution. Must use in-line 0.22 micron filter.
Midazolam	1-5	5-30	2-5 h no active metabolites Duration of action <2 h	I.M./I.V. bolus: 1-5 mg	Can be administered as a continuous infusion. Extensive distribution secondary to lipophilicity may result in prolonged elimination half-life in ICU patients.
Other Agents					
Haloperidol	10-30	20	20 h metabolized in liver and eliminated in bile and urine	0.5-2 mg mild agitation 2-5 mg moderate agitation 10-20 mg severe agitation	Potential for causing extrapyramidal reactions, however, rarely reported with I.V. haloperidol. Minimal cardiovascular effects except reports of torsades de pointes in patients with history of alcohol abuse or dilated cardiomyopathy. Reported adverse events included prolonged QT interval, atrial dysrhythmias, ventricular tachycardia, twitching, and tremors.
Propofol	30 sec	3-5	40 min	Titrate to Sedation: Initially 5 mcg/kg/min increases at 5-10 min intervals to a maximum of 50 mcg/kg/min (0.3-3 mg/kg/h)	Contraindicated in patients with known hypersensitivity to drug or components (soybean oil, egg lecithin, and glycerol). Use with caution in patients who with hyperlipidemia (increased serum triglyceride levels or serum turbidity) and patients who are hemodynamically unstable (hypovolemic or hypotensive). Significant hypotension is associated with bolus doses. Formulated in a lipid emulsion which contains 0.1 g fat (1.1 kcal) per mL. I.V. tubing must be changed every 12 hours due to potential for infection. Time to awake is minimal compared to benzodiazepines.

Comparative Dosages of Sedative Agents

Drug	Recommended Pediatric Dosage	Recommended Adult Dosage	Continuous Infusion Dosage
Benzodiazepines			
Diazepam	P.O.: 0.12-0.8 mg/kg/d in divided doses q6-8h I.M./I.V.: 0.04-0.3 mg/kg/dose q2-4h to a maximum of 0.6 mg/kg/8 h period	P.O.: 2-10 mg 2-4 times/d I.M./I.V.: 2-10 mg q3-4h prn	**Not recommended** due to poor stability
Lorazepam	I.M./P.O.: 0.05 mg/kg/dose q4-8h prn	P.O.: 1-10 mg/d in 2-3 divided doses I.V./I.M.: 1-4 mg q2-5h prn	**Not recommended** due to poor stability Maximum concentration 40 mg/1000 mL D$_5$W Bolus dose of 0.05 mg/kg (maximum 4 mg) followed by 0.5-2 mg/h
Midazolam	P.O.: <5 y: 0.5 mg/kg/dose >5 y: 0.4-0.5 mg/kg/dose Usual duration is 2 h I.M.: 0.07-0.08 mg/kg/dose I.V.: 0.035 mg/kg/dose which may be repeated up to a total dose of 0.1-0.2 mg/kg/dose **Intranasal:** 0.2 mg/kg by needleless syringe to nares over 15 sec and may be repeated in 5-15 min	I.M.: 0.07-0.08 mg/kg/dose I.V.: 0.5-5 mg/dose Usual duration is 2 h	100 mg in 250 mL D$_5$W or NS: **Children:** 1-2 mcg/kg/min titrated to desired effect (usual range 0.4-6 mcg/kg/min) **Adults:** 0.05-0.15 mg/kg loading dose followed by 0.05-0.1 mg/kg/h (1-5 mg/h) titrated to desired effect
Other Agents			
Haloperidol	6-12 y I.M./I.V.: 1-3 mg/dose q4-8h to a maximum of 0.15 mg/kg/d	I.V./I.M.: 0.5-2 mg mild agitation 2-5 mg moderate agitation 10-20 mg severe agitation Repeat dose after 30 minutes; double dose and administer after another 30 minutes and continue until calm achieved; may repeat additional doses at 6- to 12-hour intervals	Dilutions of up to 3 mg/mL in D$_5$W and up to 0.75 mg/mL in 0.9% NaCl Infusion rates of 1-40 mg/h for treatment durations of 2-12 days have been reported
Propofol	ND	Refer to continuous infusion dosage	1% concentration (10 mg/mL) Available in 100 mL bottles 5-50 mcg/kg/min (0.3-3 mg/kg/h)

SULFONAMIDE DERIVATIVES

The following table lists commonly prescribed drugs which are either sulfonamide derivatives or are structurally similar to sulfonamides. Please note that the list may not be all inclusive.

Commonly Prescribed Drugs

Classification	Specific Drugs
Antimicrobial Agents	Mafenide acetate (Sulfamylon®) Silver sulfadiazine (Silvadene®) Sodium sulfacetamide (Sodium Sulamyd®) Sulfadiazine Sulfamethizole Sulfamethoxazole (ie, Bactrim™ and co-trimoxazole) Sulfisoxazole (Gantrisin®)
Diuretics, Carbonic Anhydrase Inhibitors	Acetazolamide (Diamox®) Dichlorphenamide (Daranide®) Methazolamide (Neptazane®)
Diuretics, Loop	Bumetanide (Bumex®) Furosemide (Lasix®) Torsemide (Demadex®)
Diuretics, Thiazide	Bendroflumethiazide Benzthiazide Chlorothiazide (Diuril®) Chlorthalidone (Hygroton®) Cyclothiazide (Anhydron®) Hydrochlorothiazide (Dyazide®, HydroDIURIL®, Maxzide®) Hydroflumethiazide Indapamide (Lozol®) Methyclothiazide (Enduron®) Metolazone (Diulo®, Zaroxolyn®) Polythiazide Quinethazone Trichlormethiazide
Hypoglycemic Agents, Oral	Acetohexamide (Dymelor®) Chlorpropamide (Diabinese®) Glipizide (Glucotrol®) Glyburide (Diaβeta®, Micronase®) Tolazamide (Tolinase®) Tolbutamide (Orinase®)
Other Agents	Sulfasalazine (Azulfidine®)

PREVENTION OF BACTERIAL ENDOCARDITIS

Recommendations by the American Heart Association
(JAMA, December 12, 1990, 264:22)

Table 1. Cardiac Conditions*

Endocarditis Prophylaxis Recommended

Prosthetic cardiac valves, including bioprosthetic and homograft valves
Previous bacterial endocarditis, even in the absence of heart disease
Most congenital cardiac malformations
Rheumatic and other acquired valvular dysfunction, even after valvular
 surgery
Hypertrophic cardiomyopathy
Mitral valve prolapse with valvular regurgitation

Endocarditis Prophylaxis Not Recommended

Isolated secundum atrial septal defect
Surgical repair without residua beyond 6 months of secundum atrial
 septal defect, ventricular septal defect, or patent ductus arteriosus
Previous coronary artery bypass graft surgery
Mitral valve prolapse without valvular regurgitation†
Physiologic, functional, or innocent heart murmurs
Previous Kawasaki disease without valvular dysfunction
Previous rheumatic fever without valvular dysfunction
Cardiac pacemakers and implanted defibrillators

*This table lists selected conditions but is not meant to be all-inclusive.
†Individuals who have a mitral valve prolapse associated with thickening
 and/or redundancy of the valve leaflets may be at increased risk for
 bacterial endocarditis, particularly men who are 45 years of age or older.

Table 2. Dental or Surgical Procedures*

Endocarditis Prophylaxis Recommended

Dental procedures known to induce gingival or mucosal bleeding, including professional cleaning

Tonsillectomy and/or adenoidectomy

Surgical operations that involve intestinal or respiratory mucosa

Bronchoscopy with a rigid bronchoscope

Sclerotherapy for esophageal varices

Esophageal dilatation

Gallbladder surgery

Cystoscopy

Urethral dilatation

Urethral catheterization if urinary tract infection is present†

Urinary tract surgery if urinary tract infection is present†

Prostatic surgery

Incision and drainage of infected tissue†

Vaginal hysterectomy

Vaginal delivery in the presence of infection†

Endocarditis Prophylaxis Not Recommended‡

Dental procedures not likely to induce gingival bleeding, such as simple adjustment of orthodontic appliances or fillings above the gum line

Injection of local intraoral anesthetic (except intraligamentary injections)

Shedding of primary teeth

Tympanostomy tube insertion

Endotracheal intubation

Bronchoscopy with a flexible bronchoscope, with or without biopsy

Cardiac catheterization

Endoscopy with or without gastrointestinal biopsy

Cesarean section

In the absence of infection (for urethral catheterization, dilatation and curettage, uncomplicated vaginal delivery, therapeutic abortion, sterilization procedures, or insertion or removal of intrauterine devices

*This table lists selected conditions but is not meant to be all-inclusive.

†In addition to prophylactic regimen for genitourinary procedures, antibiotic therapy should be directed against the most likely bacterial pathogen.

‡In patients who have prosthetic heart valves, a previous history of endocarditis, or surgically constructed systemic-pulmonary shunts or conduits, physicians may choose to administer prophylactic antibiotics even for low-risk procedures that involve the lower respiratory, genitourinary, or gastrointestinal tracts.

Table 3. Recommended Standard Prophylactic Regimen for Dental, Oral, or Upper Respiratory Tract Procedures in Patients Who Are at Risk*

Drug	Dosing Regimen for Adults	Dosing Regimen for Children†
Standard Regimen		
Amoxicillin	3 g orally 1 hour before procedure; then 1.5 g 6 hours after initial dose	50 mg/kg 1 hour before procedure and 25 mg/kg 6 hours later
Amoxicillin/Penicillin-Allergic Patients		
Erythromycin	Erythromycin ethylsuccinate 800 mg, or erythromycin stearate 1 g, orally 2 hours before procedure; then half the dose 6 hours after initial dose, or	Erythromycin ethylsuccinate 20 mg/kg 1 hour before procedure and 10 mg/kg 6 hours later, or erythromycin stearate 20 mg/kg 1 hour before procedure and 10 mg/kg 6 hours later, or
Clindamycin	300 mg orally 1 hour before procedure and 150 mg 6 hours after initial dose	10 mg/kg 1 hour before procedure and 5 mg/kg 6 hours later

*Includes those with prosthetic heart valves and other high-risk patients.

†Initial pediatric doses are as follows: amoxicillin, 50 mg/kg; erythromycin ethylsuccinate or erythromycin stearate, 20 mg/kg; and clindamycin, 10 mg/kg. Follow-up doses should be half the initial dose. **Total pediatric dose should not exceed total adult dose**. The following weight ranges may also be used for the initial pediatric dose of amoxicillin: <15 kg, 750 mg; 15-30 kg, 1500 mg; and >30 kg, 3000 mg (full adult dose).

Table 4. Alternate Prophylactic Regimens for Dental, Oral, or Upper Respiratory Tract Procedures in Patients Who Are at Risk

Drug	Dosing Regimen for Adults	Dosing Regimen for Children*
Patients Unable to Take Oral Medications		
Ampicillin	I.V. or I.M. ampicillin 2 g 30 minutes before procedure; then I.V. or I.M. ampicillin 1 g or oral administration of amoxicillin 1.5 g, 6 hours after initial dose	I.V. or I.M. ampicillin 50 mg/kg 30 minutes before procedure plus gentamicin 2 mg/kg I.V. or I.M. 30 minutes before; may repeat once 8 hours after initial dose
Ampicillin/Amoxicillin/Penicillin-Allergic Patients Unable to Take Oral Medications		
Clindamycin	I.V. 300 mg 30 minutes before procedure and an I.V. or oral administration of 150 mg 6 hours after initial dose	I.V. 10 mg/kg 30 minutes before procedure and I.V. or oral administration of 5 mg/kg 6 hours later
Patients Considered High Risk and Not Candidates for Standard Regimen		
Ampicillin, gentamicin, and amoxicillin	Ampicillin: I.V. or I.M. 2 g Gentamicin: 1.5 mg/kg (not to exceed 80 mg), 30 minutes before procedure; followed by amoxicillin, 1.5 g orally 6 hours after initial dose; alternatively, the parenteral regimen may be repeated 8 hours after initial dose	Ampicillin: I.V. or I.M. 50 mg/kg 30 minutes before procedure Gentamicin: I.V. or I.M. 2 mg/kg 30 minutes before procedure, then amoxicillin 25 mg/kg orally 6 hours later
Ampicillin/Amoxicillin/Penicillin-Allergic Patients Considered High Risk		
Vancomycin	I.V. 1 g over 1 hour, starting 1 hour before procedure; no repeated dose necessary	I.V. 20 mg/kg infused slowly over 1 hour beginning 1 hour before procedure

*Initial pediatric doses are as follows: ampicillin, 50 mg/kg; clindamycin, 10 mg/kg; gentamicin, 2 mg/kg; and vancomycin, 20 mg/kg. Follow-up doses should be half the initial dose. **Total pediatric dose should not exceed total adult dose**. No initial dose is recommended in this table for amoxicillin (25 mg/kg is the follow-up dose).

Table 5. Regimens for Genitourinary/Gastrointestinal Procedures

Drug	Dosing Regimen for Adults	Dosing Regimen for Children*
Standard Regimen		
Ampicillin, gentamicin, and amoxicillin	Ampicillin: I.V. or I.M. 2 g Gentamicin: 1.5 mg/kg (not to exceed 80 mg), 30 minutes before procedure; followed by amoxicillin, 1.5 g orally 6 hours after initial dose; alternatively, the parenteral regimen may be repeated once 8 hours after initial dose	Ampicillin: I.V. or I.M. 50 mg/kg 30 minutes before procedure Gentamicin: I.V. or I.M. 2 mg/kg 30 minutes before procedure, then amoxicillin 25 mg/kg orally 6 hours later
Ampicillin/Amoxicillin/Penicillin-Allergic Patient Regimen		
Vancomycin and gentamicin	Vancomycin: I.V. 1 g over 1 hour Gentamicin: 1.5 mg/kg (not to exceed 80 mg), 1 hour before procedure; may be repeated once 8 hours after initial dose	Vancomycin: I.V. 20 mg/kg infused slowly over 1 hour beginning 1 hour before procedure Gentamicin: I.V. or I.M. 2 mg/kg 1 hour before procedure, may be repeated once 8 hours after initial dose
Alternate Low-Risk Patient Regimen		
Amoxicillin	3 g orally 1 hour before procedure: then 1.5 g 6 hours after initial dose	50 mg/kg 1 hour before procedure and 25 mg/kg 6 hours later

*Initial pediatric doses are as follows: ampicillin, 50 mg/kg; amoxicillin, 50 mg/kg; gentamicin, 2 mg/kg; and vancomycin, 20 mg/kg. Follow-up doses should be half the initial dose. **Total pediatric dose should not exceed total adult dose**.

ANTIMICROBIAL PROPHYLAXIS IN SURGICAL PATIENTS

Nature of Operation	Likely Pathogens	Recommended Drugs	Adult Dosage Before Surgery*
CLEAN			
Cardiac			
Prosthetic valve and other open-heart surgery	*S. epidermidis*, *S. aureus*, *Corynebacterium*, enteric gram-negative bacilli	Cefazolin **or** vancomycin‡	1 g I.V.
Vascular			
Arterial surgery involving the abdominal aorta, a prosthesis, or a groin incision	*S. aureus*, *S. epidermidis*, enteric gram-negative bacilli	Cefazolin **or** vancomycin‡	1 g I.V.
Lower extremity amputation for ischemia	*S. aureus*, *S. epidermidis*, enteric gram-negative bacilli, clostridia	Cefazolin **or** vancomycin‡	1 g I.V.
Neurosurgery			
Craniotomy	*S. aureus*, *S. epidermidis*	Cefazolin **or** vancomycin‡	1 g I.V.
Orthopedic			
Total joint replacement, internal fixation of fractures	*S. aureus*, *S. epidermidis*	Cefazolin **or** vancomycin‡	1 g I.V.
Ocular§	*S. aureus*, *S. epidermidis*, streptococci, enteric gram-negative bacilli, *Pseudomonas*	Gentamicin **or** tobramycin **or** combination of neomycin, gramicidin, and polymyxin B, cefazolin	Multiple drops topically over 2-24 h 100 mg subconjunctivally at end of procedure
CLEAN-CONTAMINATED			
Head and neck			
Entering oral cavity or pharynx	*S. aureus*, streptococci, oral anaerobes	Cefazolin **or** clindamycin	2 g I.V.¶ 600 mg I.V.
Gastroduodenal			
High risk, gastric bypass, or percutaneous endoscopic gastrostomy only	Enteric gram-negative bacilli, gram-positive cocci	Cefazolin	1 g I.V.
Biliary tract			
High risk only	Enteric gram-negative bacilli, enterococci, clostridia	Cefazolin	1 g I.V.
Colorectal	Enteric gram-negative bacilli, anaerobes	Oral: Neomycin plus erythromycin base Parenteral: Ceftizoxime	1 g of each at 1 PM, 2 PM, and 11 PM the day before the operation# 1 g I.V.
Appendectomy	Enteric gram-negative bacilli, anaerobes	Ceftizoxime	1 g I.V.
Vaginal or abdominal hysterectomy	Enteric gram-negative bacilli, anaerobes, group B streptococci, enterococci	Cefazolin **or** Ceftizoxime	1 g I.V. 1 g I.V.
Cesarean section	Same as for hysterectomy	High risk only: Cefazolin	1 g I.V. after cord clamping

(continued)

Nature of Operation	Likely Pathogens	Recommended Drugs	Adult Dosage Before Surgery*
Abortion	Same as for hysterectomy	First trimester in patients with previous pelvic inflammatory disease:	
		Aqueous penicillin G	1 million units I.V.
		or	
		doxycycline	100 mg P.O. 1 hour before abortion, then 200 mg P.O. 30 minutes after abortion
		Second trimester: Cefazolin	1 g I.V.

DIRTY

Nature of Operation	Likely Pathogens	Recommended Drugs	Adult Dosage Before Surgery*
Ruptured viscus	Enteric gram-negative bacilli, anaerobes, enterococci	Ceftizoxime with or without gentamicin	1 g q8h I.V. 1.5 mg/kg q8h I.V.
		or	
		clindamycin plus gentamicin	600 mg I.V. q6h 1.5 mg/kg q8h I.V.
Traumatic wound•	*S. aureus*, group A streptococci, clostridia	Cefazolin	1 g q8h I.V.

*Parenteral prophylactic antimicrobials for clean and clean-contaminated surgery can be given as a single intravenous dose just before the operation. Cefazolin can also be given intramuscularly. For prolonged operations, additional intraoperative doses should be given every 4-8 hours for the duration of the procedure. For "dirty" surgery, therapy should usually be continued for 5-10 days.

‡For hospitals in which methicillin-resistant *S. aureus* and *S. epidermidis* frequently cause wound infection, or for patients allergic to penicillins or cephalosporin.

§In addition, at the end of the operation many ophthalmologists give a subconjunctival injection of an aminoglycoside such as gentamicin (10-20 mg), with or without a cephalosporin such as cefazolin (100 mg).

¶In controlled studies, 2 g were effective, while 0.5 g was not (JT Johnson and VL Yu, *Ann Surg*, 1988, 207:108).

#After appropriate diet and catharsis.

•For bite wounds, in which likely pathogens may also include oral anaerobes, *Eikenella corrodens* (humans), and *Pasteurella multocida* (dog and cat), some *Medical Letter* consultants recommend use of amoxicillin-clavulanic acid (Augmentin®) or ampicillin/sulbactam (Unasyn®).

RECOMMENDATIONS FOR PROPHYLAXIS AGAINST TUBERCULOSIS

Multidrug-Resistant (MDR) Tuberculosis

Any patient suspected of TB should be isolated (private room, negative pressure, HCW entering should wear high-efficiency masks (disposable particulate respirators) [for details (essential): *MMWR*, 1990, 39(RR17):14].

INH Preventive Therapy

No age limit applies for these 6 groups:

1. HIV positive (risk of active disease 10%/year)

2. Household members of persons with recently diagnosed tuberculous disease (risk 2%-4% for 1st year); risk for infants and children may be twice that for adults

3. Newly infected persons; tuberculin test conversion within past 2 years (risk 3.3% 1st year)

4. Past tuberculosis, not treated with adequate chemotherapy (INH, rifampin, or alternatives)

5. Positive tuberculin reactors with chest x-ray consistent with nonprogressive tuberculous disease (risk 0.5%-5%/year)

6. Positive tuberculin reactors with specific predisposing underlying conditions: illicit injection drug use (*MMWR*, 1989, 38:236), silicosis, diabetes mellitus, prolonged adrenocorticoid rx (>15 mg prednisone qd), immunosuppressive rx, hematologic diseases (Hodgkin's, leukemia), endstage renal disease, clinical condition with substantial rapid weight loss or chronic undernutrition, previous gastrectomy (*Am Rev Resp Dis*, 1986, 134:355)

Drug Resistance

Areas of high prevalence of INH resistance include Korea and Southeast Asian countries. U.S. isolates (1991) >8% resistant to ≥1 drug, 3% resistant (R) INH + RIF. Only 11 states had INH/RIF(R) isolates (NY 40% INH/RIF(R), NJ 6%).

Dosing Recommendations

INH and rifampin should be taken in a single early morning dose on an **empty** stomach. Directly observed therapy (DOT) recommended (↑ likelihood of cure). ~20% patients noncompliant (a major cause of resistance).

Specific Circumstances/ Organism	Comments	Regimen
	Category I. Exposure (Household members and other close contacts of potentially infectious cases) (Exposee tuberculin test negative)*	
Neonate	Rx essential	INH (10 mg/kg/d) for 3 months, then repeat tuberculin test (TBnT). If mother's smear negative and infant's TBnT negative and chest x-ray (CXR) normal, stop INH. In UK BCG is then given (*Lancet*, 1990, 2:1479), unless mother HIV positive. If infants repeat TBnT positive and/or CXR abnormal (hilar adenopathy and/or infiltrate), INH + RIF (10-20 mg/kg/d) (or streptomycin). Total rx 6 months. If mother is being rx, separation from mother not indicated.

(continued)

Specific Circumstances/ Organism	Comments	Regimen
Children <5 y	Rx indicated	As for neonate first 3 months. If repeat TBnT negative, stop. If repeat TBnT positive, continue INH for total of 9 months. If INH not given initially, repeat TBnT at 3 months, if positive rx INH for 9 months (see Category II below).
Older children and adults	No rx	Repeat TBnT at 3 months, if positive rx INH for 9 months (see Category II below).

Category II. Infection Without Disease
(Positive tuberculin test)*

Regardless of age (see INH Preventive Therapy, 6 groups above)	Rx indicated	INH (5 mg/kg/d, maximum 300 mg/d for adults, 10 mg/kg/d not to exceed 300 mg/d for children). Results with 6 months rx nearly as effective as 12 months (65% vs 75% reduction in disease). *Am Thoracic Society* (6 months), *Am Acad Pediatrics* 1991 (9 months). If CXR abnormal, rx 12 months. In HIV-positive patient, rx minimum 12 months, some suggest longer (*MMWR* 1989, 38:247).
Age <35 y	Rx indicated	Reanalysis of earlier studies favors INH prophylaxis (if INH related hepatitis case fatality rate <1% and TB case fatality ≥6.7%, which appears to be the case (*Arch Int Med*, 1990, 150:2517).
INH-resistant organisms likely	Rx indicated	Data on efficacy of alternative regimens currently lacking. Regimens include ETB + RIF daily for 6 months, PZA + RIF daily for 2 months, then INH + RIF daily until sensitivities from index case (if available) known, then if INH-CR, dc INH and continue RIF for 9 months, otherwise INH + RIF for 9 months (this latter is *Am Acad Pediatrics'* 1991 recommendation).
INH + RIF resistant organisms likely	Rx indicated	Efficacy of alternative regimens is unknown; PZA (25-30 mg/kg/d P.O.) + ETB (15-25 mg/kg/d P.O.) (at 25 mg/kg ETB, monitoring for retrobulbar neuritis required), for 6 months unless HIV positive, then 12 months; PZA + ciprofloxacin (750 mg P.O. bid) or ofloxacin (400 mg P.O. bid) x 6-12 months (*MMWR*, 1992, 41(RR11):68).

INH = isoniazid; RIF = rifampin, KM = kanamycin; ETB = ethambutol; SM = streptomycin; CXR = chest x-ray; Rx = treatment.
See also guidelines for interpreting PPD in Skin Testing for Delayed Hypersensitivity in the Appendix.

*Tuberculin test (TBnT). The standard is the Mantoux test, 5 TU PPD in 0.1 mL diluent stabilized with Tween 80. Read at 48-72 hours measuring maximum diameter of induration. A reaction of ≥5 mm is defined as positive in the following: positive HIV or risk factors, recent close case contacts, CXR consistent with healed TBc. ≥10 mm is positive in foreign-born in countries of high prevalence, injection drug users, low income populations, nursing home residents, patients with medical conditions which ↑ risk (see above, preventive rx). ≥15 mm is positive in all others (*Am Rev Resp Dis*, 1990, 142:725). Two-stage TBnT: Use in individuals to be tested regularly (ie, healthcare workers). TBn reactivity may ↓ over time but be boosted by skin testing. If unrecognized, individual may be incorrectly diagnosed as recent converter. If 1st TBnT is reactive but <10 mm, repeat 5 TU in 1 week, if then ≥10 mm = positive, not recent conversion (*Am Rev Resp Dis*, 1979, 119:587).

AEROBIC CULTURE, SPUTUM

Gram's stain results more closely reflect the clinical outcome and along with the criterion of the number of neutrophils in the sputum should be laboratory basis for determining success. Other commonly recognized agents causing pneumonia are listed in the following tables.

Spectrum of Frequent Etiologic Agents in Pneumonia

Aerobic Bacteria	Anaerobes	Fungi
Gram-positive aerobes Streptococcus pneumoniae Staphylococcus aureus Streptococcus pyogenes Gram-negative aerobes Haemophilus influenzae Legionella pneumophila Escherichia coli Klebsiella pneumoniae Pseudomonas aeruginosa	Bacteroides melaninogenicus Fusobacterium Peptostreptococcus Bacteroides fragilis Actinomyces israelii	Aspergillus Coccidioides immitis Histoplasma capsulatum Blastomyces dermatitidis Cryptococcus neoformans Zygomycetes
Viruses	**Parasites**	**Other**
Respiratory syncytial virus Parainfluenza virus Influenza virus Adenovirus Enterovirus Rhinovirus Measles virus Varicella-zoster virus Rickettsia Coxiella burnetii Cytomegalovirus	Pneumocystis carinii Ascaris lumbricoides Toxocara canis and catis Filaria Strongyloides stercoralis Hookworms Paragonimus Echinococcus Schistosomes	Mycoplasma pneumoniae Chlamydia trachomatis Chlamydia psittaci Mycobacterium tuberculosis Chlamydia TWAR strains Nocardia

From Cohen GJ, "Management of Infections of the Lower Respiratory Tract in Children," *Pediatr Infect Dis,* 1987, 6:317-23, with permission.

Community-Acquired Bacterial Pneumonias: Frequency of Various Pathogens	%
Streptococcus pneumoniae	40-60
Haemophilus influenzae	2.5-20
Gram-negative bacilli	6-37
Staphylococcus aureus	2-10
Anaerobic infections	5-10
Legionella	0-22.5
Mycoplasma pneumoniae	5-15
Nosocomial Pneumonias: Frequency of Various Pathogens	**%**
Klebsiella	13
Pseudomonas aeruginosa	10-12
Staphylococcus aureus	3-10.6
Escherichia coli	4-7.2
Enterobacter	6.2
Group D Streptococcus	1.3
Proteus and Providencia	6
Serratia	3.5
Pneumococcus	10-20
Aspiration pneumonia anaerobic pneumonia*	5-25
Legionella*	0-15

*The specific incidence of pneumonias caused by *Mycoplasma, Legionella,* and anaerobes is difficult to document because of the technical problems in isolating the organisms.

From Verghese A and Berk SL, "Bacterial Pneumonia in the Elderly Medicine," 1983, 62:271-85, with permission.

INTERPRETATION OF GRAM'S STAIN RESULTS GUIDELINES

These guidelines are not definitive but presumptive for the identification of organisms on Gram's stain. Treatment will depend on the quality of the specimen and appropriate clinical evaluation.

Gram-Negative Bacilli (GNB)	**Example**
Enterobacteriaceae	*E. coli* *Serratia* sp *Klebsiella* sp *Enterobacter* sp *Citrobacter* sp
Pseudomonas aeruginosa	
Xanthomonas maltophilia	
Nonfermentative GNB	
Haemophilus influenzae	
Bacteroides fragilis group	
If fusiform (long and pointed)	*Fusobacterium* sp *Capnocytophaga* sp

Gram-Negative Cocci (GNC)	
Diplococci, pairs	*Neisseria meningitidis* *Neisseria gonorrhoeae* *Moraxella (Branhamella) catarrhalis*
Coccobacilli	*Acinetobacter* sp

Gram-Positive Bacilli (GPB)	
Diphtheroids (small pleomorphic)	*Corynebacterium* sp *Propionibacterium*
Large, with spores	*Clostridium* sp *Bacillus* sp
Branching, beaded, rods	*Nocardia* sp *Actinomyces* sp
Other	*Listeria* sp *Lactobacillus* sp

Gram-Positive Cocci (GPC)	
Pairs, chains, clusters	*Staphylococcus* sp *Streptococcus* sp *Enterococcus* sp
Pairs, lancet-shaped	*S. pneumoniae*

KEY CHARACTERISTICS OF SELECTED BACTERIA

Gram-Negative Bacilli (GNB)	**Example**
Lactose-positive	*Citrobacter* sp* (Enterobacteriaceae)
	Enterobacter sp* (Enterobacteriaceae)
	Escherichia coli (Enterobacteriaceae)
	Klebsiella pneumoniae (Enterobacteriaceae)
Lactose-negative/ oxidase-negative	*Acinetobacter* sp
	Morganella morganii
	Proteus mirabilis: indole negative
	Proteus vulgaris: indole positive
	Providencia sp
	Salmonella sp
	Serratia sp† (Enterobacteriaceae)
	Shigella sp
	Xanthomonas maltophilia
Lactose-negative/ oxidase-positive	*Aeromonas hydrophila*
	(may be lactose positive)
	Alcaligenes sp
	Flavobacterium sp
	Moraxella sp‡
	Pseudomonas aeruginosa
	Other *Pseudomonas* sp
Other	*Haemophilus influenzae* (coccobacillus)

Gram-Positive Bacilli (GPB)	
Anaerobic diphtheroids	*Propionibacterium acnes*
Bacillus sp	*B. cereus, B. subtilis* (large with spores)
Branching, beaded; partial acid-fast positive	*Nocardia* sp
CSF, blood	*Listeria monocytogenes*
Rapidly growing mycobacteria	*M. fortuitum*
	M. chelonei
Vaginal flora, rarely blood	*Lactobacillus* sp
Often blood culture contaminants	Diphtheroids (may be *Corynebacterium* sp)
Resistant to many agents except vancomycin	*C. jeikeium*
Other	*Clostridium* sp (large with spores)
	Actinomyces sp (branching, beaded)

Gram-Negative Cocci (GNC)	
Diplococci, pairs	*Capnocytophaga* sp
	Fusobacterium sp (fusiform)
	Moraxella catarrhalis
	Neisseria meningitidis
	Neisseria gonorrhoeae
Coccobacilli	*Acinetobacter* sp

Gram-Positive Cocci (GPC)	
Catalase-negative	*Streptococcus* sp (chains)
	Micrococcus sp (usually insignificant)
Catalase-positive	*Staphylococcus* sp (pairs, chairs, clusters)
Coagulase-negative	Coagulase-negative staphylococci (CNS)
Bloods	*S. epidermidis* or CNS
Urine	*S. saprophyticus* (CNS)
Coagulase-positive	*S. aureus*

Fungi	Example
Molds	
Sparsely septate hyphae	Zygomycetes (eg, *Rhizopus* sp and *Mucor*)
Septate hyphae brown pigment	Phaeohyphomycetes, for example, *Alternaria* sp *Bipolaris* sp *Curvularia* sp *Exserohilum* sp
Nonpigmented (hyaline)	Hyalophomycetes, for example *Aspergillus* sp (*A. fumigatus*, *A. flavus*) Dermatophytes *Fusarium* sp *Paecilomyces* sp *Penicillium* sp
Thermally dimorphic (yeast in tissue; mold *in vitro*)	*Blastomyces dermatitidis* *Coccidioides immitis* *Histoplasma capsulatum* (slow growing) *Paracoccidioides brasiliensis* *Sporothrix schenckii*
Yeast	*Candida* sp (germ tube positive = *C. albicans*) *Cryptococcus* sp (no pseudohyphae) *C. neoformans* *Rhodotorula, Saccharomyces* sp *Torulopsis glabrata* *Trichosporon* sp

Anaerobes

Gram-negative bacilli	*Bacteroides* sp (*B. fragilis*) *Fusobacterium* sp
Gram-negative cocci	*Veillonella* sp
Gram-positive bacilli	*Actinomyces* sp (branching, filamentous) *Bifidobacterium* sp *Clostridium* sp (spores) *Eubacterium* sp *Lactobacillus* sp *Propionibacterium acnes*
Gram-positive cocci	*Peptostreptococcus* sp

Most Common Blood Culture Contaminants

Alpha-hemolytic streptococci

Bacillus sp

Coagulase-negative staphylococci

Diphtheroids

Lactobacilli

Micrococcus sp

Propionibacterium sp

*May be lactose-negative.
†May produce red pigment and appear lactose-positive initially.
‡May be either bacillary or coccoid.

PRUDENT VANCOMYCIN USE

Recommendations of the Hospital Infection Control Practices Advisory Committee, Centers for Disease Control and Prevention, 1994

Situations in which the use of vancomycin is appropriate or acceptable:

- For treatment of serious infections due to beta-lactam resistant gram-positive microorganisms; clinicians should be aware that vancomycin may be less rapidly bactericidal than beta-lactam agents for beta-lactam susceptible staphylococci

- For treatment of infections due to gram-positive microorganisms in patients with serious allergy to beta-lactam antimicrobials

- When antibiotic-associated colitis (AAC) fails to respond to metronidazole therapy or if AAC is severe and potentially life-threatening

- Prophylaxis, as recommended by the American Heart Association, for endocarditis following certain procedures in patients at high risk for endocarditis

- Prophylaxis for surgical procedures involving implantation of prosthetic materials or devices at institutions with a high rate of infections due to MRSA or methicillin-resistant *S. epidermidis*; a single dose administered immediately before surgery is sufficient unless the procedure lasts more than 6 hours, in which case the dose should be repeated; prophylaxis should be discontinued after a maximum of two doses

Situations in which the use of vancomycin should be discouraged:

- Routine surgical prophylaxis

- Empiric antimicrobial therapy for a febrile neutropenic patient, unless there is strong evidence at the outset that the patient has an infection due to gram-positive microorganisms (eg, inflamed exit site of Hickman catheter), and the prevalence of infections due to beta-lactam-resistant gram-positive microorganisms (eg, MRSA) in the hospital is substantial

- Treatment in response to a single blood culture positive for coagulase-negative *Staphylococcus*, if other blood cultures drawn in the same time frame are negative, ie, if contamination of the blood culture is likely

- Continued empiric use for presumed infections in patients whose cultures are negative for beta-lactam-resistant gram-positive microorganisms

- Systemic or local (eg, antibiotic lock) prophylaxis for infection or colonization of indwelling central or peripheral intravascular catheters or vascular grafts

- Selective decontamination of the digestive tract

- Eradication of MRSA colonization

- Primary treatment of AAC

- Routine prophylaxis of very low birthweight infants

- Routine prophylaxis for patients on continuous ambulatory peritoneal dialysis

ANTIMICROBIAL DRUGS OF CHOICE

The following table lists the antimicrobial drugs of choice for various infecting organisms. This was published in *The Medical Letter*. Users should not assume that all antibiotics which are appropriate for a given organism are listed or that those not listed are inappropriate. The infection caused by the organism may encompass varying degrees of severity, and since the antibiotics listed may not be appropriate for the differing degrees of severity, or because of other patient-related factors, it cannot be assumed that the antibiotics listed for any specific organism are interchangeable. This table should not be used by itself without first referring to *The Medical Letter*, an infectious disease manual, or the infectious disease department. Therefore, only use this table as a tool for obtaining more information about the therapies available.

Infecting Organism	Drug of First Choice	Alternative Drugs
Gram-Positive Cocci		
Enterococcus		
endocarditis or other severe infection	Penicillin G or ampicillin with gentamicin	Vancomycin with gentamicin
uncomplicated urinary tract infection	Ampicillin or amoxicillin	Norfloxacin, ciprofloxacin, nitrofurantoin
Staphylococcus aureus or *epidermidis*		
nonpenicillinase producing	Penicillin G or V	A cephalosporin, vancomycin, imipenem, clindamycin, ciprofloxacin
penicillinase-producing	A penicillinase-resistant penicillin	A cephalosporin, vancomycin, amoxicillin-clavulanic acid, ticarcillin-clavulanic acid, ampicillin-sulbactam, imipenem, clindamycin, ciprofloxacin
methicillin-resistant	Vancomycin, with or without gentamicin and/or rifampin	Trimethoprim-sulfamethoxazole, ciprofloxacin
Streptococcus pyogenes (group A) and groups C and G	Penicillin G or V	An erythromycin, a cephalosporin, vancomycin, clindamycin
Streptococcus, group B	Penicillin G or ampicillin	A cephalosporin, vancomycin, an erythromycin
Streptococcus, viridans group	Penicillin G with or without gentamicin	A cephalosporin, vancomycin
Streptococcus bovis	Penicillin G	A cephalosporin, vancomycin
Streptococcus, anaerobic or *Peptostreptococcus*	Penicillin G	Clindamycin, a cephalosporin, vancomycin
Streptococcus pneumoniae (pneumococcus)	Penicillin G or V	An erythromycin, a cephalosporin, chloramphenicol, vancomycin
Gram-Negative Cocci		
Moraxella (Branhamella) *catarrhalis*	Amoxicillin-clavulanic acid	Trimethoprim-sulfamethoxazole, an erythromycin, a tetracycline, cefuroxime, cefotaxime, ceftizoxime, ceftriaxone, cefuroxime axetil, cefixime
Neisseria gonorrhoeae (gonococcus)	Ceftriaxone	Spectinomycin, ciprofloxacin, penicillin G, amoxicillin with probenecid, cefoxitin, trimethoprim-sulfamethoxazole, chloramphenicol
Neisseria meningitidis (meningococcus)	Penicillin G	Chloramphenicol, cefotaxime, ceftizoxime, ceftriaxone, cefuroxime, trimethoprim-sulfamethoxazole, a sulfonamide

(continued)

Infecting Organism	Drug of First Choice	Alternative Drugs
Gram-Positive Bacilli		
Bacillus anthracis (anthrax)	Penicillin G	An erythromycin, a tetracycline
Clostridium perfringens	Penicillin G	Chloramphenicol, metronidazole, clindamycin, a tetracycline
Clostridium tetani	Penicillin G	A tetracycline
Clostridium difficile	Vancomycin	Metronidazole, bacitracin
Corynebacterium diphtheriae	An erythromycin	Penicillin G
Corynebacterium, JK group	Vancomycin	
Listeria monocytogenes	Ampicillin with or without gentamicin	Trimethoprim-sulfamethoxazole
Enteric Gram-Negative Bacilli		
Bacteroides		
oropharyngeal strains	Penicillin G	Clindamycin, cefoxitin, metronidazole, chloramphenicol, cefotetan
gastrointestinal strains	Metronidazole	Clindamycin, cefoxitin, chloramphenicol, mezlocillin, ticarcillin or piperacillin, imipenem, ticarcillin-clavulanic acid, ampicillin-sulbactam, cefotetan
Campylobacter jejuni	Ciprofloxacin or an erythromycin	A tetracycline, gentamicin
Enterobacter	Cefotaxime, ceftizoxime, or ceftriaxone	Gentamicin, tobramycin, or amikacin, imipenem, carbenicillin, ticarcillin, mezlocillin, piperacillin, or azlocillin, aztreonam, ceftazidime, trimethoprim-sulfamethoxazole, ciprofloxacin, norfloxacin, chloramphenicol
Escherichia coli	A cephalosporin	Ampicillin with or without gentamicin, tobramycin, or amikacin, carbenicillin, ticarcillin, mezlocillin, piperacillin, or azlocillin, gentamicin, tobramycin, or amikacin, amoxicillin-clavulanic acid, ticarcillin-clavulanic acid, ampicillin-sulbactam, trimethoprim-sulfamethoxazole, imipenem, aztreonam, a tetracycline, ciprofloxacin, norfloxacin, chloramphenicol
Klebsiella pneumoniae	A cephalosporin	Gentamicin, tobramycin, or amikacin, amoxicillin-clavulanic acid, ticarcillin-clavulanic acid, ampicillin-sulbactam, trimethoprim-sulfamethoxazole, imipenem, aztreonam, a tetracycline ciprofloxacin, norfloxacin, chloramphenicol, mezlocillin or piperacillin
Proteus mirabilis	Ampicillin	A cephalosporin, carbenicillin, ticarcillin, mezlocillin, piperacillin, or azlocillin, gentamicin, tobramycin, or amikacin, trimethoprim-sulfamethoxazole, imipenem, aztreonam, ciprofloxacin, norfloxacin, chloramphenicol
Proteus, indole-positive (including *Providencia rettgeri, Morganella morganii*, and *Proteus vulgaris*)	Cefotaxime, ceftizoxime, or ceftriaxone	Gentamicin, tobramycin, or amikacin, carbenicillin, ticarcillin, mezlocillin, piperacillin, or azlocillin, amoxicillin-clavulanic acid, ticarcillin-clavulanic acid, ampicillin-sulbactam, imipenem, aztreonam, ceftazidime, trimethoprim-sulfamethoxazole, a tetracycline, ciprofloxacin, norfloxacin, chloramphenicol

(continued)

Infecting Organism	Drug of First Choice	Alternative Drugs

Enteric Gram-Negative Bacilli *(continued)*

Infecting Organism	Drug of First Choice	Alternative Drugs
Providencia stuartii	Cefotaxime, ceftizoxime, or ceftriaxone	Imipenem, ticarcillin-clavulanic acid, gentamicin, tobramycin, or amikacin, carbenicillin, ticarcillin, mezlocillin, piperacillin, or azlocillin, aztreonam, ceftazidime, trimethoprim-sulfamethoxazole, ciprofloxacin, norfloxacin, chloramphenicol
Salmonella typhi	Ceftriaxone	Chloramphenicol, ampicillin, amoxicillin, trimethoprim-sulfamethoxazole, ciprofloxacin
other *Salmonella*	Cefotaxime or ceftriaxone	Ampicillin or amoxicillin, trimethoprim-sulfamethoxazole, ciprofloxacin, chloramphenicol
Serratia	Cefotaxime, ceftizoxime, or ceftriaxone	Gentamicin or amikacin, imipenem, aztreonam, ceftazidime, trimethoprim-sulfamethoxazole, carbenicillin, ticarcillin, mezlocillin, piperacillin, or azlocillin, ciprofloxacin, norfloxacin
Shigella	Trimethoprim-sulfamethoxazole	Ciprofloxacin, norfloxacin, ampicillin, nalidixic acid
Yersinia enterocolitica	Trimethoprim-sulfamethoxazole	Ciprofloxacin, gentamicin, tobramycin, or amikacin, a tetracycline, cefotaxime or ceftizoxime

Other Gram-Negative Bacilli

Infecting Organism	Drug of First Choice	Alternative Drugs
Acinetobacter	Imipenem	Tobramycin, gentamicin, or amikacin, carbenicillin, ticarcillin, mezlocillin, piperacillin, or azlocillin, trimethoprim-sulfamethoxazole, minocycline, doxycycline
Aeromonas	Trimethoprim-sulfamethoxazole	Gentamicin or tobramycin, imipenem, a tetracycline
Bordetella pertussis (whooping cough)	An erythromycin	Trimethoprim-sulfamethoxazole, ampicillin
Brucella	A tetracycline with streptomycin	Chloramphenicol with or without streptomycin, trimethoprim-sulfamethoxazole, rifampin with a tetracycline
Calymmatobacterium granulomatis (granuloma inguinale)	A tetracycline	Streptomycin
Eikenella corrodens	Ampicillin	An erythromycin, a tetracycline, amoxicillin-clavulanic acid, ampicillin-sulbactam
Francisella tularensis (tularemia)	Streptomycin or gentamicin	A tetracycline, chloramphenicol
Fusobacterium	Penicillin G	Metronidazole, clindamycin, chloramphenicol
Gardnerella (Haemophilus) vaginalis	Metronidazole	Ampicillin
Haemophilus ducreyi (chancroid)	Ceftriaxone or an erythromycin	Trimethoprim-sulfamethoxazole, ciprofloxacin
Haemophilus influenzae meningitis, epiglottitis, arthritis, and other serious infections	Cefotaxime or ceftriaxone	Ampicillin plus chloramphenicol initially, cefuroxime (for pneumonia)
upper respiratory infections and bronchitis	Ampicillin or amoxicillin	Trimethoprim-sulfamethoxazole, cefuroxime, a sulfonamide with or without an erythromycin, amoxicillin-clavulanic acid, cefuroxime axetil, cefaclor, cefotaxime, ceftizoxime, ceftriaxone, a tetracycline
Legionella micdadei (*L. pittsburgensis*)	An erythromycin with or without rifampin	Trimethoprim-sulfamethoxazole
Legionella pneumophila	An erythromycin with or without rifampin	Trimethoprim-sulfamethoxazole

(continued)

Infecting Organism	Drug of First Choice	Alternative Drugs
Other Gram-Negative Bacilli *(continued)*		
Leptotrichia buccalis	Penicillin G	A tetracycline, clindamycin
Pasteurella multocida	Penicillin G	A tetracycline, a cephalosporin, amoxicillin-clavulanic acid, ampicillin-sulbactam
Pseudomonas aeruginosa		
urinary tract infection	Carbenicillin or ticarcillin	Piperacillin, mezlocillin, or azlocillin ceftazidime, imipenem, aztreonam, gentamicin, tobramycin, amikacin, norfloxacin, ciprofloxacin
other infections	Carbenicillin, ticarcillin, mezlocillin, piperacillin, or azlocillin plus tobramycin, gentamicin, or amikacin	Tobramycin, gentamicin, or amikacin with ceftazidime, imipenem, or aztreonam, ciprofloxacin
Pseudomonas mallei (glanders)	Streptomycin with a tetracycline	Streptomycin with chloramphenicol
Pseudomonas pseudomallei (melioidosis)	Ceftazidime	Chloramphenicol with doxycycline and trimethoprim-sulfamethoxazole, amoxicillin-clavulanic acid
Pseudomonas cepacia	Trimethoprim-sulfamethoxazole	Chloramphenicol, ceftazidime, imipenem
Spirillum minus (rat bite fever)	Penicillin G	A tetracycline, streptomycin
Streptobacillus moniliformis (rat bite fever, Haverhill fever)	Penicillin G	A tetracycline, streptomycin
Vibrio cholerae (cholera)	A tetracycline	Trimethoprim-sulfamethoxazole, ciprofloxacin
Vibrio vulnificus	A tetracycline	Penicillin G
Xanthomonas maltophilia (*Pseudomonas maltophilia*)	Trimethoprim-sulfamethoxazole	Minocycline, ceftazidime, ciprofloxacin
Yersinia pestis (plague)	Streptomycin	A tetracycline, chloramphenicol, gentamicin
Acid-Fast Bacilli		
Mycobacterium tuberculosis	Isoniazid with rifampin with or without pyrazinamide	Ethambutol, streptomycin, cycloserine, ethionamide, kanamycin, capreomycin
Mycobacterium kansasii	Isoniazid with rifampin with or without ethambutol or streptomycin	Ethionamide, cycloserine
Mycobacterium avium complex	Rifampin with ethambutol, ciprofloxacin, and clofazimine with or without amikacin	Ethionamide, cycloserine, rifabutin, imipenem
Mycobacterium fortuitum complex	Amikacin and doxycycline	Cefoxitin, rifampin, an erythromycin, a sulfonamide
Mycobacterium marinum (balnei)	Minocycline	Trimethoprim-sulfamethoxazole, rifampin, cycloserine
Mycobacterium leprae (leprosy)	Dapsone with rifampin with or without clofazimine	Ethionamide, protionamide
Actinomycetes		
Actinomyces israelii (actinomycosis)	Penicillin G	A tetracycline
Nocardia	A sulfonamide	Trimethoprim-sulfamethoxazole, amikacin, minocycline, trisulfapyrimidines with minocycline, ampicillin, or erythromycin, cycloserine

(continued)

Infecting Organism	Drug of First Choice	Alternative Drugs
Chlamydia		
Chlamydia psittaci (psittacosis, ornithosis)	A tetracycline	Chloramphenicol
Chlamydia trachomatis (trachoma)	A tetracycline (topical plus oral)	A sulfonamide (topical plus oral)
(inclusion conjunctivitis)	An erythromycin (oral or I.V.)	A sulfonamide
(pneumonia)	An erythromycin	A sulfonamide
(urethritis or pelvic inflammatory disease)	A tetracycline or an erythromycin	Sulfisoxazole
(lymphogranuloma venereum)	A tetracycline or an erythromycin	
Chlamydia pneumoniae (TWAR strain)	A tetracycline	An erythromycin
Mycoplasma		
Mycoplasma pneumoniae	An erythromycin or a tetracycline	
Ureaplasma urealyticum	An erythromycin	A tetracycline
Rickettsia — Rocky Mountain spotted fever, endemic typhus (murine), tick bite fever, trench fever, typhus, scrub typhus, Q fever		
	A tetracycline	Chloramphenicol
Spirochetes		
Borrelia burgdorferi (Lyme disease)	A tetracycline	Penicillin G or V, ceftriaxone, cefotaxime, an erythromycin
Borrelia recurrentis (relapsing fever)	A tetracycline	Penicillin G
Leptospira	Penicillin G	A tetracycline
Treponema pallidum	Penicillin G	A tetracycline, ceftriaxone
Treponema pertenue (yaws)	Penicillin G	A tetracycline
Viruses		
Cytomegalovirus	Ganciclovir	Foscarnet
Hepatitis B or C	Alfa-2a or -2b interferon	
Herpes simplex		
keratitis	Trifluridine (topical)	Vidarabine (topical), idoxuridine (topical
genital	Acyclovir	Vidarabine, foscarnet
encephalitis	Acyclovir	Vidarabine
neonatal	Acyclovir	Vidarabine
disseminated, adult	Acyclovir	Vidarabine, foscarnet
Human immunodeficiency virus	Zidovudine	Dideoxyinosine
Influenza A	Amantadine	
Respiratory syncytial virus	Ribavirin	
Varicella-zoster	Acyclovir	Vidarabine

RECOMMENDATIONS OF THE ADVISORY COUNCIL ON THE ELIMINATION OF TUBERCULOSIS
(*MMWR*, 1993, 42(RR-7):1-8)

Regimen Options for the Initial Treatment of TB Among Children and Adults

---

TB Without HIV Infection

Option 1

Administer daily INH, RIF, and PZA for 8 weeks followed by 16 weeks of INH and RIF daily or 2-3 times/week* in areas where the INH resistance rate is not documented to be <4%. EMB or SM should be added to the initial regimen until susceptibility to INH and RIF is demonstrated. Continue treatment for at least 6 months and 3 months beyond culture conversion. Consult a TB medical expert if the patient is symptomatic or smear or culture positive after 3 months.

Option 2

Administer daily INH, RIF, PZA, and SM or EMB for 2 weeks followed by 2 times/week* administration of the same drugs for 6 weeks (by DOT‡), and subsequently, with 2 times/week administration of INH and RIF for 16 weeks (by DOT). Consult a TB medical expert if the patient is symptomatic or smear or culture positive after 3 months.

Option 3

Treat by DOT, 3 times/week* with INH, RIF, PZA, and EMB or SM for 6 months.† Consult a TB medical expert if the patient is symptomatic or smear or culture positive after 3 months.

TB With HIV Infection

Options 1, 2, or 3 can be used, but treatment regimens should continue for a total of 9 months and at least 6 months beyond culture conversion.

---

*All regimens administered 2 times/week or 3 times/week should be monitored by DOT for the duration of therapy.

†The strongest evidence from clinical trials is the effectiveness of all four drugs administered for the full 6 months. There is weaker evidence that SM can be discontinued after 4 months if the isolate is susceptible to all drugs. The evidence for stopping PZA before the end of 6 months is equivocal for the 3 times/week regimen, and there is no evidence on the effectiveness of this regimen with EMB for less than the full 6 months.

‡DOT — directly observed therapy.

Dosage Recommendation for the Initial Treatment of TB Among Children*

Drugs	Children (daily)	Children (2 times/week)	Children (3 times/week)
Isoniazid	10-20 mg/kg Max 300 mg	20-40 mg/kg Max 900 mg	20-40 mg/kg Max 900 mg
Rifampin	10-20 mg/kg Max 600 mg	10-20 mg/kg Max 600 mg	10-20 mg/kg Max 600 mg
Pyrazinamide	15-30 mg/kg Max 2 g	50-70 mg/kg Max 4 g	50-70 mg/kg Max 3 g
Ethambutol†	15-25 mg/kg Max 2.5 g	50 mg/kg Max 2.5 g	25-30 mg/kg Max 2.5 g
Streptomycin	20-30 mg/kg Max 1 g	25-30 mg/kg Max 1.5 g	25-30 mg/kg Max 1 g

*Children ≤12 years of age.
†Ethambutol is generally not recommended for children whose visual acuity cannot be monitored (<6 years of age). However, ethambutol should be considered for all children with organisms resistant to other drugs, when susceptibility to ethambutol has been demonstrated, or susceptibility is likely.

Dosage Recommendation for the Initial Treatment of TB Among Adults

Drugs	Adults (daily)	Adults (2 times/week)	Adults (3 times/week)
Isoniazid	5 mg/kg Max 300 mg	15 mg/kg Max 900 mg	15 mg/kg Max 900 mg
Rifampin	10 mg/kg Max 600 mg	10 mg/kg Max 600 mg	10 mg/kg Max 600 mg
Pyrazinamide	15-30 mg/kg Max 2 g	50-70 mg/kg Max 4 g	50-70 mg/kg Max 3 g
Ethambutol	5-25 mg/kg Max 2.5 g	50 mg/kg Max 2.5 g	25-30 mg/kg Max 2.5 g
Streptomycin	15 mg/kg Max 1 g	25-30 mg/kg Max 1.5 g	25-30 mg/kg Max 1 g

EVALUATION AND MANAGEMENT OF EARLY HIV INFECTION

ALGORITHM 1.

Selected Elements of the Initial and Ongoing Evaluation of Adults With Early HIV Infection

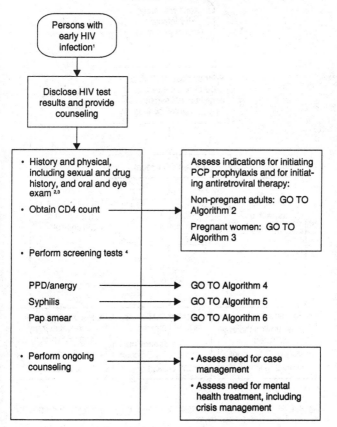

[1]Provider should review and evaluate the adequacy of HIV diagnostic tests.

[2]Appropriate immunizations should be provided (this topic was not reviewed by the HIV panel).

[3]Schedule follow-up appropriate for patient's condition.

[4]Many other screening tests were not reviewed by this panel, including toxoplasmosis, hepatitis serology, and routine laboratory tests.

Note: The algorithm presents recommendations only for the items reviewed by the HIV panel.

From U.S. Department of Health and Human Services, *Evaluation and Management of Early HIV Infection*, Clinical Practice Guideline, Number 7, 1994, 167-76.

ALGORITHM 2.

Evaluation for Initiation of Antiretroviral Therapy and PCP Prophylaxis; Men and Nonpregnant Women With Early HIV Infection

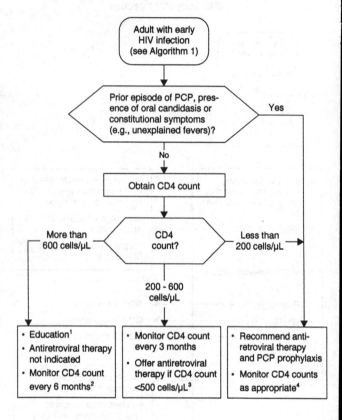

[1]Education should include a discussion of enrollment into relevant investigational drug trials for asymptomatic persons.

[2]If CD4 count has shown great variability or is rapidly declining, repeat the CD4 within 3 months.

[3]If patient develops symptoms, recommend antiretroviral therapy.

[4]If CD4 count <200 cells/μL, continued monitoring of CD4 count may be needed to determine eligibility for clinical trials, and prophylaxis for opportunistic infections other than PCP and to guide antiretroviral therapy.

Note: The algorithm presents recommendations only for the items reviewed by the HIV panel.

From U.S. Department of Health and Human Services, *Evaluation and Management of Early HIV Infection*, Clinical Practice Guideline, Number 7, 1994, 167-76.

ALGORITHM 3.

Evaluation for Initiation of Antiretroviral Therapy and PCP Prophylaxis; Pregnant Women With Early HIV Infection

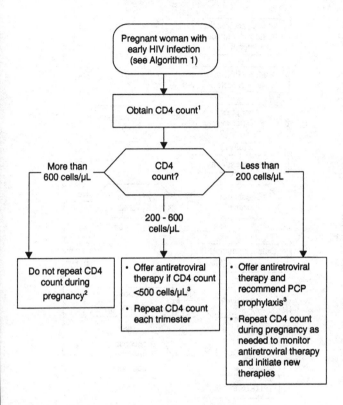

[1]CD4 count should be obtained on presentation for prenatal care; women who have received no prenatal care should have CD4 counts taken at delivery.

[2]Unless indicated by the presence of clinical symptoms.

[3]The possible benefits and risks of antiretroviral therapy to both mother and fetus should be discussed fully with the patient.

Note: The algorithm presents recommendations only for the items reviewed by the HIV panel.

From U.S. Department of Health and Human Services, *Evaluation and Management of Early HIV Infection*, Clinical Practice Guideline, Number 7, 1994, 167-76.

ALGORITHM 4.

Evaluation for *Mycobacterium* Tuberculosis Infection in Adults and Adolescents With Early HIV Infection

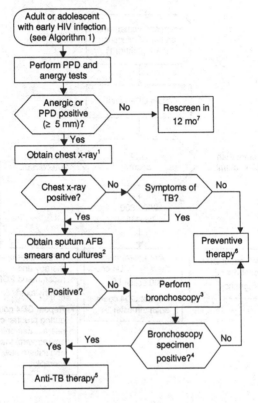

[1] Chest x-ray can be performed, using a lead apron shield, after the first trimester in pregnant women asymptomatic for TB or at any stage of pregnancy in women symptomatic for TB.

[2] At least three sputum smears and cultures should be obtained.

[3] If there is no other etiology for the abnormal chest x-ray.

[4] Both AFB smears and cultures should be obtained at bronchoscopy.

[5] Anti-TB therapy should be guided by local susceptibility patterns and modified appropriately when isolated susceptibilities become available.

[6] Preventive therapy is indicated for PPD-positive patients and should be strongly considered for anergic patients who are known contacts of patients with tuberculosis and for anergic patients belonging to groups in which the prevalence of tuberculosis is at least 10% (eg, injection drug users, prisoners, homeless persons, persons in congregate housing, migrant laborers, and persons born in foreign countries with high rates of TB).

[7] Individuals who reside in settings where TB prevalence is high should be retested in 6 months; individuals who are exposed acutely to others with suspected or confirmed TB should be retested in 3 months; anergic individuals need not be retested, except in special circumstances.

Note: The algorithm presents recommendations only for the items reviewed by the HIV panel.

From U.S. Department of Health and Human Services, *Evaluation and Management of Early HIV Infection*, Clinical Practice Guideline, Number 7, 1994, 167-76.

ALGORITHM 5.

Evaluation for Syphilis in Adults and Sexually Active Adolescents With Early HIV Infection

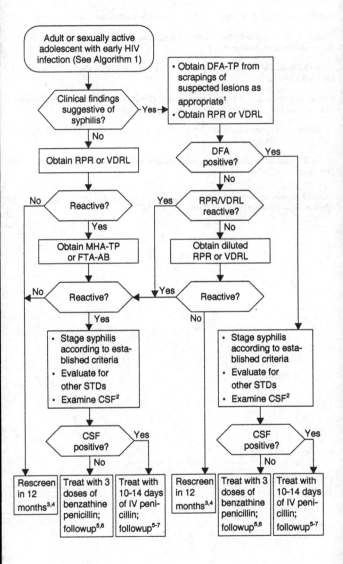

[1]If dark-field exam cannot be performed and primary syphilis is suspected, empiric treatment should be instituted.

[2]Treatment for neurosyphilis recommended if the CSF cannot be evaluated (See *Guideline for Evaluation and Management of Early HIV Infection* for recommended follow-up).

[3]Or after exposure to or diagnosis of any sexually transmitted disease.

[4]Pregnant women should be screened for syphilis at entry to prenatal care, during the third trimester, or at delivery.

[5]See *Guideline for Evaluation and Management of Early HIV Infection* for recommended follow-up.

[6]For issues specific to pregnant women, see *Guideline for Evaluation and Management of Early HIV Infection* for recommended follow-up.

[7]Alternative treatments include 10 days of I.M. procaine penicillin or 10-14 days of 1-2 g of I.M. ceftriaxone.

Note: The algorithm presents recommendations only for the items reviewed by the HIV panel.

From U.S. Department of Health and Human Services, *Evaluation and Management of Early HIV Infection*, Clinical Practice Guideline, Number 7, 1994, 167-76.

ALGORITHM 6.

Pap Smears in Women With Early HIV Infection

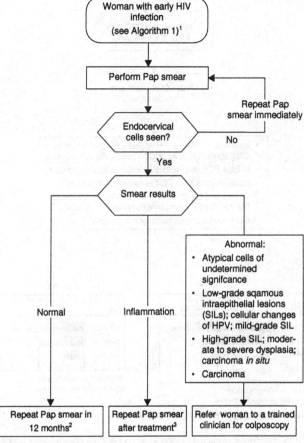

[1]Pap smears should be performed at entry to prenatal care for pregnant women and prior to discharge for women who present for delivery without prenatal care.

[2]HIV-infected women with a history of human papillomavirus (HPV) or with previous Pap smears showing squamous intraepithelial lesions should have their Pap smears repeated every 6 months.

[3]Treatment should be guided by diagnosis of the cause of inflammation.

Note: The algorithm presents recommendations only for the items reviewed by the HIV panel.

From U.S. Department of Health and Human Services, *Evaluation and Management of Early HIV Infection*, Clinical Practice Guideline, Number 7, 1994, 167-76.

ALGORITHM 7.

Evaluation for Initiation of Antiretroviral Therapy and PCP Prophylaxis; Infants and Children With Early HIV Infection

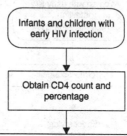

Infants and children with early HIV infection

↓

Obtain CD4 count and percentage

- Initiate antiretroviral therapy as indicated by either CD4 count (Table A) or CD4 percentage (Table B)
- Initiate PCP prophylaxis as indicated by either CD4 count (Figure A) or CD4 percentage (Figure B)[1]
- Infants and children receiving neither antiretroviral therapy nor PCP prophylaxis should have their CD4 counts and percentages monitored[2]

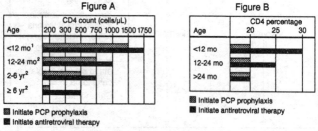

Figure A

Age	CD4 count (cells/μL)
	200 300 500 750 1000 1500 1750
<12 mo[1]	
12-24 mo[2]	
2-6 yr[2]	
≥ 6 yr[2]	

▓ Initiate PCP prophylaxis
■ Initiate antiretroviral therapy

Figure B

Age	CD4 percentage
	20 25 30
<12 mo	
12-24 mo	
>24 mo	

▓ Initiate PCP prophylaxis
■ Initiate antiretroviral therapy

Source: Figure A adapted from Centers for Disease Control, 1991

[1]Patients with prior episode of PCP should receive PCP prophylaxis regardless of CD4 count and percentage.

[2]Obtain CD4 count and percentage at 1 month of age, 3 months of age, and then at 3-month intervals through 24 months of age; thereafter obtain CD4 count and percentage every 6 months, unless values reach an age-related threshold where testing should be repeated monthly.

Note: The algorithm presents recommendations only for the items reviewed by the HIV panel.

From U.S. Department of Health and Human Services, *Evaluation and Management of Early HIV Infection*, Clinical Practice Guideline, Number 7, 1994, 167-76.

ALGORITHM 8.

Neurologic Evaluation of Infants and Children With Early HIV Infection

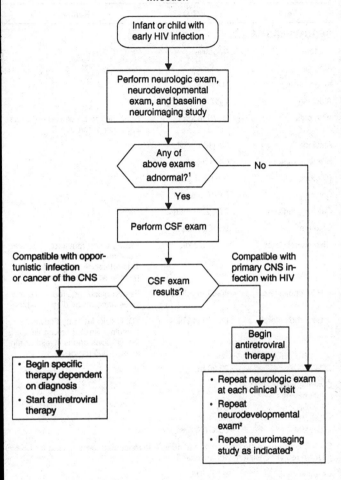

[1] Abnormal exam is defined as focal pathology, obstructive lesion, atypical CNS manifestations, or evidence of progressive neurologic disease (see *Guideline for Evaluation and Management of Early HIV Infection*),

[2] Neurodevelopmental exams should be performed at 3-month intervals up to 24 months of age, then every 6 months thereafter.

[3] Neuroimaging studies should be performed if CNS symptoms occur; such studies should be performed in conjunction with CSF analysis.

Note: The algorithm presents recommendations only for the items reviewed by the HIV panel.

From U.S. Department of Health and Human Services, *Evaluation and Management of Early HIV Infection*, Clinical Practice Guideline, Number 7, 1994, 167-76.

REFERENCE VALUES FOR ADULTS

AUTOMATED CHEMISTRY (CHEMISTRY A)

Test	Values	Remarks
SERUM/PLASMA		
Acetone	Negative	
Albumin	3.2-5 g/dL	
Alcohol, ethyl	Negative	
Aldolase	1.2-7.6 IU/L	
Ammonia	20-70 mcg/dL	Specimen to be placed on ice as soon as collected
Amylase	30-110 units/L	
Bilirubin, direct	0-0.3 mg/dL	
Bilirubin, total	0.1-1.2 mg/dL	
Calcium	8.6-10.3 mg/dL	
Calcium, ionized	2.24-2.46 mEq/L	
Chloride	95-108 mEq/L	
Cholesterol, total	≤220 mg/dL	Fasted blood required — normal value affected by dietary habits This reference range is for a general adult population
HDL cholesterol	40-60 mg/dL	Fasted blood required — normal value affected by dietary habits
LDL cholesterol	65-170 mg/dL	LDLC calculated by Friewald formula... which has certain inaccuracies and is invalid at trig levels >300 mg/dL
CO_2	23-30 mEq/L	
Creatine kinase (CK) isoenzymes		
CK-BB	0%	
CK-MB	0%-3.9%	
CK-MM	96%-100%	

CK-MB levels must be both ≥4% and 10 IU/L to meet diagnostic criteria for CK-MB positive result consistent with myocardial injury.

Test	Values	Remarks
Creatine phosphokinase (CPK)	8-150 IU/L	
Creatinine	0.5-1.4 mg/dL	
Ferritin	13-300 ng/mL	
Folate	3.6-20 ng/dL	
GGT (gamma-glutamyl-transpeptidase)		
male	11-63 IU/L	
female	8-35 IU/L	
GLDH	To be determined	
Glucose (2-h postprandial)	Up to 140 mg/dL	
Glucose, fasting	60-110 mg/dL	
Glucose, nonfasting (2-h postprandial)	60-140 mg/dL	
Hemoglobin A_{1c}	8	

(continued)

Test	Values	Remarks
Hemoglobin, plasma free	<2.5 mg/100 mL	
Hemoglobin, total glycosylated (HbA$_1$)	4%-8%	
Iron	65-150 mcg/dL	
Iron binding capacity, total (TIBC)	250-420 mcg/dL	
Lactic acid	0.7-2.1 mEq/L	Specimen to be kept on ice and sent to lab as soon as possible
Lactate dehydrogenase (LDH)	56-194 IU/L	
Lactate dehydrogenase (LDH) isoenzymes		
LD$_1$	20%-34%	
LD$_2$	29%-41%	
LD$_3$	15%-25%	
LD$_4$	1%-12%	
LD$_5$	1%-15%	

Flipped LD$_1$/LD$_2$ ratios (>1 may be consistent with myocardial injury) particularly when considered in combination with a recent CK-MB positive result.

Test	Values	Remarks
Lipase	23-208 units/L	
Magnesium	1.6-2.5 mg/dL	Increased by slight hemolysis
Osmolality	289-308 mOsm/kg	
Phosphatase, alkaline		
adults 25-60 y	33-131 IU/L	
adults 61 y or older	51-153 IU/L	
infancy - adolescence	Values range up to 3-5 times higher than adults	
Phosphate, inorganic	2.8-4.2 mg/dL	
Potassium	3.5-5.2 mEq/L	Increased by slight hemolysis
Prealbumin	>15 mg/dL	
Protein, total	6.5-7.9 g/dL	
SGOT (AST)	<35 IU/L	
SGPT (ALT)	<35 IU/L	
Sodium	134-149 mEq/L	
Transferrin	>200 mg/dL	
Triglycerides	45-155 mg/dL	Fasted blood required
Urea nitrogen (BUN)	7-20 mg/dL	
Uric acid		
male	2.0-8.0 mg/dL	
female	2.0-7.5 mg/dL	

CEREBROSPINAL FLUID

Test	Values	Remarks
Glucose	50-70 mg/dL	
Protein		
adults and children	15-45 mg/dL	CSF obtained by lumbar puncture
newborn infants	60-90 mg/dL	

On CSF obtained by cisternal puncture: about 25 mg/dL.
On CSF obtained by ventricular puncture: about 10 mg/dL.
Note: Bloody specimen gives erroneously high value due to contamination with blood proteins.

Test	Values	Remarks

URINE
(24-hour specimen is required for all these tests unless specified)

Test	Values	Remarks
Amylase	32-641 units/L	The value is in units/L and **not** calculated for total volume
Amylase, fluid (random samples)		Interpretation of value left for physician, depends on the nature of fluid
Calcium	Depends upon dietary intake	
Creatine male female	 150 mg/24 h 250 mg/24 h	 Higher value on children and during pregnancy
Creatinine	1000-2000 mg/24 h	
Creatinine clearance (endogenous) male female	 85-125 mL/min 75-115 mL/min	 A blood sample must accompany urine specimen
Glucose	1 g/24 h	
5-Hydroxyindoleacetic acid	2-8 mg/24 h	
Iron	0.15 mg/24 h	Acid washed container required
Magnesium	146-209 mg/24 h	___ do ___
Osmolality	500-800 mOsm/kg	With normal fluid intake
Oxalate	10-40 mg/24 h	
Phosphate	400-1300 mg/24 h	
Potassium	25-120 mEq/24 h	Varies with diet; the interpretation of urine electrolytes and osmolality should be left for the physician
Sodium	40-220 mEq/24 h	
Porphobilinogen, qualitative	Negative	
Porphyrins, qualitative	Negative	
Proteins	0.05-0.1 g/24 h	
Salicylate	Negative	
Urea clearance	60-95 mL/min	A blood sample must accompany specimen
Urea-N	10-40 g/24 h	Dependent on protein intake
Uric acid	250-750 mg/24 h	Dependent on diet and therapy
Urobilinogen	0.5-3.5 mg/24 h	For qualitative determination on random urine, send sample to urinalysis section in Hematology Lab
Xylose absorption test children adults	 16%-33% of ingested xylose >4 g in 5 h	

FECES

Test	Values	Remarks
Fat, 3-day collection	<5 g/d	Value depends on fat intake of 100 g/d for 3 days preceding and during collection

(continued)

Test	Values	Remarks

GASTRIC ACIDITY

Acidity, total, 12 h   10-60 mEq/L   Titrated at pH 7

BLOOD GASES

	Arterial	Capillary	Venous
pH	7.35-7.45	7.35-7.45	7.32-7.42
pCO_2 (mm Hg)	35-45	35-45	38-52
pO_2 (mm Hg)	70-100	60-80	24-48
HCO_3 (mEq/L)	19-25	19-25	19-25
TCO_2 (mEq/L)	19-29	19-29	23-33
O_2 saturation (%)	90-95	90-95	40-70
Base excess (mEq/L)	-5 to +5	-5 to +5	-5 to +5

HEMATOLOGY

Complete Blood Count

	Hgb (g/dL)	Hct (%)	MCV (fL)	MCH (pg)	MCHC (%)	RBC (x 10⁶/mm³)	RDW	PLTS (x 10³/mm³)
0-3 d	15-20	45-61	95-115	31-37	29-37	4-5.9	<18	250-450
1-2 wk	12.5-18.5	39-57	86-110	28-36	28-38	3.6-5.5	<17	250-450
1-6 mo	10-13	29-42	74-96	25-35	30-36	3.1-4.3	<16.5	300-700
7 mo - 2 y	10.5-13	33-38	70-84	23-30	31-37	3.7-4.9	<16	250-600
2-5 y	11.5-13	34-39	75-87	24-30	31-37	3.9-5	<15	250-550
5-8 y	11.5-14.5	35-42	77-95	25-33	31-37	4-4.9	<15	250-550
13-18 y	12-15.2	36-47	78-96	25-35	31-37	4.5-5.1	<14.5	150-450
Adult male	13.5-16.5*	41-50*	80-100	26-34	31-37	4.5-5.5	<14.5	150-450
Adult female	12-15*	36-44*	80-100	26-34	31-37	4-4.9	<14.5	150-450

WBC and Diff

	WBC (x 10³/mm³)	Segmented Neutrophils	Band Neutrophils	Eosinophils	Basophils	Lymphocytes	Atypical Lymphs	Monocytes	# of NRBCs
0-3 d	9-35	32-62	10-18	0-2	0-1	19-29	0-8	5-7	0-2
1-2 wk	5-20	14-34	6-14	0-2	0-1	36-45	0-8	6-10	0
1-6 mo	6-17.5	13-33	4-12	0-3	0-1	41-71	0-8	4-7	0
7 mo - 2 y	6-17	15-35	5-11	0-3	0-1	45-76	0-8	3-6	0
2-5 y	5.5-15.5	23-45	5-11	0-3	0-1	35-65	0-8	3-6	0
5-8 y	5-14.5	32-54	5-11	0-3	0-1	28-48	0-8	3-6	0
13-18 y	4.5-13	34-64	5-11	0-3	0-1	25-45	0-8	3-6	0
Adult	4.5-11	35-66	5-11	0-3	0-1	24-44	0-8	3-6	0

Sedimentation rate, Westergren
Children 0-20 mm/hour
Adult male 0-15 mm/hour
Adult female 0-20 mm/hour

Sedimentation rate, Wintrobe
Children 0-13 mm/hour
Adult male 0-10 mm/hour
Adult female 0-15 mm/hour

Reticulocyte count
Newborn 2%-6%
1-6 months 0%-2.8%
Adult 0.5%-1.5%

REFERENCE VALUES FOR CHILDREN

CHEMISTRY

Albumin	0-1 y	2-4 g/dL
	1 y - adult	3.5-5.5 g/dL
Ammonia	newborn	90-150 μg/dL
	child	40-120 μg/dL
	adult	18-54 μg/dL
Amylase	newborn	0-60 units/L
	adult	30-110 units/L
Bilirubin, conjugated, direct	newborn	<1.5 mg/dL
	1 mo - adult	0-0.5 mg/dL
Bilirubin, total	0-3 d	2-10 mg/dL
	1 mo - adult	0-1.5 mg/dL
Bilirubin, unconjugated, indirect		0.6-10.5 mg/dL
Calcium	newborn	7-12 mg/dL
	0-2 y	8.8-11.2 mg/dL
	2 y - adult	9-11 mg/dL
Calcium, ionized, whole blood		4.4-5.4 mg/dL
Carbon dioxide, total		23-33 mEq/L
Chloride		95-105 mEq/L
Cholesterol	newborn	45-170 mg/dL
	0-1 y	65-175 mg/dL
	1-20 y	120-230 mg/dL
Creatinine	0-1 y	≤0.6 mg/dL
	1 y - adult	0.5-1.5 mg/dL
Glucose	newborn	30-90 mg/dL
	0-2 y	60-105 mg/dL
	child - adult	70-110 mg/dL
Iron	newborn	110-270 μg/dL
	infant	30-70 μg/dL
	child	55-120 μg/dL
	adult	70-180 μg/dL
Iron binding	newborn	59-175 μg/dL
	infant	100-400 μg/dL
	adult	250-400 μg/dL
Lactic acid, lactate		2-20 mg/dL
Lead, whole blood		<30 μg/dL
Lipase	child	20-140 units/L
	adult	0-190 units/L
Magnesium		1.5-2.5 mEq/L
Osmolality, serum		275-296 mOsm/kg
Osmolality, urine		50-1400 mOsm/kg
Phosphorus	newborn	4.2-9 mg/dL
	6 wk - 19 mo	3.8-6.7 mg/dL
	18 mo - 3 y	2.9-5.9 mg/dL
	3-15 y	3.6-5.6 mg/dL
	>15 y	2.5-5 mg/dL
Potassium, plasma	newborn	4.5-7.2 mEq/L
	2 d - 3 mo	4-6.2 mEq/L
	3 mo - 1 y	3.7-5.6 mEq/L
	1-16 y	3.5-5 mEq/L

Chemistry *(continued)*

Protein, total	0-2 y	4.2-7.4 g/dL
	>2 y	6-8 g/dL
Sodium		136-145 mEq/L
Triglycerides	infant	0-171 mg/dL
	child	20-130 mg/dL
	adult	30-200 mg/dL
Urea nitrogen, blood	0-2 y	4-15 mg/dL
	2 y - adult	5-20 mg/dL
Uric acid	male	3-7 mg/dL
	female	2-6 mg/dL

ENZYMES

Alanine aminotransferase (ALT) (SGPT)	0-2 mo	8-78 units/L
	>2 mo	8-36 units/L
Alkaline phosphatase (ALKP)	newborn	60-130 units/L
	0-16 y	85-400 units/L
	>16 y	30-115 units/L
Aspartate aminotransferase (AST) (SGOT)	infant	18-74 units/L
	child	15-46 units/L
	adult	5-35 units/L
Creatine kinase (CK)	infant	20-200 units/L
	child	10-90 units/L
	adult male	0-206 units/L
	adult female	0-175 units/L
Lactate dehydrogenase (LDH)	newborn	290-501 units/L
	1 mo - 2 y	110-144 units/L
	>16 y	60-170 units/L

BLOOD GASES

	Arterial	Capillary	Venous
pH	7.35-7.45	7.35-7.45	7.32-7.42
pCO_2 (mm Hg)	35-45	35-45	38-52
pO_2 (mm Hg)	70-100	60-80	24-48
HCO_3 (mEq/L)	19-25	19-25	19-25
TCO_2 (mEq/L)	19-29	19-29	23-33
O_2 saturation (%)	90-95	90-95	40-70
Base excess (mEq/L)	-5 to +5	-5 to +5	-5 to +5

THYROID FUNCTION TESTS

T_4 (thyroxine)	1-7 d	10.1-20.9 µg/dL
	8-14 d	9.8-16.6 µg/dL
	1 mo - 1 y	5.5-16 µg/dL
	>1 y	4-12 µg/dL
FTI	1-3 d	9.3-26.6
	1-4 wk	7.6-20.8
	1-4 mo	7.4-17.9
	4-12 mo	5.1-14.5
	1-6 y	5.7-13.3
	>6 y	4.8-14
T_3 by RIA	newborns	100-470 ng/dL
	1-5 y	100-260 ng/dL
	5-10 y	90-240 ng/dL
	10 y - adult	70-210 ng/dL
T_3 uptake		35%-45%
TSH	cord	3-22 µU/mL
	1-3 d	<40 µU/mL
	3-7 d	<25 µU/mL
	>7 d	0-10 µU/mL

MEDIAN HEIGHTS AND WEIGHTS AND RECOMMENDED ENERGY INTAKE*

Age (y) or Condition	Weight (kg)	Weight (lb)	Height (cm)	Height (in)	REE† (kcal/d)	Average Energy Allowance (kcal)‡ Multiples of REE	/kg	/d§
Infants								
0-0.5	6	13	60	24	320		108	650
0.5-1	9	20	71	28	500		98	850
Children								
1-3	13	29	90	35	740		102	1,300
4-6	20	44	112	44	950		90	1,800
7-10	28	62	132	52	1130		70	2000
Male								
11-14	45	99	157	62	1440	1.70	55	2500
15-18	66	145	176	69	1760	1.67	45	3000
19-24	72	160	177	70	1780	1.67	40	2900
25-50	79	174	176	70	1800	1.60	37	2900
51+	77	170	173	68	1530	1.50	30	2300
Female								
11-14	46	101	157	62	1310	1.67	47	2200
15-18	55	120	163	64	1370	1.60	40	2200
19-24	58	128	164	65	1350	1.60	38	2200
25-50	63	138	163	64	1380	1.55	36	2200
51+	65	143	160	63	1280	1.50	30	1900
Pregnant								
1st trimester								+0
2nd trimester								+300
3rd trimester								+300
Lactating								
1st 6 months								+500
2nd 6 months								+500

*From *Recommended Dietary Allowances*, 10th ed, Washington, DC: National Academy Press, 1989.

†Calculation based on FAO equations, then rounded.

‡In the range of light to moderate activity, the coefficient of variation is ±20%.

§Figure is rounded.

CALCULATIONS FOR TOTAL PARENTERAL NUTRITION THERAPY — ADULT PATIENTS

Condition	Calorie Requirement (kcal/kg/d)	Protein Requirement (g/kg/d)
Resting state (adult medical patient)	20-30	0.8-1
Uncomplicated postop patients	25-35	1-1.3
Depleted patients	30-40	1.3-1.7
Hypermetabolic patients (trauma, sepsis, burn)	35-45	1.5-2

1 g protein yields 4 kcal/g
1 g fat yields 9 kcal/g
1 g dextrose yields 3.4 kcal/g
1 g nitrogen = 6.25 g protein

Electrolytes Required/Day

	mEq/d
Sodium	60-120
Potassium	60-120
Chloride	100-150
Magnesium	10-24
Calcium	10-20
Phosphate	20-50 mmol/d
Sulfate	10-24
Acetate	60-150
Bicarbonate	Should not be added

Estimated Energy Requirements

Basal Energy Expenditure (BEE)	
Harris-Benedict equation males	$BEE_{mal} = 66.67 + (13.75 \times kg) + (5 \times cm) - (6.76 \times y)$
Harris-Benedict equation females	$BEE_{fem} = 665.1 + (9.56 \times kg) + (1.85 \times cm) - (4.68 \times y)$
Total daily energy expenditure (TDE)	**TDE = (BEE) [(activity factor) + (injury factor)]**
Activity factor	Confined to bed = 1.2 Out of bed = 1.3

Injury factory	Surgery:
	  Minor operations = 1-1.1
	  Major operations = 1.1-1.2

	Infection
	  Mild = 1-1.2
	  Moderate = 1.2-1.4
	  Severe = 1.4-1.6

	Skeletal trauma = 1.2-1.35
	Head injury (treated with corticosteroids) = 1.6
	Blunt trauma = 1.15-1.35

	Burns
	  ≤20% body surface area (BSA) = 2
	  20%-30% BSA = 2-2.2
	  >30% BSA = 2.2

Estimated Fluid Requirements

30-35 mL/kg/d
or
mL/d = 1500 mL for first 20 kg of body weight + 20 mL/kg for body weight >20 kg

SKIN TESTING FOR
DELAYED HYPERSENSITIVITY

Delayed cutaneous hypersensitivity (DCH) is a cell-mediated immunological response which has been used diagnostically to assess previous infection (eg, purified protein derivative (PPD), histoplasmin, and coccidioidin) or as an indicator of the status of the immune system by using mumps, *Candida*, tetanus toxoid, or trichophyton to test for anergy. Anergy is a defect in cell-mediated immunity that is characterized by an impaired response, or lack of a response to DCH testing with injected antigens. Anergy has been associated with several disease states, malnutrition, and immuno-suppressive therapy, and has been correlated with increased risk of infection, mor-bidity, and mortality.

Many of the skin test antigens have not been approved by the FDA as tests for anergy, and so the directions for use and interpretation of reactions to these products may differ from that of the product labeling. There is also disagreement in the published literature as to the selection and interpretation of these tests for anergy assessment, leading to different recommendations for use of these products.

General Guidelines

Read these guidelines before using any skin test.

Administration

1. Use a separate sterile TB syringe for each antigen. Immediately after the antigen is drawn up, make the injection intradermally in the flexor surface of the forearm.
2. A small bleb 6-10 mm in diameter will form if the injection is made at the correct depth. If a bleb does not form or if the antigen solution leaks from the site, the injection must be repeated.
3. When applying more than one skin test, make the injections at least 5 cm apart.
4. Do any serologic blood tests before testing or wait 48-96 hours.

Reading

1. Read all tests at 24, 48, and 72 hours. Reactions occurring before 24 hours are indicative of an immediate rather than a delayed hypersensitivity.
2. Measure the diameter of the induration in two directions (at right angles) with a ruler and record each diameter in millimeters. Ballpoint pen method of measurement is the most accurate.
3. Test results should be recorded and should include the millimeters of induration present, and a picture of the arm showing the location of the test(s).

Factors Causing False-Negative Reactions

1. Improper administration, interpretation, or use of outdated antigen
2. Test is applied too soon after exposure to the antigen (DCH takes 2-20 weeks to develop.)
3. Concurrent viral illnesses (eg, rubeola, influenza, mumps, and probably others) or recent administration of live attenuated virus vaccines (eg, measles)
4. Anergy may be associated with:
    a. Immune suppressing chronic illnesses such as diabetes, uremia, sarcoidosis, metastatic carcinomas, Hodgkin's, acute lymphocytic leukemia, hypothyroidism, chronic hepatitis, and cirrhosis.
    b. Some antineoplastic agents, radiation therapy, and corticosteroids. If possible, discontinue steroids at least 48 hours prior to DCH skin testing.
    c. Congenital immune deficiencies.
    d. Malnutrition, shock, severe burns, and trauma.
    e. Severe disseminated infections (miliary or cavitary TB, cocci granu-loma, and other disseminated mycotic infections, gram-negative bacillary septicemia).
    f. Leukocytosis (>15,000 cells/mm^3).

Factors Causing False-Positive Reactions

1. Improper interpretation
2. Patient sensitivity to minor ingredients in the antigen solutions such as the phenol or thimerosal preservatives
3. Cross-reactions between similar antigens

Dosage as Part of Disease Diagnosis

Tuberculin Testing

Purified Protein Derivative (PPD)

Preparation	Dilution	Units/0.1 mL
First strength	1:10,000	1
Intermediate strength	1:2000	5
Second strength	1:100	250

The usual initial dose is 0.1 mL of the intermediate strength. The first strength should be used in the individuals suspected of being highly sensitive. The second strength is used only for individuals who fail to respond to a previous injection of the first or intermediate strengths.

A positive reaction is 10 mm induration or greater except in HIV-infected individuals where a positive reaction is 5 mm or greater of induration.

Adverse Reactions

In patients who are highly sensitive, or when higher than recommended doses are used, exaggerated local reactions may occur, including erythema, pain, blisters, necrosis, and scarring. Although systemic reactions are rare, a few cases of lymph node enlargement, fever, malaise, and fatigue have been reported.

To prevent severe local reactions, never use second test strengths as the initial agent. Use diluted first strengths in patients with known or suspected hypersensitivity to the antigen.

Have epinephrine and antihistamines on hand to treat severe allergic reactions that may occur.

Treatment of Adverse Reactions

Severe reactions to intradermal skin tests are rare and treatment consists of symptomatic care.

Skin Testing

All skin tests are given intradermally into the flexor surface of one arm.

Purified protein derivative (PPD) is used most often in the diagnosis of tuberculosis. *Candida, Trichophyton*, and mumps skin tests are used most often as controls for anergy.

Dose: The usual skin test dose is as follows:

Antigen		Standard Dose	Concentration
PPD	1 TU	0.1 mL	1 TU — highly sensitive patients
	5 TU	0.1 mL	5 TU — standard dose
	250 TU	0.1 mL	250 TU — anergic patients in whom TB is suspected
Candida		0.02 mL	
Histoplasmin		0.1 mL	Seldom used. Serology is preferred method to diagnose histoplasmosis.
Mumps		0.1 mL	
Trichophyton		0.02 mL	

Interpretation:

Skin Test	Reading Time	Positive Reaction
PPD	48-72 h	**≥5 mm considered positive for:** • close contacts to an infectious case • persons with abnormal chest x-ray indicating old healed TB • persons with known or suspected HIV infection **≥10 mm considered positive for:** • other medical risk factors • foreign born from high prevalence areas • medically underserved, low income populations • alcoholics and intravenous drug users • residents of long-term care facilities (including correctional facilities and nursing homes) • staff in settings where disease would pose a hazard to large number of susceptible persons **≥15 mm considered positive for:** • persons without risk factors for TB
Candida	24-72 h	5 mm induration or greater
Histoplasmin	24-72 h	5 mm or greater
Mumps	24-36 h	5 mm or greater
Trichophyton	24-72 h	5 mm induration or greater

Recommended Interpretation of Skin Test Reactions

Reaction	Local Reaction	
	After Intradermal Injections of Antigens	After Dinitrochlorobenzene
1+	Erythema >10 mm and/or induration >1-5 mm	Erythema and/or induration covering <½ area of dose site
2+	Induration 6-10 mm	Induration covering >½ area of dose site
3+	Induration 11-20 mm	Vesiculation and induration at dose site or spontaneous flare at days 7-14 at the site
4+	Induration >20 mm	Bulla or ulceration at dose site or spontaneous flare at days 7-14 at the site

PENICILLIN ALLERGY SKIN TESTING

The recommended battery of major and minor determinants used in penicillin skin testing will disclose those individuals with circulating IgE antibodies. This procedure is therefore useful to identify patients at risk for immediate or accelerated reactions. Skin tests are of no value in predicting the occurrence of non-IgE-mediated hypersensitivity reactions to penicillin such as delayed exanthem, drug fever, hemolytic anemia, interstitial nephritis, or exfoliative dermatitis. Based on large scale trials, skin testing solutions have been standardized.

Antihistamines, tricyclic antidepressants, and adrenergic drugs, all of which may inhibit skin test results, should be discontinued at least 24 hours prior to skin testing. Antihistamines with long half-lives (hydroxyzine, terfenadine, astemizole, etc) may attenuate skin test results up to a week, or longer after discontinuation.

When properly performed with due consideration for preliminary scratch tests and appropriate dilutions, skin testing with penicillin reagents can almost always be safely accomplished. Systemic reactions accompany about 1% of positive skin tests; these are usually mild but can be serious. **Therefore skin tests should be done in the presence of a physician and with immediate access to medications and equipment needed to treat anaphylaxis**.

History of Penicillin Allergy

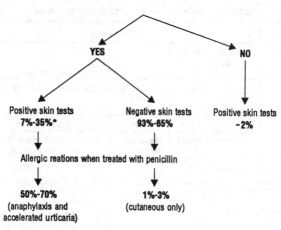

*One study found 65% positive

Prevalence of positive and negative skin tests and subsequent allergic reactions in patients treated with penicillin (based on studies using both penicilloyl-polylysine and minor determinant mixture as skin test reagents).

Penicillin Skin Testing Protocol

Skin tests evaluate the patient for the presence of penicillin IgE — sensitive mast cells which are responsible for anaphylaxis and other immediate hypersensitivity reactions. Local or systemic allergic reactions rarely occur due to skin testing, therefore, a tourniquet, I.V., and epinephrine should be at the bedside. The breakdown products of penicillin provide the antigen which is responsible for the allergy. Testing is performed with benzylpenicilloyl-polylysine (Pre-Pen®), the major determinant, penicillin G which provides the minor determinants and the actual penicillin which will be administered.

Controls are important if the patient is extremely ill or is taking antihistamines, codeine, or morphine. Normal saline is the negative control. Morphine sulfate, a mast cell degranulator, can be used as a positive control, if the patient is not on morphine or codeine. Histamine is the preferred positive control, however, is not manufactured in a pharmaceutical formulation anymore. A false-positive or false-negative will make further skin testing invalid.

Control Solutions

Normal saline = negative control
Morphine sulfate (10 mg/100 mL 0.9% NaCl, 0.1 mg/mL) = positive control

Test Solutions

Order the necessary solutions as 0.5 mL in a tuberculin syringe. **Note:** May need to order 2 syringes of each — one for scratch testing and one for intradermal skin testing.

I. **Pre-Pen®: Benzylpenicilloyl-polylysine (0.25 mL ampul) = MAJOR DETERMINANT**

    A. Undiluted Pre-Pen®
    B. 1:100 concentration
        To make: Dilute 0.1 mL of Pre-Pen® in 10 mL of 0.9% NaCl
    C. 1:10,000 concentration
        (Only necessary in patients with a history of anaphylaxis)
        To make: Dilute 1 mL of the 1:100 solution in 100 mL of 0.9% NaCl

II. **Penicillin G sodium/potassium = MINOR DETERMINANT**

    D. 5000 units/mL concentration
    E. 5 units/mL concentration
        (Only necessary in patients with a history of anaphylaxis)
        To make: Dilute 0.1 mL of a 5000 units/mL solution in 100 mL of 0.9% NaCl

III. **Penicillin product to be administered — if not penicillin G**

    F. **Ampicillin** 2.5 mg/mL concentration
        To make: Dilute 250 mg in 100 mL of 0.9% NaCl
    F. **Nafcillin** 2.5 mg/mL concentration
        To make: Dilute 250 mg in 100 mL of 0.9% NaCl

Order for placement/availability at the bedside in the event of a hypersensitivity reaction during scratch/skin testing and desensitization:

Hydrocortisone: 100 mg IVP
Diphenhydramine: 50 mg IVP
Epinephrine: 1:1000 S.C.

Scratch/Skin Testing Protocol: Must Be Done by Physician!

1. Begin with the control solutions (ie, normal saline and morphine).

2. Administer **scratch tests** in the following order (beginning with the most dilute solution):

Pre-Pen®	Syringes: C,B,A
Penicillin G	Syringes: E,D
Ampicillin/Nafcillin	Syringe: F

The inner volar surface of the forearm is usually used.

A nonbleeding scratch of 3-5 mm in length is made in the epidermis with a 20-gauge needle.

If bleeding occurs, another site should be selected and another scratch made using less pressure.

A small drop of the test solution is then applied and rubbed gently into the scratch using an applicator, toothpick, or the side of the needle.

The scratch test site should be observed for the appearance of a wheal, erythema, and pruritis.

A positive reaction is signified by the appearance within 15 minutes of a pale wheal (usually with pseudopods) ranging from 5-15 mm or more in diameter.

As soon as a positive response is elicited, or 15 minutes has elapsed, the solution should be wiped off the scratch.

If the scratch test is negative or equivocal (ie, a wheal of <5 mm in diameter with little or no erythema or itching appears), an intradermal test may be performed.

If significant reaction, treat and proceed to desensitization.

3. Administer **intradermal tests** in the following order (beginning with the most dilute solution):

Pre-Pen®	Syringes: C,B,A
Penicillin G	Syringes: E,D
Ampicillin/Nafcillin	Syringe: F

Intradermal tests are usually performed on a sterilized area of the upper outer arm at a sufficient distance below the deltoid muscle to permit proximal application of a tourniquet if a severe reaction occurs.

Using a tuberculin syringe with a 3/8-5/8 inch 26- to 30-gauge needle, an amount of each tet solution sufficient to raise the smallest perceptible bleb (usually 0.01-0.02 mL) is injected immediately under the surface of the skin.

A separate needle and syringe must be used for each solution.

Each test and control site should be at least 15 cm apart.

Positive reactions are manifested as a wheal at the test site with a diameter at least 5 mm larger than the saline control, often accompanied by itching and a marked increase in the size of the bleb.

Skin responses to penicillin testing will develop within 15 minutes.

If no significant reaction, may challenge patient with reduced dosage of the penicillin to be administered.

Physician should be at the bedside during this challenge dose!

If significant reaction, treat and begin desensitization.

PENICILLIN DESENSITIZATION

Acute penicillin desensitization should only be performed in an intensive care setting. Any remedial risk factor should be corrected. All β-adrenergic antagonists such as propranolol or even timolol ophthalmic drops should be discontinued. Asthmatic patients should be under optimal control. An intravenous line should be established, baseline electrocardiogram (EKG) and spirometry should be performed, and continuous EKG monitoring should be instituted. Premedication with antihistamines or steroids is not recommended, as these drugs have not proven effective in suppressing severe reactions but may mask early signs of reactivity that would otherwise result in a modification of the protocol.

Protocols have been developed for penicillin desensitization using both the oral and parenteral route. As of 1987 there were 93 reported cases of oral desensitization, 74 of which were done by Sullivan and his collaborators. Of these 74 patients, 32% experienced a transient allergic reaction either during desensitization (one-third) or during penicillin treatment after desensitization (two-thirds). These reactions were usually mild and self-limited in nature. Only one IgE-mediated reaction (wheezing and bronchospasm) required discontinuation of the procedure before desensitization could be completed. It has been argued that oral desensitization may be safer than parenteral desensitization, but most patients can also be safely desensitized by parenteral route.

During desensitization any dose that causes mild systemic reactions such as pruritus, fleeting urticaria, rhinitis, or mild wheezing should be repeated until the patient tolerates the dose without systemic symptoms or signs. More serious reactions such as hypotension, laryngeal edema, or asthma require appropriate treatment, and if desensitization is continued, the dose should be decreased by at least 10-fold and withheld until the patient is stable.

Once desensitized, the patient's treatment with penicillin must not lapse or the risk of an allergic reaction increases. If the patient requires a β-lactam antibiotic in the future and still remains skin test-positive to penicillin reagents, desensitization would be required again.

Several patients have been maintained on long-term, low-dose penicillin therapy (usually bid-tid) to sustain a chronic state of desensitization. Such individuals usually require chronic desensitization because of continuous occupationally related exposure to β-lactam drugs.

Reference

Stark DJ, Earl HS, Gross GN, et al, "Acute & Chronic Desensitization of Penicillin Allergic Patients Using Oral Penicillin," *J of Allergy & Clin Immunol*, 1987, 79:523-43.

Desensitization Protocol: Must Be Done by Physician!

Order for placement/availability at the bedside in the event of a hyper-sensitivity reaction during scratch/skin testing and desensitization:

Hydrocortisone: 100 mg IVP
Diphenhydramine: 50 mg IVP
Epinephrine: 1:1000 S.C.

Several investigators have demonstrated that penicillin can be administered to history positive, skin test positive patients if initially small but gradually increasing doses are given. However, patients with a history of exfoliative dermatitis secondary to penicillin should not be re-exposed to the drug, even by desensitization.

Desensitization is a potentially dangerous procedure and should be only performed in an area where immediate access to emergency drugs and equipment can be assured.

Begin between 8-10 AM in the morning.

Follow desensitization as indicated for penicillin G or ampicillin.

Ampicillin Oral Desensitization Protocol

1. Begin 0.03 mg of ampicillin.
2. Double the dose administered every 30 minutes until complete.
3. Example of oral dosing regimen:

Dose #	Ampicillin (mg)
1	0.03
2	0.06
3	0.12
4	0.23
5	0.47
6	0.94
7	1.87
8	3.75
9	7.5
10	15
11	30
12	60
13	125
14	250
15	500

Penicillin G Parenteral Desensitization Protocol: Typical Schedule

Injection No.	Benzylpenicillin Concentration (units/mL)	Volume and Route (mL)*
1†	100	0.1 I.D.
2	↓	0.2 S.C.
3		0.4 S.C.
4		0.8 S.C.
5†	1,000	0.1 I.D.
6	↓	0.3 S.C.
7		0.6 S.C.
8†	10,000	0.1 I.D.
9	↓	0.2 S.C.
10		0.4 S.C.
11		0.8 S.C.
12†	100,000	0.1 I.D.
13	↓	0.3 S.C.
14		0.6 S.C.
15†	1,000,000	0.1 I.D.
16	↓	0.2 S.C.
17		0.2 I.M.
18		0.4 I.M.
19	Continuous I.V. infusion (1,000,000 units/h)	

*Administer progressive doses at intervals of not less than 20 minutes.
†Observe and record skin wheal and flare response to intradermal dose.
Abbreviations: I.D. = intradermal, S.C. = subcutaneous, I.M. = intramuscular, I.V. = intravenous.

Penicillin Oral Desensitization Protocol

Step*	Phenoxymethyl Penicillin (units/mL)	Amount (mL)	Dose (units)	Cumulative Dosage (units)
1	1000	0.1	100	100
2	1000	0.2	200	300
3	1000	0.4	400	700
4	1000	0.8	800	1500
5	1000	1.6	1600	3100
6	1000	3.2	3200	6300
7	1000	6.4	6400	12,700
8	10,000	1.2	12,000	24,700
9	10,000	2.4	24,000	48,700
10	10,000	4.8	48,000	96,700
11	80,000	1	80,000	176,700
12	80,000	2	160,000	336,700
13	80,000	4	320,000	656,700
14	80,000	8	640,000	1,296,700

Observe patient for 30 minutes

Change to benzylpenicillin G I.V.

15	500,000	0.25	125,000	
16	500,000	0.50	250,000	
17	500,000	1	500,000	
18	500,000	2.25	1,125,000	

*Interval between steps, 15 min.

PEDIATRIC ALS ALGORITHM
BRADYCARDIA

Fig. 1: Pediatric bradycardia decision tree. ABCs indicates airway, breathing, and circulation; ALS, advanced life support; E.T., endotracheal; I.O., intraosseous; and I.V., intravenous.

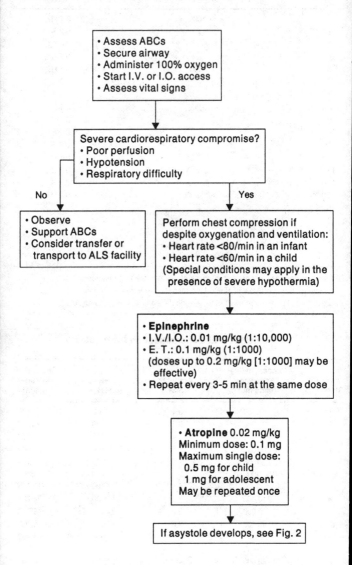

Used with permission: Emergency Cardiac Care Committee and Subcommittees, American Heart Association, "Guidelines for Cardiopulmonary Resuscitation and Emergency Care, IV: Pediatric Advanced Life Support," *JAMA*, 1992: 268:2262-75.

PEDIATRIC ALS ALGORITHM
ASYSTOLE AND PULSELESS ARREST

Fig. 2: Pediatric asystole and pulseless arrest decision tree. CPR indicates cardiopulmonary resuscitation; E.T., endotracheal; I.O., intraosseous; and I.V., intravenous.

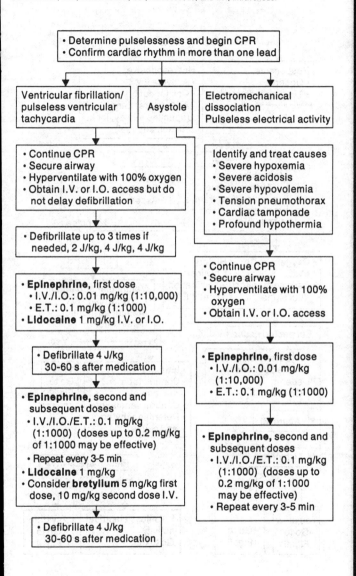

Used with permission: Emergency Cardiac Care Committee and Subcommittees, American Heart Association, "Guidelines for Cardiopulmonary Resuscitation and Emergency Care, IV: Pediatric Advanced Life Support," *JAMA*, 1992: 268:2262-75.

ADULT ACLS ALGORITHM
EMERGENCY CARDIAC CARE

Fig. 1: Universal algorithm for adult emergency cardiac care (ECC)

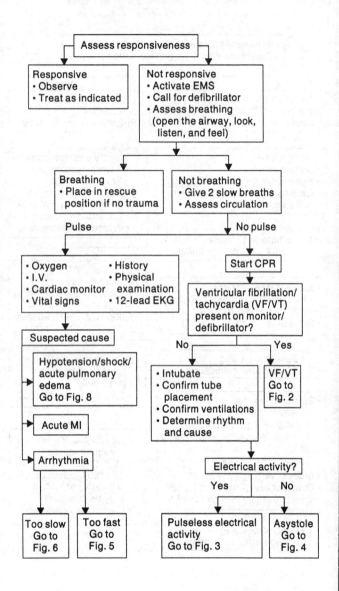

ADULT ACLS ALGORITHM
V. FIB AND PULSELESS V. TACH

Fig. 2: Adult algorithm for ventricular fibrillation and pulseless ventricular tachycardia (VF/VT)

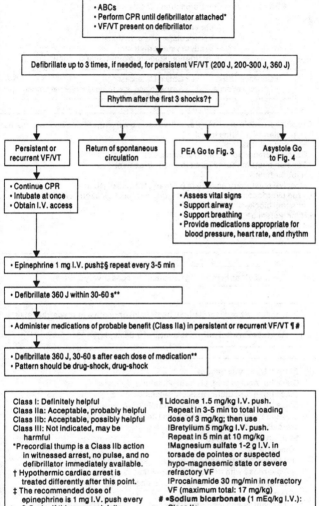

Class I: Definitely helpful
Class IIa: Acceptable, probably helpful
Class IIb: Acceptable, possibly helpful
Class III: Not indicated, may be harmful
*Precordial thump is a Class IIb action in witnessed arrest, no pulse, and no defibrillator immediately available.
† Hypothermic cardiac arrest is treated differently after this point.
‡ The recommended dose of epinephrine is 1 mg I.V. push every 3-5 min. If this approach fails, several Class IIb dosing regimens can be considered:
• Intermediate: Epinephrine 2-5 mg I.V. push, every 3-5 min
• Escalating: Epinephrine 1 mg-3 mg-5 mg I.V. push (3 min apart)
• High: Epinephrine: 0.1 mg/kg I.V. push, every 3-5 min
§ Sodium bicarbonate (1 mEq/kg) is Class I if patient has known pre-existing hyperkalemia
** Multiple sequenced shock (200 J, 200-300 J, 360 J) are acceptable here (Class I), especially when medications are delayed

¶ Lidocaine 1.5 mg/kg I.V. push. Repeat in 3-5 min to total loading dose of 3 mg/kg; then use
!Bretylium 5 mg/kg I.V. push. Repeat in 5 min at 10 mg/kg
!Magnesium sulfate 1-2 g I.V. in torsade de pointes or suspected hypo-magnesemic state or severe refractory VF
!Procainamide 30 mg/min in refractory VF (maximum total: 17 mg/kg)
•Sodium bicarbonate (1 mEq/kg I.V.): Class IIa
•If known pre-existing bicarbonate-responsive acidosis
•If overdose with tricyclic antidepressants
•To alkalinize the urine in drug overdoses Class IIb
•If intubated and continued long arrest interval
•Upon return of spontaneous circulation after long arrest interval Class III
•Hypoxic lactic acidosis

ADULT ACLS ALGORITHM
PULSELESS ELECTRICAL ACTIVITY

Fig. 3: Adult algorithm for pulseless electrical activity (PEA) (electromechanical dissociation [EMD]).

PEA includes: • Electromechanical dissociation (EMD)
- Pseudo-EMD
- Idioventricular rhythms
- Ventricular escape rhythms
- Bradyasystolic rhythms
- Postdefibrillation idioventricular rhythms

- Continue CPR
- Intubate at once
- Obtain I.V. access
- Assess blood flow using Doppler ultrasound

↓

Consider possible causes (Parentheses = possible therapies and treatments)
- Hypovolemia (volume infusion)
- Hypoxia (ventilation)
- Cardiac tamponade (pericardiocentesis)
- Tension pneumothorax (needle decompression)
- Hypothermia
- Massive pulmonary embolism (surgery, **thrombolytics**)
- Drug overdoses such as tricyclics, digitalis, beta blockers, calcium channel blockers
- Hyperkalemia*
- Acidosis†
- Massive acute myocardial infarction

↓

Epinephrine 1 mg I.V. push*‡, repeat every 3-5 min

↓

- If absolute bradycardia (<60 beats/min) or relative bradycardia, give **atropine** 1 mg I.V.
- Repeat every 3-5 min up to a total of 0.04 mg/kg§

Class I: Definitely helpful
Class IIa: Acceptable, probably helpful
Class IIb: Acceptable, possibly helpful
Class III: Not indicated, may be harmful

* **Sodium bicarbonate** 1 mEq/kg is Class I if patient has known pre-existing hyperkalemia

† **Sodium bicarbonate** 1 mEq/kg:

Class IIa
- If known pre-existing bicarbonate-responsive acidosis
- If overdose with tricyclic antidepressants
- To alkalinize the urine in drug overdoses

Class IIb
- If intubated and long arrest interval
- Upon return of spontaneous circulation after long arrest interval

Class III
- Hypoxic lactic acidosis

‡ The recommended dose of **epinephrine** is 1 mg I.V. push every 3-5 min. If this approach fails, several Class IIb dosing regimens can be considered.
- Intermediate: **Epinephrine** 2-5 mg I.V. push every 3-5 min
- Escalating: **Epinephrine** 1 mg-3 mg-5 mg I.V. push (3 min apart)
- High: **Epinephrine** 0.1 mg/kg I.V. push every 3-5 min

§ Shorter atropine dosing intervals are possibly helpful in cardiac arrest (Class IIb)

ADULT ACLS ALGORITHM
ASYSTOLE

Fig. 4: Adult asystole treatment algorithm.

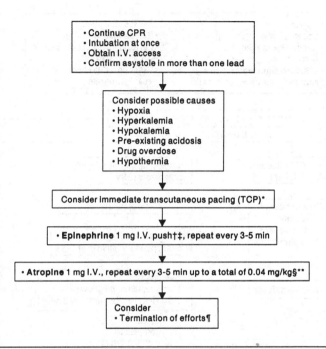

Class I: Definitely helpful
Class IIa: Acceptable, probably helpful
Class IIb: Acceptable, possibly helpful
Class III: Not indicated, may be harmful

* TCP is a Class IIb intervention. Lack of success may be due to delays in pacing. To be effective, TCP must be performed early, simultaneously with drugs. Evidence does not support routine use of TCP for asystole.

† The recommended dose of epinephrine is 1 mg I.V. push every 3-5 min. If this approach fails, several Class IIb dosing regimens can be considered:
 • Intermediate: Epinephrine 2-5 mg I.V. push every 3-5 min
 • Escalating: Epinephrine 1mg-3 mg-5 mg I.V. push (3 min apart)
 • High: Epinephrine 0.1 mg/kg I.V. push every 3-5 min

‡ Sodium bicarbonate 1 mEq/kg is Class I if patient has known pre-existing hyperkalemia

§ Shorter atropine dosing intervals are Class IIb in asystolic arrest

** Sodium bicarbonate 1 mEq/kg:
 Class IIa
 • If known pre-existing bicarbonate-responsive acidosis
 • If overdose with tricyclic antidepressants
 • To alkalinize the urine in drug overdoses
 Class IIb
 • If intubated and continued long arrest interval
 • Upon return of spontaneous circulation after long arrest interval
 Class III
 • Hypoxic lactic acidosis

¶ If patient remains in asystole or other agonal rhythms after successful intubation and initial medications and no reversible causes are identified, consider termination of resuscitative efforts by a physician. Consider interval since arrest.

Used with permission: Emergency Cardiac Care Committee and Subcommittees, American Heart Association, "Guidelines for Cardiopulmonary Resuscitation and Emergency Care, III: Adult Advanced Cardiac Life Support," *JAMA*, 1992: 268:2199-2241.

THERAPY RECOMMENDATIONS

ADULT ACLS ALGORITHM
TACHYCARDIA

Fig. 5: Adult tachycardia algorithm.

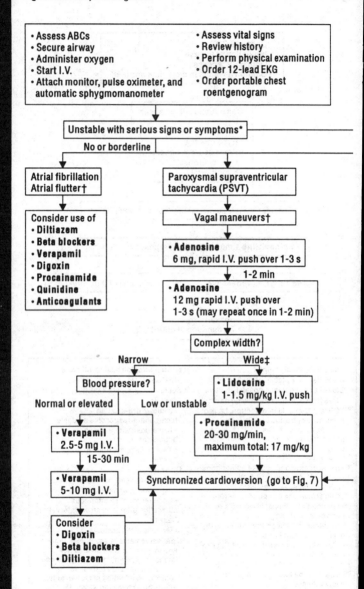

Used with permission: Emergency Cardiac Care Committee and Subcommittees, American Heart Association, "Guidelines for Cardiopulmonary Resuscitation and Emergency Care, III: Adult Advanced Cardiac Life Support," *JAMA*, 1992: 268:2199-2241.

ADULT ACLS ALGORITHM
TACHYCARDIA

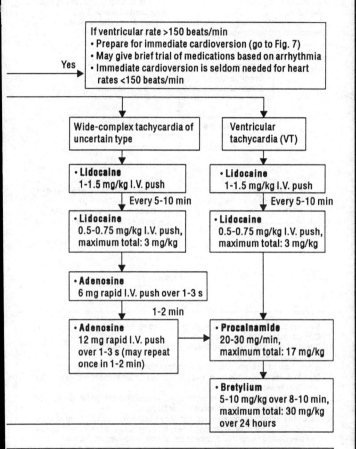

Yes →

If ventricular rate >150 beats/min
- Prepare for immediate cardioversion (go to Fig. 7)
- May give brief trial of medications based on arrhythmia
- Immediate cardioversion is seldom needed for heart rates <150 beats/min

Wide-complex tachycardia of uncertain type	Ventricular tachycardia (VT)

- **Lidocaine**
1-1.5 mg/kg I.V. push

Every 5-10 min

- **Lidocaine**
0.5-0.75 mg/kg I.V. push, maximum total: 3 mg/kg

- **Adenosine**
6 mg rapid I.V. push over 1-3 s

1-2 min

- **Adenosine**
12 mg rapid I.V. push over 1-3 s (may repeat once in 1-2 min)

- **Lidocaine**
1-1.5 mg/kg I.V. push

Every 5-10 min

- **Lidocaine**
0.5-0.75 mg/kg I.V. push, maximum total: 3 mg/kg

- **Procainamide**
20-30 mg/min, maximum total: 17 mg/kg

- **Bretylium**
5-10 mg/kg over 8-10 min, maximum total: 30 mg/kg over 24 hours

* Unstable condition must be related to the tachycardia. Signs and symptoms may include chest pain, shortness of breath, decreased level of consciousness, low blood pressure (BP), shock, pulmonary congestion, congestive heart failure, acute myocardial infarction.

† Carotid sinus pressure is contraindicated in patients with carotid bruits; avoid ice water immersion in patients with ischemic heart disease.

‡ If the wide-complex tachycardia is known with certainty to be PSVT and BP is normal/elevated, sequence can include **verapamil**.

ADULT ACLS ALGORITHM
BRADYCARDIA

Fig. 6: Adult bradycardia algorithm (with the patient not in cardiac arrest).

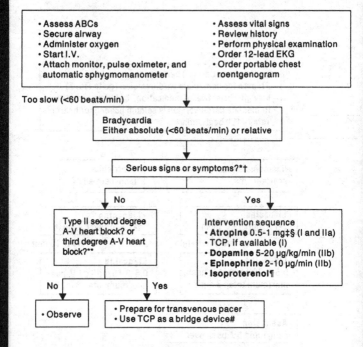

* Serious signs or symptoms must be related to the slow rate.
  Clinical manifestations include:
  Symptoms (chest pain, shortness of breath, decreased level of
  consciousness), and
  Signs (low BP, shock, pulmonary congestion, CHF, acute MI)
† Do not delay TCP while awaiting I.V. access or for **atropine** to take effect
  if patient is symptomatic.
‡ Denervated transplanted hearts will not respond to **atropine**. Go at once
  to pacing, **catecholamine** infusion, or both.
§ **Atropine** should be given in repeat doses in 3-5 min up to a total of 0.04
  mg/kg. Consider shorter dosing intervals in severe clinical conditions. It
  has been suggested that atropine should be used with caution in
  atrioventricular (A-V) block at the His-Purkinje level (type II A-V block and
  new third degree block with wide QRS complexes) (Class IIb).
** Never treat third degree heart block plus ventricular escape beats with
  lidocaine.
¶ **Isoproterenol** should be used, if at all, with extreme caution. At low
  doses it is Class IIb (possibly helpful); at higher doses it is Class III
  (harmful).
Verify patient tolerance and mechanical capture. Use analgesia and
  sedation as needed.

ADULT ACLS ALGORITHM
ELECTRICAL CONVERSION

Fig. 7: Adult electrical cardioversion algorithm (with the patient not in cardiac arrest).

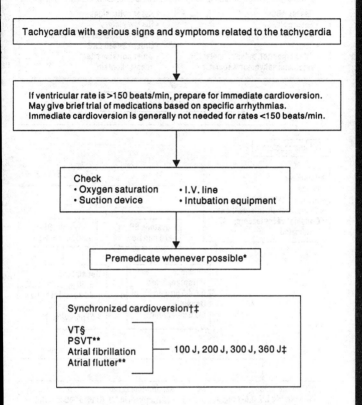

Tachycardia with serious signs and symptoms related to the tachycardia

If ventricular rate is >150 beats/min, prepare for immediate cardioversion.
May give brief trial of medications based on specific arrhythmias.
Immediate cardioversion is generally not needed for rates <150 beats/min.

Check
• Oxygen saturation   • I.V. line
• Suction device   • Intubation equipment

Premedicate whenever possible*

Synchronized cardioversion†‡

VT§
PSVT**
Atrial fibrillation   ─── 100 J, 200 J, 300 J, 360 J‡
Atrial flutter**

* Effective regimens have included a sedative (eg, **diazepam, midazolam barbiturates, etomidate, ketamine, methohexital**) with or without an analgesic agent (eg, **fentanyl, morphine, meperidine**). Many experts recommend anesthesia if service is readily available.
† Note possible need to resynchronize after each cardioversion.
‡ If delays in synchronization occur and clinical conditions are critical, go to immediate unsynchronized shocks.
§ Treat polymorphic VT (irregular form and rate) like VF: 200 J, 200-300J, 360 J.
** PSVT and atrial flutter often respond to lower energy levels (start

Used with permission: Emergency Cardiac Care Committee and Subcommittees, American Heart Association, "Guidelines for Cardiopulmonary Resuscitation and Emergency Care, III: Adult Advanced Cardiac Life Support," *JAMA*, 1992: 268:2199-2241.

ADULT ACLS ALGORITHM
HYPOTENSION, SHOCK

Fig. 8: Adult algorithm for hypotension, shock, and acute pulmonary edema.

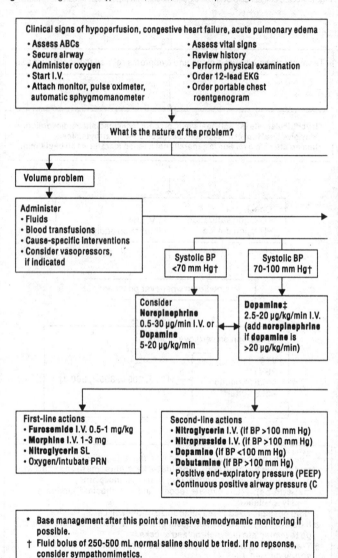

* Clinical signs of hypoperfusion, congestive heart failure, acute pulmonary edema
  * Assess ABCs
  * Secure airway
  * Administer oxygen
  * Start I.V.
  * Attach monitor, pulse oximeter, automatic sphygmomanometer
  * Assess vital signs
  * Review history
  * Perform physical examination
  * Order 12-lead EKG
  * Order portable chest roentgenogram

What is the nature of the problem?

Volume problem

Administer
  * Fluids
  * Blood transfusions
  * Cause-specific interventions
  * Consider vasopressors, if indicated

Systolic BP <70 mm Hg†

Systolic BP 70-100 mm Hg†

Consider **Norepinephrine** 0.5-30 µg/min I.V. or **Dopamine** 5-20 µg/kg/min

Dopamine‡ 2.5-20 µg/kg/min I.V. (add **norepinephrine** if dopamine is >20 µg/kg/min)

First-line actions
  * **Furosemide** I.V. 0.5-1 mg/kg
  * **Morphine** I.V. 1-3 mg
  * **Nitroglycerin** SL
  * Oxygen/intubate PRN

Second-line actions
  * **Nitroglycerin** I.V. (if BP >100 mm Hg)
  * **Nitroprusside** I.V. (if BP >100 mm Hg)
  * **Dopamine** (if BP <100 mm Hg)
  * **Dobutamine** (if BP >100 mm Hg)
  * Positive end-expiratory pressure (PEEP)
  * Continuous positive airway pressure (C

* * Base management after this point on invasive hemodynamic monitoring if possible.
* † Fluid bolus of 250-500 mL normal saline should be tried. If no repsonse, consider sympathomimetics.
* ‡ Move to dopamine and stop **norepinephrine** when BP improves.
* § Add **dopamine** when BP improves. Avoid **dobutamine** when systolic BP <100 mm Hg.

Used with permission: Emergency Cardiac Care Committee and Subcommittees, American Heart Association, "Guidelines for Cardiopulmonary Resuscitation and Emergency Care, III: Adult Advanced Cardiac Life Support," *JAMA*, 1992: 268:2199-2241.

ADULT ACLS ALGORITHM
HYPOTENSION, SHOCK

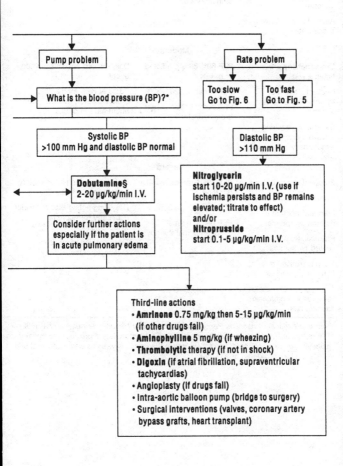

Pump problem

Rate problem

What is the blood pressure (BP)?*

Too slow
Go to Fig. 6

Too fast
Go to Fig. 5

Systolic BP
>100 mm Hg and diastolic BP normal

Diastolic BP
>110 mm Hg

Dobutamine§
2-20 µg/kg/min I.V.

Nitroglycerin
start 10-20 µg/min I.V. (use if ischemia persists and BP remains elevated; titrate to effect) and/or
Nitroprusside
start 0.1-5 µg/kg/min I.V.

Consider further actions especially if the patient is in acute pulmonary edema

Third-line actions
- **Amrinone** 0.75 mg/kg then 5-15 µg/kg/min (if other drugs fail)
- **Aminophylline** 5 mg/kg (if wheezing)
- **Thrombolytic** therapy (if not in shock)
- **Digoxin** (if atrial fibrillation, supraventricular tachycardias)
- Angioplasty (if drugs fail)
- Intra-aortic balloon pump (bridge to surgery)
- Surgical interventions (valves, coronary artery bypass grafts, heart transplant)

ASTHMA, CLASSIFICATION AND THERAPY

Classification of Asthma Severity

Clinical Features Before Treatment	Lung Function	Medication Usually Required to Maintain Control
Mild		
Intermittent, brief symptoms <1-2 times a week	PEF >80% predicted at baseline	Intermittent inhaled short-acting β-agonist only (taken as needed)
Nocturnal asthma symptoms <2 times a month	PEF variability <20%	
	PEF normal after bronchodilator	
Asymptomatic between exacerbations		
Moderate		
Exacerbations >1-2 times a week	PEF 60%-80% predicted at baseline	Daily inhaled anti-inflammatory agent
Nocturnal asthma symptoms >2 times a month	PEF variability 20%-30%	Possibly daily long-acting bronchodilator, especially for nocturnal symptoms
	PEF normal after bronchodilator	
Symptoms requiring inhaled β-agonist almost daily		
Severe		
Frequent exacerbations	PEF <60% predicted at baseline	Daily inhaled anti-inflammatory agent at high doses
Continuous symptoms	PEF variability >30%	Daily long-acting bronchodilator, especially for nocturnal symptoms
Frequent nocturnal asthma symptoms	PEF below normal despite optimal therapy	
Physical activities limited by asthma		Frequent use of systemic corticosteroids
Hospitalization for asthma in previous year*		
Previous life-threatening exacerbation*		

From *International Consensus Report on Diagnosis and Management of Asthma*, 1992.
*The potential severity — related to a patient's past history (eg, a previous life-threatening exacerbation or a hospitalization for asthma in the previous year) as well as present status — should be considered at all times.

Stepwise Approach to Asthma Therapy

Step 1: Mild	Step 2: Moderate	Step 3: Moderate	Step 4: Severe

Clinical Features Before Treatment*

- Intermittent, brief symptoms < 1-2 times a week
- Nocturnal asthma symptoms < 1-2 times a month
- Asymptomatic between exacerbations
- PEFR or FEV_1
  - ◆ > 80% predicted
  - ◆ variability < 20%

Clinical Features Before Treatment*

- Exacerbations > 1-2 times a week
- Exacerbations may affect activity and sleep
- Nocturnal asthma symptoms > 2 times a month
- Chronic symptoms requiring short-acting β-agonist almost daily
- PEFR or FEV1
  - ◆ 60-80% predicted
  - ◆ variability 20-30%

Clinical Features Before Treatment*

- Frequent exacerbations
- Continuous symptoms
- Frequent nocturnal asthma symptoms
- Physical activities limited by asthma
- PEFR or FEV_1
  - ◆ < 60% predicted
  - ◆ variability > 30%

* One or more features may be present to be assigned a grade of severity; and individula should usually be assigned the most severe grade in which any feature occurs.

Stepwise Approach to Asthma Therapy *(continued)*

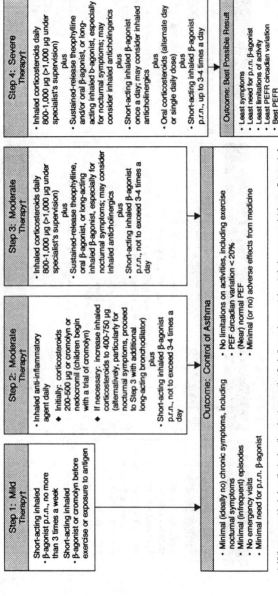

Step 1: Mild Therapy†

- Short-acting inhaled β-agonist p.r.n., no more than 3 times a week
- Short-acting inhaled β-agonist or cromolyn before exercise or exposure to antigen

Step 2: Moderate Therapy†

- Inhaled anti-inflammatory agent daily
  - ◆ Initially: corticosteroids 200-500 µg or cromolyn or nedocromil (children begin with a trial of cromolyn)
  - ◆ If necessary: increase inhaled corticosteroids to 400-750 µg (alternatively, particularly for nocturnal symptoms, proceed to Step 3 with additional long-acting bronchodilator)

  plus
- Short-acting inhaled β-agonist p.r.n., not to exceed 3-4 times a day

Step 3: Moderate Therapy†

- Inhaled corticosteroids daily 800-1,000 µg (>1,000 µg under specialist's supervision)

  plus
- Sustained-release theophylline, oral β-agonist, or long-acting inhaled β-agonist, especially for nocturnal symptoms; may consider inhaled anticholinergics

  plus
- Short-acting inhaled β-agonist p.r.n., not to exceed 3-4 times a day

Step 4: Severe Therapy†

- Inhaled corticosteroids daily 800-1,000 µg (>1,000 µg under specialist's supervision)

  plus
- Sustained-release theophylline and/or oral β-agonist, or long-acting inhaled b-agonist, especially for nocturnal symptoms; may consider inhaled anticholinergics

  plus
- Short-acting inhaled β-agonist once a day; may consider inhaled anticholinergics

  plus
- Oral corticosteroids (alternate day or single daily dose)

  plus
- Short-acting inhaled β-agonist p.r.n., up to 3-4 times a day

Outcome: Best Possible Result

- Least symptoms
- Least need for p.r.n. β-agonist
- Least limitations of activity
- Least PEFR circadian variation
- Best PEFR
- Least adverse effects from medicine

Outcome: Control of Asthma

- Minimal (ideally no) chronic symptoms, including nocturnal symptoms
- Minimal (infrequent) episodes
- No emergency visits
- Minimal need for p.r.n. β-agonist
- No limitations on activities, including exercise
- PEF circadian variation < 20%
- (Near) normal PEF
- Minimal (or no) adverse effects from medicine

† All therapy must include patient education about prevention (including environmental control where appropriate) as well as control of symptoms.

Step Up

Progress to the next higher step when control cannot be achieved at the current step and there is assurance that medication has been used correctly. If PEFR is <60% of predicted or personal best, consider a burst of oral corticosteroids and then proceed.

Step Down

Consider reducing therapy when the outcome has been achieved and sustained for several weeks or even months at the current step. Reduction in therapy is also necessary to identify the minimum therapy required to maintain control.

Advise patients of signs of worsening asthma and actions to control it.

Guidelines for the Management of Acute Asthma

Severity	Drug Therapy
	Adults and Children
Home management	Inhaled short-acting β_2-agonists (2-4 puffs every 20 minutes up to every hour) + oral corticosteroids
	Control not achieved ↓
	Nebulized β_2-agonists (3 doses over 60-90 minutes) + systemic corticosteroids
	Control not achieved ↓
Hospital care	Intensive care management

Summary of Guidelines for the Management of Chronic Asthma

Severity	Drug Therapy	
	Adults	**Children**
Mild episodic	Inhaled short-acting β_2-agonists as needed and/or before exercise and allergen exposure	
	Inhaled sodium cromoglycate before exercise and allergen exposure	
	Control not achieved ↓	
Moderate	Inhaled corticosteroids 2-4 puffs bid/qid	Sodium cromoglycate or nedocromil 2 >puffs bid/qid or 1 nebulization
	+	+
	Inhaled short-acting β_2-agonists as needed to tid/qid	
	Control not achieved ↓	
	Nocturnal episodes	
	Long-acting bronchodilators: Inhaled or oral β_2-agonists or sustained release theophylline	
	Control not achieved ↓	
Severe	Inhaled corticosteroids high dose (lowest dose for children)	
	+	
	Inhaled short-acting β_2-agonists as needed to tid/qid	
	+	
	Oral bronchodilator: Long-acting β_2-agonists or sustained release theophylline or inhaled long-acting β_2-agonists (especially for nocturnal symptoms) and/or may consider inhaled ipratropium bromide	
	Control not achieved ↓	
	+	+
	Oral corticosteroid lowest dose	Oral corticosteroid alternate day lowest dose

CONTRAST MEDIA REACTIONS, PREMEDICATION FOR PROPHYLAXIS AGAINST

(American College of Radiology Guideline for Use of Nonionic Contrast Media)

It is estimated that approximately 5% to 10% of patients will experience adverse reactions to administration of contrast dye (less for nonionic contrast). In approximately 1000-2000 administrations, a life-threatening reaction will occur.

A variety of premedication regimens have been proposed, both for pretreatment of "at risk" patients who require contrast media and before the routine administration of the intravenous high osmolar contrast media. Such regimens have been shown in clinical trials to decrease the frequency of all forms of contrast medium reactions. Pretreatment with a 2-dose regimen of methylprednisolone 32 mg, 12 and 2 hours prior to intravenous administration of HOCM (ionic), has been shown to decrease mild, moderate, and severe reactions in patients at increased risk and perhaps in patients without risk factors. Logistical and feasibility problems may preclude adequate premedication with this or any regimen for all patients. It is unclear at this time that steroid pretreatment prior to administration of ionic contrast media reduces the incidence of reactions to the same extent or less than that achieved with the use of nonionic contrast media alone. Information about the efficacy of nonionic contrast media combined with a premedication strategy, including steroids, is preliminary or not yet currently available. For high risk patients (ie, previous contrast reactors), the combination of a pretreatment regimen with nonionic contrast media has empirical merit and may warrant consideration. Oral administration of steroids appears preferable to intravascular routes, and the drug may be prednisone or methylprednisolone. Supplemental administration of H_1 and H_2 antihistamine therapies, orally or intravenously, may reduce the frequency of urticaria, angioedema, and respiratory symptoms. Additionally, ephedrine administration has been suggested to decrease the frequency of contrast reactions, but caution is advised in patients with cardiac disease, hypertension, or hyperthyroidism. No premedication strategy should be a substitute for the ABC approach to preadministration preparedness listed above. Contrast reactions do occur despite any and all premedication prophylaxis. The incidence can be decreased, however, in some categories of "at risk" patients receiving high osmolar contrast media plus a medication regimen. For patients with previous contrast medium reactions, there is a slight change that recurrence may be more severe or the same as the prior reaction; however, it is more likely that there will be no recurrence.

A general premedication regimen is

Methylprednisolone	32 mg orally at 12 and 2 hours prior to the procedure
Diphenhydramine	50 mg orally 1 hour prior to the procedure

An alternative premedication regimen is

Prednisone	50 mg orally 13, 7, and 1 hour before the procedure
Diphenhydramine	50 mg orally 1 hour before the procedure
Ephedrine	25 mg orally 1 hour before the procedure (except when contraindicated)

Indications for nonionic contrast are

Previous reaction to contrast — premedicate*
Known allergy to iodine or shellfish
Asthma, especially if on medication
Myocardial instability or CHF
Risk for aspiration or severe nausea and vomiting
Difficulty communicating or inability to give history
Patients taking beta-blockers
Small children at risk for electrolyte imbalance or extravasation
Renal failure with diabetes, sickle cell disease, or myeloma
At physician or patient request

*Life-threatening reactions (throat swelling, laryngeal edema, etc), consider omitting the intravenous contrast.

CONVULSIVE STATUS EPILEPTICUS

Recommendations of the Epilepsy Foundation of America's Working Group on Status Epilepticus
(*JAMA*, 1993, 270:854-9)

Convulsive status epilepticus is an emergency that is associated with high morbidity and mortality. The outcome largely depends on etiology, but prompt and appropriate pharmacological therapy can reduce morbidity and mortality. Etiology varies in children and adults and reflects the distribution of disease in these age groups. Antiepileptic drug administration should be initiated whenever a seizure has lasted 10 minutes. Immediate concerns include supporting respiration, maintaining blood pressure, gaining intravenous access, and identifying and treating the underlying cause. Initial therapeutic and diagnostic measures are conducted simultaneously. The goal of therapy is rapid termination of clinical and electrical seizure activity; the longer a seizure continues, the greater the likelihood of an adverse outcome. Several drug protocols now in use will terminate status epilepticus. Common to all patients is the need for a clear plan, prompt administration of appropriate drugs in adequate doses, and attention to the possibility of apnea, hypoventilation, or other metabolic abnormalities.

Precipitants of Status Epilepticus

Precipitants	Children ≤16 y, %	Adults >16 y, %
Cerebrovascular	3.3	25.2
Medication change	19.8	18.9
Anoxia	5.3	10.7
Ethanol/drug-related	2.4	12.2
Metabolic	8.2	8.8
Unknown	9.3	8.1
Fever/infection	35.7	4.6
Trauma	3.5	4.6
Tumor	0.7	4.3
Central nervous system infection	4.8	1.8
Congenital	7.0	0.8

Diagnostic Studies in Status Epilepticus*

Initial (emergent) studies

Glucose, electrolytes, BUN

Oximetry or arterial blood gases

Antiepileptic drug levels

Lumbar puncture

Complete blood count

Urinalysis

Second-phase studies (follow stabilization)

Liver function studies

Toxicology screen

EEG

Brain imaging with CT or MRI scan

---

*BUN indicates blood urea nitrogen; EEG, electroencephalogram; CT, computed tomographic; and MRI, magnetic resonance imaging.

Major Drugs Used to Treat Status Epilepticus: I.V. Doses, Pharmacokinetics, and Major Toxicities

	Diazepam	Lorazepam	Phenytoin	Phenobarbital
Adult I.V. dose, mg/kg [total dose]	0.15-0.25	0.1 [4-8 mg]	15-20	20
Pediatric I.V. dose, mg/kg [total dose]	0.1-1	0.05-0.5 [1-4 mg]	20	20
Pediatric per rectum dose, mg/kg	0.5 mg/kg (maximum 20 mg)	...	...	...
Maximal administration rate, mg/min	5	2	50	100
Time to stop status, min	1-3	6-10	10-30	20-30
Effective duration of action, h	0.25-0.5	>12-24	24	>48
Elimination half-life, h	30	14	24	100
Volume of distribution, L/kg	1-2	0.7-1	0.5-0.8	0.7
Potential side effects				
Depression of consciousness	10-30 min	Several hours	None	Several days
Respiratory depression	Occasional	Occasional	Infrequent	Occasional
Hypotension	Infrequent	Infrequent	Occasional	Infrequent
Cardiac arrhythmias	...	...	In patients with heart disease	...

Suggested Timetable for the Treatment of Status Epilepticus*

Time (min)	Action†
0-5	Diagnose status epilepticus by observing continued seizure activity or one additional seizure
	Give oxygen by nasal cannula or mark; position patient's head for optimal airway patency; consider intubation if respiratory assistance is needed
	Obtain and record vital signs at onset and periodically thereafter; control any abnormalities as necessary; initiate EKG monitoring
	Establish an I.V.; draw venous blood samples for glucose level, serum chemistries, hematology studies, toxicology screens, and determinations of antiepileptic drug levels
	Assess oxygenation with oximetry or periodic arterial blood gas determinations
6-9	If hypoglycemia is established or a blood glucose determination is unavailable; administer glucose; in adults, give 100 mg of thiamine first, followed by 50 mL of 50% glucose by direct push into the I.V.: in children, the dose of glucose is 2 mL/kg of 25% glucose
10-20	Administer either 0.1 mg/kg of lorazepam at 2 mg/min or 0.2 mg/kg of diazepam at 5 mg/min by I.V.; if diazepam is given, it can be repeated if seizures do not stop after 5 min; if diazepam is used to stop the status, phenytoin should be administered next to prevent recurrent status
21-60	If status persists, administer 15-20 mg/kg of phenytoin no faster than 50 mg/min in adults and 1 mg/kg/min in children by I.V.; monitor EKG and blood pressure during the infusion; phenytoin is incompatible with glucose-containing solutions — the I.V. should be purged with normal saline before the phenytoin infusion
>60	If status does not stop after 20 mg/kg of phenytoin, give additional doses of 5 mg/kg to a maximal dose of 30 mg/kg
	If status persists, give 20 mg/kg of phenobarbital by I.V. at 100 mg/min; when phenobarbital is given after a benzodiazepine, the risk of apnea or hypopnea is great and assisted ventilation is usually required
	If status persists, give anesthetic doses of drugs such as phenobarbital or pentobarbital; ventilatory assistance and vasopressors are virtually always necessary

*Time starts at seizure onset. Note that a neurological consultation is indicated if the patient does not wake up, convulsions continue after the administration of a benzodiazepine and phenytoin, or confusion exists at any time during evaluation and treatment. Data modified from Treiman.

†EKG indicates electrocardiogram; I.V., intravenous line.

THERAPY OF HYPERLIPIDEMIA

(*JAMA*, 1993, 269(23), 3015-23)

Risk Status Based on Presence of CHD Risk Factors Other Than Low-Density Lipoprotein Cholesterol*

Positive Risk Factors

Male ≥45 y

Female ≥55 y or premature menopause without estrogen replacement therapy

Family history of premature CHD (definite myocardial infarction or sudden death before 55 y of age in father or other male first-degree relative, or before 65 y of age in mother or other female first-degree relative)

Current cigarette smoking

Hypertension (blood pressure ≥140/90 mm Hg,† or taking antihypertensive medication)

Low HDL cholesterol (<35 mg/dL† [0.9 mmol/L])

Diabetes mellitus

Negative Risk Factor‡

High HDL cholesterol (≥60 mg/dL [1.6 mmol/L])

---

*High risk, defined as a net of two or more coronary heart disease (CHD) risk factors, leads to more vigorous intervention, shown in Figures 1 and 2. Age (defined differently for men and women) is treated as a risk factor because rates of CHD are higher in the elderly than in the young, and im men than in women of the same age. Obesity is not listed as a risk factor because it operates through other risk factors that are included (hypertension, hyperlipidemia, decreased high-density lipoprotein [HDL]cholesterol, and diabetes mellitus), but it should be considered a target for intervention. Physical inactivity is similarly not listed as a risk factor, but it too should be considered a target for intervention, and physical activity is recommended as desirable for everyone. High risk due to coronary or peripheral atherosclerosis is addressed directly in Figure 3.

†Confirmed by measurements on several occasions.

‡If the HDL cholesterol level is ≥60 mg/dL (1.6 mmol/L), subtract one risk factor (because high HDL cholesterol levels decrease CHD risk).

Initial Classification Based on Total Cholesterol and HDL Cholesterol Levels*

Cholesterol Level		Initial Classification
Total Cholesterol		
<200 mg/dL	(5.2 mmol/L)	Desirable blood cholesterol
200-239 mg/dL	(5.2-6.2 mmol/L)	Borderline-high blood cholesterol
≥240 mg/dL	(6.2 mmol/L)	High blood cholesterol
HDL Cholesterol		
<35 mg/dL	(0.9 mmol/L)	Low HDL cholesterol

*HDL indicates high-density lipoprotein.

Summary of the Second Report of the National Cholesterol Education Program (NCEP) Expert Panel on Detection, Evaluation, and Treatment of High Blood Cholesterol in Adults (Adult Treatment Panel II)

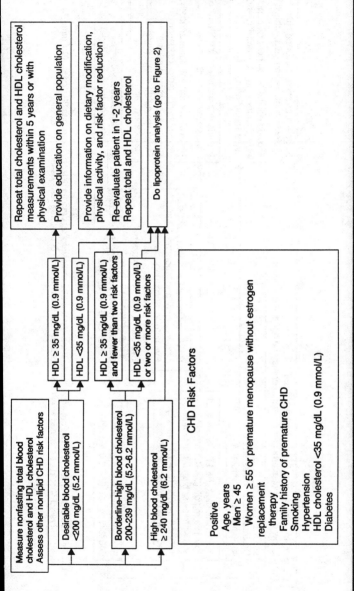

Fig. 1 - Primary prevention in adults without evidence of coronary heart disease (CHD). Initial classification is based on total cholesterol and high-density lipoprotein (HDL) cholesterol levels.

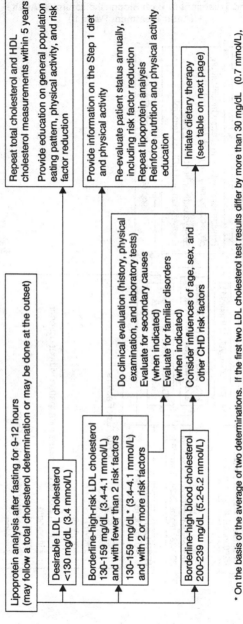

Fig. 2 - Primary prevention in adults without evidence of coronary heart disease (CHD). Subsequent classification is based on low-density lipoprotein (LDL) cholesterol level.

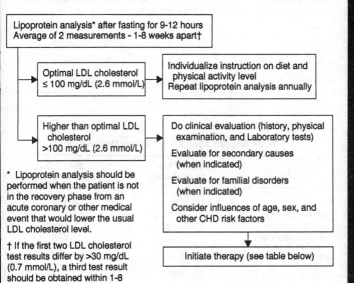

Fig. 3 - Secondary prevention in adults with evidence of coronary heart disease (CHD). Classification is based on low-density lipoprotein (LDL) cholesterol level.

Treatment Decisions Based on LDL Cholesterol Level*

Patient Category	Initiation Level	LDL Goal
Dietary Therapy		
Without CHD and with fewer than two risk factors	≥160 mg/dL (4.1 mmol/L)	<160 mg/dL (4.1 mmol/L)
Without CHD and with two or more risk factors	≥130 mg/dL (3.4 mmol/L)	<130 mg/dL (3.4 mmol/L)
With CHD	>100 mg/dL (2.6 mmol/L)	≤100 mg/dL (2.6 mmol/L)
Drug Treatment		
Without CHD and with fewer than two risk factors	≥190 mg/dL (4.9 mmol/L)	<160 mg/dL (4.1 mmol/L)
Without CHD and with two or more risk factors	≥160 mg/dL (4.1 mmol/L)	<130 mg/dL (3.4 mmol/L)
With CHD	≥130 mg/dL (3.4 mmol/L)	≤100 mg/dL (2.6 mmol/L)

*LDL indicates low-density lipoprotein; and CHD, coronary heart disease.

Classification of Serum Triglyceride Levels

Classification	Serum Triglyceride Concentration
Normal	<200 mg/dL
Borderline-high	200-400 mg/dL
High	400-1000 mg/dL
Very high	>1000 mg/dL

NCEP Stepped Approach for Dietary Modification

Nutrient	Step 1 Diet (% total kcal)	Step 2 Diet (% total kcal)
Total fat	<30	<30
saturated	<10	<7
polyunsaturated	Up to 10	Up to 10
monounsaturated	10-15	10-15
Carbohydrates	50-60	50-60
Protein	10-20	10-20
Cholesterol	<300 mg/d	<200 mg/d
Total calories	qs to maintain desirable wt	qs to maintain desirable wt

THERAPY OF HYPERTENSION

The Fifth Report of the Joint National Committee on Detection, Evaluation, and Treatment of High Blood Pressure (JNC V)
(*Arch Intern Med*, 1993:153)

Classification of Blood Pressure for Adults Aged 18 Years and Older*

Category	Systolic (mm Hg)	Diastolic (mm Hg)
Normal†	<130	<85
High normal	130-139	85-89
Hypertension‡		
Stage 1 (mild)	140-159	90-99
Stage 2 (moderate)	160-179	100-109
Stage 3 (severe)	180-209	110-119
Stage 4 (very severe)	≥210	≥120

*Not taking antihypertensive drugs and not acutely ill. When systolic and diastolic pressures fall into different categories, the higher category should be selected to classify the individual's blood pressure status. For instance, 160/92 mm Hg should be classified as stage 2, and 180/120 mm Hg should be classified as stage 4. Isolated systolic hypertension is defined as a systolic blood pressure ≥140 mm Hg and a diastolic blood pressure <90 mm Hg and staged appropriately (eg, 170/85 mm Hg is defined as stage 2 isolated systolic hypertension).

In addition to classifying stages of hypertension on the basis of average blood pressure levels, the clinician should specify presence or absence of target-organ disease and additional risk factors. For example, a patient with diabetes and a blood pressure of 142/94 mm Hg, plus left ventricular hypertrophy should be classified as having "stage 1 hypertension with target-organ disease (left ventricular hypertrophy) and with another major risk factor (diabetes)." This specificity is important for risk classification and management.

†Optimal blood pressure with respect to cardiovascular risk is <120 mm Hg systolic and <80 mm Hg diastolic. However, unusually low readings should be evaluated for clinical significance.

‡Based on the average of two or more readings taken at each of two or more visits after an initial screening.

Manifestations of Target-Organ Disease

Organ System	Manifestations
Cardiac	Clinical, electrocardiographic, or radiologic evidence of coronary artery disease; left ventricular hypertrophy or "strain" by electrocardiography or left ventricular hypertrophy by echocardiography; left ventricular dysfunction or cardiac failure
Cerebrovascular	Transient ischemic attack or stroke
Peripheral vascular	Absence of 1 or more major pulses in extremities (except for dorsalis pedis) with or without intermittent claudication; aneurysm
Renal	Serum creatinine ≥130 μmol/L (1.5 mg/dL); proteinuria (1+ or greater); microalbuminuria
Retinopathy	Hemorrhages or exudates, with or without papilledema

Recommendations for Follow-up Based on Initial Set of Blood Pressure Measurements for Adults

Initial Screening Blood Pressure (mm Hg)*		Follow-up Recommended†
Systolic	**Diastolic**	
<130	<85	Recheck in 2 y
130-139	85-89	Recheck in 1 y‡
140-159	90-99	Confirm within 2 mo
160-179	100-109	Evaluate or refer to source of care within 1 mo
180-209	110-119	Evaluate or refer to source of care within 1 wk
≥210	≥120	Evaluate or refer to source of care immediately

*If the systolic and diastolic categories are different, follow recommendation for the shorter time follow-up (eg, 160/85 mm Hg should be evaluated or referred to source of care within 1 month).

†The scheduling of follow-up should be modified by reliable information about past blood pressure measurements, other cardiovascular risk factors, or target-organ disease.

‡Consider providing advice about life-style modifications.

Pharmacologic Treatment

The decision to initiate pharmacologic treatment in individual patients requires consideration of several factors: severity of blood pressure elevation, TOD, and presence of other conditions and risk factors.

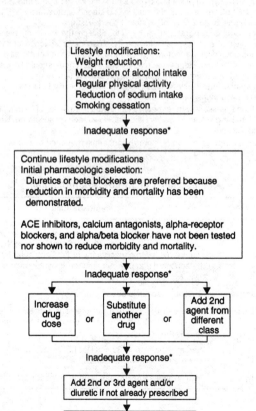

Antihypertensive Drug Therapy: Individualization Based on Special Considerations (Guidelines for Selecting Initial Therapy)*

Clinical Situation	Preferred	Requires Special Monitoring	Relatively or Absolutely Contraindicated
Cardiovascular			
Angina pectoris	β-Blockers, calcium antagonists		Direct vasodilators
Bradycardia/heart block, sick-sinus syndrome			β-Blockers, labetalol, verapamil, diltiazem
Cardiac failure	Diuretics, ACE inhibitors		β-Blockers, calcium antagonists, labetalol
Hypertrophic cardiomyopathy with severe diastolic dysfunction	β-Blockers, diltiazem, verapamil		Diuretics, ACE inhibitors, α₁-blockers, hydralazine, minoxidil
Hyperdynamic circulation	β-Blockers		Direct vasodilators
Peripheral vascular occlusive disease		β-Blockers	
After myocardial infarction	Non-ISA β-blockers		Direct vasodilators
Renal			
Bilateral renal arterial disease or severe stenosis in artery to solitary kidney			ACE inhibitors
Renal insufficiency			
Early (serum creatinine, 130-221 μmol/L [1.5-2.5 mg/dL])	Loop diuretics	ACE inhibitors	Potassium-sparing agents, potassium supplements
Advanced (serum creatinine, ≥221 μmol/L [≥2.5 mg/dL])			Potassium-sparing agents, potassium supplements

(continued)

Clinical Situation	Preferred	Requires Special Monitoring	Relatively or Absolutely Contraindicated
Other			
Asthma/COPD			β-Blockers, labetalol
Cyclosporine-associated hypertension	Nifedipine, labetalol	Verapamil,† nicardipine,† diltiazem†	
Depression		α₂-Agonists	Reserpine
Diabetes mellitus			
Type I (insulin dependent)		β-Blockers	
Type II		β-Blockers, diuretics	
Dyslipidemia		β-Blockers, diuretics	
Liver disease		Labetalol	Methyldopa
Pregnancy			
Preeclampsia	Methyldopa, hydralazine		Diuretics, ACE inhibitors
Chronic hypertension	Methyldopa		ACE inhibitors
Vascular headache	β-Blockers		

*ACE indicates angiotensin-converting enzyme; ISA, intrinsic sympathomimetic activity; and COPD, chronic obstructive pulmonary disease.
†Can increase serum levels of cyclosporine.

Management of Hypertensive Crisis: Emergencies and Urgencies*

Drug	Dose	Onset	Cautions
Parenteral Vasodilators			
Sodium nitroprusside	I.V. infusion: 0.25-10 µg/kg/min; maximal dose for 10 minutes only	Instantaneous	Nausea, vomiting, muscle twitching; with prolonged use may cause thiocyanate intoxication, methemoglobinemia acidosis, cyanide poisoning; bags, bottles, and delivery sets must be light resistant
Nitroglycerin	I.V. infusion: 5-100 µg	2-5 min	Headache, tachycardia, vomiting, flushing, methemoglobinemia; requires special delivery system due to drug binding to PVC tubing
Diazoxide	I.V.: bolus: 50-150 mg, repeated, or I.V. infusion: 15-30 mg/min	1-2 min	Hypotension, tachycardia, aggravation of angina pectoris, nausea and vomiting, hyperglycemia with repeated injections
Hydralazine	I.V. bolus: 10-20 mg I.M.: 10-40 mg	10 min 20-30 min	Tachycardia, headache, vomiting, aggravation of angina pectoris
Enalaprilat	I.V.: 0.625-1.25 mg q6h	15-60 min	Renal failure in patients with bilateral renal artery stenosis, hypotension
Parenteral Adrenergic Inhibitors			
Phentolamine	I.V. bolus: 5-15 mg	1-2 min	Tachycardia, orthostatic hypotension
Trimethaphan camsylate	I.V. infusion: 1-4 mg/min	1-5 min	Paresis of bowel and bladder, orthostatic hypotension, blurred vision, dry mouth
Labetalol	I.V. bolus: 20-80 mg every 10 min I.V. infusion: 2 mg/min	5-10 min	Bronchoconstriction, heart block, orthostatic hypotension
Methyldopate	I.V. infusion: 250-500 mg q6h	30-60 min	Drowsiness
Oral Agents			
Nifedipine (not extended release)	P.O.: 10-20 mg, repeat after 30 min	15-30 min	Rapid, uncontrolled reduction in blood pressure may precipitate circulatory collapse in patients with aortic stenosis
Captopril	P.O.: 25 mg, repeat as required	15-30 min	Hypotension, renal failure in bilateral renal artery stenosis
Clonidine	P.O.: 0.1-0.2 mg, repeated every hour as required to a total dose of 0.6 mg	30-60 min	Hypotension, drowsiness, dry mouth
Labetalol	P.O.: 200-400 mg , repeat q2-3h	30 min - 2 h	Bronchoconstriction, heart block, orthostatic hypotension

*It is sometimes appropriate to administer a diuretic agent with any of these drugs. PVC = polyvinyl chloride; I.V. = intravenous; I.M. = intramuscular; P.O. = oral.

Classification of Hypertension in the Young by Age Group*

Age Group	High Normal (90-94th Percentile) mm Hg	Significant Hypertension (95-99th Percentile) mm Hg	Severe Hypertension (>99th Percentile) mm Hg
Newborns (systolic)			
7 d		96-105	≥106
8-30 d		104-109	≥110
Infants (≤2 y)			
systolic	104-111	112-117	≥118
diastolic	70-73	74-81	≥82
Children			
3-5 y			
systolic	108-115	116-123	≥124
diastolic	70-75	76-83	≥84
6-9 y			
systolic	114-121	122-129	≥130
diastolic	74-77	78-85	≥86
10-12 y			
systolic	122-125	126-133	≥134
diastolic	78-81	82-89	≥90
13-15 y			
systolic	130-135	136-143	≥144
diastolic	80-85	86-91	≥92
Adolescents (16-18 y)			
systolic	136-141	142-149	≥150
diastolic	84-91	92-97	≥98

*Adapted from the "Report of the Second Task Force on Blood Pressure Control in Children, 1987. Note that adult classifications differ.

HEART FAILURE: MANAGEMENT OF PATIENTS WITH LEFT-VENTRICULAR SYSTOLIC DYSFUNCTION

Medications Commonly Used for Heart Failure

Drug	Initial Dose (mg)	Target Dose (mg)	Recommended Maximal Dose (mg)	Major Adverse Reactions
Thiazide Diuretics				
Chlorthalidone Hydrochlorothiazide	25 qd	As needed	50 qd	Postural hypotension, hypokalemia, hyperglycemia, hyperuricemia, rash; rare severe reaction includes pancreatitis, bone marrow suppression, and anaphylaxis
Loop Diuretics				
Bumetanide	0.5-1 qd	As needed	10 qd	Same as thiazide diuretics
Ethacrynic acid	50 qd		200 bid	
Furosemide	10-40 qd		240 bid	
Thiazide-Related Diuretic				
Metolazone	2.5*	As needed	10 qd	Same as thiazide diuretics
Potassium-Sparing Diuretics				
Amiloride	5 qd	As needed	40 qd	Hyperkalemia (especially if administered with ACE inhibitor), rash, gynecomastia (spironolactone only)
Spironolactone	25 qd		100 bid	
Triamterene	50 qd		100 bid	
ACE Inhibitors				
Captopril	6.25-12.5 tid	50 tid	100 tid	Hypotension, hyperkalemia, renal insufficiency, cough, skin rash, angioedema, neutropenia
Enalapril	2.5 bid	10 bid	20 bid	
Lisinopril	5 qd	20 qd	40 qd	
Quinapril	5 bid	20 bid	20 bid	
Digoxin	0.125 qd	As needed	As needed	Cardiotoxicity, confusion, nausea, anorexia, visual disturbances
Hydralazine	10-25 tid	75 tid	100 tid	Headache, nausea, dizziness, tachycardia, lupus-like syndrome
Isosorbide dinitrate	10 tid	40 tid	80 tid	Headache, hypotension, flushing

*Given as a single test dose initially.

Note: ACE = angiotensin-converting enzyme.

Clinical Algorithm for Evaluation and Care of Patients With Heart Failure

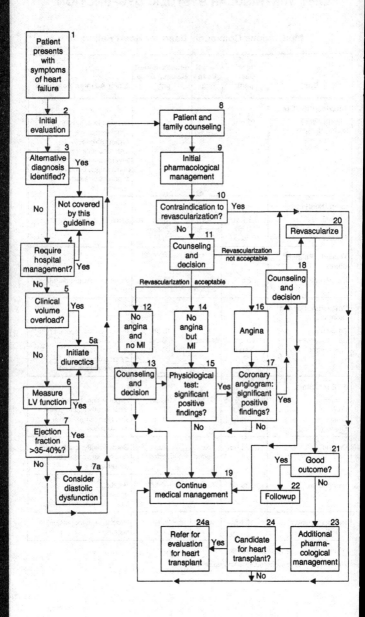

TOXICOLOGY INFORMATION

Initial Stabilization of the Patient

The recommended treatment plan for the poisoned patient is not unlike general treatment plans taught in advanced cardiac life support (ACLS) or advanced trauma life support (ATLS) courses. In this manner, the initial approach to the poisoned patient should be essentially similar in every case, irrespective of the toxin ingested, just as the initial approach to the trauma patient is the same irrespective of the mechanism of injury. This approach, which can be termed as routine poison management, essentially includes the following aspects.

- Stabilization: ABCs (airway, breathing, circulation); administration of glucose, thiamine, oxygen, and naloxone
- History, physical examination leading toward the identification of class of toxin (toxidrome recognition)
- Prevention of absorption (decontamination)
- Specific antidote, if available
- Removal of absorbed toxin (enhancing excretion)
- Support and monitoring for adverse effects

Drugs to Be Utilized in the Toxic Patient With Altered Mental Status

Drug	Effect	Comment
25-50 g **dextrose** ($D_{50}W$) intravenously to reverse the effects of drug-induced hypoglycemia (adult) 1 mL/kg $D_{50}W$ diluted 1:1 (child).	This can be especially effective in patients with limited glycogen stores (ie, neonates and patients with cirrhosis).	Extravasation into the extremity of this hyperosmolar solution can cause Volkmann's contractures.
50-100 mg intravenous **thiamine**	Prevent Wernicke's encephalopathy	A water-soluble vitamin with low toxicity; rare anaphylactoid reactions have been reported.
Initial dosage of **naloxone** should be 2 mg in adult patients preferably by the intravenous route, although intramuscular, subcutaneous, intralingual, and endotracheal routes may also be utilized. Pediatric dose is 0.1 mg/kg from birth until 5 years of age.	Specific opioid antagonist without any agonist properties.	It should be noted that some semisynthetic opiates (such as meperidine or propoxyphene) may require higher initial doses for reversal, so that a total dose of 6-10 mg is not unusual for the adults. If the patient responds to a bolus dose and then relapses to a lethargic or comatose state, a naloxone drip can be considered. This can be accomplished by administering two-thirds of the bolus dose that revives the patient per hour or injecting 4 mg naloxone in 1 L crystalloid solution and administering at a rate of 100 mL/hour (0.4 mg/hour).
Oxygen, utilized in 100% concentration	Useful for carbon monoxide, hydrogen, sulfide, and asphyxiants	While oxygen is antidotal for carbon monoxide intoxication, the only relative toxic contraindication is in paraquat intoxication (in that it can promote pulmonary fibrosis).
Flumazenil	Benzodiazepine antagonist	Not routinely recommended

TOXICOLOGY

Laboratory Evaluation of Overdose

Unknown ingestion: Electrolytes, anion gap, serum osmolality, arterial blood gases, serum drug concentration

Known ingestion: Labs tailored to agent

Toxins Affecting the Anion Gap

Drugs Causing Increased Anion Gap (>12 mEq/L)

Nonacidotic

Carbenicillin	Sodium salts

Metabolic Acidosis

Acetaminophen (ingestion >75-100 g)	Isoniazid
	Ketamine
Acetazolamide	Ketoprofen
Amiloride	Metformin
Ascorbic acid	Methanol
Benzalkonium chloride	Methenamine mandelate
Bialaphos	Monochloracetic acid
2-butanone	Nalidixic acid
Carbon monoxide	Naproxen
Centrimonium bromide	Niacin
Chloramphenicol	Papaverine
Colchicine	Paraldehyde
Cyanide	Pennroyal oil
Dapsone	Pentachlorophenol
Dimethyl sulfate	Phenelzine
Dinitrophenol	Phenformin (off the market)
Endosulfan	Phenol
Epinephrine (I.V. overdose)	Phenylbutazone
Ethanol	Phosphoric acid
Ethylene dibromide	Potassium chloroplatinite
Ethylene glycol	Propylene glycol
Fenoprofen	Salicylates
Fluoroacetate	Sorbitol (I.V.)
Formaldehyde	Strychnine
Fructose (I.V.)	Surfactant herbicide
Glycol ethers	Tetracycline (outdated)
Hydrogen sulfide	Tienilic acid
Ibuprofen (ingestion >300 mg/kg)	Toluene
Inorganic acid	Tranylcypromine
Iodine	Vacor
Iron	Verapamil

Drugs Causing Decreased Anion Gap (<6 mEq/L)

Acidosis

Ammonium chloride	Lithium
Bromide	Polymyxin B
Iodide	Tromethamine

Drugs Causing Osmolar Gap
(by freezing-point depression, gap is >10 mOsm)

Ethanol	Iodine (questionable)
Ethylene glycol	
Glycerol	Mannitol
Hypermagnesemia (>9.5 mEq/L)	Methanol
Isopropanol (acetone)	Sorbitol

Toxins Associated With Oxygen Saturation Gap
(>5% difference between measured and calculated value)

Carbon monoxide	Methemoglobin
Cyanide (questionable)	
Hydrogen sulfide (possible)	

History and Physical Examination

While the history and physical examination is the cornerstone of clinical patient management, it takes on special meaning with regard to the toxic patient. While taking a history may be a more direct method of the determination of the toxin, quite often it is not reliable. Information obtained may prove minimal in some cases and could be considered partial or inaccurate in suicide gestures and addicts. A quick physical examination often leads to important clues about the nature of the toxin. These clues can be specific symptom complexes associated with certain toxins and can be referred to as "toxidromes". See the following table.

Methods of Enhanced Elimination of Toxic Substances/Drugs

Emesis With Syrup of Ipecac

Indications

- Use within 1 hour of ingestion
- Hydrocarbons with "dangerous additives"
- Heavy metals
- Insecticides

Contraindications

- Children <6 months of age
- Nontoxic ingestion
- Lack of gag reflex
- Caustic/corrosive ingestions
- Hemorrhagic diathesis
- Sharp object ingestion
- Prior vomiting
- Ingestion of pure petroleum distillate

Dose: + 15 mL H_2O

Children: 6-12 months: 10 mL
           1-5 years: 15 mL
           >5 years: 30 mL
Adults: 30 mL

Gastric Lavage

Indications

- Use within 1 hour of ingestion
- Comatose patient with significant ingestion without contraindications
- Failure to respond to ipecac

Contraindications

- Nontoxic ingestion
- Significant hemorrhagic diathesis
- Caustic ingestions
- Usually unable to use large enough tube in children <12 years of age

Enhancement of Elimination

Only recently has this aspect of poison management received more than cursory attention in practice and in the literature. The standard practice for enhancement of elimination consisted primarily of forced diuresis in order to excrete the toxin. However, the past 10 years experience has produced a radical change in the approach to this and therefore, a more focused methodology to eliminating absorbed toxins. Essentially, there are three methods by which absorbed toxins may be eliminated: recurrent adsorption with multiple dosings of activated charcoal, use of forced diuresis in combination with possible alkalinization of the urine, and use of dialysis or charcoal hemoperfusion.

Activated Charcoal Indications

Indications

- Single dose for agents known to be bound
- Multiple dose for drugs with favorable characteristics: Small volume of distribution (<1 L/kg), low plasma protein binding, biliary or gastric secretion, active metabolites that recirculate, drugs that exhibit a large free fraction (eg, dapsone, carbamazepine, digitalis, methotrexate, phenobarbital, salicylates, theophylline, tricyclic antidepressants), unchanged, lipophilic, long half-life

Recently, multiple dosing of activated charcoal ("pulse dosing") has been advocated as a method for removal of absorbed drug. This procedure has been demonstrated to be efficacious in drugs that re-enter the gastrointestinal tract through enterohepatic circulation (ie, digitoxin, carbamazepine, glutethimide) and with drugs that diffuse from the systemic circulation into the gastrointestinal tract due to formation of a concentration gradient ("the infinite sink" hypothesis).

Toxins Eliminated by Multiple Dosing of Activated Charcoal

Amitriptyline	Methotrexate
Amoxapine	Methyprylon
Baclofen (?)	Nadolol
Benzodiazepines (?)	Nortriptyline
Bupropion (?)	Phencyclidine
Carbamazepine	Phenobarbital
Chlordecone	Phenylbutazone
Cyclosporine	Phenytoin (?)
Dapsone	Piroxicam
Diazepam	Propoxyphene
Digoxin	Salicylates (?)
Glutethimide	Theophylline
Maprotiline	Valproic acid
Meprobamate	

Contraindications

- Absence or hypoactive bowel sounds
- Caustic ingestions
- Drugs without effect: Acids, alkalis, alcohols, boric acid, cyanide, iron, heavy metals, lithium, insecticides

Dose

Children and Adults: 50-100 g initially **or** 1 g/kg weight; repeat doses of 25 g or 0.5 g/kg every 2-4 hours

Most effective at 1-hour postingestion but can remove at >1-hour postingestion

Whole Bowel Irrigation — propylene glycol based solutions

Initial dose of charcoal is necessary prior to use. Avoid pretreatment with ipecac.

Indications

- Agents not bound by charcoal
- Modified or sustained-release dosage forms
- Body packers

Contraindications

- Bowel perforation
- Obstruction
- Ileus
- Gastrointestinal bleed

Dose

Maximum of 5-10 L
Toddlers/Preschool: 500 mL/h
Adults: 1-2 L/h
Terminate when rectal effluent = infusate

Urinary Ion Trapping — to alkalinize the urine

Indications

- Salicylates
- Phenobarbital

Toxins Eliminated by Forced Saline Diuresis	Toxins Eliminated by Alkaline Diuresis
Bromides	2,4-D chlorophenoxyacetic acid
Chromium	Fluoride
Cimetidine (?)	Isoniazid (?)
Cis-platinum	Mephobarbital
Cyclophosphamide	Methotrexate
Hydrazine	Phenobarbital
Iodide	Primidone
Iodine	Quinolones antibiotic
Isoniazid (?)	Salicylates
Lithium	Uranium
Methyl iodide	
Potassium chloroplatinite	
Thallium	

Dose

Sodium bicarbonate 1-2 mEq/kg every 3-4 hours

A urine flow of 3-5 mL/kg/hour should be achieved with a combination of isotonic fluids or diuretics. Alkalinization can be achieved by administration of 44-88 mEq of sodium bicarbonate per liter to titrate a urine pH of 7.5. Although several drugs can exhibit enhanced elimination through an acidic urine (quinine, amphetamines, PCP, nicotine, bismuth, ephedrine, flecainide), the practice of acidifying the urine should be discouraged in that it can produce metabolic acidosis and promote renal failure in the presence of rhabdomyolysis.

Hemodialysis

Indications

Drugs with favorable characteristics:

- Low molecular weight (<500 daltons)
- Ionically charged
- H_2O soluble
- Low plasma protein binding (<70%-80%)
- Small volume of distribution (<1 L/kg)
- Low tissue binding

Drugs and Toxins Removed by Hemodialysis

Acetaminophen	Iodides
Acyclovir	Isoniazid
Amanita phalloides (?)	Isopropanol
Amantadine (?)	Ketoprofen
Ammonium chloride	Lithium
Amphetamine	Magnesium
Anilines	Meprobamate
Atenolol	Metal-chelate compounds
Boric acid	Metformin (?)
Bromides	Methanol
Bromisoval	Methaqualone
Calcium	Methotrexate
Captopril (?)	Methyldopa
Carbromal	Methylprylone
Carisoprodol	Monochloroacetic acid
Chloral hydrate	Nadolol
Chlorpropamide	Oxalic acid
Chromium	Paraldehyde
Cimetidine (?)	Phenelzine (?)
Cyclophosphamide	Phenobarbital
Dapsone	Phosphoric acid
Disopyramide	Potassium
Enalapril (?)	Procainamide
Ethanol	Quinidine
Ethylene glycol	Ranitidine (?)
Famotidine (?)	Rifabutin
Fluoride	Salicylates
Folic acid	Sotalol
Formaldehyde	Strychnine
Foscarnet sodium	Thallium
Gabapentin	Theophylline
Glycol ethers	Thiocyanates
Hydrazine (?)	Tranylcypromine sulfate (?)
Hydrochlorothiazide	Verapamil (?)

TOXICOLOGY

Hemoperfusion

Indications

Drugs with favorable characteristics:

- Affinity for activated charcoal
- Tissue binding
- Rate of equilibration from peripheral tissues to blood

Examples: Barbiturates, carbamazepine, ethchlorvynol, methotrexate, phenytoin, theophylline

Drugs and Toxins Removed by Hemoperfusion (Charcoal)

Amanita phalloides (?)	Meprobamate
Atenolol (?)	Methaqualone
Bromisoval	Methotrexate
Bromoethylbutyramide	Methsuximide
Caffeine	Methyprylon (?)
Carbamazepine	Metoprolol (?)
Carbon tetrachloride (?)	Nadolol (?)
Carbromal	Oxalic acid (?)
Chloral hydrate (trichloroethanol)	Paraquat
Chloramphenicol	Phenelzine (?)
Chlorpropamide	Phenobarbital
Colchicine (?)	Phenytoin
Creosote (?)	Podophyllin (?)
Dapsone	Procainamide (?)
Diltiazem (?)	Quinidine (?)
Disopyramide	Rifabutin (?)
Ethchlorvynol	Sotalol (?)
Ethylene oxide	Thallium
Glutethimide	Theophylline
Lindane	Verapamil (?)

Exchange transfusion is another mode of extracorporeal removal of toxins that can be utilized in neonatal infant drug toxicity. It may be especially useful for barbiturate, iron, caffeine, sodium nitrite, or theophylline overdose.

Criteria for Admission of the Poisoned Patient to ICU

Respiratory depression (pCO_2 >45 mm Hg)
Emergency intubation
Seizures
Cardiac arrhythmia
Hypotension (systolic blood pressure <80 mm Hg)
Unresponsiveness to verbal stimuli
Second- or third-degree atrioventricular block
Emergent dialysis or hemoperfusion
Increasing metabolic acidosis
Tricyclic or phenothiazine overdose manifesting anticholinergic signs, neurologic abnormality, QRS duration >0.12 second, or QT duration >0.5 seconds
Administration of pralidoxime in organophosphate toxicity
Pulmonary edema induced by drugs or toxic inhalation (ARDS)
Drug-induced hypothermia or hyperthermia including neuroleptic malignant syndrome
Hyperkalemia secondary to digitalis overdose
Body packers and stuffers
Concretions secondary to drugs
Emergent surgical intervention
Antivenom administration in *Crotalidae*, coral snake, or arthropod envenomation
Need for continuous infusion of naloxone

pCO_2 = carbon dioxide pressure
ARDS = adult respiratory distress syndrome

Adapted from Kulling P, Persson H, "Role of the Intensive Care Unit in the Management of the Poisoned Patient," *Med Toxicol*, 1986, 1:375-86 and Brett AS, Rothschild N, Gray R, et al, "Predicting the Clinical Course in Intentional Drug Overdose: Implication for Use of the Intensive Care Unit, *Arch Intern Med*, 1987, 147:133-7, and Callaham M, "Admission Criteria for Tricyclic Antidepressant Ingestion, *West J Med*, 1982, 137:425-9.

TOXIDROMES

Toxin	Vital Signs	Mental Status	Symptoms	Physical Exam	Laboratories
Acetaminophen	Normal	Normal	Anorexia, nausea, vomiting	RUQ tenderness, jaundice	Elevated LFTs
Cocaine	Hypertension, tachycardia, hyperthermia	Anxiety, agitation, delirium	Hallucinations	Mydriasis, tremor, diaphoresis, seizures, perforated nasal septum	EKG abnormalities, increased CPK
Cyclic antidepressants	Tachycardia, hypotension, hyperthermia	Decreased, including coma	Confusion, dizziness	Mydriasis, dry mucous membranes, distended bladder, decreased bowel sounds, flushed, seizures	Long QRS complex, cardiac dysrhythmias
Iron	Early: Normal Late: Hypotension, tachycardia	Normal; lethargic if hypotensive	Nausea, vomiting, diarrhea, abdominal pain, hematemesis	Abdominal tenderness	Heme + stool and vomit; metabolic acidosis, EKG and x-ray findings, elevated serum iron (early); child: hyperglycemia, leukocytosis
Opioids	Hypotension, bradycardia, hypoventilation, hypothermia	Decreased, including coma	Intoxication	Miosis, absent bowel sounds	Abnormal ABGs
Salicylates	Hyperventilation, hyperthermia	Agitation; lethargy, including coma	Tinnitus, nausea, vomiting, confusion	Diaphoresis, tender abdomen	Anion gap metabolic acidosis, respiratory alkalosis, abnormal LFTs, and coagulation studies
Theophylline	Tachycardia, hypotension, hyperventilation, hyperthermia	Agitation; lethargy, including coma	Nausea, vomiting, diaphoresis, tremor, confusion	Seizures	Hypokalemia, hyperglycemia, metabolic acidosis, abnormal EKG

Examples of Toxidromes

Toxidromes	Pattern	Example of Drugs	Treatment Approach
Anticholinergic	Fever, ileus, flushing, tachycardia, urinary retention, inability to sweat, visual blurring, and mydriasis. Central manifestations include myoclonus, choreoathetosis, toxic psychosis with lilliputian hallucinations, seizures, and coma.	Antihistamines Baclofen Benztropine Jimson weed Methylpyroline Phenothiazines Propantheline Tricyclic antidepressants	Physostigmine for life-threatening symptoms
Cholinergic	Characterized by salivation, lacrimation, urination, defecation, gastrointestinal cramps, and emesis ("sludge"). Bradycardia and bronchoconstriction may also be seen.	Carbamate Organophosphates Pilocarpine	• Atropine • Pralidoxime for organophosphate insecticides
Extrapyramidal	Choreoathetosis, hyperreflexia, trismus, opisthotonos, rigidity, and tremor	Haloperidol Phenothiazines	• Diphenhydramine • Benztropine
Hallucinogenic	Perceptual distortions, synthesis, depersonalization, and derealization	Amphetamines Cannabinoids Cocaine Indole alkaloids Phencyclidine	Benzodiazepine
Narcotic	Altered mental status, unresponsiveness, shallow respirations, slow respiratory rate or periodic breathing, miosis, bradycardia, hypothermia.	Opiates Dextromethorphan Pentazocine Propoxyphene	Naloxone

(continued)

Toxidromes	Pattern	Example of Drugs	Treatment Approach
Sedative/Hypnotic	Manifested by sedation with progressive deterioration of central nervous system function. Coma, stupor, confusion, apnea, delirium, or hallucinations may accompany this pattern.	Anticonvulsants Antipsychotics Barbiturates Benzodiazepines Ethanol Ethchlorvynol Fentanyl Glutethimide Meprobamate Methadone Methocarbamol Opiates Quinazolines Propoxyphene Tricyclic antidepressants	• Naloxone • Flumazenil • Urinary alkalinization (barbiturates)
Seizuregenic	May mimic stimulant pattern with hyperthermia, hyperreflexia, and tremors being prominent signs.	Anticholinergics Camphor Chlorinated hydrocarbons Cocaine Isoniazid Lidocaine Lindane Nicotine Phencyclidine Strychnine Xanthines	• Antiseizure medications • Pyridoxine for isoniazid • Extracorporeal removal of drug (ie, lindane, camphor, xanthines) • Physostigmine for anticholinergic agents

(continued)

Toxidromes	Pattern	Example of Drugs	Treatment Approach
Serotonin	Confusion, myoclonus, hyperreflexia, diaphoresis tremor, facial flushing, diarrhea	Clomipramine Fluoxetine Isoniazid L-tryptophan Paroxetine Phenelzine Sertraline Tranylcypromine Drug combinations include: MAO inhibitors with L-tryptophan Fluoxetine or meperidine Fluoxetine with carbamazepine or sertraline Clomipramine and meclobemide, Trazadol and buspirone Paroxetine and dextromethorphan	Withdrawal of drug/benzodiazepine
Solvent	Lethargy, confusion, dizziness, headache, restlessness, incoordination, derealization, depersonalization	Acetone Chlorinated hydrocarbons Hydrocarbons Naphthalene Trichloroethane Toluene	Avoid catecholamines
Stimulant	Restlessness, excessive speech and motor activity, tachycardia, tremor, and insomnia — may progress to seizure. Other effects noted include euphoria, mydriasis, anorexia, and paranoia.	Amphetamines Caffeine (xanthines) Cocaine Ephedrine/pseudoephedrine Methylphenidate Nicotine Phencyclidine	Benzodiazepines

From Nice A, Leikin JB, Maturen A, et al, "Toxidrome Recognition to Improve Efficiency of Emergency Urine Drug Screens," *Ann Emerg Med*, 1988, 17:676-80.

MANAGEMENT OF OVERDOSAGES

Poison Control Center Antidote Chart

Antidote	Poison/Drug	Indications	Dosage	Comments
Acetylcysteine (Mucomyst®)	Acetaminophen	Unknown quantity ingested and <24 hours have elapsed since the time of ingestion or unable to obtain serum acetaminophen levels within 12 hours of ingestion. >7.5 g acetaminophen acutely ingested Serum acetaminophen level >140 μg/mL at 4 hours postingestion Ingested dose >140 mg/kg	Dilute to 5% solutions with carbonated beverage, fruit juice, or water and administer orally. **Loading:** 140 mg/kg for 1 dose **Maintenance:** 70 mg/kg for 17 doses, starting 4 hours after the loading dose and given every 4 hours thereafter unless assay reveals a nontoxic serum level.	SGOT, SGPT, bilirubin, prothrombin time, creatinine, BUN, blood sugar, and electrolytes should be obtained daily if a toxic serum acetaminophen level has been determined. **Note:** Activated charcoal has been shown to absorb acetylcysteine *in vitro* and may do so in patients. Serum acetaminophen levels may not peak until 4 hours postingestion, and therefore, serum levels should not be drawn earlier.
Amyl nitrate, sodium nitrate, sodium thiosulfate (cyanide antidote package)	Cyanide	Begin treatment at the first sign of toxicity if exposure is known or strongly expected.	Break ampul of amyl nitrate and allow patient to inhale for 15 seconds, then take away for 15 seconds. Use a fresh ampul every 3 minutes. Continue until injection of sodium nitrate (3% solution) 300 mg (0.15-0.33 mL/kg over 5 minutes in pediatric patients) can be injected at 2.5-5 mL/minute. Then immediately inject 12.5 g 25% sodium thiosulfate, slow I.V. (1.65 mL/kg in children).	If symptoms return, treatment may be repeated at half the normal dosages. For pediatric dosing see package insert. Do **not** use methylene blue to reduce elevated methemoglobin levels. Oxygen therapy may be useful when combined with sodium thiosulfate therapy.

(continued)

Antidote	Poison/Drug	Indications	Dosage	Comments
Antivenin (*Crotalidae*) polyvalent (equine origin)	Pit viper bites (rattlesnakes, cotton-mouths, copperheads)	Mild, moderate, or severe symptoms and history of envenomation by a pit viper **Mild:** Local swelling, (progressive) pain, no systemic symptoms **Moderate:** Ecchymosis and swelling beyond the bite site, some systemic symptoms and/or lab changes **Severe:** Profound edema involving entire extremity, cyanosis, serious systemic involvement, significant lab changes	**Mild:** 3-5 vials of antivenin in 250-500 mL NS **Moderate:** 6-10 vials of antivenin in 500 mL NS **Severe:** Minimum of 10 vials in 500-1000 mL NS Administer over 4-6 hours. Additional antivenin should be given on the basis of clinical response and continuing assessment of severity of the poisoning.	Draw blood for type and crossmatch, hematocrit, BUN, electrolytes, CBC, platelets, coagulation profile. Do **not** administer heparin for possible allergic reaction. A tetanus shot should also be given.
Atropine	Organophosphate and carbamate insecticides, mushrooms containing muscarine (inocybe or clitocybe)	Myoclonic seizures, severe hallucinations, weakness, arrhythmias, excessive salivation, involuntary urination, and defecation	**Children:** I.V.: 0.05 mg/kg **Adults:** I.V.: 1-2 mg Repeat dosage every 10 minutes until patient is atropinized (normal pulse, dilated pupils, absence of rales, dry mouth)	Caution should be used in patients with narrow-angle glaucoma, cardiovascular disease, or pregnancy. Plasma and/or erythrocyte cholinesterase levels will be depressed from normal. Atropine should only be used when indicated; otherwise, use may result in anticholinergic poisoning. For organophosphate poisoning, large doses of atropine may be required.
Calcium EDTA (calcium disodium versenate)	Lead	Symptomatic patients or asymptomatic children with blood levels >50 μg/dL	50-75 mg/kg/day deep I.M. or slow I.V. infusion in 3-6 divided doses for up to 5 days	If urine flow is not established, hemodialysis must accompany calcium EDTA dosing. In most cases, the I.M. route is preferred.

(continued)

Antidote	Poison/Drug	Indications	Dosage	Comments
Calcium gluconate	Hydrofluoric acid (HF), magnesium	Calcium gluconate gel 2.5% for dermal exposures of HF <20% concentration S.C. injections of calcium gluconate for dermal exposures of HF in >20% concentration or failure to respond to calcium gluconate gel	Massage 2.5% gel into exposed area for 15 minutes. Infiltrate each square centimeter of exposed area with 0.5 mL of 10% calcium gluconate S.C. using a 30-gauge needle. 1 mL/kg I.V. of a 10% solution for magnesium toxicity	Injections of calcium gluconate should not be used in digital area. With exposures to dilute concentrations of HF, symptoms may take several hours to develop. Calcium gluconate gel is not currently available. Contact your regional poison control center for compounding instructions.
Deferoxamine (Desferal®)	Iron	Serum iron >350 µg/dL. Inability to obtain serum iron in a reasonable time and patient is symptomatic.	**Mild symptoms:** I.M.: 10 mg/kg up to 1 g every 8 hours **Severe symptoms:** I.V.: 10-15 mg/kg/hour not to exceed 6 g in 24 hours; rates up to 35 mg/kg have been given.	Passing of √ in rose-colored urine indicates free iron was present. Therapy should be discontinued when urine returns to normal color. Monitor for hypotension, especially when giving deferoxamine I.V.
Digoxin immune Fab (ovine), (Digibind®)	Digoxin, digitoxin, oleander, foxglove, lily-of-the-valley (?), red squill (?)	Life-threatening cardiac arrhythmias, progressive bradyarrhythmias, second or third degree heart block unresponsive to atropine, serum digoxin level >5 ng/mL, potassium levels >5 mEq/L, or ingestion of >10 mg in adults (or 4 mg in children).	Multiply serum digoxin concentration at steady-state level by 5.6 and multiply the result by the patient's weight in kilograms, divide this by 1000 and divide the result by 0.6. This gives the dose in number of vials to use. For other dosing methods, see package insert.	Monitor potassium levels, continuous EKG. **Note:** Digibind® interferes with serum digoxin/digitoxin levels.

(continued)

Antidote	Poison/Drug	Indications	Dosage	Comments
Dimercaprol (BAL in oil)	Arsenic, lead, mercury, gold, trivalent antimony, methyl bromide, methyl iodide	Any symptoms due to arsenic exposure	3-5 mg/kg/dose deep I.M. every 4 hours until GI symptoms subside and patient switched to D-penicillamine	Patients receiving dimercaprol should be monitored for hypertension, tachycardia, hyperpyrexia, and urticaria. Used in conjunction with calcium EDTA in lead poisoning.
		All patients with symptoms or asymptomatic children with blood levels >70 µg/dL	3-5 mg/kg/dose deep I.M. every 4 hours for 2 days then every 4-12 hours for up to 7 additional days	
		Any symptoms due to mercury and patient unable to take D-penicillamine	3-5 mg/kg/dose deep I.M. every 4 hours for 48 hours, then 3 mg/kg/dose every 6 hours, then 3 mg/kg/dose every 12 hours for 7 more days	
Ethanol	Ethylene glycol or methanol	Ethylene glycol or methanol blood levels >20 mg/dL	**Loading dose:** I.V.: 7.5-10 mL/kg 10% ethanol in D₅W over 1 hour	Monitor blood glucose, especially in children, as ethanol may cause hypoglycemia. Do not use 5% ethanol in D₅W as excessive amounts of fluid would be required to maintain adequate ethanol blood levels. If dialysis is performed, adjustment of ethanol dosing is required.
		Blood levels not readily available and suspected ingestion of toxic amounts	**Maintenance dose:** I.V.: 1.4 mL/kg/hour of 10% ethanol in D₅W. Maintain blood ethanol level of 100-200 mg/dL.	
		Any symptomatic patient with a history of ethylene glycol or methanol ingestion		
Flumazenil (Romazicon®)	Benzodiazepine	As adjunct to conventional management/diagnosis of benzodiazepine overdose	I.V.: 0.2 mg over 30 seconds; wait another 30 seconds, and then give an additional 0.3 mg over 30 seconds. Additional doses of 0.5 mg over 30 seconds at 1-minute intervals up to a cumulative dose of 3 mg.	Onset of reversal usually within 1-2 minutes. Contraindicated in patients with epilepsy, increased intracranial pressure, or coingestion of seizuregenic agents (ie, cyclic antidepressant).

(continued)

Antidote	Poison/Drug	Indications	Dosage	Comments
Glucagon	Propranolol: Hypoglycemic agents	Propranolol-induced cardiac dysfunction Treatment of hypoglycemia	S.C., I.M., or I.V.: 0.5-1 mg May repeat after 15 minutes	Requires liver glycogen stores for hyperglycemic response. Intravenous glucose must also be given in treatment of hypoglycemia.
Leucovorin (citrovorum factor, folinic acid)	Methotrexate, trimethoprim, pyrimethamine, methanol, trimetrexate	Methotrexate-induced bone marrow depression (methotrexate serum level >1 x 10⁻⁵ mmol/L); may also be useful in pyrimethamine-trimethoprim bone marrow depression	Dose should be equal to or greater than the dose of methotrexate ingested. Usually 10-100 mg/m²is given I.V. or orally every 6 hours for 72 hours.	Most effective if given within 1 hour after exposure. May not be effective to prevent liver toxicity. Monitor methotrexate levels. May enhance the toxicity of fluorouracil.
Methylene blue	Methemoglobin inducers (ie, nitrites, phenazopyridine)	Cyanosis Methemoglobin level >30% in an asymptomatic patient	I.V.: 1-2 mg/kg (0.1-0.2 mL/kg) per dose over 2-3 minutes. May repeat doses as needed clinically. Injection can be given as 1% solution or diluted in normal saline.	Treatment can result in falsely elevated methemoglobin levels when measured by a co-oximeter. Large doses (>15 mg/kg) may cause hemolysis.
Naloxone (Narcan®)	Opiates (eg, heroin, morphine, codeine)	Coma or respiratory depression from unknown cause or from opiate overdose	Give 0.4-2.0 mg I.V. bolus. Doses may be repeated if there is no response, up to 10 mg.	For prolonged intoxication, a continuous infusion may be used. See package insert for details or table previously presented in this text titled "Drugs to be Utilized in the Toxic Patient With Altered Mental Status.".

(continued)

Antidote	Poison/Drug	Indications	Dosage	Comments
D-penicillamine (Cuprimine®)	Arsenic, lead, mercury	Following BAL therapy in symptomatic acutely poisoned patients; Asymptomatic patients with excess lead burden; Patient symptomatic from mercury exposure or excessive levels	100 mg/kg/day up to 2 g in 4 divided doses for 5 days; 1-2 g/day in 4 divided doses for 5 days; **Children:** 100 mg/kg/day up to 1 g/day in 4 divided doses. Given for 3-10 days. **Adults:** P.O.: 250 mg 4 times/day	Possible contraindication for patients with penicillin allergy. Monitor heavy metal levels daily in severely poisoned patients. Monitor CBC and renal function in patients receiving chronic D-penicillamine therapy. Dosages given are for short-term acute therapy only.
Physostigmine salicylate (Antilirium®)	Atropine and anticholinergic agents, cyclic antidepressants	Myoclonic seizures, severe arrhythmias	**Children:** Slow I.V. push: 0.5 mg. Repeat as required for life-threatening symptoms **Adults:** Slow I.V. push: 0.5-2 mg	Dramatic reversal of anticholinergic symptoms after I.V. use. Should not be used just to keep patient awake. **Contraindications:** Asthma, gangrene; physostigmine use in cyclic antidepressant-induced cardiac toxicity it controversial. **Extreme caution** is advised — should be considered only in the presence of life-threatening anticholinergic symptoms.
	Intrathecal baclofen	Refractory seizures or arrhythmias unresponsive to conventional therapies	Same as above	
Pralidoxime (2-PAM, Protopam®)	Organophosphate, insecticides, tacrine	An adjunct to atropine therapy for treatment of profound muscle weakness, respiratory depression, muscle twitching	**Children:** 25-50 mg/kg in 250 mL saline over 30 minutes **Adults:** I.V.: 2 g at 0.5 g/minute or infused in 250 mL NS over 30 minutes	Most effective when used in initial 24-36 hours after the exposure. Dosage may be repeated in 1 hour followed by every 8 hours if indicated.
Phytonadione (vitamin K₁)	Coumarin derivatives, indandione derivatives	Large acute ingestion of warfarin rodenticides; chronic exposure or greater than normal prothrombin time	**Children:** I.M.: 1-5 mg. With severe toxicity, vitamin K₁ may be given I.V. **Adults:** I.M.: 10 mg	Vitamin K therapy is relatively contraindicated for patients with prosthetic heart valves unless toxicity is life-threatening.

(continued)

Antidote	Poison/Drug	Indications	Dosage	Comments
Protamine sulfate	Heparin	Severe hemorrhage	Maximum rate of 5 mg/minute up to a total dose of 200 mg in 2 hours. 1 mg of protamine neutralizes 90 units of beef lung heparin or 115 units of pork intestinal heparin.	Monitor partial thromboplastin time or activated coagulation time. Effect may be immediate and can last for 2 hours. Monitor for hypotension.
Pyridoxine (vitamin B$_6$)	Isoniazid monomethyl-hydrazine-containing mushrooms (Gyromitra); acrylamide, hydrazine	Unknown overdose or ingested isoniazid (INH) amount >80 mg/kg	I.V. pyridoxine in the amount of INH ingested or 5 g if amount is unknown given over 30-60 minutes.	Cumulative dose of pyridoxine is arbitrarily limited to 40 g in adults and 20 g in children.
Succimer (Chemet®)	Lead, arsenic, mercury	Asymptomatic children with venous blood lead 45-69 μg/dL. Not FDA approved for adult lead exposure or other metals.	P.O.: 10 mg/kg or 350 mg/m^2 every 8 hours for 5 days. Reduce to 10 mg/kg or 350 mg/m^2 every 12 hours for an additional 2 weeks.	Monitor liver function; emits "rotten egg" sulfur odor.

From Rush Poison Control Center, Rush-Presbyterian-St Luke's Medical Center, Chicago, IL 60612.

SERUM SALICYLATE INTOXICATION NOMOGRAM

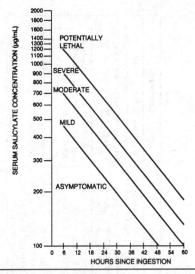

Nomogram relating serum salicylate concentration and estimated severity of intoxication at varying intervals following ingestion of a single toxic dose of salicylate. Modified from Done AK, "Salicylate Intoxication", Pediatrics, 1960, 26:800-7. © American Academy of Pediatrics, 1960.

ACETAMINOPHEN TOXICITY NOMOGRAM

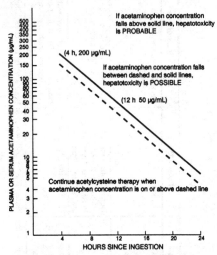

Nomogram relating plasma or serum acetaminophen concentration and probability of hepatotoxicity at varying intervals following ingestion of a single toxic dose of acetaminophen. Modified from Rumack BH, Matthew H, "Acetaminophen Poisoning and Toxicity", Pediatrics, 1975, 55:871-6,
© American Academy of Pediatrics, 1975, and from Rumack BH, et al, "Acetaminophen Overdose", Arch Intern Med, 1981, 141:380-5,
© American Medical Association.

IBUPROFEN TOXICITY NOMOGRAM

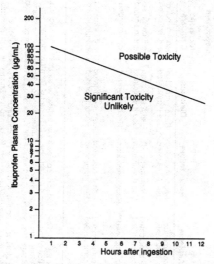

Ibuprofen nomogram, (From Hall AH, Smolinske SC, Stover B, et al, "Ibuprofen Overdose in Adults," *J Toxicol Clin Toxicol*, 1992, 30:34.)

VACCINES

Summary of ACIP Recommendations on Immunization of Immunocompromised Adults*

Vaccine†	Routine (Not Immuno-compromised)	HIV Infection or AIDS	Severely Immuno-compromised (Non-HIV related)‡	Solid-Organ Transplant Recipient Receiving Chronic Immuno-suppressive Therapy	Asplenia	Renal failure	Diabetes	Alcoholism and Alcoholic Cirrhosis
Td	Recommended	Recommended	Recommended	Recommended	Recommended	Recommended	Recommended	Recommended
MMR (MR, M, or R)	Use if indicated	Recommended/considered§	Contraindicated	Contraindicated	Use if indicated	Use if indicated	Use if indicated	Use if indicated
Hepatitis B	Use if indicated	Use if indicated	Use if indicated	Use if indicated	Use if indicated	Recommended¶	Use if indicated	Use if indicated
Hib	Not recommended	Considered#	Recommended	Recommended	Recommended	Use if indicated	Use if indicated	Recommended
Pneumococcal	Recommended if ≥65 years of age	Recommended**	Recommended**	Recommended**	Recommended**	Recommended††	Recommended	Recommended
Meningococcal	Use if indicated	Use if indicated	Use if indicated	Use if indicated	Recommended	Use if indicated	Use if indicated	Use if indicated
Influenza	Recommended if ≥65 years of age	Recommended	Recommended	Recommended	Recommended	Recommended	Recommended	Recommended

Clin Pharm, 1993; 12:675-84.

*A "recommended" entry indicates that the vaccine is recommended as part of the routine schedule or the medical condition represents an indication for use of the vaccine. A "use if indicated" entry indicates that the immunosuppression category is not a contraindication to use of the vaccine if it is otherwise indicated. A "contraindicated" entry indicates that the medical condition is an absolute or relative contraindication to use of the vaccine. A "considered" entry indicates that a decision to use the vaccine should include consideration of the individual patient's risk of disease and the likely effectiveness of the vaccine. See section on Principles for Vaccinating Immunocompromised Persons for a discussion of categories of immunosuppression.

†Td = tetanus and diphtheria toxoids adsorbed for adult use; MMR = measles, mumps, and rubella virus vaccine live; and Hib = *Haemophilus* b conjugate vaccine.

‡Severe immunosuppression can be the result of congenital immunosuppression, human immunodeficiency virus (HIV) infection, leukemia, lymphoma, aplastic anemia, generalized malignancy, or therapy with alkylating agents, antimetabolites, radiation, or large amounts of corticosteroids.

§See discussion of MMR in text.

¶Patients with renal failure on dialysis should have their anti-HB$_s$ (antibodies to hepatitis B surface antigen) response tested after vaccination, and those found not to respond should be revaccinated.

#See discussion of HIV-infected persons.

**Reimmunize every 6 years.

††Reimmunize every 3-5 years.

Summary of ACIP Recommendations on Nonroutine Immunization of Immunocompromised Persons*

Vaccine†	(Not Immuno-compromised)	HIV Infection or AIDS	Severely Immuno-compromised (Non-HIV related)‡	Solid-Organ Transplant Recipient Receiving Chronic Immuno-suppressive Therapy	Asplenia Renal failure Diabetes Alcoholism and Alcoholic Cirrhosis
Live Vaccines					
BCG	Use if indicated	Contraindicated	Contraindicated	Contraindicated	Use if indicated
OPV	Use if indicated	Contraindicated	Contraindicated	Contraindicated	Use if indicated
Vaccinia	Use if indicated	Contraindicated	Contraindicated	Contraindicated	Use if indicated
Typhoid, TY21a	Use if indicated	Contraindicated	Contraindicated	Contraindicated	Use if indicated
Yellow fever§	Use if indicated	Contraindicated	Contraindicated	Contraindicated	Use if indicated
Killed or Inactivated Vaccines					
eIPV	Use if indicated	Use if indicated	Use if indicated	Use if indicated	Use if indicated
Cholera	Use if indicated	Use if indicated	Use if indicated	Use if indicated	Use if indicated
Plague	Use if indicated	Use if indicated	Use if indicated	Use if indicated	Use if indicated
Typhoid, inactivated	Use if indicated	Use if indicated	Use if indicated	Use if indicated	Use if indicated
Rabies	Use if indicated	Use if indicated	Use if indicated	Use if indicated	Use if indicated
Anthrax	Use if indicated	Use if indicated	Use if indicated	Use if indicated	Use if indicated

Clin Pharm, 1993, 12:675-84.

*A "use if indicated" entry indicates that the immunosuppression category is not a contraindication to use of the vaccine if it is otherwise indicated. A "contraindicated" entry indicates that the medical condition is an absolute or relative contraindication to use of the vaccine. See section on Principles for Vaccinating Immunocompromised Persons for a discussion of categories of immunosuppression.

†BCG = bacillus Calmette-Guérin vaccine; OPV = oral poliovirus vaccine live; eIPV = enhanced inactivated poliovirus vaccine.

‡Severe immunosuppression can be the result of congenital immunosuppression, human immunodeficiency virus (HIV) infection, leukemia, lymphoma, aplastic anemia, generalized malignancy, or therapy with alkylating agents, antimetabolites, radiation, or large amounts of corticosteroids.

§Yellow fever vaccine should be considered for patients when yellow fever exposure cannot be avoided (see text).

Summary of ACIP Recommendations on Use of Immune Globulins in Immunocompromised Persons*

Immune Globulin	Not Immunocompromised	HIV Infected	Severely Immunocompromised†
IG	Recommended for infants and adults with contraindication to measles vaccine exposed to measles	Recommended for symptomatic patients exposed to measles regardless of immunization status	Recommended for patients exposed to measles regardless of immunization status
		Recommended for persons with exposure to hepatitis A or who will travel to HAV-endemic areas	
VZIG‡	Recommended for newborns of mothers who develop chickenpox within 5 days before and 48 hours after delivery	Recommended for susceptible infants and adults after significant exposure to V-Z	Recommended for susceptible infants and adults after significant exposure to V-Z
	Recommended for exposed newborns (≥28 weeks' gestation) of susceptible mothers		
	Recommended for exposed preterm infants (<28 weeks or <1000 g)		
	May be used for exposed susceptible adults, exposed pregnant women, and infants <28 days		
TIG	Recommended for those with serious wounds and <3 doses of tetanus toxoid	Same as for nonimmunocompromised	Same as for nonimmunocompromised
HBIG	Recommended for prophylaxis of infants born to HB_sAg^+ mothers and susceptible persons with percutaneous, sexual, or mucosal exposure to HB virus	Same as for nonimmunocompromised	Same as for nonimmunocompromised
HRIG	Recommended for postexposure prophylaxis of persons not previously vaccinated against rabies	Same as for nonimmunocompromised	Same as for nonimmunocompromised

Clin Pharm, 1993, 12:675-84.

*IG = immune globulin; VZIG = varicella-zoster immune globulin; TIG = tetanus immune globulin; HBIG = hepatitis B immune globulin; HRIG = human rabies immune globulin; HAV = hepatitis A virus; V-Z = varicella-zoster; HB_sAg + = positive for hepatitis B surface antigen; HB = hepatitis B.
†Severe immunosuppression can be the result of congenital immunosuppression, human immunodeficiency virus (HIV) infection, leukemia, lymphoma, aplastic anemia, generalized malignancy, or therapy with alkylating agents, antimetabolites, radiation, or large amounts of corticosteroids.
‡See section on Use of Immune Globulins for a discussion of issues to be considered before use of VZIG.

IMMUNIZATION GUIDELINES

Although there are small numbers of patients for whom specific vaccines are definitely contraindicated, it is likely that far greater numbers of patients fail to receive needed vaccines because of misconceptions concerning contraindications to adult immunizations. Some of the most common of these misconceptions are listed in the following table.

Conditions Which Are Not Considered to Be Contraindications to Vaccinations

- Reaction to a previous DTP dose that involved only soreness, redness, or swelling in the area of the vaccination site or temperature of less than 105°F (40.5°C)
- Mild acute illness with low-grade fever or mild diarrheal illness in an otherwise well child
- Current antimicrobial therapy or the convalescent phase of illness
- Prematurity
- Pregnancy of mother or other household contact
- Recent exposure to an infectious disease
- Breast-feeding
- A history of nonspecific allergies or relatives with allergies
- Allergies to penicillin or any other antibiotic, except anaphylactic reactions to neomycin or streptomycin
- Allergies to duck meat or duck feathers
- Family history of convulsions in persons considered for pertussis or measles vaccination
- Family history of sudden infant death syndrome in children considered for DTP vaccination
- Family history of an adverse event, unrelated to immunosuppression, following vaccination

Contraindications to Immunization

Minor illness is not a contraindication to vaccination, especially if the patient has a minor upper respiratory infection or allergic rhinitis. Delay of immunization should be considered if expected or potential vaccine side effects may accentuate or be accentuated by an underlying illness. Note that fever is not itself a contraindication to vaccination, however, if fever is associated with other signs of serious underlying illness, vaccination should be deferred until the patient has recovered. Moderate or severe illness, with or without fever, is considered a contraindication to DTP administration, as signs and symptoms associated with the underlying illness may be incorrectly attributed to the DTP vaccine.

The following conditions should be evaluated as possible contraindications to vaccination:

Vaccine	Possible Contraindications
DTP	Previous serious reaction to DTP, TD, or Td
(see *Red Book*,	Serious immunosuppressive therapy
p 366-9)	Thimerosal allergy
	Progressive neurological disorder or uncontrolled seizure disorder
	Disorders associated with conditions that predispose to either seizures or neurological deterioration
	Age 7 years or older (Td recommended)
OPV	Immunosuppression
	Immunosuppressed household contacts
	Age 18 years and older (IPV recommended)
	Pregnancy
Hib	Serious thimerosal allergy
	Serious allergic reaction to vaccine containing diphtheria toxoid
	Age 5 years and older
MMR	Serious egg allergy
	Immunosuppression
	Gamma globulin therapy within preceding 3 months
	Serious neomycin or streptomycin allergy
	Pregnancy

Table 1. **Dosage and Administration Guidelines for Vaccines Available in the United States**

Vaccine	Dosage	Route of Administration	Type
DT*	0.5 mL	I.M.	Toxoids
Td*	0.5 mL	I.M.	Toxoids
DTP*	0.5 mL	I.M.	Diphtheria and tetanus toxoids with killed *B. pertussis* organisms
DTaP (Acel-Imune®)‖	0.5 mL	I.M.	Diphtheria and tetanus toxoids with acellular pertussis
DTP-HbOC (Tetramune®)+	0.5 mL	I.M.	Diphtheria and tetanus toxoids with killed *B. pertussis* organisms and Haemophilus b conjugate (diphtheria CRM_{197} protein conjugate)
Haemophilus B conjugate vaccine	0.5 mL	I.M.	
ProHIBit® (PRP-D), manufactured by Connaught Laboratories	0.5 mL	I.M.	Polysaccharide (diphtheria toxoid conjugate)
HibTITER® (HbOC),† manufactured by Praxis Biologicals	0.5 mL	I.M.	Oligosaccharide (diphtheria CRM_{197} protein conjugate)
PedvaxHIB® (PRP-OMP),‡ manufactured by MSD	0.5 mL	I.M.	Polysaccharide (meningococcal protein conjugate)

Hepatitis B§

I.M. in the anterolateral thigh or in the upper arm; S.C. in individuals at risk of hemorrhage

Yeast recombinant-derived inactivated viral antigen

Infants born to HB_sAg-negative mothers and children <11 y■
- Recombivax HB® (MSD) 2.5 mcg (0.25 mL)
- Engerix-B® (SKF) 10 mcg (0.5 mL)

Infants born to HB_sAg-positive mothers (immunization and administration of 0.5 mL hepatitis B immune globulin is recommended for **infants** born to HB_sAg^+ mothers using different administration sites) within 12 hours of birth; administer vaccine at birth; repeat vaccine dose at 1 and 6 months following the initial dose
- Recombivax HB® (MSD) 5 mcg (0.5 mL)
- Engerix-B® (SKF) 10 mcg (0.5 mL)

Children 11-19 y
- Recombivax HB® (MSD) 5 mcg (0.5 mL)
- Engerix-B® (SKF) 20 mcg (1 mL)

Adults >19 y
- Recombivax HB® (MSD) 10 mcg (1 mL)
- Engerix-B® (SKF) 20 mcg (1 mL)

Dialysis patients and immunosuppressed patients
- Recombivax HB® (MSD) <11 y, 20 mcg (0.5 mL); ≥11 y, 40 mcg (1 mL) using special dialysis formulation

(continued)

Vaccine	Dosage	Route of Administration	Type
Engerix-B® (SKF)¶	<11 y, 20 mcg (1 mL); ≥11 y, 40 mcg (2 mL), give as two 1 mL doses at different sites		
Influenza split virus only in pediatric patients		I.M. (2 doses 4+ weeks apart in children <9 years of age not previously immunized; only 1 dose needed for annual updates)	Inactivated virus subvirion (split) (contraindicated in patients allergic to chicken eggs)
6-35 mo	0.25 mL (1 or 2 doses)		
3-8 y	0.5 mL (1 or 2 doses)		
≥9 y	0.5 mL (1 dose)		
Measles	0.5 mL	S.C.	Live virus (contraindicated in patients with anaphylactic allergy to neomycin)

Most areas: Two doses (1st dose at 15 months with MMR; 2nd dose at 4-6 years or 11-12 years, depending on local school entry requirements)

High-risk area: Two doses (1st dose at 12 months with MMR; 2nd dose as above)

Children 6-15 months in epidemic situations: Dose is given at the time of first contact with a healthcare provider; children <1 year of age should receive single antigen measles vaccine. If vaccinated before 1 year, revaccinate at 15 months with MMR. A 3rd dose is administered at 4-6 years or 11-12 years, depending on local school entry requirements.

Vaccine	Dosage	Route of Administration	Type
Meningococcal	0.5 mL#	S.C.	Polysaccharide
MMR•	0.5 mL	S.C.	Live virus
MR	0.5 mL	S.C.	Live virus
Mumps	0.5 mL	S.C.	Live virus
Pneumococcal polyvalent♦	0.5 mL (≥2 y)	I.M. or S.C. (I.M. preferred)	Polysaccharide
Poliovirus (OPV) trivalent	0.5 mL	Oral	Live virus
Poliovirus (IPV)**·†† trivalent	0.5 mL	S.C.	Inactivated virus
Rabies	1 mL	I.M.‡‡, ID§§	Inactivated virus
Rubella	0.5 mL (≥12 mo)¶¶	S.C.	Live virus
Tetanus (adsorbed)##	0.5 mL	I.M.	Toxoid
Tetanus (fluid)	0.5 mL	I.M., S.C.	Toxoid
Yellow fever	0.5 mL⚫	S.C.	Live attenuated virus

*DT & DTP for use in children <7 years of age. Td contains same amount of tetanus toxoid as DT & DTP, but a reduced dose of diphtheria toxoid. Td for use in children ≥7 years of age.

‖DTaP (Acel-Imune®) may be used only for the 4th and 5th doses for children >15 months and <7 years of age. The occurrence of fever and local reactions is lower with acellular pertussis vaccine than with whole-cell DTP.

⁺DTP-HbOC may be substituted for DTP and Haemophilus B conjugate vaccines which are administered separately, whenever recommended schedules for use of these 2 vaccines coincide. Initiate at 2 months of age for 3 doses (2 months, 4 months, and 6 months), followed by a 4th dose at 15-18 months of age. DTaP and Haemophilus B conjugate vaccine may be administered separately as an alternative to DTP-HbOC at 15-18 months of age.

†The conjugate (HbCV) vaccine is preferred over the polysaccharide (HbPV) vaccine. In children with a high risk for *Haemophilus influenzae* type b disease and HbCV is unavailable, an acceptable alternate is to give HbPV at 18 months of age with a 2nd dose at 24 months of age. Children <5 years of age who were previously vaccinated with HbPV between 18-23 months of age should be revaccinated with a single dose of HbCV at least 2 months after the initial dose of HbPV. Either HbCV or HbPV can be administered up to the 5th birthday. However they are generally not recommended for children >5 years of age.

‡PRP-OMP (PedvaxHIB®) manufactured by Merck, Sharp & Dohme is initiated at 2 months of age for 3 doses (2 months, 4 months and 12 months). If initiated at 7-11 months of age, 3 doses are administered (initial 2 doses at 2-month intervals, 3rd dose at 15-18 months of age); initiated at 12-14 months of age, 2 doses are administered at 2- to 3-month intervals between doses; initiated at 15-59 months of age, 1 dose is administered.

§Hepatitis B vaccine can be given at the same time with DTP, HbOC, polio, and/or MMR; administer 3 doses at 0, 1, and 6 months).

■Administer to newborns at 0-2 days of age before hospital discharge; repeat at 1-2 months and 6-18 months following the initial dose. If not vaccinated at birth, administer at 2, 4, and 6-18 months of age.

¶Engerix-B® — an alternate schedule for postexposure prophylaxis or more rapid induction using 4 doses at 0, 1, 2, and 12 months of age is recommended.

#Indicated in children ≥2 years of age at risk in epidemic or highly endemic areas.

•See measles.

♦Indicated for children with sickle cell disease; asplenia; nephrotic syndrome or chronic renal failure; conditions associated with immunosuppression; CSF leaks; HIV infection.

**The primary series consists of 3 doses. The first 2 doses should be administered at an interval of 8 weeks. The 3rd dose should be given at least 6 and preferably 12 months after the 2nd dose. A booster dose of 0.5 mL should be given to all children who have completed the primary series, before entering school. However, if the 3rd dose of the primary series is given on or after the 4th birthday, a 4th dose is not required before entering school. When polio vaccine is given to persons >18 years of age, IPV should be given.

††IPV is indicated for unimmunized or partially immunized patients with compromised immunity; HIV infection; unimmunized adults (>18 years of age) or adults at future risk of exposure to poliomyelitis; household contacts of an immunodeficient individual.

‡‡In infants and small children, I.M. injection can be given into the midlateral aspect of the thigh; in older children and adults, I.M. injection can be given into the deltoid muscle. Repeat doses are given on days 3, 7, 14, and 28 postexposure.

§§For pre-exposure prophylaxis against rabies for high-risk individuals, 1 mL I.M. or 0.1 mL intradermal is administered on days 0, 7, and 21 (or 28). Both I.M. and I.D. dosage forms are available.

¶¶As MMR in a 2-dose schedule.

##Adsorbed preferred to fluid toxoid because of longer lasting immunity.

➡≥9 months of age living in or traveling to endemic areas. Contraindicated in infants <4 months of age and in patients who have had an anaphylactic reaction to eggs. Increased risk of encephalitis associated with use of yellow fever vaccine in infants <9 months of age.

Note: For each vaccine, check the manufacturer's package insert for specific product information since preparations may change from time to time.

References:

ACIP, General Recommendations on Immunization, *MMWR*, 1989, 38:205-14, 219-27.

ACIP, Measles Prevention, Recommendations of the Immunization Practices Advisory Committee, *MMWR*, 1989, 38(5-9):1-18.

American Academy of Pediatrics, Report of the Committee on Infectious Diseases (Red Book), 22nd ed, 1991.

American Academy of Pediatrics, Committee on Infectious Diseases, "Acellular Pertussis Vaccines: Recommendations for Use as the Fourth and Fifth Doses," *Pediatrics*, 1992, 90:121-3.

American Academy of Pediatrics, Committee on Infectious Diseases, "Universal Hepatitis B Immunization," *Pediatrics*, 1992, 89:795-800.

Table 2. **Recommended Schedule for Active Immunization
of Normal Infants and Children****

Recommended Age	Vaccine(s)	Comments
Newborn	Hepatitis B #1	
1-2 mo	Hepatitis B #2	
2 mo	DTP1,* OPV1, HbCV1†	OPV and DTP can be given earlier in areas of high endemicity or during epidemics; DTP-HbOC can be given in place of DTP1 and HbCV1
4 mo	DTP2, OPV2, HbCV2†	6 weeks to 2 months interval desired between OPV doses; DTP-HbOC can be given in place of DTP2 and HbCV2
6 mo	DTP3, HbOC3, hepatitis B #3	An additional dose of OPV is optional in high risk areas; DTP-HbOC can be given in place of DTP3 and HbOC3
12 mo	PRP-OMP	
15 mo	MMR,‡ DTP4,¶ OPV3, HbCV3, or HbCV4§	Completion of primary series of DTP and OPV; DTP-HbOC can be given in place of DTP4 and HbCV
4-6 y	DTP5,¶ OPV4, measles	At or before school entry
11-12 y	MMR	At entry to middle school unless 2nd dose was given at 4-6 years at time of school entry
14-16 y	Td	Repeat every 10 years throughout life

**Please also refer to Hepatitis B Vaccine Guidelines in Table 1.

*DTP may be used up to the 7th birthday. The 1st dose can be given at 6th week of age, and the 2nd and 3rd doses given 4-8 weeks after the preceding dose.

†HbCV — can use either HbOC or PRP-OMP.

‡Can be given at 12 months of age in high-risk areas.

§HbCV — can use either PRP-OMP, PRP-D, or HbOC for children ≥15 months of age.

¶DTaP may be used in place of whole cell DTP only for the 4th and 5th doses for children >15 months and <7 years of age. DTaP can be given at the same time with OPV, IPV, MMR, *Haemophilus influenzae* type b conjugate vaccine, and/or hepatitis B vaccine.

References:

Centers for Disease Control, "Protection Against Viral Hepatitis: Recommendations of the Immunization Practices Advisory Committee (ACIP)," *MMWR*, 1990, 39:11.

American Academy of Pediatrics Committee on Infectious Diseases, "*Haemophilus influenzae* Type B Conjugate Vaccines: Recommendations for Immunization of Infants and Children 2 Months of Age and Older," *Pediatrics*, 1991, 88(1):169-72.

Table 3. **Recommended Immunization Schedule for Infants and Children up to the 7th Birthday Not Immunized at the Recommended Time in Early Infancy**

Timing	Vaccine(s)	Comments
First visit	DTP1, OPV1, MMR* (if child ≥15 months)	DTP, OPV, and MMR should be administered simultaneously to children ≥15 months of age
	HbCV†·‡, HBV1	DTP, OPV, MMR, and HbCV may be given simultaneously to children aged 15 months to 5 years at separate sites
2 mo after DTP1, OPV1	DTP2, OPV2, HBV2 (HbCV)‡	Second HbCV for children whose 1st dose was received when <15 months of age
2 mo after DTP2	DTP3	An additional dose of OPV is optional in high-risk areas
6 mo after HBV2	HBV3	
6-12 mo after DTP3	DTP4§ (OPV3)	OPV is given if 3rd dose was not given earlier
4-6 y	DTP5,§ OPV4 (MMR2)	Preferably at or before school entry. OTP5 and OPV4 are not needed if DTP4 and OPV3 were given after the 4th birthday. Local public health regulations may require MMR2 at school entry.
11-12 y	MMR2	MMR2 is given if 2nd dose was not given earlier
14-16 y	Td	Repeat every 10 years throughout life

*Can be given at 12 months of age to children residing in areas at high-risk for measles transmission.

†Only HbOC or PRP-OMP are licensed for use in children <15 months of age.

‡DTP-HbOC may be substituted for DTP and Haemophilus B conjugate vaccines which are administered separately, whenever recommended schedules for use of these 2 vaccines coincide. Initiate at 2 months of age for 3 doses (2 months, 4 months, and 6 months), followed by a 4th dose at 15-18 months of age. DTaP and Haemophilus B conjugate vaccine may be administered separately as an alternative to DTP-HbOC at 15-18 months.

§DTaP may be used in place of whole cell DTP only for the 4th and 5th doses for children >15 months and <7 years of age.

Table 4. **Recommended Immunization Schedule for Children >7 Years of Age Not Immunized at the Recommended Time in Early Infancy**

Timing	Vaccine(s)	Comments
First visit	Td1, OPV1, MMR, HbCV*	OPV not routinely recommended for persons ≥18 years of age
2 mo after Td1, OPV1	Td2, OPV2	OPV may be given as soon as 6 weeks after OPV1
6-12 mo after Td2, OPV2	Td3, OPV3	OPV3 may be given as soon as 6 weeks after OPV2
10 y after Td3	Td	Repeat every 10 years throughout life
11-12 y	MMR	

*Indicated only in children with a chronic illness associated with increased risk of *Haemophilus influenzae* type B disease.

RECOMMENDATIONS FOR USE OF *HAEMOPHILUS* B CONJUGATE VACCINES AND A COMBINED DIPHTHERIA, TETANUS, PERTUSSIS, AND *HAEMOPHILUS* B VACCINE
[Recommendations of the Advisory Committee on Immunization Practices (ACIP)]

Recommendations for Hib Vaccination — General

All infants should receive a conjugate Hib vaccine (separate or in combination with DTP (Tetramune®), beginning at age 2 months (but not earlier than 6 weeks). If the first vaccination is delayed beyond age 6 months, the schedule of vaccination for previously unimmunized children should be followed (see following table). When possible, the Hib conjugate vaccine used at the first vaccination should be used for all subsequent vaccinations in the primary series. When either Hib vaccines or Tetramune® is used, the vaccine should be administered intramuscularly using a separate syringe and administered at a separate site from any other concurrent vaccinations.

Schedule for Hib Conjugate Vaccine Administration Among Previously Vaccinated Children

Vaccine	Age at First Vaccination (mo)	Primary Series	Booster
HbOC/PRP-T*	2-6	3 doses, 2 mo apart	12-15 mo
	7-11	2 doses, 2 mo apart	12-18 mo
	12-14	1 dose	2 mo later
	15-59	1 dose	—
PRP-OMP	2-6	2 doses, 2 mo apart	12-15 mo
	7-11	2 doses, 2 mo apart	12-18 mo
	12-14	1 dose	2 mo later
	15-59	1 dose	—
PRP-D	15-59	1 dose	—

*Tetramune® may be administered by the same schedule for primary immunization as HbOC/PRP-T (when the series begins at 2-6 months of age). A booster dose of DTP or DTaP should be administered at 4-6 years of age, before kindergarten or elementary school. This booster is not necessary if the fourth vaccinating dose was administered after the fourth birthday. See ACIP statement for information on use of DTP and contraindications for use of pertussis vaccine.
—Not applicable.

Other Considerations for Hib Vaccination

Other considerations for Hib vaccination are discussed in the following section:

1. Although an interval of 2 months between doses of Hib vaccine in the primary series is recommended, an interval of 1 month is acceptable, if necessary.

2. Unvaccinated children aged 15-59 months may be administered a single dose of any one of the four Hib conjugate vaccines or Tetramune® (if both Hib and DTP vaccines are indicated).

3. After the primary infant vaccination series is completed, any of the four licensed Hib conjugate vaccines (or Tetramune® if both Hib vaccine and DTP vaccine are indicated) may be used as a booster dose at age 12-15 months.

4. The primary vaccine series should preferably be completed with the same Hib conjugate vaccine. If, however, different vaccines are administered, a total of three doses of Hib conjugate vaccine is adequate. Any combination of Hib conjugate vaccines that is licensed for use among infants may be used to complete the primary series.

5. Infants born prematurely should be vaccinated according to the schedule recommended for other infants, beginning at age 2 months.

6. Hib conjugate vaccines may be administered simultaneously with DTP (or DTaP) vaccine, OPV, IPV, MMR, influenza, and hepatitis B vaccines. Tetramune® may be administered simultaneously with OPV, IPV, MMR, influenza, and hepatitis B vaccines.

7. Because natural infection does not always result in the development of protective anti-PRP antibody levels, children <24 months of age who develop invasive Hib disease should receive Hib vaccine as recommended in the schedule. These children should be considered unimmunized, and vaccination should start as soon as possible during the convalescent phase of the illness.

8. Hib vaccine is immunogenic in patients with increased risk for invasive disease, such as those with sickle-cell disease, leukemia, human immunodeficiency virus (HIV) infection, and in those who have had splenectomies. However, in persons with HIV infection, immunogenicity varies with stage of infection and degree of immunocompromise. Efficacy studies have not been performed in populations with increased risk of invasive disease (see the general ACIP statement on use of vaccines and immune globulins in persons with altered immunocompetence).

9. Children who attend day care are at increased risk for Hib disease. Therefore, efforts should be made to ensure that all day-care attendees <5 years of age are fully vaccinated.

10. Rifampin chemoprophylaxis for household contacts of a person with invasive Hib disease is no longer indicated if all contacts ages <4 years are fully vaccinated against Hib disease. A child is considered fully immunized against Hib disease following a) at least one dose of conjugate vaccine at ≥15 months of age, b) two doses of conjugate vaccine at 12-14 months of age, or c) two or more doses of conjugate vaccine at <12 months of age, followed by a booster dose at ≥12 months of age. In households with one or more infants <12 months of age (regardless of vaccination status) or with a child aged 1-3 years who is inadequately vaccinated, all household contacts receive rifampin prophylaxis following a case of invasive Hib disease that occurs in any family member. The recommended dose is 20 mg/kg as a single daily dose (maximal daily dose 600 mg) for 4 days. Neonates (<1 month of age) should receive 10 mg/kg once daily for 4 days.

Contraindications and Precautions

Vaccination with a specific Hib conjugate vaccine is contraindicated in persons known to have experienced anaphylaxis following a prior dose of that vaccine. Vaccination should be delayed in children with moderate or severe illnesses. Minor illnesses (eg, mild upper-respiratory infection) are not contraindications to vaccination.

Contraindications and precautions of the use of Tetramune® are the same as those for its individual component vaccines (ie, DTP or Hib) (see the general ACIP statement on Diphtheria, Tetanus, and Pertussis: Recommendations for Vaccine Use and Other Preventive Measures for more details on the use of vaccines containing DTP).

High-Risk Groups Who Should Receive Hepatitis B Immunization Regardless of Age*

- Hemophiliac patients and other recipients of certain blood products
- Intravenous drug abusers
- Heterosexual persons who have had more than one sex partner in the previous 6 months and/or those with a recent episode of a sexually transmitted disease
- Sexually active homosexual and bisexual males
- Household and sexual contacts of hepatitis B virus (HBV) carriers
- Members of households with adoptees from HBV-endemic, high-risk countries who are hepatitis B surface antigen-positive
- Children and other household contacts in populations of high HBV endemicity
- Staff and residents of institutions for the developmentally disabled
- Staff of nonresidential day care and school programs for developmentally disabled if attended by known HBV carrier; other attendees in certain circumstances
- Hemodialysis patients
- Healthcare workers and others with occupational risk
- International travelers who will live for more than 6 months in areas of high HBV endemicity and who otherwise will be at risk
- Inmates of long-term correctional facilities

*Adapted from Report of the Committee on Infectious Disease, 1991, 246-9.

Postexposure Prophylaxis for Hepatitis B*

Exposure	Hepatitis B Immune Globulin	Hepatitis B Vaccine
Perinatal	0.5 mL I.M. within 12 h of birth	0.5 mL† I.M. within 12 h of birth (no later than 7 d), and at 1 and 6 mo‡; test for HB$_s$Ag and anti-HB$_s$ at 12-15 mo
Sexual	0.06 mL/kg I.M. within 14 d of sexual contact; a second dose should be given if the index patient remains HB$_s$Ag-positive after 3 mo and hepatitis B vaccine was not given initially	1 mL I.M. at 0, 1, and 6 mo for homosexual and bisexual men and regular sexual contacts of persons with acute and chronic hepatitis B
Percutaneous; exposed person unvaccinated		
Source known HB$_s$Ag-positive	0.06 mL/kg I.M. within 24 h	1 mL I.M. within 7 d, and at 1 and 6 mo§
Source known, HB$_s$Ag status not known	Test source for HB$_s$Ag; if source is positive, give exposed person 0.06 mL/kg I.M. once within 7 d	1 mL I.M. within 7 d, and at 1 and 6 mo§
Source not tested or unknown	Nothing required	1 mL I.M. within 7 d, and at 1 and 6 mo
Percutaneous; exposed person vaccinated		
Source known HB$_s$Ag-positive	Test exposed person for anti-HB$_s$¶. If titer is protective, nothing is required; if titer is not protective, give 0.06 mL/kg within 24 h	Review vaccination status#
Source known, HB$_s$Ag status not known	Test source for HB$_s$Ag and exposed person for anti-HB$_s$. If source is HB$_s$Ag-negative, or if source is HB$_s$Ag-positive but anti-HB$_s$ titer is protective, nothing is required. If source is HB$_s$Ag-positive and anti-HB$_s$ titer is not protective or if exposed person is a known nonresponder, give 0.06 mL/kg I.M. within 24 h. A second dose of hepatitis B immune globulin can be given 1 mo later if a booster dose of hepatitis B vaccine is not given.	Review vaccination status#
Source not tested or unknown	Test exposed person for anti-HB$_s$. If anti-HB$_s$ titer is protective, nothing is required. If anti-HB$_s$ titer is not protective, 0.06 mL/kg may be given along with a booster dose of hepatitis B vaccine	Review vaccination status#

*HB$_s$Ag = hepatitis B surface antigen; anti-HB$_s$ = antibody to hepatitis B surface antigen; I.M. = intramuscularly; SRU = standard ratio units.

†Each 0.5 mL dose of plasma-derived hepatitis B vaccine contains 10 mcg of HB$_s$Ag; each 0.5 mL dose of recombinant hepatitis B vaccine contains 5 mcg (Merck Sharp & Dohme) or 10 mcg (SmithKline Beecham) of HB$_s$Ag.

‡If hepatitis B immune globulin and hepatitis B vaccine are given simultaneously, they should be given at separate sites.

§If hepatitis B vaccine is not given, a second dose of hepatitis B immune globulin should be given 1 mo later.

¶Anti-HB$_s$ titers <10 SRU by radioimmunoassay or negative by enzyme immunoassay indicate lack of protection. Testing the exposed person for anti-HB$_s$ is not necessary if a protective level of antibody has been shown within the previous 24 mo.

#If the exposed person has not completed a three-dose series of hepatitis B vaccine, the series should be completed. Test the exposed person for anti-HB$_s$. If the antibody level is protective, nothing is required. If an adequate antibody response in the past is shown on retesting to have declined to an inadequate level, a booster dose (1 mL) of hepatitis B vaccine should be given. If the exposed person has inadequate antibody or is a known nonresponder to vaccination, a booster dose can be given along with one dose of hepatitis B immune globulin.

VACCINATIONS/IMMUNIZATIONS

Guidelines for Spacing Live and Killed Antigen Administration

Antigen Combinations	Recommended Minimum Interval Between Doses
≥2 killed antigens	None. May be given simultaneously or at any interval between doses.
Killed and live antigens	None. May be given simultaneously or at any interval between doses. (Exception: Concurrent administration of cholera and yellow fever vaccines should be avoided. Separate these vaccines by at least 3 weeks.)
≥2 live antigens	4 weeks minimum interval if not administered simultaneously. (Recent receipt of OPV is not a contraindication to MMR.) Vaccines associated with systemic reactions (cholera and parenteral typhoid or influenza and DTP in young children) should be given on separate occasions.

Passive Immunization Agents — Immune Globulins

Immune Globulin	Dosage	Route
Hepatitis B (H-BIG®)		I.M.
percutaneous inoculation	0.06 mL/kg/dose (within 24 hours) (5 mL max)	
perinatal	0.5 mL/dose (within 12 hours of birth)	
sexual exposure	0.06 mL/kg/dose (within 14 days of contact) (5 mL max)	
Immune globulin (IG)		I.M.*
hepatitis A prophylaxis	0.02 mL/kg/dose (as soon as possible or within 2 weeks after exposure) (single exposure)	
	0.06 mL/kg/dose (>3 months or continuous exposure) repeat every 4-6 months	
hepatitis B	0.06 mL/kg/dose (H-BIG® should be used)	
hepatitis C	0.06 mL/kg/dose (percutaneous exposure)	
measles†	0.25 mL/kg/dose (max 15 mL/dose) (within 6 days of exposure)	
	0.5 mL/kg/dose (max 15 mL/dose) (immunocompromised children)	
Rabies‡	20 IU/kg/dose (within 3 days)	
Tetanus (serious, contaminated wounds; <3 previous tetanus vaccine doses)	250-500 units/dose	I.M.
Varicella-zoster§ (VZIG)	Within 48 hours but not later than 96 hours after exposure	I.M.¶
	0-10 kg 125 units = 1 vial	
	10.1-20 kg 250 units = 2 vials	
	20.1-30 kg 375 units = 3 vials	
	30.1-40 kg 500 units = 4 vials	
	>40 kg 625 units = 5 vials	

*Deep I.M. in the gluteal region for large doses only. Deltoid muscle or the anterolateral aspect of the thigh are preferred sites for injection. No greater than 5 mL/site in adults or large children; 1-3 mL/site in small children and infants. Maximum dose: 20 mL at one time.

†IG prophylaxis may not be indicated in a patient who has received IGIV within 3 weeks of exposure.

‡½ of dose used to infiltrate the wound with the remaining ½ of dose given I.M. Rabies immune globulin is not recommended in previously HDCV immunized patients.

§Infants born to women who develop varicella within 5 days before or 48 hours after delivery should receive 125 units I.M. as a single dose.

¶No greater than 2.5 mL of VZIG/one injection site. Doses >2.5 mL should be divided and administered at different sites.

Guidelines for Spacing the Administration of Immune Globulin (IG) Preparations and Vaccines

Immunobiologic Combinations	Recommended Minimum Interval Between Doses

Simultaneous Administration

IG and killed antigen	None. May be given simultaneously at different sites or at any time between doses.
IG and live antigen	Should generally not be given simultaneously. If unavoidable to do so, give at different sites and revaccinate or test for seroconversion in 3 months. Example: MMR should not be given to patients who have received immune globulin within the previous 3 months.

Nonsimultaneous Administration

First	Second	
IG	Killed antigen	None
Killed antigen	IG	None
IG	Live antigen	6 weeks, and preferably 3 months
Live antigen	IG	2 weeks

*The live virus vaccines, OPV, and yellow fever are exceptions to these recommendations. Either vaccine may be administered simultaneously or any time before or after IG without significantly decreasing antibody response.

Recommended for Routine Immunization of HIV-Infected Children — United States

Vaccine	Known HIV Infection	
	Asymptomatic	Symptomatic
DTP	Yes	Yes
OPV	No	No
IPV	Yes	Yes
MMR	Yes	Yes
HbCV	Yes	Yes
Pneumococcal	Yes	Yes
Influenza	No*	Yes

*Not contraindicated.

VACCINATIONS/IMMUNIZATIONS

Immunization Side Effects

Vaccine	Side Effect	Incidence/Dose
DTP	Slight fever and irritability (within 2 days of immunization)	"Most"
	Pain and swelling at immunization site	1/2
	Continuous crying >3 hours	1/100
	Fever >105°F	1/330
	Unusual, high pitched crying	1/900
	Seizures or episodes of limpness/pallor	1/1750
	Acute encephalopathy (within 3 days of immunization)	1/110,000
	Permanent neurological sequelae*	1/310,000
DT, Td	Pain at immunization site, slight fever	"Not common"
OPV	Paralytic polio in patient immunized	1/8.1 million
	Paralytic polio in close contact of patient immunized	1/5 million
Hib	Swelling and warmth at immunization site	1/100
	Fever >101°F	2/100
	Redness at immunization site	2/100
MMR	Rash or slight fever lasting a few days 1-2 weeks following immunization	1/5
	Rash or lymphadenopathy lasting a few days 1-2 weeks following immunization	1/7
	Arthralgias, joint swelling lasting 2-3 days 1-3 weeks following immunization	1/20 (higher in adults)
	Encephalitis, seizure with fever, nerve deafness	"Very rarely"

Red Book (1991, p 355) states "The committee concludes, based on currently available data, that pertussis vaccine has not been proven to be a cause of brain damage. Although the data does not prove that pertussis vaccine will never cause brain damage, it does indicate that such occurrences are exceedingly rare."

Reportable Vaccine Side Effects

Vaccine/Toxoid	Event	Interval From Vaccination
DTP, P, DTP/poliovirus combined	A. Anaphylaxis or anaphylactic shock	24 hours
	B. Encephalopathy (or encephalitis)	7 days
	C. Shock-collapse or hypotonic-hyporesponsive collapse	7 days
	D. Residual seizure disorder	
	E. Any acute complication or sequela (including death) of above events	No limit
	F. See package insert	See package insert
Measles, mumps, and rubella; DT, Td, T toxoid	A. Anaphylaxis or anaphylactic shock	24 hours
	B. Encephalopathy (or encephalitis)	15 days for measles, mumps, and rubella vaccines; 7 days for DT, Td, and toxoids
	C. Residual seizure disorder	
	D. Any acute complication or sequela (including death) of above events	No limit
	E. See package insert	See package insert
Oral poliovirus vaccine	A. Paralytic poliomyelitis	
	– in a nonimmunodeficient recipient	30 days
	– in an immunodeficient recipient	6 months
	– in a vaccine-associated community case	No limit
	B. Any acute complication or sequela (including death) of above events	No limit
	C. See package insert	See package insert
Inactivated poliovirus vaccine	A. Anaphylaxis or anaphylactic shock	24 hours
	B. Any acute complication or sequela (including death) of above events	No limit
	C. See package insert	See package insert

Reporting of Events Occurring After Vaccination

	Vaccine Purchased With Public Money	Vaccine Purchased With Private Money
Who reports	Healthcare provider who administered the vaccine	Healthcare provider who administered the vaccine
What products to report	DTP, P, measles, mumps, rubella, DT, Td, T, OPV, IPV, and DTP/polio combined	DTP, P, measles, mumps, *Haemophilus influenzae*, hepatitis B, rubella, DT, Td, T, OPV, IPV, and DTP/polio combined
How to report	Initial report taken by local, county, or state health department. State health department completes CDC form 71.19	Healthcare provider completes Adverse Reaction Report — FDA form 1639 (include interval from vaccination, manufacturer, and lot number on form)

Where to report	State health departments send CDC form 71.19 to:
	   MSAEFI/IM (E05)
	   Centers for Disease Control
	   Atlanta, GA 30333
	Vaccine adverse event reporting
	— 1 (800) 822-7967
		Completed FDA form 1639 is sent to:
		   Food and Drug Administration
		   (HFN-730)
		   Rockville, MD 20857

Where to obtain forms	State health departments	FDA and publications such as *FDA Drug Bulletin*

MMWR, 1988, 37:197-200.

Vaccine Advice for Travelers

Vaccine	Indication	Dose	Comments
Cholera	The risk to tourists is very low	Refer to product labeling	The currently licensed parenteral vaccine (prepared from killed bacteria) has limited effectiveness, often causes reactions, and is generally not recommended for travelers
Hepatitis A immune globulin	Travelers going to areas where hygiene is poor, particularly those going outside the usual tourist routes	Adults: I.M.: 2 mL for a stay of <3 months; 5 mL for a longer stay Repeated doses every 5 months Children: 0.02 mL/kg for a stay <3 months; 0.06 mL/kg for a longer period	Administer close to the time of departure
Hepatitis B vaccine	Not ordinarily recommended for foreign travel, except for medical personnel whose work could require handling of body fluids, or for people who expect to have sexual contacts, receive medical or dental care, or stay for >6 months in areas such as Southeast Asia or sub-Saharan Africa, where hepatitis B is highly endemic	I.M.: 3 doses over 2-6 (preferable) months	Hepatitis B vaccine is less effective when injected into the gluteal area, and should be injected into the deltoid muscle
Japanese encephalitis vaccine	Travelers who anticipate spending a month or longer in rural rice-growing areas where they will be heavily exposed to mosquitoes. Countries where the disease may be a problem include Bangladesh, Cambodia, China, India, Indonesia, Korea, Laos, Malaysia, Meaner (Burma), Nepal, Pakistan, the Philippines, Singapore, Sri Lanka, Taiwan, Thailand, Vietnam, and eastern areas of Russia.	Primary series of 3 doses given over 2-4 (preferable) weeks.	Formalin-activated, purified mouse-brain-derived vaccine

(continued)

Vaccine	Indication	Dose	Comments
Measles vaccine	People born after 1956 who have not received 2 doses of measles vaccine (after their first birthday) and do not have a physician-documented history of infection or laboratory evidence of immunity should receive before traveling anywhere	Single dose of measles (or measles-mumps-rubella) vaccine at least 2 weeks before or 3 months after immune globulin	
Meningococcal vaccine	Only for tourists traveling to areas where epidemics are occurring. Epidemics occur frequently in sub-Saharan Africa from December to June, and also in northern India and Nepal. Saudi Arabia requires a certificate of immunization for pilgrims to Mecca.	Single dose	
Polio vaccine	Adult travelers to tropical or developing countries who have not previously been immunized against polio	Adults: If protection is needed within 4 weeks, a single dose of enhanced inactivated polio vaccine (eIPV) or trivalent (live) oral polio vaccine (OPV) is recommended. Travelers who have previously completed a primary series should receive a booster of OPT or eIPV.	OPV rarely can cause vaccine-induced polio, particularly in previously unimmunized adults
Rabies vaccine	Travelers with an occupational risk of exposure or those traveling for extended periods in endemic areas	3 injections of vaccine over 3-4 weeks	
Tetanus and diphtheria toxoids	Tetanus-diphtheria toxoid (Td) booster every 10 years. Especially for travelers going to developing countries and to Russia and the Ukraine, where a large outbreak of diphtheria has been occurring in recent years.		

(continued)

Vaccine	Indication	Dose	Comments
Typhoid vaccine	Travel to rural areas of tropical countries, where typhoid tends to be endemic, or to any area where an outbreak was occurring	P.O.: One capsule every other day for a total of 4 capsules, beginning at least 2 weeks before departure	Killed bacteria parenteral vaccine is not fully protective and causes 1-2 days of pain at the site of injection sometimes accompanied by fever, malaise, and headache. Live oral vaccine reported to provide equally effective, longer than parenteral vaccine and have less adverse effects. Antibiotics should be avoided, if possible, for 1 week before and 3 weeks after oral typhoid vaccine.
Yellow fever vaccine	Travelers to rural areas in the yellow fever endemic zones, which include most of tropical South America and most of Africa between 15°N and 15°S. Some countries in Africa require a certificate of yellow fever vaccination from all entering travelers. Other countries in Africa, South America, and Asia require evidence of vaccination from travelers coming from infected or endemic areas.	Boosters are given every 10 years.	Attenuated live virus vaccine

More than one vaccine can be given at the same time.
Immunocompromised or pregnant patients generally should not receive live virus vaccines, but measles vaccine is recommended for HIV-infected patients.

Prevention of Malaria[1]

	Drug	Adult Dosage	Pediatric Dosage
Chloroquine-sensitive areas			
Drug of choice:	Chloroquine phosphate[2]	300 mg base (500 mg salt) P.O., once/week beginning 1 week before and continuing for 4 weeks after last exposure	5 mg/kg base (8.3 mg/kg salt) once/week, up to adult dose of 300 mg base
Chloroquine-resistant areas[3]			
Drug of choice:[4]	Mefloquine[2,5,6]	P.O.: 250 mg once/week[7]	15-19 kg: ¼ tablet 20-30 kg: ½ tablet 31-45 kg: ¾ tablet >45 kg: 1 tablet
or	Doxycycline[2,8,9]	100 mg daily	>8 y: 2 mg/kg/d P.O., up to 100 mg/d
or	Chloroquine phosphate[2]	as above	as above
	plus pyrimethamine-sulfadoxine[10] for presumptive treatment[11]	Carry a single dose (3 tablets) for self-treatment of febrile illness when medical care is not immediately available	<1 y: ¼ tablet 1-3 y: ½ tablet 4-8 y: 1 tablet 9-14 y: 2 tablets
	or **plus** proguanil[12] (in Africa south of the Sahara)	200 mg daily during exposure and for 4 weeks afterwards	<2 y: 50 mg daily 2-6 y: 100 mg daily 7-10 y: 150 mg daily 10 y: 200 mg daily

[1]At present, no drug regimen guarantees protection against malaria. If fever develops within a year (particularly within the first 2 months) after travel to malarious areas, travelers should be advised to seek medical attention. Insect repellents, insecticide-impregnated bed nets, and proper clothing are important adjuncts for malaria prophylaxis.

[2]For prevention of attack after departure from areas where *P vivax* and *P ovale* are endemic, which includes almost all areas where malaria is found (except Haiti), some experts, in addition, prescribe primaquine phosphate 15 mg base (26.3 mg/d or, for children, 0.3 mg base/kg/d during the last 2 weeks of prophylaxis. Others prefer to avoid the toxicity of primaquine and rely on surveillance to detect cases when they occur, particularly when exposure was limited or doubtful. Primaquine phosphate can cause hemolytic anemia, especially in patients whose red cells are deficient in glucose-6-phosphate dehydrogenase. This deficiency is most common in Blacks, Orientals, and Mediterranean peoples. Patients should be screened for G-6-PD deficiency before treatment. Primaquine should not be used during pregnancy.

[3]Chloroquine-resistant *P falciparum* infections have been reported in all areas that have malaria except Central America west of Panama Canal Zone, Mexico. Haiti, the Dominican Republic, and the Middle East (including Egypt). In pregnancy, chloroquine prophylaxis has been used extensively and safely, but the safety of other prophylactic antimalarial agents in pregnancy is unclear. Therefore, travel during pregnancy to chloroquine-resistant areas should be discouraged. For chloroquine-resistant parasitemia ≥10%, exchange transfusion has been used (Miller KD, et al, *N Engl J Med*, 321:65, 1989; Saddler M, et al; Vachon F, et al; Miller KD, et al, *N Engl J Med*, 322:58, 1990).

[4]For prophylaxis where both chloroquine and pyrimethamine/sulfadoxine resistance coexist, mefloquine is the usual drug of choice. In areas with mefloquine-resistant plasmodium, such as Thailand, doxycycline is recommended.

[5]In the USA, a 250 mg tablet of mefloquine contains 228 mg of mefloquine base. Outside the USA, each 274 mg tablet contains 250 mg base.

[6]The pediatric dosage has not been approved by the FDA, and the drug has not been approved for use during pregnancy. Women should take contraceptive precautions while taking mefloquine and for 2 months after the last dose. Mefloquine is not recommended for children weighing less than 15 kg, or for patients taking beta blockers, calcium channel blockers, or other drugs that may prolong or otherwise alter cardiac conduction. Patients with a history of seizures or psychiatric disorders and those whose occupations require fine coordination or spatial discrimination should probably avoid mefloquine (*The Medical Letter*, 32:13, 1990).

[7]Beginning 1 week before travel and continuing weekly for the duration of stay and for 4 weeks after leaving.

[8]An approved drug, but considered investigational for this condition by the U.S. Food and Drug Administration.

[9]Beginning 1 day before travel and continuing for the duration of stay and for 4 weeks after leaving. The FDA considers use of tetracyclines as antimalarials to be investigational. Use of tetracyclines is contraindicated in pregnancy and in children younger than 8 years of age. Physicians who prescribe doxycycline as malaria chemoprophylaxis should advise patients to use an appropriate sunscreen (*The Medical Letter*, 31:59, 1989) to minimize the possibility of a photosensitivity reaction and should warn women that *Candida* vaginitis is a frequent adverse effect.

[10]*Fansidar* tablets contain 25 mg of pyrimethamine and 500 mg of sulfadoxine.

[11]Resistance to *Fansidar* should be anticipated in Southeast Asia, Bangladesh, Oceania, the Amazon basin, and in east Africa. Use of *Fansidar* is contraindicated in patients with a history of sulfonamide or pyrimethamine intolerance. In pregnancy at term and in infants less than 2 months old, pyrimethamine-sulfadoxine may cause hyperbilirubinema

[12]Proguanil (Paludrine® — Ayerst, Canada; ICI, England), which is not available in the USA but is widely available overseas, is recommended mainly for use in Africa south of the Sahara. Failures in prophylaxis with chloroquine and proguanil have, however, been reported in travelers to Kenya (Barnes AJ, *Lancet*, 338:1338, 1991).

CATEGORIES OF SAFE AND UNSAFE DRUGS IN ACUTE INTERMITTENT PORPHYRIA, HEREDITARY COPROPORPHYRIA, AND VARIEGATE PORPHYRIA

Unsafe	Safe
Alcohol	Acetaminophen
Barbiturates	Aspirin
Carbamazepine	Atropine
Danazol	Bromides
Ergots	Glucocorticoids
Ethchlorvynol	Insulin
Glutethimide	Narcotic analgesics
Griseofulvin	Penicillin and derivatives
Mephenytoin	Phenothiazines
Meprobamate	Streptomycin
Methyprylon	
Phenytoin	
Pyrazolones	
Succinimides	
Sulfonamide antibiotics	
Synthetic estrogens and progestins	
Valproic acid	

CYTOCHROME P-450 AND DRUG INTERACTIONS*

Drugs Causing Inhibitory and Inductive Interactions

Inhibitory (Enhancement of Interacting Drug Effect)	Inductive (Impairment of Interacting Drug Effect)
Amiodarone (Cordarone®)	Anticonvulsants
Cimetidine (Tagamet®)	Chronic ethanol use
Erythromycin	Cigarette smoking
Ethanol intoxication	Rifampin (Rifadin®, Rimactane®)
Isoniazid (Laniazid®, Nydrazid®)	
Neuroleptics	
Oral contraceptives	
Psoralen dermatologics	
Quinolone antibiotics	
Tricyclic antidepressants	

Low-Therapeutic-Index Drugs

Hepatic Oxidation (cytochrome P-450 mediated clearance)

Antiarrhythmic drugs
Anticonvulsants
Antineoplastic/immunosuppressive drugs
Oral anticoagulants
Theophylline

Drugs Metabolized by CYPIID6 That May Interact and Result in Toxicity

Tricyclic Antidepressants

Imipramine (Janimine®, Tofranil)
Clomipramine (Anafranil®)
Amitriptyline (Elavil®, Endep®)
Desipramine (Norpramin®, Pertofrane®)
Nortriptyline (Aventyl®, Pamelor®)

Phenothiazines

Perphenazine (Trilafon®)
Thioridazine (Mellaril®)

Drugs Metabolized by CYPIID6 That May Interact and Have Decreased or Altered Effect

Antiarrhythmics

Flecainide (Tambocor®)
Encainide (Enkaid®)
Propafenone (Rythmol®)
Mexiletine (Mexitil®)

β-Adrenergic Receptor Blockers

Metoprolol (Lopressor®, Toprol XL®)
Timolol (Blocadren®)

Analgesics
Codeine

Drugs That Inhibit CYPIID6

Any substrate listed in above tables
Quinidine
Haloperidol (Haldol®)

---

*From *PTT*, 1994, 19:143-50.

FEVER DUE TO DRUGS

Most Common

Cephalosporins
Iodides
Isoniazid
Methyldopa
Penicillins
Phenytoin
Procainamide
Quinidine
Streptomycin
Sulfas
Vancomycin

Less Common

Allopurinol	Hydralazine
Antihistamines	Hydroxyurea
Azathioprine	Ibuprofen
Barbiturates	Mercaptopurine
Bleomycin	Nitrofurantoin
Carbamazepine	Para-aminosalicylic acid
Cimetidine	Pentazocine
Cisplatin	Procarbazine
Clofibrate	Propylthiouracil
Colistimethate	Sulindac
Diazoxide	Streptozocin
Folic acid	Triamterene

Drug Intell Clin Pharm, Table 2, "Drugs Implicated in Causing a Fever," 1986, 20:416.

DISCOLORATION OF FECES DUE TO DRUGS

Black

Acetazolamide
Aluminum hydroxide
Aminophylline
Amphetamine
Amphotericin B
Bismuth salts
Chlorpropamide
Clindamycin
Corticosteroids
Cyclophosphamide
Cytarabine

Digitalis
Ethacrynic acid
Ferrous salts
Fluorouracil
Hydralazine
Hydrocortisone
Iodide-containing drugs
Melphalan
Methotrexate
Methylprednisolone

Phenylephrine
Potassium salts
Prednisolone
Procarbazine
Sulfonamides
Tetracycline
Theophylline
Thiotepa
Triamcinolone
Warfarin

Blue

Chloramphenicol
Methylene blue

Orange-Red

Phenazopyridine
Rifampin

White/Speckling

Antibiotics (oral)
Barium

Green

Indomethacin
Medroxyprogesterone

Pink/Red

Anticoagulants
Aspirin
Barium
Heparin
Oxyphenbutazone
Phenylbutazone
Tetracycline syrup

Yellow/Yellow-Green

Senna

DISCOLORATION OF URINE DUE TO DRUGS

Black/Brown/Dark

Cascara
Chloroquine
Ferrous salts
Metronidazole
Nitrofurantoin
Quinine
Senna

Orange/Yellow

Heparin
Phenazopyridine
Rifampin
Sulfasalazine
Warfarin

Red/Pink

Daunorubicin
Doxorubicin
Heparin
Ibuprofen
Oxyphenbutazone
Phenylbutazone
Phenytoin
Rifampin
Senna

Blue

Triamterene

Blue-Green

Amitriptyline
Methylene blue

CONTROLLED SUBSTANCES

Schedule I = C-I

The drugs and other substances in this schedule have no legal medical uses except research. They have a **high** potential for abuse. They include opiates, opium derivatives and hallucinogens.

Schedule II = C-II

The drugs and other substances in this schedule have legal medical uses and a **high** abuse potential which may lead to severe dependence. They include former "Class A" narcotics, amphetamines, barbiturates and other drugs.

Schedule III = C-III

The drugs and other substances in this schedule have legal medical uses and a **lesser** degree of abuse potential which may lead to **moderate** dependence. They include former "Class B" narcotics and other drugs.

Schedule IV = C-IV

The drugs and other substances in this schedule have legal medical uses and **low** abuse potential which may lead to **moderate** dependence. They include barbiturates, benzodiazepines, propoxyphenes and other drugs.

Schedule V = C-V

The drugs and other substances in this schedule have legal medical uses and **low** abuse potential which may lead to **moderate** dependence. They include narcotic cough preparations, diarrhea preparations and other drugs.

Note: These are federal classifications. Your individual state may place a substance into a more restricted category. When this occurs, the more restricted category applies. Consult your state law.

ORAL DOSAGES THAT SHOULD NOT BE CRUSHED

There are a variety of reasons for crushing tablets or capsule contents prior to administering to the patient. Patients may have nasogastric tubes which do not permit the administration of tablets or capsules; an oral solution for a particular medication may not be available from the manufacturer or readily prepared by pharmacy; patients may have difficulty swallowing capsules or tablets; or mixing of powdered medication with food or drink may make the drug more palatable.

Generally, medications which should not be crushed fall into one of the following categories.

- **Extended-Release Products**. The formulation of some tablets is specialized as to allow the medication within it to be slowly released into the body. This is sometimes accomplished by centering the drug within the core of the tablet, with a subsequent shedding of multiple layers around the core. Wax melts in the GI tract. Slow-K® is an example of this. Capsules may contain beads which have multiple layers which are slowly dissolved with time.

- **Medications Which Are Irritating to the Stomach**. Tablets which are irritating to the stomach may be enteric-coated which delays release of the drug until the time when it reaches the small intestine. Enteric-coated aspirin is an example of this.

- **Foul Tasting Medication**. Some drugs are quite unpleasant to taste so the manufacturer coats the tablet in a sugar coating to increase its palatability. By crushing the tablet, this sugar coating is lost and the patient tastes the unpleasant tasting medication.

- **Sublingual Medication**. Medication intended for use under the tongue should not be crushed. While it appears to be obvious, it is not always easy to determine if a medication is to be used sublingually. Sublingual medications should indicate on the package that they are intended for sublingual use.

- **Effervescent Tablets**. These are tablets which, when dropped into a liquid, quickly dissolve to yield a solution. Many effervescent tablets, when crushed, lose their ability to quickly dissolve.

Recommendations

1. It is not advisable to crush certain medications.

2. Consult individual monographs prior to crushing capsule or tablet.

3. If crushing a tablet or capsule is contraindicated, consult with your pharmacist to determine whether an oral solution exists or can be compounded.

4. Refer to individual drug monograph for crushing information.

Summary of Drug Formulations That Preclude Crushing

Type	Reason(s) for the Formulation
Enteric-coated	Designed to pass through the stomach intact with drug released in the intestines to: • prevent destruction of drug by stomach acids • prevent stomach irritation • delay onset of action
Extended release	Designed to release drug over an extended period of time. Such products include: • multiple-layered tablets releasing drug as each layer is dissolved • mixed release pellets that dissolve at different time intervals • special matrixes that are themselves inert but slowly release drug from the matrix
Sublingual buccal	Designed to dissolve quickly in oral fluids for rapid absorption by the abundant blood supply of the mouth
Miscellaneous	Drugs that: • produce oral mucosa irritation • are extremely bitter • contain dyes or inherently could stain teeth and mucosal tissue

DRUGS ASSOCIATED WITH ADVERSE HEMATOLOGIC EFFECTS

Drug	Red Cell Aplasia	Thrombo-cytopenia	Neutro-penia	Pancyto-penia	Hemolysis
Acetazolamide		+	+	+	
Allopurinol			+		
Amiodarone	+				
Amphotericin B				+	
Amrinone		++			
Asparaginase		+++	+++	+++	++
Barbiturates		+		+	
Benzocaine					++
Captopril			++		+
Carbamazepine		++	+		
Cephalosporins			+		++
Chloramphenicol		+	++	+++	
Chlordiazepoxide			+	+	
Chloroquine		+			
Chlorothiazides		++			
Chlorpropamide	+	++	+	++	+
Chlortetracycline				+	
Chlorthalidone			+		
Cimetidine		+	++	+	
Codeine		+			
Colchicine				+	
Cyclophosphamide		+++	+++	+++	+
Dapsone					+++
Desipramine		++			
Digitalis		+			
Digitoxin		++			
Erythromycin		+			
Estrogen		+		+	
Ethacrynic acid			+		
Fluorouracil		+++	+++	+++	+
Furosemide		+	+		
Gold salts	+	+++	+++	+++	
Heparin		++		+	
Ibuprofen			+		+
Imipramine			++		
Indomethacin		+	++	+	
Isoniazid		+		+	
Isosorbide dinitrate					+
Levodopa					++
Meperidine		+			
Meprobamate		+	+	+	
Methimazole			++		
Methyldopa		++			+++
Methotrexate		+++	+++	+++	++

(continued)

Drug	Red Cell Aplasia	Thrombo-cytopenia	Neutro-penia	Pancyto-penia	Hemolysis
Methylene blue					+
Metronidazole			+		
Nalidixic acid					+
Naproxen				+	
Nitrofurantoin			+ +		+
Nitroglycerine		+			
Penicillamine		+ +	+		
Penicillins		+	+ +	+	+ + +
Phenazopyridine					+ + +
Phenothiazines		+	+ +	+ + +	+
Phenylbutazone		+	+ +	+ + +	+
Phenytoin		+ +	+ +	+ +	+
Potassium iodide		+			
Prednisone		+			
Primaquine					+ + +
Procainamide			+		
Procarbazine		+	+ +	+ +	+
Propylthiouracil		+	+ +	+	+
Quinidine		+ + +	+		
Quinine		+ + +	+		
Reserpine		+			
Rifampicin		+ +	+		+ + +
Spironolactone			+		
Streptomycin		+		+	
Sulfamethoxazole with trimethoprim			+		
Sulfonamides	+	+ +	+ +	+ +	+ +
Sulindac	+	+	+	+	
Tetracyclines		+			+
Thioridazine			+ +		
Tolbutamide		+ +	+	+ +	
Triamterene					+
Valproate	+				
Vancomycin			+		

+ = rare or single reports.
+ + = occasional reports.
+ + + = substantial number of reports.

Adapted from D'Arcy PF and Griffin JP, eds, *Iatrogenic Diseases*, New York, NY: Oxford University Press, 1986, 128-30.

TRANSFER OF DRUGS INTO HUMAN MILK*

The following questions and options should be considered when prescribing drug therapy to lactating women. (1) Is the drug therapy really necessary? Consultation between the pediatrician and the mother's physician can be most useful. (2) Use the safest drug, for example, acetaminophen rather than aspirin for analgesia. (3) If there is a possibility that a drug may present a risk to the infant, consideration should be given to measurement of blood concentrations in the nursing infant. (4) Drug exposure to the nursing infant may be minimized by having the mother take the medication just after she has breast-fed the infant and/or just before the infant is due to have a lengthy sleep period.

Table 1. **Drugs That Are Contraindicated During Breast-Feeding**

Drug	Reason for Concern, Reported Sign or Symptom in Infant, or Effect on Lactation
Bromocriptine	Suppresses lactation; may be hazardous to the mother
Cocaine	Cocaine intoxication
Cyclophosphamide	Possible immune suppression; unknown effect on growth or association with carcinogenesis; neutropenia
Cyclosporine	Possible immune suppression; unknown effect on growth or association with carcinogenesis
Doxorubicin*	Possible immune suppression; unknown effect on growth or association with carcinogenesis
Ergotamine	Vomiting, diarrhea, convulsions (doses used in migraine medications)
Lithium	One-third to one-half therapeutic blood concentration in infants
Methotrexate	Possible immune suppression; unknown effect on growth or association with carcinogenesis; neutropenia
Phencyclidine (PCP)	Potent hallucinogen
Phenindione	Anticoagulant: increased prothrombin and partial thromboplastin time in one infant; not used in the United States

*Drug is concentrated in human milk.

Table 2. **Drugs of Abuse: Contraindicated During Breast-Feeding***

Drug Reference	Reported Effect or Reasons for Concern
Amphetamine†	Irritability, poor sleeping pattern
Cocaine	Cocaine intoxication
Heroin	Tremors, restlessness, vomiting, poor feeding
Marijuana	Only one report in literature; no effect mentioned
Nicotine (smoking)	Shock, vomiting, diarrhea, rapid heart rate, restlessness; decreased milk production
Phencyclidine	Potent hallucinogen

*The Committee on Drugs strongly believes that nursing mothers should not ingest any compounds listed in Table 2. Not only are they hazardous to the nursing infant, but they are also detrimental to the physical and emotional health of the mother. This list is obviously not complete; no drug of abuse should be ingested by nursing mothers even though adverse reports are not in the literature.

†Drug is concentrated in human milk.

*From "American Academy of Pediatrics Committee on Drugs: Transfer of Drugs and Other Chemicals Into Human Milk," *Pediatrics*, 1994, 93:137-50.

Table 3. **Radioactive Compounds That Require Temporary Cessation of Breast-Feeding***

Drug	Recommended Time for Cessation of Breast-Feeding
Copper 64 (^{64}Cu)	Radioactivity in milk present at 50 h
Gallium 67 (^{67}Ga)	Radioactivity in milk present for 2 wk
Indium 111 (^{111}In)	Very small amount present at 20 h
Iodine 123 (^{123}I)	Radioactivity in milk present up to 36 h
Iodine 125 (^{125}I)	Radioactivity in milk present for 12 d
Iodine 131 (^{131}I)	Radioactivity in milk present 2-14 d, depending on study
Radioactive sodium	Radioactivity in milk present 96 h
Technetium-99m (^{99m}Tc), ^{99m}Rc macroaggregates, ^{99m}Tc O4	Radioactivity in milk present 15 h to 3 d

*Consult nuclear medicine physician before performing diagnostic study so that radionuclide that has shortest excretion time in breast milk can be used. Before study, the mother should pump her breast and store enough milk in freezer for feeding the infant; after study, the mother should pump her breast to maintain milk production but discard all milk pumped for the required time that radioactivity is present in milk. Milk samples can be screened by radiology departments for radioactivity before resumption of nursing.

Table 4. **Drugs Whose Effect on Nursing Infants Is Unknown But May Be of Concern**

Psychotropic drugs, the compounds listed under antianxiety, antidepressant, and antipsychotic categories, are of special concern when given to nursing mothers for long periods. Although there are no case reports of adverse effects in breast-feeding infants, these drugs do appear in human milk and thus conceivably alter short-term and long-term central nervous system function.

Drug	Reported or Possible Effect
Antianxiety	
Diazepam	None
Lorazepam	None
Midazolam	...
Perphenazine	None
Prazepam*	None
Quazepam	None
Temazepam	...
Antidepressants	
Amitriptyline	None
Amoxapine	None
Desipramine	None
Dothiepin	None
Doxepin	None
Fluoxetine	...
Fluvoxamine	...
Imipramine	None
Trazodone	None
Antipsychotic	
Chlorpromazine	Galactorrhea in adult; drowsiness and lethargy in infant
Chlorprothixene	None
Haloperidol	None
Mesoridazine	None
Chloramphenicol	Possible idiosyncratic bone marrow supression
Metoclopramide*	None described; dopaminergic blocking agent
Metronidazole	In vitro mutagen; may discontinue breast-feeding 12-24 h to allow excretion of dose when single-dose therapy given to mother
Tinidazole	See metronidazole

*Drug is concentrated in human milk.

Table 5. **Drugs That Have Been Associated With Significant Effects on Some Nursing Infants and Should Be Given to Nursing Mothers With Caution***

Drug	Reported Effect
5-Aminosalicylic acid	Diarrhea (one case)
Aspirin (salicylates)	Metabolic acidosis (one case)
Clemastine	Drowsiness, irritability, refusal to feed, high-pitched cry, neck stiffness (one case)
Phenobarbital	Sedation; infantile spasms after weaning from milk-containing phenobarbital, methemoglobinemia (one case)
Primidone	Sedation, feeding problems
Sulfasalazine (salicylazosulfapyridine)	Bloody diarrhea (one case)

*Measure blood concentration in the infant when possible.

Table 6. **Maternal Medication Usually Compatible With Breast-Feeding***

Drug	Reported Sign or Symptom in Infant or Effect on Lactation
Acebutolol	None
Acetaminophen	None
Acetazolamide	None
Acitretin	...
Acyclovir†	None
Alcohol (ethanol)	With large amounts of drowsiness, diaphoresis, deep sleep, weakness, decrease in linear growth, abnormal weight gain, maternal ingestion of 1 g/kg daily decreases milk ejection reflex
Allopurinol	...
Amoxicillin	None
Antimony	...
Atenolol	None
Atropine	None
Azapropazone (apazone)	...
Aztreonam	None
B₁ (thiamine)	None
B₆ (pyridoxine)	None
B₁₂	None
Baclofen	None
Barbiturate	See Table 5.
Bendroflumethiazide	Suppresses lactation
Bishydroxycoumarin (Dicumarol®)	None
Bromide	Rash, weakness, absence of cry with maternal intake of 5.4 g/d
Butorphanol	None
Caffeine	Irritability, poor sleeping pattern, excreted slowly; no effect with usual amount of caffeine beverages
Captopril	None
Carbamazepine	None
Carbimazole	Goiter
Cascara None	
Cefadroxil	None
Cefazolin	None
Cefotaxime	None
Cefoxitin	None
Cefprozil	...
Ceftazidime	None
Ceftriaxone	None
Chloral hydrate	Sleepiness
Chloroform	None
Chloroquine	None
Chlorothiazide	None
Chlorthalidone	Excreted slowly
Cimetidine†	None
Cisapride	None
Cisplatin	Not found in milk
Clindamycin	None
Clogestone	None

(continued)

Drug	Reported Sign or Symptom in Infant or Effect on Lactation
Clomipramine	...
Codeine	None
Colchicine	...
Contraceptive pill with estrogen/progesterone	Rare breast enlargement; decrease in milk production and protein content (not confirmed in several studies)
Cycloserine	None
D (vitamin)	None; follow up infant's serum calcium level if mother receives pharmacological doses
Danthron	Increased bowel activity
Dapsone	None; sulfonamide detected in infant's urine
Dexbrompheniramine maleate with d-isoephedrine	Crying, poor sleep patterns, irritability
Digoxin	None
Diltiazem	None
Dipyrone	None
Disopyramide	None
Domperidone	None
Dyphylline†	None
Enalapril	...
Erythromycin†	None
Estradiol	Withdrawal, vaginal bleeding
Ethambutol	None
Ethanol	See Alcohol
Ethosuximide	None; drug appears in infant serum
Fentanyl	...
Flecainide	...
Flufenamic acid	None
Fluorescein	...
Folic acid	None
Gold salts	None
Halothane	None
Hydralazine	None
Hydrochlorothiazide	...
Hydroxychloroquine†	None
Ibuprofen	None
Indomethacin	Seizure (one case)
Iodides	May affect thyroid activity
Iodine	Goiter
Iodine (povidone-iodine/vaginal douche)	Elevated iodine levels in breast milk, odor of iodine on infant's skin
Iopanoic acid	None
Isoniazid	None; acetyl metabolite also secreted; ? hepatotoxic
K₁ (vitamin)	None
Kanamycin	None
Ketorolac	...
Labetalol	None
Levonorgestrel	...
Lidocaine	None
Loperamide	...
Magnesium sulfate	None
Medroxyprogesterone	None
Mefenamic acid	None
Methadone	None if mother receiving ≤20 mg/24 h
Methimazole (active metabolite of carbimazole)	None
Methocarbamol	None
Methyldopa	None
Methyprylon	Drowsiness
Metoprolol†	None
Metrizamide	None
Mexiletine	None
Minoxidil	None
Morphine	None; infant may have significant blood concentration
Moxalactam	None
Nadolol†	None
Nalidixic acid	Hemolysis in infant with glucose-6-phosphate dehydrogenase (G-6-PD) deficiency
Naproxen	...

(continued)

Drug	Reported Sign or Symptom in Infant or Effect on Lactation
Nefopam	None
Nifedipine	...
Nitrofurantoin	Hemolysis in infant with G-6-PD deficiency
Norethynodrel	None
Norsteroids	None
Noscapine	None
Oxprenolol	None
Phenylbutazone	None
Phenytoin	Methemoglobinemia (one case)
Piroxicam	None
Prednisone	None
Procainamide	None
Progesterone	None
Propoxyphene	None
Propranolol	None
Propylthiouracil	None
Pseudoephedrine†	None
Pyridostigmine	None
Pyrimethamine	None
Quinidine	None
Quinine	None
Riboflavin	None
Rifampin	None
Scopolamine	...
Secobarbital	None
Senna	None
Sotalol	...
Spironolactone	None
Streptomycin	None
Sulbactam	None
Sulfapyridine	Caution in infant with jaundice or G-6-PD deficiency and ill, stressed, or premature infant; appears in infant's milk
Sulfisoxazole	Caution in infant with jaundice or G-6-PD deficiency and ill, stressed, or premature infant; appears in infant's milk
Suprofen	None
Terbutaline	None
Tetracycline	None; negligible absorption by infant
Theophylline	Irritability
Thiopental	None
Thiouracil	None mentioned; drug not used in U.S.
Ticarcillin	None
Timolol	None
Tolbutamide	Possible jaundice
Tolmetin	None
Trimethoprim and sulfamethoxazole	None
Triprolidine	None
Valproic acid	None
Verapamil	None
Warfarin	None
Zolpidem	None

*Drugs listed have been reported in the literature as having the effects listed or no effect. The word "none" means that no observable change was seen in the nursing infant while the mother was ingesting the compound. It is emphasized that most of the literature citations concern single case reports or small series of infants.

†Drug is concentrated in human milk.

THERAPEUTIC CATEGORY &
KEY WORD INDEX

HYPOGLYCEMIC AGENTS, ORAL

IMMUNE GLOBULINS

IMMUNE MODULATORS

IMMUNOSUPPRESSANT AGENTS

INTERFERONS

IRON SALTS

KERATOLYTIC AGENTS

LAXATIVES, BOWEL EVACUANT

LAXATIVES, BULK-PRODUCING

LAXATIVES, HYPEROSMOLAR

LAXATIVES, LUBRICANT

LAXATIVES, MISCELLANEOUS

LAXATIVES, SALINE

LAXATIVES, STIMULANT

LAXATIVES, SURFACTANT

LEPROSTATIC AGENTS

LOCAL ANESTHETICS, AMIDE DERIVATIVE

LOCAL ANESTHETICS, ESTER DERIVATIVE

VITAMINS, WATER SOLUBLE (Continued)